AMERICAN ACADEMY OF PEDIATRICS
QUICK REFERENCE GUIDE
TO PEDIATRIC CARE

Deepak M. Kamat, MD, PhD, FAAP

Editor in Chief

Coeditors

Henry M. Adam, MD, FAAP

Kathleen K. Cain, MD, FAAP

Deborah E. Campbell, MD, FAAP

Alexander M. Holston, MD

Kelly J. Kelleher, MD, MPH, FAAP

Michael G. Leu, MD, MS, MHS, FAAP

Thomas K. McInerny, MD, FAAP

Lamia M. Soghier, MD, FAAP

Mark L. Wolraich, MD, FAAP

Beverly P. Wood, MD, MSEd, PhD, FAAP

Policy of the American Academy of Pediatrics

American Academy of Pediatrics

Elk Grove Village, Illinois

Suggested Citation: Kamat DM, Adam HM, Cain KK, et al, eds. *American Academy of Pediatrics Quick Reference Guide to Pediatric Care.* Elk Grove Village, IL: American Academy of Pediatrics; 2010.

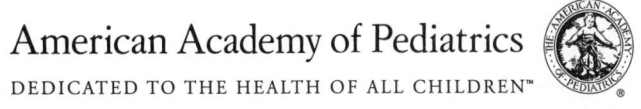

American Academy of Pediatrics

DEDICATED TO THE HEALTH OF ALL CHILDREN™

Maureen DeRosa, MPA, Director, Department of Marketing and Publications

Mark Grimes, Director, Division of Product Development

Jeffrey Mahony, Manager, Product Development

Jennifer McDonald, Manager, Online Content

Carrie Peters, Editorial Assistant

Sandi King, MS, Director, Division of Publishing and Production Services

Theresa Wiener, Manager, Editorial Production

Linda Diamond, Manager, Art Direction and Production

Kate Larson, Manager, Editorial Services

Linda Smessaert, Manager, Clinical and Professional Publications Marketing

Library of Congress Control Number: 2010901300

ISBN: 978-1-58110-371-7

Product Code: MA0530

The recommendations in this publication do not indicate an exclusive course of treatment or serve as a standard of medical care. Variations, taking into account individual circumstances, may be appropriate.

Every effort has been made to ensure that the drug selection and dosage set forth in this text are in accordance with the current recommendations and practice at the time of publication. It is the responsibility of the health care provider to check the package insert of each drug for any change in indications or dosage and for added warnings and precautions.

The mention of product names in this publication is for informational purposes only and does not imply endorsement by the American Academy of Pediatrics.

The publishers made every effort to trace the copyright holders for borrowed material. If they inadvertently overlooked any, they will be pleased to make the necessary arrangements at the first opportunity.

9-261/0210

Last digit is the print number: 9 8 7 6 5 4 3 2 1

Foreword

Medical knowledge is expanding so rapidly that busy pediatricians may find it difficult to keep up in their daily practice. *American Academy of Pediatrics Quick Reference Guide to Pediatric Care* is the go-to reference for pediatricians and their busy schedules, providing them with the information they need while seeing patients or between appointments without having to sift through paragraphs of information.

This trusted resource contains the entire Point-of-Care Quick Reference—over 240 topics—from the American Academy of Pediatrics online resource *Pediatric Care Online* at www.pediatriccareonline.org. Succinctly displayed in a bulleted format, the content covers key aspects of pediatric care: disease prevention, screening, treatment, signs and symptoms, emotional and behavioral problems, specific clinical problems, and critical situations.

In addition, 32 pages of more than 90 color images, algorithms, and graphs further enhance many of the topics, such as cardiac arrhythmias, neurocutaneous syndromes, ocular trauma, dizziness and vertigo, hematuria, preventive cardiology, and shock.

To further aid in decision-making at the point of care, the appendix houses more than 80 tools that pediatricians need most when seeing patients: formulas, reference range values, and growth charts, as well as tables for development, feeding and nutrition, immunization, medications, and obesity to name just a few.

The content in this publication was culled from the following best-selling AAP resources:

Pediatric Care Online

American Academy of Pediatrics Textbook of Pediatric Care

Red Book: 2009 Report of the Committee on Infectious Diseases, 28th Edition

Bright Futures: Guidelines for Health Supervision of Infants, Children, and Adolescents, 3rd Edition

Pediatric Nutrition Handbook

It is our hope that *American Academy of Pediatrics Quick Reference Guide to Pediatric Care* will be the standard point-of-care reference for pediatricians, pediatric residents, and medical students alike as they strive to provide the best care possible for infants, children, adolescents, and young adults.

Table of Contents

Topics

Abdominal Distention

DEFINITION

- Distention of abdomen may be from either normal causes or pathologic processes.
- Healthy infants may have variable degrees of abdominal distention caused by:
  - Aerophagia during feeding
  - Crying
  - Transient constipation
- Distention in healthy toddlers may result from:
  - Lumbar lordosis
  - Hypotonia of the abdominal rectus muscles
- Nonpathologic distention may exceed the mild distention seen with some intraabdominal cancers.

MECHANISM

- Abdominal distention may occur in:
  - Healthy infants (frequently) and children
  - Newborns and children who have intestinal obstruction
  - Infants and children who have systemic conditions
- Multiple underlying mechanisms can result in abdominal distention.
- Tympanitic distention results from accumulation of air/gas, either intraluminal or extraluminal.
  - Air swallowing (aerophagia)
  - Constipation
  - Gastrointestinal (GI) ileus
  - Gastrointestinal obstruction
  - Malabsorption
  - Peritonitis
  - Pneumoperitoneum
  - Pneumomediastinum (children on respirators)
- Distention from an intraabdominal mass
  - Constipation
  - Renal
  - Adrenal
  - Hepatic
  - Splenic/lymphatic
  - GI
  - Mesenteric/omental
  - Genitourinary (uterine, ovarian, vaginal)
- Distention from ascites
  - Urinary
  - Cardiac
  - Hepatic
  - Biliary/GI
  - Chylous
  - Idiopathic
- Distention from abdominal wall hypotonia
  - Generalized neuromuscular hypotonia
  - Rickets
  - Hypothyroidism

HISTORY

- Newborns
  - Pregnancy history of mother
    - Oligohydramnios suggests distal urinary obstruction.
    - Polyhydramnios is seen with upper GI obstruction.
- Older infants and children
  - History should establish duration and pattern of the child's distention.
    - Intermittent distention suggests intermittent GI obstruction.
    - Progressive distention suggests:
      - Intraabdominal tumor
      - Progressive hepatosplenomegaly
      - Ascites
- The primary care physician must be careful to differentiate a parent's question about whether a toddler's potbelly is normal from reports of progressive or marked distention, or palpable abdominal mass.
- Comprehensive medical and surgical history and review of systems is warranted.
  - Medication use, including herbal and alternative therapies, with particular attention to agents that can cause GI ileus and constipation
- Family history should include questions about:
  - Cystic fibrosis (meconium ileus)
  - Polycystic kidney disease
  - Metabolic diseases
  - History of fetal death or early neonatal deaths that might indicate unrecognized metabolic disease, which might produce hepatomegaly, splenomegaly, and congenital ascites
- Although rare, the presence of inherited syndromes that predispose a child to an intraabdominal cancer should be elicited.
  - In Wilms tumor, these include the WAGR syndrome (Wilms tumor, aniridia, genitourinary anomalies, and mental retardation), Denys-Drash syndrome, and Beckwith-Wiedemann syndrome.
  - Incidence of hepatoblastoma and adrenal carcinoma is increased in children with Beckwith-Wiedemann syndrome.
  - Children with DNA fragility syndromes and immunodeficient states are at risk for lymphoma and leukemia.

A

- In all female adolescents who have abdominal distention
  - A confidential history of sexual activity
  - History of the onset of puberty and menarche
- The symptoms below suggest cancer, but their absence does not exclude it.
  - Fever
  - Weight loss
  - Failure to thrive
  - Anorexia
  - Fatigue
  - Irritability
  - Bone pain
- A systematic review of symptoms referable to the intra-abdominal organs should be done.
  - Gastrointestinal obstruction
    - Vomiting
    - Pain
    - Obstipation
    - Delayed passage of meconium at birth
  - Malabsorption
    - Diarrhea
    - Greasy, bulky, malodorous stools
  - Occult hydronephrosis: possible presentations in older infants and children
    - Recurrent fever from urinary tract infection (often misdiagnosed as viral illness or otitis media)
    - Gross hematuria after minor trauma
    - Voiding difficulty in boys with posterior urethral valves

PHYSICAL EXAM

- Inspect the profile of the abdomen with the child in a supine position.
  - Note whether distention is generalized (maximal at the umbilicus) or localized.
  - Pattern and prominence of the abdominal veins should be noted.
    - Prominent superficial veins may indicate portal hypertension or obstruction to the systemic venous return.
- Imperforate anus or an incarcerated hernia will be apparent.
  - Differentiation of remaining causes of lower intestinal obstruction involves radiographic evaluation.
- Steatorrhea and growth failure with muscle wasting (a thin-limbed child with a bloated abdomen) may be associated with tympanitic distention from:
  - Fat malabsorption syndrome
  - Cystic fibrosis
  - Celiac disease

- Abdomen should be auscultated for:
  - Hyperactive bowel sounds
    - Malabsorption
    - Acute obstruction
  - Rushes
    - Incomplete obstruction
  - Absence of sounds
    - Paralytic ileus
  - Bruits
    - Vascular malformation
  - Percussion can be used to:
    - Differentiate diffuse from more focal epigastric tympani
    - Identify shifting dullness in older children
- Palpate gently for mass and tenderness.
  - Begin from the lower quadrants and progress upward so that the inferior edge of the liver and spleen are appreciated.
  - Abdomen should be assessed for focal or generalized tenderness.
    - Involuntary guarding on gentle palpation is a sensitive sign of peritoneal inflammation.
    - Rebound tenderness in young children is often falsely positive.
  - If an abdominal mass is appreciated, note:
    - Location (see list below)
    - Whether painful
    - If mobile: intraabdominal
    - If nonmobile: retroperitoneal/malignant
    - If moves with respiration: liver and spleen
    - If cystic, solid, malleable: fecal masses
    - If smooth or nodular, and whether crossing the midline: often seen with neuroblastoma
  - Renal ballottement
    - Lifting the kidney anteriorly with a finger in the costovertebral angle while palpating with the other hand can help elicit and define features of masses in the flank.
  - Rectal examination properly done can add considerable information to evaluation of:
    - Constipation
    - Anal stenosis
    - Hirschsprung disease
    - Pelvic mass
  - Hydronephrosis may manifest initially as an asymptomatic flank mass in the newborn.

- Signs of ascites
  - Infants: bilateral bulging flanks in the supine position
  - Older children: may detect shifting dullness and a fluid wave
  - Acquired umbilical hernia may indicate massive ascites.
- Genital examination
  - In girls, to exclude imperforate hymen with hydrometrocolpos, hematocolpos, and pregnancy
  - In both sexes, lower genitourinary tract malformation raises the question of upper genitourinary tract malformation.

DIFFERENTIAL DIAGNOSIS

Tympanitic abdomen in the newborn and infant

- In healthy newborns, aerophagia is common.
- An ill newborn with paralytic intestinal ileus characterized by quiet, nontender abdominal distention may have:
  - Sepsis
  - Birth asphyxia
  - Hypothyroidism
  - Electrolyte imbalance
  - Pneumonia or respiratory distress from aerophagia
- Necrotizing enterocolitis is the most common cause of acquired abdominal distention in premature infants.
- Upper GI obstruction
  - Atresias
  - Annular pancreas
  - Malrotation
- Lower GI obstruction
  - Atresias
  - Meconium ileus
  - Hirschsprung disease
  - Small left colon syndrome
  - Anorectal malformations
  - Incarcerated inguinal hernia

Tympanitic abdomen beyond the newborn period

- Constipation
- GI obstruction
  - Intraluminal
    - Pyloric stenosis
    - Intussusception
    - Bezoar
    - Meconium ileus equivalent
    - Intestinal polyps
    - Parasites (ascariasis)
    - Intrinsic tumors

  - Extraluminal
    - Postoperative adhesions
    - Appendiceal abscess
    - Meckel diverticulum
    - Abdominal or pelvic mass causing compression
    - Incarcerated hernia
  - Paralytic ileus
    - Abdominal surgery
    - Peritonitis
    - Trauma
    - Shock
    - Sepsis
    - Hypokalemia
    - Medication/anesthesia reaction
  - Fat malabsorption syndrome
  - Cystic fibrosis
  - Celiac disease

Palpable mass in the newborn and infant

- Renal or urinary tract masses account for two-thirds of neonatal abdominal masses.
  - Multicystic kidney
  - Hydronephrosis
  - Polycystic kidney disease
  - Renal vein thrombosis
  - Mesoblastic nephroma
- GI duplications
- Neuroblastoma
- Hydrometrocolpos
- Hematomas from birth trauma
  - Adrenal, hepatic, splenic
- Cysts
  - Choledochal, mesenteric, ovarian, splenic, urachal

Palpable mass beyond the newborn period

- Fecal masses from constipation
- Late presentations of congenital masses
  - Duplications
  - Mesenteric cysts
  - Choledochal cysts
  - Hematocolpos
- Cancer
  - Wilms tumor
  - Neuroblastoma
  - Hepatoblastoma
  - Ovarian tumors
  - Lymphoma (non-Hodgkin)

A

- Bezoars
- Pancreatic pseudocysts

Ascites in the newborn and infant

- Perforation in an obstructed urinary tract
  - Posterior urethral valves
- Congestive heart failure
- Liver disease
  - Congenital infection
  - Galactosemia
  - Lysosomal storage disease
- Chylous ascites from malformation or perforation of intestinal lymphatics
- Idiopathic

Ascites beyond the newborn period

- Most commonly, a consequence of chronic liver disease with cirrhosis and portal hypertension

Abdominal wall hypotonia

- Generalized hypotonia from neuromuscular disease
- Rickets
- Hypothyroidism

Peritonitis

- GI perforation
- Bacterial peritonitis
- Chemical peritonitis

Causes of distention, by location

- Epigastrium
  - Duodenal atresia
  - Pyloric stenosis
  - Malrotation
  - Gastric duplication
  - Bezoar (mass of eaten hair; usually due to a psychological disorder)
- Flank
  - Wilms tumor
  - Hydronephrosis
  - Multicystic kidney
  - Polycystic kidney
  - Neuroblastoma
  - Renal vein thrombosis
  - Adrenal hemorrhage
- Right upper quadrant
  - Choledochal cyst
  - Hepatomegaly
  - Hepatic tumors
  - Acute hydrops of the gallbladder
- Left upper quadrant
  - Splenomegaly
  - Splenic cyst
- Right lower quadrant
  - Ovarian mass
  - Intussusception
  - Appendiceal abscess
  - Crohn disease
  - Fecal mass
- Left lower quadrant
  - Ovarian mass
  - Fecal mass
- Hypogastrium
  - Hydrometrocolpos
  - Hematocolpos
  - Fecal mass
  - Presacral teratoma
  - Obstructed bladder
  - Urachal cyst

IMAGING

- Although history and physical examination may allow diagnosis, many children require radiographic imaging.
  - Choice of initial imaging technique is dictated by clinical suspicion and locally available resources and expertise.
  - Consulting with radiologist is helpful.
- In questionable cases, plain-film radiographs can confirm fecal mass; reexamination is indicated after laxative therapy to confirm that the masses are no longer present.
- Definitive radiographic evidence of necrotizing enterocolitis includes:
  - Pneumatosis intestinalis
  - Gas visible in the portal venous system of the liver

TREATMENT APPROACH

- Treating the underlying cause is the treatment for abdominal distention.

SPECIFIC TREATMENT

- Transient generalized distention due to aerophagia responds to changes in feeding technique and burping and in consoling techniques for the crying infant.

WHEN TO REFER

- Refer a child with abdominal distention to appropriate consultant if the child has:
  - Refractory vomiting
  - Moderate or severe pain that is undiagnosed

- Mass suspicious for cancer
- Urgent need for surgical or radiologic procedures

WHEN TO ADMIT

- Admit a child with abdominal distention if he or she has:
  - Refractory vomiting or dehydration
  - Peritonitis
  - Toxic or septic appearance
  - Moderate or severe pain that is undiagnosed or not well controlled
  - Mass suspicious for cancer
  - Urgent need for surgical or radiologic procedures

COMPLICATIONS

- Complications depend on the underlying cause of abdominal distention and are usually associated with delay in diagnosis and treatment.

PROGNOSIS

- Prognosis depends on the underlying cause of abdominal distention.

Abdominal Pain

DEFINITION

- Abdominal pain is defined as pain perceived to be in the area of the abdomen (between the thorax and pelvis).
- Recurrent abdominal pain is pain that occurs ≥3 times over ≥3 months that is severe enough to affect daily activities in children >3 years of age.

EPIDEMIOLOGY

- Abdominal pain is one of the most common symptoms in children and adolescents.
  - Incidence
    - Estimated to account for ~5% of unscheduled office visits
    - Each year, 4 of 1000 children undergo surgery for suspected appendicitis.
  - Prevalence
    - The precise number of children who experience acute abdominal pain is unknown.
    - For recurrent abdominal pain
      - The prevalence is estimated at 0.3–19%, although some large studies suggest 0.3–8%.
      - Higher prevalence in girls, children between 4 and 6 years of age, and in early adolescence

MECHANISM

- The mechanism for abdominal pain depends on its cause.
  - In pancreatitis, injury of the acinar cells and the premature activation of trypsinogen to trypsin in the pancreas caused by obstruction of ductal flow (in most cases) precipitate an aggressive immune response.
    - In marked contrast to adults, the causes of acute pancreatitis in children are:
      - Idiopathic causes
      - Trauma
      - Structural anomalies
      - Multisystem disease
      - Drugs and toxins
      - Viral infections
      - Hereditary causes
      - Metabolic disorders (eg, hyperlipidemia, hypercalcemia)

HISTORY

Description of pain: OLDCAR

- **O**nset/precipitating event (eg, trauma)
- **L**ocation (eg, quadrant, periumbilical)
  - Abdominal pain may be referred (eg, the cause is outside the abdomen).
    - For example, lower-lobe pneumonias may cause inflammatory irritation of the diaphragm, resulting in acute abdominal pain as the presenting symptom.
    - Pathology in the abdomen may also refer pain to other locations (eg, irritation of diaphragm may refer pain to shoulder area).
- **D**uration (eg, continuous, variable, specific time of day only, frequency)
- **C**haracter: nature, quality, severity (eg, sharp, tearing, dull, severe enough to awaken from sleep)
- **A**ssociated factors that improve or worsen (eg, activities, relationship to meals, relationship to breathing)
- **R**adiating pattern of pain
- Timing of onset and changes in intensity, location, and quality of pain over time may provide vital clues to diagnosis.
- If pain is recurrent, also consider
  - Timing of the onset of the pain in relation to other events (eg, mealtime, school)
  - Frequency of recurrence and duration of episodes
- Review of systems
  - Alarming symptoms or signs suggest a higher probability or prevalence of organic disease; these include:
    - Involuntary weight loss
    - Deceleration of linear growth
    - Gastrointestinal blood loss
    - Significant vomiting, bloody or bilious vomiting
    - Chronic severe diarrhea
    - Persistent right upper or right lower quadrant pain
    - Unexplained fever
  - Cardiopulmonary review (eg, dyspnea, tachypnea, color changes)
  - Gastrointestinal review (eg, number of bowel movements, frequency, consistency; color; whether blood is present)
  - Genitourinary review (eg, dysuria, hematuria, observed stones)
  - Neuropsychiatric review
  - Children with recurrent abdominal pain are more likely to have headache, joint pain, anorexia, vomiting, nausea, excessive gas, and altered bowel symptoms.

Medical and family history

- Trauma
- Toxin exposures, medications, diet history
- Environmental or behavioral factors (recent changes in family or school, travel, new foods)
- Sick contacts/exposure to illness, exposure to animals
- Previous abdominal surgeries
- Previous weights and growth pattern
- Family or personal history of celiac disease, inflammatory bowel disease, inherited disorders, endocrine disorders, chronic pain disorders

- For girls, obtain menstruation, gynecologic, and sexual histories.
  - Age at onset of menstruation
  - Bleeding frequency, duration, regularity, amount (number of pads/tampons and saturation)
  - Dates of previous menses
  - Concurrent symptoms (bloating, cramping, headaches)
  - Vaginal bleeding or discharge, history of tampon retention
- Perinatal history
  - Was stool passed within the first 24 hours

Personal and lifestyle factors

- Detailed discussions of personal lifestyle factors, especially in adolescents, may be conducted ideally without others present.
  - HEADSSS assessment
    - **H**ome
    - **E**ducation
    - **A**ctivities
    - **D**rugs
    - **S**uicide/depression
    - **S**exuality
    - **S**afety
  - The patient must feel comfortable discussing his or her own symptoms and concerns, even if different from those expressed by parents.
  - Assess parental expectations: The parents may want to relate some of their concerns without the child being present.

PHYSICAL EXAM

- Vital signs and anthropomorphic characteristics
  - Temperature (febrile or not)
  - Respiratory rate, oxygen saturation
  - Pain may elevate the heart rate and blood pressure.
  - Evaluate hydration status and consider orthostatic vital signs as appropriate.
  - Measure height/stature and weight; plot measurements on standardized charts.
    - Growth failure may be consistent with inflammatory bowel disease or cystic fibrosis.
- Physical examination
  - A complete physical examination is indicated.
  - Abdominal examination
    - Assess cooperation of the patient and whether the patient is distractable.
    - Palpate 4 quadrants, flank, and costovertebral angles.
    - Assess for guarding and rebound.
    - Auscultate.
    - In infants, examine the umbilicus and periumbilical area for discoloration and signs of infection.
    - Consider psoas and obdurator testing if there is clinical suspicion of appendicitis or peritonitis.
  - Cardiopulmonary examination
  - Genitourinary examination, including urethra
    - In males, examine the scrotum and inguinal canals.
    - In females, perform external examination of the vaginal orifice; consider gynecologic examination as indicated.
  - Rectal examination
  - Assess for rashes and bruises (eg, palpable purpura on buttocks and lower extremities, abdominal bruising indicative of handlebar injury)
  - Pancreatitis
    - Patients usually lie still because movement intensifies pain.
    - Examination of the abdomen may reveal decreased bowel sounds, guarding, and rebound tenderness.
    - The Gray Turner and Cullen signs—discoloration of the flanks and umbilicus, respectively—are typical of hemorrhagic pancreatitis, but are seldom present in children.

DIFFERENTIAL DIAGNOSIS

- Abdominal pain has a very broad differential diagnosis.

Acute abdominal pain

- Main causes of acute abdominal pain, by age
  - Neonate
    - Necrotizing enterocolitis
    - Spontaneous gastric perforation
    - Hirschsprung disease
    - Meconium ileus
    - Intestinal atresia or stenosis
    - Peritonitis owing to gastroschisis or ruptured omphalocele
    - Traumatic perforation of viscus (difficult birth)
  - Infant (<2 years)
    - Colic (<3 months)
    - Acute gastroenteritis or viral syndrome
    - Traumatic perforation of viscus (child abuse)
    - Intussusception
    - Incarcerated hernia
    - Volvulus (malrotation)
    - Sickling syndromes
  - School age
    - Acute gastroenteritis or viral syndrome
    - Urinary tract infection
    - Appendicitis

A

- Trauma
- Constipation
- Pneumonia
- Sickling syndromes
- Adolescent
  - Acute gastroenteritis or viral syndrome
  - Urinary tract infection
  - Appendicitis
  - Trauma
  - Constipation
  - Pelvic inflammatory disease
  - Pneumonia
  - Mittelschmerz
  - Pregnancy
  - Other gynecologic issues (dysmenorrhea, tubo-ovarian abscess)
- A rare cause of abdominal pain in children and adolescents is pancreatitis.
  - Abdominal pain is present in nearly all patients with pancreatitis and may be of sudden onset or insidious.
  - The most common location of pain is the epigastrium, but it can occur in the right or the left upper quadrant.
  - Often accompanied by vomiting, anorexia, and nausea, with food often aggravating the pain and vomiting.

Recurrent abdominal pain

- Normal examination and the absence of alarm signals point toward a functional diagnosis for abdominal pain.
- Studies have shown associations between recurrent abdominal pain and:
  - Family dynamics (eg, children living in a single-parent household are more likely to experience recurrent abdominal pain)
  - Psychological comorbidity (eg, anxiety)
  - Socioeconomic status
    - Children living in low-income, low-educated–worker families were more likely to experience pain.
- Differential diagnosis, by related symptoms/causes
  - Upper gastrointestinal inflammation
    - Gastroesophageal reflux disease
    - Peptic ulcer
    - *Helicobacter pylori* gastritis
    - Nonsteroidal antiinflammatory drug ulcer
    - Crohn disease
    - Eosinophilic gastroenteritis
    - Ménétrier disease
    - Cytomegalovirus gastritis
    - Parasitic infection (*Giardia, Blastocystis hominis*)
    - Varioliform gastritis
    - Lymphocytic gastritis or celiac disease
    - Henoch-Schönlein purpura
  - Altered bowel pattern
    - Idiopathic inflammatory bowel disorders
    - Ulcerative colitis
    - Crohn disease
    - Microscopic colitis with crypt distortion
    - Lymphocytic colitis
    - Collagenous colitis
    - Infectious disorders
    - Parasitic (*Giardia, Blastocystis hominis, Dientamoeba fragilis*)
    - Bacterial (*Clostridium difficile, Yersinia, Campylobacter,* tuberculosis)
    - Lactose intolerance
    - Complication of constipation—megacolon, encopresis, intermittent sigmoid volvulus
    - Drug-induced diarrhea, constipation
    - Gynecologic disorders
    - Neoplasia (lymphoma, carcinoma)
    - Psychiatric disorder
  - Isolated paroxysmal abdominal pain
    - Obstructive disorders
    - Crohn disease
    - Malrotation with or without volvulus
    - Intussusception with lead point
    - Postsurgical adhesions
    - Small-bowel lymphoma
    - Endometriosis
    - Infection (tuberculosis, *Yersinia*)
    - Vascular disorders
    - Eosinophilic gastroenteritis
    - Angioneurotic edema
    - Appendiceal colic
    - Dysmenorrhea
    - Musculoskeletal disorders
    - Uteropelvic junction obstruction
    - Abdominal migraine
    - Acute intermittent porphyria
    - Mental disorders (factitious disorder, conversion reaction, somatization disorder, school phobia)
    - Functional abdominal pain

- Motility disorders
  - Idiopathic gastroparesis
  - Biliary dyskinesia
  - Intestinal pseudo-obstruction
- Other
  - Obstructive disorders
  - Chronic pancreatitis
  - Chronic hepatitis
  - Chronic cholecystitis
  - Ureteropelvic junction obstruction
  - Abdominal migraine
  - Psychiatric disorder

LABORATORY EVALUATION

- Do not delay consultation for studies if surgical abdomen is suspected.
- Evaluation is guided by clinical suspicion.
- When history and physical examination indicate a dysfunctional or psychogenic cause, urinalysis should suffice as the initial laboratory study.
- Studies may include:
  - Pregnancy test for young women, especially if abdominal imaging is being considered
  - Complete blood cell count with differential
  - Serum chemistries or comprehensive metabolic panel
  - Urinalysis, urine culture
  - Stool hemoccult (guaiac)
  - Erythrocyte sedimentation rate
  - Erythrocyte smear and hemoglobin electrophoresis
  - Purified protein derivative testing for tuberculosis
  - Tests for sexually transmitted diseases
  - In patients with diarrhea:
    - Stool ova and parasite
    - Stool culture
    - *Giardia* enzyme-linked immunosorbent assay
    - *Clostridium difficile* toxin
    - Celiac panel
    - Lactose breath test
  - In patients with dyspepsia:
    - *Helicobacter pylori* serologic test
  - When hepatitis is suspected, or if direct hyperbilirubinemia is evident:
    - Liver enzymes, liver function tests
  - When pancreatitis is suspected:
    - Serum amylase and lipase
    - A >3-fold lipase increase is considered consistent with pancreatitis

IMAGING

- Imaging is guided by clinical suspicion.
  - Early diagnosis of the acute abdomen may often be made solely on clinical grounds, and imaging may not always be indicated.
  - Before abdominal imaging in young women, pregnancy status should be determined.
  - In general, the physician should consider least invasive procedures first, keeping in mind the cost of special studies in terms of pain, discomfort, and time.
- Abdominal radiographs (kidneys, ureter, and bladder)
  - May help to identify distended bowel, bowel obstruction, constipation/fecal impaction, fecaliths (associated with appendicitis), pneumonia
- Abdominal computed tomography
  - May help to identify appendicitis, peritonitis, or other anatomical pathology
- Abdominal and pelvic ultrasonography
  - Safe, noninvasive ways to assess bowel and pelvic organ structures
  - Help clarify the need for urgent surgical intervention (eg, intussusception, ovarian torsion, testicular torsion, kidney abscess)
  - May be operator dependent
  - For pancreatitis:
    - Specificity of approximately 62–67%
    - Most sensitive of available methods to appraise biliary tract for evidence of the cause of acute pancreatitis
    - Indicated when the patient has a history of major blunt trauma to stage severe pancreatitis
      - To assess for substantiation of necrosis, which is often not noted for 48–72 hours after onset
      - To learn whether noteworthy intraabdominal complications are present
- Upper gastrointestinal series
  - Should be considered in patients with recurrent vomiting to define potential anatomic abnormalities, such as gastric outlet disorder or malrotation

DIAGNOSTIC PROCEDURES

- Additional procedures can be performed as guided by clinical suspicion (eg, endoscopy and biopsy).

TREATMENT APPROACH

- In the case of acute abdominal pain, early surgical consultation should be obtained as necessary.
  - Intervention may be indicated even if imaging studies have not been obtained.
  - If a diagnosis is made, treatment is aimed at the underlying disease entity.

A

SPECIFIC TREATMENT

■ The treatment approach for acute and functional abdominal pain are quite different.

Treatment categories for acute abdominal pain

■ Acute surgical issue (manage with early surgical consultation and operative correction)
- Closed loop intestinal obstruction
- Volvulus (gastric, midgut, sigmoid)
- Incarcerated hernia (inguinal, internal, external)
- High-grade bowel obstruction
- Nonreducible intussusception
- Malrotation with Ladd bands
- Ovarian torsion
- Testicular torsion
- Acute appendicitis
- Perforated viscus with diffuse peritonitis or toxicity
- Ruptured tumor
- Ectopic pregnancy
- Trauma, especially if the patient is not hemodynamically stable

■ Acute abdominal pain that may require a combined surgical and medical approach
- Partial small-bowel obstruction
- Postsurgical adhesions
- Crohn disease
- Lymphoma
- Periappendiceal abscess
- Abdominal/peritoneal abscess
- Cholecystitis
- Gallbladder hydrops
- Pancreatitis
- Pancreatic pseudocyst
- Toxic megacolon or typhlitis
- Gynecologic issues (such as a stable patient with a tubo-ovarian abscess)

■ Acute abdominal pain to be managed medically and/or supportively
- Pregnancy
- Upper respiratory tract infection, pharyngitis
- Pneumonia
- Viral gastroenteritis, acute gastritis
- Mesenteric adenitis
- Partial bowel obstruction
- Paralytic ileus
- Intestinal gas pain
- Fecal impaction
- Meconium ileus equivalent in cystic fibrosis
- Bacterial enterocolitis
- Peptic ulcer disease
- Acute constipation
- Flare of functional abdominal pain
- Acute hepatitis
- Perihepatitis (Fitz-Hugh–Curtis syndrome)
- Inflammatory bowel disease (eg, Crohn disease, ulcerative colitis)
- Henoch-Schönlein purpura
- Hereditary angioedema
- Hemolytic uremic syndrome
- Pyelonephritis
- Renal calculi
- Dysmenorrhea
- Mittelschmerz
- Pelvic inflammatory disease
- Sickle cell crisis
- Diabetic ketoacidosis
- Poisoning
- Porphyria
- Collagen vascular disease

Treatments for functional abdominal pain

■ Treatment of functional gastrointestinal disorders, including functional abdominal pain of childhood, is becoming more common.

■ Treatments can be categorized as:
- Dietary interventions
- Psychosocial therapies
- Medical management

Dietary interventions

■ Common dietary changes include:
- High-fiber diet
- Avoidance of lactose
- Oligoantigenic diet
- Low-oxalate diet (for abdominal migraine)

■ A high-fiber diet may be suggested, primarily in constipated children, to substitute for nutrient-poor, high-fat, high-calorie diets.

■ Dietary manipulation is something that parents and children can understand, and suggesting this intervention may empower the family.

Psychosocial therapies

■ Treatment of functional gastrointestinal disorders, including functional abdominal pain of childhood, is becoming more common.

■ Specific mind-body techniques include breathing techniques, guided imagery, progressive muscle relaxation, biofeedback, hypnosis, cognitive-behavioral training, and music therapy.

 • Cognitive-behavioral therapy combines operant elements and stress management.

  – Results in short-term improvement, with more than half of patients experiencing freedom from pain

  – The child's coping skills and parent's caregiving strategies predict effectiveness.

  – Disengagement and involuntary engagement are correlated with increased anxiety, depression, and somatic symptoms.

 • Guided imagery, relaxation, biofeedback, and hypnosis show promise.

  – Reported improvement in pain, fewer school absences, better engagement in social activities, and fewer visits to physician's office may result from guided imagery and progressive-relaxation techniques taught over approximately 4 office visits.

  – Such techniques are easy to learn and teach and are office friendly, even for children.

Medical management

■ Several drugs have been used to treat recurrent abdominal pain in childhood, including:

 • Famotidine

 • Pizotifen

 • Citalopram, a selective serotonin reuptake inhibitor

  – Children who receive this agent improve in terms of abdominal pain, anxiety, depression, and functional impairment.

 • Peppermint oil

  – The only one that appears to be of specific use for abdominal pain is peppermint oil in the form of a pH-dependent, enteric-coated capsule.

■ Other medications (eg, anticholinergics, antiemetics, other antidepressants, simethicone) are commonly used but insufficiently studied.

WHEN TO REFER

■ Involuntary weight loss

■ Deceleration of linear growth

■ Gastrointestinal blood loss

■ Significant vomiting

■ Chronic severe diarrhea

■ Persistent right upper or right lower quadrant pain

■ Unexplained fever

■ Pregnancy

■ Gynecologic issues (including ectopic pregnancy, tubo-ovarian abscess)

■ Surgery required

■ Family history of inflammatory bowel disease

■ Extraintestinal symptoms

■ History of psychiatric disorder

■ Abnormal test results

■ Anemia or low mean corpuscular volume

■ Peripheral eosinophilia

■ Increased erythrocyte sedimentation rate

■ Increased transaminases

■ Increased blood urea nitrogen or creatinine

■ Hypoalbuminemia

■ Low C4 complement level

■ Intestinal infection

WHEN TO ADMIT

■ Hospitalization is required in the following circumstances.

 • Surgical or medical emergency as determined by diagnostic or therapeutic intervention

 • Inability to tolerate enteral nutrition

 • Inability to maintain hydration status

 • Diagnosis that requires observation to monitor clinical status

■ In the case of functional abdominal pain:

 • 50% of patients experience relief of symptoms during hospitalization, but the natural history of the pain does not seem to be affected.

 • As a result, hospitalization is seldom indicated, as it does not help with environmental modification and may reinforce pain behavior.

PROGNOSIS

■ Depends on the cause of the acute or recurrent abdominal pain

Acne

DEFINITION

- Acne is a disease of the pilosebaceous unit in which sebaceous glands become enlarged and increase their production of sebum.
- Increased sebaceous gland activity is necessary for acne to develop.

EPIDEMIOLOGY

- Age
  - Prevalent in a large proportion of adolescents and young adults
  - May be seen as late as the 3rd and 4th decades
- Sex
  - Found in up to:
    - 78% of premenarchal girls
    - 100% of adolescent boys

ETIOLOGY

- Hormones
  - Androgenic stimulation of sebaceous glands increases sebum production.
- Follicular obstruction
  - Keratinous impaction develops in the pilosebaceous canal, causing outlet obstruction.
  - Sebaceous and keratinous debris accumulate behind the obstruction.
- Proliferation of the anaerobic bacterium *Propionibacterium acnes*:
  - Contributes to the rupture of the dilated pilosebaceous unit
  - Results in extravasation of pilosebaceous contents into the surrounding dermis and inflammatory acne lesions

RISK FACTORS

- Adolescent age
- Increased level of circulating androgens
- Skin that is rich in sebaceous glands

SIGNS AND SYMPTOMS

- Noninflamed open and closed comedones
  - Obstruction of pilosebaceous canal causes:
    - Open comedones (blackheads)
    - Closed comedones (whiteheads)
  - Closed comedones (whiteheads) appear as dome-shaped, flesh-colored papules that are often overlooked (see Figure 1 on page F1).
  - Acne in prepubertal children is predominantly noninflammatory and easily overlooked.
- Inflammatory papules and pustules
  - Rare in young children and suggests a possible hyperandrogenic condition
  - Possible hyperandrogenic conditions include:
    - Congenital adrenal hyperplasia
    - Rare androgen-secreting tumor
  - Examine for precocious puberty in both sexes and virilization in girls.
- Cystic acne in severe cases
  - Nodules >5 mm in diameter
  - True cysts (compressible nodules under normal-appearing skin)
  - Can result in permanent acne scars
- Lesions appear most frequently on the face.
  - They also often appear on the chest and back.
  - Lower portions of the trunk, buttocks, thighs are involved less frequently.
  - Distal extremities are always spared.

DIFFERENTIAL DIAGNOSIS

Flat warts

- See Figure 2 on page F1.
- Small, flesh-colored
- Sharp, right-angled edge and finely roughened surface
- Variable in size
- Closed comedones are smooth, dome-shaped, and uniformly small.

Milia

- Small epidermal inclusion cysts
- Also confused with inflammatory pustules, especially in infants with neonatal acne

Adenoma sebaceum

- Pink papules that are occasionally confused with acne lesions
- Lesions are actually angiofibromas.
  - They are a dermal manifestation of tuberous sclerosis.
- Adenoma sebaceum lesions should be suspected if they are:
  - Clustered primarily in the center of the face
  - Persistent
  - Resistant to acne therapy

Acne rosacea

- See Figure 3 on page F1.
- An acneiform eruption that can be distinguished from acne by:
  - Background blush of erythema and telangiectasia
  - Absence of comedones
- Most often found in middle-aged adults

Steroid acne

- Can be induced by systemic or topical steroids
- Lacking in comedones
- Involutes slowly and spontaneously after discontinuation of steroids
- Acne from systemic steroids usually is:
  - Made up of numerous small, uniform-sized papules and pustules
  - Found on the upper trunk
  - Lacking in comedones

Gram-negative folliculitis

- Caused by gram-negative organisms in patients being treated for acne with systemic antibiotics
- Should be suspected in patients whose disease flares up during therapy
  - Especially when flare-up produces numerous pustules

Acne conglobata

- Unusually severe acne variant caused by:
  - Sudden deterioration of existing active acne
  - Recurrence of acne that has been quiet for many years
  - Most common in 18- to 30-year-old men
    - Lesions consist of:
      - Comedones
      - Cysts with foul-smelling seropurulent material
      - Burrowing and interconnecting abscesses, leaving irregular and disfiguring scars
    - Has been associated with systemic diseases, such as:
      - Hidradenitis suppurativa
      - Pyoderma gangrenosum
      - Renal amyloidosis
      - Musculoskeletal syndrome
    - The mainstay of treatment is isotretinoin.

Acne fulminans

- A rare and severe form of acne
  - Usually occurs in men
  - Characterized by:
    - Sudden onset of painful acne nodules
    - Rarely by ulcerative lesions
    - Systemic symptoms include fever; leukocytosis; polyarthritis; splenomegaly; erythema nodosum; and lytic bone lesions in long bones, clavicle, and sternum.
- Treatment involves a combination of systemic corticosteroids initially, followed by isotretinoin.
- Prognosis is good, although residual scarring and disfigurement may persist.

DIAGNOSTIC APPROACH

- Diagnosis is rarely difficult.
- Comedonal lesions may require closer inspection to avoid confusion with:
  - Warts
  - Milia
  - Adenoma sebaceum
  - Acne variants

LABORATORY FINDINGS

- In cases of possible hyperandrogenic condition, screening blood studies should include serum levels of:
  - Testosterone
  - Dehydroepiandrosterone sulfate
  - 17-hydroxyprogesterone
- In possible gram-negative folliculitis
  - Bacterial culture with antibiotic sensitivity studies

TREATMENT APPROACH

- Acne is important to the patient seeking help and should be managed seriously.
  - Some young people appear to be more affected psychologically than others, but no one is comfortable with acne.
- Four methods of treatment have proved effective.
  - Topical comedolytic agents
  - Topical and systemic antibiotics
  - Systemic hormonal therapy
  - Systemic retinoids
- The most traditional and effective treatment regimen is a combination of comedolytics and antibiotics.

SPECIFIC TREATMENTS

Comedolytics

- Retinoids
  - Topical retinoids help disimpact the keratinous plug in the follicular canal.
  - Topical comedolytics are available in a variety of preparations; the preparation strength reflects its irritancy and probably also its efficacy.
    - Tretinoin
      - Preparation strength depends on concentration of the drug and nature of the vehicle in which it is contained.
      - Cream in 0.025% (mildest), 0.05% (mild), 0.1% (moderate)
      - Gel in 0.01% (mild), 0.025% (moderate), 0.05% (strongest)
      - Solution in 0.05% (strongest)

- Adapalene
- Tazarotene
- Benzoyl peroxide
- Salicylic acid
- Azelaic acid
- Sodium sulfacetamide
- Most helpful in treating superficial acne lesions, including comedones and superficial papules and pustules
- Also reduce inflammatory lesions and enhance penetration of other medications
- Consensus is that in most cases, topical retinoids (alone or in combination) should be used as first-line therapy for mild-to-moderate inflammatory acne in addition to comedonal acne.
- Preferred agent for maintenance therapy
- In combination with another topical agent
  - Apply the retinoid at bedtime and the other agent each morning.
  - Adapalene
    - Gel in 0.1% and 0.3% and cream in a concentration of 0.1%.
  - Tazarotene
    - Gel and cream; each is available in concentrations of 0.05% and 0.1%.
  - Benzoyl peroxide
    - Gel in concentrations of 2.5%, 5%, and 10%
  - Salicylic acid
    - Large variety of preparations and concentrations
  - Sodium sulfacetamide
    - Lotion in 10% concentration
  - Patients are initially prescribed in the mildest preparations; potency is increased if necessary.
- Side effects
  - Skin irritation is the most common.
  - ~1% of patients develop true allergic contact dermatitis to benzoyl peroxide.
    - Requires permanent discontinuation of this agent
  - Benzoyl peroxide can bleach clothing and linens.
  - Topical retinoids may make the skin more susceptible to the effects of sunlight.
    - Patients should avoid excessive exposure to the sun and use oil-free sunscreens.

Antibiotics

- Indicated for patients who have inflammatory acne lesions
- Topical agents
  - Erythromycin
  - Clindamycin

- Combinations of benzoyl peroxide and erythromycin or clindamycin are often prescribed before oral antibiotics.
  - Benzamycin® gel (5%benzoyl peroxideand 3% erythromycin) twice daily
  - Benzaclin® gel (5% benzoyl peroxide and 1% clindamycin phosphate) twice daily
- For inflammatory lesions extensive enough to make topical therapy impractical (ie, involving the neck, shoulders, and upper trunk) or unresponsive to a topical regimen, systemic antibiotics are warranted.
  - Tetracycline is the drug of choice.
    - Proven efficacy, relative low cost, and low incidence of side effects, even over a long period
    - Should be taken on an empty stomach (on awakening or on retiring)
    - The initial dose is 500 mg orally twice daily; the dose is decreased to 500 mg once daily after sustained response is achieved.
  - Tetracycline and other drugs in the same class (ie, doxycycline and minocycline) should not be used in patients under 8 years because of dental staining.
  - Erythromycin may be used as an alternative if patient does not respond to tetracycline.
  - Doxycycline and minocycline may also be substituted.
    - Doxycycline is more likely to cause photosensitivity.
    - Minocycline is very expensive.
- Resistance to *P acnes* may affect as many as 25% of patients taking antibiotics.
  - Preventive measures should be taken.
    - Limit the use of oral antibiotics to shorter periods.
    - Combining topical comedolytics (especially topical retinoids) with topical antibiotics.
    - Avoid the use of oral antibiotics as maintenance therapy.

Systemic retinoids

- Isotretinoin
  - Reduces follicular keratinization, sebum production, and intrafollicular bacterial counts, resulting in a dramatic improvement in acne
  - Therapeutic effect usually takes several months and often persists long after the course of therapy is discontinued.
  - Historically, 6-month courses have been used, but recently some practitioners focus more on total dose given instead of duration.
    - Target is 100 to 150 mg/kg total dose.
  - Side effects are common.
    - Almost all patients experience mucocutaneous reactions (cheilitis, conjunctivitis, and dry mucous membranes of the mouth and nose).

- Extracutaneous complications also occur, including:
  - Elevation of plasma lipid levels
  - Asymptomatic vertebral hyperostoses
  - Depression and pseudotumor cerebri (rarely)
- Female patients must exercise strict birth control while taking this drug.
  - Exposure to isotretinoin in pregnancy has been associated with a 25-fold increased risk of major fetal malformations.
  - The US Food and Drug Administration requires that all patients being prescribed isotretinoin be enrolled in a national registry.
- Isotretinoin is recommended only for:
  - Patients with severe cystic and/or scarring acne (or both)
  - A minority of patients who have severe noncystic acne and have not responded to topical comedolytics and oral antibiotics

Hormonal therapy

- An excellent option for women with moderate to severe acne if:
  - Oral contraception is desired.
  - An alternative to repeated courses of isotretinoin is preferred.
  - Certain endocrine disorders are present.
- All combination contraceptives reduce free testosterone and have a positive effect on acne.
  - No single preparation is demonstrably superior.
- Contraceptives containing only progestins should be avoided because intrinsic androgenic activity may aggravate acne.

Patient compliance

- Patient compliance is the single most important aspect of successful acne treatment.
- To maximize compliance:
  - Take time at the initial visit to explain use, anticipated effects, and side effects of each medication.
    - Printed instructions are good reinforcement.
  - Medications are taken twice daily.
    - Link to an established daily routine, such as brushing the teeth.
  - The concept that the treatment will take time to be effective needs to be emphasized.
  - The most common patient questions, often unasked, pertain to diet, cleanliness, cosmetics, and picking at the lesions.

Diet

- Some evidence indicates that the usual American diet may have adverse effects on acne; however, specific foods have not been implicated.
- For most people, a sensible diet is all that is suggested.

Cleanliness

- A primary question from parents
  - The notion that acne is a function of poor hygiene should be dispelled.
- In general, cleaning agents for acne need not be recommended.
  - Most irritate the skin, unnecessarily compounding irritation caused by topical comedolytics.
- A mild soap-free cleanser is often suggested.

Cosmetics

- Cosmetics have been implicated as possibly contributing to the acne process.
- It is preferable to avoid using them.
- If used, they should be water based and applied sparingly.

Picking

- Much of skin damage in acne patients is self-inflicted.
- Picking, probing, and squeezing cause tissue damage and sometimes produce scars.
- For some patients, picking may become so obsessive that excoriations are the only lesions seen.

WHEN TO REFER

- Patients unresponsive to oral antibiotics and topical comedolytics
- Patients with cystic or scarring acne
- Young girls with acne or girls with acne and irregular menses
- Patients with acne fulminans
  - Abrupt onset of cystic acne, fever, arthralgias

FOLLOW-UP

- The first scheduled return visit should be at 2 to 3 months after the start of therapy.
  - Improvement usually occurs within this period.
  - At this visit, the acne regimen can be adjusted as necessary.
    - For example, comedolytics and antibiotics can be increased (or reduced) depending on the initial response.
- Continued improvement is to be expected with continuation of therapy.
  - For many, the dose of systemic antibiotics can be reduced gradually and eliminated after 6 to 12 months.
  - Most patients require prolonged maintenance therapy (often over years) with topical agents.
  - Some require continued topical antibiotic therapy.

COMPLICATIONS

- The major complications are the psychosocial ramifications of acne.
  - May be compounded and perpetuated by permanent scars

A

- Scars are easier to prevent than to treat.
  - The emphasis in acne is on early, aggressive medical therapy.
- Established scars are difficult to treat.
  - Acne scars are best treated when inflammatory lesions are quiescent.
  - Many patients have been disappointed with the results of dermabrasion.
    - Patients treated with isotretinoin should wait for at least 1 year before having dermabrasion.
  - Bovine collagen injections have produced short-term improvement.
    - Repeated injections are often necessary.
    - Long-term results are not yet known.
  - Laser resurfacing by experienced operators has produced some promising results.

PROGNOSIS

- With proper treatment, the prognosis for acne is good, if not excellent.
- Patients should understand that most therapy controls rather than cures acne.
- Cystic acne has been the most difficult to treat, but isotretinoin has become a powerful tool for its treatment.
  - Potential exists for prolonged remissions, sometimes lasting for years after a single course of therapy.
  - Because of serious side effects, its use is usually reserved for patients who have severe cystic or scarring acne (or both) that does not respond to standard treatment.

Acute Surgical Abdomen

DEFINITION

- Abdominal pain that may require immediate surgical intervention
- 3 major diagnoses are the most common and the most likely to cause complications if treatment is delayed.
  - Malrotation and midgut volvulus, which usually presents in the newborn period
  - Intussusception, which occurs most often in children between 2 months and 2 years of age
  - Appendicitis, which is most common in children >5 years
- There are also other causes of abdominal pain, some requiring immediate surgical intervention.
  - For a more complete list of potentially emergent diagnoses, see Differential Diagnosis.

ETIOLOGY

- Malrotation and midgut volvulus
  - At 5–6 weeks' gestation, the elongating midgut pushes out into the umbilical coelom.
  - When it returns to the abdominal cavity at 10–12 weeks' gestation, it rotates and fixes to the posterior abdominal wall.
  - The duodenum returns first and is mainly retroperitoneal.
    - It courses behind the mesenteric vessels and enters the peritoneal cavity at the duodenal jejunal junction, just to the left of L2, the ligament of Treitz.
  - The colon enters the abdomen last and rotates so that the ileocecal region is in the right lower quadrant.
  - The right and left colon are fixed to the posterior abdominal wall by avascular attachments.
  - Thus, the small-bowel mesentery is normally fixed along a line from the ligament of Treitz in the left upper quadrant just to the left of L2 to the right lower quadrant at the right sacroiliac joint.
  - This long fixation prevents the lengthy mass of small bowel from rotating with the superior mesenteric artery and vein as a center.
  - This rotation, twisting, or volvulus would obstruct blood flow to the intestine and cause gangrene.
  - If an anomaly of rotation is present, or if this long fixation does not occur, then volvulus can occur.
  - In such anomalies of rotation and fixation (usually termed *malrotation* or *nonrotation*), the avascular adhesion of the cecum still appears to occur, but:
    - The cecum is usually in the midabdomen.
    - The adhesive bands (now called *Ladd bands*) cross the duodenum to the right upper quadrant.
  - This obstruction of the duodenum in malrotation causes bilious emesis.
  - The possibility of volvulus in malrotation requires urgent intervention.

- Intussusception occurs when the terminal ileum telescopes into the right colon.
  - This causes bowel obstruction and ischemia because the mesenteric vessels are dragged along with the ileum.
  - Intussusception is most likely due to hypertrophic ileal lymphatic tissue, which acts as a food bolus that can be swallowed by the more distal bowel.
- Appendicitis is probably caused by obstruction of the lumen by feces or hypertrophic lymphatic tissue.
  - Blockage allows stasis and bacterial multiplication to occur in the closed space.

SIGNS AND SYMPTOMS

- In brief, indicators of an acute surgical abdomen include:
  - Pain lasting >1 hour that is severe enough to require analgesics
  - Bilious emesis
  - Abdominal pain of any sort lasting >6 hours
  - Obstipation
  - Localized abdominal tenderness
  - Guarding
  - Rebound
  - Guaiac-positive stools, melena, or hematochezia
- Indicators of nonsurgical problems include:
  - Diarrhea
  - Symptoms of systemic illness: headache, sore throat, and myalgia
  - Emesis precedes pain
  - High fever very early in the illness
  - No abdominal tenderness
- Physical examination
  - Inspection of the abdomen can reveal distention or a mass.
  - Palpation should begin by gently stroking all abdominal quadrants while looking at the patient's face.
    - With peritonitis, cutaneous hyperesthesia is often present, which can be determined by narrowing of the outer canthus of the eye (wincing).
  - The clinician should gently percuss the entire abdomen.
    - Pain on percussion is termed *rebound* and indicates peritonitis, which can be localized or general.
    - Other tests for rebound, such as pushing in on the abdomen and then suddenly letting go, are very painful and unnecessary.
    - Percussion can also indicate gaseous distention of the intestine by the resonant note of tympany.
  - Palpate the abdomen quadrant by quadrant while looking at the patient's face.
    - The clinician should make several passes of each quadrant, with each being deeper.

A

- Look for a mass, tenderness, and guarding.
  - When the examiner pushes on a quadrant of the abdomen over the rectus muscle and it pushes back, this is known as *guarding*.
  - Guarding cannot occur voluntarily; it indicates localized peritonitis and, most often, the need for surgery.
  - If both the right and the left rectus push back, this is known as *rigidity*, which indicates generalized peritonitis.
  - Rigidity can be performed voluntarily.
- Auscultation of the abdomen offers no useful information.
  - No data support lack of bowel sounds with an ileus or high-pitched hyperactive bowel sounds with obstruction.
- Rectal examination is useful in:
  - Pelvic abscess
  - Obtaining stool for guaic testing for intussusception
- The clinician should assess structures or organs superior and inferior to the abdomen.
  - Pneumonia, inguinal hernia, and testicular torsion can cause abdominal pain.
- Malrotation and midgut volvulus
  - Usually develops in the newborn period but can occur at any age.
  - The characteristic symptom is bilious emesis.
    - This symptom should provoke urgent gastrointestinal (GI) contrast studies.
    - Approximately one-third of all children with bilious emesis require operative intervention (although not always for malrotation and midgut volvulus).
    - Any child with bilious emesis who has abdominal pain or tenderness should have either surgery or a contrast examination.
- Intussusception
  - Most children have intermittent colicky abdominal pain.
  - Some will be lethargic.
  - The child appears well between bouts of pain (approximately 20 minutes).
  - Physical examination reveals a mass in the epigastrium and a feeling of emptiness in the right lower quadrant (signe de Dance).
  - Tenderness and guarding are present as ischemia progresses.
  - Stool is usually guaiac positive, and a currant-jelly bloody stool may be passed.
- Appendicitis
  - Early symptoms are diffuse or periumbilical abdominal pain.
  - Anorexia, nausea, vomiting, and localization of the pain to the right lower quadrant follow.
  - Physical examination reveals:
    - Fever (temperature to 38.6°C)
    - Right lower quadrant tenderness
    - Guarding

Most Common Diagnoses in Boys With a Chief Complaint of Abdominal Pain by Age[a]

<2 yr (n = 56)		2–5 yr (n = 128)		5–12 yr (n = 230)		>12 yr (n = 86)	
Diagnosis	Frequency (%)	Diagnosis	Frequency (%)	Diagnosis	Frequency (%)	Diagnosis	Frequency (%)
Abdominal pain	30 (60)	Abdominal pain	59 (46)	Abdominal pain	117 (51)	Abdominal pain	33 (38)
Constipation	9 (18)	Constipation	21 (16)	Constipation	27 (12)	Appendicitis	14 (16)
Infection	4 (8)	Infection	13 (10)	Appendicitis	24 (10)	Constipation	7 (8)
Bowel obstruction	2 (4)	Gastroenteritis	13 (10)	Gastroenteritis	14 (6)	Gastritis, esophagitis	5 (6)
Dental	1 (2)	Hematologic	4 (3)	Gastritis, esophagitis	14 (6)	Infection	4 (5)
Gastritis, esophagitis	1 (2)	Gastritis, esophagitis	4 (3)	Infection	10 (4)	Diabetes	2 (2)
Crohn disease	1 (2)	Bowel obstruction	4 (3)	Hematologic	5 (2)	Hematologic	2 (2)
Abdominal trauma	1 (2)	Appendicitis	3 (2)	Cancer	2 (1)	Cancer	2 (2)

[a] From: Klein MD, Rabbani AB, Rood KD, et al. Three quantitative approaches to the diagnosis of abdominal pain in children: practical applications of decision theory. *J Pediatr Surg*. 2001;36(9):1375-1380. Copyright © Elsevier 2001.

- Symptoms usually progress over 36 hours until perforation occurs.
  - Usually, diffuse peritonitis follows.
  - After perforation, the tenderness is no longer localized and the guarding becomes rigidity.
  - Temperature increases above 38.6°C.

DIFFERENTIAL DIAGNOSIS

Common causes of abdominal pain

- Diagnoses are listed for boys and girls with abdominal pain [(C) indicates most common causes].
- Peritoneum—inflammatory
  - Bacterial
  - Primary
  - Secondary
  - Perforated viscus
  - Stomach, duodenum
  - Appendix
  - Foreign body
- Hollow intestinal organs—inflammatory
  - Appendicitis (C)
  - Cholecystitis
  - Gastroenteritis (C)
  - Regional enteritis (C)
  - Meckel diverticulitis
  - Colitis—ulcerative, bacterial, amebic (C)
  - Typhlitis
- Hollow-intestinal organs—noninflammatory
  - Intussusception
  - Malrotation and midgut volvulus
  - Intestinal obstruction (C)
  - Inguinal hernia
  - Biliary colic
  - Peptic ulcer
  - Constipation (C)
  - Cystic fibrosis
- Enteric infections (gastroenteritis)
  - *Shigella*
  - *Salmonella*
  - *Campylobacter*
  - *Clostridium difficile*
  - Viral gastroenteritis (C)
- Unusual infections
  - Malaria
  - Tuberculosis of the spine
  - Osteomyelitis
  - Psoas abscess
  - Helminthic infestation

Most Common Diagnoses in Girls With a Chief Complaint of Abdominal Pain by Age[a]

< 2 yr (n = 25)		2–5 yr (n = 94)		5–12 yr (n = 248)		>12 yr (n = 150)	
Diagnosis	**Frequency (%)**	**Diagnosis**	**Frequency (%)**	**Diagnosis**	**Frequency (%)**	**Diagnosis**	**Frequency (%)**
Abdominal pain	11 (44)	Abdominal pain	53 (56)	Abdominal pain	126 (51)	Abdominal pain	59 (39)
Constipation	6 (24)	Gastroenteritis	9 (10)	Constipation	42 (17)	Genital, pregnancy	14 (10)
Gastroenteritis	2 (8)	Infection	6 (6)	Gastritis, esophagitis	17 (7)	Pelvic inflammatory disease	14 (10)
Infection	1 (4)	Constipation	6 (6)	Gastroenteritis	17 (7)	Urinary	10 (7)
Hematologic	1 (4)	Urinary	5 (5)	Appendicitis	12 (5)	Constipation	10 (7)
Malabsorption	1 (4)	Bowel obstruction	4 (4)	Urinary	8 (3)	Gastritis, esophagitis	9 (6)
		Gastritis, esophagitis	3 (3)	Infection	5 (2)	Appendicitis	6 (4)
		Appendicitis	3 (3)	Hematologic	4 (2)	Gastroenteritis	5 (3)

[a] From: Klein MD, Rabbani AB, Rood KD, et al. Three quantitative approaches to the diagnosis of abdominal pain in children: practical applications of decision theory. *J Pediatr Surg.* 2001;36(9):1375-1380. Copyright © Elsevier 2001.

A

- Solid viscera
  - Acute hepatosplenomegaly
  - Abscess of spleen or liver
  - Pancreatitis
  - Hepatitis
  - Fitz-Hugh–Curtis syndrome
  - Mesenteric lymphadenitis
  - Torsion of:
    - Testicle
    - Scrotal appendages
    - Omentum
    - Spleen
  - Appendix epiploica
- Gynecologic (C)
  - Salpingitis
  - Mittelschmerz
  - Ovarian cyst (usually ruptured)
  - Menstrual pain
  - Threatened abortion
  - Ectopic gestation
  - Ovarian torsion
  - Pelvic inflammatory disease
  - Endometritis
  - Endometriosis
- Urinary tract (C)
  - Pyelonephritis
  - Hydronephrosis
  - Calculi
  - Cystitis
- Trauma (C)
  - Rectus muscle tear
  - Hematoma
  - Solid-organ injury
  - Hollow-organ injury
- Trauma to a previously unsuspected mass
  - Hydronephrosis
  - Wilms tumor
- Medical diseases
  - Pneumonia
  - Sickle cell anemia (C)
  - Henoch-Schönlein purpura
  - Streptococcal pharyngitis
  - Lead poisoning
  - Green-apple bellyache
  - Hemolytic-uremic syndrome

- Diabetic ketoacidosis (C)
- Porphyria
- Hyperlipidemia
- Rheumatic fever
- Epilepsy
- Migraine
- Hemophilia
- Herpes zoster
- Systemic lupus erythematosus
- Immunosuppressed patients
  - Ischemic colitis
  - Typhlitis
  - Primary peritonitis
- Nonorganic—chronic
  - Recurrent
  - Psychogenic
  - Functional
  - Psychophysiologic

Specific considerations

- Secondary bacterial peritonitis
  - Usually caused by appendicitis
  - Can result from any hollow-organ perforation, eg, spleen, kidney
  - Peritonitis and pain from these ruptured organs are probably caused by irritation from blood and urine in the peritoneal cavity.
- Perforation of jejunum by blunt abdominal trauma
  - Radiograph of the patient's upright abdomen may not show free air, and computed tomography (CT) may show only a small amount of fluid.
  - Persistent abdominal tenderness after blunt trauma may be the only sign of perforated jejunum.
  - In children, a history of trauma may not be obvious (a fall or wrestling match) and may be difficult to elicit, particularly if the child is reluctant to admit unsafe activity to parents.
- Injury to spleen or kidney
  - May be related to previously undiagnosed enlarged kidney (hydronephrosis, Wilms tumor) or spleen (mononucleosis)
- Perforated ulcer
  - Rare in children
  - Characterized by free air on abdominal and chest radiographs
- Meckel diverticulitis is less common than bleeding from a Meckel diverticulum.
  - Signs, symptoms, and other findings are not especially different from those of appendicitis.

- Foreign bodies
  - Most, including open safety pins, will pass through a child's gastrointestinal tract without event, but perforation can occur.
- Bowel obstruction
  - Usually causes bilious emesis, abdominal pain, and distended abdomen (unless it is a high small-bowel obstruction)
  - Radiography of the upright abdomen shows distended loops of bowel with air-fluid levels and no gas in the colon or rectum.
  - Causes of bowel obstruction include adhesions from previous operation, incarcerated hernia, and congenital bands.
- Ectopic gestation
  - Can be diagnosed with a pregnancy test or ultrasonography
- Other gynecologic conditions: ovarian torsion, pelvic inflammatory disease
  - Ultrasonography is important in diagnosis.
  - Pelvic examination may reveal discharge from the cervical os or cervical motion tenderness, indicating pelvic inflammatory disease.
- Testicular disease
  - Pain is often referred to the abdomen.
  - The diagnosis can usually be made on physical examination (see Scrotal Swelling and Pain).
- Gallbladder disease
  - Right upper quadrant symptoms and signs
  - Can be confirmed by ultrasonography
- Pancreatitis
  - Usually has an underlying cause in children
  - Ultrasonography and pancreatic enzyme measurement often confirm pancreatitis.
- Torsion of spleen or omentum
  - Uncommon cause of abdominal pain
  - Can be diagnosed by ultrasonography
- Torsion of an epiploic appendage (the fat hanging off the colon)
  - Only diagnosed at laparotomy or laparoscopy
- Constipation
  - Abdominal pain caused by sensitivity of GI mucosa to distention
- Cystic fibrosis
  - Caused by meconium ileus equivalent even in older child (constipation), although intussusception occurs more frequently in patients with cystic fibrosis
- Typhlitis
  - In immunocompromised patients, indicated by right lower quadrant pain and tenderness
  - Inflammatory mass can be seen on CT and can be monitored with ultrasonography.
- Most medical diagnoses of abdominal pain can be ruled out by lack of tenderness or guarding on physical examination.
- Sickle cell crisis
  - Sickle cell anemia frequently causes abdominal pain and typical leukocyte counts of 14,000–16,000 cells/mm^3.
  - If the clinician is not sure of the diagnosis, treatment for sickle cell crisis, even including transfusion, is best.
  - If the pain resolves, the diagnosis was not appendicitis.
  - If the pain does not resolve, the patient needs to go to surgery.

DIAGNOSTIC APPROACH

- Ordering a complete blood count with differential and urinalysis is reasonable when abdominal pain is the chief symptom.
- Examination by a pediatric surgeon should be done before any other tests, including imaging studies, are ordered in the patient's best interest.
- Complete history is important in evaluating all patients with abdominal pain.
- Emphasis should be placed on eliciting:
  - Nature, location, radiation, and timing of the pain
  - Whether pain is associated with physical activity or eating
- Most patients with an acute surgical problem have anorexia and usually have nausea and vomiting.
- Generally, bowel habits are unchanged, or patients have constipation.
  - Diarrhea is unusual in diseases requiring urgent operation.
- Pain usually precedes vomiting.
- Systemic symptoms, such as headache and myalgia, are seldom present.
- Pharyngitis does not rule out a surgical problem.
- Clinicians must certainly ask specifically about genitourinary tract symptoms, other illnesses, and prior operations.
- The physical examination of the abdomen is crucial.
- Appendicitis
  - When considering appendicitis, observation is a useful diagnostic aid.
  - If appendicitis cannot be diagnosed with history, physical examination, complete blood count, urinalysis, and plain films, then 6–12 hours of observation with serial examination and a repeat leukocyte count may be diagnostic.
  - Patients with appendicitis generally worsen; those without appendicitis usually improve.
  - If observation does not clarify the diagnosis, CT is indicated.
    - Patient should have enteric preparation with contrast, or contrast should be instilled rectally so that it can reach the cecum.

- Intravenous contrast is also important because it makes the presence of inflammation much clearer.

- If a patient reports symptoms lasting >72 hours, consider perforated appendicitis with abscess or phlegmon.

LABORATORY FINDINGS

- Complete blood count with differential and urinalysis is reasonable when abdominal pain is the chief symptom, although tests may not be decisive.

- Leukocyte count
  - In acute appendicitis without perforation, the count is elevated from 9000 to 14,000 cells/mm³.
    - After perforation, the leukocyte count exceeds 14,000 cells/mm³.
  - If the bowel is perforated or gangrenous, or if an intraabdominal abscess exists, the leukocyte count will exceed 12,000 cells/mm³.

- Patients with anemia can have one of many medical conditions, such as sickle cell anemia, Henoch-Schönlein purpura, and lead toxicity.

- Urinalysis
  - High specific gravity indicates hypovolemia.
  - Ketones in urine indicate significant anorexia and emesis.
  - Leukocytes and bacteria indicate a urinary tract infection.
  - Erythrocytes indicate trauma or stone.
  - Casts may indicate glomerulonephritis that can be associated with primary peritonitis.

- Stool guaiac test
  - Most patients with intussusception will have a positive result.

IMAGING

- When appendicitis is suspected, diagnosis can often be made without resorting to imaging studies.

- When malrotation is in question, an upper GI series is the best test.

- If the patient already has signs of peritonitis and abnormal signs on plain-film radiography, then prompt operation may be appropriate.

- When intussusception is considered, contrast enema is indicated.
  - Signs of obstruction or necrotic bowel should prompt immediate surgery.

- When appendicitis is a possibility, the first imaging studies should be radiography of the chest and abdomen.
  - If the diagnosis is not clear, ultrasonography is the next step in girls, CT in boys.
  - Involving the surgeon early will allow a more prompt and accurate diagnosis.

- Plain-film radiographs of the abdomen can show:
  - Bowel obstruction

- Distended loops of bowel, air-fluid levels, absence of colonic gas

- Localized ileus, free air in the abdomen, scoliosis, or the impression of a mass

- Appendicitis
  - Scoliosis to the right, an ileus pattern, and a fecalith early in process
  - In perforated appendicitis, impression of a right lower quadrant soft-tissue mass may be present, as well as a gas pattern of bowel obstruction, with multiple loops of bowel with air-fluid levels.

- The chest radiograph may show free air under diaphragm or pneumonia.

- Ultrasonography is useful in:
  - Ovarian disease
  - Appendicitis
    - In female patients, ultrasonography can help evaluate possibility of ovarian or tubal disease.
  - Intussusception
    - Can also be diagnosed with contrast enema
  - Malrotation with midgut volvulus (reversal of the normal superior mesenteric artery and superior mesenteric vein relationship)

- CT is useful in diagnosing:
  - Appendicitis in patients with sickle cell anemia or immunocompromise (patients receiving a transplant and those being treated for cancer)
  - Appendicitis by visualization of abscess or phlegmon
  - When the diagnosis cannot be made clinically, most surgeons prefer abdominal CT with intravenous contrast and with contrast of the GI tract in which the contrast has reached the colon.

- An upper GI series is the surest way to determine malrotation.
  - Assess for the position of the ligament of Treitz.
    - Normally, the ligament of Treitz should be at the level of the pylorus and just to the left of the midline, with the second portion of the duodenum coursing posteriorly on a lateral view.
  - If the imager is inexperienced, barium enema can help find the position of the cecum, which is normally below the iliac crest and to the right of the midline (although it can occasionally be in this position in malrotation).

TREATMENT APPROACH

- Hydration
  - All patients with an acute surgical abdomen have volume depletion.
  - Administering intravenous hydration at 1.5 times the

maintenance requirement with appropriate solutions is reasonable.

- Broad-spectrum antibiotics (ampicillin, gentamicin, and metronidazole) and analgesics (morphine) are of benefit.
  - Should probably be started only after consultation with the surgeon
- Nasogastric tube
  - If a patient is vomiting or has marked abdominal distention
- No food or drink should be given until the diagnosis and disposition are decided for any patient with abdominal pain as any part of the chief symptom.

SPECIFIC TREATMENTS

Malrotation and midgut volvulus

- Once the diagnosis has been made in a patient with symptoms, surgery is urgently required to:
  - Untwist the bowel
  - Perform a Ladd procedure
- If the diagnosis of malrotation is serendipitous and symptoms are not present, a Ladd procedure should be performed to decrease the likelihood of volvulus.
  - Ladd bands are lysed, and the duodenum and colon are separated in an attempt to create a broad mesentery.
  - Appendix is removed because it will not usually be in the right lower quadrant and thus complicate any future diagnosis of appendicitis.
  - It is hoped that adhesions will be created to help decrease the chance of volvulus.

Intussusception

- Reduction can be made by contrast enema using barium, nonionic contrast, or air.
- When contrast enema reduction fails, surgery is necessary.
- The intussusception can usually be reduced surgically, or resection and anastomosis can be performed.
  - The appendix is also removed.

Appendicitis

- Once the diagnosis of appendicitis has been made:

- Surgery is indicated.
- Administering analgesics and antibiotics is reasonable.
- Surgery is performed either laparoscopically or by laparotomy, regardless of whether perforation has occurred.
- Laparoscopy is especially useful when the diagnosis remains in doubt.
  - The entire abdomen and pelvis usually can be well visualized.
  - It can reduce morbidity associated with the large incision needed in obese patients.
- Patients with symptoms of appendicitis lasting >72 hours can be treated with broad-spectrum intravenous antibiotics.
  - If their symptoms resolve in 2–3 days, they can be discharged home on antibiotics.
  - Some clinicians ask patients to return in 6–8 weeks for interval appendectomy, which can be done laparoscopically.
  - Elective laparoscopic appendectomy results in little morbidity, even after perforation.
  - Most patients will eat the evening of the operation and be discharged the next day.
  - Immediate surgery for delayed presentation of perforated appendicitis can result in a very large incision and a long, complicated hospital course.

WHEN TO ADMIT

- All patients with acute surgical abdomen need to be admitted.

WHEN TO REFER

- All patients with acute surgical abdomen need to be referred to pediatric surgeons.

COMPLICATIONS

- Intussusception
  - Recurs in 15% of cases, usually within 72 hours of the original disease
  - Treatment is the same as that in the initial occurrence.

Adrenal Dysfunction

DEFINITION

- Adrenal insufficiency
  - Syndrome characterized by wasting, hyperpigmentation, and adrenal gland atrophy
  - May be primary or secondary
  - Primary may be:
    - Congenital (congenital adrenal hyperplasia [CAH])
    - Acquired
- Adrenal hyperfunction
  - Premature adrenarche
    - Early onset of adrenal androgen secretion accompanied by pubarche
  - Cushing syndrome
    - Any form of glucocorticoid excess
  - Cushing disease
    - Glucocorticoid excess caused by adrenocorticotropic hormone (ACTH) hypersecretion
  - Adrenal medullary diseases
    - Neuroblastoma, pheochromocytoma

EPIDEMIOLOGY

- Adrenal insufficiency
  - Primary
    - Prevalence: 10 in 100,000 persons
    - Age: most prevalent in women age 25–45 years
    - Sex: The female-to-male ratio is approximately 3:1.
  - Secondary
    - Prevalence: 15–28 to 100,000 persons
  - Adrenal hyperfunction
    - Premature adrenarche
    - Most common in children with early onset of pubic and body hair growth
    - Traditional age limit has been 8 years for the onset of pubic hair in girls and 9 years in boys.
    - Lowest age limit for girls has been contested after a large cross-sectional study revealed the relatively common occurrence of either early pubic hair or breast enlargement in healthy black girls after age 6 years and in white girls after age 7 years.
  - Cushing syndrome
    - Incidence: 0.05 in 100,000 persons per year
  - Neuroblastoma
    - Most common tumor encountered in young children
    - Incidence: approximately 1 in 100,000 per year among children <15 years
    - Average age is 2 years at diagnosis in North America.
    - Mass screening of infants is done in Japan to allow earlier diagnosis.

ETIOLOGY

- Primary adrenal insufficiency
  - CAH (72%), most often caused by deficiency of enzyme 21-hydroxylase
  - Autoimmune adrenal insufficiency (13%)
  - Rare syndromes (15%)
- Secondary adrenal insufficiency
  - Abrupt discontinuation of glucocorticoid therapy is the most common cause.
  - Other pituitary hormone deficiencies cause the remainder of cases.
- Adrenal hyperfunction
  - Cushing syndrome is the most frequent noniatrogenic cause for glucocorticoid excess in adolescents.
  - Medullary disease in adolescents is most often caused by a pheochromocytoma; transmission is autosomal dominant.

SIGNS AND SYMPTOMS

Adrenal insufficiency

- Acute adrenal insufficiency
  - Hypotension and lethargy are common signs at presentation.
    - Patients and family members should be taught to recognize a change in energy level or demeanor as a potential warning sign.
    - May occur during febrile illness, especially when accompanied by dehydration, vomiting, diarrhea, or any combination of these reactions
- Primary adrenal insufficiency
  - Abdominal pain, headache, anorexia, weight loss, lethargy, postural hypotension or shock, proneness to dehydration, salt craving, hyperpigmentation, loss of axillary or pubic hair
    - Findings are nonspecific and gradual in onset.
    - Hyperpigmentation may be difficult to appreciate in dark-skinned patients; creases of the palms and of the oral mucosal surfaces are clues.
  - Hypoglycemia
    - May be present in patients who have adrenal insufficiency with or without growth hormone (GH) deficiency
    - Seldom severe enough to cause seizures
  - Gastrointestinal symptoms
    - Abdominal cramps, nausea, vomiting, and diarrhea are prominent in some patients.
  - Sexual and/or reproductive dysfunction
    - Decreased libido, potency, or amenorrhea may accompany either primary or secondary adrenal insufficiency in adolescents and adults.

- Orthostatic hypotension
  - More marked in primary than secondary adrenal insufficiency
- CAH: classic form
  - One-quarter of patients produce enough aldosterone to avoid salt-wasting crises; these patients are termed *simple virilizers.*
- CAH: nonclassic (milder) form
  - Less marked adrenal androgen excess
  - Early pubic hair and rapid advances in height in both sexes
  - Hirsutism, oligomenorrhea, or acne in adolescent girls
  - Not all persons with increased 17-hydroxyprogesterone typical of nonclassic 21-hydroxylase deficiency are symptomatic; boys are much less likely have symptoms.

■ Secondary adrenal insufficiency
  - Patients tend to be pale, in contrast to the hyperpigmentation seen in primary insufficiency.
  - Children may have delayed growth and puberty, manifestations of GH, and gonadotropin deficiencies in addition to ACTH deficiency.
  - Headaches, visual disturbances, polyuria, and polydipsia may also be seen in pituitary disorders.
    - Chronic unexplained signs or symptoms such as these should prompt consultation with a pediatric endocrinologist.

Adrenal hyperfunction

■ Prominent clinical features of adrenocortical hyperfunction in adolescents are excess central body weight gain with stunted statural growth.

■ Premature adrenarche
  - Most overweight and obese children who are growing in height at a normal pace do not have a causal underlying endocrine disease.
    - Overweight children secrete more adrenal sex hormones than lean children.
    - They may develop secondary sexual characteristics at an earlier-than-average age.
    - Obese children often show advanced bone ages, but are not usually short.
  - In most cases, children with premature adrenarche do not exhibit rapid growth in stature or advanced bone age.
  - Presence of isolated pubic hair or axillary hair with or without apocrine body odor does not necessarily presage early breast development and menstruation.
  - Endocrine evaluation should be reserved for children with:
    - Unusually early pubarche
    - Multiple signs of early puberty
    - Rapidly progressive pubertal development or statural growth (or both)

    - Nonisosexual puberty (eg, a girl with hirsutism or other signs of virilization, a prepubertal boy with gynecomastia)
■ Cushing syndrome
  - Typical appearance
    - Excess central body weight with stunted statural growth
      ■ Annual school photographs can often help reveal subtle changes in physiognomy and habitus over time.
    - Other characteristic findings are:
      ■ Easy bruisability
      ■ Broad and purplish striae
      ■ Hyperglycemia
      ■ Hypertension
  - Most obese adolescents do not have Cushing syndrome and do not require screening unless growth arrest or other suspicious signs are observed.
■ Neuroblastoma
  - Common presenting signs include:
    - Abdominal mass
    - Fever of unknown origin
    - Hematuria
    - Spinal cord compression
    - Pathological fracture
    - Hypertension
  - Metastases to liver and bone occur in approximately 50% of cases by the time of tumor detection.
■ Pheochromocytoma
  - May cause either episodic or chronic hypertension, usually accompanied by:
    - Tachycardia
    - Headaches
    - Anxiety
    - Sweating
    - Flushing
  - Weight loss may also be observed.
  - Thorough family history should be obtained for endocrine tumors, especially medullary thyroid carcinoma and hyperparathyroidism.

DIFFERENTIAL DIAGNOSIS

■ Adrenal insufficiency
  - Often goes unrecognized for extended periods
  - Findings may be mistaken for:
    - Infection
    - Malnutrition
    - Gastrointestinal disease
    - Inborn errors of metabolism

A

- Anorexia
- Chronic fatigue syndrome
- Depression

- The mild nonclassic form of CAH may be mistaken in girls for polycystic ovarian syndrome.

■ Adrenal hyperfunction

- Premature adrenarche
  - Differential diagnosis includes
    - Nonclassic forms of CAH
    - Adrenal virilizing tumors
- Pheochromocytoma
  - Differential diagnosis includes
    - Panic attacks
    - Thyrotoxicosis
    - Renovascular disease
    - Drug abuse (especially cocaine or amphetamines)

DIAGNOSTIC APPROACH

■ Diagnosis of adrenal insufficiency is frequently delayed or missed.

■ Perform laboratory studies for adrenal dysfunction in cases of unexplained, nonspecific symptoms of:

- Pain
- Salt craving
- Weight loss

LABORATORY FINDINGS

Adrenal insufficiency

■ The most commonly recognized findings by laboratory screening are:

- Hypoglycemia
- Low plasma cortisol

■ The gold standard test is a corticotropin-stimulated serum 17-hydroxyprogesterone.

- Strict quality control is important to avoid false-positive high levels generated by nonspecific measurement of cross-reacting hormones.
- Classic simple virilizing or salt-wasting CAH
  - Basal and stimulated 17-hydroxyprogesterone levels are markedly increased, generally >10,000 ng/dL (~300 nmol/L).
  - In classic CAH, cortisol levels are invariably low and fail to respond robustly to stress or exogenous stimulation.

■ Early-morning basal serum 17-hydroxyprogesterone measurements below 200 ng/dL (~6 nmol/L) usually rule out even mild forms of 21-hydroxylase deficiency.

- Nonclassic 21-hydroxylase deficiency
  - Stimulated serum 17-hydroxyprogesterone levels are moderately increased, usually >1500 ng/dL (approximately 45 nmol/L).

- Newborn screening test results from filter papers are not comparable to serum hormone levels.
  - Filter paper samples are measured differently.
  - Each state's laboratory has its own reference range for screening tests.

■ Early-morning (8:00 am) serum or salivary cortisol levels accompanied by increased ACTH may also be diagnostic.

- If zona glomerulosa function is affected, hyponatremia and hyperkalemia will be accompanied by high plasma renin activity and low serum aldosterone.
- If adrenal insufficiency results from pituitary or hypothalamic dysfunction, ACTH levels will be low.
- Diagnosis can be confirmed by absence of at least a 2-fold increment in serum cortisol 60 minutes after stimulation with a standard dose of intravenous ACTH 1-24.
- A low dose of cosyntropin can be used to test ACTH reserve in cases of suspected secondary adrenal insufficiency.

■ Patients with a known history of high-dose, long-term glucocorticoid treatment should undergo documentation of plasma cortisol level during intercurrent illness and before undergoing any surgery.

- 8:00-am level >10 mcg/dL or cosyntropin ACTH 1-24 challenge test with cortisol levels >15 to 18 mcg/dL after 30 to 60 minutes
  - These levels have been derived mainly from adult studies and may not be relevant to infants and small children.
- Insulin-induced hypoglycemia may be used to test ACTH.
  - Many clinicians are reluctant to use this test because of the danger of potential hypoglycemic seizures.
- If documentation cannot be obtained in time, treating patients with supplemental stress corticosteroid coverage in the perioperative period within 1 year of withdrawal of therapy is safest.

Adrenal hyperfunction

■ Premature adrenarche

- Mildly increased levels of dehydroepiandrosterone (DHEA) and DHEA sulfate
  - Tend to be consistent with the child's Tanner stage of pubic hair
  - DHEA sulfate has a longer half-life in the circulation and thus is not subject to circadian variability, making it a better screening tool.

■ Cushing syndrome

- Measurement of increased midnight salivary cortisol or high 24-hour urine-free cortisol, or both
  - Diagnosis may be confirmed by a nonsuppressed morning cortisol level after dexamethasone administration.

- Adrenal carcinomas (but not typically adenomas) will secrete cortisol, mineralocorticoids and androgens.
  - If adrenal carcinoma is suspected on the basis of ACTH-independent (ie, nonsuppressible) cortisol excess, request additional studies.
- Aldosterone and plasma renin activity
- DHEA sulfate
- Androgens
- Ectopic ACTH production by carcinomas is almost never seen in children.
- Pheochromocytoma
  - Diagnosis is made either by:
    - Increased 24-hour urine-free metanephrines (collected in an acid container)
    - High-performance liquid chromatography measurement of plasma-free metanephrines
  - Blood should be obtained from an indwelling venous catheter in a patient who has been fasted overnight and at rest for at least 20–30 minutes; the sample tube must be iced and processed immediately.
    - If possible, psychoactive drugs, especially tricyclic antidepressants, should be discontinued at least 2 weeks before testing.
    - Chemistry profile may demonstrate hyperglycemia.
    - Genotyping for the *RET* oncogene should be performed; if positive, other family members should be tested.
  - Screening tests for pheochromocytoma may include 24-hour ambulatory blood pressure.
- Neuroblastoma
  - Biochemical markers include:
    - Plasma and urinary dopamine
    - Vanillylmandelic acid
    - Homovanillic acid

IMAGING

- Imaging studies are required to verify clinical suspicion of adrenal tumor.
- Magnetic resonance imaging (MRI)
  - Suspected Cushing syndrome
    - Thin-slice abdominal images, including the adrenal glands
  - Carcinoma
    - Will often show a necrotic center or calcification and irregular borders, or both
  - Benign nonfunctioning adenomas
    - Typically homogeneous and more similar in density to normal adrenal tissue

- Metaiodobenzylguanidine scan
  - Norepinephrine analogue labeled with radioiodine taken up specifically by catechol-producing tumor tissue, but not normal adrenal medulla
  - Helpful in cases in which thin-slice, contrast-enhanced computed tomography (CT) or MRI fails to show a mass, yet biochemical tests and clinical findings are suggestive for pheochromocytoma
- Positron emission tomography and somatostatin analogues
  - May demonstrate masses not visible on CT or MRI
- Ultrasonography or CT
  - Used if adrenal hemorrhage is suspected
- Bone scan
  - Usually informative in neuroblastoma, revealing bone metastases, soft-tissue calcifications, or both
- Radiographs or dual x-ray absorptiometry
  - Demonstrates low bone density secondary to pituitary tumor

DIAGNOSTIC PROCEDURES

- Selective catheterization of the inferior petrosal sinuses with measurement of ACTH level on either side
  - In pituitary tumors that cannot be localized by imaging
  - Should be done at a specialized center

TREATMENT APPROACH

- Primary adrenal insufficiency
  - Prompt treatment with glucocorticoids and mineralocorticoids is life saving.
  - CAH usually requires lifelong treatment with corticosteroids titrated to maintain levels of adrenal androgen precursors in the normal to mildly increased range.
  - Adolescents should undergo gynecologic or testicular evaluation.
  - Children who do not exhibit precocious pubarche and adolescents who are not troubled with symptoms of androgen excess may not require treatment.
- Secondary adrenal insufficiency
  - The patient's growth, weight gain, vital signs, and sense of well-being should guide therapy.
- Adrenal hyperfunction
  - Provide dietary counseling and advise a rigorous exercise program to determine whether weight gain can be controlled.
  - Glucocorticoids should be tapered as soon as is practical.
  - Obtain a telephone consultation with a pediatric endocrinologist if in doubt.

A

SPECIFIC TREATMENTS

Acute adrenal insufficiency

- Children in hypotensive crisis or shock should be treated urgently.
- Individuals who cannot tolerate oral maintenance or stress doses during an illness require parenteral glucocorticoid administration.
  - Hydrocortisone suppositories are an option if parenteral administration is not feasible and if the patient does not have diarrhea.
- After emergency department evaluation, a large-bore intravenous catheter should be inserted for repletion of intravascular volume with saline solutions containing 5% dextrose.
  - More concentrated dextrose (eg, 25% dextrose in water) should be administered to treat refractory hypoglycemia.
- If acute and severe adrenal insufficiency is suspected, treatment should not be delayed for diagnostic testing.
- Stress doses of glucocorticoids should be given simultaneously with fluids.
  - Hydrocortisone is the treatment of choice because of its quick onset of action and mineralocorticoid activity.
  - Prednisone and dexamethasone are long-acting, with a slower onset of biological action.
  - Prednisone is not an ideal choice for treating acute adrenal crisis because it must be converted to prednisolone to be effective.
  - Dexamethasone does not cross-react in cortisol assays; thus, a diagnostic ACTH stimulation test may be performed immediately after administration.
- Liberal quantities of intravenous sodium chloride plus large doses of hydrocortisone will usually:
  - Restore normotension
  - Correct electrolyte abnormalities
  - Obviate need for mineralocorticoid treatment or pressor agents in the acute situation
- As vital signs stabilize, glucocorticoids and fluid infusions are tapered over several days.
- Once the patient can eat and take oral medications, oral glucocorticoids may be substituted.
- Supplemental sodium chloride may be provided if dietary salt intake is inadequate.

Primary adrenal insufficiency/CAH

- The classic form requires lifelong medical management with oral corticosteroids.
- Patients with salt wasting require both glucocorticoids and mineralocorticoids.
  - Advanced age and increasing dietary salt consumption may allow tapering or discontinuation of mineralocorticoids.
- Supplemental sodium chloride may be required for:
  - Infants who consume very little dietary sodium
  - Patients in tropical climates
  - Patients who engage in intense exercise with excessive sweat sodium losses
- Simple virilizing patients with poorly controlled disease benefit from mineralocorticoid therapy.
  - May obviate need for high-dose glucocorticoids in some
- The nonclassic form requires low-dose glucocorticoid therapy only.
- Dosing
  - Should be titrated to maintain levels of adrenal androgen precursors in the normal to mildly increased range
  - Some clinicians prefer to treat CAH with a higher dose of cortisol or a longer-acting glucocorticoid at night to suppress the early-morning ACTH-mediated adrenal androgen production.
- Maintenance glucocorticoid replacement therapy
  - Once growth is near complete, if satisfactory control of adrenal androgens is not achieved, more potent and long-acting glucocorticoids, eg, prednisone or dexamethasone, may be used.
  - In general, lower doses of glucocorticoids are required to treat Addison disease than CAH.
  - Patients with low serum sodium, high potassium, or increased plasma renin activity should receive daily oral fludrocortisone and sodium chloride supplements, adjusted to normalize these analytes.
  - DHEA is an optional hormone supplement for older women with adrenal insufficiency and low energy or libido, but no data exist on its use in adolescents.
- Adolescent girls with severe forms of CAH should undergo gynecologic examination before sexual activity.
  - Vaginoplasty may be necessary, depending on previous genital surgical procedures.
  - Psychological counseling should be provided by a professional experienced in treating this type of disorder.
- Adolescent boys should undergo careful testicular palpation and sonography to rule out testicular adrenal rests that can compromise fertility.
- Strict control of adrenal hormone levels can shrink benign tumors in many cases.

Secondary adrenal insufficiency

- Management is similar to that of primary adrenal insufficiency.
- Children who do not have precocious pubarche and adolescents who are not troubled with symptoms of androgen excess may not require treatment, or they may discontinue treatment when symptoms have abated and growth is complete.

- The patient's growth, weight gain, vital signs, and sense of well-being should guide therapy.
- Stress dosing
  - All patients with adrenal insufficiency must be informed about the need to increase their glucocorticoid dose during stress to prevent a potentially fatal adrenal crisis.
    - All such patients should wear a medical alert tag and carry an emergency medical information card to ensure that medical providers know about the underlying disorder.
  - Severe stresses, such as illness accompanied by higher fever (temperature ≥38.5°C), surgery, and major trauma, should be accompanied by tripling of oral hydrocortisone maintenance doses to prevent hypoglycemia, hypotension, and even cardiovascular collapse.
    - Supplemental parenteral hydrocortisone is suggested before general anesthesia and surgery.
    - Doses are empiric and are not determined by evidence-based guidelines. Intravenous or oral stress doses may be gradually tapered as the patient recovers until the maintenance dose is attained.
  - Mild physical stresses, such as immunizations, uncomplicated viral illnesses, low-grade fever (temperature <38.5°C), athletic activity, and emotional stress, do not usually require stress doses of glucocorticoids.

Adrenal hyperfunction

- Premature adrenarche
  - Institute dietary counseling.
  - Advise a rigorous exercise program to determine whether weight gain can be controlled.
- Telephone consultation with a pediatric endocrinologist is advised if in doubt.
- Cushing syndrome
  - If possible, glucocorticoids should be tapered as soon as practical, while substituting other therapeutic agents.
  - Patients with adrenal tumor or nodular hyperplasia as the source for cortisol excess will most often undergo adrenectomy.
  - In some patients, attenuation of cushingoid features and improvement of statural growth may take months to years.
- Cushing disease
  - Cushing disease has traditionally been treated primarily with transsphenoidal tumor resection.
  - Once ACTH levels have decreased, the patient needs long-term glucocorticoid replacement therapy.
  - Directed radiotherapy, such as gamma knife and linear accelerator techniques, can also induce gradual remission of ACTH hypersecretion.

- Medical therapy with such drugs as ketoconazole are an alternative for Cushing syndrome or Cushing disease either in the short term (eg, while waiting for radiotherapy to take effect) or long term to reduce cortisol secretion.
  - This type of treatment will not induce a permanent cure.
- Neuroblastoma
  - Medical and surgical management depends on staging risk.
  - Low-grade tumors may spontaneously regress.
- Pheochromocytoma
  - In preparation for surgery, treat for ≥1 week with a drug with both α-adrenergic blocking (eg, phenoxybenzamine) and ß-adrenergic blocking (eg, labetalol) properties.
  - α-Methyl-L-tyrosine (Demser) is also used to inhibit the rate-limiting step of catechol synthesis.
  - ~10% of pheochromocytomas are bilateral; thus, both adrenals should be explored at surgery.
  - If both adrenals are removed, substitution therapy will be required as for primary adrenal insufficiency.

WHEN TO ADMIT

- Children in hypotensive crisis or shock
  - Treat urgently in the office.
  - Transfer immediately by ambulance to the nearest emergency center.
- Extreme hypertension should prompt immediate emergency hospitalization.

WHEN TO REFER

- Referral to a pediatric endocrinologist or other appropriate specialist
  - Children with hyperglycemia (immediate referral)
  - Obese child with statural growth arrest (for more complete evaluation)
  - Children with a family history of familial tumor syndromes
    - Early detection of affected genetic status may dictate intervention before tumors develop.
- Because premature adrenarche is most often benign, telephone consultation with a pediatric endocrinologist should be considered before referral.

FOLLOW-UP

- Adrenal insufficiency
  - Monitor during therapy:
    - 17-hydroxyprogesterone, androstenedione, and testosterone
      - Attempts to suppress 17-hydroxyprogesterone to normal range usually require excessively high glucocorticoid doses and have the undesirable consequence of growth suppression and iatrogenic Cushing syndrome.

- Plasma renin activity in patients requiring mineralocorticoid replacement
- Frequent headaches, lethargy, nausea, or abdominal pain may indicate inadequate treatment; signs include orthostatic pulse or blood pressure changes.
- Measurement of ACTH is not helpful.
  - ACTH is seldom completely suppressible in patients treated for CAH.
- Testosterone is helpful in managing prepubertal children of both sexes, and adolescent girls and women.
  - Not as useful a marker of adequate therapy in adolescent boys and men
- Continuing reminders to patients, families, and medical personnel regarding the need for higher doses of glucocorticoid replacement therapy during intercurrent illness and surgery
  - Failure to increase glucocorticoid supplementation during physical stress remains a significant cause of morbidity and mortality.
  - Patients should be given letters explaining their condition and appropriate emergency management.
  - Among critically ill children, a low incremental cortisol response to ACTH does not predict mortality, although the effect of glucocorticoid treatment is not known.
- Pheochromocytoma
  - Careful long-term follow-up of patients, with regular checks of blood pressure and catechol measurements, is crucial.

PROGNOSIS

- Adrenal insufficiency
  - If unrecognized, adrenal insufficiency may produce a life-threatening crisis, with acute cardiovascular collapse.
  - Information concerning mortality in secondary adrenal insufficiency mostly comes from recent reports regarding follow-up of individuals treated with pituitary GH.
    - Up to 4-fold increase in mortality compared with the general population in children treated with pituitary GH has been reported, probably due to development of other hormone deficiencies.

- Preventable deaths were attributed to hypoglycemia or secondary adrenal insufficiency in patients of all ages and were associated with a variety of causes of hypopituitarism.
  - The death rate remained fairly constant throughout middle childhood and with advancing age (1 per 113 to 173 person-years).
- Adrenocortical hyperfunction
  - Premature adrenarche
    - A subset of girls with premature adrenarche may develop polycystic ovarian syndrome, insulin resistance, or metabolic syndrome.
  - Cushing disease
    - Surgical success largely depends on the skill of the surgeon and the nature of the lesion.
    - The cure rate ranges from 60–80%.
  - Pheochromocytoma
    - Cancer and recurrence may occur in approximately 10–15% of cases.

PREVENTION

- Adrenal insufficiency
  - To prevent mortality from adrenal crisis, among other reasons, the US and many other countries perform newborn screening.
- Adrenocortical hyperfunction
  - No strong evidence has been found to warrant preventive drug treatment in anticipation of possible polycystic ovarian syndrome in young girls with premature adrenarche.

Airways Obstruction

DEFINITION

- Airways obstruction is blockage of the airway.
- Airways obstruction may result from:
  - Aspiration of a foreign object
  - Reduction in the inner diameter of the airway
- Acute airways obstruction can occur throughout the respiratory tract.

MECHANISM

- Infants have a greater incidence of respiratory compromise compared with older children.
  - They have smaller airways diameter and increased airways resistance.
  - Connective tissue and cartilaginous structures in infants are not completely hardened.
    - Cartilaginous structures include:
      - Larynx (epiglottis, aryepiglottic folds, arytenoid cartilage, tracheal cartilage)
      - Trachea
      - Bronchi
      - Bronchioles
      - Chest wall
- In the infant and young child, the narrowest portion of the airways is the cricoid ring.
- In the older child and adolescent, the narrowest portion of the airways is the vocal cord aperture.

HISTORY

- Obtain a pulmonary history.
  - Onset of respiratory distress
    - Acute
    - Gradual
  - Duration
  - Factors that worsen or improve signs and symptoms
- Obtain a prenatal and birth history.
  - Problems during pregnancy
    - Decreased fetal movement
    - Oligohydramnios
  - Gestational age at birth
  - Type of delivery
    - Vaginal
      - Need for forceps or vacuum extraction
    - Caesarean
  - Abnormalities in presentation
    - Breech
    - Shoulder dystocia
- Resuscitation efforts required during birth
  - Intubation
  - Mechanical ventilation
  - Supplemental oxygen
- If foreign body aspiration is suspected:
  - Determine whether the event was witnessed.
  - Determine the type of object aspirated.
  - Determine what time the event occurred and how much time has elapsed.

PHYSICAL EXAM

- Determine whether the child requires emergent intervention.
  - Assess upper airways patency.
  - Assess the degree of respiratory effort.
  - Note the child's level of consciousness.
  - Observe the child's facial expression.
  - A child with incipient respiratory collapse may:
    - Have furrowed eyebrows
    - Be unable to regard and focus on the examiner
    - Appear fatigued and anxious
  - Observe for nasal flaring.
  - Note whether the child is diaphoretic.
  - Determine the effectiveness of respiratory function.
- Simple observation, without an examination, is valuable.
  - Determine the respiratory rate.
    - Note whether tachypnea is present.
    - Note whether respirations are regular or irregular.
  - Observe whether the child is using accessory muscles or has retractions.
    - Note the movement of the head and neck with respiration.
  - Note the relative ratio of inspiration to expiration.
    - Normal inspiratory:expiratory ratio is 1:2.
  - Does the child recognize his/her parents?
  - Can the child speak?
  - Can the child suck on a bottle or pacifier?
  - Listen to the quality of the child's cry.
- Perform a chest examination.
  - Observe for symmetry, pectus deformity, and size of the thorax.
  - Observe chest wall movement.
    - It may be diminished because of weak or inefficient breaths.
  - Percuss the thorax and note the presence of:
    - Localized air trapping
    - Hyperresonance

A

- Lobar consolidation
- Dullness
- Auscultate breath sounds.
  - Listen for crackles, wheezing, or stridor.
  - Note whether sounds occur on inspiration, expiration, or throughout the respiratory cycle.
  - Note distribution, pitch, and quality of breath sounds.
- Abnormal breath sounds are more prominent on the inspiratory or expiratory phase of breathing, depending on the site of the disease.
- For any rate of airflow, the degree of respiratory effort is directly proportional to the degree of obstruction.
- Complete upper airways obstruction is a medical emergency in which no effective air movement is present and child cannot:
  - Cough audibly
  - Speak
  - Produce any sound
- Children with respiratory failure have inadequate oxygenation, ventilation, or both and appear:
  - Ashen
  - Obtunded
  - Lethargic or extremely anxious
- In respiratory failure:
  - Central cyanosis may be present.
  - Chest wall movement may be diminished.
- Partial obstruction
  - Audible phonation and presence of breath sounds indicates airways patency.

DIFFERENTIAL DIAGNOSIS

Early infancy

- Laryngomalacia
  - Most common cause of stridor in an infant
    - Stridor is positional: severity is greater when the infant is supine, less when the infant is prone.
  - Onset typically within the first 2 weeks of life
    - Worsens in the first several months and resolves by 1 year of age
  - Respiratory characteristics
    - Stridor predominates on inspiration.
- Vocal cord paralysis
  - May be unilateral or bilateral
  - Often associated with birth trauma
    - Trauma associated with delivery: shoulder dystocia, forceps delivery, vacuum extraction
    - Airway instrumentation: intubation in the delivery room, mechanical ventilation

- May also result from:
  - Elevated intracranial pressure
  - Congenital Arnold-Chiari malformation
  - Intracranial mass
- When caused by birth trauma, the condition improves over time.
- Extrinsic compression of the trachea, which may be caused by:
  - Thyroglossal duct cyst
  - Ectopic thyroid tissue
  - Esophageal duplication cyst
  - Lymphoma
  - Cardiac or vascular anomaly
- Craniofacial anomalies
  - These put children at risk for chronic and severe obstruction of the upper airway.
  - Mechanical ventilation might be required in the interim.
- Tracheomalacia
  - Congenital disorder of the trachea
  - Symptoms usually appear before 2 months of age.
  - Has both inspiratory and expiratory sounds
  - Chronic wheezing is present.
    - May be misdiagnosed as asthma

Children beyond the newborn period

Acquired infectious causes of airways obstruction

- Epiglottitis (See table on following page)
  - The infectious organism is *Haemophilus influenzae* type b. Routine vaccination of children with Hib vaccine has decreased the incidence of infections with *Haemophilus influenzae* type b.
  - Age range: 2–6 years
  - Onset is rapid, over a period of hours.
  - Clinical presentation
    - Fever
    - Drooling
    - Dysphagia
    - Muffled voice
  - While epiglottitis is rare, it can result in a medical emergency.
- Laryngotracheobronchitis (croup)
  - Most common upper respiratory obstruction in childhood
  - Age range: 6 months to 3 years
    - Peak incidence in second year of life
  - Occurs most commonly in late fall and early winter
  - Worse at night

- Symptoms
  - Barky cough
  - Hoarse voice
  - High-pitched inspiratory stridor
  - Fever
- Retropharyngeal abscess
  - Most common in children between the ages of 2 and 4 years
  - Presenting symptoms:
    - Neck pain
    - Fever
    - Sore throat
  - Children may be unwilling to move the neck because of discomfort.
- Peritonsillar abscess
  - Most common deep neck infection in children and adolescents
  - Clinical presentation:
    - Severe sore throat
    - Fever
    - Muffled voice
    - Swelling of the neck accompanied by neck pain

- Bacterial tracheitis
  - Incidence is low, but illness is serious.
  - Affects children between 4 and 8 years of age
  - Distinguish from croup by patient age, severity of illness, and symptoms that worsen over time.
  - Clinical presentation
    - Fever
    - Barky cough
    - Stridor
- Laryngeal papillomatosis
  - Infection of the airways by human papillomavirus
  - Most commonly acquired as the neonate passes through the birth canal
  - Diagnosed in children between 2 and 4 years of age
  - Clinical presentation:
    - Hoarseness
    - Stridor
    - Respiratory distress in advanced cases
- Vascular anomalies, such as vascular ring
  - Structural anomalies can produce extrinsic compression of the airway, resulting in obstruction and respiratory distress.
  - With severe obstruction, infants may exhibit failure to thrive.

Comparison of Epiglottitis, Laryngotracheobronchitis, Spasmodic Croup, and Bacterial Tracheitis

Factor	Epiglottitis	Viral Croup	Spasmodic Croup	Bacterial Tracheitis
Age (yr)	2–6	0.6–2	0.5–3	4–8
Organism	*Haemophilus influenzae* type b	Parainfluenza 1,2,3	Gastroesophageal reflux	*Staphylococcus aureus, Haemophilus influenzae* type b
Season	All year	Late spring, late fall	All year	All year
Clinical Presentation	Child sitting Toxic Drooling Dysphagia Muffled voice	Child lying down Nontoxic Barking cough Hoarseness	Nontoxic Barking cough Hoarseness	Toxic Barking cough
Onset Prodrome	Rapid over a few hours	Variable; few hours to 4 days	Sudden	Variable; few hours to 5 days
Stridor	Less common	Common	Very common	Common
Fever	High	Low-grade	Afebrile	High
Chest Retractions	Less common	Common	Common	Common
Lateral Neck Film	Swollen epiglottis	Subglottic narrowing	None	Pseudomembrane in trachea
Progression	Rapid	Usually slow	Rapid	Usually slow, occasionally rapid
Recurrence	Rare	Common	Very common	Rare

A

Acquired noninfectious causes of airways obstruction

- Vocal cord dysfunction
  - Sudden onset of labored breathing with inspiratory stridor
  - Often self-limiting
- Anaphylaxis
  - If edema involves the retropharynx or larynx, the clinical presentation may be severe and life-threatening.
  - Onset of symptoms is usually sudden.
  - The patient may have urticaria and facial edema.
- Foreign body aspiration
  - Usually seen in children <3 years, with peak incidence between 1 and 2 years of age.
  - Most commonly aspirated objects include:
    - Peanuts, nuts, and seeds
    - Food particles
    - Hardware
    - Pieces of toys, eg, balloons, small marbles
  - Respiratory characteristics depend on where the foreign body is lodged.
    - Wheeze predominates on expiration.
    - Stridor predominates on inspiration.

LABORATORY EVALUATION

- C1 esterase measurement may be necessary in children with suspected angioneurotic edema.

IMAGING

- Anteroposterior or lateral neck radiograph may be required to diagnose:
  - Laryngotracheobronchitis
  - Epiglottitis
  - Retropharyngeal abscess
  - Peritonsillar abscess
- Inspiratory and expiratory radiographs may be required in the case of foreign body aspiration.

DIAGNOSTIC PROCEDURES

- Flexible bronchoscopy may be required to diagnose:
  - Laryngomalacia
  - Subglottic stenosis
  - Laryngeal cysts, webs, and hemangiomas
  - Vocal cord dysfunction
  - Epiglottic cysts
  - Laryngeal papilloma
- Rigid bronchoscopy may be required to diagnose:
  - Foreign body aspiration
  - Retained foreign body

- Suspension laryngoscopy may be required if laryngotracheoesophageal clefts are suspected.
- Fluoroscopy may be required to diagnose:
  - Foreign body aspiration
  - Laryngomalacia
- Pulmonary function testing may be necessary in children with suspected subglottic stenosis.

TREATMENT APPROACH

- Acute airways obstruction resulting in severe respiratory distress is a medical emergency and should be treated accordingly.
- In less emergent situations, the child can be treated appropriately as per the diagnosis.

SPECIFIC TREATMENTS

Anaphylaxis

- Treatment must be immediate.
- Initial therapy is intramuscular injection of epinephrine.
- After initial treatment, systemic corticosteroids should be provided.

Foreign body aspiration

- In children with severe respiratory distress, treat immediately with rigid bronchoscopic removal of the foreign body.
- Rigid bronchoscopy is preferred, as it provides control of the airway throughout the removal process.

Laryngomalacia

- The disorder improves over time.
- Infants rarely require an artificial airway.

Vocal cord paralysis

- Unilateral cord paralysis requires no specific therapy and resolves over time.
- Tracheotomy may be necessary in infants with bilateral vocal cord paralysis.

Tracheomalacia

- Use of ß-agonists may worsen the airflow obstruction.
- Medications that increase the smooth-muscle cell tone of the trachea can improve airflow.

Laryngotracheobronchitis (croup)

- Most children have an uncomplicated course and are managed without formal medical care.

Peritonsillar abscess

- See Pharyngitis and Tonsillitis.

Bacterial tracheitis

- Antibiotics and supportive care are essential.
- Some otolaryngologists recommend placing tracheotomy tubes in children with bacterial tracheitis.

Laryngeal papillomatosis

- Remove the obstructing lesions with laser ablation to prevent regrowth.
  - Recurrent ablations may be required.

Vocal cord dysfunction

- Patient education, speech therapy, and biofeedback to teach patients to control vocal cord movement have produced favorable results.
- The goal is to train the extrinsic laryngeal muscles.

WHEN TO REFER

- An otorhinolaryngologist or general surgeon should be consulted if there is a high index of suspicion for foreign body aspiration.

WHEN TO ADMIT

- Patients with severe respiratory distress requiring supplemental oxygen.
- Infants with upper airways obstruction who have difficulty drinking and maintaining hydration.
- Patients with epiglottitis, retropharyngeal abscess, or bacterial tracheitis.

FOLLOW-UP

- Patients with laryngomalacia and tracheomalacia need to be followed carefully for weight gain and improvement in symptoms.

COMPLICATIONS

- In bacterial tracheitis, complications include:
  - Toxic shock syndrome
  - Septic shock
  - Postintubation pulmonary edema
  - Acute respiratory distress syndrome
  - Subglottic stenosis

PROGNOSIS

- Prognosis depends on the cause of airways obstruction.

Allergic Rhinitis

DEFINITION

- Atopic disease caused by exposure to allergens and characterized by nasal congestion, sneezing, rhinorrhea, and pruritus
  - Seasonal variation (hay fever)
  - Year-round (perennial) form
- May exist alone or in combination with asthma or atopic dermatitis

EPIDEMIOLOGY

- Prevalence
  - Allergic rhinitis is the most common of the atopic diseases, occurring in approximately 15% of the general population.
  - The perennial form is more common than the seasonal variation
- Age
  - In children, relatively uncommon before the age of 3 years
  - Increases in frequency thereafter, reaching peak prevalence in adolescence
- Seasonality
  - Symptoms peak in spring and fall in colder climates.
  - Symptoms can occur year-round in warmer climates, with the highest levels occurring in warmer, more humid months.

ETIOLOGY

- Allergic rhinitis is caused by exposure to an allergen and subsequent sensitization in a child who has a genetic predisposition to atopy.
- Reexposure to the same allergen causes an immediate type I hypersensitivity reaction.

RISK FACTORS

- As with all atopic disease, the tendency to develop allergic rhinitis is inherited.
- Exposures: seasonal allergic rhinitis
  - Pollens
    - Wind-borne from trees and grasses in the spring
    - From weeds (especially ragweed) in the fall
    - Flower pollens rarely cause allergic problems.
    - Great variation according to location
  - Molds
    - Indoors and outdoors
- Exposures: perennial allergic rhinitis
  - Animal dander
    - Skin (dander) and saliva of household pets, such as dogs and cats
    - Rodent allergens, found predominantly in urine of vermin and pets, such as hamsters and guinea pigs
  - Dust mites
    - Major allergen in house dust and major cause of perennial allergic rhinitis
    - Prosper in warm, moist, indoor environments, colonizing pillows, mattresses, and carpets
  - Cockroaches
    - Common in urban areas

SIGNS AND SYMPTOMS

- Severity of symptoms varies depending on individual level of sensitivity and the intensity of antigen exposure.
- Younger children usually have perennial symptoms, whereas pollen sensitivity becomes more common after the age of 4 years.
- Acute seasonal variety
  - Physical examination may be striking, especially during periods of seasonal rhinitis, or unremarkable when symptoms are quiescent.
  - Pale, bluish, and boggy nasal mucosa with a clear serous discharge
  - Nasal turbinates are enlarged, sometimes enough to obstruct the airway almost completely.
  - Children who have perennial problems often have typical allergic facies.
    - Allergic shiners (dark discoloration beneath both eyes)
    - Dennie lines (extra folds below the lower eyelids)
    - Allergic crease (horizontal line across the bridge of the nose)
    - Elongated facies caused by chronic mouth breathing
  - Tonsils and adenoids often are enlarged.
  - Evidence of middle-ear effusion may be found.
  - Nasal polyps can occur but are uncommon in childhood allergic rhinitis.
- Perennial variety
  - Sufferers typically have less dramatic or fewer specific symptoms.
  - Although nasal congestion is still the most prominent symptom, children often display such symptoms as:
    - Frequent colds
    - Recurrent otitis media
    - Nasal speech
    - Mouth breathing
    - Snoring
    - Fatigue
    - Epistaxis
  - Nasal discharge is usually clear unless the child has a superimposed infection.

- Many children perform the "allergic salute," a maneuver in which they sniff and sweep the palm of their hand upward across the tip of the nose in attempt to open their nasal passages, remove secretions, or relieve nasal itching.
- Facial grimacing is used to relieve nasal itching.

DIFFERENTIAL DIAGNOSIS

- Conditions that are often confused with allergic rhinitis:
  - Recurrent upper respiratory tract infections
    - Differentiated from allergies by their intermittent course; history of contagion; and the presence of fever, purulent nasal discharge, or erythematous, inflamed nasal mucosa
    - Eosinophils will not be prominent on a nasal smear.
    - Family history for allergy is more likely to be negative.
  - Vasomotor rhinitis
    - Poorly defined condition that may begin at any age
    - Characterized by hyperreactivity of the nasal mucous membranes to a wide variety of irritant stimuli
    - The prominent symptom is usually perennial nasal obstruction that responds poorly to environmental controls or medications.
    - Usually, no family history of allergy, although other family members may report chronic nasal congestion
    - Nasal smear and skin test results are negative, serum IgE is normal, and no eye signs or other atopic manifestations are present.
  - Nonallergic rhinitis with eosinophilia
    - Affects adolescents and adults
    - Nasal smear results are positive for eosinophils, but serum IgE is normal and skin test results are negative.
  - Adenoid hypertrophy
    - Typically presents as nasal obstruction with little or no rhinorrhea
    - Commonly associated with recurrent middle ear, nasal, or sinus infections
    - In severe cases, obstruction leads to obvious changes in the structure of the face and palate caused by chronic mouth breathing.
    - Snoring is common, as is a nasal quality to the voice.
  - Nasal foreign body
  - Choanal atresia
  - Rhinitis medicamentosa
  - Cystic fibrosis
  - Nasopharyngeal tumor

DIAGNOSTIC APPROACH

- Allergic rhinitis is characterized clinically by a combination of nasal congestion, sneezing, rhinorrhea, and pruritus.
- Diagnosis of seasonal variety typically is based on the clinical presentation, physical examination, and knowledge of local pollens.
  - For local pollen counts, see American Academy of Allergy, Asthma & Immunology web site, www.aaaai.org
- Nonspecific perennial symptoms pose a more difficult diagnostic challenge.

LABORATORY FINDINGS

- Nasal smear for eosinophils
  - Simple office procedure that can help confirm the clinical diagnosis of allergic rhinitis
  - The patient blows his or her nose into plastic wrap or wax paper.
    - A cotton swab may be used to obtain secretions if the patient cannot blow.
  - Secretions are spread onto a glass slide, left to dry, and then prepared with Hansel or Wright stain.
    - If >10% of cells seen on the smear are eosinophils, an ongoing allergic process is probable.
    - Strongly positive results are most likely during heavy exposure to the allergen.
    - Concurrent nasal infection may obscure the results, and eosinophils may be absent during the off season.
    - Not recommended as a screening test for allergic rhinitis
- Leukocyte count
  - Blood eosinophilia is occasionally found.
    - >5% eosinophils on the differential leukocyte count *or*
    - >250/μL eosinophils in total
- Serum IgE
  - Elevated total serum IgE level suggests atopy, but many patients who have allergic rhinitis have a normal serum IgE level.
  - Not recommended as a screening test for allergic rhinitis
- Skin tests
  - Can detect antigen-specific IgE and identify specific allergic sensitivities in patients in whom the diagnosis is in question or who need more aggressive management
  - Should be performed by a physician who is trained in their use
  - Should be interpreted in the context of the clinical history
- Radioallergosorbent tests
  - Can detect antigen-specific IgE and identify specific allergic sensitivities in:
    - Patients in whom the diagnosis is in question
    - Patients who are in need of more aggressive management

- Higher cost and slightly lower sensitivity than skin test
- Accurate overall and can be used efficiently in the primary care physician's office as a limited screening test for allergy
  - Also will identify specific allergens to be targeted for environmental control
- When extensive laboratory testing is needed, referring the patient to an allergist will usually be more cost effective.

TREATMENT APPROACH

- Management of allergic rhinitis incorporates information from a thorough history and physical examination.
- Stepwise program of treatment typically consists of allergen avoidance measures and pharmacotherapy.
- Each child's treatment must be individualized for:
  - Age
  - Severity of symptoms
  - Specific environmental issues
  - Presence or absence of complications
  - Coexisting medical conditions

SPECIFIC TREATMENTS

Environmental control

- First line of therapy at all ages
- Particular attention should be directed to the child's bedroom and other settings where substantial amounts of time are spent.
- Dust mite allergy
  - Reduce exposure via dust mite–proof encasements for mattresses, box springs, and pillows.
  - Remove stuffed animals and similar items.
  - Hot wash bed linens every 1–2 weeks.
- Household pets
  - Ideally, pets should be removed.
- There is some benefit from keeping the pet out of the child's bedroom, using mattress and pillow encasements, removing carpets, and using an air cleaner in the bedroom.
- Pollens
  - Close windows and use an air conditioner.
  - Forced-air heating and cooling systems can be improved by adding humidifiers and air filters.
  - Keep relative humidity below 50% to discourage dust mite and mold growth.

Oral antihistamines

- First-line pharmacologic treatment
- Most effective in controlling rhinorrhea, sneezing, and pruritus
  - Less effective in relieving nasal congestion

- First-generation antihistamines: diphenhydramine, chlorpheniramine, hydroxyzine
  - Very effective, but use may be limited by their sedative side effects
  - Can impair school performance significantly
  - Many children can be treated effectively with a single bedtime dose, especially if symptoms are worse at night.
- Second- and third-generation antihistamines: loratadine, desloratadine, cetirizine, fexofenadine
  - Now approved for use in children
  - Not necessarily more potent, but lack of sedation is an important advantage

Oral decongestants

- Pseudoephedrine may have value in some children, especially when nasal congestion is a major symptom.
- Can be used either alone or in combination with an antihistamine
- Should be used with caution because some children experience significant stimulatory effects, which may produce:
  - Hyperactivity
  - Irritability
  - Sleep disturbance

Leukotriene antagonist

- Montelukast
  - Approved for treatment of both seasonal and perennial allergic rhinitis
  - Similar in efficacy to oral antihistamines
  - Generally well tolerated
  - May be particularly useful in children with coexistent asthma and allergic rhinitis

Oral corticosteroids

- Prednisone
  - Rarely, short courses may be needed for severe cases that do not respond to other therapies.
  - Topical sprays
  - Nasal corticosteroids are the most effective pharmacologic agents for allergic rhinitis.
  - Available preparations include:
    - Beclomethasone
    - Budesonide
    - Fluticasone
    - Mometasone
    - Triamcinolone
  - Mometasone and fluticasone are approved for use in patients ≥3 years of age.

- Oral corticosteroids carry the slight potential to adversely affect growth in children; therefore, they should always be used at the lowest possible dose.

Decongestant nasal sprays and other topical preparations

■ Decongestant nasal sprays
  - May provide transient relief, often followed after several days of use by rebound congestion
  - Prolonged use of nasal sprays often leads to worsening of symptoms (rhinitis medicamentosa) and should be discouraged.
■ Other topical preparations
  - Antihistamine: azelastine
    – Of similar potency to oral antihistamines; can also have sedative side effects
  - Nasalcromolyn sodium
    – A safe drug that is reasonably effective, although its usefulness is significantly limited by the need to use it 4–6 times a day
  - Ipratropium nasal spray
    – Approved for children ≥6 years of age and may be helpful in the control of rhinorrhea
    – May have a particular advantage in cases of nonallergic rhinitis in which excessive rhinorrhea is a major symptom

Immunotherapy

■ Use if clinical history and skin test results correlate.
  - Must be used selectively
  - Typically reserved only for patients in whom standard medications and avoidance measures have failed
■ 3- to 5-year course of regular injections achieves maximal benefit and minimizes the chance of relapse after discontinuing treatment.
  - Most effective in treating seasonal allergic rhinitis, with >80% of patients achieving significant relief
  - Beneficial for most cases of perennial disease
■ As treatment progresses, patients can expect a gradual decline in symptoms and reduced reliance on medication.
■ Disadvantages
  - Possible local and generalized reactions
  - Inconvenience and expense associated with regular injections

WHEN TO REFER

■ Perennial symptoms
■ Poorly controlled disease
■ Suspected complications (eg, chronic sinusitis)
■ Need for immunotherapy
■ Parental needs

COMPLICATIONS

■ Children who have allergic rhinitis may suffer early from an increased incidence of respiratory infections, acute otitis media, and eustachian tube dysfunction, leading to serous otitis media.
  - Several studies have suggested an association between allergy and chronic serous otitis media.
  - Only 1 of many risk factors
■ Acute and chronic sinusitis are common, probably the result of reduced ciliary clearance and obstruction of sinus ostia.
■ Asthma is often seen in combination with allergic rhinitis but is not viewed typically as a complication of untreated allergic rhinitis.
■ Occasional abnormal facial development, a high arched palate, and orthodontic problems from chronic mouth breathing
  - Especially in cases with associated adenoid hypertrophy

PROGNOSIS

■ Allergic rhinitis waxes and wanes over time.
■ Most children tend to improve with time, although very few (<10%) lose their symptoms completely.
■ Remission of symptoms may result from changes in environment, avoidance programs, and immunotherapy.
■ The care provider should counsel patients that allergic symptoms can be controlled but not eliminated entirely.
  - Success of any treatment depends on the patient's understanding of the causes of symptoms and compliance with the prescribed regimen.

PREVENTION

■ Prevention of recurrence involves:
  - Control of environmental factors
  - Avoidance of allergens
  - Compliance with treatment

Alopecia and Hair Shaft Anomalies

A

DEFINITION

- Alopecia
  - Loss of hair
- Hair shaft anomalies
  - Stubbly growth of broken hair rather than true alopecia

EPIDEMIOLOGY

- Sex:
  - In general, may occur in either sex
- Androgenetic alopecia
  - Age
    - 15% of adolescents >14 years of age
    - Fullest expression is most common in the mature adult.
  - Sex
    - Occurs most often in males
- Loose anagen syndrome
  - Age
    - Preschoolers between 2 and 5 years of age
  - Sex
    - Females are more often affected.

MECHANISM

- Hair loss can result from:
  - Congenital disorders
  - Hereditary disorders
  - Head trauma
  - Physical or emotional stress
  - Stress on the hair from:
    - Braiding
    - Teasing
    - Other tightly pulled hairstyles
  - Antimetabolites for treatment of cancer
- Loss can be:
  - Total
  - Thinning
    - 50% loss is necessary before the casual observer will notice hair loss.
- Phases of hair growth/loss
  - Anagen phase
    - Active hair growth over 2–6 years
  - Lanugo, the first hair made by hair follicles in utero
    - Lanugo is lost a few months after birth and is a normal process that results in a temporary near-baldness.
    - In many instances, parents are concerned with the thinning or with a localized area of loss, usually over the occiput, the result of the pressure of the head as the infant lies in the crib.
  - Telogen phase
    - Resting period of ~3 months
      - As many as 15% of scalp hairs may be in the telogen phase at any time.
      - Up to 100 hairs are lost from the scalp daily and 200 with shampooing (not apparent to casual observer).

HISTORY

- A precise, pointed history is necessary.
- When a child loses scalp hair suddenly, a toxic event should be suspected.
  - Accidental poisoning, eg, rat poison containing thallium or coumarin
  - In most instances, over several months, new hairs will replace lost hairs, unless the exposure to the toxic element is chronic.
- True congenital alopecia is rare.
  - May be inherited as an autosomal-recessive trait
  - If the loss is not due to this genetic circumstance but is congenital, it is most often evidence of a significant hereditary disorder.
- Hairs may be thin or poorly anchored to the scalp or have a variety of shaft abnormalities.

PHYSICAL EXAM

- The entire body and all its hair-bearing parts must be observed.
  - The pediatrician must not limit the examination simply to the site of hair loss.
- It is important to determine if alopecia is scarring or nonscarring.
- The texture of hair may be helpful in finding the source of difficulty.
- Appropriate diagnosis requires microscopic differentiation of the hair and its root.

DIFFERENTIAL DIAGNOSIS

Congenital alopecia

- Ectodermal dysplasia
- Skeletal defects
  - Cartilage-hair hypoplasia
  - Congenital ectodermal dysplasia
  - Orofaciodigital syndrome
- Inherited metabolic or endocrine disorders
  - Phenylketonuria
  - Homocystinuria
  - Congenital hypothyroidism

- Serious chromosomal defects
  - de Lange syndrome
  - Trisomy 13 syndrome
  - Surfeit of signs and symptoms beyond simple loss of hair

Nonscarring alopecia with hair shaft abnormalities

- Trichorrhexis nodosa
  - Common abnormality of the hair shaft characterized by:
    - Fragile, short hair with grayish-white nodules
    - Breakage of hair and short stubble over the scalp
    - White specks marking the nodes may appear after some physical and chemical injuries.
  - Usually accompanied by a history of hair straightening or repeated vigorous brushing and combing
- Monilethrix (beaded hair syndrome)
  - Scalp hairs have regularly spaced differences in their circumference, suggesting a chain of beads.
  - Fragile, short, stubble-like growth
  - Associated problems suggestive of a more widespread ectodermal defect:
    - Cataracts
    - Brittle nails
    - Faulty teeth
- Pili torti (twisted hair)
  - Fragile, short, light/"off"-colored hair appears spangled as a result of light reflection.
  - Texture is coarse and lusterless.
    - As though straight and curly hair were competing for a place in the same strand
  - Associated with Menkes kinky hair syndrome, an X-linked disease characterized by:
    - Low serum copper level
    - Progressive cerebral degeneration
    - Arterial degeneration
    - Suggestion of scurvy in the bones

Nonscarring alopecia without hair shaft abnormalities

- Alopecia areata
  - Most often seen as an acute problem
    - Sharply demarcated, round, nearly bald patches
    - Inflammatory signs are not present.
  - Patches tend to be several centimeters in diameter, usually on the scalp.
    - Possible anywhere on the body where hair is found (see Figure 4 on page F1)
    - Loss may comprise only a few patches or a total absence of body hair (alopecia universalis), including eyebrows and eyelashes.

- Sometimes salmon-colored, as a manifestation of the presumed inflammation seen histologically around the hair follicle
    - Exclamation point hairs may appear throughout the patch.
    - Hairs at the periphery of an area are plucked easily and may be particularly colorless and thin.
  - Fingernails may be pitted.
    - Possible indication of a more extensive ectodermal problem
  - Cause
    - Unknown, but may be related to a T cell–mediated autoimmune process
    - Associated with acute autoimmune thyroid disease and vitiligo
    - Possible genetic predisposition
- Androgenetic alopecia
  - Male baldness pattern
    - Begins most often with a receding hairline and some thinning over the vertex
  - Diffuse thinning with retained frontal hair in the female
  - Hairs from affected follicles do not epilate easily on pulling, but they are shorter and finer because of normal pubertal androgen increase in susceptible individuals.
  - Cause
    - Genetically determined
- Trichotillomania
  - Irregularly shaped areas of thinned stubble of varying lengths
    - Large, patchy, ill-defined patterns
    - Area of hair loss is most accessible to the probing hand.
    - May simulate alopecia areata (see Figure 5 on page F1)
  - Patient may eat hair, which can accumulate in the stomach and form a trichobezoar (hairball).
    - Abdominal pain
    - Possible acute intestinal obstruction
    - Palpable as an abdominal mass
  - Cause
    - Some children have a compulsive need to pull out their hair or even eyebrows or eyelashes.
    - May sometimes (but not always) provide a major clue to an underlying psychosocial problem
- Traumatic alopecia
  - Bizarre patterns conforming to site and method of injury
    - May be accompanied by redness and inflammation
    - Pustular involvement of the follicles is possible.

- Causes
  - Head trauma
  - Braiding
  - Constant teasing or straightening with heat or chemicals
  - Hairstyles (eg, barrettes, ponytails, braids, or cornrows) that cause constant and prolonged traction, especially along the hairline
- Telogen effluvium
  - Diffuse thinning with easy epilation from all areas of scalp
    - Nonpatterned
    - Nonscarring
  - Hair loss may increase to as much as 60%.
    - During such a period, the situation is similar to that of animals, which shed seasonally.
  - Causes
    - May be related to a history of stress
    - Prolonged fever
    - Pregnancy
    - Severe illness
- Anagen effluvium
  - Significant thinning
- Loose anagen syndrome
  - Hair appears sparse.
  - Hairs are quite easily and painlessly pulled from the scalp.
  - Individual hairs are not fragile.
  - Hair over the occiput often is matted and sticky.
  - Typically, the child's hair is said to be slow growing, seldom requiring cutting.
  - Causes
    - Hereditary factor may be involved.
    - Most cases are sporadic.

Potentially scarring alopecia without hair shaft abnormalities

- Tinea capitis and kerion
  - Presentation varies.
    - Round, minimally inflamed alopecic area with slight seborrheic scale
    - Boggy, tender often pustular, severely inflamed kerion
    - Lesions tend to be more elevated than in other forms of tinea and may be characterized by black dots.
  - Tinea capitis (see Figure 6 on page F2) should be considered:
    - When a child has patches of alopecia or stubbly hair growth
    - When alopecia is accompanied by local adenopathy
    - Even in the absence of crusting, scaling, redness, or other inflammatory signs

- Differential diagnosis includes:
  - Seborrheic dermatitis
  - Atopic dermatitis
  - Psoriasis
- Causes
  - *Trichophyton tonsurans*
  - *Microsporum canis*
  - *Microsporum audouinii*
- Kerion
  - Delayed hypersensitivity reaction to fungus
  - If unchecked, resultant scarring interferes with the regrowth of hair (see Figure 7 on page F2).
  - Early diagnosis and treatment are therefore helpful.
- Lupus erythematosus
  - Discoid variant
    - Discoid, well-demarcated erythematous plaques
    - Scale
    - Plugged follicles
    - Atrophy and/or thinning as a result of broken, fragile hair with acute flares (lupus hair)
    - Can be disfiguring to the scalp
    - With scarring, can cause permanent hair loss (see Figure 8 on page F2)
  - Systemic variant
    - Scalp may be erythematous.
    - Scarring is not characteristic.
- Acrodermatitis enteropathica
  - Abnormal zinc absorption
  - Cutaneous manifestations simulating:
    - Psoriasis
    - Epidermolysis bullosa
    - Pyoderma
    - Candidiasis
  - Zinc deficiency can result in:
    - Abdominal pain and diarrhea
    - Wispy alopecia
    - Dystrophic development of the fingernails, suggesting widespread ectodermal involvement
  - Cause
    - Autosomal-recessive

LABORATORY EVALUATION

- Light microscopy
  - Anagen hairs
    - Fat, healthy follicle bulbs
    - Attached emerging long terminal hair

- Telogen hairs
  - Small bulb
  - Attached hair with a club-shaped appearance
■ Light microscopic characteristics of various alopecias:
  - Trichorrhexis nodosa
    - Nodes along hair shaft similar to interlocking broom or brush ends
  - Monilethrix
    - Variable shaft thickness gives a beaded appearance with internodal breakage.
  - Pili torti
    - Irregularly spaced twists along the shaft appear flattened
    - In cross-section, a straight hair appears round, and a curly hair appears oval.
    - Both configurations may be seen in a single strand; this can be an important clue to Menkes kinky hair syndrome.
  - Alopecia areata
    - Exclamation point hairs from periphery of patches with poorly pigmented shaft and tapered attenuated bulb
  - Androgenetic alopecia
    - Increased telogen:anagen ratio, frontal scalp
  - Trichotillomania
    - Normal cuticle, shaft, and anagen bulb of varying lengths
  - Traumatic alopecia
    - Normal cuticle, shaft, and anagen bulb of varied lengths
  - Telogen effluvium
    - >25% of pulled hairs are telogen club hairs with no pigment
  - Anagen effluvium
    - Tapered anagen bulbs
  - Loose anagen syndrome
    - Anagen hairs have misshapen pigmented anagen bulbs with ruffled cuticle and no external root sheath.
  - Tinea capitis and kerion
    - Potassium hydroxide preparation of broken hairs (black dot hairs) reveals clusters of chains of arthrospores around or in the hair shaft and bulb.
  - Lupus erythematosus
    - Not applicable if there is scarring
    - Short, broken (frayed) anagen hairs
■ Mycologic analysis
  - *T tonsurans* indicates tinea capitis.
    - In rare cases, the endothrix fungi *M canis* and *M audouiniican* invade the hair shaft and cause breakage and stubbiness.
    - *M canis* tends to cause much more inflammation than does *M audouinii.*

- Endothrix fungal infections, but not *T tonsurans*, can produce a greenish fluorescence under Wood light in a darkened room.

IMAGING
■ Radiography
  - Congenital alopecia
    - Skeletal defects
  - Trichotillomania
    - Presence of a trichobezoar

DIAGNOSTIC PROCEDURES
■ Biopsy
  - Miniaturized anagen bulbs in androgenetic alopecia
  - Fungus *T tonsurans*

TREATMENT APPROACH
■ Treatment depends on the underlying cause of alopecia.
  - There may be helpful treatments.
  - The pediatrician's role may be only diagnostic and supportive.

SPECIFIC TREATMENT

Trichorrhexis nodosa
■ A gentle approach results in gradual improvement.
■ Eliminate any noxious exposure.

Monilethrix
■ No treatment is known.
■ Some degree of recovery may occur spontaneously, particularly after puberty or during pregnancy.

Alopecia areata
■ Spontaneous regrowth
  - About one-third of patients will regrow hair spontaneously in 6 months.
  - About one-third will regrow hair spontaneously within 5 years.
  - About one-third must be treated to stimulate hair growth.
■ Cortisone cream
  - Topical applications have been used with some success.
■ Cortisone injection
  - Direct injection into the scalp or eyebrow hair follicles can be effective.
  - The process is painful.
  - Large areas (>50% scalp hair loss) that require infiltration present difficulty.
  - Use with caution in the older, more cooperative child.

- The pediatrician must carefully assess the impact of the disease and the treatment on the child before selecting this procedure.
- The patient should be referred to a dermatologist for consideration of this intervention.

■ Oral corticosteroid therapy
- Risks serious complications, but is occasionally used

■ Minoxidil
- 5% minoxidil solution twice daily
- Can be effective for small, stubborn alopecic areas

■ Irritants
- Used for extensive alopecia
- Dinitrochlorobenzene immunotherapy
- Tars, such as short-contact anthralin
- Psoralen with ultraviolet A light (PUVA therapy)
- Use only in children >12 years.
- Should be performed only by a knowledgeable dermatologist in controlled circumstances

■ Efficacy of treatment
- Difficult to assess because of the waxing and waning nature of alopecia areata
- Pediatricians should remind patients and families that this process is nonscarring, which always has the potential for full regrowth.

Androgenetic alopecia

■ No therapy is reliably effective.

■ Some patients may be helped by:
- Topical minoxidil twice daily
- Hair transplant micrografts

■ Finasteride
- Can be given after 18 years of age in male patients
- Contraindicated in female patients because of the possibility of genital defects in exposed male fetuses if a pregnancy occurs

Trichotillomania

■ Petroleum jelly
- The primary care pediatrician can paint the attacked areas in an attempt to frustrate the habit.

■ Imipramine

■ Fluoxetine

■ Psychiatric intervention
- Without attention to the possibility of an underlying emotional issue, other treatments are temporary.
- Family structure and interaction with siblings and parents and with friends at home and at school should be explored in an effort to find stressors.
- Consulting a psychiatrist should also be considered.

■ Surgery or endoscopy
- Referral for removal of a trichobezoar

Traumatic alopecia

■ Simply discontinuing the stress will help.

■ Injured hair follicles will often require ≥3 months to return to an anagen phase.

Loose anagen syndrome

■ Management is limited to reassurance and the passage of time.

■ The hair eventually grows thicker and longer, and its pigmentation increases.

Tinea capitis

■ Griseofulvin is the standard of care.
- Topical antifungal agents do not provide adequate treatment.
- Several other systemic fungistatic agents are effective.
- The long course of oral therapy with griseofulvin (~2 months) may present difficulties with compliance in a young child.

■ Terbinafine
- This fungicidal drug appears effective when given for 2–4 weeks but is currently not approved for this use by the US Food and Drug Administration (FDA).

■ Itraconazole and fluconazole
- May be safe for short courses in children but are not FDA approved for this use
- Liquid itraconazole has been associated with diarrhea in children and with pancreatic adenocarcinoma in laboratory animals and should be avoided.

■ Prednisone
- Oral, tapered over 10 days
- Rapidly decreases tenderness and inflammation of a kerion
- Prevents widespread id reaction

■ Secondary infection
- With *M canis* or after treatment with an irritant
- Inflammation may require treatment with an antibiotic.

Lupus erythematosus

■ Discoid variant
- Early treatment with topical or intralesional steroids may prevent scarring.

■ Systemic variant
- Loss of hair is generally temporary.

Acrodermatitis enteropathica

■ Oral zinc sulfate is the treatment of choice.

■ Strategies for the patient to hide noticeable loss of hair
- Suggest that the child wear a baseball cap or other concealing adornment if appropriate.

- A hairpiece can be designed for a child.
- These steps serve in the interim while practitioners:
  - Attempt potentially helpful treatments
  - Wait expectantly if their role is diagnostic and supportive
- Management if recovery of hair is questionable
  - Work with and listen to the patient and family to:
    - Achieve an emotional balance consistent with reality
    - Adopt suitable coping mechanisms
  - Plastic surgery
    - Expertise should be sought for consideration of hair transplants and scalp reduction (for scarred areas) when possible.

WHEN TO REFER

- Rapid, diffuse hair loss
- Chronic, progressive, localized, or diffuse hair loss without regrowth
- Scarring alopecia
- Inability to grow hair as a result of breakage, loss, or abnormal texture of hair
- Appearance of scalp mass or plaque affecting localized hair loss

FOLLOW-UP

- Liver function testing
  - If antifungal medications are used for >12 weeks
  - At the start of therapy if any suggestion of preexisting liver disease exists

PROGNOSIS

- The possibility that hair will not regrow must be considered when loss:
  - Follows high fever or chronic toxicity
  - Is accompanied by scarring
  - Occurs in the areas of:
    - Nevi
    - Aplasia cutis
    - Persistent hemangioma

- Prognosis for the return of hair depends on:
  - Elimination of the toxic stimulus
  - Whether the loss is accompanied by scarring
    - Loss associated with nonscarring conditions is recoverable.
    - Loss with scarring (eg, from iatrogenic scalp injury during delivery or from a burn) is permanent.
- Alopecia areata
  - The more extensive the loss and the younger the child, the less likelihood is of a full recovery.
  - Prognosis is best when:
    - Loss is less widespread.
    - Only 1 or 2 patches are present.
  - When hair does regrow, it may initially be white.
  - Eventually, color returns, and casual observers cannot identify the formerly affected area.
- Traumatic alopecia
  - In childhood, the hair will usually return, although regrowth can be slow.
- Loose anagen syndrome
  - After recovery and even into adulthood, the hair may still pull out easily and painlessly.
- Lupus erythematosus
  - Discoid variant
    - Hair loss can be permanent.
  - Systemic variant
    - Loss of hair is generally temporary.
    - There is no scarring, unlike in discoid disease.

PREVENTION

- Hair is fragile.
  - It should be handled gently and without physical or chemical assault.
  - In children, hair is probably best left alone, except for:
    - Simple washing
    - Simple cutting to suit the fashion

Altered Mental Status

A

DEFINITION

- Consciousness
  - Awareness of self and the environment
- Coma
  - Unresponsiveness to all stimuli, including pain, with the eyes remaining closed
- Alteration of consciousness
  - Begins with becoming unaware of self
  - Followed by reduced awareness of the environment
  - Finally, an inability to be aroused
- Stages between consciousness and coma
  - A progression of symptoms is not an all-or-nothing phenomenon; rather, a continuum of levels of consciousness may exist.
    - Confusion: responses are slowed and cognitive abilities are impaired, usually accompanied by some disorientation
    - Delirium: a succession of confused and unconnected ideas, often with aggression, agitation, and combativeness, with episodes of somnolence and withdrawal
    - Lethargy: a state of profound slumber with limited movement and speech; can be awakened with moderate stimuli
    - Stupor: unresponsive except to repeated, vigorous stimuli
    - Vegetative state: loss of all cognitive neurologic function, communication, and awareness; may retain some non-cognitive functions

EPIDEMIOLOGY

- Nontraumatic coma
  - Bimodal distribution
    - Most common in infants and toddlers
    - Smaller peak in adolescence
  - Infection of the brain/meninges is the most common cause of altered mental status: more than one-third of nontraumatic cases.
  - Exposure to or ingestion of toxic substances is the next most common cause.
    - Accidental ingestion, especially in toddlers
    - Intentional ingestion in adolescents
- The overall incidence of traumatic and nontraumatic coma is similar.
  - However, the rate of traumatic injury tends to increase throughout childhood.

ETIOLOGY

AEIOU TIPS

- AEIOU TIPS is a helpful mnemonic in categorizing the etiology of altered mental status.
  - A
    - Alcohol
    - Abuse
  - E
    - Epilepsy
    - Encephalopathy
    - Electrolyte abnormalities
    - Endocrine
  - I
    - Insulin
    - Intussusception
    - Inadequate fluid
  - O
    - Overdose
    - Oxygen deficiency
    - Occult trauma
    - Obstructed ventriculoperitoneal shunt
  - U
    - Uremia
  - T
    - Trauma
    - Temperature abnormality
    - Tumor
  - I
    - Infection
  - P
    - Poisoning
    - Psychiatric
    - Postictal
  - S
    - Shock
    - Stroke
    - Space-occupying lesion (intracranial)

Commonly ingested agents that cause altered mental status

- Amphetamines
- Anticholinergics
- Anticonvulsants
- Barbiturates

- Benzodiazepines
- Clonidine
- Cocaine
- Dextromethorphan
- Ethanol
- Haloperidol
- Narcotics
- Phenothiazines
- Salicylates
- Selective serotonin reuptake inhibitors
- Tricyclic antidepressants

Infants

- Infection of the brain, meninges, or both
- Complication of congenital malformation (cardiac or central nervous system)
- Metabolic
  - Urea cycle defects
  - Organic acidemias
  - Disorders of amino acid metabolism
- Seizure
- Abuse

Children

- Infection of the brain, meninges, or both
- Seizure
- Toxin
- Trauma
- Metabolic
- Abuse
- Intussusception
- Complications from surgical correction of congenital malformations

Adolescents

- Toxin
- Trauma
- Infection
- Psychiatric
- Seizure
- Complications of surgical correction of congenital malformations
- Metabolic disorder
- Diabetic ketoacidosis is the most common metabolic disorder that occurs with alteration of consciousness.
- Can occur at any age, but is more common in adolescence

SIGNS AND SYMPTOMS

History

- Circumstances of the onset of the neurologic symptoms
  - Events and actions directly preceding the change in mental status
  - Especially for young children and children with chronic conditions, ascertain baseline state of functioning and responsiveness.
- If the alteration in consciousness occurred abruptly, consider:
  - Seizure
  - Sudden cardiac arrhythmia
  - Trauma
    - Structural lesion (epidural hematoma, cerebral contusion)
    - Nonaccidental trauma, especially if the caregiver's history is inconsistent with the clinical findings
  - Ingestion of a toxic substance
    - Ingestion in a young child may not have been witnessed.
    - A detailed list of potential poisons to which the child may have access, including prescription and nonprescription medications, should be obtained.
    - The adolescent may admit to an intentional overdose, but the history is often obscure or unobtainable.
    - In these cases, interviews with accompanying friends and family members are essential.
  - Intracranial hemorrhage
- More gradual change in mental status may suggest:
  - Infection
  - Metabolic abnormality
    - A child with diabetes may have ketoacidosis or hypoglycemia.
    - Children with a metabolic disorder or with hepatic or renal failure may develop encephalopathy.
  - Slowly growing intracranial mass
- Associated symptoms may include:
  - Weakness
  - Headache
  - Vomiting
  - Dizziness
  - Diplopia
  - Seizure-like activity
- Altered mental status preceded by headache (especially on awakening), double vision, and vomiting suggests increased intracranial pressure.

A

Physical examination

- Establish a baseline with which future examinations can be compared for improvement or deterioration of the child's clinical status.
- Regardless of the underlying cause, patients with an acute change in mental status may exhibit:
  - Reduced awareness of self
  - Reduced awareness of the environment
  - Agitation with periods of heightened mental activity
  - Inability to be aroused
- Although the child appears unresponsive in severe cases, initial changes in mental status are often subtle.
  - Changes are recognized by assessing the child's actions and responses to external and internal stimuli (behavior).
    - Appearance
    - Level of alertness
    - Speech
    - Cry
    - Gaze
    - Mood, consolability
    - Thought
    - Judgment
- Vital signs are particularly important.
  - Hyperthermia
    - Infection
    - Heatstroke
    - Some toxins (eg, cocaine, anticholinergics, phencyclidine)
  - Hypothermia
    - Exposure to cold
    - Alcohol overdose
  - Hypertension, bradycardia, irregular respirations (Cushing triad)
    - Impending cerebral herniation
    - Appear late in the course of increasing intracranial pressure
  - Abnormalities in heart rate and blood pressure
    - Fever
    - Pain
    - Arrhythmias
    - Hypovolemia
    - Myocardial injury
    - Status epilepticus
  - Abnormal respirations
    - Pain
    - Hypoxia
    - Acidosis
    - Intoxication
    - Brainstem lesions
      - In some cases, the respiratory pattern may be a clue to the level of neurologic dysfunction.
      - Posthyperventilation apnea (short apnea after deep breathing) occurs with lesions in the cerebral hemispheres.
      - As dysfunction moves rostrally from the midbrain to the medulla, the respiratory pattern progresses from Cheyne-Stokes breathing (crescendo-decrescendo hyperpnea followed by apnea) to central neurogenic hyperventilation (sustained, rapid, deep breathing).
      - Irregular, sporadic, apneustic respiration occurs with low brainstem dysfunction.
- Mouth and throat
  - Examine for signs of airway obstruction causing hypoxia.
- Head and neck
  - Bulging fontanelle and nuchal rigidity are signs of meningitis or meningeal irritation from an intracranial mass.
  - Head trauma can cause:
    - Intracerebral, epidural, or subdural bleeding
    - Contusions
    - Diffuse axonal injury
    - These conditions can lead to cerebral dysfunction, either by primary neuronal damage or the effects of cerebral herniation with brainstem compression.
- Skin examination to help identify:
  - Hypoxia
  - Anemia
  - Jaundice
  - Carbon monoxide and other poisonings
  - Trauma
  - Some infections
- Feigned coma
  - Adolescents who are pretending to be unresponsive usually:
    - Avoid hitting themselves when their hand is raised and then allowed to drop to their face
    - Resist opening their eyes
    - Close their eyes quickly and deliberately after being held open by the examiner, as opposed to true coma, during which the eyes close slowly

Neurologic examination

- Directed at determining whether the underlying cause is structural or medical
- Pupillary reflex
  - Pupils may function normally if the insult is confined to the cerebral hemispheres.
  - With thalamic/hypothalamic insult, pupils are miotic but reactive.

- With midbrain involvement, pupils may be midposition, irregular, or dilated; reflexes may be absent if oculomotor nerves are involved.
- Bilateral fixed and dilated pupils indicate massive central nervous system (CNS) dysfunction.
- A unilateral dilated pupil is a sign of uncal herniation.
- Not all abnormal pupillary response is from increased intracranial pressure.
  - Mydriasis
    - Horner syndrome
    - Exposure to anticholinergics, amphetamines, cocaine, tricyclic antidepressants
  - Miosis
    - Cold exposure
    - Exposure to opiates, ethanol, barbiturates, cholinergic agents (eg, organophosphates), clonidine
- Extraocular movements
  - Should be noted at rest
    - Deviation may mean seizure activity or a structural lesion.
  - Asymmetry suggests midbrain/upper pons involvement.
  - Absence suggests lower pons/medullary involvement.
  - Negative doll's eyes (eyes appear painted on the face because they remain stationary with respect to head movement) suggest low brainstem injury.
- Motor function
  - Spontaneous movements should be evaluated for signs of hemiparesis.
    - Structural lesion or uncal herniation
  - Tone should be assessed for flaccidity and responses to painful stimuli.
    - Patients who are unresponsive may have depressed brainstem function.
    - Those with increased tone may have diffuse cortical injury.
- Posturing
  - Poor prognostic sign
  - Decorticate posturing
    - The patient flexes the arms, wrists, and hands and adducts the upper extremities while internally rotating and plantar flexing the lower extremities.
    - Occurs as a result of diffuse damage to the cerebral cortex, white matter, and basal ganglia
  - Decerebrate posturing
    - The patient exhibits marked opisthotonus with extended arms and hands.
    - Usually the result of extensive damage involving the midbrain

DIFFERENTIAL DIAGNOSIS

- A normal level of consciousness requires functioning cerebral hemispheres and a functioning ascending reticular activating system (ARAS).
- Altered mental status can result from depression of the cerebral hemispheres, a localized abnormality of the ARAS, or global CNS dysfunction affecting both.
- Structural lesions in general produce dysfunction of the ARAS.
- Medical causes usually affect cerebral function.
- Differentiation of structural and medical causes rests on the ability to assess the function of the ARAS.
  - The ARAS is located in the vicinity of the pupillary light reflex and of the cranial nerves that control eye movements and conjugate gaze.
    - The pupillary light reflex is relatively resistant to metabolic insult.
    - Its preservation, even if sluggish, is an important way to differentiate structural from medical causes of altered mental status.
    - Asymmetric eye movements or a fixed gaze suggests a structural lesion in the region of the ARAS.
- Structural (anatomic) causes
  - Cerebrovascular accident
  - Cerebral vein thrombosis
  - Hydrocephalus
  - Intracerebral tumor
  - Subdural empyema
  - Trauma
    - Intracranial bleeding
    - Diffuse cerebral swelling
    - Shaken baby syndrome
- Structural lesions are often characterized by:
  - Unequal or unreactive pupils or inability to abduct an eye
  - Focal neurologic findings
  - Structural causes may occur without focality, such as acute bilateral cerebrovascular disease or early acute hydrocephalus.
- Medical (toxic-infectious-metabolic) causes
  - Anoxia
  - Diabetic ketoacidosis
  - Electrolyte abnormality
  - Encephalopathy
  - Hypoglycemia
  - Hypothermia or hyperthermia
  - Infection (sepsis)
  - Inborn errors of metabolism

A

- Intussusception
- Meningitis and encephalitis
- Psychogenic
- Postictal state
- Toxin
- Uremia (hemolytic-uremic syndrome)
- Medical causes usually produce:
  - Dysfunction in both cerebral hemispheres
  - Preserved pupillary reflexes
  - Nonfocal neurologic findings
  - Some medical causes may be accompanied by focal neurologic findings: eg, hypoglycemia, hypercalcemia, uremia, and a postictal state with Todd paralysis.

DIAGNOSTIC APPROACH

- In the continuum of mental status changes, initial alterations in mental status are often subtle.
  - Child- and age-specific responses to external and internal stimuli should be assessed.
- The underlying cause of altered mental status must be sought.
  - Neuroimaging of the brain
    - Fastest, most reliable test to differentiate structural from medical causes of altered mental status
  - The mnemonic AEIOU TIPS (see Etiology) is helpful when considering the major categories of illness or injury.
- Child abuse should always be considered in an infant with an altered level of consciousness and/or unexplained bruising.

LABORATORY FINDINGS

- First, determine whether the patient has life-threatening metabolic derangements.
  - Then look for the underlying cause.
- Rapid bedside glucose determination
  - Identifies hypoglycemia within minutes of clinical evaluation
  - In addition to being a common cause of altered mental status, hypoglycemia also accompanies many other underlying causes, such as diabetes, metabolic disorders, and sepsis.
- Serum chemistry panel
  - Calcium and sodium abnormalities
  - Serum bicarbonate and arterial blood gas levels
    - May show acidemia, either as a direct result of an underlying metabolic disorder or as a result of abnormal respiratory effort
  - Serum ammonia measurement
    - Important screening test for many inborn errors of metabolism
    - Mild hyperammonemia can be a nonspecific finding in children.

- Serum osmolarity
  - May be helpful if poisoning with methanol, ethylene glycol, or isopropanol is suspected
- Serum cooximetry
  - Measures carbon monoxide level
- Blood culture
  - Obtain if the child is febrile.
  - Hemoglobin levels
    - To determine whether anemia is present
  - Leukocyte count
    - May be high if the altered mental status is from an infection
- Directed drug levels
  - If ingestion of a toxic substance is considered
  - Qualitative urine toxicology screening can identify a variety of commonly ingested agents, but its usefulness is limited by the delay until results are available.

IMAGING

- The decision whether to use computed tomography (CT) or magnetic resonance imaging (MRI) depends on a variety of factors.
  - Clinical situation
  - Stability of the patient
  - Availability of the test
- CT
  - Readily available in the setting of an acute change in mental status
  - Rapidly identifies acute intracranial bleeding, masses, or contusions in emergency situations
- MRI
  - Uses no ionizing radiation and thus poses reduced risk to the developing brain
  - Provides more detail of the soft tissues and better imaging of the brain parenchyma, cerebellum, and brainstem than CT
- Plain radiography, ultrasonography
  - Diagnostic for intussusception

DIAGNOSTIC PROCEDURES

- Electrocardiography
  - Abnormalities may be seen in cardiac causes.
    - Myocarditis
    - Dysrhythmias
    - A normal electrocardiogram finding does not rule out these disorders.
  - Many serious drug overdoses have electrocardiographic findings.
    - Prolongation of the QRS interval with tricyclic antidepressants

- Ischemic changes with cocaine overdose
- QT prolongation with neuroleptic overdose (phenothiazines, thioridazine, haloperidol, chlorpromazine)
- Stool guaiac test
  - A positive result raises concern about intussusception.

TREATMENT APPROACH

- Management is similar to that of any emergency condition.
- Primary objectives
  - Stabilize the child's clinical status.
  - Correct any acute life-threatening conditions.
- Once stabilized, the child should be transported to an acute care facility for additional evaluation and management.

SPECIFIC TREATMENTS

Initial management

- ABCs—airway, breathing, circulation
  - Obstructed airway is usually identified by:
    - Stridor
    - Abnormal breathing pattern
  - Immediate maneuvers to open the airway by either:
    - Manual positioning
    - Oral airway
    - Endotracheal intubation
  - Oxygen
    - Should be routinely administered
- Peripheral intravenous (IV) catheter
  - Should be placed, as many of the causes of altered mental status require IV fluid or medication
  - Bedside blood glucose levels should be obtained immediately.
    - Hypoglycemia is readily identified and easily corrected with administration of IV dextrose.
  - Additional blood tests to help determine the underlying cause should be performed.
- Naloxone
  - Empiric administration should be considered if the underlying cause is unknown.
  - Naloxone can reverse the depressive cardiorespiratory effects of narcotic ingestion.
  - It may also be helpful in ingestions of:
    - Clonidine
    - Dextromethorphan
    - Valproic acid
    - Captopril

- A fluid bolus with normal saline should be administered if the patient has signs of poor perfusion or hypotension.
- Acid-base and electrolyte abnormalities, if present, should be corrected.

Intracranial pressure

- May be high if:
  - The patient has a history of trauma
  - The suspected cause is structural
  - Infection is present
- Head position
  - Should be elevated to 30 degrees and placed in a midline position
- Hyperventilation
  - Can be a temporizing measure to reduce intracranial pressure
- Every effort should be made to:
  - Stabilize the child as soon as possible
  - Obtain emergent CT
  - Consult with a neurosurgeon
- Obstructive hydrocephalus
  - Results from an intracranial mass lesion or obstructed ventriculoperitoneal shunt
  - May need to be relieved emergently with:
    - Ventriculoperitoneal shunt tap
    - Ventriculostomy

Medical causes

- Fever
  - May indicate an infectious origin
  - Intravenous antibiotics should be given after a blood culture is obtained.
- If meningitis is suspected:
  - Lumbar puncture can be performed to help confirm this diagnosis.
  - It should be performed if the patient is stable and does not have focal neurologic signs.
    - If the child is clinically unstable, lumbar puncture should be deferred.
  - Empiric IV antibiotics should be administered without delay.
- If herpes encephalitis is suspected:
  - Empiric acyclovir should be provided.
- Intussusception
  - Can be reduced by an air-contrast enema

A

When a clear cause cannot be identified

■ Ingestion of a toxic substance should be suspected.

  • Family members should be questioned about the availability of any medication.

    – If possible, the bottle of the medication should be checked and the remaining pills counted to estimate the maximal amount ingested.

  • For some ingestions, antidotes are available.

  • Specialists at the local poison control center can assist in the management of a suspected overdose.

  • Many children will require a dose of activated charcoal.

    – Binds the toxin and limits intestinal absorption

WHEN TO ADMIT

■ Any child with altered mental status

PROGNOSIS

■ Prognosis depends on the cause of the coma, early diagnosis, and early institution of therapy.

PREVENTION

■ Childproofing the house, obtaining appropriate vaccinations, and educating teenagers about risk-taking behaviors can prevent a significant number of cases of coma in young children and adolescents.

Amblyopia

DEFINITION

- Amblyopia
  - Poor vision resulting from blurred retinal image that disrupts normal visual development
- Strabismus
  - Ocular misalignment
    - Esotropia (eye turned in)
    - Exotropia (eye turned out)
    - Vertical (eye turned up or down)
    - Alternating
      - The child cortically turns off or suppresses images from deviated eye to prevent double vision.
      - Associated with alternating suppression and allows equal monocular visual development with no amblyopia

EPIDEMIOLOGY

- Amblyopia
  - Occurs in about 2% of the general population
  - Most common cause of decreased vision in childhood
  - Greatest susceptibility during first 3–4 months of life (critical period of visual development)
  - Can occur in older children
  - Acquired strabismus can cause less severe amblyopia up to 7 or 8 years of age.
- Visual development and amblyopia
  - Critical period: 1 week to 4 months (most susceptible to amblyopia)
  - Visual plasticity: 5 months to 8 years (susceptible to amblyopia)
  - Visually mature: 9 years to adulthood (persons do not develop amblyopia but may retain limited plasticity)

MECHANISM

- Amblyopia
  - Caused by disruption of neurodevelopment in visual areas of brain because of abnormal visual stimulation during the early developmental period
  - Structural damage in visual centers in the brain, including the lateral geniculate nucleus and visual cortex, can occur if abnormal stimulation is severe and persists during early period of visual development.
  - 2 basic forms of abnormal visual stimulation
    - Blurred retinal image (unilateral or bilateral)
    - Strabismus, with strong preference for one eye and constant suppression of deviated eye
  - Other causes of blurred images leading to amblyopia
    - Anisometropic amblyopia: Unilateral refractive error causing blurred image is a common cause of amblyopia.

- Opacity in visual axis
  - Large cataract or corneal opacity
- Severity of amblyopia depends on:
  - When the abnormal stimulus begins
  - Length of exposure to abnormal stimulation
  - Severity of image blur
    - The more severe the image blur, the earlier the onset.
    - The longer the duration of a malapropos stimulus, the more severe the effects on neurodevelopment and visual acuity.

PHYSICAL EXAM

- Inspection
  - Check symmetry: Compare fellow eyes; look at pupils, eyelids, and lid fissures.
  - Check for face turn or head tilt (compensatory mechanisms to reduce strabismus or damp nystagmus).
  - Check for ocular irritation (red eye, squinting).
  - If the timing of the onset of ocular abnormality is in question, seek family photographs for documentation.
- Ocular motility
  - Assess by having the patient follow a target right, left, up, and down, observing for full ocular rotation.
  - Patients with muscle weakness show limited eye movement.
  - Consult with an ophthalmologist if limitation of eye movement is identified.
- Preverbal children
  - Document the infant's ability to fix and follow a moving target.
    - From birth to approximately 2 months of age, ability is sporadic.
  - Test and record pupillary response, even in premature infants.
  - For infants 2–6 months old, test the ability to fix and follow on small toy or human face
    - Cover 1 of the patient's eyes and move a compelling target (eg, the examiner's face or a toy) right, left, up, and down to observe if patient's eyes accurately follow.
    - Test each eye individually (with both eyes open the eyes will track together, even if 1 eye is blind).
    - Observe for central fixation with the presence of accurate smooth pursuit (the child looks directly at the target and follows the target).
    - If the child has trouble locking on the target and appears to be looking off center, poor fixation and poor vision are indicated.

A

- Verbal children
  - By age 2.5–3 years, most children should be able to cooperate with optotype visual acuity testing using picture cards.
    - Allen cards
    - E-game
    - Wright figures
    - Snellen letters
  - Test each eye separately, ensuring that the occluded eye is covered.
  - To prevent the child from peeking, use an adhesive patch rather than a paddle occluder.
  - Examine patients with their customary eyeglasses or contact lenses.
    - If patients forget their corrective lenses, first test vision without correction and then retest using a pinhole (see under Diagnostic Procedures).
  - In children with very poor vision, measure visual acuity by the ability to:
    - Count fingers at a distance of 1–2 feet
    - See hand motions at a distance of 1 foot
    - Perceive any light

DIAGNOSTIC PROCEDURES

- Pinhole test
  - Pinholes are commercially available.
  - The pinhole test can also be done by placing several small pinholes close together in a 3- × 5-inch card.
  - If the patient's visual acuity improves after viewing through the pinhole, refractive error is probably the cause of the decreased vision.
  - The pinhole test can estimate corrected visual acuity when a patient is without customary lenses.
  - Pinholes will improve vision to approximately 20/30, even with large refractive errors.
- Cover test
  - Probably unnecessary for vision screening
    - The Bruckner test (bilateral red reflex test) and corneal light reflex test are more specific for detecting a true strabismus with a demonstrated deviation (ie, tropia).
  - Many healthy children show eye movement shift with alternate cover testing, thus making the test difficult to interpret.
  - Cover 1 eye for 3–4 seconds, then remove the cover.
  - If eye tends to drift, eye under the cover will drift.
  - If the patient has a history of intermittent strabismus (especially intermittent exotropia) but the eyes appear well aligned, the cover test may be helpful.
  - Referral to an ophthalmologist is indicated by history alone.

- Red reflex test
  - Single best vision-screening examination for infants and young children
  - Performed using direct ophthalmoscope to view the reflex off the retina
  - Bruckner test (simultaneous bilateral red reflex)
    - Hold the ophthalmoscope about 2 feet in front of the child.
    - Use the broad beam to illuminate both eyes at the same time.
    - Ask the child to look directly into the ophthalmoscope light, and dim the room lights.
    - Start with ophthalmoscope on low illumination, then slowly increase illumination until the red reflex is seen.
      - The red reflex fills the pupil, and a small white light reflex appears to reflect off the cornea.
      - The light reflex is actually a reflection from just behind the pupil, but it is commonly called the *corneal light reflex* or the *Hirschberg reflex*.
      - The Bruckner test gives both red reflex and corneal light reflex simultaneously.
  - Findings
    - The key sign of a normal red reflex test is symmetry.
    - Opacity in the optical media or large area of retinal disease will result in an abnormal red reflex.
    - Cataract can block red reflex or reflect light to give white reflex.
    - Retinoblastoma has a yellowish-white color and produces yellow reflex.
    - Anisometropia (difference in refractive error) results in unequal red reflex.
    - Strabismus causes brighter red reflex in deviated eye, and corneal light reflex will be off center.
- Corneal light reflex test (Hirschberg test)
  - Best way to assess ocular alignment
  - Hold a muscle light or flashlight at the examiner's nose and point it toward the patient's nose.
  - Have the child look directly at the light (otherwise the light will appear off center).
  - The light reflex should be symmetrically centered or slightly nasally deviated.
  - Displacement of the light reflex indicates strabismus.

SPECIFIC TREATMENT

- Amblyopia
  - Treatment strategy
    - Provide clear retinal image
    - In cases of unilateral amblyopia, force use of the amblyopic eye by occluding the good eye.

- Correct refractive errors with spectacles or contact lenses.
- Visually significant opacities, such as cataracts, must be surgically removed.
- Patients with strabismic amblyopia may or may not require optical correction, but almost all require occlusion therapy to correct ocular dominance.

WHEN TO REFER

- Poor fixation at 5–6 months of age
- Esotropia after 2 months of age
- Abnormal red reflex
- Visual acuity of 20/50 or worse in a 3- to 5-year-old
- >2-line difference between fellow eyes
- Visual acuity ≤20/40 in children ≥6 years
- Lack of full ocular rotation (eye movement in a circle)
- Strabismus, including intermittent strabismus

COMPLICATIONS

- If not treated early, amblyopia can result in permanent vision loss.
- Delay in diagnosis of disease, such as congenital cataracts, retinoblastoma, and congenital glaucoma, may result in irreversible amblyopia; vision loss; and, in the case of retinoblastoma, death.

PROGNOSIS

- The earlier the intervention, the better the prognosis for amblyopia.
- Children with visually significant congenital cataracts are best treated during the first week of life because delaying surgery until after 3–4 months carries a poor visual prognosis.

- Patients with less severe amblyopia, such as anisometropic amblyopia (difference in refractive error), have a better prognosis even when treated between 3 and 8 years of age.
  - After 8–9 years of age, prognosis is poor.
- Patients with amblyopia who are treated late can show significant improvement.
- Patients with presumed congenital cataracts who are identified after the critical period may show some visual improvement with aggressive amblyopia management.
- Suppression disrupts binocular fusion; if not corrected early, strabismus will cause loss of binocular fusion and stereopsis.

PREVENTION

- Vision screening examinations
  - Start at birth.
  - Continue as part of routine checkups.
  - Essential parts of screening: I-ARM
    - **I** = Inspection
    - **A** = Acuity
    - **R** = Red reflex
    - **M** = Motility
  - Infant screening examinations take <1 minute but can detect most eye diseases.

Amenorrhea

DEFINITION

- Amenorrhea is the absence of menses.
  - Primary amenorrhea: failure to start menstruation
  - Secondary amenorrhea: cessation of menses in an adolescent who has previously menstruated
  - Many diseases and clinical states may cause either primary or secondary amenorrhea.

EPIDEMIOLOGY

- The mean age at menarche onset in the US has decreased slightly, per national health surveys.
  - In 1973, the average age at menarche was 12.76 years.
  - Currently, the average age is 12.54 years, with some racial/ethnic variation.
  - 90% of girls will have menstruated by 13.75 years.
  - <10% menstruate before 11 years of age.
  - Menstruation usually begins approximately 2 years after breast budding.
    - The interval between the 2 events can be as short as 6 months or as long as 4 years.
  - After the onset of menarche, many teenagers will menstruate sporadically.
  - Regular monthly cycles often are not established until 1–2 years after menarche.
- Gynecologic age is important when evaluating an adolescent who seems to have secondary amenorrhea.
  - Gynecologic age is the time since onset of menarche.
  - When amenorrhea is defined as missing 3 consecutive menstrual periods in a given year, researchers found its frequency to be:
    - 12.5% of girls with a gynecologic age <1 year
    - 5.4% of girls with a gynecologic age ≥7 years
- Abrupt cessation of menstruation in a teenager who has established regular cycles is of greater concern than the absence of menses for 3–4 months in a teenager who has a gynecologic age of 6 months to 1 year.
- In adolescents, stress-related conditions are the most common cause of secondary amenorrhea, followed by pregnancy.

MECHANISM

- The ovarian cycle
  - The ovarian cycle is controlled by pulsatile gonadotropin-releasing hormone (GnRH) secretion by the hypothalamus acting on the anterior pituitary gland, stimulating the secretion of luteinizing hormone (LH) and follicle-stimulating hormone (FSH).
  - These gonadotropins bind to ovarian cells.
  - During the follicular phase, these gonadotropins stimulate follicular growth.
  - Secretion of estradiol from growing follicles results in a positive feedback loop, leading to increased GnRH secretion and a surge in LH and FSH.
  - This surge leads to ovulation and a surge in progesterone secretion.
  - As the luteal phase is entered, progesterone and estradiol provide a negative feedback effect, resulting in decreased pulsatile secretion of LH.
  - In the absence of human chorionic gonadotropin from the embryo, the progesterone level decreases and the endometrial lining is shed, resulting in menses.
- Causes of amenorrhea
  - Pregnancy
  - Disorders in the hypothalamic-pituitary-ovarian axis
  - Central nervous system (CNS) or ovarian dysfunction
  - A natural sequelae of underlying genetic processes
  - Secondary to anatomic outlet obstruction.

HISTORY

- Given the broad differential diagnosis for amenorrhea, many factors must be assessed.
- Menstrual history
  - Age at onset of menstruation
  - Bleeding frequency, duration, regularity, amount (number of pads/tampons and saturation)
  - Dates of previous menses
  - Concurrent symptoms (bloating, cramping, headaches)
- Menstrual history of mother and first-degree female relatives
- Medical and family history, including:
  - Trauma
  - Endocrine disorders
  - History of meningitis or tumor
  - Irradiation
  - Surgery
  - Weight changes and growth patterns
- Detailed discussions of personal lifestyle factors are ideally conducted without others present.
  - HEADSSS assessment
    - **H**ome
    - **E**ducation
    - **A**ctivities
    - **D**rugs
    - **S**exuality
    - **S**uicide/Depression
    - **S**afety
  - Exercise patterns
  - Body image; subtle development of physical features, such as weight gain, acne, or hirsutism

PHYSICAL EXAM

- Vital signs
  - Evaluate blood pressure.
    - High blood pressure may indicate renal disease or Cushing syndrome.
    - Low blood pressure may indicate Addison disease.
  - Plot previous growth data (especially height, weight, and body mass index).
    - Leveling of linear growth may be consistent with hypothyroidism.
    - Growth failure may be consistent with inflammatory bowel disease.
    - Short stature may be consistent with Turner syndrome.
    - Extremes of body mass index may suggest the diagnosis (eg, anorexia, female athlete triad, Cushing syndrome, Präder-Willi syndrome)
- Physical examination
  - A complete examination is indicated.
  - Examine sexual development.
    - Assess the sexual maturity of breast and genitalia.
    - Atrophied breast tissue may suggest weight loss.
    - Pelvic examination is essential to evaluate female genitalia.
      - An imperforate hymen or a transverse vaginal septum may prevent menstrual blood from escaping.
      - If the hymenal opening is patent, the examination should proceed to determine the presence of a normal vagina, cervix, and uterus.
      - If the hymenal opening is very small, the cervix and uterus can be palpated by means of a bimanual rectoabdominal examination.
      - The size of the clitoris should be noted.
        - Clitoromegaly indicates the presence of excess androgens.
    - Lack of or scant pubic hair in a girl with Tanner stage 3 to 4 breast development suggests androgen insensitivity syndrome.
  - Examine for features of genetic conditions.
    - A webbed neck, short stature, and widely spaced nipples suggest Turner syndrome.
  - Examine for features of endocrine disorders.
    - Hirsutism, receding hairline, excessive acne, moon facies, striae, thyroid abnormalities, buffalo hump
    - Acanthosis nigricans suggests insulin resistance.
    - Nipple discharge may indicate elevated prolactin levels.
  - Examine for neurological abnormalities indicative of potential CNS malformation or tumor.
    - Pupils, extraocular muscles, visual fields, smell, and cranial nerve functions
    - Funduscopy to look for papilledema
    - Reflexes
  - Examine for evidence of self-inflicted injury.
    - Cuts, burns, scars

DIFFERENTIAL DIAGNOSIS

Advice to patients

- Adolescent girls can be reassured that they should anticipate menarche 2–3 years after the initiation of puberty when:
  - Puberty starts late, but progression through puberty appears normal
  - Physical examination is also normal
  - This is especially likely with family history of late menarche in first-degree female relatives.

When to evaluate

- The point at which the clinician elects to pursue an evaluation depends on:
  - Anxiety of the patient and her family
  - Possibility of pregnancy
  - Likelihood that a potentially serious disease is responsible for the amenorrhea
- Evaluation is warranted when:
  - No signs of secondary sexual development are present by 13 years of age
    - Evaluation should include an assessment for delayed puberty.
  - Menarche has not occurred by 16 years of age, even if growth is normal and secondary sexual characteristics have developed
  - 3 consecutive menstrual cycles are absent
  - A patient who has previously menstruated has had amenorrhea for >6 months
  - Development has halted

Differential diagnosis

- The differential diagnosis for amenorrhea is broad and includes:
  - Pregnancy
  - Immature hypothalamic-pituitary-ovarian axis
    - Familial-physiologic delay
  - Suppressed hypothalamic-pituitary-ovarian axis
    - Eating disorders (including anorexia nervosa)
    - Drugs (eg, hormonal contraception, cocaine, phenothiazines)
    - Systemic factors
      - Acute illness (includes viral illness)
      - Chronic illness (includes inflammatory bowel disease, renal failure)
      - Depression

A

- Psychosocial stress
- Environmental change (eg, transitioning to college)
- High-level athletic training (eg, female athlete triad)
  - Endocrine-related cause
    - Thyroid
      - Hyperthyroidism
      - Hypothyroidism
    - Adrenal
      - Addison disease
      - Cushing syndrome
      - Late-onset congenital adrenal hyperplasia (21-hydroxylase deficiency)
      - Tumor
- CNS-related (hypothalamic, pituitary) issues
  - Developmental defects (eg, Kallmann syndrome)
  - Infiltrative disease
  - Head trauma
  - Sheehan syndrome (postpartum hypopituitarism)
  - Primary empty sella syndrome
  - Changes from prior meningitis
  - Irradiation
  - Surgery
  - Tumor (eg, prolactinoma)
- Ovarian malfunction
  - Gonadal dysgenesis
  - Ovarian failure
  - Radiation or chemotherapy
  - Ovarian removal or destruction
  - Polycystic ovary syndrome (PCOS)
  - Tumor
- Genetic conditions
  - Laurence-Moon-Bardet-Biedl syndrome
  - Präder-Willi syndrome
  - Turner syndrome
- Outlet obstruction (primary amenorrhea)
  - Uterus
    - Uterine synechiae
    - Congenital abnormalities (müllerian agenesis, androgen insensitivity)
  - Vagina, cervix, hymen
    - Agenesis
    - Imperforate hymen
    - Transverse septum

LABORATORY EVALUATION

- For primary amenorrhea
  - Consider imaging as indicated before laboratory workup.
  - Consider karyotyping and serum testosterone measurement.
- If a uterus is present, or when considering secondary amenorrhea:
  - Obtain urine pregnancy test, and consider toxicology studies.
  - If negative, obtain FSH, prolactin, and thyroid studies.
- If the FSH level is elevated, consider ovarian failure and consider karyotyping and screening for endocrinopathies.
- If the FSH level is low or normal, consider a physiologic, hypothalamic, or pituitary cause and chronic illness.
- If amenorrhea is in context of androgen excess, consider PCOS and late-onset congenital adrenal hyperplasia.
  - Serum testosterone (total and free)
  - Dehydroepiandrosterone (DHEA) and its sulfate (DHEA-S)
    - If the DHEA-S level is elevated, obtain a first morning 17-hydroxyprogesterone level.
  - Isolated elevated testosterone suggests an ovarian origin, whereas elevated DHEA-S suggests an adrenal origin.
- Assess the patient's estrogen status.
  - Measure serum estradiol levels, **or**
  - Assess by progesterone challenge or by vaginal maturation index (see Diagnostic Procedures)
- In the case of eating disorders, consider a more thorough metabolic and functional evaluation.

IMAGING

- Imaging studies may be considered as clinically indicated.
  - Consider adrenal/ovarian imaging when the patient has:
    - Evidence of virilization (eg, clitoromegaly)
    - Serum androgen levels elevated in the tumor range
  - Consider pelvic ultrasonography if:
    - Pelvic or rectoabdominal examination cannot confirm the presence of uterus
    - Bimanual examination is abnormal
  - Consider magnetic resonance imaging if:
    - Congenital abnormalities are suspected
  - Consider dual-energy x-ray absorptiometry to evaluate bone density:
    - When estrogen levels are low

DIAGNOSTIC PROCEDURES

- Assess the patient's estrogen status:
  - By progesterone challenge
    - A positive result indicates an estrogen-primed uterus.
    - Administer 10 mg of medroxyprogesterone acetate for 5–10 days.
    - Any spotting or bleeding in the week afterward is considered a positive result.
    - Some experts recommend measuring FSH before performing a progesterone challenge.
      - Women with hypergonadotropic amenorrhea will have withdrawal bleeding.
  - By vaginal maturation index
    - A vaginal maturation index is performed by:
      - Collecting cells from the upper lateral sidewall of the vaginal wall using a moistened cotton-tipped applicator
      - Rolling on a glass slide
      - Fixing by using the same technique as for Papanicolaou smear preparation
      - Samples can be interpreted on the basis of estrogen and pubertal status.

TREATMENT APPROACH

- Treatment of amenorrhea depends on the underlying cause.

SPECIFIC TREATMENT

Pharmacologic treatments

- Secondary amenorrhea and normal estrogen levels
  - Medroxyprogesterone, 5–10 mg for 12–14 days
  - Can be used every 1–3 months to stimulate withdrawal bleeding
- Sexually active patients with PCOS
  - Treat with combined contraceptives.
- Patients with PCOS may benefit from additional medications for:
  - Underlying metabolic abnormalities
  - Hirsutism, acne, or other findings associated with androgen excess

Other

- In some patients with low estrogen levels (restrictive eating disorders, female athlete triad):
  - Normalizing weight for height is important.
  - Address disordered eating and intensity of athletic training.

WHEN TO REFER

- If the amenorrhea seems to be secondary to a chronic illness that the pediatrician cannot manage
- If the pediatrician cannot offer or feels uncomfortable performing a thorough gynecologic assessment
- If long-term hormonal therapy is required
- If the patient has an eating disorder
- If evidence exists of anatomic or chromosomal abnormality
- If evidence exists of a complicated endocrine or developmental disorder
- If evidence exists of a CNS, adrenal, or ovarian tumor

WHEN TO ADMIT

- If the patient has metabolic derangements requiring close monitoring

FOLLOW-UP

- Regularly scheduled follow-up visits until menarche occurs are warranted.

Anaphylaxis

DEFINITION

- Severe allergic reaction mediated by IgE and involving ≥2 organ systems
- Anaphylactoid reactions are clinically similar but not attributable to IgE.
  - Clinical syndrome and treatment are the same as for anaphylaxis.
- Anaphylaxis may be uniphasic, biphasic, or protracted.

EPIDEMIOLOGY

- Incidence
  - 0.04% to 0.4%
  - May be higher because of underreporting and underrecognition
- Sex
  - In childhood, more likely in boys than in girls
  - In adults, more likely in women than in men
- 0.5% to 3.0% of the population experiences systemic reaction after *Hymenoptera* stings.
- Biphasic reactions occur in 4–20% of patients.
- Food-induced anaphylaxis
  - More common in children than in adults

ETIOLOGY

- Mediated through antigen-induced, IgE-mediated mast cell and basophil degranulation and histamine release
- May be induced by foods, some medications, insect stings (*Hymenoptera*), exercise

RISK FACTORS

- Atopy is a predisposing factor for food-induced anaphylaxis.
- Risk factors associated with death from anaphylaxis include:
  - Extremes of age
  - Concomitant cardiac disease
  - Asthma
  - Delay of epinephrine administration
  - Use of ß-blockers

SIGNS AND SYMPTOMS

- Respiratory
  - Bronchospasm with wheezing
  - Possibly, stridor or hoarseness
  - Cyanosis
- Upper respiratory findings
  - Nasal congestion
  - Rhinorrhea
  - Sneezing
  - Lingual and pharyngeal edema
- Cardiovascular
  - Tachycardia followed by hypotension
- Skin
  - Urticaria
  - Angioedema or flushing
  - Pruritus
  - May see only cardiovascular and no cutaneous signs or symptoms
- Lightheadedness
- Weakness and palpitations
- Sense of impending doom
- Ocular
  - Tearing
  - Conjunctival erythema
  - Edema (chemosis)
- Gastrointestinal
  - Diarrhea
  - Vomiting
- Headache

DIFFERENTIAL DIAGNOSIS

- Vasodepressor reactions, especially after an emotional stressor
  - Hypotension
  - Pallor
  - Weakness
  - Nausea
  - Bradycardia (only occurs in 5% of patients with anaphylaxis)
  - Loss of consciousness
  - Lack of skin and airway manifestations that are usually seen in anaphylactic reactions
  - Prompt recovery after assuming recumbent position
- Panic attacks
  - Palpitations
  - Flushing
  - Shortness of breath
  - Gastrointestinal symptoms
  - If accompanied by vocal cord dysfunction and stridor, panic attacks may mimic anaphylaxis.
- Systemic mastocytosis
  - Anaphylaxis may occur because mast cell lesions bind IgE and release histamine and other mast cell mediators.
  - Urticaria pigmentosa may suggest this diagnosis.

- If lesions are primarily internal
  - Total serum tryptase
    - Serum concentrations are acutely elevated in patients with anaphylaxis.
    - Concentrations are increased in mastocytosis even when patients are not acutely ill.
  - Urinary histamine metabolites
  - Genetic testing for mastocytosis
  - These tests are not useful for managing acute episodes, which are indistinguishable from anaphylaxis.
- Hypoglycemia
  - Flushing mimicking an early allergic skin reaction
  - Flushing may be associated with:
    - Tachycardia
    - Anxiety
    - Diaphoresis
    - Lightheadedness

DIAGNOSTIC APPROACH

- History and clinical assessment are far more important than laboratory testing in the initial evaluation of anaphylaxis.
- Seek history of recent food ingestion, insect sting, medication intake, and exercise.
- Food ingestion
  - Reaction can occur in first 2 hours after eating, usually within the first 30 minutes.
  - Reactions beginning up to several hours later have been reported.
  - Common allergens
    - Peanuts (62% of cases)
    - Nuts
    - Fish
    - Shellfish
    - Milk, soy, and eggs in infants and toddlers
    - In some, inhalation of offending antigen is sufficient to lead to a reaction.
- Insect sting
  - *Hymenoptera* insect sting (ie, bees, yellow jackets, hornets, wasps, fire ants)
  - History of exposure to particular insects may be important later if immunotherapy is to be considered.
  - Removing the stinger early is important to avoid further venom injection.
  - Identification of the wound or stinger helps identify the species.
    - Bees (and very rarely yellow jackets) leave a stinger; other *Hymenoptera* do not.

- Medication-induced
  - Antibiotics, most commonly penicillin
  - Aspirin and other nonsteroidal antiinflammatory agents
  - Drugs that are administered intravenously or intramuscularly are absorbed more rapidly and are associated with more frequent/severe reactions.
  - Radiocontrast media
  - Latex (becoming less common)
- Exercise-induced anaphylaxis
  - Usually occurs in teenagers and young adults
  - Prodrome of flushing and abdominal pain may occur followed by collapse during exercise.
  - Some cases occur only after ingesting foods that cross-react with pollens (eg, melons that cross-react with ragweed, apples that cross-react with birch)
  - Some have exercised-induced anaphylaxis after nonspecific food ingestion combined with exercise.
    - May follow episodes of exercise-induced urticaria

LABORATORY FINDINGS

- Histamine plasma concentration are not usually a reliable or useful marker.
- Histamine metabolites in the urine may be useful in diagnosis of systemic mastocytosis.
- Specific IgE may be useful to determine the cause.
  - Skin prick tests for specific allergens
  - Serum antigen specific IgE tests
    - Radioallergosorbent assay
    - Enzyme-linked immunosorbent assay
    - At time of presentation, these tests will not be valid because specific IgE may no longer be present.
- Serum tryptase
  - May remain elevated in blood for up to 6 hours after the event
  - Measurable for several days later in serum samples that have been refrigerated
- If cyanosis or respiratory compromise
  - Pulse oximetry
  - Arterial blood gas determinations

TREATMENT APPROACH

- Airway should be secured.
- Obtain respiratory rate, blood pressure, and pulse.
  - Place the patient in supine position with feet elevated if blood pressure is decreased.
  - If wheezing is present, balance the recumbent position with need to allow adequate air exchange.
  - Administer oxygen.

- For *Hymenoptera* sting, to slow systemic absorption of antigen and anaphylactic mediators:
  - Tourniquet applied on an extremity proximal to sting
  - Medication injection

SPECIFIC TREATMENTS

Pharmacologic therapy

- Epinephrine
  - Most important initial treatment
  - Give intramuscularly, preferably in the outer thigh, while assessment is being made.
  - The dose may be repeated as needed every 10–15 minutes.
  - Administered as a 1:10,000 solution intravenous if severe hypotension with peripheral vasoconstriction
- Fluid replacement
  - Needed for hypotension from increased vascular permeability
  - Children require up to 30 mL/kg of crystalloid solution in the first hour.
  - Adults require 1–2 L over the first hour.
- Intravenous vasopressors
  - In severe refractory hypotension, continuous infusions of either:
    - Dopamine
    - Norepinephrine
    - Epinephrine
- Inhaled albuterol
  - May be used for wheezing that is not responsive to parenteral epinephrine
- H_1 antihistamines
  - Relieve symptoms; highly effective for relieving skin manifestations and oropharyngeal angioedema
  - Not effective for treating life-threatening symptoms that do not involve the upper airway
  - Do not replace the need for epinephrine
  - First-generation H_1 antihistamines commonly cause drowsiness and may impair patient's ability to relate progress or resolution of symptoms.
  - Intravenous H_1 antihistamine (eg, diphenhydramine) combined with cimetidine (piggyback infusion) blocks both the cardiac and peripheral vascular effects of histamine.
- Adrenal corticosteroids
  - Decrease vascular permeability
  - Do not prevent biphasic reactions
- Glucagon (1 mg)
  - For patients on a ß-blocker (more frequent in adults than children)
  - For refractory hypotension

- Methylene blue
  - For severe anaphylactic hypotension
- Venom immunotherapy
  - Indicated for treatment of insect sting reactions

WHEN TO ADMIT

- Admit for:
  - Hypotension
  - Airway compromise
- Observation for up to 24 hours is recommended for biphasic reactions.
  - Cannot reliably be prevented with corticosteroids
  - Cannot be predicted

WHEN TO REFER

- Refer to an allergist for:
  - Identification of responsible agent
  - Patient education and management

FOLLOW-UP

- After an anaphylactic episode, discharge patient with epinephrine in an autoinjection device for self-administration.
  - The patient must be able to use the device.
  - The patient must understand that it should be available anywhere he/she goes.
  - The patient must understand that the devices have expiration dates and should be renewed periodically.
- Workup to identify the cause of the reaction
- Provide education on avoidance; this is particularly important for foods, insect stings, and medications.
  - In cases of exercise-induced anaphylaxis, patients should be advised to avoid exercising alone.
- Medic alert bracelet should be advised.

COMPLICATIONS

- Anaphylactic shock

PROGNOSIS

- Patients with biphasic reactions often experience recurrence of initial signs and symptoms several hours after their apparent resolution.
- Foods causing anaphylaxis in childhood are usually responsible for lifelong allergies.
  - Children are not likely to outgrow these reactions.
  - Unlike allergies to peanuts, nuts, fish, and shellfish, most children become tolerant to milk and soy with time, and some will become tolerant to eggs.

Anemia and Pallor

DEFINITION

- Anemia is a laboratory finding reflecting a decrease in red blood cell (RBC) mass below an age-appropriate normative value; this can be either:
  - Reduction in RBC number
  - Reduction in RBC mass (hematocrit)
  - Reduced hemoglobin concentration
- Anemia may be associated with pallor but is more likely to be a silent symptom.
- Pallor and anemia are clinical manifestations of an underlying disease process requiring a thorough evaluation.
- Types of anemia
  - Microcytic anemias: mean corpuscular volume (MCV) less than appropriate for age
  - Normocytic anemias: MCV within normal range for age
  - Macrocytic anemias: MCV greater than appropriate for age
- MCV changes with age; see Laboratory Evaluation for normal values.

EPIDEMIOLOGY

- Age
  - Toddlers (12–24 months) and adolescent girls account for most cases of iron-deficiency anemia.
- Race/ethnicity
  - Black persons are at greatest risk for sickle cell anemia.
  - Thalassemias occur primarily in patients of Mediterranean and Southeast Asian descent.

MECHANISM

- Sideroblastic anemia is inherited and occurs in childhood.
- Iron-deficiency anemia results from:
  - Poor iron intake
  - Poor iron absorption
  - Blood loss
    - Common causes of gastrointestinal bleeding
      - Cow milk protein allergy
      - Gastric and duodenal ulcers
      - Meckel diverticulum
      - Polyps
      - Hemorrhoids
      - Gastritis
- Thalassemias are disorders of hemoglobin production.
  - α-Thalassemia is caused by deficient production of the a chain.
  - ß-Thalassemia is caused by deficient production of the ß chain.

- Causes of microcytic anemia
  - Iron-deficiency anemia
  - Lead poisoning
  - Copper deficiency
  - Malnutrition
  - Chronic disease
  - Thalassemia
  - Hemoglobin E trait
  - Sideroblastic anemia
  - Atransferrinemia
  - Inborn errors of metabolism
- Causes of normocytic anemia
  - Infection
  - Acute blood loss
  - Renal disease
  - Connective tissue disorder
  - Hepatic disease
  - Hemolysis
  - Hypersplenism
  - Cancer
  - Aplastic anemia
  - Dyserythropoietic anemia
  - Drugs
- Causes of macrocytic anemia
  - Megaloblastic anemias from vitamin B_{12} or folate deficiency
  - Reticulocytosis
  - Postsplenectomy
  - Myelodysplastic syndrome
  - Aplastic anemia
  - Fanconi anemia
  - Diamond-Blackfan anemia
  - Persons syndrome
  - Dyskeratosis congenita
  - Paroxysmal nocturnal hemoglobinuria
  - Down syndrome
  - Hypothyroidism
  - Hepatic disease, jaundice
  - Drugs (eg, phenytoin, methotrexate)

HISTORY

- Thorough history may help identify risk as well as cause.
- Diet can identify children most likely to develop iron-deficiency anemia.

A

- Signs of systemic illness (fever, weight loss) with anemia may indicate underlying systemic disease, such as an autoimmune disorder.
- Historical factors important for diagnosis of anemia
  - Age
    - Nutritional anemias are rare in term infants but more common in infants born preterm, school-age children, and adolescents.
    - Significant anemia diagnosed in the first 6 months of life in a term infant is most likely due to a congenital anemia.
  - Sex
    - Glucose-6-phosphate dehydrogenase (G6PD) deficiency and pyruvate kinase deficiency are X-linked disorders.
  - Race/ethnicity
    - Thalassemias are more common in patients of African or Asian descent, whereas thalassemia syndromes are more common in patients of Mediterranean descent.
  - Nutrition
    - Sources of iron, folate, vitamin B_{12}, and vitamin E should be documented.
    - A history of pica suggests iron deficiency.
  - Medications
    - Phenytoin and methotrexate can induce a megaloblastic anemia.
    - Oxidants can induce hemolytic anemias
    - Sulfa drugs can produce a hemolytic anemia in patients with G6PD deficiency.
  - Family history
    - Anemia, jaundice, gallstones, cholecystitis, splenomegaly, splenectomy, or hemolytic crisis may suggest an inherited hemolytic anemia.
  - Infections
    - Infections may induce hemolysis or RBC hypoplasia or aplasia (parvovirus B19).
    - Hepatitis may induce aplastic anemia.
    - Common acute bacterial and viral infections may result in mild anemia from decreased RBC production or increased RBC destruction, or both.
      - These anemias are typically short-lived but commonly identified on routine screening.
  - Gastrointestinal
    - The gastrointestinal tract is a common source of blood loss.
    - Nutritional deficiencies may result from malabsorption syndromes.

PHYSICAL EXAM

- Most mild/moderate anemias are asymptomatic.
- Possible symptoms of anemia
  - Infants and toddlers
    - Fatigue
    - Irritability
    - Pallor
    - Increased sleep
    - Poor feeding
    - Failure to thrive
  - Older children and adolescents
    - Fatigue
    - Pallor
    - Exercise intolerance
    - Dizziness
- Headaches
- Shortness of breath
- Palpitations
- Pallor
  - Rare in mild anemias but common in children with moderate to severe anemia
  - Does not necessarily indicate a low hemoglobin level
  - Frequently only seen reliably with hemoglobin concentrations <8 g/dL
  - May be more easily identified in nail beds, mucosa, conjunctiva, and palmar creases
- Signs of hemolytic anemia
  - Splenomegaly
  - Icterus
- Signs of chronic hemolytic anemia (eg, thalassemia)
  - Frontal bossing
  - Maxillary prominence
- Leukemia or lymphoma may present with anemia with focal lymphadenopathy and hepatosplenomegaly.
- Cardiovascular signs
  - Mild to moderate decrease in RBC mass may result in pulmonary flow murmur.
  - More severe anemias may be associated with signs of congestive heart failure.

DIFFERENTIAL DIAGNOSIS

Utility of subclassification

- Subclassification of anemias as microcytic, normocytic, and macrocytic greatly reduces the differential diagnosis and limits the number of laboratory tests needed for diagnosis.

Anemia in newborns

- Classifying the cause into 1 of 3 broad classifications is helpful.
  - Blood loss
    - Twin-to-twin transfusions
    - Chronic blood loss throughout pregnancy
      - Infant may have pallor and microcytic, hypochromic anemia but appear otherwise well and hemodynamically stable.
    - Infants with acute blood loss
      - May have pallor, tachypnea, tachycardia, hypotension, and decreased tone
      - Normocytic, normochromic anemia with a reticulocytosis will be detectable soon after birth.
  - Hemolysis
    - Different maternal blood types or antigens, maternal drug use, or neonatal infections
    - Microangiopathic hemolysis may occur in infants with thrombi, disseminated intravascular coagulation, and Kasabach-Merritt syndrome (multiple cavernous hemangiomas).
  - Decreased production

Differential diagnosis of specific pathologic RBC features

- Target cells: surface-to-volume ratio is increased.
  - Thalassemia
  - Hemoglobinopathies
  - Hemoglobin C disease
  - Hemoglobin E disease
  - Hyposplenism or postsplenectomy
  - Hepatic disease
  - Severe iron-deficiency anemia
  - Abetaproteinemia
  - Lecithin or cholesterol acyltransferase deficiency
- Spherocytes: hyperdense cells with a decreased surface-to-volume ratio and an increased mean corpuscular hemoglobin concentration
  - Hereditary spherocytosis
  - Hemolytic anemia (autoimmune, ABO incompatibility, water dilution)
  - Microangiopathic hemolytic anemia
  - Hemoglobin SS disease
  - Hypersplenism
  - Burns
  - After RBC transfusions
  - Pyruvate kinase deficiency

- Acanthocytes (spur cells): cells with 10–15 spicules that are typically irregular in length, spacing, and width; cells usually smaller than normal RBCs
  - Disseminated intravascular coagulation
  - Microangiopathic hemolytic anemia
  - Hyposplenism or postsplenectomy
  - Hepatic disease
  - Hypothyroidism
  - Vitamin E deficiency
  - Abetalipoproteinemia
  - Malabsorption
- Echinocytes (burr cells): cells with 10–30 spicules that are typically of similar size and distributed evenly
  - Dehydration
  - Renal disease
  - Hepatic disease
  - Pyruvate kinase deficiency
  - Peptic ulcer disease
  - After RBC transfusion
- Pyknocytes: hyperchromic RBCs with decreased volume and distorted shape
  - Similar to acanthocytes and echinocytes
- Blister cells: contain a clear area in RBCs that contains no hemoglobin
  - Hemoglobin SS disease
  - G6PD deficiency
  - Pulmonary emboli
- Basophilic stippling: retention of RNA, resulting in fine blue inclusions in the cytoplasm
  - Iron-deficiency anemia
  - Lead poisoning
  - Hemolytic anemias
  - Pyrimidine 5'-nucleotidase deficiency
- Elliptocytes: elliptical-shaped cells
  - Hereditary elliptocytosis
  - Iron-deficiency anemia
  - Thalassemia
  - Hemoglobin SS disease
  - Sepsis
  - Megaloblastic anemia
  - Malaria
  - Leukoerythroblastic reaction
- Teardrop cells: microcytic and hypochromic cells that are teardrop-shaped
  - Normal finding in newborns

A

- Thalassemia
- Myeloproliferative diseases
- Leukoerythroblastic reaction
- Schistocytes: RBC fragments that result from trauma
  - Disseminated intravascular coagulation
  - Hemolytic anemia and microangiopathic hemolytic anemia
  - Kasabach-Merritt syndrome
  - Purpura fulminans
  - Hemolytic-uremic syndrome
  - Uremia, glomerulonephritis, acute tubular necrosis
  - Cirrhosis
  - Malignant hypertension
  - Thrombosis
  - Thrombotic thrombocytopenic purpura
  - Amylosis
  - Chronic relapsing schistocytic hemolytic anemia
  - Burns
  - Connective tissue disorders
- Stomatocyte: area of central pallor is more slitlike than round
  - Stomatocytosis (hereditary)
  - Thalassemia
- Nucleated RBCs: normal on peripheral blood smear in the first week of life only
  - Significant bone marrow stimulation
  - Congenital infections
  - Hyposplenism or postsplenectomy
  - Leukoerythroblastic reaction, particularly with severe infections and leukemias or metastatic tumors in the bone marrow
  - Megaloblastic anemia
  - Dyserythropoietic anemia

LABORATORY EVALUATION

- Tests to perform
  - Hemoglobin level and hematocrit
  - RBC morphology (see Differential Diagnosis)
  - MCV
  - Reticulocyte count
    - Elevated count implies bone marrow compensation for chronic blood loss or hemolysis.
    - Low count may suggest impaired RBC production or acute blood loss.
  - Stool guaiac tests for occult blood should be performed at several different times to capture intermittent bleeding.

- The following tests are not necessary in initial diagnosis but help identify cause.
  - Iron studies
  - Erythrocyte sedimentation rate
  - Serum bilirubin
  - Serum lactate dehydrogenase
- Normal values for hemoglobin (g/dL)/hematocrit (%)/MCV (fL), by age
  - Cord blood: 15.3/49/112
  - 1 day: 19.0/61/119
  - 1 week: 17.9/56/119
  - 1 month: 17.3/54/112
  - 2 months: 10.7/33/100
  - 3 months: 11.3/33/88
  - 6 months–2 years: 12.5/37/77
  - 2–4 years: 12.5/38/79
  - 5–7 years: 13/39/81
  - 8–11 years: 13.5/40/83
  - 12–14 years
    - Girls: 13.5/41/85
    - Boys: 14/43/84
  - 15–17 years
    - Girls: 14/41/87
    - Boys: 15/46/86
- Black children on average have normal hemoglobin values that are approximately 0.5 g/dL lower than those in white and Asian children.

IMAGING

- Chest radiograph may be required if pulmonary hemosiderosis needs to be ruled out.

DIAGNOSTIC PROCEDURES

- Bone marrow aspiration and biopsy may be required in patients with anemia suspected of having bone marrow involvement or abnormalities.

TREATMENT APPROACH

- Treatment of compensated anemia is dictated by the cause of the anemia.
- Patients with uncompensated anemia should be admitted to the hospital for observation and possible transfusion.
- Many patients with microcytic anemia or normocytic anemia have early iron-deficiency anemia, and a course of supplemental iron is appropriate.

SPECIFIC TREATMENT

- Specific treatment depends on the underlying hematologic disorder.
- For a child with hypochromic, microcytic anemia found on routine blood cell count with history of poor iron intake or excessive milk intake:
  - Give a trial of supplemental iron (3–6 mg/kg of elemental iron per day, divided into ≥2 doses) rather than drawing additional blood for analysis.
    - Reticulocyte count should increase within 5–7 days.
    - Assuming that the dietary deficiency is corrected, supplemental iron should continue for 2–3 months after the hemoglobin concentration has normalized.
- Thalassemia major requires long-term transfusion therapy.

WHEN TO REFER

- Referral to hematologist
  - Hemoglobin level <8 g/dL or hematocrit <25%
  - Anemia of unknown origin
  - When anemia is associated with disorder in leukocytes or platelets
  - If hemoglobinopathy or RBC membrane defect is suspected or confirmed
  - If no clear vitamin B_{12} or folate deficiency, for assessment of macrocytosis to rule out myelodysplasia or cancer
- Referral to a pediatric oncologist is warranted for management of most macrocytic anemias that are not related to nutritional deficiencies.

WHEN TO ADMIT

- Profound anemia (hemoglobin level <5–6 g/dL or hematocrit <15–20%)
- Uncompensated anemia or anemia associated with a rapidly decreasing hemoglobin level
- Anemia in an ill child
- Tachycardia followed by orthostasis, headache, dizziness, and hypotension

FOLLOW-UP

- Patients receiving a therapeutic trial of iron for suspected iron-deficiency anemia should be followed up at 1 week for repeated measurement of the reticulocyte count or at 1 month for hemoglobin measurement.
  - If there is no change in reticulocyte count or hemoglobin level, consider noncompliance with therapy, a problem with iron assimilation, or another diagnosis for microcytic anemia.

COMPLICATIONS

- If iron deficiency is not diagnosed and treated early, it may adversely affect the cognitive function of brain.

PREVENTION

- All infants are provided with iron-fortified food after 6 months of age.
- All infants are checked for hemoglobin and lead levels between 9 and 12 months of age.
- All children and adolescents, especially menstruating girls, need to be checked for hemoglobin and hematocrit yearly.

Animal Bites

DEFINITION

- Bites occur from dogs (most common), cats (second most common), humans, and wild animals.

EPIDEMIOLOGY

- Incidence
  - An estimated >2 million people across the US are bitten by animals annually.
  - Dog bites account for >90%; cat bites account for most of the remainder.
- Severity
  - 50% are trivial and require no medical treatment.
  - 10% are severe enough to require suturing.
  - 2% result in hospitalization.
- Age
  - Children have the greatest number of animal bites (peak age group, 5–14 years)
    - 50% of all school-age children report being bitten by an animal at some point in their life.
  - Adults are typically bitten on an extremity; children are more likely to be bitten on the head or neck.
- Sex
  - Boys are twice as likely as girls to be bitten by a dog.
  - Girls receive twice as many cat bites.
- Environment
  - Most animals live in the victim's neighborhood (75%) or home (15%).
  - Bites are usually provoked by humans.

ETIOLOGY

- Most bacteria associated with bite wounds are common organisms that reside in the animal's oral cavity or on the victim's skin and involve several pathogens.
- *Pasteurella multocida*, a gram-negative, facultative anaerobe, is found in the mouths of most dogs and cats.
  - Highly associated with cat bite infections (up to 80%) and to a lesser extent with dog bite infections (12–50%)
- Gram-negative aerobes (eg, *Pseudomonas*, *Klebsiella*, and *Enterobacter* spp) are found more often than gram-positive aerobes (eg, staphylococci, streptococci) or anaerobes (eg, *Bacteroides*, *Fusobacterium*, and *Peptococcus* spp).
- Human bites are rarely infected by *P multocida* but are often associated with gram-positive organisms, gram-negative anaerobes, or *Eikenella corrodens*.
  - Human bites can transmit HIV and hepatitis B.

RISK FACTORS

- The following factors increase the risk for infection.
  - Cat and human bites, in part because these bites more often cause puncture wounds
  - Bites to the hand
  - Waiting >24 hours to seek medical attention

SIGNS AND SYMPTOMS

- Important points to elicit while taking history
  - Length of time since injury
  - Type of animal (including domestic or wild)
  - Whether the attack was provoked or unprovoked
  - Animal's present location
  - Immunization status and health
  - Prior wound management
- Animal bites from nondomestic animals require special attention.
  - Evaluate children who may have been exposed to rabies.
  - Know when to treat.
- Human bites can transmit HIV and hepatitis B virus.
  - Test for these in situations of high risk.
- Physical examination entails a thorough musculoskeletal and neurologic examination.
  - Determine whether underlying structures were damaged.
  - Inspect wound for signs of infection.
    - Pay special attention to the hand because superficial signs of infection (redness, swelling, purulent drainage) may be absent.
  - Cellulitis
    - Due to *P multocida*
    - Generally develops rapidly, within hours of the animal bite
    - Systemic signs (fever, lymphangitis) are usually absent.
    - Development over days makes it more likely the result of gram-positive cocci or other pathogenic bacteria.
  - Cat-scratch disease is a common complication of cat bites and (less common) bites by other animals.
    - Begins with a red, painless papule at the site of recent scratch or bite
    - Within weeks: tender, enlarged, regional lymph node, usually associated with fever, malaise, and other systemic symptoms

LABORATORY FINDINGS

- Gram stain of a wound specimen is not useful.
- Cultures of infected wounds:
  - Have no growth in one-third of cases
  - Do not predict the likelihood of subsequent infection
  - May help ensure that the causative bacteria are sensitive to the antibiotic used
- Cat-scratch disease
  - Caused by *Bartonella henselae*
  - Can be diagnosed clinically or confirmed by serologic testing

IMAGING

- Radiologic studies
  - May be necessary for deep puncture wounds to determine whether the periosteum has been penetrated
  - Include the calvaria of small children who experience bites to the head.

TREATMENT APPROACH

- The initial step is meticulous wound care.
  - Gently clean the wound with soap and water.
  - Saline irrigation with a syringe and 19-gauge needle generates pressure on the tissues that facilitates cleansing and reduces risk of infection.
  - Devitalized tissue should be debrided.
  - Puncture wounds should be cleaned, but irrigation is ineffective and may result in further damage.
  - Elevation and immobilization are important for significant extremity injuries.
- The child's immunization status should be assessed and tetanus prophylaxis provided if indicated.
- Primary closure of lacerations is controversial.
  - Wounds that are clearly infected should not be closed.
  - Most noninfected lacerations can be sutured for cosmetic purposes or for hemostasis.
    - After meticulous cleansing and irrigation
    - Hand wounds are the exception, owing to great likelihood of infection and risk of serious complications from deep, closed-space infections.
    - Suturing of the hand is suggested only for large wounds.
- Prophylactic antibiotics in noninfected bite wounds is controversial.
  - They are indicated after a human or animal bite of the hand.
  - No evidence indicates that they are effective for other types of bites.

- Infected bite wounds brought to medical attention after 24 hours should be treated with antibiotics.
- For wild animal bites, consult with the local health department to determine the risk of rabies for particular geographic region.
  - Bats, skunks, foxes, raccoons, and other carnivores are considered rabid until proved otherwise by laboratory tests.
  - In the interim, or if the animal cannot be found, treatment with human rabies IgG (HRIG/RIG) and human diploid cell vaccine (HDCV) is suggested.
  - Rabies prophylaxis is now suggested after exposure to bats in a confined setting, even when no bites are visible.
    - The location of a bat bite is rarely known; HRIG/RIG dose may be given in the thigh.
    - If the bat can be captured and submitted for testing, then rabies prophylaxis can be avoided in 60% of the cases.
- Treatment approach for rabies
  - Wild carnivores
    - Begin HRIG/RIG and HDCV.
    - Submit the animal's head for testing.
  - Healthy domestic dogs and cats
    - Quarantine the animal; treat only if the animal develops symptoms.
  - Stray or sick dogs and cats
    - Submit the animal's head for testing.
    - Delay treatment until test results are known unless the clinical likelihood of rabies is high.
    - If the animal is unavailable, then complete a full series of HRIG/RIG and HDCV.
  - Rodents, rabbits
    - Unlikely to be rabid (except woodchucks)
    - Treat only if the animal acted strangely and cannot be tested.
  - Current recommendations call for most, if not all, of the HRIG/RIG dose (20 IU/kg of body weight) to be infiltrated in and around the site of the bite.

SPECIFIC TREATMENTS

- Choice of antibiotics depends on culture results or, if cultures are not available, on the likely pathogens.
- Amoxicillin/clavulanic acid (Augmentin) is an excellent choice for empirical treatment of bites from all animals.
- Intravenous antibiotics
  - Indicated in patients with:
    - Infected hand bites
    - Moderate to severe infections at other bite sites
    - Those who present with systemic symptoms, such as high fever

A

- For cat bites
  - Penicillin G for *P multocida*, plus antistaphylococcal antibiotic (eg, cefazolin or trimethoprim/sulfamethoxazole [TMP/SMX])
  - Penicillin-allergic children may be treated with azithromycin and an antistaphylococcal antibiotic.
- For dog bites
  - Ampicillin/sulbactam
  - Penicillin-allergic children may be treated with clindamycin and TMP/SMX.
- Cat-scratch disease
  - Generally self-limited and does not benefit from antibiotics
  - Large, tender, fluctuant lymph nodes may require aspiration or incision and drainage.

WHEN TO ADMIT

- Infected wounds requiring intravenous antibiotics
- Extensive facial wounds requiring skilled nursing care

WHEN TO REFER

- Complex wounds that require surgical repair
- Bites to the face or hand that require plastic surgery
- Infected wounds that do not respond to initial treatment
- Children with human bites from an adult
- Cases involving wild animal bites; consult with local health department to determine risk of rabies in a specific animal for a particular geographic region.

FOLLOW-UP

- If the animal that caused the bite is quarantined because its rabies status is unknown, then the animal and the bitten individual need close follow-up.

COMPLICATIONS

- Deep infections of tendons or bones and systemic infections can occur if animal bites go untreated.
- Major morbidity from animal bites results from direct trauma and infection.
- Dog bites can cause lacerations or avulsions if infected.
- Puncture wounds can result in deep-tissue infections.

PREVENTION

- Education about responsible pet care is important.
- Preschool-age children:
  - Should not be left alone with a pet
  - Should be advised never to tease animals, approach strange animals, or play with pets that are eating.
- Families who have children should be advised not to buy wild animals or dogs bred for aggressiveness.
- Vaccinations for pets and routine visits to the veterinarian should be encouraged.
- Families traveling with children should be on the alert for stray animals in foreign countries.
  - If the family is planning to spend an extended period in a country with endemic rabies, then prophylactic rabies vaccination should be strongly considered.

Anorexia Nervosa

DEFINITION

- Purposeful loss of weight beyond a healthy state
  - Intense fear of gaining weight or becoming fat, even though underweight
  - Disturbance in perception of body weight or shape, undue influence of body weight or shape on self-evaluation, or denial of seriousness of the current low body weight
- Restricting type: during current episode, person has not regularly engaged in binge-eating or purging behavior (ie, self-induced vomiting or the misuse of laxatives, diuretics, or enemas)
- Binge-eating or purging type: during the current episode, person has regularly engaged in binge-eating or purging behavior (ie, self-induced vomiting or the misuse of laxatives, diuretics, or enemas)

EPIDEMIOLOGY

- Sex
  - At least 0.5–1% of girls and young women
  - 0.2% of boys and young men
- Age
  - Bimodal peak of onset occurs during the adolescent years at 14.5 and 18 years.
  - Increasingly seen in both prepubertal children and adults

ETIOLOGY

- Several factors develop into an eating disorder.
  - Adolescent girls may be:
    - Culturally primed
    - Biologically at risk
    - Psychologically vulnerable in response to a particular precipitant
      - Insult by family or friends
      - Exposure to someone who has an eating disorder
      - Stressful situation
- Behavior perpetuated by:
  - Initial positive psychological feedback for improved appearance
  - Biochemical changes in response to decreased nutrition

RISK FACTORS

- Serotonergic system genetic defects relate to susceptibility.
- Low self-esteem
- Perfectionism
- Obsessiveness
- Family factors
  - History of eating disorders
  - Family dieting
  - Focus on weight in the family

- Very preterm small-for-gestational-age at infancy
- Psychiatric illnesses
  - Depression
  - Anxiety
  - Obsessive-compulsive disorder

SIGNS AND SYMPTOMS

- Concern about weight loss, vomiting, or abnormal eating attitudes noticed by family, friends, or school authorities
- Common for patients to be brought in against their will, although some may seek help willingly
- Distortion in body image
- History of binging or purging
- Overexercising
- Psychosocial changes
  - Fighting with the family
  - Withdrawing from friends
  - Performing less optimally in school
  - Improved school performance due to withdrawal from friends and family
- Symptoms of malnutrition
  - Alopecia
  - Cold hands and feet
  - Dry skin
  - Constipation
  - Fatigue
  - Absence of ≥3 consecutive menstrual cycles
  - Scaphoid abdomen
  - Muscle wasting
  - Acrocyanosis
  - Decreased subcutaneous fat
  - Lanugo hair similar to that seen in newborns
  - Ecchymoses
  - Diminished reflexes
- Weight percentage below ideal body weight (IBW)
  - Calculated by comparing current weight with the average weight expected for height, age, and sex (as determined by standard pediatric growth charts)
  - Serves as both diagnostic criterion and as gross estimate of the degree of malnutrition
    - Weight <25% below IBW: severe malnutrition
    - Weight 20% below IBW: moderate malnutrition
    - Weight not yet 20% below IBW: mild malnutrition
  - Body mass index is being used increasingly to describe nutritional status.

A

- Vital signs that show malnutrition
  - Decline in blood pressure
  - Decreased pulse
  - Cardiovascular changes
    - Decline in electrocardiogram (ECG) voltage
    - Sinus bradycardia
    - Prolonged QTc
    - Orthostatic hypotension
    - Increased vagal tone
    - Poor myocardial contractility
    - Mitral valve prolapse
    - Pericardial effusion
    - Decreased left ventricular mass

DIFFERENTIAL DIAGNOSIS

- Differential diagnosis of eating disorders includes possible causes ofweight loss or vomiting and other psychiatric causes of poor appetite.
- Medical causes
  - Cancer
  - Central nervous system tumors
  - Gastrointestinal problems
    - Malabsorption
    - Celiac disease
    - Inflammatory bowel disease
  - Endocrinologic problems
    - Diabetes mellitus
    - Hyperthyroidism
    - Hypopituitarism
  - Chronic illnesses/infections
  - Superior mesenteric artery syndrome
- Psychiatric causes
  - Depression
  - Obsessive-compulsive disorder
  - Psychosis (especially schizophrenia)
  - Patients may have concomitant depression or psychosis with anorexia; separate criteria must be used to establish each entity.
  - Sleep disorders
  - Hallucinations, delusions, or obsessions

DIAGNOSTIC APPROACH

- Distortion of body image, a hallmark of anorexia nervosa
  - Evaluate by exploring the patient's views of initial, current, and desired weight.
- Establish patient's eating and exercise patterns.

- A full psychosocial history must be obtained as part of initial evaluation to establish the diagnosis and the psychosocial severity of the disorder.
  - The patient's functioning in the family, in school, and among peers must be evaluated.
- Assess use of vomiting or medications designed to promote weight loss.
  - Diet pills
  - Laxatives
  - Diuretics
  - Ipecac
- Avoid being misled by the patient who is not completely forthright; results of physical examination and laboratory tests often suggest the true extent of the disorder.
- Initial evaluation of weight loss includes:
  - Determination of the diagnosis and its severity
  - Evaluation of other possible causes of weight loss and the effects of malnutrition
  - Analysis of the psychological context of the illness
  - Decision about treatment
- For girls, a full menstrual history should be obtained.
  - Age at menarche
  - Last normal menstrual period
  - Usual length of menses
  - Heaviness of flow
  - Presence of dysmenorrhea
  - Regularity of menses

LABORATORY FINDINGS

- Initially, laboratory results may be normal.
- Workup should include:
  - Complete blood count
    - Leukopenia
    - Occasionally thrombocytopenia
    - Rarely, severe anemia (being protected for some time from iron-deficiency anemia by the concomitant amenorrhea)
  - Serum electrolytes
    - Evidence of dehydration
      - Elevated sodium level
      - Elevated blood urea nitrogen level
    - Excessive drinking
      - Signs of hyponatremia
      - Dilute urine
    - Hypokalemia, often severe

- Nutrient values that may be altered
  - Zinc
  - Calcium
  - Magnesium
  - Copper
  - Vitamin B$_{12}$
  - Folate
- Hormone testing
  - Relative hypothyroidism caused by combination of euthyroid sick syndrome and decreased production on a hypothalamic basis can be an adaptive response to inadequate nutrition.
    - Low-normal levels of triiodothyronine, thyroxine, thyroid-stimulating hormone, or any combination
  - In patients with amenorrhea, low levels of:
    - Luteinizing hormone
    - Follicle-stimulating hormone
    - Estradiol
    - Prolactin
  - Hypercortisolemia with loss of diurnal variation
  - Low levels of insulin-like growth factor 1
- Liver and thyroid function tests
- Urinalysis for specific gravity and ketonuria is often helpful.
- ECG for persons with bradycardia

IMAGING

- Magnetic resonance imaging (MRI) of the brain, gastrointestinal series, or other tests may be considered in some cases for patients who claim to be eating well or not vomiting on purpose.
- Abnormalities may be found on computed tomography and MRI of the brain.
  - These are generally reserved for evaluating other possible causes when diagnosis is in question.
  - MRI changes including gray matter deficits and elevated cerebrospinal fluid volumes; these may not be reversible.
- Gastric emptying studies may show:
  - Delayed gastric emptying
  - Decreased gastrointestinal motility
- Bone densitometry, using dual-energy x-ray absorptiometry
  - Bone density values are correlated with body mass index, age at onset, and duration of illness.
  - Common test in evaluation of patients with eating disorders/amenorrhea of 6–12 months' duration

DIAGNOSTIC PROCEDURES

- To document orthostatic changes:
  - Patient's blood pressure and pulse should be checked in the sitting position, followed by standing for 2 minutes.
  - Significant findings, either:
    - Increase of 20 beats/min in pulse
    - Decrease of 20 mm Hg in systolic blood pressure
    - Decrease of 10 mm Hg in diastolic blood pressure

TREATMENT APPROACH

- Medical and nutritional rehabilitation are crucial.
  - Restoration of body weight to within 10% of IBW, with restoration of menses, are primary goals.
  - If malnutrition is mild to moderate (15–25% below IBW), restoration may be accomplished on outpatient basis.
  - If malnutrition is moderate to severe (>25% below IBW), treatment usually requires hospitalization.
- Medical treatment includes management of:
  - Electrolyte abnormalities
  - Cardiovascular issues
  - Endocrine disorders
  - Other organ system dysfunction
  - These are managed simultaneously with or aided by nutritional rehabilitation.
- Nutritional therapy
  - Daily intake of 3 substantial meals and 3–4 snacks is usually sufficient to bring about required weight gain.
  - At inpatient units, meals are generally provided as part of a strict regimen, and snacks generally consist of high-calorie supplements.
  - Too-rapid weight gain is associated with severe metabolic abnormalities in some patients (refeeding syndrome).
  - Slow refeeding and phosphorus supplementation are required in patients with severe malnutrition to prevent this syndrome (which can involve cardiac failure, hemolysis, coma, and death).
- Behavioral therapy is normally a necessary component of treatment.
  - The goal is to offer external positive and negative reinforcements to replace specific internal sensors that usually control appetite and weight gain but are missing.
  - Not intended to be definitive but to stabilize weight and diet in a more medically healthy patient
  - Inpatient treatment
    - Strict plans on some psychiatric units involve removal of privileges (using the phone, television, and regular clothing) if weight goal is not achieved each day.

– Less strict plan used on some adolescent medicine units

  ▪ Includes phases of treatment, moving from 1 phase to another based on achievement of progressively higher weight goals

  ▪ Each phase incorporates additional daily privileges (eg, mobility on the unit, exercise, meals, snacks, passes), so that improved weight and eating patterns lead to additional privileges/responsibilities.

  ▪ If the patient does not respond to such a phased system, an all-liquid diet, provided by mouth or, more rarely, nasogastric tube, may be substituted.

- Outpatient treatment

  – Use of monetary or similar rewards may not be strong enough to overcome the fear of eating.

  – Fear of hospitalization itself may be the sole motivation.

▪ A team approach is needed to treat disease; this may consist of:

- Primary care physician
- Psychiatrist
- Psychologist or social worker
- Nutritionist
- The exact combination is determined by local expertise, availability, and preference.
- Team meetings or discussions are held frequently to prevent miscommunication that can sabotage treatment.

▪ The team may use multimodal therapy, including:

- Medical management
- Nutritional rehabilitation
- Behavior therapy
- Individual psychotherapy
- Family and group therapy
- Psychopharmacology
- Such multimodal therapy holds the best promise for successful treatment.
- Degree to which each of these approaches is incorporated varies with both:

  – The preferences of the treatment team

  – The requirements of the individual patient

- Each of these approaches may be used for inpatients, day-program patients, and outpatients.

SPECIFIC TREATMENTS

Pharmacologic therapy

▪ Selective serotonin reuptake inhibitor (SSRI) antidepressants

- Helps with concurrent psychiatric disorder
- Helps treat obsessive-compulsive symptoms

- Only physicians familiar with psychopharmacologic agents should prescribe these as part of the treatment, given the potential for SSRIs to increase risk of suicide in a minority of children and adolescents.

- Not effective in promoting weight gain or treating symptoms of depression or obsessive-compulsive disorder when body weight is low

▪ Atypical antipsychotic agents at low doses can improve weight gain and treat symptoms of depression and obsessional thoughts.

▪ Menses restoration

- Generally requires an estradiol level >30 mg/dL
- Estrogen replacement has not been shown to reverse or prevent bone loss.

Dietary plan

▪ In outpatients

- May be developed on the basis of the patient's and the family's prior eating habits or on a specific dietary plan offered by the physician or a nutritionist

- Should be specific so that ambiguities that can lead to family fighting are avoided

- Should provide 2000–3000 calories a day

  – Some may be supplied as high-calorie supplements.

- Should be balanced and include foods from each of the major food groups

- Weight gain should be 1–2 pounds per week (inpatient gains may be 2–4 pounds per week).

- Compliance with the dietary regimen may be evaluated by having the patient keep a diet diary; however, many patients do not keep these records accurately and honestly.

Individual psychotherapy

▪ An essential part of treatment

▪ Exploration of underlying psychological features and determination of possible mechanisms for change are appropriate for most patients.

▪ Because anorexia often serves as a defense against other difficult aspects of life, psychological change is acknowledged as the necessary precursor to significant improvement.

▪ No single type of therapy is better than others.

▪ Associated with improved weight gain and psychosocial function

Family therapy

▪ Important, especially for younger patients

▪ Family sessions, arranged in varying combinations to include parents and siblings, generally focus on disordered communication patterns that often accompany the disorder.

▪ Resolving specific conflicts arising from the eating disorder itself becomes important.

- Course of the disorder is more difficult for adolescents whose families are unable or unwilling to make necessary changes in their customary patterns of communication and parenting.
- Outpatient treatment in which families provide and supervise all meals is increasingly used for younger patients with anorexia nervosa, with positive results.

Group therapy

- For mild anorexia, may be only approach used
- Groups may focus on psychotherapeutic approach or more specifically on behavioral changes.
- The risk of patients learning bad habits from one another is outweighed by benefit derived; this is especially true for patients who have had social difficulties during adolescence.

WHEN TO ADMIT

- Any ≥1 of the following should prompt admission.
  - Severe malnutrition (weight <75% IBW)
  - Dehydration
  - Electrolyte disturbances
  - Cardiac disturbances
  - Physiologic instability
    - Bradycardia
    - Hypotension
    - Hypothermia
    - Orthostatic changes
  - Arrested growth and development
  - Failure of outpatient treatment
  - Acute food refusal
  - Acute medical complication of malnutrition
    - Syncope
    - Seizures
    - Cardiac failure
    - Pancreatitis
  - Acute psychiatric emergencies
    - Suicidal ideation
    - Acute psychosis
  - Comorbid diagnosis that interferes with the treatment of the eating disorder
    - Severe depression
    - Obsessive-compulsive disorder
    - Severe family dysfunction

WHEN TO REFER

- A team approach is most often used.
- Refer to a dietician if the primary care physician or staff does not have the expertise or time to set a nutritional plan with the patient.
- Refer to a psychotherapist if:
  - The patient is open to therapy.
  - The patient cannot attain goals set by the physician, even if the patient is resistant.
- Refer for psychopharmacologic evaluation if:
  - Both the physician and the therapist believe the patient might benefit from medication
  - Patient is binging and open to medication
  - Obsessive-compulsive symptoms are interfering with treatment
- Refer to adolescent medicine if:
  - The physician is not comfortable treating the patient.
  - The physician cannot provide sufficient time for patient needs.
  - The patient does not adhere to the physician's treatment plan.

COMPLICATIONS

- Acrocyanosis
- Dry skin
- Lanugo
- Ecchymosis
- Fatigue
- Muscle wasting
- Decreased subcutaneous fat
- Decreased deep-tendon reflexes
- Constipation
- Delayed gastric emptying
- Delayed gastric motility
- Orthostatic hypotension
- Bradycardia
- Mitral valve prolapse
- Pericardial effusion
- Electrocardiographic abnormalities
- Decreased left ventricular mass and contractility
- Psychomotor retardation
- Growth delay
- Pubertal delay
- Amenorrhea
- Osteopenia, osteoporosis
  - 3-fold increase in the long-term risk of fracture development

A

PROGNOSIS

- Adolescents with severe anorexia nervosa have a protracted disease course; recovery estimates 10–15 years later vary from 76% to 24%.
- Estimated 50% of patients do well in the long term.
- 30% show varying degrees of improvement.
- 20% do poorly despite adequate treatment.
- Patients who are younger or have milder disease fare better.
- Predictors of poorer outcome
  - Older age
  - Vomiting
  - Premorbid personality problems
  - Any particular patient with these may do well with treatment.
- Mortality is higher than in any other psychiatric illness, up to 5% per decade after the onset of the eating disorder.

PREVENTION

- Best preventive strategies are not clear.
- Early case detection is most effective.
  - The earlier an eating disorder is treated, the easier the treatment will be and the less entrenched the disease becomes.
  - Families, friends, school personnel, and health professionals must be vigilant for signs and symptoms of an eating disorder so that early treatment can be initiated.

- Programs are geared toward teenage boys and girls, primarily in school settings.
  - Aimed at maintaining a healthy body image and healthy eating
  - Work to promote self-esteem without relation to weight
  - Seem to succeed in terms of increasing awareness and knowledge about eating disorders
  - Effectiveness is debatable.
- Programs focused on building self-esteem are being explored.
- Classroom interventions
  - Staff training throughout the school
  - Informal discussions between staff and students
  - Integration of material about eating issues into the curriculum
  - More intensive work with persons at high risk
  - Changes within the school with respect to cafeteria food and physical education
  - Referrals and outreach (both within the school and the community)

Anuria and Oliguria

DEFINITION

- Oliguria is decreased urine output.
  - Infants: <0.5 mL/kg per hour for 24 hours
  - Older children: <500 mL/1.73 m² body surface area per day
- Anuria is absence of any urine output.
  - Normal, healthy newborns may have no urine output for 24 hours after birth.
- Oliguria is much more common than anuria but can lead to anuria, resulting in serious renal damage that requires specialized care.

EPIDEMIOLOGY

- Incidence of oliguria or anuria is unknown in previously healthy children.
- In hospitalized patients
  - Oliguric acute renal failure (ARF) occurs in:
    - 10% of newborns in the intensive care unit
    - 2–3% of older children requiring intensive care
    - 8% of patients undergoing cardiac surgery
- Prevalence of ARF in newborns
  - Prerenal: 85%
  - Renal: 11%
  - Postrenal: 3%
- Prevalence of ARF in older children
  - Prerenal: 66%
  - Renal: 33%
  - Postrenal: <1%

ETIOLOGY

Causes of oliguria, anuria, and ARF

- Common causes of oliguria, anuria, or ARF are best defined in relation to the patient's age.
- Prerenal ARF caused by dehydration is the most common cause of oliguria/anuria (70% of community-acquired cases of ARF and up to 60% of hospital-acquired cases).
- Renal ARF caused by intrinsic renal damage can be categorized into 3 types.
  - *Acute tubular necrosis* (ATN) results from prolonged ischemia or drug- or toxin-mediated renal tubular injury (reversible).
  - *Glomerular lesions* may occur with postinfectious glomerulonephritis.
  - *Vascular lesions* may occur with hemolytic-uremic syndrome or Henoch-Schönlein purpura.

- Postrenal ARF
  - Mechanical or functional obstruction to urine flow
    - May be in lower urinary tract, eg, posterior urethral valves
    - May be bilaterally in the upper tract, eg, bilateral uretero-pelvic junction obstruction (rare)
  - Unilateral obstruction can cause ARF in patients with only 1 functioning kidney.
  - More common in newborns than in older infants

Most common causes of oliguria and anuria in neonates and children

- Neonates
  - Prerenal
    - Perinatal asphyxia
    - Respiratory distress syndrome
    - Hemorrhage
    - Sepsis or shock
    - Congenital heart disease
    - Dehydration
    - Drugs (indomethacin, maternal use of ACE inhibitors or nonsteroidal antiinflammatory drugs)
  - Renal
    - Acute tubular necrosis
    - Exogenous toxins (aminoglycosides, amphotericin B)
    - Endogenous toxins (hemoglobin, myoglobin, uric acid)
    - Congenital kidney diseases
    - Vascular (renal vein thrombosis, renal artery thrombosis)
  - Postrenal
    - Posterior urethral valves
    - Meatal stenosis
    - Bilateral ureteral obstruction
    - Neurogenic bladder
- Children
  - Prerenal
    - Dehydration
    - Hemorrhage
    - Burns
    - Third-space loss (surgery, trauma, nephrotic syndrome)
    - Renal loss (diabetes mellitus, diabetes insipidus, diuretics)
    - Shock
    - Decreased cardiac output
  - Renal
    - Acute tubular necrosis
    - Glomerulonephritis

A

– Exogenous toxins (aminoglycosides, amphotericin B)

– Endogenous toxins (hemoglobin, myoglobin, uric acid)

– Vascular (hemolytic-uremic syndrome, vasculitis)

• Postrenal

– Posterior urethral valves

– Meatal stenosis

– Bilateral ureteral obstruction

– Neurogenic bladder

RISK FACTORS

■ Common underlying comorbid conditions

• Neurologic conditions

– Compromised thirst mechanism

– Serious disability and total dependence on others for nutrition and hydration, eg, patients with severe cerebral palsy

• Renal diseases that impair ability to concentrate the urine, eg, salt-losing nephropathy or chronic renal failure

• Gastrointestinal conditions that cause hypoalbuminemia and decreased intravascular volume, eg, celiac disease or hepatic failure

• Endocrine disease, such as:

– Diabetes insipidus, associated with increased hypotonic urine output

– Diabetes mellitus, associated with osmolar diuresis

• Hematologic conditions that impair urine concentration mechanism

■ Oncologic emergencies, eg, tumor lysis syndrome (causes renal failure, particularly if patient is not well hydrated)

■ Therapy that may predispose to renal failure because they impair renal autoregulation in the presence of mild renal insufficiency or dehydration

• Nonsteroidal antiinflammatory drugs

• Angiotensin-converting enzyme inhibitors

• Aminoglycosides

• Radiologic contrast media

SIGNS AND SYMPTOMS

■ Clinicians need to search for specific signs of underlying renal disease.

• Severe anemia due to hemolytic-uremic syndrome

• Butterfly rash on face/musculoskeletal involvement in systemic lupus erythematosus

• Purpuric rash over buttocks and extensor surface of lower extremity in Henoch-Schönlein purpura.

• Palpable kidney may be due to:

– Renal vein thrombosis

– Polycystic kidney disease

– Multicystic dysplastic kidney

– Hydronephrosis

■ Palpable bladder with weak urine stream or dribbling suggests obstruction.

■ Sacral tuft of hair or myelomeningocele may be seen with neurogenic bladder (can cause obstructive uropathy/postrenal oliguria or anuria).

■ Symptoms of prerenal cause

• Vomiting

• Diarrhea

• Hemorrhage

• Sepsis

• Decreased oral intake

• Increased thirst

• Palpitations

• Fatigue

• Clinical signs of dehydration

• Weight loss

■ Symptoms of hypovolemia (ie, prerenal pathology)

• Tachycardia

• Dry mucous membranes

• Sunken eyes

• Orthostatic blood pressure changes

• Decreased skin turgor

• Hypotension

■ Symptoms of intrinsic renal disease

• Gross hematuria

– Pharyngitis or impetigo a few weeks before the onset of gross hematuria

• Hypertension

• Edema

• Bloody diarrhea

– Often precedes hemolytic-uremic syndrome

• Younger children, particularly infants: signs of congestive heart failure

– Hepatomegaly

– Gallop rhythm

– Pulmonary edema

■ Symptoms of systemic vasculitis (eg, systemic lupus erythematosus)

• May see history of fever, joint pains, and skin rash

■ Recurrent sinusitis or lower respiratory tract infections may suggest Wegener granulomatosis.

■ Hemoptysis may indicate pulmonary-renal syndrome, due to either:

• Goodpasture syndrome

• Microscopic polyangiitis

DIAGNOSTIC APPROACH

- Thorough history and physical examination are important in identifying the cause of oliguria or anuria.
  - Comprehensive physical examination is key to assessing severity of the disease process and possible cause.
  - In prerenal and postrenal ARF, early diagnosis and prompt treatment often result in quick recovery.
- Detailed history of recent or ongoing long-term medication use is important for excluding possible interstitial nephritis.
- In neonates, history of umbilical artery catheterization implies renal artery thrombosis.
- Family history is helpful in diagnosing such conditions as diabetes insipidus and polycystic kidney disease.

LABORATORY FINDINGS

- Risk factors, history, and results of physical examination will help in the selection of appropriate laboratory tests.
- Urinalysis is the most important noninvasive diagnostic test.
  - Thorough examination of a freshly voided or bladder-catheterized urine sample helps distinguish prerenal from renal causes.
    - Normal or near-normal urinalysis, with few cells, few or no casts, or little or no proteinuria, is seen in prerenal disease, obstruction, and some cases of acute tubular necrosis.
    - A sample showing muddy-brown granular casts and epithelial cell casts strongly suggests acute tubular necrosis.
    - Erythrocyte casts are diagnostic of glomerulonephritis.
    - Proteinuria indicates glomerular disease.
- Urinary indices important for diagnosis of oliguria
  - Urinary sodium
    - <10 mEq/L in oliguria resulting from intravascular volume depletion
    - Neonates: prerenal disease is associated with urine sodium concentration <20–30 mEq/L.
  - Specific gravity
    - >1020 in prerenal oliguria
  - Creatinine
    - Urine/plasma creatinine ratio >40 in prerenal oliguria
    - Urine/plasma creatinine ratio <20 if renal cause
  - Osmolality
    - Urine/plasma osmolality >1.5 in prerenal oliguria
    - Urine/plasma osmolality <1.5 if renal cause
- Fractional excretion of sodium
  - <1% suggests reabsorption of almost all filtered sodium in response to decreased renal perfusion (prerenal).
  - In acute tubular necrosis: >2%

- Blood urea nitrogen (BUN) and serum creatinine
  - In prerenal oliguria, increased BUN level is marked and the BUN/serum creatinine ratio is >20.
  - BUN/creatinine ration of 10–15 suggests intrinsic renal damage.

IMAGING

- Renal ultrasonography
  - Generally not indicated in children with prerenal failure from dehydration who respond promptly to fluid resuscitation
  - Provides important information regarding
    - Kidney size and echogenicity
    - Renal blood flow
    - Collecting system
    - Urinary bladder
  - Children with intrinsic causes
    - Echogenic and slightly enlarged kidneys
  - Bilateral hydronephrosis or hydroureteronephrosis and bladder wall thickening indicate obstruction of bladder outlet causing postrenal oliguria/anuria.
  - Ultrasonography can detect congenital disorders, such as polycystic kidney disease and multicystic dysplastic kidney.
- Doppler examination of renal blood flow is helpful in diagnosing renal vascular thrombosis.

CLASSIFICATION

- Prerenal: dehydration is the most common cause of oliguria/anuria in children.
- Renal: intrinsic renal disorders, such as acute tubular necrosis and glomerulonephropathies
- Postrenal: obstruction to urinary flow in posterior urethral valves in boys

TREATMENT APPROACH

- Major goal of treatment of prerenal oliguria/anuria is to restore intravascular volume.
- Oliguria/anuria due to intrinsic renal conditions needs to be managed by a pediatric nephrologist.
- Urology needs to be consulted in patients with postrenal obstructive lesions.

SPECIFIC TREATMENTS

- A dehydrated child with oliguria/anuria should receive a fluid bolus of normal saline or lactated Ringer's solution at 20 mL/kg to restore fluid volume.
  - Depending on response, another bolus may be needed.
- Estimation of volume status is needed to begin and continue fluid therapy.

A

- Amount is assessed by history and physical exam that includes assessment of:
  - Body weight
  - Anterior fontanelle in infants
  - Heart rate
  - Mucous membranes
  - Skin turgor
  - Capillary refill
  - Peripheral edema
  - Blood pressure
- Children with oliguria and volume overload may:
  - Benefit from furosemide
  - Require fluid restriction
  - Need blood pressure and acid-base monitoring
- Children with oliguria due to obstruction may require urinary catheterization.
  - Relief of obstruction may be followed by postobstructive diuresis and may need fluid/electrolyte replacement.

WHEN TO ADMIT
- See When to Refer.

WHEN TO REFER
- Refer to a nephrologist or admit (or both) if child has any of the following:
  - Persistent oliguria or anuria despite adequate fluid challenge in a dehydrated child

- Persistent oliguria or anuria that continues after removal of the offending nephrotoxins
- Oliguria or anuria associated with:
  - Swelling
  - Hypertension
  - Gross hematuria
  - Abnormal blood chemistry
  - Severe systemic signs or symptoms
- Urology referral for oliguria or anuria caused by obstructive uropathy

PREVENTION
- The key to preventing oliguria or anuria is adequate hydration in at-risk patients.
  - Patients who have just undergone surgery
  - Patients receiving nephrotoxic medications
    - Amphotericin B
    - Acyclovir
    - Radiocontrast agent
  - Patients at risk of tumor lysis syndrome
  - Patients at risk of pigment nephropathy caused by hemoglobinuria or myoglobinuria

Apparent Life-Threatening Event

DEFINITION

- An apparent life-threatening event (ALTE) is:
  - Frightening to the observer, who may fear the infant has died
  - Characterized by some combination of:
    - Apnea
    - Color change
    - Marked change in muscle tone
    - Choking
    - Gagging
- ALTE replaced the terms:
  - *Aborted crib death*
  - *Near-miss sudden infant death syndrome (SIDS)*
  - Change corrects erroneous implication of an association between ALTE and SIDS.
- Pathologic apnea
  - Respiratory pause
    - Prolonged, lasting ≥20 seconds **or**
    - Associated with cyanosis, pallor, hypotonia, or bradycardia
  - Central apnea
    - No respiratory effort for 20 seconds, or shorter if associated with hypoxemia or bradycardia
  - Obstructive apnea
    - Respiratory effort in thoracic or abdominal impedance tracings, or both
    - No airflow in nasal and end-tidal carbon dioxide tracings
  - Mixed apnea
    - Central and obstructive events at the same time
- Periodic breathing (common in young infants)
  - Breathing pattern:
    - ≥3 respiratory pauses >3 seconds
    - <20 seconds of respiration between pauses

EPIDEMIOLOGY

- Frequency and prevalence are unknown.
  - Estimates:
    - 0.21% of all children and 0.6% of all patients <1 year seeking care at an emergency department
    - 9.4 per 1000 live births
- Age
  - Median age at presentation of infants with an ALTE ranges between 7 and 8 weeks of age.
- Sex
  - Relatively equal distribution

ETIOLOGY

- A variety of different disorders can lead to an ALTE.
- Up to 50% of cases of ALTE remain unexplained and are considered idiopathic.

RISK FACTORS

- Premature birth
  - Approximately one-third of patients with an ALTE
- Previous ALTE
  - 19% of patients

SIGNS AND SYMPTOMS

History

- Detailed history and description of the infant at the time of the ALTE are particularly important.
  - Most infants appear normal by the time of evaluation.
- Perinatal history
  - Full-term or premature birth
  - Pregnancy or perinatal complications
- Medical and surgical history
  - Previous evaluations and treatments
  - Prior hospitalizations
  - Medications
- Sleep and feeding habits
  - Breastfeeding versus bottle feeding
  - Usual amount and frequency of feedings
  - Usual behavior and temperament
- Family history
  - Siblings with ALTE, SIDS, or early death
  - Family history of genetic, metabolic, cardiac, or neurologic problems
- Parental or caretaker history
  - Smoking or drinking habits
  - Recent medical problems and treatments
- Usual sleep conditions
  - Sleep position when placed down for sleep and when found
  - Sleeping attire
  - Bedding materials
- Other conditions
  - Clothing
  - Room temperature
  - Use of pacifiers

Circumstances and characteristics of the ALTE

- Preceding events
  - Recent fever or illness
  - Medications for the infant and others in the home

- Immunizations
- Sleep deprivation
- Change in daily life routine
■ Place and time
  - Exact place in which the ALTE occurred, eg:
    – Child's bed
    – Parent's bed
    – Parent's arms
    – Bathroom
    – Sofa
    – Car
  - Time of event
  - Time since last feeding
  - Estimated time to recover from the ALTE
  - Estimated duration of event
■ Witnesses and interventions
  - Who discovered or witnessed the ALTE
  - Reason that led to the discovery of the ALTE (noise, unusual cry)
  - Any interventions performed, eg:
    – Gentle stimulation
    – Shaking
    – Cardiopulmonary resuscitation
  - Child's response to the intervention
■ Description of infant during ALTE
  - State of infant when event began: asleep or awake
  - If asleep:
    – Child's body position
    – Type of bedding
    – Face covered or free
  - If awake, was the child:
    – Being fed
    – Being handled
    – Crying
    – Being bathed
  - Child's appearance when found
    – Consciousness
    – Muscle tone
    – Color
    – Respiratory effort
      ■ Choking
      ■ Gasping
    – Emesis
    – Sweating

- Limb or eye movements
- Pupil size
- Skin or rectal temperature

Physical examination

■ Detailed physical examination is essential to uncover any clues to the underlying cause.
■ The clinician should:
  - Pay particular attention to abnormalities that may account for the infant's symptoms
    – Neurologic
    – Respiratory
    – Cardiac
  - Note any evidence of physiological compromise, eg:
    – Mental status changes
    – Cyanosis
    – Apnea

DIFFERENTIAL DIAGNOSIS

■ Differential diagnosis focuses on determining the underlying condition associated with the ALTE.
■ Gastrointestinal
  - Gastroesophageal reflux disease (GERD) (31%)
    – Diagnosis most often associated with an ALTE
    – Its precise role is debated.
    – GERD is common in the general population; the physician should not assume a causal relationship when it is discovered in an infant with a history of an ALTE.
■ Neurologic
  - Seizures (11%)
■ Respiratory
  - Lower respiratory tract infections (8%)
    – Pertussis
    – Respiratory syncytial virus infection
■ Cardiovascular
  - Cardiac arrhythmias
  - Persistent ductus arteriosus
■ Endocrine, metabolic
  - Inborn errors of metabolism
■ Infectious
  - Urinary tract infections
■ Neoplastic
  - Brain tumor
■ Drug-related
  - Opioid-related apnea

- SIDS
  - Apnea is not predictive of or a precursor to SIDS.
    - ALTEs are not near-miss SIDS cases.
    - Apnea appears to resolve at an age before most SIDS deaths occur.
  - Infants with an ALTE are:
    - 1–3 months younger than infants who die of SIDS
    - More likely to be found during the daytime or while sleeping supine at the time of the event
  - <7% of patients with SIDS have a history of an ALTE.
  - Although the SIDS mortality rate markedly decreased between 1986 and 1994, the mean annual admission rate for ALTEs did not change significantly.
- Other
  - Child abuse should be considered in children with a history of:
    - Recurrent cyanosis
    - Apnea
    - ALTE witnessed only by a single caretaker or in a family with previous unexplained infant deaths
    - Clinicians must be vigilant to avoid stigmatizing or adding to the distress of families.
  - Factitious illness

DIAGNOSTIC APPROACH

- ALTE:
  - Describes a clinical syndrome rather than a specific diagnosis
  - Is a common, nonspecific disorder of the young infant
    - Usually self-limited
    - May be potentially serious and life threatening
- No single accepted standard for evaluation
  - Thorough clinical assessment is most likely to lead to a diagnosis of the underlying problem.
    - Detailed history
    - Physical examination
  - Diagnostic studies and observation should be based on the findings of the clinical assessment.
    - If enough tests are performed, the increasing likelihood of false-positive results will diminish their diagnostic value.

LABORATORY FINDINGS

- The yield of most studies is low.
  - Even if a positive result is found, the question of a causal relationship still remains.

- Consider in infants with no identified cause after clinical assessment:
  - Complete blood count
  - Urinalysis and culture
  - Blood culture
- Additional studies to consider after an initial period of observation:
  - Metabolic studies
    - These studies may not be available in all hospitals.
    - A pediatric specialist may need to be consulted to interpret the results.
  - Tests for respiratory pathogens as indicated
  - Toxicology screen
  - Child abuse

IMAGING

- Consider in infants with no identified cause after clinical assessment.
  - Usually after an initial period of observation
- Chest radiography
- Skeletal survey
  - Child abuse
- Upper gastrointestinal series
  - Not sensitive for diagnosing GERD, but may be useful for identifying intestinal obstruction that contributes to GERD
    - Volvulus
    - Gastric outlet obstruction
- Brain neuroimaging
  - Child abuse
- Gastroesophageal reflux study

DIAGNOSTIC PROCEDURES

- Electrocardiography
  - Child with a witnessed seizure
  - Consider in infants with no identified cause after clinical assessment.
- Continuous cardiorespiratory (CR) monitoring with pulse oximetry
  - Detects:
    - Apnea
    - Bradycardia
    - Hypoxemia
- Polysomnography (PSG)
  - Suspected hypoxemia or hypercarbia associated with an atypical ALTE
  - Prolonged clinical course

- Recurrent or severe episodes
- Obstructive apnea
  - Repeat PSG may be necessary to determine when and if intervention is needed.
- If CR monitoring in the inpatient unit fails to provide a clear diagnosis
  - Central apneas (no respiratory effort for 20 seconds, or shorter if associated with hypoxemia or bradycardia)
  - Obstructive apneas (respiratory effort in thoracic or abdominal impedance tracings, or both, with no airflow in nasal and end-tidal carbon dioxide tracings)
  - Mixed apneas (central and obstructive events at the same time)
  - Episodes of periodic breathing
- Pneumography
  - Unattended studies that collect data on respiratory effort with:
    - Thoracic impedance monitor
    - Nasal flow
    - Oxygenation
    - Cardiac rhythm
  - But not:
    - Sleep staging
    - Carbon dioxide signal
    - Abdominal effort
  - Pneumography generates more technical artifacts and is less informative than PSG.
    - Should be limited to medical centers where PSG is unavailable
- 24-hour pH probe or milk scan by ^{99m}technetium
  - If GERD is the suspected cause of an ALTE
  - Up to 89% of infants with an ALTE may have a positive milk scan.
    - Only 41% of these infants have a correlating clinical diagnosis.
- Dilated funduscopic examination
  - Child abuse

TREATMENT APPROACH

- A period of observation with continuous CR monitoring in the hospital when a benign cause of ALTE is not evident:
  - Gathers additional information
  - Directs appropriate diagnostic studies
- Education and guidance should be provided to the guardian.
- Monitoring in the home setting after hospitalization detects recurrence.

SPECIFIC TREATMENTS

Hospital admission

- Hospital admission may not be required if:
  - The ALTE appears to be benign.
  - The patient is normal when evaluated immediately after the event.

Hospitalization with CR monitoring

- Required if:
  - The episode was significant.
  - The child required intense stimulation.
  - Physical examination reveals an abnormality.

Intensive care unit admission

- If the witnessed event or a review of the history suggests severe CR compromise
- Treatment directed at the underlying diagnosis determined by the evaluation should be started.
  - For example:
    - Antibiotics for suspected bacterial infection
    - Anticonvulsants for an infant with seizures
    - Medications for GERD

Stimulants

- Caffeine may correct periodic breathing associated with hypoxemia.

Preparation for discharge home

- Once the infant has been stabilized, consideration should be made for home CR monitoring.
  - Particularly for infants with an ALTE of unknown cause

WHEN TO ADMIT

- History, examination, or diagnostic studies suggest physiologic compromise.

WHEN TO REFER

- Suspected:
  - Seizure disorder
  - Hypoxemia
  - Hypercarbia
  - Cardiac dysrhythmia
- Vascular ring identified
- Congenital facial anomalies with obstructive apnea
- Evidence of child abuse
- Atypical manifestation

FOLLOW-UP

- Home CR monitoring
  - An ALTE is an indication for home monitoring.
    - Episodes of periodic breathing and obstructive apnea events will not be captured on home CR monitoring unless a secondary effect of these events on heart rate occurs.
  - Review of results
    - CR monitor results should be reviewed by a practitioner or specialist who is trained in their review.
    - Physician should establish a specific plan for periodic review.
    - In most cases, results should be reviewed monthly if the guardian has no concerns about the baby, or sooner if guardian reports ≥1 significant events.
  - Discontinue when:
    - No further physiologically significant events have occurred
    - No further objective evidence of pathologic events for ≥6 weeks
- Parents and caregivers should be counseled on:
  - Cardiopulmonary resuscitation for infants
    - In case further ALTEs occur after discharge
  - Practicing safe sleeping techniques (see Prevention)
  - Avoiding passive smoke exposure

PROGNOSIS

- Morbidity and mortality vary according to underlying diagnosis.
  - Mortality of infants with apnea of infancy
    - 0–6%
    - In healthy term and premature infants, apnea events become rare by 43 weeks' postmenstrual age.

- ALTE recurrence rate
  - 0–24%
- Long-term outcomes for infants with an unexplained ALTE
  - Unpredictable
  - Severe event requiring resuscitation, recurrent ALTE, or seizure disorder:
    - >25% risk of death
    - However, normal cognitive and behavioral outcomes have been reported up to 10 years after an ALTE.

PREVENTION

- Parents and caregivers should be counseled on:
  - Safe sleeping tips
    - Infants should be placed on their backs to sleep.
    - Redundant soft bedding and soft objects in the infant's sleeping environment should be avoided.
    - Adults and infants sleeping in the same bed is discouraged.
    - Excessive clothing and extreme room temperatures should be avoided.
  - Passive smoke exposure
    - Should be avoided during fetal and postnatal development

Appendicitis

DEFINITION

- Ischemia and inflammation of the vermiform (worm-shaped) appendix, which leads to local peritoneal inflammation
- Without surgical intervention, the appendix will eventually rupture, causing peritonitis.

EPIDEMIOLOGY

- Age
  - Rare in the first 2 years of life, accounting for <2% of childhood cases, but morbidity is high
  - More common after age 10
- Sex
  - Boys and girls are affected equally before puberty.
  - After age 15, twice as many boys are affected as girls.
- Seasonality
  - Increased incidence in spring and autumn

ETIOLOGY

- Appendicitis is always initiated by obstruction of the appendiceal lumen; the cause is:
  - Usually, a fecalith or lymphoid hyperplasia
  - Rarely, a parasite, tumor, or foreign body
  - Rarely, inspissated secretions in cystic fibrosis
- Organisms cultured from the peritoneal cavity after perforation include:
  - Aerobic bacteria; the most common organisms are:
    - *Escherichia coli*
    - *Staphylococcus aureus*
    - *Enterococcus organisms*
  - Anaerobic bacteria; the most common species are:
    - *Bacteroides*
    - *Clostridium*

RISK FACTORS

- Family history of appendicitis
  - Unclear whether related to genetics or diet

SIGNS AND SYMPTOMS

- Pain
  - Dull, steady, periumbilical at onset
  - If sufficient to awaken patient from sleep, may indicate acute appendicitis
  - Patients may be most comfortable lying supine with their legs flexed.
  - After 4–6 hours, it may shift to the right lower quadrant, but location may vary.
- Anorexia
  - Consistent, though not invariable finding
- Vomiting
  - 1 or 2 episodes, but not preceding pain
- Bowel habits
  - Usually unchanged
- Low-grade fever
  - Rarely above 100.3°F (37.9°C) before perforation
- In infants thought to have abdominal pain symptoms:
  - Vomiting and fever
  - Colicky appearance
  - Abdominal distention
  - Diffuse tenderness is likely; infants are rarely seen before perforation.

DIFFERENTIAL DIAGNOSIS

- Most common conditions that must be differentiated
  - Gastroenteritis
    - Abdominal examination is generally benign.
    - Vomiting and diarrhea usually occur before onset of pain.
  - Constipation
    - Pain is usually diffuse.
    - The patient often has a history of constipation.
    - Abdominal flat-plate roentgenogram can help in the diagnosis.
    - A small Fleet enema is often diagnostic and therapeutic.
  - Urinary tract infection
    - Urinalysis will help rule this out.
  - Diabetic ketoacidosis
    - Urinalysis will help rule this out.
  - Sickle cell crisis
  - Right lower-lobe pneumonia
    - May generate referred pain to the right lower quadrant of the abdomen
    - Examine the lungs to rule out.
  - Primary peritonitis
  - Inflammatory bowel disease
    - Check for an elevated erythrocyte sedimentation rate (ESR).
    - With appendicitis, ESR is usually normal.
- Gynecologic conditions
  - Pelvic examination is indicated for any adolescent girl who has abdominal pain.
  - A thorough history, pelvic examination, and appropriate diagnostic studies can rule out:
    - Pelvic inflammatory disease
    - Ovarian torsion
    - Ruptured ectopic pregnancy

- Dysmenorrhea
- Mittelschmerz
- Ruptured corpus luteum cyst

■ Unusual conditions that are indistinguishable from or mimic appendicitis
  • Henoch-Schönlein purpura
  • Hemolytic-uremic syndrome
  • Rocky Mountain spotted fever

■ Surgical emergencies that mimic appendicitis and may be ruled out only in the operating room
  • Meckel diverticulitis
  • Intestinal adhesions
  • Intussusception
  • Necrotizing enterocolitis

DIAGNOSTIC APPROACH

■ To differentiate appendicitis from other disorders:
  • A thorough history, especially of pain, is invaluable.
  • A period of observation can safely differentiate surgical and nonsurgical conditions.
    - Appendix rarely perforates within 24 hours of the onset of pain.
  • Perforation of the appendix may be associated with an initial decrease in pain.
    - Symptoms worsen within a few hours.

■ In any infant thought to have abdominal pain, consider appendicitis.
  • With a high index of suspicion, surgery must be performed immediately to prevent or manage perforation.

■ Physical examination
  • A gentle, nonthreatening approach is most effective.
  • Assess for peritoneal signs, such as pain on walking or coughing.
  • If the patient can jump up on the examining table, he or she does not usually have appendicitis.
  • Abdominal tenderness
    - Always present
    - Often greatest at the McBurney point (two-thirds of the distance on a direct line from the umbilicus to the anterosuperior iliac spine)
  • There may be hyperesthesia of the skin overlying the painful area.
  • Rebound abdominal tenderness (particularly referred to the right lower quadrant) is common.
  • Pain in the right lower quadrant may be accentuated when the inflamed appendix is located retrocecally, by:
    - Placing the patient in the left decubitus position and extending the right leg at the hip, placing tension on the

right psoas muscle, the origins of which underlie the appendix (psoas sign)
    - Placing the patient supine and internally rotating the flexed right hip, extending the right internal obturator muscle, the origins of which also underlie the appendix (obturator sign)
  • When the inflamed appendix is located anteriorly, pain in the right lower quadrant may be accentuated when the patient is asked to sit up from a supine position while pressure is placed against the forehead.
  • Bowel sounds may be diminished or hyperactive.

■ Rectal examination often reveals right-sided tenderness.

■ Pelvic examination should be performed for any adolescent girl with abdominal pain.

■ Without surgical intervention, appendicitis eventually will lead to rupture and peritonitis.

LABORATORY FINDINGS

■ Blood count and urinalysis
  • The leukocyte count is most often 10,000–20,000 cells/μL.
  • Slight increase in the number of neutrophils, particularly young forms

IMAGING

■ Clinical decision rules are used to:
  • Aid in the diagnosis of appendicitis
  • Avoid overuse of imaging studies

■ Consultation with a pediatric surgeon may:
  • Minimize the need for imaging studies
  • Reduce rates of perforation and negative appendectomy

■ Radiography
  • Abdominal roentgenograms are occasionally helpful.
  • Absence of abnormalities on images does not rule out appendicitis.
  • Suggestive features include:
    - Calcified appendicolith
    - Air-filled appendix
  • In neonates, diagnostic signs include:
    - Appendicolith
    - Free peritoneal fluid
    - Bowel wall edema
    - Rarely, free air

■ Ultrasonography and computed tomography (CT)
  • Recently have been used to establish the diagnosis in equivocal cases
  • In 1 study, selective use of CT and ultrasonography:
    - Decreased incidence of perforated appendicitis from 35.4% to 15.5%
    - Decreased the rate of removing a normal appendix (a negative appendectomy) from 14.7% to 4.1%

A

TREATMENT APPROACH

- Nonsurgical management
  - For patients who have symptoms for ≥5 days and a palpable mass consistent with an appendiceal abscess, many surgeons prefer initial nonsurgical management.
  - This approach lowers the incidence of diffuse peritonitis and associated complications precipitated by surgical manipulation during acute inflammatory stages.
- Surgical management
  - Incidence of rupture increases dramatically 24–36 hours after the onset of abdominal pain.
  - Delaying surgery >36 hours results in at least a 65% incidence of perforation.
  - Once the diagnosis is made, the patient must be prepared for immediate surgery.
  - Laparoscopic appendectomy is being performed at many institutions.

SPECIFIC TREATMENTS

Nonsurgical management

- For patients who have symptoms for ≥5 days and a palpable mass consistent with an appendiceal abscess, many surgeons prefer initial nonsurgical management.
  - Treatment with broad-spectrum antibiotics for 14 days
    - Initiated in the hospital and completed at home
    - If the clinical condition allows and barring interim complications, the child returns in 6–8 weeks for elective appendectomy.

Surgical management

- Nothing is given by mouth.
- A nasogastric tube is inserted and placed on low suction if the child is vomiting.
- Intravenous hydration is started (eg, 10 mL/kg/h of lactated Ringer's solution).
- Fever may be controlled with acetaminophen given by rectum.
- Broad-spectrum antibiotics are administered intravenously before surgery.
  - For example, ampicillin, gentamicin, and clindamycin or acephalosporin
  - Antibiotics have been shown to reduce morbidity even in nonperforated cases.
- Appendectomy is performed as soon as the patient's condition has been stabilized.

WHEN TO ADMIT

- Hospitalize for inpatient observation if the diagnosis cannot be excluded.
- Hospitalize for appendectomy if the diagnosis of appendicitis is made.

- Average hospital stay is approximately 2 days.
  - Significantly longer in cases of perforation

WHEN TO REFER

- Refer to surgery immediately whenever appendicitis is suspected.

FOLLOW-UP

- In nonsurgical management
- Antibiotics, initiated in the hospital and completed at home
- Subsequent elective appendectomy in 6–8 weeks

COMPLICATIONS

- Complications that increase morbidity include:
  - Peritonitis
  - Postoperative abscess
  - Prolonged ileus
  - Perforation
    - Significantly increases risk of postoperative adhesive small-bowel obstruction
- Recent studies have shown that female infertility is not a long-term complication of a ruptured appendix.

PROGNOSIS

- For uncomplicated appendicitis treated with prompt surgical intervention:
  - Mortality is much less than 1%.
  - Long-term morbidity is primarily the risk of adhesive small-bowel obstruction.
- The incidence of perforated appendicitis exceeds 30%, despite increasing use of radiographic imaging.
- For infants <2 years of age:
  - Incidence of perforation approaches 100%.
  - Morbidity is high.
- A ruptured appendix increases the risk of mortality in:
  - Infants
  - Older children with delayed diagnosis who develop sepsis
- A higher index of suspicion on the part of families and pediatricians may:
  - Lead to earlier diagnosis of the condition
  - Reduce incidence of appendiceal perforation and its morbid complications

PREVENTION

- The risk of appendicitis may be reduced with a high-fiber diet.

Asthma

DEFINITION

- Asthma is a chronic lung disease characterized by 3 features.
  - Airway obstruction that is at least partially reversible
  - Airway hyperreactivity or hyperresponsiveness to a variety of external stimuli
  - Chronic inflammation of the airway

EPIDEMIOLOGY

- Prevalence
  - 15 million people in the US have asthma.
  - Asthma affects 5 million children or adolescents.
    - This represents between 3% and 7% of the children in the US.
  - Asthma prevalence in children <5 years has increased 160% in the past 2 decades.
- Age
  - In 80% of patients with asthma, onset of symptoms began before 5 years of age.
- Childhood asthma is responsible for:
  - 13 million physician visits
  - 200,000 hospitalizations
  - 10 million lost school days
  - 550,000 emergency department visits
  - 8 million prescriptions
- The number of deaths from childhood asthma has doubled in the past 2 decades.

ETIOLOGY

- Typically, an external trigger initiates the inflammatory cascade.
  - This trigger may be identifiable.
  - Common triggers include:
    - Viral respiratory infections
    - Exercise
    - Irritants, such as tobacco smoke
    - Allergens
      - Animal dander
      - Dust
      - Dust mites
      - Cockroaches
      - Food, eg, nuts, food additives
      - Mold
    - Change in the weather, particularly cold air
    - Emotional expression, such as laughter or anger
    - Gastroesophageal reflux disease
- The immediate response to the trigger exposure is bronchospasm and bronchoconstriction.
  - Airway constriction leads to cough, wheezing, and shortness of breath.

- Immediate decrease in forced expiratory volume (FEV_1)
  - This returns to normal 4–8 hours after exposure.
- A second, more severe decrease in FEV_1 occurs 8–24 hours after trigger exposure.

RISK FACTORS

- The most common cause of wheezing in infants and young children is upper respiratory tract infections.
- The strongest predictor of wheezing continuing into asthma is atopy.
- Allergens and irritant exposures increase the risk for asthma.
  - Cockroach allergy in children living in urban areas
  - Exposure to maternal smoking
- Prematurity increases risk for asthma.
- Risk factors for asthma
  - Major criteria
    - Parent with asthma or atopic dermatitis
  - Minor criteria
    - Allergic rhinitis
    - Wheezing apart from colds
    - Eosinophilia ≥4%
  - Children at increased risk for asthma between 6 and 13 years of age are those with:
    - 1 of the 2 major criteria **and**
    - 2 of the 3 minor criteria **and**
    - Wheezing
- The number of deaths from childhood asthma has doubled in the past 2 decades.
  - Risk factors associated with asthma deaths include:
    - History of sudden, severe exacerbations
    - Prior admission to the intensive care unit
    - Prior intubation for asthma
    - Within a 12-month period:
      - ≥2 hospitalizations or
      - ≥3 emergency department visits
    - Use of >1 canister per month of inhaled short-acting ß-agonist
    - Long-term use of oral corticosteroids
    - Difficulty perceiving airflow obstruction or its severity

SIGNS AND SYMPTOMS

- A detailed medical history should be obtained from the patient and family.
  - Ask about symptoms, such as cough, wheezing, shortness of breath, or chest tightness.
    - Frequency
    - Severity

A

- Are the symptoms made worse by triggers?
  - Identify triggers, if possible.
- Are the symptoms worse during the day or night?

■ Physical examination should focus on the upper respiratory tract, chest, and skin.

- Look for signs of allergic disease.
  - Conjunctivitis
  - Allergic shiners
  - Pale boggy turbinates
  - Rhinorrhea
  - Polyps
  - Transnasal crease
- Physical signs **not** usually associated with asthma include:
  - Failure to thrive
  - Cyanosis
  - Clubbing

DIFFERENTIAL DIAGNOSIS

■ Gastroesophageal reflux

■ Not all wheezes indicate asthma.

■ Other diagnoses to consider:

- Cystic fibrosis
- Foreign body aspiration
- Vocal cord dysfunction
- Airway lesions
  - Airway stenosis
  - Tracheal webs
  - Tracheobronchomalacia
- Vascular rings
- Mediastinal masses
- Gastroesophageal reflux or recurrent aspiration
- Heart failure
- Immunodeficiency
- Parasitic diseases
- Bronchiolitis caused by viral pathogens

DIAGNOSTIC APPROACH

■ For a diagnosis of asthma, the following must be present.

■ Recurrent, episodic symptoms of airflow obstruction

- Cough
- Wheezing
- Shortness of breath
- Chest tightness

■ Airway flow obstruction or limitation that is at least partially reversible

- In older children, spirometry before and after bronchodilator use can determine this.

- In younger children, assess by a positive response to a ß-agonist.

LABORATORY FINDINGS

■ In general, laboratory evaluation is peripheral to the diagnosis.

- Testing for immunoglobulin E level and allergies may be useful so that appropriate treatment can be started.
- Complete blood count with differential may indicate an allergic or immunologic condition.

IMAGING

■ Chest radiography

- May be useful to rule out other conditions, such as foreign body aspiration

DIAGNOSTIC PROCEDURES

■ Spirometry is the gold standard for measuring severity of obstructive airway disease.

- Should be performed on any child ≥5 years of age who can perform the test
- Spirometry is preferred over peak flow monitoring.
  - Peak flow measurements reflect large airway function.
- Measurements to assess:
  - FEV_1
  - Forced vital capacity
  - Forced midexpiratory flow rate
  - Examination of flow volume loop
- Perform at baseline and then annually.
- Determines airflow obstruction and whether this airflow obstruction is reversible

■ Pre- and post-bronchodilator spirometry is recommended.

- Confirm the diagnosis
- Classify disease severity

■ Objective measures of lung function are useful:

- To diagnose airflow obstruction
- To determine the reversibility of airflow obstruction
- To assess daily variation and monitor changes over time
- To manage exacerbations in severe airway obstruction

■ Peak flow meters are useful as monitoring tools.

- They lack sensitivity for diagnostic use.
- Reference values vary, depending on the brand of the peak flow meter.
- As a monitoring tool, peak flow measurement can assist the clinician to:
  - Determine whether airway narrowing is occurring before the patient becomes symptomatic.
  - Monitor the effect of medication addition or withdrawal
  - Determine when to seek help

– Determine the effect of triggers

– Determine changes in lung function

CLASSIFICATION

- National Heart, Lung, and Blood Institute Guidelines for Asthma Severity
  - Mild intermittent asthma
    - >80% FEV_1 and peak expiratory flow rate (PEFR) before bronchodilator use
    - <12% and 20% change, respectively, after bronchodilator use
  - Mild persistent asthma
    - >80% FEV_1 and PEFR before bronchodilator use
    - >12% and 20% change, respectively, after bronchodilator use
  - Moderate persistent asthma
    - 60–80% FEV_1 and PEFR before bronchodilator use
  - Severe persistent asthma
  - <60% FEV_1 and PEFR before bronchodilator use
- Symptom class: current clinical features
  - Intermittent asthma
    - Intermittent symptoms (wheeze, cough, dyspnea) <2 times/week
  - Brief exacerbations (from a few hours to a few days)
  - Nighttime asthma symptoms <2 times/month
  - Mild persistent asthma
    - Intermittent symptoms (wheeze, cough, dyspnea) >2 times/week but <1 time/day
    - Exacerbations that may affect activity and sleep
    - Nighttime asthma symptoms >2 times/month but <1 time/week
  - Moderate persistent asthma
    - Symptoms (wheeze, cough, dyspnea) daily
    - Exacerbations >2 times/week; may last days and affect activity
    - Nighttime asthma symptoms >1 time/week
  - Severe persistent asthma
    - Continuous symptoms
    - Frequent exacerbations
    - Frequent nighttime asthma symptoms
    - Physical activities limited by asthma symptoms
- Patients with intermittent asthma experiencing severe exacerbations requiring hospitalization should be treated as having moderate persistent asthma (category 3 above).
- Children requiring intensive care should be treated as having severe persistent asthma (category 4 above).
  - These children should be referred to an asthma specialist.

- Classification can change over time.
  - Ongoing review of symptoms and treatment plan every 1–6 months is helpful.

TREATMENT APPROACH

- Therapy has 5 major goals.
  - Prevent chronic and troublesome symptoms
  - Maintain normal or near-normal pulmonary function
  - Maintain normal activity levels, including exercise
  - Prevent exacerbations
  - Provide optimal medical regimen with minimal or no adverse side effects
- There are 4 interventions to achieve these goals.
  - Objective measurements of lung function
    - Spirometry
    - Peak flow monitoring
  - Pharmacologic therapy
    - Relieve obstruction and provide quick relief of symptoms.
      - Short-acting ß-agonists
      - Systemic corticosteroids
      - Anticholinergic agents
    - Treat underlying inflammation.
      - Long-acting ß-agonists
      - Inhaled corticosteroids
      - Nonsteroidal antiinflammatory agents
      - Leukotriene (LT) modifiers
      - Theophylline
  - Environmental control of allergies and irritants
  - Patient education

SPECIFIC TREATMENTS

Short-term pharmacologic therapy

- Quick relief of symptoms
- Short-acting ß-agonists are the most well known in this category.
  - Bronchodilate
  - Bronchoprotect
  - Can prevent exercise-induced bronchospasm
  - Most common side effects
    - Tachycardia
    - Tremor
    - Headaches
    - Palpitations
    - Hypokalemia
    - Hyperglycemia

A

- **Examples**
  - Albuterol
    - Oral solution: 2 mg/5 mL
    - 0.1–0.2 mg/kg, 3 times/day
    - Do not exceed 12 mg/day.
  - Albuterol (Proventil HFA, Proair HFA)
    - Metered-dose inhaler (MDI): 108 mcg/puff
    - 2 puffs, 15 minutes before exercise
    - 2 puffs, 3–4 times/day, as needed
  - Albuterol (Ventolin HFA)
    - MDI: 100 mcg/puff
    - 2 puffs, 15 minutes before exercise
    - 2 puffs, 3–4 times/day, as needed
  - Albuterol (AccuNeb)
    - Nebulizer solution: 0.63 mg/3 mL; 1.25 mg/3 mL
    - 0.63 to 1.25 mg, 3–4 times/day, for ages 2–12 years
  - Albuterol sulfate
    - Nebulizer solution: 2.5 mg/3 mL; 0.083% (unit dose)
    - 0.05 mg/kg (min: 1.25 mg; max: 2.5 mg), 3–4 times/day
  - Levalbuterol (Xopenex)
    - Nebulizer solution: 0.31 mg/3 mL; 0.63 mg/3 mL; 1.25 mg/3 mL
    - 0.31–0.63 mg, 3 times/day, for maintenance
    - 1.25 mg, 3 times/day, for acute bronchospasm and patients who are unresponsive to lower dose
  - Levalbuterol (Xopenex HFA)
    - MDI: 45 mcg/puff
    - 1–2 puffs up to every 4 hours
  - Pirbuterol (Maxair)
    - MDI: 200 mcg/puff
    - 2 puffs 3–4 times/day, as needed
- **A short course of oral corticosteroid is a quick-relief medication.**
  - Broad antiinflammatory effects
  - Usually given for 3–10 days to:
    - Gain initial control of asthma
    - Speed resolution of moderate to severe persistent exacerbations
  - Methylprednisolone (Medrol)
    - Tablets: 4, 6, 8, 16, 24, 32 mg
    - Short-course (3–10 days)
      4 burst: 1–2 mg/kg/day (max: 60 mg/day)
  - Prednisolone
    - Tablet: 5 mg
    - Short-course (3–10 days)
      4 burst: 1–2 mg/kg/day (max: 60 mg/day)
  - Prednisolone (Pediapred)
    - Liquid: 5 mg/5 mL
    - Short-course (3–10 days)
      4 burst: 1–2 mg/kg/day (max: 60 mg/day)
  - Prednisolone (Prelone syrup)
    - Liquid: 15 mg/5 mL
    - Short-course (3–10 days)
      4 burst: 1–2 mg/kg/day (max: 60 mg/day)
  - Prednisolone (Orapred ODT)
    - Chewable tablet 10, 15, 30 mg
    - Short-course (3–10 days)
      4 burst: 1–2 mg/kg/day (max: 60 mg/day)
  - Prednisone (Prednisone)
    - Tablet: 1, 2.5, 5, 10, 20, 50 mg
    - Liquid: 5 mg/5 mL
    - Short-course (3–10 days)
      4 burst: 1–2 mg/kg/day (max: 60 mg/day)
  - Prednisone (Prednisone Intensol)
    - Liquid: 5 mg/5 mL
    - Short-course (3–10 days)
      4 burst: 1–2 mg/kg/day (max: 60 mg/day)
- **Anticholinergic agents, in combination with a ß-agonist, have a positive effect on acute asthma exacerbations.**
  - The most common agent is ipratropium.
    - Decreases vagal tone, leading to bronchodilation
    - Blocks reflex bronchoconstriction to irritants
    - Has no effect on the early- or late-phase response
    - Acts an additive to a ß-agonist
  - Ipratropium bromide (Atrovent HFA)
    - MDI: 17 mcg/puff
    - Nebulizer solution: .20 mg/mL; 0.02% (ampule)
    - 1–2 puffs 4 times a day or 1 ampule 4 times a day
    - 0.25–2 mg/kg or every other day in single dose as needed for long-term control up to a maximum of 60 mg/day
  - Ipratropium bromide/albuterol (DuoNeb)
    - Nebulizer solution: 0.20 mg/mL/2.5 mg albuterol (ampule)
    - 1 ampule 4 times a day
    - 0.25–2 mg/kg or every other day in single dose as needed for long-term control up to a maximum of 60 mg/day

Long-term pharmacologic therapy

- Treat the underlying inflammatory disorder.

Inhaled corticosteroids

- Inhaled corticosteroids are the most effective long-term antiinflammatory medications currently available.
  - Available in variety of delivery formats:
    - MDI

- Dry powder inhaler (DPI)
- Nebulizer
- Improves long-term symptoms in pulmonary function
- Reduces the need for quick-relief medications
- Major issues and concerns
  - Growth delay
  - Ocular problems, such as cataracts and potential glaucoma
  - Thrush
  - Contraindicated during certain infections (herpes simplex)
- Budesonide inhalation suspension (Pulmicort Flexhaler)
  - Approved for nebulization by the US Food and Drug Administration
  - May be used in infants as young as 12 months.
  - DPI: 90 mcg/inhalation
    - Low dose: 2–4 inhalations/day, once daily or divided twice daily
    - Medium dose: 6–8 inhalations/day, divided twice daily
  - DPI: 180 mcg/inhalation
    - Low dose: 1–2 inhalations/day, once daily or divided twice daily
    - Medium dose: 3–4 inhalations/day, divided twice daily
    - High dose: 8 inhalations/day, divided twice daily
- Budesonide (Pulmicort respules)
  - Liquid: 0.25 mg/2 mL; 0.5 mg/2 mL
    - Low dose: 0.5 mg, once or twice daily
    - High dose: 1.0 mg, once or twice daily
- Beclomethasone dipropionate (QVAR HFA)
  - MDI: 40 mcg/puff
    - Low dose: 1–4 puffs/day, divided twice daily
    - Medium dose: 4–8 puffs, divided twice daily
  - MDI: 80 mcg/puff
    - Low dose: 1–2 puffs/day, divided twice daily
    - Medium dose: 2–4 puffs/day, divided twice daily
    - High dose: 8 puffs/day, divided twice daily
- Flunisolide (AeroBid, AeroBid M)
  - MDI: 250 mcg/puff
    - Low dose: 2–4 puffs/day, divided twice daily
    - Medium dose: 4–6 puffs/day, divided twice daily
    - High dose: 8 puffs/day, divided twice daily
- Fluticasone propionate (Flovent)
  - MDI: 44 mcg/puff
    - Low dose: 2–4 puffs/day, divided twice daily
  - MDI: 110 mcg/puff
    - Medium dose: 2–4 puffs/day, divided twice daily

- MDI: 220 mcg/puff
  - Medium dose: 2 puffs/day, divided twice daily
  - High dose: 3–8 puffs/day, divided twice daily
- DPI: 50 mcg/inhalation
  - Low: 2–4 inhalations/day, divided twice daily
- DPI: 100 mcg/inhalation
  - Medium: 2–4 inhalations/day, divided twice daily
- DPI: 250 mcg/inhalation
  - Medium: 2 inhalations/day, divided twice daily
  - High: 3–8 inhalations/day, divided twice daily
- Mometasone furoate (Asmanex Twisthaler)
  - DPI: 220 mcg/inhalation
    - Low dose: 1 inhalation/day, at night
    - Medium dose: 2–3 inhalations/day, once (at night) or divided twice daily
    - High dose: 4 inhalations/day, divided twice daily
- Triamcinolone (Azmacort)
  - MDI: 200 mcg/puff
    - Low dose: 4–8 puffs/day, divided 3–4 times/day
    - Medium dose: 8–12 puffs/day, divided 2–4 times/day
    - High dose: 12–16 puffs/day, divided twice daily

Combination inhaled corticosteroids and long-acting ß-agonists

- Fluticasone propionate and salmeterol (Advair)
  - DPI
    - 100 mcg/50 mcg inhalation
      - Low dose: 1 inhalation, twice daily
    - 250 mcg/50 mcg inhalation
      - Medium dose: 1 inhalation, twice daily
    - 500 mcg/50 mcg inhalation
      - High dose: 1 inhalation twice daily
  - MDI
    - 45 mcg/21 mcg puff
      - 2 puffs, twice daily
    - 115/21 mcg/puff
      - 2 puffs, twice daily
    - 230/21 mcg/puff
      - 2 puffs, twice daily

Nonsteroidal anti-inflammatory agents

- Cromolyn sodium (Intal)
  - Mast-cell stabilizer
  - Decreases early- and late-phase response after allergen challenge
  - Has a good safety profile

- Can be dispensed as a nebulizer solution or
  - Nebulizer: 20 mg/2 mL in an ampule
    - 1 ampule, 3–4 times/day
  - MDI: 1 mg/puff
    - 1–2 puffs, 3–4 times/day
    - This dose may be inadequate to affect airway hyperresponsivenss.
- Nedocromil
  - Has a good safety profile
  - Poor patient compliance with this medication due to its unpleasant taste.
  - MDI: 1.75 mg/puff
    - 1–2 puffs, 2–4 times/day

LT modifiers

- Block synthesis of LTs or block LTD4 receptors
- Can be administered orally
- Improve symptoms and pulmonary function
- Can negatively affect the pharmacokinetics of certain medications
- Montelukast (Singulair)
  - Sprinkles: 4 mg for ages 12–23 months
  - Tablet
    - 4 mg, chewable, for ages 2–4 years
    - 5 mg, chewable, for ages 6–14 years
    - 10 mg, for ages >14 years
  - 1 tablet or packet in the evening for all dose formulations
- Zafirlukast (Accolate)
  - Tablet
    - 10 mg for ages 7–11 years
    - 20 mg for ages ≥12 years
  - 1 tablet, twice a day; take 1 hour before or 2 hours after meals.
- Zileuton (Zyflo Filmtab)
  - 600 mg for ages ≥12 years
  - 1 tablet, 4 times/day

Long-acting ß-agonists

- Relax the bronchial smooth muscle
- Only available as DPIs
- Salmeterol (Serevent diskus)
  - DPI: 50 mcg/blister
  - 1 inhalation, twice daily
- Formoterol (Foradil aerolizer)
  - DPI: 12 mcg/capsule
  - 1 capsule inhaled twice daily, or 15 minutes before exercise

- Sustained-release albuterol (VoSpire ER)
  - Tablet: 4 mg, 8 mg
  - Maximal dose:
    - 6–12 years: 4 mg, twice daily
    - ≥12 years: 8 mg, twice daily

Theophylline

- Use has diminished in children with asthma owing to need for frequent monitoring and side effects, some of which are life threatening.
- Uniphyl, Theo-24
  - Capsules: 100, 125, 200, 300, 400, 600 mg
  - Starting dose: 10 mg/kg/day
- Elixophyllin
  - Liquid: 80 mg/15 mL
  - Maximal dose (for children <1 year of age): $(0.2 \times \text{age in weeks}) + 5 = \text{mg/kg/day}$
- Theo-Dur
  - 50, 75, 125, 200 mg sprinkles
  - Maximal dose (for children ≥1 year of age): 16 mg/kg/day, not to exceed the adult maximum of 800 mg/day.

Omalizumab

- Anti–immunoglobulin E humanized monoclonal antibody
- Only prescribed by asthma specialists

WHEN TO ADMIT

- Admission may be required when:
  - The child does not respond to ß-agonist therapy.
  - The child has peak flows <50% of personal best after ß-agonist therapy.
  - The child has difficulty breathing, as evidenced by:
    - Chest and neck pulling in
    - Hunched posture
    - Trouble walking or talking
    - Stopping playing or inability to restart
    - Gray or blue lips or fingernails

WHEN TO REFER

- Refer the child to an asthma specialist when:
  - The child has had a life-threatening exacerbation.
  - The child has been admitted to an intensive care unit.
  - Goals of asthma therapy are not being met after 3–6 months of treatment.
  - Signs and symptoms are atypical.
  - Severe persistent asthma is present.
  - The child requires >2 bursts of oral corticosteroids per year.

FOLLOW-UP

- Factors that influence adherence to asthma therapy
  - Medication characteristics
    - Taste
    - Dosing schedule
    - Side effects
    - Expense
  - Patient variables
    - Apathy
    - Misperception of disease severity
    - Failure to obtain medication
  - Physician factors
    - Poor communication
    - Failure to monitor patients regularly
    - Incorrect medication and dose level
- To assess medication compliance:
  - Determine what factors may have prevented proper use of prescribed medications.
    - Bothered by taste
    - Cost
    - Concern about side effects
    - Denial
    - Difficulty remembering or organizing medications
    - Difficulty tolerating side effects
    - Difficulty using delivery system
    - Difficulty with school
    - Unable to understand how medicine works
    - Inconvenient or inappropriate dosing schedule
    - Embarrassment
    - Fear of addiction
    - Lack of parental supervision
    - Language difficulties
    - Rebellion
    - Unable to refill prescription on time
    - Inadequate transportation to health services
    - Inadequate transportation to the pharmacy
- To promote successful disease management:
  - The clinician should use a friendly manner and be attentive.
  - The patient should be supported and praised for success.
  - Elicit family concerns and allay their fears.
  - Ongoing education should be provided to reinforce the medication regimen and technique of administration.
    - Keep the therapy as simple as possible.
      - Limit number of medications.
      - Limit number of doses.

- Communicate with school personnel.
  - Have a plan for the child with asthma.
  - The child should be allowed to carry and use a short-acting ß-agonist for quick relief of symptoms.

COMPLICATIONS

- There are 5 questions to ask when the patient does not respond to reasonable therapy.
  - Is it asthma?
    - Anatomic lesions or other medical conditions should be ruled out.
  - Is the patient adherent to the medication regimen?
  - Is the patient's technique for medication delivery appropriate?
  - Did the patient run out of medication and not realize it or say so?
  - Is there a continual exposure present that is causing problems for the patient?
- A referral or second opinion should be considered if the desired effect is not being achieved.

PREVENTION

- Warning signs and symptoms that a patient may experience before an asthma attack
  - Chest pain
  - Irritable
  - Fatigue
  - Quiet
  - Eczema flare-up
  - Fever
  - Scratchy throat
  - Heartburn, gastroesophageal reflux
  - Heart palpitations
  - Decreased exercise tolerance
  - Mood changes
  - Runny or stuffy nose
  - Headaches
  - Wheezing
  - Cough
  - Loss of appetite
  - Trembling hands
  - Watery eyes
  - Dark circles under eyes

Atopic Dermatitis

DEFINITION

- Atopic dermatitis (AD) is a multifactorial dermatologic condition involving chronic inflammation of the skin.
- Sometimes referred to as *eczema*, a general term to describe skin that is erythematous, scaling, vesicular, and crusting.
- May be the initial condition signaling the progression to further allergic disease, known as the *atopic march*
- Associated immunoglobulin E (IgE)-mediated diseases
  - Allergic rhinitis
  - Asthma
  - Food allergies

EPIDEMIOLOGY

- Prevalence
  - >10% of infants and young children may be affected.
  - ~5% of adolescents are affected.
  - In 2007, 18 million Americans had a self-reported diagnosis, with more than one-third having the diagnosis confirmed by a physician.
- Age
  - Predominantly disease of infancy and childhood
  - Onset occurs in first year of life in the majority of affected individuals.
- Sex
  - Both sexes are affected equally.

ETIOLOGY

- The exact cause is unknown, but genetic and environmental factors play a role.
- Involves:
  - Dysfunction of the epidermal barrier and
  - Dysfunction of the immune system
    - Abnormal IgE-mediated (type I) reaction
    - Abnormal cell-mediated (type IV) reaction
- The hygiene hypothesis states that decreased exposure to microbes stunts immunologic maturation of Th1 cells.
- Other cells implicated in the development of AD
  - Macrophages
  - IgE-bearing Langerhans cells
  - Eosinophils
  - Mast cells
  - Resulting inflammatory reactions lead to disruption of the epidermis.
- Potential antigenic triggers
  - Airborne allergens (dust mites, cat and dog dander, molds, pollen)
  - Foods (especially milk, eggs, peanuts)
  - Infectious agents
  - Contact allergens
- Psychological stress may exacerbate AD.

SIGNS AND SYMPTOMS

Acute dermatitis

- Associated with:
  - Severe pruritus
  - Redness
  - Vesicles
  - Exudation
  - May have subacute pattern of pruritus, redness, and scaling

Chronic lesions

- Marked by:
  - Excoriations
  - Lichenification (thickened skin and deeper or exaggerated skin lines)
  - Postinflammatory hypopigmentation or hyperpigmentation

Infantile AD

- Eruption of erythematous papules on facial cheeks and extensor surfaces of arms and legs
- Dry hair, scaly scalp (often)

Childhood AD

- Begins at approximately 3 years and lasts through puberty
- The areas most affected include:
  - Antecubital and popliteal folds
  - Neck
  - Flexor surfaces of wrists and ankles
  - More subacute and chronic dermatitis.

Adult AD

- Additional clinical signs include:
  - Diffuse involvement of the body
  - Xerosis
  - Lichenification
  - Central facial pallor

Other clinical manifestations

- Keratosis pilaris
  - Characteristic goose flesh appearance secondary to multiple, small, skin-colored or mildly erythematous keratotic papules located on upper arms, thighs, and facial cheeks
- Lichen spinulosus
  - Tiny hairlike spines top the small papules that occur in crops on various locations
- Pityriasis alba
- Dennie-Morgan folds

- Urticaria
- Hyperlinear palms
- Juvenile plantar dermatosis
  - Mainly affects the feet, rarely the hands
  - Produces shiny, fissured skin on the plantar surfaces
- Nummular eczema
- Cataracts

DIFFERENTIAL DIAGNOSIS

- Seborrheic dermatitis
- Seborrhea is associated with scaling, commonly on the scalp, forehead, and around the eyebrows.
- Can be accompanied by pruritus
- Contact dermatitis (allergic and irritant forms)
  - Diagnosis often requires positive exposure history to the potential offending agent.
  - Limited in distribution on the body to the area of contact
  - More likely to have acute onset and localized appearance
- Psoriasis
- Scabies
- Dermatophyte infection
- Systemic immunologic or metabolic disorders
  - Wiskott-Aldrich syndrome
  - Leiner disease
  - Histiocytosis X
  - Ataxia telangiectasia
  - Ahistidinemia
  - Agammaglobulinemia
  - Hartnup disease
  - Hurler syndrome
  - Eosinophilic gastroenteritis
  - Acrodermatitis enteropathica
  - Phenylketonuria

DIAGNOSTIC APPROACH

- Diagnosis is determined solely by history and clinical examination.
- Criteria for diagnosis (patient characteristics to look for)
  - Major criteria (all must be present)
    - Pruritus
    - Typical morphology and distribution
      - Facial and extensor involvement during infancy and early childhood
      - Flexural lichenification and linearity by adolescence
    - Chronic or recurring dermatitis

- Minor criteria (≥2 must be present)
  - Personal or family history of atopy (eg, asthma, allergic rhinoconjunctivitis, atopic dermatitis)
  - Immediate skin test reactivity
  - White dermatographism or delayed blanch to cholinergic agents
  - Anterior subcapsular cataracts
- Associated conditions (≥4 must be present)
  - Xerosis, ichthyosis, hyperlinear palms
  - Pityriasis alba
  - Keratosis pilaris
  - Facial pallor, infraorbital darkening (allergic shiner)
  - Dennie-Morgan fold
  - Elevated serum IgE level
  - Keratoconus
  - Nonspecific hand dermatitis
  - Recurring cutaneous infections
- Patients may have AD and not meet these criteria.

LABORATORY FINDINGS

- No routine laboratory studies are needed for diagnosis.
- Specific tests to rule out other disorders, on a case-by-case basis
  - If infections are recurrent, consider an immunodeficiency workup.
- Bacterial cultures of encrusted or exudative skin lesions/nares to detect staphylococcal organisms are warranted when:
  - Secondary infection is suspected
  - Improvement is not noted with standard therapy
- Patch testing may be considered to pinpoint potential antigenic triggers, which may add a component of contact dermatitis.
- Skin biopsy may be necessary when the definitive diagnosis is in question.

TREATMENT APPROACH

- Treatment of uncomplicated cases
  - Treatment to relieve dryness, inflammation, and pruritus and eradicate secondary bacterial infections
  - Daily applications of emollients (cream or ointment), especially after brief warm baths
    - Ointments are better than emollients in more severe cases.
    - If discomfort (stinging sensation) occurs or if ointment feels too occlusive (eg, in humid weather), creams can be substituted.

A

- Bathing should last no longer than 5 minutes.
  - Mild soaps or nondetergent cleansers are recommended.
  - Pat dry with a towel and apply emollient immediately to all skin.
  - Apply prescription topical medicines to affected areas.
- Inflammation is best treated with corticosteroids.
  - Generally, ointments tend to work better than creams.
    - Ointments remain the choice for chronic dermatitis in which dryness and lichenification predominate.
  - Creams
    - Sometimes preferred for cosmetic appeal
    - Can be used for acute weeping, erythematous lesions
- Treatment of complicated cases
  - If flares continue despite compliance with medication and appropriate skin care, a secondary infection may be responsible that requires treatment.
  - Many patients have significant colonization with *Staphylococcus aureus.*
    - If *S aureus* superinfection occurs, hospitalization for aggressive care and intravenous antibiotics may be required.
    - Skin cultures may help identify appropriate antibiotic sensitivities.
    - Application of nasal mupirocin may be necessary to eradicate bacterial carriage.
  - May also require treatment for herpes simplex virus, human papillomavirus (HPV), and molluscum contagiosum

SPECIFIC TREATMENTS

Steroids

- Low-potency topical agents, such as 1% hydrocortisone or desonide:
  - Can be used for mild disease, even on the diaper area and face
  - Twice-daily dosing should be limited to a 2-week course or less.
- Mid- to high-potency steroids, such as triamcinolone or fluocinonide:
  - Can be used in more severe cases on the trunk and extremities
- Strong, halogenated steroids:
  - Should not be applied to the face, axillae, or groin
  - Oral systemic steroid taper should rarely be prescribed.
- Most worrisome side effects
  - Dermal and epidermal atrophy
  - Suppression of the pituitary-adrenal axis
  - Applying topical steroids to the occluded groin area of a diapered child increases the risk of systemic side effects.

Nonsteroidal immunomodulators and other topical medications

- Topical tacrolimus and pimecrolimus
  - Approved for children ≥2 years of age
  - Most efficacious in mild to moderate disease
  - Alternatives to topical steroids
  - Can be applied to the face
  - Theoretical risk of cancer
- Other topical medications, coal tar and doxepin, are not routinely prescribed by pediatricians.

Pharmacologic therapy

- Antihistamines may help relieve pruritus, especially if dermatitis accompanies allergic rhinitis, urticaria, and sleep disturbance.
  - Nonsedating antihistamines, such asloratadine, can be used daily.
  - The sedating antihistamines, hydroxyzine and diphenhydramine, are most useful at bedtime.
- Efficacy of alternative medicine, such as herbal or probiotic supplementation, remains unknown.

Behavior modification

- Teach the child to rub rather than scratch.
- Have the child wear mittens or socks on his or her hands when in bed at night to reduce the itch-scratch cycle.
- Trim the fingernails frequently to avoid trauma and infection.

Diet

- Dietary management is controversial, and changes should be made judiciously.
- Peanuts, milk, and eggs are the most common food culprits.
- If food allergies are highly likely, as determined by a pediatric allergist, then strict avoidance of foods that serve as antigenic triggers should be encouraged; the most common are:
  - Cow milk
  - Hen eggs
  - Soy
  - Peanuts
  - Tree nuts (and seeds)
  - Wheat
  - Fish and shellfish

Secondary infections

- Topical or oral antibiotics
  - Cephalexin
  - Dicloxacilli
  - Amoxicillin-clavulanate
  - Azithromycin
  - Clindamycin
  - Mupirocin(topical)

- HPV treatments
- Vesicants
- Immunomodulators
- Cryotherapy
- Ablation with carbon dioxide laser
- Molluscum contagiosum treatments
  - Manual expression
  - Cryotherapy
  - Topical application of cantharidin or imiquimod
- Widespread herpes infection requires treatment with intravenous acyclovir.

Aggressive interventions for severe cases

- Prescribed at the discretion of the skin experts
  - Systemic immunomodulators
  - Ultraviolet light therapy

WHEN TO ADMIT

- Severe cases requiring systemic immunomodulation
- Extensive secondary bacterial infection requiring intravenous antibiotics
- Widespread herpes infection (eczema herpeticum, Kaposi varicelliform eruption)

WHEN TO REFER

- Recalcitrant cases should be referred to a dermatologist or allergist.
- Secondary HPV or molluscum contagiosum infections should be referred to a dermatologist for aggressive treatment.

COMPLICATIONS

- *S aureus* superinfection
  - Hospitalization for aggressive care and intravenous antibiotics may be required.
  - Skin cultures may help identify antibiotic sensitivities.
  - Application of nasal mupirocin may be necessary to eradicate bacterial carriage.
- Herpes infection, known as eczema herpeticum or Kaposi varicelliform eruption:
  - Requires treatment with intravenous acyclovir.
- HPV infection
- Molluscum contagiosum infection

PREVENTION

- AD cannot be prevented, but meticulous adherence to proper skin care can control symptoms and secondary infection.
- Moisturization of the skin with daily applications of emollients, especially after bathing, is crucial to keep the skin hydrated.
- Prophylactic avoidance of food allergens, both for lactating mothers and infants via exclusive breastfeeding in the first 6 months of life, may be helpful in families with a strong family history of atopy.

Attention-Deficit/Hyperactivity Disorder

DEFINITION

- Attention-deficit/hyperactivity disorder (ADHD) is a common neurodevelopmental disorder in children and adolescents.
- Frequently diagnosed in children with academic under-achievement or behavioral problems
- Hallmarks are hyperactivity, impulsivity, and inattention that are beyond normal developmental expectations for a child's age.
- Core symptoms interfere with attainment of many normal developmental milestones (academic, fine-motor, and social and adaptive skills).

EPIDEMIOLOGY

- Prevalence
  - 6.8% of school-age children
- Sex
  - Diagnosed in boys 3 times more than in girls (9.2% vs 3.0%)
- Age
  - Rates of diagnosed ADHD increase with age up to 9 years of age.
  - Rates level off or decline, depending on whether youth are taking medications.
- Race/ethnicity
  - Diagnosed in white children at a greater rate than in black or Hispanic children (8.6% vs 7.7% and 3.7%, respectively).

ETIOLOGY

- Whether the symptoms of ADHD represent a unique disor-der or merely one end of the continuum of age-appropriate behavior is unclear.
- Data supporting ADHD as a unique disorder
  - Cohort studies have consistently shown similar long-term outcomes for youth identified with ADHD (predictive validity).
  - Twin studies suggest a genetic predisposition.
  - Genetic studies have shown higher rates of gene alterations involving dopamine neurotransmission in people with ADHD.
  - Brain imaging and physiologic studies suggest a neuro-developmental process leading to ADHD.
- Psychosocial and environmental factors may contribute.

RISK FACTORS

- Coexisting conditions
  - Oppositional defiant disorder (average prevalence rate, 35.2%)
  - Conduct disorder (25.7%)
  - Mood disorders

- Anxiety disorders (25.8%)
- Depressive disorders (18.2%)
- Learning disabilities (12–50%)

SIGNS AND SYMPTOMS

- *Diagnostic and Statistical Manual of Mental Disorders, Fourth Edition (DSM-IV)* criteria for diagnosis
  - Either 1 or 2 of the following 3 overarching criteria
    - 1. ≥6 of the following symptoms of inattention, persistent for ≥6 months, to a degree that is maladaptive and inconsistent with developmental level
      - Often fails to give close attention to details or makes careless mistakes in school work, work, or other activities
      - Often has difficulty sustaining attention in tasks or play activities
      - Often does not seem to listen when spoken to directly
      - Often does not follow through on instructions and fails to finish schoolwork, chores, or duties in the workplace (not caused by oppositional behavior or failure to understand instructions)
      - Often has difficulty organizing tasks and activities
      - Often avoids, dislikes, or is reluctant to engage in tasks that require sustained mental effort (eg, school-work, homework)
      - Often loses things necessary for tasks or activities (eg, toys, school assignments, pencils, books, tools)
      - Is often easily distracted by extraneous stimuli
      - If often forgetful in daily activities
    - 2. ≥6 of the following symptoms of hyperactivity or impulsivity have persisted for ≥6 months to a degree that is maladaptive and inconsistent with developmental level
      - Often fidgets with hands or feet or squirms in seat
      - Often leaves seat in classroom or in other situations in which remaining seated is expected
      - Often runs about or climbs excessively in situations in which doing so is inappropriate (in adolescents or adults, may be limited to subjective feelings of restlessness)
      - Often has difficulty playing or engaging in leisure activities quietly
      - Is often on the go or often acts as if driven by a motor
      - Often talks excessively
      - Often blurts out answers before the questions have been completed
      - Often has difficulty awaiting his or her turn
      - Often interrupts or intrudes on others (eg, butts into conversations or games)

- Some hyperactive-impulsive or inattentive symptoms causing impairments were present before 7 years of age.
- Some impairment from the symptoms is present in ≥2 settings (eg, at school [or work] or at home).
- Clear evidence exists of clinically significant impairment in social, academic, or occupational functioning.
- Symptoms do not occur exclusively during the course of:
  - A pervasive developmental disorder
  - Schizophrenia
  - Other psychotic disorder
- Symptoms are not better accounted for by another mental disorder, such as:
  - Mood disorder
  - Anxiety disorder
  - Dissociative disorder
  - Personality disorder
- The *DSM-IV* criteria do not account for differences in presentation by age, sex, or race/ethnicity; clinicians must exercise judgment in their use of the criteria.
- Any symptoms suggestive of possible harm to self or others warrant immediate evaluation by a skilled clinician.

DIFFERENTIAL DIAGNOSIS

- Conditions that may mimic or co-occur with ADHD
  - Developmental differences or normal variants
    - Normal variation
    - Giftedness
    - Sociocultural differences in expectations or parenting, or both
  - Medical disorders
    - Medication side effects
    - Substances of abuse
    - Hearing impairment
    - Visual impairment
    - Obstructive sleep apnea
    - Toxins (eg, chronic lead exposure or acute lead intoxication; chronic iron-deficiency anemia)
    - Thyroid disorders
    - Chronic disease complications
  - Neurologic or developmental disorders
    - Learning disabilities
    - Pervasive developmental disorders
    - Tic disorders (Tourette syndrome)
    - Communication disorders
    - Processing disorders
    - Mental retardation

- Neurodevelopmental syndromes (eg, fetal alcohol syndrome, fragile X syndrome)
- Cerebral palsy
- Seizure disorders (petit mal or developmental delays)
- Sequelae of central nervous system trauma or infection
- Neurodegenerative disorders
- Motor coordination disorders
- Psychosocial or environmental problems
  - Stress in family situation (marriage, separation or divorce, birth of sibling, death)
  - Stress in environment (new home, new school)
  - Family dysfunction
  - Parenting dysfunction
  - Neglect, abuse, or both
  - Parental psychopathology
  - Parental substance abuse
  - Inappropriate educational program
- Emotional or behavioral disorders
  - Oppositional defiant disorder
  - Conduct disorder
  - Depressive disorders
  - Anxiety disorders
  - Bipolar disorder
  - Obsessive-compulsive disorder
  - Posttraumatic stress disorder
  - Adjustment reaction
  - Schizophrenia

DIAGNOSTIC APPROACH

- No biological marker or gold standard diagnostic test exists that can reliably identify persons with and without ADHD.
- Ascertain whether any other disorders or factors exist that may better explain a child's symptoms and impairment.
  - Such conditions may:
    - Be the primary cause of the child's behavioral and attention difficulties
    - Increase the child's level of impairment if comorbid with ADHD
  - Evaluation can be streamlined through a complete history and thorough physical examination.
- The AAP recommends that children age 6–12 years should undergo evaluation for ADHD if they exhibit any of the following.
  - Inattention
  - Hyperactivity
  - Impulsivity

A

- Academic underachievement
- Behavior problems
- Diagnosing ADHD is complicated by the fact that presentations of ADHD can vary substantially.
- Core symptoms result in 3 distinct subtypes of ADHD recognized in the *DSM-IV Text Revision (TR)*:
  - Predominantly inattentive subtype (ADHD-IA)
  - Hyperactive/impulsive subtype (ADHD-HI)
  - Subtype that includes a combination of both inattentive and hyperactive/impulsive features (ADHD-CT)
  - In addition, many conditions can coexist with ADHD, further adding to variation in presentation.
- Essential step: comprehensive history, with particular attention to:
  - Presenting complaint
  - Development
  - School history
  - Family history
  - Social history
- Physical examination (usually normal)
  - Can help identify other problems that may contribute to or represent the cause of behavior problems
  - May allow the opportunity to assess a child's mental status and interaction with caregivers
- Several excellent ADHD rating scales for parent and teacher respondents are commercially available to clinicians.
  - Vanderbilt Rating Scales
    - Available in the public domain at no cost
  - ADHD Rating Scale
  - Conners' Rating Scales
  - Swanson, Nolan, and Pelham (SNAP) Rating Scales
- There are often co-occurring behavioral or developmental conditions; all youth undergoing an evaluation for ADHD should be assessed for these conditions.
  - Take a complete history.
  - Several ADHD ratings scales (ie, Vanderbilt, Conners' Rating Scales and SNAP-IV) include items that query for symptoms of depression or anxiety, oppositional-defiant, and conduct disorders.
  - Rating scales exist that specifically target the assessment of particular conditions including depression, anxiety, and disruptive behaviors.
    - Center for Epidemiological Studies Depression Scale for Children
    - Multidimensional Anxiety Scale for Children
    - Eyberg Child Behavior Inventory

- Questionnaires that review *DSM-IV TR* criteria for most common childhood mental health disorders in 1 instrument
  - Child Symptom Inventory
  - DISC Predictive Scales
- Algorithm to assess ADHD
  - **Step 1:** Patients with behavior problems or academic difficulties undergo a complete physical examination, including hearing and vision assessments, and are given assessment materials.
    - Assessment materials may contain:
      - Pediatric intake history form
      - Request for school records
      - Behavior rating scales
      - Educational materials
  - **Step 2:** Once the results and assessment materials have been reviewed, patients may be scheduled for an evaluation.
    - Number of visits needed to complete an evaluation depends on the complexity of symptoms and amount of time available at each visit.
    - The time reported to complete the overall evaluation, review background records, provide patient and family education, and establish a treatment plan may be 90–240 minutes.
    - Offices have found multiple solutions for obtaining assessment materials and completing an evaluation, including:
      - Use of written assessment or computerized packets
      - Longer appointments scheduled at designated times (eg, evenings, Saturday mornings, one particular clinic session every other week)
      - Partnerships with local schools
      - Use of affiliated health care personnel, including social workers or mental health professionals
    - ADHD toolkit includes:
      - Vanderbilt Rating Scales (both parent and teacher initial assessment and follow-up forms)
      - Sample cover letter to assist physicians in creating an office-based system for efficiently evaluating a child for ADHD.
- Clinicians should obtain data from schools on children's level of functioning and academic achievement.
  - Results of multidisciplinary evaluations
  - Individual educational programs (IEPs)
  - Achievement test results
  - Grades
  - Written or verbal teacher narratives

- Many ADHD rating scales use teacher versions that can be used to facilitate endorsement of diagnostic criteria or to assess for other conditions by school or after-school personnel.
- If the child is home schooled or heavily involved in after-school activities, clinicians may want to obtain information from adults overseeing these programs (coaches, religious educators, after-school caregivers, and tutors).

LABORATORY FINDINGS

- Blood lead levels and thyroid hormone levels are infrequently abnormal in youth with ADHD.
  - There is little evidence that these tests adequately discriminate between youth with and without ADHD.

IMAGING

- Youth with ADHD often have abnormalities on brain imaging or electroencephalography.
  - Abnormalities are not consistent.
  - Do not usually represent clinically significant findings
  - Do not adequately discriminate youth with and without ADHD

CLASSIFICATION

- ADHD can be classified as the following 3 types.
  - Predominantly inattentive subtype (ADHD-IA)
  - Hyperactive/impulsive subtype (ADHD-HI)
  - A combination of both inattentive and hyperactive/impulsive features (ADHD-CT)

TREATMENT APPROACH

- ADHD is a chronic condition that requires ongoing, collaborative care.
  - ADHD affects youth across multiple domains of functioning, and understanding the implications across these domains is important.
  - Parents are important partners in treatment because they ultimately implement any program.
  - Youth with ADHD are often cared for by a spectrum of health and school professionals; the child eventually has to take all of this over.
  - Strategies include educational and support groups, such as:
    – Children and Adults with ADD
    – Learning Disabilities Association
- The AAP recommends that clinicians, parents, and the child, with school personnel, identify specific target outcomes in functioning that they hope to affect with treatment.

- 3 broad treatment modalities have been recommended, most often combined (multimodal treatment).
  - Medications
  - Psychosocial interventions directed at the child in the home and school
  - Classroom assistance
  - Solid evidence exists for the use of stimulant medication, behavioral-modification strategies, and their combination.
- If psychostimulants are used, medication choice, dose, and time interval must be carefully titrated to meet the individual child's needs.
  - Several trials may be necessary before the most effective medication type and dose with the fewest side effects are identified.
  - It is important to document changes in ADHD symptoms and target outcomes, and the development of any side effects.
- Behavioral-management interventions that seek to improve parenting practices, school function, and peer relationships decrease ADHD symptoms and impairment.
  - Parent training programs
  - Youth-focused intensive summer camp programs
  - Behavioral consultation in the classroom
- School-based services are a critical part of a comprehensive management plan.
  - Communication with school personnel is essential for diagnosing ADHD and for optimal titration of medication.
  - Evidence exists for effectiveness of highly structured behavioral-management strategies implemented by school staff, such as:
    – Daily report cards
    – Point or token systems with primary outcomes of:
      - Following classroom rules
      - Complying with teacher requests
      - Improving peer interactions
      - Increasing classwork productivity
  - Comorbid learning disabilities can be identified by school staff.
    – Specific learning interventions require an IEP, as stipulated under the Individuals with Disabilities Education Act (IDEA).
    – Learning disabilities coexistent with ADHD usually fall into the category of language-based disorders of learning or impaired mathematics performance.
- It is important to educate school personnel about ADHD-associated behaviors.
  - Motor challenges, including dysgraphia, with resultant poor handwriting
  - Problems related to poor visual-motor abilities (eg, copying materials off of a board or textbook onto paper)

A

- Inconsistent performance
- Delayed acquisition of core reading and math skills
- Low productivity
- Delay in rapid retrieval of facts
- Difficulty with higher-level problem solving involving multiple steps
- Impaired reading comprehension
- Poor meta-cognitive abilities (eg, organization, time management, breaking tasks down into smaller components)

■ Most alternative treatment approaches lack real evidence for or against their use.
  - Dietary recommendations
  - Ocular training
  - Hypnotic and biofeedback regimens

SPECIFIC TREATMENTS

General

■ Psychostimulants (methylphenidate, dextroamphetamine, and mixed salts ofamphetamine) with careful medication management:
  - Address core symptoms and improve sustained attention, organization, and motor inhibitor control
  - Decrease disruptive behaviors (eg, fidgetiness, impulsive interrupting, aggression, relational interactions, oppositionality)
  - Increase the accuracy of performance and improve short-term memory, reaction time, and seatwork computation; however, the effect is smaller than that seen for behavioral challenges
  - Are effective for about 70%; increases to >90% if an alternative stimulant is tried after initial failure
  - Children starting on medication should have a complete medical history taken (including a family history of heart disease or arrhythmias, as well as symptoms of shortness of breath, chest pain, dizziness, or palpitations on exertion) and a physical examination.

Stimulant medications, dosing, and duration of effects

■ Dextroamphetamine/levoamphetamine
  - Adderall (scored tablet)
    - Start with 5 mg 1–2 times per day and increase by 5 mg each week until good control is achieved.
    - Maximal recommended dose: 40 mg
    - Duration of effect: 4–6 hours
  - Adderall RX (capsule; sprinkle-able)
    - Start at 5 mg in the morning and increase by 5 mg each week until good control is achieved.
    - Maximal recommended dose: 30 mg
    - Duration of effect: 10–12 hours

■ Dextroamphetamine
  - Dexedrine (tablet) or Dextrostat (scored tablet)
    - Start with 5 mg 1–2 times per day and increase by 5 mg each week until good control is achieved.
    - Maximal recommended dose: 40 mg
    - Duration of effect: 4–6 hours
  - Dexedrine Spansules (sustained-release capsule)
    - Start with 5 mg once daily and increase by 5 mg each week until good control is achieved.
    - Duration of effect: 6–10 hours

■ Methylphenidate
  - Ritalin or Methylin (scored tablet, chewable, or oral solution)
    - Start with 5 mg 1–2 times per day and increase by 5 mg each week until good control is achieved.
    - May need a third reduced dose in the evening
    - Maximal recommended dose: 60 mg
  - Focalin (scored tablet)
    - Start with 2.5 mg 1–2 times per day and increase by 2.5 mg each week until good control is achieved.
    - May need a third reduced dose in the evening
    - Maximal recommended dose: 30 mg
    - Duration of effect: 4–5 hours
  - Ritalin-LA (capsule; sprinkle-able), Ritalin-SR (tablet), Metadate-ER (tablet), Metadate-CE (capsule; sprinkle-able)
    - Start with 10–20 mg in the morning and increase each week until good control is achieved.
    - Alternatively, titrate using short-acting methylphenidate and then switch over to a longer-acting form.
    - May need a second dose or regular methylphenidate dose in the evening
    - Maximal recommended dose: 60 mg
    - Duration of effect: 6–10 hours
  - Focalin XR (capsule; sprinkle-able)
    - Start with 5 mg in the morning and increase by 5 mg each week until good control is achieved.
    - Maximal recommended dose: 30 mg
    - Duration of effect: 8–10 hours
  - Concerta (capsule; noncrushable)
    - Start at 18 mg in the morning and increase by 18 mg each week until good control is achieved.
    - Maximal recommended dose: 72 mg
    - Duration of effect: 8–12 hours
  - Daytrana (patch)
    - Worn daily for 9 hours; replace once a day in the morning

- Skin sensitization as compared with contact rash may occur rarely; the US Food and Drug Administration advisory board recommends oral methylphenidate use before the patch.
    - 12 hours
- Lisdexamfetamine
    - Vyvanse (sprinkle in water and immediately drink)
        - Start at 30 mg in the morning and increase by 20 mg each week until good control is achieved.
        - Maximal recommended dose: 70 mg
        - Duration of effect: 12 hours

Risks

- Common side effects
    - Headaches
    - Stomachaches
    - Insomnia
    - Anorexia
    - Possible growth delay (approximately 1 cm in height lost per year)
    - Irritability
    - Emotional lability or constriction
    - Compulsive picking of the nose or skin
    - Possible high abuse potential
- Other safety concerns
    - Cardiovascular
        - Elevations in heart rate and blood pressure
        - Rare events, such as stroke, myocardial infarction, and sudden death, particularly in youth with preexisting cardiac disease
        - Youth should be monitored for the emergence of hypertension
    - Psychiatric concerns
        - New onset or acute exacerbation of aggressive symptoms
        - Rare hallucinogenic symptoms, particularly visual hallucinations related to bugs

Management of side effects

- General
    - For mild side effects, allow 7–10 days for tolerance to develop.
    - Evaluate time-action, and determine whether timing of administration can be adjusted to minimize side effects.
    - Determine whether side effects are related to other disorders or current environmental stressors and adjust accordingly.
    - If these strategies fail, consider an alternative stimulant.

- Weight loss or anorexia
    - Administer medication during or after a meal.
    - Try calorie enhancement strategies, such as high-protein instant breakfasts or protein bars.
    - Get eating started with any highly preferred food before giving regular foods.
    - Allow grazing in the evening when appetite suppression wanes.
    - Change stimulant medications.
    - Consider drug holidays.
- Dizziness
    - Monitor blood pressure and pulse.
    - Encourage adequate hydration.
    - If dizziness is associated only with peak drug effect, try a longer-acting preparation.
- Insomnia or nightmares
    - Establish bedtime routine.
    - Omit or reduce the last dose or change to the standard, short-acting version if the patient is using longer-acting preparation.
    - Administer medication earlier in the day.
    - Try a different stimulant.
    - Give "Sleep Problems" handout (sample available at www.dbpeds.org).
    - Consider additional medication as a last resort.
- Dysphoric mood/emotional constriction
    - If the problem occurs during peak drug effect, reduce the dose or switch to a longer-acting preparation.
    - Evaluate when it occurs.
    - Try a different stimulant.
    - Consider comorbid anxiety or depression disorders requiring alternative or adjunctive treatment.
    - Consider additional medication as a last resort.
- Rebound
    - Try to decrease precipitous drop in blood levels by:
        - Using a stepped-down dose at the end of the day
        - Increasing morning long-acting dose
        - Adding a smaller dose of short-acting medication toward the end of the day
    - Switch to a longer-acting preparation.
    - Combine longer-acting and short-acting preparations.
    - Overlap stimulant dosing.

A

- Tics
  - Conduct drug trial at different doses, including no medication, to be sure that tics are drug related.
  - For mild tics that abate after 7–10 days, reconsider risk versus benefit and negotiate a new informed consent with the parent or guardian.
  - Conduct a drug trial to see whether tics abate with another stimulant.
  - Consider a nonstimulant treatment, such asclonidine, alone or in combination with a stimulant.
  - Refer to a mental health specialist or neurologist skilled in the management of tics.
- Psychosis
  - Discontinue stimulant treatment.
  - Assess for presence of coexisting bipolar or thought disorder.
  - Consider alternative treatments, or referral to mental health specialist.

Other medications

- Other medications used as second-line treatment of ADHD:
- Selective norepinephrine reuptake inhibitor (atomoxetine)
  - Common side effects
    - Stomachache
    - Nausea
    - Appetite suppression
    - Weight loss
  - Warnings have surfaced regarding aggression, suicidality, reversible hepatotoxicity, and cardiac effects
- Tricyclic antidepressants (desipramine, nortryptiline)
  - Low toxic-to-therapeutic ratio has limited widespread use
- Atypical antidepressants (bupropion)
  - Suggested as an option in youth with comorbid depression
- α-Agonists (clonidine and guanfacine)
  - Moderate effects on hyperactivity and impulsivity, aggression, and tics
  - Given their effect on the cardiovascular system, care must be taken to avoid stopping these medications abruptly, which might result in rebound hypertension.
  - Sedation, particularly with clonidine, can be a significant problem.

Behavioral techniques

- In combination with medication, may allow reduction of the medication dose.
- Therapeutic benefits of stimulant medication usually occur during the day, whereas behavioral interventions may be used in the late afternoon or evening in place of an additional dose of medication.

- Disruptive disorders that commonly co-occur with ADHD have been shown to respond to behavioral modification.
- Psychosocial treatment may help to enhance parents' positive perception of their children and of their own parenting abilities.
- Results for medication last only as long as a youth continues to take the medication, whereas behavioral interventions may extend over time.
- Medications may be more expensive than behavioral interventions in the long run.
- Specific techniques
  - Positive reinforcement
    - Provide rewards or privileges contingent on the child's performance.
  - Time-out
    - Remove access to positive reinforcement contingent on performance of unwanted or problem behavior.
  - Response cost
    - Withdraw rewards or privileges contingent on the performance of unwanted or problem behavior.
  - Token economy
    - Combining positive reinforcement and response cost.
    - The child earns rewards and privileges contingent on performing desired behaviors and loses rewards and privileges based on undesirable behavior (eg, working toward a prize).

WHEN TO ADMIT

- The core symptoms of ADHD should not necessitate admission to a medical or psychiatric hospital.
- Indications for admission result from:
  - Symptoms related to mental health conditions that may co-occur with ADHD
  - Adverse event secondary to medication used to treat ADHD
  - A medical condition resulting from the core symptoms of inattention, hyperactivity, or impulsivity associated with ADHD (eg, accidental injury)

WHEN TO REFER

- Refer to a mental health or school-based professional if:
  - A comorbid condition is suspected
  - A clinician is not equipped to evaluate sufficiently for these types of disorders in the office setting
  - Results of assessment are discrepant or complicated clinical picture exists and the primary care physician is uncomfortable continuing evaluation
  - Psychological testing is needed
  - Intensive parent training in behavior modification is needed

- Coexisting conditions that are unresponsive to treatment for ADHD are present (oppositionality, depression, and anxiety may improve with treatment of ADHD core symptoms)
  - Psychosocial or pharmacologic interventions for a coexisting mental health disorder
  - Significant familial stress or psychopathology
    - Domestic violence
    - Substance abuse
- A mental health resource list can help identify local mental health care providers on the family's insurance plan who can evaluate the youth for possible comorbid mental health disorders.
- Bright Futures provides a template for mental health referrals that can be used to structure referral information.
- For school referrals, parents should be directed to draft a letter requesting a multidisciplinary evaluation, including psychoeducational testing, if the history suggests a possible learning disability, such as:
  - Reading disorder (dyslexia)
  - Mathematics disorder (dyscalculia)
  - Disorder of written expression
  - Communication disorder
- Public schools are required to respond to family requests for evaluations within a specified period (determined by school district policies).
- Children attending private schools or those who are home schooled are eligible to receive an evaluation through their local school district.
- Families may be referred to independent psychologists for psychoeducational evaluations through their insurance plans.
  - Clinicians should inquire whether the local school district accepts outside evaluations before making any referrals.

FOLLOW-UP

- Youth functioning should be systematically monitored over time to evaluate whether target outcomes are achieved or adverse side effects to treatment develop.
  - If targeted outcomes are not met, the clinician, parents, and school personnel should collaboratively determine:
    - Validity of the diagnosis
    - Adherence to all components of the treatment plan
    - Possibility of previously unidentified coexisting conditions
  - The ADHD toolkit includes sample management plans and follow-up assessment forms to assist clinicians in monitoring treatment.

- Once a child is stable on a medication, AAP treatment guidelines recommend an office visit every 3–6 months to reassess
  - Academic performance
  - Behavior
  - Side effects
- More intensive visits may be necessary around predictable periods of change.
  - Entry into middle or high school
  - Onset of puberty
- Trials off medication are important to conduct but should be scheduled so as to not overlap with
  - Beginning of school terms
  - Examinations
  - Family stressors
- Families, youth, and clinicians should consider carefully using medication in the afternoons and evenings, on weekends, and during the summer.
  - Take into account:
    - Severity of a youth's dysfunction
    - Effect on family and peers
    - Cultural expectations
    - Presence of any decrease in weight or height velocity
- School-based services
  - Youth can access school-based services through local public school system
    - Individual teachers will often modify curriculum or classroom environment to address a child's needs.
    - Many schools have an interdisciplinary council (eg, student study team, multidisciplinary assessment team) that informally reviews a child's academic performance and behavior and suggests possible remediation.
    - Through Section 504 of the Rehabilitation Act, school systems are mandated to provide accommodations in the mainstream classroom.
    - Under IDEA, school systems provide a continuum of special education services, ranging from accommodations in the mainstream classroom to a special day class in a public or private, nonpublic placement.
    - Youth with ADHD often qualify for special education services because of a coexisting specific learning disability, language disorder, or severe emotional disturbance.
      - Organizational difficulties may require:
        - Supervision of the writing of homework assignments in a planner
        - Extra set of books at home
        - Assistance breaking large projects into small steps

A

- Approaches to problems with handwriting
  - Access to a computer for written work
  - Copies of teacher lectures
  - Electronically recorded textbooks
  - If behavior interferes with the child's academic performance or the ability of other children in the classroom to learn, then a behavioral intervention plan is necessary that delineates:
    - What behaviors a youth displays
    - Factors that escalate or dampen the behavior
    - Appropriate behavioral interventions
- Consideration should be given to the appropriate educational placement of a child.
  - Mainstream classroom with or without assistance from a resource specialist
  - Special day class
  - Private nonpublic placement
- Sample letters requesting a 504 plan or IEP, as well as additional information on these programs, are available in the ADHD toolkit and on the Bright Futures Web site.
- Concerns exist that these accommodations may lead to youth who feel entitled to extra assistance and will not be able to function adequately in college or the workplace setting.
  - Accommodations must be provided within the context of teaching the child to understand his or her own strengths and weaknesses
  - The child needs to develop compensatory strategies for addressing their areas of challenge.

PROGNOSIS

- Youths with ADHD who have been monitored into adolescence demonstrated increased risk for:
  - Poor academic attainment
  - Impaired familial and peer functioning
  - Lower self-esteem
  - Substance abuse
  - Delinquency
  - Driving-related accidents
- Treatment may ameliorate some risks, particularly for substance abuse.
- Age-dependent decline appears to exist in apparent symptoms as children grow older.
  - Hyperactivity and impulsivity tend to remit at a greater rate than inattention.
- As many as 70% of children and adolescents continue to be symptomatic in adulthood, but outcomes are improved with:
  - Familial stability and support
  - Ongoing therapeutic relationships with a health care professional
  - Higher IQ

Autism

DEFINITION

- Autism is a neurobiological developmental disorder characterized by:
  - Developmental delays in language and communication
  - Abnormalities in language
  - Impairments in social behavior
  - Narrow repertoire of interests
  - Ritualized behavior

EPIDEMIOLOGY

- Prevalence
  - 100–200 per 100,000 children
  - More common in boys than in girls

ETIOLOGY

- No known, single cause has been found.
- There is increasing evidence for a genetic link.
  - May affect neurologic development as early as the prenatal period

RISK FACTORS

- Medical and genetic conditions associated with autism
  - Fragile X syndrome
  - Cornelia de Lange syndrome
  - Tuberous sclerosis

SIGNS AND SYMPTOMS

History

- Medical history
  - Birth and neonatal history
  - History of seizures
  - Hyperactivity (extreme)
  - Pica
  - Family history of autism or mental retardation
- Developmental history
  - Milestones may be delayed.
  - Regression in development can occur.
- Psychosocial history
  - Irritability
  - Self-injury possible
  - Feeding or sleeping problems frequent

Physical examination

- Head circumference
  - Sometimes larger than in nonautistic children

- Motor impairments may include:
  - Hand flapping
  - Hypotonia
  - Limb apraxia
- Rule out tuberous sclerosis.
  - Neurocutaneous disorder affecting the brain and other organs
  - Present in 0.4–3% of children with autism
  - Expose to ultraviolet light and observe for ash-leaf–shaped depigmented macules; this is diagnostic.

Screening and evaluation standardized instruments

- Autism Diagnostic Interview: Revised
  - For children 18 months to adulthood
  - Semistructured parent interview provides comprehensive information.
  - Requires specialized training to administer
  - >1 hour required to complete
- Autism Diagnostic Observation Schedule
  - For children 18 months to adulthood
  - A trained examiner observes child-adult interactions and codes behaviors.
  - Requires specialized training to administer
  - 30 minutes to complete
- Modified Checklist for Autism in Toddlers
  - For children 18 months old to 30 months old
  - Parent or teacher questionnaire
  - Widely used in research and clinical settings for screening
  - Lacks specificity as a diagnostic measure
  - 5 minutes to complete
- Pervasive Developmental Disorders Behavior Inventory
  - For children 18 months to 12.5 years
  - Parent or teacher questionnaire
  - Comprehensive; may be sensitive to treatment effects
  - 30–45 minutes to complete
- Social Responsiveness Scale
  - For children 4–18 years
  - Parent or teacher questionnaire
  - Emphasizes social disability
  - 20 minutes to complete

DIFFERENTIAL DIAGNOSIS

- Autism spectrum disorders (ASDs)
  - Autistic disorder
    - Child meets full diagnostic criteria for:
      - Language (delayed or impaired)
      - Social interaction (impaired)
      - Repetitive, restricted behaviors

- Asperger disorder
  - Typical language development is present.
  - Impaired social interactions
  - Repetitive, restricted behaviors
- Pervasive developmental disorder not otherwise specified
  - Child presents with language delays; impaired social interaction; or restricted, repetitive behaviors.
  - However, these symptoms are not present to the degree that would warrant a more specific diagnosis.
- Pervasive developmental disorders that are not ASDs
  - Childhood disintegrative disorder
    - Children experience a period of developmental regression after at least 2 years of normal development.
  - Rett syndrome
    - Deceleration of head growth before 48 months
    - Loss of purposeful hand movements before 30 months
    - Development of stereotyped hand movements
    - Severe language and cognitive delays
    - Associated with mutations of the *MECP2* gene on the X chromosome
      - More common in girls than boys
- Developmental language disorder
  - Delays in receptive or expressive language skills
  - Social interaction skills are not impaired.
  - Children do not demonstrate repetitive, restricted behaviors.

DIAGNOSTIC APPROACH

- Diagnosis is not straightforward.
  - There is no single biological marker, laboratory test, or procedure to identify autism.
- Primarily a behavioral diagnosis, based on:
  - Comprehensive history
  - Direct observation
  - Standardized assessment
- Comorbid conditions with autism
  - Mental retardation
    - Reported in approximately 70% of children with autism
    - Children with autism and mental retardation have the poorest prognosis.
  - Seizures
  - Gastrointestinal problems
  - Sleep difficulties
  - Behavioral problems
    - Pica
    - Self-injury
    - Aggression

LABORATORY FINDINGS

- There is no single test for autism.
- Lead screening
  - Pica is a common comorbidity that is associated with lead toxicity.
- DNA analysis and karyotype testing
  - To rule out fragile X syndrome
- Metabolic and genetic testing should be considered in children with:
  - Unusual and dysmorphic features
  - Seizures
  - Abnormal growth
- Electrophysiologic testing is needed only in patients with:
  - Suspected seizure disorder
  - Severe sleep problems
  - Developmental regression

IMAGING

- No imaging evaluation procedures are needed in routine evaluation for autism.
- Standard assessment should be considered in children with co-occurring neurologic findings, including:
  - Seizures
  - Asymmetric motor functioning
  - Cranial nerve dysfunction
  - Severe headache

TREATMENT APPROACH

- General approach for managing ASDs
  - Screen to identify children at risk.
  - Refer to a specialist for evaluation.
  - Manage medical comorbidities.
  - Prescribe and manage psychopharmacologic medications.
  - Refer for psychosocial interventions.

SPECIFIC TREATMENTS

Psychopharmacologic treatment

- Behavioral problems present in autism can be partially managed with medication.
- Risperidone
  - Atypical antipsychotic
  - Used to treat irritability, aggression, self-injury, and tantrums
  - Approved by the US Food and Drug Administration for use in autism
- Fluoxetine, sertraline
  - Selective serotonin reuptake inhibitors
  - Used with limited success for rigidity and anxiety

- Stimulants, atomoxetine
  - Designed to improve attention and limit distractibility
  - Used with limited success

Psychosocial interventions

- Early intervention is critical.
  - Children age 2–7 years
- Highly intensive, behaviorally oriented programs
  - Known by several names
    - Applied behavior analysis
    - Discrete trial training
    - Intensive behavioral intervention
    - Early intensive behavioral intervention
  - Programs ideally offered for:
    - At least 2 years
    - 40 hours per week
    - One-on-one behavioral instruction
  - The literature is mixed, but targeted outcomes include:
    - Age-level functioning
    - Normal intelligence
    - Average adaptive behavior
    - Regular educational placement

WHEN TO ADMIT

- Severe malnutrition related to restricted food interests
- Evaluation for gastrointestinal problems
- Evaluation for seizure disorder
- Evaluation for sleep disorder
- Life-threatening self-injurious behavior or aggression
- Psychopharmacologic toxicity

WHEN TO REFER

- Refer to a developmental specialist if, at the age of 18–24 months, any of the following are present.
  - The child does not engage in simple pretend play.
  - The child does not point to objects of interest.
  - There is an inability to direct the child's attention.
  - The child has little interest in other children.
  - The child cannot follow simple instructions.
  - There is little or no expressive language, including:
    - Single words by 18 months
    - Phrases by 24 months

PROGNOSIS

- Prognosis has improved over the past 3 decades.
- For children with developmental disabilities
  - Increased availability of community special education services since the early 1980s
  - Decreased institutionalization
  - Increased access to learning experiences
- Parents, teachers, and health professionals have learned to advocate for children with developmental disabilities.
- Research into autism is a federal research priority.

A

Back Pain

DEFINITION

- Pain or discomfort in the region from the upper thoracic vertebra (T1) and shoulder girdle to the sacrum and surrounding musculature
- Patients may have a specific sense of localization (eg, to a muscle group or vertebral body), or sense the pain as diffuse or deep and difficult to localize.

EPIDEMIOLOGY

- Prevalence
  - Back pain is uncommon in pediatrics.
- Age
  - Most studies have shown that back pain increases with age.
    - <10% of preteens report back pain.
    - Nearly 50% of 18- to 20-year-olds have ≥1 episode of lower back pain.
  - A 6-year study in a tertiary orthopedic setting found:
    - Back pain constituted <2% of referrals in children age 15 years or younger, but roughly half of these children had serious underlying diseases.
  - From early adolescence onward:
    - Back pain becomes more common.
    - Back pain is more likely to be related to injury or repetitive stress.

MECHANISM

- Back pain has many potential mechanisms.
- In the context of febrile illness, strongly consider an infectious, inflammatory, or neoplastic process.
- Back pain may also be secondary (eg, to vasoocclusive changes from sickle cell disease, or a progressive anatomic or structural issue).
- Consider musculoskeletal and trauma-related causes, and that in older children pain may be functional.

History

History should ascertain:

- Description of pain: OLDCAR
  - **O**nset/precipitating event (eg, trauma)
  - **L**ocation (eg, midline, paraspinal)
  - **D**uration
  - **C**haracteristics, nature, or quality (continuous or not, severity, whether present when awakening from sleep)
  - **A**ssociated factors which improve or worsen (eg, activity)
  - **R**adiating pattern of pain
- Related neurologic findings

- Changes in urination or defecation
- Whether fever is present
  - Exposures to infectious agents (eg, tuberculosis)
  - Signs of systemic illness
    - Weight loss
    - Bone pain in other locations
    - Bruising
    - Organomegaly
    - Adenopathy
- Specific activities, especially those that require spinal extension (gymnastics, football); history of training
- Changes in activities, such as walking, play, sports activities
- Growth patterns/recent growth spurt
- Consider an evaluation of family and social factors if functional pain is in the differential diagnosis.
- Special considerations
  - Confirm pain history with others (parents, coaches, school personnel).
  - Children may minimize pain because of fear of procedures.
  - Children and adolescents usually do not use pain symptoms for secondary gain.

PHYSICAL EXAM

Physical examination considerations

- Vital signs
  - Temperature (febrile or not)
  - Pain may elevate the heart rate and blood pressure.
- Spinal examination
  - Palpate for step-offs.
  - See whether there is midline or paraspinal tenderness.
  - Straight leg-raising test
    - A positive result is highly suggestive of nerve root compression.
    - Using cervical flexion to accentuate the patient's symptoms may add to the test's sensitivity.
    - Any reproduction of the patient's usual symptoms during testing before 60 degrees of hip flexion, or marked asymmetry, should be considered a positive result.
    - Pain after 60 degrees or limited to the posterior thigh is more likely caused by hamstring tightness.
  - May evaluate for scoliosis
  - In case of trauma, check ABCs, C-spine, ribs, pelvic

stability and implement C-spine and other precautions as needed

- Neurologic evaluation: Evaluate the following at or below the suspected level of the lesion:
  - Motor function (including symmetry, strength, gait, coordination)
  - Sensation
  - Reflexes
  - Rectal sphincter tone
- Evaluate the skin for evidence of bruising or trauma.
- Check for the presence of organomegaly or lymphadenopathy.

Physical considerations particular to adolescents

- Look for excessive lordotic curvature, especially in children who perform repetitive spinal extension (eg, gymnasts, football linemen).
- Look for evidence of connective tissue disorders.
  - Hyperextensibility
  - Marfanoid body habitus
    - Joint hyperextensibility
    - Pectus excavatum
    - Pes planus
    - Dislocated lenses
    - Hernia
    - Arachnodactyly
    - Scoliosis
- Stork test: can pain be reproduced reliably by hyperextension of back while standing on one leg?
- Waddell test: presence of ≥3 of the following 5 criteria may help determine whether significant psychologic stress is associated with chronic low back pain.
  - Inappropriate tenderness that is superficial or widespread
  - Pain on pressing the top of the head or on passive rotation of shoulders and pelvis
  - Distraction signs, such as inconsistent performance between straight-leg raising in the seated and supine positions
  - Strength and sensory loss patterns that do not fit a directional distribution
  - Overreaction during the physical examination

DIFFERENTIAL DIAGNOSIS

All children

- Be aware of the relatively higher risk of serious underlying disease in younger children, even those without specific physical findings.
- Back pain before adolescence is uncommon.
- The combination of fever and back pain strongly suggests an infectious, inflammatory, or neoplastic process in all age groups.
- Fever in the setting of conditions below should prompt aggressive diagnostic evaluation for cancer.
  - Weight loss
  - Bone pain in other locations
  - Bruising
  - Organomegaly
  - Adenopathy
- Neurologic symptoms along with back pain may indicate lumbar disk herniation or other nerve compression.
- Idiopathic scoliosis usually does not cause back pain; thus, scoliosis with pain should raise concern for spinal tumor.

Infants (through 3rd or 4th year of life)

- Infants are not always capable of localizing or complaining about pain in the back.
- Differential diagnosis includes:
  - Diskitis
    - Unexplained fever or toxicity *and*
    - Refusal to walk or stand
  - Leukemia
  - Lymphoma
  - Vasoocclusive crisis
  - Vertebral osteomyelitis/epidural abscess, in a child with sickle cell disease
  - Trauma (especially intentional injury)
  - Pyelonephritis

Children

- Pyelonephritis
  - Consider with fever; costovertebral angle tenderness; dysuria; polyuria; urinary urgency; or cloudy, dark, or pink/red-tinged urine.
- Diskitis
  - Unusual, if not rare, condition
  - Most common in children <10 years
  - Typical discomfort in an upright posture
  - Refusal to walk or pain when bending forward
  - Even in the absence of fever, a child (especially preschool age) who refuses to walk should be evaluated for diskitis.
- Tethered cord
  - Back pain when walking may be the only sign at presentation.
  - Sacral dimple of unclear depth, hairy patch, or discoloration
  - Bowel or bladder issues
  - Lower extremity weakness
- Vertebral osteomyelitis

- Usually affects school-age children and teenagers
- Causes severe back pain and systemic symptoms
■ Ankylosing spondylitis
  - Consider with a family history of rheumatoid disease.
■ Vasoocclusive crisis
  - Consider in patients with sickle cell disease.
■ Leukemia, lymphoma
■ Primary vertebral tumors
  - Ewing sarcoma
  - Aneurysmal bone cyst
  - Benign osteoblastoma
  - Osteoid osteoma
■ Spinal tuberculosis (Pott disease)
  - Rare in US children; mainly occurs in children where tuberculosis is endemic
  - Consider if back pain is accompanied by low-grade fever.
■ Muscular or ligamentous strain in this age group should be considered only after a thorough diagnostic evaluation.

Adolescents

Acute pain (<3 weeks)
■ Lumbar disk disease
■ Muscle or ligament strain
■ Sciatica/piriformis syndrome
■ Vertebral osteomyelitis
■ Epidural abscess
■ Spinal tuberculosis
■ Pyelonephritis
  - Consider with fever; costovertebral angle tenderness; dysuria; polyuria; urinary urgency; or cloudy, dark, or pink/red-tinged urine.

Chronic pain (≥3 weeks)
■ Spondylolysis
  - One of the most common identifiable causes of low-back pain in this age group
  - Athletes participating in gymnastics, dance, cheerleading, football, and diving are at highest risk.
■ Spondylolisthesis (anterior movement of vertebral body on top of another, usually L5 on S1)
  - A result of bilateral spondylolysis
  - One of the most common identifiable causes of low-back pain in this age group
■ Scheuermann kyphosis (thoracolumbar spinal deformity with localized vertebral body changes)
■ Facet or vertebral dysfunction
■ Sacroiliac dysfunction

■ Lumbar disk disease
  - Especially in athletes or others with cumulative trauma
■ Spinal stenosis
■ Spondyloarthropathy
■ Tumor or cancer
  - Osteoid osteoma and osteoblastoma
    - Consider in cases of nocturnal back pain, even if relieved by nonprescription analgesics.
■ Muscular or ligamentous strain
  - Typical presentation
    - Lower back pain ≤3 weeks' duration
    - With or without recollection of an acute injury
  - Pain is exacerbated by lifting, stooping, and exercising.
  - May be caused by repetitive strain coupled with genetic predisposition and environmental factors, such as:
    - Studying or reading while sitting at a desk
    - Carrying an excessively heavy backpack (10–20% of body weight)
■ Functional (nonorganic) pain
■ Ankylosing spondylitis

LABORATORY EVALUATION
■ Complete blood count
■ Uric acid
■ Lactate dehydrogenase level
■ Erythrocyte sedimentation rate
■ Urinalysis and culture (if considering nephrolithiasis, urine calcium and creatinine)

IMAGING
■ Imaging is guided by clinical suspicion; options include:
■ Radiographs of the spine (anteroposterior [AP], lateral, oblique views)
■ Computed tomography (CT)
■ Magnetic resonance imaging (MRI)
■ Nuclear medicine imaging (bone scans)
■ Single-photon emission computed tomography (SPECT)
■ By suspected diagnoses:
■ Muscle or ligament strain
  - Studies not routinely indicated
■ Compression fracture (eg, after trauma such as motor vehicle accident, or athletic injury)
  - Spinal radiography (AP, lateral)
■ Diskitis

- Spinal radiography
- MRI as indicated
- Osteoid osteoma or osteoblastoma
  - Spinal radiography
    - Primary vertebral tumors almost always will be visible.
  - CT is the definitive study.
  - If radiography is inadequate, consider bone scan, CT, or MRI.
- Scheuermann disease
  - Spinal radiography (lateral)
    - Diagnosis is confirmed by anterior wedging of ≥3 contiguous vertebrae, by ≥5 degrees.
  - Consider oblique views, as associated with spondylolysis
- Spondylolysis
  - Spinal radiography (AP, lateral, oblique)
    - "Scotty dog with a collar" can be seen on the oblique view.
    - Normal radiography may not rule out the diagnosis.
  - Consider SPECT if the diagnosis is highly suggested.
  - A positive radiograph and negative SPECT indicates that spondylolysis not metabolically active (may not be the cause of back pain).
  - Back pain on extension with normal radiographs and positive SPECT usually indicates facet or vertebral dysfunction
- Spondylolisthesis
  - Spinal radiography (lateral)
    - Used to diagnose anterior slippage and to stage treatment
    - Rarely, may reveal congenital absence of a lumbosacral articular process

DIAGNOSTIC PROCEDURES

- In the case of vertebral osteomyelitis/epidural abscess, consider aspiration and culture.

TREATMENT APPROACH

- Consider whether pain is acute (<3 weeks) or chronic.
  - Acute pain, especially with a history of musculoskeletal injury, may be managed conservatively.
- Chronic pain demands further investigation.
- Back pain that results from an underlying disorder will probably require treatment of the primary condition, in addition to treatment of pain.
- Psychosocial or nonorganic causes should be considered if:
  - Thorough diagnostic evaluation of chronic back pain is unrevealing *and*

- Usual management involving exercise and stretching is not beneficial.
- As children and adolescents usually do not use pain symptoms for secondary gain, do not assume that pain is feigned; rather, assume that it represents a very real physical symptom rooted in psychologic or emotional distress.
  - This distress can be addressed openly by the clinician.
  - After diagnosis, remember to reconsider organic causes, especially if symptoms continue to evolve.

SPECIFIC TREATMENT

Diskitis

- Treatment depends on cause.
- Most experts recommend:
  - If bacterial cause, parenteral followed by oral antibiotics
  - Rest and pain management

Vertebral osteomyelitis/epidural abscess

- Prompt orthopedic surgery consultation
- Antibiotics (ensure staphylococcal coverage)
- Rest and pain management

Ankylosing spondylitis

- Best coordinated by a pediatric rheumatologist
- Antiinflammatories
- Physical and occupational therapy

Vasoocclusive crisis

- Careful evaluation and reassessment for acute chest syndrome and other related complications
- Hydration, red blood cell transfusion as indicated
- Pain management
- Physical therapy as indicated

Cancer, including leukemia, lymphoma, Ewing sarcoma

- Manage with a pediatric oncologist.

Osteoid osteoma

- Nonsteroidal antiinflammatory agents (NSAIDs)
- Refer to pediatric orthopedic surgery for possible excision

Musculoskeletal back pain

- For acute pain, think PRICEMMMS (**P**rotection, **R**est, **I**ce, **C**ompression, **E**levation, **M**edication, **M**otion, **M**odalities, **S**trength)
- For chronic pain, heat may be helpful.
- Discourage bed rest, as this may delay recovery.
- Teach proper posture.
- Pain-free activity may be resumed gradually.

B

- Backpack weights should not exceed 15–20% of the person's body weight.
- Exercises may be helpful.
  - Stretch after warming the muscles by gentle exercise
    - Improve flexibility of lower back and hamstrings
  - Strengthen core musculature (abdomen, hips, and back)
    - Abdominal muscle strengthening reduces pelvic tilt and decreases the tendency toward lordosis.
    - Strengthening spinal extensor muscles (eg, by raising the torso and head off the floor/exercise ball while lying prone) is recommended, as decreased strength and endurance of these muscles is associated with lower back pain.
  - May use an exercise ball or Pilates instruction
- Full sit-ups with fixed feet and bent knees should be discouraged.
  - Uses hip flexors rather than abdominal muscles
  - Increases intervertebral disk pressure
- Continuous frequency ultrasonography and massage may be helpful.

Spondylolysis

- Treatment is controversial and may be best managed with a pediatric sports medicine specialist or orthopedic surgeon.
- Provide symptomatic relief.
- Thoracolumbar bracing to prevent extension has been shown to be helpful; bracing should be used up to 6 months or until the patient is pain-free with extension.
- Some experts advocate restricting extension activities without a brace.
- Consider the Williams program: physical therapy that promotes abdominal strengthening and hamstring stretching.
- Bone stimulators have been used as adjunctive therapy.

Scheuermann disease

- Treatment is usually conservative.
  - Physical therapy: strengthening and stretching exercises
  - Avoid painful activities.
  - Analgesic medication if needed
- Thoracolumbar bracing and surgery may be indicated if kyphosis exceeds 60 degrees.
- Refer patients in whom conservative management fails, those

with intractable pain, or those in whom kyphosis progresses to orthopedic surgery (pediatric or spinal).

WHEN TO REFER

- Prompt and urgent evaluation and referral are needed when back pain is accompanied by:
  - Radicular pain down the leg
  - Numbness or tingling
  - Bowel or bladder problems
  - Erectile dysfunction
  - Loss of sphincter tone on rectal examination
  - High clinical suspicion of vertebral osteomyelitis/epidural abscess
- Consider referral for:
  - Ankylosing spondylitis
    - Refer to pediatric rheumatology.
  - Leukemia, lymphoma, and Ewing sarcoma
    - Refer to pediatric oncology.
  - Osteoid osteoma
    - Refer to pediatric orthopedic surgery.
  - Spondylolysis
    - Refer to a pediatric sports medicine specialist or orthopedic surgery.
  - Scheuermann disease
    - Refer to orthopedic surgery (pediatric or spinal) if patients in whom conservative management fails, those with intractable pain, or those in whom kyphosis progresses or when diagnosis and evaluation are outside of scope of expertise

WHEN TO ADMIT

- Admit patients with back pain with associated fever or neurologic findings or when prompt and thorough diagnostic assessment cannot be completed as an outpatient.

PROGNOSIS

- Prognosis depends on the underlying etiology of back pain.

PREVENTION

- Muscular low back pain prevention measures
- Proper posture
- Backpack should not exceed 15–20% of body weight.
- Stretch to improve flexibility of lower back and hamstrings
- Exercise to strengthen core musculature (abdomen, hips, and back)

Bacterial Skin Infections

DEFINITION

- Bacterial infections of the skin are common and most often caused by gram-positive bacteria
  - *Staphylococcus aureus*
  - Group A streptococci
- The clinical disease that results depends on the infection's location in the skin.

ETIOLOGY

Impetigo

- *S aureus* is the major cause of impetigo in childhood.
  - Responsible for virtually 100% of bullous impetigo
  - Causes approximately 75% of nonbullous impetigo
- The remainder of cases is caused by group A ß-hemolytic *Streptococcus*.

Pyoderma

- Presumably, trauma to the skin results in inoculation, followed by infection.
- Frequently extends through the epidermal layer into the underlying dermis
- The process may start with small erythematous papules and rapidly proceed through vesicular, pustular, and crusted stages.
  - May be clinically confused with impetigo
- Streptococcal pyoderma is more common in warm, humid environments.
  - Higher humidity favors survival of group A streptococci on normal skin.

Folliculitis

- Infection of the hair follicles, caused almost exclusively by *S aureus*
  - In rare cases, the infection is caused by gram-negative organisms.
  - Occurs occasionally in patients whose acne is being treated with antibiotics
  - Moderately common, primarily affecting older children and young adults
- *Pseudomonas aeruginosa* is the usual cause of hot tub folliculitis.
  - Pruritic papules and pustules on the trunk and proximal extremities
  - Usually clears without treatment, although antipruritics can be used

Furuncles and abscesses

- Pus-filled nodule or boil resulting from unchecked folliculitis
- Almost always caused by *S aureus*
- Many clinicians use the terms *furuncle* and *abscess* interchangeably.

- Abscesses are collections of pus in the dermis and deeper skin tissues.
  - They do not originate from a primary folliculitis.
  - Bacteria may be inoculated into the skin and underlying soft tissue by traumatic injury, including surgery.
  - Most skin abscesses are caused by *S aureus*, but gram-negative and anaerobic organisms also can be causes.

Cellulitis

- Deep, locally diffuse infection of the skin with systemic manifestations and life-threatening potential
- *S aureus* and group A streptococci more commonly are responsible for cellulitis of the extremities.
  - On an extremity, the bacteria presumably have been externally inoculated into the deep dermal tissue.
  - The portal of entry is often undetectable clinically.
  - A hematogenous or lymphangitic source is also possible and may explain the development of cellulitis in cases in which overlying skin is unbroken.
- *S aureus* and group A streptococci are the most common cause of perianal dermatitis.
  - Two-thirds of these patients have positive pharyngeal cultures.
- Preseptal (periorbital) cellulitis is likely to be caused by:
  - *Streptococcus pneumoniae* in younger children
  - Group A streptococci in older children
- In rare cases, other aerobic and anaerobic bacterial organisms, as well as deep fungal agents, such as *Cryptococcus neoformans*, can cause cellulitis.
  - These infections usually occur in immunosuppressed individuals.
- Before the introduction of protein-conjugated *Haemophilus influenzae* type b (Hib) vaccines in 1988, Hib was a frequent cause of facial cellulitis (buccal cellulitis).
- The incidence of invasive infections from this organism in the US has decreased by 95%.
- Now occurs primarily in:
  - Undervaccinated populations
  - Infants who have not completed the primary Hib vaccine series
- Almost 90% of cases of facial cellulitis in the post-Hib vaccine era are related to:
  - Trauma
  - Dental infection
  - Sinus infection

B

Community-associated methicillin-resistant *S aureus* (MRSA) infections

- The prevalence of community-associated MRSA is increasing.
- The most frequently reported presentation is furunculosis, followed by skin abscesses and cellulitis.
- Less frequent are bullous and nonbullous impetigo, nodules, pustules, and scalded skin syndrome.

RISK FACTORS

- Uncontrolled diabetes
- Immunodeficiency involving reduced neutrophil number and function

SIGNS AND SYMPTOMS

Impetigo

- History
  - The patient usually has no history of preceding trauma to the skin.
  - Mild to moderate itching may be associated with lesions.
  - Other family members also may be affected.
- Physical findings
  - Most commonly found on the face
  - Lesions may be single or multiple and scattered elsewhere on the body as well.
  - Usually yellow- or honey-colored crusts that when removed reveal a pink, superficially eroded, glistening base
    - A culture sample should be obtained from this base.
  - Intact bullae, if present, contain deceptively clear fluid.
  - Blisters break easily, leaving behind a superficially denuded skin surface covered with a thin, brown, varnish-like crust surrounded by a thin rim of loose, ragged epidermis that represents the remnants of the blister roof.
    - Surrounding erythema is minimal.
    - Regional lymphadenopathy is rare.

Pyoderma

- History
  - May occur in epidemics among children of lower socioeconomic status who live in crowded conditions in a warm, humid environment
  - In contrast to impetigo, lesions occur most commonly on the lower extremities.
  - Usually preceded by trauma such as a scratch or insect bite
  - Family members may be affected.
- Physical findings
  - Early lesion is a pustule with surrounding erythema.
  - Typically, the more advanced lesion of ecthyma is seen.

- Lesion appears as a thick, usually brown crust surrounded by erythema.
  - When the crust is removed, an actual ulcer is revealed.
- Regional adenopathy is often present.

Folliculitis

- History
  - Appears most commonly as a chronic eruption unaccompanied by symptoms
  - Occasionally, a patient has mild discomfort or pruritus.
- Physical findings
  - Lesions are usually located on the buttocks and upper portion of the thighs.
  - Scattered individual small papules and pustules
  - On close inspection, hairs can be seen growing out of the very center of many of the lesions.

Furuncles and abscesses

- History
  - A history of trauma may be elicited but often is not, especially with furuncles.
  - Immunodeficiency states and diabetes may predispose certain patients to bacterial skin infections.
  - The typical patient with a furuncle or abscess has no underlying medical disease.
- Physical findings
  - Furuncles and abscesses are fluctuant masses filled with pus.
  - Often begin as hard, tender, red nodules that become more fluctuant and painful with time
  - Abscesses tend to be larger and deeper than furuncles.
  - The 2 lesions may be difficult to differentiate clinically.

Cellulitis

- History
  - Children often feel and appear ill.
  - Fever may precede clinical skin signs.
  - May complain of pain in the affected area; patients who have perianal cellulitis often have pain on defecation
  - Symptoms of accompanying otitis media may be present in buccal cellulitis.
- Physical findings
  - Fever at the time of presentation is common.
  - The area of involved skin shows the classic signs of inflammation.
    - Redness
    - Swelling
    - Heat
    - Tenderness

DIFFERENTIAL DIAGNOSIS

Impetigo

- Herpes simplex virus (HSV) infection is the condition most often confused with impetigo.
- Clinical clues that suggest herpes rather than impetigo
  - Intact vesicles are more likely in HSV infection.
  - As vesicles age, they become cloudy and ultimately result in crusts that also may be honey colored.
  - The crusted phase most often causes the diagnostic confusion.
- HSV infection tends to be a recurrent condition.
  - Recurrence is not the case with impetigo.
- When an impetiginous pustule is unroofed, it is noticeably filled with pus.
  - A herpetic lesion may appear to be pus filled, but when it is unroofed, only a scant amount of clear fluid is found.
- In impetigo, Gram staining shows numerous gram-positive cocci.
  - In HSV infection, Wright staining of a scraping from the base of a crust or a vesicle reveals multinucleated giant cells.

Pyoderma

- Ecthyma gangrenosum is an uncommon but serious manifestation of sepsis in immune-compromised hosts.
  - Most frequently associated with *P aeruginosa* infection
  - Can be seen with other gram-negative organisms or even with fungi
- Clinical features that help differentiate this lesion from ecthyma
  - Location: ecthyma gangrenosum is often on the upper extremities or in the inguinal or axillary folds.
  - Lesion's appearance: a deeper ulcer is covered with a tightly adherent, black (gangrenous) crust.
  - Host: seriously ill, usually immunocompromised patient with other signs of sepsis

Folliculitis

- Clinically, folliculitis is caused by gram-negative organisms and differs from staphylococcal folliculitis in its distribution.
  - Lesions occur primarily on the face and shoulders, often concentrated in the perioral and perinasal areas.
  - Hot tub folliculitis usually appears on the lower trunk on areas most exposed to the contaminated water in the tub.
- Keratosis pilaris is another common follicular disorder.
  - Exhibits as tiny, rough, scaling papules on back of the upper parts of the arms, buttocks, and thighs
  - Although its distribution may be similar to that of staphylococcal folliculitis, the appearance of the lesions is not.
    - In keratosis pilarsis the lesions are smaller, more numerous, and scaling, but not pustular.

Cellulitis

- Erysipelas
  - A form of cellulitis caused most commonly by group A streptococci
  - Infection is limited to the upper dermis.
  - Erysipelas has raised and sharply demarcated borders.
  - Bedside differentiation of erysipelas from cellulitis is sometimes difficult.
    - Not particularly useful clinically since therapeutic considerations are the same for both conditions
- Severe, local, confluent contact dermatitis may sometimes be confused with cellulitis.
  - Both may show marked erythema of the skin.
  - Important differences from contact dermatitis
    - The complaint is of itch rather than pain.
    - The skin usually is not tender.
    - The patient is not febrile.
    - The presence of vesicles also favors contact dermatitis.
    - Vesicles and bullae may sometimes occur in erysipelas or cellulitis as the condition evolves.

Perianal dermatitis

- Originally thought to be cellulitis, but now known to be a more superficial infection
- May be misdiagnosed as candidiasis or diaper dermatitis
- Bright-pink erythema and pain or tenderness of the involved skin suggest bacterial infection.
  - A swab culture usually shows *S aureus* or group A streptococci.
  - Laboratory personnel must be aware that they are to look for these organisms; otherwise, they will look for enteric flora with a culture from this site.

Necrotizing fasciitis

- A fulminant skin infection most often caused by group A streptococci.
  - Flesh-eating bacteria
  - Warm, violaceous, exquisitely tender, and markedly edematous (orange peel–like) skin with indiscriminate edges.
  - Systemic toxicity is often seen.
    - Fever
    - Leukocytosis
    - Thrombocytopenia
    - Hypocalcemia
    - Hyponatremia
  - Systemic antibiotics are an adjunct to prompt surgical debridement.

Erythema infectiosum

■ Fifth disease, caused by parvovirus B19

■ Erythema of the cheeks, with a slapped-cheek appearance

■ Important diagnostic differences between erythema infectiosum and cellulitis

• Involvement is bilateral.

• The site is not usually very tender.

• The patient does not appear toxic.

• The patient may be mildly febrile.

LABORATORY FINDINGS

■ Impetigo

• Gram stain of either the clear blister fluid or serum underlying the crusts shows gram-positive cocci.

• Cultures grow *S aureus* or *Streptococcus pyogenes*.

■ Pyoderma

• Culture sample taken from the base of the denuded ulcer usually grows group A ß-hemolytic streptococci.

• *S aureus* is occasionally recovered concomitantly, thought to be a secondary invader.

■ Folliculitis

• Culturing is not usually necessary in the typical case.

• If presentation is atypical and laboratory confirmation is desired, then the contents of a fresh pustule should be cultured.

■ Furuncles and abscesses

• Gram stain of the pustular material may identify the bacterial cause.

• For precise identification, cultures are required.

– For anaerobic cultures: aspirate the pus, seal the syringe, and deliver to the laboratory.

– If insufficient material is available to aspirate, a swab culture can be used for anaerobic and aerobic cultures.

– Blood culture results rarely are positive in patients with furuncles or abscesses.

■ Not indicated unless the patient shows signs of sepsis

■ Cellulitis

• Leukocytosis is a common finding.

• Causative pathogen is usually assumed from history and physical examination.

• Identifying it by culture is difficult.

• Blood cultures are positive in <5% of cases.

• Many advocate culturing the skin directly.

– Prepare the skin with an antiseptic.

– Introduce an 18- or 21-gauge needle into the deep dermis and aspirate.

– If no material is obtained, inject 0.5 to 1 mL of non-bacteriostatic saline and re-aspirate.

– All aspirates should be Gram stained and cultured.

– Causative organism is identified in approximately 25% of cases.

– Skin aspiration is best in special cases.

■ Immunocompromised host

■ Cellulitis that is not responsive to empiric therapy

■ Cellulitis secondary to an unusual exposure, such as an animal bite

– In neonates or undervaccinated hosts with facial cellulitis, lumbar puncture with culture of cerebrospinal fluid may disclose unsuspected meningitis.

SPECIFIC TREATMENTS

Impetigo

■ Topical and systemic antibiotics can be used to treat impetigo.

■ Mupirocin topical antibiotic ointment has been reported to equal or exceed the efficacy of oral erythromycin in the treatment of bacterial impetigo.

• A cream form is also available.

• Topical mupirocin should be considered whenever feasible because it can be effective in treating impetigo caused by MRSA.

• Infected area should be washed carefully and crusts gently removed, if possible, 3 times daily before antibiotic cream or ointment is applied.

■ Traditional topical preparations that contain bacitracin or neomycin, either alone or in combination

• Poorly absorbed, thus not particularly effective

■ Systemic antibiotics should be used for more extensive lesions.

• Clindamycin might be an appropriate choice in the era of MRSA.

– Studies of this approach have not been published.

• Traditional choices in the pre-MRSA era

– Erythromycin

– Penicillinase-resistant penicillin(eg, dicloxacillin)

– Amoxicillin-clavulanic acid

– Cephalexin

– These agents would still be appropriate for treatment of disease caused by methicillin-sensitive *S aureus* or *S pyogenes*.

• Treatment course should be 7–10 days.

• Patients with more extensive disease who fail traditional empiric antibiotic therapy should have cultures and susceptibility studies performed.

Pyoderma

- Antibiotics are the treatment of choice, but route of administration is debated.
- Prophylactic topical agents, such as mupirocin, may be applied to scratches or insect bites to prevent the development of pyoderma.
- Systemic antibiotics are recommended for streptococcal infections, particularly if the infection is extensive.
  - Injectable benzathine penicillin G
    - A 7- to 10-day course of oral penicillin or erythromycin is preferred if the patient is likely to be adherent to the prescribed regimen.
  - Penicillin treatment occasionally fails.
    - Most likely because of the persistence of coexisting penicillinase-producing *S aureus* organisms

Folliculitis

- Mild staphylococcal folliculitis can be managed by having the patient use an antiseptic cleanser (eg, chlorhexidine) or antibacterial soap containing triclosan or triclocarban.
  - Use daily or every other day for at least several weeks.
  - For more extensive involvement a 7- to 10-day course of systemic antibiotics (eg, erythromycin or dicloxacillin) is suggested in addition to the topical regimen.

Furuncles and abscesses

- Very small furuncles can be treated with moist heat, which promotes drainage.
- For larger furuncles, incision and drainage is the appropriate therapy.
- For furuncles <5 cm in diameter, incision and drainage alone results in complete healing in most cases.
- For abscesses >5 cm or patients with surrounding cellulitis or signs of systemic illness, systemic antibiotics should be used.
- If lesions are seen early in their development, then systemic antibiotics may result in involution, obviating the need for incision and drainage.
  - Dicloxacillin, cephalexin, and erythromycin were considered the antibiotics of choice.
  - They need to be reevaluated in light of MRSA in furunculosis.
    - Most community-associated MRSA isolates are susceptible to trimethoprim-sulfamethoxazole.
    - Many are sensitive to clindamycin.
    - Clindamycin has excellent penetration into the infected tissues.
    - Some erythromycin-resistant strains of MRSA have inducible resistance to clindamycin.
  - It is important to know local susceptibility patterns.
- Culture results from abscesses may help in the ultimate selection of the appropriate antibiotic.

Cellulitis

- Systemic antibiotics are the mainstay of therapy.
- Mild cases of cellulitis on an extremity may be treated with:
  - Oral antibiotic
  - Warm soaks
  - Outpatient follow-up in several days
- Cellulitis of the extremity most often is caused by gram-positive organisms; thus, the following are appropriate.
  - Erythromycin
  - Dicloxacillin
  - Cephalexin
- More seriously ill patients should be hospitalized for parenteral antibiotic therapy.
  - Infants and young children, patients with predisposing medical conditions, such as diabetes mellitus
  - Patients with immunodeficiencies or on immunosuppressive therapies
  - Patients in whom sepsis is suspected
- Community-associated MRSA strains are generally more susceptible to non–ß-lactam antibiotics than are nosocomial MRSA strains.
  - Clindamycin
  - Trimethoprim-sulfamethoxazole
- Some erythromycin-resistant strains develop resistance to clindamycin during treatment.
  - The microbiology laboratory should provide results of a D-test for strains resistant to erythromycin.
  - If the D-test is negative, then clindamycin can be used.

WHEN TO ADMIT

- Cellulitis with suspected sepsis or suspected underlying serious infection
- Invasive infections (necrotizing fasciitis)
- Staphylococcal scalded skin syndrome
- Toxic shock syndrome

WHEN TO REFER

- Preseptal cellulitis
- Treatment failure
- Recurrent bacterial skin infections

FOLLOW-UP

- Impetigo
  - Exclusion from school
    - A child may be asked to leave school until the infection is treated.
    - The period of infectiousness of impetigo is unknown.

– Most child-care centers and schools recommend exclusion as long as open lesions persist.

– 24 hours after appropriate therapy has been initiated, the child can probably return to school without posing a significant risk to other children.

COMPLICATIONS

Impetigo

■ If the infection does not respond rapidly to therapy, it may be caused by an antibiotic-resistant strain.

- In such cases, initial culture and susceptibility results serve as a guide in selecting an alternate antibiotic.

■ Historically, differentiating between staphylococcal and streptococcal impetigo was considered to be important.

- There was a belief that glomerulonephritis was a sequela of streptococcal impetigo.

- Evidence now shows that treatment of streptococcal skin infections does not alter the risk of glomerulonephritis.

Pyoderma

■ Cellulitis may develop if the infection extends into larger and deeper areas of skin and subcutaneous tissue.

■ Some strains of group A streptococci produce the toxin responsible for scarlet fever.

■ Acute glomerulonephritis may follow streptococcal infection of the skin.

- Caused by only a few nephritogenic serotypes (49, 55, and 57) of pyoderma-inducing streptococci

- The usual period from onset of infection to development of glomerulonephritis is 18–21 days.

■ Skin infection with streptococci never leads to acute rheumatic fever.

Furuncles and abscesses

■ Recurrent furunculosis

- Consider an underlying immunodeficiency (rare).

- Many patients harbor *S aureus* in a sequestered mucocutaneous site, most commonly in the anterior nares.

  – Apply mupirocin to the external nares twice daily for 5 days.

  – Repeat the process monthly or every 2 months.

  – This decreases recurrences by approximately one-half.

- Some recommend an every-other-day total-body scrub with an antiseptic cleansing agent, such as chlorhexidine, or antibacterial soap containing triclosan or triclocarban

  – Overuse may dry the skin, harming skin integrity.

- Some advocate the addition of a small amount of bleach to the bath water.

  – Anecdotally, this approach shows some promise.

  – No studies evaluating its efficacy have been conducted.

- Most oral antibiotics do not eradicate nasal carriage of *S aureus*, but clindamycin is an exception.

- In cases that are refractory to all previously described methods, a single oral dose of clindamycin, given daily for 3 months, may be effective at eliminating recurrences.

■ In rare cases, a staphylococcal abscess may be the focus of toxin production.

- Can result in:

  – Staphylococcal scalded skin syndrome, most commonly seen in infants and neonates

  – Toxic shock syndrome

  – Staphylococcal scarlet fever

Cellulitis

■ In some instances, findings that are clinically diagnosed as cellulitis may actually be a clue to underlying, deeper-seated infection.

- Cellulitis of the periorbital tissues may be secondary to sinusitis.

- Abdominal wall cellulitis may hide an underlying peritonitis.

- Redness, warmth, and swelling of tissues overlying bones or joints may indicate septic arthritis or osteomyelitis.

- Facial cellulitis may be caused by an undiagnosed dental abscess.

- Redness of the neck is sometimes a clue to underlying deep neck space infections.

- Inflammation of the skin of the sacrum might be from an infected pilonidal cyst.

- Redness of the pinna or postauricular area may point to malignant otitis externa or mastoiditis.

■ Uncomplicated cellulitis was once a serious, life-threatening disease, but antibiotics have now reduced the fatality rate to nearly zero in otherwise healthy patients.

PROGNOSIS

■ Impetigo

- With appropriate antibiotic therapy, prompt healing is expected.

- Bacteriologic cures occur within 7–10 days.

■ Pyoderma

- In most patients, the lesions heal uneventfully.

- Because they are deeper, streptococcal lesions often take longer than staphylococcal lesions to heal.

- Bacteriologic cures are usually accomplished within 1 week.

  – If prompt response is not achieved, then secondary infection from a penicillinase-producing staphylococcal strain should be considered, particularly if penicillin was used for treatment.

  – Erythromycin-resistant strains of group A streptococci may be encountered.

- Folliculitis
  - Most patients respond to treatment.
  - If not, bacterial culture should be performed to rule out infection by gram-negative organisms or MRSA.
  - Some patients are plagued with recurrences, for which a more prolonged course of antibiotic therapy is recommended.
  - In rare cases, the follicular infection extends deeply, producing a furuncle.
- Furuncles and abscesses
  - Untreated lesions often rupture and drain spontaneously.
  - After either surgical or spontaneous drainage, uneventful healing is the rule.
  - Larger lesions may leave scars.

- Cellulitis
  - With appropriate antibiotic therapy, fever usually resolves within 24 hours.
  - If it does not, then a change in antibiotic therapy should be considered, optimally guided by early culture and bacterial sensitivity results.
  - The skin reaction resolves more slowly than does fever, sometimes taking ≥1 week to subside completely.

Brain Tumors

DEFINITION

- Brain tumors include tumors of the brain parenchyma, cranial nerves, meninges, and the pituitary gland and immediate surrounding structures.
- Although they are rare, they are the second most common cancer and most common solid tumor in childhood.

EPIDEMIOLOGY

- Incidence
  - Primary brain and central nervous system (CNS) tumors in the US
    - 4.3 cases per 100,000 person-years
    - 3410 new cases diagnosed in 2005
    - Incidence appears to be increasing.
- Age
  - Incidence is inversely proportional to age.
  - Highest in children 0–4 years of age (5.0 cases/100,000 person-years)
  - Lowest in patients 10–19 years of age (3.9 cases/100,000 person-years)
- Sex
  - Incidence slightly higher in boys than in girls
    - Higher proportion of medulloblastoma and germ cell tumors in boys

ETIOLOGY

- Brain tumors arise from persistence of:
  - Embryologic precursors of neurons (primitive neuroectodermal tumors)
  - Glial elements that provide structural and nutritional support to the neurons (astrocytomas and oligodendrogliomas)
  - Lining cells, such as:
    - Arachnoid (meningioma)
    - Nerve sheath (schwannoma)
    - Pituitary gland (pituitary adenomas)
    - Intracranial rests (craniopharyngiomas)

RISK FACTORS

- Proven risk factors include:
  - Previous therapeutic radiotherapy
    - Therapy for acute lymphoblastic leukemia, including radiotherapy, increases risk for second malignant neoplasms, including CNS tumors.
  - Predisposing genetic syndromes
    - Neurofibromatosis types 1 and 2
    - Tuberous sclerosis types 1 and 2
    - von Hippel-Landau syndrome
    - Li-Fraumeni syndrome
    - Nevoid basal cell carcinoma syndrome
    - Turcot syndrome
    - Ataxia-telangiectasia syndrome
    - Gardner syndrome
    - Down syndrome
  - Maternal diet
    - Strong protective dose-response relations observed for maternal consumption of:
      - Fruit
      - Vegetables
      - Vitamin C
      - Nitrate
      - Folate
- Children with primary CNS neoplasms without a documented genetic syndrome have increased risk of a second CNS neoplasm.

SIGNS AND SYMPTOMS

General information

- Symptoms often appear weeks to months before diagnosis is made.
  - Interval between onset of symptoms and diagnosis is approximately 9 weeks.
  - Correlate with patient's age and location/histologic type of the tumor
    - In infants, increased intracranial pressure (ICP) may exhibit with nonspecific signs.
      - Drowsiness or lethargy
      - Irritability
      - Vomiting
      - Abnormal tilting of the head
      - Developmental stagnation or regression
    - In older children, the following may occur before overt symptoms (eg, headache, vomiting) develop.
      - Declining academic performance
      - Fatigue
      - Emotional, appetite, or personality changes

Characteristics of symptoms

- Children will typically have a progression of symptoms and physical findings that may not correlate with grade of underlying disease.
  - Manifestations depend on:
    - Site of tumor origin
    - Child's age and developmental level
    - Existence of accompanying hydrocephalus

Specific symptoms

- The most typical symptom is headache, which may be:
  - Frontal
  - Occipital
  - Unilateral
  - Diffuse in location
  - Exacerbated by Valsalva maneuvers
- Vomiting
  - May be the result of increased ICP or, less commonly, direct irritation of the vagal nuclei or the floor of the 4th ventricle
  - May be associated with morning or waking headaches
  - May relieve the headaches
  - Some infants will appear to be failing to thrive as a result of vomiting caused by the increased ICP.
- Seizures are not frequently observed in children with brain tumors.
- More specific symptoms may help localize the tumor.
  - Infratentorial tumors
    - Clumsiness
    - Worsening handwriting
    - Scanning speech
    - Ataxia
  - Infiltrating brainstem glioma
    - Ataxia
    - Diplopia (due to 6th-nerve palsy)
    - Headache
    - Vomiting
  - Supratentorial tumors, cerebral hemispheres
    - Hemiparesis (muscle weakness)
    - Personality changes
    - Focal weakness
    - Language dysfunction
    - Visual field defects
    - Sensory changes
  - Disease along optic nerve
    - Visual loss or visual field defects
  - Tumors near the optic chasm or hypothalamus
    - Hormonal changes such as growth failure or precocious puberty
  - Tumors of the hypothalamus, diencephalic syndrome in infants, characterized by:
    - Failure to thrive
    - Emaciation
    - Euphoric mood

- Pineal tumors and tumors involving midbrain tectum, Parinaud syndrome
  - Paralysis of upward gaze
  - Convergence-retraction nystagmus
  - Lid retraction
  - Light-near dissociation of the pupils
- Tumors involving suprasellar and hypothalamic region
  - Precocious or delayed puberty
  - Growth failure
  - Hypothyroidism
- Macrocephalyin infants
  - Head circumference measurements that cross percentile lines on standard chart
  - Bulging of the fontanel
  - Split cranial sutures
  - Lack of upgaze
  - Alteration in tone
- Symptoms warranting evaluation for brain tumor in patients with headache
  - Presence or onset of neuralgic abnormality
  - Ocular findings, such as:
    - Papilledema
    - Decreased visual acuity
    - Loss of vision
  - Vomiting that is either:
    - Persistent
    - Increasing in frequency
    - Preceded by recurrent headaches
  - Changes in character of headache
    - Increased severity or frequency
    - Begins awakening child from sleep
  - Recurrent morning headaches or headaches that repeatedly awaken the child from sleep
  - Child with short stature or deceleration of linear growth
  - Diabetes insipidus
  - Neurofibromatosis

DIFFERENTIAL DIAGNOSIS

- Space-occupying lesions and causes of increased ICP
  - Arteriovenous malformations
  - Subdural hematoma, effusion, or empyema
  - Abscess
  - Infarction
  - Hemorrhage
  - Demyelination

- Pseudotumor cerebri
- Hemiplegic migraine
- Todd paralysis
- Venous sinus thrombosis

DIAGNOSTIC APPROACH

- In addition to a thorough history, complete neurologic examination, including the fundus, is required to reveal both localizing and nonlocalizing findings.
- Neurologic findings, with or without complementary history, are required for further investigation and for referring the child to a specialist.
- Repeated neurologic examinations are ideal because signs are frequently progressive in situations in which the diagnosis remains in question.

LABORATORY FINDINGS

- In tumors of pituitary gland the involving the pituitary stalk and hypothalamus, endocrine function should be evaluated before surgery.
- If the pituitary stalk or posterior portion of gland is involved, electrolytes and osmolality measurements can help diagnose diabetes insipidus.
- Patients with nongerminomatous germ cell tumors (choriocarcinoma, yolk-sac tumors, embryonal cell tumors, and the mixed variety) can excrete:
  - α-Fetoprotein
  - ß-Human chorionic gonadotropin
  - Alkaline phosphatase
  - These markers are most easily found in cerebrospinal fluid, but they may also be detected in serum.
- HIV serologic testing may be useful if primary CNS lymphoma is suspected (although this is rare in children).

IMAGING

- Computed tomography (CT) is widely available and has short imaging times, requiring less sedation in young children.
  - First modality to be used
  - Initial scan can provide important immediate information about:
    - Presence of hydrocephalus
    - Cerebral edema
    - Midline shifts
    - Risk of uncal herniation
  - Tumors of the brainstem, posterior fossa, and mesial temporal lobe structures may not be clearly visible.

- Magnetic resonance imaging (MRI)
  - Modality of choice for definitive diagnosis of CNS neoplasms
  - More sensitive than CT for most brain tumors
  - Best for tumors of the brainstem, posterior fossa, mesial temporal lobe, and spinal column
  - If seizures with a focal onset are present, either simple partial (focal) seizures or partial seizures with secondary generalization, contrast-enhanced MRI should be used to evaluate the patient for a tumor.

DIAGNOSTIC PROCEDURES

- Diagnosis using histologic evaluation of biopsy material
  - Best way to diagnose some tumors, when a biopsy sample can be obtained without substantial morbidity
  - Biopsy samples of tumors situated in the deep gray masses (eg, the thalamus and basal ganglia) are often obtained by means of a stereotactic navigation system.
  - Diffuse pontine gliomas and tectal plate gliomas are never sampled for biopsy because of:
    - Risk of damaging essential structures
    - Predictable histologic appearance and clinical course
  - Visual pathway glioma and intrinsic pontine gliomas seldom need pathologic corroboration of a diagnosis.

CLASSIFICATION

- World Health Organization classification (published in 2000) has >120 entries.
  - Integrates histopathologic criteria with factors that are:
    - Clinical
    - Epidemiologic
    - Radiologic
    - Biological
    - Molecular genetic
    - Predictive
  - Continues to evolve, with new diagnoses continually being added
  - 4 malignancy grades or estimates of malignant potential
  - Distinction between malignant and nonmalignant tumors may not always reflect the clinical course of the disease.
  - Terms such as *benign* or *malignant* have been replaced by *low-grade* or *high-grade* because the former terms can be misleading.
    - Prognosis for some high-grade tumors is better than for some low-grade tumors.

TREATMENT APPROACH

- Treatment usually requires a multidisciplinary team approach with physicians from:
  - Neurosurgery
  - Neurology
  - Oncology
  - Pathology
  - Radiology
  - Radiation oncology
  - Endocrinology
  - Ophthalmology
- Treatment outcomes are better when care is provided at a specialized tertiary-care cancer center.
  - The AAP released a statement outlining the guidelines for facilities, capabilities, and available personnel.
  - Patients benefit from an experienced team of:
    - Pharmacologists
    - Nurses
    - Neuropsychologists
    - Audiologists
    - Nutritional experts
    - Child life specialists
    - Physical, occupational, and speech therapists
    - Social workers
- Children should be considered for enrollment into a clinical trial whenever one is available.

SPECIFIC TREATMENTS

Surgery

- Presurgical corticosteroid therapy is essential if the patient has brain edema and increased ICP.
  - Methylprednisolone reduces capillary permeability in tumor and adjacent brain tissue.
  - Methylprednisolone often results in rapid or marked resolution of edema, with corresponding improvement of symptoms, and a more relaxed brain during the operative procedure.
- Excision removes the tumor and resolves the surrounding edema.
  - Use of stereoscopic microscopes coupled with real-time surgical navigation systems is the most striking advance.
    - Navigation system permits an operative burr hole to be placed with high precision and allows tumor resection through small openings.
    - Modern microscopes allow the surgeon to distinguish between healthy brain and tumor, yielding a greater likelihood of total resection.

- Electrophysiologic monitoring during surgery contributes to safer and bolder approaches.
- Intraoperative MRI shows promise in selected cases, but its use is limited by high cost and often considerably longer operating times.
- For pilocytic astrocytoma, the strategy of choice is gross total resection.
- For other tumors, debulking of the primary tumor allows more effective chemotherapy and radiotherapy.
  - Chemotherapy improves survival from CNS tumors.

Radiotherapy

- Radiotherapy is an important treatment for all but the youngest patients.
  - In very young patients, new treatment protocols with intensive chemotherapy with stem cell rescue should replace radiotherapy (since the latter has long-term consequences).
- Radiotherapy
  - Best therapy for many tumors, but may result in growth/intellectual development failure, and increased risk of another cancer
  - Treatment planning requires balancing cure rates with profound morbidity and late effects.
  - Current radiotherapies allow small-volume or local irradiation while sparing surrounding tissues and essential structures.
    - External-beam
    - 3-dimensional
    - Intensity-modulated radiotherapy
    - Stereotactic radiosurgery and gamma-knife surgery

WHEN TO ADMIT

- Patients with signs of increasing ICP
  - Admit urgently for evaluation and imaging.
  - CT scanning can provide immediate information about:
    - Ventricular size
    - Volume of the normal cisternal spaces
    - Shifting of normal brain structures
    - Degree of ICP
- Progressive life-threatening symptoms that require urgent consult with neurosurgeon
  - Increasing blood pressure and decreasing heart rate
  - 6th-nerve palsy
  - Occipital headaches caused by irritation of posterior roots of the cervical cord
  - Symptoms may quickly progress to neck stiffness and opisthotonus (body spasm in which the head and heels are bent backward and the body is bowed forward).

- Patients with supratentorial mass lesions may exhibit pupillary dilatation, often unilateral initially, from uncal herniation.
  - May culminate in tonsillar herniation, which is a potential sequela of an untreated posterior fossa mass lesion, obstructive hydrocephalus, or both

WHEN TO REFER

- Children require further evaluation because of:
  - History that suggests brain tumor
  - Focal findings at physical examination
- Oncologists, neurologists, and neurosurgeons prefer early referrals if neoplasm is suspected.
  - Tumor will be smaller and easier to resect, causing less damage to adjacent brain tissue.

COMPLICATIONS

- An untreated posterior fossa mass lesion, or obstructive hydrocephalus, or both may lead to tonsillar herniation.
- Radiation therapy may result in failure of growth or intellectual development and increased risk of another cancer.

PROGNOSIS

- Except for medulloblastoma and nongerminomatous germ cell tumors, recent advances have only modestly affected outcomes.
- Survival depends on many factors.
  - Histology
  - Tumor behavior, size, and location
  - Patient age
- Children who survive may experience substantial morbidity.

Bronchiolitis

DEFINITION

- Bronchiolitis is a common, acute viral lower respiratory tract illness of children, occurring during the first 2 years of life.
- In bronchiolitis, acute inflammation of the airways results in:
  - Wheezing
  - Hyperinflation
  - Tachypnea

EPIDEMIOLOGY

Prevalence

- An increasing cause of hospitalization among infants in the US
- An appreciable and escalating economic burden to the health care system
- In 1 review of a private group practice, bronchiolitis caused 4% of hospitalizations among pediatric patients of all ages.

Incidence

- Annual reported rate of hospitalizations attributable to respiratory syncytial virus (RSV) among infants varies from 500 to 4100 per 100,000 infants.
- Recent population-based studies in the US estimate annual RSV-associated hospitalization rates of approximately 1300 per 100,000 children <12 months.
  - >3 times that associated with parainfluenza virus
  - >6 times that attributable to influenza
- Annual rates of hospitalization for bronchiolitis and RSV in other countries reported at 1900 to 2200 per 100,000 children <12 months.
- Rate of outpatient visits attributable to bronchiolitis or RSV is less well studied.
  - May be many times higher than that for hospitalized patients
- Mortality estimates due to bronchiolitis by Centers for Disease Control and Prevention
  - In children <5 years from 1979 to 1997
    - Average of 95 cases annually
    - Range of 66 to 127 cases each year
    - Highest in those <1 year
- Deaths in infants associated with RSV have more recently been estimated to be <500 per year.

Seasonal pattern

- Well-defined in temperate climates
- Reflects the activities of its viral agents, particularly RSV
- Yearly outbreaks of bronchiolitis occur during the winter to spring, when RSV is epidemic in the community (see Figure 9 on page F2).
- In Monroe County, New York, the greatest number of cases is reported during the yearly January-to-February peak of RSV activity.
  - Lesser peaks are observed:
    - During the fall, when parainfluenza virus type 1 is present in the community
    - During the spring, concurrent with the major activity of parainfluenza virus type 3

Age

- Occurs primarily in children within the first 2 years of life.
- >80% of bronchiolitis cases occur during the first year of life.
- Peak attack rate generally occurs:
  - Between 1 and 10 months of age
  - Between 2 and 6 months of age in hospitalized children
- In ambulatory children, the peak attack rate occurs in the second 6 months of life.

Sex

- Boys are approximately 1.5 times more likely than girls to develop bronchiolitis.
- Anatomic and physiologic differences, such as airway tone, may partly explain the male preponderance.

Genetic factors

- May predispose an infant to more severe bronchiolitis
- The following may predispose a patient to more severe disease.
  - Polymorphisms in genes coding interleukins
  - Tumor necrosis factor
  - Other immune mediators
  - An atopic family history
  - Predisposition to hyperreactivity of the airways
  - Native American ancestry

ETIOLOGY

- Bacteria were once thought to be the cause of bronchiolitis.
- Respiratory viruses are now recognized as the major agents of bronchiolitis.
- RSV
  - The most frequently identified cause of bronchiolitis
  - Accounts for approximately 50–85% of cases.
- Parainfluenza viruses (predominantly parainfluenza virus type 3)
  - The next most common agents
- In Monroe County, New York, RSV was isolated from 55% and parainfluenza virus type 3 from 11% of the cases of bronchiolitis examined in pediatric practices.

B

- Less common causes of bronchiolitis:
  - Rhinoviruses
  - Enteroviruses
  - Influenza viruses
  - Adenoviruses
  - Human metapneumovirus (hMPV)
    - Responsible for 4–10% of lower respiratory tract illnesses in hospitalized children
    - Approximately 3% of the outpatient respiratory illnesses
    - Epidemiologic characteristics and clinical manifestations of bronchiolitis caused by hMPV appear to be very similar to bronchiolitis from RSV.
- Children with bronchiolitis may be infected by >1 virus type simultaneously, usually by viruses that tend to have concurrent or overlapping seasons of circulation.
- Most frequently, the dual infections are caused by:
  - RSV with parainfluenza viruses type 3
  - hMPV 3
  - Influenza
- Respiratory distress arises from:
  - Inflammation of the epithelium
  - Obstruction of the medium and small bronchi and bronchioles
- The viral infection causes:
  - Increased mucus production
  - Edema
  - Necrosis of the bronchiolar epithelium, which is sloughed into the lumen of the small airways
- Because resistance to the flow of air is related inversely to the radius of the lumen, the small diameter of the bronchioles makes the infant particularly vulnerable to obstruction caused by the edema and inflammatory exudate.
- Peripheral to the sites of partial obstruction, air becomes trapped by a process similar to that of a ball valve mechanism.
- During inspiration, the negative intrapleural pressure allows air to flow past the site of partial obstruction.
- On expiration, the positive intrathoracic pressure decreases the diameter of the bronchiolar lumen.
- This causes:
  - An increase in the degree of obstruction
  - Hyperinflation of the lung
- If the inflammation progresses, complete obstruction can occur, and when the trapped air is absorbed, multiple areas of focal atelectasis result.

RISK FACTORS

- Genetic factors may predispose an infant to more severe bronchiolitis.
  - Polymorphisms in genes coding interleukins
  - Tumor necrosis factor
  - Other immune mediators
  - An atopic family history
  - Predisposition to hyperreactivity of the airways
  - Native American ancestry
- Low socioeconomic status
- Exposure to tobacco smoke
- Not being breastfed
- Contact with other young children
  - ≥1 siblings
  - Day care attendance
- Increased risk of bronchiolitis that is severe or requires hospitalization has been associated with:
  - Young age, particularly within the first several months of life
  - Prematurity
  - Low birth weight
  - Cardiopulmonary disease
  - Immunodeficiency

SIGNS AND SYMPTOMS

- Fluctuation of physical findings on examination is characteristic.
- Acute onset of wheezing
  - Auscultation usually reveals wheezing with or without crackles, but findings may vary from hour to hour.
  - Decrease in the auscultatory findings accompanied by increasing respiratory distress may indicate progressive obstruction to the flow of air in the small airways and impending respiratory failure.
- Increased respiratory rate is almost always evident.
  - Tachypnea must be judged on the basis of age.
    - Overall respiratory rate:
      - 50 breaths per minute in full-term newborns
      - 40 breaths per minute at 6 months
      - 30 breaths per minute at 1 year of age
  - Tachycardia commonly accompanies tachypnea.
- Acute inflammation of the airways
- Infants with bronchiolitis typically have a recent history of signs compatible with a common cold:
  - Rhinorrhea
  - Nasal congestion

- A low-grade fever
- Cough
  - More common as infection spreads to the lower respiratory tract
  - Followed by tachypnea
- Fever (in about 50% of infants at diagnosis)
- Clinical appearance
  - Infant may appear irritable, lethargic, or anxious.
  - Signs of increased work of breathing and airway obstruction
  - Flaring of the nasal alae and expiratory grunting
  - Retractions of the chest wall in the subcostal, intercostal, and suprasternal areas
  - Use of the accessory muscles of respiration
  - Prolonged expiration that may be difficult to detect in a young infant who has a rapid respiratory rate
  - Impeded flow of air on inspiration (to a lesser extent)
  - Hyperinflation
    - Increased diameter of the chest
    - Hyperresonance on percussion
  - Liver and spleen may become easily palpable from the downward placement of overinflated lungs.
- Clinical findings may develop from acute complications during the infant's course.
  - Apnea
    - First manifestation of illness in 10–20%
    - Risk of apnea greatest in:
      - Infants of premature gestation
      - Postconceptional age <44 weeks
  - Otitis media
    - Present in 3–30% of infants
    - May be caused by the infecting virus, bacteria, or both
  - Risk of dehydration from:
    - Paroxysms of coughing that trigger vomiting
    - Decreased fluid intake resulting from congested nasal passages
    - Respiratory distress
    - Tachypnea
    - Fever
  - Aspiration
    - Seen frequently in infants hospitalized with RSV bronchiolitis
    - Correlated with an increased risk of subsequent hyperactive airway disease
    - Abrogated by the prophylactic administration of therapy for aspiration

DIFFERENTIAL DIAGNOSIS

- Asthma
  - Wheezing and respiratory distress are associated with both bronchiolitis and asthma in young children.
  - In a single episode, differentiating these 2 entities is often not possible.
  - Both asthma and bronchiolitis may be engendered by viral infection.
    - Differentiation is confounded by the possibility of a link between them.
    - RSV infection in infancy may lead to subsequent wheezing associated with asthma.
  - Previous wheezing episodes and family history of atopy are more suggestive of asthma.
- Gastroesophageal reflux
  - The infant may exhibit episodes of wheezing clinically identical to bronchiolitis.
  - History of the timing of feeding and frequency of wheezing, and lack of upper respiratory tract signs typical of a viral infection, are helpful in differentiating.
- Other entities that may result in wheezing and respiratory distress in the bronchiolitic age group include:
  - Obstruction from an aspirated foreign body
  - A vascular ring
  - Retropharyngeal abscess
  - Significantly enlarged adenoids (rarely)
- Wheezing may also occur in:
  - Congestive heart failure
  - Chronic lung disease (eg, with prematurity or cystic fibrosis)

DIAGNOSTIC APPROACH

- Diagnosis of bronchiolitis is usually based on clinical history and physical findings.
  - Features that strongly support the diagnosis include:
    - Illness occurring during a community outbreak of a major viral agent, mainly RSV
    - Young age (especially <12 months)
    - No prior episode of wheezing
  - Assess risk factors for the development of more severe disease, especially:
    - Presence of prematurity
    - Cardiopulmonary disease
    - Immunodeficiency
    - Other underlying diseases
  - Recent history of signs compatible with a common cold

B

- Fever
  - Commonly present during the prodromal period and usually not high
  - By the time the child exhibits bronchiolitis associated with RSV, only ~50% are febrile.

LABORATORY FINDINGS

- Laboratory diagnostic tests
  - Not routinely recommended for normal infants at first episode of wheezing
  - Except in atypical cases or with abrupt clinical changes, such tests as leukocyte count, arterial oxygen saturation, serum chemistries, and cultures to rule out bacterial infection are generally not helpful or necessary.
- Pulse oximetry
  - Not shown to improve outcomes for infants with bronchiolitis
  - Use in hospitalized patients has been associated with:
    - Lower threshold for hospitalization
    - Higher rates of admission to intensive care units and mechanical ventilation
- Viral identification
  - Not routinely recommended
  - Assays to identify the specific virus may be warranted:
    - In more severely ill children in whom specific antiviral therapy for RSV or influenza is considered
    - In determining feasible infection control procedures, such as cohorting
  - Laboratory assays most commonly used to determine the viral causes are:
    - Isolation in tissue culture
    - Rapid antigen detection assays
  - Most of respiratory viruses causing bronchiolitis are identifiable in cell culture within 3–7 days.
  - Sensitivity of viral isolation techniques are variable among laboratories and highly dependent on expertise.
- Rapid viral diagnostic techniques
  - Have variable sensitivities
  - Should be used only when the virus is prevalent in the community, preferably during peak period of activity
    - Positive predictive value is low when little circulation of the virus occurs in the area.
    - False-positive rate increases as the incidence of the disease in the community falls.
  - Detect within hours some types of viruses in respiratory secretions that commonly cause bronchiolitis

- Rapid antigen detection kits are generally not available for the parainfluenza viruses.
- Recent increased use of reverse transcriptase polymerase chain reaction has demonstrated high sensitivity and improvement over viral isolation.
- Antibody determinations on acute and convalescent sera in young infants are rarely helpful because of:
  - Time required to obtain a convalescent serum
  - Presence of passive maternal antibody
  - Diminished antibody response of young infants to the viral respiratory agents causing bronchiolitis

IMAGING

- Imaging may be helpful when:
  - Diagnosis is not clear
  - Course is not as expected
- It should not be used routinely when:
  - The child was previously normal
  - Diagnosis can be made based on clinical and historical findings
  - Monitoring the course of an infant with bronchiolitis
  - Making admission or discharge decisions
- Findings on chest radiography:
  - Are commonly relatively benign
  - Do not correlate with severity of illness
- Classical findings
  - Increased bronchovascular markings radiating out from the hila
  - Scattered small areas of atelectasis
    - May be mistakenly interpreted as pneumonic infiltration and bacterial infection
- In prospective studies of children with suspected lower respiratory tract infection, those evaluated with chest x-rays:
  - Were more likely to receive antibiotics
  - Did not have improved outcome or reduced duration of illness

TREATMENT APPROACH

- Little agreement exists as to the value and use of therapeutic modalities.
- Management consists primarily of:
  - Supportive care, including adequate rest
  - Comfort
  - Hydration
  - Antipyretics, if necessary

SPECIFIC TREATMENTS

Congestion of nasal passages and upper airway

- May be alleviated by gentle nasal suctioning and positioning
- Mist therapy has not been shown to be beneficial.

Supplemental oxygen

- For the severely affected child who is hospitalized
  - Supplemental oxygen, as indicated by repetitive readings indicating inadequate oxygen saturation
  - No consensus as to the level of oxygen saturation that indicates the need for supplemental oxygen
- Recent bronchiolitis guidelines from the AAP recommend:
  - Initiating supplemental oxygen when the oxyhemoglobin saturation is persistently <90%
  - Consider discontinuing supplemental oxygen when the level is persistently ≥90%

Common therapies

- Frequently used, especially in first-time wheezers, although evidence showing benefit is lacking
- Corticosteroids
- Antivirals
- Antibiotics
- Bronchodilators
  - Studies evaluating their use in bronchiolitis have given variable and contrasting results.
  - Most controlled trials and reviews of ß-adrenergic agents have shown:
    - No consistent clinical benefit in children hospitalized with their first episode of wheezing
    - Transient or short-term clinical benefit in outpatients when evaluated by varying clinical score systems
  - AAP recommends that bronchodilators not be used routinely in the management of bronchiolitis, but a carefully monitored trial of inhaled α- or ß-adrenergic agents is an option.
    - Bronchodilators should be continued only if a beneficial clinical response is clearly documented.
- Corticosteroids
  - In some facilities, the majority of infants with bronchiolitis are treated with systemic glucocorticosteroids.
  - Meta-analyses have not shown consistent or statistically significant benefit in clinical scores, rates of hospitalization, or outcome.
  - The largest multicenter double-blind randomized trial was conducted in 20 emergency departments and completed in 2006.
    - Children 2–12 months of age with a first episode of wheezing from moderate to severe bronchiolitis received >3 respiratory seasons
      - Single dose of oral dexamethasone (1 mg/kg) *or*
      - Placebo
    - No significant difference was observed in the requirement for hospitalization.
    - The same lack of benefit was observed in subgroups of children with asthma or with family history of asthma.
  - AAP recommends that corticosteroid medications not be used routinely for care of infants with a first episode of bronchiolitis.
- Antivirals
  - Few antivirals are potentially useful against the viral agents that cause bronchiolitis.
  - Antivirals for influenza have not been approved as therapy for young infants nor evaluated in bronchiolitis.
  - Inhaled ribavirin (a synthetic nucleoside)
    - Only agent currently approved for the treatment of RSV lower respiratory tract disease in infants
    - Not recommended routinely to treat children with bronchiolitis
    - Generally should only be considered for use in infants at high risk for severe disease
    - Expensive, difficult to administer to ventilated patients
    - Benefits in clinical outcome are controversial.
    - Use should be decided on an individual basis after consideration of relative benefit to cost.
- Antibiotics
  - Should not be used unless:
    - Bacterial infection is documented *or*
    - Evidence strongly indicates concurrent presence of a bacterial infection.
  - Bacterial infection is uncommon in bronchiolitis and RSV lower respiratory tract disease.
- Chest physiotherapy, including percussion and vibratory techniques:
  - Have shown no clinical value
  - Are not recommended

WHEN TO ADMIT

- Oral intake is inadequate.
- Child appears toxic or has marked tachypnea or lethargy.
- Respiratory distress is rapidly progressive.
- History suggests apneic episodes.

B

WHEN TO REFER

- Episodes of bronchiolitis or wheezing are recurrent or started at birth.
- Wheezing continues despite clinical improvement.

COMPLICATIONS

- Apnea
  - Initial manifestation of illness in 10–20% of infants
  - Most at risk of apnea
    - Infants of premature gestation
    - Infants whose postconceptional age is <44 weeks
  - Subsequent prognosis for children with apnea associated with RSV infection is generally good.
  - Does not appear to be associated with increased risk of subsequent apnea, even during subsequent viral infections
- Otitis media
  - Present in 3–30% of infants
  - May be caused by infecting virus, bacteria, or both
- Risk of dehydration from:
  - Paroxysms of coughing that trigger vomiting
  - Decreased fluid intake resulting from congested nasal passages
  - Respiratory distress
  - Tachypnea
  - Fever
- Aspiration
  - Frequent among infants hospitalized with RSV bronchiolitis
  - Correlated with increased risk of subsequent hyperactive airway disease
  - Shown to be abrogated by prophylactic administration of therapy for aspiration

PROGNOSIS

- Most infants improve appreciably within several days.
- Cough and other signs resolve gradually over 1–2 weeks.
- Most hospitalized children are discharged after 3–7 days.
- Radiographic resolution of atelectasis may require several weeks.

- In ambulatory children
  - Median duration has been reported to be 12 days for children <24 months.
  - 18% are symptomatic after 3 weeks.
  - 9% are symptomatic after 4 weeks
- Clinical course tends to be more prolonged in:
  - Young infants
  - Those with underlying conditions
  - Those who acquired the infection nosocomially
- Some studies suggest increase in severity of infection when 2 viruses are present; others do not.
- Despite the increase in hospitalizations, mortality associated with bronchiolitis and RSV has declined.
- Recurrent wheezing
  - The most frequent sequelae of bronchiolitis, especially that caused by RSV
  - Reported in 30–50% of the children hospitalized for bronchiolitis
  - Episodes tend to occur most frequently during the first 2 years after the initial bronchiolitis.
  - Most of these children subsequently improve and become asymptomatic.
- Lung function abnormalities may persist beyond 10 years, despite clinical improvement.
  - Significantly reduced mean expiratory flow rates and increased risk of bronchial hyperreactivity during adolescence have been demonstrated.
  - One episode of bronchiolitis and less severe bronchiolitis not requiring hospitalization have not been associated with later pulmonary abnormalities.
- Relationship between bronchiolitis in early infancy and subsequent hyperreactive airway disease is unclear and confounded by the increasing recognition that asthma or reactive airway disease is a heterogeneous group of disorders with variable pathogenesis.
  - Some follow-up studies have shown that, by school age, risk of hyperreactive airway disease is not greater than in children with no history of bronchiolitis.
- Prognosis for children with apnea associated with RSV infection is generally good.
  - Does not appear to be associated with increased risk of apnea later, even during subsequent viral infections

Bulimia Nervosa

DEFINITION

- Eating disorder involving recurrent episodes of binge eating, along with purging behaviors

EPIDEMIOLOGY

- Prevalence
  - Up to 15% of adolescents report binge eating, purging, or both.
- Sex
  - 2% of female adolescents meet the full diagnostic criteria for bulimia nervosa.
  - 0.3% of male adolescents meet the full criteria.
- Age
  - Symptoms peak at 2–4% among white Western girls and women aged 17–25 years.
  - Modal age of onset is 18–19 years.
  - Occurs rarely in patients <14 years

ETIOLOGY

- Behavior may begin in response to a particular precipitant.
  - Insult by family or friends
  - Exposure to another individual with an eating disorder
  - Stressful situation
- Behavior perpetuated by:
  - Positive psychological feedback that initially accompanies perceived improved appearance
  - Biochemical changes that occur in response to decreased nutrition

RISK FACTORS

- Extreme or frequent dieting
- Early menarche
- Early sexual experiences
- Very early or late puberty and early sexual experiences in boys
- Personal and parental obesity
- Urbanization: occurs at a rate 5 times higher in large cities than in rural areas
- Childhood sexual abuse, especially when psychiatric comorbidity is present
- Premorbid negative self-evaluation
- Stressful life events
- Parental/family factors
  - Parental alcoholism
  - Low parental contact
  - High parental expectations
  - High levels of family conflict
  - Inadequate expression of emotions
  - Lack of parental warmth and care
  - Inappropriate parental control
  - Family history of affective disorders or eating disorders
  - Likely genetic factors

SIGNS AND SYMPTOMS

- Recurrent episodes of binge eating, characterized by both of the following:
  - Eating, in a discrete period (eg, within any 2-hour period), more food than most people would eat during a similar period/under similar circumstances
  - Sense of lack of control over eating during the episode (eg, the person feels that she or he cannot stop eating or control what/how much she or he is eating)
- Compensatory behavior to prevent weight gain (at least twice a week for 3 months)
  - Self-induced vomiting
    - Hands should be examined for the Russell sign (ie, irritation on the dorsum of the joints of the fingers used to induce vomiting).
    - Erosion of tooth enamel as a result of vomiting
    - Parotid enlargement
  - Misuse of laxatives, diuretics, enemas, or other medications
  - Fasting
  - Excessive exercise
- Symptoms of malnutrition
  - Cold hands and feet
  - Hair loss
  - Irregular menses
- Symptoms related to purging
  - Heartburn
  - Hematemesis
  - Constipation
  - Diarrhea
- Vital signs: begin initial physical examination with measurements of weight, height, blood pressure, and pulse.
  - Indicators of diet pill use
    - Tachycardia
    - Hypertension
  - Indicators of stimulant laxative or diuretic use
    - Tachycardia
    - Hypotension
  - Excessive exercise may result in significant bradycardia with resting heart.
  - If dehydration needs to be ruled out, measure blood pressure for orthostatic changes (see Diagnostic Procedures).

DIFFERENTIAL DIAGNOSIS

- Other medical causes of weight loss or vomiting
  - Cancer
  - Central nervous system tumors
  - Gastrointestinal problems
    - Malabsorption
    - Celiac disease
    - Inflammatory bowel disease
  - Endocrinologic problems
    - Diabetes mellitus
    - Hyperthyroidism
    - Hypopituitarism
  - Chronic illnesses and chronic infections
  - Superior mesenteric artery syndrome
- Psychiatric causes of weight loss
  - Depression
  - Obsessive-compulsive disorder
  - Psychosis (especially schizophrenia)
  - Sleep disorders
  - Hallucinations, delusions, or obsessions

DIAGNOSTIC APPROACH

- History should include:
  - Frequency of binging and purging
  - Maximum, minimum, and usual weight
  - Establish the patient's eating and exercise patterns.
  - Establish vomiting habits.
- Evaluate any medications designed to promote weight loss.
  - Diet pills
  - Laxatives
  - Diuretics
  - Ipecac
- Avoid being misled by the patient; physical examination and laboratory tests suggest the true extent of the disorder.
- The patient may be underweight, overweight, or normal weight.
- Specific abnormalities on physical examination are rarely found; more subtle changes in vital signs, physical examination, and laboratory tests should be sought.
- Full psychosocial history must be obtained to establish diagnosis and the psychosocial severity of the disorder.
  - Patient's functioning in the family, in school, and among peers
  - Possible psychiatric symptoms
    - Sleep disorders
    - Hallucinations, delusions, or obsessions

- Psychosocial changes
  - Fighting with the family
  - Withdrawing from friends
  - Performing less optimally in school, or improved school performance as withdrawal from friends and family intensifies
  - If additional psychiatric symptoms are found, the possibility of an additional diagnosis should be pursued.

LABORATORY FINDINGS

- Blood tests
  - Complete blood cell count with differential
  - Electrolytes and serum chemistries
  - Lipid studies
  - Liver function tests
  - Amylase (levels are elevated)
- Urine tests
  - Urinary pH may be elevated.
  - Urinalysis may reveal:
    - Elevated specific gravity in dehydration
    - Elevated ketones in starvation
    - Increased pH in presence of vomiting
- Hormone tests, if menstrual periods are problematic
  - Thyroid function tests
  - Luteinizing hormone
  - Follicle-stimulating hormone
  - Estradiol
  - Prolactin (if amenorrheic)
- Echocardiography
  - If potassium levels are abnormal
  - If history of ipecac use
- Bone density test for osteopenia
  - If oligomenorrheic or amenorrheic

IMAGING

- Magnetic resonance imaging of the brain, gastrointestinal series, or other tests may be considered in some cases for patients who claim to be eating well or not vomiting on purpose.

DIAGNOSTIC PROCEDURES

- To document orthostatic changes:
  - Check blood pressure and pulse with patient in the sitting position, followed by standing for 2 minutes.
  - Significant changes:
    - Increase of 20 beats per minute in pulse
    - Decrease of 20 mm Hg in systolic blood pressure
    - Decrease of 10 mm Hg in diastolic blood pressure

TREATMENT APPROACH

- Cognitive-behavioral therapy, followed by introduction of medication if necessary, has been suggested as a logical treatment approach.
- Treatment may be difficult for any single professional; a team approach is most often used, consisting of:
  - Primary care physician
  - Psychiatrist
  - Psychologist or social worker
  - Nutritionist
- The exact combination should be determined by local expertise, availability, and preference.
  - Team meetings/discussions should be held frequently to prevent miscommunication that can sabotage the treatment.
- Multimodal therapy
  - Medical management
  - Nutritional rehabilitation
  - Behavior therapy
    - May be difficult when treating in the outpatient setting
    - Classic approaches may not be effective because vomiting cannot be measured readily.
    - Cognitive-behavioral approaches allow patients to understand and participate in their own behavioral therapy.
      - Diaries
      - Modification of daily patterns to effect change
  - Individual psychotherapy
    - Essential part of treatment for most patients
    - Exploration of underlying psychological features and determination of mechanisms for change
    - Psychological change is generally acknowledged to be a necessary precursor to significant improvement.
  - Family therapy
    - Important component of treatment, especially for younger patients
    - Family conflicts and problems play a major role in symptom continuation.
    - Sessions arranged in varying combinations to include parents and siblings
    - General focus on disordered communication patterns
    - Resolution of specific conflicts arising from the eating disorder itself is important.
    - The course of the disorder is much more difficult for adolescents whose families are unable or unwilling to make needed changes in their customary patterns of communication and parenting.
  - Group therapy
    - For college-aged patients, may be the only approach used
    - Groups may focus on either:
      - Psychotherapeutic approach
      - Behavioral changes
    - Benefits outweigh the risks of learning bad habits from others in the group.
- Psychopharmacology
- The degree to which each of these is used varies by preferences of the treatment team and requirements of the individual patient.
- Each of these approaches may be used for inpatients, day-program patients, and outpatients.
- If hospitalization is necessary for uncontrolled binge or purge cycles, abnormal electrolytes, or unstable vital signs, then supervision after meals, locked bathrooms, and restricted access to food are often needed.

SPECIFIC TREATMENTS

Dietary plan

- An appropriate meal pattern may be developed on the basis of the patient's and family's prior eating habits or a specific dietary plan offered by the physician or nutritionist.
- The plan should be specific so as to avoid ambiguities that can lead to family fighting.
- The plan should provide 2000–3000 calories daily.
  - Some may be supplied as high-calorie supplements.
  - A similar dietary plan without high-calorie supplements may be offered to healthy-weight bulimic patients, who require nutritional adjustment rather than nutritional rehabilitation.
  - Caloric requirements depend on need for weight gain, loss, or maintenance.
- Because caloric restriction may spark binge eating, a nonrestrictive well-balanced diet should be implemented.
- The diet should be balanced and include foods from each major food group.
- Outpatient gains should be 1–2 pounds per week.
- Inpatient gains may be 2–4 pounds per week.
- Compliance may be evaluated with a diet diary, but many patients do not keep records accurately and honestly.

Psychopharmalogic treatments

- Selective serotonin reuptake inhibitor (SSRI) antidepressants
  - Can treat concurrent psychiatric disorder
  - May diminish the urge to binge and purge and help treat obsessive-compulsive symptoms

- Only physicians familiar with the use of these should prescribe them, given concerns about associated increased risk of suicide in a minority of children and adolescents.
- Not effective in treating symptoms of depression or obsessive-compulsive disorder when body weight is low
- Atypical antipsychotic agents at low doses can improve weight gain and treat symptoms of depression and obsessional thoughts.
  - Other antidepressant medications, roughly equivalent to SSRIs
    - Tricyclics
    - Monoamine oxidase inhibitors
    - Fluoxetine at 60 mg per day
    - Anticonvulsants— see modest changes in symptoms
- To restore menses:
  - Generally requires estradiol level >30 mg/dL

WHEN TO ADMIT

- ≥1 of the following:
  - Severe malnutrition (body weight < 75% ideal)
  - Dehydration
  - Electrolyte disturbances
  - Cardiac disturbances
  - Physiologic instability
    - Bradycardia
    - Hypotension
    - Hypothermia
    - Orthostatic changes
  - Arrested growth and development
  - Failure of outpatient treatment
  - Acute food refusal
  - Uncontrollable binging and purging
  - Acute medical complication of malnutrition
    - Syncope
    - Seizures
    - Cardiac failure
    - Pancreatitis
  - Acute psychiatric emergencies
    - Suicidal ideation
    - Acute psychosis
  - Comorbid diagnosis that interferes with treatment
    - Severe depression
    - Obsessive-compulsive disorder
    - Severe family dysfunction

WHEN TO REFER

- Refer to a dietician if the primary care physician or staff does not have the expertise or time to set a nutritional plan.
- Refer to a psychotherapist if:
  - The patient is open to therapy.
  - The patient cannot attain goals set by the physician, even if the patient is resistant to psychotherapy.
  - Refer for psychopharmacologic evaluation if both the physician and the therapist believe that patient might benefit from medication if:
    - The patient is binging and open to medication.
    - Obsessive-compulsive symptoms are interfering with treatment.
- Refer to adolescent medicine if:
  - The physician is not comfortable treating the patient.
  - The physician does not have the time to treat.
  - The patient does not adhere to the physician's treatment plan.

COMPLICATIONS

- Hypertension or hypotension
- Electrolyte abnormalities
- Dehydration
- Erosion of dental enamel
- Calluses on the dorsum of the hand
- Parotid enlargement
- Acute pancreatitis
- Acute gastric dilatation or rupture
- Mallory–Weiss tears
- Gastric and esophageal irritation
- Gastric and esophageal bleeding
- Gastroesophageal reflux disease
- Barrett esophagus
- Aspiration pneumonia
- Diarrhea, constipation, steatorrhea
- Emetine cardiomyopathy
- Menstrual irregularity
- Polycystic ovarian syndrome
- Osteopenia, osteoporosis

PROGNOSIS

- Approximately 50% of patients recover.
- 30% experience relapse.
- 20% continue to meet the full criteria for bulimia nervosa 5 years after diagnosis.

PREVENTION

- Programs geared toward both teenage boys and girls, primarily in school settings
  - Aimed at maintaining healthy body image, healthy eating
  - Try to promote self-esteem without relation to weight
  - Succeed in terms of increasing awareness and knowledge about eating disorders
  - Effectiveness is debatable.
- Programs focused on building self-esteem/comprehensive school-based approach
  - Classroom interventions
  - Staff training throughout the school
  - Informal discussions between staff and students
  - Integration of material about eating issues into the curriculum
  - More intensive work with persons at high risk
  - Changes in the school with respect to cafeteria food and physical education
  - Referrals and outreach, both within the school and to the community
- Early case detection and treatment are the most effective preventive measures.
  - Treatment will be easier.
  - Disease will be less entrenched.
  - Families, friends, school personnel, and health professionals must be vigilant for signs of an eating disorder so that early treatment can be initiated.

Cancers in Childhood

DEFINITION

- Solid tumors seen in children include:
  - Wilms tumor: malignant renal tumor
  - Neuroblastoma: arises from fetal neural cells that normally develop into the sympathetic nervous system
  - Retinoblastoma: congenital malignant tumor of the retina
  - Rhabdomyosarcoma: tumor that can occur almost anywhere, including sites not normally containing skeletal muscle; can be aggressive and disseminate early
  - Germ cell tumors and teratomas: growths arising from primordial germ cells
  - Ewing family of tumors: Ewing sarcoma of bone, extraosseous Ewing tumor, and peripheral primitive neuroectodermal tumors (PNETs)
    - Malignant tumors that usually arise in bone but may also occur in soft tissues
    - PNET of the chest wall is referred to as *Askin tumor*.
  - Osteosarcoma: bone tumor
  - Non-Hodgkin lymphoma (NHL): heterogeneous group of cancers arising from lymphocytes and lymphoid precursors
    - Migratory; occur at variable sites
    - Lymphoblastic lymphoma (30% of cases)
    - Anaplastic large-cell (10%)
    - Burkitt (40%)
    - Diffuse large B-cell (20%)
  - Hodgkin disease: cancer of the lymphoreticular system characterized by multinucleated giant cells, known as *Reed-Sternberg cells*

EPIDEMIOLOGY

Wilms tumor

- Prevalence
  - Most common abdominal tumor of childhood (5–6% of pediatric cancers)
- Incidence
  - 600–700 new cases diagnosed each year in the US
- Age/sex/race
  - Patients usually 2–5 years of age
  - Rare in teenagers
  - Bilateral disease more common in younger patients and in girls
  - Occurs more often in black patients than in white patients

Neuroblastoma

- Prevalence
  - Second most common abdominal tumor of childhood; most common extracranial solid tumor
  - Most common cancer of infants, accounting for more than one half of cancer cases in infants
  - Accounts for 7% of all children with a cancer diagnosis
  - Accounts for 15% of childhood cancer mortality
- Age/race
  - 90% of patients are <5 years.
  - 97% of patients receive a diagnosis before 10 years of age.
  - Approximately 9.7 white children and 7.4 black children per million in the US diagnosed yearly (800–900 new cases/year)

Retinoblastoma

- Prevalence
  - Unilateral disease is a sporadic form of the tumor in 90% of patients with this presentation; the other 10% have familial retinoblastoma.
  - Bilateral disease present in 30–40% of patients.
- Incidence
  - 350 children in the US annually
- Age
  - Diagnosed in 95% before age 4 years; median age of diagnosis is 2 years
  - Bilateral disease occurs at an earlier age.

Rhabdomyosarcoma

- Prevalence
  - Accounts for 2–4% of childhood cancers and 5–15% of childhood solid tumors
- Incidence
  - Annual incidence among children (≤18 years of age) in the US is 4.5 per million.
  - 400 new cases diagnosed each year
- Age/sex/race
  - 40% are <5 years.
  - 47% are 5–14 years.
  - The remainder are >15 years.
  - Incidence is greater in boys than in girls.
  - More common in white patients than in black patients

Germ cell tumors/teratomas

- Prevalence
  - 3% of tumors in children
  - Sacrococcygeal teratoma: benign in 80% of patients; occurs in 1/35,000 live births
- Incidence
  - Annual incidence of 4 cases per million children <15 years
- Age/sex
  - Incidence or sacrococcygeal teratoma is greatest in adolescents and very young children.
  - Sacrococcygeal teratoma is more common in girls than in boys (2:1 to 4:1).

Ewing family of tumors

- Prevalence
  - 3% of childhood cancers
- Age/race
  - Most common bone tumor in children <10 years
  - Peak incidence between 11 and 17 years (7 per million per year)
  - Ewing sarcoma is extremely rare in patients <5 years, as well as in black and Asian persons.

Osteosarcoma

- Prevalence
  - Most common bone tumor in children: 8.7 per million
  - Comprises 60% of malignant bone tumors
- Incidence
  - Approximately 400 patients diagnosed per year in the US
- Age/sex
  - Peak incidence is at age 14.5 for boys and 13.5 for girls, corresponding to growth spurts, although disease can occur before puberty and after the adolescent growth spurt.
  - Male-to-female ratio of approximately 1.5:1

NHL

- Prevalence
  - Accounts for approximately 10% of childhood cancer cases
  - 60% of lymphomas are NHLs.
- Age/sex
  - Incidence low in children <5 years and then increases
  - More common in boys than in girls (2:1 to 3:1)
  - Greatest sex difference in Burkitt lymphoma; male-to-female ratio is approximately 4.5:1

Hodgkin disease

- Prevalence
  - 6% of cancers in children
- Incidence
  - 600 cases diagnosed in the US each year
- Age/sex/race
  - Two age peaks: 15–30 years of age and late adulthood
  - Extremely rare before 5 years
  - Male predominance throughout preadolescent age range; thereafter, incidence approximately equal in both sexes
  - In older teenagers and young adults, disease is most common among white persons.

ETIOLOGY

- Wilms tumor
  - Anomalies are reported in 13–28% of affected patients.
    - Most involve the genitourinary (GU) tract.
    - Hemihypertrophy is second in frequency, sometimes noted as a component of the Beckwith-Wiedemann syndrome (excessive growth of many body organs).
  - 33% of children with the sporadic form of congenital aniridia have Wilms tumor.
  - Syndromes are associated with germ-line mutations of the *WT1* gene, located at 11p13.
    - WAGR syndrome: association of Wilms tumor, aniridia, GU abnormalities, and mental retardation
    - Denys-Drash syndrome: association of Wilms tumor with ambiguous genitalia and diffuse glomerular disease
  - A second Wilms tumor suppressor locus may be at 11p15; this is also the locus for the familial form of Beckwith-Wiedemann syndrome.
  - Loss of heterozygosity at 1p and 16q has been identified.
- Neuroblastoma
  - May be related to abnormal maturation of fetal neural crest cells
  - Possible prezygotic germinal mutation
- Retinoblastoma
  - Two independent mutations occur in a single retinal cell.
  - Possibly due to abnormalities of chromosome 13q14
  - Possible role of human papillomavirus in sporadic retinoblastoma
- Rhabdomyosarcoma
  - The cause is unknown.
  - Possibly due to mutations in at 11p15 and to chromosomal translocation, t(2:13)
- Germ cell tumors/teratomas
  - Aberrant path of migration: extragonadal germ cell tumors along the dorsal wall of the embryo in midline sites (sacrococcygeal, retroperitoneal, mediastinal, and pineal regions)
  - Association with a family history of twinning resulted in early theories suggesting that teratomas were abortive attempts at the development of twins.
- Ewing family of tumors
  - Chromosomal translocation, t(11:22) and gene fusion rearrangements
- Osteosarcoma
  - Abnormality at the *Rb* gene; mutation or loss of *RB1* gene
  - Inactivation of *p53* tumor suppressor gene
  - Other chromosomal abnormalities

- NHL
  - Epstein-Barr virus (EBV) or other viral infection may be a contributing factor.
  - Immunodeficiency
    - Defect of T-cell regulation
  - Genetic
    - Chromosomal aberrations in Burkitt lymphoma
    - Several specific, nonrandom chromosomal abnormalities have been reported in lymphoblastic lymphoma and large-cell lymphomas.
- Hodgkin disease
  - Possible genetic role
  - Possible environmental role
  - EBV may play a role.
  - Underlying immunodeficiency may be involved.

RISK FACTORS

- Wilms tumor
  - May occur in siblings, cousins, and parent-child pairs, particularly in association with specific congenital anomalies and bilateral disease
  - Genetic predisposition (15–20% of cases)
- Neuroblastoma
  - Reported to occur with increased incidence in patients with Hirschsprung disease
- Lymphomas
  - Immunosuppressive therapy for renal, cardiac, or bone marrow allografts
- Osteosarcoma
  - Irradiation to the bone, usually for treatment of cancer
  - Presence of 1 tumor already
  - Hereditary retinoblastoma

SIGNS AND SYMPTOMS

Wilms tumor

- Painless mass that is usually firm, occasionally lobulated, and confined to one side of the abdomen
- Occasionally:
  - Rapid abdominal enlargement
  - Anemia
  - Hypertension (perhaps because of a sudden subcapsular hemorrhage)
- Malaise
- Abdominal pain
- Hematuria
- Fever

Neuroblastoma

- Presenting features largely depend on the location of the tumor.
  - Large, firm, irregular abdominal mass that may cross the midline is often the first sign of disease.
  - Disturbances of bowel or bladder function, possibly from compression by a pelvic mass
  - Cough or respiratory distress, thoracic mass
  - Horner syndrome or heterochromia iridis
  - Dumbbell-shaped mass along backbone, neuroblastomas that arise in the paravertebral ganglia and grow into the intervertebral foramina
- Spinal cord compression may cause pain, extremity weakness, paralysis, or incontinence (difficult to assess if the patient is still in diapers).
  - Cord compression is an emergency requiring surgical decompression, radiation, or chemotherapy to prevent paraplegia.
- If there is hepatic involvement in infants, marked abdominal distention may be followed by respiratory compromise.
- Bluish skin nodules are sometimes noted in infants who have neuroblastoma.
  - Palpation causes erythematous cutaneous flush, lasting for 2–3 minutes, followed by vasoconstriction and blanching.
- Pain, if bone involvement in skull, orbit, or proximal long bones
- Raccoon-like appearance if there is orbital involvement
- In infants with intracranial disease, separation of cranial sutures
- Fever
- Malaise
- Failure to thrive
- Opsoclonus-myoclonus (rapid, dancing-eye movements) is an unusual symptom.

Retinoblastoma

- Abnormal red reflex (leukocoria)
  - *Leukocoria* (cat's-eye reflex) describes a whiteness detected in the pupillary area caused by a large retrolental mass.
- Strabismus
- In rare cases, pain in the eye

Rhabdomyosarcoma

- Disturbance of a normal body function (due to tumor)
- Pain at site of tumor
- Orbital tumor
  - Swelling
  - Proptosis
  - Discoloration
  - Limitation of extraocular motion

- Head and neck tumor
  - Hoarseness
  - Difficulty swallowing
  - Nasopharyngeal polyps
  - Nasopharyngeal obstruction
  - Decreased hearing acuity
  - Persistent otitis
  - Sinusitis, bloody nasal discharge
  - Parotitis
  - Cranial nerve palsies
  - Headache
  - Vomiting
  - Diplopia
- Retroperitoneal tumor
  - Mass or partial or complete bowel obstruction
- GU tumor
  - Vaginal bleeding
  - Pelvic or perineal masses
  - Hematuria
  - Urinary frequency
  - Urinary retention
  - May be extruded from the bladder or female genital tract
- Paratesticular
  - Hydrocele
  - Incarcerated hernia
  - Testicular torsion or testicular mass
- Pain, difficulty, or refusal to ambulate resulting from bone metastases
- Fever
- Fatigue
- Weight loss

Germ cell tumors/teratomas

- Sacrococcygeal tumors
  - Mass between the anus and the coccyx
  - Abnormality of the overlying skin may be noted.
  - Intrapelvic tumor may be associated with an external tumor or may be noted by urinary or rectal obstruction.
- Ovarian tumors
  - In infants, present as abdominal mass
  - Older girls
    - Abdominal pain
    - Nausea
    - Vomiting
    - Constipation

- Urinary tract obstruction
- Palpable mass noted in 50%
- Acute abdominal pain
- Vaginal tumors in girls <3 years may cause bloody vaginal discharge.

- Testicular tumors
  - Symptom-free scrotal masses
  - Torsion in an undescended testis may result in acute abdominal pain.
- Retroperitoneal teratomas
  - In children >2 years
    - Anorexia
    - Vomiting
    - Abdominal pain
- Tumors of the anterior mediastinum
  - Coughing
  - Wheezing
  - Dyspnea
  - Chest pain
- Intrapericardial tumors
  - Heart failure and cardiac tamponade
- Cranial tumors
  - In infants
    - Hydrocephalus
    - Intracranial pressure
  - Teenagers
    - Headaches
    - Lethargy
    - Vomiting
    - Diabetes insipidus
    - Seizures
    - Visual disturbance, especially loss of upward gaze

Ewing tumors

- Pain
- Swelling
- Symptoms may initially be attributed to trauma.
- Palpable mass (in 60% of patients)

Osteosarcoma

- Bone pain is ubiquitous.
- Palpable masses
- Swelling
- Limited motion
- Fractures (rare)

NHL

- Localized lymphadenopathy
- Patients with mediastinal masses: history of cough and, occasionally, acute respiratory distress
  - Obstruction can occur during evaluation, even in patients who have few symptoms, particularly with administration of sedation.
  - Obstruction may involve the lower airway, beyond the reach of an endotracheal tube, resulting in an inability to effectively ventilate the lungs.
- Abdominal mass that may involve the ileocecal region, mesentery, ovaries, or retroperitoneum is seen in 30–40% of patients
- Large-cell lymphomas may produce peripheral adenopathy.

Hodgkin lymphoma

- Bone pain is ubiquitous and commonly associated with trauma.
- Palpable masses
- Swelling
- Limited motion
- Weight loss/other systemic effects are rarely seen; if present, overt metastasis is likely.
- Fractures (uncommon)
- Cough, chest pain, and dyspnea may occur with extensive pulmonary metastases.

DIFFERENTIAL DIAGNOSIS

Differential diagnosis of abdominal and pelvic tumors

- Wilms tumor
  - Age: preschool
  - Clinical signs: unilateral flank mass, aniridia, hemihypertrophy
  - Lab findings: hematuria
- Neuroblastoma
  - Age: preschool
  - Clinical signs: gastrointestinal (GI) or GU obstruction, raccoon eyes, opsoclonus-myoclonus, diarrhea, skin nodules (infants)
  - Lab findings: increased vanillylmandelic acid, increased homovanillic acid, increased ferritin, stippled calcification in mass
- NHL
  - Age: >1 year
  - Clinical signs: intussusception in those >2 years
  - Lab findings: increased urate
- Rhabdomyosarcoma
  - Age: Any

  - Clinical signs: GI or GU obstruction, sarcoma botryoides, vaginal bleeding, paratesticular mass
  - Lab findings: none
- Germ cell or teratoma
  - Age: preschool, teens
  - Clinical signs
    - Girls: abdominal pain, vaginal bleeding
    - Boys: new-onset testicular mass, hydrocele, sacrococcygeal mass or dimple
  - Lab findings: increased human chorionic gonadotropin (hCG), increased a-fetoprotein (AFP)
- Hepatoblastoma
  - Age: birth to 3 years
  - Clinical signs: large, firm liver
  - Lab findings: increased AFP
- Hepatoma
  - Age: school age, teens
  - Clinical signs: large, firm liver; hepatitis B, cirrhosis
  - Lab findings: increased AFP

Differential diagnosis of head and neck tumors

- NHL
  - Age: >1 year
  - Clinical signs: lymphadenopathy not responsive to antibiotics, immunodeficiency, EBV (in Africa)
  - Lab findings: increased urate
- Hodgkin disease
  - Age: >10 years
  - Clinical signs: lymphadenopathy not responsive to antibiotics; weight loss, night sweats, fever, pruritus
  - Lab findings: increased erythrocyte sedimentation rate (ESR)
- Rhabdomyosarcoma
  - Age: all
  - Clinical signs: orbital mass, hoarseness, persistent otitis, sinusitis
  - Lab findings: none
- Neuroblastoma
  - Age: preschool
  - Clinical signs: heterochromia iridis, Horner syndrome, opsoclonus-myoclonus, raccoon eyes, skin nodules (infants)
  - Lab findings: increased homovanillic acid, vanillylmandelic acid, or both in urine; calcification
- Retinoblastoma
  - Age: preschool

- Clinical signs: cat's-eye reflex, strabismus, family history
- Lab findings: calcification

Differential diagnosis of tumors of the extremities

- Ewing sarcoma
  - Age: ≥5 years
  - Clinical signs: pain, swelling; genitourinary or skeletal anomaly; weight loss, fever; malaise (metabolic)
  - Imaging: onionskin appearance on roentgenography
- Osteogenic sarcoma
  - Age: teens
  - Clinical signs: pain, swelling; familial retinoblastoma; prior radiation to bone; Paget disease
  - Imaging and lab findings: Codman triangle (cortical elevation, new bone formation); sunburst ossification of soft tissue; soft-tissue mass; increased alkaline phosphatase level
- Lymphoma
  - Age: all
  - Clinical signs: pain
- Fibrosarcoma
  - Age: infants, teens
  - Clinical signs: painless mass; prior radiation; plastic implant
- Rhabdomyosarcoma
  - Age: all
  - Clinical signs: mass
- Synovial sarcoma
  - Age: teens
  - Clinical signs: mass
  - Laboratory findings: calcification (40%)

Differential possibilities

- Retinoblastoma
  - Coats disease
  - Retrolental fibroplasia
  - Persistent hyperplastic primary vitreous
  - Toxoplasmosis
  - *Toxocara canis* infection
  - Other causes of severe uveitis
- Germ cell tumors/teratomas
  - Sacrococcygeal masses: meningocele
  - Abdominal or pelvic masses
    - Neuroblastoma
    - Wilms tumor
    - Rhabdomyosarcoma
    - Lymphomas
    - Hydronephrosis
    - Benign ovarian cysts
    - Constipation
    - Splenomegaly
  - Anterior mediastinal tumors
    - T-cell lymphoma
    - Leukemia
    - Thymoma
  - Intrascrotal mass
    - Testicular torsion
    - Epididymitis
    - Testicular infarction
- Ewing sarcoma
  - Osteosarcoma
  - Osteomyelitis
  - Benign bone tumors
  - Bone cysts
  - Lymphoma
  - Leukemia
  - Neuroblastoma
  - Rhabdomyosarcoma
- NHL
  - Other causes of cervical adenopathy
    - Hodgkin disease
    - Neuroblastoma
    - Leukemia
    - Nasopharyngeal carcinoma
    - Rhabdomyosarcoma
    - Thyroid carcinoma
  - Anterior mediastinal masses
    - T-cell leukemia
    - Thymoma
  - Abdominal masses
    - Constipation
    - Splenomegaly
    - Wilms tumor
    - Rhabdomyosarcoma
    - Neuroblastoma
    - Lymphoma (rare bone tumor)

C

DIAGNOSTIC APPROACH

- Wilms tumor
  - Begin with history and physical examination.
  - Pay particular attention to the associated congenital anomalies and the family history.
- Neuroblastoma
  - Initial physical examination followed by imaging and biopsy
- Retinoblastoma
  - Examination under anesthesia after dilating the pupils is necessary to evaluate the retina.
  - Enucleation may be necessary for diagnosis and treatment when disease is unilateral.
  - The extent of local disease (extension beyond the globe or optic nerve infiltration) is assessed at the time of enucleation.
  - For high-risk patients, bone marrow and cerebrospinal fluid specimens are obtained for evidence of dissemination.
- Rhabdomyosarcoma
  - Initial evaluation should include complete history and physical examination.
  - Follow with roentgenography, computed tomagraphy (CT) or magnetic resonance imaging (MRI), and in some instances (eg, GU tract) ultrasonography of involved and adjacent areas.
  - Biopsy of the lesion establishes the diagnosis and should be performed before extensive resection.
- Germ cell tumors/teratomas
  - Identified through physical examination
    - In cases of sacrococcygeal mass or abdominal pain, particular attention should be paid to the abdominal and rectal examination.
  - Pelvic examination (under anesthesia in young girls) is necessary if ovarian or vaginal tumor is suspected.
- Ewing sarcoma
  - Radiograph should be obtained if:
    - Mass is overlying bone *or*
    - In the presence of bone pain not characteristic of trauma (by lack of history or duration of symptoms)
  - Possibility of bone marrow involvement should be evaluated by bilateral bone marrow aspirates and biopsies.
  - Identification of micrometastases in the bone marrow by polymerase chain reaction may identify high-risk patients without other evidence of metastases.
  - Cerebrospinal fluid should be examined in patients who have parameningeal tumors.
  - Biopsy of the lesion is necessary to establish the diagnosis.
    - If possible, tissue should be obtained from soft tissue rather than from cortical bone to reduce potential for pathologic fracture.

- Osteosarcoma
  - Biopsy should be performed by an orthopedic surgeon.
  - CT or MRI is used to define extent of primary lesion.
- NHL
  - Complete resection of diseased area is not necessary.
  - Lumbar puncture should be performed with cytocentrifugation of cerebrospinal fluid to detect meningeal involvement.
- Hodgkin disease
  - Begin assessment with complete history and thorough physical examination.
    - Particular attention should be paid to B disease symptoms.
  - Lymphatic areas to be evaluated include Waldeyer ring and the cervical, supraclavicular, axillary, and inguinal lymph nodes.
    - Node size and presence of tenderness should be noted and recorded carefully.
  - A thorough abdominal examination should be performed, particularly to evaluate liver and spleen size; retroperitoneal lymph nodes are not palpable.
  - Bone marrow biopsies should be performed in all but those with stage IA or IIA disease.
  - Define subdiaphragmatic involvement when radiotherapy is the primary therapeutic modality.

LABORATORY FINDINGS

- Wilms tumor
  - Laboratory studies should include a complete blood count, urinalysis, and renal and liver function tests.
  - In some cases, polycythemia or hypocalcemia is present.
- Neuroblastoma
  - Evaluate amplification of the N-*myc* oncogene (poor prognosis); a DNA index >1 indicates disease that is sensitive to chemotherapy (good prognosis).
  - The following are confirmatory in patients who have a small round blue cell infiltrate in bone marrow:
    - Increased levels of vanillylmandelic acid and homovanillic acid in 24-hour urine samples
    - Increased vanillylmandelic acid–creatinine or homovanillic acid–creatinine ratios in spot urine samples
    - Ferritin and lactic dehydrogenase levels predict a poor prognosis if increased.
- Germ cell tumors/teratomas
  - Serum AFP and ß-hCG should be assayed before surgery.
  - Detection of AFP or ß-hCG improves ability to monitor the disease status.
    - Rate of disappearance after resection reflects adequacy of the tumor removal.
    - With response to chemotherapy, levels decrease.
    - A significant increase suggests disease recurrence.

- Osteosarcoma
  - Baseline lactic dehydrogenase and alkaline phosphatase levels should be obtained.
  - Osteoid found within a sarcomatous tumor is a characteristic histologic pattern.
  - Osteosarcoma in the child or adolescent is usually a high-grade tumor characterized by osteoblasts that demonstrate pleomorphism and bizarre mitoses.
- NHL
  - Enzyme studies (terminal deoxynucleotidyl transferase) or gene rearrangement studies may be helpful as are cytogenetic studies, if possible.
- Hodgkin disease
  - Blood cell counts may show:
    - Anemia (caused by hemolysis or chronic disease)
    - Abnormal neutrophil count
    - Thrombocytopenia
  - Increased ESR, serum copper level, and ferritin level (in some patients)
  - Serum hepatic alkaline phosphatase isoenzyme may be increased.

IMAGING

Wilms tumor

- Plain-film radiography of the abdomen may show:
  - Coarse calcifications, unlike the fine, stippled pattern commonly seen in neuroblastoma
  - A mass effect may be noted.
- Chest radiograph should be obtained; it may demonstrate pulmonary nodules.
- Ultrasonography is often performed first.
  - Particularly helpful in evaluating the renal vein, vena cava, and the right side of the heart for tumor spread.
- Abdominal CT with contrast
  - Studies may reveal an intrarenal mass displacing and distorting the collecting system of the involved kidney.
  - Tumors may be very large.
  - Minimal kidney parenchyma may be identified.
- Chest CT
  - Should be performed before surgery to detect small pulmonary metastases
  - Postoperative atelectasis can obscure metastatic nodules.
- Liver metastases may be diagnosed either by ultrasonography or by CT.
- Intravenous pyelography generally is not indicated.
- MRI may occasionally be indicated to define the extent of the tumor.
- Bone scans indicated if there is clear cell sarcoma of the kidney (which often spreads to bone).

Germ cell tumors/teratomas

- CT of benign germ cell tumors often reveals calcifications.
- Chest CT and bone scan should be performed to detect pulmonary and bony metastases.
- Teratoma frequently shows cystic and solid, including fat, components on radiologic examination.
- Malignant germ cell tumors often have areas of hemorrhage and necrosis.

Neuroblastoma

- Radiologic examination of the area of primary disease, as well as of areas to which neuroblastoma metastasizes
- CT of the abdomen, pelvis, and chest
  - In cases with cervical masses, CT should include this area.
- MRI should be performed on any patient with intervertebral lesions, because paravertebral lesions may extend into the intervertebral foramina.
- Skeletal survey and a bone scan should be performed to detect bony lesions.
  - Radiography is useful for detecting small lytic lesions at the end of bones.
  - Bone scan helps identify lesions of the skull and tubular bones.
- Positron emission tomography (PET) may also be helpful.

Retinoblastoma

- Ultrasonography is useful to evaluate the mass, particularly if the fundal examination is obscured by hemorrhage or retinal detachment.
- Calcification may be apparent on radiography, ultrasonography, or CT.
- CT helps demonstrate the extent of intraocular disease and may detect possible extraocular extension.
- MRI can help to evaluate the tumor involvement with the optic nerve, the subarachnoid, and the brain.

Rhabdomyosarcoma

- In GU disease, cystourethrography and barium enema may be needed.
- Dental films may be helpful.
- Bone surveys, bone scans, and chest and abdominal CT are necessary to assess for metastatic disease.
- Basal skull erosion may be seen on CT.
- If spinal cord symptoms present, spinal MRI is necessary.

Ewing sarcoma

- CT and MRI are necessary to determine the extent of the primary lesion.
  - Radiography often shows a destructive lesion in the diaphysis.
  - An onionskin appearance arises from periosteal elevation and subperiosteal new bone formation associated with tumor extension through the cortex.

- A mottled pattern may be seen as a result of bone destruction, sclerosis, and cystic formation.
- Associated soft-tissue mass occurs in >50% of patients who have primary tumors of long bones.
- Radionuclide bone scanning can detect primary/metastatic lesions.
- CT of the chest is necessary to determine whether pulmonary lesions are present.

Osteosarcoma

- Radiographs of involved bone may show:
  - Bony destruction with periosteal new bone formation
  - Characteristic sunburst appearance
  - Soft-tissue swelling
  - Necrosis, fibrosis, and calcification
- The extent of the primary lesion is defined further by CT or, preferentially, by MRI.
- Metastatic disease in the lung should be sought by CT (present in 80% of patients with metastases).
- Bone scans can be helpful for outlining primary tumor and detecting multiple primary lesions and metastasis.
- PET may be helpful.

NHL

- Imaging studies should include chest radiograph and CT of the chest and abdomen in all patients.
- Bone scans and gallium scans can be helpful in selected patients, although positron emission tomography (PET) is also being used.

Hodgkin disease

- Chest radiograph and CT of the chest and abdomen
- Gallium scanning
- PET is becoming routine, although it may be most applicable for monitoring response and recurrence as opposed to staging.
- Bone scan should be considered in advanced disease, particularly in the presence of bone pain or increased serum alkaline phosphatase level.

DIAGNOSTIC PROCEDURES

- Wilms tumor
  - Tumor staging upon surgery: favorable histology (FH) or unfavorable histology (UH)
    - FH indicates absence of unfavorable features.
    - UH indicates presence of focal or diffuse anaplasia, defined by the presence of gigantic polypoid nuclei in the tumor sample.
- Neuroblastoma: biopsy and histology
  - In localized disease, a biopsy specimen must be obtained from primary tumor.

- In metastatic disease, neuroblastoma cells can be identified in the primary tumor or in areas of metastases, including the bone, bone marrow, or liver.
- Neuroblastoma produces small round cells with scant cytoplasm that must be differentiated from lymphoma, leukemia, Ewing sarcoma, and retinoblastoma.
- Osteosarcoma: biopsy and histology
  - The biopsy site is of critical importance and should be performed by an orthopedic surgeon with experience in oncology.
  - Osteoid found in a sarcomatous tumor is the characteristic histologic pattern.
  - Osteosarcoma in the child or adolescent is usually a high-grade tumor characterized by osteoblasts that demonstrate pleomorphism and bizarre mitoses.
  - Necrosis, fibrosis, and calcification may be noted.
- NHL
  - Surgical biopsy
    - If adenopathy is present, removal of the most suspicious node is suggested.
    - Biopsy may be contraindicated if large mediastinal masses pose an imminent possibility of airway obstruction, unless endotracheal intubation will ensure airway patency.
    - If distal end of endotracheal tube lies proximal to the mass, localized radiation to the mediastinum may be necessary before specimen is obtained.
    - Alternative sites for obtaining specimens must then be considered.
- Hodgkin disease biopsy
  - Histology defines the 4 subtypes:
    - Nodular sclerosing subtype
      - Has collagenous bands that divide the lymphoid tissues into nodules and the presence of a lacunar variant of the Reed-Sternberg cell
    - Lymphocyte-predominant subtype
      - Characterized by destruction of the lymph node architecture, with cellular proliferation of benign-appearing lymphocytes
      - Reed-Sternberg cells are rarely found in the absence of fibrosis.
      - Disease is usually localized.
    - Mixed-cellularity subtype
      - Lymph node architecture is not preserved.
      - Approximately 10 Reed-Sternberg cells are seen per high-power field, often with interstitial fibrosis.
      - Necrosis is not pronounced.

– Lymphocyte-depleted subtype

- Characterized by presence of fibrosis, necrosis, and abnormal cells (but only a rare lymphocyte)
- Rare in children

CLASSIFICATION

Staging of Wilms tumor

- Stage I: Tumor is limited to the kidney and completely resected.
- Stage II: Tumor extends beyond the kidney but is completely resected. Isolated tumor spill may exist confined to the flank.
- Stage III
  - Residual, nonhematogenously spread tumor is confined to the abdomen.
  - Unresectable tumors
- Stage IV: Hematogenous metastases are present.
  - Lung (only site in 80% of patients who have metastases)
  - Liver
  - Lymph node
  - Less commonly, bone, brain, and other sites
- Stage V: Bilateral renal involvement is present; for treatment purposes, each side is staged.

Neuroblastoma: International Neuroblastoma Staging System

- Stage 1: tumors with complete gross resection and microscopically negative ipsilateral and contralateral lymph nodes
- Stage 2: tumors are unilateral tumors with complete or incomplete gross resections but, at the most, only ipsilateral microscopically positive lymph nodes.
- Stage 3: includes tumors that cross the midline or unilateral tumors that have contralateral lymph node involvement
- Stage 4: metastatic disease
- Stage 4S (for special): tumors in infants <1 year who have stage 1 or 2 primary tumors with dissemination limited to liver, skin, or bone marrow

Germ cell tumors

- Low risk: stage I testicular and ovarian tumors
- Intermediate risk: stage II–IV testicular, stage II–III ovarian, stage I–II extragonadal malignant germ cell tumors
- High risk: stage III–IV extragonadal tumors

NHL: Murphy staging system

- Stage I: single tumor, nodal or extranodal
- Stage II
  - ≥2 nodal or extranodal sites, both on the same side of the diaphragm
  - GI tumors with only mesenteric nodes involved

- Stage III
  - Involve both sides of the diaphragm
  - Extensive abdominal disease
  - Paraspinal or epidural tumors
  - Any primary intrathoracic tumors
- Stage IV
  - CNS or bone marrow involvement

Hodgkin disease: Ann Arbor staging system

- Stage I
  - Involvement of 1 lymphatic region only
- Stage II
  - Involvement of ≥2 lymphatic regions on the same side of the diaphragm
- Stage III
  - Involvement on both sides of the diaphragm, including nodal regions, the spleen, or both
  - The Cotswold modification further divides stage III on the basis of specific subdiaphragmatic nodal sites involved.
    - Stage III_X for bulky mediastinal disease
    - Stage III_E for involvement of a single nodal site that is contiguous with a known nodal site of disease
- Stage IV
  - Involvement of extranodal organs, such as lungs, liver, bone marrow, kidneys, bone, or skin, in addition to lymph nodes

TREATMENT APPROACH

Wilms tumor

- Initial approach is complete resection by nephrectomy.
  - Requires meticulous and gentle surgical techniques to prevent tumor from spilling
  - Large transabdominal incision facilitates full exploration and excision.
  - Entire ureter is removed, and lymph nodes are sampled.
- For bilateral disease, chemotherapy is suggested after bilateral biopsy rather than immediate resection of the most involved site.
- Second-look excision of residual disease may be accomplished by partial nephrectomies, when possible.
- Tumors deemed unresectable by clinical and radiologic evaluation are sampled initially, with second-look resection performed after adequate chemotherapy-induced shrinkage.
- Patients with underlying syndromes, such as WAGR, should be considered for partial nephrectomies because of high risk of renal failure.
- Risk of renal failure is <0.6% in patients with sporadic disease; routine use of partial nephrectomies in this population not usually called for.

Neuroblastoma

- Sensitive to both chemotherapy and radiotherapy
- Surgery
  - Surgery alone may suffice for localized disease; minimal residual disease may regress spontaneously.
  - Complete removal of the tumor offers best chance of cure in higher-risk patients, but often only a diagnostic biopsy is feasible.
  - Surgical reduction after initial cytoreductive therapy may increase the likelihood of cure.
- Chemotherapy
  - Main therapeutic technique
  - Combination therapy is used most intensively in more advanced stages of disease.
  - Intensive regimens are at the limits of bone marrow tolerance.
- Myeloablative therapy
  - Followed by purged autologous stem cell transplantation to restore hematopoiesis improves event-free survival
  - Cis-retinoic acid improves survival for high-risk patients, regardless of whether stem cell transplantation was used.
- Radiation
  - May facilitate surgical resection of residual disease or may reduce risk of recurrence in surgically unresectable disease
  - Emergent situations may be treated with radiation, for example:
    - Large mediastinal mass resulting in respiratory compromise
    - Dumbbell lesion protruding into the intervertebral foramen that causes cord compression
  - Total-body irradiation may be a component of the preparative regimen used before hematopoietic stem cell transplantation.

Retinoblastoma

- Treatment is individualized on the basis of extent of disease and the possibility of preserving vision.
- Enucleation is used for unilateral sporadic disease where large lesions and compromised vision, with removal of the longest segment of the optic nerve possible.
- External-beam radiotherapy
- Plaque brachytherapy
- Cryotherapy
  - For small lesions, most commonly in patients who have hereditary bilateral disease
- Photocoagulation
  - For small lesions, most commonly in patients who have hereditary bilateral disease

- Chemotherapy
  - To allow local therapy to preserve vision
  - Significant tumor shrinkage can be achieved, but local therapy is required for cure.
  - May prevent pineoblastoma, a usually fatal second cancer in patients with hereditary retinoblastoma

Rhabdomyosarcoma

- Requires multitherapeutic approach: chemotherapy, surgery, radiation
- The initial surgical procedure should be diagnostic biopsy.
- Wide resection of the primary tumor, including surrounding normal tissue, is preferable if excessive functional or cosmetic morbidity can be prevented.
- Complete resection is correlated with a better outcome but is possible in only approximately 20% of patients.
- Biopsy should be performed on large regional nodes.
- Second-look surgery after chemotherapy
  - May allow resection with reduction of surgical morbidity
  - Provides assessment of therapeutic response by determining the presence of viable tumor
  - Potentially reduces the dose of radiotherapy
- Chemotherapy
  - Required in all cases
  - Regimens are determined by risk group (based on stage, group, histology, and age).
- Radiation
  - Portals should include the entire extent of tumor volume.
  - Required for patients with embryonal histology and residual disease after surgery and for all patients with alveolar histologic features
  - High doses (60–65 Gy) control local residual disease but have greater morbidity; lower doses result in an increased recurrence rate.

Germ cell tumors/teratomas

- Chemotherapy is effective in most cases.

Ewing sarcoma

- Local therapy alone with either surgery or radiotherapy is unlikely to be curative.
- Chemotherapy cures most localized sarcoma and improves outcome for metastatic disease.
- Choice of radiation or surgery for local control is based on likelihood of preserving function.
- Surgery
  - Functionally expendable bones should be removed.
  - Aggressive surgical procedures, including limb-sparing excisions, are frequently performed.
  - Surgical resection may improve prognosis.

- Radiotherapy
  - Required for local control and will improve prognosis when resection with appropriate margins is not achieved or when the tumor is unresectable
  - Preoperative radiotherapy may provide benefit.
  - Local failure rate is 22.5%, with higher failure rates for central versus noncentral tumor sites.
  - Patients receiving radiotherapy are a negatively selected group with unfavorable tumor sites or size.
  - Radiotherapy may also be helpful for treatment of pulmonary or osseous metastases.
- Chemotherapy
  - Effective for extraosseous Ewing sarcoma and peripheral PNETs

Osteosarcoma

- Surgery
  - Amputation has the same survival rate as limb salvage.
  - A portion of bone with tumor is removed and replaced by a prosthesis, bone graft, or composite.
    - Performed only if the vascular and neurologic integrity of the limb is not compromised
  - Preoperative chemotherapy may reduce the mass enough to make such surgery possible.
  - For lesions of the humerus, any preservation of hand function greatly improves quality of life.
  - In cases of pulmonary metastasis, surgical resection of nodules may result in long-term survival, even if multiple surgeries are required.

NHL

- Chemotherapy for all cases
  - Treatment regimens differ for lymphoblastic lymphoma versus nonlymphoblastic lymphoma; histologic class predicts efficacy.
  - Localized nonlymphoblastic lymphoma can be treated with short-course, low-intensity chemotherapy.
  - Localized lymphoblastic lymphoma requires maintenance therapy.
  - High-risk patients with lymphoblastic lymphoma are treated with protocols like those used for acute lymphoblastic leukemia.
  - Leukemia-like therapy may also be beneficial for patients with anaplastic large-cell lymphoma.
- Radiotherapy
  - Helpful in treating emergent situations, such as:
    - Airway compromise
    - Spinal cord compression
    - Overt meningeal involvement

- Patients with stage III or IV lymphoblastic lymphoma may benefit from prophylactic cranial radiation.
- Plays a role in treating patients:
  - Who do not achieve complete remission after standard chemotherapy
  - Who require bone marrow transplantation or palliative therapy

Hodgkin disease

- Responds to radiation and/or chemotherapy
- Choosing the appropriate therapeutic plan necessitates assessing risk of recurrence and potential risk for long-term ill effects.
- Chemotherapy
  - ABVE-PC (adriamycin [doxorubicin], bleomycin, vincristine, etoposide, prednisone, and cyclophosphamide)
  - Add appropriate additional chemotherapy regimens for patients who do not have a good initial response.
  - Cures with chemotherapy alone, even in higher-stage disease, have been described; should define patients who can avoid any radiation
  - Chemotherapy with radiotherapy: considerations
    - Age and skeletal maturity of the patient (likely effects on the developing child)
    - Extent of disease present (how much therapy is necessary)
    - Symptoms that might predict a poor prognosis
    - Response to initial therapy

SPECIFIC TREATMENTS

Wilms tumor

- Actinomycin D and vincristine are the mainstays of chemotherapy.
  - Shorter-duration therapy (6 months) with single high doses of actinomycin D results in the same outcome as multiple smaller doses, with less toxicity and cost.
- Addition of doxorubicin and 10 Gy of radiation to vincristine and actinomycin D improves prognosis for stage III–V FH tumors and for stage II–IV tumors with focal anaplasia.
- Cyclophosphamide as a fourth agent can benefit stage II–IV tumors with diffuse anaplasia.

Retinoblastoma

- Vincristine, carboplatin, and etoposide
- Periocular carboplatin has been used in specific clinical situations.
- Emerging therapy includes transpupillary thermotherapy with or without adjuvant chemotherapy.
- Cyclosporin with chemotherapy overcomes multidrug resistance and may improve long-term response to chemotherapy.

C

Rhabdomyosarcoma

- Vincristine
- Actinomycin D
- Cyclophosphamide

Germ cell tumors/teratomas

- Methotrexate for gestational choriocarcinomas and testicular germ cell tumors
- Ovarian tumors responded to vincristine, actinomycin D, and cyclophosphamide.
- Vinblastine and cisplatin in testicular germ cell tumors of young men
- Standard therapy with cisplatin, etoposide, and bleomycin for intermediate-risk patients
- Higher doses of cyclophosphamide with surgery and standard 3-drug regimen are being studied for high-risk patients.

Ewing sarcoma

- Standard chemotherapy: vincristine, doxorubicin, and cyclophosphamide alternating with etoposide and ifosfamide

Osteosarcoma

- High-dosemethotrexate, doxorubicin, and cisplatin are standard therapy for osteosarcoma.

Neuroblastoma

- Cyclophosphamide, doxorubicin, cisplatin, epipodophyllotoxin, and vincristine

NHL

- Cyclophosphamide, vincristine, prednisone, methotrexate, doxorubicin, cytosine arabinoside, etoposide, and ifosfamide

Hodgkin disease

- ABVE-PC (adriamycin [doxorubicin], bleomycin, vincristine, etoposide, prednisone, and cyclophosphamide)
- Full-dose radiotherapy (35–45 Gy) is standard therapy for adults with low-stage (I, II, and III) disease.
  - Involved fields and 1 field beyond the area of proven disease are treated.
  - Skeletal and soft-tissue growth, especially in the neck and clavicular areas, are severely compromised when used in children.
  - Low-dose radiotherapy (20–25 Gy) to involved fields only, and not extended fields, in conjunction with chemotherapy results in fewer and less severe late effects from the radiation.

WHEN TO ADMIT

- Patients whose bone marrow has been infiltrated may have pancytopenia and thus be at risk of infection, bleeding, and congestive heart failure as a result of anemia.

- In cases of increased uric acid (risk of urate nephropathy), hyperkalemia, hypocalcemia, or hyperphosphatemia:
  - Medical management includes allopurinol or urate oxidase, urinary alkalinization, and binders of potassium and phosphate.
  - Dialysis may be necessary.
  - If delayed arrival to the medical center is anticipated, allopurinol should be started by the referring physician when tumor with a large cell burden is suspected.
    - Leukemia, Burkitt lymphoma, bone marrow involvement
    - Neuroblastoma, Ewing sarcoma, or rhabdomyosarcoma

WHEN TO REFER

- Begin with referral to a pediatric oncologist, even if the initial procedure indicated is surgical.
  - Recognition of potential cancer is essential to ensure that inappropriate therapy will not be administered.
  - The oncologist will advise on radiation and chemotherapy.
- Services at pediatric referral hospitals often ease the pain of being diagnosed with a life-threatening disease.
  - Pediatric social workers, child life workers, and nurses experienced in dealing with children/adolescents with cancer are available.
  - For patients far from a center, initiating therapy at referral medical center and administering a portion of the subsequent treatments/evaluations closer to home, is often possible.
- A local oncologist can assist in giving chemotherapy to children far from a center, but pediatric oncologists at the referral medical center should be involved in:
  - Choosing therapeutic regimen
  - Evaluating major problems
- Emergencies that require immediate referral to a pediatric oncologist include:
  - Cord compression
  - Incontinence
  - Loss of reflexes in the lower extremities
  - Decreased ability to use the lower extremities
  - Decreased rectal sphincter tone
- Refer if there is potential for mediastinal mass or symptoms of superior vena cava syndrome.
  - Swelling, plethora, and cyanosis of the face, neck, and upper extremities
  - Engorged vessels
  - Cough and wheezing
  - Chest pain
  - Headache
  - Diaphoresis
  - Changes in vision

FOLLOW-UP

General

- Maintenance of a relationship with the patient and family is essential.
  - Children receiving treatment for cancer should continue to see their primary pediatrician for well-child visits.
  - Immunizations are delayed until 1 year after therapy is terminated because live vaccines may cause disease, and inactivated vaccines rarely result in a normal immune response.
    - Exception: inactivated influenza vaccine; patient's family should also be immunized
  - The pediatrician should remain involved in continuing developmental issues that are at times exacerbated by the cancer treatment.

Wilms tumor

- During therapy, monitor for disease recurrence at the primary site (usually, with abdominal ultrasonography).
- Medical care should be sought promptly for unexplained masses, pain, or other symptoms.
  - CT may be indicated.
  - Lungs are usually evaluated with chest radiograph.
- Some patients may be followed up with CT of the chest and abdomen at increasing intervals until approximately 5 years after diagnosis.
- Contact sports are often discouraged, although evidence for significant risk of renal injury is lacking.
  - Some experts suggest a kidney guard for particularly active children, if only to serve as a reminder of the need for caution.
- Renal function should be monitored.

Retinoblastoma

- After treatment, follow closely for evidence of recurrence and for second cancers.
  - Examine under anesthesia:
    - Every 2–3 months during the first year
    - Every 3–4 months during the second year
    - Every 6 months thereafter until age 6
- After enucleation, a prosthesis is necessary.
- After radiation, monitor hypothalamic-pituitary axis function.

Neuroblastoma

- Most tumors recur while patients are receiving therapy or shortly afterward.
- Close follow-up with physical examination and radiologic studies should continue after completing therapy.
- Urinary catecholamine levels may be useful in the surveillance of patients who had increased values at diagnosis.
- Patients should be monitored for late toxicities of chemotherapy and radiotherapy.

- High-dose therapy associated with autologous hematopoietic stem cell procedures may result in significant late effects, for example:
  - Hearing loss
  - Renal insufficiency
  - Growth impairment
  - Gonadal failure

Rhabdomyosarcoma

- Follow closely for evidence of recurrent disease for at least 3–5 years after diagnosis.
- CT or MRI of the primary site, chest CT, and bone scans are used for surveillance.
- Radiotherapy often results in unacceptable cosmetic effects in patients who have orbital tumors.
  - For patients with orbital or other tumors of head or face who received radiation to the sinuses, hypothalamus, and pituitary gland
    - Sinusitis is a common symptom.
    - Hormone levels (eg, growth hormone, gonadotrophins) may need monitoring.
- Patients should be monitored for any potential late effects of chemotherapeutic agents.

Teratoma

- Malignant evolution may occur years after removal of an apparently benign tumor, particularly in the sacrococcygeal area.
  - Complete excision of the coccyx is often suggested, with close follow-up.
- Relapse may occur as many as 10 years after diagnosis.
- Late-brain metastases are possible.
- Close follow-up care is essential.
  - Frequent physical examinations and radiologic evaluations
  - Monitoring of AFP and ß-hCG levels, if levels are high at diagnosis
  - Salvage therapy may prolong survival or even provide a cure.
- Late effects of chemotherapy should be monitored (see Complications).

Ewing sarcoma

- Follow closely for evidence of recurrent disease for at least 5 years after diagnosis.
- Bone films should be obtained periodically.
- Patients with lower-extremity lesions whose growth is incomplete should be monitored for evidence of leg-length discrepancies; they may require arresting growth in the opposite limb.
- Monitor for potential late effects of specific chemotherapeutic agents (see Complications).

Osteosarcoma

- Imaging of the primary tumor site, bone scans, and chest CTs semiannually for 5 years and then at least chest radiographs annually until 10 years after diagnosis to monitor for recurrent disease.

- Orthopedic evaluation and monitoring for late effects of the chemotherapeutic agents

Hodgkin disease

- Monitor for evidence of recurrent disease for as long as 10–15 years after original diagnosis.
  - Thorough physical examination
  - Complete blood cell count
  - Sedimentation rate
  - Chest radiograph

- Patients should undergo annual mammographic examinations beginning 8 years after therapy or at age 25 years.

- Thyroid function should be assessed for at least 15 years.
  - Thyroid replacement therapy is suggested when the level is increased.

- Menstrual history should be elicited at each visit to check effects of radiation infertility, if relevant.

- Patients who have had a splenectomy are at risk for overwhelming infection.
  - Empirical treatment with intravenous antibiotics is recommended for fever (>101°F).

Other care of survivors

- Neurocognitive function and school performance will be affected in many who are going through or who have undergone treatment.
  - Education specialists, pediatric oncological nurse practitioners, or both can be extremely helpful to child and child's teachers by:
    - Explaining diagnosis and treatment to school administrators and teachers and, when appropriate, to classmates
    - Defining the problems/limitations child will have in keeping up with schoolwork during periods of intensive treatment
    - Providing or arranging (through the school system) for lessons and special tutoring during prolonged hospitalizations and recovery periods at home
  - Legal protection in case of discrimination in the work place is available to survivors through the Americans with Disabilities Act, and advocacy resources exist at both the community and national levels.
  - Pediatricians must be advocates.

COMPLICATIONS

All cancers

- Recurrence from second cancer is possible for all tumors.

Wilms tumor

- Scoliosis
  - Major problem following treatment with moderate-dose radiation (30–40 Gy), particularly if all vertebrae were not included in the field
  - Less severe with lower-dose radiation (10 Gy) and irradiation of the entire width of the vertebrae adjacent to the renal bed
  - Alterations of vertebral growth and tethering caused by hypoplasia of soft tissues may still result in some degree of curvature.

- Close observation of patients who received irradiation, particularly during growth spurt in puberty, is necessary. Hypoplasia with a decrease in adipose tissue occurs in the radiation field and is accentuated by obesity.

Long-term side effects of chemotherapy

- Chemotherapeutic agents, their possible side effects, and techniques used for follow-up are listed.

- Anthracyclines (eg, doxorubicin)
  - Cardiac: myocardial damage, congestive failure, arrhythmias
    - History: exercise intolerance, palpitations; electrocardiography (QTc interval); echocardiography scheduled based on age, dose, and radiation exposure; Holter monitor; exercise electrocardiography; exercise nuclear angiography

- Bleomycin
  - Pulmonary: fibrosis, impaired diffusion capacity, exacerbated by increased oxygen (eg, anesthesia)
    - History: shortness of breath, dyspnea on exertion, cough; chest radiograph and pulmonary function tests (with diffusion capacity) at baseline and with symptoms

- Cyclophosphamide, ifosfamide
  - Gonadal: infertility, sterility, early menopause
    - History: menses, question of fertility; luteinizing hormone (LH), follicle-stimulating hormone (FSH), testosterone or estradiol during pubertal development or if fertility problems or amenorrhea (or both) exists; semen analysis (as required to conceive)
  - Bladder: hemorrhagic cystitis
    - Urinalysis annually
  - Marrow: secondary acute myeloblastic leukemia
    - Complete blood cell count annually

- Lomustine
  - Pulmonary, gonadal
    - Pulmonary and gonadal evaluation
- Cisplatin
  - Kidney: decreased glomerular filtration rate
    - Serum creatinine at baseline and per guidelines
    - Creatinine clearance at baseline and per guidelines
  - Ears: hearing loss (high frequency)
    - Audiography at baseline and per guidelines
- Methotrexate
  - Liver dysfunction
  - Central nervous system (CNS): learning impairment (high intravenous dose)
    - Liver function tests
- 6-Mercaptopurine, 6-thioguanine, actinomycin D
  - Liver dysfunction
    - Liver function tests

Long-term side effects of radiation

- The site of side effects, risks, and monitoring techniques are listed.
- Cranium and nasopharynx
  - Cataracts
    - Physical examination
  - Impaired growth
    - Growth charts (bone age, growth hormone, organ system function as appropriate)
  - Learning impairment
    - Monitoring school function; neuropsychological evaluation
  - Abnormal dentition formation
    - Dental evaluation
  - Overt or compensated hypothyroidism
    - Free thyroxine and thyroid-stimulating hormone
  - Hypothalamic dysfunction (decreased growth hormone; decreased gonadotropin, hyperprolactinemia)
    - Growth; pubertal, menstrual, and fertility history (growth hormone, LH, testosterone, estrogen, prolactin levels)
  - Hearing (especially with cisplatin)
    - Audiography
- Neck and mandible
  - Hypoplasia of bone or soft tissues
    - Examination of area
  - Dentition: abnormal formation, abnormal salivary function
    - Dental evaluation

- Hypothyroidism
  - Free thyroxine and thyroid-stimulation hormone
- Thorax
  - Hypoplasia (includes impaired chest wall growth)
    - Examination of area
  - Lungs: fibrosis, decreased capacity
    - History, pulmonary function tests, chest radiograph at baseline and as appropriate
  - Cardiac: pericardial and valvular thickening; possibility of early myocardial infarction
    - History, electrocardiography, and echocardiography are scheduled on the basis of age, dose, and radiation exposure.
  - Breasts: impaired growth, possibility of increased malignancy
    - Breast self-examination and early mammograms start 8 years after therapy or at age 25 years.
- Abdomen/pelvis
  - Hypoplasia (including scoliosis)
    - Examination of area, radiograph of spine during puberty
  - Liver (if in field)
    - Liver function tests
  - Kidney (if in field)
    - Serum creatinine, urinalysis protein (24-hour collection for creatinine, protein)
  - Gonads (if in field)
    - Pubertal, menstrual, and fertility history, LH, FSH, estradiol or testosterone levels during puberty; if fertility is doubtful, semen analysis
  - GI tract
    - Nutritional history
- Extremities
  - Hypoplasia
  - Examination

Other risks

- The most prominent toxicity from chemotherapy is myelo-suppression, which can rapidly result in septic shock.
  - Recognize the risk of fever and refer to a pediatric oncologist immediately.
  - If the cancer center is at a distance, be prepared to obtain proper culture specimens and initiate antibiotic therapy (usually anaminoglycoside and semisynthetic penicillin or a fourth-generation cephalosporin).

- Patients with indwelling central venous catheters have increased risk for septicemia.
  - Have blood drawn for culture, and consider therapy with antibiotics if fever develops.
- Varicella is a major threat to immunocompromised patients.
  - If exposed by a sibling or close playmate, the patient should receive varicella-zoster immunoglobulin within 4 days of the exposure.
  - Should chickenpox occur, treat with acyclovir or related new-generation antiviral drugs, often as an inpatient, and withhold chemotherapy.

PROGNOSIS

Wilms tumor

- Prognosis is determined by histopathologic factors of the tumor.
- Prognosis also depends on stage of disease at diagnosis.
  - More patients with UH tumors die compared with those with FH tumors.
  - UH tumors, particularly diffuse anaplasia, confer worse prognosis.
  - Most relapses occur within 2 years of diagnosis.
  - The 2-year relapse-free survival for stage I–III disease with FH findings is approximately 91%.
  - The 2-year relapse-free survival rate is 84% for stage IV disease and FH features.
  - Patients with diffuse anaplasia have a poor prognosis, with survival rates 4 years after diagnosis of:
    - 59% with stage II disease
    - 45% with stage III disease
    - 7% with stage IV disease
  - 4-year event-free survival is 74.9% for patients with focal anaplasia.
- Patients who relapse have a better prognosis if initial management did not include radiotherapy or doxorubicin.
- Fertility is preserved in most patients, although a risk of ovarian failure exists with whole-abdomen radiotherapy.

Neuroblastoma

- Patients <1 year of age do much better than those >2 years of age.
- Patients who have stage 1, 2, or 4S neuroblastoma with favorable biological features have survival rates >90%.
- Long-term survival for patients with stage 3 neuroblastoma:
  - Patients <1 year of age have survival rate of 100% at 4 years.
  - Patients with favorable biology have survival rate of 90% at 4 years.
- Intensive multiagent chemotherapy appears to result in improved cure rates.

- In studies of patients with stage 4 disease treated with stem cell transplants, event-free survival is 23–47% at 3–6 years.
- Skeletal disease and persisting bone marrow involvement are predictive of poorer outcome; patients who have complete response to chemotherapy benefit most from transplantation.

Retinoblastoma

- Survival is excellent; >85% have no recurrence, and survival from primary tumor is >95%.
- Hereditary retinoblastoma carries a high incidence of second cancer.
  - 50% of cases occur within the radiation field.
  - Osteosarcoma or other sarcomas are particularly common.
  - Patients irradiated when <1 year are at increased risk.
    - One-third have a second cancer within 15 years.
    - Two-thirds have a second cancer by 30 years.
  - Avoiding radiotherapy may reduce but not eliminate this risk.

Rhabdomyosarcoma

- Survival is determined by site and stage.
- Overall survival: 73% at 5 years from diagnosis.
- Prognosis is particularly good (90–95% long-term survivors) for:
  - Orbital tumors
  - Nonbladder and nonprostate GU tract tumors
  - Localized tumors that can be resected fully
- Patients with stage IV (metastatic) disease who are <10 years and have embryonal histology have a better prognosis than older patients who have stage IV disease.
- 80% of recurrences occur within 2 years of treatment.
  - Local relapse is most common, although distant spread to the lungs, CNS, lymph nodes, bone, liver, bone marrow, and soft tissues does occur.
- Metastatic disease at diagnosis
  - 25–30% of these patients will survive 5 years from diagnosis.
  - Hematopoietic stem cell transplant or the use of new agents may offer hope to these patients.
- 20% who experienced relapse have favorable features, with 50% 5-year survival; the other 80% of patients have only 10% 5-year survival (if poor stage).

Germ cell tumors/teratomas

- 3 prognostic groups for patients >1 year:
  - Stage III disease (more than microscopic residual disease), sacrococcygeal or mediastinal primaries, and AFP level >10,000 ng/mL: 43% 3-year disease-free survival

- Stage I disease (complete resection) or stage II disease (microscopic residual), testicular, ovarian, perineal, or retroperitoneal primary tumor, and AFP level <10,000 ng/mL: 100% 3-year disease-free survival
- The remaining patients were in an intermediate-prognosis group and had 81% disease-free survival.
- Prognosis is improved for patients treated with cisplatin versus carboplatin.
- Event-free survival rates >80% and up to 100%
- Teratoma prognosis depends on its degree of maturity and age.
  - Sacrococcygeal teratomas are usually benign in children <2 months; thereafter, likelihood of malignant evolution increases rapidly.
    - This may be the reason that intrapelvic teratomas that are not detected early often are found to be malignant.
  - Mediastinal teratomas behave benignly in children and young teenagers; in older patients, they are more aggressive.
  - Cervical and intracranial teratomas in infants are usually benign; those in adolescents and adults are often malignant.
  - Immature teratomas can be treated with surgery alone, with event-free survival rates of 97.8%, 100%, and 80% for patients who have ovarian, testicular, and extragonadal tumors, respectively.
- For patients who experience relapse, cisplatin-based chemotherapy offers an excellent chance of cure.

Ewing sarcoma

- Older age is associated with worse prognosis.
- Metastatic disease is present in 20–25%.
- Histologic response of marked tissue necrosis after chemotherapy indicates better prognosis.
- 5-year disease-free survival is approximately 75% for nonmetastatic disease.
- Event-free survival of 12–24% is seen in patients with metastatic disease.
- Outcome after relapse is very poor; there are few survivors among patients who have relapse >2 years from initial diagnosis or who have relapse with lung metastases only.

Osteosarcoma

- Adjuvant chemotherapy improves long-term disease-free survival if osteosarcoma is nonmetastatic (survival rates of 65–75%).
- Outcome after preoperative chemotherapy is similar to or better than with immediate surgical excision.
- The alkaline phosphatase level has been shown to have independent prognostic significance.
- Other factors
  - Patients who have distal tumors may have better outcomes than those who have proximal or central-axis tumors.
  - Age (outcome improves with older patients)

- Presence of metastatic disease
  - Pulmonary metastases are associated with better prognosis than bone metastases.
  - Unilateral disease or <8 nodules may carry a better prognosis; survival of 65–75%, compared with 25–35% for other patients with pulmonary involvement.
  - Prognosis for bone metastases at diagnosis or relapse is grim.

NHL

- Prognosis is excellent for most children: >95% survival for those with localized disease and 80–90% survival for patients who have high-risk disease (advanced stage, a large mediastinal mass, more than 4 sites of involvement, and B symptoms).
- Worse prognosis with Burkitt and bone marrow and CNS involvement, mediastinal diffuse large B-cell lymphoma, and some patients with widespread anaplastic large-cell lymphoma
- Histologic findings are of prognostic significance for outcome.
- Age and sex may affect prognosis, even within histologic subtypes.
- Other prognostic factors include lactic dehydrogenase and, as with other types of cancer, response to therapy.
- New intensive chemotherapy or bone marrow transplantation regimens should improve survival in patients whose prognosis is poor or who experience relapse.

Hodgkin disease

- Radiotherapy alone may cure up to 70% with stage I or IIA disease and 50% with IIB or IIIA disease.
- Subsequent chemotherapy enables 50% who experience relapse after radiotherapy.
- With combined-modality therapy, 5-year disease-free survival is 90–100% for localized disease and 80–90% for advanced-stage disease.
- High-risk features
  - Advanced-stage disease
  - Large mediastinal mass
  - ≥4 sites of involvement
  - B symptoms
- Patients whose disease progresses or relapses
  - Cure may be accomplished with intensive chemotherapy and radiation or with stem cell transplantation.
  - Salvage rates >60%
  - Patients whose diseases progress while in therapy have a poorer prognosis than those who experience relapse after treatment.

PREVENTION

- Diet, particularly folic acid intake, and breastfeeding may protect against development of neuroblastoma.

Cardiac Arrhythmias

DEFINITION

- Cardiac arrhythmias comprise a spectrum of variations to normal heartbeat.
- Normal rhythm variations
  - A wide range of normal heart rates is present in young persons.
- Premature (early) beats
  - Usually benign arrhythmias that occur as:
    - Premature atrial contractions (PACs)
    - Premature ventricular contractions (PVCs)
  - Couplet
    - 2 premature beats in a row
  - Bigeminal or trigeminal rhythm
    - Every second or third beat is a premature impulse.
- Supraventricular tachycardia (SVT)
  - Tachycardia with origin above the ventricles
- Atrial flutter
  - Primary atrial reentrant tachycardia
  - Atypical form (intraatrial reentrant tachycardia)
- Atrial fibrillation
  - Irregular tachycardia with variable atrioventricular conduction
  - Types
    - Lone (idiopathic, no underlying cause)
    - Underlying heart disease
- Ventricular tachycardia (VT)
  - ≥3 repetitive excitations arising from the ventricles
- Conduction abnormalities
  - First-degree atrioventricular (AV) block
  - Second-degree AV block
    - Wenckebach block or Mobitz type I
    - Mobitz type II
  - Complete AV block
- Sudden cardiac death

EPIDEMIOLOGY

- Prevalence
  - PACs
    - Seen in 50–75% of pediatric patients
  - PVCs
    - Less common than PACs
    - On Holter monitoring, seen in up to 25% of healthy infants, children, and adolescents
  - SVT
    - Up to 1 in 250 children
      - Reentrant: >90% of pediatric SVT
      - Automatic: <10% of pediatric SVT
  - Wolff-Parkinson-White (WPW) syndrome:
    - 0.15% in the general population with or without SVT
  - Atrial flutter
    - Bimodal distribution in newborn infants and in older children
  - Atrial fibrillation
    - Less common than other arrhythmias
    - Incidence in adolescence may be underestimated.
  - VT
    - Rare in the newborn and young infant
  - Sudden cardiac death
    - 1:100,000
    - Beyond infancy, 25% of sudden deaths in the young occur during exercise.
  - Long QT syndrome (LQTS)
    - 10:100,000
    - May be underestimated because of incomplete genetic ascertainment
- Age
  - Arrhythmias in the young are common.
    - Usually benign
    - May be life-altering or fatal
  - Arrhythmias may begin at any age.
    - In utero up to the later teenage years
    - Higher incidence in early infancy and mid-adolescence
  - Sudden cardiac death
    - Most common in mid-adolescence
- Sex
  - No sex preference

MECHANISM

- Premature beats
  - May arise in the atria, the AV junction, or the ventricles
- SVT
  - Early infancy
    - Usually initiated by PAC or sinus tachycardia
    - AV reentry tachycardia through an accessory pathway (preexcitation)
  - Childhood and adolescence
    - PVCs and sinus pauses with junctional escape beats are additional initiators.
    - AV nodal reentry tachycardia using the fast and slow pathways in the AV nodal region
  - Primary atrial tachycardias
    - Automatic SVT
    - Atrial flutter
    - Atrial fibrillation

- Conduction abnormalities
  - Second-degree AV block
    - Type I
      - Predominance of vagal tone
      - Block is in the AV node.
    - Type II
      - Block is more distally located in the bundle of His.
  - Complete AV block
    - Acquired
      - Usually results from conduction system injury
    - Congenital complete atrioventricular block (CCAVB)
      - Fetus exposed to antibodies in a mother with autoimmune disease between 15 and 24 weeks of gestation
- Sudden cardiac death
  - Ion channel cardiac disorder that prolongs repolarization
  - Genetic basis
    - Romano-Ward form (95% of patients)
    - Jervell and Lange-Nielsen syndrome (5%)

HISTORY

- Thorough family history focuses on:
  - Sudden death
  - Premature death
  - Syncope
  - Recurrent arrhythmias
- Typical symptoms of cardiac dysfunction
  - Palpitations
  - Lightheadedness
  - Syncope
  - Visceral chest pain
  - Dyspnea
- Nonspecific signs and symptoms of arrhythmia
  - Depend on age of the patient and the rate and type of rhythm disturbance
    - Fatigue
    - Malaise
    - Poor feeding
    - Nausea
    - Pallor
- Premature beats
  - The majority have no obvious incitant.
  - Observed most often in healthy children and adolescents
  - Associated with:
    - Myocarditis
    - Hypertrophic cardiomyopathy
    - Dilated cardiomyopathy

- Ventricular dysfunction
- Congenital cardiac malformations
- Sympathomimetics
- Stimulant drugs
- Electrolyte imbalances
- Intracardiac catheters
- SVT
  - Onset
    - First 4 months of life (~50%)
    - 1–5 years : usually electrically quiescent
    - >5 years: associated with high probability of recurrence
  - WPW syndrome
    - May be inherited in an autosomal-dominant fashion
- Risk factors for atrial flutter
  - Cardiomyopathy
  - Previous repair of complex congenital heart malformations lesions (Fontan procedure) (see Figure 10 on page F3)
- Risk factors for atrial fibrillation:
  - Structural heart disease
  - Cardiomyopathies
- VT
  - Risk factors
  - Myocarditis
  - Repaired and unrepaired congenital cardiac lesions
  - Cardiomyopathies
  - LQTS, short QT syndrome
  - Catecholamine use
  - Exercise-induced VT
  - Marked electrolyte imbalances
  - Use of street drugs (eg, cocaine)
  - Associated conditions
    - Ventricular tumor
    - Mitochondrial fatty acid beta-oxidation disorders in neonates
    - In general, VT is a marker for myocardial disease.
- Conduction abnormalities
  - Risk factors in acquired conduction abnormalities
    - Conduction system injury during repair of congenital cardiac malformations (most commonly)
    - Myocarditis
    - Lyme disease
  - Risk factors in CCAVB
  - Complex structural heart disease (~50% of affected patients)
  - Levo-transposition of the great vessels
  - Complex AV septal defects

- Immune-mediated block in utero from mother with overt or occult autoimmune disease (~50% of affected patients)
  - <5% of infants born to mothers who have autoimmune disease develop CCAVB
  - If a mother bears 1 child who has CCAVB, the risk in future pregnancies is 15%.
- Prolonged QT interval (up to 25%)
- Fetal hydrops
- Premature birth
- Congestive heart failure
- Ventricular ectopy
- Atrioventricular valve insufficiency
- Low or decreasing ventricular rate (≤55 bpm in a neonate)
- Risk factors in sudden cardiac death
  - Repaired complex congenital heart malformations
  - Cardiomyopathies
  - Myocarditis
  - Drugs that prolong the QT interval
    - Cisapride
    - Imipramine
    - Pentamidine
  - Congenital coronary artery anomalies
    - Especially origin of the left main coronary artery from the right sinus of Valsalva
  - Acquired coronary artery anomalies
- Kawasaki disease
- Primary arrhythmias
  - LQTS
  - WPW syndrome
  - Catecholamine-sensitive polymorphic VT
- Associated conditions
  - Congenital deafness (Romano-Ward form)

PHYSICAL EXAM

Normal rhythm variations in childhood

- Sinus arrhythmia (phasic respiratory variations of sinus rate with inspiratory slowing and expiratory acceleration)
- Fast heart rates
  - Sinus tachycardia at rates of 230–250 bpm during infancy have been documented.
  - A rate >200 bpm in a teenager who is not involved in maximal exertion would be abnormal.
- Slow heart rates/sinus bradycardia
  - Sinus rate below that expected for a patient's age
  - Greater reason for alarm than fast rates
  - Sinus rate below 100 bpm in an awake neonate is abnormal.
  - During sleep, rates down to 80 bpm are common.

- Brief dips into the 60–80 bpm range are also observed in sleeping neonates during normal, vagally induced episodes of junctional rhythm.
- A highly conditioned adolescent endurance athlete may have a resting heart rate ≤40 bpm.

Premature beats

- PACs
  - Usually asymptomatic to the patient
  - Characterized by premature P waves with an axis and morphology different from the sinus P waves
  - Usually occur with normally conducted QRS complexes
  - If wide beats are also noted, the apparently prolonged QRS beats are likely to be aberrant PACs.
    - Premature atrial and ventricular contractions rarely occur together, especially in the newborn period.
  - Sign of blocked atrial bigeminy in a newborn infant
    - Slowing of the heart rate sufficient to alter feeding and arousal time
- PVCs
  - Benign if:
    - No evidence for heart disease
    - QTc is normal (≤0.44 seconds)
    - Family history is not adverse
    - PVCs are uniform in appearance
    - PVCs are either suppressed or not aggravated with exercise
  - Worrisome if:
    - Answer to any of the above questions is positive
  - New appearance of PVCs in the setting of a febrile illness should raise the question of myocarditis.

SVT

- May be noted incidentally
- Commonly associated with signs and symptoms of congestive-heart failure
  - Tachycardia
  - Tachypnea
  - Dyspnea
  - Truncal diaphoresis
  - Diminished pulses
  - Pallor
  - Hepatomegaly
  - Poor feeding
  - Palpitations
  - Chest pain
  - Nausea
  - Respiratory distress
  - Syncope (rarely)

- Infants
  - 25% of infants are in congestive heart failure with tachycardia of 24 hours' duration.
  - 50% of infants have heart failure after SVT for 48 hours.
- Children >5 years
  - Usually can communicate their distress soon after onset of SVT
  - Hence, the relative paucity of congestive heart failure caused by SVT in older pediatric patients
- Duration
  - Ranges from a few seconds to several hours
- Heart rate
  - Infants: 230–300 bpm but usually between 260 and 280 bpm
  - Older patients: 180–240 bpm

Atrial flutter

- Newborn infants
  - Atrial rate typically between 350 and 500 bpm
  - 2:1 atrioventricular conduction and brief interruptions caused by higher degrees of AV block
  - Congestive heart failure may be seen.
  - Not as dramatic as in infants who have the usual variety of SVT
  - Structural cardiac problems are uncommon.
- Onset in utero
  - Fetal hydrops may develop.
- Atypical form (intraatrial reentrant tachycardia)
  - Slower atrial rate
  - Heart rate of 100–140 bpm in a patient with risk factors should prompt investigation.

VT

- Signs and symptoms
  - Rate >120 bpm or 25% faster than sinus rate
  - Congestive heart failure
  - Chest pain
  - Dyspnea
  - Palpitations
  - Fatigue
  - Reduced exercise capacity
  - Pallor
  - Presyncope
  - Syncope
- VT is confirmed by the presence of atrioventricular dissociation.
  - Similar but isolated PVCs and fusion beats in sinus rhythm assist in establishing the diagnosis
  - Cardiac output frequently is compromised to a greater degree than in SVT.

- Heart rate may be extremely rapid (up to 500 bpm) and slightly irregular.
- All wide QRS tachycardias should be considered VT until proven otherwise
- Benign forms of VT
  - Accelerated ventricular rhythm
    - ≤120 bpm, or <25% faster than the basic sinus rate
  - Right ventricular outflow tract
  - Idiopathic left VT

Conduction abnormalities

- First-degree AV block
  - Prolongation of the PR interval beyond the upper limit of normal for age, with all impulses conducted
  - Benign finding
  - Seen with:
    - Congenital cardiac malformations (especially AV septal defects)
    - Electrolyte disorders
    - Rheumatic fever
    - Myocarditis
    - Congenital muscular disorders
    - Patients receiving antiarrhythmic drugs
- Second-degree AV block
  - Type I
    - Progressive prolongation of the PR interval until a dropped ventricular beat (nonconducted P wave) occurs
    - Generally benign unless syncope occurs
    - Normal finding in:
      - Healthy children during sleep
      - Highly conditioned athletes at rest
  - Type II
    - Intermittent loss of AV conduction without preceding lengthening of the PR interval
    - Implies an abnormal conduction system
  - Complete AV block
    - No atrial impulses are conducted to the ventricles

Sudden cardiac death

- Exertion or emotional stress triggers 1 of the following:
  - Syncope
  - Atypical seizures
  - Cardiac arrest
- Long QT3 subtype events
  - Predominantly occur at rest
  - Physical examination is usually normal.
  - Bradycardia may be the only sign.

DIFFERENTIAL DIAGNOSIS

- Premature beats
  - Escape or late beats occurring when higher pacemaker cells fail to produce an impulse at the expected interval
- VT
  - SVT with persistent aberrancy (see Figure 11 on page F3) is uncommon.
  - SVT with antegrade conduction across an accessory pathway (see Figure 12 on page F4) is uncommon.
- LQTS
  - Electrolyte abnormalities
    - Hypokalemia
    - Hypocalcemia
    - Hypomagnesemia
  - Myocardial ischemia or injury
  - Acute central nervous system events
  - Cardiomyopathy

IMAGING

- Echocardiography
- Used to assess cardiac structure and function when new PVCs are seen in the setting of a febrile illness where underlying disease may be subtle
- Used in SVT to identify:
  - Subtle congenital cardiac defects in patients with WPW syndrome
  - Ebstein malformation of the tricuspid valve
  - Levo-transposition of the great vessels

DIAGNOSTIC PROCEDURES

12-lead electrocardiography (ECG)

- Must be obtained when an arrhythmia is being considered
  - Rhythm alterations may be quite subtle and not always identified on a rhythm strip.
  - ECG will detect chamber enlargement.
  - Calculate corrected QT interval: QTc = QT interval (seconds) / $\sqrt{}$preceding RR interval (seconds)
- Analyze arrhythmia in an organized fashion.
  - Is the rhythm fast or slow?
  - Is the rhythm regular or irregular?
  - Are the QRS complexes narrow or wide?
  - What is the relationship between the P waves and the QRS complexes?
- Sinus bradycardia
  - Neonates and infants: <100 bpm, awake
  - Children to 3 years: <100 bpm
  - Children 3–9 years: <60 bpm

- Adolescents 9–16 years: <50 bpm
- Adolescents >16 years: <40 bpm
- PACs
  - If PAC occurs when 1 of the bundle branches is refractory:
    - The premature beat will be conducted down the other bundle branch.
    - The result is an aberrant PAC with QRS morphology wider than and different from sinus QRS complexes (see Figure 13 on page F4).
  - If both bundle branches are refractory:
    - PAC will not be conducted to the ventricles (blocked PAC).
    - PAC may reset the sinus node, with a resultant pause greater than the previous RR interval.
  - T waves
    - Usually smoothly inscribed
    - Consistent sharp deflections in the T waves may represent P waves (see Figure 14 on page F4).
- Wandering atrial pacemaker related to alterations in vagal tone
  - Usually noted with slower heart rates and characterized by different P wave morphologies
- QRS morphology of PVCs
  - Different from sinus QRS beats
  - Occur before the next expected sinus beat
  - Not preceded by a premature P wave
  - QRS duration may be only slightly prolonged.
  - Uniform PVCs
    - Similar morphology in contrast to multiform beats
  - Late PVCs
    - Hybrid or fusion beat with morphology intermediate between the sinus QRS and PVC
- SVT
  - QRS complexes are usually narrow but may be transiently wide at initiation, especially with aberrant left bundle branch morphology in early infancy (see Figure 11 on page F3).
  - Wide QRS tachycardias should be considered ventricular in origin until proven otherwise.
  - Careful attention should be paid to the T waves for sharp deflections representing retrograde conduction from the ventricles to the atria via an accessory pathway (see Figure 15 on page F4).
  - WPW syndrome warrants further (echocardiographic) investigation.
    - Shortened PR interval
    - Delta wave
    - Wide QRS

- Atrial flutter
  - Newborn infants
    - Rapid saw-tooth pattern with inverted P waves in the inferior limb leads
  - Atypical form (intraatrial reentrant tachycardia)
    - Distinct P waves separated by isoelectric periods
- VT
  - QRS complexes differ from the sinus QRS complexes
    - Typically wide
    - Young infants are an exception; minimal QRS prolongation (0.08–0.09 seconds) may be seen.
- Sudden cardiac death
  - Marked prolongation of QTc intervals
  - QTc interval >460 ms = LQTS
  - QTc interval 440–460 = borderline
- During administration of adenosine
  - Detect rare conversion to a more malignant arrhythmia
  - Once conversion to a sinus rhythm is achieved, 12-lead ECG should be repeated to look for evidence of preexcitation.

Ambulatory (Holter) monitoring

- Criteria for diagnosis of sinus bradycardia
  - Neonates and infants: <60 bpm, sleeping, <80 bpm, awake, quiet
  - Children 2–6 years: <60 bpm
  - Children 7–11 years: <45 bpm
  - Adolescents >11 years: <40 bpm
  - Athletes: <30 bpm

TREATMENT APPROACH

- Empirical therapy without detecting arrhythmia does not meet the current standard of practice.
- Young children
  - Drug treatment for 6–12 months followed by observation
  - Pacemaker implantation for complete AV block
- Older children and adolescents
  - Depending on clinical and nonclinical factors
    - No therapy
    - Drug therapy
    - Ablation
    - Pacemaker

SPECIFIC TREATMENT

Premature beats

- PACs
  - Therapy not necessary unless:
    - PACs initiate SVT.
    - PACs block impulses in a newborn infant dependent on heart rate to maintain adequate cardiac output.
  - If suppressive therapy is required:
    - Digoxin
    - Propranolol
- PVCs
  - Neither treatment nor curtailment of exercise is required, even if a bigeminal rhythm is present.
  - If worrisome PVCs are present, the need for therapy should be determined by a pediatric cardiologist.

SVT

- Young children
  - Cardiogenic shock:
    - Direct current synchronized cardioversion
      - 0.5–2 watt-seconds or J/kg with the largest paddles allowing effective chest contact
    - Adenosine
      - Administered via intravenous bolus, if venous access is available
      - Follow with a second doubled if the first dose is ineffective.
      - Should be administered with ECG monitoring
      - Effective in approximately 90% of episodes
    - Procainamide
      - Use if adenosine is ineffective, or if SVT quickly recurs
      - Can be administered intravenously to infants and young children after appropriate loading, with a subsequent repeat trial of adenosine.
      - If conversion does not ensue, aprocainamide level should be obtained 4 hours into the infusion (therapeutic range, 4–8 µg/mL).
  - Intravenous verapamil and propranolol
    - Suppressive therapy with propranolol is appropriate in WPW syndrome.
    - These agents are contraindicated in children <1 year.
  - Digoxin and verapamil
    - Should be avoided in SVT
    - May shorten the antegrade refractory period of the accessory pathway, allowing more rapid conduction to the ventricles
      - Potentially fatal if atrial fibrillation develops
    - If preexcitation is not present, either agent can be used to prevent recurrence.

- ß-Blockers
  - Should be avoided in the presence of congestive heart failure, sick sinus syndrome, or a history of bronchospasm
- Other medical therapies
  - Use if the above agents are ineffective.
  - All require hospitalization for drug initiation.
    - Flecainide
    - Sotalol
    - Amiodarone
- Ablation
  - Not recommended during the first 2 years of life
    - Resultant myocardial scar may grow with the patient and become a subsequent nidus for malignant, often drug-refractory arrhythmias.

■ Older children and adolescents
- Therapeutic choices depend on:
  - Frequency
  - Ease of conversion of episodes
- No therapy other than self-conversion via a Valsalva maneuver or headstand
- Drug therapy with consideration of:
  - Duration
  - Compliance
  - Cost
- Radiofrequency ablation
  - At least 90% successful, but with a chance of a later recurrence
  - If the patient with SVT will undergo surgery for a cardiac defect, preoperative assessment and ablation should be considered to reduce arrhythmia-related postoperative morbidity and potential mortality.

Atrial flutter

■ Digoxin
- One-third of very young patients respond in utero or postnatally.
■ Electrical cardioversion
- Required in about two-thirds of patients
■ Long-term therapy
- Usually unnecessary because recurrences are rare

VT

■ Acute management
- Depends on the patient's clinical status
  - Rate and duration of VT
  - Presence of structural cardiac lesions
  - Prior myocardial dysfunction

- Hemodynamic compromise
  - Electrical cardioversion with 1–2 watt-seconds/kg
- If reasonable clinical stability is present:
  - Intravenous lidocaine
  - Procainamide
  - Magnesium
  - Amiodarone
■ Long-term suppressive therapy
- Predicated on:
  - Risk of recurrence
  - Morbidity and mortality of the type of VT
  - Risk-benefit ratio of treatment
- Common antiarrhythmic agents to prevent VT recurrence:
  - ß-Blockers
  - Sotalol
  - Amiodarone
- Other treatments:
  - Implantation of an automatic cardioverter-defibrillator
  - VT ablation
■ Benign forms of VT
- Accelerated ventricular rhythm
  - Requires observation only (see Figure 16 on page F5).
- Right ventricular outflow tract tachycardia

Conduction abnormalities

■ First-degree AV block
- No therapy is required.
■ Second-degree AV block
- Type I
  - No therapy is required in most cases.
- Type II
  - Ongoing medical surveillance
  - Potential need for pacemaker implantation
■ Complete AV block
- Early pacemaker implantation is advised in infants with:
  - Risk factors
  - Symptoms of inadequate cardiac output
- Isoproterenol
  - Infuse if necessary to increase the heart rate while awaiting pacemaker therapy
  - Should not delay implantation
- If not in infancy, pacemaker insertion in adolescence is usually necessary depending on:
  - Symptoms
  - Ventricular rate
  - Stability of the ventricular escape rhythm

Sudden cardiac death

- LQTS
  - For any child or adolescent who collapses suddenly with no discernible cardiac output:
    - Rapid resuscitation
    - Early defibrillation
  - ß-Blocker therapy
  - Cardiac pacing
  - Left stellate ganglionectomy
  - Implantation of cardioverter-defibrillator
  - Avoidance of:
    - Competitive sports
    - Drugs capable of prolonging the QTc
    - Sympathomimetics
    - Rapid correction of electrolyte abnormalities

WHEN TO REFER

- Arrhythmias associated with presyncope, syncope, chest pain, or a sense of doom
- Underlying heart disease
- Family history of premature (before age 35 years) sudden cardiac death
- Persistent or repetitive bradycardias or tachycardias
- Premature ventricular beats that increase with exercise

WHEN TO ADMIT

- Arrhythmias associated with syncope or low cardiac output
- Symptomatic high-grade AV block
- Difficult-to-control SVT, atrial flutter
- VT
- LQTS with syncope, aborted sudden death

FOLLOW-UP

- Premature beats
  - Frequent PVCs
    - Long-term yearly follow-up
    - Watch for arrhythmia-induced ventricular dilatation.
    - Watch for ventricular dysfunction.
- SVT
  - Infants should be observed after treatment in view of the risk of later recurrence.

PROGNOSIS

- SVT
  - SVT onset during the first 4 months of life
    - 60% will have recurrences.
    - >90% will be free of clinical episodes of tachycardia by 1 year of age.
      - As many as one-third of these children may have a recurrence at a mean age of 8 years.
  - SVT onset at ≥5 years
    - Chance of recurrent episodes of tachycardia is 75–80%.
  - WPW syndrome/preexcitation
    - Substantially increased risk of sudden death
  - Automatic ectopic tachycardias
    - Often incessant and relatively drug resistant
    - Tachycardia-induced cardiomyopathy is possible if conversion is not achieved.
- Atrial flutter
  - Atypical form
    - If conversion to and maintenance in a sinus rhythm cannot be achieved, morbidity is substantial, with 4- to 5-fold increase in risk for sudden death
- VT
  - Benign forms
    - Substantial incidence of spontaneous resolution in childhood
- Conduction abnormalities
  - Second-degree AV block
    - Type I: little risk of progression to complete block
    - Type II: progression to higher levels of AV block occurs
  - Complete AV block
    - 20% mortality risk
- Sudden cardiac death
  - Annual mortality after onset of symptoms in untreated young patients
    - 1–5%
    - Nearly 10% risk of sudden death as the initial symptom
  - Highest risk for sudden death in patients with:
    - History of syncope
    - QTc more than 530 ms
  - LQTS
    - Cumulative probability of a cardiac event (predominantly syncope) in patients who are genotyped LQT1, 2, and 3 by 15 years of age
      - 10% LQT3
      - 69% LQT1

– Jervell and Lange-Nielsen syndrome
  ■ Substantially higher incidence of sudden death compared with Romano-Ward variant
– Rarely, may be a cause of sudden infant death syndrome

PREVENTION

■ Conduction abnormalities
  ● LQTS
    – Automatic external defibrillators
      ■ Availability in some school systems has already begun to decrease the incidence of sudden cardiac death in the young.

– Risk reduction may be achieved by asking 2 critical questions in pre-sports clearance evaluations.
  ■ Has the patient ever passed out, had visceral chest pain, or experienced symptomatic palpitations during strenuous exercise?
  ■ Has any family member died suddenly and unexpectedly before the age of 35 years?
  ■ An affirmative answer to either question should prompt a cardiologic referral before participation in competitive sports.

Cardiovascular Screening

BACKGROUND

- Congenital and acquired heart diseases are common chronic disorders in children.
- Heart disease in children is often undetected until a child develops symptoms.
  - Heart failure
  - Sudden death
  - Exception: diseases contracted shortly after birth that produce severe symptoms
- Pediatric heart diseases are a heterogeneous group of conditions.
  - Individual diseases are not common.
- However, as a group, pediatric heart diseases raise questions about need for universal screening.
- Congenital structural lesions, when undetected, often result in sudden death.
  - Screening may be most important for lesions associated with sudden death.
  - Occur in 0.8–1% of all births
- Improved screening strategies have resulted in higher incidence of cardiomyopathies (1.13 new cases per 100,000 births).
- Hypertrophic cardiomyopathy (HCM) is:
  - Defined as unexplained left-ventricular hypertrophy in the absence of a hemodynamic cause
  - The most common cause of sudden cardiac death in healthy, often athletic adolescents
- Rhythm disturbances of concern are:
  - Long QT syndrome (LQTS)
    - Inherited disorder of cardiac ion channels
  - Brugada syndrome
  - Both syndromes predispose affected individuals to sudden death from ventricular tachycardia.
- Arrhythmogenic right-ventricular dysplasia (ARVD)
  - Also referred to as *arrhythmogenic right-ventricular cardiomyophathy*
  - Includes rhythm abnormality and cardiomyopathy
    - Accounts for 5% of cases of sudden death in North America.
- Acquired conditions can also be severe and lead to sudden death or heart failure.
  - Infectious
    - Myocarditis
    - Vasculitis
    - Pericarditis
    - Endocarditis
  - Toxic
    - Adriamycin
    - Thalassemias
    - Medications
  - Vascular
    - Atherosclerosis
  - No overall incidence and prevalence data are available for acquired conditions.
- Incidence of sudden cardiac death
  - Approximately 1 death in 200,000 high school athletes per year
    - Devastating effect on public and survivors when a young person in dies unexpectedly
    - An even larger number of youth with these conditions will be disabled by heart failure.

GOALS

- Clinicians should maintain a high level of alertness in their practices for these potentially life-threatening cardiac conditions by conducting a thorough history, physical examination, and laboratory evaluation.
- Cardiovascular screening depends on a high index of suspicion of disease in young children.
  - Those who appear healthy and fit, with normal clinical examinations, are the most difficult to refer for further assessment.
  - The risk of sudden cardiac death associated with many of the clinically relevant cardiac diseases is not known.
- Some subpopulations may be particularly vulnerable or require additional consideration.
  - Screening methods include:
    - Fetal screening
    - Infant screening
    - Hypertension screening
    - Screening of young athletes

GENERAL APPROACH

- Many recommend wide-scale screening for cardiovascular disease in childhood, because of:
  - Devastating consequences
  - Hidden nature of the disease
  - Relatively common occurrence of different cardiovascular conditions
  - Prolonged asymptomatic period

- To identify the many types of cardiac conditions, echocardiography and electrocardiography (ECG) would be necessary for all children and adolescents.
  - Cost would be prohibitive.
  - ECG may generate a large number of false-positive results.
  - Comprehensive assessments such as these are probably not indicated.
- Office tools readily available to all practitioners for evaluating cardiovascular health in children
  - Positive communication skills
  - Growth curves and documentation of normal developmental milestones
  - Accurate scales and a stadiometer (or a tape measure) to measure height
  - Tape measure for head circumference and wing span
  - Accurate blood pressure cuffs, with a range of appropriate-size cuffs
    - An oscillometric cuff is easier to use on infants and small children.
    - Aneroid cuffs are portable.
      - May be more reliable, particularly in older children who may be hypertensive
  - Pulse oximeter
  - Body mass index (BMI) calculator
    - US Centers for Disease Control and Prevention (CDC) guidelines for the normal range of BMI by sex and age
    - To calculate BMI: weight (in kilograms) divided by height (in meters) squared
    - Printed tables are available from the CDC.
  - Clinical examination by observation, palpation, and auscultation
  - Access to radiographs, ECG, and echocardiography
  - Blood biomarkers may be useful in distinguishing heart diseases from other causes of distress.
    - Interpretation of results may require discussion with a subspecialist who uses these tests with greater frequency.
  - In some tertiary care centers, thorough clinical screening may allow the identification of the affected individual and genotype.
    - Genetic testing of individual family members may be necessary.
  - Should provide sufficient clues to heart disease to prompt referrals to a pediatric heart specialist
- These tools and a high index of suspicion can identify some cases of occult cardiovascular disease in children and adolescents.

SPECIFIC INTERVENTIONS

Fetal screening

- A fetal diagnosis of complex congenital heart disease may prompt delivery at a tertiary care center.
  - Cost/benefit ratio is unknown.
- Advance knowledge of an infant's cardiac defect may allow the family more time to process the disease emotionally.
  - The emotional effect of this advance knowledge is difficult to assess.
- Indications for fetal echocardiography include:
  - Obvious structural abnormality visualized on routine fetal sonography
  - Perceived rhythm abnormality
  - Sibling with congenital heart defect or cardiomyopathy
  - Known fetal chromosomal abnormality
  - Family history of syndromes or heart disease
  - Maternal lupus or phospholipid antibodies
  - Maternal diabetes
  - Maternal exposure to infectious diseases
  - Multiple spontaneous abortions
  - Known teratogens and toxins

Neonatal and infant screening (general)

- Most neonates have not been screened by fetal echocardiography.
  - Screening all fetuses is presently not cost effective.
  - Current efforts rely on standard tools to make a diagnosis.
  - An abnormal screening result should prompt referral to a pediatric heart specialist.
- Pediatricians screen most infants in the immediate newborn period.
  - First 2 weeks and again at 2 months of life
- Detecting lesions that are dependent on the ductus arteriosus is critical.
  - Critical coarctation
  - Pulmonary atresia
  - Hypoplastic and left-heart syndrome
  - Presentation is often nonspecific.
  - Coarctation may occur surreptitiously with a cranky infant who is mildly tachypneic and diaphoretic.
    - The infant may appear septic.
  - Other ductal-dependent lesions lend themselves to cyanosis.
    - May be readily apparent
      - Less so in the darker-skinned infant and anemic infant

- The 2-month screening is particularly important in detecting left-to-right shunts.
  - The patient's pulmonary vascular resistance drops maximally at that point.
- A detailed family history is important.
  - Pregnancy history
  - Known heart disease before age 50 years
  - Heart murmur that required treatment
  - Sudden infant death in prior pregnancies
  - Abrupt deaths under the age of 50 years
    - Ask about automobile crashes or swimming deaths.
      - May give clues to a family history of LQTS or Brugada syndrome
  - Deafness at birth
    - An association exists with the Jervell and Lange-Nielsen form of LQTS and abnormalities of ion flux into the organ of Corti.
  - Seizures
    - Possibly caused by ventricular tachycardia
  - Potassium abnormalities
    - Associated with LQTS
  - Developmental delays, physical handicaps, or syndromes
  - Diabetes
  - Thyroid disease, lupus, rheumatoid arthritis
    - May have associations with pericarditis, cardiomyopathies, and atrioventricular block
  - Enlarged heart
    - Cardiomyopathy
  - Use of a pacemaker or antiarrhythmic
  - Tall family members
    - Indicates connective tissue disease
  - Deaths due to aneurysm
    - Indicates connective tissue disease and familial aortic aneurysm
  - Obesity
  - Kidney disease or kidney transplantation
    - Applicable when screening for systemic hypertension

Screening infants using the medical history and review of systems

- Signs of a possible cardiac lesion, although nonspecific:
  - Poor Apgar score
  - Tachypnea
  - Cyanosis at birth

- In the review of systems, indications that cardiac disease and congestive heart failure (CHF) are present
  - Any indications of poor or lengthy feeding
  - Tachypnea
  - Dyspnea
  - Diaphoresis with feeding
- Reflux
  - Common in infants
  - Persistent reflux with sweating and pallor or cyanosis may be indication that a heart lesion is present with associated CHF caused by:
    - Diminished gut perfusion
    - Hepatosplenomegaly
    - Or both
- Cranky, colicky infant who is also pale, tachypneic, or not growing may have CHF or intermittent arrhythmia.
- Frequent upper respiratory symptoms are often an indication of pulmonary edema.
  - Dyspnea
  - Tachypnea
  - Wheezing
  - Caused by CHF or congenital heart disease associated with immune deficiency
- The clinician should ask how well the patient sleeps.
  - An infant with heart failure or arrhythmia may sleep restlessly.

Screening infants using the physical examination

- Vital signs are crucial.
  - If the infant is cyanotic or dusky, obtain pulse oximetry.
  - Assess upper- and lower-extremity pulses, including the femoral pulse, to assess for coarctation of aorta.
    - Comparing upper- and lower-extremity pulses simultaneously during the physical examination may increase accuracy.
      - Coarctation is the most frequently missed cardiac lesion.
  - 4-extremity blood pressures are less sensitive and specific for diagnosis of coarctation of aorta than formerly thought.
    - Obtaining 4-extremity blood pressures at least once in all infants is still good practice.
- A flat or declining growth curve may indicate failure to thrive.
  - May be a sign of CHF
  - Infants and children with cyanotic and valvular heart disease may continue to grow along a normal curve.

C

- Head, ears, eyes, nose, and throat
  - Should be referred to a pediatric cardiologist if:
    - Any jugular venous distention
    - Brisk carotid upstroke
    - Cranial bruit
    - Neck webbing prompts suspicion of Noonan or Turner syndrome.
    - A bifid uvula prompts suspicion of Loeys-Dietz syndrome.
      - With a predilection toward bicommissural aortic valves, aortic root dilatation and, ultimately, dissection
- Chest
  - A precordial bulge can indicate cardiomegaly.
  - Pectus excavatum and carinatum may signal the presence of a connective tissue disorder.
  - Marfan syndrome
- Lungs
  - Pulmonary edema
    - Persistent, recalcitrant wheezing
    - Frequent respiratory symptoms
- Cardiac system
  - Many children have innocent murmurs.
    - Soft or musical and systolic in nature
    - Some of these murmurs are even continuous.
      - Disappear when the child is supine
    - Murmurs that require referral
      - Present in diastole or continuously
      - Harsh and loud
      - Persistent systolic murmurs
      - Clicks
      - Snaps
      - Rubs
      - Third and fourth heart sound gallop rhythms
- Abdomen
  - Organomegaly is suspicious for CHF and storage diseases.
    - Associated with cardiomyopathy
- Extremities
  - Clubbing is a sequela of cyanotic disease.
  - Arachnodactyly is associated with Marfan syndrome.
  - Genetic syndromes
    - Polydactyly
    - Clinodactyly
    - Absent radii

Appearance as a screening tool in infants

- Is the child dysmorphic?
- Does the child have similarities in appearance to either parent?
  - The clinician should not use this look-alike phenomenon to exclude syndromes.
  - Parents may not realize they have a syndrome if it has never been diagnosed.
    - A parent with bad acne may in fact have tuberous sclerosis.
  - If the child is dysmorphic, and if a syndrome is suspected:
    - Heart disease should be considered as an associated issue
    - A very strong association exists between structural heart abnormalities or cardiomyopathies and syndromes or chromosomal abnormalities.

Screening infants with noninvasive tools

Chest radiography

- Allows assessment of:
  - Visceral situs
  - Pulmonary blood flow patterns
  - The shape and size of the cardiac silhouette
- The following are associated with some forms of cardiac disease.
  - Dextrocardia
  - Situs inversus
  - Increased cardiopulmonary blood flow
  - Cardiomegaly
    - Volume or pressure overload lesions
    - Cardiomyopathies
    - Myocarditis
    - Ebstein anomaly
    - Pericardial effusions
- The side of the aortic arch may be inferred.
  - A right-sided aortic arch is seen in 10% of the population.
  - More common with conotruncal defects, such as tetralogy of Fallot
  - A right-sided arch may also be seen in persons with a double aortic arch.
    - Produces a vascular ring
- The thymic sail should be obvious in newborns and neonates.
  - If it is absent, consider:
    - DiGeorge syndrome
    - Conotruncal defects

■ The pulmonary blood flow pattern is important because Kerly B lines may confirm the suspicion of:

- Pulmonary edema consistent with shunt lesions

- Cardiomyopathy

- Myocarditis

- Chronic lesions may produce hyperinflation and flattened diaphragms.

Barium esophagography (barium swallow)

■ Readily accessible

■ Does not require sedation

■ Excellent screening tool for vascular rings and slings

■ Less expensive than magnetic resonance imaging

■ Indentation of the esophagus indicates abnormal vasculature.

■ The test is indicated for:

- Stridorous infants

- Infants with reflux

- Any infant in whom the suspicion of right-sided aortic arch is raised

■ Direct imaging techniques are required to make a definitive diagnosis.

■ In all cases, requires further investigation by a pediatric cardiologist

ECG

■ Relatively insensitive, nonspecific screening tool for structural heart defects

■ Important screening tool for rhythm disturbances

■ Inexpensive

■ Readily accessible

■ Provides baseline information regarding heart lesions

■ Use of the ECG as a routine screening tool is not universally established.

- Has been adopted in some parts of Europe

■ In newborns suspected of having heart disease, attention must be paid to the QRS axis and the T-wave morphology.

- A superior axis may suggest the presence of major cardiac defects.

  – Atrioventricular septal defect

  – Tricuspid atresia

  – Some forms of double-outlet right ventricle

- The persistence of an upright T wave in V1 beyond the first week of life usually indicates significant right-ventricular hypertrophy.

  – In the context of cardiac or pulmonary disease

- If the heart rhythm is not sinus, heart disease should be considered.

- If degrees of atrioventricular block are found, maternal systemic lupus must be considered.

■ Greatly elevated (sinus) heart rates may be present in patients with CHF.

■ Extremely low heart rates (not sinus) may be consistent with atrioventricular block.

■ If a superior QRS vector is found, it may be:

- Normal variant

- Sign of preexcitation

- Indication of Noonan syndrome

- Indication of a more complex lesion

  – Atrioventricular canal

  – Tricuspid atresia

■ Configuration of the P waves and QRS complexes is important.

- Ventricular preexcitation patterns may be present within families.

  – Wolff-Parkinson-White syndrome

  – Ebstein anomaly

  – Wolff-Parkinson-White syndrome is also seen with left-ventricular noncompaction-type cardiomyopathy.

■ Diagnosis of Brugada syndrome depends on the appropriate analysis of the QRS complex.

- Including ST-segment elevation in the right precordial leads

■ rSR' patterns may be a normal variant evident of:

- Right-ventricular hypertrophy

- Initial sign of an atrial septal defect

- More pronounced right bundle-branch block patterns, which are not surgically induced, may be present in:

  – Mitochondrial dystrophies (Kearns-Sayre syndrome)

  – Arrhythmogenic right-ventricular dysplasia

  – Beckwith-Wiedemann syndrome

  – Some septal defects

  – May also be present in familial right bundle-branch block

    ■ Generally benign

■ Ventricular hypertrophy as indicated by ECG should prompt referral for echocardiography.

■ Right- and left-ventricular hypertrophy may be signs of:

- Cardiomyopathy lesions

- Shunt lesions

- Pressure overload lesions

- However, voltage is not uniformly accurate in predicting disease.

  – If increased voltage is combined with a strain pattern, cardiac disease is likely.

- Certain ECGs are considered pathognomonic for disease.
  - Pompe disease
    - Massively increased voltage
    - Strain pattern
    - Shortened PR interval
  - Many patients with severe left-ventricular noncompaction-type cardiomyopathy have a similar pattern of severe ventricular hypertrophy on ECG.
    - Pathognomonic for this disease and of strain
      - With or without evidence of preexcitation

Serum markers of heart disease

- Cardiac enzymes and B-type natriuretic peptide (BNP) levels are routinely used in screening symptomatic adults for cardiac ischemia or heart failure.
  - Their use as screening tools has not been established for diagnosing heart disease in children.
    - They serve as secondary tools that aid in defining the severity of the disease.
- Troponin I and troponin T are components of the cardiomyocyte.
  - May be released during myocyte degradation
  - Have been useful in identifying adults with ischemic heart disease
  - Use of troponin analysis in children is less clear.
  - Active release of troponins may be more consistent with acute myocarditis than chronic dilated cardiomyopathy.
- BNP is released from the ventricle during times of cardiac stress.
  - Appears to correlate well with heart failure in adults and children
  - A linear correlation of BNP with degree of heart failure appears to exist.
  - The specific level of BNP may be predictive of adverse cardiac events in children.
- Other biomarkers are presently being investigated as possible indications of heart disease.
- More conventional markers of disease are nonspecific and not very useful in screening for heart disease.
  - C-reactive protein
  - Sedimentation rate
  - Blood chemistry
  - Complete blood counts

Echocardiography

- Echocardiographic screening in every newborn is not cost effective.
- Expensive

- Time consuming
- Indiscriminate performance of echocardiography may create more anxiety than comfort among practitioners and parents.
  - The finding of a tiny patent ductus arteriosus or patent foramen ovale on routine echocardiography often results in:
    - Unnecessary follow-up
    - Increased parental anxiety
    - Increased medical expenditures
- Appropriate echocardiographic screening of children with heart murmurs is determined by a thorough clinical examination.
  - Reported to be 80% sensitive in identifying pathologic heart disease when performed by general pediatricians
    - Sensitivity increases to 96% when a pediatric cardiologist performs the examination.
- Screening echocardiography may be warranted:
  - In neonates with siblings with complex congenital heart disease
  - If maternal exposure to toxins or potential teratogens is suspected
  - For infants born to mothers with gestational diabetes
  - Any neonate with genetic syndrome

Screening for cardiovascular disease in children in adolescents

- In the US, structural heart disease is frequently diagnosed early in life.
  - Some occult cardiac defects and cardiomyopathies may not come to light until children grow and their physiologic features change.
    - Bicuspid aortic valve
    - HCM
    - ASDs
    - Partial anomalous pulmonary veins
    - Coronary artery anomalies

History

- History of present illness
- Family history
- Medical history
- Review of systems
- History of multiple family members with diabetes may indicate a predisposition for:
  - Acquired heart disease
  - Metabolic or mitochondrial cardiomyopathy

- Underlying heart defect may be suspected if a patient:
  - Is hospitalized yearly for respiratory infections
    - A frequent presentation of:
      - ASDs
      - Pulmonary vein anomalies
      - Dilated cardiomyopathies
  - Has sedentary lifestyle (doesn't have the energy to play)
- Symptoms of chest pain and palpitations are often nonspecific in growing children and adolescents.
  - Warrant evaluation for heart disease in appropriate cases
- Presyncope should be thoroughly evaluated.
  - A history of syncope warrants screening for cardiovascular disease.
- In a child with a heart murmur, ask whether this murmur is new.
  - May help differentiate between innocent and pathologic murmurs
- Coarctation of the aorta may sometimes occur beyond infancy.
  - Physical examination in suspected cases should include:
    - Palpation of femoral pulses
    - Measurement of upper- and lower-extremity blood pressure
- In addition to the history, questions to ask of children and adolescents include:
  - What grade are you in, and how are you doing in school?
    - Chronically ill children tend to have more difficulty concentrating on school activities.
  - Do you participate in activities outside of school? What type?
    - Some children do not have the energy to participate in activities.
  - How well do you sleep at night? How many pillows do you use for sleeping? Has anyone ever told you that you snore? Are you sleepy during the day? Do you nap?
    - These questions are useful in identifying sleep apnea, which has been linked with:
      - Systemic hypertension
      - Severe sinus bradycardia with obstruction
      - Cor pulmonale
  - How often and how much do you eat?
    - This question may be difficult for some children and adolescents to answer.
      - The question may be further refined by asking what the patient has had to eat today.
    - A chronically ill child may have high caloric needs.
    - A patient with organomegaly caused by CHF, storage disease, or both may have early satiety and abdominal pain.

Screening for systemic hypertension, obesity, and metabolic syndrome as precursors to cardiovascular disease

- Cardiac risk factors are additive risk factors for future cardiac disease.
  - Systemic hypertension
  - Obesity
    - With or without metabolic syndrome
  - Obstructive sleep apnea caused by obesity

Blood pressure screening

- Mass screening is important but may produce a variety of false-positive results.
- Repeated testing and questioning may be necessary to obtain true-positive results.
- Additional questions for patients
  - How and when were you diagnosed with high blood pressure?
  - Have you had any tests for your high blood pressure?
  - Have you gained or lost weight recently? How much and over what period?
  - What are your favorite foods? How often do you eat out?
  - What are your favorite drinks? How much water do you drink in a day?
  - What medicines (prescription and over the counter) are you taking?
  - Do you take any dietary supplements, such as creatine, protein shakes, or MetRx?
    - Anabolic steroids will cause acne and blood pressure elevation.
  - How active are you? Is your exercise limited? By what?
  - Do other people in your family have high blood pressure? Does anyone have kidney dialysis, transplants, or diabetes?
  - How do you sleep at night? Do you snore? How many pillows do you use under your head when sleeping?
  - Do you ever have trouble with palpitations, breathing difficulties, fainting, or dizziness?
- If the initial blood pressure is taken in an outer room and it is elevated:
  - The patient should be allowed to lie down in the examining room for at least 5 minutes.
    - Blood pressure assessment is then repeated.
- The readings are compared with those recently established by the Task Force for Systemic Hypertension in Children.
  - Using sex, height, and weight percentiles
- If 3 readings on different visits are consistently >97th percentile:
  - The patient should be referred to a subspecialist.
    - Pediatric cardiologist
    - Nephrologist

Obesity and comorbid conditions

■ Childhood obesity has become increasingly prevalent.

■ Once an individual has been identified as obese by BMI:

- Associated comorbid conditions should be assessed by history and physical examination.

- Appropriate referrals can be made.

  – Nutritionists

  – Behavioral modification specialists

  – Physical therapists

  – Exercise or rehabilitative programs

  – Pulmonology or sleep specialists

  – Endocrinologists

■ ECGs should be obtained in obese children with:

- Systemic hypertension

- Obstructive sleep apnea

- Hyperlipidemia

- Any obese child who is seeking exercise clearance

- The presence of obesity may preclude a reliable ECG.

  – The layer of adipose may provide voltage insulation, arbitrarily decreasing the total voltage.

- The presence of any of the following should prompt further investigation.

  – Right-ventricular hypertrophy (may be seen with cor pulmonale caused by obstructive sleep apnea)

  – Left-ventricular hypertrophy

  – Bundle-branch blocks

  – Ischemic changes

■ Obese children with systemic hypertension and obstructive sleep apnea should have echocardiography.

- Echocardiography is technically challenging in obese individuals.

  – Resolution is often poor.

- Although some studies have reported increased left-ventricle mass in obese individuals, obese children have not been thoroughly assessed.

  – Lack of increased left-ventricle mass or left-ventricle hypertrophy on the echocardiogram should not be a measure of comfort.

■ Obesity may first occur as an endothelial disease.

- Therefore, newer noninvasive imaging modalities may be in order.

  – Carotid or intimal thickening

  – Vascular reactivity studies

■ Individuals with obesity or systemic hypertension should have blood tests, including:

- Metabolic profile

- Liver function tests

- Complete blood cell count with differential

- Thyroid function tests

- Aldosterone, uric acid testing

  – If systemic hypertension or as a baseline marker

- Insulin level testing (likely to be elevated)

- Glycated hemoglobin test

- Glucose tolerance testing if diabetes is suspected

- C-reactive protein testing as a nonspecific marker for cardiac inflammatory disease

- Fasting lipid profile

- BNP assessment: often performed at baseline

  – Serial follow-up in patients with suspected or proven cardiomyopathy

  – Obese individuals have been documented to have lower BNP levels.

  – A false-negative result may occur.

Athletic screening: ruling out sudden death

■ Genetic diseases, such as HCM, Marfan syndrome, and ARVD, may be suspected in individuals on the basis of family history, medical history, and current illness history.

■ However, many diseases that cause sudden cardiac death are relatively silent.

- History and physical examination alone cannot guarantee identification of many critical cardiovascular abnormalities that may occur in young athletes.

  – Even with the addition of noninvasive screening (echocardiography and ECG performed in populations of 250–2000 athletes, followed up over 1 year), very few definitive examples of lethal cardiovascular abnormalities have been detected.

- Given the expense, time, and labor intensiveness of genetic molecular screening for the widely heterogeneous cardiovascular diseases, screening blood testing for mutations is untenable.

Echocardiography

■ Can diagnose HCM in young athletes

- Most common cause of sudden cardiovascular death in young athletes

- Other relevant abnormalities associated with sudden cardiac death may also be identified.

  – Valvar heart disease (mitral valve prolapse, aortic valve stenosis)

  – Aortic root dilatation

  – Left-ventricular dysfunction (myocarditis or dilated cardiomyopathy)

- Some relevant diseases may occasionally be missed even with echocardiographic assessment.
  - Coronary anomalies
  - Early coronary diseases
  - ARVD
- Cost efficiency must be considered in mass screening.
  - Cost range: $600–$2000
  - Institutions cannot be expected to bear the expense of these screening programs.
  - Additional emotional, financial, and medical burdens exist because of false-negative and false-positive results

ECG

- More practical and cost-efficient than echocardiography for population-based screening
- Is abnormal in 75–95% of patients with HCM
- Will usually assist in identifying LQTS and Brugada syndrome
  - Not all affected relatives within a family with LQTS will exhibit an ECG abnormality.

- Some patients with coronary anomalies have normal ECGs; therefore, ECG does not have the same power as the echocardiogram as a preliminary screening tool.
  - It has a relatively low specificity because of the frequency with which ECG alterations may occur in normal athletic physiologic circumstances.
    - False-positive results complicate its use as a primary screening tool, anticipating that 20–25% of all athletes will exhibit these abnormalities, prompting further echocardiographic study.
    - Elite athletes without structural cardiac abnormalities are likely to exhibit ECG abnormalities most consistent with HCM and ARVD.
- If an abnormality is identified, refer for a full evaluation by a pediatric cardiologist.

Cerebral Palsy

DEFINITION

- Cerebral palsy (CP) is a clinical descriptive term for a heterogeneous group of conditions classified according to type, distribution, and severity of motor abnormality.
- Describes a group of disorders of the development of movement, posture, and coordination
  - Motor disorder often accompanied by disturbances of any of the following, alone or in combination:
    - Sensation
    - Cognition
    - Communication
    - Perception
    - Behavior
  - Can also be accompanied by a seizure disorder
  - Can include impairment in the musculoskeletal system, most commonly:
    - Contractures (eg, equinus deformity)
    - Torsional changes in long bones (eg, femoral and tibial torsion)
    - Joint instability (eg, hip displacement)

EPIDEMIOLOGY

- Prevalence
  - Approximately 2–2.5 cases/1000 live births in developed countries
  - Has generally remained stable over the past 20 years
  - More common with lower birth weight and lower gestational age
    - In 1 survey, children born weighing <1000 g constituted 0.2% of survivors but accounted for 8% of children who had CP.
  - Prevalence of CP in very low birth weight infants and those born at <32 weeks' gestation decreased from 6% of live births in 1980 to 4% in 1996.
- In the US, 59% of children with CP attend a special school versus 0.5% without CP.
- Use of health care services for children with CP versus without (over 12 months; 100 children each group)
  - 16 versus 3 visits to a physician
  - 29 versus 4 hospital admissions
  - 108 versus 20 hospital days

ETIOLOGY

- A definite cause cannot be identified for many cases.
  - When a cause can be identified, it is usually of prenatal origin.
  - Intrapartum events play a limited role.
    - Neither sophisticated fetal monitoring nor a higher rate of cesarean deliveries has reduced the occurrence of CP.

- Each form of CP can be caused by a multitude of conditions, and a single etiologic factor (eg, meningitis) can lead to different forms of CP.
- Caused by nonprogressive disturbances affecting the brain in its early development (fetal, infantile, and early childhood)
- The timing of insult to the brain may affect manifestation.
  - Disturbances between 24 and 28 weeks' gestation are more likely to produce spastic diplegia or tetraplegia (quadriplegia).
  - Those occurring at term are more likely to produce dyskinesia.
- In approximately 10%, the cause is thought to be postneonatal (after 28 days).
  - Infection (eg, meningitis, encephalitis)
  - Asphyxia
  - Unintentional injury

RISK FACTORS

- Associated conditions
  - Periventricular leukomalacia (necrosis of white matter near the lateral ventricles)
  - Hydrocephalus
  - Congenital malformations
  - Newborn encephalopathy (recurrent seizures, hypotonia, coma)
- Low birth weight
- Low gestational age
- Multiple pregnancies (in mother)
- Isolated risk factors are poor predictors of CP, especially in full-term infants.
  - Fetal bradycardia
  - Neonatal acidosis
  - Intraventricular hemorrhage in the absence of periventricular leukomalacia
  - Low Apgar scores
  - Prenatal maternal chorioamnionitis

SIGNS AND SYMPTOMS

- Although the brain lesion or anomaly, once recognized in early childhood, is no longer progressive, clinical signs change, especially in the first several years of life.
  - Abnormal patterns emerge as the damaged nervous system matures.
    - For example, a child destined to have spastic quadriplegia:
      - Is often hypotonic in early infancy
      - At 6 months, may develop adduction of the thumb (palmar thumb)

- Followed in a month or 2 by scissoring of the legs when held upright
- By 9 months, may have diffuse spasticity and hyperactive deep-tendon reflexes
- Dyskinetic patterns may not be obvious until approximately 18 months.
- Ataxia may be apparent even later.

■ Early signs
  - Difficulty feeding because of abnormal oral-motor patterns
    - Tongue thrusting
    - Tonic bite
    - Oral hypersensitivity
  - Irritability
  - Delayed milestones, such as head control

DIFFERENTIAL DIAGNOSIS

Possible diagnoses

■ Neurodegenerative disorders
■ Inborn errors of metabolism
  - Some rare inborn errors of metabolism (arginase deficiency and glutaric aciduria) may mimic CP.
  - These cause progressive deterioration, whereas CP does not.
■ Developmental or traumatic lesions of the spinal cord
■ Severe neuromuscular disease
  - Hypotonia in association with weak muscles and depressed tendon reflexes suggests a neuromuscular disease.
  - Many children with both spastic and extrapyramidal CP are hypotonic in early infancy.
■ Movement disorders
■ Spinocerebellar degeneration
  - Repeated examinations are necessary to rule out a progressive degenerative condition.
■ Neoplasms
■ Hydrocephalus
■ Subdural hematoma
■ Dopa-responsive dystonia
  - Rare but treatable form of dystonia
  - May begin with toe-walking and difficulties with gait
  - Responds dramatically to administration of levodopa
  - In most instances, no history can be found of a preexisting condition that would be consistent with CP.
■ Hereditary spastic diplegia
  - Consider in a child with a parent who has CP and has late-onset spastic diplegia with no preceding history of prenatal or neonatal problems

Categorization by type, distribution, and severity of motor abnormality

■ CP can be simplified into 3 categories.
  - Spastic (involving the pyramidal tracts)
  - Dyskinetic (involving the extrapyramidal tracts)
  - Mixed (involving both)
■ Spastic CP
  - Associated with neurologic signs, including:
    - Hyperreflexia
    - Clonus
    - Extensor plantar response
    - Co-contractures
    - Persistent primitive reflexes
    - Abnormal postural control
  - Abnormalities impair normal movements, such as gait and the manipulation of objects, in complex ways.
    - Movement is often stiff, and patterns of movement, such as fisting of hands, retraction of shoulders, scissoring of legs, and toe-walking are often abnormal.
    - Hypotonia of the trunk and neck is common.
  - 3 types of spasticity
    - Diplegia
      - The legs are affected with general sparing of the arms.
      - Children with hydrocephalus are more likely to develop spastic diplegia.
    - Quadriplegia
      - All 4 limbs are significantly and functionally impaired, with the legs more severely involved than the arms.
      - More likely to be intellectually disabled (64% have an IQ <50) and have seizures (56%)
      - More likely to have feeding difficulties, severe joint contractures, and scoliosis
    - Hemiplegia
      - Only 1 side is involved, with the arm usually more impaired than the leg.
■ Dyskinetic CP
  - Dyskinesia includes the involuntary movements of athetosis, chorea.
  - Dystonia
    - Sustained muscle contractures that lead to abnormal posture and twisting
  - Ataxia
    - Incoordination of movement and impaired balance and may be associated with an intention tremor

C

C

DIAGNOSTIC APPROACH

- A direct link between the type of CP and its cause cannot be established without using diagnostic evaluations, such as cranial ultrasonography or magnetic resonance imaging (MRI), and even then, one is often not found.
- The mean age at which CP is diagnosed is 10 months.
  - Therefore, in addition to formal developmental screening recommended for all children, those at risk for CP should have:
    - Regular careful physical examinations
    - Special attention to neurologic status
- Early diagnosis is aided by:
  - History of abnormal pregnancy, labor, delivery, or neonatal period
  - Report of serious acute illness and trauma
- Should evaluate:
  - Primitive reflexes (eg, the asymmetric tonic neck response)
  - Postural responses
    - Delayed
    - Righting the head when tilted to the side
  - Muscle tone (abnormal)
  - Motor milestones
  - Neurobehavioral responsiveness
- Routine screening for metabolic and genetic disorders is not recommended unless the child has atypical features, such as unusual facial features, or a progressive condition.

IMAGING

- Neuroimaging techniques may aid in understanding of structural abnormalities and timing of lesions.
  - Ultrasonography
  - Computed tomography
  - MRI
- Neuroimaging may demonstrate:
  - Periventricular leukomalacia
  - Postischemic necrosis
  - Cerebral dysgenesis
  - Hydrocephalus
  - Porencephaly
  - Tumor
  - Prenatal ischemic injury
  - Leukodystrophy

DIAGNOSTIC PROCEDURES

- Electroencephalography
  - Important part of diagnosis and management of associated seizures
    - Continuous electroencephalographic monitoring with videography may help differentiate seizures from other movement disorders.
  - Not helpful in diagnosis of CP
- Evaluation of altered gait and feeding disorders may require special diagnostic studies.
  - Gait analysis
    - Using videography, electromyelography, and sensors
    - Has improved the orthopedic care given to these children
  - Videofluoroscopic swallowing studies

CLASSIFICATION

- Gross motor function classification system
  - Most common system for classifying severity
  - 5-level system to classify severity of motor involvement based on functional abilities and need for assistive technology and wheeled mobility

TREATMENT APPROACH

- The goal is for the patient to be as independent as possible and to participate in family and community activities with nonaffected peers.
  - Opportunities for participation may be limited, but the physician should:
    - Try to identify opportunities
    - Encourage child to participate in any and all activities that are available
- Multiple interventions are possible.
  - Muscle strengthening
  - Orthotics (eg, ankle-foot orthoses)
  - Oral medication
  - Botulinum toxin injections (with or without serial casting)
  - Intrathecal baclofen pump
  - Selective dorsal rhizotomy
  - Orthopedic surgery
- The best approach requires input of child and family with a team of clinicians (therapists, orthotists, surgeons, nurses, physicians, and social workers).
- Families often turn to alternative therapies.
  - The primary care physician should inquire about them and be aware of:
    - Their nature
    - Possible interactions with medications
    - Potential for harm

- Adults with CP
  - The 3 most important issues are:
    - Communication skills
    - Self-care
    - Mobility
  - Interventions (eg, medications, surgery, braces, or adaptive equipment) should focus on these issues.

SPECIFIC TREATMENTS

Medications

- Oral medications can reduce spasticity but have potential adverse effects.
  - Diazepam
  - Oral baclofen
  - Tizanidine
  - Dantrolene
- No controlled studies have documented improvement in functioning from these medications.
- Intramuscular botulinum toxin is effective in children with functional spasticity in transiently reducing spasticity in individual limbs.
- Drooling can be treated with:
  - Scopolamine (available as transdermal patch and tablet)
  - Glycopyrrolate
  - Botulinum toxin injections into salivary glands

Surgical procedures

- Selective dorsal rhizotomy and intrathecal baclofen reduce spasticity and increase range of motion.
- Orthopedic procedures, such as tenotomies, tendon releases, and transfers, are necessary to address soft-tissue and bone problems.
- Drooling may be managed with surgical removal of the salivary glands.

Physical modalities

- Constraint therapy produces anatomic changes in the brain on functional MRI.
  - Cannot improve selective motor control, difficulties with balance, and weakness
  - Immobilizing the better upper extremity in children with hemiplegia while providing therapy to enhance the function of the affected/worse arm and hand improves function.
- Strength training can improve function.
- Various casting and splinting techniques to maintain muscle length and inhibit increased tone may be helpful.
- After orthopedic surgery, therapy should be started to maximize range of motion and skills.

Assistive devices

- To assist motor activities
  - Switches that improve ability to control the environment
  - Computers
  - Small electric motors
- Communication augmentation
  - Speech synthesizers
  - Symbol charts
  - Spelling boards
- Simple enhancements to improve quality of life
  - Ramps
  - Accessible showers
  - Assistive devices, such as a pencil holder or mouth-activated switch
- The Individuals with Disabilities Education Act requires that school-aged children with disabilities be assessed for the utility of assistive devices and be given the support needed to use them effectively.
- Gaining access to these services requires:
  - Coordination of care
  - Knowledge of the resources available in the community
  - Referral to experts
  - Financial assets
- The physician is obliged to ensure that these services are available to the patient and the family.

Alternative treatments

- The following may offer functional benefits.
  - Equine-assisted therapy (hippotherapy)
  - Acupuncture
- Hyperbaric oxygen
  - Does not appear to improve function
- Electrical stimulation
  - Evidence for effectiveness is inconclusive.

Treatment for specific conditions

Impaired growth

- Evaluating growth impairment includes:
- Evaluation of dietary intake and feeding
  - Assess the child's seating and posture during meals.
  - Assess swallowing mechanism.
    - Can be aided by a videofluoroscopic swallow study using foods of different consistencies
    - Videofluoroscopic swallow study can assess risk of aspiration.
    - Assistance of feeding specialists is invaluable.

C

- Evaluation for gastroesophageal reflux using:
  - pH probe
  - Endoscopy with biopsy
  - Barium swallow or radionuclide gastric-emptying study
- Provide special seating devices to maintain the child in an upright, neutral position.
- Thickened feedings
- Gastrostomy tube, with or without fundoplication
  - Usually improves weight gain and general health
  - May not improve longitudinal growth

Impaired communication

- Augmentative communication aids have been used, but few studies on these have been done.

Impaired cognition

- Early intervention referral for young children
- Special education program for school age
- Formal educational testing

Weakness or impaired mobility

- Orthoses/braces
- Walker
- Wheeled mobility and strength training
- Constraint therapy for hemiplegia

Joint contractures

- Range of motion
- Orthoses
- Surgery

Scoliosis

- Orthoses
- Surgery

Sexual functioning

- Education
- Adaptive devices

Dental caries, malocclusion

- Repair of dental caries
- Orthodontia

Seizures

- Medication
- Surgery

Impaired vision/hearing

- Assistive devices
- Surgery

WHEN TO ADMIT

- Children who aspirate food or saliva or have inadequate nutrition:
  - Demonstrate increased susceptibility to acute illnesses (eg, pneumonia)
  - Should be hospitalized if severely ill or cannot be managed at home
- Hospitalize for most major surgeries, such as complex orthopedic procedures.

WHEN TO REFER

- In US, all infants with CP between birth and 3 years of age should be referred to an early intervention program.
  - Mandated under the Individuals with Disabilities Education Act
  - Special education
  - Physical, occupational, and speech therapies
  - Adaptive equipment
  - Training for mobility and living skills
  - Communication
  - Therapies may not change the basic disorder significantly.
    - However, therapists may help the families by:
      - Teaching them how to position and handle their infant
      - Providing more opportunity for play and learning
      - Facilitating feeding and the parent-child relationship
- Children with moderate or severe CP:
  - Should be referred to an interdisciplinary clinic, if one exists
    - If not, referral to an orthopedist, physical therapist, and health care provider (developmental pediatrician, neurologist, pediatric rehabilitation specialist) who can manage spasticity, other abnormalities of tone, and optimize functioning
- The primary care physician should coordinate referrals.
  - Ensure that the child is receiving coordinated, comprehensive care.
- The family should have early professional support to help them cope with the crisis of diagnosis.
- Specific referrals
  - Speech therapist, audiologist
    - Augmentative communication aids
  - Education specialist, psychologist, school advocate
    - Early intervention
    - Special education
    - Formal educational testing

- Orthopedist, orthotist, physical therapist, equine specialist, occupational therapist
  - Orthoses/braces
  - Walker
  - Wheeled mobility and strength training
  - Hippotherapy
  - Constraint therapy for hemiplegia
- Physical therapist, orthopedist, orthotist
  - Range of motion, orthoses, surgery
- Orthopedist, orthotist
  - Orthoses, surgery
- Gynecologist, urologist, psychologist
  - Sex education
  - Adaptive devices
- Dentist, pedodontist, orthodontist
  - Repair of dental caries, orthodontia
- Neurologist
  - Seizure medication, surgery
- Ophthalmologist, otolaryngologist
  - Vision/hearing assistive devices, surgery
- Financial counselor, care coordinator, specialty program
  - Financial counseling, care coordination, transportation
- Social worker, psychologist, specialty program, care coordinator
  - Parent support group, counseling, support

FOLLOW-UP

- Careful monitoring of physical growth is critical.
  - Monitoring weight for length rather than weight alone is important.
  - Reliable measures are often impossible to obtain.
    - Tibial length is used as a proxy for height.
- Long-term planning and preparation are required to help children make the transition from adolescence to adulthood, particularly when the child has multiple needs.

COMPLICATIONS

- Osteoporosis
  - Common in patients with severe quadriplegia and immobility
- Impaired self-care/hygiene
  - Due to gross motor and fine-motor abnormalities and associated conditions, such as drooling
- Dental disease
  - Malocclusion
  - Dental caries

- Seizures
  - Often, onset in first 2 years of life
- Inhibited physical growth
- Failure to thrive
  - Especially those with dyskinesia or spastic quadriplegia
  - Feeding difficulties/recurrent vomiting may be associated with aspiration.
- Language abnormality (from aphasia to poor articulation)
- Specific learning disabilities, such as visuospatial impairment, are common in a child with a normal range of intelligence.
- Cognitive impairment (75% of cases)
  - 40% are intellectually disabled.
    - Mildly in approximately one-third of cases
    - Moderately or worse in one-third
- Impaired mobility
- Impairment in gastrointestinal functioning, such as gastroesophageal reflux disease
- Impairment in growth
- Impaired vision
  - Strabismus
  - Refractive error
  - Nystagmus
- Behavioral problems

PROGNOSIS

- Survival depends on the severity of CP.
  - A 2-year-old child with severe CP is expected to have a 40% chance of living to age 20 years.
  - A child with mild CP has a 99% chance.
- Greatest risk for early death if child has all of the following:
  - Intellectual disability
  - No independent mobility (ie, rolling), limited spontaneous movement
  - Can be fed only by gastronomy tube
- Prognostication before child's second birthday may be difficult, except at the extremes of involvement.
- Prognosis for functioning is related to:
  - Clinical type of CP
  - Pace of motor development
  - Evolution of infantile reflexes
  - Intellectual abilities
  - Sensory impairment
  - Emotional-social adjustment

- Prognosis for walking
  - Patients who sit unsupported by 24 months and crawl by 30 months are more likely to walk independently.
  - Retention of obligatory primitive reflexes at 18 months of age makes independent ambulation unlikely.
  - Virtually all with hemiplegia learn to walk, as do many with dyskinesia or ataxia.
- Individual achievement is related to many factors.
  - Intelligence
  - Physical functioning
  - Ability to communicate
  - Personality attributes
  - Major factors in adjustment as adults
    - Availability of training, jobs, sheltered employment
    - Counseling
  - A supportive family and availability of specialist medical care are other important factors.

PREVENTION

- Prevention of prematurity
- In some instances, CP may be prevented by:
  - Reducing occurrence of injuries during childhood
  - Minimizing periventricular leukomalacia in premature infants
    - Improving circulation
    - Countering effects of excitatory neurotransmitters (eg, head cooling in newborn who has had a hypoxic or ischemic event)

Chest Pain

DEFINITION

- Chest pain is defined as discomfort in the thoracic region.

EPIDEMIOLOGY

- Most cases are due to trauma to the musculoskeletal wall.
- Pulmonary disease accounts for one-fifth of cases.
- The rest are due to psychiatric causes, gastrointestinal disorders, or cardiac disease.
  - Undiagnosed cardiac disease causes chest pain in <5% of patients.
  - Excluding children with preexisting heart disease, cardiac abnormalities are found in <1% of patients.
- Approximately 15% of cases remain idiopathic.

MECHANISM

- Pulmonary conditions
  - Children with asthma may have chest pain from excessive coughing and overuse of their intercostal muscles.
- Gastrointestinal conditions
  - Acid reflux to the esophagus can mimic the pain of angina and can cause both acute and chronic chest pain.
- Cardiac conditions
  - Aortic stenosis and idiopathic hypertrophic cardiomyopathy can cause chest pain as a result of the heart's inability to increase the cardiac output with exercise.
    - These are the most important lesions that cause left ventricular outflow obstruction.
    - These disorders cause syncope and chest pain with exertion.
    - Mild aortic stenosis does not cause chest pain.
  - Pericarditis can result from either an infectious agent or an autoimmune process.

HISTORY

- A detailed history includes:
  - The child's response to the pain.
    - If possible, children should describe the pain in their own words.
    - They should be asked what they think is causing the pain.
  - The location, duration, radiation, and quality of the pain.
  - Aggravating and alleviating factors
  - Any associated signs and symptoms
  - Any history of trauma, even if it occurred 1–3 months earlier
- To many adolescents, chest pain is synonymous with heart disease; therefore, this issue should be addressed.
  - If no cardiac cause is discovered, the physician should unequivocally state to the adolescent and the family that the heart is normal.

- The quality of pain can help determine its source.
  - Deep, poorly localized pain that radiates to the neck or shoulders is characteristic of visceral pain.
  - Superficial sharp pain that is exacerbated by lifting or movements of the torso suggests musculoskeletal pain.
  - Peripheral pain that increases with inspiratory efforts originates from pleural inflammation.
  - Sharp pain that decreases when the child leans forward is characteristic of pericardial inflammation.
  - Pain that occurs with exercise points toward respiratory or cardiac conditions.
  - Pain that awakens the child from sleep is never psychological.
- Common, uncommon, and rare causes of chest pain and associated signs and symptoms
  - Musculoskeletal
    - Costonchondritis (common): localized, superficial, reproducible pain over costochondral junction
    - Exercise, overuse, muscle strain (common): reproducible pain with use of involved muscle group
    - Protracted coughing or vomiting (common): intercostal muscle tenderness
    - Trauma: localized pain; pain with movement of involved areas
    - Stitch (common): sharp, crampy costal pain that occurs with running
    - Precordial catch (uncommon): transient, stabbing pain at left sternal border; relieved by forced inspiration
  - Pulmonary
    - Asthma (common): associated with cough, shortness of breath, wheezing, abnormal pulmonary function tests; relief with inhaled bronchodilators
    - Exercise-induced bronchospasm (common): abnormal findings on exercise tests; improvement with bronchodilators
    - Pneumonia (common): crackles, fever, cough
    - Pleural effusion (uncommon): pleural rub, fever, decreased breath sounds
    - Pneumothorax (uncommon): sudden pain, referred shoulder pain, dyspnea
    - Pulmonary embolus (rare): contraceptive use or recent abortion, pleuritic pain
  - Gastrointestinal
    - Esophagitis (common): retrosternal pain; relief with antacids
    - Gastroesophageal reflux (common): retrosternal burning pain; worse after eating and when reclining; relief with antacids

- Cardiac
  - Hypertrophic cardiomyopathy (rare): syncope, family history, systolic ejection murmur
  - Pericarditis (rare): associated fever with acute onset of pain; pain increases with movement; narrow pulse pressure, distant heart sounds; alleviated by leaning forward
  - Myocarditis (rare): precedent viral illness, anorexia, shortness of breath, third heart sound or gallop, cardiomegaly
- Nonorganic
  - Psychogenic (common): normal physical examination, trouble sleeping, family or school problems, life stresses, family history of chest pain, other somatic symptoms
  - Hyperventilation (common): associated light-headedness, paresthesias, underlying anxiety

PHYSICAL EXAM

- Findings that suggest musculoskeletal and chest wall conditions
  - Signs of trauma, such as bruising
  - Swelling over joints
  - Splinting or an abnormal breathing pattern
  - Reproduction of point tenderness at the origin of the spontaneous pain is the strongest evidence favoring the diagnosis of chest wall disease.
    - Each rib cartilage should be palpated with only 1 finger or with the child's finger.
  - Pain from the thoracic cage that can be elicited by movements of the torso or by flexion of the arms is highly suggestive of a musculoskeletal chest wall injury.
- Findings that suggest a parapneumonic effusion
  - Fever, tachypnea, tachycardia, pleural friction rub and/or crackles, and dullness to percussion
- Findings that suggest a spontaneous pneumothorax
  - Dyspnea, shoulder pain, and tachypnea
- Findings that suggest a cardiac source
  - Any new clicks, rubs, or systolic murmur or change in a previous murmur
- Findings that suggest myocarditis or pericarditis
  - An ill appearance, fever, dyspnea, changes in the pain associated with the respiratory cycle
  - A third heart sound or gallop can be heard in myocarditis and congestive heart failure.
- Findings that suggest a hyperventilation syndrome
  - Carpopedal spasm
  - Paresthesias
- Adolescents with gynecomastia or breast pain may experience chest pain that is easily discernible on inspection and palpation of the developing breast tissue.

DIFFERENTIAL DIAGNOSIS

Musculoskeletal conditions
- Costrochondritis (common)
- Exercise, overuse, muscle strain (common)
- Protracted cough or vomiting (common)
- Trauma
- Stitch (common)
- Precordial catch (uncommon)

Pulmonary conditions
- Asthma (common)
- Exercise-induced bronchospasm (common)
- Pneumonia (common)
- Pleural effusion (uncommon)
- Pneumothorax (uncommon)
- Pulmonary embolus (rare)

Gastrointestinal conditions
- Esophagitis (common)
- Gastroesophageal reflux (common)

Cardiac conditions
- Hypertrophic cardiomyopathy (rare)
- Pericarditis (rare)
- Myocarditis (rare)

Nonorganic
- Psychogenic (common)
- Hyperventilation (common)

LABORATORY EVALUATION

- Screening laboratory tests are usually not helpful in establishing a specific diagnosis.
- A thorough history and physical examination should guide the clinician in ordering tests.

IMAGING

- In most cases, chest radiographs will only confirm what is suspected clinically.
- A chest radiograph is indicated if the provider suspects:
  - Pericarditis
  - Pneumonia
  - Pleural effusion
  - Other pulmonary disease

DIAGNOSTIC PROCEDURES

- In most cases, electrocardiography will only confirm what is suspected clinically.
- If the pain occurs with exercise, exercise testing or spirometry may help uncover underlying asthma or exercise-induced bronchospasm.

■ To confirm the diagnosis of exercise-induced or cold air–induced bronchospasm:

- Exercise testing
- Cold air challenge
- A therapeutic trial of bronchodilators

TREATMENT APPROACH

■ It is important to define whether the chest pain is secondary to an underlying abnormality, psychogenic, or idiopathic.

■ Treatment of psychogenic chest pain should be focused on:

- The family's understanding of the cause of the pain
- Reassurance that no long-term sequelae exist
- Acknowledging that the pain is real to the child

■ Children with idiopathic chest pain may benefit from a trial of antacids or histamine$_2$-blockers because the clinical presentation of esophagitis can be nonspecific.

SPECIFIC TREATMENT

■ Exercise-induced bronchospasm

- Treatment with bronchodilators will help these children participate in sports and allow them to lead normal, active lives.

■ Hyperventilation syndrome

- For a child with an acute episode, the treatment is to have the child breathe into a paper bag to relieve the hypocapnia.
- Resolution of the chronic problem is based on techniques to allow children to understand the nature of their anxiety and regain control of their emotional state.

WHEN TO REFER

■ Signs and symptoms that accompany chest pain and warrant referral or hospitalization

- Symptoms
  - Chest pain with exercise
  - Palpitation
  - Syncope
  - Fever, chills, weight loss, malaise, anorexia
  - History of Kawasaki disease, Turner syndrome, Marfan syndrome, sickle cell disease, or cystic fibrosis
  - Recent elective abortion, calf pain, oral contraceptive use
  - Family history of hypertrophic obstructive cardiomyopathy or unexplained syncope
  - Pica, foreign body aspiration
  - Conversion disorder

■ Signs

- Cyanosis, toxic appearance, or respiratory distress
- Murmur that increases with Valsalva maneuver
- Pleural or pericardial friction rub
- Pulsus paradoxus
- Cardiac clicks, thrills, gallop, or third heart sound

■ A pediatric cardiologist should see children with chest pain and a family history of sudden death.

■ If palpitations or chest pain occur infrequently or are not associated with exercise, referral for Holter monitoring is indicated.

■ For children with severe psychiatric problems, referral to a psychiatrist may be necessary.

WHEN TO ADMIT

■ Children with chest pain rarely require hospitalization because chest pain is usually benign, self-limited, and not associated with severe intrathoracic illness.

■ Children with the following should be hospitalized:

- Myocarditis
- Pericarditis
- Empyema
- Pneumothorax
- Significant thoracic trauma
- Acute chest syndrome
- Esophageal foreign bodies
- Coronary artery anomalies or other cardiac lesions
- Myocardial ischemia
- Chest pain and palpitations
- Cyanosis
- Distress

FOLLOW-UP

■ Patients with psychogenic or idiopathic chest pain should be followed up at regular intervals.

PROGNOSIS

■ Prognosis depends on the cause of the chest pain.

Chickenpox

DEFINITION

- Chickenpox (varicella) is a childhood viral disease characterized by a pruritic vesicular rash that appears in crops.
  - "Chicken" is believed by some to derive from a likeness to the chickpea *Cicer arietinum*, or from the French for chickpea, *pois chiche*.
  - Others postulate that the name may come from the Old English word for itch, *gican*.
- It is highly contagious and has been regarded as relatively benign, inasmuch as complications are rare in healthy children.

EPIDEMIOLOGY

- Incidence
  - Until 1995 (before the vaccine era), ~4 million chickenpox cases occurred yearly in the US
  - By 2000
    - Incidence decreased overall by 71–84% in populations with varicella immunization coverage rates for 1- to 3-year-olds of 74–84%.
    - Incidence decreased in every age group, with the greatest decrease (83–90%) seen in the 1-to 4-year-old group.
    - Incidence continued to be highest in children age 1–4 years and those age 5–9 years.
  - By 2001
    - The rate of varicella-related hospitalizations in the US had declined by 75% overall, with <3800 such hospitalizations.
    - A reduction was seen in all age groups but was greatest for young children.
    - Deaths in the US caused by varicella dropped by 66% overall to an all-time low of 26.
    - The drop in mortality rates was most pronounced in children age 1 to 4 years (92%) and those age 5 to 9 years (89%) but was evident in all age groups, except for persons >50 years.
  - Epidemics occur every 2–3 years and are distributed worldwide.
- Prevalence
  - Historically, 80–90% of children are infected by 9–10 years of age.
  - In tropical climates, 40–90% of children enter adulthood without contracting the disease.
    - Much larger pool of susceptible persons in older age groups
- Seasonality
  - Occurs throughout the year, with most cases during the winter and spring months
- Historic case-fatality rates from chickenpox (pre-vaccine era)
  - 5 per 100,000 infants
  - 1 per 100,000 1- to 14-year-olds
  - 3 per 100,000 15- to 19-year-olds
  - 25 per 100,000 30- to 49-year-olds
  - Higher rates in neonates, immunocompromised patients, and older adults
  - 10,000 hospitalizations annually, predominantly in children
  - Annual deaths ranged from 40–150.
    - Most (80%) occurred in children in the early 1970s.
    - The majority (54%) occurred in adults in the early 1990s.
  - From 1990–1994, an average of 50 annual pediatric deaths were attributed to varicella.
    - >90% of deaths occurred in children with no risk factors for severe varicella.

ETIOLOGY

- Caused by the varicella-zoster virus, a DNA virus and member of the herpesvirus family
  - The virus causes both chickenpox and herpes zoster.
  - Herpes zoster is a reactivation (after a latent phase) of the initial varicella infection.
- One of the most contagious viral infections to cause disease in humans (only known natural host).
  - Slightly less contagious than measles and smallpox
- Varicella virus
  - Gains entry into the susceptible individual through respiratory tract or conjunctiva via droplet or airborne transmission
  - Migrates to regional lymph nodes, where primary replication occurs
  - Primary viremia spreads the virus to internal organs approximately 4–6 days later, where secondary replication occurs.
  - Secondary viremia spreads the organism to the skin and is followed by clinical chickenpox.
    - Viremia has been documented in blood-borne monocytes 9–12 days after exposure, 1–5 days before onset of the rash.
    - Appearance of the rash in crops may be the result of intermittent secondary viremia.

RISK FACTORS

- Exposure to varicella-zoster virus
- Infection is thought to be spread by:
  - Respiratory secretions
    - Airborne particles from patients can transmit infection before onset of rash.
  - Contact with the vesicular fluid of chickenpox or herpes zoster
  - Indirect contact (fomite transmission)
    - Rare because of the lability of the varicella-zoster virus

- Transmission from pregnant woman to her fetus or newborn
  - Transplacentally acquired antibody to varicella-zoster virus is partially protective.
  - Chickenpox can occur in young infants born to immune mothers.
- Communicability period
  - From 1 or 2 days before the onset of the rash until 5 days after the onset or until all vesicles have crusted
  - Most vesicles have lost virus particles after 5 days.
  - Incubation period is between 10 and 21 days and averages 14–15 days.
- With household exposure, clinical disease will develop in approximately 90% of susceptible contacts after 1 incubation period.
  - Secondary household cases are often more severe.

SIGNS AND SYMPTOMS

Young children

- Mild malaise
- Low-grade fever (varies from none to 102°F [38.9°C])
  - May continue until vesicles cease to appear
- Fever followed in a few hours to days by a macular rash
  - Usually begins on the scalp, neck, or upper portion of the trunk
- Macules progress to a papular, vesicular, pruritic rash (usually within 12–24 hours).
  - Rash spreads centrifugally and involves all areas of the skin in severe cases.
  - Lesions occur more frequently in areas of irritation or dermatitis or in skin folds.
  - Occasionally appears as a macular rash in the diaper area or on the trunk and remains for 1 or 2 days before becoming vesicular.
  - Papular lesion contains a minute vacuole.
  - Fluid accumulates in the vacuole.
    - Causes vesicle to appear on a reddened base
    - Produces the classic "dewdrop on a rose petal" lesion
- Vesicles appear in crops.
  - A new crop occurs every 1–2 days over the next 2–5 days.
  - 2–4 crops during the illness
  - Typically produces a total of 250–500 lesions
- Vesicles turn to pustules and then crust over.
  - Crusts develop and may remain attached for 1–2 weeks.
  - Vesicles are pruritic, and excoriations are common.
  - Vesicles may occur on the mucous membranes.
    - Mouth
    - Conjunctiva
    - Esophagus
    - Trachea
    - Rectum
    - Vagina
  - On mucous membranes, the roof of the vesicle sloughs to leave a shallow ulcer.
- Total length of illness: 5–10 days

In older children and adults

- Irritability
- Listlessness
- Headache
- Chills
- Anorexia
- Myalgia
- Fever
  - Usually present
  - Higher and more prolonged than in young children
- More severe rash than in young children

In immunized children

- Milder systemic symptoms
- Lesions
  - Fewer (usually <50)
  - Less pruritic
  - Crust over faster
- Lesions may appear only as papules that never vesiculate.
- Children with typical, mild breakthrough varicella are also approximately half as likely to transmit the disease to household contacts.

DIFFERENTIAL DIAGNOSIS

- Smallpox (variola)
  - Historically the most important disease to be differentiated from chickenpox
  - Has again become a concern because of its possible use in bioterrorism
  - Clinical smallpox prodrome is typically more severe than that of chickenpox.
  - In varicella lesions, all stages of evolution are present at once.
  - In smallpox, most of the lesions are present in a uniform stage of development.
    - Lesions progress together from macules to papules to deep-seated vesicles and crusting.
    - Involvement of palms and soles is much more typical of smallpox.

- Vaccinia (cowpox)
  - Produces a vesicular rash resulting from exposure to infected livestock
  - When smallpox vaccine use was commonplace, resulted from direct contact with a smallpox vaccination
- Disseminated herpes simplex
  - History and progression of the diseases usually differentiate these 2 entities.
  - Confusion ordinarily arises only in newborns.
    - Disseminated herpes is rare in normal children.
  - Tzanck test will be positive in both diseases, but direct fluorescent antibody testing, culture, and polymerase chain reaction are specific.
- Rickettsialpox
  - Vesicles are deeper and are at a uniform stage of development.
  - Prodrome is more severe.
- Other viruses (especially coxsackievirus and echovirus)
  - Can produce vesicular exanthema that usually do not crust
  - Course is distinctly different.
  - Tzanck test is negative in these infections.
- Stevens-Johnson syndrome
  - Clinical course is different.
  - Rashes develop differently.
  - Tzanck test will be negative.
- Contact dermatitis
  - May produce a rash similar to that of chickenpox (including pruritus)
  - Different distribution and evolution
- Insect bites and scabies
  - May cause confusion if they are vesicular
- Bullous impetigo (especially staphylococcal skin infection)
  - May produce bullae that resemble chickenpox

DIAGNOSTIC APPROACH

- Chickenpox is usually diagnosed clinically.
  - History of exposure in the previous 10–21 days

LABORATORY FINDINGS

- Leukocyte counts and other laboratory test results are usually normal in uncomplicated varicella.
- Tzanck test (scraping of the base of a vesicle and staining with Giemsa or Wright stain)
  - Positive for multinucleated giant cells in varicella-zoster virus infections.
  - Herpes simplex types 1 and 2 also produce a positive Tzanck test.

- Varicella-zoster virus–specific direct fluorescent antibody testing of vesicle scrapings
  - Can provide specific diagnostic confirmation within hours
- Vesicle fluid can also be cultured for varicella-zoster virus.
  - Growth may take weeks.
- Polymerase chain reaction
  - Superior to viral culture in identification of varicella virus from vesicles
  - Can distinguish eruptions due to wild-type and vaccine virus
- Viral titers during acute and convalescent stages
  - Can document a recent infection if obtained early in the illness (preferably day 1 or 2)
  - Higher titers are noted during convalescence 2–6 weeks later.
- Commercially available antibody tests
  - Perform well for detection of serologic responses to infection
  - Not as sensitive for detecting vaccine-induced antibody response

TREATMENT APPROACH

- In most cases, treatment focuses on:
  - Control of fever
  - Relief of prodromal symptoms
  - Measures to control pruritus

SPECIFIC TREATMENTS

Fever and prodromal symptoms

- Acetaminophen
- Ibuprofen may increase risk of necrotizing fasciitis and other secondary bacterial infections.
  - This association has not been firmly established.
- Aspirin
  - Should be avoided in any child with chickenpox because of its association with Reye syndrome

Pruritus

- Oral antihistamine (eg, diphenhydramine)
  - Uncommon but reported encephalopathic side effects of diphenhydramine may mimic neurologic complications of varicella.
- Calamine lotion
- Cetaphil lotion
- 0.25% menthol lotion
- Baking soda or oatmeal preparations (Aveeno) in a warm bath to relieve discomfort
  - Daily baths also help prevent bacterial superinfection.

- Children's nails should be kept clean and trimmed to help discourage scratching.
  - Gloves or socks on the hands may be required.

Superinfection

- Usually a result of group A streptococci or *Staphylococcus aureus*
- Superinfection of a few lesions can be treated topically with mupirocin ointment.
- Superinfection of many lesions or of lesions in difficult areas (eg, around nares or the mouth) can be treated systemically.
  - First-generation cephalosporin (eg, cephalexin, cefadroxil) or other antibiotics that are active against streptococci and staphylococci
  - Where clindamycin-susceptible, methicillin-resistant *S aureus* is endemic, clindamycin may be an appropriate choice.

Antiviral agents

- Acyclovir
  - Effective in treating varicella infections in healthy children and adolescents
  - Not routinely recommended in healthy preadolescent children
  - Recommended (by intravenous route) for treatment of immunocompromised children who develop varicella infection
  - Increasingly, children infected with HIV, particularly those who have higher CD4 percentages, have been treated successfully for primary varicella with oral acyclovir.
  - When instituted within 24 hours of the onset of rash, treatment has resulted in modest reductions in:
    - Duration of illness
    - Number of cutaneous lesions
    - Fever
    - Systemic symptoms
  - Should be considered in adolescents because they are at greater risk for more severe disease
  - Can be considered for other nonimmunocompromised children who are at increased risk of more severe varicella, including:
    - Chronic lung disease
    - Chronic skin disorders
    - Those on salicylate therapy
    - Those taking aerosolized or low-dose systemic corticosteroids
    - Secondary household cases
  - In 1 study, treatment of the index case with acyclovir did not change the transmission rate to other susceptible household contacts.

- Valacyclovir and famciclovir
  - Licensed for treatment of zoster in adults
  - No studies and no pediatric formulations exist on which to base recommendations for use in children.

Hospitalization

- Should be avoided whenever possible because hospital epidemics can occur even when the strictest isolation procedures are followed
- Generally, disease is spread by:
  - Infection of staff members who were thought to be immune
  - Airborne spread of the virus through ventilation systems
- When unavoidable, hospitalization requires strict isolation.
- Hospitalization on an adult ward that has no immunosuppressed patients may reduce chance of spread where effective strict isolation is not available.
- All health care workers should have immunity to varicella verified at the time of hire.

WHEN TO ADMIT

- Varicella pneumonia
- Moderately to severely immunosuppressed host
- Moderate to severe bacterial complications
- Chickenpox in neonates
- Encephalopathy

WHEN TO REFER

- Immunodeficient children
- Pregnant women

COMPLICATIONS

Secondary bacterial infection

- Most common complication of chickenpox
- Children <5 years appear to be at increased risk.
- Symptoms begin, on average, 4 days after appearance of the varicella rash, often with a secondary fever.
- Superficial bacterial skin infections remain most common, but invasive group A streptococcal infections have become increasingly important.
- Infections are usually caused by group A streptococci or *S aureus* and include:
  - Impetigo
  - Cellulitis
  - Abscess
  - Necrotizing fasciitis
  - Myositis
  - Gangrene
  - Arthritis

- Osteomyelitis
- Pneumonia
- Empyema
- Conjunctivitis
- Toxic shock syndrome (usually streptococcal)
- Sepsis
- Erysipelas

■ Occasionally, lesions are bullous as a variant of the disease itself, but these are more often caused by staphylococcal superinfection.

- Can lead to complications in neonates, immunocompromised children, older adults
- Bullous lesions caused by *S aureus* may begin on the second or third day of the rash and show as bullous impetigo.

Neurologic complications

■ Second most common complication of varicella

■ Mortality from neurologic complications reached approximately 10% overall.

■ Most deaths occurred among cases of encephalitis, some of which may have represented unrecognized Reye syndrome.

■ Acute cerebellar ataxia (ACA)

- Most common neurologic complication
- Occurs in 1 in 4000 cases of chickenpox
- The average age is 4 years; the great majority of cases is seen in those <5 years.
- Onset of symptoms usually occurs 1–2 weeks after onset of varicella, from 2–21 days after the appearance of the rash.
  - May precede the rash (rare)
- Clinical features of varicella-related ACA are:
  - Acute onset of vomiting
  - Ataxic gait disturbance without major disturbance in mental status
  - Dysmetria (68%)
  - Trunk ataxia (74%)
  - Fever (5–10%)
  - Nystagmus (5–10%)
- Laboratory studies usually reveal:
  - Normal peripheral leukocyte count
  - Normal to mildly elevated cerebrospinal fluid protein level
  - Cerebrospinal fluid pleocytosis in 50%
- Between 95% and 100% of normal children who have varicella-related ACA recover completely with only supportive care.
  - Many cases are mild enough that hospitalization is not necessary.
  - Recovery usually takes place within the first 3 months.

- Some concern exists for longer-lasting subtle behavioral and learning difficulties.
- These need further study with controlled comparisons.

■ Encephalitis

■ Seizures

- Many may be febrile seizures.
  - In 1 series, 12 of 23 patients who had varicella and seizures had concomitant fever.
  - In older series

■ Aseptic meningitis

■ Myelitis

■ Peripheral neuropathy

Immunocompromised children

■ Usually have the most severe symptoms

- Higher fever and more prolonged vesicular eruption

■ Neonates are at greatest risk of death from chickenpox.

■ All complications are increased in this population.

- Varicella pneumonia is the most common cause of death.

■ Progressive varicella

- Seen in immunocompromised children or those being treated with immunosuppressive therapy
- Develops in up to 30% of immunocompromised children
- Varicella-zoster virus spreads to the:
  - Lungs
  - Liver
  - Pancreas
  - Central nervous system
- Vesicles may be larger and hemorrhagic.

■ Children with HIV (especially those with very low CD4 percentages)

- Most do not develop severe acute varicella.
- Many experts use high-dose oral acyclovir to manage selected children infected with HIV and who have relatively normal CD4 values.
- Others manage all children with HIV as being at increased risk of severe disease.

■ Children who receive systemic steroid therapy for diseases other than cancer

- Children who receive >2 mg/kg or 20 mg prednisone (or equivalent) for >2 weeks should be considered at increased risk for more severe involvement and complications.
  - Possibly attributable to the potentially immunocompromising effect of non-oncologic conditions for which steroids are prescribed
- Inhaled corticosteroids do not appear to increase risk, but definitive data are lacking.

Congenital and neonatal varicella

- In primary maternal varicella during the first 2 trimesters of pregnancy
  - Varicella-zoster virus can cross the placenta.
  - Leads to congenital varicella syndrome in 2%
  - Affected infants have:
    - Skin lesions in a dermatomal distribution (76%)
    - Neurologic defects (60%)
    - Eye diseases (51%)
    - Skeletal anomalies (49%)
- Maternal infection during the late third trimester of pregnancy
  - May result in transplacentally acquired varicella in the newborn
  - Neonatal varicella is seen in 24% of infants of mothers with chickenpox in the 2 weeks before delivery.
  - Risk of death seems to be small if:
    - Onset of maternal rash occurs >5 days before delivery.
    - Rash initiates in infants <4 days.
    - This reprieve is probably attributable to maternally transferred immunity.
  - 20–30% neonatal mortality occurs if:
    - Maternal rash emerges between 4 days before and 2 days after delivery,
    - Newborn rash begins at 5–10 days of age
- Risk is uncertain for infants who are nursing when the mother contracts chickenpox.
- Herpes zoster in pregnant women appears to confer minimal risk of infection to the fetus.
  - In 1 series of 366 women with herpes zoster in pregnancy, no infants had evidence of intrauterine infection.

Reye syndrome

- Acute illness occurring almost exclusively in children, characterized by encephalopathy and fatty degeneration of the liver
- Case-fatality rate is 30% overall.
  - Reaches 43% for children <5 years
- In 1980, the association between Reye syndrome and use of aspirin during varicella or influenza illnesses was first reported.
  - This report led to:
    - 1980—advisory from the Centers for Disease Control and Prevention (CDC)
    - 1982—Surgeon General advisory
    - 1986—mandatory warning labels of all aspirin-containing medications, cautioning physicians and parents to avoid using salicylates in children with varicella or influenza-like illnesses

- The annual number of reported cases of Reye syndrome in the US has decreased.
  - 555 cases in 1980
  - No more than 36 cases per year from 1987–1993
  - No more than 2 cases per year from 1994–1997
- Given its rare occurrence, any child suspected of Reye syndrome should be evaluated thoroughly for the presence of another metabolic disorder.
- Aspirin should be avoided in any child who has chickenpox.

Varicella pneumonia

- Occurs most often among adults, adolescents, and immunocompromised children
  - In children, occurs in <1 per 10,000 cases of chickenpox
  - In adults, it may be present in 30–50% of cases of varicella.
    - More recent studies estimate 5–10%
- One of the more common causes of death from varicella
  - Mortality is 10–20%, higher among severely immunodeficient patients.
- Onset typically occurs:
  - 5–6 days after onset of rash in immunodeficient persons
  - Within the first 3 days of rash onset in immunocompetent hosts (adults)
- Manifestations include:
  - Abnormal chest radiograph findings
  - Cough
  - Rales
  - Tachypnea
  - Hemoptysis
  - Chest pain
  - Cyanosis
  - Respiratory failure
- Chest radiographs typically show diffuse, reticulonodular densities of various sizes, best viewed in the lung periphery.
  - As disease progresses, nodules may enlarge and coalesce into extensive infiltrates.
- Treatment with intravenous acyclovir is recommended.

Hematologic complications

- Thrombocytopenia
  - Most common hematologic abnormality seen with varicella
  - May occur with:
    - Invasive secondary bacterial infection
    - Sepsis, where it is associated with more severe illness and worse outcome

- In the absence of secondary bacterial infections, varicella may produce thrombocytopenia (or pancytopenia) that is attributed to:
  - Infection-related suppression
  - Antibody-mediated destruction (idiopathic thrombocytopenic purpura) of platelets
  - Onset occurs from 3 days to 3 weeks after the chickenpox rash appears.
- The following have been described with varicella infection:
  - Febrile purpura
  - Malignant chickenpox with purpura
  - Postinfectious purpura
  - Purpura fulminans
  - Henoch-Schönlein purpura

Hepatitis

- Hepatitis may appear on second to fourth day after rash appears; marked by:
  - Onset of abdominal pain
  - Vomiting
  - Continued fever
- Liver function tests become abnormal but return to normal with resolution of abdominal symptoms.
- No progression to classic Reye syndrome
- Blood ammonia level is normal.
  - Some experts believe that some of these cases may represent low-grade Reye syndrome.
  - A study of 39 children who had uncomplicated chickenpox found:
    - 47% had a mildly increased level of aspartate aminotransferase (serum glutamic-oxaloacetic transaminase).
    - 29% had significantly increased aspartate aminotransferase levels.

Zoster (shingles)

- Reactivation of varicella-zoster virus that has remained dormant after clinical chickenpox
  - Virus resides in the dorsal nerve ganglia.
  - Virus is reactivated by periods of decreased host immunity or other unknown stimuli.
  - During reactivation, rash covers the dermatome corresponding to infected nerve root.
  - Disseminated zoster can occur, involving multiple dermatomes.
- Has been described in all age groups, including in infancy after prenatal exposure to varicella from maternal chickenpox
- Young children, especially those <1 year of age, have increased incidence of zoster later in life.

- Immunocompromised children are at greater risk.
  - 27% of children infected with HIV with primary varicella after 1 year of age; zoster an average of 2 years later
  - Significantly fewer children with leukemia (25 cases per 1000 person-years)
  - 70% of children whose CD4 percentage was <15% at the time of varicella infection

Other complications

- Appendicitis
- Myocarditis
- Arthritis (viral)
- Nephritis
- Orchitis
- Splenic hemorrhage and rupture
- Pancreatitis
- Pericarditis
- Parotitis (rare)
- Papillary conjunctivitis (most common ophthalmologic complication)
- Keratitis
- Uveitis
- Optic neuritis
- Chorioretinitis

PROGNOSIS

- Complications are rare in healthy children.
- Little scarring occurs unless the lesions become superinfected or are continually traumatized.
- Areas where chickenpox lesions have occurred may remain hypo- or hyperpigmented months after rash has resolved.

PREVENTION

Varicella vaccine

- A live-attenuated varicella virus vaccine licensed by the US Food and Drug Administration in 1995 is effective in preventing varicella infection in most recipients.
- Recommended doses
  - Susceptible immunocompetent children ≥1 year should receive 2 doses: one at 12 months and one at 4–6 years.
  - Susceptible adolescents ≥13 years should receive 2 doses of the vaccine at least 1 month apart.
  - *Susceptible* is defined as a lack of reliable history of chickenpox.
  - A positive serologic result excludes the need for vaccination.
    - Routine serologic confirmation of susceptibility in adolescents is not likely to be cost effective.

- Effectiveness
  - Studies have suggested vaccine effectiveness as follows:
    - 44–88% complete prevention of chickenpox
    - 86–90% prevention of moderate or severe chickenpox
  - Risk factors for breakthrough disease included:
    - Immunization at <15 months of age
    - Longer elapsed time since immunization
    - Oral steroid use
    - Receipt of measles-mumps-rubella vaccine <28 days before varicella vaccine
  - Limited data (from Japan) demonstrate persistence of humoral and cell-mediated immunity following vaccination for up to 20 years.
  - The contribution of boosting by continued circulation of wild-type varicella to maintaining immunity is unknown.
- Adverse events
  - Mild (2–5 lesions on average) maculopapular or varicelliform rash at the injection site or other sites in the month following vaccination
    - Seen in 7–8% of vaccinated healthy children
    - When tested by polymerase chain reaction, the majority of rashes occurring within 2 weeks of varicella immunization are determined to be from natural infection.
  - Modified chickenpox (shorter duration, fewer lesions, less fever) occurs at a rate of approximately 2–3% per year among vaccinees.
    - Associated with low 6-week postvaccination varicella zoster virus antibody titers
  - Other, more serious but much less common adverse events occur at lower frequencies than would be expected following natural infection.
    - Encephalitis
    - Ataxia
    - Erythema multiforme
    - Pneumonia
    - Thrombocytopenia
    - Seizures
    - Herpes zoster
- Precautions
  - Transmission of vaccine virus to susceptible contacts is extremely rare and has occurred only in the presence of a vaccine-associated rash.
  - Vaccinees who develop a rash should avoid direct contact.
  - Immune globulin or other blood products (except washed red blood cells) may interfere with the immune response to varicella vaccination.
    - Vaccine should be deferred for 3–11 months after receipt of blood products, depending on the dose and type of blood product use.
  - Salicylates should not be given for 6 weeks following vaccination; there is a theoretical risk of Reye syndrome.
  - Measles-mumps-rubella vaccine and varicella vaccine should not be given <28 days apart; it may be given simultaneously, eg, as MMR-V, without reducing efficacy.
- Contraindications
  - Because the varicella vaccine is an attenuated-live virus vaccine, it is not generally recommended for use in pregnant women or in immunocompromised children, including those with:
    - Congenital immunodeficiencies
    - Severely symptomatic HIV infection
    - HIV infection with CD4 percentages <15%
    - Blood dyscrasias
    - Leukemia
    - Lymphoma
    - Immunosuppressive therapy for cancer
    - High-dose steroid therapy (equivalent of prednisone 2 mg/kg/day or 20 mg/day)
- Special considerations
  - Children with leukemia
    - For children whose leukemia is in remission and with a break in chemotherapy before and after vaccination, the 2-dose varicella vaccine was safe, immunogenic, and completely effective in clinical trials.
    - 50% developed a mild rash in the month following vaccination.
    - They were less likely to develop zoster than were comparable leukemic children who had natural varicella infection.
    - Not currently licensed or routinely recommended for susceptible children who have leukemia, but children may be eligible to receive the vaccine through a research protocol.
  - Children with HIV
    - Varicella vaccine should be considered for children who have asymptomatic (CDC class N) or mildly symptomatic (CDC class A) HIV infection and whose CD4 percentages are ≥25%.
    - Eligible children infected with HIV should receive 2 doses of varicella vaccine ≥3 months apart.
    - The Advisory Committee on Immunization Practices has made provisional recommendations to broaden the group of eligible HIV-infected children who should receive the 2-dose varicella vaccine series to include:
      - Symptomatic involvement ranging from asymptomatic to moderately symptomatic (class N, A, or B) and
      - CD4 percentages ≥15%

■ Varicella vaccine after exposure

- Nonpregnant, healthy adults and children ≥1 year of age (without contraindication to the vaccine)
  - May be vaccinated within 3 days and perhaps up to 5 days after exposure
- Recommended for vaccine-eligible patients who received VariZIG, intravenous immunoglobulin, oracyclovir prophylaxis unless varicella disease has occurred
- To minimize potential interference with vaccine response by passive antibody from these products, delay vaccine by:
  - 5 months after VariZIG
  - 8 months after 400-mg/kg intravenous immunoglobulin

MMR-V vaccination

■ In 2005, varicella vaccine with the measles-mumps-rubella vaccine as a combination product (MMR-V) was licensed for use based on its safety and immunogenicity in children.

■ In 2007, the Provisional Advisory Committee on Immunization Practices recommended a routine second dose of varicella vaccine for all children to help reduce breakthrough disease.

- The second dose to be routinely given between 4 and 6 years of age
  - Single injection of MMR-V at 12–15 months
  - Repeated at 4–6 years for optimal protection against all 4 viral exanthema
- The second varicella vaccine dose can be given as soon as 3 months after the initial dose.
- The dose does not need to be repeated if 2 doses are given at least 28 days apart.

Public health

■ Easiest prevention strategy in institutions, such as hospitals, schools, or child care facilities

- Isolation or exclusion of the child who has chickenpox
  - Not always effective because the disease is contagious 1–2 days before the appearance of the rash
  - Generally, isolation is not feasible for preventing household contamination.

Immunoglobulin

■ Varicella-zoster immunoglobulin (VZIG)

■ Until recently, the most common and recommended method of postexposure prophylaxis for susceptible, high-risk patients

■ When administered within 72–96 hours of a known or anticipated exposure, can prevent or modify disease in children and adults

■ Despite VZIG prophylaxis, varicella may occur up to 28 days after exposure.

■ Because widespread vaccine use has reduced the need for VZIG, the manufacturer halted production in 2005.

■ VariZIG (investigational)

- A purified human immune globulin preparation with high antivaricella antibody titers (similar to VZIG)
- Recommended in place of VZIG
- Can be obtained through an expanded access protocol

■ IVIg

- Recommended dose: 400 mg/kg intravenously
- If VariZIG cannot be obtained, IVIg is the best alternative for:
  - Exposed neonates
  - Immunocompromised patients
  - Susceptible pregnant women
  - Other susceptible patients

■ Postexposure prophylaxis with VariZIG or IVIg

- Recommended for susceptible individuals at high risk of severe varicella, including:
  - Children who are infected with HIV
  - Other immunocompromised children
  - Pregnant women
  - Newborn infants whose mothers develop varicella eruption from 5 days before until 2 days after delivery.
  - Hospitalized premature infants >28 weeks' gestation whose mothers are susceptible (these infants have been deprived of active transport of maternal antibody that takes place in the final trimester)
  - Hospitalized premature infants <28 weeks or <1000 g, regardless of maternal susceptibility
- May be repeated following reexposure to varicella >3 weeks after initial dose (if varicella has not developed)
- May be considered for susceptible adolescents and adults because these age groups are at higher risk of severe disease compared with younger children
  - Alternative preventive strategies (immunization oracyclovir) may be more appropriate for this group.

Acyclovir

■ Acyclovir

- 10-day course at a dose of 40–80 mg/kg/day (divided into 4–5 doses) up to adult dose of 800 mg 5 times daily, beginning 10 days after exposure
- Can be used to prevent or attenuate chickenpox in high-risk outpatients beyond the newborn period
- This use is not approved by the US Food and Drug Administration.
  - Use is based on small studies.
  - Potential effect on the immune response has not been fully evaluated.

Chronic Fatigue Syndrome

DEFINITION

- Chronic fatigue syndrome (CFS) describes an illness characterized by prolonged periods of debilitating fatigue for which no definitive cause is known.
- Although the Centers for Disease Control and Prevention has created a working definition of CFS, it is not a well-defined clinical entity.

EPIDEMIOLOGY

- Prevalence
  - 20–200 cases of CFS-like illness per 100,000 persons
  - Cases of CFS have been reported to occur both sporadically and epidemically.
- Age
  - The majority of reported cases are in persons 35–40 years of age.
  - Adolescents with CFS have been described.
- Sex
  - Predominantly seen in females
- Race
  - White women from upper socioeconomic groups are most commonly affected.
  - Minorities, the indigent, and people living in developing countries are strikingly underrepresented.
    - Whether this reflects a bias in patient selection or predisposing factors remains to be determined.

ETIOLOGY

- No specific causative agents or characteristic pathophysiologic models have been identified.
- Causative factors under consideration for CFS are likely to interact in differing degrees in each individual.
  - Infectious agents
  - Other medical and immunologic conditions
  - Psychological factors

RISK FACTORS

- Depression
  - Both a risk factor and a reaction to CFS
- Additional adolescent-specific risk factors include:
  - School performance anxiety
  - Overprotection and overindulgence associated with difficulty in mother-teen separation
    - Infection or other stressor serves as a model for persistent symptoms that may become a mechanism to maintain overprotective environment or avoid school.
- Other possible risk factors
  - Low blood pressure (postural orthostatic tachycardia syndrome [POTS])
  - Hormonal factors (eg, depressed cortisol responses)

SIGNS AND SYMPTOMS

- Primary manifestation is severe fatigue.
  - >6 months in duration
  - Limits individual to activity <50% of the premorbid level
- Associated symptoms
  - Sore throat
  - Low-grade fever (oral temperatures of 37.5°C to 38.6°C)
  - Painful lymph nodes
  - Unexplained generalized weakness, myalgias, or arthralgias (or both)
  - Prolonged fatigue after exercise
  - Headache
  - Difficulty concentrating or memory loss
  - Sleep disturbances (hypersomnia or insomnia)
- Onset
  - Most patients describe sudden onset with an initial mononucleosis- or influenza-like illness.
  - Many describe a history of atopy, multiple allergies, or both.
- History
  - Question the patient about the nature and duration of symptoms.
  - Identify possible exposures to ill persons that might suggest an alternative diagnosis.
  - Obtain personal and social history.
    - Family dynamics
    - Prior level of functioning
    - Response to illness
    - Family history of psychiatric illness
    - Psychological or marital problems
      - Common psychological issues include internalizing symptoms and feeling different from others.
- Physical examination, with a goal of eliminating other causes of the patient's symptoms
  - Mild inflammation of the pharynx
  - Cervical or axillary lymphadenopathy
  - Low-grade temperature elevation in up to 50% of cases

DIFFERENTIAL DIAGNOSIS

- The following should suggest an alternative diagnosis.
  - Enlarged lymph nodes (>2 cm)
  - Weight loss >10% of body mass index without dieting
  - Focal neurologic abnormalities
- Differential diagnoses
  - Cancer
  - Autoimmune disease
  - Localized infection (eg, sinusitis, occult abscess)

- Chronic or subacute infection (eg, Lyme disease, endocarditis, tuberculosis, mononucleosis)
- HIV infection
- Fungal disease (eg, candidiasis, histoplasmosis, coccidioidomycosis, blastomycosis)
- Parasitic disease(eg, toxoplasmosis, giardiasis)
- Chronic inflammatory disease (eg, sarcoidosis, Wegener granulomatosis)
- Endocrine disease (eg, hypothyroidism, Addison disease, diabetes, hypoglycemia)
- Neuromuscular disease (eg, myasthenia gravis, multiple sclerosis)
- Drug dependency
- Side effects of chronic medications or other toxic agents (eg, chemical solvent, heavy metal, pesticide)
- Psychiatric disorder
- Total allergy syndrome
- Other poorly defined CFS-like conditions
  - Neurasthenia, myalgic encephalomyelitis, postviral syndrome, fibromyalgia

DIAGNOSTIC APPROACH

- Focus on excluding all other diagnoses and making an extensive differential diagnosis.
  - Physical examination
  - Laboratory tests
  - Chest and sinus radiographs
  - Cardiologic evaluation may be useful in patients with dizziness.

LABORATORY FINDINGS

- No specific laboratory tests exist that can be used to diagnose CFS.
- Primary aim of laboratory evaluations is to eliminate other conditions.
- Suggested battery of screening tests
  - Complete blood count and differential
    - Erythrocyte sedimentation rate
    - Serum electrolytes
    - Creatinine
    - Blood urea nitrogen
    - Glucose
  - Liver enzyme and function tests
  - Thyroid function tests
  - Tuberculin skin test with controls

- Alkaline phosphatase
- Antinuclear antibodies
- Rheumatoid factor
- HIV antibody
- Additional tests (eg, Lyme disease test, viral serologies) may be indicated based on history and physical examination.
- Immunologic testing is generally not warranted.
  - Abnormalities are rare and opportunistic infections do not occur in CFS.

IMAGING

- Chest and sinus radiography
  - Used to eliminate other causes of symptoms
- Magnetic resonance imaging
  - In some patients with CFS, increased white matter on T2-weighted scans suggestive of:
    - Possible infiltration of the perivascular spaces
    - Focal demyelination
    - Disease of the small blood vessels of the cerebral white matter
  - The significance of these finding is uncertain.

DIAGNOSTIC PROCEDURES

- Head-upright or tilt-table testing
  - Used to assess the role of POTS
  - Appropriate for the subset of patients in whom dizziness is a significant symptom

TREATMENT APPROACH

- A coordinated approach minimizes doctor shopping, unnecessary testing, and unconventional therapies.
  - Provide counseling and symptomatic relief for depression, sleep disorders, and musculoskeletal pains.
  - Offer emotional support with involvement of a social worker, psychologist, or psychiatrist as needed.
  - Identify and eliminate secondary gain from continuing to contribute to the illness.
  - Devise programs with the patient to increase school (or work) attendance and exercise capability gradually.
- No specific therapy for CFS has been proven to be effective.

SPECIFIC TREATMENTS

- Confirm the diagnosis of CFS and acknowledge the symptoms as real.
- Explain and explore the potential relationship to psychological symptoms.
  - Use team approach and coordinate services.

- Stress-coping skills
  - Modify lifestyle.
  - Develop a realistic schedule.
    - Work with school on gradual return to classes, home tutoring, and neuropsychometric testing.
  - Develop a graduated exercise program.
- Cognitive-behavioral approaches
  - Pay attention to sleep patterns and nutrition.
  - Increase activity gradually.
- Psychological support
  - Individual therapy and family therapy
  - Decrease secondary gain
- Symptom-based management
  - In documented POTS, dietary (eg, increased salt intake) or pharmacologic management (or both) may be beneficial.
    - Medications, such as fludrocortisone, propranolol, or midodrine
    - Therapy for neurally mediated hypotension has been only of partial benefit, even in adolescents whose tilt-table tests are abnormal.
  - Immunoglobulin injections have been reported to be beneficial in a study of patients with CFS.
    - Subsequent studies failed to confirm this observation.

WHEN TO REFER

- To resolve issues relating to possibility of ongoing infection or inflammation
- Multiple specialists may become involved and multiple laboratory tests may be ordered.
  - Symptoms are often extensive and varied.
  - Coordinate a team approach to avoid redundant or unnecessary testing.

- To provide a higher level of supportive care or counseling than can be provided in the office setting
  - Especially if the individual is cannot attend school or participate in normal activities

FOLLOW-UP

- Periodic physical examinations
  - Monitor for other possible conditions.
  - Monitor physical symptoms and psychological issues.
- Provide ongoing guidance and continued reassurance.
- Be aware of untested fad therapies that the patient may investigate.
  - Megavitamin treatment
  - Immune modifiers (eg, Ampligen, thymic extract, interleukin-2)
  - Magnesium sulfate
  - Liver extract injections
  - Anti-*Candida* diets
  - Colonic irrigation
  - Removal of dental fillings

PROGNOSIS

- Most patients report improvement or resolution of symptoms over 2–3 years.
- Few patients report progressive symptoms, although symptoms may wax and wane.
- With better definition of the nature of CFS, additional therapeutic approaches may become available.

Cleft Lip and Cleft Palate

DEFINITION

- Clefts of the lip and/or palate
  - May occur in isolation or may have several associated anomalies representing a syndrome
- Clefts are divided into 4 groups by an early classification system.
  - Soft palate clefts alone
  - Clefts of both the hard and soft palate
  - Complete unilateral clefts of the lip and palate
  - Complete bilateral clefts of the lip and palate
- Complete cleft of the primary palate with a degree of skin bridging the superior aspect of the lip is termed a *Simonart band.*
- Pierre Robin sequence consists of micrognathia, glossoptosis, and upper airway obstruction, with or without cleft palate, or any combination.

EPIDEMIOLOGY

- Prevalence
  - Cleft lip with or without cleft palate occurs in ~1 in 700 new births.
  - Isolated cleft palate occurs in ~1 in 1000 new births.
- Race/ethnicity
  - Patients of Asian descent: 2.1 in 1000
  - Black patients: 0.41 in 1000
  - White patients: 1.3 in 1000
- Sex
  - Cleft lip and palate are more common in boys than girls (2:1).
  - Isolated cleft palate occurs twice as often in girls than boys.
- Location
  - Clefts are more common on the left side.
  - Unilateral cleft lips occur much more commonly than bilateral cleft lips (4:1).
  - Frequency of orofacial clefting between cleft lip to cleft palate and cleft lip and palate is 1:1.2:2.5.

ETIOLOGY

- Cleft is caused by failure of penetration or fusion of the mesenchymal masses of the 5 facial prominences.
  - Isolated failure of fusion of the medial nasal prominence with the maxillary prominence on 1 side results in a unilateral cleft lip.
  - Bilateral cleft lip results from failure of both medial nasal prominences to fuse with the maxillary prominence.
  - Palatal clefts result from incomplete fusion of the lateral palatine processes with the nasal septum.
- Clefting may be associated with other conditions meeting the criteria of a syndrome; >300 syndromes are associated with clefting.

- Most common syndromes
  - Van der Woude syndrome
  - Velocardiofacial syndrome
  - Pierre Robin sequence
  - Goldenhar syndrome
  - Treacher Collins syndrome
  - Down syndrome
  - Stickler syndrome
- Most clefts are nonsyndromic and multifactorial in nature or a result of changes at a major single-gene locus.
  - Candidate genes
    - TGF alpha and beta
    - *MSX-1*
    - Retinoic acid receptor alpha
    - Homeobox gene
    - Distal-less homeobox 2
    - B-cell leukemia or lymphoma 3

RISK FACTORS

- Environmental agent exposure
  - Agents found to increase rate of clefting during first trimester of pregnancy
    - Corticosteroids
    - Ethanol
    - Ionizing radiation
    - Phenytoin
    - Isotretinoin
    - Diazepam
    - Methotrexate
  - Exposures to caffeine and tobacco are theorized to increase risk.
- Infections in first trimester of pregnancy, including rubella and toxoplasmosis
- Family risk for cleft lip/cleft palate
  - No family history of cleft lip or cleft palate: 0.1%/0.04%
  - Unaffected parents with 1 previously affected child: 4%/2%
  - Unaffected parents with 2 previously affected children: 9%/1%
  - 1 affected parent: 4%/6%
  - 1 affected parent and 1 previously affected child: 17%/15%

IMAGING

- Diagnosis of cleft lip or palate can be reliably established by prenatal ultrasonography.
  - Transvaginal ultrasonography can detect a cleft lip by 13–16 weeks of gestation.
  - Clefts of secondary palate can be diagnosed at 19 weeks of gestation using real-time magnetic resonance imaging.

TREATMENT APPROACH

- Treatment by age
  - Repair in utero: no current safety and ethical standards
  - Newborn: Establish airway stability and feeding optimization.
  - First 3–4 months of age:
    - Audiologic evaluation
    - Ear-nose-throat evaluation for middle ear abnormalities
    - Possible orthodontic evaluation for use of presurgical orthopedics
  - 3–4 months of age: surgical management with lip repair
  - Around 1 year of age: palate repair
  - 2–4 years of age: speech evaluation and therapy, with or without possible surgical management of velopharyngeal insufficiency
  - Late childhood and teen years, on as-needed basis:
    - Alveolar bone grafting
    - Lip and nose revisions
    - Orthodontics
    - Orthognathic surgery
- Care is usually coordinated through multidisciplinary team following guidelines of the American Cleft Palate-Craniofacial Association.
  - Plastic surgeon
  - Speech therapist
  - Audiologist
  - Otolaryngologist
  - Oral surgeon
  - Dentist, orthodontist
  - Nurse
  - Social worker or psychologist
- Nutritional care
  - A nurse is usually the feeding expert who monitors the nutritional status of the infant carefully to ensure adequate caloric intake.
  - Other feeding specialists may include:
    - Occupational therapists
    - Lactation consultants
    - Speech therapists
  - Neonates with cleft of the primary palate (lip and alveolar ridge) can usually feed using a regular bottle or breastfeed without significant difficulty.
  - Infants with a cleft of the secondary palate (hard and soft palate) usually require special bottles.
    - Haberman feeder (Medela)
    - Pigeon nurser (Respironics)
    - Mead Johnson nurser
    - Infant may have to be fed with a syringe (Breck feeder) or nasogastric tube.
  - Infants with cleft of the secondary palate are unlikely to be able to breastfeed.
    - If the mother wishes to attempt breastfeeding, a lactation consultant with experience in cleft feeding should be consulted.
    - Infants should be monitored closely by a primary care physician, cleft-team nurse, and surgeon, with frequent weight checks.
    - Receiving human milk is desirable, even if by bottle; a hospital-grade breast pump (Medela) can be provided.
  - Many centers fit infants with cleft of the secondary palate with a feeding plate that is custom fabricated by a dentist or orthodontist.
    - Decreases nasal regurgitation and irritation
- Evaluation/treatment for middle ear disease
  - Common (90%) with secondary palate cleft; results in limited drainage of middle ear through the eustachian tube and potentially causing conductive hearing loss (50%)
  - Patients are monitored closely for middle ear effusion and hearing impairment.
  - Almost universally treated with myringotomy tubes to prevent chronic hearing loss and cholesteatoma
    - Tubes are generally placed at around 3 months of age.
- Presurgical orthopedics to align the alveolar segments and facilitate the lip repair
  - Passive (nasoalveolar molding appliance)
    - Many centers use a standard in which the cleft of the lip is narrowed, the cleft nostril is elevated into a more normal configuration, and the alveolar ridges become aligned.
    - Active (Latham appliance)
    - Performed by a pediatric dentist or orthodontist who monitors the child weekly, progressively modifying the appliance from birth to the time of lip repair as the child grows

SPECIFIC TREATMENTS

Primary lip repair

- Usually performed between 3 and 4 months of age
- Timing of lip repair, 10-10-10 rule:
  - 10 weeks of age
  - 10 g of hemoglobin
  - Weight of 10 lb
- Surgical techniques include:
  - Rotation advancement repair (Millard)
  - Triangular flap repair (Tennison-Randall; less common)

- Additional primary cleft rhinoplasty at the time of the lip repair results in enhanced nasal aesthetic outcomes.
- The alveolus may also be repaired at time of the lip repair (gingivoperiosteoplasty), providing the framework/potential for ossification of the cleft alveolar arch.
- Lip adhesion in the first few weeks of life, before formal lip repair, molds the alveolar ridges, especially when used with a dental plate, in preparation for lip repair several weeks later.

Cleft palate repair (palatoplasty)

- Usually performed between 9 and 12 months of age (although protocols vary widely).
- Repair around 1 year of age is desirable to maximize normal speech development; however, repairing too early might result in poor maxillary growth.
- 2 most common procedures
  - Furlow double-opposing Z-plasty
  - Intravelar veloplasty technique of levator muscle reorientation
- Flaps used to repair the hard palate include the von Langenbeck and Veau-Wardill-Kilner techniques.
- Subperiosteal release of the floor of the mouth
- Tracheostomy for the most severe cases

Pierre Robin sequence

- Infants with a small mandible and upper airway obstruction:
  - Should be placed in the prone position to allow the tongue to fall forward out of the pharynx
  - Should be kept on a pulse oximeter to assess oxygen saturation level in the blood
  - If this is not adequate to alleviate obstruction/maintain saturations >94%:
    - A nasal trumpet may be placed (12 or 14 French).
    - If necessary, the infant may be bag ventilated with a jaw thrust, nasal trumpet, or oral airway in place and endotracheal or nasotracheal intubation carried out in a controlled environment by medical staff.
    - If necessary, the tongue may be pulled forward with a piece of gauze between the fingers or, rarely, a towel clamp.
- Further workup
  - 3-dimensional craniofacial computed tomography to evaluate the size of the mandible and the position of the tongue in the pharynx and to rule out choanal atresia and other anomalies
  - Nasoendoscopy to evaluate the position of the tongue in the pharynx with spontaneous respirations
  - Direct laryngobronchoscopy to rule out other airway anomalies (laryngomalacia or tracheomalacia)
  - Evauation for gastroesophageal reflux disease and treatment as necessary

- Polysomnography, if the child is stable enough
- Feeding assessment: Children may have to be fed via nasogastric tube or syringe until more definitive treatment is carried out.
- Indications for surgical intervention
  - Continued upper airway obstruction/oxygen desaturation such that the baby cannot be taken out of the prone position
  - Need for nasal trumpet or intubation
  - Abnormal apnea-hypopnea index on sleep study
  - Inability to be fed with a bottle
  - Failure to thrive
- Surgery
  - Mandibular distraction osteogenesis
    - Involves lengthening the mandible using internal or external devices
    - The mandible is distracted 1.0–1.5 mm/day until in a normal or overcorrected position and airway obstruction/feeding difficulties are alleviated.
    - Regenerated bone consolidates in 6–8 weeks, and distractors are removed.
    - Complications
      - Device failure
      - Possible tooth bud damage
      - Possible inferior alveolar nerve paresis
      - Poor scar formation
    - Future mandible growth is unknown at this time.
  - Tongue-lip adhesion
    - Suturing a flap of muscle and mucosa from undersurface of the tongue to a similar flap on the inner surface of the lower lip
    - Complications include dehiscence, inability to feed with a bottle, and failure to alleviate upper airway obstruction.
    - Reversed at 9–12 months of age to allow normal oral-motor coordination for speech and swallowing, once the mandible has grown sufficiently so that the tongue base no longer obstructs the airway
    - Cleft palate is repaired during tongue-lip adhesion reversal operation as well.

WHEN TO ADMIT

- Poor weight gain and dehydration in an infant who has feeding difficulty due to cleft palate

WHEN TO REFER

- Prenatally
  - Refer to plastic surgery, otolaryngology, genetics, and nursing specialists to provide appropriate council for what is to be expected postnatally.

- From birth until 3–4 months of age
  - Audiologic evaluation
  - Ear-nose-throat evaluation for middle ear disease
  - Possible orthodontic evaluation for the use of presurgical orthopedics
  - Surgical management follows with lip and nose repair
- 1 year of age
  - Palate repair
- 3–6 years of age
  - Speech evaluation and therapy with or without possible surgical management of velopharyngeal insufficiency
- Late childhood and teen years
  - Alveolar bone grafting as needed
  - Lip and nose revisions as needed
  - Orthodontics and orthognathic surgery as needed

FOLLOW-UP

- A child with a cleft should be followed up closely from before birth through adulthood by a multidisciplinary team.
  - Evaluate annually and until the management plan is completed in the child's late teens/early twenties.
  - The goal is to achieve normal function, characterized by:
    - Normal occlusion
    - Normal speech and hearing
    - Growth that is as normal as possible and optimal form, characterized by normal lip, nose, and facial aesthetics
- Speech
  - Even after palatoplasty, some children will have velopharyngeal insufficiency or incompetence (cleft palate speech), due to either:
    - Muscular incoordination (as is frequently the case in velocardiofacial syndrome)
    - Short palate
  - Speech should be assessed by a speech therapist in children 18–24 months of age to establish a diagnosis of velopharyngeal insufficiency.
    - Velopharyngeal insufficiency is often treated with speech therapy with or without surgical management.
    - The most common surgical techniques include a pharyngeal flap or sphincter pharyngoplasty, when the patient is 3–6 years of age.
    - These partly obturate the oronasopharynx, resulting in decreased air escape through the nose and thus necessitating careful monitoring of the airway.

- Lip and nose revisions
  - Before starting school (4–5 years): intermediate revisions
  - When growth is completed (14 years for girls, 16 years for boys)
    - A final septorhinoplasty or lip revision, or both
    - Reconstruction of deviated nasal septum and asymmetric nasal bones or lip (or both)
- Orthodontics/cleft alveolus management
  - May be started as early as 4 years and continued through the teen years
  - Teeth adjacent to the cleft site may be missing, misshapen, or misaligned; teeth may need to be passively molded or extracted.
  - If no gingivoperiosteoplasty was performed or gingivoperiosteoplasty failed, orthodontics are performed before secondary alveolar bone grafting.
    - Involves harvest of cancellous bone from the iliac crest, grafted into the alveolar cleft site
      - Allows complete ossification of the alveolar arch
      - Allows eruption of the canine tooth
    - Some surgeons advocate primary bone grafting in infancy (using a small piece of rib), although most perform alveolar bone graft as needed, between 7 and 9 years (mixed dentition period).
- Orthognatic (jaw) surgery
  - Sometimes needed to align the jaws in a normal occlusal relationship
  - Maxillary advancement (LeFort I osteotomy)
    - School-aged children, by distraction osteogenesis
    - Teenagers, advancement osteotomy with rigid titanium plate fixation
    - In some cases the mandible is set back to meet the maxilla.
  - Factors considered in timing orthognathic surgery
    - Upper airway obstruction
    - Sleep apnea
    - Malocclusion
    - Articulation errors
    - Masticatory problems caused by malocclusion
    - Psychosocial effects of facial disharmony
  - Final prosthodontic care, including dental implants or bridges, may be needed for missing or malformed teeth around the cleft site in the late teenage years.

PROGNOSIS

- Successful treatments result in a well-adjusted child with normal facial appearance, dental occlusion, speech, and hearing.

Colic

DEFINITION

- Inconsolable crying that:
  - Occurs for >3 hours per day **and**
  - Occurs >3 days per week **and**
  - Lasts >3 weeks

EPIDEMIOLOGY

- Prevalence
  - Colic is extremely common, affecting 20% of babies.

ETIOLOGY

- The exact cause of colic is unknown.
- Various causative theories have been suggested, including:
  - Food allergy
  - Gastrointestinal tract immaturity
  - Parental stress
  - Infant temperament

RISK FACTORS

- Parental stress or anxiety may lead to, or aggravate, colic.
- Family history of colic in a sibling.

SIGNS AND SYMPTOMS

- Colic presents as bouts of crying, fussing, or irritability that may develop into agonized screaming.
- The infant may draw up his/her knees against the abdomen, as if in pain.
- Symptoms follow the typical crying curve.
  - Crying bouts begin in the second week.
  - Crying peaks at 6 weeks.
  - Usually resolves by 4 months of age
  - Crying bouts are more common in the evening hours.
- It has been suggested that colic represents the upper end of the continuum of normal crying.
- Babies seem inconsolable during these crying periods.
  - Feeding, diaper changes, and soothing techniques are not effective in halting the crying.

DIFFERENTIAL DIAGNOSIS

- Crying in the newborn can be a sign of any number of disease processes; thus, they must be excluded before colic can be diagnosed.
- Gastroesophageal reflux disease
  - Presents with episodes of fussiness
  - Often accompanied by emesis which occurs soon after feeding
- Milk protein intolerance
  - Crying accompanied by diarrhea or hematochezia

- If the mother used alcohol or other drugs during pregnancy, the infant may be excessively fussy.
- All of the following typically present with persistent, rather than paroxysmal, symptoms.
  - Corneal abrasion
  - Hair tourniquet
  - Acute abdominal processes that constitute medical emergencies and symptoms including anorexia or vomiting
    - Volvulus
    - Intussusception
    - Incarcerated hernia
  - Infectious processes, usually accompanied by fever
    - Otitis media
    - Urinary tract infection
    - Meningitis
  - Inflicted injuries
    - Fractures
    - Intracranial bleeding

DIAGNOSTIC APPROACH

- A complete history is essential.
  - Parents may state that the baby is fussy and has excessive gas.
  - They may be concerned that the infant is in pain.
  - Ask:
    - When did symptoms begin?
    - How often do they occur?
    - During what part of the day do the symptoms occur?
    - How long do the symptoms last?
    - What have you done to try to ameliorate the symptoms?
    - What interventions, if any, are effective?
  - Obtain a history of the pregnancy.
    - Determine whether there was any maternal alcohol or drug use.
    - Determine whether there were any infections during pregnancy.
  - Family history
    - Metabolic or allergic disorders
    - Sibling with colic
  - Social history
    - Assess parental anxiety regarding real or perceived health concerns.
    - Ask who in the family is responsible for caregiving.
    - Ask what types of supports for caregiving are available to the family.

- Review of systems
  - Inquire about organic signs and symptoms of irritability, including:
    - Fever
    - Lethargy
    - Vomiting
    - Diarrhea
    - Hematochezia
  - Review feeding techniques and history.
    - For formula-fed infants
      - Ensure that formula is being prepared correctly.
      - Assess whether the baby is being overfed or underfed.
    - For breastfed infants
      - Assess the mother's supply of milk.
      - Review how often and for how long the baby is fed.
- Physical examination
  - Generally serves to exclude pathologic abnormalities
  - In most cases, physical examination will be normal.
  - Acute abdominal processes, otitis media, and hair tourniquet can all be excluded by physical examination.
  - Determine weight, length, and head circumference and plot on a growth chart.
    - Poor growth suggests inadequate nutrition or other organic causes for crying.
    - Increasing head circumference suggests hydrocephalus or abuse.

LABORATORY FINDINGS

- Laboratory testing is seldom indicated.
  - Should be reserved for cases in which an organic cause is suspected
- Unnecessary laboratory testing should be avoided because it may convey to the parents the message that the baby is ill.

TREATMENT APPROACH

- Management primarily involves parental education and support.
  - Teach the parents that the baby is not sick.
  - Excessive crying is not harmful.
    - Use the baby's normal growth and results from the physical examination to reinforce this.
  - Reassure parents about their abilities as caregivers.
  - Emphasize that they are not to blame for the baby's symptoms.
- Acknowledge the parents' frustration.
  - Inform them that the office will provide support.

SPECIFIC TREATMENTS

- Teach parents to respond to the baby's fussiness with a predictable set of responses.
  - Having a plan to use during fussy periods can be reassuring.
- First, make sure the baby is not hungry, soiled, or tired.
  - Soothe the baby by encouraging:
    - Nonnutritive sucking
    - Swaddling
    - Gentle rocking or swinging
- It is acceptable to allow the infant to cry for a short period.
  - Allows the parents to regroup
  - Provides the baby with some time to blow off steam
- Educate parents about infant crying.
  - Most parents are surprised to learn how much healthy babies cry.
  - Highlight the differences among healthy babies.
    - Some babies are just naturally fussier.
  - The mnemonic PURPLE, from the Period of PURPLE Crying program (aimed at preventing shaken baby syndrome), can be used to remind parents of the pattern of normal, healthy infant crying that can cause stress and frustration in caregivers.
    - **P**: peak pattern
    - **U**: unexpected timing of episodes
    - **R**: resistance to soothing
    - **P**: pain-like face, even though baby is not in pain
    - **L**: long bouts of crying
    - **E**: evening cluster of symptoms
- Parents should be encouraged to:
  - Take care of themselves
  - Get adequate rest
  - Enlist family members or friends to take over from time to time to reduce caregiver stress
- Few medical interventions are helpful for colic.
  - If indicated by history, changing to hypoallergenic formula may be considered.
  - For breastfeeding mothers, consider an elimination diet.
  - If symptoms suggest reflux, treat for gastroesophageal reflux disease.
- Pharmacologic therapies have been found to be unhelpful, and possibly harmful.
  - Simethicone is not effective in symptom reduction.
  - Dicyclomine, an anticholinergic, is effective.
    - The manufacturer has advised against its use in children <6 months of age.

- Herbal tea made of chamomile, vervain, licorice, fennel, and balm-mint has been shown to be effective.
  - Large volume of fluid, 120 mL/3 times a day
  - May cause potential harm, such as hyponatremia or decreased milk intake

WHEN TO ADMIT

- In the vast majority of cases, colic can be successfully managed in the outpatient setting.
- If the history is confusing or suggests more serious symptoms, admission for observation may be necessary.

WHEN TO REFER

- Referral to specialists in developmental or behavioral medicine may be useful if the parents are extremely anxious or in need of additional reassurance.
- Be alert to parents who are overwhelmed by the infant's crying and may be in danger of harming the infant.
  - In this case, referral to children's services may be necessary.

FOLLOW-UP

- Support the parents until they are comfortable managing their child's symptoms.
- Very anxious parents may be offered a return office visit in 1 week.

- Provide support through telephone contact a few days after the initial visit.
- Excessive crying may be a stimulus for shaken baby syndrome.
  - Provide support and education to the parents, and carefully assess the baby at follow-up visits.

PROGNOSIS

- Prognosis is generally good.
- Symptoms usually decrease dramatically by 4 months of age.
- The presence of colic in an infant does not necessarily predict a more difficult temperament in an older baby.
- Excessive parental anxiety and frustration may lead to later parent-child interaction problems, such as:
  - Prolonged night waking
  - Overfeeding
  - Vulnerable child syndrome

Common Cold

DEFINITION

- Colds are viral infections of the upper respiratory tract.
- Mucosal surfaces that are lined with respiratory epithelium are involved.
  - Potentially affected areas include:
    - Nasal passages
    - Sinuses
    - Eustachian tubes
    - Middle ear spaces
    - Conjunctivae
    - Nasopharynx

EPIDEMIOLOGY

- Distribution
  - Worldwide
- Incidence
  - More frequent during cooler months in temperate climates
  - Northern hemisphere
    - Peaks in early fall
    - Remains high during winter
    - Decreases in spring
- Age
  - Adults and children
  - Most common in preschool-age children, who experience 6–8 colds per year (4 times adult rate)
  - Frequent infection in the preschool years might decrease the frequency of colds in the school years.
- Race or ethnicity
  - All ethnic groups

ETIOLOGY

- >100 different infectious agents can cause cold symptoms.
  - Most frequent cause
    - Rhinoviruses and small RNA viruses of the picornavirus family (autumn)
  - Frequent cause
    - Coronavirus (winter)
  - Less frequent causes
    - Influenza virus (winter)
    - Respiratory syncytial virus (winter)
    - Parainfluenza virus (winter)
  - Occasional causes
    - Enterovirus (all seasons)
    - *Mycoplasma pneumoniae* (all seasons)
    - Metapneumovirus (autumn and winter)

- Exposure to a cold environment:
  - Does not cause a cold
  - Does not decrease immunity that may potentially allow a viral infection to begin
- Infection begins most commonly after self-inoculation of a virus onto the individual's own nasal or conjunctival mucosa.

RISK FACTORS

- Exposure to nasal secretions
  - Virus easily spread by way of fingers and hands to objects, such as clothing or environmental surfaces
    - Children then acquire and self-inoculate their respiratory tracts by picking their noses or rubbing their eyes.
  - Inhalation of virus-containing aerosols
    - An effective means of virus acquisition
- Chronic stress
  - Colds are more likely in chronically stressed adults after inoculation by rhinovirus.
    - Whether this is the case in children is unknown.
- Crowds
  - Colds occur more commonly in children who:
    - Attend child care centers
    - Are exposed to other school-aged children versus those who spend most of their time at home

SIGNS AND SYMPTOMS

- Infants
  - Fever
  - Irritability
  - Changes in feeding pattern
  - Changes in sleep patterns
  - Mild diarrhea occasionally
  - Respiratory syncytial virus and parainfluenza viruses
    - Croupy cough
    - Bronchiolitis
- Children
  - Usually afebrile
  - Stuffy nose
  - Watery nasal discharge
    - Becomes more purulent within 3–4 days
  - Sneezing after a few days
  - Dry cough by third or fourth day
  - Rhinovirus infection
    - Generalized symptoms are uncommon.

- Adenoviral and other viral infections
  - Headache
  - Malaise
  - Myalgia
  - Pharyngitis
  - Gastrointestinal symptoms
- Duration of symptoms
  - Generally ~1 week
    - However, mild rhinorrhea and dry cough may persist for 2–3 weeks.
    - Cilia necessary for proper function of the respiratory epithelium may take as long as 3 weeks to return to their normal state.
  - When the symptoms are prolonged, a secondary infection may be present if:
    - Fever persists or is prominent.
    - Ear pain or a productive cough develops.
- Ear and lung examinations are essential for a child whose cold has persisted longer than expected.

DIFFERENTIAL DIAGNOSIS

- Allergy
  - Similar symptoms may be caused by seasonal allergy or allergy associated with nasal eosinophilia.
- Non–cold-causing viruses
  - Cold symptoms are associated with significant:
    - Pharyngitis
    - Rash
    - Other systemic symptoms
  - Streptococcal pharyngitis
    - Not usually associated with rhinorrhea or cough
- ß-Hemolytic streptococcal infection
  - Occasionally causes persistent purulent nasal discharge in children <2 years
  - Usually associated with mild excoriations around the nares
- Nasal foreign body
  - Unilateral nasal discharge must be evaluated carefully to exclude nasal foreign body.
- Drug use
  - Older children with persistent symptoms
  - Irritation and swelling of the nasal passages from inhalation of:
    - Cocaine
    - Medicated nasal sprays

- *Bordetella pertussis* infection
  - Should be considered in a child with persistent cough
  - Children who have been partially immunized may not have the characteristic whoop.
- Concurrent bacterial infection
  - If a cold causes the usual symptoms for 5–7 days:
    - Concurrent bacterial infection is unlikely.
  - Purulence used to be interpreted as indicating a bacterial infection (eg, sinusitis).
    - Little evidence is available to support this impression.

DIAGNOSTIC APPROACH

- Diagnosis is based on clinical grounds.
- No routine tests exist to diagnose the common cold.

LABORATORY FINDINGS

- Viral cultures
  - Expensive and generally unnecessary

IMAGING

- Routine use of imaging is unnecessary.
  - Radiologic finding of opacification of the sinuses has not correlated with the clinical indications of sinusitis in adults.
- Chest radiograph
  - Confirms diagnosis of pneumonia as a complication of a protracted cold

TREATMENT APPROACH

- Most remedies give marginal, if any, symptomatic relief.
  - In many cases, they are potentially quite harmful.
  - Acetaminophen or ibuprofen can be used to treat fever in older children.
  - Oral decongestants may be used in older children.
- Infants should receive nothing more than saline nose drops.

SPECIFIC TREATMENTS

Infants

- Most pediatricians advise against using any cold remedies for infants.
  - At most:
    - Saline nose drops and bulb syringe to aspirate secretions
    - Cool-mist vaporizer to humidify room air

Children

- Acetaminophen or ibuprofen for malaise and fever
  - Some studies suggest that ibuprofen may lead to:
    - Shorter period of viral shedding
    - Better neutralizing antibody response

- Aspirin should be avoided; it is associated with Reye syndrome.
- Decongestants or antihistamines
  - Preschoolers
    - Studies have not demonstrated a beneficial effect singly or in combination.
  - Older children and adolescents
    - May use an oral decongestant (eg, pseudoephedrine hydrochloride) alone or with an antihistamine
    - Provides symptomatic relief with low possibility of side effects
  - Nasal spray or drops containing vasoconstrictors, such as oxymetazoline hydrochloride
    - Use should be discouraged.
    - High incidence of rebound nasal congestion after only a few days of use.
  - Corticosteroid or atropine-like nasal sprays
    - Have not been evaluated in children
- Mast-cell stabilizers (eg, nedocromil, sodium cromoglycate)
  - Their place in pediatric care is not clear.
- Zinc lozenges
  - Efficacy to reduce the duration of cold remains controversial.
- Antirhinoviral drugs
  - Studies are still too preliminary to judge their therapeutic potential.
- Vitamin C supplementation
  - Has not been proven efficacious; should be discouraged
- Antibiotics
  - Many parents will request that the physician prescribe antibiotics.
  - Discouraging antibiotic use is particularly important when bacterial infection is unlikely.
    - Evidence indicates increasing drug resistance among some bacterial pathogens.
- Alternative therapies
  - *Echinacea*
    - A recent randomized clinical trial showed no benefit to the use of extract of *Echinacea purpura* in treating children 2–11 years of age at the onset of their colds.
  - *Echinacea angustifolia*
    - A randomized clinical trial in adults using *E angustifolia* extract showed no benefit in treating experimental rhinovirus infection.

WHEN TO ADMIT

- Patients who develop pneumonia secondary to bacterial infection may need to be hospitalized if home therapy is ineffective or inappropriate.

COMPLICATIONS

- Otitis media
  - Most common in younger children
  - May be acute
  - Common cold can cause eustachian tube dysfunction.
- Pneumonia
- Secondary bacterial sinusitis
  - Uncommon and overdiagnosed
    - Fever
    - Headache
    - Purulent nasal discharge
- Lower respiratory tract infection (rare)
  - May progress topneumonia
    - Cough
    - Tachypnea
    - Fever (usually)
  - Origin may be viral or a secondary bacterial infection.
- Reactive airway disease
  - Role of rhinovirus infection as a trigger of exacerbation is well documented.
  - Wheezing or a prolonged cough after a cold should alert the clinician to this possibility.

PREVENTION

- Frequent hand washing with soap and water by the patients and their caregivers may prevent the spread of infection.

Complementary and Alternative Medicine

BACKGROUND

- Interest in complementary and alternative medicine (CAM) has redefined modern Western medicine.
  - Widely used by the public and increasingly available at conventional hospitals:
    - Acupuncture
    - Biofeedback
    - Guided imagery
    - Hypnotherapy
    - Herbs
    - Dietary supplements
    - Massage
    - Chiropractic
  - Formal definitions of health care quality now acknowledge the importance of respecting:
    - Spirituality
    - Culturally based healing traditions
- CAM includes all of the following that are not considered part of conventional medicine as practiced in the US
  - Health care systems
  - Therapies
  - Products
  - These can be used:
    - To supplement conventional care (complementary)
    - In place of conventional care (alternative)
- *Integrative medicine* is the preferred term.
  - Incorporates both conventional medicine and complementary and alternative therapies for which sufficient evidence of safety and efficacy exists
- Consortium of Academic Health Centers for Integrative Medicine
  - Consists of 36 prominent medical schools
  - Further defines integrative medicine as "the practice of medicine that reaffirms the importance of the relationship between practitioner and patient, focuses on the whole person, is informed by evidence, and makes use of all appropriate therapeutic approaches, health care professionals and disciplines to achieve optimal health and healing."

GOALS

- New competencies in pediatric care are necessary because of:
  - Tremendous growth in demand for CAM
  - Parental use of the Internet and mass media for health information
- Pediatricians should be able to:
  - Inquire regarding CAM use
  - Counsel on CAM from an evidence-based perspective
  - Partner with and refer appropriately to CAM practitioners

- Pediatricians do not need to:
  - Be content experts on CAM
  - Reject their training in biomedicine or critical thinking
- CAM emphasizes the:
  - Centrality of the therapeutic relationship
  - Importance of prevention
  - Healing power of nature

GENERAL APPROACH

- Strengthen the physician-patient relationship with:
  - Honest dialogue
  - Nonjudgmental manner
  - Compassion
  - Attention
- Use the best of scientifically based medical therapies whenever appropriate.
- Use appropriate complementary and alternative approaches when they enhance conventional medicine.

SPECIFIC INTERVENTIONS

Mind-body medicine

- Includes all therapies that activate the following factors, which can have significant mediating effects (positive and negative) on health outcomes
  - Emotional
  - Mental
  - Social
  - Spiritual
  - Behavioral
- Therapies include:
  - Relaxation
  - Stress management
  - Yoga
  - Hypnosis
  - Guided imagery
  - Biofeedback
  - Spirituality/prayer
    - The most prevalent complementary therapies in the US
    - May or may not involve formal religion
    - Frequently important in medical decisions
    - Closely linked to successful coping, faster recovery, and higher quality of life
    - Many patients may want help with meaning, hope, or overcoming fears.
    - Unmet spiritual needs are associated with despair and increased mortality.
    - Parents often have significant spiritual needs around the life-threatening illness or death of a child.

- Meditation
- Music therapy
  - Increases oxygen saturation and weight gain, decreases salivary cortisol and distress behaviors in premature infants
  - Intraoperative and postoperative music reduces pain and pharmaceutical requirements in surgical patients, including the use of sedatives and analgesics.
  - Reduces pain and suffering, improves mood and attitude in pediatric oncology patients
  - Reduces patient anxiety and depression in intensive care units
  - Improves the quality of life in dying patients
- Support groups
- Psychological therapies
  - Cognitive-behavioral therapy
- Mind-body therapies are recognized as safe and effective for many pediatric conditions, including:
  - Headaches
  - Asthma
  - Enuresis
  - Sleep problems
  - Pain
  - Stress
- Nonphysician providers of mind-body therapies
  - Psychologists
  - Nurses
  - Social workers
  - Chaplains
  - Music therapists

Biologically based therapies

- Includes all therapies that use natural products to modulate physiologic function
  - Herbs
  - Vitamins
  - Other supplements
- Dietary supplements can be sold without premarket approval and do not require a specific postmarketing study.
  - Only functional foods can claim specific health benefits.
    - Such approvals require significant supporting clinical data and US Food and Drug Administration approval.
- Commonly used herbal therapies and their uses
  - Aloe (*Aloe vera*)
    - Burns
    - Minor wounds
    - Skin irritations
    - Aphthous stomatitis

- Constipation
- Gastric and duodenal ulcers
- Astragalus (*Astragalus* species)
  - Immune booster
- Calendula (*Calendula officinalis*)
  - Skin soother
- Cascara (*Rhamnus purshiana*)
  - Constipation
- Cayenne (*Capsicum frutescens*)
  - Pain (topical)
  - Postherpetic neuralgia (topical)
  - Migraine (nasal spray)
  - Cluster headache (nasal spray)
- Chamomile (*Matricaria recutita*)
  - Sedative
  - Colic
  - Antiinflammatory
  - Antispasmodic
- Clove oil (*Syzygium aromaticum*)
  - Teething pain
- Coffee (*Coffea* species)
  - Stimulant
  - Attention-deficit/hyperactivity disorder
  - Bronchodilator
- Dandelion (*Taraxacum officinale*)
  - Mild diuretic
  - Liver tonic
- Dill (*Anethum graveolens*)
  - Antispasmodic
  - Colic
  - Flatulence
- Echinacea (*Echinacea* species)
  - Immune stimulation
  - Antiinflammatory
- Ephedra (ma huang) (*Ephedra* species)
  - Vasoconstriction
  - Allergy
  - Upper respiratory infection
  - Asthma
  - Appetite suppressant
- Evening primrose oil (*Oenothera biennis*)
  - Eczema
  - Premenstrual syndrome
- Feverfew (*Tanacetum parthenium*)

- Migraine
- Rheumatoid arthritis
- Garlic (*Allium sativum*)
  - Antimicrobial
  - Cholesterol lowering
- Ginger (*Zingiber officinale*)
  - Antiemetic
  - Antinausea
- Ginkgo (*Ginkgo biloba*)
  - Enhances blood flow past clogged arteries
  - Prevents memory loss
  - Attention-deficit/hyperactivity disorder
- Ginseng (*Panax* species)
  - Stimulant
  - Adaptogen
  - Enhances endurance and performance
- Hawthorn (*Crataegus oxycantha*)
  - Cardiac stimulant; enhances cardiac contractility
- Hops (*Humulus lupulus*)
  - Sedative
- Kava kava (*Piper methysticum*)
  - Anxiolytic
- Lavender (*Lavendula* species)
  - Sedative
- Licorice (*Glycyrrhiza* species)
  - Antiinflammatory
  - Antiviral
  - Demulcent
- Milk thistle (*Silybum marianum*)
  - Hepatoprotection against cirrhosis, hepatitis
- Oats (*Avena sativa*)
  - Antipruritic
  - Eczema
  - Varicella
- Pine bark extract (*Pinus* species)
  - Antioxidant
  - Attention-deficit/hyperactivity disorder
- Rhubarb root (*Rheum officinale*)
  - Constipation
  - Chronic renal failure
- St John's wort (*Hypericum perforatum*)
  - Depression
  - Antiviral

- Skullcap (*Scutellaria* species)
  - Sedative
- Slippery elm bark (*Ulmus fulva*)
  - Demulcent
  - Pharyngitis
- Tea tree oil (*Melaleuca alternifolia*)
  - Topical antimicrobial
  - Acne
  - Minor skin infections, eg, fungal and yeast infections
- Thyme (*Thymus vulgaris*)
  - Antimicrobial
  - Expectorant
  - Colds
  - Sore throat
  - Cough
- Valerian (*Valeriana officinalis*)
  - Sedative
- Witch hazel (*Hamamelis virginiana*)
  - Topical antiseptic
  - Antiinflammatory
- Licensed practitioners who promote use of herbal medicine:
  - Naturopaths
    - Not all naturopaths are graduates of accredited naturopathic medical schools.
    - International Board Certified Lactation Consultants frequently prescribe herbs to nursing mothers, eg, galactagogues to stimulate milk production.
  - Chiropractors

Manipulative and body-based methods

- Includes all therapies that focus on:
  - Manipulation
  - Compression
  - Stretching of skin, muscles, joints
  - Touch
- Activates a variety of mechanisms that support and promote health, including:
  - Mechanical
    - Enhances blood flow to the muscles and soft tissues and enhances lymphatic flow
  - Immunologic
    - Enhances specific immune cell functions, such as natural killer cell activity
  - Neurologic
    - Triggers relaxation response
    - Lowers sympathetic nervous system arousal, reduces serum cortisol

- Enhances endogenous serotonin and dopamine levels
  - Modulates pain perception
- Energetic
  - Provides balance
  - Improves the flow of life force energy (*chi*)

■ Chiropractic
  - Chiropractors are licensed in all 50 US states.
  - Their services are widely covered by insurance, including Medicaid.
  - Most chiropractic schools now offer courses in pediatric care.
  - In children, chiropractors tend to use:
    - Few radiographs
    - Lighter force when making adjustments
    - A device called an *activator* to make adjustments
    - Special pediatric tables or treat the children in their parents' laps

■ Osteopathy
  - Osteopaths are licensed in all 50 US states.
  - Their services are widely covered by insurance, including Medicaid.
  - Doctors of osteopathy are considered mainstream physician practitioners.
  - Graduates of osteopathic medical schools can enter pediatric residency programs.

■ Massage
  - One of the oldest health care practices
  - Among the most popular options selected by pediatric and adolescent patients
  - Can include many different techniques and forms that require more substantial training
    - Structural integration (Rolfing)
    - Movement integration (Feldenkrais technique, Alexander technique)
    - Pressure point techniques (shiatsu, acupressure)
    - Craniosacral therapy
    - Reflexology
  - May be enhanced through the use of clinical aromatherapy
    - Therapeutic application of essential oils distilled from plants
    - Topical oils that enhance blood flow and engender a sense of warmth are often added (eg, lemongrass, black pepper oil).
    - Specific scents can have application to specific symptoms, such as lavender or chamomile for relaxation, ginger or spearmint for nausea, and peppermint or lemon for fatigue.

- The appropriate amount of massage has not yet been measured.
- Therapy is provided most often by parents or other family members.
  - Family members frequently appreciate the chance to learn a skill that can contribute to the comfort and well-being of the patient.
- Massage therapists are licensed in all 50 US states.
  - Training and licensure requirements vary.
  - The largest professional national organization is the American Massage Therapy Association.

Alternative medical systems

■ Based on comprehensive theories and healing traditions found outside conventional Western biomedicine
  - Restoration of the body and mind through:
    - Lifestyle
    - Diet
    - Exercise
    - Herbal medicines
    - Spiritual practices

■ Ayurveda
  - From the Indian subcontinent

■ Acupuncture
  - One component of traditional Asian medicine systems
    - Vital energy, chi (qi), is thought to circulate through the body in channels called *meridians*.
    - When the circulation of chi is blocked or disrupted, disease is present.
    - When the flow is balanced, harmonized, and restored, the patient returns to health.
    - Acupuncture—insertion of needles into key points on known meridians—is one means of restoring flow of chi.
  - Among major teaching hospitals with a pediatric pain service, 33% offer acupuncture therapy to treat chronic pain.
    - Therapy can be taught to and performed by parents and children for home treatments.
    - Care must be taken to present it in a nonthreatening light.
    - Use of the term *acupoint stimulation* avoids eliciting fear of needles.
  - Acupoint stimulation can be achieved by:
    - Massage
    - Comfortable electrical stimulation
    - Stickers with beads
    - Very thin (>30 gauge) nonhollow acupuncture needles

- After comfort and trust is established with a noninvasive approach, many children and teens will agree to needle insertion.
  - Performed correctly, acupoint stimulation is virtually painless and well tolerated by older children.
  - Immediate benefits are rarely seen.
  - Acupuncturists often ask patients to commit to 4 to 6 visits before deciding to stop treatment.
- Homeopathy
  - System of medical treatment invented in the early 1800s by Samuel Hahnemann, for whom Hahnemann Medical School was named.
    - Homeopathy was frequently taught and practiced in US medical schools until rigorously criticized in the Flexner Report (1910).
    - Almost 2 million visits were made to homeopathic practitioners in the US in 1997.
  - Homeopathy is based on 2 principles.
    - Law of Similars
      - A remedy that would cause a symptom in a healthy person is used to treat the same symptom in a sick person.
      - Example: A remedy made from the poison ivy plant (*Rhus toxicum*) might be used to treat a child with eczema.
    - Law of Dilutions
      - The more a remedy is diluted, the more powerful it becomes.
      - Homeopaths think that these highly diluted solutions contain an energy, or information, that the patient uses to heal symptoms.
      - They report that the right remedy may worsen symptoms briefly before they improve.
      - Many physicians think that the remedies are simply placebos that trigger the patient's psychoneuroimmunologic healing systems.
      - Randomized controlled trials suggest activity exists for remedies for diarrhea and otitis media but not for attention-deficit/hyperactivity disorder.
  - Side effects
    - Serious side effects from homeopathic treatment are exceedingly rare.
      - Far less common than side effects from standard over-the-counter and prescription medications
  - An estimated 12,000 homeopaths practice in the US
    - 50% lay practitioners
    - 35% chiropractors
    - 10% physicians
    - 5% other health professionals

- Most states allow certified health professionals to practice acupuncture or homeopathy.
  - Certification boards for health care professionals:
    - Physicians and doctors of osteopathy (American Institute of Homeopathy)
    - Chiropractors (National Board of Homeopathic Education)
    - Naturopaths (Naturopathic Academy of Homeopathic Physicians)
  - Non-health care professionals
    - Registered with the North American Society of Homeopaths

Energy therapies

- Includes all therapies that affect physiologic function by the modulation of hypothesized energy fields
  - Spirit
  - Chi
  - Energy
  - Life force
- Practitioners transmit bioenergetic healing energy through their hands to foster healing.
  - Actual touching does not always take place.
  - Includes therapies that use measurable electromagnetic fields to relieve the underlying causes of unexplained pain, eg, magnet therapies
- Therapeutic Touch
  - 5-step process of healing outside of a specific religious faith or belief
    - Having a clear and conscious intent to be helpful and heal
    - Being centered in a peaceful state of mind
    - Using hands to assess the patient's energy (typically moving the hands 1–3 inches away from the body in a slow downward sweep from the head to the toes)
    - Using hands to help restore the patient's energy to a balanced, harmonious, peaceful state
    - Releasing the patient to complete the healing process while the healer returns to the healer's own centered, peaceful state of mind
  - Primary clinical benefits
    - Increased relaxation
    - Diminished anxiety
    - Diminished pain
    - Enhanced sense of well-being
  - Therapeutic Touch is taught in nursing schools across the US
    - Nursing practice in many hospitals, including children's hospitals, includes policies and procedures for performing Therapeutic Touch.

■ Healing Touch

■ Reiki

  • Similar to Therapeutic Touch; from a Japanese tradition

  • Typically provided by lay practitioners outside of medical settings

  • Practitioners are trained by a Reiki master through apprenticeship and spiritual and energetic initiation.

How to talk with patients about CAM

Concerns

■ Physicians

  • Families who use CAM may be dissatisfied with mainstream medical care.

  • Patients may abandon effective therapies in favor of unproved alternatives.

    – Data do not support these concerns.

    – Families who seek out CAM rarely abandon their pediatrician.

■ Families

  • Therapies that are consistent with their:

    – Values

    – Worldview

    – Culture

  • Therapists who:

    – Respect them as individuals

    – Offer time and attention

    – Offer compassion and hope

    – Provide comprehensive primary care

  • Additional information in areas over which they may exert some control:

    – Healthy lifestyles

    – Dietary supplements

    – Environmental therapies

The medical interview

■ Ask all patients about CAM.

  • Use a manner that is:

    – Seamless

    – Structured

    – Positive

    – Nonjudgmental

  • Begin new patient interviews with questions, such as:

    – Number of meals eaten together as a family

    – Fun things the family does together

    – Hopes and dreams for the child

    – Aspects of the child of which they are most proud

  • At each return visit, a helpful question would be to also ask:

    – "Since the last visit, which other health professionals has your child visited?"

  • Listen for understanding rather than agreement or disagreement.

Social history

■ Diet

■ Exercise

■ Environment

  • ACHHOO mnemonic for potential exposure site to known toxins

    – **A**ctivities

    – **C**ommunity

    – **H**ousehold

    – **H**obbies

    – **O**ccupation

    – **O**ral behaviors

■ Illness care at home

  • Foods

  • Teas

  • Rubs

  • Prayers or rituals that are helpful for the patient's family

■ Any mind-body therapies used to:

  • Manage stress

  • Reduce chronic symptoms

  • Promote well-being

■ Academic history, including:

  • Learning style

  • Friends

  • Hobbies

  • Extracurricular activities

■ Questions regarding spirituality as appropriate and ethical:

  • FICA mnemonic:

    – **F**aith or belief—What is your faith or belief?

    – **I**mportance and influence—Is faith important in your life? How?

    – **C**ommunity—Are you part of a religious community?

    – **A**wareness and addressing—What would you want me as your physician to be aware of? How would you like me to address these issues in your care?

  • HOPE mnemonic:

    – **H**ope—What are your sources of hope, meaning, strength, peace, love, and connectedness?

    – **O**rganization—Do you consider yourself part of an organized religion?

- **P**ersonal spirituality and practices—What aspects of your spirituality or spiritual practices do you find most helpful?
- **E**ffects—How do your beliefs affect the kind of medical care you would like me to provide?
- SPIRIT mnemonic:
  - **S**piritual belief system—What is your formal religious affiliation?
  - **P**ersonal spirituality—Describe the beliefs and practices of your religion or spiritual system that you personally accept or do not accept.
  - **I**ntegration within a spiritual community—Do you belong to a spiritual or religious group or community? What importance does this group have for you?
  - **R**itualized practices and Restrictions—Are there specific practices that you carry out as part of your religion/spirituality (eg, prayer or meditation)?
  - **I**mplications for medical care—Would you like to discuss religious or spiritual implications of health care?
  - **T**erminal events planning—As we plan for your care near the end of life, how does your faith affect your decisions? Are there particular aspects of care that you wish to forgo or have withheld because of your faith?
- The following guidelines should be kept in mind when discussing spirituality:
  - The physician's role is not to provide answers but to support the search for answers.
  - Anticipate the presence of spiritual concerns with every illness—those of the patient, the family, and care team members.
  - Comprehend how the patient's and the family's faith or spirituality can be a resource during illness.
  - Seek to understand how the patient's or the family's cultural and spiritual worldview influence understanding of the disease, the appropriate treatment, and the recovery process.
  - Determine what effect, positive or negative, the patient's or the family's spiritual orientation or interpretation has on perceived needs.
  - Partner with, and refer to, chaplains or the patient's or the family's preferred spiritual care provider for assistance with significant spiritual concerns.
- Medical history
  - Do you use multivitamins?
  - Do you use over-the-counter medications?
    - Example: for pain
  - Do you use herbal medicines?
    - Example: *Echinacea* or chamomile
  - Do you take specific vitamins and minerals?
    - Example: Vitamin C or calcium

- Do you take dietary supplements?
  - Example: fish oil
- Follow-up questions:
  - What brand?
  - What dose?
  - How often?
  - What directions are you following?
  - What goals are you hoping to achieve by taking it?
  - Are you using any other remedies now?
- Identify patients at risk for:
  - Interactions with prescription medications
  - Excessive bleeding during surgery
  - Highest risk associated with:
    - Anticoagulants
    - Hypoglycemics
    - Antidepressants
    - Sedative-hypnotics
    - Antihypertensives
    - Medications with narrow therapeutic windows (eg, digoxin, theophylline)
- Ask patients to bring all remedies with them to every visit, so that:
  - Chart can be updated
  - Use is monitored

How to counsel families about CAM

- Goals
  - Strengthen the physician-patient relationship through honest dialogue that is:
    - Clinically responsible
    - Ethically appropriate
    - Legally defensible
- Follow 3 steps when patients or families report seeing other health professionals and describe current CAM use.
  - 1—Determine whether the use of CAM:
    - Represents a rejection of standard care for a serious or life-threatening disease for which a reasonable chance exists of cure or will delay proven treatment
      - In such cases, the first step is to protect the child while understanding the parents' goals.
      - Reporting requirements for abuse and neglect may apply.
      - Parental inclusion of CAM does not in itself constitute neglect.
  - 2—Determine whether the CAM therapies used are known to be unsafe or ineffective.

- If yes:
  - The physician's responsibility is to counsel from the documented evidence that the therapy should be stopped.
  - Resistance to such advice may place the parents at risk for charges of neglect or abuse.
- If no:
  - Monitor as clinically appropriate.
  - Offer to talk with other therapists involved in the child's care to maintain coordinated, comprehensive care.
  - Offer to learn more to help answer the family's questions.
  - Offer additional information and resources to address family's questions about CAM.
- Document the following in the medical record:
  - Therapy used and the goal of the therapy
  - Patient or family preferences and expectations regarding the therapy
  - Provider of the therapy, location, contact information, and treatment plan (as known by the family)
  - Review of the safety and efficacy issues of the therapy from the medical literature
  - Results of counseling including plan for monitoring CAM treatment and its results
  - Advice provided or resources recommended for further information
- 3—Ensure that the patient and family's decision to use CAM without a referral is:
  - Based on a fully informed judgment
  - Documented as verbal consent, including what options have been discussed, offered, tried, refused

How to partner with and refer to CAM practitioners

- Document the following in the medical record.
  - Parity of evaluation
    - Medical history and physical examination as thorough as for conventional care
  - Informed consent
    - Review of diagnosis
    - All medical options for that diagnosis
    - Discussion of risks and benefits of recommended treatments, including potential interference with ongoing conventional care
    - Any applicable financial interests
  - Treatment plan objectives and goals (expected favorable outcomes and monitoring plan for duration of treatment)
    - Physicians must be able to demonstrate a basic understanding of the medical scientific knowledge connected with the CAM.
- Physicians should only refer to:
  - Licensed or otherwise state-regulated health care practitioners
  - CAM practitioners with the requisite training and skills
    - Some credentialed practitioners exist in conventional settings.
- When making referrals for children with complex chronic illness or chronic pain:
  - Carefully prioritize and schedule necessary conventional therapies.
  - Coordinate care with all subspecialists.
  - Consider time and expenses of families who are vulnerable as they seek any available therapies for children.
  - Set appropriate expectations.
  - Support appropriate hope.
  - Avoid overscheduling and overtreating children.
- Physicians are not liable for negligence on the part of a CAM provider unless the physician:
  - Delayed necessary conventional treatment
  - Knew the provider was not competent to provide the therapy
  - Hired the CAM provider or provided joint treatment with the provider

Conduct Disorders

DEFINITION

- Conduct disorders encompass a range of repetitive and persistent patterns of behavior.
  - In all, basic rights of others or major age-appropriate societal norms or rules are violated.
- Terms used and misused for children and adolescents with these behaviors
  - Conduct disordered
  - Oppositional
    - Conduct disorder is more serious than oppositional behavior.
  - Violent
  - Delinquent
  - Sociopathic
  - Psychopathic
  - Antisocial

EPIDEMIOLOGY

- Conduct disorder
  - Prevalence: approximately 5% (5000 per 100,000)
  - Sex: 3:1–4:1 ratio of boys to girls
- Oppositional disorder
  - Prevalence: higher than that of conduct disorder but declines substantially between early childhood and school age compared with other age groups
  - Sex: 3:1 or 4:1 ratio of boys to girls

ETIOLOGY

- Genetics seem to play a role that has not been defined specifically.
  - The genetics of alcohol and substance use, depression, and impulsivity are better defined by and relate to aspects of conduct disorder.
  - Other neuronal substrates to these behaviors, such as autonomic underarousal, may also have genetic roots.

RISK FACTORS

- Comorbid or co-occurring conditions
  - Learning disabilities
    - Increased risk of school dropout and running away when coexisting with oppositional or conduct disorder
  - Attention deficit/hyperactivity disorder (ADHD)
    - Increased risk of unintentional injury when oppositional or conduct disorder coexists with the impulsivity of ADHD
  - Depression
    - Increased risk of suicidal behavior when coexisting with oppositional or conduct disorder
  - Substance use
    - Increased risk of unintentional injury when oppositional or conduct disorder coexists with alcohol use, especially in adolescence
  - Anxiety
- Familial factors
  - Insecure early attachment between young child and caretaker
  - Harsh discipline, abuse, or neglect
  - Family dysfunction, marital conflict, domestic violence
  - Mental illness in parents, especially depression
  - Paternal criminality
  - Financial stresses, low income
  - Frequent family moves
  - Birth of a sibling
- Characteristics of the child
  - Rigid temperament
  - Poor fit between child's temperament and parenting styles
  - Academic difficulties
  - Struggles concerning autonomy
- Poor social environment, negative peer group influences (such as gangs)

SIGNS AND SYMPTOMS

- Pediatricians commonly hear about conduct-disordered and oppositional children from parents who are frustrated and angry.
  - Examples of parental behavioral concerns
    - "Jimmy runs out of the house while I am telling him not to."
    - "Sally will not stay in her room for a time out."
    - "My husband and I cannot get Billy to sit down and start his homework."
    - "Jason lied to me about where he was."
    - "Peter used my credit card to buy a violent video game on the Internet."
    - "Tom drove the car, despite having only a learner's permit, to see his girlfriend, even though he was grounded."
    - "Mike may be using and even selling marijuana to his friends."
    - "Jared is getting into fistfights at school."
  - A wide range of behaviors can raise the concern of oppositional or conduct disorder.
  - Even the simplest symptoms require thoughtful assessment.
    - Is refusing to go to school an issue of anxiety, emerging learning disabilities, fear of a bully, a consequence of rejection by peers, oppositional behavior, or a reaction to parental conflict?

- Thorough history assessment of each behavior and its circumstances is critical.
  - For many children, the behavior is not the core problem but is the solution that emerges to the child feeling overwhelmed, frustrated, or angry.
  - Although parents will have worries of delinquency or even criminality, the focus of primary care efforts will be a review of risk factors.
  - Pediatricians should assess the severity, frequency, and context of the behavior.
    - What family, personal, and social risk factors may be underlying the behavior?
    - What is the parental reaction, and do any legal ramifications exist?
    - Given the complexity of the behavior and likely contributing circumstances, no easy questionnaires or tools have been developed that substitute for interviews of the child and family.
  - Hierarchy of behavior severity: reactive, nonviolent, proactive nonviolent, reactive violent, and proactive violent
    - In general, reactive behavior, such as arguing or losing one's temper after feeling unfairly punished or exhausted by a long school day, is less serious than proactive anger.
    - A younger child occasionally blaming others or even lying as a means of coping is not as serious as a more consistent pattern of annoying or blaming others.
    - Reacting to bullying with violence or destroying property as part of a group prank is very different from proactively initiating fights, using weapons, or acting out cruelty.
    - Behaviors exhibited as part of a group are, in general, not as serious as acts performed alone.
  - Problem behaviors can be conceptualized as related to:
    - Property (vandalism, theft, fire setting)
    - Interpersonal aggression (bullying, cruelty, fighting, assault)
    - High personal risk (truancy, substance use, running away from home)
- Comprehensive mental health evaluation
  - Required in a patient with persistent, escalating, violent, and remorseless behavior
  - Behaviors are most worrisome if they are severe, repeated, done alone, and done without remorse.

DIFFERENTIAL DIAGNOSIS

- Differential diagnosis focuses on separating common behaviors from serious disorders that portend long-term risk.
- Some forms of aggressiveness are part of a developmental trajectory to autonomy and independence.
  - They are often socially sanctioned, as in competitive sports, academics, and dating.

- Such aggression is often socially accepted and achievement oriented.
- Oppositional behavior for many children is a sign of or a solution to a hidden problem.
  - Disrupting a class may be:
    - A solution to an underlying fear of appearing stupid, a sign that the child needs treatment for learning problems or ADHD
    - A reaction to tension or violence in the home
  - Violating rules to see a girlfriend or boyfriend may be:
    - Simply oppositional
    - A reasonable attempt to assert autonomy in the face of overly restrictive parents
  - Sensible in the context of a private adolescent crisis
- Diagnostic criteria for conduct disorder
  - Presence of ≥3 of the following criteria in the past 12 months, with ≥1 criterion present in the past 6 months:
    - Often bullies, threatens, or intimidates others
    - Often initiates physical fights
    - Has used a weapon that can cause serious physical harm to others (eg, a bat, brick, broken bottle, knife, gun)
    - Has been physically cruel to people
    - Has been physically cruel to animals
    - Has stolen while confronting a victim (eg, mugging, purse snatching, extortion, armed robbery)
    - Has forced someone into sexual activity
    - Has deliberately engaged in fire setting with the intention of causing serious damage
    - Has deliberately destroyed others' property (other than fire setting)
    - Has broken into someone else's house, building, or car
    - Often lies to obtain goods or favors or to avoid obligations (ie, cons others)
    - Has stolen items of nontrivial value without confronting a victim (eg, shoplifting, but without breaking and entering; forgery)
    - Often stays out at night despite parental prohibitions, beginning before age 13 years
    - Has run away from home overnight at least twice while living in parental or parental surrogate home (or once without returning for a lengthy period)
    - Is often truant from school, beginning before age 13 years
  - The disturbance in behavior causes clinically significant impairment in social, academic, or occupational functioning.

- Specify the severity.
  - Mild: few, if any, conduct problems in excess of those required to make the diagnosis and conduct problems cause only minor harm to others
  - Moderate: the number of conduct problems and effect on others is between mild and severe
  - Severe: many conduct problems in excess of those required to make the diagnostic or conduct disorder problems that cause considerable harm to others
- Diagnostic criteria for oppositional defiant disorder
  - A pattern of negativistic, hostile, and defiant behavior lasting ≥6 months, during which ≥4 of the following are present:
    - Patient often:
      - Loses temper
      - Argues with adults
      - Actively defies or refuses to comply with adults' requests or rules
      - Deliberately annoys people
      - Blames others for his or her mistakes or misbehavior
      - Is touchy or easily annoyed by others
      - Is angry and resentful
      - Is spiteful or vindictive
  - A criterion is met only if the behavior occurs more frequently than typically observed in individuals of similar age and developmental level.
  - The disturbance in behavior causes clinically significant impairment in social, academic, or occupational functioning.

DIAGNOSTIC APPROACH

- Thorough history that includes assessment of each behavior and its circumstances
  - Severity
  - Frequency
  - Context
- Close analysis of risk factors
  - Concomitant conditions
  - Family dynamics and social issues
- Comprehensive mental evaluation in the face of persistent, escalating, violent, and remorseless behavior

TREATMENT APPROACH

- Initial goals
  - Increase safety.
    - Seek to have guns or life-threatening medications removed from the home.

- Decrease the level of tension, discord, and stress.
  - Consider structured family agreements or having the child stay with another caretaker.
  - Involve social services if immediate threat to family, child, or others.
- Long-term goals
  - Family and behavior interventions (especially parent training) to:
    - Eliminate the conduct disordered behavior
    - Help the patient make amends
    - Relieve underlying stressors or comorbid conditions
    - Restore trust
    - Build on the child's adaptive strengths in school, activities, with friends, and in the family
- Conduct disorder is more serious than oppositional behavior.
  - Maintaining an appropriate sense of optimism is important because most adolescents with disturbing behaviors emerge as productive adults.
    - However, the risks for self-injury, injury to others, academic discipline, and intervention by legal authorities are real, with serious consequences.
- Mild-to-moderate, short-term defiant behaviors
  - These may yield to the pediatrician's assessment and recommendations.
- Persistent, escalating, violent, and remorseless behaviors
  - Psychosocial and behavioral treatments
  - Appropriate use of medication to treat associated conditions, such as depression, ADHD, or anxiety

SPECIFIC TREATMENTS

Non-pharmacologic management

- Actions and considerations that may be helpful in initial management if conduct-disordered behavior is a serious concern:
  - Patient safety
    - Does the child experience abuse or violence from peers or gang members?
    - Does the child exhibit self-destructive behaviors, including use of substances?
    - Does the child exhibit suicidal risk caused by depression, severe embarrassment, or shame, intensified by a sense of being trapped with no escape and no solution?
    - Does the child have access to guns or life-threatening medications?
  - Family safety
    - Does the home have guns, patterns of domestic violence, or patient-initiated violence to parents or peers?
    - Does the child's home life have escalating, physical confrontations between the child and the parent as part of the emerging behavior?

– Consider structured family agreements or having the child stay with a relative or friend.

- Support structure

  – Provide access to mental health consultation for patient, parent, or family work.

  – Determine the need for other urgently needed services, such as legal representation, liaison with school guidance or probation officer, or state department of social services.

- Limit setting and negotiation

  – Suggest limit setting that decreases stress, for example:

    ▪ Limiting contact to provocative peers

    ▪ Limiting access to substances (or substance abuse treatment)

    ▪ Tracking where the patient is when not in school

- Building on strengths

  – Reinforce any positive supports, such as:

    ▪ Areas of competence

    ▪ Relationship with a caring adult (coach, teacher, parent, sibling, grandparent)

    ▪ Behaviors that will elicit parental praise

- Establishing rules

  – Encourage consistency and unanimity of parental discipline and overall response to conduct-disordered behaviors.

  – Support by a behavioral psychologist is often critical.

- School interventions

  – Help the child reduce academic stress with the help of the school psychologist or guidance counselor, through a teacher conference, by eliminating a stressful class, or by implementing an education plan.

  – Consider whether school-based peer pressures, such as bullying, threats, humiliation, or clique or gang group behavior, are contributing factors.

  – If others are involved, the clinician should support contacting the relevant parents.

- Legal interventions

  – Facilitate parents contacting a lawyer or public defender to deal with potential legal issues, arrests, or pressure from local law enforcement.

  – Lawyers may appropriately engage police who are assigned as youth officers, work with probation departments, or negotiate with the court and local agencies to ensure the availability of services in the context of legal proceedings.

- Specialty mental health interventions: parent training

- Department of social services referral if there is danger to child or family

  – A comprehensive plan often must be mobilized to provide safety.

– Consider referral to the local department of social services to coordinate legal, mental health, and school resources.

Drug treatment

■ Risperidone

- Antipsychotic drug prescribed off-label to address violent conduct-disordered behavior

- Use of this potent and complex medication should not be initiated without a comprehensive treatment plan and collaboration with a child and adolescent psychiatrist.

■ Treat underlying concomitant conditions/risk factors, such as ADHD.

PROGNOSIS

■ We do not know which patients will have lifelong problems.

- The specific profile of causes and symptoms that are prognostic for a persistent course is not well defined.

- Oppositional and conduct-disordered symptoms at any age cause dysfunction in the child and family and are potentially dangerous to others.

- Most children who demonstrate oppositional behavior do not progress to conduct disorder as adolescents.

- More serious conduct disorders do not necessarily lead to criminality, addiction, or lifelong disorders.

■ Early childhood

- Oppositional disorder declines substantially between early childhood and school age compared with other age groups.

■ School age and adolescence

- Aggressive behavior seems to decline after early childhood but is more stable and worrisome when evident in school age and adolescence.

  – The younger the patient, the more violent the behavior, and the less the child experiences remorse or guilt, the more serious the eventual prognosis.

- Adolescents who demonstrate a sense of feeling connected to a school, team, peers, or family probably have a better prognosis than those who are isolated, unfeeling, or alone.

■ Late adolescence

- Period of another substantial decline in conduct disorder

- A distinct subsample becomes criminal.

■ Protective factors that probably improve prognosis

- Adaptable temperament

- Higher IQ

- Competence in ≥1 area (eg, academic, social, athletic)

- Warm relationship with a parent or adult

- Opportunities to connect to the community (eg, clubs, teams)

- Financial resources to facilitate opportunities

PREVENTION

- Encouraging efforts focused on high-risk populations
  - Early identification of at-risk infants
    - Postpartum home visits or screening in child care settings for young mothers who are vulnerable to depression, domestic violence, conflictual relationships, or using harsh disciplinary techniques
    - Identifying and providing services for school-aged children who demonstrate aggression, bullying, learning disabilities, and ADHD
    - Identifying high-risk adolescents who might be failing in school, depressed, using substances, or fighting
  - Broad-based prevention efforts
    - Comprehensive services for abused and neglected children
    - Community efforts directed against substance use or development of gangs
    - Adequate opportunities for connecting children and adolescents to their community through sports, activities, and religious affiliation
    - Access to mental health services when needed

- Financial pressures on community services and schools have decreased preventive services.
  - Pressures to control health care spending have lowered the priority of mental health services for children and families.
  - An adolescent with conduct disorder who elicits mental health, social service, school-based, and legal attention costs the community $70,000 over a 7-year period.
    - Despite this high cost, prevention, early intervention, and mental health services in most communities are poorly funded.
    - Primary care pediatricians shoulder more of the burden for mental health problems, such as oppositional and conduct disorders.

Congenital and Acquired Heart Disease

DEFINITION

Congenital defects

- Intracardiac shunting lesions
  - A defect or hole in the septum separating the 2 ventricles that allows blood to traverse from one side of the heart to the other
  - Shunting can be:
    - Left side of the heart to the right
    - Right side of the heart to the left
    - Bidirectional
  - Right heart
    - Systemic veins, inferior vena cava (IVC), and superior vena cava (SVC)
    - Atrium
    - Ventricle
    - Great artery/pulmonary artery
  - Left heart
    - Pulmonary veins
    - Atrium
    - Ventricle
    - Great artery/aorta
- Left-to-right shunting lesions
  - Ventricular septal defect (VSD)
  - Atrial septal defect (ASD)
  - Patent ductus arteriosus (PDA)
  - Atrioventricular septal defects (AVSDs)
  - Arteriovenous malformations
- Right-to-left shunting lesions
  - Tetralogy of Fallot
  - Eisenmenger syndrome
    - Untreated septal defect
  - Pulmonary hypertension
  - Pulmonary atresia
    - No prograde flow across the pulmonary valve
  - Ebstein anomaly
  - Anomalous pulmonary venous return (PVR)
    - Total
    - Partial
  - Dextrorotation
    - Rightward transposition of the great arteries
- Left-sided obstructive lesions
  - Characterized by impedance to blood flow from the systemic ventricle (generally the left) to the body
  - Aortic stenosis
  - Coarctation of the aorta

- Complete mixing lesion/single-ventricle heart
  - Arterial oxygen saturation (SaO_2) is the same in both the aorta and the pulmonary artery.
    - Hypoplastic left heart syndrome
    - Tricuspid atresia

Acquired heart disease

- Infectious
  - Infectious endocarditis (IE)
    - Bacterial infection of the endocardium or endothelium of the heart
  - Myocarditis
    - Generalized inflammation of the cardiac muscular walls
  - Pericatrditis
    - Inflammation of the pericardium
    - Both the parietal and the visceral layers of the pericardium are inflamed.
- Cardiomyopathies
  - Any structural or functional abnormality of the ventricular myocardium that is not associated with congenital heart disease or diseases of the coronary arteries, cardiac valves, or pulmonary vasculature
    - Dilated cardiomyopathy (DCM)
    - Hypertrophic cardiomyopathy (HCM)
    - Restrictive cardiomyopathy (RCM)
    - Miscellaneous cardiomyopathies

EPIDEMIOLOGY

Congenital defects

- Only 5–8 of 1000 live births are affected by a congenital heart lesion.
- Left-to-right shunting lesions
  - Ventricular septal defects (VSD)
    - One of the most common types of congenital heart disease
    - Nearly 20% of patients in heart disease registries have a solitary VSD.
  - PDA
    - Most commonly encountered in premature infants
  - AVSDs
    - Nearly 50% of all patients with trisomy 21 have congenital heart disease.
    - Nearly 50% are AVSDs (also known as *atrioventricular canal defects* or *endocardial cushion defects*).
- Right-to-left shunting lesions
  - Tetralogy of Fallot
    - One of the most commonly encountered cyanotic heart defects, occurring in 0.33 per 1000 live births and comprising approximately 7% of heart defects

- Dextrorotation
  - The most common type of cyanotic heart disease

Acquired heart disease

- Infectious
  - IE
    - Prevalence has increased substantially over the past 2 decades.
  - Myocarditis
    - In a 10-year study of 14,000 cardiac patients between 1954 and 1977, myocarditis was diagnosed in 0.5% of patients at presentation and another 2–5% at autopsy.
    - Nearly 20% of pediatric sudden deaths may be related to myocarditis.
- Cardiomyopathies
  - DCM
    - Accounts for 60–70% of pediatric cardiomyopathies
    - Prevalence: 5–20 cases/1,000,000 persons
  - HCM
    - Second most common form of cardiomyopathy (20–30%) in children
    - Prevalence: 4–6/1,000,000 persons
  - RCM
    - Rarest form of cardiomyopathy in children
  - Miscellaneous cardiomyopathies
    - Arrhythmogenic right-ventricular dysplasia (ARVD) and mitochondrial and noncompaction cardiomyopathies comprise only 2–3% of pediatric cardiomyopathies.

ETIOLOGY

Intracardiac shunting lesions

- In all shunting lesions, the volume of shunted blood depends on the size of the defect.

Left-to-right shunting lesions

- VSD
  - Left-sided heart pressure generally exceeds that on the right side.
  - Blood will preferentially shunt from left to right and is added directly to the pulmonary circulation.
  - In the case of large VSDs, this addition of blood results in left-ventricle volume overload.
    - Over time, the left heart will dilate to accommodate this increased volume.
    - Abnormal mechanical stresses inherent in the chronically volume-loaded, dilated ventricle can lead to myocyte dysfunction and heart failure.

- ASD
  - In addition to pressure, a difference in chamber compliance is the dominant force directing blood from left to right.
  - The highly compliant right atrium becomes a sink for blood draining into the smaller, less-compliant left atrium by the pulmonary veins.
    - This additional blood volume is routed into the right ventricle, resulting in right-heart dilation over time.
- PDA
  - When the ductus arteriosus does not involute shortly after birth, it is a potential source of shunting from the aorta to the pulmonary arteries once PVR decreases.
- AVSDs
  - Partial type (primum type ASD with a cleft mitral valve)
  - Complete type (single atrioventricular valve spanning the entire width of the heart)
    - Variability in the attachment of the atrioventricular valve leaflets to the interventricular septum
    - Can result in a significant left-to-right shunt volume
- Arteriovenous malformations
  - Direct connection between the arterial and venous vascular systems results in:
    - Shunting of blood to the right heart
    - Possible high-output, left-sided heart failure
  - Common locations in children
    - Cerebral
    - Abdominal

Right-to-left shunting lesions

- Oxygen-poor blood is shunted to the oxygen-rich systemic blood.
  - Systemic peripheral cyanosis is the key difference between left-to-right and right-to-left shunting lesions.
  - As with left-to-right shunting lesions, the volume of shunted blood depends on:
    - Size of the defect
    - Pressure gradient across it
- Tetralogy of Fallot
  - May occur as a result of disproportionate segregation of the truncus arteriosus into the pulmonary artery and aorta
  - Shunting of right-ventricular blood through the VSD into the aorta produces systemic, peripheral cyanosis.
  - Tetralogy spell (Tet spell), a hypercyanotic event, occurs when systemic vascular resistance decreases, resulting in an increased right-to-left shunt.
- Eisenmenger syndrome
  - Unrepaired VSDs or large ASDs with secondary pulmonary hypertension

- Significant shunting and progressive cyanosis occur once the pulmonary artery, and therefore right-ventricular, pressures are higher than the systemic blood pressure.
- Pulmonary hypertension
  - Isolated or idiopathic pulmonary hypertension
    - No septal defects through which blood can shunt right to left
  - Pulmonary hypertensive crisis (transient, severe elevation of pulmonary artery pressures) causes markedly decreased right-ventricular and then left-ventricular output.
- Pulmonary atresia
  - Blood entering the right ventricle is regurgitated through the tricuspid valve back into the right atrium, where it mixes with SVC and IVC blood.
    - The increase in blood volume increases right atrial pressure, resulting in shunting of blood across the patent foramen ovale to the left atrium.
- Ebstein anomaly
  - Tricuspid valve insufficiency
    - Course of blood flow is much the same as in pulmonary atresia with intact ventricular septum.
  - With worsening tricuspid valve incompetence, the effectively smaller right ventricle is less able to propel blood across the pulmonary valve, which is usually narrowed or stenotic, or both.
    - Blood instead returns to the right atrium and crosses the patent foramen ovale.
- Total anomalous PVR
  - Occurs when the pulmonary veins do not connect with the posterior wall of the left atrium but instead form a confluence that then drains via a vertical vein indirectly to the right atrium
  - Within the heart, blood is shunted from the right atrium across an obligate ASD into the left atrium.
    - This provides the only source of systemic cardiac output.
- Partial anomalous PVR
  - Anomalous return of ≥1 pulmonary veins to the right heart
- Dextrorotation
  - Embryologic defect of the conotruncus
    - The aortic valve lies rightward and anterior of the pulmonary valve instead of rightward and posterior, as in the normal heart.
    - Pulmonary and systemic circulations are in parallel rather than in series.
    - The body relies on both intra- and extracardiac shunting to provide oxygenated blood to the tissues.

Left-sided obstructive lesions

- Aortic stenosis
  - A large portion of fetal cardiac output is provided by ductal flow from the pulmonary artery to the descending aorta.
    - The transition to postnatal circulation occurs with closure of the ductus arteriosus.
    - In the newborn with severe or critical aortic stenosis, this process is associated with a significant decrease in systemic blood flow.
- Coarctation of the aorta
  - In neonates, occurs as either a discrete narrowing or a diffuse hypoplasia of the transverse and isthmic aortic arch
    - Discrete coarctation can occur in virtually any portion of the aorta but is typically found near the insertion of the ductus arteriosus (juxta-ductal).
  - In adolescents, a discrete, relatively undersized segment of the aorta that did not continue to grow at a rate commensurate with the remainder of the aorta
    - The coarctation is bypassed by collateral arteries.
- Complete mixing lesion/single-ventricle heart
  - Systemic and pulmonary venous blood volumes drain into a single ventricle to produce a partially desaturated blood volume perfusing both the body and the lungs.
    - The same physiologic mechanism and management is applicable to essentially all variations of the single-ventricle heart.
  - Hypoplastic left-heart syndrome (HLHS)
    - Group of cardiac anomalies characterized by underdevelopment of the aortic arch, aortic valve, mitral valve, and left ventricle
    - Used herein as the prototype for single-ventricle heart
  - Tricuspid atresia
    - The single ventricle is a left ventricle generally connected to the aorta.

Acquired heart disease

- Infectious
  - IE
    - Generally associated with a procedural or surgical intervention
    - Spontaneous IE does occur but is exceedingly rare without predisposing risk factors.
    - Staphylococci, streptococci, and enterococci are the most common pathogens because of their ability to interact with platelets and resist the host's immune response.
  - Myocarditis
    - Viral infiltration of myocytes and the associated immune-mediated cell lysis
    - Enteroviruses, particularly the coxsackievirus B3 and B4 serotypes, and adenovirus are most frequently involved.

- Pericarditis
  - Infectious causes: enteroviruses (especially coxsackievirus B), influenza, cytomegalovirus, Epstein-Barr virus; *Staphylococcus aureus*, *Streptococcus pyogenes*, *Streptococcus pneumoniae*
  - Noninfectious causes: rheumatic fever, autoimmune diseases, postcardiac surgery, uremia, cancer
- Cardiomyopathies
  - DCM
    - A viral cause is identified in 2–15% of cases of biopsy-proven myocarditis.
    - The remaining cases are classified as idiopathic but are probably genetic.
    - Regardless of cause, the progressive cardiac dysfunction associated with DCM is probably related to the remodeling response of the heart after an inciting injury.
  - HCM
    - Genetic basis; multiple familial forms
    - 40–50% have a point mutation on chromosome 14q1.
  - RCM
    - Thought to have both genetic and nongenetic causes
  - Miscellaneous cardiomyopathies
    - ARVD: dysplasia of the right ventricle develops from fatty deposits within the ventricular walls.
    - Mitochondrial cardiomyopathies: maternally inherited
    - Left-ventricular noncompaction cardiomyopathy: deep crevices or trabeculations within the left ventricle reduce cardiac function.

RISK FACTORS

Congenital defects

- Down syndrome
  - 40–60% of children with Down syndrome are born with some form of congenital heart disease.
  - Patients with Down syndrome comprise ~9% of the pediatric cardiologist's practice.
- Williams syndrome
  - Supravalvar obstruction
- Turner syndrome
- Coarctation of aorta
- Noonan syndrome
- Pulmonary valvular stenosis

Acquired heart disease

- IE
  - Congenital heart defects (~90% of cases)
    - Risks of IE in the preoperative state of congenital heart defects
      - Tetralogy of Fallot: >30%

- VSD: 12–14%
- PDA: 8%
- Aortic stenosis: 2%
- Pulmonary stenosis: 1%
  - Indwelling venous catheters without associated structural heart disease
- Myocarditis
  - Frequently associated with infectious pericarditis
    - More so with viral than with bacterial agents
- Pericarditis
  - Autoimmune disease
  - Uremia
- HCM
  - Noonan syndrome
  - Friedreich ataxia
- RCM
  - Sarcoidosis
  - Amyloidosis
- Mitochondrial cardiomyopathies
  - Other muscle, liver, neurologic, and developmental abnormalities
- Left-ventricular noncompaction cardiomyopathy
  - Mitochondrial, metabolic, and systemic (Barth syndrome) disorders

SIGNS AND SYMPTOMS

Cardiac murmur

- Audible blood flow through the heart or vascular system that can be auscultated in a normal heart, resulting from hyperdynamic function or a thin chest wall
- Diastolic murmur
  - Generally indicates an abnormality
- Systolic murmur
  - May be either:
    - Normal (functional)
    - Pathologic
- Regardless of the timing, location, or cause of the murmur, its frequency and pitch depend on:
  - Size of the opening through which the blood flows
  - Pressure gradient across it

VSDs and ASDs

- Smaller ASDs and VSDs
  - May not be detected prenatally
    - Usually detected by the presence of a murmur, with or without the signs of heart failure

- The timing of presentation depends on the size of the defect and whether the infant has fully transitioned from fetal circulation.
- A small VSD will produce a high-pitched, holosystolic murmur that continues from the onset of ventricular systole through the closure of the atrioventricular valves (obscuring the first heart sound), to the closure of the semilunar valves.
- In some patients, PVR never decreases after birth or decreases at a slower rate and then increases.
  - These patients will have few or no symptoms of pulmonary overcirculation.
  - As a result, they may not be brought to a physician's attention.
  - Elevated PVR produces elevated pulmonary artery pressures and commensurate pulmonary hypertension (mean pulmonary pressures >25 mm Hg at rest).
- Large VSDs
  - Produce a softer holosystolic murmur because the pressures of the 2 ventricles more closely approximate one another
    - This murmur will be loudest at the left lower sternal border and may be best described as a mid-frequency blowing murmur.
  - A neonate with a large VSD may demonstrate poor weight gain and lethargy as PVR decreases, increasing the gradient for shunting the left ventricle to the right
    - If untreated, heart failure (marked pulmonary over-circulation) may ensue.
- ASD
  - Auscultation differs significantly from that of a VSD.
  - The lack of a marked pressure gradient between the 2 atria does not produce a murmur at the site of shunting.
    - Rather, the murmur of an ASD is due to excess volume traversing the pulmonary valve, commonly described as a relative pulmonary stenosis.
    - It is described as a mid-frequency systolic ejection murmur best auscultated at the upper left sternal border and will commonly radiate to the lung fields bilaterally.
  - ASD may remain asymptomatic for many years.
  - Pulmonary edema symptoms
    - Typically do not develop until the pulmonary artery blood flow has doubled in volume

PDA

- Auscultation
  - Machinery murmur (continuous, undulating)
    - Heard during both systole and diastole
    - As the ductus arteriosus begins to close, the murmur is higher in pitch
  - Murmur is best auscultated in the left upper sternal border of the chest; it may radiate to both lung fields.

- Other signs
  - Worsening chronic lung disease
  - Poor renal perfusion
  - Hemodynamic instability
  - Intraventricular hemorrhage
  - Necrotizing enterocolitis

Tetralogy of Fallot

- Commonly detected by prenatal ultrasonography between 18 and 22 weeks' gestation
- Clinical presentation can vary greatly, depending on:
  - Degree of pulmonary stenosis
  - Presence of pulmonary atresia
- Newborns
  - Cyanosis
  - Audible murmur
    - Systolic murmur may be appreciated at the left upper sternal border and is produced by the narrowing of the right-ventricular outflow tract (RVOT).
    - Grade (I–VI/VI) and quality (harsh or soft) depend on the degree of obstruction.
  - In the newborn with tetralogy of Fallot and pulmonary atresia:
    - RVOT murmur is replaced by a flow murmur through the ductus arteriosus, the only source of pulmonary blood flow.

Eisenmenger syndrome

- Physical examination of patient with pulmonary hypertension caused by Eisenmenger syndrome may be virtually indistinguishable from that of a simple ASD or VSD.
  - A subtle difference may be a loud pulmonary valve component of the second heart sound.

Pulmonary hypertension

- Idiopathic pulmonary hypertension or pulmonary hypertension secondary to bronchopulmonary dysplasia
  - Cyanosis (from intrapulmonary or right-left atrial level cardiac shunting)
  - Loud pulmonary valve component of the second heart sound without an associated cardiac murmur
    - In the absence of pulmonary or tricuspid insufficiency
  - Equal ventricular pressures in Eisenmenger syndrome secondary to a VSD will not produce an audible murmur.

Dextrorotation

- Can be diagnosed prenatally
  - Neonates are cyanotic at birth without associated respiratory distress.
    - Physical examination will be remarkable for cyanosis and possibly a ductal murmur.
    - Should otherwise be normal for a newborn

- SaO$_2$ will not increase significantly with supplemental oxygen (failed hyperoxia challenge test).
- Care should be taken to assess lower-extremity pulses.
  - Coarctation of the aorta can be associated with dextro-looped transposition of the great arteries (d-TGA).
  - Prostaglandin E$_1$ infusion should be initiated once this defect is suspected.

Aortic stenosis

- Valvar aortic stenosis can occur in isolation or be associated with either subvalvar or supravalvar obstruction.
- With few exceptions, the presentation and alteration of cardiovascular physiologic characteristics are very similar among the 3 defects.
- Mild to moderate stenosis
  - Cardiac murmur may be the only sign of an abnormality in the newborn.
    - Ejection click followed by a harsh systolic ejection murmur
    - Best auscultated at the right upper sternal border
  - Additional signs and symptoms may not develop until childhood.
    - Particularly in the pediatric population, mild to moderate aortic stenosis will not produce exercise intolerance, chest pain, syncope, or shock.
    - As a result, these patients are often referred to a pediatric cardiologist after the characteristic murmur is heard during a routine physical examination.
- Severe or critical aortic stenosis will develop in the newborn as heart failure or clinical extremus.
  - Signs and symptoms of congestive heart failure will ensue.
    - Diaphoresis with feeding
    - Irritability
    - Lethargy
    - Fatigue
    - Acyanotic, but ashen pallor
    - Harsh cardiac murmur
    - Diminished or absent peripheral pulses

Coarctation of the aorta
- Auscultation
  - Systolic murmur is loudest at the left upper sternal border.
  - Murmur generally radiates to the back, medial to the left scapula.
- Neonates
  - Patient presentation tends to have a bimodal distribution.
    - Cases with diffuse arch hypoplasia are typically diagnosed shortly after birth.
    - Cases with an isolated discrete narrowing may not be diagnosed until later in infancy or childhood.

- This lesion may not be detected by prenatal ultrasonography.
  - Therefore, palpation of the femoral pulses becomes a crucial part of the newborn examination.
  - When not palpable in an otherwise healthy-appearing infant, both upper-extremity and 1 lower-extremity blood pressure should be obtained.
- Blood pressure
  - Must be checked in both arms; the left subclavian artery may arise either proximal or (more rarely) distal to the coarctation site.
  - In the legs, a single-leg blood pressure should be adequate.
- Determining presence of a PDA is of critical importance.
  - Because of the presence of ductal tissue in the aorta, coarctation cannot definitively be ruled out until the ductus has closed.
  - If the ductus is closed and a blood pressure gradient on cuff or narrowing on echocardiography is not found, then a hemodynamically significant coarctation does not exist.
  - If there is concern about the existence of a coarctation, the patient should not be discharged until the ductus arteriosus has completely closed or close follow-up has been arranged.
- Adolescents
  - Distinctly different presentation from that in infants
    - Multiple collateral arteries connect the aorta proximal and distal to the obstruction, thus bypassing the coarctation.
    - Intercostal arteries supplying the collateral artery system can become extensive and produce indentations or notching of the ribs.
  - Patients exhibit systolic murmur, upper-extremity hypertension, or both.
  - Upper- and lower-extremity blood pressures
    - May be a more accurate modality than Doppler flow for determining the clinical coarctation gradient

HLHS
- Newborns with HLHS can achieve normal birth weight and gestational age.
  - Fetal circulation can be adequately supplied by the right ventricle.
- Timing of diagnosis
  - Unless HLHS is diagnosed prenatally, the newborn with HLHS may not be immediately recognized.
    - Some of these patients do not receive a diagnosis for several weeks.
    - Such patients typically present with pulmonary over-circulation and systemic shock.

– Profound systemic cyanosis may not occur until the SaO_2 falls below approximately 85% (possibly lower in dark-skinned children).

- Auscultation
  - Cardiac murmur is commonly not present or appreciated.
- Palpation of femoral pulses
  - Critical step in every newborn's routine evaluation
  - Commonly decreased in the newborn with HLHS
    – These pulses will become progressively weaker as the ductus arteriosus closes.
    – If aortic atresia exists, then all 4 extremity pulses will diminish with ductal closure.

Tricuspid atresia

- Patients have a similar physiologic display to those with HLHS.
  - Several anatomic variants exist.

IE

- Clinical course
  - Typically indolent
  - In rare cases, can cause cardiogenic shock
- Patients may have:
  - Recurrent low-grade fever (90%)
  - Arthralgia (25%)
  - Gastrointestinal discomfort (15%)
  - Fatigue
  - Rigors
  - Other nonspecific findings
- Physical examination may be significant for:
  - New cardiacmurmur (rare)
  - Splenomegaly (55%)
  - Neurologic changes (20%)
- Classically described findings are rare in children.
  - Osler nodes (tender subcutaneous nodules on pads of fingers)
  - Janeway lesions (nontender hemorrhagic macules on palms or soles)
  - Roth spots (pale centered oval hemorrhages on retina)
  - Splinter hemorrhages in the nail beds
- Duke criteria for diagnosis of IE
  - Criteria are met if a patient demonstrates:
    – Both major criteria
    – 5 of the 6 minor criteria
    – 1 major and 3 minor criteria
    – Overall, the minor criteria are often used when diagnosing pediatric IE

Myocarditis

- Clinical presentation
  - Ranges from mild electrocardiographic (ECG) abnormalities in an otherwise asymptomatic child to fulminant congestive heart failure
- Less fulminant presentations
  - More typical in older children
  - 7–10 days after a viral upper respiratory infection or gastroenteritis
- Severe, fulminant onset
  - Cardiogenic shock may be present.
- Signs and symptoms
  - Fever
  - Malaise
  - Chest pain
  - Dyspnea
  - Pallor
  - Poor perfusion
- Auscultation
  - Muffled heart sounds
  - Gallop rhythm
  - Suggestive of congestive heart failure

Pericarditis

- History
  - Viral upper respiratory infection 10–14 days before the development of pericarditis is common.
- Physical examination
  - Pain in the left side of the chest
    – Worse in the supine position or with deep breathing
    – Relieved on sitting or leaning forward
    – May radiate to the left shoulder or to the neck
  - Fever (especially with bacterial pericarditis)
  - Signs of low cardiac output
    – Hypotension
    – Tachypnea
    – Tachycardia
    – Dyspnea
    – Pale, gray (sometimes mottled) pallor
    – Clammy skin
  - Auscultation
    – Pericardial friction rub (a biphasic sound) is the cardinal sign of early pericarditis.
    – With further accumulation of pericardial fluid, the friction rub may disappear and the heart sounds may become muffled.

C

- With the onset of cardiac tamponade:
  - Venous return during inspiration is compromised, resulting in a paradoxic rise in the jugular venous pressure (Kussmaul sign).
  - Cardiac output and systolic blood pressure decreases (pulses paradoxicus).
- Symptoms and signs depend on:
  - Fluid volume within the pericardial space
    - The pericardial fluid can be serous, serofibrinous, hemorrhagic, or purulent in nature.
  - Rapidity with which the fluid collects
    - Rapid collection of fluid, as occurs in bacterial infections, may cause severe circulatory compromise (cardiac tamponade).
    - A gradually developing pericardial effusion allows the pericardium to stretch, and therefore the increase in the pericardial pressure is slower and more readily tolerated.
  - Myocardial function
    - If myocardial function is depressed, even a gradual increase in pericardial fluid and pressure may cause significant circulatory compromise.

DCM

- Clinical presentation
  - Varies from progressive exercise intolerance with pulmonary congestion to systemic decompensation with complete cardiovascular collapse
  - Diagnosis typically does not occur until the cardiac reserve is exhausted or is nearly exhausted.
    - Often diagnosed after the patient experiences an acute viral illness that elevates resting metabolism enough to exceed the failing heart's compensatory mechanisms
- Physical examination
  - Consistent with congestive heart failure in symptomatic patients
    - Tachycardia
    - Cachexia
    - Sallow color
    - Tachypnea
    - Orthopnea (older children)
    - Hepatomegaly and weakened peripheral pulses may be found with severe cardiac dysfunction.
  - Auscultation
    - Gallop
    - Early systolic, regurgitant murmur of mitral regurgitation

HCM

- Presentation
  - Variable
    - Asymptomatic to congestive heart failure

- Classic presentation
  - Syncopal patient with a loud cardiac murmur
- Physical examination
  - Typically normal
  - Progressive exercise intolerance
- Auscultation
  - Harsh systolic ejection murmur at the left sternal border with radiation to the neck
  - If present, this murmur is accentuated when a squatting patient is asked to stand.
- History
  - Family history is critical.
    - Nearly one-half of all patients with HCM will have a first-degree relative with HCM or with a history of syncope or sudden death.

Miscellaneous cardiomyopathies

- ARVD
  - Patients typically present with dysrhythmias.
- Mitochondrial cardiomyopathies
  - Often present early in life
  - Hypertrophied or (less commonly) dilated, poorly functioning heart
- Left-ventricular noncompaction cardiomyopathy
  - Cardiac dysfunction has a varying age of onset.
    - Newborn period to adulthood

DIFFERENTIAL DIAGNOSIS

- Peripheral pulmonary branch stenosis
  - Accompanied by a physiologic murmur
    - Short, relatively high-pitched II/VI systolic ejection murmur
    - Auscultated equally on both sides of the sternum with diffuse radiation to both lung fields
  - Characteristic of the natural transition period from fetal to postnatal circulation
    - Does not require urgent consultation
  - Most physicians are concerned that they may be missing the murmur produced by pulmonary stenosis.
    - This murmur is distinct from that of peripheral pulmonary stenosis in both its severity and focality.
    - Peripheral pulmonary branch stenosis is a softer, less intense murmur that is equally audible throughout the chest.
  - A murmur produced by significant valvar pulmonary stenosis will be:
    - Harsh in character
    - At least grade III on a severity scale of I to VI
    - Often preceded by a valve click

– Best auscultated at the left sternal border, but will radiate to both lung fields

■ Cyanosis

   ● In most of these situations, a cardiac lesion is not the cause.

      – Pulmonary disease is more commonly the culprit.

   ● Verify that cyanosis is truly present.

      – Acrocyanosis is a frequent occurrence in newborns, particularly in the setting of volume depletion or cool extremities.

      – Full-body cyanosis can occur in several scenarios, including respiratory distress syndrome.

■ Pediatric hypertension

   ● Any evaluation should include investigation for coarctation of the aorta.

■ RCM

   ● Care must be taken to distinguish RCM from constrictive pericarditis.

DIAGNOSTIC APPROACH

■ In all heart lesions, the severity of the obstruction determines:

   ● Age at presentation

   ● Clinical manifestations

■ Foremost diagnostic tools

   ● History and physical examination

      – Signs of low cardiac output

   ● Imaging

      – Electrocardiography

      – Chest radiography

      – Echocardiography

■ All patients with Down syndrome should be evaluated by a pediatric cardiologist within the first month of life.

LABORATORY FINDINGS

■ IE

   ● Blood cultures

      – Identical bacterial pathogens are identified before IE is diagnosed.

■ Myocarditis

   ● The following may be elevated.

      – Erythrocyte sedimentation rates

      – C-reactive protein

      – Leukocyte count

      – Platelet count

   ● Measures of cardiac cell damage to establish that myocyte injury has occurred and monitor progress

      – Troponin-I

      – Creatinine kinase–MB fraction

■ Verify the cause.

      – Serum viral cultures

      – Serologic titer assays

      – Polymerase chain reaction amplification of the viral genome

■ Pericarditis

   ● Determine the cause with:

      – Total cell count

      – Differential cell count

      – Glucose

      – Protein concentration

      – Gram stain

      – Acid-fast stain

      – Cultures (with viral polymerase chain reaction as indicated)

      – Cytologic assays

IMAGING

■ Chest radiography

   ● VSD and ASD

      – Generally noncontributory in diagnosing left-to-right shunt lesions before the onset of pulmonary overcirculation and the resulting pulmonary edema

      – Once pulmonary overcirculation has developed, the cardiac silhouette will gradually increase in area and pulmonary vascular markings will become substantially more prominent.

      – Can also be used to help assess effectiveness of medical management, such as diuretic therapy.

   ● Tetralogy of Fallot

      – The classic radiographic finding is the boot-shaped cardiac silhouette.

      – Relative right-ventricular hypertrophy in the healthy newborn often results in the erroneous reading of a boot-shaped cardiac silhouette on initial chest radiographic examination.

   ● Ebstein anomaly

      – Marked cardiomegaly from right-atrial dilation

   ● Dextrorotation

      – The classic radiographic finding for d-TGA is the *egg on a string*.

      – The great arteries are often oriented parallel (the string) instead of perpendicular, removing the aortic and pulmonary knobs.

      – This great artery orientation can also create a mesocardiac orientation of the cardiac silhouette producing an egg-shaped silhouette.

C

- Aortic stenosis
  - Chest radiography is helpful only if pulmonary edema has developed because of left-heart failure.
  - The anteroposterior projection of the cardiac silhouette is usually not particularly helpful.
- Coarctation of the aorta
  - In the adolescent with long-standing, unrepaired coarctation, rib notching may be seen from engorgement of the intercostal blood vessels.
- HLHS
  - Unless pulmonary overcirculation occurs, radiography is unlikely to contribute to the diagnosis, except possibly to differentiate a cardiac from a pulmonary source of cyanosis.
- Myocarditis
  - Global cardiac enlargement and increased pulmonary vascularity with varying degrees of edema
- Pericarditis
  - May be normal when the pericardial effusion is small
  - With a large effusion, the heart looks enlarged and has a globular appearance.
  - The pulmonary vascular marking may be prominent in patients with tamponade.
- Dilated cardiomyopathy
  - Cardiomegaly with or without increased pulmonary vascular markings
- Echocardiography
  - VSD and ASD
    - Two-dimensional echocardiography will show a defect in the interatrial or interventricular septum and allow for determination of cardiac function.
    - Doppler flow velocities across the defect can estimate pressure differences between the respective chambers.
    - Together, this information can help guide timing and type of surgical correction, if indicated.
  - Right-to-left shunting lesions
    - Two-dimensional and Doppler echocardiograms define cardiac anatomy, function, and direction of blood flow across any cardiac defects.
    - Doppler flow velocity across the RVOT allows estimation of outflow gradient, degree of obstruction, and any evidence of branch pulmonary artery stenosis.
  - Dextrorotation
    - Two-dimensional echocardiography will confirm the diagnosis and can evaluate the extent of intra- and extracardiac shunting.
    - ASD size, direction of ductus arteriosus shunting, and presence of a VSD are important components of intercirculatory mixing.

- Aortic stenosis
  - Two-dimensional echocardiography is adequate to diagnose aortic stenosis.
  - Hyperdynamic systolic function of a hypertrophied left-sided ventricle may be found.
  - A bicuspid aortic valve will be present in nearly 60% of cases.
  - Doppler flow can approximate the systolic flow gradient across the obstructed region.
  - In the setting of subvalvar aortic stenosis, flow acceleration begins below the valve and can be associated with aortic regurgitation.
  - Supravalvar aortic stenosis is commonly seen with Williams syndrome and should prompt a search for the associated lesion of pulmonary branch stenosis.
  - In the neonate with aortic stenosis, patency of the ductus arteriosus and its direction of flow are important to help plan an appropriate management strategy.
- Coarctation of the aorta
  - To determine whether the coarctation is ductal dependent and to evaluate for other left-sided obstructive lesions
  - Used to diagnose the presence of a hypoplastic aortic arch or discrete narrowing of the aorta
- HLHS
  - Confirmatory study
  - The sonographer should document presence or absence of PDA and flow through aortic and mitral valves, estimate the left-ventricular volume, determine size of the ascending aorta and ASD, and characterize the aortic arch and coarctation.
  - Size and competency of the pulmonary and tricuspid valves, and right-ventricular function are critical information to obtain to stratify surgical morbidity and mortality risks.
- IE
  - Transthoracic echocardiography
    - Excellent specificity, but poor sensitivity limits its role in the diagnosis of IE
  - Transesophageal echocardiography
    - Preferred visual diagnostic modality
    - Sensitivity of 80–90%
    - Should be strongly considered in highly suggestive cases even if transthoracic echocardiography is negative
- Myocarditis
  - Global cardiac chamber enlargement with atrioventricular valve regurgitation and poorly contracting ventricles

- Pericarditis
  - Most frequently used to assess the size of a pericardial effusion, which can occur with pericarditis
  - Very useful in detecting evidence for cardiac tamponade and associated conditions (ie, myocarditis)
- DCM
  - Confirms diagnosis
  - Dilated cardiac chambers, atrioventricular valve regurgitation, and depressed systolic function are nearly universal findings.
- HCM
  - Diagnostic method of choice
  - Type of hypertrophy (concentric versus asymmetric)
  - Ratio of interventricular septum to left-ventricular posterior wall thickness (>1.5 is diagnostic)
  - Presence of LVOT or RVOT obstruction
  - Systolic anterior motion of the anterior mitral valve leaflet
- RCM
  - Distinguish RCM from constrictive pericarditis
  - Echocardiogram shows normal ventricular size and function associated with dilated atria caused by the ventricular diastolic dysfunction.
- ARVD
  - Echocardiogram is diagnostic.
- Kawasaki disease
  - Evaluate for coronary artery aneurysms
  - Confirm diagnosis
- Computed tomography, magnetic resonance imaging
  - Pericarditis
    - If echocardiogram is inconclusive
    - Pericardial effusion is suspected to be loculated or hemorrhagic
    - Distinguish from RCM

DIAGNOSTIC PROCEDURES

- ECG
  - VSD and ASD
    - ECG can be normal for age in patients with both ASDs and VSDs.
    - As chamber dilation or hypertrophy occurs, however, signs of ventricular or atrial enlargement may develop.
    - Classic finding for patients with ASDs is an rSR' in lead V1 from volume overload of the right ventricle.
    - ECG may be helpful for identifying the onset of pulmonary hypertension by the gradual development of right-ventricular hypertrophy.
    - Patients with complete ASD defect generally demonstrate a northwest, superior QRS axis and some element of ventricular hypertrophy.

- AVSD
  - Left axis deviation
  - Northwest QRS axis
  - Small Q wave in lead aVL
- Tetralogy of Fallot and pulmonary hypertension
  - Right-axis deviation
  - Tall R waves in the early or right-sided precordial leads
- Pulmonary atresia
  - Hypoplastic ventricles
  - Decreased voltage in left or right precordial leads
  - Abnormal QRS axes
- Ebstein anomaly
  - Right atrial enlargement
- Dextrorotation
  - ECG generally unremarkable for a newborn
  - Will not offer added information unless other cardiac defects exist
- Aortic stenosis
  - ECG findings depend on disease severity.
  - In the newborn with critical stenosis:
    - ST-segment elevation or depression, T-wave inversion, and sinus tachycardia may be present.
    - Right-ventricular hypertrophy is usually noted.
    - Voltage criteria for left-ventricular hypertrophy may already be present or develop quickly.
  - Mild-to-moderate disease will probably demonstrate voltage criteria for left-ventricular hypertrophy, but ST- or T-wave changes are less likely.
- Coarctation of the aorta
  - ECG is unlikely to contribute to the diagnosis unless left-ventricular hypertrophy or strain is present.
- HLHS
  - A healthy newborn pattern of right-ventricular hypertrophy with a right-axis deviation may be more pronounced.
  - A distinguishing feature may be a relative paucity of left-ventricular forces.
- Myocarditis
  - A pathognomonic electrocardiographic finding is decreased precordial voltages consistent with a loss of functioning myocardium.
  - This finding can generally be differentiated from pericarditis by the absence of diffuse ST-segment elevation commonly present.
  - First-, second-, and third-degree atrioventricular block may develop, as well as wide-complex ventricular tachycardias.

- Pericarditis
  - Low-voltage QRS complexes with substantial pericardial effusion
  - Changes caused by associated myocarditis, such as diffuse ST elevation in initial stages
  - Gradually, the ST segment begins to normalize, with decrease in the T-wave amplitude eventually leading to T-wave inversion.
  - These ECG changes may resolve completely, with the exception of T-wave abnormalities, which may persist for long periods.
- DCM
  - May show biventricular hypertrophy by voltage criteria with ST-segment and T-wave abnormalities
- HCM
  - ECG is abnormal in 90–95% of cases.
  - Large voltages in the precordial leads suggest biventricular hypertrophy, ST-segment elevation and depression, T-wave inversion, and abnormally deep Q waves.
  - Occasional delta wave of Wolff-Parkinson-White syndrome
  - Tendency for frequent episodes of ventricular tachycardia and ST-segment elevation on ECG during exercise
- Cardiac catheterization
  - May be required with total anomalous PVR or partial anomalous PVR
    - Particularly in cases of complex anatomy
  - The diagnosis can be difficult to confirm by echocardiography.
  - Distinguishes RCM from constrictive pericarditis
- Endomyocardial biopsy
  - Required for the definitive diagnosis of myocarditis
- Pericardiocentesis
  - Diagnostic and therapeutic
    - Pericardial fluid collection is large or rapidly increasing.
    - Bacterial pericarditis or when tuberculous pericarditis is suspected
  - Drains the fluid to minimize the potential for clinical decompensation from tamponade
  - Allows possible etiologic diagnosis

CLASSIFICATION

- 6 grades of systolic or diastolic murmur severity
  - Grade I
    - Barely audible and may require several cardiac cycles to detect
  - Grade II
    - Soft, but easily audible

- Grade III
  - Moderately loud murmur without a thrill
- Grade IV
  - Loud murmur with a thrill
- Grade V
  - Loud murmur heard with the stethoscope barely off the chest
- Grade VI
  - Loud murmur heard without the stethoscope touching the chest

TREATMENT APPROACH

- Prevention of disease progression
  - Consultation with a pediatric cardiologist if pathologic entity is suspected
- Determining whether surgical intervention is required
  - Preoperative management to maximize survival and minimize morbidity and mortality
  - Maintaining cardiovascular stability
  - End-organ perfusion and oxygen delivery
  - Multidisciplinary approach

SPECIFIC TREATMENTS

VSD and ASD

- Patients with known septal defects should be monitored closely for:
  - Weight gain
  - Development
  - Clinical status
- Any signs of respiratory distress or failure to thrive will generally occur during the first 6 months of life.
  - Reevaluation by the pediatric cardiologist is indicated.
- Medical management
  - Temporary improvement of complications may be achieved with:
    - Diuretics
    - Afterload reduction
- Definitive prompt closure of an ASD or VSD
  - Indicated when signs of pulmonary overcirculation develop

PDA

- In a healthy infant
  - Outpatient follow-up
    - Most PDAs close within days to months postnatally.
- Indocin
  - Standard treatment
    - If contraindicated or unsuccessful, PDA can often be ligated in the neonatal intensive care unit.

- Coil embolization
  - Indicated if persistent into childhood
  - Performed in the catheterization laboratory
- Surgical closure
  - In the presence of decreased renal perfusion or pulmonary overcirculation

AVSD

- Surgical repair
  - Indicated for complete AVSD, includes:
    - Patch closure of the ASD and VSD
    - Creation of 2 functioning atrioventricular valves from the single, frequently regurgitant common atrioventricular valve
    - Performed between 3 and 6 months of age to minimize the potential for irreversible pulmonary hypertension
  - Postoperative outcomes depend on:
    - Severity of any residual atrioventricular valve regurgitation
    - Presence of pulmonary vascular disease
  - Partial AVSD
    - Can generally be repaired later in life (first few years)
    - Low risk of pulmonary vascular obstructive disease

Arteriovenous malformations

- Coil embolization
  - May reduce or reverse heart failure in many cases

Tetrology of Fallot

- Tet spell (hypercyanotic spell)
  - Uncommon, but can be fatal if not treated urgently
    - Supplemental oxygen
    - Fluid boluses
    - Anxiolytics
    - Sedatives
    - Knee-to-chest positioning
    - Phenylephrine
- Tetralogy of Fallot without pulmonary atresia
  - Neonatal intensive care unit monitoring
    - Until ductus arteriosus (if present) closes
    - Patients who can produce pulmonary blood flow to maintain SaO_2 >80% may be discharged from the hospital and allowed to grow.
  - Surgical repair
    - Tet spell is a semi-urgent indication for repair.
    - In the absence of earlier unacceptable cyanosis (SaO_2 <75%), elective repair is performed at age 4–6 months.
    - Operative correction consists of patching the VSD and correcting the obstruction to pulmonary blood flow.

- Resection or division (or both) of RVOT muscle bundles is performed first through the right atrium to remove this source of impedance.
- The VSD is then patched.
- Finally, depending on pulmonary artery anatomy, a patch is placed:
  - Supravalvar (main pulmonary artery)
  - Subvalvar (infundibular or outflow region)
  - Transvalvar (across the pulmonary valve annulus and extending into the supra and subvalvar regions)
- In many cases, a pulmonary valvectomy is performed during these repairs.
  - Patients are left with some degree of pulmonary insufficiency.
- Tetralogy of Fallot with pulmonary atresia
  - Prostaglandin E_1 infusion
    - Maintains ductal patency until surgical repair
  - Surgical repair
    - If pulmonary artery size is favorable (>3 mm in diameter):
      - Complete repair can be performed in the neonate.
    - If pulmonary artery size is unfavorable (<3 mm in diameter):
      - An aortopulmonary shunt is placed to allow pulmonary artery growth until complete repair is performed later.
    - Patients without confluent pulmonary arteries who rely instead on multiple aortopulmonary collaterals
      - The collateral arteries can be unifocalized through a single or staged procedure to a conduit arising from the right ventricle.

Eisenmenger syndrome

- Surgical closure of the septal defect
  - Will worsen the outcome if pulmonary hypertension is not addressed first
  - If not reversed, pulmonary hypertension can be fatal.
- Multiple approaches to decreasing pulmonary artery pressure and right-to-left shunting
  - Calcium-channel blockers
  - Nitric oxide donors
  - Endothelin receptor antagonists
  - Inhaled oxygen therapy
  - Continuous infusions of prostacyclin (severe cases)
    - If the pulmonary vasculature proves to be reactive with these measures, surgical intervention may be considered.
- Lung transplantation
  - May be the only other therapeutic option if the pulmonary vasculature does not respond to medications to decrease pulmonary hypertension

Pulmonary atresia

- Opening pulmonary valve
  - Balloon dilation or radiofrequency ablation to perforate through the valve cusps.
    - This approach is controversial and, in many institutions, surgical valvotomy is preferred.
  - If right-heart structures are significantly affected, the single-ventricle treatment route must be used.
    - Surgical specifics will be determined by the presence or absence of sinusoids.

Ebstein anomaly

- Treatment consists of monitoring until the ductus arteriosus closes and PVR decreases.
  - At that time, the degree of forward pulmonary blood flow can be reassessed.
  - If pulmonary blood flow is adequate to produce SaO_2 >75–80%, the infant may be discharged from the hospital.
    - PVR should continue to decrease with a commensurate increase in systemic SaO_2.
- Single-ventricle palliative surgery
  - Consider in infants with insufficient pulmonary blood flow.

Total anomalous PVR

- Surgical correction
  - Infracardiac drainage frequently becomes obstructed at some point along the extended, tortuous course of the vertical vein into the liver.
    - When present, constitutes a surgical emergency
  - Surgical correction for uncomplicated total anomalous PVR consists of reanastomosis of the pulmonary venous confluence to the posterior wall of the left atrium.
    - Common postoperative complications
      - Obstruction at the site of the anastomosis
      - Pulmonary vein stenosis
      - Left-atrial dysrhythmias

Partial anomalous PVR

- Surgical correction may not be necessary unless symptoms develop (ie, exercise intolerance).
  - Unless ≥1 of the pulmonary veins returns anomalously, this anomaly rarely becomes hemodynamically significant.

Dextrorotation

- Preoperative management
  - Complex to manage in the newborn period
  - The most important component is maintaining adequate atrial-level shunting.
    - Although the presence of a VSD is important when considering surgical options, ventricular-level shunting does not usually contribute a significant amount of intracardiac mixing in the newborn period.

- Prostaglandin E_1 infusions
  - Many patients with d-TGA have already begun receiving prostaglandin E_1 infusions at the time of diagnosis after failing the hyperoxia challenge.
  - Dosing ranges from 0.02–0.2 mcg/kg per minute.
    - Higher doses inherently increase the side effect profile.
    - PDA diameter cannot generally be titrated by changing infusion doses.
    - Once open, only doses of 0.01–0.02 mcg/kg per minute are usually required to maintain patency.
  - May be discontinued after assessing for paradoxical cyanosis (as seen with persistent fetal circulation), SaO_2, and arterial oxygen content
    - Arterial oxygen content >30 mm Hg (typical fetal partial pressure of oxygen in arterial blood) with a corresponding SaO_2 >75–80%, in the absence of metabolic acidosis, is predictive of adequate atrial-level mixing.
    - If these conditions are not met and the newborn demonstrates any signs of respiratory distress or pulmonary edema with marked cyanosis, the ASD is probably restrictive and needs to be enlarged.
  - Side effects of prostaglandin E_1
    - Apnea (prophylaxis with caffeine or aminophylline may decrease risk)
    - Irritability
    - Hyperthermia
    - Jitteriness
    - Decreased leukocyte function
    - High probability of intubation
- Catheterization procedures
  - Balloon septostomy (Rashkind procedure)
  - Blade septostomy
  - Radiofrequency ablation of the atrial septum
    - These procedures increase blood exchange and systemic oxygen delivery.
    - These life-saving interventions can be associated with significant risks of morbidity and mortality.
- Surgical correction
  - Arterial switch (Jantene) operation
    - Surgical option of choice for most patients with d-TGA
    - Technically complex operation
      - Once the patient is placed on cardiopulmonary bypass, the aortic and pulmonary arteries are transected above their native valves.
      - The surgeon removes the coronary arteries from the aortic root (arising from the right ventricle) by cutting small buttons of tissue surrounding the coronary artery's ostium.

- Similar-sized buttons of tissue are removed from the pulmonary artery (arising from the left ventricle), and the coronary arteries are sutured into the native pulmonary artery root (arising from the left ventricle).

- The aorta is freely mobile within the thorax and is easily sutured to the exposed pulmonary artery root.

- The main and branch pulmonary arteries remain attached to the lungs and are subsequently more restricted in their range of motion.

- To minimize surgical stretch and subsequent obstruction, the Lecompte maneuver is performed, which drapes the main and branch pulmonary arteries over the ascending aorta instead of underneath.

- Abnormal coronary artery anatomic configuration
  - Occurs in ~30% of all patients with d-TGA
  - This abnormality can produce one of the major complications of the arterial switch operation.
    - A single coronary artery origin necessitates flipping of the button before reimplantation and is often associated with kinking and compromise of coronary artery flow.
  - Although no coronary pattern precludes a switch, transmural (coursing through the arterial wall) coronary artery anatomy and others may increase the risk of the procedure.
    - Alternative surgical approaches may be necessary.
  - Discordant annulus size of the great arteries can also produce difficulty.
    - Not usually a contraindication to an arterial switch

- Surgical outcomes
  - An overall mortality rate of 7% was reported in 1 study of 223 patients with d-TGA after the arterial switch operation.
    - Coronary artery pattern was not associated with an increased risk of death.
    - However, 2 studies with a total of 1263 patients demonstrated a rate of coronary artery events between 7% and 8% over 15 years of follow-up.
  - Abnormal coronary artery vasomotor function has been demonstrated in asymptomatic children after arterial switch.
  - Patients require close postoperative follow-up.

Aortic stenosis

- If diagnosed prenatally or shortly after birth in an otherwise healthy, stable newborn:
  - Careful monitoring alone is justified.
  - Timely intervention on rapidly progressive stenosis can be planned before congestive heart failure and systemic shock occur.

- Right-to-left shunting through the ductus arteriosus suggests ductal-dependent systemic cardiac output (in the absence of persistent fetal circulation).
  - Patient should remain monitored in the hospital until a final decision regarding the need for intervention is reached.

- Balloon valvuloplasty
  - Standard of care for valvar aortic stenosis
    - Equally effective with less morbidity and mortality vs surgical valvotomy
    - In most cases, aortic valvotomy results in some degree of aortic insufficiency.
    - Degree of insufficiency is usually mild and is well tolerated for many years.
  - Indications for nonemergent balloon valvuloplasty
    - Progressively severe left-ventricular hypertrophy with a transvalvar gradient >50 mm Hg
    - Most cardiologists would also intervene in the presence of:
      - Syncope
      - Exercise intolerance
      - Chest pain
      - Abnormal exercise stress test

- Surgical intervention
  - Indications
    - Stenosis is accompanied by significant valvar insufficiency.
    - More than moderate insufficiency develops after a balloon procedure.
  - Surgical options
    - Valve replacement with a prosthetic mechanical valve
    - Cadaveric homograft
    - Porcine xenograft
    - Pulmonary valve autograft (Ross procedure)
  - Important considerations
    - Patient age
    - Size
    - Lifestyle
    - Future adherence to an anticoagulation regimen

- Subaortic stenosis
  - With the exception of an absent valve click, subaortic stenosis is clinically indistinguishable from valvar stenosis.
    - However, blood flow velocity becomes accelerated before reaching the aortic valve and gradually damages the leaflets over time, which can result in progressive valvar regurgitation.

C

- Surgical resection of this subaortic region is indicated to:
  - Relieve obstruction
  - Prevent progressive aortic valve damage and resultant insufficiency
  - In general, surgical resection is performed with the onset of any degree of aortic insufficiency or gradients between 20 and 40 mm Hg.
- The decision to intervene is difficult.
  - Recurrence after resection is common.
  - Significant valve damage cannot be accurately predicted.
  - The rate of progression of subaortic stenosis is insidious and is not associated with acute cardiovascular decompensation.
- Progressive valvar damage may ultimately require valve repair or replacement.
  - Homograft valve
  - Artificial valve
  - Autograft valve via the Ross procedure
- Supravalvar aortic stenosis (least common form)
  - When surgery is indicated:
    - Patch aortoplasty of the narrowed region is corrective.
      - Reduces the coronary artery perfusion pressure and can produce coronary artery ischemia

Coarctation of the aorta

- Initial treatment
  - Infusion of prostaglandin E_1 to maintain ductal patency or regain it
  - Patient should receive no enteral feeds.
    - Possible intestinal underperfusion
  - Renal function should be monitored closely.
- Discharged newborn or ductus closed at home insidiously, resulting in a coarctation
  - Shock is likely to be present from poor lower-body perfusion.
  - Patients should be treated similarly but will also require:
    - Frequent blood gas monitoring for assessment and correction of acidosis
    - Possible mechanical ventilation
    - Upper- and lower-extremity blood pressures to track the success of the prostaglandin infusion in regaining ductal patency
  - If the clinician cannot reestablish adequate lower-body perfusion:
    - Emergent intervention may be required.
- Balloon dilation
  - Gradient >20 mm Hg is generally considered the clinical indication for intervention.
- Balloon dilatation results in splitting or tearing of intimal or proximal medial tissue planes.
  - Will often be repeated 2–3 times to ensure adequate luminal diameter
- Stent placement during balloon dilatation reduces the rate of restenosis and provides significant relief from obstruction in adults.
- Metallic stent placement is not recommended in young children; the artificial stent will not grow with the rapidly growing patient.
- Surgical management (standard of care)
  - Discrete coarctations
    - Subclavian flap repair
      - The subclavian artery closest to the coarctation (generally the left) is ligated distally and filleted open.
      - The coarctation region is also filleted open.
      - The flap of subclavian artery tissue is then rotated and sutured in place.
      - Less likely to result in aneurysmal dilatation of the segment of aorta, but can be associated with a mild growth retardation and loss of strength in the respective arm
    - Patch aortoplasty
      - Use of a Dacron patch to open the coarctation
  - Coarctation associated with isthmic hypoplasia
    - Coarctation segment resection with extended end-to-end reanastomosis
  - Coarctation associated with a diffuse segment of transverse arch hypoplasia
    - Not generally amenable to an extended end-to-end reanastomosis, except in specific circumstances

HLHS

- Prostaglandin E_1 infusion
  - Should be started immediately if HLHS is suspected
    - Starting doses can vary widely based on clinical status, but all can result in apnea.
  - If cardiac lesion is strongly suspected, beginning prostaglandin E_1 infusion should not be held until a pediatric cardiology consult can be obtained.
- Arterial and venous catheters
  - Should be inserted if possible, when diagnosis is confirmed
- Parameters directing management:
  - Renal function (assessed by urine output and serum creatinine)
  - Blood pressure
  - SaO_2
  - Arterial blood gases

- Strategies to provide adequate pulmonary and systemic blood flow
  - Hypoxia
    - Producing subambient oxygen by increased nitrogen infusion into the inhaled gas mixture
  - Hypercarbia
    - Increasing carbon dioxide content of inhaled gas mixture
  - Permissive hypercapnia
    - When patient is intubated, decreasing minute ventilation with resultant pulmonary vasoconstriction
  - Decreasing systemic vascular resistance with vasodilatory medications
    - Milrinone
    - Phenoxybenzamine
- Surgical intervention
  - Surgical options depend on how blood flow is provided to the lungs and body.
  - The strategy for all single-ventricle hearts is based on 2 simple premises, regardless of which ventricle is hypoplastic.
    - A single ventricle cannot perform the function of 2 ventricles indefinitely.
    - PVR is elevated initially after birth and, in most cases, does not decrease completely until 2–6 months of age.
    - The physiologic characteristic does not change regardless of which ventricle is hypoplastic.
  - First-stage palliative surgery (Norwood procedure)
    - Produces a neoaorta from the main pulmonary artery and the hypoplastic ascending aorta
    - Necessary but suboptimal
    - PVR does not fully decrease for several months and requires systemic blood pressures to overcome elevated pulmonary artery pressures.
    - The right ventricle is then obligated to perform as both a right and a left ventricle and is also volume overloaded from shunt-mediated pulmonary overcirculation.
  - Second-stage palliative surgery
    - Performed once PVR decreases
    - Decreases the work of the single ventricle by removing the need for active pumping of the pulmonary blood supply
    - The Glenn procedure connects the SVC to the pulmonary artery, and the previously placed shunt or conduit is ligated.
    - Pulmonary blood flow is provided passively from the SVC into the low-resistance and low-pressure pulmonary arteries.
    - Systemic SaO_2 after the Norwood and Glenn procedures will generally remain 75–85%, and patients typically have a higher hemoglobin concentration than acyanotic children.
  - Third-stage palliative surgery
    - Fontan procedure
    - Baffles the IVC to the pulmonary artery, routing all systemic venous return directly into the lungs
    - Oxygen-rich blood s separated from oxygen-poor blood.
    - Systemic SaO_2 is typically near normal (>90%).

Tricuspid atresia

- Surgical correction
  - Less complicated than with HLHS correction because it does not require formation of a neoaorta
    - Aortopulmonary shunt is placed to provide pulmonary blood flow.
  - Glenn and Fontan surgeries are the same as for HLHS.

IE

- A prolonged course of intravenous antibioticsis given to eradicate the high concentration of organisms deeply embedded in the fibrin-platelet matrix.
  - Duration of intravenous therapy will vary between 2 and 6 weeks, depending on bacterial speciation and antimicrobial sensitivity.
    - Blood cultures should be repeated during and after antibiotic therapy to ensure proper choice and duration.
  - For a complete review of the suggested regimen of antibiotic therapy, see the American Heart Association's recommendations for IE therapy in adults.
- Once the patient has received adequate therapy and demonstrated several negative blood cultures, the infection can generally be considered cleared.
  - If no evidence exists of congenital heart disease or significant valvar derangement, then continued evaluation by a pediatric cardiologist may not be indicated.

Myocarditis

- Treatment is largely supportive.
  - Although antiviral medications, corticosteroids, and intravenous γ-globulin are administered, limited and somewhat controversial data exist to support their use.
- Milder cases
  - Bed rest
  - Hospitalization until the patient's cardiac status returns to baseline
- More severe cases
  - Aggressive diuresis
  - Inotropy
  - Chronotropy
  - Afterload-reducing medications
  - Antiarrhythmic agents
  - Ventilator support

C

- Mechanical circulatory support
  - Extracorporeal membrane oxygenation
  - Ventricular assist devices
- Patients who survive the initial phase
  - Many will require long-term medical therapy.
    - Diuresis
    - Afterload reduction
    - Long-term antiarrhythmic medications
    - Automatic implantable cardioverter defibrillators (ICDs)
    - ß-Blockers (experimental)
- When patients do not respond adequately to medical or mechanical support
  - Cardiac transplantation is the only alternative for long-term survival in appropriately selected patients.

Pericarditis

- Management of pericarditis depends on:
  - Size and cause of the effusion
  - Effect on cardiac function
- Purulent pericarditis
  - Urgent decompression
    - Life-saving in patients with cardiac tamponade
    - Necessary for suspected purulent pericardial effusion
  - Percutaneous pericardiocentesis or surgical drainage
    - Large-bore pericardial drain or a surgically created pericardial window
    - Permits continuous drainage of purulent material
    - Prevents development of tamponade
  - Intrapericardial infusion of a fibrinolytic agent
    - Streptokinase decreases the recurrence of pericardial effusion.
  - Antibiotics
    - Given intravenously for 4–6 weeks
  - Partial or total pericardiectomy
    - Often necessary after treatment of purulent effusions to prevent development of constrictive pericarditis
- Viral pericarditis
  - No treatment other than a short course of antiinflammatory medication, such as ibuprofen.
- Pericarditis associated with other conditions
  - Treatment of the underlying condition leads to the resolution of the pericardial effusion.
    - Patients should be treated aggressively for all episodes of strep pharyngitis and receive appropriate procedural antibiotic prophylaxis.
  - Corticosteroids
    - Can be considered for persistent or refractory viral or secondary pericarditis

DCM

- Pharmacologic intervention
  - Treats the symptoms of congestive heart failure
  - Blunts the neurohumoral cascade
  - Aggressive diuresis
    - Spironolactone
    - Reduces pulmonary edema, hepatic congestion, excessive intravascular volume expansion
  - Angiotensin-converting enzyme inhibitors, angiotensin receptor blockers
    - Decrease morbidity and mortality
    - Use is discouraged in the acute, decompensated period.
  - ß-Blocker therapy
    - One of the few medical interventions for congestive heart failure that has evidence supporting its use in both adults and children
  - Anticoagulation therapy
    - Aspirin
    - Warfarin
    - Commonly used to reduce the risk of thrombus formation
- Cardiac resynchronization therapy
  - Pacing modality used in patients with DCM and heart failure refractory to conventional medical management
    - Synchronizes ventricular wall motion
    - Improves diastolic filling and systolic ejection fraction
    - Reduces symptoms
    - Further research is needed to determine efficacy in patients without intraventricular conduction delay or with nonsinus rhythms.
    - Use in children is limited by lack of controlled study data.
- Severe cases
  - Ventricular assist devices
  - Extracorporeal membrane oxygenation
  - Cardiac transplantation
    - May be indicated in appropriately selected patients if other treatment regimens are unsuccessful

HCM

- Symptomatic relief
- Minimizing the risk of fatal arrhythmias
  - Exercise stress tests
  - 24-hour Holter monitoring to help stratify risk of ventricular tachycardia and sudden death
  - Asymptomatic, nonsustained ventricular tachycardia on Holter monitor increases risk of sudden death 8–10 times.

- Pharmacologic intervention
  - ß-Blockers
    - Indicated for patients who have symptoms or left-ventricular outflow tract obstruction at rest.
  - If ß-blockers are poorly tolerated:
    - Calcium-channel blockers have been shown to produce similar effects.
  - Amiodarone
    - Indicated when tachycardia is present
  - Prophylactic implantation of an automatic ICD is strongly recommended for patients with:
    - Left ventricular wall thickness >3.0 cm
    - Family history of death related to HCM
    - Unexplained syncope
    - Nonsustained ventricular tachycardia on Holter monitor
  - Automatic ICD implantation as secondary prevention in patients with:
    - Aborted sudden death
    - Documented ventricular tachycardia or fibrillation
    - Malignant ventricular ectopy
    - Now considered the standard of care
- Surgical myomectomy
  - Reduction of flow gradient in patients whose symptoms are related to their degree of left-ventricular outflow tract obstruction
  - Brock or Morrow procedure
    - Reserved for symptomatic, medically refractory patients with an ventricular outflow tract gradient >50–60 mm Hg
    - 10-year survival rate approximately 86%
    - Intraoperative mortality rate can approach 5%.
- Medical septal reduction
  - Alternative to surgical myomectomy to improve left-ventricular outflow tract obstruction
    - Infusion of desiccated alcohol into the septal perforating coronary vessels in the interventricular septum
  - Performed under transesophageal echocardiographic guidance in the cardiac catheterization laboratory
  - Advocated for patients with HCM who are failing medical management
    - Has been used with a resting ventricular outflow tract gradient as low as 40 mm Hg
  - Reduces the morbidity and mortality compared with surgery; however, risk is increased in:
    - Coronary artery dissection
    - Uncontrolled myocardial infarction
    - Complete heart block (5–10% risk) requiring pacemaker placement

RCM

- Generally unresponsive to conventional medical therapy
- Patients should be referred for heart transplantation once the diagnosis is made.
  - Pulmonary hypertension that is unresponsive to pulmonary vasodilators is the most commonly cited problem preventing heart transplantation in these patients.

Miscellaneous cardiomyopathies

- ARVD
  - Treatment is directed at preventing life-threatening arrhythmias
    - Medications
    - Automatic ICDs
- Kawasaki disease
  - In the absence of cardiac involvement at either presentation or a 2- to 4-week follow-up appointment, further evaluation by a pediatric cardiologist is probably unnecessary.

Orthotopic heart transplantation (OHT)

- Standard therapy for end-stage congenital and acquired heart disease
- Indications for OHT
  - Infants
    - >75% of all recipients <1 year undergo OHT because of surgically irreparable congenital heart disease.
    - 17% of cardiomyopathy-related heart failure and dysrhythmias unresponsive to medical therapy result in OHT.
  - Adolescents
    - ~25% of 11- to 17-year-old OHT recipients have surgically irreparable congenital heart disease.
    - 62% of cardiomyopathy-related heart failure and dysrhythmias unresponsive to medical therapy result in OHT.
- Contraindications
  - Absolute
    - Significantly elevated PVR
    - Elevated PVR unresponsive to vasodilatory therapy (ie, oxygen and nitric oxide)
    - Active cancer
    - Hepatic cirrhosis
  - Relative
    - Bacterial or viral infection
- The decision to proceed with OHT should be made on the basis of the individual patient's clinical status.
  - Cardiac catheterization
    - Determine hemodynamics and PVR.

- Complete antiviral antibody titer panel
  - Exclude infection and guide use of antiviral medications postoperatively.
    - Herpes simplex virus
    - Cytomegalovirus
    - HIV
    - Epstein-Barr virus
    - Hepatitis A, B, and C
- Panel reactive antibody testing
  - Assess the amount of circulating preformed antibodies in the recipient's serum.
  - May limit acceptable donor organs
- Social screening
  - Evaluate a potential recipient's emotional coping skills.
- Financial screening
  - Verify that the financial burden of transplantation is minimized.

■ Transplant status classification
- Strongly influences the expected waiting time for the recipient
  - Transplant status can change at any time if the clinical condition improves or worsens.
- UNOS (United Network for Organ Sharing) status Ia
  - Generally several days to months before receiving a heart transplant, assuming survival is possible for this period
  - Patient must be inotrope dependent and hospitalized.
- UNOS status II
  - Depending on weight and blood type, infants >6 months can expect to wait up to several months.
  - Adolescents may require as long as 2 years before a suitable heart is located.

■ Surgical procedure
- The donor heart is harvested in its entirety, with the exception of a cuff of posterior left atrial wall, which contains the pulmonary veins.
- Once the recipient is placed on cardiopulmonary bypass, the heart is removed in a reciprocal fashion.
- Anastomosis of the donor heart to the recipient is performed by either a biatrial or a bicaval (SVC-IVC) connection.

■ Postoperative management
- Unique challenge of managing a patient with a denervated heart that has been ischemic for as long as 4 hours
- Heart rate
  - Dependent on the intrinsic sinoatrial nodal rate
  - Not influenced by the Valsalva maneuver, carotid massage, or atropine

- The resting heart rate of a transplanted heart is typically higher than that in normal controls.
  - However, it is frequently abnormally slow in the immediate postoperative period.
- Isoproterenol
  - Can be titrated to produce the desired heart rate
- As the transplanted heart begins to recuperate from the surgical insult, heart rate and cardiac output will increase to meet the patient's needs.

- Immunosuppressive medications
  - Typically started soon after the transplantation is complete
  - The dosage is gradually decreased with time after transplantation.
    - Calcineurin inhibitor (ie, tacrolimus or cyclosporine) plus
    - Antimetabolite (ie, mycophenolate mofetil or azathioprine) plus
    - Corticosteroids
  - Side effects
    - Cyclosporine and tacrolimus: hypertension, nephrotoxicity, and derangement of the lipid profile (especially cyclosporine)
    - Azathioprine: neutropenia and hepatotoxicity
    - Mycophenolate: lymphopenia and gastrointestinal distress (may require dose adjustment)
    - Side effects of corticosteroids have been well described.

WHEN TO ADMIT

■ Same as when to refer (see next section)

WHEN TO REFER

■ Diminished or absent femoral pulses

■ PDA murmur in the presence of decreased renal perfusion or pulmonary overcirculation

■ Coarctation of the aorta
- Pulses absent or thready
- Lower-extremity blood pressures >15 mm Hg less than upper extremities

■ Cyanotic heart lesion is suspected
- Persistent hypoxemia (<70–80 mm Hg) despite adequate oxygen therapy
- Failure of the hyperoxia challenge

■ Progression of cardiomyopathy
- Murmur
- New gallop
- Abnormal ECG or chest radiograph

- Indicators of declining cardiac function
  - Weight loss or a plateau in weight gain
  - Missed developmental milestones
  - Fatigue
  - Activity intolerance
  - Personality changes
- OHT recipients who:
  - Are febrile, immunosuppressed without obvious, treatable cause
    - The transplant cardiologist should be involved to minimize the chance that graft rejection will be misinterpreted as a common, benign infectious illness.
  - Show signs of rejection
    - New-onset fatigue
    - Shortness of breath
    - Exercise intolerance
    - Low-grade fever
    - Vomiting
    - Diarrhea
  - Have unexplained abdominal distention, pain, or vomiting
    - Should prompt evaluation for an ileus or intussusception
    - May also be a sign of intestinal angina caused by decreased cardiac output
  - Have no chest pain
    - Absence of pain should not be comforting to the physician.
    - A denervated transplanted heart will not become significantly tachycardic in response to fever or pain.
    - A heart rate increase of only 10 beats per minute may indicate imminent cardiovascular collapse.

FOLLOW-UP

- Aortic stenosis
  - Once the infant is home, most pediatric cardiologists will arrange biweekly or monthly visits for the first 6 months of life.
  - During this rapid phase of somatic growth, changes in clinical status or aortic stenosis gradient can occur quickly.
  - When neonatal intervention is required, frequent return visits may occur for at least the first 6 months of life.
- After valve repair
  - Patients must be proactively managed in the postoperative cardiac intensive care unit.
- Coarctation repair
  - Complications include paradoxic hypertension or systemic blood pressure higher than preoperative measures.
    - ß-Blockers are often used to treat hypertension in the immediate postoperative period.
    - When hypertension persists beyond the first few postoperative days, an giotensin-converting enzyme inhibitors offset the renin-mediated phase of hypertension.
- Monitoring for rejection after OHT
  - Potentially life-threatening situation
    - Cellular rejection can begin within the first 5–7 days after transplantation
    - Highest incidence during the first 3 post-OHT months
  - Patients may exhibit:
    - Malaise
    - Anorexia
    - Gastrointestinal distress
    - Low-grade fever
    - Nonspecific changes in sleeping patterns
  - If significant rejection is present, physical examination will reveal:
    - Hepatomegaly
    - Mild elevation in heart rate from baseline
    - Possibly a new murmur or gallop
  - Patients require prompt evaluation and assessment.
    - Echocardiography to assess cardiac function
    - Endomyocardial biopsy if indicated
  - If disease proves the presence of rejection:
    - Pulse steroids are administered.
    - Maintenance immunosuppressive regimen will usually be augmented.
  - Repeat biopsy
    - Necessary to verify effective treatment for the rejection episode
  - Interventions (ie, scheduled vaccinations) that might upregulate the immune response
    - Delay for approximately 3 months after resolution of the episode.
  - Frequent blood monitoring of OHT recipients
    - Immunosuppressive agent side effects, such as neutropenia and hepatotoxicity

COMPLICATIONS

- Complications of OHT
  - First 6 months
    - Bacterial infections in 52% of patients
    - Opportunistic infections in 15% of patients
  - After 6 months
    - Immunosuppressive medications are decreased to maintenance dosing.
    - Predominant infectious organisms shift from bacterial to viral (83% of infections).

- Specific microbes parallel those afflicting the general, nonimmunosuppressed pediatric population.
- Long-term complications
  - Posttransplantation lymphoproliferative disease
    - Abnormal growth of lymphoreticular cells in immunosuppressed patients
    - Occurs in approximately 5–10% of pediatric OHT recipients
    - Has been linked to primary posttransplant Epstein-Barr virus infection
    - Most forms can be treated solely by a decrease in immunosuppression.
    - Some forms will require chemotherapy and possibly surgical resection.
  - Posttransplantation coronary vasculopathy
    - Progressive intimal and medial thickening of the transplanted heart's coronary arteries, with loss of coronary flow reserve and eventual luminal obliteration
    - Risk increases with each episode of rejection, certain infections (ie, cytomegalovirus), original harvest time, and associated donor ischemic time; it is also increased in the presence of abnormal lipid profiles.
    - Statins (ie, pravastatin, atorvastatin) have been recommended in OHT recipients.
    - Freedom from posttransplantation coronary vasculopathy decreases with time from transplantation and with each decade of life after which transplantation occurs.
  - Newer immunosuppressant agents (ie, sirolimus) have shown initial promise as potential treatments for posttransplantation coronary vasculopathy; however, retransplantation is the only definitive therapy.
- Immunization
  - Live viral vaccines
    - Should not be given
    - The immunosuppressed patient's response to vaccinations will be blunted, particularly during the early post-OHT period.
    - Any systemic antigenic response may precipitate a rejection episode.
  - Nonlive vaccinations
    - Should be given approximately 3 months after transplantation to minimize rejection
- Immunosuppression
  - Predisposes these patients to serious infectious complications
    - However, deficiency in these medications places them at significant risk for rejection.

PROGNOSIS

- VSDs and ASDs
  - Natural history
    - Regardless of the mechanism, the PVR will reflexively increase in proportion to the degree of shunt volume (in ASD and VSD) and pressure (in VSD) to reduce stress on the arteriolar walls.
      - Over time, these pulmonary arterioles can become quite hypertrophied and cannot vasodilate.
      - This irreversible state of pulmonary arteriolar vasoconstriction results in pulmonary hypertension and eventual pulmonary vascular obstructive disease.
    - Small defects in the muscular portion of the interventricular septum often close spontaneously.
      - VSDs in other regions of the interventricular septum close less commonly.
    - The natural history of secundum-type ASDs depends largely on the initial defect size.
      - Nearly 85% <5 mm in diameter resolve spontaneously.
      - <2% resolve when they are >8 mm in diameter.
  - Patients at risk for pulmonary vascular obstructive disease
    - Those in whom VSDs neither close spontaneously nor are associated with pulmonary overcirculation
    - Those with an unrepaired defect and persistently elevated PVR (eventually can become irreversible)
      - As early as 6 months of age, particularly in patients with trisomy 21 syndrome
      - As early as 1 year in children without Down syndrome
      - When pulmonary artery pressures exceed those of the left ventricle, the direction of shunted blood will become right to left, producing peripheral cyanosis (Eisenmenger syndrome).
  - Surgical mortality rates
    - <1% for both ASDs and VSDs
    - Device closure vs surgical correction of ASDs
      - Failure rate requiring surgical repair occurs in 4% of patients with devices.
      - Device-related complication rate, 7.2%; surgical complication rate, 24%
    - Device closure of VSDs
      - Currently being performed in limited situations
      - Success rates have been reported to be 99% but have been associated with a nearly 50% serious complication rate.

- Tetralogy of Fallot
  - Surgical outcomes
    - Pulmonary valvectomy performed during repairs leaves patients with some degree of pulmonary insufficiency.
      - Progressive RV dilation associated with pulmonary insufficiency is one of the sources of long-term morbidity in these patients.
    - Unifocalization of collateral arteries
      - 10- and 20-year actuarial survival rates of 86% and 75%, respectively
      - Freedom from repeat surgery is 55% and 29% at 10 and 20 years, respectively.
- Pulmonary hypertension
  - Can be fatal if not reversed
  - Patients are at a significantly elevated risk for right-ventricular failure and sudden death.
- Ebstein anomaly
  - Long-term outcomes are related to severity of disease (degree of cyanosis) at presentation.
  - Severely hypoplastic lungs will preclude cardiac palliation.
    - Most of these infants die shortly after birth.
- Anomalous pulmonary venous return
  - Natural history of prolonged untreated obstruction of the anastomosis or pulmonary veins
    - Irreversible pulmonary venous obstructive disease
    - Pulmonary vascular disease
    - Eventual right-heart failure
- Aortic stenosis
  - Progression rate
    - Unpredictable during the first 6 months of life
      - Final valvar gradients are poorly predicted by initial gradients.
    - Slower and more predictable after the first year
  - Patients not requiring intervention before 6 months of life are less likely to:
    - Develop heart failure
    - Become critically ill during the follow-up period
  - After neonatal intervention:
    - Frequency of restenosis is 15–30%.
    - Aortic valvotomy results in mild aortic insufficiency, which is well tolerated for many years.
  - Subaortic stenosis
    - Recurrence rate is 20–30% after resection.
  - Supravalvar aortic stenosis
    - Insidious disease progression marked by significantly elevated coronary artery perfusion pressures

- Coarctation of the aorta
  - 5–25% rate of recoarctation, depending on surgical procedure
  - The restenosis rate is <20% after balloon dilation.
    - Associated transverse arch hypoplasia is associated with a higher rate of reintervention.
  - Repair during or after adolescence is associated with a higher rate of persistent hypertension.
- HLHS
  - Sequelae include:
    - Cardiac dysrhythmias
    - Cerebrovascular accidents with seizures
    - Myocardial ischemia
    - Pleural effusions
  - Patients may require multiple cardiac catheterizations.
  - Survival
    - Improved survival after the Fontan procedure has been shown to be strongly correlated with shorter cardiopulmonary bypass and aortic cross-clamp times.
    - When the condition results in end-organ damage or a delay in surgical intervention, morbidity and mortality increase significantly.
    - Long-term prognostic data are lacking.
    - A palliative approach for single-ventricle physiological arrangement may ultimately serve as an extended bridge to cardiac transplantation.
      - 20–30% of patients after undergoing the Fontan procedure develop heart failure, resulting either in successful OHT or death.
  - Neurodevelopmental outcomes
    - A majority of postoperative 8- to 9-year-olds had cognitive scores similar to those in the general population, but approximately 18% had IQ scores <70.
    - Some children have also had developmental motor delay and behavioral problems, including obsessive-compulsive disorder and attention-deficit/hyperactivity disorder.
- Tricuspid atresia
  - A single left ventricle is intuitively advantageous over a single right ventricle.
    - However, the data have failed to demonstrate any differences in long-term survival.
- IE
  - Survival
    - Before the era of antibiotics, IE was universally fatal.
    - Today, survival has increased by 70–80%.

- Long-term prognosis
  - Primarily determined by the presence of complications
  - If treatment is initiated early, valvar damage, heart failure, embolic events, and heart block can be prevented.
  - Prognosis is more guarded if IE involves a prosthetic valve or *Staphylococcus*.
- Myocarditis
  - Although its incidence is low in the pediatric population, accurate and timely diagnosis is critical for improving the related morbidity and mortality.
  - Mortality rates vary inversely with age of onset.
    - Nearly 75% of all newborns and infants who develop myocarditis will die of it.
    - In older children with less fulminant disease, the mortality rate is approximately 25%, with 50% exhibiting a complete recovery and another 25% becoming asymptomatic but having persistent abnormal cardiac function.
- Pericarditis
  - The pathologic course depends on the virulence of the offending organism.
- DCM
  - If unchecked, this change in myocardial structure and function can become irreversible.
- HCM
  - Morbidity
    - Ischemia-induced arrhythmias are the most likely source.
  - Mortality
    - Ventricular fibrillation is the most common cause of death in undiagnosed adolescents and young adults.
    - Overall risk of sudden death, 1–2% per year (may be as high as 4–5% in adolescents)
- RCM
  - Prognosis is poor.
  - Elevated left-ventricle end-diastolic pressures usually result in pulmonary hypertension and pulmonary vascular disease.
  - Death occurs within 1–4 years of diagnosis in symptomatic patients.
    - Pulmonary hypertensive crisis
    - Sudden death

- ARVD
  - Patients <30 years are at high risk for life-threatening ventricular tachycardias.
- OHT
  - Survival
    - Overall 50% survival at 13 years after transplantation
    - Younger age at transplantation is associated with longer survival and decreased need for retransplantation.
  - Quality of life
    - Although transplantation is a formidable treatment strategy for most patients and their parents, approximately 90% of OHT recipients surveyed at 1, 3, and 5 years after transplantation report excellent quality of life with no activity limitations.
    - Transplantation seems to be an acceptable treatment for patients with irreparable congenital or acquired heart disease.
  - Access to treatment
    - OHT is limited by the number of available donor hearts.
    - Approximately 20–30% of patients die while awaiting a suitable donor.

PREVENTION

- To ensure that no unnecessary or unknown risks are taken, exercise intensity, duration, and participation in any type of athletic event must be discussed among the:
  - Health care team (including cardiologist and pediatrician)
  - Patient
  - Family
- IE
  - Prevention is an integral step in caring for persons at risk.
    - Good oral hygiene
    - Appropriate antibiotic prophylaxis
    - Inappropriate prophylaxis can pose more risk than benefit when considering hypersensitivity reactions to antibiotics.
    - Avoid unnecessary interventions.

Constipation

DEFINITION

- Constipation
  - Infrequent elimination of large or hard stools that cause straining or pain
- Chronic constipation in childhood not caused by an organic lesion may also be called:
  - Dysfunctional stool retention
  - Psychogenic constipation
  - Idiopathic constipation
  - Functional constipation
- One expert consensus defined constipation as any of the following:
  - Passage of hard, scybalous, pebblelike, or cylindrical cracked stools
  - Straining or painful defecation
  - Passage of large stool that may clog the toilet
  - Stool frequency <3 times per week, unless breastfed
- Can present as pain, fecal soiling, urinary tract infection, or enuresis

EPIDEMIOLOGY

- Prevalence
  - Common among children of the industrialized world
  - Among referral populations
    - >90% of childhood constipation is functional.
    - 50–90% will be cured.
- Age
  - Of toddlers, 16–37% suffer constipation at some time.

MECHANISM

Normal colonic function

- Focal circular contractions
  - Impede progress of luminal contents
  - Allow solutes and water to be absorbed from liquid ileal effluent
- Progress of a relatively dehydrated fecal stream is achieved by contractile waves.
- Bolus of stool
  - Propelled to next colonic segment
  - Ultimately, stool arrives at the rectum.
- Defecation
  - Coordinated sequence of neuromuscular events
  - Involves reflexive and conscious components
  - At rest, continence is maintained by:
    - Involuntary resting tonic contraction of smooth muscle cuff of internal anal sphincter
    - Posterior turn of anal canal in relation to anterior angulation of rectal vault
  - When stool arrives in rectal ampulla, it causes:
    - Distention of rectal walls
    - Relaxation of internal anal sphincter, which lowers the pressure of the anal canal and allows the stool bolus to descend to the anal canal (rectoanal inhibitory reflex)
  - Control of defecation is a critically important social achievement in early childhood.
  - Voluntary (and learned) contraction of striated muscle of external sphincter and puborectalis sling muscles increases pressure in anal canal and makes the exiting angle more acute.
  - The Valsalva maneuver in combination with relaxation of the external anal sphincter and puborectalis sling permits defecation to proceed.

Constipation

- Functional
  - Stool is most often withheld in response to the rectoanal inhibitory reflex.
  - The cause is not clear, but functional constipation may result from several distinct pathophysiologic events, including:
    - Disorder of dynamics of defecation
    - Problem with rectal sensation
    - Disorder of colonic transit, leading to impacted, overly desiccated stool in colon
- Withholding
  - Commonly recognized clinical scenarios that result in constipation include:
    - Painful anal fissures
    - Perianal streptococcal cellulitis
    - Traumatic toilet-training experiences
    - Transient periods of dehydration, illness, or immobility
  - Stool withholding may figure prominently in the perpetuation of constipation after pain or an aversive experience.
  - Withholding behavior in the toddler or child is strongly self-reinforcing.
    - Avoidance of painful bowel movements makes the stool harder and more painful to pass.
    - Parental concern may unwittingly reinforce withholding behavior
  - Lack of privacy commonly found in some school lavatories can engender withholding by older children.
  - Studies have documented abnormalities in the dynamics of defecation.
    - Most common is paradoxical contraction of the external anal sphincter and the puborectalis sling in response to the rectoanal inhibitory reflex, also called:
      - Rectoanal pelvic floor dyssynergia
      - Abnormal defecation dynamics

■ Anismus

- Dyssynergia is considered to be a learned phenomenon.

- Painful defecation and withholding antedate the clinical presentation of constipation by 1–5 years.

- In a significant subset of children who experience persistent constipation, withholding becomes entrenched and particularly difficult to unlearn.

■ Sensory abnormalities

• Megarectum

- The rectum is dilated, with chronic impaction.

- Associated with increase in sensory threshold to minimal rectal distention

- Associated with increase in minimal volume required to initiate the urge to defecate

• May persist for several years

• May contribute to relapses

■ Slow transit of fecal stream through colon

• Occurs predominantly in young women

• Can occur in children

• Unclear whether this is a primary problem or acquired epiphenomenon of more distal difficulties with defecation

• Not easily differentiated clinically from normal-transit constipation

• A unique therapeutic approach has not emerged.

■ Dietary factors

• Dietary fiber is believed to have an important role in promoting regular bowel habit.

• Decreased fiber intake as a risk factor for childhood constipation has been documented, but overlap exists in fiber intake between cases and controls.

• In infancy, the transition from breast milk or formula to whole cow's milk or periods of excess protein intake are associated with constipation.

• It is a myth that iron-containing formulas cause constipation.

HISTORY

■ Description of stools that child passes

• Frequency

• Consistency

• Caliber

■ History of stool withholding (a positive history strongly supports functional constipation)

■ Age of child at onset

• If a newborn, whether child passed meconium in first day of life

■ Toilet-training experience

• Whether traumatic

• Critical in toddlers and preschool children

■ Diet history—how constipation began

• With transition to cow's milk

• During periods of high protein intake

• With excessive cow's whole milk consumption

■ Complications

• Fissures

• Bleeding

• Abdominal pain

• Anorexia

• Enuresis

• Urinary tract infection

• Distention and vomiting (not caused by functional constipation)

■ Prior evaluation and treatment

• Over-the-counter medicines

• Home remedies

• Alternative therapies

• Culturally specific therapies

- Can be part of treatment plan if they pose no harm

■ Change in urinary voiding pattern (possible occult spinal process affecting sacral nerves)

• Stream

• Continence

■ Family history of:

• Heritable conditions

• Functional constipation

■ Specific questions to address differential diagnosis of:

• Hirschsprung disease

• Endocrine, metabolic, and neurologic disease

■ In infants

• Delayed passage of meconium

PHYSICAL EXAM

Infants

■ An empty rectum raises the possibility of Hirschsprung disease, particularly in conjunction with any or all of following:

• History of delayed passage of meconium

• Explosive gush of stool on withdrawal

• Hard impacted mass palpated in the pelvis or lower abdomen

■ In infants with delayed passage of meconium

• Anorectal manometry

• Rectal suction biopsy

• Unprepared barium enema

• Sweat test

- Impactions
  - Unusual
  - May indicate Hirschsprung disease
- External examination of perineal area
  - Establish the normal placement of anal orifice.
  - Look for:
    - Anal fissure
    - Skin tag
    - Normal anal wink
- Examine lower extremities for:
  - Tone
  - Strength
  - Symmetry
  - Reflexes
- Examine spine for:
  - Dimple
  - Hair tuft
  - Vertebral anomalies

Children

- Check the child's growth parameters.
  - Recent growth velocity
  - For growth failure, failure to thrive, or short stature, consider:
    - Thyroid function tests
    - Celiac panel
    - Sweat test
- Assess physical appearance.
  - The child should appear well and not wasted or malnourished.
  - Abdomen should not be distended.
- Examination should establish presence or absence of fecal impaction in lower quadrants or the hypogastric area.
- External examination of perineal area
  - Establish normal placement of anal orifice.
  - Look for:
    - Soiling
    - Fissures
    - Skin tags
    - Normal anal wink in response to touch
- Rectal examination, with patient's cooperation
  - With functional constipation, desiccated stool is found in the rectal vault.
  - Megarectum
    - In older children with long-standing constipation:
      - Chronic rectal distention may efface the internal sphincter along the rectal wall.

- Anal canal will feel foreshortened.
  - In children who soil from chronic constipation:
    - The disorder is sensory.
    - Tone of the internal sphincter should be normal.
  - Older child with functional constipation
    - The rectum may be empty if the child has just defecated.
    - Carefully consider the possibility of Hirschsprung disease.
  - Be alert for extrinsic mass compressing the rectum (rare).
  - Patulous anus is indicative of a neurologic lesion or sexual abuse.
- Neurologic examination
  - Explicitly assess lower extremities for:
    - Tone
    - Strength
    - Symmetry
    - Reflexes
  - Analyze the patient's gait.
- Examine spine for:
  - Signs of spina bifida occulta
  - Dimple
  - Hair tuft
  - Palpable vertebral deformity

DIFFERENTIAL DIAGNOSIS

Functional constipation

- Despite the large number of possible diagnoses, at least 90% of affected children have functional constipation.
- Infants
  - Parental definition of constipation in the first 6 months may be incorrect.
  - In otherwise healthy breastfed infants:
    - Stool consistency rather than frequency is a critical determinant of constipation.
    - Straining and grunting (turning deep red) in producing a soft stool of average caliber is normal.
    - Mushy stool once a week requires no intervention.
  - Functioning rectoanal inhibitory reflex
    - Manometric studies have documented this at birth.
    - Likely represents unsuccessful attempts to coordinate voluntary with involuntary defecation
  - Treatment is required for the constipated infant who:
    - Strains with production of a desiccated plug of stool followed by loose stool
    - Produces consistently desiccated stool of pebbly consistency

- Toddlers
  - History of stool withholding is critical for both diagnostic and therapeutic purposes.
  - Parents of toddlers are:
    - Usually aware the child is constipated
    - Frequently do not recognize stool withholding
  - During typical withholding, the child may:
    - Hide quietly
    - Cling to an inanimate object
    - Squeeze buttocks together
  - Variations of stool-withholding behavior
    - Crouching
    - Dancing or walking on tiptoes
    - Crying out in anticipation of pain
  - Episodes of withholding:
    - Are misinterpreted by the parents as attempts to defecate
    - Generate great concern in the parent
- Children
  - Once the child has attained privacy in the bathroom:
    - Parents are not likely to be involved in toilet routine.
    - Constipation becomes occult.
  - Incomplete evacuation is common in school-age children; typical scenario:
    - Child goes to the bathroom with regular or increased frequency.
    - Child passes only a small, hard piece of desiccated stool.
    - Child emerges from bathroom not terribly bothered.
    - Parent inquires, "Did you go?" Child answers, "Yes." Thus both parties are happy.
    - Pattern is punctuated episodically by the passage of massive bowel movements.
  - Many children do not seem terribly bothered by their constipation.
  - Children are often brought in, not for constipation itself, but for:
    - Soiling
    - Recurrent abdominal pain
    - Blood streaks seen on stool
    - Excessive flatus
    - Anorexia
  - Pelvic floor dyssynergia in children with stool withholding:
    - Can affect urinary voiding dynamics
    - Predisposes child to enuresis or urinary tract infection
- Findings that support the diagnosis of functional constipation
  - Onset after infancy
  - Presence of stool-withholding behavior
  - Episodic passage of large-caliber stools

- Absence of red flags
  - Failure to thrive (weight loss, poor growth)
  - Vomiting
  - Abdominal distention
  - Persistent anal fissures, perianal disease
  - Persistent blood in stool or guaiac-positive stool
  - Delayed passage of meconium
  - Weak urinary stream, diurnal enuresis

Anal and rectal disorders

- Anal fissure
  - May induce self-perpetuating cycle of withholding, worsening constipation, and reinjury
- Anterior ectopic anus
  - Occasionally, the anal orifice is misplaced anteriorly, so that the stool bolus must turn anteriorly at the perineum.
  - Parents may report seeing a perineal bulge when the infant attempts to defecate.
  - Consider surgical reconstruction in children who fail to improve with medical therapy.
- Anal stenosis
  - Characterized by straining during the production of small-caliber stools
  - Frequently diagnosed during infancy
  - Digital examination shows that the anal canal is narrow and not distensible.
- Rectal duplication
- Anal trauma (abuse)
- Extrinsic masses, though rare, may intermittently or partially obstruct the rectum.
- Rectal duplication cyst
- Pelvic mass, such as neuroblastoma, presacral teratoma, ovarian tumor, hematocolpos

Neurologic

- Hirschsprung disease
  - The most common reason to consider Hirschsprung disease is failure of treatment for functional constipation.
    - Appropriate in early infancy, when functional constipation is unusual and easily treatable
    - In the toddler and the school-age child, more likely to reflect the complexity and duration of intervention required rather than a missed diagnosis of Hirschsprung disease
    - Findings with a very high negative predictive value for Hirschsprung disease:
      - Almost all children with functional constipation withhold stool in response to the rectoanal inhibitory reflex.
      - This reflex is absent with Hirschsprung disease.

- Hirschsprung disease should be considered in any child with refractory constipation who has had any of the following:
  - Failure to pass meconium in the first 24 hours of life
  - Onset of constipation before 3 months of age
  - Symptoms of intestinal obstruction at any time (distention, pernicious emesis)
  - Lifelong dependence on laxatives, enemas, or mechanical manipulation to initiate defecation
  - History of enterocolitis in early infancy (sometimes misdiagnosed as gastroenteritis)
- Spinal cord lesions
  - Affect the second, third, and fourth sacral nerves
  - Associated with both sensory and motor deficits affecting defecation
  - Trauma to sacral cord, intraspinal and extraspinal tumors, and congenital malformations can tether the spinal cord.
  - Consider when constipation is accompanied by abnormalities in bladder function or gait.
  - Consider when visible abnormalities or palpable deformities of the lumbosacral spine exist.
- Cerebral palsy
- Neuromuscular diseases with hypotonia
- Refractory constipation
  - Frequently multifactorial and difficult to treat
  - Prevalent in children with:
    - Cerebral palsy
    - Muscular dystrophy
    - Generalized hypotonia
- Pseudo-obstruction syndromes
  - Characterized by intermittent episodes of functional intestinal obstruction
  - Affects the neuromuscular function of the colon

Metabolic and endocrine
- Hypothyroidism
- Diabetes insipidus
- Hypercalcemia
- Hypokalemia

Medication and toxin related
- Antihistamines
- Anticholinergics
- Anticonvulsants
- Opioids
- Bismuth, aluminum hydroxide
- Tricyclic antidepressants
- Iron preparations (**not** iron-fortified formulas)

- Plumbism
- Infant botulism

Miscellaneous
- Celiac disease and cystic fibrosis should be considered in children with:
  - Poor growth in weight or height
  - Recurrent respiratory symptoms
  - Anemia
  - Hypoproteinemia
- Cow's milk allergy
  - For treatment-resistant chronic constipation, soy milk has been used as a substitute.
  - In study of 65 children, 44 had a positive response when soy milk replaced cow milk.
  - Replacing cow milk with soy milk is controversial.
- Scleroderma
- Systemic lupus erythematosus

LABORATORY EVALUATION
- Routine laboratory tests
  - Not indicated in evaluating for functional constipation
- Tests to consider
  - Thyroid function tests
  - Serum calcium
  - Potassium
  - Lead
  - Celiac panel
  - Sweat test

IMAGING
- Plain abdominal radiographs:
  - Often do not have significant diagnostic value
  - In functional constipation, should show dilated, enlarged rectum
  - In Hirschsprung disease, should show empty rectum
  - Can be used:
    - Selectively for confirmation that palpable abdominal mass is a fecal impaction
    - For a questionable diagnosis in a child unable to cooperate with rectal examination
- Barium enema:
  - In functional constipation, should reveal diffusely dilated colon and rectum
  - In Hirschsprung disease, should reveal distal spasm, proximal dilatation

- Magnetic resonance imaging of lumbosacral spinal cord for:
  - Hair tufts, lipomas, hemangiomas overlying the lumbosacral spine
  - Abnormalities of gait
  - Abnormalities of urination
  - Absent anal wink
  - Absent cremaster reflex

DIAGNOSTIC PROCEDURES

- Rectal manometry
  - Functional constipation: rectoanal reflex present
  - Hirschsprung disease: rectoanal reflex absent

TREATMENT APPROACH

- Goals of treatment
  - Establish a pattern of soft bowel movements with ≥3 per week.
  - Wean the child from pharmacotherapy.
  - Have the child and family manage problem on their own with diet and behavioral modification.
- Involves parental education, laxatives, diet, behavioral modification
- Considerations
  - Age of patient
  - Duration of symptoms and treatment
    - Transient constipation lasting several days
      - Typically can be managed with 1 to a few days of laxative use and dietary change
    - Functional constipation
      - Patients are affected for weeks to months before seeking medical attention.
      - Requires a phased approach and months of treatment
      - In older children, may require 1–2 years of laxative therapy

SPECIFIC TREATMENT

Infants

- Before the introduction of solids, add undigestible, osmotically active carbohydrates to formula/breast milk.
  - Dark corn syrup or malt soup extract
  - Dose: 2–6 teaspoons per day, divided among several bottles
- Once juice and infant food are introduced:
  - Give apple or prune juice and fruits.
- Infant glycerin suppositories
  - Can be used at the beginning of therapy to remove a desiccated rectal plug
  - Should not be the mainstay of therapy because infants can become dependent on rectal stimulation

- 2 studies have established the efficacy of polyethylene glycol (PEG).
- Constipated infants should not be treated with mineral oil: risk of pneumonia from aspiration
- Treat externally visible anal fissures with petroleum jelly.

Toddlers and older children

- Functional constipation
  - Highly successful treatment adopted widely by pediatric gastroenterologists with published guidelines
  - Divided into 3 phases
    - Education and disimpaction
    - Maintenance
    - Weaning
  - Controlled studies have not documented greater improvement with biofeedback training than with standard treatment regimens.
- Education
  - Parents need to know:
    - Constipation frequently engenders withholding.
    - Withholding is self-perpetuating.
    - Toddlers may require several months of laxative that produces soft stools before they abandon withholding.
    - Long-term nonstimulant laxatives are safe, based on innumerable studies.
    - Nonstimulant laxatives that do not engender laxative dependence include:
      - Mineral oil
      - Milk of magnesia
      - PEG
      - Lactulose
    - Reluctance to medicate children leads to premature discontinuation of therapy.
    - The limited use of senna, an anthraquinone-stimulant laxative, is acceptable as:
      - Adjunct to an osmotic agent
      - Rescue therapy for children who have transient relapses
    - Experts discourage the prolonged use of stimulant laxatives (senna, bisacodyl).
    - No proof exists that prolonged use of mineral oil impairs fat-soluble vitamin absorption.
  - Parents should be instructed to:
    - Ignore withholding events as they would a temper tantrum
    - Talk directly to toddlers and engage them in the therapeutic program.
    - Say, "I want you to push the poo-poo out of your body; don't hold it in. That's how you will get better, and it will stop hurting."

- Disimpaction
  - The goal of disimpaction is to remove all hard-formed stools throughout colon.
  - Treatment begins with disimpaction for the patient who:
    - Has had months to years of symptoms
    - Has an impaction on examination
  - For older children:
    - Defer disimpaction until the weekend.
    - Treat with mineral oil to lubricate impacted stool.
  - Fiber is withheld during the disimpaction phase.
  - Enemas
    - Once a day for 3–6 days
    - Simple, effective, and safe (with important caveats)
    - Dose guidelines should be followed.
    - In the rare event of failure to pass stool following an enema, the child needs medical attention.
    - Sodium phosphate enemas are contraindicated in children who:
      - Weigh <10 kg
      - Have cardiac or renal impairment or electrolyte disorders
      - May have any form of intestinal obstruction
  - Oral route versus enemas
    - Oral PEG has been used successfully for disimpaction.
    - Choice should be made with the child's and family's input.
  - Laxative doses
    - Rectal
      - Hypertonic sodium phosphate enema: 3 mL/kg/dose, once daily via rectum for 1–6 days
      - Mineral oil enema: 30–60 mL, once daily via rectum for 1–6 days
    - Oral
      - PEG electrolyte-free: 1.5 g/kg/day, maximum 100 g for 3 days
      - Mineral oil: 30 mL/year of age to maximum 8 oz twice daily for 3 days
      - PEG with electrolytes: 10-40 mL/kg/hr, via nasogastric tube (maximum 2 L/h) until stool effluent clear
- Maintenance
  - Follows disimpaction and incorporates laxative use, dietary advice, behavioral modification
  - Laxative choice
    - Less important than close follow-up for dose adjustment
    - Mineral oil

- Contraindicated for children <2 years or at risk for pulmonary aspiration
- Parents should be counseled explicitly never to force a child to take mineral oil.
  - PEG
    - Cautions for mineral oil also apply for PEG.
    - PEG is an osmotic laxative widely used to treat functional constipation.
    - Polymer of ethylene glycol that is not absorbed or fermented by colonic bacteria
    - Fairly tasteless, water-soluble powder that can be disguised when mixed into a child's drink
    - Pediatric studies have established clinical tolerance, effective dose, and absence of unanticipated or serious adverse effects.
    - In a study comparing low-dose PEG with lactulose, no difference was found between the prevalence of abnormal electrolyte or nutritional parameters.
    - Despite its popularity, it is unclear whether PEG is better and safer than other commonly used laxatives.
    - For severe pulmonary edema from PEG aspiration, bronchoalveolar lavage has been used successfully.
  - Dietary fiber
    - Addition of fiber is widely advocated as an adjunct.
    - A randomized controlled trial has shown benefits of fiber supplement when prescribed with laxative.
    - Dietary changes that increase child's fiber intake
      - Whole-grain breads and cereals
      - Increased fruit and vegetable intake
  - Behavioral modification
    - Toddlers
      - Focus on replacing stool-withholding behavior with deliberate attempts to defecate.
      - Defer toilet-training efforts until the child stops withholding.
    - Older children
      - Have the child sit on the toilet after meals for 5–10 minutes to capitalize on the gastrocolic reflex
      - Reward success by use of a star chart.
      - Child should be rewarded for the targeted behavior: sitting
    - Physician
      - Titrate laxative dose to achieve desired effect (soft bowel movement every day)
      - Work in partnership with the child and parents, who should report to physician frequently

- Laxative Doses (oral)
  - PEG electrolyte-free powder: 0.8g–1.5g/kg/day
  - Mineral oil: 1–3 mL/kg/day
  - Milk of magnesia: 1–3 mL/kg/day
  - Lactulose 10 g/15 mL: 1 mL–2 mL/kg/day
  - Senna syrup 218 mg/5 mL: 10–20 mg/kg/dose at bedtime
- Weaning
  - Laxative therapy should not be stopped abruptly.
  - Some toddlers can be weaned after 6–12 weeks of maintenance treatment.
  - In older children, weaning may take 6–12 months.
  - Daily laxative dose can be decreased in 1 of 2 ways.
    - Decrease to 75%, 50%, and 25% of initial dose over successive months
    - Give a full dose every second day for 6–8 weeks, then every third day for another 6–8 weeks.
  - Efforts should be redoubled to:
    - Increase fiber intake
    - Foster compliance with behavioral program
  - Older school-age children should:
    - Be encouraged to practice self-monitoring of frequency and adequacy of bowel movements
    - Have a rescue plan (enema, suppository, or stimulant laxative) for a transient relapse
    - Consider no stool for >3 days a transient relapse
- Common reasons for treatment failure of functional constipation
  - Inadequate disimpaction
  - Failure to escalate laxative dose to achieve 1–2 soft stools per day
  - Premature discontinuation because of the widely held notion that laxatives are addictive
  - Relying on dietary fiber alone

WHEN TO REFER

- Abnormal diagnostic studies
- Findings that are inconsistent with functional constipation
  - Growth failure
  - Distention
  - Vomiting
  - Bleeding
- Treatment is complicated by other significant problems.
  - Behavioral
  - Emotional

- Parenting
- Mental health issues
- Toileting is the focus of a power struggle.
- Refer to pediatric gastroenterologist
  - Infant who is refractory to treatment
  - Child who is refractory to treatment or cannot wean from laxative therapy after 12 months
- If Hirschsprung disease is suspected:
  - Consult with surgeon and radiologist
  - Decide on initial diagnostic test (rectal biopsy is the gold standard)

WHEN TO ADMIT

- Constipation associated with obstruction or enterocolitis
- Failure of disimpaction as an outpatient

FOLLOW-UP

- Toddlers and older children
  - Follow-up by phone within 2 days of starting therapy.
    - Ascertain whether the child is still passing hard stools.
    - Titrate laxative dose to induce a daily soft bowel movement.
    - Determine whether disimpaction is complete.
  - Question to determine whether disimpaction was thorough.
    - Disimpaction failure is a common therapeutic mistake.
    - Initial disimpaction failure undermines successful treatment because maintenance-dose laxatives will not penetrate or remove impaction.
    - Failure should prompt a revisit to consider:
      - Abdominal or rectal examination *and/or*
      - Abdominal radiography
    - Children who have extremely hard or treatment-resistant impactions can be admitted for nasogastric administration of PEG.
  - Remain optimistic and involved, because improvement beyond 12 months of therapy is well documented.

PREVENTION

- Dietary fiber is believed to have an important role in promoting regular bowel habit.
- Sufficient fluid intake to prevent dehydration

Contact Dermatitis

DEFINITION

- Contact dermatitis is inflammation of the skin secondary to contact with an offending agent.
- 2 broad types
  - Irritant contact dermatitis
  - Allergic contact dermatitis

EPIDEMIOLOGY

- Prevalence
  - Represents 6–10% of visits to dermatologists' offices
  - Allergic contact dermatitis may account for at least 20% of all childhood dermatitis.
- Affects both sexes, all ages, and all races
  - Irritant contact dermatitis is more common than allergic contact dermatitis in very young children.
- Regional differences can exist, depending on the allergens or irritants in the environment.

ETIOLOGY

- Irritant contact dermatitis
  - Result of skin exposure to substances that cause an inflammatory reaction that is not immune mediated
  - Irritant agents may be present in the home, child care center, or school (eg, harsh detergents and cleaning materials).
  - Diaper dermatitis is common.
    - Urine, feces, and persistent moisture macerate the occluded skin of the perineum.
    - Typically does not involve the infant's skin creases
      - If the femoral creases or anal area is involved, infection is likely to be candidal.
  - Can be caused by airborne agents (dust or volatile chemicals)
    - These are often missed but must be considered in all cases.
    - Solvent/aerosol sniffers are susceptible to irritant contact dermatitis secondary to the airborne agent.
- Allergic contact dermatitis
  - Delayed hypersensitivity reaction, caused by primed T cells, producing a cascade of cytokines and chemotactic factors leading to dermatitis
  - *Anacardiaceae* is a family of plants that cause allergic contact dermatitis.
    - Poison ivy
    - Poison oak
    - Poison sumac
    - Japanese lacquer tree

- Cashew nut tree (allergen in the nutshell)
- Mango (allergen in rind, leaves, or sap)
- Rengas tree
- Dermatitis appears within 48 hours of exposure in a previously sensitized individual.
  - Allergic reaction to nickel is common and the most frequently positive patch test allergen in North America.
    - Body piercing
    - Metallic areas of clothing, such as snaps and zippers
  - Other allergens are becoming more important.
    - Topical antibiotic preparations, such as those containing neomycin
    - Hair dye products that contain paraphenylenediamine
    - Latex (eg, in children who have repeated exposure to latex in the clinical settings)

RISK FACTORS

- Patients with a history of atopic dermatitis are likely to have contact dermatitis.

SIGNS AND SYMPTOMS

- Clinical presentation of both types of contact dermatitis can be similar.
  - Range of responses:
    - Eczematous changes of the skin
    - Pink, scaling, irritated plaques
    - Severe vesiculobullous eruptions characterized by blistering changes of the skin and severe pruritus
- Irritant contact dermatitis
  - Can lead to lichenification
    - Accentuation of skin lines, often with hyperpigmentation, and an almost hardening of the skin
  - Acute irritant dermatitis occurs minutes to hours after exposure.
    - Intensity of the reaction, related to:
      - Nature of the chemical
      - Concentration
      - Duration of contact
    - Conditions that foster a more severe reaction
      - Wet skin
      - Skin under friction, occlusion, or pressure
  - Solvent sniffers
    - Irritant dermatitis of the arms and chest
    - Eczematous changes found mostly around the nose and mouth

C

- Allergic contact dermatitis—reactions can be:
  - Bullous
  - Purpuric
  - Lichenoid
  - Papular
  - Urticarial
  - Pigmented
  - Hypopigmented
  - From plants, ie, poison ivy
    - Linear arrays of vesicles where plant has come in contact with the skin
    - The genitals in young boys may be affected, because they transfer the allergen to this area when voiding.

DIFFERENTIAL DIAGNOSIS

- Atopic dermatitis
- Seborrheic dermatitis
- Tinea
- Psoriasis
- Rare conditions that can mimic diaper dermatitis
  - Acrodermatitis enteropathica from zinc deficiency
  - Letterer-Siwe disease

DIAGNOSTIC APPROACH

- The child or parent may be aware immediately of an offending agent.
- Use of a diary to chart symptoms and associated activities and exposures is recommended.
- If the irritant dermatitis is acute, identifying the culprit is often easy, given that it may be only a single agent.
- In chronic cases, multiple offenders are often present.
- Initial episode of allergic contact dermatitis may be easily identified because:
  - The rash usually is localized to a specific area.
  - The history of the offending agent can be ascertained.

DIAGNOSTIC PROCEDURES

- Patch testing
  - Application of suspected allergens to intact uninflamed skin
    - Substances are usually applied to the back and left on for 48 hours.
    - After 48 hours, patches are removed and coded sites are evaluated for the presence of a reaction.
      - Erythema *or*
      - Bullae
    - Some positive reactions may not show for up to 7 days; reevaluate at 5 and 7 days.

- Commercially available patch testing system (23 common allergens) can be performed easily in the dermatologist's office.
- In more extensive patch testing, individually prepared aluminum chambers with multiple allergens can be placed and then applied with hypoallergenic tape to the back.
- Photopatch testing to detect contact photoallergy is available.
  - The patch is applied, and after 24 hours the area is exposed to ultraviolet A light.
  - The patch is read 48 hours later.

TREATMENT APPROACH

- Uncomplicated cases (for both irritant and allergic contact dermatitis)
  - Topical steroids and emollients for milder disease
    - Elimination of the offending agent and liberal application of emollients is curative for mild irritant contact dermatitis.
  - Systemic medications, including oral corticosteroids and antihistamines for more dramatic presentations
    - Topical steroids are effective in allergic contact dermatitis, but less so for irritant dermatitis.
- Identifying the causative factors so that they may be avoided is accomplished by good history taking.
  - In chronic cases, a parent or older patient may need to keep a diary.
- Complicated cases that may require skin biopsy
  - Patient who has not responded to treatment in 1 month
  - Patient with involvement of a large body surface
  - Patient displays severe reactions (such as bullae)

SPECIFIC TREATMENTS

- Treatment of diaper dermatitis
  - Gentle application of protective barrier ointments, eg, zinc oxide and petrolatum
  - Lowest-potency corticosteroids
    - Can be used in severe cases 2–3 times daily for a limited time (3 days, no longer than 2 weeks)
    - Long-term exposure should be avoided in the occluded diaper area.
  - Care of diaper area
    - Bathing in water with minimal use of nondetergent soaps, followed by liberal use of emollients
    - Barrier ointments should be used with each diaper change, with care not to produce excess friction.
    - Involved areas should be kept dry and free of urine and stool.
    - Caregivers should be encouraged to change the diaper frequently, as often as every ≥2 hours.

- Commercial cleansing wipes, if used, should be fragrance-free and alcohol-free.
- Topical antifungal agents
  - Work well for secondary candidal infection of the diaper area
  - Should be considered in irritant rashes that are present for >3 days.
- Treatment of allergic contact dermatitis, specifically, *Rhus* dermatitis
  - Washing the skin and other items that may have come in contact with the plant
  - If patient develops skin lesions, systemic antihistamines are usually needed.
    - Topically, mild to moderate strength (class 7 to 4) steroids are appropriate
    - Topical pramoxine (an antihistamine) is safe and can be used over large areas of the body 2–3 times a day.
    - If lesions are limited but very pruritic, a more potent topical steroid cream (class 1 or 2) can be applied for no more than 2 weeks.
    - If lesions are more extensive, systemic steroid therapy for 2 weeks at a beginning dose of 0.5–1.0 mg/kg, followed by a rapid taper over the subsequent 2 weeks, is justifiable.
      - Should not have quick bursts of systemic steroids, because this is often associated with rebound of the rash
- In rare or severe cases, systemic steroids can be given for 2 weeks at a dose of 0.5–1.0 mg/kg with a rapid wean.

WHEN TO ADMIT

- If contact dermatitis is severe, such as seen in a generalized contact dermatitis or systemic contact dermatitis
  - Generalized contact dermatitis may occur if a patient is exposed to the smoke of a burning antigen (ie, various plants, such as those from the *Rhus* family).
  - Systemic contact dermatitis occurs when a patient is repeatedly exposed to a substance via an oral, intramuscular, or intravenous route that cross-reacts with an allergen.
- Patients experiencing any:
  - Fever
  - Chills
  - Nausea
  - Vomiting
  - Hypotension

- Secondary bacterial infection may require intravenous antibiotics if large body-surface involvement exists.
- Although rare, secondary infection with herpes virus may require intravenous antivirals.

WHEN TO REFER

- Presumed irritant contact dermatitis (including diaper dermatitis) that has persisted for ≥1 month despite aggressive topical treatment
  - Refer to a dermatologist.
- Involvement of a large body surface area or severe reactions (eg, bullae) or an atypical presentation
  - Refer to a dermatologist for skin biopsy.
- Patients in need of patch testing
  - Refer to a dermatologist or qualified pediatric allergist.

COMPLICATIONS

- Repeated episodes of irritant contact dermatitis that compromises the protective skin barrier may create a fertile environment for subsequent allergic contact dermatitis.

PREVENTION

- Irritant contact dermatitis
  - Maintain the skin barrier.
    - By maintaining a healthy stratum corneum
    - By keeping skin well hydrated (but not overly) and well moisturized
  - Avoid irritants.
    - Parents and older children must be educated about common irritants (soaps/detergents, especially those with fragrance and dyes).
    - Formaldehyde, formaldehyde releasers, and other clothing treatments can aggravate the skin; clothing should be washed before wearing.
- Allergic contact dermatitis
  - Identify trigger factors.
  - Educate the parent and older child about avoidance of triggers.
    - Patients and their families should be taught to identify a poison ivy plant so that it can be avoided and removed, if possible.
    - Commercial nickel spot tests are available from several sources.
      - Patients may identify the presence of nickel in metal items with which they may come in contact.

Contagious Exanthematous Diseases

DEFINITION

- Exanthem, meaning to bloom or to break out, refers to an eruption or rash that is usually associated with fever.
  - Generally implies that the eruption is infectious in origin
- These eruptions are extremely common in children, and rashes for different diseases may appear similar.

EPIDEMIOLOGY

- Enteroviral exanthems
  - The most common cause of exanthems in children
  - Typically occur in the late summer and early fall
  - Associated with epidemics of aseptic meningitis
- Roseola (exanthem subitum)
  - Occurs year-round
  - Limited to children between 6 months and 3 years of age
- Infectious mononucleosis
  - Occurs in approximately 15% of children
- *Mycoplasma pneumoniae* infection
  - Cutaneous signs are a minor manifestation of mycoplasmal infections.
- Mumps
  - Exanthem develops in <10% of persons infected.
  - Clinical mumps develops in approximately 60% of infected persons.
  - The remaining 40% have inapparent infections, without salivary gland swelling.

ETIOLOGY

- Exanthems may be caused by infection with:
  - Viruses
  - Bacteria
  - *Rickettsia* species
  - *Mycoplasma* species
  - Fungi
- Many serotypes of echoviruses and coxsackieviruses are associated with rashes.
  - Transmission is via the fecal-oral route.
- Roseola transmission is via secretions, usually from an asymptomatic contact.
- Erythema infectiosum is caused by infection with human parvovirus-B19.
  - Infection is spread by respiratory tract droplets.
- Rubella is transmitted through direct or droplet contact from nasopharyngeal secretions.
- Infectious mononucleosis is the exanthem of the Epstein-Barr virus.

- Measles (rubeola) is highly contagious and transmitted via respiratory droplets.
- Mumps transmission is through direct contact via the respiratory route.

SIGNS AND SYMPTOMS

Enteroviral exanthems

- Typically, these rashes are generalized maculopapular types that have discrete lesions similar to those of rubella or roseola.
- 2–3 days of fever precedes eruption.
  - Generally, prodromal fever is much lower than that of roseola.
- Vesicular lesions have been observed in coxsackievirus A5, A9, and A16 infections.
  - Hand-foot-mouth disease commonly is seen with coxsackievirus A16 infection.
    - Manifests as vesicles on the palms and soles
    - Oral ulcerations of enteroviral herpangina typically occur in the back of the mouth; this feature can distinguish it from the more diffuse lesions of primary herpes stomatitis.

Roseola (exanthem subitum)

- Human herpesvirus-6 is the infectious agent.
- 3 or 4 days of high fever (104–105°F [40–40.6°C])
- Abrupt resolution of fever
- Eruption of a pink maculopapular rash
  - Begins on the neck and spreads to the trunk and extremities
  - Face usually spared
- Lesions are discrete and last for 1 or 2 days.
- Usually, the child has no other manifestation of illness.
- The child does not appear as ill as the severity of the fever might imply.

Erythema infectiosum (fifth disease)

- Rash without fever or other systemic signs
- Fever can occur in 15–30% of patients.
- Rash occurs 7–10 days after nonspecific symptoms.
  - Malaise
  - Myalgias
  - Headache
- Rash erupts as a bright-red erythema of the cheeks ("slapped-cheek") and forehead.
  - Many large maculopapular lesions coalesce to form a confluent red rash.
  - Lesions are hot to the touch, palpable, and nontender.
  - Circumoral pallor

- Second stage: after 1 day, maculopapular rash appears on the proximal extremities.
  - Spreads gradually to the trunk and distal extremities
  - Leaves a lacelike appearance as it clears
  - Lasts 2–4 days
- Third stage: rash may reappear transiently when the skin is traumatized by pressure, sunlight, or extremes of hot and cold.
- Arthritis and arthralgia, which often occur in adults, are infrequent findings in children.
- Mild myelosuppression typically goes unnoticed in normal individuals.
  - A life-threatening aplastic crisis may occur in patients with shortened red cell survival, such as occurs in sickle cell disease or hereditary spherocytosis.

Rubella

- Also known as *German measles* or *3-day measles*
- The period of maximal communicability is just before and up to 1 week after onset of the rash.
- Incubation period is 2–3 weeks; disease peaks at 16–18 days.
- Clinical illness is mild and brief.
- Rash is the first sign of infection.
  - A pink, maculopapular eruption begins on the face and spreads downward to the trunk and extremities.
  - Lesions remain discrete and pink, in contrast with the raised, confluent, and deep-red lesions of rubeola.
- Facial rash clears as the extremity rash erupts.
- Rash has cleared by the third to the fifth day.
- Fever is very mild, between 99°F and 101°F (37.2°F and 38.3°C).
  - Lymphadenopathy
    - Posterior auricular and suboccipital chains are most commonly involved.
    - Tender at the onset of rash, with tenderness resolving rapidly over 2–3 days
    - Although lymphadenopathy is an important sign of rubella infection, it is not specific.
  - Tiny reddish spots may occur on the soft palate, which are indistinguishable from those of scarlet fever or rubeola.

Infectious mononucleosis

- The rash is pink to red and macular or maculopapular.
- The lesions are discrete and have no specific distinguishing characteristic.
  - Disease is most often diagnosed on the basis of other signs of infectious mononucleosis and confirmed by the peripheral blood smear and serologic tests.

- Administration of ampicillin (and sometimes other penicillins) results in approximately 50% of patients developing a much more intense rash.
  - This ampicillin-associated rash is deep red and confluent, giving it a morbilliform appearance.
  - Rash resolves spontaneously within a week.
  - The appearance of such a rash in a patient treated for presumptive group A streptococcal pharyngitis is cause to reconsider the diagnosis.
  - Reassure parents that rash does not represent penicillin hypersensitivity.

Measles (rubeola)

- The most serious of the childhood exanthems because of morbidity of the acute infection and potential for producing permanent sequelae.
- Incubation period: 10–11 days
- Prodromal illness
  - Increasing fever
  - Cough
  - Conjunctivitis
  - Coryza
- By the fourth day
  - Fever is high (104°F [40°C]).
  - A deep-red macular rash erupts, beginning on the face and neck and spreading down the trunk and extremities.
  - Appearance is similar to that of rubella.
  - The lesions on the face and upper portion of the trunk soon become confluent to produce the characteristic morbilliform rash.
  - Rash in rubella tends to remain discrete.
- By the sixth day
  - Fever subsides.
  - The rash begins to fade, leaving a faint brown stain in the skin.
  - A fine desquamation ensues.
- Children are usually very ill but recover rapidly after the eighth or ninth day and are most often back to normal in a few days; hence, the moniker *10-day measles*.

Atypical measles

- Occurs in some children who were exposed to wild measles virus and had been immunized with inactivated measles vaccine
- May have 2–3 days of fever and headache followed by a rash erupting on wrists and ankles
- Rash may be maculopapular, purpuric, petechial, or vesicular.
- Marked myalgia, with swelling of the hands and feet, may also occur.
- Pneumonia is common.
- Inactivated measles vaccine is no longer available in the US

M pneumoniae infection

- A maculopapular eruption may appear on the trunk and extremities of 10–15% of persons infected with *M pneumoniae*.
- These infections are more commonly associated with allergic-type eruptions.
  - Urticaria
  - Erythema multiforme
  - Vesicles
  - Bullae
- Patients frequently have had a prodromal illness of fever, headache, malaise, and cough.
- Disease may escape physical diagnosis, only to crop up on the chest radiograph as an incidental finding.

Mumps

- Exanthem is uncommon, but when present, lesions are maculopapular, pale pink, discrete, and concentrated on the trunk.
- Virus more typically involves salivary glands, testicles (after puberty), pancreas, and meninges.
- Incubation period of 16–18 days
- Illness begins with 1 or 2 days of anorexia, headache, and mild to moderate fever that usually lasts 2–5 days.
- This is followed by discomfort when chewing and pain around the ear.
- Diffuse but noticeable enlargement and tenderness of the parotid gland is usually present.
  - Swelling extends anterior to the ear and below the ramus of the mandible posteriorly to the mastoid bone, usually obliterating the angle of the jaw.
    - Rarely, only 1 parotid gland is involved.
    - Submandibular salivary glands rather than the parotids may be involved.
  - Lymph nodes are more discrete and generally submandibular in location.
  - Erythema accompanying the parotitis is commonly seen around the opening of the Stensen duct.

Scarlet fever

- Rash (scarlatina) is caused by a circulating erythrotoxin produced by certain strains of streptococci and staphylococci.
  - Characterized by a fine papular eruption on an erythematous base
- Generalized erythema of the skin is present, even including areas that are not yet involved with the papular rash.
  - Concentrated on the trunk and proximal extremities
  - Feels rough to the touch, similar to fine sandpaper
  - Commonly associated with prominent erythema of the lips, soles, and palms

- Transverse red streaks (Pastia lines) are sometimes present, usually in the antecubital space.
- Desquamation of involved skin typically occurs in the recovery phase.
- On the tongue, prominent papillae appear on a very red base, giving a "strawberry tongue" appearance.
- If streptococci are the source of the erythrogenic toxin, the pharynx is the usual site of focal infection.
  - Other focal infections (eg, vaginitis, cellulitis) may also be found.
- When staphylococci are the source of erythrogenic toxin, the infective focus is usually some site other than the pharynx, eg, infected surgical or traumatic wounds.

DIFFERENTIAL DIAGNOSIS

- Clinical manifestations other than the rash must often be explored to distinguish one disease from another.
  - Incubation period
  - Prodromal symptoms and signs
  - Patient age
  - Immunization history
  - Contact history
  - Distribution and progression of the rash
  - Evidence of other organ involvement
  - Pathognomonic signs, such as peeling or Koplik spots
- Certain allergic and immune-complex diseases, such as childhood arthritis, can mimic infectious exanthems.
- Kawasaki disease must be carefully differentiated from scarlet fever.
  - Coronary artery disease may complicate untreated Kawasaki disease.
    - Cutaneous manifestations overlap those of scarlet fever.
    - Can usually be distinguished by additional signs
      - Discrete bulbar conjunctivitis without exudate
      - Cracking of the lips
      - Lymphadenopathy, usually solitary, unilateral, and >1.5 cm in diameter
      - Induration with erythema of palms and soles
      - Meatitis
      - Children are profoundly irritable.
      - Fever persists for more than 1 week (5 days of fever is necessary for diagnosis).
    - As in scarlet fever, patients have erythema of the palms and soles.
      - Striking desquamation is evident during the second and third weeks of the disease.

- Measles (rubeola)
  - The exanthem of measles is pathognomonic.
  - Koplik spots begin approximately 2 days before the rash erupts and increase in number until the first or second day of the exanthem.
    - Tiny bluish-white spots on an erythematous base
    - Cluster adjacent to the molars on the buccal mucosa
  - The combination of Koplik spots, fever, cough, conjunctivitis, and morbilliform rash is sufficient to make a firm clinical diagnosis of measles.

LABORATORY FINDINGS

- Clinical suspicion of erythema infectiosum (fifth disease) confirmed by
  - Testing for anti–parvovirus B19 immunoglobulin M in the immunocompetent patient
  - Through polymerase chain reaction testing in the immunocompromised patient
  - Dot-blot hybridization of serum specimens may have adequate sensitivity for patients with HIV.
- Rubella
  - Virus grown from the pharynx within 5 days of the onset of the rash
  - Serological diagnosis is made by demonstrating antibody titer increase between acute and convalescent serum samples obtained 2 weeks apart.
  - Serologic tests
    - Traditional hemagglutination-inhibition antibody titers
    - Enzyme immunoassays

SPECIFIC TREATMENTS

Erythema infectiosum (fifth disease)

- Supportive care is sufficient for most patients.
- Patients in aplastic crises may require transfusion.
- In immunodeficient patients with chronic infection, intravenous immune globulin therapy should be considered.
- Transmission of parvovirus B19 may be decreased through the use of routine infection control measures.

M pneumoniae infection

- Macrolide antibiotics may be used to treat *M pneumoniae* infections.

Measles and its complications

- Vitamin A supplementation should be considered for patients 6 months to 2 years of age who are hospitalized

Scarlet fever

- Treatment should be directed toward eradication of the focal infection.

- Streptococcal infections
  - Penicillin
  - Erythromycin
- Staphylococcal infections
  - Cephalexin
  - Amoxicillin-clavulanate
  - Dicloxacillin
  - Oxacillin

WHEN TO ADMIT

- Patients with measles may need to be hospitalized in an isolation room.
- Patients who have developed severe complications such as pancreatitis in mumps, pneumonia in measles due to contagious exanthematous diseases.

FOLLOW-UP

- All children who have measles should have careful follow-up, and the examiner should have a high degree of suspicion for secondary bacterial pneumonia.

COMPLICATIONS

- Rubella
  - The major serious complications of rubella virus result from fetal infection.
    - High probability that infection in the first trimester of gestation will result in fetal infection with multiorgan involvement
  - Complications are rare in children.
    - Transient arthritis develops in approximately 15% of adolescents and young adults that rarely becomes chronic.
- Measles (rubeola)
  - Induces inflammation throughout the respiratory tract and respiratory complications are common
    - Otitis media (treat as usual)
    - Pneumonia may be either a primary measles pneumonia or a superimposed bacterial pneumonia.
    - Croup
  - Subacute sclerosing panencephalitis, also known as *Dawson encephalitis*, is the major complication of persistent measles virus infection.
    - Occurs in approximately 1 per 1000 cases
    - Commonly results in death or permanent neurologic sequelae
  - Signs and symptoms of subacute sclerosing panencephalitis
    - Headache
    - Vomiting
    - Drowsiness

- Personality changes
- Seizures
- Coma
- Cerebrospinal fluid reveals pleocytosis and elevated protein levels
- Some have only mild disease and recover in a few days; others have a fulminant course

- Mumps
  - Meningoencephalitis is estimated to occur in 10% of all cases of mumps.
  - Characterized by
    - Headache
    - Nausea
    - Vomiting
    - Mild nuchal rigidity
  - It may occur before, during, or after the parotitis phase of the disease.
  - Follows a course similar to the aseptic meningitis that is caused by other viruses.
  - Usually has no sequelae.
  - Orchitis is uncommon in children.
    - Unilateral involvement of the testes and epididymis is observed in approximately 25% of male patients who are infected with mumps virus after puberty.
    - Patients who have orchitis are usually quite ill.
      - Sterility rarely occurs.
  - The pancreas and other exocrine glands are rarely involved.
  - Late neurologic complications include nerve deafness and very rare postinfectious encephalitis.

PREVENTION

- Prevention can be achieved by utilizing appropriate infection control procedures.
- Many of the contagious exanthematous diseases such as measles, mumps, and rubella can be prevented by vaccination.

Conversion Reactions and Hysteria

DEFINITION

- Conversion reactions are medical complaints or symptoms associated with unconscious distress.
- They are a way of communicating the uncomfortable, or "a psychic mechanism whereby an idea, fantasy, or wish is expressed in bodily rather than in verbal terms and is experienced by the patient as a physical symptom rather than as a mental symptom."
- The terms *conversion symptom*, *conversion reaction*, and *conversion disorder* often are used interchangeably.
- Somatic or functional complaints differ from conversion symptoms.
  - Patients with somatic or functional complaints are aware of emotional distress associated with the symptom.
  - Patients with conversion symptoms are not cognizant of any associated emotional distress.

EPIDEMIOLOGY

- Prevalence
  - Specific overall prevalence of conversion symptoms in children and adolescents is not known.
  - 5–13% suggested by available data
  - Lack of more definitive data reflects the difficulty in ascertaining whether a somatic complaint represents a conversion symptom.
- Gender
  - 2 to 3 times more common in girls
- Age
  - May appear as early as 7 or 8 years of age
  - Appears to be more common among adolescents than among younger children
    - Adolescents more often have alarming somatic complaints, such as chest pains and fainting spells.
    - Younger children frequently suffer from more indolent complaints, such as sporadic abdominal pains.
- Socioeconomic status
  - No correlation apparent
- Less sophisticated patients tend to have rare or very unusual and physiologically unexplained symptoms.
  - Therefore, the more classic conversion symptoms (eg, paralysis, blindness) are less likely to be seen in Western societies.
  - Practitioners in Western societies are more likely to diagnose conversion symptoms in patients presenting with chronic abdominal pain or chronic headaches.
- Can appear as a group phenomenon, often referred to as *epidemic hysteria*.
  - Episodes of epidemic hysteria appear to have several characteristics in common:
    - Audiovisual cues (eg, seeing ambulances arrive to care for accident victims) seem to be important precipitators.
    - Adolescent girls are involved more often than adolescent boys.
    - Reaction is more likely if it is initiated by a group member identified either as a leader (of a large sub-group) or an authoritative outsider.
    - Episodes are likely to involve larger numbers of adolescents if adults are not present.
  - For example, adolescent girls swooning and fainting at rock concerts
    - In this situation, the unacceptable wish relates to sexualized thoughts involving rock stars.
  - Other examples are explained less easily.
  - Entire school populations may be involved in mass conversion reactions.

ETIOLOGY

- A conversion symptom serves as a form of decompression whereby unpleasant effects associated with acknowledgment of the wish are dissipated through the use of a somatic symptom.
  - The idea or wish is psychologically threatening to individuals or unacceptable for them to express directly.
  - Because the wish is completely unconscious, patients in no way relate any psychological stigmata to the somatic complaint.
- Conversion symptoms have no organic basis by themselves.
  - May be perpetuated by biochemical or physiological body changes, known as *conversion complications*
  - Can include changes such as
    - Muscle atrophy caused by longstanding paralysis
    - Respiratory alkalosis secondary to acute hyperventilation
    - Body activity (ie, gestures) used to express ideas during verbal interaction
- Some somatic complaints can result directly from emotional upsets:
  - Headaches
  - Nausea
  - Vomiting
- Anxiety often is associated with
  - Palpitations
  - Sweating
  - Tremulousness
- Depression often is exhibited by
  - Fatigue
  - Weakness

SIGNS AND SYMPTOMS

- All body systems may be invoked in a conversion reaction.
  - Any bodily process that can be perceived by the individual can serve as the focus for conversion symptoms.
  - Body activity (ie, gestures) is used to express ideas during verbal interaction.
  - Developmentally, infants express feelings and communicate through visible behavior long before spoken language becomes their dominant mode of communication.
  - Common conversational phrases frequently allude, metaphorically, to the intermixing of emotion and body functioning.
    - "I'm fed up."
    - "He is a pain in the neck."
- Typical symptoms include:
  - Paresthesia
  - Anesthesia
  - Diffuse pain
  - Paralysis
  - Tremors
  - Weakness of an extremity
  - Hyperventilation
  - Dizziness
  - Vomiting
  - Nausea
  - Visual problems
- Sensory system symptoms typically are not distributed in the correct pattern of innervation of the implicated cutaneous nerves.
- Abdominal pain
  - Common conversion symptom in children and young adolescents
  - An extensive investigation of 100 children who had abdominal pain showed an organic cause in only 8 cases.
  - Another study revealed abdominal pain in 14% of the children studied.
    - Highest incidence in children 9 years of age
    - Lowest incidence in those 16–17 years of age
  - Recurrent abdominal pain and its causes remain controversial.
  - Recurrent abdominal pain may indicate emotional concerns of which patient is unaware.
- Somatic symptoms of relatives or close friends can serve as the source of a patients' complaints.
  - Patients' interpretation of another person's symptom provides a model.
  - When the symptom is adapted from one observed in another person, that person frequently evokes strong feelings in patients.

- Patients express guilt about their feelings or impulses toward that person and may take the other's symptoms.
  - A form of self-punishment and psychological expression of the patient's forbidden idea or wish.
- Adolescents who have conversion symptoms frequently display characteristic patterns of behavior, sometimes designated as traits of the hysterical personality, including
  - Egocentricity
  - Labile emotional states (quick shifts from sadness to elation or from anger to passivity)
  - Dramatic, attention-seeking behavior
  - Sexual provocativeness (displayed in gestures and in dress)
- Patients who have such characteristics also
  - Usually are demanding
  - Display an air of pseudomaturity
  - Are dependent in personal interactions
- Their personal relationships, however, are rarely intimate or satisfying.
- Many aspects of the hysterical personality are seen in adolescent patients who have conversion symptoms, but also are demonstrable in adolescents who do not have such symptoms.
  - Therefore hysterical behavior traits alone in adolescents are not synonymous with conversion symptoms.
  - In isolation, these traits are not indicative of a psychopathologic condition.

DIFFERENTIAL DIAGNOSIS

- Other psychosomatic disorders at times may be confused with conversion symptoms.
- Hypochondriasis
  - Common, especially in adolescents
  - Patients view their symptoms with extreme concern.
  - Patients lack the apparent indifference seen in those who have conversion symptoms.
  - Patients who have conversion symptoms frequently seem relieved by consideration of an organic cause.
  - Patients who have hypochondriasis become more concerned if an organic diagnosis is suggested; they suspect and fear a serious or fatal disease.
  - Neither type is reassured more than transiently by being informed that there is no disease.
- Malingering
  - Uncommon in adolescents
    - May be seen in institutionalized adolescents
    - May be seen in adolescents in restrictive situations (eg, military service)
  - May be seen as an appropriate means of avoiding threatening or unpleasant circumstances

- Attempts to feign illness often are naive, especially in younger patients.
- Many of these individuals appear to be accident prone.
- May submit to painful procedures readily and without objection
- Malingering adolescents are aloof and hostile to the physician, delaying discovery of their deception.
- Patients who have conversion symptoms are often normal in their fear of invasive medical procedures.
  - May appear charming and garrulous with the physician
- Both malingerers and patients who have conversion symptoms may have parents with an unconscious psychological need to have their children be ill, therefore reinforcing symptoms.
■ Somatic delusions
- Symptoms of psychosis
- Usually not confused with conversion symptoms
- Other signs of severe mental illness usually are present:
  - Inability to relate to peers
  - Visual or auditory hallucinations
  - Stereotypical behaviors
- The symptoms described sometimes are intermittent and often extremely bizarre.
  - For example, patients who have somatic delusions may express the conviction that their heart is shriveling or that something is wrong with the blood that is running from the head to the leg.
■ Psychophysiological symptoms
- May occur when conversion symptoms have failed to dissipate anxiety
- Continuing anxiety activates biological systems (especially the autonomic nervous system), resulting in physiological changes such as
  - Tachycardia
  - Hyperperistalsis
  - Vasoconstriction
- Patient's cognizance of these changes is exhibited by
  - Palpitations
  - Diarrhea
  - Sweating
- In this situation, the symptom itself has no organic symbolic meaning and results from a reaction to actual body changes.
- Therefore psychophysiological symptoms can occur when conversion symptoms have failed.
- Similarly, conversion symptoms can replace psychophysiological symptoms.

DIAGNOSTIC APPROACH

Evaluating somatic complaints

■ Evaluation of any patient who has a somatic complaint not easily explained by another medical condition should always include consideration of the possibility of a conversion symptom.
■ Evaluation of any somatic complaint should involve inquiry into areas that reveal the patient's baseline emotional functioning:
- Family
- School attendance and performance
- Peer relationships
■ Advise both parents and patient that having feelings about somatic complaints is acceptable.
- If the physician communicates an appreciation of the role of emotions in physical disease, then the family may volunteer information more readily about psychosocial functioning.
- Both family and patient may be more accepting of primary emotional involvement if permission for expressing feelings is given early in the physician-patient relationship.
- Eventual diagnosis involving emotional aspects of health may be more acceptable if the family has been prepared for the possibility.
- Focusing only on physical diagnosis intimates to parents that psychological involvement is unlikely, unimportant, and improbable.
- Turning to psychological issues after all physical tests prove unremarkable implies to parents that this tack was chosen as a last resort because the physician was unable to ascertain an organic cause.
- A concurrent physical-psychological diagnostic approach not only prepares the physician to consider the problem with some psychotherapeutic intent, but also may save the family time and money by avoiding multiple laboratory tests.
■ From the outset, parents and patient should
- Be told that the body has physical ways of responding to emotional stress.
- Be encouraged to suggest diagnostic tests and possible diagnoses for consideration by the physician.
- Understand that the goal is to help maintain normal daily functioning in school and with peers even though symptoms may persist.
- Understand that referral to a trained psychiatric professional may be necessary if progress is not made.
■ A thorough history may not only elicit symptom inconsistencies in the present illness, but may also reveal a record of inexplicable or recurrent bouts of illness associated with life events, such as
- Chronic abdominal pain that occurs only on school days

C

- Somatic complaints associated with stressful social events
- Documentation of abdominal surgery with equivocal findings

Diagnostic criteria

- Diagnosis of a conversion reaction should never be one of exclusion and should follow specific diagnostic criteria:
  - The symptom has symbolic meaning to the patient.
  - The patient frequently exhibits characteristic interpersonal behaviors.
  - Reporting symptom has a characteristic style.
  - The symptom helps patients cope with their environment (secondary gain).
  - Health issues and symptoms frequently are used in family communication.
  - Symptoms occur at times of stress.
  - The symptom has a model or representation in the patient's life.
  - History and physical findings often are inconsistent with anatomic and physiological concepts.
  - No one criterion can be confirmatory; each patient who has a conversion symptom may not display every criterion.

Approach to patient interview

- Nondirective interviewing proves more rewarding than direct questioning.
  - For example, asking patients to describe the pain ("Tell me how it feels.") almost always provides insight into the emotions that patients associate with symptoms.
  - Suggestions ("Is it dull or sharp pain?") limit possible responses.
- If patients spontaneously offer information about recent events, then the interviewer should look for relationship of changes to patient's life.
  - However, care should be taken to avoid suggesting a cause-and-effect relationship between feelings and symptoms.
  - Patients who have conversion symptoms have no conscious knowledge of such an association, so the suggestion may alienate them and prevent establishment of trust.
- Patients who have a conversion symptom often describe their problem in a distinctive way.
  - The account frequently is dramatic.
  - Pain may be described as "thousands of burning needles thrust into my leg" or "a giant spike being driven into my chest."
  - Because they are suggestible, any symptom description alluded to by the physician may be adopted readily and thereafter reported.

- The conversion symptom has a specific, but unconscious, symbolic meaning to the patient.
  - Often related to an unconscious wish, and physical impairment serves to prevent acting out the wish
    - For example, the adolescent boy who has hand paralysis may have anxieties about masturbating.
  - The family or clinician may not always be aware of the symbolic meaning of the symptom.
  - Cognizance of the presence of the symbolic meaning may be intellectually rewarding for the physician; ignorance of the specific symbolism does not prevent adequate treatment.
- Conversion symptoms are adopted unconsciously in an attempt to reduce unpleasant affects such as
  - Anxiety
  - Depression
  - Guilt
- Therefore, although patients may describe incapacitating pain, they often affect an air of unconcern.
  - Psychiatrists refer to this as *la belle indifference.*

Primary and secondary gain

- The extent to which the conversion symptom diminishes the unpleasant affect and symbolically communicates the forbidden wish for the patient is referred to as the *primary gain.*
- Patients who have conversion reactions are often stubborn in their belief that the symptom is caused by organic problems, reflecting denial of the underlying emotional problem.
  - Conversely, insistence (especially by an adolescent) that a symptom is psychological in origin may indicate denial of a physical problem.
  - Therefore, differentiating between conversion symptoms and physical disease in adolescent patients cannot depend solely on the patient's emotional response.
- Conversion symptoms not only effect a primary gain for patients, but also help them cope with the environment.
- The conversion symptom achieves a secondary gain for patients.
  - For example, a conversion symptom defending against homosexual thoughts may be an excuse from attending school, where anxiety may have been intensified.
- Limitations imposed by symptom may contradict verbalized wishes to participate in activities but, nevertheless, remove the patient from potentially threatening social interactions.
- Interference with daily activities may provide secondary gain of attention and more frequent expressions of love from parents and friends.
  - The situation may be resistant to change, not only because the symptom is reinforced continually, but also because the symptom meets parents' psychological needs.

– Symptom may provide the parents with a reason for inappropriately attending to or infantilizing their child.

- Consequently, patients and entire families may fall into a vicious circle of dependence on the symptom.

■ Demonstration of a secondary gain does not ensure a diagnosis of conversion.

- To an extent, all illness is involved with some secondary gain.
  - Bedridden patients must accept increased attention to cope with their physical confinement.
  - Therefore, a degree of secondary gain is necessary for adequate adaptation to disability.
- In conversion symptoms, secondary gain not only intensifies symptoms, but may also be associated with further occurence of a somatic complaint.
- Perpetuation depends on concern from others, thus conversion symptom is more readily exhibited in the presence of individuals meaningful to the patient.

■ Children and adolescents who develop conversion symptoms are often overprotected and become extremely dependent on their parents.

- Daily familial communication may have been invested heavily in somatic complaints.
  - Children may recognize how often activities may have been canceled because of health complaints by other family members.
- Therefore, patient's symptoms may conform to the unspoken interactional family rules.
- Family members indirectly reinforce patient problems, although parents may assume an air of indifference with respect to the patient's symptoms.

Identifying precipitating events

■ Precipitation of a conversion symptom may be related to specific stressful events, such as

- A change of school
- Final examinations
- New social experiences
- Parental conflict
- Unresolved grief reactions
  - For instance, loss of a parent through death, divorce, or moving

■ Both adolescent and adult patients experience pseudo-seizures more often in families in which an unspeakable dilemma was present.

- Often associated with a fear of physical or sexual assault
- Even though other family members were aware of the specific problem, they often underestimated the severity of trauma.

■ Because the association between conflict and conversion reaction is unconscious, a history is helpful only if the interviewer elicits details about daily activities.

- The stressful event precipitating a conversion symptom often becomes apparent only after many visits.

■ Symptom selection is based on the unconscious remembrance of the patient's own body function or understanding of symptoms in others.

- The patient's conversion symptom may appear quite dissimilar to that displayed by the other (often a parent or a close relative) because the patient's perception of disease governs the display of symptoms.
- Parents and relatives often misinform children and adolescents about diseases, fearing that the truth would be too frightening.
- Such misinformation may actually potentiate fantasies and result in the development of a symptom quite different from the model.

■ Choice of symptom may be based on a previous physical illness.

- Thus patients who have a history of seizures may, after many years of adequate anticonvulsant control, have atypical and physiologically unexplainable seizures.
- Because the somatic complaint expressed by the patient is based on a model symptom, a physical disease often is mimicked.
- Close scrutiny of the symptom's history and description often reveals anatomic and physiological discrepancies.
  - The child or adolescent who has a stocking anesthesia—an anesthesia confined to a specific area of an extremity without any relationship to cutaneous nerve innervation—demonstrates an example of symptom inaccuracy.
  - It is based on the concept of the patient's own body rather than on anatomic principles.

TREATMENT APPROACH

■ In essence, treatment of the patient begins before a definitive diagnosis is made.

■ The initial interaction between the physician and the patient is critical to the degree of success achieved.

■ Before embarking on a treatment plan, the physician must be satisfied with the completeness of the medical evaluation.

- Common sense should dictate when the physician believes that further organic tests will be futile.
- Patient and family can often sense physician uncertainty, especially if the family is averse to accepting a psychological diagnosis.
- A prudent step is to ask the family what additional tests they expect and what other diagnoses they have considered.

- Treatment goals must be realistic.
  - Conversion symptoms seldom disappear completely.
  - However, adolescents often acquire increased coping skills so that
    - Daily function is unimpaired.
    - Dependence on secondary gain is minimized.
- Care of the adolescent patient who has a conversion reaction involves
  - Establishing a renegotiable number of regular visits
  - Encouraging the patient to discuss daily activities and interrelated feelings
  - Meeting with parents regularly to provide emotional support and counseling
  - Knowing that palliation rather than a cure may be the end goal
- Although patients who have conversion symptoms are suggestible, reassurance that the symptom will go away rarely is effective and does not contribute to psychological investigation of the symptom.
- On the contrary, suggesting that the symptom will persist allows time to work out a therapeutic relationship and sometimes has a paradoxical effect.
  - Because the symptom is unlikely to disappear after 2 or 3 visits, patients will retrospectively view the physician's suggestion as sound.
  - Trust in the physician will be reinforced, and patients may be more comfortable communicating information about their feelings.
  - Anxiolytic medications may reduce transiently attendant anxiety in some cases; however, medication as the sole therapy rarely results in lasting improvement.
    - Medication does not relieve the underlying conflict responsible for the symptom and another symptom eventually may appear.
    - There is a risk that medication side effects may become the model for new conversion symptoms, or new symptoms may be confused with side effects.
  - When physicians feel comfortable acting as both therapist and provider of acute medical care, occasions may arise when a teenager has a new physical symptom or complaint that requires attention.
    - If the physician suspects a physical illness unrelated to the conversion symptom, then whatever evaluation that is indicated must be performed, including a full or partial physical examination.
    - Overzealous search for disease should be avoided.
- The patient who has a conversion symptom usually will not outgrow it in the short term.

WHEN TO REFER

- Referral to mental health professionals is indicated
  - If symptoms continue to interfere with the patient's daily activities or functioning, such as
    - School attendance
    - Participation in extracurricular activities
    - Involvement with peers
  - If the family believes that inadequate progress has been made after an agreed-on duration of therapy
  - If the patient's symptom creates uncomfortable feelings in the pediatrician
    - For example, situations involving seductive adolescent behavior in association with a conversion symptom
  - If the patient or family member is a social acquaintance or a relative of the pediatrician
    - Dealing with the emotional problems of friends' or relatives' children is inappropriate.
    - Personal details of family or sexual functioning often may be required in the evaluation and may jeopardize the social relationship.
    - Failure or hesitancy to obtain appropriate data may jeopardize subsequent resolution of the problem.
- In all cases when referral is suggested, parental and patient compliance with the referral is improved if the possibility has been mentioned as a contingency early in the evaluation.
- The pediatrician should help families understand that seeing a psychiatrically trained professional does not connote "craziness."
  - Suggest that a mental health professional can help teenagers understand feelings about prolonged or unusual symptoms better than can most pediatricians.
  - Recommend a specific counselor rather than offering a list of suggested therapists.
    - Before the name of the therapist is given, verify that the counselor feels comfortable with the referral and has time available.
- After the referral is made, continued contact with the family concerning the conversion symptom promotes adherence with therapy.

FOLLOW-UP

- The number of anticipated follow-up sessions should be discussed with the family.
  - The number of sessions should be flexible so that it can be renegotiated if necessary.
  - Follow-up sessions with teenagers can usually be limited to 15–20 minutes every 2–4 weeks.
  - More frequent visits may be necessary if symptoms interfere with school attendance, peer relationships, or family functioning.

- During follow-up sessions, teenagers should be encouraged to talk about their daily life (eg, school, friends, family, dating).
  - If the teenager volunteers information about recurrence of the somatic complaint, the physician should inquire about events that were transpiring concurrently and feelings that accompanied these events.
- Having the adolescent keep a symptom diary may be helpful.
  - The patient records
    - When the symptom occurred
    - What was happening at the time the symptom began
  - This record may illustrate the association of the symptom with feelings or emotionally charged life events.
- For physicians with sufficient expertise, follow-up visits with parents should take place every 4 to 6 weeks.
  - Such meetings may
    - Elicit persistent or new concerns that parents may have
    - Attempt to assess the parents' reaction to continuing complaints
  - Emphasize the validity of the teenager's concerns so that misconceptions about the symptom being faked are dispelled.
  - Offer positive reinforcement so that parents believe they are doing what is best for their child.

- Selected follow-up sessions with parents should include the teenager to
  - Demonstrate to the patient that confidentiality is not being violated
  - Offer the physician an opportunity to observe parent-adolescent interaction

PROGNOSIS

- The prognosis for patients who have conversion reactions is unknown.
- Many patients who have conversion symptoms have an encouraging future.
- For some patients, adolescent conversion symptoms mark the beginning of a lifelong course of conversion illness.
- In a report of 74 children who had psychogenic pain, many were judged to be improved after several years regardless of whether professional intervention took place.
- In a 7-year follow-up of patients hospitalized with conversion, 23 of 41 patients
  - No longer suffered from presenting physical symptom
  - Were free of underlying stress
  - Had experienced no symptom substitution or new associated complaint

Cough

DEFINITION

- Cough can be described as a forceful exhalation.
  - Generally results from acute viral infection and is therefore self-limited
  - May be the harbinger of a more serious problem
- Cough can be exceedingly disruptive to the child and family.
  - It can lead to significant anxiety for all involved parties.
  - Allaying this anxiety through appropriate diagnosis and management is of prime importance.

EPIDEMIOLOGY

- Cough is one of the most common complaints of children.

MECHANISM

- The primary purpose of cough is to facilitate removal of inhaled irritants and secretions from the airway.
- 3 classic phases of the cough sequence
  - Inspiratory phase
    - Deep inspiration ending in glottic closure
    - Compressive phase
    - Intrathoracic pressure increases as a result of coordinated contraction of the expiratory muscles.
  - Expiratory phase
    - Glottis opens rapidly, leading to the sudden, sometimes explosive, release of the pent-up intrathoracic air (ie, cough).
    - Secretions and irritants are expelled from the airway.
    - Incomplete or inefficient removal of these materials will result in recurrence of the cough sequence, as will ongoing irritation or inflammation.

HISTORY

Accurate description of the cough

- Pattern and progression of symptoms
  - Duration
  - Frequency of discrete cough episodes
  - Quiet periods between cough (daily cough vs days or weeks between cough episodes)
  - Quality
  - Timing
  - Triggers

Age at onset

- Chronic or recurrent cough that begins in early infancy, especially in children <3 months
  - Congenital or anatomic origin
  - Requires a more aggressive approach toward evaluation

- Cough that begins relatively suddenly in toddlers
  - Foreign body aspiration
  - Requires active approach toward testing (bronchoscopy)
- Cough beginning at >6 months of age
  - May suggest airway hyperreactivity
- Cough beginning relatively suddenly in adolescents
  - Especially at times of psychosocial stress, might indicate a psychogenic origin

Family history

- Especially helpful with chronic symptoms
- Allergies, atopy, or asthma
  - Makes these diagnoses far more likely in the child with chronic or recurrent cough
  - History of asthma or atopy in first-degree relatives increases the risk of asthma in the child by 2-fold to 4-fold.
- Family history of early childhood death related to infection
  - Makes an immune deficiency more likely

Neonatal history

- Preterm infants are more likely than full-term infants to have:
  - Persistent airways hyperreactivity
  - Laryngotracheomalacia
  - Gastroesophageal reflux
- Central nervous system sequelae are likely in infants with:
  - Poor Apgar scores
  - Perinatal hypoxia
  - Difficult postnatal course
  - Suck or swallow dysfunction increases the risk of aspiration.
- Congenital abnormalities (eg, diaphragmatic hernia)
  - Pulmonary hypoplasia
  - Chronic respiratory dysfunction
  - Recurrent pneumonia

Environmental history

- Smokers in the household
  - Associated with significantly more respiratory infections and asthma symptoms in children
- Exposure to molds
  - Household water leaks
  - Decaying garbage
  - Ineffective cleaning of bathroom tile
- Dust mites
  - Old mattresses
  - Stuffed animals
  - Forced air heating systems
- Roaches

- Mice
- Pets
- Exposure to other children
  - At school
  - At child care
  - Babysitters
  - Siblings

PHYSICAL EXAM
- Physical examination plays a critical role in:
  - Pinpointing the origin of the cough
  - Identifying signs of a more serious underlying chronic condition
- Nasal mucosa
  - Nasal speculum examination
    - Color and quality of mucosa
    - Presence or absence of nasal secretions helps determine whether the cause of the cough is upper airway disease.
    - Rhinitis
      - Pale, boggy, swollen nasal mucosa
    - Sinusitis (when symptoms are prolonged)
      - Associated maxillary or frontal sinus tenderness
      - Pharyngeal drip with a cobblestone appearance (lymphoid hyperplasia) further supports the diagnosis of sinusitis.
      - Halitosis may also be present.
    - Chronic pharyngeal inflammation
      - In the absence of other signs of acute infection, suggests gastroesophageal reflux
- Oral mucosa
  - Ulcerations or thrush suggest an immune deficiency.
  - Cough paroxysms triggered by a tongue depressor support the diagnosis of pertussis.
- Signs of an acute infectious process
  - Fever
  - Adenopathy
  - Pharyngitis
  - Rash
    - These do not necessarily rule out a predisposing condition, especially when the pattern of illness suggests chronicity or frequent recurrence.
- Thorough assessment of other body systems
  - Important in judging whether a more global workup is necessary
  - Clues to a more severe underlying process
    - Growth failure
    - Poor developmental milestone achievement
    - Clubbing
    - Heart murmur
    - Hepatosplenomegaly
    - Chronic lymphadenopathy
- Respiratory system
  - Stridor, inspiratory rhonchi, or wheeze
    - Suggest upper and large central airway disease
  - Rales, expiratory rhonchi, and wheeze
    - Indicative of lower or distal airway inflammation
  - Change in the quality of air exchange
    - Can be an early finding in asthma and other diseases of airway obstruction
  - Accurate lower airway examination depends on the cooperation of the patient.
    - Wheeze and distal airway sounds can be masked by a patient's vocalization or crying.
    - A force of airflow insufficient to uncover milder changes may mask both inspiratory and expiratory findings in infants and children who do not take deep breaths on command.
  - Every effort should be made to place the child at ease during the examination.
    - Game-playing can be helpful.
      - Blowing on a feather
      - Blowing up a balloon
    - In younger children and infants:
      - The examiner can mimic a forced expiratory maneuver by firmly but gently compressing the anterior-posterior chest wall inward once the child has begun voluntary exhalation.
      - This approach will frequently uncover milder degrees of wheezing not appreciated with passive breathing.
      - The examiner should allow the child to begin exhalation passively before performing this maneuver to ensure that the glottis is relaxed.

DIFFERENTIAL DIAGNOSIS
- Acute vs chronic (>3 weeks' duration) cough
  - Chronic cough requires a more extensive evaluation plan.
- Upper, lower, or mixed airway origin
  - Upper airway cough
    - Croupy
      - Young children with asthma (disease of the lower airway) may initially exhibit a croupy cough.
    - Throaty
    - Honking
    - Foghorn

- Lower airway cough
  - Productive with expectoration of sputum is classically the result of bacterial pneumonia.
    - Children with severe chronic sinusitis (disease of the upper airway) will frequently cough and expectorate or swallow thick sputum that may be blood tinged.
- Cough character can be a useful starting point.
  - Paroxysmal
    - Pertussis
  - Staccato
    - *Chlamydia* infection
  - Barking
    - Laryngotracheal infection
  - Throat clearing
    - Postnasal secretions
  - Honking
    - Psychogenic cough
      - Occurs during the daytime
      - Increases when more attention is paid to it
      - Does not limit or change with physical activity
  - Cough during feeding
    - Suggests swallowing dysfunction
    - Tracheoesophageal fistula with aspiration
  - Cough after feeding
    - Spitting up, retching, or arching of the back
    - Gastroesophageal reflux
  - Associated fever
    - Respiratory tract infection
  - Cough worsening with exercise
    - Suggests reactive airway disease
    - Asthma
  - Night cough
    - Postnasal drip
    - Allergy
    - Sinusitis
  - Previous episodes, especially with seasonal variation
    - Allergy
  - Chronic cough with poor weight gain
    - More severe systemic illness
    - Cystic fibrosis
    - Immune deficiency

LABORATORY EVALUATION

- Acute cough rarely needs extensive laboratory assessment.
- Hematologic tests
  - Complete blood count with differential
    - May help distinguish a bacterial from a viral cause if infection is suspected
    - Localized infections, such as sinusitis, are not always accompanied by an elevated leukocyte count with a left shift.
    - Total eosinophil count may be an important clue to the atopy.
    - Elevated immunoglobulin E level further corroborates the diagnosis of allergy and suggests the possibility of asthma.
- Nasal smear
  - Positive for eosinophils
    - Corroborates the diagnosis of allergy and suggests the possibility of asthma
  - Increased polymorphonuclear leukocytes on nasal smear may suggest rhinosinusitis.
    - However, the result is difficult to quantify, and test may be misleading.
- Tuberculin skin test
- Immunologic studies
- α_1-Antitrypsin levels
- Sweat chloride

IMAGING

- Computed tomography of the sinuses
  - Confirms the diagnosis of sinusitis
- Chest radiography
- Barium swallow
  - In infants
    - Anatomic causes of partial obstruction
    - Tracheoesophageal fistulae
    - Vascular rings
  - Modified for aspiration
  - Standard for gastroesophageal reflux
    - ~40% false-negative rate

DIAGNOSTIC PROCEDURES

- Pulmonary function tests
  - Distinguish between:
    - Upper and lower airways disease
    - Obstructive vs restrictive changes

- Children must be old enough to exhale fully and inhale forcefully on command.
- Test should be reproducible to ensure accuracy and reliability of results.
- Airway tests
  - Changes on the inspiratory loop of the flow-volume curve
    - Upper airway obstruction
  - Changes in the FEV_1/FVC ratio or the forced midexpiratory flow rate over the middle half of the FVC (FEF 25–75%)
    - Airway obstruction consistent with distal disease
  - Reversibility of these changes (20% improvement) with a ß2-agonist confirms asthma and leads to effective therapy.
- pH probe monitoring
  - The gold standard for diagnosing gastroesophageal reflux
    - Reserve for patients in whom primary empiric treatment fails
- Bronchoscopy
  - Cough that begins relatively suddenly in toddlers
    - To confirm foreign body aspiration
  - Useful to diagnose structural abnormalities of both the upper and lower airways
    - Should be considered in patients with chronic symptoms not responsive to empiric treatment
  - If an upper airway origin is likely, flexible bronchoscopy can make a definitive diagnosis.
    - The bronchoscopist must always look beyond the vocal cords in this setting.
    - Lesions at the level of the thoracic inlet can exhibit as findings suggestive of upper airway obstruction.
- Sweat test

TREATMENT APPROACH

- Treatment is based on the underlying disorder.
  - Empiric therapy, based on primary assessment, can be a reasonable starting point.
- Detailed history and physical examination are usually sufficient to reach an accurate presumptive diagnosis.
  - Response to empiric therapy will confirm this assessment.
- The cough as a symptom of an underlying condition should be discussed with the patient and family.
  - Treatment of the underlying disorder (if necessary) should always be the primary focus.
  - In some conditions, cough is an important component of the body's natural response to the primary illness.
    - Suppressing the cough, in the absence of effective therapy for the primary disorder, may worsen the problem.

- The decision to use a cough medicine as an adjunct to the treatment of the primary disease is left to the primary care physician and family.
  - When cough is limiting or otherwise debilitating the patient, symptomatic treatment may be reasonable.
  - Cold and cough medicines should not be used in children <2 years of age because of serious side effects. Further, they are generallly ineffective in children <6 years.

SPECIFIC TREATMENT

Expectorants

- Despite widespread use, expectorants have not been shown to decrease cough in children.
- Guaifenesin (formerly glyceryl guaiacolate)
  - May be used to make secretions more fluid and reduce sputum thickness
  - Useful when drainage of secretions is important, as with sinusitis
- Saline solutions
  - Safe adjunct to primary therapy
  - Water is the most effective expectorant because expectorants work by increasing the fluid content of secretions.
  - Administration via nasal spray, inhalation, or orally
- Older expectorants
  - Potassium iodide
  - Ammonium chloride
  - No longer prescribed to children because of their adverse effects when used at effective doses

Mucolytic agents

- Acetylcysteine
  - Previously used as a mucolytic agent to help liquefy thick secretions, especially in such diseases as cystic fibrosis
  - Its propensity for inducing airway reactivity and inflammation has made it less popular.

Cough suppressants

- Peripheral agents
  - Can be effective in transiently decreasing cough severity and frequency
  - Demulcents (eg, throat lozenges) soothe the throat.
  - Topical anesthetics can be sprayed or swallowed; effects are short-lived, as oral secretions rapidly wash them away.
- Centrally acting agents
  - Narcotics
    - Effective narcotic agents commonly used in children include hydrocodone and codeine.
    - The metabolic clearance pathway of codeine in infants is immature and data for adults should not be extrapolated to children, particularly those <2 years.

– Hydrocodone has a greater risk of dependency and no demonstrated advantage.

– They should be used in older children with appropriate instructions and caution to avoid overuse or abuse.

- Nonnarcotic medications

  – Dextromethorphan

  – Despite evidence in adults, proven efficacy data in children are lacking.

Decongestants (pseudoephedrine)

- Topical or systemic
- Decreases nasal mucosal swelling
- Facilitates sinus drainage
- May work well in combination with expectorants to optimize treatment of chronic sinusitis
- Care should be taken in the use of these agents because:
  - When used in excess, they have been shown to lead to tachyarrhythmias.
  - Topical nasal decongestants can cause rhinitis medicamentosa.
  - They have not been studied in younger children.
  - They should be avoided in children <2 years.
  - Use should always be limited to short periods to minimize these risks.

Antihistamines

- Can be helpful in the treatment of cough triggered by allergy
- Minimal effect when cough is the result of viral or bacterial infection

- May be detrimental because they can increase the thickness of secretions.
  - First-generation histamine$_1$-receptor antagonists may decrease nasal drip by exerting an anticholinergic effect.
- Diphenhydramine may have a modest direct effect on the medullary cough center.
  - The clinical benefits of these findings are unclear.

Bronchodilators

- Therapeutic trial of treatment with a ß$_2$-agonist may be a reasonable first step in suspected airway hyperreactivity.

WHEN TO REFER

- When cough persists despite adequate therapy
- When cough recurs more than every 6–8 weeks
- When associated with failure to thrive
- When associated with other systemic illness

WHEN TO ADMIT

- When the patient has respiratory distress
- When the infant cannot feed
- When associated with bacterial pneumonia not responsive to an oral antibiotic trial

Cross-Sex Behavior and Gender Identity Disorder

DEFINITION

- Gender-variant behavior
  - Display of behaviors, attitudes, or interests outside the cultural norm for the child's biological (genetic/anatomic) sex
    - Boys who prefer playing house, enjoy dressing up in their mother's clothes or trying on their makeup, prefer long hair, and are more stereotypically feminine in their mannerisms and speech
    - Girls who avoid wearing girls' clothes, enjoy more physically aggressive play with boys, prefer short hair, and have the stereotypic mannerisms of a tomboy
- Gender identity is a person's deepest inner sense of being female or male, often established by age 2–3 years.
  - Incongruent with biological sex for some
  - Different concept from sexual orientation
- *Transsexual* or *transgender* refers to an inner identity of the opposite gender or a sense of gender separate from female or male.
  - Transsexual persons
    - Gender identity does not match biological gender.
    - Seek to physically change their bodies to be consistent with their inner sense of gender
  - Cross-dressers (transvestites), drag kings and queens, and persons who perceive themselves to be of both genders
  - Individuals who are simply gender nonconforming in terms of attitudes, interests, and behaviors
  - Transgender individuals often refer to themselves as *trans*, *TG*, or *T*.
  - Many experience significant gender dysphoria: persistent discomfort with the gender assigned at birth and accompanying societal gender role expectations.
  - Transition occurs when transgender individuals gradually let go of the need to conform to societal expectations of their biological gender and increasingly present themselves in a manner consistent with their gender identity.
    - Male-to-female (MTF) and female-to-male (FTM) transgender describe the direction of transition from biological gender to gender identity.
    - The transition process may include hormone treatment and sex-reassignment surgery.
- One of the most debated issues related to gender expression and gender identity during childhood and adolescence is whether gender nonconformity, gender-variant behaviors, and transgenderism are causes for concern.
  - Is it a pathological abnormality or simply part of the continuum of normal human development?
    - Similar debates occurred around homosexuality until it was officially removed from the American Psychiatric Association's list of mental disorders in 1973.

- Gender identity disorder (GID): Although controversial, transsexualism is listed in the fourth edition of the *Diagnostic and Statistical Manual of Mental Disorders* (*DSM-IV*) under the diagnostic category of *gender identity disorder*. See Diagnosis for listing of 4 criteria for diagnosis of GID.

EPIDEMIOLOGY

- Prevalence
  - Occasional or single gender-variant behaviors among elementary school children are common.
  - During development of the Child Behavior Checklist, mothers of 4- to 5-year-old children reported:
    - 6% of boys and 11.8% of girls sometimes or frequently behaved in a manner more typical of the opposite sex.
    - 1.3% of boys and 5.0% of girls sometimes or frequently wished to be the opposite sex.
  - The prevalence of transgenderism is uncertain.
    - Few people seek hormonal and surgical sex reassignment.
    - Some transgender individuals do not have access to, or do not want, sex-reassignment treatments.

ETIOLOGY

- No clear biological marker for GID has yet been found.
- Possible causes for development of gender-variant behavior and transgender identity
  - Animal studies suggest an influence of prenatal hormones.
    - Studies of girls exposed to large levels of androgens prenatally (congenital adrenal hyperplasia) found that the girls had more masculine gender roles than those of peers.
    - Exposure to subtle changes in prenatal androgens during fetal psychosexual development may result in gender-variant behavior and transgender identity.
  - Some studies, mostly in boys, have found an association between GID and:
    - Handedness
    - Sibling sex ratio
    - Birth order
    - Birth weight
- Psychosocial theories (controversial)
  - Familial, particularly parental, psychopathology
  - Predisposal because of aberrant parenting practices
  - These theories are criticized because they appear to identify presumed negative factors (eg, parental failure to discourage a son's feminine behaviors) that might be modified through family therapy to prevent undesirable gender-variant behaviors in a child.

RISK FACTORS

- Any gender-variant child or adolescent raised in a society that enforces a binary view of gender will predictably experience discomfort related to gender expression and identity.

- Given the overt discrimination and violence against transgender individuals in US society, distress or impairment in social and other areas of function should be expected.

- Evidence suggests that transgender individuals growing up in more accepting societies experience less discomfort and distress related to gender identity and gender role than those in the US.

SIGNS AND SYMPTOMS

- 4 criteria for diagnosis of GID
  - Evidence of strong and persistent cross-gender identification (eg, desire to be or insistence that one is of the other sex)
  - Persistent discomfort with assigned sex or a sense of inappropriateness of assigned gender role for that sex
  - No concurrent physical intersex condition (eg, androgen insensitivity syndrome, congenital adrenal hyperplasia)
  - Evidence of clinically significant distress or impairment in social, occupational, or other important areas of functioning

- Based on these criteria, GID would not be diagnosed in a child or adolescent with gender-variant behaviors who identifies with the gender assigned at birth.

- Some signs include:
  - Wearing clothes or exhibiting behaviors or interests typical of the opposite gender
    - This may or may not relate to the child's gender identity.
  - Some may have begun the transition process.
    - Come to the clinic displaying dress, hairstyles, makeup, and mannerisms usually associated with the opposite gender but consistent with gender identity
      - Occasionally wear non–gender-defining street clothes but underwear appropriate for gender identity
  - Patients who have begun transition hormone treatment may show:
    - Evidence of breast development (MTF)
    - Appearance of facial hair (FTM)
    - Other expected changes of estrogen and testosterone treatment (see Specific Treatments)
  - Significant discomfort related to pubertal changes, which feel alien to gender identity
    - MTF-transgender adolescents may tuck their genitals, placing them between their legs so they are less visible.
    - FTM-transgender youths may wear chest binders or baggy tops to make their breasts less visible.

- Comorbid mental health problems, including:
  - Depression
  - Separation anxiety
  - Behavior problems
  - Distress/mental health problems that may result from stigmatization, peer rejection, and discrimination
- Results of violence/fear for own safety
- Sexually transmitted infections (STIs)
  - Can result from promiscuity (eg, in runaways)
- Multisubstance use

DIAGNOSTIC APPROACH

- Physicians should not presume the sexual orientation or gender identity of any patient.

- Many transgender youths hide their true gender identity; the physician must watch for:
  - Fears of primary care physician (PCP) disapproval
  - Uncertainty about confidentiality
  - Confusion about the meaning of their emerging feelings
- Mistaken assumptions
  - That no children in a practice are dealing with issues of gender identity
  - That significant gender-variant behavior in childhood accurately predicts sexual orientation
  - That transgender youths are gay, lesbian, or bisexual
    - An MTF-transgender adolescent who falls in love with a boy is considered heterosexual.
  - That gender identity predicts sexual orientation
- It is important to make distinctions between sexual orientation and gender identity for the provision of care.
- PCPs should reflect on their own feelings about gender-variant behaviors/gender identity issues.
  - Discomfort or disapproval will diminish the ability to care for these patients.
  - Should receive training about transgender health issues
  - Need to provide care that addresses the patient's needs in a compassionate and comprehensive manner
- At a well-child visit, beginning in early childhood:
  - Ask parents how they think their child is developing compared with other children.
  - Ask parents and child how the child is getting along with siblings and peers.
  - See whether the child appears happy.
  - All parents should be asked whether they have concerns with child's sexual development or gender expression.
    - Many parents are hesitant but relieved when the PCP brings the topic up.

- If a child with gender-variant behavior is happy and safe and parents have no concerns, no reason exists to question further.
- If parents express concerns, the PCP should ask what they have noticed or heard from the child and what their concerns or fears might be.
- PCPs may gently question a gender-variant child:
  - To see whether the child feels safe from teasing at home and school
  - About the child's feelings of being more like a girl or a boy inside
- Care must be taken to avoid conveying that anything is wrong with a child because of gender variance.
- At each well-teen visit
  - Initiate a discussion of sexuality, including sexual orientation and gender identity.
    - In broader context of HEEADSSS (home, education, eating, activities, drugs, sexuality, safety, and suicide) interview
    - Acknowledge that sexual feelings can be confusing.
    - Ask about attractions (sexual orientation), and ask, "And how about inside? Does it seem to feel more like a girl or a boy or maybe somewhere in between?"
    - Let the patient know that you are available to talk.
- For adolescents who acknowledge transgender identity:
  - Thank them for their trust.
  - Reassure them about confidentiality.
  - Ask what they know about gender identity and what it means to be transgender.
  - Ask if they have told others about their inner feelings of gender.
    - Have they been scolded, teased, harassed, or ridiculed?
  - With whom do they spend time, and what kinds of things do they do together?
  - Have they been in relationships, and have they been healthy ones?
  - Have they been sexually active, and do they use safe-sex practices?
    - Ever been pregnant
    - Ever impregnated anyone
    - Ever had an STI
    - How many different sexual partners and their gender
    - Ever been touched sexually or forced to have sex without permission

- Recommendations for examination
  - Prior to examination, discuss the rationale for suggesting areas that might be uncomfortable for a transgender adolescent, eg, breast and genital examinations.
  - Explain that the intent is to make the examination as comfortable as possible and to elicit the patient's guidance in how best to accomplish this task.
  - Inform patients that they have a right to refuse any part of the examination.
  - Ask transgender patients what words they would like used in referring to various body parts.
    - *Genitals* instead of *penis* or *vagina*
    - FTM-transgender patient, *chest* rather than *breast*
  - MTF-transgender patients should be treated like other female patients.
  - FTM-transgender patients should be treated like other male patients.
  - Drape the patient in a gown to minimize exposure.
  - Acknowledge that anatomic gender may suggest gender-specific evaluation, such as breast, testicular, or pelvic examination, is appropriate.
    - Most transgender patients agree to a suggested examination if the medical rationale is presented in a factual and respectful manner.
    - Invite questions/input on how to make the examination as comfortable as possible.
- Questions to ask transgender individuals
  - Have you run away from home or dropped out of school?
  - Have you needed to sell your body, deal drugs, or engage in other illegal activities to survive?
  - Have you been involved with child welfare or juvenile justice system, and how have you been treated within that system?
  - Have you ever used drugs or contemplated suicide?
  - How has your physical health been, and do you have any health needs you believe are not being addressed?
  - Finally, have you begun transition process, MTF or FTM?
    - Have you chosen a new name, and would you like the PCP to call you by that name?
    - Have you begun to cross-dress?
    - Have you begun hormone therapy?
      - If so, where have you obtained hormones?
    - Have you injected silicone?
    - Have you thought about sex-reassignment surgery or other transition-related procedures?

LABORATORY FINDINGS

■ No special laboratory evaluation is needed when there is an unremarkable history and normal physical examination.

■ Laboratory evaluation of transgender adolescents should be based on:
- Accurate and comprehensive history, including sexual and other risk behaviors
- Physical examination

■ Evaluation for STIs if engaged in sexual activity

TREATMENT APPROACH

■ There is a growing belief that gender-variant children should be permitted to express gender-variant behaviors and identities freely and without shame.
- Some investigators believe that a GID diagnosis has been used as an indirect means of treating children to prevent development of a later homosexual orientation.
- Much research pathologizes gender-variant behavior and transgenderism.
  - Has not invited study subjects into a discussion of what research questions are important and how study results are to be interpreted and used
- By trying to answer the question, "What went wrong?" the focus on individuals and their families is likely misdirected.
  - The most important questions may be found by observing gender-variant children and families within the context of a disapproving and often violently retributive society.

■ The goal of care is to promote optimal:
- Physical development
- Emotional development
- Social development
- Well-being
- PCPs are challenged to achieve this goal within a context of nonacceptance and stigmatization by many in society.

■ PCPs should focus on risks that transgender youths face, but also identify specific strengths.

■ Listen carefully to understand patients' unique experience and needs; counseling of gender-variant and transgender youths will address:
- Self-acceptance and validation of gender expression and identity
- Safety
- Ways to connect to support groups
- Self-disclosure or coming out
- Healthy relationships and sexual decision making
- Optimism for the future

■ Acknowledge the controversy around the use of GID as a diagnostic category.
- Inform the patient that many professionals disagree that being transsexual or transgender is a disorder.
- Reassurance of health rather than disorder

■ Provide transgender youths with information on sexual orientation, gender identity, and being transgender.
- Assure that confusion about being gay, bisexual, straight, transgender, or a combination of these is normal.
- Connect ethnic and other minority youths who are transgender to appropriate supportive resources within their communities.

■ Check on safety.
- At home, school, or church; within the peer group; and within the broader community
- Work to help identify and implement appropriate strategies to end violence.
  - Tell patients they should expect safety and respect.
  - Offer to join with them where they experience violence, including the home and school, to work out a plan to end violence immediately and completely.
  - If necessary, call on state child protective services or advocacy organizations, such as the American Civil Liberties Union.

■ Never reveal gender identity to the parents without the permission of the child unless risk of harm exists.

■ Help adolescents decide whether they are ready to come out to family or friends, and help them choose:
- Appropriate time
- Appropriate place
- Approach for disclosure

■ Create a safe, accepting clinical setting where patients and families know they can discuss gender identity/expression.
- Specific messages can be provided through clinic posters and brochures.
- History taking and anticipatory guidance should include issues of child and adolescent sexuality and gender.
- After patients have identified themselves as transgender, use pronouns consistent with patients' gender identity; ask what name they would like to be called by clinic staff.
  - Medical records must retain patients' legal names, but add "Also Known As [preferred name]" to front of the chart; staff members should use these names with patients.
  - Patients should use either a unisex restroom or a restroom consistent with their gender identity while in the clinic.
  - Transgender patients should be seen alone and their confidentiality respected.

– Ask patients how they want gender identity recorded in the chart, if at all, because records containing confidential information may be accessible to parents.

SPECIFIC TREATMENTS

Suppression of puberty

- In cases where physical changes of puberty are very distressing to transgender youths, protocols exist to suppress progression of puberty.
  - Allows time for later decisions about hormone therapy or surgery
  - Gonadotropin-releasing hormone analogue
    – For patients ≥12 years of age with a sexual maturity rating of 2 or 3
    – If the adolescent later decides not to pursue hormone therapy or surgical sex reassignment, suppression can be discontinued.
    – If at age 16 years adolescent wishes hormone treatment, estrogen or testosterone can be added to gonadotropin-releasing hormone analogue to initiate pubertal changes consistent with gender identity.

Elective process for transition after GID diagnosis

- Transition represents emotional, psychological, social, physical, and legal processes that transgender persons experience to assume a body and role consistent with gender identity.
- PCPs play an important role in facilitating the patient's transition FTM or MTF, either by referring patients or by providing transition medical care and counseling themselves.
  - Pediatric PCPs generally refer transgender patients for transition-related care and counseling but retain a central role as PCP.
  - Providers of transition medical care and supportive counseling to transgender patients can be located through local gay, lesbian, bisexual, and transgender centers or national organizations, such as the Gay and Lesbian Medical Association.
    – Adolescent medicine
    – Family practice
    – Internal medicine physicians
    – Mental health care providers
- 3 stages
  - Real-life experience consistent with gender identity
  - Hormones of the desired gender
  - Surgery to change genitalia and other sexual characteristics
- Requirements for initiating hormone treatment
  - Minimum age of 16 years (preferably with parental consent if <18 years)

- Involvement of mental health professional with both patient and family for ≥6 months
- Letter authorizing hormone treatment from patient's therapist to physician
- Plan for monitoring by physician and therapist of adaptation to physical and psychosocial changes

- Transition is not the same for everyone.
  - Some individuals are satisfied to live their lives consistent with their gender identity in a social sense but have no urge to initiate hormone therapy or undergo surgery.
  - Others seek hormone treatment but think that surgical alteration is unnecessary.
  - Others choose partial surgical gender reassignment.
    – Many FTM transgender individuals choose mastectomy but not genital reconstruction.
  - The transition process is not necessarily linear.
    – Some individuals move back and forth between feeling more feminine or masculine.
      ▪ May present themselves differently to the world at different times
    – This fluidity of identity should be expected and supported by the PCP.

Hormone treatments for transition

MTF transition

- Estrogen
  - Oral, injectable, transdermal forms
  - Expected changes
    – Breast development
    – Softening of skin
    – Increase in subcutaneous fat and its redistribution to the thighs and buttocks
    – Diminished body hair
    – Fewer erections
    – Testicular atrophy
    – Possible infertility
  - Possible, sometimes permanent changes
    – Decreased libido
    – Weight gain
    – Emotional changes
  - Medical contraindications to estrogen treatment in adolescents are rare.
- Antiandrogens, such as spironolactone, may be added to:
  - Suppress the action of endogenous testosterone
  - Augment breast development
  - Soften facial and body hair

C

FTM transition

- Testosterone
  - Injection, patch, and topical gel forms
  - Expected changes
    - Increased facial and body hair
    - Clitoral enlargement
    - Cessation of menses
    - Possible infertility
    - Increased acne
    - Male-pattern baldness
    - Deepening of voice
    - Redistribution of fat and increased muscle mass
  - Possible changes
    - Increased libido
    - Mood changes
    - Increased weight
    - More prominent veins
    - Coarser skin
    - Mild breast atrophy

Other treatments

- Occur post-adolescence (expensive and seldom covered by insurance)
  - MTF-transgender individuals
    - Reconstructive surgery
    - Orchiectomy
    - Vaginoplasty
    - Breast augmentation
    - Tracheal shaving
    - Facial reconstruction
    - Electrolysis or other hair-removal procedures
  - FTM-transgender individuals
    - Chest reconstruction surgery
    - Hysterectomy, oophorectomy
    - Genital reconstruction
    - Voice therapy
  - Professional guidance in how to present themselves to the world
  - Discussing these or making appropriate referrals should be part of the PCP's anticipatory guidance.

WHEN TO REFER

- When an adolescent has acute or recurrent suicidal ideation
- When an adolescent is engaged in multiple high-risk behaviors

- When the PCP believes that time, expertise, or comfort is insufficient to provide care and counseling to gender-variant children and transgender youths
- Referral should be made only to health care providers and counselors who have:
  - Experience in working with gender-variant children and transgender youths *and*
  - Who accept gender variance as normal
- Referrals for therapy to change a child's or adolescent's gender expression or gender identity are unethical and potentially harmful.

FOLLOW-UP

- Refer parents to Web sites, mailing lists, and brochures geared to parents of gender-variant children.
- Discuss gender variance and its possible causes with parents.
  - Many, but not all, boys with gender-variant behaviors identify themselves as homosexual as they grow older.
  - Most, but not all, girls with gender-variant behaviors identify themselves as heterosexual or bisexual as they grow older.
  - A few may eventually seek hormone therapy or surgery to make their biological gender more consistent with their inner gender identity.
  - Recommend that parents avoid efforts to change a child's behavior to conform to stereotypic notions of appropriate behaviors.
- Review the Children's National Medical Center Guidelines with parents.
  - Love and accept your child.
  - Do not allow societal expectations to come between you and your child.
  - Create a safe space, especially in the child's home.
  - Seek out socially accepted activities (sports, arts, hobbies) that respect the child's interests while helping the child fit in socially.
  - Validate the child's interests.
  - Speak openly and calmly about gender variance in positive terms, and listen as child expresses feelings of being different.
  - Seek out supportive resources (books, videos, Web sites, support groups).
  - Talk about gender variance with other significant people in the child's life.
    - Siblings
    - Extended family members
    - Babysitters
    - Family friends

- Prepare for bullying.
  - Let the child know that he or she does not deserve to be hurt.
  - Be aware of behaviors that suggest that bullying may be occurring.
    - School refusal
    - Crying excessively
    - Complaining of aches and pains
- Be the child's advocate.
  - Parents should insist on acceptance, respect, and safety wherever their child is.
  - Parents may need to educate school staff and others about the special experience and needs of gender-variant children.
- Advise parents to avoid these pitfalls.
  - Avoid finding fault.
    - No blame exists.
    - The child's gender variance came from within, not from them as parents.
    - Blame will get in the way of enjoying their child.
  - Do not pressure the child to change, because this will cause much pain and harm.
  - Do not accept bullying as just the way things are.
    - No one has the right to torment or criticize others because they are different.

COMPLICATIONS

- Many transgender individuals experience daily verbal, physical, and sexual harassment.
  - Often not addressed, or even encouraged, by teachers, counselors, or school staff
  - Most schools have no policies prohibiting harassment or bullying based on gender identity.
- Broader societal forms of discrimination
  - Common forms of identification and personal records usually reflect biological sex rather than gender identity.
    - Fear, embarrassment, and potential humiliation accompanying presentation of these documents to others may prevent transgender individuals from applying for school, a job, or health care.
- Rejection or violence within families lead many to be thrown of the home out or to run away.
  - Youths often survive by exchanging sex for money, drugs, or shelter.
  - At high risk for STIs, infection with HIV, physical and sexual assault
  - Multisubstance use

- May be sheltered by transgender adults; often a conduit to:
  - Commercial sex work
  - Substance use
  - Underground acquisition of transition hormones or injectable silicone
- Many attempt suicide.

PROGNOSIS

- Boys with GID
  - Most eventually self-identify as homosexual or bisexual and no longer report gender dysphoria.
  - A small percentage later self-identify as heterosexual and report no gender dysphoria.
  - Approximately 15% continue to experience discomfort with their biological sex and self-identify as transgender.
- Girls with GID
  - Most eventually self-identify as heterosexual or bisexual.
  - A small percentage report being homosexual.
  - Only a small percentage continue to have gender dysphoria.
- Most children with significant gender-variant behaviors eventually identify themselves as gay, lesbian, or bisexual.
  - Most experience significant confusion and distress.
  - In our society, many feel overwhelming shame, anger, self-hatred, and despair.
  - Often experience profound isolation that intensifies feelings of confusion and distress
- Discrimination, stigma, violence
  - Completing the developmental tasks of childhood/adolescence related to identity and self-esteem is enormously difficult.
  - Many are viewed by their families with shame and disgust; they often are forced to renounce their declared inner sense of being female or male.
  - Many run away from or are thrown out of their homes.
  - Many end up in the child welfare or juvenile justice systems.
    - Harassment/abuse often continues in these settings, perpetrated by other youths and by staff members.
- PCPs should challenge the belief of many transgender adolescents that their futures will be significantly limited by their gender identity.
  - Although some communities are more accepting of transgender people than others, many transgender adults lead happy, healthy, and productive lives.
  - Although growing up transgender is often challenging, the future should be seen as hopeful and exciting.
  - If provided with loving, supportive validation, they can expect to grow into happy, healthy, and productive adults.

Croup (Acute Laryngotracheobronchitis)

DEFINITION

- Viral croup, also known as *acute laryngotracheobronchitis*, is an age-specific viral syndrome characterized by acute laryngeal and subglottic swelling, resulting in:
  - Hoarseness
  - Cough
  - Respiratory distress
  - Inspiratory stridor
- *Spasmodic croup* is a term sometimes used to denote afebrile episodes of croup that may be recurrent.
- In the past, membranous croup *was* commonly referred to as *diphtheria*.
  - Until the 20th century, considered the cause of most croup cases
  - Occasionally, the term *membranous croup* is still used for crouplike cases caused by bacteria.

EPIDEMIOLOGY

- Prevalence
  - Accounts for approximately 10–15% of respiratory tract disease in children
- Incidence
  - 7 per 1000 children <6 years of age annually in a prepaid group practice in Seattle
    - Between 1 and 2 years of age, this incidence approximately doubled.
  - In a Chapel Hill, North Carolina, practice, the annual incidence per 100 children for all ages was 1.82 for boys and 1.27 for girls
    - The attack rate during the 2nd year of life was 4.7 per 100 children per year.
  - Hospital admissions from croup in the US have been declining since the 1990s, despite concurrent increase in the population of young children.
    - Most likely explained by the improved and more widely used therapeutic modalities of corticosteroids and nebulized epinephrine
- Age
  - Primarily in children between 3 months and 3 years of age
  - Peak incidence between 6 and 24 months
  - A 14-year Canadian study showed that the rates of hospitalization for croup were highest in the 1st year of life.
- Sex
  - Boys seem to be more susceptible to croup than girls.
  - Among both hospitalized and ambulatory croup cases, the ratio of boys to girls is approximately 2:1.
- Seasonality
  - Seasonal patterns of croup correlate closely with activity of the major viral agents causing the syndrome (see Etiology).

ETIOLOGY

- Inflammation at the subglottic area can cause marked airflow obstruction.
- The anatomy of the cricoid and thyroid cartilage make this area the narrowest and least distensible part of the larynx.
- Inflammation, however, commonly affects the conducting airways at all levels.
- Airway hyperreactivity resulting from allergens may play a role in predisposing these children to repetitive bouts of croup.
- Most frequent cause
  - Parainfluenza types 1 and 2: biennial epidemics in the fall
  - Parainfluenza type 3: annual spring outbreaks, extending into summer, early fall
- Frequent cause
  - Influenza A: epidemic, winter
  - Influenza B: epidemic, winter
  - Respiratory syncytial virus: epidemic, winter and spring
- Less common
  - Human metapneumovirus: winter and spring
  - Adenoviruses: endemic
  - Picornaviruses: fall, spring-summer
  - Coronaviruses: winter and spring
- The age predilection of viral croup can be partly explained by the anatomic features of the airway.
  - Smaller airways are prone to greater degrees of obstruction from inflammation of the lining membranes.
    - Resistance to airflow is inversely related to the 4th power of the radius of the airway.
    - Subglottic trachea of a young child is relatively smaller and more pliable than that of an older individual.
  - Narrowing that occurs with inspiratory effort may therefore be exaggerated in a young child with croup.
  - In addition, obstruction above the subglottic area, as may occur with nasal congestion, increases collapsing force, and increased respiratory rate associated with crying or anxiety may compromise ventilation further.

RISK FACTORS

- Respiratory syncytial virus tends to cause croup in younger children, primarily in the 1st year of life.
  - Often results in prolonged symptoms and hospitalization
- Parainfluenza viruses cause croup predominately in toddlers but may infect younger or school-age children.
- Genetic, immunologic, and other mechanisms are likely to contribute to the development and severity of croup.
  - Atopy or hyperreactivity of the airways has been suggested as playing a role in spasmodic or recurrent croup.
  - Higher incidence of a family history of allergy and positive skin tests for allergens in such children.

- The role of genetic and anatomic factors is supported by studies of lower respiratory tract disease, in which children enrolled at birth were monitored through 13 years of age with periodic pulmonary function tests and markers of atopy.
  - The group with wheezing had significantly lower indices of intrapulmonary airway function as infants, before any lower respiratory tract illness, and increased risk of persistent wheezing in later life.
  - Among children who subsequently developed croup without wheezing or those who never developed croup, premorbid inspiratory resistance was significantly higher.

SIGNS AND SYMPTOMS

- Viral croup typically includes signs of an upper respiratory tract infection for 1–2 days.
- This period is followed by characteristic cough, indicating the progression of infection.
  - Cough may be spasmodic, with a deep brassy or harsh barking quality.
- Laryngitis with a raspy-sounding voice may develop.
- Fever is commonly present, particularly with influenza and parainfluenza viral infections.
  - Temperature often reaches 103°F–104°F.
  - Patients with higher temperatures and more toxic appearance should be suspected of having bacterial tracheitis.
- Child may awaken at night with:
  - Spasms of the cough
  - Acute onset of respiratory distress and inspiratory stridor
- On physical examination, distress is most evident during inspiration.
  - Each inspiratory effort is marked audibly by the stridulous sound and accentuated visibly by retractions of accessory chest wall muscles.
  - Suprasternal, supraclavicular, and particularly substernal retractions are characteristic of the inspiratory obstruction.
  - Distress may be marked by asynchronous movements of the chest wall and abdomen.
- Respiratory rate is increased but usually not >50 breaths/min.
  - Unlike bronchiolitis , in which respiratory distress may be accompanied by respirations of 80–90 breaths/min
- Auscultation of the chest reveals prolonged inspiration, often accompanied by coarse crackles.
  - Wheezes and rhonchi may also be heard on expiration.
  - With more severe obstruction, breath sounds may be diminished.
- Cyanosis may occasionally be noted, particularly around the lips and nail beds.

- Varying intensity of respiratory distress is characteristic.
  - In some children, the symptoms appear to abate on waking in the morning but may worsen again as the day progresses.
  - For most, signs of croup extend over 3 or 4 days, but upper respiratory tract signs and cough may last longer.
  - In a few children, respiratory distress may be unremitting or associated with significant pneumonitis and hypoxemia.

DIFFERENTIAL DIAGNOSIS

- Viral croup must be differentiated from the 2 bacterial causes of stridor.
  - Bacterial tracheitis
  - Epiglottitis, which may be fatal without immediate therapy
    - Rare since conjugated *Haemophilus influenzae* type b vaccines became available
- Differentiating characteristics of epiglottitis
  - Rapidly progressive and unrelenting course, drooling, toxic appearance
  - Coryza and barking cough characteristic of viral croup usually are not present with epiglottitis.
- Infectious causes of stridor
  - Epiglottitis
  - Bacterial tracheitis
    - The second emergent entity that needs to be differentiated from viral croup
    - Relatively uncommon and may affect children of any age, sometimes occurring after an episode of viral croup
    - Onset is acute with respiratory stridor, high fever and, often, copious and purulent secretions.
    - The child appears toxic, and respiratory obstruction rapidly progresses, often necessitating tracheal intubation.
    - Most often involved are *Staphylococcus aureus* and group A ß-hemolytic streptococci.
    - Diagnosis may be confirmed by direct laryngoscopy, which shows purulent secretions and inflammation in the subglottic area.
    - Sometimes, lateral neck radiography reveals an area of subglottic narrowing with a shaggy membrane.
  - Human papillomavirus (acquired perinatally)
  - Retropharyngeal and parapharyngeal abscess
    - May occasionally have features similar to croup
    - Should be especially considered in a child with a history of a penetrating pharyngeal injury, eg, by a fishbone
    - Usually preceded by mild pharyngitis and more gradual in onset than croup
    - The child may be febrile, with sore throat and difficulty in swallowing.

- Stridor is not usually present until disease has markedly progressed.
- Important differential findings include muffled voice, head held in a position allowing extension of the neck, resistance to oropharyngeal examination, and progressive drooling and visible asymmetry to the wall of the posterior oropharynx.
- Diphtheria may be excluded by:
  - History of adequate immunizations
  - Absence of characteristic gray pharyngeal or laryngeal diphtheritic membrane
- Other infectious agents that may mimic croup are now rare.
- Noninfectious causes of stridor, many of which can be differentiated by thorough history
  - Foreign body aspiration
    - Abrupt onset of stridor
    - Respiratory distress
    - Lack of preceding respiratory symptoms
    - Fever
    - History of previous choking on food or foreign body
  - Acute edema of upper respiratory tract caused by an allergic reaction
    - May cause abrupt swelling and severe respiratory distress with stridor
    - Lack of previous respiratory signs
    - Concurrent onset of other manifestations of allergic reaction, eg, swollen lips and tongue and urticaria
  - Vocal cord paralysis
  - Angioneurotic edema of upper airway
  - Hypocalcemic tetany
  - Congenital malformations of upper airway
  - Laryngotracheal malacia, web, cleft
  - Vascular ring
  - Tracheal stenosis
  - Hemangioma, cyst of larynx or trachea
  - Cystic hygroma
  - Trauma

DIAGNOSTIC APPROACH

- Croup is usually diagnosed on the basis of characteristic clinical findings and a compatible history.
- History is integral in:
  - Diagnosing viral croup
  - Assessing the severity of the illness on which the management depends

- Carefully obtain:
  - Prodromal signs
  - Characteristics of the onset of illness
  - Course of the development of the respiratory signs
- A child may be at an increased risk for severe disease if there is evidence of:
  - Atypical onset
  - Rapidly progressive illness
  - History of recurrent episodes of illness with respiratory distress
  - Underlying condition

LABORATORY FINDINGS

- Laboratory testing is usually not necessary for most outpatients.
- Testing may upset the child, causing an increased respiratory effort, further subglottic narrowing, and obstruction to airflow.
- In severe cases, measurement of oxygen saturation may detect hypoxemia.
- If the child's appearance or history, suggests dehydration, serum chemistries may be warranted.
- Leukocyte count and differential are not usually helpful.
  - Total leukocyte count may be normal or low from viral infection.
  - However, a shift to the left with increased number of neutrophils and band forms may also occur in more distressed and hypoxemic children or, infrequently, may suggest bacterial infection.
- Multiple laboratory assays are available to determine the specific viral agent; however, specific diagnosis of the viral agent usually is not necessary.
  - Viral isolation
  - Rapid antigen detection techniques, such as immunofluorescence assays and enzyme immunoassays
  - Methods to detect viral RNA, as by reverse transcriptase polymerase chain reaction
- In some instances, determination of the specific viral cause may help determine infection control procedures or need for antiviral therapy.

IMAGING

- Imaging is not usually necessary in diagnosing or managing children with viral croup.
- In some atypical cases or those likely to be confused with other syndromes characterized by stridor, diagnosis may be aided by:
  - Lateral inspiratory and expiratory radiography
    - May show distension of the hypopharynx

- Posteroanterior radiography of the neck
  - The air shadow of the larynx narrows, resembling an hourglass or a steeple, in the subglottic region as a result of the characteristic inflammation inspiratory lateral view.
  - However, in some instances, the radiograph is not interpretable, or the classic signs may not be evident.

TREATMENT APPROACH

- The first phase of management is to evaluate which children may be managed at home and which require hospitalization.
- Severity is often difficult to determine in this fluctuating disease, and no clinical signs are consistently prognostic of a complicated course.
- Clinical scoring systems, such as the Westley croup score, have been used to aid in the decision as to which children should be hospitalized (see table Clinical Scoring System for Croup).
- Toxic appearance, dehydration, and fatigue are indications for hospitalization.

SPECIFIC TREATMENTS

Supportive care

- Supportive care is of prime importance for both outpatients and hospitalized patients.
- The child should be made comfortable to avoid unnecessary anxiety and fatigue.
- Fluids should be encouraged.
- Antipyretics may be given for fever and to diminish the associated increased respiratory rate and fluid requirements.
- Few other home therapies have proved beneficial; however, because of the variable nature of croup, several unverified therapies may appear to work.

Humidified air

- Water particles from such devices as vaporizers, home-devised mist tents, and showers are generally too large to reach the lower respiratory tract.
  - They generally humidify primarily the anterior nares and oropharynx.
  - Hot water poses the potential hazard of accidental burns
- Cool mist may help cool the airway and may be beneficial to some children with croup.
- Studies in children of the efficacy of humidified air in treating croup are few and involve small numbers of patients; nevertheless, no significant benefit has been shown.

Nebulized epinephrine

- Nebulized epinephrine has been shown to be beneficial for children with more severe croup.

Clinical Scoring System for Croup[a]

Category		Score
Level of Consciousness	Normal (including sleep)	0
	Disoriented	5
Cyanosis	None	0
	Cyanosis with agitation	1
	Cyanosis at rest	2
Stridor	None	0
	When agitated	1
	At rest	2
Air Entry	Normal	0
	Decreased	1
	Markedly decreased	2
Retractions	None	0
	Mild	1
	Moderate	2
	Severe	3

[a] From: Westley CR, Cotton EK, Brooks JG. Nebulized racemic epinephrine by IPPB for the treatment of croup: a double-blind study. *Am J Dis Child.* 1978;132(5):484–487. Copyright ©1978 American Medical Association. All rights reserved.

- Clinical improvement occurs in most cases by reducing degree of stridor and retractions.
- Epinephrine causes diminished subglottic swelling via stimulus of α- and ß-adrenergic receptors.
  - Results in decreased blood flow and swelling in the upper respiratory tract
- Racemic epinephrine, which contains both D and L isomers, has been preferably used because it was believed to reduce adverse effects.
  - However, controlled evaluation of the 2 isomers indicated no difference in effect or in adverse reactions.
- Nebulized epinephrine should be used with the understanding that:
  - Amelioration of the clinical signs is transient, and the child again may worsen within 2 to 3 hours.
  - Arterial oxygen saturation is not affected.
  - Nebulized epinephrine should be used only for children with moderately severe or severe croup.
    - These children should usually be concurrently treated with corticosteroids.

C

Corticosteroid therapy

- The major advance and mainstay in the management of both ambulatory and hospitalized children with viral croup is the use of systemic or nebulized corticosteroids.
  - Multiple well-designed trials have shown that both systemic and nebulized corticosteroid therapy has resulted in significant clinical improvement, decreased hospitalization, and fewer follow-up visits.
  - A recent Cochrane systematic review of 31 studies involving 3736 children found:
    - Significant clinical improvement in the Westley score at 6–12 hours.
    - Benefit by 24 hours was no longer significant.
    - Clinical efficacy did not differ significantly according to the agent or route of administration.
    - Conclusion
      - Dexamethasone and budesonide show clinical benefit as early as 6 hours after administration.
      - Treatment was associated with fewer and shorter hospital stays, return visits, and need for other therapies.
      - Dexamethasone was also effective for mild cases of croup.

Antibiotic therapy

- Because croup is of viral etiology, antibiotics are rarely indicated.
- Secondary or concurrent bacterial infection is unusual, and antibiotics should be reserved for such documented cases.

WHEN TO ADMIT

- When the child appears toxic, lethargic, in respiratory distress, or dehydrated
- When the onset of illness was sudden, with rapid progression of symptoms
- When signs of respiratory distress are unresponsive to outpatient drug therapy

WHEN TO REFER

- When the child has a wheezing condition predisposing to more severe croup
- When the child has history of recurrent episodes of croup
- When the episode of croup occurs during the neonatal period
- When symptoms progress despite supportive care at home

Cystic and Solid Masses of the Face and Neck

DEFINITION

- Cystic lesions are either congenital cysts or vascular malformations.
  - Traumatic hematomas and abscesses may appear to be cystic.
- Solid neck masses usually consist of inflammatory lymph nodes or, rarely, neoplastic lesions.

ETIOLOGY

- Thyroglossal duct cysts
  - Result from failure of the embryologic thyroglossal duct to degenerate during the fifth week of gestation, leaving a fistula, sinus tract, or cyst at the midline of the neck just below the hyoid bone.
- Branchial cleft cysts
  - Congenital remnants of the lateral 4 branchial pouches and clefts
- Causes of cervical lymphadenopathy include:
  - Viral infections of the upper respiratory tract
  - Bacterial infections
  - HIV infection
  - Kawasaki disease
  - Systemic disorders, such as systemic lupus erythematosus, juvenile idiopathic arthritis, sarcoidosis, and histoplasmosis

SIGNS AND SYMPTOMS

History

- The physician should determine:
  - Whether the neck mass was observed at birth
    - Lymph nodes >1 cm rarely appear at birth, whereas many congenital cysts are noted in the newborn period.
    - Some congenital cysts may not be noted until childhood or beyond and are detected only when they become infected.
  - Whether it has increased or decreased in size
  - Whether it has changed color
  - Whether the lesion has drained or opened
- Any history of pain or tenderness is important.
  - Congenital cysts are nontender unless they become infected.
  - Inflamed lymph nodes are tender and painful.
  - Pain during eating suggests parotid gland involvement.
- Infectious processes and cancer may be suggested by:
  - History of fever
  - Other systemic symptoms such as loss of appetite, weight, fatigue, etc.

Physical examination

- The first step in the physical examination is to determine whether abnormalities exist in other parts of the body.
  - Other cysts
  - Lymphadenopathy
  - Hepatosplenomegaly
  - Skin lesions
  - Signs of infection
- The exact anatomic location of the neck mass must be determined.
  - Midline masses usually are associated with a thyroid abnormality.
  - A mass along the anterior edge of the sternocleidomastoid muscle that moves with swallowing or that has a sinus opening to the surface of the overlying skin is likely to be a branchial cleft cyst.
  - The clinician should note whether the mass is in a typical location of a lymph node (see Figure 17 on page F5).
- Characteristics of the mass must be determined.
  - Consistency, color, and firmness
  - Presence of tenderness
  - Size
  - Whether the mass moves or is fixed
    - Masses that move with swallowing or with tongue protrusion suggest a thyroglossal duct cyst.
      - These lesions may be tethered to the foramen cecum by the thyroglossal duct remnant.
    - Both cysts and benign lymph nodes are freely mobile.
    - Malignant lesions are more likely to be fixed to underlying structures.
- Neoplasms may be suspected.
  - Rapidly growing, painless neck masses are worrisome because they may be neoplastic.
  - Additional signs associated with a neoplastic process include:
    - Fixation of the mass to subcutaneous tissue
    - Firm consistency
    - Size >3 cm
    - Presence of constitutional symptoms
    - Supraclavicular nodes are the most likely neck mass to be malignant and should always be investigated.

DIFFERENTIAL DIAGNOSIS

- Major challenges in the differential diagnosis are:
  - Differentiating congenital masses from lymph nodes
  - Determining the type of congenital lesion
- Most neck masses encountered by pediatricians are lymph nodes, not cysts.

- Knowing the location of the different groups of lymph nodes within the anterior and posterior anatomic triangles of the neck is crucial.
- Figure 17 on page F5 shows the location of the major groups of lymph nodes, the sternocleidomastoid muscle, and the typical locations of congenital cysts encountered most frequently.

Congenital cysts

Thyroglossal duct cysts

- Account for >70% of congenital cysts of the neck
- Are not often detected at birth but usually are noted first after 2 years of age
- May show initially as an inflamed, tender mass
- When not infected, they are smooth, firm, mobile, and nontender and move upward with tongue protrusion or with swallowing.
- Differential diagnosis includes:
  - Sebaceous cysts
  - Epidermal cysts
  - Submandibular lymph nodes
  - Lipomas

Branchial cleft cysts

- Account for >20% of congenital cysts of the neck
- Most branchial cleft cysts arise from the second cleft or pharyngeal pouch.
- They appear as a small dimple or opening anterior to the middle portion of the sternocleidomastoid muscle.
- The cyst, located just under the skin, is nontender, firm, and mobile.
- A small sinus, which occasionally drains fluid to the surface of the overlying skin, may be present; a long fistulous tract may extend from it to the tonsil bed.
- Branchial cleft cysts without sinuses often are unnoticed until later childhood, when they become infected.
- Infected cysts can easily be confused with lymphadenitis.

Vascular malformations and other lesions

- Account for 4–5% of congenital cysts of the neck

Other lesions

- Other lesions included in the differential diagnosis
  - Sternocleidomastoid muscle masses associated with torticollis
  - Small cystic hygromas
  - Epidermoid cysts
  - Neurofibromas
  - Lipomas
  - Ectopic thyroid gland
- Other congenital masses occur rarely in the head and neck.

Cystic hygromas

- Congenital, avascular masses derived from congenital obstruction of lymphatic vessels
- Usually multilocular, fluid-filled, soft, compressible, painless masses located in the posterior triangle just behind the sternocleidomastoid muscle and in the supraclavicular fossa
- Occur infrequently in the axilla, on the trunk, or on the extremities
- In older children, when they occur within the subcutaneous tissues, they may be mistaken for a lipoma or a hemangioma.
- Usually can be transilluminated
- May grow rapidly because of accumulation of lymph
  - Can reach an enormous size, compressing important structures and obstructing the airway
- Although diagnosis usually is obvious during the physical examination, smaller cystic hygromas may resemble hemangiomas or other cysts.

Cavernous hemangiomas

- Vascular lesions within the subcutaneous tissues
  - May appear in any part of the body
  - May be difficult to differentiate from congenital cysts
- Often noted in the newborn period
- Enlarge, sometimes rapidly, during the first year of life
- Usually regress spontaneously by school age
- The skin overlying these vascular lesions often is bluish.
- Less firm, more diffuse, and more easily compressible than cystic masses (except for cystic hygromas)
- Unlike cystic hygromas, cavernous hemangiomas do not transilluminate, and their size may increase with crying or straining.

Epidermoid cysts

- Relatively common masses that may arise from an embryologic or fusional defect
- Usually located at midline on the face, most often at the level of the eyebrows
- These small cysts feel doughy and smooth and contain sebaceous material, sometimes even hair, cartilage, or bone.
- One-third are present at birth; the remaining two-thirds appear by school age.

Preauricular cysts and sinuses

- The most common anomalies arising from an embryologic fusion failure of precursor tissues that develop into the external ear
- The sinuses are pinhole-size pits.
  - Usually located anterior to the helix
  - May contain a short sinus tract

- Preauricular cysts often are bilateral.
- They are inherited in an autosomal-dominant manner, with incomplete penetrance, and are found more commonly in blacks than in whites.
- They are a far more common cause of preauricular lesions than are first branchial cleft cysts and sinuses, which are located in the same area.
- Hearing deficit may be associated with these lesions, but their prevalence is unknown.

Solid neck masses

- Cervical lymph nodes
  - Often palpable in normal children
  - Can be distinguished by location, size, shape, consistency, and mobility
  - Enlarged cervical lymph nodes (>1 cm) should be defined further by:
    - Their association with surrounding nodes or generalized adenopathy
    - The presence of an infection of the head or pharynx
    - Localized signs of inflammation and erythema
  - Cervical adenitis typically develops as a swollen, tender, erythematous mass in a child with fever.
    - *Staphylococcus aureus* and *Streptococcus pyogenes* account for 80% of acute unilateral cervical adenitis and usually respond to oral antibiotics, such as a penicillin or cephalosporin.
  - Chronic inflammation of the lymph nodes can be seen with infections such as cat-scratch disease, atypical mycobacterium, and toxoplasmosis.
- Cancer
  - Malignant tumors often are found as a single supraclavicular mass or as multiple or matted masses crossing into both the anterior and the posterior triangles.
  - >25% of children with cancer have a tumor of the head or neck.
  - The most common neck cancers include:
    - Hodgkin and non-Hodgkin lymphoma
    - Lymphosarcoma
    - Rhabdomyosarcoma
    - Fibrosarcoma
    - Thyroid tumors
    - Neuroblastoma

DIAGNOSTIC APPROACH

- Because the causes of neck masses range widely from common inflamed lymph nodes and cysts to rare neoplasms, an orderly approach to the workup and management of a neck mass is needed.
  - The mass must be defined as lateral or midline.

- The exact anatomic position of the mass must be determined.
- Localizing a lateral neck mass further into either the anterior cervical triangle (anterior to the sternocleidomastoid muscle) or the posterior cervical triangle is helpful.

LABORATORY FINDINGS

- A complete blood count and blood culture can sometimes be helpful in assessing a tender, erythematous mass.
- Erythrocyte sedimentation rate may be helpful in differentiating inflammatory or malignant lesions from other lesions, such as cysts.
- Thyroid hormone should be measured if the thyroid gland is enlarged.

IMAGING

- Ultrasonography or computed tomography can determine whether the mass is cystic or solid or whether it extends to deeper structures within the neck.
- Thyroglossal duct cysts
  - Unless normal thyroid tissue is palpable, the presence of the thyroid gland should be confirmed by ultrasonography or technetium scan.
    - What may seem to be a thyroglossal duct cyst may actually be an ectopic thyroid gland; removal would leave the child dependent on thyroid hormone supplementation for life.
- Cystic hygromas
  - Ultrasonography reveals fluid and multiple cystic components, confirming the diagnosis.

DIAGNOSTIC PROCEDURES

- Biopsy (needle or excision) of the lesion may be necessary to establish the diagnosis, especially when a malignant lesion is being considered.

TREATMENT APPROACH

- For children with enlarged cervical lymph nodes and evidence of infection, antibiotic therapy is recommended.
  - The child should be evaluated further and monitored closely until the enlarged node has resolved if:
    - Adenopathy is persistent
    - Inflammation is not present
    - Any characteristics are worrisome (eg, the node is >3 cm, immobile, associated with systemic symptoms, or in an abnormal location)
- Congenital cysts and masses
  - Should be monitored closely by the primary care physician
  - Acute bacterial infections should be treated with systemic antibiotics.

C

- Thyroglossal duct cysts, branchial cleft cysts, cystic hygromas, and epidermal cysts should be referred to a surgeon who is experienced at excising these congenital lesions.
  - Elective surgery before an infection develops is preferable because excision of an entire sinus tract, fistula, or embryologic connection is more difficult after an infection.
  - However, many primary care physicians and surgeons prefer to delay surgery until the child is beyond infancy and can better tolerate the procedure.
- Hemangiomas can be observed without referral unless they begin to impinge on vital structures.
  - Hemangiomas that interfere with physiologic functions (eg, blocking the vision, interfering with eating) may be:
    - Treated with glucocorticoid steroids
    - Referred to a surgeon for management

SPECIFIC TREATMENTS

- Thyroglossal duct cysts
  - Because the likelihood of infection is high, thyroglossal duct cysts should be removed surgically.
- Cystic hygromas
  - Because spontaneous regression is rare and the risk of compression of vital upper airway structures is high, surgical removal is indicated.
  - Several procedures often are necessary to remove large lesions completely.
- Cavernous hemangioma
  - Surgery is indicated only for masses that compress vital structures or that cause severe disfigurement.
- Epidermoid cysts
  - Because these cysts may become infected and may form deep tracts, surgical excision is indicated.
- Cervical lymph nodes
  - Lymph node aspiration usually is reserved for patients whose disease does not respond to initial therapy.
  - Incision and drainage may be needed for masses that become fluctuant.

WHEN TO ADMIT

- Infected mass that is unresponsive to oral antibiotics
- Worrisome mass requiring immediate intervention and imaging
- Mass that compromises the airway or other vital structures

WHEN TO REFER

- Congenital cysts or tracts
  - All congenital cysts or tracts should be removed.
- Mass that does not resolve with antibiotic therapy (≥2 weeks)
- Mass in the thyroid gland
- Mass in the parotid gland
- Rapidly enlarging mass (>3 cm)
- Mass that is fixed or lymph nodes that are matted
- Mass in an area that causes concern (eg, supraclavicular)
- Abnormal chest radiograph
- Systemic signs and symptoms (eg, fever, weight loss, easy fatigability, hepatosplenomegaly)

FOLLOW-UP

- All cystic and solid masses of neck require close follow-up to make sure that they are not enlarging rapidly and interfering with physiologic functions, such as vision, eating, and speaking.

COMPLICATIONS

- Interference with physiologic functions, such as vision, eating, or speaking
- Compromise of vital structures, such as airways or the carotid artery

PROGNOSIS

- For children with enlarged cervical lymph nodes and evidence of infection:
  - Antibiotic therapy should improve the condition within 7 days.
  - The condition should resolve completely over the next few weeks.
- Cystic lesions have a good prognosis after surgical removal.
- Prognosis for malignant diseases depends on the type of disease and the extent of spread.

Cystic Fibrosis

DEFINITION

- Cystic fibrosis (CF) is an autosomal-recessive disease.
  - Involves both exocrine and endocrine gland dysfunction
  - Involves multiple organ systems, especially the pancreas and lungs

EPIDEMIOLOGY

- Prevalence
  - CF occurs with a frequency of approximately 1:3600 live births in the white population.
    - It is the most common inherited fatal disease in this group.
  - Frequency in other ethnic groups
    - 1:29,000 in black persons
    - 1:6500 in Hispanic persons
- Age
  - The mean age at diagnosis is 3.3 years.
  - The median age at diagnosis is 6 months.
  - 75% of children with CF receive a diagnosis by 2 years of age.
  - When CF was first described in 1938, the median survival for children with CF was <1 year.
  - Today, the predicted median survival for people with CF in the US is >36 years.
    - This demonstrates how dramatically the face of this disease has changed over a relatively short period.

ETIOLOGY

- Mutation of the cystic fibrosis transmembrane-conductance regulator (CFTR) gene causes a change in structure of the CFTR glycoprotein and results in the development of CF.
- The CFTR glycoprotein is located in numerous organs throughout the body, including:
  - Lungs
  - Upper respiratory tract
  - Sweat glands
  - Pancreas
  - Intestines
  - Liver
  - Reproductive tract
- Ineffective mucociliary clearance and other changes predispose CF airways to infection.
- *Pseudomonas aeruginosa* has become the primary pathogen in this disease.
- *Staphylococcus aureus* and *Haemophilus influenzae* are important bacterial pathogens.

- Initially, nonmucoid environmental strains of *P aeruginosa* are detected in patients.
  - The CF airway environment leads to a transition to mucoidy and to a biofilm mode of growth.
    - Accelerates the rate of decline in lung function
- Despite the chronic nature of the airway infection, ongoing neutrophilic inflammation is typical.
  - DNA released from dying neutrophils increases the viscosity of the airway secretions.
  - Impaired ciliary function and tenacious secretions lead to stasis, and the distal airways become plugged.

RISK FACTORS

- Mutation of the CFTR gene
  - >1000 known mutations of the CFTR gene have been found.
  - The birth of a child with CF is often the first knowledge parents have that they carry a mutation.
- Those in the carrier state are asymptomatic.

SIGNS AND SYMPTOMS

Respiratory symptoms

- Patients with CF most commonly have respiratory symptoms.
- Recurrent pulmonary infections in 49% of patients at presentation
- Failure to thrive or malnutrition in 40%
- Steatorrhea or abnormal stools in 32%
- Meconium ileus or intestinal obstruction in 20%
- Family history of CF in 15%

Pulmonary symptoms

- The common pulmonary symptoms at presentation include:
  - A recurrent cough (most common) that is productive of purulent sputum
    - The cough may initially be dry but becomes progressively productive of purulent sputum.
    - Over-the-counter therapies are generally ineffective.
    - Antibiotic treatment produces only transient, partial improvement in the cough.
    - The cough is present both day and night and may be exacerbated by physical activity or by crying in infants.
  - Difficult-to-control wheezing
    - Some children with CF also have asthma.
  - Nasal polyps
  - Recurrent otitis media
  - Sinusitis
  - Pneumonia
- Vitamin deficiency, specifically deficiencies in the fat-soluble vitamins A, D, E, and K

C

- Other manifestations of CF that may trigger initial patient encounters include:
  - Salt loss syndrome
  - Nasal polyps
  - Hepatobiliary disease
  - Impaired fertility
  - Failure to thrive
  - Irritability
  - Vomiting
  - Salt crystals are sometimes caked on the skin

Gastrointestinal manifestations

- In the pancreas, abnormal electrolyte secretion from the epithelial cells lining the pancreatic ducts results in:
  - Dehydration of the ductal secretions
  - Blockage of the pancreatic ducts
  - Destruction of the pancreatic acini
    - Pancreatic enzyme secretion is significantly decreased.
  - Bicarbonate secretion from the pancreatic ducts is also reduced.
    - In 85–90% of patients with CF, this further decreases the effectiveness of the pancreatic enzymes, known as *pancreatic insufficiency* (PI).
  - PI results in the malabsorption of:
    - Fat
    - Proteins
    - Carbohydrates
    - The fat-soluble vitamins A, D, E, and K
  - Children with PI have difficulty growing and gaining weight.
  - Optimization of nutritional status is also essential to maintaining pulmonary function.
- Patients with PI are at risk for intestinal dysfunction.
  - 20% of infants with CF have meconium ileus.
    - Obstruction of the distal ileum with thick, inspissated, poorly hydrated material
  - Clinically, newborns exhibit:
    - Delayed passage of meconium
    - Abdominal distention
    - A bubbly or granular-appearing material in the region of the terminal ileum on radiography
  - In older children and adults partial or complete obstruction of the small or large intestine may be caused by:
    - Poor hydration of intestinal contents
    - Decreased secretion of pancreatic enzymes
    - Inspissated intestinal secretions
    - Fecal stasis

- Distal intestinal obstruction syndrome (DIOS) may develop as an acute event or may occur chronically, with the following symptoms:
  - Vomiting
  - Abdominal distention
  - Crampy abdominal pain
  - Possibly, a mass in the abdomen, most often in the right lower quadrant.
  - Patients may continue to pass stool around a partial obstruction.
  - Regions of stool retention may serve as lead points for intussusception.
  - Some patients experience rectal prolapse secondary to difficulty passing stool and from increased intraabdominal pressure from coughing.
- Symptomatic liver disease is an uncommon manifestation of CF, with characteristic pathologic findings of:
  - Focal biliary cirrhosis with edema
  - Chronic inflammatory cell infiltration
  - Bile duct proliferation with patchy accumulation of eosinophilic material in the intrahepatic ducts
- The localization of CFTR to the apical membrane of the intrahepatic bile duct cells suggests that a reduction in CFTR activity in CF may result in dehydration and increased viscosity of the bile.
  - May be a key factor in the pathophysiological features of the hepatic disease
  - Prolonged jaundice can occur in neonates.
  - Some patients may develop fatty infiltration of the liver.
  - The characteristic liver lesion in CF is focal or multilobular cirrhosis.
    - Hepatomegaly is detected on examination.
    - The secondary development of splenomegaly suggests the possibility of portal hypertension.
    - Other features of portal hypertension, such as variceal bleeding, have been reported in CF but are relatively rare.

DIFFERENTIAL DIAGNOSIS

- The differential diagnosis includes:
  - Asthma
  - Environmental allergies
  - Immunodeficiency syndromes
  - Ciliary agenesis or dyskinesia
  - α_1-Antitrypsin deficiency
  - Foreign body aspiration

DIAGNOSTIC APPROACH

General

- In the majority of cases, no known family history of CF is found.
- Parents often report that their child has had:
  - Recurrent pneumonia
  - Sinusitis
  - Bronchitis
  - Otitis media
  - Pneumonia and atelectasis may have occurred repeatedly in the same area of the lung.
  - A history of nasal polyps without a concomitant history of nasal allergies
  - Changes to the child's nail beds consistent with clubbing
- From the gastrointestinal standpoint, infants with CF are often voracious feeders despite having poor weight gain.
  - The infants' stools are frequent, bulky, loose, and foul-smelling.
    - The stools are so voluminous that they may overflow the diaper.
  - Grease may be seen in the stool; absorbed in the diaper; or, in the case of older children, seen in the toilet bowl.
  - Abdominal cramping and bloating after eating are common.
  - Foul-smelling flatulence may be described.
- Test for CF:
  - Any neonate born with meconium ileus with delayed passage of meconium
  - Any infant or child with rectal prolapse

Vital signs

- Respiratory rates and heart rates should be monitored relative to age-appropriate normal values.
- Fever and exacerbation or progression of the underlying lung disease may elevate both values.
- Oxygen saturation should be assessed at each visit.
- Overnight pulse oximetry or polysomnography should be considered to evaluate for nocturnal hypoxemia and hypercarbia in patients with more advanced disease.

Growth parameters

- At all ages, pay particular attention to growth parameters.
  - Weight, height, head circumference, and weight for length in children ≤2 years
  - Weight, height, and body mass index in children >2 years
  - The child's height percentile should be compared with the height percentile predicted from the parental height.

- Concern should arise whenever a child:
  - Fails to gain weight
  - Loses weight
  - Crosses percentiles for height or weight

Head and neck

- Otoscopic examination should be performed at all visits to assess for otitis media.
- Audiometry should periodically be performed if a child has recurrent otitis media or is exposed to frequent doses of aminoglycosides.
- Nasal mucosa should be inspected for discharge, swelling of the tissue, or polypoid tissue.
- Palpation of the sinuses should be performed.
- Examination of the oropharynx should include assessment of the tonsils and the posterior pharynx.
  - Children with CF have similar risk for adenotonsillar hypertrophy as children without CF.
- The posterior pharynx should be checked for exudates emanating from the nasopharynx.

Chest and lungs

- Coughing frequency and the productivity of the cough should be assessed.
- The child's ability to communicate without coughing, becoming dyspneic, and using accessory muscles is indicative of the status of the lung disease.
- Auscultation of the lungs may reveal clear breath sounds.
  - With exacerbation of the underlying lung disease, wheezing, rhonchi, or crackles may be heard.
  - As the patient's pulmonary status worsens, these findings may not change with antibiotic therapy.
    - Any clearing that does occur may be short lived.
- As the lung disease progresses, breath sounds may become globally decreased.
- Tubular breath sounds may be heard in areas of severe tissue destruction or bronchiectasis and fibrosis.
- Unilaterally decreased breath sounds should raise concern about development of pneumothorax, particularly in association with an acute onset of dyspnea.
- Progression of the obstructive component of CF lung disease is increasing hyperinflation of the lungs.
  - The chest may take on a barrel shape with an increased anterior–posterior diameter.
- Progression of the fibrotic component of the lung disease results in tachypnea and decreased vital capacity.

Heart

- Fixed splitting of the first and second heart sounds, with increased loudness of the second heart sound, may be heard with progression of the lung disease and development of cor pulmonale.

C

Abdomen

- Infants often have protuberant abdomens.
  - Distention of the abdomen with pain on palpation may be noted in children with acute intestinal obstructions.
- The frequency and distribution of bowel sounds should be assessed by auscultation.
- Palpation should be performed to assess for:
  - Retention of stool, most commonly in the left lower quadrant
  - Tenderness
  - Hepatomegaly
  - Splenomegaly

Genitourinary tract

- Tanner staging should be performed:
  - By direct inspection
  - By having the child indicate his or her developmental status from a series of pictures
- Girls should be questioned about:
  - Onset of menstruation
  - Regularity of cycles
  - Associated symptoms
- All sexually active girls should undergo annual pelvic examination.

Extremities

- Joints should be examined for swelling that may be caused by CF-related arthropathy.
- The digits and nail beds should be examined for clubbing and cyanosis.
- Edema may arise from hypoproteinemia, especially in:
  - Newly diagnosed malnourished infants
  - Patients with end-stage lung disease
  - Patients with cor pulmonale

LABORATORY FINDINGS

General

- Laboratory tests
  - Increased:
    - Serum pH
    - Bicarbonate levels
  - Decreased serum levels of:
    - Sodium
    - Chloride
    - Potassium
- The diagnosis of CF requires:
  - Either 2 positive sweat tests *or*
  - Genotype analysis revealing 2 CFTR mutations known to cause CF

- Plus 1 of the following:
  - Chronic sinopulmonary disease
  - Gastrointestinal or nutritional abnormalities
  - Obstructive azoospermia in boys
  - Salt loss syndrome
  - CF in a first-degree relative

Sweat testing

- The pilocarpine iontophoresis technique of Gibson and Cooke is the gold standard for the diagnosis of CF.
  - Pilocarpine stimulates the secretion of sweat.
  - The volume of sweat and concentration of chloride secreted are then measured.
  - Sweat testing should be performed in accordance with the Clinical and Laboratory Standards Institute (formerly National Committee for Clinical Laboratory Standards) guidelines.
  - Normal chloride values are <40 mEq/L.
  - Values of 40–60 mEq/L are considered borderline.
  - Repeat sweat testing or genetic testing is required to make a definitive diagnosis.
- For some borderline cases, referral to specialized centers may be needed to confirm or rule out CF.
  - For example, a borderline sweat test result with identification of only 1 CFTR mutation
  - Assess CFTR function by measuring nasal potential difference.
  - Abnormal results on 2 nasal potential difference tests are indicative of CF.
- Chloride values >60 mEq/L are considered diagnostic of CF.
  - Many possible causes of false-positive sweat tests exist.
    - Laboratory error
    - Untreated adrenal insufficiency
    - Autonomic dysfunction
    - Ectodermal dysplasia
    - Glucose-6-phosphate deficiency
    - Hypothyroidism
    - Malnutrition
    - Mucopolysaccharidosis
    - Glycogen storage disease (type 1)
    - Fucosidosis
    - Hereditary nephrogenic diabetes insipidus
    - Mauriac syndrome
    - Pseudohypoaldosteronism
    - Familial cholestasis
  - A repeat confirmatory sweat test should be performed together with genetic mutation analysis.
  - Sweat testing should not be performed before 48 hours of age.

- False-negative values can result from edema, malnutrition, and laboratory error.
- Several CFTR mutations that cause CF can also result in a false-negative sweat test.
- When genetic testing is done to resolve borderline sweat testing or when genetic testing alone is performed:
  - The presence of 2 mutations known to cause CF is required to make the diagnosis.
  - DNA from blood or buccal swabs can be used for genetic testing.

Newborn screening

- Newborn screening for CF is being widely adopted in the US.
  - Evidence of moderate benefits and low risk of harm are justification for screening.
  - Recommended by an expert panel convened by the Centers for Disease Control and Prevention and the Cystic Fibrosis Foundation
  - Evidence exists to support the efficacy of newborn screening in the areas of:
    - Improved nutritional status
    - Cognitive development
    - Economic benefit
    - Improved survival
  - The impact of newborn screening on pulmonary status varies.
  - The benefit of improved height and weight status on pulmonary status is well known.
    - Believed to outweigh variability in data concerning pulmonary outcomes for newborn screening
- Newborn screening for CF is typically a 2-tier test.
  - The first tier involves measuring serum immunoreactive trypsinogen (IRT) levels.
    - IRT values are elevated in newborns with CF.
      - Except in infants with meconium ileus, when IRT levels are low
      - All infants with meconium ileus should undergo sweat testing or genetic analysis.
  - The second tier of testing varies among states.
    - May use either repeat IRT measurement or limited genetic mutation analysis.
    - Sweat to confirm results of newborn screening.
- If the child has signs and symptoms consistent with CF, sweat testing or genetic analysis should be performed regardless of newborn screening results.

Microbiological assessment

- Cultures to assess lower respiratory tract flora should be obtained at least quarterly in clinically stable patients and when there is any change in clinical status.
  - An expectorated sputum sample is the usual source.
  - Throat swab or cough swab is often obtained in infants and young children who cannot expectorate.
  - Not necessarily predictive of lower-airway pathogens
- In young children, *S aureus* and *H influenzae* are the most common organisms.
- With advancing age, *P aeruginosa* becomes the predominant pathogen.
- Other pathogens can also infect the lungs in CF.
  - *Burkholderia cepacia* complex
  - *Stenotrophomonas maltophilia*
  - The prevalence of methicillin-resistant *S aureus* has been increasing over the past decade.
- Specialized media are recommended to ensure isolation of pathogens.
  - *P aeruginosa* is best detected using MacConkey agar.
  - *S aureus* on mannitol salt agar or Columbia or colistin–nalidixic acid
  - *H influenzae* on horse blood or chocolate agar
  - *B cepacia* complex is best determined using *B cepacia*–selective agar, oxidation-fermentation polymyxin bacitracin lactose agar, or *Pseudomonas cepacia* agar.
- Antimicrobial susceptibility testing should be determined using an agar-based diffusion assay.
  - Use E-tests (antibiotic-impregnated strips) or antibiotic discs rather than automated commercial systems.
  - Organisms in the *B cepacia* complex and other unidentified gram-negative rods should be further evaluated at a reference laboratory.
    - For instance, Cystic Fibrosis Foundation–sponsored *B cepacia* laboratory at the University of Michigan

IMAGING

- Chest radiography should be performed every 2–4 years in clinically stable patients.
  - Annually in patients with declining pulmonary function
  - As clinically indicated at times of pulmonary exacerbation in all patients
  - Bronchial wall thickening, together with hyperinflation caused by small-airway obstruction, are the first changes noted.
    - Bronchiectasis develops with time.
    - Acute or chronic infiltrates may be noted depending on the patient's clinical status.

– The progression of radiographic changes varies among patients and does not necessarily correlate with abnormalities in lung function tests.

  ▪ Pulmonary function may be relatively well maintained even as radiographic changes may be fairly advanced.

▪ Lateral chest radiographs should be examined for fractures at least annually if patients are ≥8 years of age and at risk for bone disease because these patients are:

  • Malnourished

  • Have severe pulmonary disease

  • On chronic glucocorticoid therapy

  • Have delayed puberty

  • Have low levels of 25-hydroxy vitamin D

▪ Children with these risk factors for bone disease who are ≥8 years of age should undergo a dual-radiograph absorptiometric scan to measure bone density.

▪ All children with CF should have bone densitometry performed by their 18th birthday.

▪ Chest CT may detect structural changes in the lung before symptoms are present.

  • Enthusiasm for periodic chest CT has been limited by concerns about the radiation exposure.

  • No current formal recommendations have been made for routine CT in patients with CF.

▪ Abdominal ultrasonography should be performed:

  • If liver function test results change

  • If hepatomegaly or splenomegaly is detected

▪ Fetal ultrasonography may reveal hyperechoic bowel.

  • Intestinal manifestations of CF may be present even before birth.

  • Suggests retention of mucus material in the intestine.

▪ In older patients, as in meconium ileus, bubbly, granular material can be detected by radiography in the region of intestinal obstruction.

DIAGNOSTIC PROCEDURES

▪ Bronchoscopic studies of infants with CF reveal that neutrophil and proinflammatory (interleukin-8) mediator levels are increased even though children appear clinically well.

▪ Spirometry should be performed every 3–6 months and as needed on the basis of the patient's pulmonary status.

  • Most children <6 years cannot perform the test reliably.

    – Infant pulmonary function testing is available at many CF centers.

  • It may be difficult to get a reliable, reproducible effort, especially when the child is first learning to perform the test.

  • Best performed with supervision of a certified respiratory therapist trained to work with children.

• The changes seen in pulmonary function are obstructive in nature secondary to plugging of the small airways with thick secretions.

• Severity of pulmonary disease is categorized on the basis of percentage predicted forced expiratory volume in 1 second (FEV_1).

  – Normal lung function is defined as an FEV_1 >90%.

  – Mild disease is 70–89%.

  – Moderate disease is 40–69%.

  – Severe disease is <40%.

• <20% of children have moderate to severe lung disease.

• One measure of the health of the small airways is a forced expiratory flow of 25–75%.

  – The average amount of air expelled over the middle half of all the air expelled during spirometry

  – Clinicians should consider this value, particularly in younger children.

  – Researchers have suggested that changes may be seen in a forced expiratory flow of 25–75% before FEV_1.

TREATMENT APPROACH

▪ The improved survival for patients with CF seen over recent decades is likely to continue.

  • Greater understanding of the pathobiological characteristics of the disease

  • Significant increase in therapeutic options

▪ The challenge to the practitioner treating CF is in choosing the best, most appropriate combination of therapies for the individual patient that are aimed at maintaining optimal health status.

▪ Consultation with a regional CF care center and physicians who are experienced with the nuances of CF care is strongly recommended.

▪ More specific therapies aimed at the basic defect in CF are being developed.

  • The ultimate goal is delivery of a therapy to infants with CF that will provide them with long and healthy lives.

▪ All children with diagnosed CF and those who have clinical stigmata of CF but equivocal diagnostic test results should be referred to a local CF care center for evaluation by professionals who are highly experienced in the management of CF.

▪ A team of individuals that can provide counseling, support, and education to families of newly diagnosed children comprises:

  • Pediatrician, most often a pediatric pulmonologist

  • Nurse

  • Respiratory therapist

  • Dietician

  • Social worker

- Pulmonary and gastrointestinal therapies can be initiated.
- Children should be seen at least quarterly in the CF care center.
  - The adequacy of their therapies, as well as their growth, nutrition, and pulmonary function, can be assessed and therapies adjusted accordingly.
- CF social workers are an invaluable resource for families.
  - Help families deal with the psychological and financial aspects of raising a child with CF
  - Work with the child over the years to help him or her develop into an adult capable of managing the disease independently
- CF centers also can make available to patients clinical trials of novel therapies.
  - The CF center should not be considered a replacement for the general pediatrician.
  - The child absolutely must continue to receive routine well-child care.
  - CF centers generally have physicians available at all times to consult on medical management issues relating to CF.
  - A list of accredited CF care centers in the US can be accessed at www.cff.org.

SPECIFIC TREATMENTS

Pulmonary therapy

- From the moment that CF is diagnosed in a child, the family should be counseled to minimize environmental tobacco smoke exposure.
- Children, especially adolescents, should be educated about the detrimental effects of tobacco smoke and illegal inhalants on their lungs.
- Annual influenza vaccination is recommended for children with CF who are >6 months of age and for their families.
- The cornerstone of pulmonary therapy for children and adults with CF is chest physiotherapy (CPT).
  - Patients are prescribed a daily regimen of CPT to help them mobilize and expectorate the thick, tenacious secretions in their airways.
  - Frequency of therapy is generally increased during times of acute exacerbations.
  - Numerous airway clearance techniques are available for CPT.
    - Manual percussion with postural drainage
    - Autogenic drainage
    - An inflatable vest that vibrates the chest at different frequencies
    - Several handheld devices (eg, Flutter/Acapella) and therapies (eg, positive expiratory pressure) are also available.

- Clearance techniques are designed to shear the mucus off the airways and provide back-pressure to stent the airways open so that secretions may be expelled.
- Each technique has specific advantages; no single technique is superior.
- To optimize adherence, choice of therapy should be based on the method that is:
  - The most effective for that patient
  - The best fit for the family's lifestyle
- Physical activity and regular exercise should be recommended as an integral part of the regimen.
- Bronchodilators are often given before CPT to maximally dilate the airways and help facilitate clearance of the secretions.
  - Patients with CF have a variable response to ß-agonists.
    - Some patients exhibit a transient decline in pulmonary function, most likely secondary to collapse of bronchiectatic airways.
  - Patients with CF should be assessed for bronchodilator response by pulmonary function testing.
    - Therapy should be adjusted accordingly.
    - Long-acting ß-agonists, however, may be beneficial in some patients with CF and asthma.
- The chronic inflammatory process in CF lung disease has led to considerable interest in anti-inflammatory therapies.
  - Alternate-day prednisone therapy has been shown to improve lung function in patients with chronic *P aeruginosa* infection.
    - An increased incidence of growth retardation, glucose abnormalities, and cataracts have dampened enthusiasm for this therapeutic approach.
  - Inhaled steroids and leukotriene modifiers are attractive alternatives and are widely prescribed.
    - Their use should be limited to patients with concomitant asthma, because evidence of efficacy for CF treatment is lacking.
  - High-dose ibuprofen has been shown to decrease the rate of decline in lung function and the need for hospitalization, primarily in patients with CF who have mild lung disease.
    - The requirements for a pharmacokinetic study to determine the optimal dose of ibuprofen and concerns about safety have limited penetration of this therapy into clinical practice.
- Dornase alpha, a recombinant human deoxyribonuclease, was developed for nebulization into the airways.
  - It cleaves the viscous DNA released by dying neutrophils as part of the exaggerated inflammatory response characteristic of CF lung disease.

C

- Deoxyribonuclease treatment improves the rheologic properties of the sputum.
  - It enables the patient to expectorate the sputum more easily.
  - It is generally administered once a day.
- A multicenter study of dornase alpha revealed an improvement in lung function and a decrease in the frequency of pulmonary exacerbations with chronic use.
  - This therapy has been widely adopted in the treatment of CF.

■ Inhaled hypertonic saline is the newest therapy in the CF armamentarium.

- Inhaling a highly concentrated (7%) saline solution may increase the osmotic load and stimulate water movement into the airways.
- Improved hydration of the secretions results in better mucociliary clearance.
- A 48-month trial of 7% saline inhaled twice daily revealed improved pulmonary function and fewer pulmonary exacerbations compared with controls who inhaled 0.9% saline twice daily.
  - Some patients may experience wheezing with the medication; this can be attenuated by pretreatment with a bronchodilator.

■ Long-term daily antibiotic therapy is not well supported by evidence in the literature.

- Either to prevent the initial infection or to treat chronic bacterial infection
- Generally recommended for treating acute exacerbations when bacterial burden increases and patients develop associated symptoms, such as:
  - Increased cough frequency and sputum production
  - Declining pulmonary function with or without radiographic changes
- Macrolide antibiotics and inhaled tobramycin are used for treating chronic *P aeruginosa* infection.
  - Research has shown that 3-times-weekly administration of azithromycin has a positive impact on lung function, weight, and the frequency of pulmonary exacerbations in older children and adults.
  - A high-dose preparation of tobramycin given twice daily in alternating months reduced the need for hospitalization and improved pulmonary function.
  - These therapies are widely used in CF.

■ When patients experience an exacerbation of bronchopneumonia or an apparent viral respiratory illness, antibiotic therapy directed against the most recently cultured pathogen is recommended.

- If the patient does not have respiratory distress or hypoxemia, then oral outpatient therapy may be initiated.
- Hospitalization, intravenous antibiotics, and aggressive chest physiotherapy are recommended when patients show an acute worsening of their respiratory status, hypoxemia, or respiratory distress.

■ *P aeruginosa* is routinely treated with 2 antipseudomonal antibiotics.

■ Duration of antibiotic therapy depends on the severity of the exacerbation.
  - Generally 10 days or longer, based on the response to treatment

■ As lung disease progresses, intervals of stability between exacerbations may become shorter.

- Patients may require supplemental oxygen therapy because of progressive hypoxemia.
- Noninvasive ventilation may be instituted when evidence exists of carbon dioxide retention or sleep-disordered breathing.

■ Lung transplantation is a final therapeutic option for the treatment of progressive, severe lung disease.

- It is an inherently risky procedure with a 5-year posttransplantation survival rate of approximately 50–60%.
- Referral for lung transplantation should be made when other therapeutic options are exhausted.
- Survival models have been developed that facilitate calculation of a patient's predicted survival without transplantation.
  - Aids selection of patients most likely to gain a survival advantage from the procedure
  - Patients should be made aware that the complicated medical regimen they follow to treat their CF-related lung disease will be replaced by a transplant medical regimen that is often equally complicated.
  - Contraindications to lung transplantation
    ■ Active tuberculosis
    ■ HIV
    ■ Hepatitis B
    ■ Significant psychosocial dysfunction that precludes adherence to the posttransplantation medical regimen

Gastrointestinal therapy

■ Nutritional therapy is a cornerstone of good CF therapy.

■ Patients should be evaluated at least annually by a dietitian who is knowledgeable about CF.

■ Frequent nutritional problems faced by both adults and children with CF

- Lack of appetite caused by intercurrent illness
- Inability to consume the increased number of calories needed to:
  - Sustain normal growth
  - Make up for lost weight
  - Achieve catch-up growth

- Infants and children with CF who have PI should receive at least 120–130% of the recommended daily allowance of age-appropriate calories.
  - Fat intake should make up 35–40% of the daily required calories, compared with <30% in people without CF.
  - Caloric requirements are higher when acute illness or exacerbation of the pulmonary disease is present and when catch-up growth is needed.
  - Modifications are initially made to increase the caloric density of the child's regular diet.
  - High-calorie, high-fat supplements in the forms of shakes and formulas are also recommended.
  - Supplementation via nasogastric or gastrostomy tube is recommended, if the child cannot orally consume the daily requirement of calories.
- The following are usually adequate to prevent salt loss syndrome:
  - Increased consumption of salty foods in older children
  - Addition of salt to the formula for infants
- Patients with CF-related diabetes (CFRD) should *not* be placed on a diabetic diet.
  - A significant reduction in caloric intake might compromise the patient's overall nutritional status.
  - Patients are taught how to distribute carbohydrates more equally throughout the day.
- Pancreatic enzyme supplements are given with each fat-containing meal or snack.
  - The recommended dose for infants is 2000–4000 units of lipase per 120 mL of formula or per breastfeeding.
  - A powdered enzyme preparation is often used for infants, but it is not enteric coated.
    - Much of the dose may be destroyed in the stomach.
    - Infants are at risk for ulceration of oral mucosa if enzymes are not completely cleared from the oral cavity.
    - Low-dose, enteric-coated enzyme preparations can be administered to infants.
      - Mix with a small amount of applesauce or other nonalkaline food.
  - Brand-name enteric-coated enzymes should be used exclusively.
    - Enteric coating keeps enzymes from being destroyed by stomach acids.
    - Generic preparations should be avoided.
      - Lack of standardization of the enzyme dose
    - Enzyme dosing is initially based on the patient's weight.
      - Subsequently adjusted based on clinical symptoms of continued malabsorption.
        - Frequency and consistency of stools
        - Perceived greasiness of stools
        - Abdominal cramping

- Enzyme therapy for children <4 years should be initiated at a dose of 1000 units of lipase per kilogram per meal.
- Therapy for children ≥4 years should be initiated at a dose of 500 units of lipase per kilogram per meal.
- To reduce the risk of fibrosing colonopathy, doses should generally be kept to:
  - <2500 units of lipase per kilogram per meal *or*
  - <4000 units of lipase per gram-fat per day

Vitamin supplements

- Children with CF should receive a standard, age-appropriate dose of non–fat-soluble multivitamins.
  - Children with PI should also receive supplements of vitamins A, D, E, and K.
    - Vitamin K is supplemented at higher levels in patients:
      - With liver disease with abnormalities in clotting
      - Receiving prolonged antibiotic therapy
  - Special high-dose preparations of these vitamins are available for patients with CF.
- Dosages for vitamin supplementation
  - 0–12 months:
    - Vitamin A: 1500 IU
    - Vitamin E: 40–50 IU
    - Vitamin D: 400 IU
    - Vitamin K: ≥0.3 mg
  - 1–3 years:
    - Vitamin A: 5000 IU
    - Vitamin E: 80–150 IU
    - Vitamin D: 400–800 IU
    - Vitamin K: ≥0.3 mg
  - 4–8 years:
    - Vitamin A: 5000–10,000 IU
    - Vitamin E: 100–200 IU
    - Vitamin D: 400–800 IU
    - Vitamin K: ≥0.3 mg
  - >8 years:
    - Vitamin A: 10,000 IU
    - Vitamin E: 200–400 IU
    - Vitamin D: 400–800 IU
    - Vitamin K: ≥0.3 mg
- Acid blockers should be used as needed to treat gastro-esophageal reflux.
  - Common in patients with CF
  - Acid suppression may be beneficial for optimization of pancreatic enzyme function.

- Findings during examination should raise concern about the possible development of cirrhosis.
  - Elevated liver enzyme levels and abnormal liver function tests
  - Detection of hepatomegaly or splenomegaly (or both)
  - Order abdominal ultrasonography.
  - Ursodeoxycholic acid has been shown to benefit patients with cholestatic diseases.
    - For example, primary biliary cirrhosis
    - Often administered in patients with CF who have hepatobiliary disease:
      - In an effort to improve bile flow and to limit further liver damage
- Liver transplantation is a therapeutic option when end-stage liver disease develops.

WHEN TO ADMIT

- Pulmonary exacerbations
  - Characterized by:
    - Increased cough
    - Sputum production
    - Decline in pulmonary function
  - Associated symptoms may include:
    - Fever
    - Wheezing
    - Dyspnea
    - Malaise
    - Weight loss
  - Acute changes in the chest radiograph may or may not be seen.
  - The patient should be admitted for intravenous antibiotic therapy if response to oral antibiotic therapy is inadequate.
  - If the patient is hypoxemic, he or she should be admitted to the hospital for further management.
- Major hemoptysis
  - Hemoptysis over 3–7 days of more than:
    - 240 mL in 24 hours
    - >100 mL per day
- Pneumothorax
  - Patients will likely require a chest tube if:
    - Respiratory distress or
    - Pneumothorax occupying at least 20% of the pleural space
  - Other patients should be observed until the pneumothorax is clearly stable or resolving.

- Hospitalized patients should have frequent blood glucose measurements.
  - Altered glucose metabolism may be present only during times of acute illness or stress, particularly in patients receiving supplemental feedings via gastrostomy tube.

WHEN TO REFER

- All children with CF should be referred to a local CF center for ongoing care.

FOLLOW-UP

- Recommended monitoring of patients with an established diagnosis of CF.
- The Cystic Fibrosis Foundation recommends that patients with CF should have annually:
  - A complete blood count with:
    - Differential
    - Fat-soluble vitamins
      - Retinol
      - α-Tocopherol
      - 25-hydroxy vitamin D
    - Albumin and prealbumin
    - Prothrombin time
    - Liver enzymes
- Patients ≥14 years should be screened for CFRD on an annual basis.
- Patients should have at least annual measurement of renal function, particularly those who:
  - Are receiving long-term inhaled aminoglycoside therapy
  - Receive frequent courses of intravenous aminoglycosides
- All patients should receive a complete physical examination annually.
  - Including hearing and vision screening
  - Particularly relevant for patients receiving multiple courses of aminoglycosides because of potential ototoxicity

COMPLICATIONS

Respiratory

- Hemoptysis and pneumothorax are both common complications of CF lung disease.
  - Patients with CF may have blood-streaked sputum.
    - If the volume of blood expectorated is large, treatment should be initiated.
      - Bed rest
      - Intravenous antibiotics
      - Cessation of any medications with anticoagulant properties

- Bronchial artery embolization may be required if the bleeding does not resolve or becomes life threatening.
  - Resection of the bleeding segment is the therapeutic option of last resort.
- Pneumothorax occurs annually in approximately 1% of patients with CF.
  - Patients with respiratory distress or with a pneumothorax occupying at least 20% of the pleural space will likely require a chest tube.
    - If the pneumothorax does not resolve with chest tube placement, pleurodesis may be required.
- Children with CF are predisposed to recurrent and chronic sinusitis despite normal nasal mucociliary clearance.
  - Hypoplasia of the sinuses is a common finding.
  - Polyps may obstruct the nasal passages and contribute to the development of sinusitis.
  - The etiology of polyposis is unknown; it does not appear to be associated with allergies.
- Death most commonly results from respiratory failure and cor pulmonale caused by recurrent or chronic pulmonary infections.

Gastrointestinal

- In newborns, complications may occur because of meconium ileus.
  - Volvulus
  - Intestinal atresia
  - Meconium peritonitis
- DIOS is a common complication of CF.
  - Patients with vomiting, crampy abdominal pain, and decreased stool output should be evaluated for intestinal obstruction by imaging.
  - If DIOS is diagnosed:
    - Oral intake should be withheld.
    - Intravenous fluids or total parenteral nutrition should be initiated.
  - Obstruction may be relieved with a Gastrografin enema or oral or nasogastric administration of osmotic laxatives (polyethylene glycol).
  - Surgical intervention may be needed.
  - Other diagnostic considerations for these symptoms include:
    - Appendicitis
    - Pancreatitis
    - Cholecystitis
    - Intussusceptions
    - *Clostridium difficile* colitis
- Liver disease leads to death in a small minority of the patient population.

Nutritional

- Patients with CF are prone to the development of CFRD, particularly in their late teens and adulthood.
  - CFRD results primarily from a relative insulin deficiency caused by gradual destruction of the islet cells in the pancreas.
  - CFRD is associated with increased morbidity and mortality.
  - Patients may have the classic symptoms of diabetes.
    - Polyuria
    - Polydipsia
    - Weight loss
  - Many have minimal symptoms.
  - An element of insulin resistance has been reported.
- Patients with CFRD:
  - Rarely develop diabetic ketoacidosis.
  - But are at risk for other complications of diabetes.
    - Retinopathy
    - Renal dysfunction
    - Neuropathy
- CFRD should be considered as a possible cause of:
  - Poor growth
  - Delayed puberty
  - Increased frequency of pulmonary exacerbations
  - Unexplained decline in pulmonary function

Bone density

- Osteopenia and osteoporosis are relatively common in adolescents and adults with CF, for several reasons.
  - Failure to thrive
  - Delayed pubertal development
  - Liver disease
  - Physical inactivity
  - Malabsorption of:
    - Calcium
    - Magnesium
    - Vitamins D and K
  - Steroid use may further exacerbate these problems.
- Patients with decreased bone mineral density are predisposed to atraumatic fractures, especially of spine and ribs.
- Patients may experience transient arthritis.
  - Monoarticular, pauciarticular, or polyarticular
  - Knees, ankles, wrists, and proximal interphalangeal joints of the hands are most often affected.

C

Endocrine

- Pubertal development is often delayed in both boys and girls with CF.
  - Delayed or blunted pubertal development results from:
    - Poor nutrition and decrease in glucose tolerance, accompanied by delayed increase in sex hormone levels
- Female infants with CF have excessive cytoplasmic and extracellular mucus.
  - Can continue into childhood
  - Thickened cervical secretions may reduce fertility.
- Girls may have abnormal menstrual cycles.
  - Possible primary and secondary amenorrhea
  - Increasing numbers of successful pregnancies are occurring as the population with CF ages.
- Boys with CF may have reduced testicular and epididymal size and reduced testosterone levels.
  - In most boys, bilateral absence of the vas deferens occurs secondary to obstruction and subsequent resorption of the structure.
    - Results in infertility
    - Assisted reproductive technologies have been developed and used to treat infertility in men with CF.

PROGNOSIS

- A vicious cycle of infection and inflammation develops in the lungs of patients with CF.
  - Typically punctuated by acute exacerbation, eventually leading to bronchiectasis
  - Damages and destroys the airways
- In general, a good correlation exists between pancreatic status and genotype.
  - Patients with 2 severe mutations, such as $\Delta F_{508}/\Delta F_{508}$, are generally pancreatic insufficient.
  - Patients with 1 or 2 mild mutations are much more likely to be pancreatic sufficient; they are at increased risk of pancreatitis.
  - Individuals who are pancreatic sufficient generally have better clinical outcomes than patients with PI.

Dehydration

DEFINITION

- Dehydration is a condition in which pure water loss occurs.
- Volume depletion or hypovolemia is a condition in which extracellular fluid is lost.
- These terms are used interchangeably.

EPIDEMIOLOGY

- Incidence
  - Diarrheal illness, the most common cause of dehydration
    - Globally, 2.5 million deaths annually from diarrheal illnesses
  - Gastroenteritis
  - >200,000 hospital admissions annually in the US
  - >1.5 million outpatient visits annually in the US

ETIOLOGY

- Infectious processes include:
  - Viral agents
    - Rotavirus
    - Norwalk agent
    - Enteric adenovirus
    - Uncommon viral agents
      - Calicivirus
      - Astrovirus
  - Bacterial agents
    - *Salmonella* spp
    - *Shigella* spp
    - *Campylobacter jejuni*
    - Uncommon bacterial agents
      - *Yersinia enterocolitica*
      - *Vibrio cholerae*
      - *Escherichia coli*
      - *Clostridium difficile*
  - Parasitic agents
    - *Giardia lamblia*
    - Uncommon parasitic agents
      - *Entamoeba histolytica*
      - *Cryptosporidium*
- Noninfectious causes include:
  - Osomotic agents
    - Laxatives or cathartics that contain high concentrations of sugars
    - Obstructive processes in the gastrointestinal tract
    - Occasionally, vomiting as a sign of elevated intracranial pressure

- Nondiarrheal causes of water and electrolyte loss
  - Losses through the skin
    - Losses with fever usually are in the range of a 10–15% increase in insensible losses for each 1°C rise in temperature above 38°C
  - Losses through the respiratory system (ie, increase in insensible losses)
  - Renal losses
    - Diuretic use or abuse
    - Diabetes mellitus
    - Chronic renal disease, obstructive uropathy
  - Water deficit
    - Nephrogenic diabetes insipidus
    - Central diabetes insipidus
  - Increased insensible losses
    - Premature infants
    - Radiant warmers
    - Phototherapy
    - Tracheostomy, tachypnea
  - Inadequate intake of water
    - Ineffective breastfeeding
    - Child abuse
  - Water and sodium deficits
    - Burns
    - Excessive sweating
  - Miscellaneous
    - Surgical drains
    - Third spacing

RISK FACTORS

- Very young children are at risk because of:
  - Higher surface area-to-volume ratio
  - Proportionally higher rate of insensible losses
  - Inability to communicate
  - Inability to actively seek fluids to replenish their losses

SIGNS AND SYMPTOMS

- Volume depletion (see table Degree of Dehydration)
  - Measured as change in body weight from baseline
  - Pre-illness weight is used to determine degree of weight loss due to the fluid deficit.
    - If pre-illness weight is unavailable, use:
      - Pulse rate
      - Blood pressure
      - Urine output
      - Skin turgor

Degree of Dehydration

Parameter	Degree of Dehydration		
	Mild	**Moderate**	**Severe**
Weight loss (%)—infants	5	10	15
Weight loss (%)—children	3	6	>9
Skin color	Pale	Gray	Mottled
Skin turgor	May be normal	Decreased	Tenting
Mucous membranes	Slightly dry	Dry	Dry, parched, collapse of sublingual veins
Eyes	Normal	Decreased tears	Sunken, absence of tears
Central nervous system	Alert but thirsty	Irritable	Lethargic, grunting, coma
Pulse	Normal and strong	Rapid and slightly weak	Significantly tachycardic, and very weak to not palpable
Capillary refill	Normal (<2 sec)	2–4 sec	>4 sec
Blood pressure	No change	Orthostatic decrease	Shock
Urine	Normal to mildly reduced	Significantly reduced	Anuria
Volume of deficit—infants	50 mL/kg	100 mL/kg	150 mL/kg
Volume of deficit—children	30 mL/kg	60 mL/kg	>90 mL/k

- Dehydration is categorized as:
  - Mild (3–5% volume loss)
  - Moderate (6–9% volume loss)
  - Severe dehydration (≥10% volume loss)

DIFFERENTIAL DIAGNOSIS

- In children who only have vomiting (without diarrhea)
  - Appendicitis
  - Intussusception
  - Volvulus
  - Pyloric stenosis

DIAGNOSTIC APPROACH

- 5-point assessment
  - Volume deficit
    - History
    - Physical examination
  - Osmolar disturbance
    - Serum sodium
    - Serum osmolality
  - Acid-base disturbance
    - Blood pH
    - Partial pressure of carbon dioxide
    - Serum bicarbonate
  - Potassium
    - Serum potassium
  - Renal function
    - Blood urea nitrogen
    - Creatinine
    - Urine specific gravity

LABORATORY FINDINGS

- Laboratory tests to assess clinical condition and origin of dehydration are usually not needed in children with mild or moderate dehydration.
- For moderate to severe dehydration
  - Serum electrolytes
    - Sodium
    - Potassium
    - Chloride
    - Bicarbonate
  - Blood urea nitrogen
  - Serum creatinine
  - Urine specific gravity
  - Serum glucose (finger-prick at the bedside)
- Laboratory testing is less useful in assessing the degree of volume depletion.
- Serum bicarbonate (<17 mEq/L) differentiates moderate or severe hypovolemia from mild hypovolemia.
- Serum sodium measurements to determine type of dehydration
  - Isonatremic (135–145 mEq/L)

- Hyponatremic (<130 mEq/L)
- Hypernatremic (>150 mEq/L)
■ Serum potassium
  - Falsely elevated when acidosis causes a shift from the intracellular compartment
  - Low because of losses in the gastrointestinal tract
■ Urine osmolality and specific gravity
  - May be high (often >450 mOsm/kg)
  - May be low if the patient has lost renal concentrating ability
    – Osmotic diuresis
    – Diabetes insipidus
■ Bacterial cultures for children with:
  - Ill appearance
  - Fever
    – ≥38°C in infants <3 months
    – 39°C in children >3 months
  - Bloody or mucoid stools
  - Travel or exposure history suggestive of enteric pathogens
■ Routine stool cultures should be discouraged.
■ Studies for rotavirus antigen are needed only rarely.

CLASSIFICATION

■ Dehydration is categorized as:
  - Mild (3–5% volume loss)
  - Moderate (6–9% volume loss)
  - Severe dehydration (≥10% volume loss)

TREATMENT APPROACH

■ Rapid repletion of fluids:
  - Restores circulating volume
  - Reverses acidosis
  - Improves perfusion and end-organ function
  - Administer fluid rapidly and with the intent to restore the entire deficit in 4–6 hours.
■ Dehydration resulting from gastroenteritis
  - Oral rehydration on an outpatient basis
  - Little laboratory evaluation is necessary.
■ Proper dietary management is essential to minimize:
  - Severity of symptoms
  - Duration of symptoms
■ Most dehydrated children can be rehydrated successfully without resorting to parenteral (intravenous or intraosseous) therapy.
  - Parenteral therapy is reserved for severe or unusual cases.

■ Combined use of an oral rehydration solution (ORS) and an appropriate regimen of refeeding is referred to as *oral rehydration* therapy (ORT).

SPECIFIC TREATMENTS

Oral rehydration

■ First choice for the conscious child who has mild or moderate dehydration (see table Fluid Therapy for Dehydration).
■ Fluid absorption can be promoted by enteral administration of properly designed fluids, even in the face of ongoing losses.
■ ORS
  - Fluid designed to promote water and electrolyte absorption through the co-transport system in the gut
  - A physiologically appropriate ORS contains:
    – 70–90 mEq/L sodium
    – ≤25 g/L glucose
  - An ORS typically contains:
    – 20 mEq/L potassium
    – 30 mEq/L of base in the form of citrate
  - The World Health Organization formula published in 2002 specifies:
    – 13.5 g/L carbohydrates
    – 75 mEq/L sodium
    – 20 mEq/L potassium
    – 30 mEq/L of bicarbonate base
    – Osmolarity of 245 mOsm/kg of water
  - The World Health Organization and the United Nations Children's Fund recommend the following properties for an ORS for global use:
    – Total osmolality 200–310 mmol/L
    – Equimolar concentrations of glucose and sodium
    – Glucose concentration ≤20 g/L (111 mmol/L)
    – Sodium concentration 60–90 mEq/L
    – Potassium concentration 15–25 mEq/L
    – Citrate concentration 8–12 mmol/L
    – Chloride concentration 50–80 mEq/L
  - Juices, soft drinks, and punches usually contain much higher concentrations of sugars and almost no sodium; they are inappropriate for use as an ORS.
    – The higher sugar concentrations in these fluids may exacerbate diarrhea by presenting a large osmotic load in the intestinal lumen.
  - An ORS can be used to restore both fluid and electrolyte balance in children who have a wide range of initial serum sodium values.

Fluid Therapy for Dehydration

Degree of Dehydration[a]	Signs	Rehydration Phase (First 4 Hours; Repeat Until No Signs of Dehydration Remain)	Maintenance Phase[b] (Until Illness Resolves)
Mild (3–5%)	Slightly dry mucous membranes, increased thirst	ORS, 60 mL/kg[c]	Breastfeeding, undiluted lactose-free formula, half-strength cow's milk, or lactose-containing formula
Moderate (6–9%)	Sunken eyes, sunken fontanelle, loss of skin turgor, dry mucous membranes, decreased urine output	ORS, 80 mL/kg	Same as above
Severe (>10%)	Signs of moderate dehydration, plus ≥1 of the following: rapid thready pulse, hypotension, cyanosis, rapid breathing, delayed capillary refill, markedly reduced or absent urine output, lethargy, coma	Intravenous or intraosseous isotonic fluids (0.9% saline or lactated Ringer's solution), 20 mL/kg over 1 hr; repeat until pulse and state of consciousness return to normal, then 50-100 mL/kg of ORS based on remaining degree of dehydration[d]	Same as above

Abbreviation: ORS, oral rehydration solution.

[a] Percent of total body weight lost.

[b] In addition to the rehydration amounts shown, replace ongoing stool losses and vomitus with ORS, 10 mL/kg for each diarrheal stool and 5 mL/kg for each episode of vomitus.

[c] If no signs of dehydration are present, the rehydration phase may be omitted. Proceed with maintenance therapy and replacement of ongoing losses.

[d] While parenteral access is being sought, nasogastric infusion of ORS may be begun at 30 mL/kg per hour, provided that airway protective reflexes remain intact.

- Types of ORS
  - Premixed liquids
    - Most widely available commercially in the industrialized world
    - Contain 50–70 mEq/L sodium
    - Appropriate for the mildly dehydrated child
  - Significantly dehydrated infants and children need a solution with 70–90 mEq/L.
  - Packets of oral rehydration salts for preparation of a solution containing 90 mEq/L of sodium are available for mixing with 1 L of water to provide an inexpensive and reliable alternative.
    - These packets always should be distributed with a 1-L bottle to promote proper mixing.
  - Juices, punches, and other soft drinks are inappropriate for children who have diarrhea because of the high osmotic load they introduce into the intestines.
  - See table Solutions Commonly Used in Children Who Have Diarrhea for commonly available solutions and their compositions.
- Rehydration phase
  - Fluids are best administered initially by a parent using a needle-less syringe to introduce the solution into the child's mouth.
    - Infants: 1 tsp (5 mL) per minute

    - Toddlers: 10 mL per minute
    - Older children: 15 mL per minute
  - At a steady rate of administration, provides 300, 600, and 900 mL/h, respectively
  - Generally replaces the calculated deficit within 4–6 hours
  - The child should be reassessed frequently.
  - Rehydration phase should be completed in the office, clinic, or emergency department before the child is sent home.
- Vomiting
  - Usually not a contraindication to ORT
  - Even when vomiting occurs, steady fluid replacement is continued orally.
  - Children usually do not discharge their entire stomach contents when they vomit.
  - As dehydration and tissue acidosis are corrected, the frequency and severity of vomiting are generally reduced.
- Maintenance
  - After 4 hours, reassess the child's state of hydration using the original clinical criteria.
    - If dehydration is still detectable, repeat the rehydration phase based on the remaining calculated volume deficit.
    - If rehydration is complete, begin the maintenance phase.
  - Continued administration of ORS in ad libitum quantities

- Alternate between ORS and breast milk, formula, or other appropriate feedings.
- Resume regular feedings.
- Strong evidence suggests that both the volume and duration of diarrhea are reduced when children are fed immediately following rehydration.

Parenteral and enteral rehydration

■ Parenteral administration of initial rehydration fluids
- For patients who have severe dehydration (shock) fluids are administered
  - Intravenously
  - Intraosseously when line placement proves difficult
- Rapid boluses of 0.9% sodium chloridein in itial volumes of 20 mL/kg for ≤20 minutes
- Severely dehydrated patients may require 60–100 mL/kg before the restoration of circulating volume is apparent.

■ Enteral fluid therapy may begin immediately if:
- The patient is conscious
- Airway protective reflexes are intact

■ Fluids are given either by mouth or nasogastric tube.

Emergency department

■ Children who seek treatment at emergency departments may represent a distinct group of patients.
- Often have seen a primary care physician earlier in the illness
- Physician may have attempted oral rehydration.

■ Use of ORT in the emergency department is strongly encouraged.
- Should always be attempted in the mild and moderately dehydrated child

■ ORT in children who are sick enough to come to the emergency department is likely to be unsuccessful.
- Intravenous treatment probably will be required, especially in the older (school-age) child in whom vomiting is the most prominent feature.
- Such children are often too exhausted to continue with efforts to drink.
- Reasonable to approach with a brief trial of ORT followed, if necessary, by a brief course of intravenous fluids and subsequent reintroduction of liquids and solids

WHEN TO ADMIT

■ Persistently abnormal mental status
■ Persistently abnormal electrolyte levels
■ Chronic diarrhea (>14 days)
■ Other medical problems, eg, short-gut and inflammatory bowel disease
■ Hydration status that cannot be restored or maintained after 6 hours of outpatient treatment

COMPLICATIONS

■ Inadequately treated dehydration can lead to:
- Full-blown shock
- Multiorgan dysfunction syndrome
- End-organ damage to the kidneys, liver, and brain
- Death

■ Mild overhydration results from aggressive oral hydration.
- Some transient periorbital puffiness
- 2–3% weight gain
- These complications are self-limited and of no clinical consequence.

Solutions Commonly Used in Children Who Have Diarrhea

Solution	Glucose/Phenol (g/L)	Sodium (mEq/L)	Base (mEq/L; Citrate or Bicarbonate)	Potassium (mEq/L)	Osmolality (mmol/L)
Physiologically Appropriate Solutions					
Pedialyte	25	45	30	20	270
Ricelyte	30[a]	50	30	25	200
Rehydralyte	25	75	30	20	310
WHO and UNICEF oral replacement solution	20	90	30	20	310
Physiologically Inappropriate Solutions					
Cola	700	2	13	0.1	750
Apple juice	690	3	0	32	730
Gatorade	255	20	3	3	330

Abbreviations: UNICEF, United Nations Children's Fund; WHO, World Health Organization.
[a] Rice syrup solids.

D

- Hypokalemia results from the loss of total body potassium as a consequence of the increased aldosterone activity in the kidney.
  - Common in severe dehydration
  - As sodium is avidly retained, potassium is lost in the urine.
  - Hypokalemia can result in ileus.
    - May impair fluid and electrolyte absorption from the intestines
  - ORS containing 20 mEq/L potassium chloride can restore potassium balance.
- Elevated aldosterone levels caused by hypovolemia may cause:
  - Renal potassium loss
  - Circulatory collapse
  - Shock
  - Irreversible organ damage
  - Death

PROGNOSIS

- Prognosis is excellent for appropriately treated diarrheal dehydration.
- Typical episodes of gastroenteritis last 3–7 days.

PREVENTION

- Extreme consequences may be prevented by early and aggressive fluid therapy.
- Risking overhydration is better than being exceptionally cautious with fluid administration.

Dental Stains

DEFINITION

- Extrinsic stains
  - Teeth stained from external deposits on their surface layer
  - Usually removable by careful daily brushing and professional oral prophylaxis (scaling)
- Intrinsic stains
  - Staining substance is incorporated into the deep structures of the tooth (enamel, dentin, or both).
  - Cannot be removed by scaling

MECHANISM

Green color

- Several teeth; gingival third of crowns; extrinsic stain
  - Chromogenic bacteria in plaque biofilm
  - Associated with poor oral hygiene

Orange color

- Less common than green stain
- Several teeth; gingival third of crowns; extrinsic stain
  - Chromogenic bacteria in plaque biofilm
  - Associated with poor oral hygiene

Black color

- Less common than green and orange stains
- Several teeth; gingival third of crowns; extrinsic stain
  - Chromogenic bacteria in plaque biofilm
  - Associated with poor oral hygiene
- Several teeth; extrinsic stain
  - Oral medications, especially iron
- ≥1 teeth; occlusal or interproximal surfaces; hard, shiny
  - Arrested dental caries

Brown/black color

- Several teeth; occlusal pits and fissures or smooth surfaces
  - Accumulation of tin or staining of demineralized enamel after strontium fluoride topical treatment

Pink color

- Single tooth; entire crown
  - Posttraumatic change
  - Within 1–2 days, bleeding into dentin; changes to gray in 1–3 weeks
  - After several months: internal resorption of dentin

Gray color

- Several teeth; linear pattern or entire crown, depending on stage of tooth development
  - Tetracycline incorporation in tooth and subsequent oxidation by sunlight
  - Exhibits other colors

- All primary and permanent teeth; entire crown
  - Dose-dependent and duration-linked
  - Caused by the incorporation of tetracycline into the mineral complex at the dentinoenamel junction during odontogenesis
  - If tetracycline was ingested by the mother during pregnancy or by the child in the first months after birth, the primary teeth will be affected.
  - Permanent teeth will be stained if drug ingestion occurs between 3 months and 7–8 years of age.
    - The result may be yellow, gray, or brown tooth discoloration in a linear pattern that, without restoration, may be quite disfiguring.
- All primary and permanent teeth; entire crown
  - Dentinogenesis imperfecta (autosomal dominant)
- Single tooth; entire crown
  - Posttraumatic change
  - Within 1–3 weeks: hemosiderin pigment in dentin
  - After several months: pulpal necrosis

Yellow color

- Several teeth; entire crown
  - Natural color of permanent compared with primary teeth
- Several teeth; linear pattern or entire crown
  - Tetracycline
  - Systemic infection
- All primary and permanent teeth; entire crown
  - Amelogenesis imperfecta (various inheritance patterns)
- Single tooth; entire crown
  - Posttraumatic change
  - Pulpal obliteration by dentin
- Several teeth; gingival third of crown; extrinsic stain
  - Food debris and chromogenic bacteria in plaque biofilm
  - Associated with poor oral hygiene
- Several teeth; extrinsic stain; part of or entire crown
  - Tea
  - Coffee
  - Cola
  - Tobacco

Yellow/brown color

- Several teeth
  - Premature birth; enamel disturbance
  - Hypoplasia and hypocalcification
- ≥1 teeth; ≥1 surfaces with cavitations
  - Advanced active dental caries

- Brown color
  - Several teeth; entire crown
    - Amelogenesis imperfecta
    - Dentinogenesis imperfecta
    - Premature birth
    - Jaundice
  - Individual teeth; localized area
    - Turner hypoplasia secondary to infection
    - Brown or yellow/brown discoloration of a single tooth associated with hypoplasia of the enamel
    - Occurs in a tooth undergoing odontogenesis at the time of illness
    - Hypocalcified or hypoplastic area
    - Traumatized primary tooth affecting permanent crown
  - Several teeth; linear or generalized distribution; associated hypoplasia
    - Fluorosis; systemic infections
    - Especially with high fever; nutritional deficiencies
  - Several teeth; generalized or linear
    - Tetracycline
  - Several teeth; ≥1 surfaces; loss of tooth structure
    - Advanced active dental caries

Red/brown color

- Several teeth; primary and permanent; generalized
  - Porphyria

Blue color

- Several teeth; extrinsic stain; part of or entire crown
  - Berries

Blue/green or yellow/green color

- All primary teeth; entire crown
  - Bilirubin pigments incorporated into dentin
  - Erythroblastosis fetalis
  - Biliary atresia
  - Neonatal hepatitis

White or cream color

- Several teeth; linear or entire crown
  - Fluorosis
  - Systemic infection
- All primary and permanent teeth; entire crown
  - Amelogenesis imperfecta
- Individual teeth; localized area
  - Turner hypoplasia
- ≥1 teeth; occlusal or gingival third of smooth surface
  - Early active dental caries
  - Demineralization of enamel

- Several teeth; any surface; extrinsic stain
  - Plaque biofilm and food debris (materia alba)
  - Removed easily with gauze

HISTORY

- Parental concerns
  - Changes in tooth color are often the cause of much anxiety.
  - Concerns are frequently first brought to the pediatrician.
- Extrinsic stains
  - Oral hygiene habits
  - Ingestion of staining substances, especially liquid iron preparations
  - Frequent prolonged exposure to chlorinated swimming pools
- Intrinsic stains
  - Medical history: neonatal
    - Erythroblastosis fetalis
    - Biliary atresia
    - Hepatitis
  - Medical history: childhood
    - Porphyria
    - Tooth trauma and associated bleeding into dentin
    - Active dental caries
    - Local infection
    - Excessive fluoride intake
    - Tetracycline exposure

PHYSICAL EXAM

- Erythrodontia caused by deposition of red-brown porphyrin pigments into the tooth structure is readily apparent in ultraviolet light, if not in daylight.

DIFFERENTIAL DIAGNOSIS

- Normal tooth color varies greatly:
  - From 1 tooth to another
  - From 1 individual to another
  - Between the usual blue-white of primary dentition and the yellowish ivory of permanent teeth
- Cyanoticcongenital heart disease
  - As many as 50% of such children may have dull, pale, bluish-white teeth.
    - Color of teeth resembles skim milk.
- Amelogenesis imperfecta, dentinogenesis imperfecta
  - Inherited disorders associated with hypoplastic enamel and yellow, opalescent, blue-gray, or brown-violet tooth color

TREATMENT APPROACH

- Allay parental anxieties.
- Consider referring a child with extrinsic or intrinsic stains.

SPECIFIC TREATMENT

Chromogenic bacteria in plaque biofilm

- Oral prophylaxis
- Preventive education

Discoloration from oral medications

- Oral prophylaxis after discontinuing medication

Dental caries

- Arrested
  - Dental evaluation, observation, or restoration
- Advanced, active
  - Restoration

Accumulation of tin

- No treatment, or aesthetic restoration

Staining of demineralized enamel after topical fluoride treatment

- No treatment, or aesthetic restoration

Posttraumatic change

- None, or observation
- Minor resorption
  - Endodontics
- Severe resorption
  - Extraction
- Pulpal necrosis
  - Endodontic treatment or extraction
- Pulpal obliteration by dentin
  - Observation or esthetic restoration

Tetracycline incorporation in tooth

- Esthetic restoration
- Endodontic therapy and bleaching

Fluorosis

- Esthetic restoration

Systemic infections

- Esthetic restoration

Nutritional deficiencies

- Esthetic restoration

Dentinogenesis imperfecta

- Esthetic improvement
- Protection from wear—prosthetic coverage

Amelogenesis imperfecta

- Esthetic restoration
- Protection from occlusal wear

Tea, coffee, cola, tobacco use

- Oral prophylaxis
- Avoid excessive use of substance

Premature birth; enamel disturbance

- Hypoplasia and hypocalcification
- No treatment

Turner hypoplasia secondary to infection

- No treatment, or esthetic restoration

Hypocalcified or hypoplastic area

- No treatment, or esthetic restoration

Porphyria

- No treatment, or esthetic restoration

Bilirubin pigments incorporated into dentin

- No treatment
- Generally fades
- Permanent teeth are not affected if the condition does not continue.

WHEN TO REFER

- Consider referring a child with extrinsic or intrinsic stains.
  - Simple office dental procedures and preventive education can resolve all extrinsic staining problems.
  - Esthetic improvement is possible with the majority of intrinsic discoloration.

PROGNOSIS

- Extrinsic stains
  - Discoloration will usually resolve with:
    - Oral prophylaxis
    - Avoidance of the staining substance
- Intrinsic stains
  - Major restoration of dental surfaces may be required to restore normal appearance.

PREVENTION

- Extrinsic stains
  - Good oral hygiene
  - Oral prophylaxis
  - Avoidance of staining food and beverages
  - Children who are receiving liquid medications, especially iron preparations
    - Staining may be completely prevented if medication is administered through a straw from the onset.

- Competitive swimmers
  - Professional oral prophylaxis is protective.
- ■ Intrinsic stains
  - Avoidance of excessive fluoride intake
    - Fluoride content >1.5 parts per million (ppm) results in hypoplastic enamel, with characteristic dull, opaque, white mottled patches in the permanent teeth.
    - If the amount of fluoride consumed is >5 ppm, the teeth will show a blotchy brown or black/brown color that is highly disfiguring and requires extensive restoration of dental surfaces.
- Tetracycline should be avoided in:
  - Pregnant or lactating women
  - Children <8 years of age

Developmental Surveillance and Intervention

BACKGROUND

- Developmental screening and surveillance helps families:
  - Optimize their children's acquisition of skills
  - Understand behavior
  - Facilitate learning
- For children with developmental differences or delays, universal or focused screening provides an opportunity for:
  - Early identification
  - Referral for intervention
- Growth, development, and behavior are inextricably linked.
  - Screening needs to consider the whole child.
    - Social and emotional development in the context of family and community
- Approximately 16% of children have developmental or behavioral disabilities.
  - Speech and language delays
  - Intellectual disabilities or deficits
  - Learning disabilities
  - Emotional problems
    - Even at preschool age, 13% of children have mental health problems.
    - 5% of 4- to 17-year-olds in the US (2.7 million children) have severe emotional or behavioral difficulties.
- Risk factors for developmental delay or behavioral disabilities
  - Poverty
  - Maternal depression
  - Substance abuse
  - Domestic violence
  - Foster care placement
  - Premature birth or prolonged neonatal intensive care unit course
- Despite the medical community's knowledge of prevalence and risk, detection of developmental and behavioral problems before school age is very poor (~30%).
  - Lack of detection eliminates the possibility of early intervention.
  - By contrast, 70–80% of children with developmental disabilities are correctly identified when standardized screening tests are used.
  - Reasons given for not screening include:
    - Screening takes too long.
    - Tools are difficult to administer.
    - Children may not cooperate.
    - Reimbursement is limited.
  - Perceived barriers to screening
    - Time
    - Cost
    - Staff
    - Language availability
    - Practicality
  - Waiting to screen until a problem is observable is pointless.
    - Time for intervention has been lost.
    - Informal checklists, used by many primary care physicians, have no validated criteria for referral and result in missed referral opportunities.

GOALS

- Creating collaborative relationships that link the:
  - Family
  - Practice
  - Community
    - Counselors
    - Agencies
    - Early intervention programs
    - Child care
    - Head Start
    - Schools
- Early identification:
  - Allows referral and early intervention even for children with developmental diagnoses that cannot be cured or completely remediated
  - Improves function for the child and family
  - Can save up to $100,000 per student in special-education costs over the course of the child's education
- The primary care physician does not need to become an expert at diagnosing and managing developmental and behavioral disorders.
  - However, the physician is a:
    - Resource for referrals for further assessment and interventions
    - Partner in finding information
    - Sounding board
    - Facilitator to negotiate the system
- If a screen has an at-risk score:
  - For more detailed assessment to confirm or rule out a diagnosis, the primary care physician refers (generally outside the practice) to:
    - Developmental and behavioral pediatrician
    - Infant-toddler specialist
    - Psychologist
    - Speech and language pathologist
    - Physical therapist

- The primary care physician screens periodically (surveillance).
  - Surveillance increases the sensitivity and accuracy of the assessment of the child's skills and progress.

GENERAL APPROACH

- Developmental and behavioral screening
  - Early identification of potential problems or delays
  - Review of appropriate expectations at a given developmental age
    - Facilitates understanding of the child's behavior
    - Potentially facilitates use of appropriate discipline by parents
    - Leads to referring children with at-risk scores to early intervention services
- Psychosocial screening can cover risk factors.
  - Family relationships
  - Maternal depression
  - Domestic violence
  - Substance abuse
  - Unstable housing
  - Financial resources
    - Must be considered individually for a realistic care plan
- The screen:
  - Provides a template for anticipatory guidance
  - Facilitates patient flow
    - Reduces "doorknob concerns" as the physician leaves the examination room
    - Improves patient and physician satisfaction

SPECIFIC INTERVENTIONS

Screening tools for primary care practice

- Types of developmental screening tools
  - Direct elicitation
  - Interview
  - Parent questionnaires
- Advantages of parent questionnaire
  - Family-centered process
  - Does not require staff administration; only scoring and recording
  - Can be completed while the parent is in the waiting room or examination room
    - Some tools are available in an online version that can be completed by the family before the visit.
      - Removes the problem of trying to elicit skills from young child in a foreign environment

- Parents' concerns are accurate indicators of true problems, particularly for:
  - Speech and language
  - Fine-motor skills
  - Hearing
  - General function
- Parent estimations correlate well with developmental quotients for:
  - Cognitive skills
  - Motor skills
  - Self-help skills
  - Academic skills
- Disadvantages to a parent questionnaire
  - Recall (eg, milestones) is unreliable.
  - Staff time for scoring, transcribing, and filing depends on how the questionnaire is administered.
  - Parental reading skills may be a concern.
    - Parents can be asked if they would like to complete the screen independently.
    - The provider can offer to have someone go through the screen with the parent.

Screening schedule

- Screens can be interwoven into the schedule of well-child visits and the growing relationship with the family.
  - Primary screens should be routine for all families.
  - Secondary screens are used as indicated.
- 1-week, 1-month visits
  - Primary screen
    - Psychosocial
  - Pertinent issues
    - Support
    - Housing
    - Transportation
    - Peak crying in second month
  - Parenting
    - Newborn care
    - Feeding
    - Sleep
    - Reading cues
    - Soothing strategies
- 2-month visit
  - Primary screen
    - Maternal depression (Edinburgh Postnatal Depression Scale)

- Pertinent issues
  - Socioeconomic
  - Family relationships
  - Attachment
- Parenting
  - Sleep
  - Reading cues
- **4-month visit**
  - Primary screen
    - Maternal depression
  - Pertinent issues
    - Socioeconomic
    - Family relationships
    - Attachment
    - Reaching
    - Rolling
    - Social smile
  - Parenting
    - Sleep
    - Reading cues
- **6-month visit**
  - Primary screens
    - Mental health
    - Substance abuse
    - Domestic violence
  - Pertinent issues
    - Emergent motor skills
    - Emergent social skills
    - Mobility
  - Parenting
    - Sleep
    - Book sharing
    - Age-appropriate expectations
  - Secondary screen
    - Ages and Stages Questionnaire Social-Emotional (ASQ SE), if indicated
- **9-month visit**
  - Primary screens
    - ASQ
    - Parents' Evaluation of Developmental Status (PEDS)
  - Pertinent issues
    - Emerging stranger anxiety
    - Mobility
    - Feeding self

- Parenting
  - Sleep
  - Book sharing
  - Discipline
- **12-month visit**
  - Primary screens
    - ASQ
    - PEDS (if not at 9 months)
  - Pertinent issues
    - Emerging language
    - Joint attention
    - Mobility
  - Parenting
    - Sleep
    - Book sharing
    - Discipline
    - Toilet training
  - Secondary screens
    - ASQ SE
    - Temperament and Atypical Behavior Scale (TABS)
    - Brief Infant Toddler Social Emotional Assessment (BITSEA)
- **15-month visit**
  - Primary screens
    - Psychosocial mental health
    - Substance abuse
    - Domestic violence
  - Pertinent issues
    - Language
    - Home environment
  - Parenting
    - Sleep
    - Book sharing
    - Discipline
    - Toilet training
- **18-month visit**
  - Primary screen
    - ASQ
    - PEDS
  - Pertinent issues
    - Language
    - Independence
    - Ambivalence

- Parenting
  - Sleep
  - Book sharing
  - Discipline
  - Toilet training
- Secondary screens
  - ASQ SE
  - TABS
  - BITSEA
  - Modified Checklist forAutismin Toddlers (MCHAT)

■ 24-month visit
- Primary screen
  - ASQ/PEDS (if not at 18 months)
  - Psychosocial
- Pertinent issues
  - Language
  - Independence
  - Ambivalence
- Parenting
  - Interaction with peers
  - Discipline
  - Toilet training
  - Book sharing
- Secondary screens
  - ASQ SE
  - TABS
  - BITSEA
  - Eyberg Child Behavior Inventory
  - MCHAT

■ 30- or 36-month visit
- Primary screen
  - ASQ
  - PEDS (if not at 30 months)
- Pertinent issues
  - Communication
  - Social skills
- Parenting
  - Book sharing
- Secondary screens
  - ASQ SE, etc

■ 48-month visit
- Primary screen
  - ASQ
  - PEDS

- Pertinent issues
  - School readiness
  - Communication
  - Social skills
  - Early graphomotor
- Parenting
  - Book sharing
- Secondary screens
  - ASQ SE
  - TABS
  - Eyberg Child Behavior Inventory
  - Pediatric Symptom Checklist (PSC)

■ 60-month visit
- Primary screen
  - ASQ
  - PEDS
- Pertinent issues
  - School readiness
  - Communication
  - Social skills
  - Early graphomotor
- Parenting
  - Book sharing
- Secondary screens
  - ASQ SE
  - TABS
  - Eyberg Child Behavior Inventory
  - PSC

■ 6- to 18-year visits
- Primary screen
  - PSC
- Pertinent issues
  - Learning
  - Peers
  - Self-esteem
- Parenting
  - Building self-esteem
  - Making good choices
- Secondary screens
  - Attention-deficit/hyperactivity disorder
  - Depression
  - Anxiety

Developmental and behavioral screens

- Excluded tests
  - Poor validation or sensitivity and specificity
    - Prescreening Developmental Questionnaire
    - Denver Developmental Screening Test II
    - Developmental Indicators for the Assessment of Learning III
    - Gesell Developmental Observation Test
- Effective screens, with sensitivity and specificity of at least 70–80% (details below subject to change)
  - ASQ
    - Type: parent questionnaire
    - Age: 4 mo–5 yr
    - Staff required: paraprofessional
    - Cost: $199.00/kit
    - Refills, copies: ok to copy
    - Time: 3 min to score
    - Languages: English, Spanish, French, Korean
    - Reading level: 4th–6th grade
  - Bayley Infant Neurodevelopmental Screener (BINS)
    - Type: direct elicitation
    - Age: 3–24 mo
    - Staff required: master's or equivalent
    - Cost: $195.00/kit
    - Refills, copies: refills of score sheet
    - Time
      - 20–30 min to administer
      - 10 min to score
    - Languages: English
  - PEDS
    - Type: parent questionnaire
    - Age: 0–8 yr
    - Staff required: paraprofessional
    - Cost
      - $69.95 manual
      - $30.00 kit
    - Refills, copies: refills at $30.00/50 sheets
    - Time: 5 min to score
    - Languages: English, Spanish, Vietnamese, Hmong, Somali
    - Reading level: 5th grade
  - PEDS DM
    - Type: parent questionnaire
    - Age: 0–7 to 11 yr
    - Staff required: paraprofessional
    - Cost
      - $275.00/starter kit
      - Extra: laminated questionnaire book $110.00 each
    - Refills, copies: refills for record form $32/100 sheets
    - Time: 5–10 min to score
    - Languages: English, Spanish
    - Reading level: 3rd–4th grade
  - IDI
    - Type: parent questionnaire
    - Age: 3–18 mo
    - Staff required: paraprofessional
    - Cost: $14.00/pad (25 sheets)
    - Refills, copies
      - Refills: $14.00
    - Time: 10 min to score
    - Languages: English, Spanish
  - BRIGANCE
    - Type: direct elicitation
    - Ages
      - 0–23 mo
      - 2–2.5 yr
      - 3–4 yr
    - Staff required: professional
    - Cost: for each age range: $110.00/manual, $148.00/120 data sheets
    - Refills, copies: refills at $148.00/120 sheets
    - Time: 10–15 min to administer
    - Languages: English, Spanish

Social-emotional screens

- Secondary screens help the primary care physician make decisions about referrals and types of interventions.
  - The primary care practice may opt not to do secondary screening.
  - Patients can be referred for further assessment when the primary screen indicates an at-risk area.
- A secondary screen can be performed at a follow-up visit:
  - With the primary physician
  - By a care manager
  - By a social worker in the practice
  - For example, MCHAT can be used if a child has indicators of risk on the communication portion of the primary screen.

- ASQ SE
  - Type: parent questionnaire or interview
  - Age: 6–60 mo
  - Cost: $125/kit
  - Refills, copies: free to copy
  - Time: 10 min
  - Languages: English, Spanish
  - Reading level: 4th–6th grade
- TABS
  - Type: parent questionnaire or interview
  - Age: 11–71 mo
  - Cost: $85/kit
  - Refills, copies: $25 for pad of 50 sheets
  - Time: 5 min
  - Languages: English, Spanish
  - Reading level: 3rd grade
- BITSEA
  - Type: parent questionnaire or interview
  - Age: 12–36 mo
  - Cost: $99.00/kit
  - Refills, copies: $35 for 25 sheets
  - Time: 7–10 min
  - Languages: English, Spanish, French, Dutch, Hebrew
- Eyberg Child Behavior Inventory
  - Type: parent questionnaire or interview
  - Age: 2–16 yr
  - Cost: $147/kit
  - Refills, copies: $29 for pad of 25 sheets
  - Time: 5 min
  - Languages: English
  - Reading level: 6th grade
- PSC
  - Type: parent questionnaire or interview
  - Age: 4–18 yr
  - Cost: free, downloadable

- Refills, copies: free to copy
- Time: 5 min
- Languages: English, Spanish, Chinese

Office process

- Assess protocols for developmental screening already in use in the practice.
- Map the workflow to include:
  - Physician
  - Nursing staff
  - Office manager
  - Tailor the workflow to the practice.
- Select tool or tools.
- Identify system supports for:
  - Parent education
  - Referral
  - Community services
- Meet with key partners.
  - Invite community partners to a lunch meeting at the practice.
  - Share screening plans.
  - Align goals.
- Establish a process for:
  - Referral
  - Communication
  - Orient all staff members to new procedures.
- Billing issues
  - The American Medical Association *Current Procedural Terminology* code for screening tools is 96110.
    - Can be billed with a well-visit code
    - Can be billed with an evaluation and management code
    - 0.36 relative value units

Diabetes Mellitus

DEFINITION

- Diabetes mellitus
  - Heterogeneous group of conditions with diverse under-lying pathophysiologic factors that result in elevated blood glucose levels
- Type 1 diabetes (T1D)
  - Elevated blood glucose level caused by an absolute insulin deficiency
  - Type 1A
    - Classic form caused by autoimmune destruction of the pancreatic ß cells
  - Type 1B
    - Non–immune-mediated severe insulin deficiency caused by such conditions ascystic fibrosis or pancreatectomy
- Type 2 diabetes (T2D)
  - Caused by a relative insulin deficiency, peripheral resistance to the action of insulin, or both
- Maturity-onset diabetes of the young (MODY): defect in pancreatic ß cells

EPIDEMIOLOGY

- Prevalence
  - T1D
    - 12 per 100,000 person-years for individuals <20 years
    - Worldwide incidence of T1D increasing
  - T2D
    - Increasing in recent years, especially among specific ethnic groups
  - MODY
    - 5% of all cases of diabetes
- Race or ethnicity
  - T1D
    - Northern Europeans have a much higher risk than individuals from most Asian countries.
  - T2D
    - Incidence in African Americans, Hispanics, and Native Americans is increasing.
- Age
  - T1D
    - Occurs at any age, including in the neonatal period
  - T2D
    - Occurring in younger children as obesity becomes more common
    - Most common in children during puberty, a time of relative insulin resistance

ETIOLOGY

- T1D: absolute deficiency of insulin
  - Precise cause is elusive; probably a combination of:
    - Genetic factors
      - Strongest associations have been found with the genes encoding human leukocyte antigen (HLA) molecules on chromosome 6.
      - Other HLA molecules appear to offer protection against the development of diabetes.
      - Genetic factors do not account for all of the risk, and other factors must play a role.
    - Environmental factors
      - Environmental exposures have been implicated in the development of T1D in genetically susceptible individuals.
      - Congenital rubella syndrome confers added risk to the development of T1D.
      - A link with viral infections has not been proved.
      - There is no association between T1D and immunization status.
    - Dietary factors
      - Definitive data regarding dietary antigen exposure are lacking.
    - Antibodies
      - Islet cell antigens
      - Glutamic acid decarboxylase
      - Insulin
      - Whether these antibodies are causal or simply a marker of disease is unclear.
- T2D: relative deficiency of insulin or peripheral resistance to insulin, or both
  - The definite etiology is not known.
    - Environment (increased prevalence of obesity)
    - Genetic (strong family history)
- MODY
  - Defect in pancreatic ß cells
  - Autosomal-dominant inheritance

RISK FACTORS

- T1D
  - Genetic factors
    - Strongest associations have been found with the genes encoding HLA molecules on chromosome 6.
  - Environmental factors
    - Environmental exposures
    - Congenital rubella syndrome

- T2D
  - Obesity
  - Family history of T2D

SIGNS AND SYMPTOMS

- T1D
  - Acute or subacute onset of symptoms (days to weeks)
    - Abdominal pain
    - Headache
    - Nausea
    - Polyuria
    - Polydipsia
    - Significant weight loss despite an increasing appetite
- Severe ketoacidosis
  - Tachypnea
  - Fruity odor to the breath
- Severe diabetic ketoacidosis
  - Altered mental status
  - Seizures
- Physical examination
  - May be helpful in the case of suspected diabetes but will not substitute for laboratory confirmation of the diagnosis
  - T1D and T2D have no pathognomonic physical findings.
  - Physical findings are consistent with the degree of insulin deficiency and the duration of the disorder.
    - Dehydration
    - Tachycardia in some cases
- T2D
  - More insidious than T1D in onset
    - Patients may be asymptomatic.
    - Polyuria
    - Polydipsia
  - Signs of insulin resistance
    - Acanthosis nigricans
    - Weight loss may be apparent, but patients are invariably obese at the time of diagnosis.
    - Hypertension
- MODY
  - Clinical course varies considerably among the different forms.
  - Suspect if:
    - T2D develops at a young age in a thin individual.
    - Family history is suggestive of autosomal-dominant inheritance.
  - The specific type of MODY should be characterized if the diagnosis is made or suspected.

DIFFERENTIAL DIAGNOSIS

- Hyperglycemia from any cause can lead to symptoms related to an osmotic diuresis.
- Glycosuria: Glucose may be seen in the urine of some normoglycemic individuals, and glycosuria alone should not be used to diagnose diabetes mellitus.
- Causes other than diabetes mellitus that may lead to glycosuria
  - Diabetes
    - Neonatal diabetes
    - Gestational diabetes
  - Endocrinopathies
    - Cushing syndrome
    - Growth hormone excess
    - Pheochromocytoma
    - Glucagonoma
    - Somatostatinoma
  - Drugs
    - Glucocorticoids
    - Diazoxide
    - Glucagon
    - Cyclosporin
    - Phenytoin
    - Niacin
    - Antipsychotics
    - Calcium-channel blockers
    - Pentamidine
    - L-Asparaginase
  - Other
    - Cystic fibrosis
    - Pancreatitis
    - Pancreatectomy
    - Wolfram syndrome
    - Stiff man syndrome
    - Anti-insulin receptor antibodies

DIAGNOSTIC APPROACH

- Criteria for diagnosis
  - Symptoms of diabetes
    - Polyuria
    - Polydipsia
    - Unexplained weight loss
  - Causal (ie, any time of day without regard to time since the last meal) plasma glucose level ≥200 mg/dL *or*
  - Fasting (≥8 hours) plasma glucose level ≥126 mg/dL *or*

- Plasma glucose level ≥200 mg/dL 2 hours after an oral glucose challenge
  - Glucose load should contain 75 g of glucose for adults or 1.75 g/kg in children (maximal dose, 75 g).
- T2D can be asymptomatic, and the diagnosis may be made only as a result of screening.

LABORATORY FINDINGS

- Plasma glucose level
  - ≥126 mg/dL after an 8-hour fast is diagnostic.
- Oral glucose tolerance test
  - More costly and labor intensive than plasma glucose level
  - May identify some individuals with diabetes who have a fasting plasma glucose level <126 mg/dL
- Blood and urine ketone levels
  - Traditionally associated with T1D but occasionally present in patients with T2D
- Insulin and C-peptide concentrations
  - Generally low in established T1D
  - Elevated in T2D
- Antibody measurements (T1D)
  - Sensitivity and specificity are not sufficient to warrant routine clinical use.
  - Antibodies can be elevated in patients who may not develop disease for many years or ever.

CLASSIFICATION

- T1D
  - Type 1A
  - Type 1B
- T2D
- MODY
  - Type 1
    - Hepatocyte nuclear factor-4-α defect
  - Type 2
    - Glucokinase defect
  - Type 3
    - Hepatocyte nuclear factor-1-α defect
  - Type 4
    - Insulin promoter factor-1 defect
  - Type 5
    - Hepatic transcription factor-2 defect
  - Type 6
    - Neurogenic differentiation factor defect

TREATMENT APPROACH

- Therapy must be tailored to the specific underlying pathophysiologic condition.
  - Individualized patient education and support is imperative for success.
- T1D requires an integrated multidisciplinary team.
  - Physicians
  - Nurses
  - Diabetes educators
  - Dietitians
  - Social workers
  - Psychologists
- Insulin therapy
  - Required in patients with T1D
  - May not always be necessary for children with T2D
  - Safe and effective choice if it is not initially clear whether the patient has T1D or T2D
- Diabetes caused by excess glucocorticoids or other medications
  - Dose reduction or elimination of the drug (if possible) may be all that is required.

SPECIFIC TREATMENTS

Patient education

- Critical to safe and successful diabetes management
- Must be developmentally appropriate
  - Teenagers should be able to assume more responsibility for their care than young children.

T1D

- The goal is to safely achieve as near euglycemia as possible while minimizing adverse events, primarily hypoglycemia.
  - Glycemic control improves outcomes with regard to:
    - Microvascular complications
    - Macrovascular complications
    - Reduction in progression of diabetic retinopathy
- American Diabetes Association (ADA) age-adjusted guidelines for glycemic control
  - Age 0–6 years
    - Premeal plasma glucose 100–180 mg/dL
    - Bedtime or overnight plasma glucose 110–200 mg/dL
    - Hemoglobin (Hb) A_{1c} <8.5% (but >7.5%)
    - Less tight control is recommended for younger children.
      - Risks of hypoglycemia may be greater.
      - Advantages of very tight control have not been proven.
  - Age 6–12 years
    - Premeal plasma glucose 90–180 mg/dL
    - Bedtime or overnight plasma glucose 100–180 mg/dL
    - HbA_{1c} <8%

- Age 13–19 years
  - Premeal plasma glucose 90–130 mg/dL
  - Bedtime or overnight plasma glucose 90–150 mg/dL
  - HbA_{1c} <8%
- Adults
  - Premeal plasma glucose 90–130 mg/dL
  - HbA_{1c} <7%
- Lower HbA_{1c} values may be safely obtained in select patients in whom the risk of severe hypoglycemia is deemed low.
- Pregnancy
  - Postprandial glucose targets are widely used in the management of diabetes during pregnancy.
    - These targets are not commonly used outside pregnancy because their value has not been studied rigorously in children.

T2D

- Treatment options available for patients with T2D are more diverse than for those with T1D.
  - Although many effective medications with a variety of mechanisms of action are available, few are indicated for the treatment of T2D in children.
  - Therapy must be tailored to fit the clinical situation of the patient.
- Weight loss and exercise
  - Can significantly improve insulin sensitivity in T2D
  - Appropriate in the asymptomatic patient with a normal or near-normal HbA_{1c} level
  - May be adequate for maintenance of glycemic goals in patients who will adhere to dietary and exercise guidelines
  - Lifestyle modification intervention has been shown to reduce development of T2D in adults by 58% over 2.8 years of follow-up.
- Pharmacologic intervention
  - Consider for patient with:
    - Symptomatic hyperglycemia
    - Significantly elevated HbA_{1c} level
  - No pharmacologic intervention is a substitute for lifestyle intervention and medical nutrition therapy.
  - Insulin
    - The only medication approved for the treatment of diabetes in children at all ages
    - Most children with T2D can improve glycemic control with less intensive programs than are needed for patients with T1D.
    - Once- or twice-daily, intermediate- or long-acting insulin may be sufficient.

- Metformin
  - The only oral agent approved for use in children
  - Advantages
    - Safe and effective in lowering HbA_{1c} levels when used appropriately
    - Does not induce hypoglycemia when used alone
    - Weight stabilization or mild weight loss
  - Gastrointestinal disturbance is the major side effect.
    - Largely prevented by slow titration of the dose
  - Contraindications
    - Significant liver disease or renal impairment

Specific insulin programs

- All patients taking insulin will need to have an individualized plan for:
  - Type and dose of insulin
  - Timing of injections
  - Frequency of home glucose monitoring
- Typical doses of insulin in children
  - 0.5–1 unit of insulin per kg per day
  - During puberty, children require higher insulin doses to achieve the same control.
  - For patients with T1D
    - Intermediate- or long-acting insulin is used as the basal insulin.
    - A short-acting insulin bolus is used to control the post-meal glucose increase (see Figure 18 on page F5).
- Short-acting
  - Regular
    - Onset: 30 minutes
    - Peak: 2–4 hours
    - Duration: 4–6 hours
  - Lispro
    - Onset: <15 minutes
    - Peak: 1 hour
    - Duration: 3–4 hours
  - Aspart
    - Onset: <15 minutes
    - Peak: 1 hour
    - Duration: 3–4 hours
  - Glulisine
    - Onset: <15 minutes
    - Peak: 1 hour
    - Duration: 3–4 hours

- Intermediate-acting
  - NPH
    - Onset: 2–4 hours
    - Peak: 4–6 hours
    - Duration: 10–16 hours
  - Lente
    - Onset: 3–4 hours
    - Peak: 6–10 hours
    - Duration: 10–20 hours
- Long-acting
  - Glargine
    - Onset: 2–3 hours
    - Peak: none
    - Duration: ≥24 hours
  - Detemir
    - Onset: 1–2 hours
    - Peak: 3–9 hours
      - Higher doses result in delayed peak and longer duration of action.
    - Duration: 6–23 hours
      - Higher doses result in delayed peak and longer duration of action.
- Split-mixed program
  - Commonly used in younger patients in whom fewer injections may be desirable
  - A short-acting and an intermediate-acting insulin are mixed.
    - Given as a single injection before breakfast and again before the evening meal
    - Higher doses are required in the morning compared with the evening.
  - Typical ratio
    - 2/3 to 3/4 of the total daily dose given in the morning and the remainder in the evening
    - ~2/3 of the morning dose is intermediate-acting insulin.
      - The rest is short-acting insulin.
    - Equal amounts of intermediate- and short-acting insulin are given with the evening meal.
  - Prevention of hypoglycemia
    - A snack at bedtime can prevent nighttime hypoglycemia.
    - The intermediate-acting insulin will have its peak action in the early morning hours.
    - The evening dose of intermediate-acting insulin can be given at bedtime to help prevent this complication.

- Limitations
  - Achieving adequate glycemic goals is sometimes not possible.
  - Program requires patients to be on a fixed diet with respect to timing and nutrient content at each meal.
- Multiple daily injection (MDI) program
  - Intermediate- or long-acting insulin as the basal insulin
  - Short-acting insulin as a bolus with each meal
    - Requires 3–4 (or more) injections each day.
    - More flexibility in timing and content of meals than split-mixed programs
  - Basal insulin
    - Constitutes approximately half of the total daily dose
    - Usually given in the evening
  - The amount of short-acting insulin given with each meal depends on the amount of carbohydrate consumed at that meal.
    - If the patient has been prescribed an exchange diet with a fixed amount of carbohydrate for each meal, the dose of insulin will be the same from day to day.
    - Patients who vary carbohydrate consumption will need to adjust insulin accordingly.
- Continuous subcutaneous insulin injection (CSII) program
  - Cartridge filled with short-acting insulin serves as both the basal and bolus insulin.
    - Insulin is delivered through tubing connected to a flexible plastic cannula, which is inserted subcutaneously.
  - Advantages
    - Pump can be concealed under a person's clothing.
    - Multiple basal rates can be programmed for patients whose basal insulin requirements are not constant throughout the day.
    - This feature is not available with a split-mixed or MDI program.
    - Tubing and cannula are changed every 2–3 days, significantly reducing the number of injections required.
    - There may be a slight improvement in HbA_{1c} in patients treated with CSII compared with MDI.

Meal plan
- Carbohydrate ingestion is a major determinant of blood glucose concentration.
- Matching the amount of food intake with the appropriate amount of insulin requires knowledge of:
  - Onset
  - Peak
  - Duration of action of the various types of insulin available

- No single meal plan has been shown to be superior.
  - As children grow and vary their activity levels, caloric requirements can change significantly.
  - Advice from a dietitian experienced in the management of children with diabetes is necessary.
    - Plans require specific education.
    - Patients must be able to assess the nutrient content of foods.
    - Patients must understand how nutrition affects the management of their disease.
- Exchange diet
  - Patient eats a consistent amount of nutrients at a consistent time of day.
    - Example: 45 g of carbohydrate for breakfast, 60 g for lunch, and 60 g for dinner
    - Fat and protein may also be prescribed for each meal.
    - The patient is expected to eat according to this pattern each day.
  - Foods are categorized according to nutrient content.
    - This list is used to create a meal.
    - Foods with equivalent nutrient content can be exchanged for each other to introduce variety in the diet.
    - Snacks are usually incorporated into this diet depending on the individual patient's needs and preferences.
  - Advantages
    - Nutrient intake is consistent.
    - Allows insulin dosing also to be consistent
    - Can be used for patients on split-mixed, MDI, or CSII programs
- Carbohydrate counting
  - More complex than exchange diet, but increasingly popular
    - Patients must be familiar with the carbohydrate content of each food.
  - For each unit of carbohydrate taken, a specific amount of insulin must be given to maintain euglycemia.
    - Typical ratio may be 1 unit of short-acting insulin for each 15 g of carbohydrate eaten.
    - Ratio is adjusted for each patient.
    - Ratio may vary based on time of day for a given individual.
  - Advantages
    - Can be used for patients on an MDI or CSII insulin regimen
    - Carbohydrate counting allows more flexibility in the timing and content of each meal.
  - Caveats
    - Patients can take more insulin to maintain glycemic control while overeating.
    - Carbohydrate counting must be a part of an overall meal plan so that overeating does not lead to obesity or contribute to hyperlipidemia.
    - Carbohydrate counting requires specific education and a motivated patient and family to be implemented correctly.
  - Contraindications
    - Patients on a split-mixed insulin program
    - Insulin doses in a split-mixed program cannot easily be adjusted to account for the dietary variability of carbohydrate counting.

Exercise

- Exercise can be performed safely.
  - Children should not be discouraged from participating in sports because of diabetes.
  - However:
    - Attention to the effects of activity on glucose levels can assist in preventing hypoglycemia during or after exercise.
    - Hypoglycemia may occur if changes are not made in the amount of food eaten or insulin taken.
    - The effect of exercise may be sustained and lead to delayed hypoglycemia.
- Planned activity—2 methods of preventing hypoglycemia:
  - Reduce the dose of short-acting insulin given at the previous meal.
  - A snack can be given just before or during the activity.
- Unplanned activity
  - A snack is the only option.
- Blood glucose level
  - Should be checked before and again after exercise to determine the effect of the activity on glucose concentrations
  - If the activity is prolonged (>45–60 minutes), level should be checked:
    - Periodically during the activity
    - Again at night
  - Documenting the effect of exercise on the patient's glucose level is the only way to make appropriate decisions to prevent hypoglycemia.

Illness

- Illness can have a notable affect on blood glucose values.
  - Hypoglycemia or hyperglycemia may result.
    - Dependent on the severity of the illness and the amount of food eaten
- Regardless of food intake, insulin is necessary in health or illness.
  - A common error made is the omission of insulin injections because the child is not eating.

- Although the dose may change, some insulin should be given even if the child cannot eat.
- Practical guidelines can assist in appropriate care during illness and avoidance of hospitalization.
  - Never completely omit insulin.
  - Monitor and record blood glucose concentrations every 2–4 hours.
  - Monitor urine ketone concentrations frequently, even if the blood glucose level is not significantly elevated (>250 mg/dL).
    - Some patients with T1D can develop ketosis in the absence of hyperglycemia when ill.
  - Encourage adequate hydration.

WHEN TO ADMIT

- Admit when diabetic ketoacidosisis present.
- Consider admitting patients with:
  - Newly diagnosed T1D
  - Severe hypoglycemia or dehydration

WHEN TO REFER

- Refer when:
  - T1D is newly diagnosed
  - A multidisciplinary diabetes program is needed and not available

FOLLOW-UP

- Monitoring
  - Appropriate insulin dosing cannot be accomplished without adequate blood glucose monitoring.
    - Simply checking the glucose concentration is not enough.
    - Glucose values must be recorded in a log and reviewed on a regular basis to determine whether insulin doses need to be adjusted.
  - Frequency
    - Patients with T1D and some patients with T2D treated with insulin
      - Before meals
      - Bedtime
      - Occasionally at night
    - T2D treated with lifestyle modification or oral agents
      - Less frequent monitoring is required.
    - Additional glucose determinations may be needed during:
      - Illness
      - Exercise
      - Symptoms of hyperglycemia or hypoglycemia

- Home management
  - Many good home glucose monitors are available.
  - All of these monitors should be checked periodically for accuracy.
  - Patients should receive training on proper technique.
  - Data from many home glucose meters and insulin pumps can be transferred to a computer to assist in tracking glycemic control.
- Adjusting
  - Adjusting insulin doses is necessary to maintain good glycemic control.
    - Adjustment is based on patterns of blood glucose concentrations recorded in the log
    - Generally made as a 10% increase or decrease.
  - The purpose of an adjustment is to prevent future abnormal glucose levels.
    - Primary care physicians should commonly ask patients to look for a 3-day trend of hyperglycemia before making an adjustment.
    - Example: A patient consistently has glucose values before his or her evening meal that are higher than the goal range.
      - An increase in the short-acting insulin before the noon meal would be made.
  - Many variables exist that cannot be accounted for, therefore:
    - Patients should be informed that their blood glucose concentration will not always fall in the normal range.
      - For some people, this circumstance can be discouraging and lead to improper insulin adjustments.
      - For others, lack of education or fear of hypoglycemia leads to improper dose adjusting.
  - Primary care physicians must be clear about the difference between insulin adjustments and supplements.
- Supplementing
  - Used to correct a glucose concentration outside the goal range
    - The supplement (either adding or subtracting insulin) is used to correct the abnormal glucose.
    - The bolus dose of short-acting insulin is used to account for the food that will be eaten at a meal.
  - Example: A patient has a blood glucose level that is below the goal range before breakfast.
    - Insulin would be subtracted from the morning bolus dose of short-acting insulin.
  - Example: Glucose is above the goal range before a meal.
    - Supplemental insulin may be added to the bolus dose of short-acting insulin at that meal to correct the hyperglycemia.

D

COMPLICATIONS

- Both T1D and T2D greatly increase the risk of:
  - Blindness
  - Chronic kidney disease
  - Neuropathy
  - Cardiovascular disease
  - Stroke
  - Risks can be attenuated in adolescents and adults treated with intensive diabetes management.
  - Screening for chronic complications must be performed to intervene early to reverse or slow disease progression.
- Hypoglycemia
  - Common complication of treatment
    - Blood glucose levels should be checked to confirm symptoms are due to low blood glucose level.
    - Some symptoms of hypoglycemia are nonspecific.
    - Unnecessary treatment should be avoided.
    - Children <5 or6 years at the time of diagnosis:
      - At particularly high risk of frequent hypoglycemia, cognitive impairment
  - Mild hypoglycemia
    - Symptoms
      - Shakiness
      - Nervousness
      - Tachycardia
      - Sweating
- Older children are generally able to recognize symptoms.
- Younger children may not be able to recognize or effectively communicate these symptoms.
- Primary care physicians must be responsible for identifying hypoglycemia.
- Parents frequently report unusual behavior and irritability as signs of hypoglycemia in younger children.
- Management of mild hypoglycemia
  - 10–15 g of carbohydrate will correct the situation.
  - Glucose level should be rechecked in 15–20 minutes to be certain hypoglycemia has resolved.
  - Glucose tablets and gels are available and easy to carry.
  - Some form of carbohydrate should always be available to the patient.
- Severe hypoglycemia
  - Defined as an episode requiring assistance for treatment
  - Symptoms
    - Neurologic symptoms can include confusion or loss of consciousness.
    - Symptoms markedly increase with lowering of the HbA_{1c} level (see Figure 19 on page F5).

- Management of severe hypoglycemia
  - In an unconscious patient, severe hypoglycemia may be treated with glucagon or intravenous glucose.
  - Training on proper use of glucagon should be provided to individuals caring for the patient (parents, school nurses, older siblings, others).
  - Glucagon is reserved for patients with severe hypoglycemia who cannot ingest carbohydrates.
  - Response is short-lived; as soon as practical, the patient should eat.
  - Nausea frequently accompanies glucagon administration.
- After hypoglycemia treatment, cause of hypoglycemia should be considered.
  - If no cause is readily apparent, the insulin dose should be adjusted the next day to avoid additional hypoglycemia.
    - This advice is in contrast to monitoring glucose trends before making adjustments to prevent hyperglycemia.
  - One episode of unexplained hypoglycemia should prompt an insulin adjustment.
  - Less tight glycemic control should be considered for patients with frequent severe hypoglycemia and associated long-term neurologic consequences.
- Diabetic retinopathy
  - Screening is recommended for all individuals with diabetes.
  - Retinopathy within the first 3 years of diagnosis is unusual for a child.
    - Especially if the child is <10 years
  - Ophthalmologic evaluation for patients with T1D
    - Starts between 3 and 5 years after the initial diagnosis
    - Annual follow-up thereafter
- Diabetic nephropathy
  - Leading cause of chronic kidney disease and need for dialysis
  - Uncommon in the young patient or the patient with newly diagnosed T1D
  - Screening should start at age 10 years in children who have had T1D for ≥5 years.
    - Random urine sample to determine the microalbumin-to-creatinine ratio
    - Ratio of ≥30 mg/g (albumin to creatinine) is considered abnormal, and further testing may be indicated.
    - Because other factors may contribute to albuminuria, including exercise, 2–3 abnormal determinations may need to be obtained to confirm the diagnosis.
- Hyperlipidemia
  - Screening is also recommended at or shortly after the initial diagnosis of T1D in all patients.
  - Lifestyle and pharmacologic intervention may be required.
    - Depending on the lipid profile and additional risk factors

- Autoimmune disorders
  - Thyroid disease (~17% of patients)
    - Screening should begin at or shortly after diagnosis of T1D.
    - Measurement of sensitive thyroid-stimulating hormone
    - Annual screening thereafter
  - Celiac disease
    - Patients with T1D are at risk.
    - Screening by measuring tissue transglutaminase antibodies or endomysial antibodies
    - Normal total immunoglobulin A concentrations should also be documented.

PROGNOSIS

- T1D
  - Fatal disease until the discovery of insulin
    - Progressive metabolic abnormalities, including ketoacidosis, would eventually lead to death.
    - With the availability of insulin for clinical use in the early 1920s, patients were able to survive the more immediate threat of severe acidosis.
  - Uncorrected severe hyperglycemia and metabolic acidosis can lead to neurologic sequelae.
    - Seizures
    - Coma
  - Antibodies predict progression in high-risk individuals with HLA susceptibility or a family history of diabetes.
    - Islet cell antigens
    - Glutamic acid decarboxylase
    - Insulin

- MODY
  - Clinical course can range from mild to progressive disease with the development of microvascular complications.

PREVENTION

- Recognizing early symptoms of diabetes may help prevent:
  - Severe diabetic ketoacidosis
  - Potentially fatal outcomes
- Criteria for Screening High-Risk Children for Diabetes
  - Overweight (body mass index >85th percentile for age and sex)
  - *Plus* any 2 risk factors:
    - Family history of T2D in a first- or second-degree relative
    - High-risk race or ethnicity (Native American, African American, Latino, Asian American, or Pacific Islander)
    - Signs of insulin resistance or associated conditions
      - Acanthosis nigricans
      - Hypertension
      - Dyslipidemia
      - Polycystic ovarian syndrome
    - Maternal history of diabetes or gestational diabetes
  - Age to initiate screening
    - 10 years
    - Onset of puberty if <10 years
  - Frequency: every 2 years
  - Preferred screening test: plasma glucose after an 8-hour fast

Diabetic Ketoacidosis

DEFINITION

- Diabetic ketoacidosis (DKA) is the metabolic consequence of insulin deficiency.
  - Biochemical hallmarks of DKA
    - Hyperglycemia
    - Acidosis

EPIDEMIOLOGY

- Age
  - Adolescents
- Sex
  - More prevalent in girls
- Race and ethnicity
  - Although DKA is more common with type 1 diabetes (T1D) than type 2 diabetes (T2D), Hispanic and African-American youths are more prone than other populations with T2D to develop DKA.

ETIOLOGY

- DKA results from a lack of insulin.
- The following counterregulatory hormones may have elevated levels and contribute to hyperglycemia:
  - Glucagon
  - Catecholamines
  - Cortisol
- Fat stores are broken down in the absence of adequate insulin action, leading to:
  - Ketone body formation
  - Metabolic acidosis

RISK FACTORS

- Diabetes
  - T1D
    - Poor glycemic control (higher hemoglobin A_{1c} level)
    - High reported daily insulin doses
    - Omission of insulin
    - Previous episode of DKA (frequently)
    - Coexisting psychiatric disorders
    - Lower socioeconomic status (underinsured)
    - Adolescent age (especially girls)
  - T2D
    - Historically, less commonly associated than T1D with DKA
    - However, patients with T2D may have DKA.

- Other factors
  - Illness
  - Trauma
  - Alcohol
  - Medications
  - Pancreatitis
- Family history
  - Positive in most patients with T2D
  - Negative in most patients with T1D

SIGNS AND SYMPTOMS

- Symptoms vary and are consistent with the degree of metabolic disturbance.
  - Polyuria
  - Polydipsia
  - Enuresis in previously continent children
  - Dehydration
    - Can be severe if the child has limited access to fluids or is vomiting
    - Signs include tachycardia and weight loss.
    - Most patients with moderate to severe DKA are at least 5–10% dehydrated.
    - True dehydration (intracellular and extracellular fluid loss) rather than simple hypovolemia (intravascular fluid loss) is the rule.
    - Few patients become hypotensive.
  - Fatigue
    - May be evident even before significant dehydration and acidosis
  - Weight loss
    - May be difficult to quantify unless a recent accurate weight is available
    - Polyphagia may be evident early but is typically replaced with a loss of appetite as ketosis and metabolic acidosis worsen.
    - Abdominal pain
    - Vomiting
- Initial assessment
  - Cardiovascular status (heart rate, blood pressure, perfusion)
  - Respiratory status
    - Address immediately if compromise is present.
    - Rapid, deep respirations (Kussmaul breathing)
    - Fruity breath odor may be detected with release of acetone.

- Signs of neurologic dysfunction
  - Confusion
  - Altered sensorium
  - Cerebral edema: consider in all patients with DKA who exhibit signs or symptoms of neurologic compromise
- Severity of disease assessment
  - Sensorium
    - Mild: alert
    - Moderate: drowsy, lethargic
    - Severe: obtundation, coma
  - Hyperpnea
    - Mild: normal respiration
    - Moderate: modest increased respiration
    - Severe: frank Kussmaul respiration
  - Hydration
    - Mild: no dehydration
    - Moderate: mild to moderate dehydration (3–5%)
    - Severe: severe dehydration (>5%)
  - Plasma bicarbonate level
    - Mild: >16–18 mEq/L
    - Moderate: 10–16 mEq/L
    - Severe: <10 mEq/L
  - Anion gap
    - Mild: <20 mEq/L
    - Moderate: 20–25 mEq/L
    - Severe: >25 mEq/L
- Special considerations in infants and young children
  - Young patients cannot verbalize symptoms.
  - Infants' inability to access fluids freely may mask polyuria.
    - Increased urine production may be difficult to judge on the basis of how wet infants' diapers are or how frequently the diapers need to be changed.
  - Parents are less likely to recognize symptoms of hyperglycemia and DKA in children <2 years.
    - May delay diagnosis of diabetes
    - More children in this age group have DKA at initial diagnosis compared with older children.

DIFFERENTIAL DIAGNOSIS

- Coexisting illness should be considered if:
  - The patient is in shock.
  - Lactic acidosis or hemodynamic instability is present.
    - Sepsis or poor perfusion may coexist with DKA.
  - Ketoacidosis does not improve or worsens with insulin administration.

DIAGNOSTIC APPROACH

- 2 biochemical requirements for diagnosis of DKA
  - Blood glucose level >200 mg/dL
  - Metabolic acidosis with a venous pH <7.3 or bicarbonate level <15 mEq/L
  - Although these criteria will identify most patients, glucose concentration ≤200 mg/dL does not always rule out DKA.
- During initial assessment, precipitating factors associated with the episode should be identified.
- DKA is present at the time of initial diagnosis in many patients with T1D.

LABORATORY FINDINGS

- Sodium
  - Estimated depletion per kg body weight
    - 6 mEq/kg (range, 5–13 mEq/kg)
  - Accurate assessment of sodium concentration is necessary to determine appropriate fluid management.
  - Apparent hyponatremia (pseudohyponatremia)
    - Some laboratory methods take this into account when measuring sodium (eg, direct potentiometry using an ion-selective electrode).
    - Primary care physicians need to know the method being used by the laboratory to determine whether pseudohyponatremia is contributing to this biochemical abnormality.
- Potassium
  - Estimated depletion per kg body weight
    - 5 mEq/kg (range, 4–6)
  - Must be monitored closely and replaced appropriately
  - At initial evaluation, potassium levels are typically normal or elevated because of acidemia.
  - When treatment begins, total body potassium is depleted, even with hyperkalemia
    - Profound hyperkalemia or hypokalemia may lead to cardiac arrhythmias.
- Phosphorus
  - Estimated depletion per kg body weight
    - 3 mEq/kg (range, 2–5)
  - Patients with DKA may have profound hypophosphatemia.
    - This may become apparent only during therapy.
- Other biochemical features of DKA
  - Estimated water depletion per kg body weight
    - 60–100 mL/kg
  - Estimated chloride depletion per kg body weight
    - 4 mEq/kg (range, 3–9)

D

D

- Other laboratory tests
  - Renal function
  - Blood urea nitrogen (BUN)
  - Creatinine
    - Values are typically elevated in a pattern consistent with a prerenal state.
  - Insulin and C-peptide concentrations are generally low in patients with newly diagnosed T1D.
  - Antibody levels against islet cell antigens and insulin
    - Frequently elevated at time of diagnosis
    - Not useful in diagnosis or management of DKA

IMAGING

- Brain imaging
  - Order promptly if symptoms of cerebral edema are encountered at any time during the treatment of DKA.

DIAGNOSTIC PROCEDURES

- Cultures
  - Blood
  - Urine
    - Glucose
    - Ketones
  - Cerebrospinal fluid
- Electrocardiography
  - Obtain in patients with significantly elevated potassium concentrations to determine whether cardiac abnormalities are present.

TREATMENT APPROACH

- Treatment approach depends on severity of DKA.
  - Mild
    - Patients with established diabetes can be managed in the outpatient setting if they can maintain oral intake.
  - Moderate to severe
    - Medical emergency requiring meticulous attention to optimize outcomes
    - Early recognition and appropriate intervention are imperative.
- Principles of managing DKA are the same whether the underlying diagnosis is T1D or T2D.
  - Correction of metabolic disturbances
  - Prevention of potential complications
  - Mandatory insulin administration
  - Fluid and electrolyte replacement
  - Treatment of concomitant conditions
- No single protocol will be appropriate for all patients.

SPECIFIC TREATMENTS

Fluid replacement

- Initial fluid replacement
  - Patients with moderate to severe DKA are generally considered to be 5–10% dehydrated.
  - 10–20 mL/kg intravenous (IV) fluid is suggested for initial fluid replacement.
    - Isotonic solutions such as lactated Ringer's solution or 0.9% saline
  - Additional fluid resuscitation may be required in some patients.
    - Caution must be used, especially in patients with possible cerebral edema.
  - Aggressive fluid resuscitation is rarely required.
  - The goal of initial fluid resuscitation is not to replace the entire fluid deficit.
    - Rehydration should take place over 36–48 hours.
    - Less aggressive rates of fluid replacement have been associated with more rapid correction of acidosis.
    - Gradual rehydration may reduce the risk of cerebral edema compared with more aggressive fluid administration.
  - Fluid therapy (even before insulin) will reduce the blood glucose concentration.
- After initial fluid bolus
  - Content of IV fluid should be changed to:
    - Address additional electrolyte abnormalities
    - Prevent hyperchloremic metabolic acidosis that may occur if isotonic saline solutions are continued
    - Add potassium to the IV solution when:
      - Potassium concentration is normal or low *and*
      - Urine flow has been established.
  - Rehydration should take place over ≥48 hours.
    - Rate of fluid administration should rarely exceed 1.5–2 times the maintenance fluids.
    - Urinary losses should not be added to the calculated fluid requirement.
- Transition to oral intake after correction of acidosis
  - IV fluids should be reduced or discontinued.

Insulin therapy

- IV insulin
  - Preferred route of administration for regular insulin
    - Subcutaneous (SC) and intramuscular delivery are used initially only if IV access is impossible.
  - Can be titrated frequently if necessary

- SC delivery
  - Consider converting to SC insulin when:
    - The serum bicarbonate level is >16–18 mmol/L (or pH >7.3).
    - The patient can begin oral intake.
  - Child with previous diagnosis of diabetes
    - Home insulin regimen may serve as a guide in choosing:
      - Initial SC insulin doses
      - Type of program to use (split-mixed vs multiple daily injection)
  - Child with newly diagnosed diabetes
    - 0.5–1.0 units/kg per day in divided doses
  - Adjust dose on the basis of:
    - Meal plan
    - Level of activity
    - Pubertal status (insulin requirement is increased during puberty)
- Dosing
  - Initial infusion rate
    - 0.1 unit/kg per hour of IV regular insulin
    - Ketosis and metabolic acidosis will not correct without adequate insulin administration.
    - A constant insulin infusion rate should be used.
    - Rate of insulin infusion may need to be increased in some children if ketoacidosis does not improve or worsens.
    - Metabolic acidosis often corrects many hours after euglycemia has been restored.
  - Blood glucose concentration
    - Should not be used alone to determine when to discontinue or decrease rate of infusion
  - Addition of glucose to IV fluids
    - When blood glucose level falls below 250–300 mg/dL
    - An infusion of 5% dextrose may be sufficient for many patients.
    - Higher rates of dextrose infusion may be required to prevent hypoglycemia while ketoacidosis is resolving.

Electrolytes

- Sodium
  - Sodium depletion is addressed with isotonic solutions suggested for initial fluid management.
  - Correction factors for hyponatremia
    - Add 1.6 mEq/L to the measured sodium concentration for every 100 mg/dL that the glucose concentration is over the normal range.
    - Other researchers have suggested that a correction factor of 2.4 mEq/L is more appropriate than 1.6 mEq/L.
    - Excessive isotonic sodium chloride should not be given; hyperchloremic metabolic acidosis may result.
  - Sodium concentrations should be monitored closely.
    - Failure of the sodium concentration to increase during treatment of DKA may be associated with higher risk of cerebral edema.
- Potassium
  - Before insulin therapy, potassium concentrations may be elevated, normal, or low, depending on:
    - Severity of DKA
    - Duration of DKA
    - Gastrointestinal losses caused by vomiting
  - After initiation of insulin therapy, potassium concentrations invariably decline as acidosis resolves and may become normal or low.
  - Potassium should be replaced after:
    - Initial isotonic fluid bolus has been given.
    - Serum potassium concentration becomes normal or low.
    - Urine output is established.
  - Dosing
    - Add 20 mEq/L potassium acetate and 20 mEq/L potassium phosphate to 0.45% saline.
    - The combination of salts prevents excess chloride while replacing potassium and phosphorus.
    - This solution is safe and an effective means to prevent profound hypokalemia.
  - Potassium levels should be monitored closely and therapy adjusted according to individual patient needs.
- Phosphorus
  - Phosphate concentrations may vary before initiation of insulin therapy.
  - Phosphate replacement in patients with DKA has *not* been shown to:
    - Provide clinically important improvements in outcome
    - Eliminate significant complications
  - However, possibility of a decrease in oxygen delivery to tissues is present.
  - Dosing
    - Add 20 mEq/L potassium acetate and 20 mEq/L potassium phosphate to 0.45% saline (as for potassium replacement).
    - The combination of salts prevents excess chloride while replacing potassium and phosphorus.
  - If phosphate therapy is used:
    - Serum calcium concentrations should be monitored because hypocalcemia may occur.

D

D

■ Bicarbonate

- Data are lacking to support use of bicarbonate therapy for patients with mild to moderate DKA.

- Even for patients with severe DKA, bicarbonate therapy has not been proven beneficial.

- Use of bicarbonate in patients with DKA may not be appropriate because:

  - Ketoacidosis can be completely corrected by the administration of IV fluids and insulin.

  - Bicarbonate will add sodium that may not be required.

  - Bicarbonate therapy may cause paradoxical central nervous system acidosis.

  - Bicarbonate therapy has been associated with an increased risk of cerebral edema.

- Despite these concerns, some patients may benefit from cautious alkali administration.

  - Patients with cardiovascular dysfunction caused by severe acidosis and/or hyperkalemia

WHEN TO ADMIT

■ Patients with moderate to severe DKA

■ Patients with dehydration or those who cannot maintain adequate oral intake

■ All patients with newly diagnosed diabetes regardless of severity of ketoacidosis

WHEN TO REFER

■ When facilities to provide frequent patient assessment (clinical and laboratory) are not available

■ When a physician experienced in the diagnosis and treatment of DKA is not available

FOLLOW-UP

■ Monitoring

- Frequent monitoring of patient's response to therapy is imperative to assess whether change in treatment is required.

- Hourly measurement
  - Glucose

- Measure every 2–4 hours:
  - Electrolytes
  - Bicarbonate
  - Ketones
  - pH

- Severe DKA
  - More frequent monitoring (every 2 hours)

- When improvement in ketoacidosis has been established
  - Less frequent monitoring (every 4 hours)

COMPLICATIONS

■ Cerebral edema

- Affects ~1% of children

  - Some studies suggest an increased incidence of subclinical cerebral edema when imaging criteria are used to diagnose the condition.

- Consequences are severe.

  - 20–25% mortality rate

  - A significant proportion of survivors will have permanent neurologic consequences.

- High index of suspicion should be maintained for early identification of this potentially fatal condition.

  - Clinical findings suggestive of cerebral edema should prompt emergent assessment.

  - Frequent neurologic examinations should be performed in children with DKA in an attempt to identify and intervene early.

  - Cerebral edema can be present before therapy for DKA.

    ■ Prevention of DKA may be the only effective strategy to prevent this potentially devastating complication.

- Symptoms of cerebral edema attributed to increased intracranial pressure

  - Decreased level of consciousness

  - Elevated blood pressure

  - Bradycardia

  - Nonspecific symptoms, such as headache

- Risk factors for cerebral edema:

  - Lower partial pressure of arterial carbon dioxide at presentation

  - Severity of dehydration (higher initial BUN)

  - Smaller increase in serum sodium during treatment

  - New-onset diabetes

  - Treatment with bicarbonate

  - Younger age

  - Longer duration of symptoms before presentation

- Management of cerebral edema associated with DKA

  - Reduce rate of fluid administration.

  - IV mannitol may be given and repeated after 2 hours if clinically indicated.

  - Hypertonic saline has been suggested as an alternative to mannitol.

  - If intubation is required, hyperventilation should be avoided.

    ■ Has been associated with worse outcomes

- Hypoglycemia
- Venous thrombosis
  - Especially in children with a central venous catheter
- Seizures
- Coma

PROGNOSIS

- The reported mortality rate in children with DKA is low (<0.5%).
  - Most deaths occur in patients who develop clinically apparent cerebral edema.
  - In adults, coexisting conditions, such as myocardial infarction, contribute to a larger percentage of the mortality associated with DKA.

PREVENTION

- Most children with established diabetes develop DKA because of omission of insulin.
  - Failure to recognize the need for insulin during illness
    - This common mistake can be prevented by providing adequate education to the patient and family.
    - Insulin need may be greater during illness.
  - Financial constraints
  - A small percentage of patients with diabetes accounts for a disproportionate number of episodes of DKA.
    - Interventions targeted at this high-risk population would seem appropriate.
- Patients with newly diagnose ddiabetes
  - Raising public awareness of symptoms of diabetes may be a cost-effective way to prevent DKA.

D

Diaper Rash

DEFINITION

- Diaper rash is not a single disorder, but rather a reaction of the skin to a host of factors, both local and systemic.
- On occasion, it may result from serious illness.

EPIDEMIOLOGY

- Prevalence
  - The most common skin disorder of infants and toddlers
  - Occurs in 1 of 4 infants
    - In a survey of suburban infants, 25% had some diaper dermatitis and 4% had a severe rash.
- Age
  - The greatest frequency occurs between 9 and 12 months of age.

ETIOLOGY

- 4 factors have been associated with the occurrence of diaper rash (see Figure 20 on page F6).
  - Wetness of the skin
  - Elevated pH of the skin
  - Fecal enzymes (especially proteases and lipases)
  - Microorganisms, especially *Candida albicans*
- Wet skin
  - Has a reduced ability to withstand frictional forces
- Elevated pH and fecal enzymes
  - Increase permeability
  - The normal pH of the skin is between 4.5 and 5.5.
  - Elevated pH:
    - Has been associated with more severe diaper rash
    - Increases activity of fecal proteases and lipases
    - Decreases normal skin microflora
  - Ammonia once was believed to be the primary irritant causing diaper rash but is no longer considered to be the major factor.
  - Fecal proteases and lipases along with moisture:
    - Lead to maceration of the skin
    - Increase permeability to such substances as bile salts, which worsen the inflammation
- *Candida albicans*
  - The most important microorganism found on the skin of infants who have diaper rash
  - Produces a protease that penetrates the skin and can:
    - Cause a primary infection
    - Be a secondary invader in systemic conditions, such as seborrheic dermatitis
    - Be found in many infants who have nonspecific diaper rash

- Even a small number of *Candida* organisms can cause significant infection.
- In 1 survey, candidal species were isolated from one-half of the mouths of healthy infants.
  - Infants who routinely sucked a pacifier had a higher rate of oral candidal carriage.
- Use of oral or parenteral antibiotics
  - Can increase the number of *Candida* organisms on the skin and frequency of stools
- *Staphylococcus aureus*
  - Has been isolated as a secondary invader of systemic illness, such as atopic dermatitis
  - Although present on skin, it does not appear to be a common primary pathogen in other forms of diaper rashes.

RISK FACTORS

- Historical factors that may help determine the contributors to diaper rash include:
  - Duration of the rash
  - Frequent bowel movements, eg, in infants with gastroenteritis or taking antibiotics
  - Presence of increased enzymes, yeast, pathogenic bacteria
  - Type of diaper
    - Diapers made of water-absorbent gel material keep skin drier and decrease the occurrence of diaper rash.
  - Frequency of changing: wet skin
    - In 1 study, infants whose diapers had been changed ≥8 times during the day had fewer rashes than those changed less often.
  - Method of laundering cloth diapers
  - Use of outer coverings, such as plastic or rubber pants
  - Past illness (especially dermatologic, allergic, and infectious)
  - Medication use (eg, antibiotics) that include the therapy for the rash
  - Exposure to contagious disease (eg, scabies, varicella)
  - Presence of systemic symptoms
  - Family history of illness (eg, psoriasis, allergy)

SIGNS AND SYMPTOMS

- Diaper rashes can be classified into 3 distribution patterns by appearance and location.
  - This approach has limitations.
    - A single agent (eg, *C albicans*) can lead to different presentations.
    - A single presentation may be caused by many agents (either alone or in concert).

- Diaper dermatitis from any cause
  - Can become secondarily infected with *Staphylococcus* or *Streptococcus*, leading to impetigo, bullous impetigo, or staphylococcal scalded skin
- Some diaper rashes do not fit any of these patterns, eg, that due to herpes simplex virus infection

■ First pattern
- Chafing or irritant dermatitis (see Figure 21 on page F6)
  - Erythematous desquamative rash involving the convex surfaces that touch the diaper and spare the inguinal folds
  - Erythema is mild, with or without papules.
  - Skin has a shiny, glazed appearance.
  - Meatitis may be seen in boys.
  - Rashes that have persisted for >72 hours are usually found to have significant *Candida* involvement.
- Atopic dermatitis
  - Eczematoid appearance with lichenification (thickening), pruritus, and atopic dermatitis elsewhere should help substantiate this diagnosis.
  - Uncommon in children <6 months

■ Second pattern
- Involves skinfolds and spares convex surfaces (see Figure 22 on page F7)
- Rashes involving the perianal area only
  - Are common in the neonatal period
  - May result from irritation by diarrhea
  - Are especially common in children whose diarrhea is secondary to disaccharidase deficiency
  - May be caused by infection with *C albicans*
- Intertrigo
  - Causes moist, macerated symmetric eruptions in skinfolds and creases
  - Commonly becomes infected secondarily by *C albicans*, especially when satellite lesions are present
- Classic primary candidal (monilial) diaper rash
  - Bright red confluent lesions, often with raised borders
  - Occasional pustular-vesicular satellite lesions on the trunk and legs
  - Other areas, eg folds of the neck, the postauricular area, and the oral mucosa (thrush), may be involved.
  - Usually painful and tender
  - In 1 study, rashes least like that shown in Figure 22 on page F7 were more likely to be associated with *Candida* organisms.

- Langerhans cell histiocytosis
  - May have the same distribution as *Candida* infection but is more papular, hemorrhagic, and more likely to be eroded
  - Fails to respond to conventional therapy
  - Constitutional symptoms (such as malaise) and abnormal physical findings (such as hepatosplenomegaly) may be present.
- Seborrheic dermatitis
  - Characterized by erythematous, often salmon-colored, patches with greasy scale that involve the convexities and creases (see Figure 23 on page F7)
  - May be difficult to distinguish from psoriasis, which has a deeper red color

■ Third pattern (see Figure 24 on page F7)
- Erythema in this distribution has been termed *tide mark dermatitis*.
- Believed to be related to frequent cycles of wetting and drying
- Irritation from diapers that are too tight (constrictive) and that may have an elastic band can lead to a similar rash.

DIFFERENTIAL DIAGNOSIS

■ Serious, systemic illness must always be considered in the child with:
- An atypical or a severe rash
- Failure to respond to customary therapy

■ Some conditions may occur or begin with greater intensity in the diaper area and may change morphologically.
- Such predilections probably represent the Koebner (isomorphic) response.
  - Skin lesions of a systemic illness concentrate on areas previously inflamed by other factors, such as friction.
- Conditions include:
  - Seborrhea
  - Atopic dermatitis
  - Hand-foot-and-mouth disease
  - Primary herpes simplex virus infection
  - Psoriasis
  - Varicella
  - Miliaria
  - Scabies

■ Less common causes of diaper rash include:
- Infectious or presumed infectious
  - Herpes simplex virus: Vesicular; may be associated with immunosuppression
  - Cytomegalovirus: Usually associated with immunosuppression

D

– Kawasaki disease: red, desquamating perineal eruption associated with fever, often during the first week after syndrome onset

– Syphilis: May have other manifestations of secondary syphilis

– Trichophyton: Extremely uncommon; annular scaly patches

• Neoplastic

– Histiocytosis (Letterer-Siwe disease): Resembles seborrhea plus reddish-brown papules

• Nutritional and metabolic

– Zinc deficiency (acrodermatitis enteropathica): Mimics monilial rash; vesicular eruptions elsewhere

• Presumed iatrogenic

– Granuloma gluteale infantum: May be secondary to use of halogenated steroid creams

• Genetic

– Wiskott Aldrich syndrome: Thrombocytopenia and recurrent infections in boys

■ Severe, persistent, and recurrent infections with *Candida* organisms

• May (rarely) result from immunodeficiency, including HIV infection or diabetes mellitus

■ Children who are immunosuppressed from HIV infection or neoplasia (or its treatment):

• May have diaper rash from such organisms as herpes simplex virus or cytomegalovirus

• If an immunosuppressed child has a serious or unresponsive diaper rash, then aggressive pursuit of an etiologic agent, including skin biopsy, should be considered.

■ Child abuse (including sexual abuse) or neglect

• Should be suspected in the child who has lesions in the diaper area (especially burns) that are inconsistent with the history provided.

LABORATORY FINDINGS

■ Laboratory tests are not indicated for most diaper rashes.

■ Tests that may be helpful in identifying the cause of a diaper rash include:

• Potassium hydroxide preparation and a fungal culture of skin scrapings for *Candida* organisms

• Bacterial culture for *Staphylococcus* organisms

• Mineral oil slide preparation for scabies

• Serum zinc level (to rule out acrodermatitis enteropathica)

• Serologic tests for syphilis

IMAGING

■ Radiography of the skull and long bones may be helpful for evidence of child abuse.

DIAGNOSTIC PROCEDURES

■ Skin biopsy

• Rarely, may be useful in cases in which the diaper rash is atypical or unresponsive to therapy

TREATMENT APPROACH

■ The initial step should be to minimize contact with soiled diapers.

• Most clinicians recommend that during therapy:

– Diapers should be changed frequently (≥8 times a day), using breathable diapers with absorbent gel material.

– Stool should be wiped off the skin as soon as possible.

– Plastic pants that retain water should not be used.

– Breaks from wearing diapers should be offered as much as possible.

■ Commercial disposable baby wipes, which typically contain water, an emollient, and surfactants:

• Are less irritating than cotton washcloths

• May be better for cleaning intertriginous areas

• Are well tolerated by children with atopic dermatitis

■ Systemic conditions such as scabies, atopic dermatitis, and varicella

• Most can be managed as they are for other parts of the skin.

• Seborrheic dermatitis is an exception (see Specific Treatments).

■ Many more children have been harmed by well-intended diaper rash therapies than have ever been harmed by the rash itself.

• Boric acid, mercury compounds, and pentachlorophenol have led to illness and death in infants.

• Talcum powder never should be used.

– Provides no protection

– Is abrasive

– Inhalation of a large quantity can produce serious or fatal pulmonary damage.

• Topical steroids present numerous dangers.

– In a nationally representative survey, 16% of diaper rashes were treated with a combination of nystatin and triamcinolone, a mid-potency steroid that should not be used in the diaper area.

– In a survey of pediatricians, 23% who prescribed clotrimazole-betamethasone dipropionate (Lotrisone) did so for diaper dermatitis.

– Betamethasone dipropionate is a high-potency steroid and is not indicated for the diaper area.

• Hair dryers may cause perineal burns and should never be recommended to dry the skin in the diaper area.

- Products containing iodochlorhydroxyquin, such as Vioform or Iodo Plain, should never be used.
  - Systemic absorption may lead to optic atrophy and neuropathy.

SPECIFIC TREATMENTS

Irritant diaper dermatitis

- Usually, the only interventions needed are:
  - Frequent diaper changes
  - Skin washing with plain water or disposable baby wipes
  - Allowing the skin to dry between diaper changes
- Scrubbing the rash or diaper area should be discouraged.
- Diapers with absorbent gel materials:
  - Have been shown to decrease wetness in the diaper area
  - May hasten the disappearance of a diaper dermatitis
- Barrier pastes and ointments
  - Form a resistant covering over the skin surface and decrease friction
  - Insufficient evidence available to support use of one product over another.
- Cloth diapers
  - Rinsing in methylbenzethonium chloride (Diaparene), a bacteriostatic agent, or in a vinegar solution (1 ounce in 1 gallon of water) has been shown to reduce recurrences.
  - Elimination of fabric softeners and changing detergents
    - May be effective in some cases
    - Is not scientifically documented as beneficial
- 1% hydrocortisone
  - May promote healing in cases of significant inflammation
  - Steroids that are more potent than 1% hydrocortisone should never be used in the diaper area because diapers form an occlusive dressing.
    - Long-term use may lead to skin atrophy, telangiectasis, granuloma gluteale, striae and, possibly, Cushing syndrome.
- Topical antibiotics
  - May be used to prevent stricture in meatitis
  - Antibiotic solutions available in ophthalmologic containers can be used.
- Miconazole in a zinc oxide-petrolatum base
  - One study showed it was more effective in eliminating moderate to severe diaper rashes (even without direct evidence of candidiasis) than the base alone.
- Agents to acidify urine (cranberry juice, vitamin C), cornstarch, and ointments that contain vitamins A and D
  - Widely used
  - No experimental evidence supports their efficacy.

Seborrheic dermatitis

- Because the diaper area is often infected secondarily with *Candida* organisms, measures to treat yeast must be undertaken as well.
- For this and other diaper rashes in which *Candida* organisms are present
  - Topical nystatin, miconazole, clotrimazole, haloprogin, or ketoconazole should be applied for 5–10 days.
  - Such agent as miconazole and clotrimazole have the advantage of requiring only twice-daily application.
  - 1% hydrocortisone may be used simultaneously to decrease inflammation.
    - Steroids that are more potent than 1% hydrocortisone should never be used in the diaper area because diapers form an occlusive dressing.
    - Long-term use may lead to skin atrophy, telangiectasis, granuloma gluteale, striae and, possibly, Cushing syndrome.
- Gentian violet
  - Effective, but is extremely messy
  - Rarely if ever indicated
- Oral nystatin
  - Effectiveness in the therapy of candidal diaper rash is uncertain.
  - In a controlled study, recurrence of candidal diaper rash was not decreased significantly.
  - In another controlled trial, oral fluconazole was more effective than nystatin in eliminating oral *Candida* in infants who had oral thrush.
- Oral fluconazole
  - Effective for candidal diaper rash in the absence of thrush
  - Can be used if other therapies have failed

WHEN TO ADMIT

- Systemic illness that cannot be treated safely at home
- Severe illness, such as septicemia

WHEN TO REFER

- The rash has not responded to conventional treatment in several weeks or is worsening.
- The rash is nodular.
- Abuse is suspected.

PREVENTION

- The following measures should prevent many diaper rashes.
  - Frequent diaper changes
  - Cleansing the diaper area promptly
  - Avoidance of plastic or rubber pants

D

- Airing the diaper area
- Careful diaper selection
  - Disposable diapers that contain absorbent gel are associated with the lowest incidence of diaper rashes in otherwise healthy children and those who have atopic dermatitis.
  - Breathable covers are associated with lower counts of *Candida* and reduced occurrence of diaper rash.
  - A recent Cochrane review concluded that not enough evidence from quality randomized controlled trials exists to choose one type of disposable diapers over another.
- Use of barrier creams and ointments

- Breastfeeding
  - Lower levels of enzymes in infant stools, lower urinary pH, and fewer diaper rashes
- Educating caregivers
  - Physician should educate parents about commonly used home remedies that might be harmful.
- Parents who usually use cloth diapers may consider using commercial diapers:
  - That contain absorbent gel materials when their children are at increased risk for diaper rash
  - During travel away from home

Diarrhea and Steatorrhea

DEFINITION

- Diarrhea
  - Increased stool frequency
  - Stools with increased water content
- Steatorrhea
  - Excess fat in the stool

EPIDEMIOLOGY

- Incidence
  - 1 or 2 episodes per year in US children in the first few years of life, on average

MECHANISM

- The pathophysiologic mechanisms for diarrhea fall into 4 basic groups.
  - Osmotic diarrhea
    - The ingestion of a poorly absorbable, osmotically active substance and its presence in the bowel lumen create an osmotic gradient that encourages movement of water into the lumen and subsequently into the stool.
  - Diarrhea resulting from secretion or altered absorption of electrolytes
    - Secretory diarrhea occurs when a physiologic electrolyte secretory process is pathologically stimulated.
      - A net increase in luminal electrolytes and, subsequently, a secondary increase in water occur.
    - Diarrhea also may result from a decrease in active electrolyte absorption in the absence of any change in secretory function.
  - Exudative diarrhea
    - A break in the integrity of the mucosal surface of the intestine can result in water and electrolyte loss, driven by hydrostatic pressure in blood vessels and lymphatics.
  - Diarrhea resulting from abnormal intestinal motility
    - The intestine has a cyclical, orderly pattern of motility.
    - Increased, decreased, or disordered movement can lead to diarrhea.
- Each mechanism has unique clinical characteristics and requires a different therapeutic approach.
  - Frequently, >1 mechanism of diarrhea will be involved in an episode of diarrhea.
  - This variation will be apparent in the evaluation.
- Steatorrhea signifies an excess of fat in the stool and is a symptom of malabsorption.
  - Absorption of fat by young infants varies with the type of fat that is fed and with the maturity of the infant.
    - Normal premature infant: as little as 65–75% of dietary fat
    - Term infants: 90% of dietary fat
    - Neonates absorb vegetable fat much more efficiently than butterfat.
    - Neonates absorb human milk fat best of all.
  - By comparison, older children and adults typically absorb ≥95% of the fat in a normal diet.

HISTORY

- During initial evaluation, establish:
  - Length of illness
  - Characterization of stools
    - Frequency
    - Looseness (watery vs mushy)
    - Presence of gross blood
  - Oral intake
    - Diet
    - Quantity of fluids and solids taken
  - Presence of vomiting
  - Associated symptoms
    - Fever
    - Rash
    - Arthralgia
  - Urine output
    - Frequency
    - Qualitative amount
  - Possible exposure to diarrheal illness

PHYSICAL EXAM

- Determine hydration status.
  - Mild dehydration: 3% in infants and 5% in older children
    - Dry mouth
    - Absence of tears
  - Moderate dehydration: 6% in infants and 10% in older children
    - Dry mouth
    - Absence of tears
    - Sunken eyes
    - Sunken fontanelle
    - Poor skin turgor
  - Severe dehydration: >9% in infants and ≥15% in older children
    - Shock
- Assess body weight.
  - A recorded weight is essential.
    - Can be compared with previous weights
    - Can be used to reevaluate the child's state of hydration during the illness
  - Infants should be weighed at least daily.

■ Assess:
  • Vital signs
  • Alertness
  • In infants, vigor of suck
■ Measurement of stool output
  • If the urine is collected in a urine bag, diapers can be weighed before and after stools to give an accurate measure of stool output.

DIFFERENTIAL DIAGNOSIS

Steatorrhea

■ Cystic fibrosis
■ Congenital pancreatic insufficiency with cyclic neutropenia (Shwachman-Diamond syndrome)
■ Intestinal lymphangiectasia
■ Abetalipoproteinemia
■ Transient steatorrhea following acute enteritis
■ Celiac disease
■ Pancreatic insufficiency, as detected by measurement of stool elastase or serum trypsinogen

Acute diarrhea

Neonates

■ Neonates with acute diarrhea must be considered differently from older infants and children.
  • Lower tolerance to associated fluid shifts
  • Greater likelihood of severe infection or congenital anomaly
■ Signs of necrotizing enterocolitis should raise concern.
  • Gastric retention (frequently bilious)
  • Distention
  • Occult or bright-red blood in the stool
  • More common in premature infants
  • The presence of pneumatosis intestinalis, gas in the portal vein, or free intraperitoneal gas seen on abdominal radiographs supports the diagnosis.
■ Epidemics of diarrhea associated with rotavirus, enteropathogenic *Escherichia coli*, *Salmonelleae*, and other organisms, including *Klebsiella* organisms, have been reported in nurseries.
■ Onset of diarrhea associated with initial feedings
  • Consider congenital digestive defects, especially sugar intolerance.
■ Hirschsprung disease
  • May produce acute diarrhea and enterocolitis in the neonatal period
  • Should be considered, especially in the infant who has not passed meconium in the first 24 hours

■ Bloody diarrhea
  • May result from cow's milk or soy protein intolerance
  • May develop as early as the first few days of life
  • Resolution and exacerbation on removal and reintroduction of cow's milk or soy formula, as well as an atopic family history, are clues to the diagnosis.

Older infants and children

■ Enteric infection
  • *Salmonella* organisms
  • *Yersinia enterocolitica*
  • *Campylobacter, Giardia, Cryptosporidium,* and *Cyclosporaorganisms*
  • *Clostridium difficile* toxin
    – The cause of most cases of pseudomembranous colitis
    – May be associated with chronic childhood diarrhea in the absence of colitis
  • Enterotoxin C *E coli*
    – In older infants and children, associated with watery stools
    – No evidence of mucosal invasion (ie, no high fever or blood in the stool)
  • Rotavirus
  • Adenovirus
■ Parenteral diarrhea
  • Diarrhea in association with extraintestinal infections, most notably otitis media and pyelonephritis
  • The mechanism is obscure.
  • Associated viral enteritis in some cases of otitis media
  • Certain antibiotics, especially ampicillin, have been associated with transient diarrhea.
  • Less common but of greater danger is antibiotic-associated pseudomembranous colitis.
    – May occur acutely or as a more chronic illness lasting 1–2 months
■ Bacteria
  • *Shigella*
    – Patients appear severely ill.
    – May have meningismus or seizures
    – Stools tend to be foul smelling.
    – Hemolytic-uremic syndrome (although *E coli* is the more common cause)
  • *Campylobacter*
    – Evidence of infection before the onset of neurologic symptom in up to 40% of cases of Guillain-Barré syndrome
  • *Yersinia* (less common in the US)

- *E coli*
  - Produces diarrhea by several pathogenic mechanisms
  - Enteroadherent, enteroinvasive, enterohemorrhagic, and enteroaggregative forms can all be associated with blood in the stool.
  - Hemolytic-uremic syndrome results largely from entero-hemorrhagic *E coli* (especially serotype O157:H7).
- Parasites
  - *Entamoeba histolytica*
  - *Giardia lamblia*
- Food-borne spread of organisms or toxins
  - Improperly prepared poultry and eggs are the major source for both campylobacteriosis and salmonellosis.
  - The major source for *E coli* O157:H7 infection is ground beef.
  - Preventive measures include:
    - Safe food-handling practices
    - Pasteurization of in-shell eggs
    - Irradiation of ground meat and raw poultry
  - Explosive diarrhea after ingesting seafood is likely to be due to infection with *Vibrio* species.

Chronic diarrhea

Infants

- Chronic nonspecific diarrhea (toddler's diarrhea, irritable colon of childhood)
- Protracted diarrhea of infancy
  - Poorly understood
  - Previously called *intractable diarrhea of infancy*
  - Probably represents the final pathway for multiple causes
    - Gastrointestinal infections
    - Food intolerances
  - Defined somewhat arbitrarily as occurring in infants younger than 3 months and persisting for longer than 2 weeks
  - In the past, associated with high mortality from irreversible diarrhea and related malnutrition
    - Outcome has improved markedly with the advent of elemental diets and total parenteral nutrition.
  - Now rare and related to more specific causes, such as microvillus inclusion disease
- *C difficile* infection
- Hirschsprung disease
  - Accounts for approximately 25% of intestinal obstructions in newborns
    - Almost invariably fail to pass meconium early
    - Persistent obstipation and recurrent abdominal distention

- Usually have a history of the absence of stools in the first 24 hours of life
- These features may be overlooked, and infants may subsequently have chronic diarrhea.
- The diarrhea is secondary to enterocolitis.
  - The enterocolitis can be a surgical emergency that demands rapid diagnosis and treatment.
- Infants with Hirschsprung disease require decompression colostomy to remove risk of perforation of the colon.
- Cystic fibrosis
  - Although cystic fibrosis is thought of primarily as a respiratory disease, some infants and children have malabsorption and little history of respiratory symptoms.
  - Patients typically have voracious appetites.
  - Diagnosis must be confirmed by sweat electrolyte studies or genetic testing.
- Celiac disease (gluten-sensitive enteropathy)
  - Much more common than previously recognized
  - In infancy, celiac disease becomes apparent 1 to several months after the introduction of gluten-containing products (eg, wheat, rye, barley) into the diet.
  - Diagnosis should be confirmed by small-bowel biopsy.
  - *Giardia* infection can produce small-bowel malabsorption that mimics celiac disease.
- Carbohydrate (monosaccharide or disaccharide) intolerance
  - Usually secondary to other gastrointestinal disorders
  - Extent of symptoms varies in response to quantity of the offending sugar in the diet.
  - Age at presentation varies with the age at which the sugar is introduced into the diet.
- Congenital deficiency of trypsinogen, the zymogen precursor of the pancreatic protease trypsin (very rare)
- Infection
  - Urinary tract infection
  - *Candida*
    - Rare cause of diarrhea in immunocompetent individuals
    - The incidental finding of *Candida* is so common that the clinician must be cautious before identifying it as the cause of diarrhea.
    - A dramatic response to treatment for *Candida* would support this diagnosis.
  - *Salmonella* infection may be associated with persistent diarrhea in infants.
  - *Yersinia enterocolitica* enteritis has been associated with a chronic relapsing diarrhea, although not commonly in the US.
    - The microbiology laboratory must look specifically for this organism, or it will be missed.

- *Campylobacter* enteritis also may have a protracted course.
- Persistence of rotavirus excretion has been identified in immunocompromised individuals but also rarely in immunocompetent children after severe gastroenteritis.

■ Parasites
- *G lamblia*
  - Principal parasitic cause in US
  - May be associated with watery diarrhea and crampy abdominal pain
  - May be epidemic
- *Cryptosporidium*
  - Causes diarrhea in immunocompetent individuals
- *Cyclospora*
- *Blastocystis hominis*
- *Dientamoeba fragili*
  - Amebic dysentery may be indistinguishable from colitis of inflammatory bowel disease and must be considered along with bacterial colitis before inflammatory bowel disease can be diagnosed.

■ Food allergy
- 6–8% of children have dietary protein hypersensitivity during the first 5 years of life.
- Hypersensitivity to cow's milk protein is most common.
- Symptoms resolve by 3 years of age in 85% of children.
- Consider in an infant with chronic diarrhea with any of the following manifestations
  - Occult or gross blood in the stool (colitis)
  - Protein-losing enteropathy
  - Peripheral eosinophilia
  - Other extraintestinal manifestations of allergy (eg, eczema, hives, or asthma)
- Most food allergic reactions include immediate gastrointestinal hypersensitivity.
  - Nausea
  - Abdominal pain
  - Vomiting within 1–2 hours
  - Diarrhea in 2 hours
- Implicated food proteins include:
  - Milk
  - Egg
  - Peanut
  - Soy
  - Cereal
  - Fish
- Eosinophilic (allergic) gastroenteropathy
  - Characterized by infiltration of the stomach and intestine with eosinophils and often a peripheral eosinophilia

- Symptoms include vomiting, abdominal pain, growth failure, and diarrhea (often with gross blood).
  - May respond to elimination diet, but corticosteroid treatment may be necessary
  - Dietary protein enterocolitis is most common in the first year of life.
- Diet-induced proctitis
  - Gross blood in stool
  - Diarrhea in the first few days to months of life
  - Symptoms usually resolve within 72 hours with removal of the offending food allergen.
  - Bloody diarrhea can develop in some infants while they are nursing.
    ■ Resolution when cow's milk is removed from the mother's diet or when a protein hydrolysate formula is substituted for nursing suggests an allergic basis.

■ Short-bowel syndrome
- Chronic malabsorption and diarrhea follow extensive resection of the small intestine.
- Begins most commonly in the newborn period in association with necrotizing enterocolitis or a congenital anomaly involving small intestine (eg, gastroschisis, intestinal atresia, malrotation with secondary midgut volvulus)
- Total parenteral nutrition (TPN) may be required for the first several years of life.

■ Intestinal lymphangiectasia
- Protein-losing enteropathy
- Steatorrhea
- Lymphocytopenia
- Chronic diarrhea
- Sometimes, hypogammaglobulinemia and hypoalbuminemia, usually with peripheral edema
- Primary intestinal lymphangiectasia
  - Appears to be a developmental anomaly of unknown origin
  - Often associated with lymphatic abnormalities of the extremities
- Secondary lymphangiectasia may result from:
  - Chronic volvulus secondary to malrotation with malfixation of the bowel
  - Constrictive pericarditis
  - Tumor
  - Lymphatic malformation
  - Elevated right atrial pressure associated with the Fontan procedure for congenital heart disease
  - Any other factor that leads to obstruction of intestinal lymphatic flow

- The diagnosis is suggested by:
  - History of chronic diarrhea and poor growth
  - Peripheral edema
  - Hypoalbuminemia
  - Hypogammaglobulinemia
  - Lymphocytopenia
- Acrodermatitis enteropathica
  - Rare familial disease
  - Typically appears when breastfed infants are weaned
  - Associated with a zinc deficiency, possibly secondary to malabsorption
  - Nutritional zinc deficiency (eg, TPN without zinc supplementation orcystic fibrosis) may produce a syndrome similar to acrodermatitis enteropathica.
- Factitious diarrhea
  - More common than pediatricians recognize
  - Laxative abuse may be suspected when an infant has persistent diarrhea that does not seem to fit any known pattern.
    - Surreptitious administration of laxative to an infant indicates the caretaker's psychosocial dysfunction.
  - Stool osmolality well below 290 mOsm/L can occur only by surreptitious dilution of stool with water.
  - Factitious diarrhea occurs among teenage girls who take laxatives surreptitiously to lose weight.
- Hormonal
  - Adrenal insufficiency
    - Adrenogenital syndrome
    - Adrenal hemorrhage
  - Hyperthyroidism
  - Vasoactive intestinal polypeptide–secreting tumors of the pancreas (rare)
  - Congenital thyrotoxicosis
  - Ganglioneuroma and ganglioneuroblastoma
    - Associated with chronic secretory diarrhea
    - Usually abdominal but also reported in the mediastinum
    - Catecholamine-secreting, but prostaglandins or vasoactive intestinal polypeptide may be the mediator of the diarrhea
    - Diarrhea usually resolves abruptly when a tumor is found and is completely excised.
- Immunodeficiency states
  - AIDS
    - A major cause of immunodeficiency in childhood
    - Its first manifestation may be diarrhea.

- In addition to the organisms the clinician usually considers in individuals with persistent diarrhea (especially *Giardia*), cytomegalovirus, *Mycobacterium avium-intracellulare, Cryptosporidium parvum, Isospora belli,* and *Enterocytozoon bieneusi* must also be considered.
- Astrovirus, calicivirus, and adenovirus have been associated with diarrhea in HIV-infected individuals and may be more important than rotavirus as agents of AIDS diarrhea.
- HIV may be a primary pathogen in the bowel of these patients as well.
- Lactose intolerance occurs commonly in individuals with AIDS, presumably as a result of injury to small-bowel mucosa.
- Pancreatic insufficiency with steatorrhea also has been noted in these patients.
- Cytomegalovirus
- Inborn disorders of immunity
  - Severe combined immunodeficiency
  - Wiskott-Aldrich syndrome
- Late-onset, variable hypogammaglobulinemia
- Pure T-cell abnormalities (DiGeorge syndrome and other T-cell deficiencies)
- Selective IgA deficiency
  - Patients have an increased risk of celiac disease.
- Chronic parasitic, adenovirus, or rotavirus infection can be seen with immunodeficiencies.
- Chronic granulomatous disease of childhood
  - Perianal fistulas or gastric outlet obstruction may be seen.
  - May initially be mistaken for Crohn disease
- Children who have received organ transplants
  - The clinician must consider the full range of enteric infections associated with immunosuppression.
  - Tacrolimus toxicity
  - Lymphoproliferative disease
- Graft-versus-host disease
  - Common cause of diarrhea in bone marrow transplant recipients
- Autoimmune enteropathy
  - Chronic diarrhea beginning in the first year of life
  - Often associated with failure to thrive
  - Extraintestinal autoimmune disorders (eg, diabetes mellitus, arthritis, thrombocytopenia, hemolytic anemia) are common.
  - Rule out celiac disease, food allergy, and gastrointestinal infection.
  - Response to immunosuppressive therapy confirms the diagnosis.

- Immunodysregulation, polyendocrinopathy, enteropathy, X-linked syndrome (IPEX)
- Idiopathic intestinal pseudoobstruction
  - A group of rare disorders characterized by widespread gastrointestinal dysmotility
  - In early infancy
    - Vomiting and diarrhea
    - Diarrhea may alternate with constipation.
  - In older children
    - More insidious presentation
    - A long history of constipation may precede the onset of diarrhea.
  - Intermittent or constant abdominal distention
  - Roentgenographic findings of bowel dilation with disordered motility
  - Urinary bladder dysfunction often is present.
  - Bacterial overgrowth is an important cause of diarrhea in this disorder.
- Microvillus inclusion disease (rare)
  - Familial enteropathy
  - Present from birth
  - Causes severe intractable secretory diarrhea with malabsorption
  - The most common cause of intractable diarrhea in the neonatal period
  - Several families have been identified with >1 child with this disorder.
- Tufting enteropathy
- Congenital disorders of electrolyte absorption
  - Congenital chloride-losing diarrhea and congenital sodium-secretory diarrhea (very rare)
    - Autosomal-recessive
    - Associated with maternal polyhydramnios
- Congenital disorders of glycosylation
  - Exhibit in the first year of life, often with multisystem dysfunction
  - Hepatic, neurologic, cardiac, and optic manifestations
  - Can be associated with chronic diarrhea or severe protein-losing enteropathy, or both
  - Screening for this diagnosis has been performed with serum transferrin isoelectric focusing.
- Lactase deficiency
- Disaccharide intolerance
- Chronic constipation with overflow diarrhea
- Monosaccharide intolerance
- Eosinophilic (allergic) gastroenteritis

- Postenteritis bile acid malabsorption
- Congenital deficiency of enterokinase
- Neural crest tumor and carcinoid
- Intestinal stricture or blind loop
- Pancreatic insufficiency with neutropenia
- Trypsinogen or enterokinase deficiency
- Congenital chloride-losing diarrhea
- Congenital sodium-secretory diarrhea
- Abetalipoproteinemia
- Intestinal pseudoobstruction
- Ileal bile salt receptor defect

Infant of a drug-addicted mother

- Diarrhea may be a prominent manifestation of neonatal drug abstinence syndrome.
- This diagnosis should be considered in newborns with persistent diarrhea, especially when other symptoms of neonatal drug withdrawal are present.

Older children

- Irritable bowel syndrome
- Inflammatory bowel disease: Crohn disease or ulcerative colitis
- Chronic constipation

Diarrhea that usually occurs without blood in stool

- Viral enteritis C rotavirus
- Orbivirus
- Noroviruses (includes Norwalk virus)
- Other caliciviruses
- Enteric adenovirus
- Astrovirus
- Sapoviruses
- Enterotoxin C *E coli*
- *Klebsiella* organisms
- Cholera
- *Clostridium perfringens*
- *Staphylococcus* organisms
- *Bacillus cereus*
- *Vibrio* species
- Parasitic *Giardia, Cryptosporidium, Cyclospora, Dientamoeba fragilis,* and *Blastocystis hominis* organisms
- Extraintestinal infection C
- Otitis media
- Urinary tract infection
- Antibiotic-induced
- *C difficile* toxin (without pseudomembranous colitis)

Diarrhea that commonly is associated with blood in stool

- *Shigella, Salmonella,* and *Campylobacter* organisms
  - With symptoms of colonic involvement (tenesmus, urgency, and crampy lower abdominal pain)
  - With *C difficile* toxin–associated pseudomembranous colitis
  - Symptoms of dysentery may be less striking with *Salmonella.*
  - When the *Shigella* is an enterotoxin-producing organism, watery diarrhea may precede the onset of dysentery.
- *Yersinia enterocolitica*
- Invasive *E coli*
- Gonococcus (venereal spread)
- Enteroadherent *E coli*
- Enteroaggregative *E coli*
- *Aeromonas hydrophilia*
- *Plesiomonas* shigelloides
- Cytomegalovirus (especially in immunocompromised individuals)
- Amebic dysentery
- *Trichuris trichiura* (whipworm)
- Hemolytic-uremic syndrome (enterohemorrhagic *E coli*— *E coli* O157:H7 and other Shiga toxin-producing *E coli*)
- Henoch-Schönlein purpura
- Pseudomembranous enterocolitis (*C difficile* toxin)
- Ulcerative or granulomatous colitis (acute presentation)
- Necrotizing enterocolitis (neonates)

LABORATORY EVALUATION

Stool evaluation

- Smear for leukocytes to establish presence of colitis
- Polymorphonuclear leukocytes
  - Usually account for at least 60–80% of the cells
  - The presence of only occasional cells is considered a negative finding.
- Leukocytes are found in high numbers, frequently in sheets, in both infectious and noninfectious colitis.
- Absence of leukocytes in grossly bloody diarrheal stool occurs with enterohemorrhagic *E coli* infection but should also direct attention to such entities as intussusception and Meckel diverticulum when these diagnoses seem clinically appropriate.
- Amebic colitis also may not be associated with leukocytes in the stool, although the trophozoites and numerous red blood cells may be visible on a saline wet mount preparation of the stool.
- Invasive bacterial diarrhea frequently is associated with a peripheral blood leukocytosis.

- Culture stool if blood or leukocytes are noted in the stool and the child is severely ill.
- Ova and parasites
- *C difficile* toxin assay
- Occult blood
- Reducing substances
- Urine specific gravity and volume
  - May be deceptive because of poor concentration by the kidneys in the presence of malnutrition and total body hypokalemia
- Complete blood count
- Blood urea nitrogen and serum electrolyte levels if hydration status is in question
- Urinalysis
- If the child is lethargic or has had a seizure
  - Culture for sepsis
  - Blood urea nitrogen and creatinine
  - Serum electrolyte and glucose levels
  - Cerebrospinal fluid
- For a child with chronic diarrhea who has been fed recently, the presence of reducing substance or an acid stool pH (<5.3) suggests carbohydrate malabsorption.
- Stool pH is not a good measure of the effect of diarrhea on total body acid-base balance.
- If stool concentration of sodium and potassium minus chloride is greater than the plasma bicarbonate level, then the infant is losing bicarbonate.
- Leukocytes or gross blood in stool usually indicates colonic inflammation.
- Occult blood in stool suggests loss of blood across the mucosa anywhere in the gastrointestinal tract.
- Hypernatremia indicates more severe dehydration than suggested on physical examination.

IMAGING

- Flat-plate radiograph of the abdomen
  - In Hirschsprung disease, may show a dilated colon with absence of air in the rectum
  - Toxic megacolon may also be seen in infectious colitis or in chronic inflammatory bowel disease in infancy.
  - Air-fluid levels throughout the bowel
    - Common in infants with gastroenteritis
    - Not helpful in defining a cause
- Barium enema under low pressure in the unprepared patient may show the narrow distal segment of rectum.
  - Delayed radiograph (24–48 hours after the barium enema) may show the transition zone of Hirschsprung disease.

DIAGNOSTIC PROCEDURES

- Protracted diarrhea of infancy
  - Small-bowel biopsy specimen may show patchy villous shortening with a decreased villus/crypt ratio and marked inflammation, as well as a damaged surface epithelium.
    - However, the results of the small-bowel biopsy also may be normal.
  - Similarly, a rectal biopsy specimen may show evidence of inflammation, including crypt abscesses, or it may be normal.
  - Presence or absence of these biopsy findings may not correlate with severity of the clinical syndrome.
  - Affected infants are severely malnourished and have low serum protein and hemoglobin levels.
  - Several stools should be collected for culture, examination for parasites, and *C difficile* toxin assay when indicated.
    - Blood and urine cultures should also be ordered.

TREATMENT APPROACH

- Fluid and electrolyte management
  - Commercial oral rehydration solutions (ORS) provide more sodium and lower carbohydrate concentration than traditional clear liquids.
  - Human milk contains low concentrations of sodium (6–7 mEq/L).
  - Supplemental rehydration solution should be used when diarrhea is persistent or severe.
  - Electrolyte content in diarrheal stool varies widely.
    - Highest concentrations occur in secretory diarrheas, such as cholera.
  - Fecal sodium levels
    - Range from 40–100 mEq/L
    - Occasionally as high as 150 mEq/L.
  - In rotavirus diarrhea, fecal sodium concentration typically is 20–40 mEq/L.
- ORS
  - Infants with diarrhea can usually drink large volumes of salty-tasting liquids ad libitum appropriate for the stool output.
  - Episodes of diarrhea in previously healthy, well-nourished children are often mild.
    - Nevertheless, use of ORS to replace diarrheal loss is encouraged in infants.
- Liquids can be offered ad libitum.
  - Smaller volumes per feeding may be tolerated better when diarrhea is associated with vomiting.

- Guidelines for rehydration
  - The most recent World Health Organization recommendation is for a lower osmolarity (245 mOsm/L) solution for rehydration (containing 75 mEq/L sodium and 75 mmol/L glucose).
  - Continuing regular feedings with supplemental ORS is generally tolerated and thought to lead to quicker recovery.
  - Vomiting usually is not a contraindication for oral rehydration.

SPECIFIC TREATMENT

Fluid and electrolyte management of acute diarrhea
General rules

- Oral rehydration therapy with ORS containing glucose-electrolytes is the preferred treatment of fluid and electrolyte loss, except as noted below.
  - These solutions generally contain 25 g/L glucose (or ≥30 g/L rice starch), 45–90 mEq/L sodium, 20–25 mEq/L potassium, and 30 mEq/L bicarbonate.
  - The higher sodium concentration is appropriate for rehydration.
  - The lower concentration is usually adequate for rehydration with mild diarrhea and is appropriate for maintenance.
- Moderate-to-large stool output should be replaced with ORS at 10 mL/kg per stool, if losses cannot be estimated.
- Losses from emesis should be replaced with ORS at 2 mL/kg per episode of emesis or replace estimated losses.
- The use of ORS is labor intensive.
  - If a caregiver is not available to give small amounts of fluid frequently, then intravenous therapy may be necessary.
  - If the child is not severely dehydrated, oral rehydration may be completed at home with close follow-up.
    - Otherwise, intravenous fluids should include replacement of deficit, ongoing losses, and maintenance fluids.
- ORS therapy is effective for hypernatremic dehydration, as well as for hyponatremic and isotonic dehydration.
- Age-appropriate feedings should be continued during acute diarrhea, except as noted below.
  - Formula should be offered full strength.
  - Diet may be better tolerated if fatty foods and foods high in simple sugars (eg, undiluted juices and soft drinks) are avoided.
- Breastfeeding should be continued when possible.
- A lactose-free diet is generally unnecessary.
  - If stools worsen on reintroduction of lactose (human milk, cow's milk, or lactose-containing formula), lactose intolerance should be considered.
  - If stools become acidic and contain reducing substances, lactose intolerance is likely.

No dehydration

- Continue age-appropriate feeding.
- Use ORS only to replace excessive stool output.

Mild-to-moderate dehydration (3–10% of body weight)

- Correct dehydration with 50–100 mL/kg ORS over 3–4 hours.
- Replace continuing losses from stool and emesis with additional ORS. (See section below on special considerations for vomiting.)
- Reevaluate hydration and replacement of losses at least every 1–2 hours.
  - This process may require medical supervision (emergency department, hospital outpatient unit, or physician's office).
- Once dehydration is corrected, begin feeding and continue to correct losses as above.

Severe dehydration (>10%)

- Resuscitate with intravenous or intraosseous normal saline or lactated Ringer's solution 20 mL/kg of body weight over 1 hour.
  - Monitor vital signs closely.
  - Repeat until pulse and state of consciousness return to normal.
  - Larger volumes and shorter periods of administration may be required.
  - Delay giving intravenous potassium until urine output is established.
- Determine serum electrolyte levels.
- Lack of response to initial resuscitation suggests an underlying problem, such as:
  - Septic shock
  - Toxic shock syndrome
  - Myocarditis
  - Myocardiopathy
  - Pericarditis
  - Persistently poor urine output may be a sign of hemolytic-uremic syndrome.
- ORS may be initiated when the child's condition has stabilized and mental status is satisfactory.
  - An intravenous line should be maintained until no longer needed. (See section below on special considerations for vomiting.)
- Feeding may be restarted when rehydration is complete.

Special considerations

- Vomiting
  - Vomiting occurs commonly during acute gastroenteritis.
  - Children who are dehydrated and vomit usually tolerate ORS.
  - Intractable, severe vomiting, unconsciousness, and ileus are contraindications to ORS.
  - ORS should be started at 5 mL every 1–2 minutes.

- Vomiting usually decreases as dehydration improves.
  - Larger amounts can be given at less frequent intervals.
- A nasogastric tube can be used for continuous ORS infusion for persistent vomiting or feeding refusal secondary to mouth ulcers.
  - Do not use in a comatose child or one who has ileus or intestinal obstruction.
- Intravenous fluids should be used if ORS treatment is unsuccessful.
- Refusal to take ORS
  - Children who are not dehydrated may not take ORS because of the salty taste.
    - However, dehydrated children generally take it well.
  - Giving ORS in small amounts at first allows child to become accustomed to the taste.
  - ORS can be frozen in ice-pop form.
- Hyponatremia and hypernatremia must be corrected slowly to prevent complications of the central nervous system.
- Oral solutions are better tolerated and result in fewer central nervous system complications than intravenous solutions in infants with hypernatremia.
- Potassium should not be added to intravenous fluids until adequate urine output is established.

Acute gastroenteritis

- Indications for medications in the treatment of acute gastroenteritis in infants and children are limited.
- There is no apparent rationale for medications that slow gut motility (diphenoxylate, loperamide, andanticholinergics).
- Slowing intestinal transit with drugs may allow greater mucosal contact with pathogens and thereby permit local mucosal invasion.
- Bismuth subsalicylate, which may decrease the duration of diarrhea, has been shown to be a safe adjunct to oral rehydration but is not used routinely.
- Antibiotics are useful in specific situations.
  - *Shigella* dysentery
  - *Yersinia* or *Campylobacter* gastroenteritis
  - Pseudomembranous colitis
  - *Salmonella* infections in infants <6 months
  - *Salmonella* infections in older patients who have enteric fever, typhoid fever, or complications of bacteremia
  - *Campylobacter* gastroenteritis must be identified very early for antibiotics to shorten the illness.
  - For the individual patient, the presence of an *E coli* serotype previously labeled enteropathogenic correlates poorly with the presence of diarrhea and is not alone an indication for antibiotic treatment.
- *Lactobacillus* or other probiotics may be useful to prevent infectious diarrhea but are probably not effective as treatment.

Rotavirus

- The current approach to treatment is to restart the previous full-strength formula and solids early after the onset of diarrhea.
- If diarrhea recurs on the introduction of lactose-containing formula, then the child may have transient lactose intolerance.
  - In this situation, a lactose-free formula should be offered.
  - Transient lactose intolerance usually lasts only ≤1 week but can, at times, persist for months.

Severe dehydration and shock

- Rapid intravenous administration of 10–20 mL/kg of isotonic fluid or colloid is required initially.
- May need to be repeated early

Chronic diarrhea

Infants (general)

- Restrict frequency of feedings, whether liquids or solids, in an effort to decrease stimulation of the gastrocolic reflex.
  - In the toddler, 3 meals and a bedtime snack with nothing by mouth in between
- Restrict volumes of fluids ingested when excessive.
- Avoid excessive intake of juices.
- Reassure parents of the benign nature of this entity.
- High-fat diet may be helpful in some children.
  - Probably is of less importance
- Cholestyramine (2 g by mouth 1–3 times daily) is also effective at times.
  - Duration of use should be restricted because of potential for interference with fat-soluble vitamin absorption.
- This condition is self-limited and typically resolves by 3.5 years of age.
  - The only danger is that well-intentioned parents may restrict oral intake to clear liquids repeatedly in an effort to treat the child; this action may result in poor weight gain.
- Bile acid malabsorption is an occasional sequela of gastroenteritis that can produce persistent, watery diarrhea.
  - Will respond to cholestyramine therapy

Protracted diarrhea of infancy

- Nutritional rehabilitation should begin at once.
  - The best choices are either enteral alimentation with an elemental or modular formula or TPN, peripheral or central.
    - Elemental formulas are composed of predigested components in fixed proportions.
    - Modular formulas allow the clinician to vary the components.

- In many instances, enteral nutrition is tolerated best by the continuous drip method, and recovery may be more rapid when enteral alimentation is used.
  - Nevertheless, unsuccessful attempts at enteral feeding necessitate initiation of TPN in some infants.
- Initial treatment with TPN and a gradually increasing, continuous enteral drip is a good approach to patients who do not tolerate an elemental diet alone.
- Stool output and weight gain may be measured to assess the infant's response.
  - During treatment, further workup as indicated
    - Upper gastrointestinal series with small-bowel radiography
    - Barium enema
    - Small-bowel biopsy
      - If disaccharidase levels are abnormal on small-bowel biopsy, then disaccharides should be avoided.
    - Proctoscopy

Malabsorption syndromes

- Oral enzyme supplements are available for both lactase and sucrase deficiency.
- Congenital deficiency of enterokinase is reversed with very small amounts of pancreatic replacement.

Intestinal lymphangiectasia

- Treatment includes the dietary use of medium-chain triglycerides and avoidance of long-chain fat.
- Protection from and early treatment of infection also are important.

Autoimmune enteropathy

- Immunosuppressive therapy

Irritable bowel syndrome

- Increased fiber in the diet
- Anticholinergics
- Amitriptyline for diarrhea-predominant irritable bowel syndrome

WHEN TO REFER

- Persistent diarrhea when the workup for routine infectious causes is negative
- Steatorrhea
- Diarrhea or steatorrhea (or both) causing weight loss or failure to thrive
- Diarrhea associated with fever, chronic anemia, or abdominal pain without an obvious explanation

WHEN TO ADMIT

- Acute or chronic diarrhea with mild to moderate dehydration that cannot be managed successfully with outpatient rehydration solution

- Dehydration >10% of body weight

- Diarrhea with intractable vomiting

- Severe electrolyte imbalance, including hypernatremic dehydration or serum potassium level <3.0 mEq/L

- Laboratory evidence suggesting hemolytic-uremic syndrome

- Chronic diarrhea or steatorrhea (or both) with persistent signs of malnutrition that is unresolved with outpatient management

FOLLOW-UP

- Patients undergoing rehydration therapy should be monitored frequently and need close follow-up.

COMPLICATIONS

- Chronic diarrhea can lead to failure to thrive.

PREVENTION

- Acute gastroenteritis caused by rotavirus can be prevented by oral rotavirus vaccine during infancy.

D

Disorders of Sexual Development

DEFINITION

- Patients with ambiguous genitalia have *disorders of sexual development* (DSD).
  - Previously termed *intersex conditions*
- The nomenclature used to describe atypical sexual differentiation has changed.
  - Patient advocacy groups were concerned that the terminology was pejorative
- Historically, the term *male pseudohermaphrodite* was used to describe the patient with incompletely masculinized external genitalia possessing XY chromosomes and a typical number of autosomes (also known as *46, XY* karyotype).
  - These conditions are now denoted as *46, XY DSD.*
- The term *female pseudohermaphrodite* was used to describe the patient with *46, XX* karyotype and with masculinized external genitalia.
  - Currently, these disorders are denoted as *46, XX DSD.*
- In some rare cases, a patient has both ovarian and testicular tissue.
  - These patients had been called *true hermaphrodites* in the past.
  - They are now considered to have *ovotesticular DSD.*

EPIDEMIOLOGY

- 46, XX disorders of sexual development
  - Occurs in 1 in 14,000 white infant births
  - Late-onset, or nonclassical, 21-hydroxylase deficiency usually occurs in childhood or the teenage years.
  - Defects in 11ß-hydroxylation are rarer than defects in 21-hydroxylation, occurring in roughly 1 in 100,000 white infant births.
    - Occurs more frequently in children of Middle Eastern descent
- Disorders of gonadal differentiation (sex chromosome disorders of sexual development)
  - Klinefelter syndrome
    - Most common form of primary hypogonadism in males
    - Incidence of 1 in 1000 males
  - Turner syndrome (syndrome of gonadal dysgenesis)
    - Occurs in 1 in 2500 live-born female infants
    - Occurs in a greater percentage of conceived pregnancies
      - ~15% of first-trimester spontaneous abortions have an *XO* karyotype.
    - Cardiac involvement is common.
      - ~10% of patients have coarctation of the aorta leading to hypertension in the upper extremities.
      - An even greater percentage of patients have bicuspid aortic valves, which increases their risk for subacute bacterial endocarditis.

- In some cases, short stature may be the sole phenotypic manifestation of the syndrome.
- 90% of infants with ambiguous genitalia have congenital adrenal hyperplasia.
  - >50% of these patients experience significant sodium loss.
- Rarely, disorders of either testicular or ovarian differentiation may lead to gonadal dysgenesis and thus anomalous sexual development.

ETIOLOGY

- Disorders of sexual development arise from chromosomal, gonadal, or anatomic abnormalities in the pathway of sexual differentiation.
- Incomplete masculinization of a fetus with testes may result from
  - Decreased synthesis or secretion of testosterone or dihydrotestosterone (DHT)
  - Peripheral tissue resistance to androgen action
  - Defective production or action of antimüllerian hormone (AMH)
- *46, XX DSD* may result from abnormally high levels of androgen from either a fetal or exogenous source.

46, XX disorders of sexual development

- ~90% of cases of congenital adrenal hyperplasia (CAH) are caused by 21-hydroxylase deficiency.
- Virilization of a female fetus results from excess androgen exposure from either a fetal or maternal source.
- Timing is important.
  - If the female fetus is exposed to elevated androgen levels after the 8th week of gestation but before the 13th week, the vaginal opening may fuse posteriorly and appear slitlike.
  - Females with CAH will have posterior fusion of the labia and not clitoromegaly, given their high circulating androgen levels between weeks 8 and 12.
  - Exposure to androgen after the 12th week of gestation (eg, exogenous administration to the mother) will result in clitoromegaly without fusion of the labioscrotal folds.
- Fetal sources of androgen excess
  - CAH
    - Overproduction of adrenal androgens by the female fetus may occur in virilizing CAH.
    - Group of disorders in which a biochemical defect in cortisol synthesis leads to hyperplasia of the adrenal gland resulting from compensatory elevation in adrenocorticotropic hormone (ACTH)
    - These disorders are inherited in an autosomal-recessive manner.
    - The degree and timing of virilization, as well as the presence or absence of salt wasting, depend on the specific genetic lesion (see table Differential Diagnosis of Adrenal Enzyme Defects).

Differential Diagnosis of Adrenal Enzyme Defects[a]

Deficiency	Newborn Phenotype	Postnatal Virilization	Other
StAR (also called lipoid congenital adrenal hyperplasia)	Infantile female	–	Salt loss
3ß-Hydroxylase	Ambiguous in *XY* and *XX*	+	Salt loss
17α-Hydroxylase (P450c17)	Infantile female	–	Delayed puberty
11ß-Hydroxylase (P450c11 ß)	Male in *XY*, ambiguous in *XX*	+	Hypertension
21 Hydroxylase (P450c21)	Male in *XY*, ambiguous in *XX*	+	Salt loss
18 Hydroxylase (P450c11B2)	Normal	–	Salt loss

Abbreviations: HT, hypertension; StAR, steroidogenic acute regulatory protein function.
[a] From: Styne D. *Pediatric Endocrinology*. Philadelphia, PA: Lippincott Williams & Wilkins; 2004.

- P450c21 hydroxylase converts 17-hydroxyprogesterone (17-OHP) to II-deoxycortisol.
  - Deficiency in this enzyme leads to extreme elevation in 17-OHP levels.
  - Defects in 21-hydroxylase will lead to low aldosterone and cause renal salt wasting and potassium retention in approximately 50% of patients.
- P450c11 hydroxylase deficiency typically results in:
  - Hypertension in either gender as a result of elevated levels of 11-deoxycorticosterone
  - Virilization of the female fetus as a result of increased adrenal androgen production
- 3ß-Hydroxysteroid-dehydrogenase deficiency causes mineralocorticoid, glucocorticoid, and sex-steroid deficiency.
  - Genetic females may be phenotypically normal or have varying levels of clitoromegaly or labial fusion.
  - Virilization occurs in genetic females because of increased levels of dehydroepiandrosterone (DHEA) and its sulfate (DHEA-S).
  - Peripheral conversion of DHEA to testosterone may cause virilization in females.
  - May be a common cause of late-onset CAH
  - Salt loss, as a result of aldosterone deficiency, occurs to varying degrees.
- Aromatase deficiency
  - In rare cases, deficiency in the enzyme aromatase caused by mutations in the *CYP19* gene may lead to virilization of the female fetus and often of the mother during pregnancy.
  - Aromatase catalyzes the conversion of androgen to estradiol.
  - Deficiency leads to elevated levels of androstenedione and testosterone and low levels of estrogens.

- Maternal or exogenous sources of elevated androgen levels
  - Maternal use of androgenic steroids, such as danazol or certain progesterone compounds, during pregnancy may lead to virilization of the female fetus.
  - Exposure to these compounds during weeks 8–12 of gestation may lead to significant ambiguity.
    - Later exposure may result only in an enlarged clitoris.
  - In rare instances, maternal CAH or a virilizing maternal tumor of ovarian or adrenal origin may lead to masculinization of the fetus.
  - Luteomas of pregnancy have been reported to cause genital ambiguity in the newborn.
    - More commonly, result only in maternal virilization

46, XY disorders of sexual development

- Luteinizing hormone (LH) receptor defects
  - Testosterone secretion is controlled by human chorionic gonadotropin (hCG) early in gestation and LH from the fetal pituitary later in gestation.
  - Failure of hCG or LH to stimulate testosterone production at the critical times is due to mutations in the LH/hCG receptor. This will result in incomplete masculinization of a male fetus.
  - This failure may occur in the situation of Leydig cell agenesis or hypoplasia.
  - Stimulation testing with hCG will result in little or no increase in androgen levels.
  - Basal and stimulated LH levels are typically elevated.
- Androgen biosynthesis defects
  - Enzyme defects in the pathways of testosterone biosynthesis may result in incomplete virilization of the male fetus.
    - Some of the defects affect synthesis of corticosteroids and are thus forms of CAH.

- The initial conversion of cholesterol to delta-5-pregnenolone requires the enzyme P450scc (side chain cleavage), as well as the steroidogenic acute regulatory protein, which transports cholesterol to the inner mitochondrial membrane where P450scc is located.
  - Owing to low testosterone levels, patients with steroidogenic acute regulatory protein or P450scc enzyme deficiencies have:
    - Lipid-laden adrenal glands
    - Adrenal insufficiency
    - Sexual infantilism in males
- 3ß-Hydroxysteroid dehydrogenase deficiency may result in:
  - Mineralocorticoid
  - Glucocorticoid
  - Sex-steroid deficiencies
- 17-Hydroxylase deficiency caused by a defect in the *CPY17* gene results in deficiencies in cortisol and testosterone and thus can result in an incompletely masculinized *46, XY* fetus.
  - Excess of the mineralocorticoid deoxycorticosterone leads to:
    - Hypertension in both sexes (caused by increased salt and water resorption)
    - Hypokalemia
    - Suppression of aldosterone production
- Enzyme defects affecting testosterone biosynthesis without affecting corticosteroid production are described.
  - In a male fetus, 17,20 lyase (also called *17,20 desmolase*) deficiency and 17ß-hydroxysteroid dehydrogenase-3 deficiency will lead to an incompletely masculinized phenotype without any abnormalities related to mineralocorticoid or glucocorticoid effects.
  - Virilization may occur at puberty in either condition.
  - Gynecomastia may occur at puberty in those with 17,20 lyase deficiency.

Defects in androgen action

- Syndrome of complete androgen resistance (androgen insensitivity syndrome or testicular feminization) results from a defect in the androgen receptor.
- Affected individuals are phenotypic females with a *46, XY* karyotype and bilateral testes that secrete elevated levels of testosterone.
- At puberty, LH increases and leads to elevations in testosterone, some of which is converted peripherally to estrogens.
- Incomplete forms of androgen resistance are caused by mutations in the androgen receptor.

5α-reductase-2 deficiency

- Mutations in the *SRD5A2* gene coding for 5α-reductase-2, an enzyme that converts testosterone to dihydrotestosterone, lead to deficiency of DHT.
  - At birth, affected males may have ambiguous genitalia or be phenotypically female as a result of decreased conversion of testosterone to DHT in the sexual skin during the critical times of male genital development.
  - These patients have well-developed wolffian ducts (given that these structures are testosterone and not DHT responsive) and absent müllerian structures (given that AMH is produced from the normal testes).
  - During puberty, virilization occurs with growth of the phallus and testes, probably secondary to expression of a different form of the 5α-reductase enzyme (type 1) in the liver and other tissues at that time, with subsequent increases in circulating DHT levels.

Disorders of gonadal differentiation (ses chromosome disorders of sexual development)

- Turner syndrome (syndrome of gonadal dysgenesis)
  - Classic manifestations of Turner syndrome are linked to the absence of the *SHOX* gene on the X chromosome.
- Other disorders of gonadal development
  - Additional disorders of testicular development may be caused by:
    - Complete *XY* gonadal dysgenesis (Swyer syndrome)
    - Partial gonadal dysgenesis
    - Gonadal regression
  - *Gonadal dysgenesis* is descriptive and bears no etiologic relationship to the syndrome of gonadal dysgenesis or Turner syndrome.
  - 15–20% of these cases are caused by mutations in the *SRY* gene.
  - Partial gonadal dysgenesis in *46, XY* individuals leads to variable amount of testosterone and AMH production.
  - Anorchia must be considered in all phenotypic male patients with bilaterally nonpalpable testes.
  - Gonadal dysgenesis may occur in patients with a *46, XX* karyotype who may have streak gonads and sexual infantilism, but none of the other characteristics of Turner syndrome.
  - Genetic abnormalities, such as translocation of the *SRY* gene, can result in a *46, XX* genotypic patient developing testicular instead of ovarian tissue.

SIGNS AND SYMPTOMS

History

■ Evaluation of an infant with a disorder of sexual differentiation must include a detailed obstetric and family history.

■ The patient's mother should be asked about medication use and symptoms of virilization during pregnancy.

● May occur in aromatase deficiency or with androgen-secreting maternal ovarian or adrenal tumors

■ Family history should not focus solely on genital abnormalities but should include

● History of consanguinity

● Unexplained neonatal deaths, especially in apparently phenotypic males

● Infertility

● Disorders of puberty

■ Many conditions associated with ambiguous genitalia are sporadic or inherited in an autosomal-recessive manner.

Physical examination

■ Initial physical examination should begin with an assessment of the general health of the patient and an evaluation for malformations or dysmorphic features.

■ Physical findings in patients with DSD may range from an apparently normal phenotype to complete ambiguity.

■ Unstable vital signs or hypoglycemia with no apparent cause should raise concern about cortisol deficiency associated with CAH.

■ Typically, shock in patients with CAH does not develop until day 4–5 of life.

■ Patients with ambiguous genitalia may benefit from earlier diagnosis of salt loss and signs of cortisol deficiency than phenotypically normal patients.

■ Midline abnormalities, such as cleft palate, may be associated with hypopituitarism and low gonadotropin levels, leading to microphallus.

■ Increased skin pigmentation caused by elevated levels of ACTH occurs well after the newborn period and thus is not helpful in early diagnosis.

■ Stretched penile length in a term male infant should be >2 cm.

● Average length is ~3.5 cm.

■ A normally formed phallus and scrotum indicate that testosterone production in the critical window of male differentiation was appropriate.

■ Micropenis (penile length <2 cm) often indicates gonadotropin deficiency and may be a sign of hypopituitarism.

● Congenital growth hormone deficiency can also cause microphallus.

● Proper examination technique is critical, as an infant with chordee or a generous suprapubic fat pad may be thought mistakenly to have micropenis.

■ Position of the urethral meatus should be noted.

● Sometimes requires observation of urination

● A urogenital sinus can be mistaken for the urethra.

● Indentation at the end of the glans penis can be mistaken for the penile urethra.

■ The labioscrotal folds should be examined for:

● Degree of fusion

● Symmetry

● Rugosity

● Color

■ Presence or absence of a vaginal opening should be established.

■ Gonads, when palpable bilaterally, are most often testes, but might be ovaries or ovotestes as well.

■ A unilaterally palpable and symmetrical gonad may be a testis, an ovotestis, or an ovary.

■ Sweeping the fingers down the path of the inguinal canal with soap may allow palpation of gonads that might not otherwise be located.

■ If gonads are palpable, then the infant is not a virilized female with CAH, because these patients have nonpalpable gonads (ovaries) that are normally situated in the pelvis.

DIFFERENTIAL DIAGNOSIS

■ Differential diagnosis of the infant born with developmental anomalies of the external genitalia is extensive, given the complicated process of human sexual differentiation.

■ See table Differential Diagnosis of Adrenal Enzyme Defects.

46, XX disorders of sexual development

■ Late-onset, or nonclassical, 21-hydroxylase deficiency begins with excessive or premature acne and sexual hair.

● May be associated with increased growth and bone age advancement

■ 17-Hydroxylase deficiency

● Females are phenotypically normal at birth but will not progress through pubertal changes.

● Primary amenorrhea may be the presenting feature.

■ 3ß-Hydroxysteroid dehydrogenase deficiency

● Genetic females may be phenotypically normal or have varying levels of clitoromegaly or labial fusion.

● Varying degrees of salt loss, as a result of aldosterone deficiency

■ Aromatase deficiency

● Females may exhibit mild virilization in addition to osteopenia and delayed bone age (given the estrogen deficiency).

46, XY disorders of sexual development

- 3ß-Hydroxysteroid dehydrogenase deficiency
  - Affected males may be incompletely masculinized at birth.
  - Often experience salt loss or adrenal crisis in infancy
  - May experience gynecomastia around the time of puberty
  - Elevated levels of enzyme substrates, such as DHEA and delta-5-pregnenolone
- Aromatase deficiency
  - Males with aromatase deficiency will be tall and have delayed bone age and osteoporosis caused by estrogen deficiency.

Defects in androgen action

- Development of female secondary sexual characteristics
  - Pubic and axillary hair is sparse, if present at all.
  - Menarche cannot occur.
- Incomplete forms of androgen resistance have great phenotypic variability.
  - External genitalia may range in appearance from completely ambiguous to mildly hypoplastic male genitalia with a small but normally formed phallus.
  - Hypoplastic wolffian duct structures are typically present.
  - Müllerian derivatives are absent because of production of AMH.
  - At puberty, virilization is usually incomplete.
  - Gynecomastia often becomes apparent.
  - Axillary and pubic hair is normal in amount and distribution.
- External genitalia are phenotypically female, given the inability of the tissue to respond to dihydrotestosterone.
- Müllerian structures, such as the cervix and uterus, are absent or hypoplastic.
  - Production of AMH by the fetal Sertoli cells is normal.
  - The vagina ends in a blind pouch.

5α-reductase-2 deficiency

- Secondary sexual characteristics, such as increased muscle mass and voice deepening

Disorders of gonadal differentiation (sex chromosome disorders of sexual development)

- Klinefelter syndrome
  - Before puberty, patients have:
    - Decreased upper segment to lower segment ratios
    - Small testes
    - Increased incidence of developmental delay (mainly in the areas of speech and language)
    - Behavioral problems
  - Puberty is not usually delayed because Leydig cell function is characteristically less affected than seminiferous tubule function.

- Testosterone is often adequate to stimulate pubertal development.
  - Serum gonadotropin levels increase after the onset of puberty, as the testes become firm and rarely grow >3.5 cm in diameter.
  - After the onset of puberty, histologic changes of seminiferous tubule hyalinization and fibrosis, adenomatous changes of the Leydig cells, and impaired spermatogenesis occur.
  - Gynecomastia is common.
  - Variable degrees of male secondary sexual development
- Turner syndrome (syndrome of gonadal dysgenesis)
  - Turner syndrome (45, XO karyotype) is associated with:
    - Sexual infantilism
    - Short stature
    - Characteristic female phenotype often includes webbing of the neck
  - Patients have streak gonads consisting of fibrous tissue without germ cells.
  - Pubic hair may appear late and is usually sparse.
    - Adrenarche progresses even in the absence of gonadarche.
  - Serum gonadotropin concentrations are extremely high between birth and age 4 years.
    - Decrease toward the normal range in prepubertal patients and then increase again dramatically after age 10 years
  - Because of decreased ovarian secretion of estrogens, puberty does not usually begin spontaneously.
    - Patients have no pubertal growth spurt and reach a mean final height of 143 cm.
    - Growth hormone function is usually normal.
  - Various mosaic forms have been identified, with such karyotypes as 45, X/46, XX, or 45, X/46, XY.
  - These patients may have any phenotype varying from normal female to normal male to manifestations of many of the features of Turner syndrome.
    - Some have apparently normal gonadal function.
    - Others have abnormality of 1 X chromosome, such as a ring X, or other abnormalities, which are out of the scope of this chapter.
- Other disorders of gonadal development
  - In complete gonadal dysgenesis, 46, XY karyotype individuals fail to develop normal testes.
  - Instead, they have:
    - Gonadal streaks
    - Müllerian duct development
    - Wolffian duct regression
    - Female external genitalia
  - Usually associated with ambiguous genitalia and partial development of both the wolffian and müllerian ducts

- In gonadal regression or vanishing testes syndrome, the testes are lost after the external genitalia and internal structures have formed.
- These *46, XY* individuals will be phenotypically male except for absence of both testes.
- Patients may phenotypically resemble those with Klinefelter syndrome.

■ Ovotesticular disorders of sexual development
- Patients with ovotesticular DSD have both ovarian and testicular tissue present.
- The majority of patients have a *46, XX* phenotype, and the remainder have a *46, XY* karyotype or *46, XX/46, XY* chimerism.
- Great phenotypic variability exists in both the internal and external genitalia in these patients.

DIAGNOSTIC APPROACH

■ Diagnostic algorithms for evaluation of infants with indeterminate gender, as well as some infants with relatively subtle genital findings are shown in Figures 25 and 26 on page F8 and F9.

■ In males, even very mild hypospadias can be considered to represent incomplete masculinization.
- Most uncomplicated cases do not need diagnostic evaluation.
- More severe degrees of hypospadias, especially when a testis is not palpable, should raise concern about an identifiable abnormality.
- In an apparently phenotypic female, mild clitoromegaly may represent
  - Severe undervirilization in a genetic male who has undescended testes
  - Masculinization of a female fetus

■ Specific recommendations for which genital findings should elicit concern for a sexual development disorder
- An apparent male born at term with the following characteristics:
  - Bilateral nonpalpable testes
  - Micropenis
  - Perineal hypospadia
  - Single undescended testis with hypospadia of any degree
- An apparent female with the following characteristics:
  - Clitoral hypertrophy of any degree
  - Posterior labial fusion (but not just labial adhesions)
  - Inguinal or labial mass
- All infants with truly ambiguous genitalia and thus indeterminate gender
- Infants with family history of DSD or discordance between apparent gender and a previously obtained prenatal karyotype

- Because the testes do not normally descend until ~34 weeks of gestation, significantly preterm males with nonpalpable testes alone do not necessarily require evaluation.

■ No individual patient should be assumed to have virilizing adrenal hyperplasia.

■ Newborn screening should eliminate cortisol and aldosterone deficiency in diagnostic time.

■ Diagnosis of P450c11 hydroxylase deficiency is usually made after the discovery of elevated levels of 11-deoxycortisol (compound S).

■ Diagnosis of aromatase deficiency is made around the time of puberty.

■ Defects in androgen action are suggested by elevated levels of testosterone.

■ 5α-reductase-2 deficiency
- Ovotesticular disorders of sexual development
  - Ovotesticular DSD should be considered in all patients with DSD.
  - A *46, XX/46, XY* karyotype or a bilobate gonad in the inguinal region or labioscrotal folds should raise suspicion.

LABORATORY FINDINGS

■ Basic serum chemistries should be obtained immediately to evaluate for salt wasting or hyperkalemia associated with CAH.
- Abnormalities may take days to become apparent.

■ Normal electrolyte values in the few days after birth do not exclude salt losing.

■ Karyotype will establish whether the patient is genotypically XX or XY (or other) and should always be performed.
- Results from an urgently ordered karyotype can be available within ~3 days in some cytogenetics laboratories.

■ Endocrine testing generally consists of measurement of:
- 17-OHP
- Testosterone
- DHT
- Androstenedione
- Follicle-stimulating hormone
- LH
- AMH

■ Tests should be performed in a national specialty laboratory with pediatric standards rather than the local laboratory.
- Most local laboratories are unlikely to have pediatric standards or appropriately sensitive techniques.
- On the basis of these results, additional tests may be performed.

■ In the first weeks after birth, measurement of testosterone may reveal the amplitude of the episodic spike of testosterone.

■ After this period, hCG administration will help determine whether functional Leydig cells are present (given that functional cells will secrete testosterone in response to the hCG).

■ Serum testing of the steroid hormones involved in the pathways for cortisol and testosterone is indicated in many cases because the forms of CAH rarer than 21-hydroxylase deficiency will not cause elevations in 17-OHP levels.

■ In some cases, stimulatory testing with ACTH is necessary.

■ Newborn screening for 21-hydroxylase deficiency (but not other forms of CAH) is currently done in 46 states.

- Testing is required but not yet implemented in 3 of the 4 remaining states.

- Results can be returned several days after the specimens are drawn.

- Available within the first week of life, but not always before clinical symptoms develop

- This screening test is most helpful in diagnosing the condition in males who appear normal but are affected.

■ 5α-reductase-2 deficiency

- Laboratory testing reveals abnormally high testosterone/DHT ratios with normal to elevated testosterone and low to undetectable DHT.

■ Confirmatory testing via mutation analysis of the 5α-reductase-2 gene is currently only available as a research tool.

IMAGING

■ Imaging is useful to determine internal anatomy.

■ Ultrasonography

- Determination of the presence and appearance of müllerian structures

  – Lack of müllerian structures implies that AMH was produced from testicular tissue and that the underlying problem is an abnormality of testosterone or DHT synthesis or action.

- Renal problems (eg, in Frasier syndrome)

- Visualization of the adrenal glands

- Visualization of the gonads

  – Magnetic resonance imaging may be required, particularly if the gonads are intraabdominal.

- Defects in androgen action

  – Shown by absence of the corpus and cervix and the presence of testes

TREATMENT APPROACH

■ A team to address the multiple issues surrounding management of patients with DSD may include:

- Endocrinologist

- Urologist and/or pediatric surgeon and/or plastic surgeon

- Gynecologist

- Neonatologist

- Geneticist

- Ethics specialist

- Psychologist or psychiatrist

- Social worker

■ Gender assignment should be avoided after delivery and during evaluation.

- The infant should be referred to using gender-neutral terms such as *your baby* or *the baby* rather than *he* or *she* .

■ Goal is to establish a diagnosis as rapidly as possible.

■ Gender assignment should occur with the participation of the family.

- The family must realize that not all patients with a given abnormality identify themselves in the same way.

- Considerations may need to include cultural practices.

■ Factors to consider include:

- Underlying diagnosis

- Fertility

- Capacity for sexual function

- Appearance of the genitalia

- Surgical options

- Potential hormonal therapies

■ Surgical issues include:

- Preventing patient dissatisfaction with genital reconstruction discordant with his/her gender identity

- Timing and feasibility of surgery

- Potential for malignant degeneration of a gonad in certain disorders of sexual development involving Y chromosome material

  – In the case of a streak gonad of an *XY* cell line, the gonad should be removed at the time of diagnosis.

  – In androgen resistance syndrome, the testis may be brought into the scrotum, where it can be observed for potential cancer.

■ Long-term psychological support is required for the majority of patients with DSD.

- Help should be provided by a mental health professional, preferably experienced in DSD.

- National and local support groups are available for families.

■ *Gender identity* is the personal conception of oneself as male or female.

- It is distinct from sexual orientation and gender role.

- Influences on gender identity include:

  – Hormonal effects (specifically androgen effect on the prenatal brain)

  – Brain structural differences

  – Assigned sex of rearing

  – Sex-steroid effects at the time of puberty

- Some patients who are assigned a particular gender are later dissatisfied.
- Outcome data for gender identity in DSD are relatively sparse; the largest study to date showed that:
  - Genetic males with active prenatal androgen effects should be raised as males.
  - Female infants virilized as a result of CAH should be given a female gender assignment.
- Gender identity outcomes are more difficult to predict in other disorders.

SPECIFIC TREATMENTS

Equivocal cases

- A trial of testosterone injections (eg, 25 mg of testosterone enanthate intramuscularly every month for 3 months) is given in some equivocal cases to assess whether phallus size responds to androgen, eliminating substantial androgen resistance.
  - The effect of this cannot be assessed for several months.

Defects in androgen action

- Removal of the testicular tissue is indicated, given the increased risk of neoplasm after puberty.
  - The timing of removal is controversial.
  - After removal of the testes, estrogen replacement is provided.

5α-reductase-2 deficiency

- Some patients change gender identity from female to male at the time of puberty.

Disorders of gonadal differentiation (sex chromosome disorders of sexual development)

- Turner syndrome (syndrome of gonadal dysgenesis)
  - Growth hormone treatment increases growth rate and adult stature.
  - Estrogen treatment is initiated in adolescence in these patients to allow feminization.

WHEN TO ADMIT

- Patients with significant electrolyte abnormalities, such as hyponatremia and hyperkalemia
- Patients with dehydration
- Patients with hypoglycemia

WHEN TO REFER

- All patients with ambiguity of the external genitalia should be evaluated immediately by an experienced multidisciplinary team that includes a pediatric endocrinologist.
- This process necessitates transfer of the patient to a medical center with a neonatal intensive care unit and the appropriate pediatric subspecialists.

- The patient should never be sent home and referred to subspecialty care as an outpatient.
- Indications for referral include:
  - In a male infant born at term
    - Bilateral nonpalpable testes
    - Micropenis
    - Perineal hypospadias
    - Single undescended testes with hypospadias of any degree
  - In a female infant
    - Clitoral hypertrophy of any degree
    - Posterior labial fusion (not adhesion)
    - Inguinal or labial mass

COMPLICATIONS

- DSD is considered an endocrine emergency.
  - In the majority of cases, the genital findings may be accompanied by:
    - Life-threatening electrolyte abnormalities
    - Hypotension
    - Shock
- The psychological stress to the family cannot be overstated.
- In its most serious form, cortisol and aldosterone deficiency are severe enough to result in:
  - Severe hyponatremia
  - Hyperkalemia
  - Dehydration
  - Hypotension
  - Shock
  - Death
- Male infants die more frequently than female infants.
  - As a result of their visibly normal phenotype at birth, the condition is not suspected.
- Female infants with virilization are usually evaluated quickly.
- Disorders of gonadal differentiation (sex chromosome disorders of sexual development)
  - In Klinefelter syndrome, the risk of breast cancer is increased.

Disseminated Intravascular Coagulation

DEFINITION

- Disseminated intravascular coagulation (DIC) is a pathologic syndrome that arises from a heterogeneous group of medical disorders.
  - Simultaneous activation of both clotting and fibrinolysis, resulting in severe bleeding
  - DIC is always a secondary phenomenon and not a disease entity in its own right.
- Because of variable clinical manifestations and heterogeneity of primary disorders, DIC is also known as:
  - Consumptive coagulopathy
  - Hemorrhagic syndrome
  - Defibrination syndrome
  - Consumptive thrombohemorrhagic disorder

EPIDEMIOLOGY

- Prevalence
  - Seen in ~0.4–1% of hospitalized children
  - Infection is a contributing factor in almost 95% of children with DIC.
  - Multiorgan dysfunction is present in almost 85%.
- Incidence by underlying disease process is unknown.

ETIOLOGY

- The normal physiology of coagulation is disturbed by the simultaneous action of 4 mechanisms.
  - Increased thrombin generation
  - Suppressed physiologic anticoagulant pathways
  - Activation and subsequent impairment of fibrinolysis
  - Activation of the inflammatory pathway
- Steps in DIC
  - During an inciting event (eg, sepsis), monocytes and endothelial cells are injured by toxic substances elaborated during the disease process.
  - They generate tissue factor, which activates the coagulation cascade.
  - Continuous activation of coagulation leads to unregulated or explosive generation of thrombin.
    - Depletes clotting factors and platelets
    - Activates the fibrinolytic system
  - Activation of clotting leads to generalized fibrin deposition and microthrombi formation.
  - Microthrombi deposit in various organs, leading to tissue ischemia and multiorgan failure.
  - Deposition of fibrin in microvasculature leads to mechanical fragmentation of erythrocytes, causing microangiopathic hemolytic anemia.

- Impaired anticoagulant pathway function can amplify thrombin generation and contribute to fibrin formation.
  - Plasma levels of antithrombin are reduced in patients with sepsis, and significant depression of the activated protein C system may occur.
  - Initial hyperfibrinolytic response causes clot lysis, contributing to cutaneous hemorrhages and bleeding into internal organs.

RISK FACTORS

- Sepsis
- Trauma
- Systemic inflammatory syndrome

SIGNS AND SYMPTOMS

- Clinical manifestations are bleeding and/or thrombosis
- Bleeding
  - Typically acute and occurs from multiple sites
  - Bleeding from venipuncture sites and intravascular access sites (intraarterial lines or surgical wounds) is an important early indication of DIC.
  - Mucocutaneous bleeding is common.
    - Petechiae
    - Purpura
    - Epistaxis
    - Gum bleeding
    - Bleeding after tracheal suctioning
    - Gastrointestinal bleeding
    - Hematuria
  - In advanced cases, internal bleeding in the brain, lung, heart, and gastrointestinal system may constitute a medical emergency.
    - Increased intracranial pressure
    - Brain herniation
    - Respiratory compromise
    - Possibly, shock
- Thrombosis
  - Generalized microvascular thrombosis may produce:
    - Purpura fulminans
    - Peripheral acrocyanosis
    - Pregangrenous changes in digits, genitalia, and nose
  - Microvascular thrombosis further contributes to multiorgan failure and hemodynamic instability.

DIFFERENTIAL DIAGNOSIS

- Fulminant hepatic failure
  - Synthesis of coagulation proteins and inhibitors of coagulation is affected.
  - Associated hypersplenism contributes to thrombocytopenia.
  - Bleeding manifestations predominate.
  - The main treatment strategy is supportive care and blood component therapy.
- HELLP (hemolysis, elevated liver function tests, and low platelets) syndrome
  - Commonly associated with pregnancy
  - Clinical and laboratory features are similar to DIC, but hypertension is relatively common.
- Chronic DIC (Trousseau syndrome)
  - Rare in children
  - Commonly associated with certain types of cancer
    - Mucinous adenocarcinomas
    - Ovarian cancer
    - Pancreatic tumors
  - Exhibits as migratory thrombophlebitis, arterial and venous thrombosis, hemorrhagic diathesis, and laboratory values consistent with DIC
  - Treated with long-term anticoagulation with heparin therapy
- Massive transfusion
  - Defined as replacement of >1 blood volume in 24 hours or replacement of 50% of total blood volume within 3 hours
  - Prolonged prothrombin time (PT) and partial thromboplastin time (PTT), decreased fibrinogen level, and thrombocytopenia are seen.
  - Management
    - Bleeding associated with hemostatic failure can be managed first with prompt transfusion with cryoprecipitate and fresh-frozen plasma (FFP).
    - Platelet transfusion may be required if bleeding persists.
    - Recombinant factor VIIa is effective in management of excessive perioperative bleeding.
- Thrombotic thrombocytopenic purpura (TTP)
  - Symptoms
    - Fever
    - Thrombocytopenia
    - Microangiopathic hemolytic anemia
    - Renal failure
    - Neurologic signs

- Tests (PT, activated PTT [aPTT]) and fibrin degradation products are usually normal.
- Treated with plasmapheresis and supplementation of ADAMTS13 protease through FFP infusion
- Hemolytic-uremic syndrome is a triad of microangiopathic hemolytic anemia, thrombocytopenia, and renal insufficiency.
  - Clinically similar to TTP and is often confused with DIC
  - Occurs in children <3 years; acute mortality, 3–5%
  - Laboratory findings include microangiopathic hemolytic anemia (hemoglobin level <10 g/dL) and negative direct antiglobulin (Coombs) test.
  - Presence of schistocytes and helmet cells on a blood smear suggests mechanical trauma.
  - Typical findings accompanying hemolysis
    - Increased indirect bilirubin
    - Decreased haptoglobin
    - Increased lactate dehydrogenase values
    - Thrombocytopenia, approximately 40×10^3 cells/mcL (40×10^9 cells/L)
    - Urinalysis shows hematuria and proteinuria.
    - Elevated blood urea nitrogen and creatinine concentrations
    - Albumin level may be decreased.
  - Management is primarily supportive and includes renal replacement therapy.

DIAGNOSTIC APPROACH

- DIC is a clinical diagnosis based on laboratory results in a patient with a clinical condition known to be associated with DIC (listed below).
- A practical approach is to categorize and understand the clinical presentations of DIC, by:
  - Rate of progression (acute or chronic)
  - Extent (localized or systemic)
  - Chief clinical manifestations (thrombotic or hemorrhagic, with or without progressive organ dysfunction)
- Conditions associated with DIC
  - Sepsis or severe infection
    - Viruses (eg, HIV, cytomegalovirus, varicella, hepatitis)
    - Fungal (eg, *Histoplasma*)
    - Parasitic (eg, malaria)
  - Trauma
    - Polytrauma
    - Neurotrauma
    - Fat embolism
  - Organ failure
    - Severe pancreatitis
    - Liver cell failure

- Cancer
  - Acute promyelocytic leukemia
  - Lymphoproliferative disorders
  - Hemophagocytic lymphohistiocytosis
  - Solid tumors
- Obstetric calamities
  - Dead fetus syndrome
  - Abruptio placentae
  - Amniotic fluid embolism
- Vascular abnormalities
  - Kasabach-Merritt syndrome
  - Large vascular aneurysms
- Immunologic conditions
  - Systemic lupus erythematosus
  - Autoimmune hemolytic anemia
  - Crohn disease
  - Ulcerative colitis
  - Transfusion reactions
  - Transplant rejections
- Miscellaneous
  - Snake bites
  - Recreational drugs
  - Poisoning
  - Burns
  - Massive transfusions

LABORATORY FINDINGS

- Laboratory tests should show evidence of consumptive coagulopathy with activation of the fibrinolytic cascade.
  - Laboratory values change rapidly based on clinical status and may create confusion in patient management.
  - Such changes make diagnosis at an early stage particularly difficult.
- Complete blood cell count may show moderate or severe thrombocytopenia with or without anemia.
  - Thrombocytopenia
    - Present in approximately 50% of patients
    - Suggests consumption of platelets
- Blood smear
  - Presence of fragmented erythrocytes (schistocytes) confirms the diagnosis of microvascular angiopathy.
- Screening tests for extrinsic/intrinsic coagulation cascade
  - PT and aPTT are prolonged in 50–60% of patients.
  - Concentrations of fibrinogen-fibrin degradation products and D-dimers are increased in most patients.

- Prothrombin fragment 1.2 and TAT complexes are the most sensitive tests for diagnosis.
- The International Society for Thrombosis and Hemostasis Scientific Standardization, Subcommittee on DIC, proposed a scoring system based on a 5-step algorithm, assigning a score based on severity of abnormality for each of the following.
  - Platelet count
    - $>100 \times 10^9$ cells/L = 0
    - $<100 \times 10^9$ cells/L = 1
    - $<50 \times 10^9$ cells/L = 2
  - Elevated levels of fibrin-related markers
    - No increase = 0
    - Moderate increase = 2
    - Strong increase = 3
  - Prolonged PT
    - <3 seconds = 0
    - ≥3 seconds but <6 seconds = 1
    - ≥6 seconds = 2
  - Fibrinogen level
    - >1 g/L = 0
    - <1 g/L = 1
  - Total score of 5 or more is considered compatible with DIC.
  - The algorithm should be applied only if an underlying disorder known to be associated with DIC is present.

TREATMENT APPROACH

- The fundamental principal of DIC treatment is the specific and vigorous treatment of the underlying disorder.
  - In some cases, DIC completely resolves within hours after resolution of the underlying condition, eg:
    - Placental abruption
    - Intrauterine fetal death
  - In some cases, supportive measures are required to control DIC until the underlying condition is resolved, eg:
    - Use of all-trans-retinoic acid and chemotherapy for treating acute promyelocytic leukemia and DIC

SPECIFIC TREATMENTS

Blood component treatment

- Low levels of platelets and coagulation factors may increase risk of bleeding.
- Rational therapy in bleeding patients or patients at risk for bleeding who have significant depletion of the following substances is treatment with:
  - FFP
  - Fibrinogen
  - Cryoprecipitate *or*
  - Platelets

- Blood component therapy should not be instituted on the basis of laboratory results alone; it is indicated only if:
  - Active bleeding is present.
  - The patient requires an invasive procedure.
  - The patient is otherwise at risk for bleeding complications.
- Large volumes of plasma may be necessary to correct the coagulation defect.

Anticoagulants

- Heparin or other anticoagulants to inhibit thrombin generation
- However, the beneficial effect of heparin on clinically important outcomes has never been demonstrated.
- Safety is debatable.
- Therapeutic doses of heparin are indicated in:
  - Clinically overt thromboembolism
  - Chronic DIC
  - Extensive fibrin deposition, as seen in purpura fulminans or acral ischemia

Restoration of coagulation pathways

- Recombinant activated protein C has been used in patients with sepsis.
  - Bleeding is the only recognized adverse effect.
  - Maintaining the platelet count above 30×10^9 cells/L is prudent during this therapy.
  - The dose is 24 mcg/kg/hour.

Other agents

- Recombinant factor VIIa is effective for certain situations.
  - Volume overload, persistent bleeding: give 75 mcg/kg every 2 hours
  - To inhibit fibrinolysis in patients with severe hemophilia A with inhibitors: high doses of recombinant factor VIIa (250 mcg/kg every 2–4 hours)

Supportive therapy

- Multiorgan support may be required.
  - Ventilatory support
  - Circulatory resuscitation or inotropic agents
  - Hemodialysis
- Blood product support may be needed if there is evidence of active bleeding.
  - Platelets if platelet count is $<50 \times 10^9$ cells/L.

- FFP if clotting times are prolonged
  - Dose: 15 mL/kg
- Cryoprecipitate to keep fibrinogen level >100 mg/dL
  - Dose: 1-1.5 bags/10 kg
- Packed red blood cell transfusion
  - Dose: 10 mL/kg
- Recombinant VIIa for intractable bleeding or volume overload
  - Dose: 75 mcg/kg every 2 hours
- Recombinant human activated protein C in desperate situations
  - Severe sepsis and multiple organ failure
  - Platelet count must be $>50 \times 10^9$ cells/L.
  - Dose: 24 mcg/kg/hour for 24–72 hours

WHEN TO ADMIT

- Most children with DIC:
  - Are already in the intensive care unit because of their underlying disease *or*
  - Require admission because of the disease complications that can occur

WHEN TO REFER

- All patients with DIC need to be treated with the help of hematologists.
- They also need to be treated in critical care units, where they can be monitored closely.

FOLLOW-UP

- Frequent monitoring is needed.
  - Clinical monitoring
  - Monitoring of PT, aPTT, fibrinogen level, and platelet count up to several times per day
  - Monitoring of D-dimer levels daily is usually adequate.

PROGNOSIS

- Associated comorbid conditions that determine outcome
  - Multiorgan dysfunction
  - Respiratory failure

Dizziness and Vertigo

DEFINITION

- Dizziness and vertigo are very different symptoms with different clinical implications.
- Dizziness
  - Term commonly used by patients to describe subjective symptoms such as faintness, giddiness, light-headedness, or unsteadiness
  - Patients with simple dizziness do not describe the room spinning around them, and do not have nystagmus.
- Vertigo
  - Sensation of rotation, spinning or whirling motion
  - True vertigo is accompanied by nystagmus.

EPIDEMIOLOGY

- The causes of vertigo in children are very different from those in adults.
  - Acute episodic vertigo
    - The type most commonly encountered by pediatricians
    - Usually not accompanied by hearing loss
  - Benign paroxysmal positional vertigo (BPPV)
    - Extremely common in adults but rare in children
  - Benign paroxysmal torticollis of infancy
    - Begins in infancy, and generally resolves spontaneously by 2–3 years of age
  - Benign paroxysmal vertigo of childhood
    - Considered a migraine variant
    - Typically seen in children <5 years
  - Ménière disease
    - Rare in young children
    - Usually occurs after 11 years of age

MECHANISM

- The mechanisms for dizziness and vertigo depend on their underlying etiology.

HISTORY

- Vertigo can be differentiated from dizziness based on 3 elements in the history:
  - Whether the vertigo is acute or chronic
  - Whether episodes are recurrent
  - Whether it is accompanied by hearing loss
- History should ascertain:
  - Description of events
  - Onset/precipitating event (eg, trauma, standing up, change in head position, excessive strain/exertion such as flying, diving, coughing, sneezing)
  - Characterization in patient's words (eg, "room spinning")
  - Context (eg, vision changes, hearing changes, medicine or toxin exposure)
  - Associated events
    - Aura
    - Scintillating scotomas
    - Oral paresthesias
    - Tinnitus
    - Drop attacks
    - Seizures
    - Loss of consciousness
    - Altered mental status
  - Observations from others, including:
    - Eye deviations
    - Nystagmus
    - Unsteady gait or evidence of dysequilibrium
    - Loss of consciousness
  - When young children cannot describe dizziness or vertigo, observers tend to apply these terms to a child who is unsteady while standing
- Medical history/review of systems
  - Hearing loss, recent illnesses, history of trauma or blood loss
  - Medication history
  - Cardiac symptoms, including:
    - Palpitations
    - Chest pain
  - Neurologic symptoms, including:
    - Headache
    - Motion sickness
  - Family history, including:
    - Neurofibromatosis
    - Seizures
    - Migraines
    - Syncope
    - Sudden death
  - In adolescents, as indicated, consider a full HEADSSS assessment
    - **H**ome
    - **E**ducation
    - **A**ctivities
    - **D**rugs
    - **S**exuality

- **S**uicide/Depression
- **S**afety
- Alternatively, at a minimum, the following:
  - Home situation
  - Educational status
  - Sexual history and last menstrual period
  - Stressors

PHYSICAL EXAM

- Vital signs
  - Temperature
  - Heart rate
  - Blood pressure
  - Orthostatic vital signs
  - It may be useful to compare weight with previous weights when assessing hydration status
- Physical exam
  - Mental status
  - Volume status
  - Assess for anemia (eg, pale conjunctiva)
  - Examine head and neck, and pay particular attention to ears.
    - Vesicles may suggest herpes zoster (Ramsay-Hunt syndrome).
    - A distorted tympanic membrane may be seen with otitis media, cholesteatoma, and perilymph fistula.
    - Two useful maneuvers that may help in the diagnosis of perilymph fistula are:
      - Application of pressure to the tragus to occlude the external auditory canal
      - Pneumatic otoscopy
      - Both may induce nystagmus or vertigo and transiently worsen hearing loss.
  - Complete examination of the cardiac and neurologic systems
  - The Dix-Hallpike maneuver (Nylan-Barany test) can help localize the source of nystagmus or vertigo.
    - To provoke an episode, the child is moved rapidly from a sitting to supine position with the head 45 degrees below the edge of the table and turned 45 degrees to 1 side.
    - The ear that is facing the floor when the nystagmus is elicited is the affected side.
  - Nystagmus that resolves when the child fixates on an object is suggestive of a peripheral or vestibular disease.
    - Persistent nystagmus suggests central nervous system disorders.

DIFFERENTIAL DIAGNOSIS

- Most episodes of dizziness and vertigo can be diagnosed by history and physical examination alone.
- See table Differential Diagnoses of Dizziness and Vertigo for suggested diagnoses based on history.

Dizziness

- See Figure 27 on page F10 for suggested evaluation.
- Middle ear disease
  - Middle ear effusion may cause deterioration in vestibular balance and motor function.
  - If not self-limited, symptoms usually resolve after placement of tympanostomy tubes.
- Pre-syncope and syncope related to:
  - Fever
  - Dehydration
  - Orthostatic hypotension
  - Vasovagal episodes
  - Cardiac arrhythmias
- Anemia
  - From acute or chronic blood loss
  - From a congenital condition such as sickle cell disease
- Cardiovascular
  - Any heart disease or arrhythmia that affects cardiac output
  - Hypertension
- Hypoglycemia
- Endocrine cause, such as:
  - Hyperthyroidism
  - Hypothyroidism
  - Addison disease
- Ocular disorders, such as:
  - Refractive errors
  - Astigmatism
  - Amblyopia
  - Strabismus
- Acute cerebellar problems, especially in young children
  - Postviral acute cerebellar ataxia
  - Posterior fossa tumors
- Medications such as:
  - Aminoglycosides
  - Phenytoin
  - Loop diuretics
  - Nonsteroidal antiinflammatory drugs
- Pregnancy
- Anxiety or panic attacks

Differential Diagnoses of Dizziness and Vertigo

Information		Possible Diagnoses
Family History	Neurofibromatosis	– Acoustic neuroma
	Seizure disorder	– Seizure
	Migraine	– Benign paroxysmal torticollis of infancy – Benign paroxysmal vertigo of childhood – Migraine
	Unexplained syncope or sudden cardiac death	– Dysrhythmias
	Anxiety, panic disorders	– Anxiety
Medication History	Aminoglycosides, loop diuretics, phenytoin, nonsteroidal antiinflammatory drugs, chemotherapeutic agents, quinine	– Ototoxicity – Intoxication
Medical History	Acute or chronic blood loss	– Anemia
	Palpitation or chest pain	– Dysrhythmias – Anxiety, panic disorder
	Recent life stressor	– Anxiety
	Last menstrual period	– Pregnancy
	Motion sickness	– Benign paroxysmal vertigo of childhood – Migraine
	Recent upper respiratory infection	– Vestibular neuritis
	Fever	– Otitis media – Labyrinthitis
	Ear trauma, barotrauma	– Perilymph fistula
	Headache	– Migraine – CNS disease
	Head trauma	– Temporal bone fracture – Labyrinth or brain stem concussion – Cerebellar contusion – Perilymph fistula
	Neurologic deficits	– CNS tumor – Multiple sclerosis
	Hearing loss	– Cholesteatoma – Acoustic neuroma – Temporal bone fracture – Perilymph fistula – Labyrinth concussion – Labyrinthitis – Ramsay-Hunt syndrome – Ménière disease
	Triggered by change in head position	– Benign paroxysmal positional vertigo – Perilymph fistula – Vestibular neuritis – Acute labyrinthitis
	Loss of consciousness or altered mental status	– Seizure – Dysrhythmias – Vasovagal syncope – CNS disease – Hypoglycemia

Abbreviation: CNS, central nervous system.

Vertigo

- See Figure 28 on page F11 for suggested evaluation.
- Acute episodic or recurrent vertigo
  - Usually not accompanied by hearing loss
  - Migraine headaches and related syndromes
    - Benign paroxysmal torticollis of infancy is thought to be a migraine variant.
      - Episodes of recurrent head tilt for hours or days, often associated with vomiting, agitation, pallor, and ataxia
    - Benign paroxysmal vertigo of childhood also is considered a migraine variant.
      - Sudden onset of extreme unsteadiness and inability to stand, usually with nystagmus and sometimes with vomiting
      - Episodes last seconds to minutes
      - Family history of migraines; many develop typical migraines later in life.
    - Basilar artery migraines
      - Scintillating scotomas or visual obscuration, oral paresthesias, tinnitus
      - Occasionally *drop attacks* with or without loss of consciousness
      - Often followed by a pounding headache
  - Seizures that are associated with vertigo are followed by an alteration in or loss of consciousness.
  - Perilymph fistula
    - Abnormal connection between inner and middle ear spaces, which may be congenital or acquired by trauma
  - Benign paroxysmal positional vertigo
    - Acute episodes of severe vertigo precipitated by a change in head position
    - Associated with nystagmus, nausea, and vomiting, but not hearing loss
- Acute febrile vertigo
  - Usually associated with severe otitis media leading to labyrinthitis.
    - Patients uncomfortable, with ear pain and severe vertigo
    - Usually with nausea, vomiting, and nystagmus
  - Vestibular neuritis
    - Consider if vertigo preceded by viral illness.
    - Not associated with hearing loss
- Acute vertigo related to head or ear trauma
  - May be associated with hearing loss
  - May create perilymph fistula
- Chronic persistent vertigo
  - Especially if accompanied by neurologic signs
  - Usually is indicative of central nervous system disease

- Menière disease
  - Vertigo
  - Fluctuating hearing loss
  - Pressure in the ear
  - Tinnitus
- Central nervous system tumors
- Acoustic neuromas (seen in neurofibromatosis type II)
- Demyelinating disorders
- Degenerative disorders
- Multiple sclerosis
  - In adolescents, particularly girls, ataxia as part of multiple sclerosis may be described as dizziness.

LABORATORY EVALUATION

- Laboratory testing has a limited role in the evaluation of dizziness and vertigo.
- Evaluation is guided by clinical suspicion, and may include:
  - Blood glucose and chemistries
  - Complete blood count
  - Metabolic panel
  - Thyroid function tests
  - Medication levels
  - In girls, pregnancy testing

IMAGING

- Imaging is guided by clinical suspicion.
  - MRI of brain or other neuroimaging may be helpful.

DIAGNOSTIC PROCEDURES

- Diagnostic procedures may be obtained as guided by clinical suspicion.
  - Electrocardiogram
    - Consider especially if history suggests syncope or pre-syncope.
  - Electroencephalogram
  - Audiometry and electronystagmogram
    - Consider in evaluation of vertigo

TREATMENT APPROACH

- Treatment is aimed at the underlying disease entity.

SPECIFIC TREATMENT

- Vestibular suppressants may be used to relieve the symptoms of vertigo and nausea.
  - Diazepam
  - Meclizine (for children >12 years)
  - Dimenhydrinate

- Orthostatic hypotension with dizziness
  - Hydrate appropriately with IV fluids as needed.
  - Provide reassurance and education.
    - Caution against rising suddenly.
    - Educate about necessity of putting the head lower than the heart when symptoms occur.
- Labyrinthitis
  - Treat with antibiotics
- Migrainous vertigo
  - Treatment is symptomatic and targeted to the treatment of migraines.
- Panic attack or significant stress presenting with dizziness
  - Further history should be obtained, including any suicidal ideation.
  - Referral for counseling should be considered.
- Postinfectious vestibular neuritis
  - Treatment is symptomatic and supportive.
  - Evidence suggests that prednisone may be helpful.

WHEN TO REFER

- Acute ataxia
- A clear history of vertigo, especially with other neurologic signs or after head or barotrauma
- Suspected perilymph fistula or cholesteatoma
- Suspected seizure
- Complicated migraine

WHEN TO ADMIT

- Bacterial or suppurative labyrinthitis
- Head trauma with temporal bone fracture
- Space-occupying lesions
- Potentially life-threatening cardiac dysrhythmias
- Labile hypertension

Down Syndrome

DEFINITION

- Down syndrome (DS) is a constellation of abnormalities caused by triplication or translocation of chromosome 21.

EPIDEMIOLOGY

- Prevalence
  - ~1 in 732 births in the US

ETIOLOGY

- DS is caused by a chromosomal aberration, trisomy 21.
  - Most individuals (95%) with trisomy 21 have 3 free copies of chromosome 21.
  - In approximately 5% of patients, 1 copy of chromosome 21 is translocated to another chromosome, most often chromosome 14 or 21.
  - The DNA sequence of chromosome 21 is now known, and >100 genes have been identified.

RISK FACTORS

- Advanced maternal age
  - The likelihood of bearing a fetus with DS increases with maternal age >35 years.

SIGNS AND SYMPTOMS

Common features

- All characteristic features may or may not be present.
  - Presence of 8 of the features is diagnostic for DS.
    - A child can have fewer characteristics and still have DS.
    - A child can have some of the characteristics and not have DS.
- Head
  - Brachycephaly (flat occiput)
- Eyes
  - Inner epicanthal folds
  - Upward slanting palpebral fissures
- Face
  - Flat appearing, low nasal bridge
  - Small shell-like ears with small or no earlobes
  - Brushfield spots (speckling of the iris)
- Fingers and toes
  - Single-flexion crease on fifth finger and incurving of the fifth finger
  - 4-finger sign (simian crease)
    - Present in 50% of children with DS and 15% without DS
    - Transverse palmar lines
  - Brachydactyly (short fingers)
  - Wide space between the first and second toes

- Heart (commonly, congenital defects)
  - Endocardial cushion defects
  - Ventricular septal defects
- Neck
  - Short
  - Superabundant skin at nape
- Neuromuscular system
  - Absent or diminished Moro reflex
  - Muscular hypotonia
  - Joint hyperflexibility
- Tongue
  - Excessive protrusion

History and physical examination, by age

- Newborn to 1 month of age
  - History
    - Feeding pattern
    - Stooling pattern
  - Physical examination
    - General physical examination
    - Neurologic examination
  - Signs of congenital heart defects:
    - Ocular examination for congenital cataracts
  - Signs of gastrointestinal malformation:
    - Vomiting
    - Weight loss
    - Absence of stools
  - Signs of cardiac malformation:
    - Cyanosis
    - Murmur
    - Irregular heart rate
  - Signs of cataracts:
    - Absent red reflex
- Infants 1–12 months of age
  - History
    - Parents' concerns
    - Otitis media
    - Upper respiratory tract infection
    - Nutritional intake/feeding
  - Physical examination
    - Plot growth on a DS growth chart; consider possibility of celiac disease in infants with DS, failure to thrive, or diarrhea.
    - Cardiac assessment
    - Neurologic examination

- Ocular examination: strabismus, cataract, nystagmus
- Tympanic membranes: otitis media, upper respiratory tract infection
- Audiologic screening
- Administer age-appropriate immunizations.

■ Children 1–5 years of age
  ● History
    - Parental concerns about the child's behavior and school program.
    - Symptoms of a vision or hearing disorder
    - Snoring, restless sleep, and sleeping positions
    - The primary care physician should ask about the child's snacks and the amount of time the child spends watching television.
  ● Physical examination
    - Height and weight plotted on a DS growth chart
    - Obesity may become a problem at ~5 years of age.
    - Ears should be examined for impacted cerumen that can cause moderate hearing loss.
    - Eye examination should be performed to detect cataracts.
    - Vision screening should be performed yearly or more often, if indicated.

■ Children 5–13 years of age
  ● History
    - Parental concerns about the child's behavior and school program
    - Symptoms of a vision or hearing disorder
    - Snoring, restless sleep, sleeping positions, sleep apnea
    - Skin problems, such as dryness
  ● Physical examination
    - Height and weight plotted on a DS growth chart
    - Body mass index/obesity
    - Neurologic examination
    - Vision screening
    - Hearing screening

■ Adolescents 13–21 years of age
  ● History
    - Answer the parents' questions.
    - Education or behavioral problems
    - Ensure that the child is up to date on immunizations.
  ● Physical examination
    - Height and weight plotted on a DS growth chart
    - Body mass index/obesity
    - Gynecologic examination (consider referral)
    - Neurologic examination for long-tract signs
    - Vision screening
    - Hearing screening

■ Young adults
  ● History
    - Evaluate the family's concerns.
    - Ask about symptoms of dementia and mental disorders.
  ● Physical examination
    - Gynecologic examination, Papanicolaou smear
    - Testicular and breast examination
    - Neurologic examination

DIAGNOSTIC APPROACH

■ Accurate and prompt diagnosis can often be accomplished at the bedside.
  ● When 8 of the many characteristics commonly associated with DS are present, the diagnosis is relatively simple.
  ● 1 or 2 physical findings are not diagnostic of DS.
■ Chromosomal analysis is required to confirm diagnosis.
  ● Every newborn clinically suspected of having DS requires chromosomal analysis.
  ● Confirmation of DS diagnosis by chromosomal analysis helps the parents accept the clinical diagnosis.
    - Physicians should share the suspected diagnosis of DS with the family as soon as possible.

LABORATORY FINDINGS

■ Chromosomal analysis
  ● Required to confirm DS diagnosis
  ● Complements a detailed family history
  ● Forms the basis of genetic counseling of the parents on the risk of recurrence
■ Thyroid screening
  ● Newborn and annually thereafter
    - Serum-free thyroxine
    - Free triiodothyronine
    - Thyroid-stimulating hormone
■ Serum immunoglobulin A antigliadin antibody and anti–tissue transglutaminase antibody levels
  ● Screen for celiac disease.
■ Complete blood count
  ● Newborns
    - Blast cells in the peripheral blood smear and normal neutrophil and hemoglobin levels indicate transient leukemia.
    - All newborns with transient leukemia need follow-up with the hematologist every 3 months for review of the peripheral blood smear.
  ● Adolescents

IMAGING

- Cervical spine radiography (flexion and extension)
  - Should be interpreted by an experienced radiologist
  - Indicated in:
    - Children with signs of atlantoaxial instability
    - Patients who wish to participate in contact sports in school or Special Olympics
  - The natural history of atlantoaxial instability and subluxation remains poorly understood.
    - Whether only 1 set of cervical spine radiographs is necessary or whether these films need to be repeated is unclear.
    - Cervical spine radiographs may be unreliable in identifying all children at risk.
- Cervical spine computed tomography
  - Child with normal radiographs but abnormal neurologic examination results
- Echocardiography
  - To check for mitral valve prolapse in young adults
- Pelvic ultrasonography
  - Gynecologic examination by age 17 years
- Mammography
  - Baseline at age 35 years
  - Follow-up is based on the physical examination and family history.

TREATMENT APPROACH

- Early detection and correction of medical problems (preventive management)
  - The usual preventive interventions and anticipatory guidance given to other children and families
  - Additional evaluation and close monitoring of problems specific to children with DS
    - Growth: failure to thrive and growth retardation
    - Dental: malaligned teeth and periodontal disease
    - Ophthalmologic: refractive errors, strabismus, myopia, and cataracts
    - Otologic: chronicotitis media, and hearing loss
    - Respiratory: obstructive sleep apnea
    - Cardiac: congenital heart defects
    - Endocrine: hypothyroidism and diabetes mellitus
    - Gastrointestinal: constipation and congenital intestinal obstruction
    - Neurologic: delayed development, intellectual disability, seizures, and depression
    - Immune: immunologic disorders and leukemia

SPECIFIC TREATMENTS

Newborn to 1 month of age

- Provide a gentle and hopeful delivery of diagnosis to the family.
  - Avoid discussion over the telephone.
    - Inform both parents together.
    - Meet in a quiet and private place where the physician and parents will not be interrupted.
  - Provide current information to the family.
    - Be hopeful.
    - Provide name and telephone number of a local DS support group (National Down Syndrome Congress)
  - Discuss future expectations briefly.
    - Discuss potential medical problems.
    - Point out that many children who have DS are healthy and participate in most of the usual childhood activities.
    - Inform that the average life span of those who have DS is 55 years.
    - Discuss the plan to identify and manage medical problems.
  - Allow time for the parents to respond, voice concerns, raise questions, and express feelings:
    - Anger
    - Guilt
    - Sorrow
  - Provide written information about DS.
    - Parents find that having something to read after their discussion with the physician is useful.
    - Most information >5 years old should be considered outdated.
  - Suggest consultation with a geneticist.
    - Reinforces the discussion provided by the pediatrician
    - Provides information about additional resources, such as literature and support groups
    - Educates the family about prenatal detection and the risk of recurrence
  - Arrange for a follow-up meeting with the family.
    - Give time to begin adjusting to the new information and to formulate questions.
    - Offer to meet extended family members to answer questions.
- Adoption
  - Most families accept a child born with DS.
  - Some families have greater initial difficulty and require more extended counseling.
    - In rare cases, a family cannot accept a child with DS.
    - In this event, adoption should be discussed.

- In many instances, families are waiting to adopt children with DS.
  - Call the Down Syndrome Adoption Exchange (914/428-1236) for more information.
- Oral motor problems
  - Mild feeding problems include weak sucking, fatigue during feeding, and uncoordinated breathing.
    - Usually resolve in 2–3 weeks
  - Measures parents can take to help simplify feeding
    - Make sure the child is fully awake when fed at night.
    - Clear mucus from the baby's nose before feeding so that breathing will be easier.
    - Support the infant's chin during feeding.
  - The primary care physician should monitor the weight and caloric intake carefully.
    - If feeding problems are particularly severe or do not resolve with these interventions, consider referral to an oral motor (swallowing) specialist.
- Breastfeeding problems
  - Most infants who have DS can breastfeed successfully.
  - If breastfeeding appears to be going poorly:
    - Primary care physician should arrange a visit to review the infant's weight gain and the mother's breastfeeding technique.
  - For particularly severe problems:
    - Referral to a lactation specialist may help.
    - Bottle feeding may be needed.
- Constipation
  - Stool softeners
  - If an infant has constipation despite adequate intake and does not respond to stool softeners:
    - Evaluation for Hirschsprung disease should be considered.

Infants 1–12 months of age

- The parents' anxiety and questions decrease with time.
  - For the initial few months, they need to be able to depend on the primary care physician to be available.
    - Set aside a period each week, perhaps half a day, for consultation and family education.
    - Keep this time free of acute-care office visits.
  - Consider reliance on a nurse practitioner to help meet extra educational and health care needs.
  - Set up a medical record with special sections for:
    - Problems
    - Procedures (date, site, and result of all special medical procedures completed)
    - Consultants involved in the child's care (with emergency telephone numbers)

- An updated, 1-page medical summary to be used for emergency admissions and consultations
- A flowchart of significant laboratory data and medications
- Provide special check-out instructions for covering or on-call physicians.
  - Especially those outside the office and not familiar with the patient
- Discuss with the family:
  - Enrollment in an early education program
  - Supplemental Security Income (SSI) and other government programs that help families financially with the extra costs of a special needs child
- Tongue protrusion
  - Factors that produce tongue protrusion include a small oral cavity and mouth breathing.
    - Behavior management techniques can be used.
    - Oromotor exercises may alleviate tongue protrusion.
- Controversial therapies
  - Discuss whether the family is contemplating:
    - Tongue resection
      - Improvement in speech has not been observed.
      - Primary care physician should try to inform families about risks and benefits of any surgical procedures.
    - Megavitamin supplements
      - Preparations high in vitamins and minerals initially seemed to result in increased intelligence scores.
      - However, no studies to date have replicated these results.
      - Because side effects from megavitamin regimens have been reported, unproved megavitamin and mineral therapies should be avoided.
      - Routine nutritional screening should be performed at health assessment visits and vitamins prescribed when warranted by standard criteria.

Children 1–5 years of age

- Behavioral problems
  - Many children who have DS do not fit the stereotype of being placid or compliant.
    - Parents may not volunteer information about obstinacy or noncompliance.
  - When the child seems to have a behavioral disorder:
    - A thorough history should be obtained.
    - Parents should be asked about changes in the environment or their expectations.
    - A complete physical examination should be performed.
    - Laboratory tests should be obtained, if warranted, to identify medical problems that may lead to behavior disorders.

– A trial of behavior management should be initiated for mild problems.

■ Learning problems

● School learning problems require further evaluation.

– They often come to the physician's attention when children with DS are placed in mainstream classes.

● Review the current individual educational program.

– Ensure that appropriate developmental testing has been completed.

– Parents should have had an opportunity to provide information in the individual educational program process.

● History should be reviewed thoroughly.

– Ensure that the parents' and teachers' expectations are appropriate for the child's developmental age.

● Medical problems that can affect learning and behavior should be identified.

Children 5–13 years of age

■ Obesity

● Preventive approach:

– Monitor the child's diet.

– Promote regular exercise.

– Screen yearly for hypothyroidism.

■ Hyperactivity

● Parents or teachers may bring up symptoms of hyperactivity.

– Thoroughly assess to identify medical problems associated with inattention.

– Behavior-management techniques and classroom adaptations should be tried before resorting to medications.

Adolescents 13–21 years of age

■ Physical, emotional, and educational needs in adolescents with DS require a special approach.

● During the annual health assessment visit, the primary care physician should discuss with the family the child's:

– Health

– Educational program

– Behavioral problems

– Prevocational experience and training

■ Sexuality

● Many adolescents who have DS receive some formal education about sexuality in school.

– Primary care physicians should ensure that this education is complete and discuss this with the family.

● When a young woman who has DS becomes pregnant, the father of the woman's child is usually a close relative.

– Families need to know about birth control options and routine procedures for safeguarding their adolescent.

● Families usually have many questions about a teenager's sexuality but often do not ask the primary care physician about them.

– Sexual interests of their children

– Level at which they experience sexual feelings

– How to deal with masturbation

– How to answer questions about wanting to give birth

– Management of menstrual hygiene

● Sterility

– Although young men who have DS are usually sterile, a small number of girls and women have given birth to children.

– Families may ask about sterilization procedures for both young men and young women.

– In most states, performing sterilization procedures is difficult because of the difficulty in obtaining consent.

■ Smoking and drug abuse

● Adolescents who have DS need education about smoking and drug abuse.

● If at all possible, they should:

– Have well-balanced diets

– Continue regular exercise

– Be involved in appropriate social activities

■ Prevocational experiences

● When possible, adolescents with DS should also have opportunities for prevocational experiences, such as volunteer work that can provide adequate supervision.

● The school curriculum should make the transition to planning for a life vocation.

– Psychoeducational testing is often helpful to determine the individual's aptitudes and job interests.

■ Behavioral problems

● Assess any changes or regression in self-care skills.

– Family may report important information about withdrawal or loss of interest in recreational activities.

● Some emotional disorders are characterized by:

– Excessive anger

– Frustration

– Aggressive behaviors

● Other signs of a possible disorder

– Self-injurious behavior (hitting or biting themselves)

– Crying spells

– Refusal to participate in self-care activities

● When evaluating a patient who has a sudden increase in behavioral problems:

– The primary care physician should look for underlying medical problems.

D

– Changes in vision or hearing may result in withdrawal or temper tantrums.

– Hypothyroidism can cause lethargy and lack of interest in activities.

– Alzheimer disease may (rarely) appear in adolescence.

– Psychological testing that includes an assessment of self-care skills should be performed.

■ Community living arrangements

● The primary care physician needs to discuss with the family a long-term plan for the adolescent's living arrangements.

● Most communities have a spectrum of community living facilities, for example:

– Small, heavily supervised group homes

– Apartments that have minimal supervision

● Families need to make living arrangements 2 or 3 years before they anticipate need.

– Most community facilities will have waiting lists.

Young adults

■ Primary care physicians often continue to monitor and treat adolescents into the early adult years.

● Families are often attached to the primary care physician and ask about continuing care.

● This discussion can center on aspects of preventive medical care for the young adult.

■ Adults with DS require the same annual health assessment as any other adults.

● Limited expressive speech may not allow accurate history.

● Medical problems may be seen as behavioral problems.

■ Immunizations should be reviewed and kept current.

● Hepatitis B and pneumococcal vaccines should be considered for adults at special risk.

■ Vocational training

● Young adults should be enrolled in vocational training to enhance skills for either a community job or workshop placement.

– The program should include some basic educational activities for continued improvement in skills.

■ Community living arrangements

● The primary care physician should ask about:

– Family or community living arrangements

– Future living arrangements if the adult with DS continues to live at home

– Plans for guardianship and wills and trusts

● Young adults should be guided to:

– Voter registration

– Selective Service System (men)

■ Health education

● Drug and alcohol abuse

● Smoking

● Sex

WHEN TO REFER

■ Newborn to 1 month of age

● All infants

– Cardiology consultation

– Genetics consultation

● Leukocoria/lens opacity

– Ophthalmology assessment

● Transient myeloproliferative disease

– Hematology consultation every 3 months

● Severe constipation

– Pediatric gastroenterology evaluation

● Families who have serious difficulty adapting to their newborn

– A family counselor may be needed.

■ Infants 1–12 months of age

● Severe constipation not responding to dietary control

– Pediatric gastroenterology evaluation

● Chronic middle ear effusions

– Consultation with an ear, nose, and throat specialist

● Ophthalmology consultation

– At 6 months

● All infants should be referred to an early intervention program.

■ Children 1–5 years of age

● Infantile spasms

– Immediate referral to a pediatric neurologist

● Neck pain, loss of bladder and bowel control, and gait disturbance

– Immediate pediatric neurosurgery consultation

● Disruptive behavior or excessive short attention span

– Evaluation by developmental or behavioral specialists

● Chronic middle ear effusions and symptoms of obstructive sleep apnea

– Require a consultation with an ear, nose, and throat specialist

● Ophthalmology evaluation

– Every 2 years from 12 months of age

● Behavior specialist

– Severe behavioral problems

– Persistent behavioral problems with no medical cause

- Children 5–13 years of age
  - Audiology evaluation
    - Annual
  - Ophthalmology evaluation
    - Annual
  - Symptoms of obstructive sleep apnea
    - Require a consultation with an ear, nose, and throat specialist.
  - Normal cervical spine radiograph results but abnormal neurologic examination results
    - Referral to a neurosurgeon or orthopedic physician experienced with DS
- Adolescents and young adults
  - Gynecologic evaluation by age 17 years
    - Pelvic examination
    - Birth control options
    - Seek a specialist with experience in evaluating women with developmental disabilities.
  - Sexual issues
    - Referral to community resources should be considered if the primary care physician's expertise or the school curriculum needs to be complemented.
  - Neurologic evaluation
    - Teenagers who have lost skills with no obvious medical explanation
  - Financial and custody issues
    - The Arc (formerly known as The Association for Retarded Citizens) has local branches around the country.
  - Psychiatric evaluation
    - Recommended for all adolescents with severe behavioral disturbances
  - Ophthalmologic evaluation
    - Annual
  - Audiologic evaluation
    - Annual

FOLLOW-UP

Newborn to 1 month of age

- The primary care physician should arrange a visit with the parents and child 1–2 weeks after discharge.
  - This meeting provides time for further discussion with the family and for a follow-up medical assessment.
  - Karyotype results may not be available at discharge from the hospital.
    - Recurrence risk of DS in future pregnancies and prenatal diagnosis should be discussed when the karyotype is available.

Infants 1–12 months of age

- Psychosocial concerns—habilitation
  - Refer the parents to an infant education program.
  - Continue educating the family about DS, and review risk of DS in future pregnancies.

Children 1–5 years of age

- Eye examination every 2 years
- Hearing test every 6 months till age 3 years, annually thereafter
- Dental examination
  - Twice a year
  - Children with DS have higher risk of periodontal disease.
- Psychosocial concerns—habilitation
  - Discuss behavioral management and sibling adjustments.
  - Review:
    - The child's education program
    - Dietary habits and physical activity pattern
    - Risk of DS recurrence and prenatal diagnosis

Children 5–13 years of age

- Eye examination every year
- Hearing test every year
- Dental examination
  - Twice a year
  - Children with DS have higher risk of periodontal disease.
- Psychosocial concerns—habilitation
  - Review:
    - Dietary habits and physical activity pattern
    - The child's education program
    - Psychosexual development, menstrual hygiene, and fertility
    - Review risk of DS in future pregnancies
  - Discuss:
    - Respite and long-term care plans, guardianship, and financial arrangements with the family
    - Age-appropriate social skills, self-help skills, and the development of a sense of responsibility
- If the child has normal neurologic examination and cervical radiographs are normal, he or she may participate in all sports.

Adolescents 13–21 years of age

- Eye examination every year
- Hearing test every year
- Dental examination
  - Twice a year
  - Children with DS have higher risk of periodontal disease.

- Psychosocial concerns—habilitation
  - Check to see whether the patient is obtaining vocational training.
  - Have the patient continue speech therapy.
- Family concerns
  - Ask about community living plans for the patient.
  - Discuss:
    - Enrolling the patient in Medicaid and SSI if eligible
    - Sexuality, including preventing pregnancy
  - Help the parents teach their child to avoid smoking and abusing drugs.
  - Facilitate transfer to adult medical care.

Young adults

- Cardiologic examination
- Eye examination every 2 years
- Hearing test every 2 years
- Dental examination
  - Twice a year
  - Children with DS have higher risk of periodontal disease.
- Cervical spine examination at age 30 years
- Psychosocial concerns—habilitation
  - Inquire about the patient's exercise and recreational activities.
  - Urge the patient and family to continue with vocational and adult education programs to allow better job placement.
  - When appropriate, check to see whether patient has registered to vote and (for young men) has registered with the Selective Service System.
- Family issues
  - Remind the family to update their estate planning and wills.
  - Evaluate the patient for community living if not already in this type of setting.
  - Check on patient's eligibility for Medicaid and SSI.

Atlantoaxial instability

- Excess mobility of the atlantoaxial joint without neurologic complications
- If atlantoodontoid distance is >5 mm and neurologic examination results are normal:
  - Patient should be monitored yearly with repeated neurologic examinations.
  - Sports that place the child's neck in extreme extension (tumbling, gymnastics, diving) should be avoided.
- Careful monitoring during intubation for induction of anesthesia is needed if surgery is performed.

COMPLICATIONS

- Acquired hypothyroidism
  - 9–35% of individuals with DS
- Atlantoaxial instability
  - ~15% of children with DS
- Atlantoaxial subluxation
  - Backward movement of the odontoid process of the axis, compressing the spinal cord and resulting in the signs and symptoms of cord compression
    - Neck pain
    - Head tilt
    - Progressive weakness and loss of bladder or bowel control
  - Neurologic examination reveals:
    - Long-tract signs, such as increased deep-tendon reflexes in the lower extremities
    - Positive Babinski sign
    - Ankle clonus
  - Although rare, it is life threatening.
- Cardiac malformations
  - Increased incidence
- Cataracts
  - Absent red reflex
- Congenital hearing loss
  - 15% of children with DS
- Gastrointestinal problems
  - Celiac disease
  - Gastrointestinal malformations
  - Duodenal atresia
    - 2–15% of cases
- Infection
  - Increased susceptibility
- Leukemia
  - Increased incidence
- Mitral valve prolapse
  - Develops in ~50% of adults with DS
- Obesity
  - Increased risk in those with:
    - Greater hypotonia
    - Shorter stature
    - Preschool-age children
    - Adolescents
- Transient leukemia (transient myeloproliferative disease)
  - 10% of newborns with DS

PROGNOSIS

- Newborn to 12 months of age
  - The first year of life holds the highest probability of death for children with DS who have an additional anomaly.
    - ~78% survive with an additional anomaly.
    - 96% survive without an anomaly.
- Cardiac malformation
  - Survival of children with cardiac malformations has improved.
    - Only 8–9% mortality in children with DS and heart defects is now reported.
- Leukemia
  - As a cause of death, <10% of cases
  - Transient leukemia (transient myeloproliferative disease)
    - 10% of newborns with DS
    - Most infants with transient leukemia go into spontaneous remission and recover by 3 months of age.
    - 20% develop life-threatening complications.
    - Of those who recover, ~20% develop acute megakaryocytic leukemia (a type of acute myelogenous leukemia) in the first 4 years of life.
      - Cure rate for acute megakaryocytic leukemia is >80%.
- Children 1–5 years of age
  - >50% have serious medical disorders.
  - 2% of children with DS have Hirschsprung disease.
- Life expectancy
  - Average life expectancy in adults with DS has increased into the middle 50s.
  - Some are alive in their 60s.

PREVENTION

- Recent advances have improved noninvasive techniques for identifying fetuses with DS.
  - Regardless of maternal age, this screening should to be offered to all pregnant women.
- Screening using a combination of maternal age and multiple serum markers
  - α-Fetoprotein, unconjugated estriol, human chorionic gonadotropin, and dimeric inhibin A in the second trimester of pregnancy
    - Detects 75% of fetuses with DS
    - False-positive rate of 5%
- Screening during the first trimester at 10–14 weeks using:
  - Fetal nuchal translucency, maternal serum free ß-human chorionic gonadotropin and pregnancy-associated plasma protein-A
    - Improves detection rate to 89%
    - False-positive rate of 5%
  - First-trimester screening may become the standard method of screening in the future.
- Risk of DS in subsequent pregnancies
  - For nondisjunction trisomy 21, ~1 in 100 for women <35 years
    - Age-related for older women
  - A higher recurrence risk may exist for the translocation types of DS if the mother has a balanced translocation.

Drowning and Near Drowning

DEFINITION

- Drowning is death caused by suffocation within 24 hours after submersion in a liquid medium.
  - It is an important cause of accidental death among children and adolescents.
- Near drowning is an event that a person has survived through resuscitative efforts.

EPIDEMIOLOGY

- Incidence
  - In the US, approximately 1400 drowning deaths occur each year in patients <19 years.
  - For every submersion injury resulting in death within 24 hours, 4 hospital admissions and 14 emergency department (ED) visits occur.
- Groups most at risk
  - Children <5 years
  - Boys age 5–19 years
- Age
  - Toddlers are more likely than older children to experience submersion injuries.
  - Older children and adolescents may experience submersion injuries during a diving accident.
  - Adolescent drowning incidents are often associated with drinking alcohol or using drugs.
- Bathtub submersion injuries
  - More common in children <1 year who are left in the care of an older sibling or who are without adult supervision
  - May be associated with scald burns from hot water or child abuse

ETIOLOGY

- Events in submersion injury
  - The child initially panics, then holds breath and loses consciousness.
  - The child may lose cough and gag reflexes, then aspirate large amounts of water.
  - This produces anoxia, resulting in decreased oxygen delivery to the tissues.
  - The heart rhythm becomes abnormal, with fibrillation and finally asystole.
  - The child's core temperature drops.
- The type of fluid aspirated affects circulatory volume and electrolyte balance.
  - Fresh water
    - Hypotonic
    - Rapidly absorbed across the alveoli
    - May result in increased blood volume, hemodilution, reduced serum electrolytes, and hemolysis
  - Salt water produces:
    - Hemoconcentration
    - Decreased blood volume
    - Elevated serum electrolytes
  - Most children aspirate <4 mL/kg of fluid.
  - There is little clinical relevance to the type of water in which the child is submerged.
- Most patients who experience near drowning are intravascularly hypovolemic as a result of capillary leak from asphyxia.
  - Effects on the body may be on a single system or may be multisystem.
- In addition to hypovolemia, near drowning may cause serious injury.
  - Pulmonary injury with surfactant washout and aspiration of gastric contents or contaminated water contents
  - Central nervous system (CNS) injury resulting from anoxic or ischemic events
  - Myocardial injury
  - Renal impairment
  - Injury to the gut mucosa
  - Liver function abnormalities

RISK FACTORS

- Conditions predisposing children to submersion injuries
  - Underlying seizure disorders
  - Occult cardiomyopathy
  - Alterations in the conduction system

SIGNS AND SYMPTOMS

- Effects on lungs
  - Hypoxia and hypercarbia
  - Aspiration pneumonia or simple pulmonary edema that may progress to acute respiratory distress syndrome
    - The patient may have apnea or agonal respirations.
    - The patient may have difficulty with airway protection.
  - Understanding the mechanism enables the astute clinician to act to prevent further hypoxic or anoxic injury.
- Cardiovascular effects
  - Cardiovascular instability
  - Hypotensive shock
  - Metabolic acidosis
    - Pulmonary vascular resistance may be increased and further potentiate metabolic acidosis.
  - If cardiovascular instability continues, the clinician must consider sepsis or further myocardial dysfunction.

- CNS effects (ultimate complication)
  - Severity is determined by the duration of hypoxia and hypotension.
  - After loss of consciousness, blood flow to the CNS may be increased and result in:
    - Reperfusion injury
    - Marked decrease in cerebral blood flow
  - The patient may have severe CNS injury even after:
    - Restoration of cardiac output
    - Normalization of blood pressure
    - Adequate oxygenation
- Other systems
  - Gastrointestinal system
    - Rectal discharge of material sloughed from the intestinal mucosa mixed with blood is commonly associated with severe hypoxic-ischemic injury after perfusion to the gastrointestinal tract becomes severely reduced.
    - Followed by gut necrosis
  - Hematopoietic system (disseminated intravascular coagulation)
  - Hypoxic-ischemic injuries may result in:
    - Coagulopathy
    - Renal failure
    - Predisposition to infection

LABORATORY FINDINGS

- Periodic review of blood tests is important for changes in:
  - Hematocrit
  - Coagulation profile
  - Leukocyte count
- Review of liver and renal function studies helps ascertain whether other organs have been injured.

IMAGING

- Before transfer to a pediatric intensive care unit (PICU)
  - Radiographic studies to confirm:
    - Placement of the endotracheal tube
    - Placement of vascular access catheters
    - Contour of the lungs
- If indicated, the physician may order head computed tomography to evaluate the brain and to determine whether traumatic head injury has occurred.

TREATMENT APPROACH

- Approach after significant submersion injury involves at least 4 phases.
  - Initial lay person rescue at the scene
  - Emergency medical team or paramedic response
  - Stabilization in the ED
  - Care in the PICU

Initial rescue

- Identify the problem.
- Call 911.
- Remove the child from the water.
- Clear the airway and perform CPR until emergency medical team arrives.
  - Effective CPR at the scene is a major determinant of success.
  - Note the time that CPR was initiated.
  - If possible, note the duration of submersion and temperature of the water.

Emergency response

- At the scene, an effort should be made to resuscitate the child to restore cardiac output, oxygenation, and acid-base status.
  - Ignore the down time that the child may have had during this initial resuscitative phase.
  - Assessing patency of the airway is critical, as is clearing airway of any debris before attempting to ventilate the patient with either a bag-mask device or intubation in the field.
  - Try to protect:
    - Airway from aspiration of stomach contents
    - Lungs from aggressive positive pressure ventilation, which may produce overdistention of the lungs and possibly barotrauma.
- Once heart rate is established and adequate chest wall rise is observed, the child should be transported to the closest ED that deals with children.

Stabilization

- In the ED, the child should be in a room large enough to accommodate the many interventions required.
  - Careful examination
  - Further stabilization
  - Vascular access
  - Gastric decompression
  - Bladder catheterization
  - Appropriate respiratory support
- Vital signs, including temperature, should be assessed.
- The child's cardiorespiratory status should be monitored, including:
  - Continuous electrocardiographic monitoring
  - Recording of oxygen saturation
  - If possible, intermittent recording of blood pressure
- If the child is spontaneously moving and breathing, close observation and monitoring are required to ensure that response to the submersion injury is not delayed.

D

■ Children may be discharged after 4–8 hours if they:
  ● Are well saturated in room air
  ● Have age-appropriate responses
  ● Have a normal Glasgow Coma Score
■ Children need to be admitted if they:
  ● Require significant amounts of oxygen
  ● Have abnormal sensorium
■ Imaging studies may be required to make certain that internal organs are not adversely affected.
■ Before transferring the child to the PICU:
  ● His or her neurologic condition must be carefully determined.
  ● The cervical spine must be cleared.
  ● All lines and tubes must be stabilized to make certain that the child cannot dislodge them.
■ Patients should be assessed to ensure that no pneumothorax or other evidence of air leak exists.

PICU

■ Closely monitor:
  ● All aspects of vital signs
  ● Oxygen saturation
  ● End-tidal carbon dioxide (if child is intubated)
■ If the child is intubated, an arterial line should be positioned.
■ If the child requires cardiovascular support with inotropes, a central venous catheter should be placed.
■ Management is aimed at:
  ● Restoring cardiac output
  ● Minimizing brain injury
  ● Preventing catastrophic complications
■ Neurointensive care support is often required.
  ● Aggressive management of intracranial hypertension (with osmotic agents, hypothermia, hyperventilation, steroids, or barbiturate-induced coma) have not proven to have much benefit.
    – Such interventions may increase risk for nosocomial infections, pulmonary insufficiency, and cardiac dysfunction.
■ Efforts should be made to assess the degree of neurologic injury over the first 24–48 hours.
  ● Electroencephalography may help identify electrical seizures.
  ● Seizure activity should be treated quickly and aggressively.
  ● Patients should receive sedation only if clinically indicated.
  ● Severity of encephalopathy is the main determinant of outcome.

SPECIFIC TREATMENTS

Initial management

■ If spontaneous respirations are present, the clinician should first administer oxygen.
■ If the child cannot protect the airway, intubate with an endotracheal tube of appropriate size.
■ Initial ventilatory settings
  ● Require enough tidal volume (6–10 mL/kg) or inspiratory pressure to allow adequate rising of the chest wall.
  ● Higher tidal volumes may be associated with lung injury.
  ● Positive end-expiratory pressure (4–8 cm H_2O) must be used to help alveolar distention.
  ● An age-appropriate respiratory rate and a fraction of inspired oxygen of 1.0 should be provided.
■ The child should undergo chest radiography to assess degree of lung injury and to make certain that the endotracheal tube is correctly placed.
■ Patients who were intubated in the field:
  ● Need thorough evaluation in the ED before being extubated
  ● At most institutions, patients:
    – Remain intubated and mechanically ventilated
    – Get transferred to the closest PICU
  ● The stomach must be decompressed with a nasogastric tube.
  ● A bladder catheter must be placed to measure urine output.
  ● Appropriate vascular access lines must be inserted.
■ Patients who were not intubated in the field but have poor oxygenation
  ● Positive-pressure ventilation is indicated if signs indicate increased work of breathing or if there is a high oxygen requirement.
    – The child should then be intubated with an appropriately sized endotracheal tube.
  ● The child should be placed on an appropriate ventilator setting for the underlying condition.
■ To facilitate intubation, the physician may administer a muscle relaxant and an analgesic-amnesic agent.

Cardiovascular management

■ Vascular volume should be restored with an isotonic solution (10–20 mL/kg).
■ The patient should be warmed to prevent hypothermia, which is associated with abnormal cardiac rhythms.
■ Treatment for reduced myocardial contractility
  ● The patient may require inotropic support via a proximal port.
    – Dopamine
    – Epinephrine
    – Dobutamine

- A central venous catheter and arterial line should be inserted.
  - A double-lumen catheter should be used for central venous access.
  - A distal port should be used to transduce the central venous pressure (CVP).
- Lines may be inserted into 1 of several vessels.
  - Subclavian
  - Internal jugular
  - External jugular
  - Femoral
- The child will require continuous monitoring of vital signs and CVP.
  - CVP monitoring enables assessment of volume status, which helps guide fluid administration.
  - An arterial line enables continuous monitoring of the mean arterial pressure, which should be kept in the correct range for age.
  - If patient continues to struggle with high CVP and poor cardiac output, the clinician should consider placing a pulmonary artery catheter to measure the wedge pressure (a reflection of true CVP).
- Normalization of blood gases by various ventilatory strategies is preferred to hyperventilation.
- Support of cardiovascular system with inotropes as needed to maintain
  - Adequate blood pressure
  - Blood flow to vital organs

Other care

- Nutritional support is provided as:
  - Parenteral nutrition *or*
  - Enteral nutrition if the intestinal tract can tolerate feeds
- Minimization of stress ulcers in the gastric mucosa is vitally important.
  - Agents may be used to maintain a gastric pH >5.
- Antibiotics to treat suspected or proven infections
  - Victims are susceptible to bacterial infections due to aspiration of water.
  - Bacterial infections may result from complications of mechanical ventilation or vascular access attempts.
  - Initiating empiric antibiotic treatment may be reasonable.
- Unusual forms of ventilatory support
  - High-frequency ventilation for acute pulmonary injury
  - Inhaled nitric oxide for severe hypoxia-induced respiratory failure
  - Extracorporeal oxygenation
    - Used for rewarming
    - In theory, allows the lungs to rest and prevent barotraumas associated with high airway pressures

WHEN TO ADMIT

- Children with significant respiratory distress requiring oxygen
- Children with abnormal sensorium
- Children with abnormalities on coagulation, liver, and renal function studies

WHEN TO REFER

- All patients with near drowning should be referred to an ED (preferably a children's ED) for complete physical, laboratory, and imaging evaluation.

FOLLOW-UP

- The health care team should provide resources to the family as needed.
  - Support for sustaining the child in a long-term care facility
  - Support after a child's death
    - A palliative care team or another specialist may provide bereavement support for the family.

PROGNOSIS

- Most important for positive outcome is:
  - Return of normal neurologic function within 24–72 hours
  - Successful resuscitative measures at the scene
    - If the child is conscious on arrival at hospital, the chance of intact survival is excellent.
    - Pulmonary injury can be managed successfully with new approaches to mechanical ventilation.
- The worst prognosis is associated with continued need for resuscitation in the ED, despite age, duration of submersion, pH at the time of care, or body temperature.
- Other poor prognostic findings
  - Continuation of CPR beyond 25 minutes
  - Fixed, dilated pupils
  - Seizures
  - Flaccidity
  - Glasgow Coma Score <5
  - Decreased cerebral blood flow
- Cold-water submersions that produce severe hypothermia may influence outcome.
- Outcome after submersion injuries will be determined within the first 24–72 hours.
- If neurologic function has not recovered after 48–72 hours, the child is not likely to recover neurologic function.
  - This must be explained to the child's parents within 12–24 hours after the child's admission to PICU.

- A multidisciplinary meeting (neurologists, primary care physician, PICU nurses, and a social worker assigned to the case) should be held with the family to explain in detail the potential outcomes of prolonged coma.
  - The child may regain much, but not all, of previous neurologic function.
  - The child may experience less severe neurologic sequela.
  - The child may remain in a vegetative state or may experience brain death.
- Parents need to make informed decisions about aggressive approaches to care.
  - Technology-based ongoing support
  - Long-term mechanical ventilation
  - Tracheostomy
  - Gastrostomy feeds
  - Fundoplication
  - Placement in a long-term or chronic care facility or nursing the child at home
- Parents may wish to attempt extubation, thinking that if recovery of breathing without mechanical ventilation does not happen, the physician will reintubate.
  - Provides more time to come to a consensus about what to do next
- If the medical team has established that the most likely outcome is severe encephalopathy or a persistent vegetative state, the parents may request extubation and natural death.
- A do-not-resuscitate order on record ensures that no further heroic efforts will be undertaken to save the child.

PREVENTION

- Primary care physicians need to educate families during routine office visits about pool safety.
- Swimming pools
  - Should not be built until children in the household are >5 years
  - Parents should never leave children alone in or near the pool, even for a moment.

- A fence should be erected to separate house from pool.
  - The fence should be ≥4 feet high around all 4 sides of the pool.
  - The fence should completely separate pool from the house and play area of the yard.
  - Gates should auto-close and auto-latch, with latches higher than children's reach.
- Parents should consider a safety cover.
  - A power safety cover that meets the standards of the American Society for Testing and Materials adds to the protection of children but should not be used in place of a fence between house and pool.
- Even fencing and a power safety cover will not prevent all drownings.
- Keep rescue equipment (eg, a shepherd's hook, life preserver) and a telephone by the pool.
- Remove all toys from the pool after use so children are not tempted to reach for them.
- After children are done swimming, the pool should be secured so they cannot get back into it.
- Do not let children use air-filled swimming aids.
  - They are not a substitute for approved life vests.
  - They can be dangerous.
- Know CPR.
  - Anyone watching young children around a pool should learn CPR and be able to rescue a child if needed.
- Parents should stay within an arm's length of child.
- Teaching a child how to swim does not mean that he/she is safe in water.

Drug Eruptions

DEFINITION

- Systemically administered drugs can cause almost any kind of rash.
- The types of skin reactions caused by drugs include:
  - Most common
    - Morbilliform (measles-like) eruptions
    - Urticaria
    - Erythema multiforme (EM)
      - An acute, self-limited eruption of symmetrical erythematous macules and papules that can evolve into target lesions
      - Best viewed as a separate entity from Stevens-Johnson syndrome (SJS) and toxic epidermal necrosis (TEN)
  - Most severe
    - SJS
      - The major form of EM
      - SJS and TEN, also known as *Lyell syndrome,* are 2 ends of a more severe process involving the acute onset of mucocutaneous necrosis.
      - SJS produces more focal skin necrosis than TEN, with ≥2 mucosal sites involved.
    - TEN
      - Extensive areas of epidermal necrosis and resulting denudation
  - Other
    - Erythema nodosum
    - Vasculitis
    - Photosensitivity reactions
    - Acneform eruptions
    - Alopecia
    - Blistering disorders
    - Fixed drug eruptions
    - Lichenoid reactions
- Drug rash with eosinophilia and systemic symptoms (DRESS), formerly known as *drug hypersensitivity syndrome*
  - Characterized by the clinical triad of fever, rash, and internal organ involvement (most commonly hepatitis, nephritis, pneumonitis, or myocarditis)

EPIDEMIOLOGY

- DRESS
  - The incidence of DRESS with anticonvulsants has been estimated at 1 in 10,000 exposures.

ETIOLOGY

Morbilliform eruptions

- Caused by a wide variety of agents, most commonly among recipients of:

- Aminopenicillins
  - 4.4–8.0 per 100
- Sulfonamides
  - 2.5–3.7 per 100
- Ampicillin
  - 3.3 per 100
- Semisynthetic penicillins
  - 2.9 per 100
- Blood
  - 2.2 per 100
- Cephalosporins
  - 2.1 per 100
- Erythromycin
  - 2.0 per 100
- Penicillin G
  - 1.6 per 100
- Allopurinol
  - 0.8 per 100
- Nonsteroidal antiinflammatory drugs (NSAIDs)
  - 0.3–0.69 per 100
- Barbiturates
  - 0.4 per 100
- Diazepam
  - 0.04 per 100

Urticaria

- Drug-induced hives can be mediated immunologically by either:
  - Immediate immunoglobulin (Ig) E reactions, usually within hours
    - More common than delayed reactions
  - Delayed immune complexes that result in serum sickness-like reactions after 7–10 days
- A precise cause is not usually found among patients with hives.

DRESS

- Associated with the use of:
  - Aromatic anticonvulsants (phenytoin, carbamazepine, phenobarbitone)
  - Sulfonamides
  - NSAIDs
  - Ranitidine
  - Calcium-channel blockers
  - Allopurinol
  - Thalidomide
- Cross-reactivity with structurally related drugs is common.

EM

- Most often occurs in association with recurrentherpes simplex virus (HSV) types I and II
  - ~50% of patients had an HSV lesion a few days to 2 weeks before EM
  - In the rest a cause generally cannot be identified.
- Circulating immune complexes have been detected in patients who have EM, consistent with the concept that the disorder is an immunologic reaction
- Other infectious agents that have been rarely implicated in EM include *Histoplasma capsulatumvirus*, and possibly Epstein-Barr virus.

SJS and TEN

- Medications are the most common cause.
- Antibiotics (especially sulfonamides), anticonvulsants, and NSAIDs have been most commonly implicated.
- Infections, particularly with *Mycoplasma pneumoniae*, have also been implicated in SJS.

RISK FACTORS

- DRESS
  - First-degree relatives with this syndrome

SIGNS AND SYMPTOMS

Morbilliform eruptions

- Onset is not usually immediate but begins within several days to 1 week after drug initiation.
- Itching is usually present, but it is not helpful as a diagnostic marker.
- Eruption is generalized and consists of brightly erythematous macules and papules that tend to be confluent over large areas.
- It usually starts proximally and proceeds distally.
  - Legs are typically the last to be involved and the last to clear.
  - Palms and soles are affected.
- Most drug eruptions are not accompanied by an elevation in body temperature.

Urticaria

- Hives appear as edematous plaques.
  - Often have pale or dusky centers and red borders
  - Frequently assume geographic shapes
  - Sometimes confluent
  - May be scattered, but are usually generalized
- By definition, an individual hive is transient, lasting <48 hours, although new hives may develop continuously.
- Itching is almost always present.
- Obstructed airway or urticaria with significant edema suggests anaphylaxis.

- Fever, lymphadenopathy, and arthralgia often accompany hives in serum sickness reactions, for which the 2 most common causes are:
  - Drugs, especially antibiotics
  - Viral hepatitis
- Hives are skin lesions that are recognized more easily than described.

DRESS

- Occurs within 8 weeks of initiating medication use
- Clinical manifestations include:
  - Fever early in the course
  - Diffuse macules
  - Papules or pustules that can progress to an exfoliative dermatitis mimicking SJS or TEN
  - Eosinophilia
  - Atypical lymphocytosis
- The severity of skin involvement does not correlate with the extent of internal organ involvement.

EM

- HSV lesions a few days to 2 weeks earlier
- Occasionally preceded by a febrile prodrome
- Characterized by a variety of lesions, including:
  - Erythematous plaques
  - Blisters
  - Targetoid lesions, sometimes confused with hives
    - Hives have only 2 zones of color: a central pale area surrounded by an erythematous halo.
    - The target lesion requires 3 zones: a central dark area or blister, surrounded by a pale zone, surrounded by a peripheral rim of erythema.
    - True target lesions are diagnostic for EM.
    - Seen more often on the palms and soles but may occur anywhere
- Typically, EM is a strikingly symmetrical eruption, most frequently seen on the dorsal hands and forearms and often involving palms, neck, face, and trunk.
- Lesions can be quite numerous, often exceeding 100.
- Lesions may appear grouped on the elbows or knees.
- Koebner phenomenon can be observed: after cutaneous trauma, target lesions may appear in the affected areas.
- Mild, discrete oral erosions occur in more than half of patients but are usually few in number and can be relatively asymptomatic.

SJS and TEN

- SJS and TEN are usually preceded by a prodrome of up to 2 weeks of influenza-like symptoms followed by the abrupt onset of skin eruption.

- When these conditions are drug related, eruption typically begins 7–21 days after initiation of the causative drug.
- Eruption is initially macular or morbilliform, tender, dusky, and erythematous and widespread in distribution.
- Skin strips off easily with minor friction (positive Nikolsky sign).
- Lesions gradually coalesce, and flaccid bullae develop.
- Bullae easily rupture and detach, leaving necrotic sheets of epidermis with a moist, bright red base.
- Similar lesions are also typically seen on mucous membranes, usually involving >2 mucosal sites.
- Thick, hemorrhagic crusts may appear on the lips.
- When up to 10% of the body surface area is involved, the eruption is termed *SJS*.
- When >30% is involved, it is termed *TEN*.
- When 10–30% is involved, the eruption is termed *SJS-TEN* overlap.
- Constitutional symptoms occur.
  - Fever
  - Arthralgia
  - Malaise
  - Lymphadenopathy
  - Occasional symptoms of an upper respiratory infection
  - Rarely, hepatitis, nephritis, and myocarditis

DIFFERENTIAL DIAGNOSIS

- A general principle of dermatologic diagnosis is: For any rash, think of drugs.

Morbilliform eruptions

- Patients receiving >1 drug present a problem.
- The 2 variables to consider are:
  - The temporal relationship between the administration of the drug and the onset of the rash
  - The likelihood that a given medication can cause a drug eruption (see Etiology)
- Morbilliform eruptions have been reported in patients with Epstein-Barr virus infection taking amoxicillin; their pathogenesis remains to be elucidated.
- Major differential diagnosis for morbilliform eruption
  - Drug reaction
    - May be more erythematous and confluent, but not always
    - Presence of eosinophilia favors a drug-related cause.
  - Viral exanthem
    - Clinically indistinguishable from a drug eruption
  - Toxic erythema, eg, scarlet fever, staphylococcal-induced scarlatiniform eruptions, Kawasaki disease (possibly)

- Distinguishing features
  - Sandpaper-like roughened texture of the rash and mucous membrane involvement (scarlet fever and Kawasaki disease)
  - Fever
  - Focus of infection
  - Lymphadenopathy
- Postinflammatory desquamation from the skin of the hands and feet often follows the rash of toxic erythema, but this sign is not specific.
  - Drug eruptions and viral exanthems can involve hands and feet, particularly palms and soles in drug eruptions.

Urticaria

- Differential diagnosis of urticaria may be approached in 2 ways.
  - From the causes of hives per se
    - Usually the cause of hives cannot be determined; when found, it is usually drug-related.
    - Other causes include infection, physical stressors (eg, cold, pressure, sunlight), emotions, and foods.
- From consideration of the cause of lesions sometimes mistaken as hives
  - Includes those seen in EM and juvenile idiopathic arthritis
  - In juvenile idiopathic arthritis, lesions are transient but differ in:
    - Size (only 2–3 mm)
    - Color (typically salmon)
    - Timing (usually appear with fever spikes)

EM

- Skin reactions most commonly considered in the differential diagnosis are:
  - Giant urticaria
    - Individual hives last <48 hours; the lesions in EM persist much longer.
  - Subacute cutaneous lupus erythematosus
  - Viral exanthems
    - Usually monomorphous and tend to be less red, more confluent, and more centrally distributed than EM
  - Vasculitis
    - Purpura is the distinguishing feature of vasculitic lesions.
  - Staphylococcal scalded-skin syndrome (SSSS)
  - Other blistering eruptions
- Recurrent EM caused by HSV can be mistaken for photosensitive disorders because it can be triggered by significant sun exposure.
  - Polymorphous light eruption
  - Juvenile spring eruption

SJS and TEN

- The skin in SSSS is diffusely red and tender and exhibits a Nikolsky sign.

DIAGNOSTIC APPROACH

- Morbilliform eruptions
  - Presumptive diagnosis is made based on clinical data.
- Urticaria
  - Drug history is the most important but also the most difficult to obtain, at least among outpatients.
  - Whenever a drug is suspected, persist in eliciting a medication history to be sure no drugs are invariably overlooked.
  - Many patients and their parents consider over-the-counter medications unimportant.
    - Ask about specific medications to help jog their memories.
    - NSAIDs cause hives in some and can aggravate them in others who have urticaria, regardless of its cause.
    - Aspirin can cause hives but is not widely used in children because of the risk of Reye syndrome.
- SJS and TEN
  - History of all medications should be elicited.

LABORATORY FINDINGS

Morbilliform eruptions

- No laboratory test can identify the responsible drug and are not usually helpful.
- Peripheral blood eosinophilia is sometimes present and may heighten the suspicion for a drug reaction.

Urticaria

- May be accompanied by eosinophilia
- In afebrile patients, laboratory tests are rarely helpful in eliciting a cause and are of no help in implicating a specific drug.
- To evaluate for hepatitis, obtain liver function tests in patients who have hives and fever.

DRESS

- Abnormal liver function test results

EM

- Laboratory evaluation usually is not helpful, although leukocytosis can be seen.
- For herpes simplex disease, if vesicular lesion is still present:
  - Base can be scraped for HSV direct fluorescent antibody.
  - Fluid can be cultured for HSV or examined for multinucleated giant cells (Tzanck preparation).

SJS and TEN

- *M pneumoniae* infection can be confirmed further by:
  - Cold agglutinin
  - IgM antibodies to *Mycoplasma*

- Complete blood count may show leukocytosis.
- Urinalysis may show hematuria or proteinuria.

IMAGING

- SJS and TEN
  - Chest radiograpy is appropriate to screen for pulmonary involvement, including that caused by *M pneumoniae*.

DIAGNOSTIC PROCEDURES

- EM
  - When the diagnosis is in doubt, skin biopsy can exclude conditions that mimic EM.
    - Lupus erythematosus
    - Vasculitis
- SJS and TEN
  - Skin biopsy helps distinguish SSSS from SJS.
    - Histologically, the level of the blister is intraepidermal in SSSS.
    - In SJS and TEN, the blister is subepidermal.

TREATMENT APPROACH

Morbilliform eruptions

- When an offending agent is identified, its use should be discontinued.
- If a patient is taking several drugs and causative agent cannot be identified:
  - The number of drugs administered should be reduced to an absolute minimum.
  - Whenever possible, any remaining possible offending agents should be changed to alternative agents.
- Drug eruption may clear even when use of the offending agent is continued; however, continued use of the drug is unwise if an alternative is available.

Urticaria

- Use of any suspected medication should be discontinued.

DRESS

- Immediate withdrawal of all suspected medications
- Supportive care of symptoms

EM

- No convincing evidence has been found that medical therapy favorably alters the course of EM.
- Treating a precipitating infection seems appropriate, even though no proof exists that it alters the course of the skin reaction.

SJS and TEN

- Use of any drug suspected of causing the reaction should be discontinued.
- Underlying infection should be treated.

D

- Supportive measures are vitally important.
  - Restore and maintain fluid and electrolyte balance.
  - Prevent secondary infection.
  - Relieve pain.

SPECIFIC TREATMENTS

Morbilliform eruptions

- Therapy is directed toward symptoms.
- Antihistamines are used most commonly for the pruritus.
- Topical agents are usually confined to moisturizers, which are most helpful during the desquamative phase of the reaction.
- Although topical steroids may be of some value in controlling pruritus, systemic steroids are rarely required.

Urticaria

- Symptoms are usually treated with antihistamines given on a regular, rather than an as-needed schedule.
  - Hydroxyzine is the preferred agent; give every 6 or 8 hours.

DRESS

- Systemic corticosteroids are generally used in more severe cases involving significant exfoliative dermatitis, pneumonitis, or hepatitis.

EM

- Acyclovir begun after the onset of EM has not proven to be effective.
- Treatment of symptoms also can be helpful.
  - Antihistamines may reduce the sensation of stinging and burning.
  - Antacid suspensions applied topically may alleviate oral ulcers.
- Children with frequently recurring EM caused by HSV may be good candidates for prophylactic acyclovir for 6–12 months.
- Systemic prednisone is sometimes used early in the course of patients who have severe EM.

SJS and TEN

- Erythromycin is recommended for *M pneumoniae* infections, although treatment may not alter the course of the skin disease.
- Supportive care
  - Patients with severe oral involvement may be unable to eat and drink.
  - When skin involvement is extensive, transcutaneous fluid loss increases and replacement volumes must be adjusted accordingly.
  - Fluid replacement poses a unique challenge for patients with SJS and TEN.
    - Surface area in patients with SJS and TEN may change, thus altering their fluid requirements.

- Fluid intake may need frequent adjustment to maintain constant urine output while avoiding fluid overload, which can lead to pulmonary edema, acute respiratory distress syndrome, and death.
- Some experts recommend inserting a nasogastric tube on admission to maximize oral intake and decrease the need for intravenous fluids or parenteral nutrition, thus decreasing risk of fluid overload if the course becomes complicated.
- Parenteral nutrition requires a central venous line, with attendant risks of sepsis and other line-associated complications.

- Local therapy with antiseptics and dressings may help prevent secondary infection.
  - Patients who have severe involvement may require treatments similar to those for burn patients.
  - Silver nitrate–impregnated dressings have been shown to be particularly helpful without causing further epidermal detachment on removal.
- Systemic analgesics are used for pain.
- Topical anesthetics may be used intraorally to provide temporary relief for patients who have painful mouth lesions.
  - "Magic swizzle," containing 1 part each of diphenhydramine hydrochloride elixir, aluminum and magnesium hydroxide (Maalox), and viscous lidocaine 2%, is one agent.
  - Be aware of the potential for systemic effects from lidocaine when ordering this agent for young children.
- Use of systemic steroids is controversial.
  - They have been used frequently in SJS and TEN, but with mixed success.
  - One retrospective study found that children treated for SJS with systemic steroids required a longer hospital stay and had more complications (eg, infection, gastrointestinal bleeding) than untreated patients.
- Intravenous immunoglobulin may hasten the course of this disorder by blocking apoptosis of epidermal cells.
  - However, published reports have been mixed.
  - Well-controlled, prospective, multicenter studies are needed to confirm efficacy and safety and to determine optimal dosing guidelines.

WHEN TO ADMIT

- Admit patients with SJS and TEN.

WHEN TO REFER

- Recurrent EM
- Drug hypersensitivity reactions with multiorgan involvement
- Early diagnosis and management of SJS and TEN with referral to a tertiary-care center may:
  - Lessen morbidity and mortality
  - Improve the outcome

FOLLOW-UP

- SJS and TEN
  - Early ophthalmic evaluation is warranted because of mucous membrane involvement.

COMPLICATIONS

Morbilliform eruptions

- The complications of skin rashes are primarily cutaneous.
- When large areas of skin are inflamed, body heat increases and water is lost.
  - These changes might be a problem for patients who are seriously ill.
- Continuing use of an offending agent in the setting of a drug eruption can result in 2 types of consequences.
  - Cutaneous
    - Possible progressive worsening of the rash may result (rarely) in SJS or TEN.
  - Renal
    - Allergic interstitial nephritis is an uncommon development usually associated with penicillins and cephalosporins and only rarely with other drugs.

Urticaria

- In rare cases, can be accompanied by anaphylactic reactions

SJS and TEN

- Oral mucous membrane involvement can produce painful erosions, restricting intake and resulting in dehydration.
- Similar lesions in genital mucous membranes can cause dysuria and urinary retention.
- Internal organs are affected less often.
  - TEN can affect the respiratory system and may lead to:
    - Patchy pulmonary disease
    - Bronchiolitis obliterans
    - Respiratory failure
  - TEN can affect the gastrointestinal tract.
    - Esophageal involvement can lead to dysphasia, malnutrition, and strictures.
    - Involvement of the small intestine can lead to abdominal pain and diarrhea.
- Conjunctivitis can produce residual ophthalmic complications, including
  - Keratitis sicca
  - Corneal ulceration or scarring
  - Permanent visual impairment
  - Blindness

PROGNOSIS

Morbilliform eruptions

- Eruptions gradually clear after the use of responsible agent is discontinued, usually 1–2 weeks.
- Eruption may worsen for several days after use of the offending drug has been stopped.

Urticaria

- Drug-induced hives usually clear within several days after use of the responsible medication is discontinued.

EM

- Patients with mild forms of EM usually recover uneventfully within 2–3 weeks.
- EM recurs in 10–20% of patients and is particularly common in patients with milder disease that is precipitated by recurrent HSV infection.

SJS and TEN

- Disease can last as long as 4–6 weeks in patients with severe involvement.
- Patients with these disorders may die because of extensive loss of skin integrity or complications from involvement of other organ systems.
  - Mortality rates of up to 30% have been reported.
  - A severity-of-illness score for TEN predicts a patient's risk of death according to the presence or absence of 7 risk factors
    - Age >40 years
    - Presence of cancer
    - Heart rate >120 beats/min
    - Extent of skin involvement >10% on admission
    - Blood urea nitrogen level >28 mg/dL
    - Serum glucose level >252 mg/dL
    - Serum bicarbonate level <20 mM

PREVENTION

Morbilliform eruption

- If a responsible drug has been identified:
  - The patient should be advised about the allergy.
  - The medical record should be clearly labeled, even though not all of these reactions reflect true allergy.

Urticaria

- If a specific agent has been identified, the patient must be alerted to avoid that drug in the future.
- Most hives are IgE mediated and a repeat challenge with the responsible drug is more likely to result in an anaphylactic response than it would following a morbilliform eruption.

Drug Overdose

DEFINITION

- Drug overdose occurs when a child ingests or is given an amount of a substance that exceeds the recommended dose.

EPIDEMIOLOGY

- Prevalence
  - In 2004, the American Association of Poison Control Centers tabulated 2,473,570 case reports of human exposure to potentially toxic substances among the 292.2 million people they serve.
  - 51.6% were <6 years.
  - 39.1% were ≤2 years.
- Incidence
  - Annually, 1.4 million children ≤12 years are exposed to drugs that are potentially toxic.
  - In 2002, these exposures resulted in 29 deaths.
- Toxic exposure, by patient age
  - Pharmaceutical agents
    - <6 years: 504,725
    - 6–9 years: 168,053
  - Nonpharmaceutical agents (chemicals, plants, gases)
    - <6 years: 725,941
    - 6–19 years: 188,002
- Deaths, by patient age
  - <6 years: 25
    - Reflects unintentional ingestions
  - 6–12 years: 4
  - 13–19 years: 48
    - Reflects suicidal events

ETIOLOGY

- Most drug overdoses do not affect the upper airway (larynx, trachea) but interfere with air exchange by either depressing the central nervous system or paralyzing neuromuscular transmission.

RISK FACTORS

- The most common drug overdoses causing death are analgesics, antidepressants, and over-the-counter cough and cold preparations.
- For some compounds, therapeutic mistakes may play a significant role.
  - Many acetaminophen poisonings are caused by errors in 1 of the following:
    - Inappropriate dosing
    - Unintentional multiple overdosing
    - Ingestion of acetaminophen along with another hepato-toxic drug
    - Administration of adult rather than pediatric preparations
    - Concurrent administration of an over-the-counter fixed-dose combination product that also contains acetaminophen
    - Supervision of medication administration by another child

SIGNS AND SYMPTOMS

- Vomiting
- Altered mental status (lethargic or aggressive)
- Pale looking or cyanotic
- Suppressed or labored breathing
- Sometimes, hypotension
- Constricted (opiates, phenothiazines) or dilated (anticholinergics, amphetamines) pupils

DIFFERENTIAL DIAGNOSIS

- Other conditions can mimic signs and symptoms of drug overdose.
- Head trauma is a consideration in patients who have alterations in sensorium.
  - Adolescents who have head trauma may have ingested ethanol.
  - Head injury with drug overdose in a child may indicate child abuse.
- Near-drowning victims may have ingested ethanol.
- Use of illicit drugs can alter mental status and should be considered.
- General urine toxicologic screens ordered in an emergency department will test for:
  - Tetrahydrocannabinol (marijuana)
  - Cocaine
  - Opioids
  - Benzodiazepines
  - Barbiturates
  - Phencyclidine
- Spontaneous intracranial hemorrhages in pediatric patients are rare.
  - Usually produce focal neurologic signs rather than global depression of consciousness
- Metabolic conditions, such as:
  - Diabetes mellitus
  - Hypoglycemia
  - Addisonian crisis
- Infections of the central nervous system, particularly viral encephalitis

- Most difficult is the patient who has a psychiatric illness and who may develop tremors, hallucinations, or hysterical paralysis.
  - Precise and rapid laboratory analyses are most important in ruling out drug ingestion.
  - If the patient is having a reaction to prescribed psychoactive medications, management is identical to that for overdose, with special attention to child's emotional needs.

DIAGNOSTIC APPROACH

- As much information as possible should be gathered immediately.
- The person or persons who brought the child to the hospital or office should be detained.
- If initial contact is by telephone:
  - The caller's name and telephone number should be obtained.
  - The caller should be instructed to proceed immediately with the child to the hospital.
- Obtaining the precise description of the ingested drug is important, including, if known:
  - Name
  - Dose
  - Pharmacy of origin
  - Prescription number
  - Parents should be instructed to bring the actual container when they come with the patient.
- An attempt should be made to determine the amount of drug ingested.
  - Determination is frequently impossible; if obtained, it is occasionally misleading.
  - Maximal exposure is assumed unless a precise tablet count or liquid amount is available.
- As always with an acute, life-threatening event, the patient's airway, breathing, and circulation should be promptly assessed.
- General homeostatic support
  - Thermal monitoring is an important aspect of management in drug overdose.
    - Centrally and peripherally induced hypothermia is a common problem.
    - Hyperthermia can occur with salicylate, atropine, or selective serotonin reuptake inhibitor poisoning.
  - Monitoring fluid and electrolyte homeostasis is important.
    - Amount of maintenance fluids required depends on changes in the vital and physical signs.
  - Central venous pressure and arterial pressure should be monitored to assess vascular volume and tone.
  - Respiratory function and oxygenation (with pulse oximetry) require monitoring.

- Intracranial pressure may need to be assessed to determine the need to treat cerebral edema.
- The need for peritoneal dialysis, hemodialysis, charcoal perfusion, or exchange transfusion to remove the ingested drug must be considered.

LABORATORY FINDINGS

- Assays must be available for:
  - Blood
  - Urine
  - Gastric contents for:
    - Barbiturates
    - Antidepressants
    - Phenytoin
    - Iron
    - Digoxin
    - Salicylate
    - Acetaminophen
    - Narcotics
    - Alcohol
    - Cocaine
    - Propoxyphene
- Rapid drug screens should be available and quantitative analyses should follow as quickly as possible.

IMAGING

- Flat-plate radiographic examination of the abdomen may be required to identify radiopaque tablets (eg, iron) or foreign bodies.
- Computed tomography of the head should be performed if intracranial hemorrhage is suspected after amphetamine or cocaine ingestion.
- Chest radiography is needed if narcotic-induced pulmonary edema or aspiration is suspected.

TREATMENT APPROACH

- Major considerations are:
  - Expertise of the physician in the management of drug overdose
  - Available hospital support facilities
  - It is best to decide early in the clinical course whether special facilities will be needed.
  - It is preferable to transfer a stable patient earlier than a critically ill child requiring mobile life support later.
- Frequent and open communication with the patient's family should be maintained.
  - Parents are in constant need of counseling, especially with regard to any feelings of guilt they may be experiencing.

- Adolescents with intentional drug overdoses often have complex psychosocial problems that typically require psychiatric consultation.
- Steps to treat the patient with a drug overdose
  - Stabilize the patient.
  - Identify the drug ingested and determine the amount ingested.
  - Contact the local poison control center for toxicology data and information regarding the signs and symptoms and clinical course.
    - The toll-free telephone for poison control centers in the US is 800/222-1222.
  - Use gastrointestinal decontamination (see Specific Treatments).
  - If a specific antidote exists, administer it.
    - All staff members must know the precise location of antidotes within the hospital.
  - Provide supportive care in an intensive or intermediate care unit as appropriate.
  - Meet social service needs as indicated (eg, drug ingestion by a toddler as a symptom of chaotic family structure or by an adolescent as a symptom of depression or as a suicidal gesture).
  - Provide counseling concerning the institution of poison-control measures in the home.

SPECIFIC TREATMENTS

Gastric decontamination

- Gastric decontamination procedures have undergone recent changes in recommendations.
- Before 2003, the AAP recommended that ipecac syrup be kept in the home to administer to children on the direction of a physician or poison control center.
  - This policy has been reversed because research has shown that ipecac:
    - Does not completely remove an ingested substance from the stomach
    - Has side effects of its own (including lethargy)
    - May be given inappropriately by caregivers
    - Does not improve health outcomes or reduce utilization of emergency services
- Gastric lavage may still be used on occasion in an emergency setting for patients who have ingested a near-lethal or lethal amount of a toxic agent within the prior 1–2 hours.
- Activated charcoal is now considered the best method of gastrointestinal decontamination.
- Gastrointestinal fluid obtained by any decontamination method should be saved for drug analysis.

- Activated charcoal
  - Dose: 1 g/kg, usually administered via nasogastric tube
  - Use of a cathartic remains controversial, with no firm evidence supporting this measure.
  - Among the few compounds that appear not to be adsorbed by the charcoal are acids, alkalis, and iron salts.
- For substances that are poorly adsorbed by charcoal, whole-bowel irrigation (with a polyethylene glycol–electrolyte solution [Colyte or Golytely])
  - Dose: 25 to 40 mL/kg/hour
  - May be especially helpful in treating for overdoses of increasing numbers of delayed-release drugs

Antidotes

- Specific antidotes exist for some drugs but, unfortunately, not for most (see table Common Antidotes).
- For those without antidotes
  - Intensive supportive care
  - Treatment of signs and symptoms as they develop (eg, hypotension and hypertension, thermal instability, cardiac arrhythmias)
- Acetaminophen
  - Diagnostic findings requiring treatment: history of ingestion and toxic serum level
  - Antidote: N-acetylcysteine
  - Dosage: 140 mg/kg PO, then 70 mg/kg every 4 hr PO × 17
- Anticholinergics, antihistamines, atropine, phenothiazines, tricyclic antidepressants
  - Diagnostic findings requiring treatment: supraventricular tachycardia (hemodynamic compromise); unresponsive ventricular dysrhythmia, seizures, pronounced hallucinations or agitation
  - Antidote: physostigmine
  - Dosage: in children, 0.5 mg IV slowly (over 3 minutes) every 10 minutes as needed
- Benzodiazepines
  - Diagnostic findings requiring treatment: drowsiness, ataxia, hallucinations, confusion, agitation, respiratory depression, hypotension
  - Antidote: flumazenil
  - Dosage: 0.01 mg/kg IV every min × 1–5 doses; maximum, 0.2 mg/dose
- Cholinergics
  - Diagnostic findings requiring treatment: cholinergic crisis—salivation, lacrimation, urination, defecation, convulsions, fasciculations
  - Antidote: atropine sulfate, physostigmine, insecticides
  - Dosage: 0.05 mg/kg/dose (usual dose 1–5 mg; test dose for child 0.01 mg/kg) every 4–6 hr IV or more frequently as needed

D

Common Antidotes[a]

Drug	Diagnostic Findings Requiring Treatment	Antidote	Dosage
Acetaminophen	History of ingestion and toxic serum level	N-acetylcysteine	140 mg/kg/dose PO, then 70 mg/kg/dose every 4 hr PO × 17
• Anticholinergics • Antihistamines • Atropine • Phenothiazines • Tricyclic antidepressants	– Supraventricular tachycardia (hemodynamic compromise) – Unresponsive ventricular dysrhythmia, seizures, pronounced hallucinations or agitation	Physostigmine	Child: 0.5 mg IV slowly (over 3 min) every 10 min as needed
Benzodiazepines	Drowsiness, ataxia, hallucinations, confusion, agitation, respiratory depression, hypotension	Flumazenil	0.01 mg/kg IV every min × 1–5 doses; max 0.2 mg/dose
Cholinergics	Cholinergic crisis: salivation, lacrimation, urination, defecation, convulsions, fasciculations	– Atropine sulfate – Physostigmine – Insecticides	0.05 mg/kg/dose (usual dose 1–5 mg; test dose for child 0.01 mg/kg) every 4–6 hr IV or more frequently as needed
Carbon monoxide	Headache, seizure, coma, dysrhythmias	Oxygen, hyperbaric oxygen	100% oxygen (half-life 40 min); consider hyperbaric chamber
Cyanide	Cyanosis, seizures, cardiopulmonary arrest, coma	Amyl nitrite	Inhale pearl every 60–120 sec
		Sodium nitrite (3%)	0.27 mL (8.7 mg)/kg (adult: 10 mL [300 mg]) IV slowly (Hb ≥10 g/dL)
		Sodium thiosulfate (25%)	1.35 mL (325 mg)/kg (adult: 12.5 g) IV slowly (Hb ≥10g/dL)
		Also consider hyperbaric chamber	
Ethylene glycol	Metabolic acidosis, urine calcium oxalate crystals	Fomepizole	15 mg/kg IV over 30 min
		Ethanol (100% absolute, 1 mL–790 mg)	1 mL/kg in 5% dextrose in water IV over 15 min, then 0.16 mL (125 mg)/kg/hr IV; maintain ethanol level of 100 mg/dL
Iron	Hypotension, shock, coma, serum iron >350 mg/dL (or greater than iron-binding capacity)	Deferoxamine	• Shock or coma: 15 mg/kg/hr IV for 8 hr • No shock or coma: 90 mg/kg/dose IM every 8 hr
• Phenothiazines • Chlorpromazine • Thioridazine	Extrapyramidal dyskinesis, oculogyric crisis	Diphenhydramine (Benadryl®)	1–2 mg/kg/dose (max: 50 mg/dose) every 6 hr IV, PO
Methanol	Metabolic acidosis, blurred vision; level >20 mg/dL	Fomepizole	15 mg/kg IV over 30 min
		Ethanol (100% absolute)	1 mL/kg in 5% dextrose in water over 15 min, then 0.16 mL (125 mg)/kg/hr IV
• Methemoglobin • Nitrate • Nitrites • Sulfonamide	Cyanosis, methemoglobin level 30%, dyspnea	Methylene blue (1% solution)	1–2 mg (0.1–0.2 mL)/kg/dose IV; repeat in 4 hr if necessary

Common Antidotes^a, _continued_

Drug	Diagnostic Findings Requiring Treatment	Antidote	Dosage
• Narcotics • Heroin • Codeine • Propoxyphene	Respiratory depression, hypotension, coma	Naloxone (Narcan®)	0.1 mg/kg up to 0.8 mg initially IV, if no response give 2 mg IV
• Organophosphates • Malathion • Parathion	Cholinergic crisis: salivation, lacrimation, urination, defecation, convulsions, fasciculations	Atropine sulfate	0.05 mg/kg/dose (usual dose 1–5 mg; test dose for child 0.01 mg/kg) every 4-6 hr IV or more frequently as needed
		Pralidoxime	After atropine, 20–50 mg/kg/dose (max: 2000 mg) IV slowly (<50 mg/min) every 8 hr IV as needed × 3

Abbreviations: Hb, hemoglobin; IV, intravenously; PO, orally.

^a Reprinted with permission from SLACK Incorporated: Barkin RM. Toxicologic emergencies. _Pediatr Ann._ 1990(11);19:629–633.

■ Carbon monoxide
- Diagnostic findings requiring treatment: headache, seizure, coma, dysrhythmias
- Antidote: oxygen, hyperbaric oxygen
- Dosage: 100% oxygen (half-life 40 minutes); consider hyperbaric chamber

■ Cyanide
- Diagnostic findings requiring treatment: cyanosis, seizures, cardiopulmonary arrest, coma
- Antidote
  - Amyl nitrite: inhale pearl every 60–120 seconds
  - Sodium nitrite (3%): 0.27 mL (8.7 mg)/kg (adult: 10mL [300 mg]) IV slowly (hemoglobin level ≥10 g/dL)
  - Sodium thiosulfate (25%): 1.35 mL (325 mg)/kg (adult: 12.5 g) IV slowly (hemoglobin level ≥10 g/dL)
  - Also consider hyperbaric chamber.

■ Ethylene glycol
- Diagnostic findings requiring treatment: metabolic acidosis, urine calcium oxalate crystals
- Antidote
  - Fomepizole: 15 mg/kg IV over 30 minutes
  - Ethanol (100% absolute, 1 mL–790 mg): 1 mL/kg in 5% dextrose in water IV over 15 minutes, then 0.16 mL (125 mg)/kg/hr IV; maintain ethanol level of 100 mg/dL

■ Iron
- Diagnostic findings requiring treatment: hypotension, shock, coma, serum iron level >350 mg/dL (or greater than iron-binding capacity)
- Antidote: deferoxamine
- Dosage
  - Shock or coma: 15 mg/kg/hour IV for 8 hours
  - No shock or coma: 90 mg/kg/dose IM every 8 hours

■ Phenothiazines, chlorpromazine, thioridazine
- Diagnostic findings requiring treatment: extrapyramidal dyskinesis, oculogyric crisis
- Antidote: diphenhydramine (Benadryl)
- Dosage: 1–2 mg/kg (maximum, 50 mg/dose) every 6 hours IV, PO

■ Methanol
- Diagnostic findings requiring treatment: metabolic acidosis, blurred vision; level >20 mg/dL
- Antidote
  - Fomepizole: 15 mg/kg IV over 30 minutes
  - Ethanol (100% absolute): 1 mL/kg in 5% dextrose in water over 15 minutes, then 0.16 mL (125 mg)/kg/hour IV
- Dosage: 1–2 mg/kg/dose (maximum, 50 mg/dose) every 6 hr IV, PO

■ Methemoglobin, nitrate, nitrites, sulfonamide
- Diagnostic findings requiring treatment: cyanosis, methemoglobin level ≥30%, dyspnea
- Antidote: methylene blue (1% solution)
- Dosage: 1–2 mg/kg/dose (maximum, 50 mg/dose) every 6 hours IV, PO

■ Narcotics: heroin, codeine, propoxyphene
- Diagnostic findings requiring treatment: respiratory depression, hypotension, coma
- Antidote: Naloxone (Narcan)
- Dosage: 0.1 mg/kg up to 0.8 mg initially IV; if no response, give 2 mg IV

■ Organophosphates: malathion, parathion
- Diagnostic findings requiring treatment: cholinergic crisis—salivation, lacrimation, urination, defecation, convulsions, fasciculations

- Antidote
  - Atropine sulfate: 0.05 mg/kg/dose (usual dose, 1–5 mg; test dose for child 0.01 mg/kg) every 4–6 hr IV or more frequently as needed
  - Pralidoxime: after atropine, 20–50 mg/kg/dose (maximum, 2000 mg) IV slowly (< 50 mg/min) every 8 hours IV as needed × 3

WHEN TO ADMIT

- Any patient strongly suspected of ingesting a toxic or lethal dose of any substance
- An unstable patient
- Any patient requiring gastrointestinal decontamination, intravenous therapy, hemoperfusion, or charcoal perfusion, even if clinically well
- A patient in an environment suggesting child abuse

WHEN TO REFER

- Ingestion of any substance unfamiliar to the primary care physician
- Any patient who may require a therapy unfamiliar to the primary care physician

COMPLICATIONS

- Many poisoned patients require ventilator therapy for such complications as:
  - Pneumothorax
  - Oxygen toxicity
  - Airway infections
  - Nosocomial infections, especially hypostatic pneumonia
  - Urinary tract infection (secondary to catheter placement)
  - Septicemia from vascular catheters
  - Thrombotic and embolic episodes (from vascular catheters)

- Permanent central nervous system damage sometimes follows periods of hypoxia or hypoglycemia, usually before therapy is instituted.
- Skin, mucous membrane, and deeper-tissue injuries often result from acids, substances containing lye, or corrosives.
- Specific compounds can cause permanent organ damage.
- Hazards of treatment for drug overdose include:
  - Overtreatment
    - Occurs when errors are made in assessing the amount of drug ingested
  - Wrong treatment
    - A nontoxic ingestion may be inappropriately treated with potentially toxic antidotes.
    - Mistakes may be made in identifying the drug ingested.
  - Insufficient period of observation
  - Failure to appreciate drug ingestion as an indication of child neglect or abuse
    - Should be particularly suspected in a child <12 months admitted with accidental ingestion or the child who has a history of repeated drug ingestions

PROGNOSIS

- Prognosis depends on the drug ingested, early identification, and treatment at facilities equipped with managing toxic ingestions.

PREVENTION

- Preventive measures, such as child-resistant bottle tops, are effective in eliminating acute, single-dose, unintentional exposures.

Dysmenorrhea

DEFINITION

- Dysmenorrhea (painful menstruation) is a syndrome characterized by
  - Varying degrees of crampy, lower abdominal pain
  - Nausea
  - Vomiting
  - Urinary frequency
  - Low back pain
  - Diarrhea
  - Fatigue
  - Thigh pain
  - Nervousness
  - Dizziness
  - Sweating
  - Headache
- Pain typically begins just after menses and lasts approximately 1–2 days.
  - Can also begin 1–2 days before onset of menses and last up to 4 days into menstruation
  - Cramps may be more severe among teenagers who smoke.

EPIDEMIOLOGY

- Prevalence
  - At least 40–60% of adolescent girls suffer some degree of discomfort during menstruation.
  - ~15% report severe symptoms.
  - 14% report frequently missing school as a result of menstrual symptoms.
- Age
  - Incidence increases with gynecologic age (as does the percentage of ovulatory cycles).
    - Up to 31% of girls report dysmenorrhea in their first year of menses vs 78% in their fifth year.

MECHANISM

- Increased amounts of prostaglandins E_2 and $F_{2\alpha}$ in the endometrium lead to:
  - Smooth-muscle contractions
  - Vomiting
  - Diarrhea
- Correlates with the clinical observation that women who have anovulatory cycles usually do not have dysmenorrhea
  - Adolescent girls typically develop dysmenorrhea 1–2 years after menarche, correlating with the onset of ovulatory cycles.
- The increase in prostaglandin synthesis may be related to changes in serum progesterone levels not seen in anovulatory women.

- Women experience dramatic response with use of prostaglandin synthetase inhibitors or oral contraceptive pills (OCPs), which inhibit ovulation.
- Increased levels of prostaglandin activity are associated with increased uterine tone and high-amplitude myometrial contractions that result in reduced uterine blood flow and onset of pain.

HISTORY

- Assessment of a teenager with dysmenorrhea should include:
  - Complete menstrual history
  - Timing of cramps or pain
  - Episodes of missed school or other activities
  - Ability to participate in social events
  - Presence of nausea, vomiting, diarrhea, dizziness, or other symptoms
  - Medications used, including doses
  - Factors that improve or worsen symptoms
  - Family history of dysmenorrhea or endometriosis
- Consider the possibility that the patient has another, unstated purpose in seeking care.
  - Reluctance to attend school
  - History of physical or sexual abuse
  - Significant psychosocial problems
  - Secretly sexually active and seeking to obtain OCPs for the purpose of contraception
- Causes of secondary dysmenorrhea
  - Can usually be excluded by careful history and physical examination
  - Underlying pathologic conditions should be anticipated when:
    - Pain begins after 20 years of age.
    - There is a history of surgery related to the genitourinary or gastrointestinal tract.
    - Pain is dull and constant rather than crampy.

PHYSICAL EXAM

- Physicians differ in their opinions regarding what examination is necessary to evaluate a patient with dysmenorrhea; in general:
  - For a nonsexually active teenager with mild to moderate menstrual cramps relieved by nonsteroidal antiinflammatory drugs (NSAIDs)
    - Only an external genital examination to rule out hymenal abnormalities is indicated.
  - If dysmenorrhea is unresponsive to NSAIDs:
    - Initiate OCPs for a few cycles without first performing a pelvic examination.

- For a sexually active teenager or for one who is having significant pain that is unresponsive to NSAIDs
  - A thorough pelvic examination is necessary.
  - If pelvic examination is not possible, rectoabdominal examination will provide some useful information about the presence of masses or adnexal tenderness.

DIFFERENTIAL DIAGNOSIS

Primary dysmenorrhea

- Most affected teenage girls have primary dysmenorrhea.
  - Not associated with pelvic or other pathologic conditions
- Secondary dysmenorrhea always should be considered when the patient is evaluated.

Secondary dysmenorrhea

- Endometriosis
  - Functional endometrial glands and stroma are located outside the normal anatomic location in the uterus
  - Therapy with NSAIDs and OCPs fails.
  - A family history of endometriosis can often be elicited.
  - Signs and symptoms
    - Pain may be acyclic rather than cyclic.
    - Menstrual bleeding may be irregular.
    - Gastrointestinal symptoms may be present.
    - May be associated with dyspareunia, tenesmus, and rectal pain
    - Most adolescents generally have normal examinations.
      - Endometriosis can be difficult to detect on clinical grounds alone.
  - Some studies of teenagers with chronic pelvic pain show that 25–38% of those undergoing laparoscopy have endometriosis.
  - In other studies, 52–73% of teenagers with chronic pelvic pain have evidence of endometrial implants.
  - May be difficult to manage
  - Increases risk for infertility
- Pelvic inflammatory disease (PID)
  - Can cause dysmenorrhea acutely
  - Women often develop chronic pelvic pain as a consequence.
  - Even with assurances of confidentiality, some young women may still not admit to sexual activity.
    - Clinicians must maintain a high index of suspicion if historical and physical examination findings suggest PID.
  - A pelvic examination that reveals cervical motion tenderness, adnexal tenderness, or masses strongly suggests PID.
  - Should be treated according to standard antibiotic regimens (see Sexually Transmitted Infections)

- Follow-up is critical; once infected, young women are at risk for:
  - Further episodes of PID
  - Chronic pelvic pain
  - Ectopic pregnancy
  - Infertility
- Outflow tract obstruction
  - Teenagers with a history of genital tract surgery, including abortions, may have outflow tract obstruction.
  - A variety of müllerian anomalies with incomplete obstruction of the outflow tract also produce dysmenorrhea.
  - Depending on the type of obstruction, a pelvic mass may be palpable.
  - Outflow obstruction is possible (eg, a uterus with a blind horn) if:
    - The cervical os is stenotic.
    - The cervix or uterus feels atretic or abnormally shaped.
- Endometrial polyps or fibroids
  - Rare in women <20 years
  - Should be anticipated if menstrual bleeding is:
    - Heavy
    - Prolonged
    - Associated with the passage of clots
  - Unclear whether these entities alone cause dysmenorrhea

LABORATORY EVALUATION

- If sexually active, evaluate for:
  - Sexually transmitted infections
  - Pregnancy

IMAGING

- Pelvic ultrasonography
  - May be useful in defining uterine and vaginal abnormalities associated with obstruction
  - Not helpful in the detection of pelvic or abdominal adhesions or endometriosis

DIAGNOSTIC PROCEDURES

- Confirmation of endometriosis requires laparoscopy.
  - Should be performed by a gynecologist experienced in evaluating adolescents because the lesions of endometriosis in adolescents may differ from the typical lesions seen in adults

TREATMENT APPROACH

■ Treatment of primary dysmenorrhea is likely to include drug therapy.

■ Valuable opportunity to teach the patient about her body

  ● The patient may not understand fully the physiologic mechanisms of menstruation.

  ● The patient may have inaccurate beliefs passed on from mother to daughter.

SPECIFIC TREATMENT

Primary dysmenorrhea

■ NSAIDs

  ● Teenagers who have very mild discomfort benefit from almost any analgesic.

  ● Prostaglandin synthetase inhibitors in the form of NSAIDs are the treatment of choice for most young women with dysmenorrhea.

  ● Dosage and timing vary from patient to patient.

    – Establishing prior use of specific medications as well as doses is important, given that most patients use them suboptimally.

      ■ In 1 study, 57% of adolescents used medications less often than the maximal daily frequency.

      ■ Advising patients of the range of correct doses is important.

  ● Most effective if started at the first sign of menstrual bleeding

    – Women who experience significant nausea with menses may benefit from starting treatment at the earliest symptom of menses, even before bleeding occurs.

  ● Some need medication only for part or all of the first day of menstruation; others require medication for ≥4 days.

  ● Ibuprofen (200–800 mg every 6–8 hours) and naproxen sodium (550 mg immediately and then 275 mg every 6–8 hours) are highly effective.

  ● Mefenamic acid blocks the effect of prostaglandin at the end-organ level and inhibits its production.

    – Can be used in an initial dose of 500 mg, followed by 250 mg every 6 hours

    – Note that there is a black box warning.

  ● Response to different NSAIDs varies.

    – If the patient does not respond to a particular NSAID (eg, ibuprofen), another (eg, naproxen sodium) should be tried

  ● Between 70% and 80% of girls will respond to NSAID therapy.

■ OCPs

  ● OCPs used in the same way as for contraception usually provide relief.

  ● OCPs work by suppressing ovulation and decreasing endometrial prostaglandin production.

  ● Patients should be told that 2–3 cycles may elapse before maximal effect.

  ● If the patient is sexually active, OCPs can be continued on a routine basis.

  ● For the nonsexually active teenager, therapy can be reassessed at 6- to 12-month intervals.

  ● After 3 cycles, adolescent patients using OCPs with 20 μg of ethinyl estradiol and 100 mg of levonorgestrel experienced significant relief of dysmenorrhea compared with those using placebo.

■ Other hormonal contraceptives

  ● In a study of adolescent girls using a contraceptive patch, dysmenorrhea:

    – Decreased in 39%

    – Increased in 11%

    – Resulted in no change in 50%

  ● Depot medroxyprogesterone acetate (DMPA)

    – Used to prevent ovulation and menstrual flow when OCPs are not tolerated or estrogen is contraindicated

  ● Extended oral contraceptive regimen in which OCPs are taken for up to 12 consecutive weeks, followed by 1 hormone-free week

  ● DMPA and extended OCP regimens:

    – Decrease dysmenorrhea

    – Decrease the frequency of menses

■ Other treatments

  ● Some authorities remain skeptical of alternative treatments, and efficacy is unproved.

  ● Other experts recommend:

    – Heat

    – Pelvic exercise

    – General exercise

    – Biofeedback

    – Relaxation therapy

    – Massage

    – Vitamin E

    – Various herbal remedies

  ● Magnesium has been shown to be beneficial in some studies.

  ● Patient should be encouraged to:

    – Exercise

    – Eat a well-balanced diet

– Decrease stress

– Decrease caffeine consumption

– Stop smoking if applicable

WHEN TO REFER

■ The clinician feels uncomfortable prescribing OCPs for the treatment of primary dysmenorrhea.

■ The patient does not respond to NSAIDs and OCPs.

■ The clinical presentation or course suggests that the patient has secondary rather than primary dysmenorrhea.

■ The patient is sexually active and the clinician feels uncomfortable performing a pelvic examination.

WHEN TO ADMIT

■ With PID, some clinicians recommend hospitalization of adolescents for treatment.

■ Others recommend hospitalization under some but not all circumstances (see Sexually Transmitted Infections).

FOLLOW-UP

■ Reevaluate after 2–3 menstrual cycles to determine the effectiveness of the treatment.

Dysphagia

DEFINITION

- Dysphagia is defined as difficulty with swallowing.
  - Derives from the Greek *dys* (difficulty) and *phagia* (to eat)
  - It is not synonymous with *odynophagia*, which refers to painful swallowing.

EPIDEMIOLOGY

- Prevalence
  - Minor feeding problems are reported in 25–35% of normal young children
  - Major feeding disorders observed in 40–70% of:
    - Infants born prematurely
    - Children with chronic medical problems

MECHANISM

- Normal development of swallowing
  - Sucking reflex
    - Present as early as 18 weeks' gestation
    - Initially disorganized
    - Organized and efficient for feeding by 34–36 weeks' gestation.
  - For the infant born at term, the suck reflex is mature and efficient for liquid feedings.
  - Early infancy
    - Development of a more rapid suck rate and higher suck pressure
    - Tongue movements are differentiated and become more coordinated, preparing the infant for pureed food by 5–6 months of age.
  - Later infancy
    - Sensory experience with food increases.
    - Oral motor skills expand to handle more textured food.
    - Gag reflex decreases to allow swallowing of an increasing amount of food with more texture.
  - By age 2 years
    - Chewing and tongue movements become more proficient.
- Normal phases of swallowing
  - Oral
    - Food is mixed with saliva and chewed if needed.
    - A single bolus of food is collected between the roof of the mouth and tongue.
    - The bolus is propelled to the posterior of the tongue and then to the pharynx.
    - In infants and young children, the suckling swallow allows liquid to fall from mouth into the pharynx.
  - Pharyngeal
    - Reflexive swallow stimulated by the presence of food on the posterior tongue.

- The soft palate rises to keep food out of the nasal passage.
- The larynx moves up and forward, closing the glottis.
- The vocal cords come together.
- The epiglottis closes over the airway.
- Respirations cease.
- Food is propelled further by contraction of the pharyngeal muscles and relaxation of the upper esophageal sphincter.
  - Esophageal
    - Esophageal peristalsis moves the food down the esophagus into the stomach through the relaxed lower esophageal sphincter.
    - Lower esophageal sphincter then returns to the closed tonic state to prevent regurgitation of gastric contents.

HISTORY

- Emphasis should be placed on:
  - Birth history
  - Neurodevelopmental history
  - Medical comorbid conditions
  - Detailed feeding history
    - Current diet
      - Texture
      - Route of administration
      - Meal duration
      - Specific food aversions
    - Age at which oral feeding commenced
    - Exposure to taste and textures during sensitive periods
    - Aversive experiences
    - Method of delivering tube feeds
      - Prolonged tube feeding in infancy or childhood can lead to long-term feeding difficulties.
- General symptoms
  - Feeding difficulties
  - Food refusal
  - Failure to thrive
  - Sensation of food stuck in the throat or chest
- Additional symptoms
  - Drooling
  - Difficulty initiating swallowing
  - Change in dietary habits
  - Aversion to certain food textures
  - Unexplained weight loss
  - Change in voice
  - Recurrent coughing
  - Noisy breathing during feeding

D

- Symptoms of specific dysphagias
  - Oral phase
    - Failure to initiate or maintain sucking
    - Prolonged feeding time
    - Drooling
  - Oral hypersensitivity
    - Exaggerated gag reflex
    - Difficulty making the transition to textured foods
    - Sensitivity to touch in and around mouth
  - Oral hyposensitivity
    - Retaining food in the mouth
    - Increased drooling
  - Pharyngeal phase
    - Coughing
    - Choking
    - Noisy breathing during feeding
    - Nasopharyngeal reflux
  - Esophageal phase
    - Spitting up or vomiting
    - Irritability or arching during feeding
    - Preference for liquid food
    - Sensation of food stuck in the throat

PHYSICAL EXAM

- Document any orofacial malformation.
  - Mechanical or obstructive factors generally result in dysphagia for solids.
  - Micrognathia and glossoptosis seen in Pierre Robin sequence may cause feeding difficulty.
  - Cleft lip and palate, including submucous cleft, are important causes of dysphagia.
  - Choanal stenosis may cause difficulty feeding in newborns because of obligate nasal breathing.
- Neurologic examination
  - Assess muscle tone and strength.
  - Evaluate cranial nerve function.
  - Dysphagia for liquids is more pronounced in patients with neurologic disorders.
- Clinical feeding evaluation
  - Performed by an experienced occupational therapist or speech pathologist
  - Includes assessment of:
    - Posture
    - Positioning
    - Oral structure and function
    - Patient motivation
    - Interaction between the infant and feeder

- A variety of foods, positions, and adaptive utensils may be used during the examination.

DIFFERENTIAL DIAGNOSIS

Utility of specific symptoms

- Specific symptoms observed during feeding can help identify the underlying disorder.
  - Gagging, coughing, or emesis
    - Structural or neurologic disorder
  - Repeated swallowing after feeding, fussiness, crying, regurgitation, or nausea
    - Gastroesophageal reflux disease
    - Requires further investigation

Oropharyngeal dysphagia

- Oropharyngeal dysphagia should be considered in young children with:
  - Recurrent aspiration
  - Unexplained respiratory symptoms
    - Coughing
    - Chronic congestion
    - Recurrent choking
    - Acute life-threatening events
    - Recurrent pneumonia
    - Chronic lung disease

Causes of dysphagia

- Prematurity
  - Birth weight <10th percentile for gestational age is a risk factor for dysphagia and feeding difficulties.
- Congenital abnormalities of the nasal and oral cavity
  - Cleft lip or palate
  - Choanal atresia or stenosis
  - Craniofacial anomalies
    - Apert syndrome
    - Crouzon syndrome
    - Möbius sequence
    - Pierre Robin sequence
    - Treacher Collins syndrome
  - Congenital nasal masses
    - Dermoids
    - Encephaloceles
- Congenital anomalies of the larynx, trachea, and esophagus
  - Laryngomalacia
  - Laryngeal clefts
  - Laryngeal stenosis and webs
  - Vocal cord paralysis
  - Tracheoesophageal fistula

- Esophageal atresia
- Esophageal duplication
- Vascular rings
  - Double aortic arch
  - Right aortic arch with left ligamentum from a descending aorta
  - Innominate artery tracheal compression
- Infection
  - Acute pharyngitis or tonsillitis
  - Peritonsillar and retropharyngeal abscesses
  - Epiglottitis
  - Esophagitis (cytomegalovirus, herpesvirus, *Candida albicans*)
- Inflammatory causes
  - Esophagitis secondary to gastroesophageal reflux disease
  - Eosinophilic esophagitis
    - Should be considered in the differential diagnosis of children with unexplained:
      - Oral aversion
      - Feeding difficulties
      - Poor weight gain
- Neurologic or neuromuscular disorders
  - Hypoxic-ischemic encephalopathy
  - Head trauma
  - Cerebral palsy
  - Congenital malformations
    - Arnold-Chiari malformation
    - Absent corpus callosum
  - Degenerative diseases of white and gray matter
  - Brainstem tumors
  - Syringomyelia
  - Infantile spinal muscular atrophy (Werdnig-Hoffmann disease)
  - Diseases of the neuromuscular junction
    - Myasthenia gravis
    - Guillain-Barré syndrome
    - Botulism
  - Muscle disorders
    - Congenital myopathies
    - Mitochondrial diseases
    - Glycogen storage diseases
    - Congenital muscular dystrophy
    - Myotonic dystrophy
- Trauma
  - External trauma
  - Intubation injury
  - Caustic ingestion

- Neoplasms
  - Hemangioma
  - Lymphangioma
- Miscellaneous
  - Foreign body aspiration
  - Achalasia (esophageal motor dysfunction)
  - Epidermolysis bullosa

LABORATORY EVALUATION

- Complete blood count
  - Useful as a screening test for infectious or inflammatory conditions
- Serum protein and albumin
  - Useful for nutritional assessment
- Chromosomal karyotyping, metabolic analysis, specific DNA tests
  - May be required for a specific diagnosis as directed by physical and neurologic examination

IMAGING

- Chest radiography
  - Suspected pneumonia or chronic lung disease
- Magnified airway radiography
  - Infants or children with recurrent stridor or upper airway obstruction
- Computed tomography or magnetic resonance imaging of the brain
  - May be especially helpful in patients with suspected central nervous system injury or structural abnormalities
- Upper gastrointestinal barium study
  - Assess anatomic or structural abnormalities
    - Strictures
    - Fistulae
    - Masses
    - Intestinal rotational anomalies
  - Usually more sensitive than endoscopy in the evaluation of suspected:
    - Achalasia
    - Vascular rings, which appear as a persistent indentation of the esophagus
- Videofluorographic swallowing study (VFSS)
  - Gold standard for assessment of the oral and pharyngeal stages of swallowing
    - Also known as the *modified barium study*
  - Conducted jointly by a radiologist and a speech pathologist or occupational therapist
  - The child drinks or eats foods mixed with barium while radiographic images are observed and recorded.

D

- Provides evidence of all categories of oropharyngeal swallowing dysfunction:
  - Inability or excessive delay in initiation of pharyngeal swallowing
  - Aspiration of food
  - Nasopharyngeal regurgitation
  - Residue of food in the pharyngeal cavity after swallowing
- Allows for testing of the efficacy of compensatory:
  - Dietary modifications
  - Postures
  - Swallowing maneuvers

DIAGNOSTIC PROCEDURES

- Fiberoptic endoscopic evaluation of swallowing (FEES)
  - Permits observation of the pharyngeal phase of swallowing
    - Laryngeal penetration
    - Aspiration
  - A fiberoptic endoscope is introduced into the nose and advanced into the laryngopharyngeal area
    - Swallowing assessment is performed with liquids and a variety of textures, if developmentally appropriate.
    - Typically, dye is added to the food to provide better visualization and to determine residual pooling of food versus saliva.
  - Combined with laryngopharyngeal sensory testing:
    - Has shown that patients with a higher laryngopharyngeal sensory threshold are more likely to experience laryngeal penetration and aspiration during a feeding assessment.
    - Ability to initiate airway closure with stimulation demonstrates airway protection.
    - FEES and sensory testing may be particularly valuable for the evaluation of swallowing safety in children who refuse to ingest adequate amounts of barium to perform VFSS.
- Esophagastroroduodenoscopy
  - Confirms or establishes diagnosis of dysphagia of esophageal origin
    - When appropriate, used to implement therapy
  - Endoscopic and histologic features are required for the diagnosis of eosinophilic esophagitis.
    - Normal appearance of the esophagus during endoscopy does not exclude histopathological esophagitis.
    - Subtle mucosal changes, such as erythema and pallor, may be observed in the absence of esophagitis.
    - During endoscopy, esophageal biopsy should be performed to detect microscopic esophagitis and to exclude causes of esophagitis other than gastroesophageal reflux.

- Particularly useful in evaluating suspected:
  - Strictures
  - Webs
  - Mucosal inflammatory lesions
  - Specific infections
- Esophageal manometry
  - Standard test for disorders of esophageal motility
  - Especially useful in:
    - Establishing a diagnosis of achalasia
    - Detecting esophageal motor abnormalities associated with autoimmune diseases
- Esophageal pH probe study
  - Valid and reliable measure of acid reflux
    - Establishes the presence of abnormal acid reflux
    - Determines whether a temporal association exists between acid reflux and frequently occurring symptoms
    - Assesses the adequacy of therapy in patients who do not respond to treatment with acid suppression
- Scintigraphy
  - Useful in the evaluation of gastric emptying
  - Can demonstrate episodes of aspiration detected during a 1-hour study or on images obtained up to 24 hours after the test feeding is administered
  - Its role in diagnosing gastroesophageal reflux disease in infants and children is unclear.
- Children with suspected neuromuscular disorders may need:
  - Electromyography
  - Nerve conduction studies
  - Muscle biopsy

TREATMENT APPROACH

- Goals
  - Reduce aspiration
  - Improve ability to eat and swallow
  - Optimize nutritional status
- Detect and treat:
  - Surgically or endoscopically treatable structural abnormalities
  - Inflammatory conditions
    - Reflux esophagitis
    - Eosinophilic esophagitis
  - Infections
  - Underlying systemic conditions
- Management of associated disorders
  - Associated disorders may also need to be specifically managed.
- Management often involves a multidisciplinary approach.

SPECIFIC TREATMENT

Normalization of posture and tone

- Head and trunk control are crucial to the development of oral motor skills.
  - Children with neurologic abnormalities frequently have poor head control and poor trunk stability.
- As a basis for improved oral motor function, occupational and physical therapy can be used to improve:
  - Head control
  - Neck and trunk tone
  - Posture

Adaptation of food and feeding equipment

- Change the attributes of food and liquids.
  - Bolus volume
  - Consistency
  - Temperature
  - Taste
- Adjustments in feeding schedule
  - May be beneficial for children receiving continuous tube feeds with supplemental food orally
  - The feeds can be changed gradually to bolus feeds to stimulate the child's appetite.
- Rate of feeding
  - Should be paced to allow sufficient time to swallow before giving another bite
- Bottle or utensils
  - May be changed according to the child's needs

Oral motor therapy

- Focuses on improving the oral phase of feeding
- May include stimulation with:
  - Stroking
  - Stretching
  - Brushing
  - Icing
  - Tapping
  - Vibrating areas of the face and mouth

Nutritional support

- The child's nutritional needs must be met for adequate growth.
  - Supplemental feedings through a nasogastric tube or a percutaneous endoscopic gastrostomy may be necessary.
    - The presence of a feeding tube is not a contraindication to therapy.
    - Many children with feeding disorders have neurologic or anatomic abnormalities that cannot be corrected, making oral feeding difficult or unsafe

Synchronized neuromuscular electrical stimulation to cervical swallowing muscles (VitaStim therapy)

- Improves oral intake in adults
- Helps restore normal swallowing mechanism in adults
- Empirical data are lacking to support its use in children.

WHEN TO REFER

- Referral is warranted:
  - When symptoms are persistent
  - When the cause of dysphagia is unclear
  - On evidence of aspiration
- Referral to a pediatric dysphagia center, if available, provides the most complete method to establish a diagnosis and develop a management plan.
  - Members of the team vary from center to center and usually include a:
    - Gastroenterologist
    - Otolaryngologist
    - Physical medicine and rehabilitation specialist
    - Surgeon
    - Occupational therapist
    - Pediatric dietitian

WHEN TO ADMIT

- Severe feeding difficulties
- Malnutrition
- Failure to thrive
- Dehydration
- Aspiration

FOLLOW-UP

- Patients who are undergoing therapy for dysphagia should be monitored closely for appropriate weight gain.

COMPLICATIONS

- Undernutrition
- Failure to thrive

PREVENTION

- Early recognition, diagnosis, and intervention are necessary, especially in children born prematurely, those with anatomic abnormalities, and those with neuromuscular disorders.

Dyspnea

DEFINITION

- Dyspnea is the feeling of not being able to satisfy air hunger.
- It is a symptom and describes the sensation of breathlessness caused by an underlying disorder.

MECHANISM

- Dyspnea is most commonly seen with exercise because of the increased work of breathing necessary to keep up with increased metabolic demands.
- The sensation is probably transmitted from stretch receptors in the chest wall muscles to the central nervous system (CNS).
- The transmission is processed in the CNS, causing the individual to experience the sensation of dyspnea with exercise.
- In normal breathing, respiratory muscles work only during inspiration, and the diaphragm does most of the work.
  - The work of inspiration is the sum of the work necessary to overcome the elastic forces of the lung, the tissue viscosity of the lung and chest wall, and airway resistance.
  - When any of these factors is increased, the work of inspiration must increase.
  - The accessory muscles of inspiration (the sternocleidomastoid, anterior serratus, and external intercostal muscles) are recruited to accomplish this task.
    - Contraction of these muscles causes forceful expansion of the thorax, resulting in an unusually large negative intrathoracic pressure.
    - This negative pressure draws in the soft tissues of the chest wall and creates a classic sign of dyspnea: retractions.
    - Retractions may be seen in the suprasternal, infrasternal, intercostal, subcostal, and supraclavicular areas.
  - Alternatively, the rate of breathing is increased, resulting in the second classic sign of dyspnea: tachypnea.
- Little energy is expended during normal expiration.
  - Relaxation of the diaphragm, elastic recoil of the lungs and chest wall, and compression of the lungs by the intra-abdominal organs force air from the lungs.
  - In obstructive airway disease, the force generated by these processes may not be great enough to effect adequate expiration.
  - In a child with tachypnea, the elastic recoil may not be fast enough to allow adequate exhalation between breaths.
  - In either instance, accessory muscles of expiration are used.
    - Abdominal recti muscles contract and force the abdominal contents against the diaphragm to compress the lungs.
    - Internal intercostal muscles contract to pull the ribs downward and to create a positive intrathoracic pressure to force the air from the lungs.
    - Contractions of these muscles provide the most important expiratory sign of dyspnea.

- Although dyspnea is a respiratory symptom, it may be caused by primary disorders in other body systems.

HISTORY

- Obtain a complete description of the dyspnea.
  - Onset
    - Sudden, suggesting inhaled foreign body or lung collapse
    - Evolving over time, suggesting asthma or diabetic ketoacidosis
  - Duration
  - Frequency of attacks
  - Any identifiable trigger event
- Quantify the severity of the dyspnea.
  - Ask how daily activities are restricted by shortness of breath.
- Ask whether the dyspnea changes according to patient's position.
  - Dsypnea that is worse when the patient lies with the affected side down:
    - Suggests unilateral lung disease
  - Dyspnea that worsens when the patient is recumbent:
    - Suggests left ventricular failure, obstructive airway disease, or muscle weakness
  - Dyspnea in the upright position that is relieved by lying down:
    - Suggests intracardiac, vascular, or parenchymal lung shunts
- Ask about associated symptoms.
  - Cough
  - Wheezing
  - Sputum production
  - Pleuritic pain
- History (patient and family) of:
  - Allergies
  - Respiratory illness
  - Medications
  - Environmental exposure

PHYSICAL EXAM

- A complete physical examination is necessary, with special attention paid to the cardiac and respiratory systems.
- Observe for retractions in the following areas.
  - Suprasternal
  - Infrasternal
  - Intercostal
  - Subcostal
  - Supraclavicular

- Observe for tachypnea.
  - Measure the respiratory rate.
- Observe for nasal flaring and grunting.
- Observe the abdominal and intercostal muscles during expiration.
- Assess the ratio of inspiration to expiration.
  - In normal respiration, they are of equal length.
  - If inspiration and expiration are equally prolonged, a fixed obstruction may be present.
  - If inspiration is longer than expiration, extrathoracic obstruction may be present.
    - Inspiratory stridor is likely to be present in this setting.
  - If expiration is longer than inspiration, intrathoracic obstruction may be present.
    - If the large airways are involved, rhonchi are present.
    - If the small airways are involved, the patient will be wheezing.
- Observe for signs of chronic lung or heart disease.
  - Barrel chest
  - Clubbing
  - Cyanosis
  - Paradoxical pulse
- Palpate the chest.
  - Tactile fremitus can be a sign of pulmonary consolidation or pleural effusion.
- Percuss the chest.
  - Assess for effusions, consolidation, and abnormal diaphragmatic excursion.
- Auscultate the chest.
  - Listen for rales, rhonchi, and wheezing.
  - Assess for changes in whispered pectoriloquy and egophony.

DIFFERENTIAL DIAGNOSIS

Nonrespiratory causes of dyspnea

General

- Dyspnea is a respiratory symptom, but it may be caused by primary disorders in other body systems.
- The child's age is important.
  - Various disorders occur with different frequencies at different ages.

Exercise-induced dyspnea (EID)

- If EID is severe or occurs after only minimal exertion, further evaluation is warranted.
- Asthma is the most common cause.
- Other causes of EID

- Vocal cord dysfunction
- Exercise-induced laryngomalacia
- Exercise-induced hyperventilation
- Skeletal deformities (eg, scoliosis) that restrict the airway

Vascular pulmonary disease

- Characterized by a decrease in the size of the pulmonary vascular bed.
- Usually due to persistent pulmonary hypertension
- Can also be a result of:
  - Thromboembolitic disease
  - Obliteration (vasculitis)
  - Destruction (emphysema)
- Cardiac findings in pulmonary edema
  - Accentuated P_2
  - Paradoxical splitting of the 2nd and 3rd heart sound
  - Pulmonary injection click
  - Right ventricular heave

Cardiac disease

- Congenital structural anomalies in the heart
- Pump failure (myocarditis or cardiomyopathy)
- Restrictive pericarditis
- Arrhythmia

Hematologic disease

- Severe anemia
  - Chronic or acute
  - Congenital or acquired
- Tissue hypoxia
- Dyspnea

Metabolic disease

- Disorders that increase the body's rate of metabolism and oxygen consumption (eg, hyperthyroidism or fever) can result in dyspnea.
- Disorders that increase production of hydrogen ion and carbon dioxide (eg, diabetic ketoacidosis or aspirin poisoning) can result in dyspnea-like breathing.
- Muscle enzyme deficiencies can result in increased acid production and decreased work tolerance.
- In chronic renal failure, the kidney cannot remove acid from the blood, resulting in dyspnea.

Obesity

- Dyspnea occurs because of increased metabolic requirements for a given amount of work.

Pregnancy

- Dyspnea is normal in pregnancy.
  - Rarely severe and rarely occurs at rest

D

- Dyspnea as a result of cardiac disease in pregnancy begins during the second half of pregnancy and is worst during the 7th month.

Intravenous drug use

- Heroin can cause bronchospasm.
- Heroin and other opioids can precipitate pulmonary edema.
- Infection in intravenous drug users
  - Community-acquired pneumonia is the most common.
  - Opportunistic pulmonary infections
  - Tuberculosis
  - Bacterial endocarditis
  - Talc granulomatosis

Psychogenic causes

- Stress or hysteria
  - Dyspnea does not improve with rest and may worsen.
  - The patient has chest pain.
  - The patient sighs frequently.
  - Paradoxical adduction of the vocal cords has been reported.

Causes of obstructive pulmonary disease

- Obstructive pulmonary disease is characterized by airway narrowing.

Newborns

- Choanal atresia or stenosis
- Dermoid cyst
- Encephalocele
- Nasolacrimal duct cyst
- Hemangioma
- Vocal cord paralysis
- Pierre Robin syndrome
- Ankyloglossia (tongue tie)
- Pertussis
- Tracheal stenosis (postintubation)

Infants

- Foreign body
- Vascular ring
- Tracheal web
- Bronchiolitis
- Asthma
- Cystic fibrosis
- Bronchomalacia
- Pyogenic thyroid
- Accessory thyroid

Children and adolescents

- Foreign body (airway or esophagus)
- Asthma

- Adenopathy
  - Lymphoma
  - Systemic lupus erythematosus
  - Tuberculosis
  - Sarcoidosis
- Croup
- Epiglottitis
- Retropharyngeal abscess
- Enlarged tonsils or adenoids
- Cystic fibrosis
- Anaphylaxis
- Tumors
  - Laryngeal
  - Vocal cord
  - Tracheal
  - Mediastinal
- Vocal cord polyp
- Laryngeal trauma
- Supraglottitis
- Diphtheria
- Bacterial tracheitis
- Ingestion of caustic substance
- Crack cocaine
- Trauma
- Environmental or occupational inhaled toxin exposure

Causes of restrictive pulmonary disease

Cardinal features of restrictive pulmonary disease

- Reduction in lung volume and pulmonary compliance
- Rapid, shallow respirations are usually present.

Newborns

- Hyaline membrane disease
- Hypoplastic lungs
- Pulmonary agenesis
- Eventration of the diaphragm
- Meconium aspiration
- Pneumonia (group B streptococci or gram-negative organisms)
- Diaphragmatic paralysis
- Osteogenesis imperfecta
- CNS depression
  - Hypoxia
  - Congenital
  - Maternal drugs
- Congenital myasthenia gravis
- Aspiration

- Pulmonary edema
- Septicemia
- Congenital heart disease

Infants

- Pneumonia
  - Bacterial
  - Viral
  - Aspiration
- Bronchopulmonary dysplasia
- Wilson-Mikity syndrome
- Hamman-Rich syndrome
- Pulmonary edema
- Infantile botulism
- Congenital lobar emphysema

Children and adolescents

- Skeletal
  - Kyphoscoliosis
  - Ankylosing spondylitis
  - Pectus excavatum
  - Crush chest injury
- Parenchymal
  - Pneumonia
  - Hypersensitivity pneumonitis
  - Systemic lupus erythematosus
  - Scleroderma
  - Fibrosis
  - Toxin inhalation
  - Granulomatous disease
  - Drugs (eg, antineoplastic agents, narcotics)
  - Carcinoma
  - Fat embolus
  - Pneumothorax
  - Pneumomediastinum
- Smoke inhalation
- Pulmonary infarction
- Pulmonary edema
  - Congestive heart failure
  - Sepsis
  - Intracranial disease
  - Croup
  - Epiglottitis
- Neuromuscular
  - Cord transection
  - Myasthenia gravis
  - Muscular dystrophy

- Multiple sclerosis
- Guillain-Barré syndrome
- Pickwickian syndrome
- Toxins
- Pleural effusion
  - Pneumonia
  - Cancer
  - Cardiac disease
  - Hepatic disease
  - Renal disease
  - Rheumatologic disease
- Hypoproteinemia
- Renal failure
- Tumor
- Pulmonary infarction

LABORATORY EVALUATION

- Most useful laboratory tests include:
  - Complete blood count
  - Peripheral blood smear
  - Arterial blood gas measurement
  - Normal with mild obstructive disease
  - Hypoxemia is the first abnormality seen in progressive disease, followed by hypocapnia, then hypercapnia.
  - Hypoexmia and hypocapnia in restrictive pulmonary disease
  - Vascular pulmonary disease shows reduced blood flow through the lungs, resulting in arterial hypoxemia and hypercapnia.
  - Hematologic disease may not show hypoxemia when assessed by arterial blood gas measurement.

IMAGING

- Chest radiograph in obstructive pulmonary disease
  - May reveal hyperinflation
- Chest radiograph in restrictive pulmonary disease
  - Decreased lung volume
  - Pleural thickening and effusions
  - Increased interstitial markings
  - Parenchymal consolidation
  - Skeletal deformities
  - Abnormal movement of the diaphragm
- Chest radiograph in pulmonary edema
  - Increased right ventricular size
  - Enlargement of the pulmonary artery
  - Alterations in pulmonary blood flow

DIAGNOSTIC PROCEDURES

- Use pulse oximetry as a quick, noninvasive means to measure arterial saturation.
- Pulmonary function tests may be useful but may not be immediately available for an acutely ill patient.
- Laryngoscopy, bronchoscopy, and esophagoscopy may be useful to identify a radiolucent foreign body.

TREATMENT APPROACH

- Severe dyspnea is a medical emergency.
  - If not treated promptly, the child may progress to respiratory failure and death.
- Dyspnea in chronic illness
  - There may be no satisfactory therapy for the underlying disease.
  - Relieving the dyspnea can still improve functional ability and quality of life.

SPECIFIC TREATMENT

Severe dyspnea

- Assess the adequacy of the airway.
- Remove foreign bodies, if present.
- Treat bronchospasm with ß-agonists.
- In the postemergent period, evaluate the efficacy of ventilation.
  - If the child cannot effect adequate ventilation, consider the need for mechanical ventilation.
- Assess the heart, peripheral circulation, intravascular volume status, and blood oxygen-carrying capacity.
  - Treat with vasopressors, fluids, blood transfusion, or diuretics, as appropriate.
- Administer oxygen until the cause of dyspnea is known.

Dyspnea in chronic illness

- Sedatives and narcotics can be used to reduce minute ventilation.
- Prostaglandin inhibitors and ß-agonists may blunt the feeling of dyspnea without affecting ventilation.
- Theophylline may improve diaphragmatic contractility.
- Continuous supplemental oxygen reduces ventilatory drive.
- Exercise and proper nutrition can maintain or increase inspiratory muscle mass.

Psychogenic dsypnea

- Calm reassurance
- Occasionally, mild sedation
- Psychotherapy and hypnosis may be required to reduce stress and gain insight in to the cause of the dyspnea.

WHEN TO REFER

- Chronic pulmonary disease
- Congenital or acquired heart disease
- Metabolic disease
- Conditions requiring endoscopy or surgical procedures

WHEN TO ADMIT

- Respiratory failure
- Impending respiratory failure
- Hypoxia while breathing room air

PROGNOSIS

- Prognosis depends on the underlying cause.

Dysuria

DEFINITION

- Pain or burning associated with urination that stems from irritation of the bladder, the urethra, or both

MECHANISM

- Dysuria is a result of any condition that leads to inflammation, irritation, or obstruction of the urinary tract.
- Typically stems from a common disorder, such as:
  - Urinary tract infection (UTI)
  - Urethritis
  - Chemical irritation
  - Trauma

HISTORY

- A thorough history is essential.
- Dysuria is rarely the only symptom.
  - Ask about associated symptoms.
- Ask about family history of nephrolithiasis or other genitourinary problems.
- Nonspecific symptoms not related to the genitourinary system
  - Any of the following suggest a systemic inflammatory condition.
    - Conjunctival erythema
    - Oral lesions
    - Joint pain or swelling
    - Generalized rash
  - Recent fever indicates a systemic infectious condition.
- Specific symptoms related to the genitourinary system
  - Hematuria
  - Malodorous urine
  - Frequency
  - Urgency
  - Incontinence
  - Refusal to void
  - Ask about exposure to chemicals, such as:
    - Detergents
    - Perfumed soaps
    - Bubble baths
    - Medications
- History of voiding dysfunction
  - Delayed toilet training
  - Enuresis
  - Constipation
- Sexual history
  - Ask whether the patient is sexually active.
  - Ask about sexual trauma, masturbation, or abuse.

PHYSICAL EXAM

- Perform routine physical examination.
  - Presence or absence of fever may be indicative of the cause of dysuria.
    - Pyelonephritis: fever usually present and temperature >38.5°C
    - Cystitis: only occasionally produces fever
    - Infectious, chemical, or traumatic urethritis: no febrile response
  - If there is a history of voiding dysfunction, observe the lower back for midline defects.
  - Evaluate the integrity of the lower motor neuron reflex arcs.
    - Check the neurologic integrity of the lower extremities.
    - Elicit the bulbocavernosal reflex.
- Physical examination of the genitourinary tract
  - Palpate the abdomen.
    - Costovertebral tenderness suggests pyelonephritis.
    - Suprapubic tenderness suggests cystitis.
    - Enlarged kidneys or bladder suggests urethral obstruction.
  - Examine the genital area and observe for:
    - Labial adhesions
    - Vesicles
    - Ulcerations
    - In girls, observe for urethral prolapse.
      - Reddened or dark circumferential protrusion of the mucosa from the urethral orifice
  - In boys, note whether the child is circumcised.
    - Note the size and location of the meatus.
  - Observe for vaginal discharge or urethral discharge.
    - Character of the discharge can help to identify the specific pathogen.
      - Cheesy discharge is found in candidal vaginitis.
      - Green discharge is associated with gonorrhea.

DIFFERENTIAL DIAGNOSIS

UTI

- Most common cause of dysuria
- Patient may report suprapubic pain.
- Fever, if present, is usually low grade.
- Children <5 years with their first UTI should be evaluated for congenital anatomic abnormalities.
- Pyelonephritis is suggested by the presence of systemic features.
  - Fever
  - Chills
  - Vomiting

- Flank pain
- Costovertebral angle tenderness

Urethritis

- May result from:
  - Infection
  - Trauma
  - Allergy
  - Foreign body
- Urethral discharge or blood spots on the underwear may be present.
- Infectious urethritis in children is uncommon.
  - May occur in sexually active adolescents
  - May occur in children who have been sexually abused by an infected adult
  - *Neisseria gonorrhoeae* and *Chlamydia trachomatis* are the most common pathogens.
  - Vesicles or genital ulcers may be present in cases of herpes simplex virus infection.

Irritants and trauma

- Local irritants may produce mild erythema.
  - Bubble baths
  - Detergents
  - Perfumed soaps
- Trauma may cause dysuria.
  - Sexual abuse
  - Voluntary sexual activity
  - Masturbation

Vulvovaginitis

- Erythema and inflammation of the vaginal mucosa
- Vaginal discharge is present.
  - Varies from scant whitish to green
  - Foul smelling
- Causes include poor hygiene, allergy, or infection.
  - Pathogens include group A *Streptococcus* and *Shigella*.
    - Vulvar bleeding may be present.
  - *Candida albicans*
    - Usually occurs after recent antibiotic use, in patients with diabetes, and in patients who wear diapers.
    - Pruritusis usually present.

Dysfunctional voiding

- Dyscoordination between the bladder and bladder outlet that results in inefficient bladder emptying
- Neuropathic disorders
  - Spina bifida
  - Transverse myelitis
  - Spinal cord trauma

- Nonneuropathic disorders
  - Functional problems with micturition
- Patients may experience:
  - Incontinence
  - UTIs
  - Constipation

Less common causes of dysuria

- Pelvic inflammatory disease (in sexually active adolescent girls)
  - Fever
  - Abdominal pain
  - Pelvic discomfort
- Balanitis and balanoposthitis
  - Inflammatory lesions of the glans penis or glans penis and prepuce
  - Most common in uncircumcised young boys
  - Infection results from smegma trapped beneath the foreskin.
  - May be a result of trauma or poor hygiene
- Pinworms
  - Caused by *Enterobius vermicularis* parasite
  - Anal pruritus is the symptom, but young children may incorrectly describe this as dysuria.
- Labial adhesions in prepubertal girls may cause:
  - Dysuria
  - Postvoid dribbling
  - UTIs
  - Easy to visualize on inspection
- Urethral strictures
  - Acquired
    - Result of urethral instrumentation, trauma, or inflammation
  - Congenital
  - Symptoms include retention, dysuria, or a weak urinary stream.
- Meatal stenosis (circumcised boys)
  - Typically an upward, deflected, difficult-to-aim urinary stream
  - May be accompanied by:
    - Dysuria
    - Urgency
    - Frequency
    - Prolonged urination

- Urethral prolapse
  - Occurs primarily in black girls
  - Presenting age is 4 years.
  - Vaginal bleeding is the most common symptom.
- Hypercalciuria
  - Patients report:
    - Urinary frequency
    - Hematuria
    - Recurrent UTIs
    - Dysuria

Systemic causes

- Stevens-Johnson syndrome
- Behçet syndrome
- Reiter syndrome
- Varicella

LABORATORY EVALUATION

- Perform a urethral smear and urine culture if urethritis is suspected.
- If vaginal discharge is present, examine sample for:
  - pH
  - Wet preparation
  - Potassium hydroxide
  - Gram stain
  - Culture

IMAGING

- Retrograde urethrography or cystoscopy can confirm a diagnosis of urethral strictures.

TREATMENT APPROACH

- The overall goal is to identify the cause of dysuria and treat appropriately.

SPECIFIC TREATMENT

- Cystitis and UTI—see Urinary Tract Infections
- Suspected sexual abuse
- Antibiotic treatment of vaginitis—see Vaginal Discharge
- Dysfunctional voiding due to neurologic conditions—see Anuria and Oliguria
- Pelvic inflammatory disease and sexually transmitted infections—see Sexually Transmitted Infections
- Labial adhesions
- Balanitis and balanoposthitis
  - Warm soaks
  - Appropriate antibiotic therapy
- Meatal stenosis
  - Refer to a pediatric urologist.
  - Surgical meatomy is the recommended treatment.
- Urethral prolapse
  - Medical treatment
    - Sitz baths
    - Antibiotics
    - Estrogen cream
  - Surgery is recommended if medical treatment fails.

WHEN TO REFER

- Voiding dysfunction
- Nephrolithiasis
- Girls <5 years with a UTI for the first time
- Boys of any age with a UTI
- Genitourinary tract anomalies

WHEN TO ADMIT

- Systemic inflammatory or infectious cause of dysuria
- Suspicion of sexual abuse

Edema

DEFINITION

- Edema is the accumulation of fluid in the interstitial tissues.
  - Results from disruption of forces that control normal fluid movement out of and into capillaries
  - May result from many different disease states
  - Diagnosis of the underlying cause is generally apparent, but it may be subtle.
  - Intervention may initially need to be supportive.
    - Once a patient is stable, efforts to treat the underlying cause of the edema should be pursued.
    - Services of a specialist may be required.

MECHANISM

- Fluid distribution between the intravascular compartment and the interstitial compartment results from the interplay of:
  - Oncotic pressure
  - Hydrostatic pressure
  - Capillary membrane permeability
  - Disruption of these forces can result in edema.
    - Sodium concentration is usually the ultimate controller of this fluid movement.
- An increase in capillary membrane permeability is often the result of cytokines released from inflammation.
  - Infections and burns tend to cause localized edema.
  - An allergic reaction may cause more generalized edema.
  - Hereditary angioedema can cause localized edema of the gastrointestinal tract and larynx.
  - Trauma causes local edema.
- A decrease in the capillary oncotic pressure can be caused by decreased levels of protein (usually from albumin in the blood).
  - Decreased synthesis of albumin occurs
    - In patients with cirrhosis
    - As a result of malnutrition or intestinal malabsorption
- Protein loss by the kidneys in nephrotic syndrome may also contribute to edema.
  - Albumin levels <2 mg/dL are usually associated with generalized edema.
  - The mechanism of edema formation with decreased oncotic pressure results in extravasation of fluid into the interstitium.
    - It also results in poor kidney perfusion.
    - Activates renin-aldosterone secretion and results in:
      - Increased sodium reabsorption
      - Fluid retention
      - Increased capillary hydrostatic pressure
    - All of which compounds the formation of edema.

- Systemic venous hypertension can be the result of:
  - Heart failure
  - Constrictive pericarditis
  - Cardiomyopathy
  - Tricuspid valvular disease
  - Cirrhosis
  - All of these conditions increase the capillary hydrostatic pressure and result in edema from increased extravasation of fluid into the interstitium.
    - Left-ventricular heart failure results in pulmonary edema.
    - Right-ventricular heart failure results in venous congestion, hepatomegaly, and peripheral edema.
- Localized edema may result from
  - Increased venous pressure with deep-vein thrombosis
  - Compression of the inferior vena cava or iliac vein by a tumor
  - Increased venous pressure raises the capillary hydrostatic pressure.
- All of the conditions below lead to increased plasma volume through a similar mechanism:
  - Renal disease
    - Glomerulonephritis
    - Nephrotic syndrome
    - Renal failure
  - Heart failure
  - Liver disease
    - Cirrhosis
  - Increased sodium reabsorption in the kidney leads to increased water reabsorption and increased plasma volume.
    - Activation of the renin-angiotensin-aldosterone system
    - Sympathetic nervous stimulation can also result in increased sodium reabsorption in the kidney.
- Increased interstitial hydrostatic pressure, although rare, may result from lymphatic obstruction.
  - By a tumor or large lymph nodes
  - From damage to the lymphatic system by radiation or surgery
  - From parasitic infections such as filariasis

HISTORY

- A detailed history must be obtained to discover the cause of the edema.
- The time course of the edema—whether its onset is recent or chronic—is particularly important.
  - If chronic, then the parents and child may report:
    - Weight gain
    - Tight clothing
    - Snug-fitting shoes
  - Parents may have attributed findings to normal growth.

- History of a recent illness, such as pharyngitis, is important for the diagnosis of glomerulonephritis.
- Other systemic complaints may be present, which may indicate the presence of heart failure and pulmonary edema.
  - Shortness of breath
  - Tachypnea
  - Cough
- Ascites, a form of localized edema, is seen with liver failure or cirrhosis and with some congenital liver malformations.
- The child's nutritional status should be assessed.
  - Malnutrition may result in hypoalbuminemia, which can result in edema.

PHYSICAL EXAM

- Edema may be generalized or localized.
  - If localized, edema is very apparent when it affects an extremity.
    - Deep-vein thrombosis
    - Cellulitis
    - Burn
  - Edema may be more occult.
    - Pulmonary edema from left-ventricular heart failure
    - Ascites from liver disease
  - Generalized edema may include scrotal or labial edema.
    - Findings related to generalized edema may depend on whether the patient has been lying down (sacral edema) or standing (feet and lower legs).
    - Chronic edema may result in bedsores.
- Physical examination should begin with close observation of the vital signs.
  - Tachypnea may indicate pulmonary edema.
  - Increased blood pressure may be present in glomerulonephritis and renal failure.
  - Fever and localized edema may be present with cellulitis.
  - Periorbital edema is generally found with nephrotic syndrome and glomerulonephritis.
  - Crackles or rales may indicate the presence of pulmonary edema.
  - A gallop may indicate heart failure.
  - With ascites, the following may be present:
    - Abdominal distention
    - Shifting dullness
    - A fluid wave
  - A distinction may be made between pitting and nonpitting edema.
    - *Nonpitting edema* is often the result of lymphedema.
    - *Pitting edema* is the result of increased membrane permeability, increased hydrostatic pressure, or decreased oncotic pressure.

DIFFERENTIAL DIAGNOSIS

- Renal causes of edema
  - Nephrotic syndrome
    - The presence of proteinuria with low serum albumin is highly suggestive of nephrotic syndrome.
  - Glomerulonephritis
    - Assess for the presence of:
      - Red cell casts
      - Hematuria
      - Cola-colored urine
  - C3 levels may be needed to help distinguish between the types of glomerulonephritis.
  - For nephrotic syndrome, levels of C3, C4, or antinuclear antibody can help exclude lupus or membranoproliferative glomerulonephritis.
  - Bilateral hydronephrosis in an infant boy with edema may be the result of posterior urethral valves.
  - Congenital renal anomalies may produce ultrasound results of small or malformed kidneys and clinical findings of renal failure.
  - Children with undiagnosed reflux nephropathy may have severe hydronephrosis and renal failure.
- Cardiovascular causes of edema
  - Congestive heart failure
  - Deep-vein thrombosis
  - Embolic disease
  - Vasculitis
  - Constrictive pericarditis
- Hematologic causes of edema
  - Severe anemia can result in edema, especially in a newborn.
  - Edema can be the result of:
    - Hemolysis from ABO blood type or Rh incompatibility
    - Glucose-6-phosphate dehydrogenase deficiency
- Endocrine or metabolic causes of edema
  - Thyroid disease
  - Starvation
  - Hereditary angioedema
- Gastrointestinal causes of edema
  - Cirrhosis
  - Protein-losing enteritis
  - Cystic fibrosis
  - Celiac disease
  - Enteritis
  - Lymphangiectasis
  - Lymphatic abnormalities
  - Milk protein allergy
  - Inflammatory bowel disease

E

- Hypoalbuminemia without proteinuria suggests:
  - Synthesis defect found with chronic liver disease.
  - A protein-losing enteropathy.
- Prothrombin time is a good marker of the liver's ability to synthesize protein.
  - Should be assessed when hypoalbuminemia is present without proteinuria.
- Liver function tests may also provide helpful information.
  - Analysis of stool α1-antitrypsin will help diagnose protein-losing enteropathy.
- Venous thrombosis
  - If venous thrombosis is suspected, then coagulation studies should be conducted.
    - Especially if no predisposing factor, such as an indwelling catheter is present.
    - A Doppler ultrasound examination should be performed to assess the blood flow in the area that may be affected by the thrombosis.
- Enteropathy
  - The presence of increased fat in fecal matter strongly suggests intestinal malabsorption.
  - Determining which intestinal disorder may be the cause of the hypoalbuminemia requires further testing and consultation with a gastroenterologist.
    - Cystic fibrosis
    - Inflammatory bowel disease
    - Milk protein allergy
    - Enterokinase deficiency
    - Celiac disease
    - Intestinal lymphangiectasia

LABORATORY EVALUATION

- Initial testing may include:
  - Urinalysis
  - Complete blood count
  - Electrolytes with blood urea nitrogen and creatinine
  - Liver function tests (liver enzymes as well as serum albumin, prothrombin time and partial thromboplastin time)
  - Testing for fecal fat is appropriate if intestinal malabsorption is suspected.
    - α1-antitrypsin may be helpful for diagnosing protein-losing enteropathy.
  - With angioedema levels of C1 esterase inhibitor are low.
    - Whether hereditary or acquired
  - When serum albumin is normal, depending on the clinical circumstance, thyroid function tests may be required.

IMAGING

- When serum albumin level is normal, depending on the clinical circumstance, chest x-ray may be required.
- Renal and abdominal ultrasound examination may be appropriate.
  - Bilateral hydronephrosis is usually demonstrated on a renal ultrasound.

DIAGNOSTIC PROCEDURES

- When serum albumin is normal, depending on the clinical circumstance, electrocardiogram may be required.

TREATMENT APPROACH

- Initial management involves determining whether the patient should be admitted to the hospital.
  - Many causes of edema require admission, including:
    - Presence of respiratory distress that results from airway swelling as in angioneurotic edema
    - Heart failure with pulmonary edema
    - Previously undiagnosed renal failure
    - Acute glomerulonephritis
    - Nephrotic syndrome
    - Oliguria from renal failure or poor renal perfusion
    - Previously unrecognized cirrhosis
    - Respiratory distress resulting from the ascites
    - Localized edema that results from venous thrombosis or lymphatic obstruction
  - Admission is needed to assess and treat the underlying cause.
- Ongoing management depends on the underlying cause of the edema.

SPECIFIC TREATMENT

General

- Most patients with renal disease benefit from a low-sodium diet.
- Fluid restriction may help, but should be used cautiously on an individual-patient basis in consultation with a nephrologist.
- Diuretics may be needed but should be used cautiously.
- If plasma volume is decreased, then fluid expansion with colloid followed by diuretics may be necessary.

Anemia

- Severe anemia may need to be treated with transfusion.
  - A hematologist should be consulted if the cause of the anemia is not readily apparent.

Ascites

- A low-sodium diet is generally helpful.
- Diuretics may be beneficial, especially spironolactone.
- When possible, treating the underlying cause of the ascites is critical.

Heart failure

- Treating heart failure may require inotropic medications.
  - Digoxin
  - Dobutamine
  - Angiotensin-converting enzyme inhibitor may help with afterload reduction.
  - If congenital heart disease is the cause of heart failure, surgical repair of the underlying structural lesion is the ultimate treatment.

Venous thrombosis

- When venous thrombosis is present, anticoagulation therapy may be indicated.
  - Consultation with a hematologist and possibly a vascular surgeon may be necessary.
  - In the absence of an obvious predisposing factor, investigation for an underlying coagulopathy is appropriate.

Enteropathy

- For patients with enteropathy, treatment depends on the cause.
  - A gastroenterologist should be consulted.

Hypothyroidism

- Generally, myxedema is found with hypothyroidism.
  - Responds to treatment with thyroid hormone replacement

WHEN TO REFER

- Many disorders that cause edema may require the assistance of a specialist.
- A referral to a specialist should be considered if evidence exists of
  - Liver disease (ie, ascites)
  - Renal disease (glomerulonephritis, nephritic syndrome)

- Anemia
- Protein depleting enteropathy or increased fecal fat with malabsorption with secondary hypoalbuminemia
- Heart failure

WHEN TO ADMIT

- Many of the causes of edema are serious medical problems that require admission.
  - This approach may initially be for support.
  - Once a diagnosis is established and the patient is stable, further treatment usually continues on an outpatient basis with assistance of a specialist.
- Any of the following may require admission:
  - Respiratory distress
  - Heart failure
  - Renal failure
  - Acute glomerulonephritis or nephrotic syndrome
  - Oliguria from renal failure should result in emergent admission.
  - Edema caused by previously unrecognized cirrhosis
  - Localized edema that results from venous thrombosis or lymphatic obstruction
  - Anemia severe enough to require a transfusion

PROGNOSIS

- Prognosis depends on the underlying cause and the appropriateness of treatment.

E

Encopresis

DEFINITION

- Soiling
  - Voluntary or involuntary passage of feces into the clothing
- Retentive encopresis
  - Leakage of fecal material involuntarily from an impaction
- Nonretentive encopresis
  - Passage of normal bowel movement into underwear rather than the toilet

EPIDEMIOLOGY

- Prevalence
  - ~2% of children in kindergarten and first grade are affected.
- Sex
  - Boy-to-girl ratio is 3:1.

ETIOLOGY

- Organic basis for retentive encopresis in <5% of cases
  - Constipating medication
  - Constipating diet
  - Chronic anal fissure
  - Perianal cellulitis
  - Hypothyroidism
  - Anal or rectal stenosis
  - Pelvic mass
  - Hirschsprung disease
- Most children who hold back stool do so:
  - In an attempt to avoid the pain associated with passage
  - Because they are enmeshed in a control issue with a parent
- Approximately 10–20% of children with encopresis are not constipated.
  - Preschoolers often resist bowel training deliberately.
  - School-aged children postpone bowel movements (BMs).
    - They do not want to leave some enjoyable activity (eg, video games).
    - They do not want to use public toilets (eg, school bathrooms).

SIGNS AND SYMPTOMS

- Patient or parent reports:
  - Constipating medication
  - Constipating diet
- Findings on physical examination
  - Chronic anal fissure
  - Perianal cellulitis
  - Delayed linear growth
    - Indicates hypothyroidism
- Mass on rectal examination
  - Dilated rectum packed with stool (often 6–10 cm across)
  - Impacted stool usually has the consistency of wet clay.
- Rectal ampulla empty, rectum tight
  - Hirschsprung disease
- Retentive encopresis
  - Palpable abdominal mass
    - Usually involves only the rectosigmoid area but may extend throughout the colon
    - Midline, suprapubic, irregular, and moveable
    - Can be missed if the rectus abdominis muscles are not relaxed
    - Protuberant abdomen may be caused by backup of gas and stool
  - Fecal matter protruding from the anal opening
- Nonretentive encopresis
  - Normal abdominal examination
  - Rectal vault contains:
    - Stool of normal caliber
    - Nothing, if the child has evacuated recently

DIFFERENTIAL DIAGNOSIS

- Retentive encopresis
  - Symptoms of constipation
  - Soiling many times per day
  - Small stools
  - Loose stools
  - Need for laxatives, suppositories, or enemas
  - Abdominal mass present
  - Abdominal distention
  - The anal canal may be full
  - Rectum packed with stool
  - Periodic pain or crying with BMs
  - Blood on the toilet tissue
  - Passage of a huge BM that clogs the toilet
  - Posturing that suggests deliberate holding back
- Nonretentive encopresis
  - No constipation
  - Soiling once per day
  - Stool of normal size
  - Stool of normal consistency
  - No need for laxatives, suppositories, or enemas
  - No abdominal mass
  - No abdominal distention
  - Empty anal canal
  - Normal rectum

DIAGNOSTIC APPROACH

- Thorough history to distinguish between retentive and nonretentive encopresis
- Review diet.
  - Milk products
  - Fruit juice
  - Fiber
- Question child's use of the toilet.
  - How many times per day?
  - Is sitting spontaneous or prompted by parents or teachers?
- If the stool pattern is unknown, the parent should be sent home with a soiling diary to complete for the child.

LABORATORY FINDINGS

- Urinalysis
  - For nitrite and pyuria
    - To screen for urinary tract infection, especially if associated with enuresis
- Culture for group A *Streptococcus* if abnormal perianal erythema is present
- Thyroid function tests if warranted

IMAGING

- Plain film, postvoiding, supine abdominal radiography
  - Needed to determine whether the patient is impacted (eg, abdominal fullness but empty rectum)
  - For a sexually abused child who might be emotionally traumatized by a rectal examination
  - If child refuses rectal examination
- Radiologic findings
  - Grossly dilated rectum
  - Granular stool
  - Increased stool in the transverse and descending colon
- Barium enema
  - Only if Hirschsprung disease is strongly suspected
  - For children with repeated treatment failures, to reassure the family (and physician) that some rare diagnosis has not been overlooked

DIAGNOSTIC PROCEDURES

- Rectosigmoid manometric study
  - In suspected Hirschsprung disease

CLASSIFICATION

- Soiling
- Retentive encopresis
- Nonretentive encopresis

TREATMENT APPROACH

- Retentive and nonretentive encopresis must be addressed separately.
- Retentive encopresis
  - Hyperphosphate enemas (1 daily for 2 or 3 days) to remove impaction
  - Mineral oil, polyethylene glycol, or lactulose for 3 months to keep the stools soft
  - Senna laxatives if stool softeners are ineffective
  - Sitting on the toilet for 10 minutes after meals
  - Nonconstipating high-fiber diet
    - Such foods as popcorn, grains, fruits, and vegetables
  - Limited consumption of milk products
    - ~10% of children with impactions are drinking great amounts of milk (>32 oz per day).
    - Milk intake can be limited to 16 oz per day in children >1 year.
    - Fluid requirements for these children can be met with fruit juices.
      - Pear, peach, and prune juices have high sorbitol content that can increase the frequency of stools.
- Nonretentive encopresis
  - Medications are not needed.
  - Stop all reminders, lectures, or punishments.
  - Give incentives for BMs into the toilet.
  - For soiling, insist on immediate cleanup.
  - Refer treatment failures.

SPECIFIC TREATMENTS

Retentive encopresis

Disimpaction

- The traditional approach is daily sodium phosphate enema for 2 or 3 days.
  - Excessive doses of phosphate enemas can cause tetany, dehydration, or death.
  - If the child refuses an enema, administer high-dose mineral oil or polyethylene glycol (Miralax) orally for ~4 days.
- These approaches may be combined, starting with mineral oil or polyethylene glycol orally and followed by enemas on day 3.
- Occasionally, enemas must be administered in the office or clinic.

Stool softeners

- First line of therapy for constipation
- Appropriate for long-term treatment
- Administered orally
- Begun as soon as the impaction is eliminated

- Goal is the passage of 1 or 2 normal-sized BMs per day.
- Continued for 3 months
  - It takes 3 months for bowel diameter and tone to return to normal.
- Mineral oil
  - 1–2 mL/kg twice daily
  - Adolescents: 60 mL/dose (max 8 oz/day)
  - Contraindicated in children who:
    - Have gastroesophageal reflux or vomiting
    - Are not yet walking
  - Emulsified derivatives of mineral oil taste better but are more expensive.
- Lactulose
  - 0.5–1.0 mL/kg twice daily
  - Adolescents: 15 mL twice daily (max 3 oz/day)
- Polyethylene glycol (Miralax)
  - 0.5 g/kg/day
  - Adolescents: 17 g/day
- Milk of magnesia
  - 1–2 mL/kg/dose
  - Adolescents: 30–60 mL

Stimulant laxatives

- Recommended if stool softeners are not effective
  - Usually needed for children who deliberately hold back BMs or for those who have developed megarectum and megacolon (see table Medications for Constipation)
- Treatment failure and recurrence usually are due to undermedicating.
  - Increase dose if child is not having a normal-sized BM daily.
  - Some children temporarily require doses that exceed the standard dose recommended by textbooks and the package insert.
  - Children can be tapered off laxatives successfully, even after 6 months.
  - Continue medications until the child has gone ≥1 month without any soiling.
  - Taper medications gradually over 1–2 months.
- Senokot (senna)
  - <5 years: 1–2 tsp syrup/day
  - ≥5 years: 2–3 tsp syrup
  - Adolescents: 1 tbsp/day (max 2.5 tbsp or 8 tablets)
- Fletcher's Castoria
  - <5 years: 1–2 tsp/day
  - ≥5 years: 2–3 tsp
  - Adolescents: 2 tbsp max

- Ex-Lax (senna)
  - >5 years: 1 square/day
  - Adolescents: 2 squares
- Dulcolax, 5-mg tablet
  - >5 years: 5 mg/day
  - >12 years: 10 mg (2 tablets)
  - Adolescents: 4 tablets max
- Rectal suppositories
  - Glycerin suppository
    - 1 or 2 suppositories
  - Dulcolax, 10-mg suppository
    - >2 years: 1 suppository
- Enema for disimpaction
  - Mineral oil enema
    - 1–2 oz/20 lb of body weight/day
    - Adolescents: 4 oz
  - Sodium phosphate enema (Fleet)
    - 1 oz/20 lb of body weight/day
    - Adolescents: 4 oz (max 8 oz)

Oral disimpaction

- Mineral oil
  - 1 oz per year of age/day
  - Max dose: 8 oz/day
- Polyethylene glycol (Miralax)
  - 0.5 g/kg 3 times daily
  - Max 25 g, or 1.5 capful 3 times daily

Toilet habits

- The child must sit on the toilet for ≥10 minutes once a day with a timer.
  - The gastrocolic reflex takes effect 20–30 minutes after a meal (especially breakfast).
  - Should be used to advantage
  - Any treatment that neglects this opportunistic timing will fail.
- Children who have been impacted for many months have no urge to defecate.
  - The defecation urge may not return until the rectum is kept empty for 1–2 weeks.
  - Child should be instructed to flex the hips to open the rectum, to use a footstool for leverage, and to apply some pressure to the abdomen while pushing down.
  - If they have no BM for 24 hours, then these children need to sit on the toilet more often and longer each time.
  - Soiling (leakage) requires:
    - Sitting on the toilet
    - Cleanup

Medications for Constipation

Medication		Dosage	Comments
Stool Softeners	Mineral oil	• 1–2 mL/kg per dose twice daily • Adolescents: 60 mL/dose (max 8 oz/day)	• Do not use in children who have gastroesophageal reflux or vomiting or who are not yet walking. • Emulsified types (Petrogalar, plain Agoral, Kondremul) taste better.
	Lactulose	• 0.5–1.0 mL/kg per dose twice daily • Adolescents: 15 mL twice daily (max 3 oz/day)	This is a prescription item.
	Polyethylene glycol (Miralax)	• 0.5 g/kg per day • Adolescents: 17 g/day	This is a prescription item.
	Milk of Magnesia	• 1–2 mL/kg per dose • Adolescents: 30–60 mL	1 Milk of Magnesia tablet = 2.5 mL liquid.
Stimulant laxatives	Senokot (senna)	• <5 yr: 1–2 tsp syrup/day • >5 yr: 2–3 tsp syrup/day • Adolescents: 1 tbsp/day (max 2.5 tbsp or 8 tablets)	1 tablet = 3 mL granules = 5 mL syrup.
	Fletcher's Castoria	• <5 yr: 1–2 tsp/day • >5 yr: 2–3 tsp/day • Adolescents: 2 tbsp max	—
	Ex-Lax (senna)	• >5 years: 1 square/day • Adolescents: 2 squares	Chewable squares
	Dulcolax, 5-mg tablet	• >5 yr: 5 mg/day • >12 yr: 10 mg (2 tablets)/day • Adolescents: 4 tablets max	Liquid form not available
Rectal suppositories	Glycerin suppository	1 or 2 suppositories	
	Dulcolax suppository, 10 mg	>2 yr: 1 suppository	
Enema for disimpaction	Mineral oil enema	• 1–2 oz/20 lb of weight daily • Adolescents: 4 oz	Squeeze-bottle size: 4.5 oz
	Sodium phosphate enema (Fleet)	• 1 oz/20 lb of weight/day • Adolescents: 4 oz (max 8 oz)	Squeeze-bottle size: 2.25 oz children, 4.5 oz adult
Oral disimpaction	Mineral oil	• 1 oz/yr of age daily • Max dose: 8 oz/day	—
	Polyethylene glycol (Miralax)	• 0.5 gm/kg per dose 3 times daily • Max 25 g or 1.5 caps 3 times daily	—

E

- Preschoolers and toddlers:
  - May refuse to sit on the toilet
  - May hold back stools when forced to sit on the toilet
  - The goal is to produce a BM daily.
    - Pediatricians and parents need to lower their expectations.
    - The child can be told that the "poop wants to come out every day and it needs your help."
    - Going in the diaper is fine.
      - The child is not put back in diapers full-time.
      - The diaper is made available when child needs to release a stool.
    - This approach prevents the child from bladder control regression.

Nonretentive encopresis

- Stool softeners, laxatives, and enemas are not needed.
- For children who simply postpone BMs:
  - Admonition "to find a toilet whenever you feel rectal pressure" or "don't make your body wait" usually removes the symptom.
- Stop all reminders, lectures, or punishments.
  - Parents should be reassured that nothing more can be taught to their child.
  - To eliminate the control issue, the parents should be told to let the child decide when the need exists to go to the bathroom.
    - Reminders, inquiries, and lectures are a form of pressure, and pressure does not work.
  - Parents should not threaten punishment.
    - Many young children try to hold back all BMs to avoid punishment for soiling.
    - Parents should be told about the importance of not punishing their child for soiling.
    - Child should be reassured that soiling will no longer incur punishment.
- Give incentives for BMs into the toilet.
  - Immediate positive feedback, such as praise, a hug, or a sticker/stars on a chart
  - Major incentives may be offered to achieve breakthrough with some children who have never had a BM into a potty chair or toilet.
- Soiling should not be ignored.
  - Immediate cleanup
  - Parents should help the child change clothes.
  - Changing should be a neutral, timely interaction.

- Most children with nonretentive encopresis are resistant to toilet training.
- If initial behavioral methods above are not helpful, more intensive psychological or family interventions are needed.

WHEN TO ADMIT

- Hospitalization rarely is needed for children with constipation.
- For severe impactions involving the entire colon, possible hospitalization for polyethylene glycol-electrolyte solution by nasogastric tube for 8–24 hours

WHEN TO REFER

- Refer to a mental health professional in the following situations:
  - Nonretentive encopresis unresponsive to pediatric management
  - Child >5 years who refuses to sit on the toilet
  - Child who refuses to take medications
  - Child >8 years with nonretentive encopresis
  - Child with nonretentive encopresis who deliberately passes BMs on family possessions or at school (overt anger)
  - Child who is depressed
  - Severely disturbed parent-child relationship

FOLLOW-UP

- Follow up ~1 week into treatment.
  - >30% still will be impacted.
  - Some children need enemas in the office.
- If a child still is impacted at the follow-up examination, a more detailed explanation of the disimpaction process is necessary.
- Repeat abdominal examination even if patients report that the child is having normal BMs and no soiling.
  - Children who have an impaction can keep themselves clean temporarily by making a superhuman effort at control and sitting on the toilet several times a day.

COMPLICATIONS

- Secondary emotional problems
  - Shame
  - Constant fear of exposure
  - Many children with encopresis are scapegoated at home, teased by peers, and ostracized at school.

PROGNOSIS

- 99% of children who have mainly pain-related impaction are cured by pediatric management.
- ~70% of children who have psychogenic impaction are successfully treated by the pediatrician.
  - The remainder need to work with a mental health professional
- Nonretentive encopresis
  - Good results if the problem is recent
  - Poor results if the problem is long-standing (>5 years)
- In mildly resistant children, primary care management can achieve a 90–95% cure rate.
- Children who have severe resistance need early referral.

PREVENTION

- Back-up plans for preventing relapses
  - Increased dose of stool softener or laxative if >48 hours without a normal-size BM

- Child is at risk for recurrent impaction if soiling occurs more than twice over a few days.
  - Double dose of laxative, a suppository, or an enema
    - Merely mentioning an enema sometimes results in the child sitting on the toilet and producing a BM.
  - For older children who are cooperative about sitting on the toilet, sitting there for 10 minutes out of every hour will usually relieve an early impaction.
  - The family should be made to realize that soiling always means that the rectum is full and the impaction is returning.
- Primary care interventions may fail due to:
  - Rectal hyposensitivity acquired from prolonged stretching of the rectum
  - Inability to relax the external anal sphincter caused by voluntary attempts to prevent stool leakage or pain
  - Both of these conditions usually recede once stool impaction is permanently resolved with more aggressive interventions.

Enterovirus Infections

DEFINITION

- Enteroviruses are *Picornaviridae*, small RNA viruses.
- Traditionally classified into 3 groups:
  - Polioviruses
  - Coxsackieviruses
  - Enteric cytopathogenic human orphan viruses (echoviruses)
- Classification is based on disease produced in humans and animals.
- Modern molecular genetic analysis has allowed a better understanding of the relationships among the various enterovirus serotypes.
  - The current taxonomy divides the enteroviruses into 4 species: human enterovirus A, B, C, and D (see table Classificaton of Enteroviruses).
  - Except for those reclassified as nonenteroviral, individual serotypes have retained their traditional names.
  - Newly identified enteroviruses are designated by number, starting with EV68 up to the most recently identified EV101.

EPIDEMIOLOGY

- Prevalence
  - In the US, ~15 million cases of symptomatic enterovirus infections occur every year.
  - ≥90% of infections are clinically silent.
  - Reinfection is common.
  - Nonpolio enteroviruses are the major cause of hospitalization in febrile infants <3 months of age.
    - Resulted in hospitalization in 2% of infants in the first month of life
    - Accounted for 82% of admissions for suspected sepsis
- Paralytic disease with wild-type poliovirus has been eradicated in the Western Hemisphere.
  - No cases have occurred in the US since 1979.
  - Outbreaks continue in parts of South Asia and Africa.
- Enteroviruses and parechoviruses are the most commonly identified viral infections in neonates, with mortality as high as 10%.
- The economic impact of enteroviral aseptic meningitis is estimated to be >$1.5 billion annually.
- Host
  - Age correlates inversely with the severity of clinical disease.
    - An individual becomes immune to an increasing number of serotypes over several seasons.
    - Neonates may develop fatal sepsis rapidly.
    - Most older children and adults have mild or no symptoms.
  - Some enteroviral syndromes are severe at any age.
    - Poliomyelitis
    - Acute hemorrhagic conjunctivitis
    - Myocarditis
  - In childhood, boys seem to suffer more infections and more diseases than girls.
  - Individuals with humoral immunodeficiencies may have chronic, debilitating infection.
    - Except for poliovirus, enteroviral infection does not seem to pose a particular threat to individuals who have cancer or AIDS.
    - Recipients of bone marrow transplants may experience severe or prolonged infection.

Classification of Enteroviruses[a,b]

Traditional Taxonomy	Current Taxonomy
Polioviruses • PV1–3	Human enterovirus A (HEV-A) • CAV2–8, 10, 12, 14, 16; EV71, 76, *89–91*
Coxsackie A viruses • CAV1–22, 24	Human enterovirus B (HEV-B) • CAV9; CBV1–6; E1–7, 9, 11–21, 24–27, 29–33; EV69, 73–75, 77–78, *79–88, 100–101*
Coxsackie B viruses • CBV1–6	Human enterovirus C (HEV-C) • CAV1, 11, 13, 17, 19–22, 24; PV1–3
Echoviruses • E1–7, 9, 11–21, 24–27, 29–33	Human enterovirus D (HEV-D) • EV68, 70
Numbered enteroviruses • EV68–71	

[a] Enterovirus 79–101, which are not yet included in the International Committee on Taxonomy of Viruses classification, are shown in italics. The gaps in numbering result from changes in classification.

[b] From: Khetsuriani N, LaMonte-Fowlkes A, Oberste MS, et al, Centers for Disease Control and Prevention. Enterovirus surveillance—United States, 1970-2005. *MMWR*. 2006;55(No SS-8):1–20.

- Virus
  - Most enteroviral syndromes are not serotype specific.
  - Several different types may produce the same clinical disease.
  - A single serotype may produce varying clinical syndromes in different seasons and communities, or even in different individuals infected at the same time and place.
  - The common pattern is endemic infection caused by several concurrently circulating enterovirus types.
    - The predominant serotypes may vary yearly, by locality, and within the same year.
    - The pattern of clinical syndromes changes over the enterovirus season.
  - Pandemic illness is unusual but not unknown.
- Environment
  - Enterovirus infections are seasonal, although sporadic cases are noted in all seasons.
    - Occur from June through October in the northern hemisphere
    - In tropical regions, infection is noted throughout the year, with increased incidence during rainy periods.
  - Crowding, poor sanitation, and low socioeconomic conditions increase incidence of infection.

ETIOLOGY

- Enterovirus infection is initiated by viral replication in the lymphoid tissues of the oropharynx and intestines (days 1–3).
- Virions spread to the reticuloendothelial system at 3–5 days.
- The reason why serotypes have a tropism for certain tissues, such as poliovirus for the neurons of the brain and spinal cord, is unknown.

SIGNS AND SYMPTOMS

Natural history

- >90% of enterovirus infections are not apparent.
- When symptoms do occur, a variety of host factors and viral factors determine the clinical disease.
  - Nearly all protean syndromes associated with enteroviruses have been noted with numerous serotypes.
  - Certain diseases are associated more frequently with specific serotypes, eg, coxsackievirus A16 is the likely etiologic agent of an outbreak of hand-foot-mouth disease.
  - In the US, 15 serotypes accounted for almost 85% of all enterovirus identification reports over 1970 to 2005.
- Patient is symptom free for 1–3 days after infection.
  - A minor viremia follows.
  - The patient is contagious at 3–5 days.
    - Symptoms of disease are not yet apparent.
    - In subclinical infection, the process is halted at this point by host defenses.

- Subsequently, a major viremia results in viral dissemination to secondary organs.
  - Skin
  - Heart
  - Liver
  - Pancreas
  - Adrenal glands
  - Central nervous system
- This phase is often recognized clinically as a nonspecific febrile illness.
  - In poliomyelitis, it is the phase of minor illness.
  - In a very small percentage of cases, viral replication continues, producing clinical syndromes of enterovirus infection, such as poliomyelitis, herpangina, or pleurodynia.

Nonspecific febrile illness

- Can be caused by any of the enteroviruses
- Lasts ≥7 days
- Increases in late summer and early fall
- A child may have several episodes of enterovirus-induced febrile illness within the same season.
- Most frequent presenting symptoms
  - Fever
  - Irritability
  - Lethargy
  - Myalgia
  - Malaise
  - Poor feeding
  - Diarrhea, vomiting, sore throat, or upper respiratory tract symptoms may be present but are not severe.
  - Concomitant aseptic meningitis in infants is common and is not predicted by clinical symptoms.
  - The illness occasionally takes a biphasic course.
    - Relapse of fever associated with irritability within 1 or 2 days sometimes results in a second hospital admission for the same illness.

Respiratory tract disease

- Nonexudative pharyngitis with or without lymphadenopathy is common.
  - Major cause of summertime sore throat
  - May be the initial manifestation of more severe disease that appears after an apparent recovery period of 1–3 days
- Other respiratory syndromes are less common and are generally mild.
  - Bronchitis
  - Croup
  - Pneumonia

E

Enanthem and exanthem diseases

- Hand-foot-mouth syndrome
  - Toddlers
  - School-age children
- Hallmark signs
  - Relatively painless vesicles on a red base
    - Buccal mucosa
    - Tongue
    - Hands
    - Feet
- May spread to extremities and buttocks
- Patients usually have a low-grade fever and a sore throat.
  - Recovery within 1 week

Gastrointestinal disease

- Enteric disease is not a prominent clinical syndrome.
- Gastrointestinal symptoms are occasionally seen, but almost always with other signs of systemic enterovirus infection.
  - Nausea
  - Vomiting
  - Abdominal pain
  - Constipation
  - Diarrhea
  - Peritonitis
- Hepatitis or pancreatitis is usually part of a generalized enterovirus syndrome.

Acute hemorrhagic conjunctivitis

- Epidemic disease
- Marked by sudden onset of:
  - Severe eye pain
  - Photophobia
  - Tearing
  - Subconjunctival hemorrhage
  - Swelling
- Lasts 7–10 days
- Most often observed in middle-age individuals
  - Epidemics in schools have been noted.
- Neurologic sequelae may be seen in adults.
- Clinical improvement may take several months.

Aseptic meningitis

- Enterovirus infection is the major cause in countries that immunize against mumps.

- Most cases are sporadic, but epidemic aseptic meningitis does occur.
  - Usually associated with person-to-person spread
    - Summer camps
    - Playgrounds
    - Child care centers
- Typically occurs in school-age children
- Symptoms
  - Headache
  - Nuchal rigidity
  - Fever
  - Photophobia
  - Pharyngitis
  - Rash
  - Meningismus may be subtle or absent in up to 50% of patients.
- Infants often have nonspecific symptoms.
  - Fever or febrile seizures
  - Poor feeding
  - Cough or congestion
  - Diarrhea
  - Rash
- Course is usually mild.
  - Adults and older children may have headache severe enough to require narcotic analgesia.
  - Most patients recover within 2 weeks, but relapses may occur.
  - Early information suggested that as many as 10% of survivors of aseptic meningitis that occurred before 3 months of age suffered long-term neurologic sequelae, eg, speech and language delays.
    - Recent prospective outcome studies dispute this claim.
  - Older children recover completely.

Paralytic disease

- All cases of poliovirus infection acquired in the US since the 1990s were associated with vaccine-derived poliovirus strains and occurred in:
  - Young adults
  - Immunodeficient individuals
  - Unimmunized individuals
- Live polio vaccine has not been used in the US since 2000.
  - Any case of vaccine-derived or wild-type poliovirus infection is likely to have been imported and should be reported immediately to public health authorities.

Perinatal infection

- Enterovirus infection in neonates may occur as any of the syndromes seen in older children.

- Premature infants and newborns born without specific passively acquired maternal antibody may have a fulminant, rapidly fatal disease.

  - Begins as a syndrome of lethargy and poor feeding, with or without fever, indistinguishable from early bacterial sepsis

  - Progression is swift.

  - Multiorgan involvement

    - Hepatitis

    - Pancreatitis

    - Coagulopathy

    - Myocarditis

    - Encephalitis

- The virus in neonates is most often transmitted from mother to infant at or near the time of delivery.

  - Nursery outbreaks with fatal cases have been reported.

- Myocarditis and pericarditis occur, with a high mortality rate as part of the generalized disease of newborns.

  - <50% of older children and adults who have myocarditis die; severe sequelae have been reported.

- Orchitis and parotitis occasionally occur in association with coxsackievirus B infection and are differentiated from mumps only by laboratory studies.

Unusual enterovirus syndromes

- Encephalitis often occurs in severely ill neonates.

- Chronic meningoencephalitis in patients with hypogammaglobulinemia

- Dancing eyes-dancing feet (opsoclonus-myoclonus) syndrome

DIFFERENTIAL DIAGNOSIS

- Herpangina

  - Commonly diagnosed in a young child

    - Fever

    - Sore throat

    - Pain on swallowing

  - Enanthem may be noted early; it is soon succeeded by small vesicles or tiny white papules and then by ulcers.

    - Tonsils

    - Pharynx

    - Soft palate

  - Herpangina is differentiated from herpes simplex stomatitis by:

    - Milder fever

    - Primarily posterior oropharyngeal involvement

    - Epidemic seasonal occurrence

- Epidemic pleurodynia or Bornholm disease

  - Coxsackievirus B serotypes

  - Fever

  - Severe pain in the intercostal and abdominal muscles occurs in spasms lasting minutes to hours.

  - Succeeding episodes are milder than the first and may occur days or months later.

  - Rarely, symptoms are severe enough to prompt exploratory laparotomy.

- A variety of exanthems may be the sole or major manifestation of enterovirus infection.

  - Classic macular blanching

  - Rubella-like rash

  - Boston exanthem

    - Begins on the face and trunk and spreads to the extremities

  - Distinguished from rubella by lack of posterior auricular and suboccipital adenopathy

  - Unusual enterovirus rashes may be maculopapular, vesicular, roseola-like, urticarial, or petechial.

    - When such exanthems occur in conjunction with other enterovirus syndromes, such as aseptic meningitis, illness may be mistaken for a more serious disease, such as meningococcal meningitis.

- Meningitis-like illness

  - Diagnostic dilemmas are common.

  - Lyme meningitis occurs in a similar age group and during the same season as enteroviral meningitis and can usually be distinguished by symptoms not seen in enteroviral disease.

    - Presence of cranial neuropathy

    - Papilledema

    - Erythema migrans

  - West Nile virus infection in children is clinically indistinguishable from enteroviral meningitis.

    - Differential diagnosis depends entirely on virologic evaluation.

- Paralytic disease

  - Asymmetrical weakness, paralysis, or both, without sensory loss, differentiates enteroviral paralysis from Guillain-Barré syndrome.

    - Guillain-Barré syndrome is a life-threatening disease, usually involving paralysis of primary and accessory respiratory muscles or inflammation of the bulbar respiratory center.

  - Recovery of muscle function may continue for several months.

  - Infection with other enterovirus serotypes may also result in paralysis.

E

- Nonpolio enterovirus and West Nile virus associated paralysis are more common than classic poliovirus-associated disease.
- Postpolio syndrome is seen decades after the initial infection.
  - A syndrome of progressive weakness and fatigue
  - Occurs in long-term survivors of paralytic poliomyelitis
  - Previously affected muscles are denervated as overburdened motor neurons eventually wear out.
    - Long-term outcome is unknown.
    - Most patients have only modest decline in function even >50 years after infection.
    - Associated fatigue may adversely affect the quality of life.
- Parechovirus infection
  - Enteroviruses 22 and 23 have been reclassified as HPeV1 and HPeV2.
    - They share many clinical and epidemiologic features with the enteroviruses.
  - Disease appears in an endemic pattern.
  - Summer-fall seasonality
  - Most infections are reported in very young children.
    - Necrotizing enterocolitis
    - Nursery outbreaks
    - Neonatal sepsis syndrome
    - Febrile seizures
    - Paralysis
    - Rash
    - Respiratory illness
  - Death may occur in up to 10% of patients with recognized HPeV1 infection.
    - Asymptomatic disease is common.
    - >95% of adults show serologic immunity.

LABORATORY FINDINGS

- When obtaining specimens, understand the concept of permissive versus nonpermissive sites.
  - Permissive sites may harbor enteroviruses and may persist for weeks to months after infection, eg, nasopharynx, feces.
    - Identification of an enterovirus from a permissive site may be completely unrelated to the illness under investigation.
    - Vague, nonspecific symptoms or highly unusual or rare syndromes may be completely unrelated to enterovirus shed in the gastrointestinal tract.
    - Many disease associations with enteroviruses are

probably explained by such incidental enterovirus identification.
  - Classic enterovirus disease during a known epidemic season is interpreted more easily.
  - Isolating an enterovirus from the stool of an infant who has fever and cerebrospinal fluid (CSF) pleocytosis in the summer, without any other pathogen isolated, is presumptive evidence of enteroviral meningitis.
- Nonpermissive sites are those from which virus is identified only during periods of disease, eg, blood, spinal fluid, skin vesicle.
  - Shedding of virus in these sites is usually brief.
  - Finding an enterovirus in a nonpermissive site is strong evidence that the virus is related to the concurrent clinical illness.
- Almost all enterovirus serotypes can produce any enterovirus syndrome.
  - No disease is associated uniquely with any enterovirus serotype.
  - An enterovirus usually does need not be identified beyond its actual presence.
    - Enterovirus presence from a nonpermissive site is sufficient to diagnose the origin of the illness.
  - In rare cases, both enteroviral and bacterial pathogens may be present in blood or spinal fluid.
  - Symptoms associated with the bacterial agent are more severe than those with the viral agent and dictate clinical management.
- Virus isolation
  - Enteroviruses are isolated readily in cell cultures.
    - A positive culture can be noted as early as 18 hours.
    - Culture typically requires 2–5 days.
  - Suckling mouse inoculation is the only available method of isolating most coxsackievirus A serotypes.
    - It is expensive and difficult to obtain.
  - Viruses may be isolated from:
    - Throat swabs
    - Feces
    - CSF
    - Blood or serum
    - Skin vesicles
    - Tissue obtained at autopsy
  - Specimens from several sites increase diagnostic yield.
    - Predicting the pathologic stage of infection and, thus, the most likely source of the virus, is not always possible.

- Aseptic meningitis
  - Cerebrospinal fluid (CSF) analysis shows moderate pleocytosis with a predominance of lymphocytes, normal glucose levels, and slightly increased protein levels.
    - Predominant polymorphonuclear cell type
    - Cell counts >1000 cells/mm³
    - The percentage of mononuclear cells tends to increase over time.
    - In some children, the polymorphonuclear predominance persists for several days.
  - In 20–50% of cases of proven aseptic meningitis in infants < 30 days of age, pleocytosis is minimal or absent.
  - Other laboratory studies on CSF, such as C-reactive protein level or leukocyte aggregation, show too broad an overlap to distinguish reliably from bacterial meningitis.
  - Results of rapid virus identification techniques may reduce empirical use of antibiotics and the length of hospitalization.

SPECIFIC TREATMENTS

- Intravenous immunoglobulin has been successful in eradicating chronic enterovirus infections in some patients with immunodeficiency diseases.
- Neonates with severe disseminated disease have been treated with infusions of intravenous immunoglobulin up to 1 g/kg and of specific serotype high antibody titer maternal plasma, with no discernible benefit.
- Pleconaril is a novel oral antiviral drug.
  - Active against picornaviruses, including enteroviruses
  - In clinical trials, infants, older children, and adults who have enterovirus-associated aseptic meningitis treated with pleconaril had a shorter illness and returned to normal activity sooner.
    - Older children reported a marked decrease in headache apparent as early as 24 hours after the initiation of treatment.
  - Pleconaril is available for compassionate use.
  - Effective in stopping replication of virus in immunodeficient individuals
  - Well tolerated
    - Few or no side effects are attributed to the drug.
  - Clinical enterovirus isolates resistant to pleconaril have not been detected.

WHEN TO ADMIT

- Neonates and infants <90 days with suspected enteroviral syndromes in whom systemic bacterial disease is not yet ruled out
- Disease significant enough to require subspecialty expertise, especially cardiac, immunologic, or neurologic disease
- Any enteroviral syndrome that has a rapidly progressive or atypical course
- Older children who have aseptic meningitis who require symptomatic treatment for severe headache or dehydration

WHEN TO REFER

- Neonates with any evidence of disseminated or rapidly progressive enterovirus-like infection
- Immunocompromised individuals who have chronic enterovirus-like syndromes
- Normal hosts who have atypical progression of enteroviral disease, especially those with neurologic or cardiac involvement

COMPLICATIONS

- Poliovirus infections lead to permanent paralysis of muscles innervated by affected neurons.
- Aseptic meningitis may lead to neurologic sequelae, such as speech and language delay.
- Enteroviral infections in neonates may be fatal.

PROGNOSIS

- Prognosis in neonates with enteroviral infection without passive immunity from mother is poor.

PREVENTION

- Attenuated live or killed poliovirus vaccines are the only preventive enterovirus preparations currently available.
  - Enhanced-potency inactivated poliovirus vaccine is the only choice for routine immunization in the US.
- In the prevaccine years, 0.2 mL/kg of pooled immune serum globulin given intramuscularly prevented or ameliorated poliovirus infection and might be indicated:
  - In nursery epidemics
  - For infants of mothers who develop a probable enterovirus disease within a few days of delivery

E

Enuresis

DEFINITION

- Urinary incontinence occurring when a child:
  - Is at least 5 years old *and*
  - Urinates in bed or on clothes
    - At least twice per week
    - For at least 3 consecutive months
- Variations
  - Diurnal
  - Nocturnal
    - Monosymptomatic nocturnal enuresis (MNE): no day-time symptoms to suggest lower urinary tract disorders
    - Polysymptomatic: associated with additional symptoms
      - Urgency
      - Frequency
      - Dribbling
      - Daytime enuresis
  - Primary
    - Children who have never had a period of sustained dryness
  - Secondary
    - Children who have been dry in the past
      - At least 6 months with nocturnal enuresis
      - At least 3 months with diurnal enuresis

EPIDEMIOLOGY

- Prevalence
  - Nocturnal
    - ~20% of children at 5 years of age
    - 6%–10% by age 7
    - 1%–3% persisting into late teens
  - Diurnal
    - 10% of 5-year-olds at least once every 2 weeks
  - Primary
    - Twice as common as secondary enuresis
- Sex
  - Nocturnal
    - 2–3 times more common in boys than in girls
  - Diurnal
    - More likely in girls than in boys
- Age
  - By 5 years of age, 24-hour/day bladder control should be achieved.
  - Children who are mentally disabled should reach a mental age of 4 years before they are considered enuretic.

ETIOLOGY

- Monosymptomatic nocturnal enuresis (MNE)
  - Relative nocturnal polyuria that exceeds the child's bladder capacity
    - In children with enuresis, bladder capacity has been found to be smaller at night compared with normal controls.
  - In some children with MNE, secretion of antidiuretic hormone is decreased at night, resulting in increased urine production.
  - Some children with MNE are more difficult to arouse from sleep than normal controls or children with primary nocturnal enuresis.
- Diurnal enuresis
  - Anatomic abnormalities
    - Urethral obstruction
    - Congenital (posterior urethral valves)
    - Acquired (foreign body)
    - Ectopic ureter in girls
  - Lesions involving the spinal cord
  - Vaginal reflux of urine
    - Girls who do not open the labia during voiding develop leakage of urine on standing.
  - Holding urine
    - Common in preschoolers and older children at school

RISK FACTORS

- Nocturnal enuresis
  - Family history
    - Strong hereditary component
    - Concordance rate of 19%–36% for dizygotic and 46%–68% for monozygotic twins
  - Sleep disorders
    - Obstructive sleep apnea (33%)
      - Resolves in 61% and decreases in 23% within 9 months after tonsillectomy and adenoidectomy
    - Nocturnal hypercalciuria
    - Aquaporin-2 dysfunction
  - Developmental/psychological factors
    - Delayed speech
    - Delayed walking
    - Early toilet training
    - Poor self esteem
    - Chronic anxiety

E

■ Diurnal enuresis

- Urinary tract infection
  - Cystitis causes spontaneous detrusor contractions
  - More common in children who have abnormal genitourinary anatomy

SIGNS AND SYMPTOMS

History

■ Determine nocturnal or diurnal enuresis

- Does the wetting occur during the day, the night, or both?
- How often does wetting occur and at what times?
- How often does the child void during the day and during the night?

■ Determine primary or secondary enuresis

- What age did the wetting start?
- Has the child ever been dry?
- Has the child had any dry spells?
  - How long did dry spells last?
- What has been done about the symptom before this evaluation?

■ Social situation

- How does the family handle wet nights?
  - Does the child wear pull ups or is a plastic sheet used?
  - Who is responsible for laundering sheets and clothing?
  - Do siblings tease the child?
  - Is the child punished for wetting?
- Any recent traumatic events or changes in social situation?

■ Fluid intake before bedtime

- How much and when does the child drink after supper?

■ Sleep habits

- Is the child difficult to wake from sleep?
- Are there any signs of obstructive sleep apnea (mouth breathing, snoring, and restless sleep)?

■ Daytime symptoms

- Urinary frequency (normal = 4–7 times per day)
- Urgency
- Dysuria
- Dribbling between voids
- Straining with voids
- Constipation

■ Medical history including a thorough perinatal history

- Spina bifida or meningomyelocele
- Delayed developmental motor milestones

- Spinal trauma
- Psychological issues
  - Attention deficit disorder
  - Depression
  - Conduct disorder
  - Feelings about the enuresis
  - Motivation for doing something about it
- History of enuresis in 1 or both parents

Physical examination

■ Physical exam is often normal.

■ Examination should be thorough with focus on signs that may indicate any of the causes of enuresis.

- Abnormal vital signs and growth parameters may indicate chronic disease.

■ Complete neurologic examination

- Gait
- Muscle tone and strength
- Deep-tendon reflexes
- Sensory abnormalities

■ Spinal examination may reveal subtle signs of spinal dysraphism

- Dimples
- Hair tuft
- Skin discoloration

■ Abdominal examination

- Distended bladder
- Constipation

■ Rectal examination

- Fecal impaction
- Decreased rectal tone

■ Flank examination

- Lower abdominal tenderness may indicate urinary tract infection.

■ Genitourinary examination

- Rash
- Adhesions
- Trauma
- Foreign body
- Vulvitis
- Vaginitis

DIFFERENTIAL DIAGNOSIS

- Focuses on excluding underlying disorders:
  - Urinary tract infection
  - Renal masses or renal diseases
  - Neurologic disorders
    - Neurogenic bladder
    - Detrusor instability
    - Spinal cord conditions
  - Structural genitourinary tract defects
    - Ectopic ureter
    - Posterior urethral valves
  - Constipation
  - Endocrine disorders
    - Diabetes mellitus
    - Diabetes insipidus
  - Hypercalciuria
  - Sickle cell disease
  - Drugs
    - Caffeine
    - Methylxanthines
  - Sexual abuse

DIAGNOSTIC APPROACH

- Diagnosis depends on a thorough history and physical examination.
- Imaging is indicated
  - In the presence of daytime symptoms
  - If initial laboratory evaluation, physical examination are abnormal

LABORATORY FINDINGS

- Urinalysis
  - Useful in MNE
  - Renal pathologic abnormality
    - Proteinuria
    - Hematuria
    - Red blood cell casts
  - Diabetes mellitus
    - Glucosuria
  - Diabetes insipidus, psychogenic polydipsia
    - Low specific gravity
- Urine culture
  - Diagnostic for urinary tract infection

IMAGING

- Ultrasound
  - Prevoid and postvoid renal and bladder
- Voiding cystourethrogram, urodynamic studies if ultrasound result is abnormal
- Spine MRI
  - To rule out possible spinal dysraphism

CLASSIFICATION

- Diurnal
- Nocturnal
  - MNE: no daytime symptoms to suggest lower urinary tract disorders
  - Polysymptomatic: associated with additional symptoms
    - Urgency
    - Frequency
    - Dribbling
    - Daytime enuresis
- Primary
  - Children who have never had a period of sustained dryness
- Secondary
  - Children who have been dry in the past

TREATMENT APPROACH

- Treat any underlying cause(s).
- Consider treatment of MNE in children 6–8 years of age.
  - Conservative measures
  - Careful/detailed explanation to parents and child
  - Alarm therapy is most effective.
- Pharmacotherapy depends on underlying cause.

SPECIFIC TREATMENTS

General

- Treat any underlying organic causes.
- If both daytime and nighttime symptoms are present, daytime symptoms should be treated first.
- Good voiding hygiene and habits should be reinforced.
- Primary and secondary nocturnal enuresis are treated similarly.
- In children <8
  - Conservative measures
    - Pull-ups
    - Plastic-lined bed sheets

- MNE
  - Treatment should be considered in a child 6–8 years of age.
    - Provide careful and detailed explanation of the condition to both parents and child in language that is easily understood.
    - Expect relapses.
  - The combination of a motivated child and a cooperative family is the best predictor of a positive outcome.
  - Alarm therapy should be considered in most patients 8 or older

Nonpharmacologic therapy

- Conservative measures to minimize nocturnal polyuria:
  - Decrease fluid intake several hours before bedtime.
  - Void before bed to minimize nocturnal bladder volume.
  - Consider awakening the child to urinate before the parents go to bed.
  - Encourage the child to void often during the day and take the time to empty the bladder completely.
- Charts for positive reinforcement
  - Children fill out a chart depicting wet and dry nights symbolically, such as stars or the sun for dry nights and a cloud for wet nights.
- Enuresis alarm therapy
  - In some families, alarms may increase parental annoyance and place the child at risk for physical or emotional abuse.
  - Many children will not initially awaken with the alarm and need a parent to assist in awakening.
  - Relapses occur and do not preclude future success.
  - Despite the evidence supporting the efficacy of alarm therapy, it is prescribed to <5% of children
- Dry bed training
  - Effective, comprehensive program combining:
    - Enuresis alarms
    - Positive practices
    - Waking routines
    - Personal cleanliness routine after enuresis
    - Bladder training

Pharmacotherapy

- Desmopressin (DDAVP)
  - First-line treatment often together with alarm therapy for MNE
  - Efficacy
    - Produces faster improvement (2–3 months) by itself than alarm therapy alone
    - Not as effective as alarms over long term
    - Up to 80% relapse rate when desmopressin is stopped
    - Thus, if used, should be done so in conjunction with alarms

- Side effects
  - Nausea
  - Vomiting
  - Abdominal pain
  - Headache
  - Facial flushing
  - Elevated blood pressure
  - Chest pain
  - Tachycardia
  - Hyponatremia from water intoxication
- If treatment is successful, a 1-week interruption every 3 months is recommended to see if enuresis has resolved.
- Some patients who do not respond to the usual dose of DDAVP may respond when the dose is doubled.
- If no response occurs to medication alone, alarm therapy should be considered.
- Oxybutynin
  - Useful in treating daytime enuresis caused by detrusor overactivity
    - May be of benefit to enuretic children with restricted bladder capacity caused by bladder overactivity
  - Efficacy
    - Ineffective as a single agent for primary enuresis
    - Combined therapy with oxybutynin and desmopressin produces more rapid results for nocturnal enuresis than single therapy with either desmopressin or imipramine.
  - Also used to treat:
    - Urge syndrome
    - Hinman syndrome
    - Neurogenic bladder
  - Side effects
    - Nausea
    - Vomiting
    - Abdominal pain
    - Diarrhea
    - Constipation
    - Urinary retention
    - Dry mucous membranes
    - Blurred vision
- Imipramine/tricyclic antidepressants
  - Efficacy
    - Minimal effectiveness in treatment of MNE
    - Relapse is common.

- Side effects
  - Potential for lethal effects in the setting of accidental or intentional overdose
    - Clinicians must use caution in prescribing these agents.
    - Families must be aware of dangerous potential of overdose and need for safe storage and supervision.
  - Nausea
  - Vomiting
  - Constipation
  - Blurred vision
  - Urinary retention
  - Cardiac arrhythmias
  - Hypotension

WHEN TO REFER

- Abnormal urinalysis findings suggestive of a metabolic disorder
- Concerns of neurologic bladder dysfunction
- Failure to respond to appropriate therapy

- Presence of any structural urinary tract abnormalities on imaging studies
- History of:
  - Recurrent urinary tract infections
  - Significant constipation and encopresis

PROGNOSIS

- Nocturnal enuresis
  - Annual spontaneous resolution rate is approximately 15%.
  - With alarm therapy
    - Long-term cure rate of MNE with alarm therapy
      - 25% by 2 months
      - 50% by 3 months
      - 90% by 6 months
    - 47% remain dry long term after alarm therapy is stopped.
    - Alarm therapy is not only a management modality but also a cure.

Envenomations

DEFINITION

- *Venoms* are complex chemical mixtures designed either for defending or for hunting.
  - Various venom delivery systems exist.
  - Most systems consist of specially evolved exocrine gland mechanisms to make and store venom and a sophisticated delivery apparatus.
- *Stings* are delivered through a posterior structure (stinger) and are primarily defensive.
- *Bites* refer to injection through structures associated with the mouth that are primarily for handling prey.
- *Envenomation* is the injection of venom through a bite or sting.

EPIDEMIOLOGY

- Incidence
  - In 2005 the American Association of Poison Control Centers National Poison Database reported 2,547,394 exposures.
  - 82,151 (3.2%) were a result of a bite or sting.
  - Of the 1460 total deaths recorded in the database, 7 (0.5%) were from bites and stings, and none involved children.
- Prevalence
  - Bites and envenomations ranked number 10 in all age groups in the National Poison Database but did not make the top 20 in children <6 years.

Hymenoptera

- Prevalence
  - Systemic reactions occur in <5% of patients.
  - Large local cutaneous reactions occur in 2.3–18.6% of the general population.
  - Biphasic anaphylactic reactions, characterized by the return of symptoms 6–10 hours after initial symptoms resolve, occur in up to 20% of patients.
  - Death by honeybee or wasp envenomation is rare, especially in children.
  - IgE-mediated type 1 anaphylaxis, although uncommon, is usually responsible for related deaths.
  - Massive envenomation involving hundreds of stings may also result in death.
  - Hymenoptera envenomation is the second-leading cause of anaphylactic reactions, after penicillin.
    - It accounts for more deaths in the US than any other envenomation.
- Fire ants
  - Fire ant envenomations are becoming an increasingly important concern in the US.
  - Systemic allergic reactions occur in ≤16% of patients treated for fire ant stings.
  - Serious reactions, including anaphylaxis, occur in ≤2%.
  - The literature suggests a 20–30% annual attack rate in areas where imported fire ants are endemic.
  - The highest sting rate (close to 50%) occurs in persons <20 years.

Arachnids

- Approximately 50 spider species are of medical importance.
  - Most are venomous and can cause serious injury.
  - Fatalities from spider bites are rare.
- Scorpion envenomation may be life threatening in children.
  - Systemic manifestations tend to be more common in children <10 years.

Snakes

- Envenomations by snakes in North America are overwhelmingly caused by indigenous Crotalinae, also called *pit vipers*.
  - ~20–25% of pit viper bites are dry, meaning they do not result in envenomation.
- Coral snakes constitute <1% of envenomations.
- Nonindigenous snakes in zoos or kept as exotic pets are responsible for a small percentage of envenomations.
- All sea snakes are venomous; none inhabit the coastal waters of North America.
- Most bites in the US occur in the Southwest.
- Body area
  - Most bites are inflicted on the upper extremity, including fingers, hand, and arm.
  - Less commonly affected sites are the leg, foot, and torso.
- Mortality
  - The number of deaths from snakebite in the US ranges from 0 to 14 per year.
  - Most snakebite deaths are associated with absence of medical care, errors in medical management, or presence of an underlying medical condition.
  - Children are at increased risk for serious sequelae because of their lower body mass and relatively high venom dose compared with adults.

ETIOLOGY

Hymenoptera

- In the US, Hymenoptera are responsible for most insect stings.
  - Family Apidae (honeybees)
  - Family Bombidae (bumblebees)
  - Superfamily Vespidae (paper wasps, white-faced hornets, yellow hornets, and yellow jackets)
  - Superfamily Formicidae (harvester ants and native and imported fire ants)

- All Hymenoptera possess a stinger located posteriorly.
- Reactions may be either a direct effect of the venom or an IgE–mediated allergic reaction.

Winged Hymenoptera

- The sting apparatus, or aculeus, of wasps (vespids) and honeybees resembles a stylet with 2 shafts that pulls the stinger deep into the flesh.
- Unlike the honeybee, the vespid sting stylet is less likely to remain in the victim.
- Honeybees die after stinging; because vespids can withdraw their stingers, they can sting multiple times.
- Venoms of the winged Hymenoptera contain many different protein components that account for the observed reactions.

Ants

- Fire ants bite the skin of their victims with their mandibles, then arch their bodies to inject venom through a lancet-shaped stinger located at the distal end of their abdomen.
  - If undisturbed, they will sting repeatedly in a circular pattern, using their mandibles as a pivot, injecting venom with each sting.
- Harvester ants also bite the skin with their mandibles and envenomate their victim through a sting.
  - Their venom contains a larger fraction of protein constituents than fire ant venom and is more similar to other Hymenoptera venoms.

Arachnids

- Class Arachnida includes 2 orders: Araneae (spiders) and Scorpionidae (scorpions).
- Envenomations can result in significant morbidity, but deaths are rare.

Spiders

- A diverse group with approximately 40,000 species worldwide
- In North America, spiders most commonly involved in human exposures are:
  - Loxosceles species (brown recluse spider, also known as the *violin spider* or *fiddleback spider*); 11 species in the US, usually the Southeast and Southwest
  - *Latrodectus* species (black widow spider)
  - Tarantulas

Scorpions

- *Centruroides exilicauda*, or the black scorpion, is the only medically relevant species of scorpion in the United States.
  - Found in Arizona and adjacent southwestern states
- Its venom is a potent neurotoxin that activates neuronal sodium channels and results in excessive firing of affected neurons, including both the adrenergic and parasympathetic systems.

Snakes

- Venomous snakes of North America can be divided into 2 families: Viperidae (subfamily Crotalinae) and Elapidae.
  - Crotalinae, also called *pit vipers*, includes rattlesnakes, water moccasins or cottonmouths, copperheads, pygmy rattlesnakes, and massasauga rattlesnakes.
  - Elapidae includes coral snakes, as well as nonindigenous cobras and mambas.

Crotaline snakes (pit vipers)

- Their highly mobile, retractable, hollow fangs function like a hypodermic needle.
  - Usually penetrate to subcutaneous tissue, whereas the fangs of larger snakes penetrate dermal or subcutaneous structures and deposit venom into the muscle
- Venom is generally absorbed through the lymphatic system.
- Crotaline venom is a complex mixture of biologically active proteins and peptides capable of damaging vascular endothelial cells.
  - This leads to increased permeability to plasma and erythrocytes into the extravascular space and ultimately can result in hypotension and shock.
  - Venom is spread throughout the body as a result of the action of hyaluronidase and its integrity-reducing effect on connective tissue.
- Pit viper venoms are designed to immobilize and digest prey; prominent effects include:
  - Direct tissue injury resulting from enzymatic degradation
  - Local inflammatory responses exaggerated by metalloproteinases
  - Increased intracellular calcium in skeletal muscle, resulting in prolonged contraction and necrosis
  - Increased permeability of erythrocyte membranes, changing their morphology and potentially causing hemolysis
  - Damage to mast cell membranes, causing histamine release
  - Isolated defibrination caused by coagulopathy following fibrinolysis and thrombin-like peptide actions
  - Thrombocytopenia resulting from platelet aggregation at sites of tissue injury and from a direct effect of venom on individual platelets, particularly from rattlesnake venom.
  - Neurotoxins are present in varying degrees, notably in the Mojave and timber rattlesnakes, and can produce weakness, paralysis, and myokymia.
- The notion that juvenile rattlesnakes are more dangerous than adult snakes is a misconception.

Coral snakes

- Coral snakes tend to be small, secretive, and mild-mannered unless provoked.
- Coral snakes lack facial pits, are diurnal, and have fixed fangs and nearly round pupils.

- Bites may produce superficial scratches or definite fang marks; retroverted teeth gnaw or chew on their prey, making coral snakes difficult to shake off.

- Local tissue injury is uncommon.

- Venom causes paresthesias and paralysis by inhibiting acetylcholine receptors at the neuronal synapse.

RISK FACTORS

- An amount of venom that would not harm an adult may be disastrous for a child.

Hymenoptera

- The risk of a systemic reaction appears to be increased:
  - In patients with a history of multiple stings
  - In patients who are stung within a few weeks of a previous sting

- In patients with a history of anaphylaxis, the risk of anaphylaxis with subsequent stings is 35–60%.

- Atopic patients do not appear to be at greater risk of systemic complications, but the severity of their symptoms may be greater.

- History of a large local reaction does not reliably predict progression to systemic complications.
  - Risk of subsequent anaphylaxis after a large local reaction is approximately 5–10%.

- Children are at high risk because of their failure to perceive the risk and inability to escape.

Winged Hymenoptera

- Yellow jacket wasps are common near exposed food and garbage.

- If disturbed, any wasp or bee will sting in self-defense.

- Eyes, mouth, and nostrils may be selectively targeted.

Fire ants

- Trespassing into their territory or disturbing a nest will incite aggressive, swarming behavior, often resulting in multiple stings.

- Ants do sometimes attack victims indoors, especially following heavy rains.

Arachnids

- Most spiders are not aggressive and only bite in self-defense when:
  - Humans invade their territory.
  - The spider becomes lost in such items as bedclothes.

- Tarantulas kept as pets pose a risk to the unsuspecting child.

- *Loxosceles* (brown recluse spider) bites are usually the result of accidental contact.

- Scorpion stings usually result from accidental contact with a scorpion trapped in linen or clothing or during outdoor play.

Snakes

- The typical snakebite victim is a young white adult male who is bitten while handling or playing with a snake.

- Alcohol consumption increases risk.

- Most bites are inflicted on an upper extremity, including fingers, hand, and arm.

SIGNS AND SYMPTOMS

Winged Hymenoptera

- Local
  - The nonallergic reaction is a direct result of envenomation through mast cell degranulation and the production of a wheal-and-flare response causing:
    - Erythema
    - Swelling
    - Pain
    - Itching
  - In conjunction with these reactions, some patients may experience:
    - Headache
    - Nausea
    - Malaise
  - Skin and soft-tissue necrosis in the weeks after a Hymenoptera sting have also been reported.
  - Corneal stings
    - May result in damage through toxic and immunologic reactions
    - Stingers retained in the eye may cause corneal edema with striate and toxic keratopathy.
    - Immunologic reactions can result in extensive inflammation, uveitis, and inflammatory glaucoma.

- Systemic
  - Common systemic manifestations include:
    - Urticaria
    - Angioedema
    - Wheezing
    - Shortness of breath
    - Stridor
    - Nausea
    - Vomiting
    - Diarrhea
    - Abdominal pain
    - Malaise
    - Dizziness
    - Anaphylaxis

- Dysphagia
- Dysarthria
- Hoarseness
- Weakness
- Confusion
- Effects on the hematologic system include:
  - Hemolysis with associated hemoglobinuria and hemoglobinemia
  - Thrombocytopenia
  - Disseminated intravascular coagulation
- Multiple stings from Africanized bees may cause:
  - Hemolysis
  - Thrombocytopenia
  - Rhabdomyolysis (skeletal and myocardial)
  - Acute tubular necrosis
- Systemic symptoms typically develop within 24 hours, although delayed onset (2–6 days) has been reported.

Fire ants

- Local
  - Stings tend to be multiple and cause immediate local burning and itching.
  - Soon after, the area becomes erythematous and raised.
  - This reaction usually subsides after 30–60 minutes.
  - The classic pathognomonic finding of small, sterile pustules developing 4–24 hours later is more common with stings of imported fire ants.
    - Pustules may occur in rings or lines consistent with fire ant stinging behavior.
    - Pustules usually resolve over 3–10 days.
  - Some patients develop a large local reaction similar to that of other Hymenoptera stings.
  - The initial wheal-and-flare reaction evolves into an erythematous, pruritic, warm, indurated area around the sting site.
  - Large local reactions may progress over 48 hours and may not subside for 7 days.
  - The pathophysiologic mechanism of large local reactions is not clear and may be confused with cellulitis.
- Systemic allergic reactions are similar to those associated with other insects and include:
  - Bronchospasm
  - Angioedema
  - Urticaria
  - Pruritus
  - Laryngeal edema
  - Hypotension

- Anaphylaxis
- Seizures
- Mononeuritis
- Guillain-Barré syndrome
- Serum sickness
- Nephritic syndrome
- Worsening of preexisting cardiopulmonary disease
- Direct systemic toxic effects of fire ant venom are not well understood.
- No deaths have been attributed to date to fire ant venom.

Harvester ants

- Unlike imported fire ants, harvester ants do not leave characteristic skin lesions.
- Their sting resembles that of other insects and may be associated with allergic reactions.

***Loxosceles* (brown recluse spider)**

- Local, cutaneous
  - The bite itself does not cause much discomfort and may go unnoticed.
  - A minor stinging or burning sensation may be felt at the site.
  - Erythema, pruritus, pain, and edema typically develop within 2–8 hours.
  - Symptoms may be followed in the next 24–48 hours by a blue-gray halo surrounding the erythematous center.
  - Vesicles or bullae containing serous or hemorrhagic fluid soon follow.
  - Local ischemia and necrosis result in formation of a black eschar within 7–10 days of the bite.
  - This necrotic area may expand slowly for weeks, especially in fatty areas that have delicate blood supplies such as the abdomen, buttocks, and thighs.
  - The eschar is shed after 2–5 weeks, and an ulcer remains that may take weeks to months to heal.
- Systemic manifestations of the bite are less common.
  - The most common symptoms are:
    - Fever
    - Chills
    - Malaise
  - Symptoms usually occur within 24 hours of the bite and also may include
    - Nausea
    - Vomiting
    - Diarrhea
    - Arthralgia
    - Urticaria or maculopapular rash

- Hemolytic anemia
- Disseminated intravascular coagulation
- Jaundice
- Renal failure
- Transverse myelitis
- Seizures
- Shock

Latrodectus (black widow spider)

- Local
  - A bite may go unnoticed or may be experienced as a pinprick or burning sensation.
  - 2 small puncture lesions may be visible.
  - Within 30 minutes, pain develops at the site and in the regional lymph nodes.
  - Central pallor at the bite site with surrounding erythema has been described.
  - Inflammatory response is mild.
  - An unusual reaction may include compartment syndrome, which may improve after antivenin administration.

- Systemic
  - The onset of systemic symptoms is frequently sudden, with crampy, skeletal muscle pains in the legs, abdomen, back, and chest and associated autonomic dysfunction.
  - The most frequent systemic signs and symptoms are:
    - Generalized abdominal pain or back pain
    - Local or extremity pain
    - Hypertension
    - Diaphoresis
    - Isolated abdominal or chest pains
    - Nausea
    - Vomiting
    - Tachycardia
    - Restlessness
    - Salivation
    - Bronchorrhea
    - Priapism
    - Urinary retention
    - Periorbital edema
    - Tremor
    - Convulsions
    - Muscle symptoms
    - Target-shaped skin lesions
    - Irritability
    - Agitation

- Abdominal rigidity may mimic peritoneal irritation.
- Respiratory paralysis, heart failure, and myocarditis have been reported.
- Patients who do not receive antivenin may experience protracted symptoms that may last for several days to 1 week, including:
  - Fatigue
  - Weakness
  - Paresthesias
  - Generalized aches
  - Diaphoresis
  - Headache
  - Sleeplessness
  - Excessive sweating
  - Impotence
  - Mental status changes
  - Transient hemiparesis

Tarantulas

- Most bites are no more severe than a bee sting.
- Occasionally result in local erythema, swelling, and pain
- Nausea and vomiting may occur.
- Some genera (*Lasiodora*, *Grammostola*, *Acanthoscurria*, and *Brachypelma*) can release urticaria-producing hairs from their abdomen by rubbing their hind legs on the area.
  - Can result in local histamine release with mild pruritus
  - Itching can last for weeks.
  - Hairs may cause considerable itching and discomfort in eyes or airways.

Scorpions

- Not all stings result in clinical evidence of envenomation.
- Patients may have both adrenergic and cholinergic symptoms.
- Local
  - Pain at the sting site with or without paresthesias is common.
  - In mild envenomations, pain may be the only symptom and may account for such manifestations as unexplained crying in infants.
  - Local erythema and swelling may surround a small puncture wound, but the sting site is often unidentifiable.
  - Paresthesias and pruritus are frequent.
- Systemic
  - Manifestations can be dramatic and usually develop within 60 minutes of sting.
    - Tachycardia or bradycardia
    - Central nervous system dysfunction, a finding that is rare in adults

- Severe hypertension in one third to two thirds of the victims
  - Can be associated with acute hypertensive encephalopathy
  - May not respond to medical management
- Heart failure
- Acute lung injury
- Pulmonary edema
- Neurologic toxicity includes excessive cholinergic stimulation resulting in salivation, sweating, and vomiting.
- Profound sialorrhea
- Skeletal muscle findings include twitching or jerking of the extremities, which may be severe enough to be mistaken for seizure activity.
- Rhabdomyolysis
- Nystagmus
- Seizures and agitation

Crotaline snakes

- Local
  - Presence of ≥1 fang marks, typically with ragged edges that may be obscured as a result of trauma resulting from first-aid attempts
  - Pain in >90% of envenomations
  - Edema
  - Ecchymosis
  - Erythema develops 15 minutes to 4 hours after the bite.
  - Hemorrhagic toxins in pit viper venom may cause blood to ooze from the puncture sites, and hemorrhagic bullae may develop.
  - Muscle necrosis
  - Lymphangitis and lymphadenopathy with tender regional lymph nodes and warmth in the injured body part as a result of lymphatic spread of venom
- Systemic
  - Malaise
  - Weakness
  - Lightheadedness
  - Diaphoresis
  - Visual disturbances
  - Nausea
  - Vomiting
  - Syncope
  - Myokymia
  - Perioral paresthesias
  - Metallic or minty taste

- More severe systemic effects include:
  - Altered sensorium
  - Acute respiratory distress syndrome
  - Respiratory depression
  - Hemodynamic instability leading to circulatory collapse
  - Renal failure
- A consumptive coagulopathy is frequently present in serious envenomations and is characterized by:
  - Hemolysis
  - Unmeasurable international normalized ratio (INR) and activated partial thromboplastin time
  - Hypofibrinogenemia
  - The presence of fibrin degradation products
  - Thrombocytopenia (<20,000 cells/mm)
  - Generalized hemorrhage
- When combined with defibrination, venom-induced thrombocytopenia may appear as disseminated intravascular coagulation.
- Mojave rattlesnake venom may cause more neurotoxicity, specifically myokymia, than the venom of other rattlesnakes.

Coral snakes

- Local
  - Erythema and local pain are transient or absent.
  - Most patients have evident fang marks.
- Systemic
  - May be delayed for 12 hours
  - May appear suddenly
  - May include bulbar paralysis with:
    - Ptosis
    - Dysphagia
    - Dysarthria
    - Excessive salivation
    - Paresthesias
    - Euphoria or apprehension
    - Drowsiness
    - Dizziness
    - Weakness
    - Confusion
    - Nausea
    - Vomiting
    - Diaphoresis
    - Muscle tenderness or fasciculations
    - Tremors

- Altered sensorium
- Drowsiness
- Ophthalmoplegias that cause visual disturbances
- These manifestations may be followed by:
  - Seizures
  - Respiratory paralysis
  - Pulmonary hemorrhage
- It can be unclear which findings are the result of the venom itself and which are the result of hypoxia.

DIFFERENTIAL DIAGNOSIS

Hymenoptera

Flying Hymenoptera

- Differential diagnosis of the local reaction includes:
  - Other arthropod envenomations
  - Puncture wounds with reactive erythema or cellulitis
  - Simple cellulitis
- Differential diagnosis of systemic reactions include:
  - Any other cause of allergic reaction
  - Reactive airway disease
  - Infectious processes
- Other causes of stridor, wheezing, and allergic reaction should be considered if a sting site cannot be identified.
- A stinger may sometimes be found at the sting site, which usually indicates a honeybee sting or, in some cases, a yellow jacket sting.
- Most patients cannot reliably identify the insect that stung them.

Fire ants

- Large local reactions must be carefully examined to differentiate them from cellulitis.
- Absence of lymphadenopathy and lymphangitis supports the diagnosis of large localized reaction.

Arachnids

- Differential diagnosis includes:
  - Other arthropod bites
  - Skin infections
  - Injury caused by chemical and physical agents

Loxosceles *(brown recluse spider)*

- In the absence of a definitive history of spider bites, other diagnostic possibilities must be considered, such as:
  - Emboli
  - Thrombi
  - Focal vasculitis

- Envenomation by other insects or reptiles
- Fat herniation with infarction
- Pressure sore
- Pyoderma gangrenosum
- Poison oak or ivy
- Cutaneous manifestation of gonorrhea orherpes simplex
- Diabetic ulcer
- Purpura fulminans
- Erythema nodosum
- Erythema multiforme
- Stevens-Johnson syndrome
- Abusive or self-inflicted trauma
- Cutaneous anthrax has been misdiagnosed as *Loxosceles* envenomation.
- Other species of spiders have been implicated in the cause of necrotic skin lesions similar to *Loxosceles*.
  - *Argiope* (orb weaver spider)
  - *Chiracanthium* (sac spider)
  - *Lycosa* (wolf spider)
  - *Phidippus* (jumping spider)
  - *Tegenaria agrestis* (hobo spider)
- The temptation to diagnose all necrotizing skin lesions as *Loxosceles* bites should be avoided.
- Positive identification of the spider is important not only for correct diagnosis but also to understand true clinical course of *Loxosceles* envenomation.

Latrodectus *(black widow spider)*

- Causes of acute abdominal pain should be part of the differential diagnosis.
- Close resemblance of the autonomic hyperactivity seen after black widow spider bites and those seen in organophosphate poisoning

Scorpions

- 2 factors make establishing the correct diagnosis difficult.
  - The sting site may not be identifiable
  - The child may not be able to communicate the history of a sting clearly.
- Some of the differential diagnostic possibilities are:
  - Seizure disorder
  - Intraabdominal process
  - Phenothiazine or cholinergic poisoning
  - Allergic reaction
- Asthma has been misdiagnosed in some children with wheezing and respiratory distress.

- Progression of symptoms is not predictable.
  - Progression to serious symptoms usually occurs in <5 hours, if at all.
  - Numbness, tingling, and pain may persist for 2 weeks.
  - Duration of symptoms has been found to be inversely related to the age of the patient.

Snakes

- The helpfulness of identifying the type of snake is controversial.
- The bite reflex in recently killed or decapitated snakes can remain intact, rendering them capable of biting even when they are dead.
- If medically necessary, a herpetologist from a zoo or aquarium may be able to help with positive identification.

LABORATORY FINDINGS

Hymenoptera

- No specific laboratory test is useful in the acute management of Hymenoptera stings.

Arachnids

- *Loxosceles* (brown recluse spider)
  - No current clinical laboratory study can confirm the presence of arachnid venom–related necrosis.
  - Several research tests, including enzyme-linked immunosorbent assay and passive hemagglutination inhibition test, have been studied but are not in clinical use.
  - Complete blood count, coagulation profile, electrolytes, and renal function should be monitored in systemic illness.
- *Latrodectus* (black widow spider)
  - No specific laboratory test helps establish a diagnosis.
  - Leukocytosis and hyperglycemia are common.
  - Creatine phosphokinase may be increased as a result of increased muscle activity.
  - Serum calcium levels are normal.
- Scorpions
  - No confirmatory laboratory test exists.
  - Leukocytosis, cerebrospinal fluid pleocytosis, and increased creatine phosphokinase have been reported.

Snakes

- Crotaline snakes (pit vipers)
  - Only of minor assistance to asses severity
  - May be useful in determining whether envenomation has occurred
  - Tests include:
    - Complete blood count with differential
    - Erythrocyte morphology (to assess for spherocytosis)

- INR and prothrombin time
- Plasma thromboplastin time
- Fibrinogen level
- Fibrin-split products
- Platelet count
  - If these studies reveal any abnormalities, or if the patient has clinical symptoms, then envenomation must be assumed and the clinician should perform:
    - Analysis of electrolytes
    - Blood urea nitrogen
    - Blood type and cross-match
    - Urinalysis
- Coral snakes
  - Do not mandate routine laboratory screening
  - If respiratory insufficiency is suspected, obtain:
    - Transcutaneous pulse oximetry
    - Arterial blood gases

IMAGING

- Rarely indicated, except in the case of a scorpion sting, where echocardiography can reveal hypodynamic ventricular motion with decreased systolic performance

DIAGNOSTIC PROCEDURES

- Rarely indicated, except in the case of a scorpion sting, where electrocardiographic changes are common and include:
- Ischemic electrocardiographic pattern
- Nonspecific ST-T changes or ST elevation or depression consistent with myocardial infarction

TREATMENT APPROACH

- The primary care clinician must be aware of local venomous species and be able to recognize and treat the injuries caused by them.
- In North America, venomous species include:
  - Arthropods
    - Bees
    - Wasps
    - Hornets
    - Ants
  - Arachnids
    - Spiders
    - Scorpions
  - Snakes
    - Pit vipers
    - Coral snakes

SPECIFIC TREATMENTS

Winged Hymenoptera

- Stinger removal
  - Traditional teaching advocates stinger removal by scraping with a hard-edged object, such as a credit card, to prevent pressure on the venom sac.
  - However, experimental data show that removal of the stinger with the fingers does not increase envenomation.
  - Rapid removal of the stinger by any means is most effective in minimizing envenomation.
  - Removal of bee stingers embedded for >1 minute will not reduce envenomation; most venom empties from detached honeybee stings within 10–20 seconds.
- Nonallergic local reactions
  - Nonallergic local reactions require symptomatic treatment, including:
    - Cool compresses (ice should not be placed directly on the skin)
    - Elevation
    - Local wound care
  - No further evaluation is necessary.
  - If local itching is bothersome
    - An oral histamine-1 (H_1) antagonist, such as diphenhydramine, may help.
  - Local allergic reactions require similar care as nonallergic reactions.
  - For very large cutaneous reactions
    - Prednisone (0.5–2 mg/kg/day given in 1–4 doses for 3–5 days) may be useful.
- Acute management of corneal bee sting includes:
  - Preventing secondary infection with broad-spectrum topical antibiotics
  - Reducing inflammation with topical corticosteroids
  - Treating anterior uveitis
  - Early detection and treatment of inflammatory glaucoma
  - Providing pain relief
  - Surgical removal of the embedded stinger is controversial.
  - Pulse corticosteroids may prevent permanent loss of vision.
- Medications
  - Mild systemic allergic reactions
    - Diphenhydramine or another H_1-antihistamine
    - Supportive care
    - Observation
  - Severe systemic allergic reactions
    - Epinephrine
      - 0.01-mL/kg dose of 1:1000 aqueous epinephrine solution is injected subcutaneously.
      - The original dose should not exceed 0.3 mL, but may be repeated in 15 minutes.
      - Susceptible individuals should carry epinephrine self-administered kits when they go outdoors.
      - After kit is used, medical help should be sought because the effect of the drug is short lasting.
    - H_1-antagonists
    - Corticosteroids
    - Intensive supportive care
  - Severe systemic reactions from direct toxic effects of massive envenomation require:
    - Intensive supportive care
    - Therapy similar to that for anaphylactic reactions
    - Careful monitoring for:
      - Rhabdomyolysis
      - Thrombocytopenia
      - Cardiac arrhythmias
      - Renal failure
      - Possible dialysis

Fire ants

- Mild local reactions are treated conservatively with
  - Cool compresses
  - Oral antihistamines
  - Wound care
- Large local reactions may require oral antihistamines and systemic corticosteroids.
- Systemic allergic reactions are treated similarly to those from any cause.
- Epinephrine is the mainstay of therapy, coupled with:
  - H_1-antagonists
  - Systemic corticosteroids
  - Vigorous supportive care as appropriate

Harvester ants

- Treatment is the same as that for other Hymenoptera stings.

Loxosceles (brown recluse spider)

- Management is controversial.
- Serial observation, wound cleansing, cool compresses, splinting of the affected extremity, and tetanus prophylaxis are often-suggested measures.
- Symptomatic relief with antipruritics and analgesics may be useful in some cases.

- Different therapies have been proposed, including:
  - Systemic corticosteroids
  - Antibiotics
  - Antihistamines
  - Colchicine
  - Dapsone
  - Electric shock
  - Hyperbaric oxygen
  - Metronidazole
  - Surgical excision
  - Skin graft
- Delay surgical repair of skin defects until necrotic demarcation is discrete and no further spread occurs, which takes about 8 weeks.

Latrodectus *(black widow spider)*

- Most black widow spider bites require only:
  - Cool compresses
  - Elevation of the affected extremity
  - Tetanus update (if needed)
  - Analgesics
- In more severe cases, suggested treatments include:
  - Oxygen
  - Cardiac monitoring
  - Intravenous access
- Muscle cramps may be relieved with opiates and muscle relaxants.
  - The following have been used, with varying results:
    - Diazepam
    - Methocarbamol
    - Calcium gluconate (the efficacy of 10% calcium gluconate has been questioned)
- Patients who do not receive antivenin will gradually improve over the next 12–48 hours.
  - Some patients may experience protracted symptoms.
- *Latrodectus* antivenin of equine origin neutralizes venom from all related species.
  - Patients should be tested for horse serum hypersensitivity before administration to prevent death from anaphylaxis.
  - Consider in cases of:
    - Severe envenomation with evidence of respiratory distress, marked hypertension, and cardiovascular compromise
    - Pregnancy
    - Protracted symptoms that do not respond to analgesic sand muscle relaxants

- Response is usually dramatic after antivenin infusion.
- Administration of antivenin may decrease length of hospital stay and prevent lingering neurologic complications.

Tarantulas

- Local wound care and a tetanus update are all that is needed in most cases.
- Antihistamines and oral analgesics may be helpful.
- Adhesive tape or irrigation with saline solution may be used to remove the urticaria-producing hairs from the skin.

Scorpions

- There is no standard therapy.
- Treatment is primarily supportive, with the use of cold compresses and analgesics.
- Severe cases require aggressive supportive therapy.
- Antihypertensives have been used, including:
  - Calcium-channel blockers
  - Hydralazine
  - Prazosin
  - Captopril
- Afterload reducers are front-line therapeutic agents for hypertension, including:
  - Angiotensin-converting enzyme inhibitors
  - Calcium-channel blockers
  - Prazosin
- Concern about reflex tachycardia has led some clinicians to favor prazosin and captopril.
- The use of diuretics for pulmonary edema is controversial.
- Atropine may be used with caution if cholinergic symptoms become severe.
  - Atropine may improve hypersecretion, obviating the need for more aggressive therapy.
- Treatment should be guided by thorough hemodynamic monitoring.
- Benzodiazepines are generally administered for seizures and agitation.
- Corticosteroid therapy has been shown to be of no benefit.
- Currently, no scorpion antivenin is approved by the US Food and Drug Administration.
- Clinical trials are ongoing of an equine-derived antigen-binding fragment (Fab_2) antivenin.

Snakes

- First aid
  - Observe the approximate size and characteristics of the snake only if this can be done without danger of remaining within striking range.
  - Move the patient as little as possible.
  - Mark the victim's skin with a pen to indicate the area of swelling and the time and repeat every 15 minutes.

- Remove rings, watches, and constrictive clothing.
- Immobilize the affected limb by splinting as if for a fracture, keeping the limb below the level of the heart.
- Regardless of early symptoms, transport the victim to the nearest medical facility at a safe speed.
- Avoid use of:
  - Ice (tissue damage)
  - Aspirin (anticoagulation)
  - Alcohol or sedative drugs (vasodilation)
  - Stimulants, such as caffeine (acceleration of venom absorption)
- As soon as possible, start basic life support, including volume expansion and Trendelenburg position for patients with hypotension.
- Patients should be kept as calm as possible during transport because agitation hastens venom distribution.
- Controversial forms of first aid
  - Incision and suction should not be performed.
  - Constricting bands that impede blood or lymph flow should not be used.
  - Loose-fitting bands placed in an effort to reduce lymphatic flow have been advocated but have not been shown to be of clear benefit.
  - Although the routine use of an extractor device for field care is not advocated, patients with an extractor or suction device in place should not remove it until they arrive at a health care facility.
- In-hospital care
  - Medical history of known envenomations should include
    - Size and species of the snake
    - Circumstances of the bite (eg, through clothing, alcohol related)
    - Number of bites and body area affected
    - First-aid methods used
    - Time of bite and transport time
    - Previous snakebite history
    - Allergy to horse- or sheep-derived products (eg, drugs, food, animal products)
    - Tetanus immunization status
  - Coexisting medical conditions, with special attention paid to the cardiovascular, pulmonary, and neurologic systems, should be factored into clinical management.
  - Snakebites from exotic (nonindigenous) species, which usually occur in zoo employees or in those illegally keeping the snake as a house pet, should be part of the history-gathering process.
  - Clinical presentation and medical management of an exotic bite may differ from bites of North American poisonous snakes.

- Local therapy
  - Local wound care includes:
    - Gentle irrigation
    - Nonconstrictive immobilization
    - Elevation of the bitten extremity
    - Close observation
  - Circumferential measurements at several points along the affected limb should be performed at baseline and regularly repeated.
  - Intercompartmental pressures should only be measured when the patient's symptoms are consistent with compartment syndrome.
  - In cases of suspected compartment syndrome, clinical diagnosis requires objective evidence of increases in compartment pressure to >30 mm Hg.
  - Fasciotomy has not been shown to be beneficial; it may lengthen hospitalization and cause significant long-term morbidity.
  - Digital dermotomy may be indicated on clinical grounds.
- Use of antivenin
  - Crotaline polyvalent immune Fab (ovine) antivenin (CroFab)
    - CroFab has replaced the horse serum–based antivenin ACP as the drug of choice.
    - CroFab is a purified ovine polyvalent Fab immunoglobulin fragment product produced by immunizing sheep with venoms of 4 crotaline snakes.
    - Indicated in treatment of patients with minimal or moderate North American crotaline envenomation
    - Administer within 6 hours.
    - Delayed use of CroFab has been reported with successful correction of significant toxicity incurred after crotaline envenomation.
  - Antivenom use should proceed simultaneously with supportive therapy.
- Steps in using antivenin
  - Prepare to manage anaphylaxis.
    - Anaphylactic reaction to CroFab is uncommon but has been reported.
    - All patients receiving antivenin should be monitored, and 2 sites for intravenous access should be considered—1 for the antivenin and 1 for emergency drugs and fluids.
    - Intravenous epinephrine, diphenhydramine, and plasma expanders, as well as cardiorespiratory support, must be readily available.

- Test for sensitivity.
  - Skin testing is not needed for the administration of CroFab.
  - Pretreatment with epinephrine, H_1-receptor antagonists, and H_2-receptor antagonists, or corticosteroids is not routinely recommended unless the patient has a history of hypersensitivity.
- Start the infusion.
  - Dosing is based on estimated venom injected; no dose adjustment is required for children.
  - Each vial of CroFab is reconstituted with 10 mL of sterile water for injection.
  - After reconstitution, the entire dose (4–6 vials) is diluted in 250 mL of 0.9% sodium chloride and mixed by swirling gently.
  - Use reconstituted and diluted product within 4 hours.
  - Dose should be infused intravenously over 60 minutes with careful observation for allergic or anaphylactoid reactions.
- Repeat infusion.
  - If initial control is not achieved, the loading dose of 4–6 vials should be repeated until initial control of envenomation syndrome has been achieved.
  - After initial control has been achieved, giving additional 2-vial doses every 6 hours for 3 doses is recommended.
  - Additional doses may be necessary, as guided by clinical status and consultation with a clinician experienced in treating snakebite or a regional poison control center.
- CroFab is administered with the goal of achieving initial control, defined as the reversal or marked attenuation of all effects of venom.
  - This process encompasses 3 general areas.
    - Coagulation abnormalities
    - Systemic effects
    - Local effects (progression of swelling)
  - Volume depletion should be aggressively treated before initiating antivenin therapy because of the risk of rapid vasodilatation and third-space fluid loss associated with anaphylaxis.
  - Anaphylaxis associated with antivenin therapy should be treated in the standard manner.
- Antivenom use in copperhead bites
  - Envenomations by copperheads are not considered to be as serious as rattlesnake or cottonmouth bites.
  - Clinically significant local effects may occur, suggesting that these bites should be cautiously managed.
  - Copperhead victims treated with CroFab had marked improvement in local tissue effects, but clinical failures and recurrence of local effects also occurred.

- The use of CroFab in copperhead bites has been shown to halt local tissue effect.
  - More data are needed to define the role of CroFab for treatment of copperhead envenomation.
  - The suggested dosing of CroFab in copperhead envenomation is a single loading dose.
  - Additional maintenance doses after initial control did not reduce incidence of recurrent swelling in 1 study.
  - After administering the loading dose, monitor patient for progressive swelling, coagulopathy development, and systemic effects.
  - The need for additional antivenin should be evaluated on a case-by-case basis, and poison control center consultation is advised.
- Antivenom use in children
  - CroFab use in children 14 months to 13 years of age has been found to be safe and effective.
  - Children with crotaline envenomation may be more likely to experience serious effects as a result of the larger ratio of venom to serum volume.
  - Any child with a crotaline envenomation that meets the criteria for antivenin therapy should receive the same dosing regimen as adults.
  - Weight-based dosing is not appropriate for antivenin neutralization because the dose should reflect venom load, not patient size.
- Additional therapeutic measures
  - Pain control
    - Adequate pain control allows rehabilitation to begin as early as possible to prevent contractures.
    - Opioid analgesics should be used cautiously if the venom is known to have neurotoxicity (eg, Mojave rattlesnake).
    - Nonsteroidal antiinflammatory agents should be used with caution, especially in patients with evidence of coagulopathy.
  - Infection control
    - Infection is rare in the absence of severe necrosis.
    - Good wound care is usually sufficient to prevent secondary infection.
    - Antibiotic prophylaxis is not currently suggested.
  - Corticosteroids
    - They should not be routinely administered to snakebite victims.
    - They are efficacious in patients who develop serum sickness after antivenin administration.
  - Tetanus prophylaxis
    - *Clostridium tetani* are not part of the mouth flora of snakes.
    - Updating the patient's tetanus immunization is the only necessary intervention.

Coral snakes

- First aid
  - Do not use cryotherapy, incision and suction (including the Sawyer extractor), or constricting bands.
  - Australian pressure mobilization technique has been used.
    - Wrapping the entire bitten extremity with a crepe bandage, elastic bandage, or article of clothing as tightly as possible, then splinting it
- Use of antivenin
  - Antivenom effective against Eastern and Texas coral snake venom is used if a patient has definitely been bitten or if any signs or symptoms develop.
  - Guidelines are based on the judgment that risks of intravenous hyperimmune horse serum are offset by potential prevention of respiratory paralysis if therapy is not immediately administered.
  - Skin testing is of little benefit in making therapeutic decisions.
  - 3–5 vials of antivenin are mixed in 250–500 mL of normal saline, and 1–2 mL is given intravenously over 3–5 minutes.
  - The medical team must be prepared for anaphylaxis and have necessary drugs and equipment at bedside.
  - If the patient does not show any signs of an allergic reaction, then the remainder of the solution is infused slowly as tolerated.
  - An additional 3–5 vials of antivenin-saline mixture may be infused if signs and symptoms do not abate.
  - >10 vials of antivenin are rarely required for coral snake envenomations.
- Additional therapeutic measures
  - Prophylaxis for infection and tetanus as for pit viper bites is not indicated.
  - Additional measures may become necessary if aspiration pneumonia develops.
  - Patients should be aware that muscular weakness may persist for 3–6 weeks.
- Supportive therapy
  - Elective intubation before impending respiratory paralysis tends to prevent aspiration pneumonia and should be performed if any signs of bulbar paralysis develop.
  - Patient should receive cardiac and pulse oximetry monitoring (if not intubated), and intravenous access should be established.

Nonindigenous snakes

- If a bite from an exotic species is suspected, the suggested approach includes:
  - Local wound care
  - Supportive care
  - Consultation with experts at a regional poison control center

WHEN TO ADMIT

- Hymenoptera
  - Severe systemic allergic reactions or severe systemic reactions caused by massive envenomation
- *Loxosceles* (brown recluse spider)
  - Secondary infection requiring intravenous antibiotics
  - Inability to provide adequate wound care at home
  - Severe systemic symptoms
- *Latrodectus* (black widow spider)
  - Severe systemic symptoms
  - After use of antivenin
- Tarantulas
  - Significant comorbidity
  - Inability to tolerate oral fluids
- Scorpions
  - Cardiac or neurological toxicity
  - Severe systemic signs or symptoms
- Pit vipers
  - Chance of envenomation
- Coral snakes
  - Chance of envenomation
  - All victims of potential coral snake envenomation should be admitted to an intensive care unit and monitored closely for a minimum of 12 hours.
    - Effects of envenomation may develop precipitously hours after a bite and are not easily reversed once they occur.
  - If the snake cannot be found, then victims of bites suspected to be from coral snakes should be admitted to the hospital for 12 hours of observation.

WHEN TO REFER

- Concerns about allergic reactions, mostly from insects, result in referrals to allergy and immunology specialists.
- Hymenoptera
  - Children who experience extracutaneous systemic reactions should be referred to an allergist for risk analysis and possible venom immunotherapy.
- Fire ants
  - Patients who have experienced severe allergic reactions to stings should be referred to an allergist or immunologist for venom immunotherapy assessment.
- *Loxosceles* (brown recluse spider)
  - Surgical intervention necessary for wound care
- *Latrodectus* (black widow spider)
  - Before administration of antivenin
- Tarantulas
  - Hairs in eyes that are not easily removed

- Scorpions
  - Considered use of antivenin
- Pit vipers
  - Considered use of antivenin
  - Surgical intervention necessary for wound care
- Coral snakes
  - Patients who experience full-thickness tissue damage may require referral to a surgeon.
  - Physical or occupational therapy may be needed to encourage joint mobilization of the affected extremity.
  - Anticipated need for airway control or intensive care unit monitoring

FOLLOW-UP

Hymenoptera

- Patients with systemic reactions who respond completely to therapy in the emergency department should be observed for 6–8 hours after the sting for a possible delayed anaphylactic episode.
- Patients with severe symptoms, including airway, cardiovascular, or pulmonary compromise, or persistent symptoms should receive a short course of corticosteroids.
- At the time of discharge after a systemic reaction, all patients should be given a prescription for a self-administered epinephrine kit.
  - Patient or caretaker should be instructed in its proper use before discharge from the emergency department.
  - They should be encouraged to wear a Medic Alert bracelet indicating allergy to insect stings.
- Patients should be taught how to prevent further stings.
- The perception that children generally outgrow Hymenoptera sting allergies is not always true.

Snakes

- After pit viper envenomation, all patients should be observed in the emergency department for a minimum of 8 hours.
  - Patients who remain asymptomatic and whose coagulation study results are normal may be discharged with instructions to return if symptoms develop.
  - Symptomatic patients and all patients treated with antivenin should be admitted to the intensive care unit.
- Preservation of joint mobility and muscle strength is a goal after pit viper envenomation.
  - Pain control may be needed in the weeks after discharge.
  - If the patient received antivenin, then serum sickness should be discussed.
    - The patient should be taught how to monitor for this syndrome.

COMPLICATIONS

Winged Hymenoptera

- Severe neuroophthalmic complications include:
  - Optic neuritis
  - Loss of vision
  - Cataracts
- Respiratory and cardiovascular complications are observed more often in adults than children.
- In rare cases, serum sickness, vasculitis, encephalopathy, neuritis, and renal disease with or without rhabdomyolysis have been observed.
- Renal failure or death may occur when 20–200 wasp stings or 150–1000 or more honeybee stings have been inflicted.

Fire ants

- Secondary bacterial infections from excoriation and open erosions are not uncommon after fire ant stings.
  - These infections are usually minor and localized.
- Sepsis may result from superinfected lesions.

Snakes

- Shock
  - Patients may have a marked decrease in intravascular volume as a result of:
    - Hemorrhage
    - Third-space fluid loss
    - Vomiting
    - Diaphoresis
  - Crystalloid replacement should begin immediately in envenomated patients.
  - In the case of hypotension caused by extravascular fluid shifts or hemorrhage, antivenin therapy should be considered.
- Fluid and electrolyte abnormalities
  - May be caused by extensive third-space fluid loss
  - Electrolyte and urine output monitoring with fluid and electrolyte replacement with crystalloid is essential.
- Hematologic complications
  - Treatment of thrombocytopenia and anemia (caused by hemolysis) may require multiple transfusions.
  - Transfusions of fresh-frozen plasma and cryoprecipitate may be required in severely envenomated patients.
  - Therapy with blood products is rarely effective in the absence of antivenin therapy.
  - Treatment with coagulation factors may worsen coagulopathy by adding more substrate for unneutralized venom, thus increasing the levels of degradation products, which are also anticoagulants.

- Thrombocytopenia often corrects with antivenin therapy alone, and clotting factor levels rarely improve when blood products are provided without antivenin.
- Disseminated intravascular coagulopathy caused by snakebite does not respond to heparin; antivenin is the treatment of choice.
- Recurrence phenomena
  - Worsening status caused by return of venom effect after it has been successfully abated with antivenin
  - *Local recurrence* is return of swelling after initial control is achieved.
  - *Coagulopathic recurrence* is return of thrombocytopenia or hypofibrinogenemia after initial control is achieved.
    - All CroFab recipients should be reevaluated at least once during the 5 days after antivenin treatment.
    - The decision to administer additional antivenin in patients who develop delayed coagulopathy must be made on a case-by-case basis.
  - An isolated hematologic abnormality after envenomation poses a low risk for significant bleeding.
  - *Multicompartment coagulopathies* (critically abnormal INR, activated partial thromboplastin time, fibrinogen, platelets) may represent a risk for bleeding and may warrant additional antivenin consideration.
  - Conservative management for this scenario may be adequate; clinicians should consult with someone experienced in treating crotaline envenomations or with a regional poison control center.
- Serum sickness
  - Delayed reactions to antivenin are thought to be the result of serum sickness–like reactions attributable to immune complexes due to an immune response against antivenin proteins.
  - May occur 7–21 days after completion of treatment
  - Few patients require hospitalization.
  - Oral corticosteroids (prednisone) should be prescribed at the first signs (usually urticaria and pruritus) and should be continued for 24 hours after all symptoms have subsided and then tapered over 72 hours.
  - If necessary, diphenhydramine or hydroxyzine may be added to control pruritus.

PREVENTION

Hymenoptera

- Do not disturb nests or hives—have someone else remove them.
- Do not wear perfume, cologne, scented sunscreens, or hairspray when outdoors.
- Use footwear when outside.
- Avoid garbage sites, orchards, fields of clover, and flowerbeds.
- Be extra careful when gardening, and cover the hands and body.
- For patients receiving immunotherapy, avoid trips outdoors if medical help is not readily available or until maintenance immunotherapy is established.
- Install screens on windows and doors to prevent insects from entering the home.

Spiders

- Prevention is mostly focused on caution in areas inhabited by spiders.
- A clean house greatly decreases the risk of spider bite.
- Wear long-sleeved shirts and gloves when outside gardening or long pants tucked into socks when hiking.
- Insect repellents that contain meta-N,N-diethyltoluamide (DEET) or picaridin offer some protection.

Snakes

- Children should not approach, disturb, play with, capture, or kill any snake.
- Snakes frequently can be found under rocks, boulders, fallen trees, fences, rubbish piles, and boats that have been left on shore for several hours; in tall grass and heavy underbrush; or sunning themselves on logs, boulders, trees, walls, or cliffs.
- The striking distance of a snake is roughly half its length.
- The striking reflex remains intact for up to 1 hour after the snake has died.
- Rattlesnakes are nocturnal feeders and are active after dark.
  - Never gather firewood after dark.
  - Camp should be set up on open ground.
  - Camp should not be set up near wood, rubbish piles, swampy areas, or the entrance of a cave.
- Once someone is bitten, everyone present should get away from the snake as quickly as possible.
  - The benefit of identifying the snake is small compared with the risk of additional bites.

Epistaxis

DEFINITION

- Defined as acute bleeding from the nostril, nasal cavity, or nasopharynx
  - Relatively common and usually self-limited occurrence in childhood
  - Can be extremely distressing to children and parents when profuse or recurrent
  - Can at times be a sign of a more serious condition
- Anterior epistaxis
  - Accounts for >90% of epistaxis in children
  - Almost all the blood exits anteriorly through the nares.
  - Much easier to visualize and control than posterior bleeding
- Posterior epistaxis
  - Most of the blood flows into the nasopharynx and mouth, making the degree of bleeding difficult to assess.
  - Bleeding generally much more profuse than anterior bleeding
  - More likely than anterior bleeding to lead to hemodynamic instability

EPIDEMIOLOGY

- Incidence
  - 5–14% of Americans have a nosebleed each year.
    - Approximately 10% of those affected seek care from a physician.
- Prevalence
  - In a study of the epidemiology of epistaxis in US emergency departments (EDs) from 1992–2001:
    - Approximately 1 in 200 of all ED visits were for epistaxis.
    - Peaks were found in children <10 years and in older adults age 70–79 years.
    - 83% of cases were from atraumatic causes.
    - A higher proportion of visits occurred during the winter months.
  - Likelihood of experiencing ≥1 nosebleed during childhood
    - ~30% of children from birth to age 5 years
    - 56% of children age 6–10 years
    - 64% of children age 11–15 years
- Sex
  - More common in boys than in girls
- Age
  - Bimodal distribution, with peaks in children <10 years and in adults >50 years
  - Rare under age 2 years
  - Peaks between age 3 and 8 years
  - Infrequent after puberty

MECHANISM

- Blood supply to the nose originates in both the internal and the external carotid arteries.
- Nosebleeds are usually classified as anterior or posterior on the basis of the location of the vessels that are the source of the bleeding (see Definition).
- Anterior epistaxis
  - Kiesselbach plexus is primary source.
    - Made up of anastomoses of vessels in the anterior 2–3 cm of the nasal septum, just 0.5 cm from the tip of the nose
    - Also known as *Little area*
    - Rich vasculature under thin mucosa
    - Area most exposed to trauma and dry air
- Posterior epistaxis
  - Woodruff plexus, specifically the sphenopalatine, is the primary source.
    - Convergence of the sphenopalatine, posterior nasal, and ascending pharyngeal arteries, located over the posterior middle turbinate

HISTORY

- Evaluation should begin with a careful history and physical examination.
- Note season and associated environmental conditions.
- History of nose picking or blunt trauma
- Unilaterality
  - May suggest a local anatomic cause
- Unilateral foul-smelling discharge in a young child
  - May indicate a retained foreign body
  - One-half of children treated in an ED for intranasal foreign body admitted placing the object in the nose; therefore, young children should be questioned.
- Unilateral progressive obstruction
  - Suggests a mass
- Presence and character of any associated rhinorrhea
  - Clear, watery rhinorrhea with associated sneezing suggests allergic rhinitis .
  - Mucosal discharge with cough suggests upper respiratory infection.
- Degree of chronicity
  - May suggest an inherited systemic cause
- History of petechiae or easy bruising or other mucosal bleeding (eg, menorrhagia, postsurgical)
  - May point to a bleeding disorder
- Associated fever or pallor
  - May suggest leukemia

- History of medication use
  - Particularly aspirin or nonsteroidal antiinflammatory drugs (NSAIDs)
- Family history of bleeding symptoms or diagnosed disorder
  - Useful in identifying children with a bleeding diathesis
- Migraine headaches
  - A recent study showed a significant association between migraine headaches and recurrent epistaxis, suggesting a common pathogenesis.

PHYSICAL EXAM

- Blood pressure and pulse if the history suggests significant acute or chronic blood loss
- Careful examination of the nose
  - Attempt to identify the source of any active bleeding.
  - Note any discharge, obstructing mass, or foreign body.
- The neck should be examined for the presence of a mass.
- The skin should be checked for petechiae or unusual location or number of ecchymoses.
- If the child is ill, perform a full examination, including a search for lymphadenopathy and hepatosplenomegaly.

DIFFERENTIAL DIAGNOSIS

Local causes

- >1 factor often plays a role in the bleeding.
  - Trauma from nose picking or rubbing
    - Accounts for most cases in children, particularly in association with inflammation from infection or allergy
  - Blunt external trauma
    - Generally acute and self-limiting
    - Should prompt evaluation for fractures of the facial bones and an anterior septal hematoma
  - Trauma from a foreign body
    - Occasional cause in toddlers
    - Often results in unilateral bleeding accompanied by foul-smelling or bloody discharge
  - Upper respiratory infection and allergic rhinitis
    - Resultant rhinorrhea leads to digital manipulation or forceful sneezing and nose blowing.
    - Vascular congestion and mucosal irritation promote easy injury to the blood vessels of the anterior septum.
    - Association in children of positive allergy skin tests and recurrent epistaxis
  - Low environmental humidity, especially in winter months
  - Deviated nasal septum
    - Can contribute to recurrent epistaxis by causing a change in normal airflow, leading to mucosal drying and irritation

- Intranasal drugs (steroids, cocaine)
- Neoplasms
  - Uncommon in children but should be considered in certain circumstances
  - Polyps in children are usually associated with cystic fibrosis.
  - Juvenile nasopharyngeal angiofibroma
    - Benign vascular tumor originating in the lateral nasopharynx
    - Occurs only in male adolescents because of its hormonal sensitivity
    - Recurrent epistaxis is the most frequent presenting symptom.
    - Unilateral progressive obstruction or discharge are clues to the diagnosis.
  - Rhabdomyosarcoma of the nasal cavity or nasopharynx
    - A rare malignant cause of severe episodic epistaxis
    - May be associated with signs of eustachian tube dysfunction, such as unilateral middle ear effusion
  - Nasal hemangioma
    - Rare
    - Should be considered in infants
  - Nasopharyngeal carcinoma
    - Extremely uncommon but serious disease in children
    - Epistaxis is the presenting symptom in approximately 50% of children.
    - Nearly always accompanied by a neck mass or neck pain

Systemic causes

- Should be considered whenever nosebleeds are recurrent or persistent in the absence of any obvious local cause
- Epistaxis scoring system (see table Epistaxis Scoring System)
  - Frequency, duration, amount, age at onset, and bilateral epistaxis have been used to determine which patients should be evaluated for an underlying bleeding disorder.
- Hematologic disorders (congenital or acquired)
  - Platelet disorders
  - Coagulation defects
  - Thrombocytopenia
    - Almost always accompanied by petechiae or ecchymoses
    - Idiopathic thrombocytopenic purpura
      - Most common cause of isolated thrombocytopenia in otherwise healthy children
      - Presents as acute mucosal hemorrhage, often epistaxis, in approximately 30% of patients
      - Bleeding is rarely severe.

Epistaxis Scoring System[a]

Component		Score[b]
Frequency	5–15/yr	0
	16–25/yr	1
	>25/yr	2
Duration	<5 min	0
	5–10 min	1
	>10 min	2
Amount[c]	<15 mL	0
	15–30 mL	1
	>30 mL	2
Epistaxis history and age[d]	33%	0
	33–67%	1
	>67%	2
Site	Unilateral	0
	Bilateral	2

[a] From: Katsanis E, Luke K, Hsu E, et al. Prevelance and significance of mild bleeding disorders in children with recurrent epistaxis. *J Pediatr.* 1988;113(1):73–76. Copyright © Elsevier 1988.
[b] Mild=0–6; severe=7–10
[c] Estimate of average blood loss per episode, based on fractions or multiples of teaspoons, tablespoons, or cups.
[d] Proportion of the child's life that nosebleeds have been recurrent (>5/yr).

- Can be an adverse reaction to a variety of medications, including anticonvulsants, such as carbamazepine and chemotherapeutic agents
- Leukemia
  - Epistaxis is rarely the first symptom.
  - Should be considered in an ill-appearing child with epistaxis, especially with fever, pallor, lymphadenopathy, or hepatosplenomegaly
- Platelet dysfunction from aspirin or NSAIDs can predispose the individual to epistaxis.
- Bernard-Soulier syndrome
  - Disorder of platelet aggregation
  - Occasional diagnosis in children evaluated for isolated epistaxis

- Primary coagulation defects
  - May result in persistent and long-standing epistaxis
  - Positive family history is often present.
  - Up to one-third of children with isolated recurrent epistaxis have a diagnosable coagulopathy.
  - Von Willebr and disease (VWD)
    - The most commonly identified inherited coagulopathy
    - 60% of patients with VWD have recurrent epistaxis.
    - Other mucosal bleeding (eg, menorrhagia or post-surgical or postdental extraction) is also a common symptom in older children and adolescents.
  - Hemophilia
    - Much less common
    - In mild cases, may cause isolated epistaxis (factor VII, VIII, IX, or XI deficiency)
- Acquired coagulopathies
  - Unlike adults, rare cause of epistaxis in children
  - Include various liver diseases (eg, chronic active hepatitis) with consequent depletion of clotting factors
  - An acquired form of VWD has been described in children receiving valproic acid.
- Vascular abnormalities
  - Osler-Weber-Rendu disease (hereditary hemorrhagic telangiectasia)
    - Autosomal-dominant disorder of the blood vessel walls
    - Characterized by the progressive development of cutaneous and mucosal telangiectasias
  - >90% of affected patients have recurrent and progressively worsening epistaxis.
  - Present at a mean age of 12 years
  - Gastrointestinal bleeding and pulmonary arteriovenous malformations occasionally also occur in childhood.
- Primary isolated hypertension
  - Has not been clearly associated with epistaxis in children, except in the context of renal failure

LABORATORY EVALUATION

- The need for and extent of laboratory testing should be guided by history and physical examination.
- Frequent and prolonged episodes may warrant ruling out anemia caused by blood loss.
- Complete blood count
  - Always indicated in the presence of petechiae or unusual ecchymoses to rule out thrombocytopenia
  - Will help rule out leukemia in an ill child with pallor, fever, lymphadenopathy, or hepatosplenomegaly

- Prothrombin time and partial thromboplastin time
  - Useful as initial screening tests for VWD
    - Results may be within the normal range in some patients with VWD.
    - Further evaluation with von Willebrand factor studies may be necessary.

IMAGING

- Rarely indicated
- Plain films can rule out associated fracture of the facial bones in the setting of blunt trauma.
- Computed tomography should be considered if a mass is thought to be present.

DIAGNOSTIC PROCEDURES

- Identifying the source of posterior bleeding must be done by an otolaryngologist using a flexible fiberoptic nasopharyngoscope.
  - Sedation may be required for younger patients.
  - Endoscopic visualization may also reveal such causes as foreign bodies, tumors, or sinusitis.
  - In older, more cooperative patients, a rigid endoscope may be used.
- Cauterization of a posterior bleeding site can be performed under general anesthesia.
  - Posterior packing can be done with gauze or even urinary catheter balloons.
    - Other types of packing include premade nasal tampons or balloons.

TREATMENT APPROACH

- Management can be divided into 3 general phases.
  - Initial first aid measures
    - Often performed at home
    - Should also be the first line of treatment on presentation to the physician
    - Parents should be educated about the home management of an acute nosebleed.
  - Acute management of persistent bleeding
    - May be initiated by a pediatrician in an office or ED
    - May have to be continued by an otolaryngologist if initial measures are unsuccessful
    - May involve medical or surgical intervention
  - Long-term preventive treatment of recurrent epistaxis
    - Including evaluation and treatment of underlying causes
- Once acute episode of epistaxis has resolved:
  - Look for predisposing factors or causes.
  - Implement respective preventive strategies or specific management.

- If allergic rhinitis is a factor:
  - Appropriate testing and medical management are indicated.
  - Treat with inhaled topical nasal steroids.
  - For sinusitis, oral antibiotics are prescribed.
- Management of recurrent nosebleeds
  - Common challenge for physicians
  - No consensus on the frequency or severity of episodes that warrant medical intervention
  - Common interventions for less severe cases include:
    - Cautery with silver nitrate
    - Antibiotic nasal creams
    - Nasal saline spray
    - Coating of the interior nose with ointments, such as petroleum jelly
  - Less frequently advocated topical agents include:
    - Oxymetazoline
    - Desmopressin
    - Antifibrinolytics
    - Fibrin sealants (most recently)
  - More invasive measures rarely indicated in children:
    - Arterial embolization for refractory bleeding
    - Arterial ligation for recurrent epistaxis
  - A recent Cochrane review of the literature on interventions for recurrent idiopathic epistaxis in children (<16 years) exposed the lack of evidence for current treatments.
    - No single treatment (neomycin-chlorhexidine antiseptic cream, silver nitrate cautery, petroleum jelly) was found to be superior to another or to no treatment.
    - No serious adverse effects were experienced.
      - Silver nitrate cauterization caused pain in children despite topical anesthesia.
    - High-quality studies are needed to ascertain which, if any, of these remedies are most effective.

SPECIFIC TREATMENT

First aid measures

Direct pressure

- Many health care providers and patients are unaware of the proper spot for applying direct pressure to the nose to stop a nosebleed.
  - Vast majority of bleeding episodes originate anteriorly, in the Little area.
  - Apply pressure to the alar nasi using the first and second fingers.
  - Pressure should be held by pinching the nostrils without interruption for 5–10 minutes.

- The child should sit up with the head bent forward slightly.
  - Minimizes blood dripping posteriorly and being swallowed, which can cause nausea and hematemesis
- Some providers suggest placement of ice packs on the forehead, bridge of the nose, nape of the neck, or upper lip to promote vasoconstriction.
  - Only theory supports this practice.

First aid in the health care setting

- Initial treatment measures should occur simultaneously with assessment and history taking.
- Basic equipment should be readied.
  - Examination
    - Flashlight or
    - Otoscope with speculum or
    - Headlight and nasal speculum suction
  - Vasoconstriction
    - Oxymetazoline or
    - Phenylephrine or
    - Epinephrine (1:1000)
  - Topical anesthesia
    - 4% lidocaine or
    - 3–5% cocaine ethyl chloride solution
  - Hemostasis
    - Silver nitrate sticks
    - Vaseline strip gauze
    - Oxycellulose sponges or
    - Gelatin sponges or
    - Nasal tampons
  - Additional items
    - Antibiotic ointment or cream
    - Cotton pledgets, gauze
    - Gown, gloves, mask
- Most anterior nosebleeds in children will stop after basic first aid.
- If bleeding persists, then additional measures are available.
  - As in any acute situation, an initial ABCD assessment should be made.
  - Evaluation for major hemorrhage includes evaluating for tachycardia, hypotension, and orthostasis.
- Attempt to locate the source of bleeding.
  - Bleeding has often stopped by the time medical attention is sought.
  - The child should be asked to blow out all clots.
    - If this is not possible, blood in the nose can be suctioned out.

- To try to visualize the source of bleeding, use:
  - A flashlight, while applying gentle upward pressure to the nasal tip or
  - An otoscope with speculum or
  - A headlight and nasal speculum
- Inspect the anterior septum first.
- Anterior bleeding on the septum, or lateral wall, should be evident by:
  - Active bleeding
  - Clots
  - Crusts
  - Ulcerations
  - Prominent blood vessels
- If an anterior source is not found and posterior bleeding is suspected, an otolaryngologist should be consulted immediately.
  - Posterior bleeding is usually profuse and difficult to stop.

Topical vasoconstrictors

- Use if anterior bleeding has not ceased with application of pressure alone.
- Oxymetazoline, phenylephrine, or epinephrine (1:1000) can be applied with a cotton pledget to:
  - Shrink the nasal mucosa to improve visualization
  - Possibly slow down or stop the bleeding
- Pressure, again by pinching, should be applied for another 5–10 minutes.

Chemical cauterization

- Next step to attempt to stop persistent hemorrhage
  - Local anesthesia with 4% lidocaine should be administered with a cotton pledget for 5 minutes to reduce the discomfort of cauterization.
  - Insert and open a nasal speculum.
  - Using adequate lighting, apply silver nitrate on applicator sticks to the bleeding point.
    - Can be rolled over the site for several seconds
    - May have to be repeated several times to achieve hemostasis
    - Silver nitrate does not work well in pools of blood; therefore, suction may be necessary to keep the area dry.
    - A gray eschar will form at the cautery site.
    - Remove excess silver nitrate with cotton or gauze to minimize dispersion by nasal secretions and resulting injury to intact mucosa.
  - Caution should be used to avoid cauterizing too large or too deep an area or both sides of the septum.
    - Can lead to septal perforation

- After cauterization
  - Prescribe antibiotic cream or ointment to apply to the area twice a day for 5 days to prevent crusting and infection.
  - Hydration with saline or ointment should continue until healing is complete (approximately 1–3 weeks).
  - Nasal trauma and forceful nose blowing should be avoided.
- Otolaryngologists may use electrocautery as another hemostatic measure.
  - Cannot be performed with topical anesthesia alone

Nasal packing

- Nasal packing may be required if anterior bleeding persists despite direct pressure or nasal cautery.
  - Packing is uncomfortable, requires subsequent removal (usually after 2–3 days), and can cause additional mucosal injury.
  - All types of packing and sponges should be impregnated or coated with antibiotic ointment to prevent toxic shock syndrome, a reported complication of anterior and posterior nasal packing.
- Petroleum jelly gauze
  - Layered into the anterior nose
  - Provides a tight pack
- Oxycellulose or gelatin sponges
  - Absorbable and do not require later extraction
  - Do not apply a great deal of pressure to the bleeding site but are usually adequate for most nosebleeds
- Commercially available nasal tampons made of a dehydrated polyvinyl polymer sponge:
  - Are inserted dry and then expand with blood or added saline partially to fill the nasal cavity
  - Come in many sizes and can be cut to fit a child's nasal cavity
  - Must be removed, usually after 3–5 days, and have a tendency to adhere to the nasal lining
- Prophylactic antibiotics
  - No clear evidence exists to prove that they reduce the incidence of serious infection.
  - Studies have shown that they reduce gram-negative bacterial growth.
  - Common practice is to prescribe them for any patient with nasal packing.
  - May also help prevent sinusitis that can result from stasis of nasal secretions when packing is in place
  - Recommended antibiotics include:
    - First-generation cephalosporins *or*
    - Penicillins with activity against penicillinase-producing organisms

WHEN TO REFER

- Ear, nose, and throat
  - Urgent referral
    - Profuse, uncontrollable bleeding
    - Inability to locate source of bleeding
    - Posterior bleeding
    - Assistance with anterior packing
    - Recurrence of bleeding after initial ED measures
  - Nonurgent referral
    - Removal of anterior packing
    - Recurrent epistaxis
    - Evaluation for structural lesions (ie, granulomas, tumors, polyps)
    - Treatment of specific lesions
- Hematology
  - Abnormal coagulation laboratory profile
  - Severe, persistent, or recurrent bleeding
  - Bleeding from >1 site, based on history or physical examination
  - Bleeding that required blood transfusion or iron therapy
  - Family history of coagulopathy

WHEN TO ADMIT

- Airway compromise or hemodynamic instability on presentation

FOLLOW-UP

- Posterior nasal packing in place
  - Must be monitored in an intensive care unit for airway obstruction and respiratory compromise

PREVENTION

- In a dry environment
  - Normal saline nasal spray to humidify the nasal cavity
    - Spray should be used 4–5 times a day.
  - Home humidifier
  - Increased moisture:
    - Helps prevent the accumulation of crusts, which are often the impetus for nose picking
    - Keeps scabs soft, allowing them to stay in place longer, promoting healing of underlying mucosal injury
- Local trauma should be minimized.
  - Discourage nose picking, forceful rubbing, or blowing of the nose.
  - Trim fingernails.

Esophageal Caustic Injury

DEFINITION

- Caustic injury of the esophagus is a major, but preventable, pediatric health concern.
- Injuries continue despite federal legislation mandating preventive packaging and labeling, injury-prevention programs, and laws restricting potency and availability of caustic substances.

EPIDEMIOLOGY

- Prevalence
  - 20% of caustic ingestions result in esophageal injury.
  - In 2003 cleaning substances were the second most frequent substance involved in pediatric exposures (9.7% of the total).
- Age
  - 39% of exposures occur in children <3 years.
  - 52% occur in those <6 years.
- Sex
  - Among victims <13 years, most caustic injuries occur in boys.
  - This sex association is reversed during adolescence, when intentional suicide attempts are more prevalent.

ETIOLOGY

- Many household agents can cause caustic exposures.
- Acids and alkalis both can induce pylorospasm, resulting in pooling of the agent in the gastric antrum and extensive damage to this area.

Acids

- Hydrochloric acid
  - Swimming pool cleaners
  - Toilet bowl cleaner
  - Metal cleaner
- Hydrofluoric acid
  - Rust remover
- Sulfuric acid
  - Automotive batteries
  - Drain cleaners
- Acids have rapid esophageal transit and previously were thought to cause more damage to the stomach or intestine.
- Recent studies have revealed that acids cause extensive esophageal injury as well.
- Acids cause coagulation necrosis, resulting in superficial eschar formation, which may limit penetration into deeper tissues.

Alkalis

- Ammonia
  - Toilet bowl cleaners
  - Hair dyes
  - Floor strippers
  - Glass cleaners
- Sodium hydroxide
  - Anhydrous Benedict's reagent tablets
  - Detergents
  - Laundry powders
  - Paint removers
  - Drain cleaners
  - Button batteries
  - Oven cleaner
- Sodium borates, carbonates, and phosphates
  - Detergents
  - Electric dishwasher detergents
    - Liquid laundry detergents and dishwasher solutions usually cause mild esophageal injury that heals without complication.
  - Water softeners
- Sodium hypochlorite
  - Bleaches
    - Household bleaches rarely have been associated with severe esophageal injury because of their low concentration of sodium hypochlorite.
  - Household cleaners
  - Mildew remover
- Solid alkalis, such as anhydrous Benedict's reagent tablets and batteries, tend to lodge and cause focal burns and perforations at point of impaction.
- Strong alkalis cause liquefaction necrosis.
  - This allows penetration of the corrosive agent transmurally through esophagus and into adjacent mediastinal tissues.
  - Heat production and small-vessel thrombosis resulting from the reaction compound initial damage.
- Ensuing inflammatory reaction can result in:
  - Gangrene
  - Perforation
  - Mediastinitis
  - Fibrosis
  - Severe contracture of the esophagus
- *Lye* is the lay term for the alkaline agent found in most cleaning substances.
  - Liquid lye is the most common cause of esophageal caustic injury and associated with the greatest morbidity.

- Lye is odorless, tasteless, and viscous, which facilitates ingestion by children and suicidal teens and adults.
- High viscosity retards transit through the esophagus.
  - Tissue injury is rapid in the first few minutes, but lye can continue causing further injury for hours.

■ Lesions caused by lye injury occur in 3 phases.

- Acute necrotic phase
  - Usually lasts 24–96 hours after ingestion
  - An intense inflammatory reaction surrounds nonviable tissue.
- Ulceration and granulation phase
  - Begins 3–5 days after injury
  - Superficial necrotic tissue sloughs and is replaced by an ulcerated and inflamed granulation bed.
  - Healing tissue lacks collagen deposition and has very little tensile strength.
  - Although perforation can occur at any point during the first 2 weeks after injury, during this phase (10–12 days) the esophagus is most vulnerable.
- Scarring and cicatrization phase
  - Begins during the third week after injury
  - Wound contracture may lead to stricture formation and alteration of lower esophageal sphincter pressure, leading to gastroesophageal reflux.

SIGNS AND SYMPTOMS

■ No single symptom, sign, or combination has been found to predict accurately the degree of esophageal injury after corrosive ingestion.

■ Symptoms
- Searing or burning pain of mouth and lips
- Drooling or hypersalivation
- Difficulty with swallowing

■ Absence of pain does not exclude significant injury.

■ Epiglottic or vocal cord edema may result in:
- Stridor
- Dysphonia
- Aphonia

■ Substernal or back pain usually results from esophageal disruption and mediastinitis.

■ Acute epigastric pain may indicate gastric perforation.

■ Presence of fever is strongly correlated with significant injury.

■ Absence of oral burns does not exclude an esophageal burn injury.
- 20–45% of patients with esophageal burns have no evidence of oral burns.

■ Oropharyngeal damage does not reliably indicate esophageal involvement.
- 70% of persons with oropharyngeal injuries do not have esophageal lesions.

■ Bleeding can result from mucosal sloughing, with persistent ooze from the exposed submucosa or muscularis.
- Life-threatening hematemesis from development of an aortoesophageal fistula is rare.

DIFFERENTIAL DIAGNOSIS

■ Every attempt should be made to identify the agent ingested.
- In the case of young children, parents are usually aware of the offending agent and often bring the container to the emergency department.
- With suicidal intent, the caustic agent may be unknown.

IMAGING

■ Chest radiography may identify:
- Concomitant aspiration
- Subcutaneous cervical emphysema
- Pneumomediastinum, corroborating perforation

■ Circumferential burns limit full visualization.
- Contrast radiography with water-soluble medium followed by thin barium may be required for identification of grade III injuries (see Figure 29 on page F11).

DIAGNOSTIC PROCEDURES

■ Laryngoscopy
- After the patient is stabilized, the airway and gastrointestinal tract are inspected.
- Initial examination should include laryngoscopy.
- Evidence of a supraglottic or epiglottic burn indicates a risk for airway obstruction and requires endotracheal intubation.

■ Endoscopy
- Once upper airway integrity is confirmed, endoscopy should be performed to establish extent of injury.
  - Done even in the absence of oropharyngeal burns
- >50% of victims of caustic ingestion have no evidence of damage to the gastrointestinal tract.
- Many have extensive esophageal damage in the absence of oropharyngeal lesions.
- Presence of a third-degree burn to the hypopharynx precludes advancement of the endoscope beyond that level.
- Flexible esophagoscopy is preferred to minimize risk of iatrogenic perforation.
  - Most endoscopists will advance the scope only to the level at which maximal injury is encountered.
  - Others advocate full examination of stomach and, if possible, duodenum.

- Endoscopy allows examination of superficial mucosa only, making it difficult to differentiate between grade IIb and III lesions.

CLASSIFICATION

- The degree of injury can be graded similarly to that of thermal skin burns and holds similar prognostic implications.
  - Grade 0: normal
  - Grade I: mucosal hyperemia and edema
  - Grade IIa: mucosal hemorrhage, exudate, superficial ulceration, sloughing, and pseudomembrane formation
  - Grade IIb: same as IIa, plus deep discrete or circumferential ulcerations
  - Grade IIIa: deep ulcerations and necrosis, massive hemorrhage, obliteration of the lumen, charring, and perforation
  - Grade IIIb: extensive necrosis

TREATMENT APPROACH

- Therapy depends on the grade assigned at endoscopy.
  - No injury or grade I injuries
    - Usually admitted and observed for 24–48 hours
  - More severe injuries
    - Admitted to pediatric intensive care unit for monitoring and management
- Emergency management
  - Close attention to the ABCs (airway, breathing, and circulation)
    - Stridor or aphonia indicate laryngoepiglottic injury and may require urgent orotracheal intubation for airway protection.
    - Occasionally, severe laryngeal destruction necessitates emergency cricothyroidotomy or tracheostomy.
  - Adequate vascular access to allow for correction of hypovolemia or hypotension
  - Nasogastric tube placement is not recommended routinely because it may be associated with subsequent stricture formation.
  - Initial orders include:
    - Nothing by mouth
    - Proper fluid resuscitation
    - Nutritional support through total parenteral nutrition
    - Pain management
- Antimicrobial therapy
  - After disruption of the mucosal barrier by caustic ingestion, bacterial translocation and secondary bacterial invasion are likely.
    - Rationale for early institution of prophylactic antibiotic therapy
      - However, controlled trials do not support antibiotic use.
      - Most experts no longer advocate empirical antibiotic therapy.
  - Vigilance for mediastinitis or systemic infection must be maintained.
  - Reserve appropriate antimicrobials for any evidence of local or systemic infection.
- Nutrition
  - Parenteral nutrition for patients with grade II and III injuries
  - Oral feedings are withheld until dysphagia of initial phase has regressed and no evidence exists of clinical or radiographic deterioration.
- Proton pump inhibitors should be prescribed.
  - Loss of lower esophageal sphincter tone occurs secondary to corrosive esophageal injury.
  - Acid reflux can exacerbate underlying injury and accelerate stricture formation.
- Use of corticosteroids to limit fibrosis after caustic injury has debatable efficacy.
  - Most studies demonstrate lack of proven benefit.
  - Potential side effects argue against routine use.
- Gastric lavage and emetics should be avoided, because of:
  - Risk of reexposing esophagus to ingested corrosive agent
  - Threat of aspiration
  - Possibility of propagation of injury beyond level of the pylorus
- Any attempt to neutralize an ingested caustic agent poses additional danger, because resultant exothermic reaction frequently exacerbates the primary burn injury.
- Activated charcoal is not recommended, is ineffective, and obscures endoscopic visualization.
- Placement of a nasogastric tube should be deferred because of risk of esophageal perforation.

SPECIFIC TREATMENTS

Surgical management

- Surgical management is required for:
  - Severe corrosive injuries
  - Intractable esophageal strictures
- Surgical options include:
  - Bypass with placement of an esophageal substitute
  - Resection
  - Both bypass and resection
  - Esophagoplasty (see Figure 30 on page F11)

- Decisions regarding surgical management are based on:
  - Age
  - General health
  - Severity and extent of stricture
  - Risk of long-term complications
- Early surgical intervention is vital and can be life saving.
- Bypass with complete esophageal resection is the preferred approach, because
  - The retained proximal esophagus may distend, forming a mucocele or abscess.
  - The distal esophagus may develop reflux esophagitis, ulceration, and hemorrhage.
  - The retained esophagus is at increased risk for malignant transformation.
- Resection is not without risk.
  - Extensive dissection necessary to remove damaged esophagus can result in significant morbidity.
- Accepted procedures to replace injured esophagus include:
  - Colonic interposition
  - Gastric advancement
  - Gastric tube esophagoplasty
  - Jejunal interposition
- Esophagoplasty with a colonic patch over less extensive but persistent strictures has been used to manage focal strictures.
- Full and immediate resection of devitalized tissue is necessary to prevent expansion of corrosive injury.
- Delay in diagnosis of esophageal perforation can be fatal; a high index of suspicion in grade II and III injuries must be maintained.
- Immediate surgery is required for:
  - Peritonitis
  - Pneumoperitoneum
  - Clinical deterioration, evidenced by refractory acidosis, neurologic decline, or coagulopathy
- Complete surgical exposure of the foregut—esophagus, stomach, and duodenum—is necessary to assess extent of the damage and allow resection.
- Full-thickness injury to stomach or duodenum invariably predicts severe esophageal injury.
  - An indication for complete esophagogastrectomy
- Full-thickness circumferential injury to esophagus carries a 20% mortality rate, mandating surgical resection.

Esophageal dilation

- Conservative management, including later esophageal dilation, may be considered for short segments of full-thickness esophageal mucosal damage.
- If any question persists after initial exploration, then a second-look operation (often within 24 hours) is required.

- Primary treatment with esophageal dilation offers a satisfactory outcome for most otherwise healthy children with grade IIa injuries.
- Repeated dilation rarely is successful for the most severe corrosive strictures; early surgical resection is associated with a better outcome.
- Because risk of perforation is highest in the first weeks after injury, most experts advocate waiting 6 weeks before initiating dilation.
- Dilation can be accomplished by 2 methods.
  - Pulsion dilation
    - Graded bougies are passed over endoscopically or radiographically placed guide wires.
    - This technique is difficult with tortuous or complicated strictures and warrants fluoroscopic guidance.
  - Radial dilation
    - Uses endoscopically or radiographically controlled balloon dilation
- The goal is dilation of the stricture to 18 mm, the diameter required for normal swallowing.
  - Typically performed every other week
  - ≥3 dilations usually are required.
- Esophageal rupture is a potentially fatal complication of dilation and warrants immediate surgical repair.
  - Incidence is 17–32%.
- Serial dilations are complicated by dysphagia between treatments, which may precipitate pulmonary aspiration.
- An adequate lumen is usually attained within 6 months to 1 year, with progressively longer intervals between dilations.
- Esophageal replacement should be considered if dilation is ineffective beyond 1 year.

WHEN TO ADMIT

- All patients with esophageal caustic injury should be hospitalized.

WHEN TO REFER

- All patients need referral to gastroenterologists and surgeons for evaluation of extent of damage and for management.

FOLLOW-UP

- Strictures after grade I and IIa injuries are rare, and follow-up contrast esophagography is unnecessary.
- After grade IIb and III injuries, barium esophagography for early detection of stricture development is performed 2–4 weeks later.
  - Early stricture detection is important because less mature strictures are more responsive to dilation.
- Long-term follow-up of children who have grade II and III burns is warranted, regardless of their symptoms.

- Esophagography and surveillance esophagoscopy should be performed annually or biannually.

COMPLICATIONS

- Long-term complications of corrosive ingestions include:
  - Stricture formation
  - Gastric outlet obstruction
  - Esophageal carcinoma
- Gastric outlet obstruction
  - Occurs in ~9% of corrosive ingestions
  - Is characterized by early satiety and weight loss
  - Can occur years after initial injury
  - Follows acid or alkaline ingestions with equal frequency
  - Is treated surgically
    - Balloon dilation of the pylorus, pyloroplasty, and Billroth I reconstruction are all effective.
    - Selection of operation depends on findings at laparotomy and surgeon preference.
- Esophageal carcinoma
  - Where native esophagus is retained, risk of postcorrosive esophageal carcinoma is estimated to be 1000- to 3000-fold higher than the incidence in the general population.
  - ≤3% of patients with esophageal carcinoma have a history of corrosive ingestion.
    - These squamous cell carcinomas usually originate in mid-esophagus.
  - Because local dissemination occurs infrequently, the potential for curative resection is slightly improved over that for primary esophageal cancer.
  - The interval between burn injury and development of carcinoma ranges from 10–70 years, with a mean of 50 years.

PROGNOSIS

- Long-term morbidity after corrosive esophageal ingestion correlates with the grade of injury.

PREVENTION

- Proposed interventions to prevent stricture formation have not demonstrated a proven benefit.
  - Esophageal dilation to prevent adhesion formation in the injured segment
  - Intraluminal stenting
  - Prolonged esophageal rest (maintenance of nothing-by-mouth status; total parenteral nutrition)
  - Multiple animal studies with a variety of agents (heparin, epidermal growth factor, caffeic acid phenethyl ester) have demonstrated varying degrees of success, but none of these agents have been studied in humans.

Extremity Pain

DEFINITION

- Extremity (limb) pain is pain present in ≥1 of the arms or legs.

EPIDEMIOLOGY

- Incidence
  - Up to 16% of school-age children report at least 1 episode of activity-limiting extremity pain annually.
- Prevalence
  - Between 6% and 7% of pediatric office visits are related to extremity pain.

MECHANISM

- The mechanism for extremity pain depends on its etiology.

HISTORY

- Description of pain: OLDCAR
  - **O**nset/precipitating event (eg, trauma, only at night)
    - Trauma accompanied by an audible pop or snap suggests a dislocation, sprain, or fracture.
  - **L**ocation/distribution of pain (eg, specific joints)
    - Referred pain is common in children; thus, the location of pain may be deceiving.
      - Joint pain may refer to the bones and joints adjacent to the presenting symptom.
      - Hip pathology may present as knee pain (eg, as in slipped capital femoral epiphysis [SCFE]).
      - Spine pathology may present as lower-extremity pain or gain disturbance.
    - Migrating extremity pain is less likely to occur after trauma and is more typical of systemic illness.
    - Multiple joint involvement may also suggest reactive arthritides or rheumatologic conditions, such as lupus and juvenile idiopathic arthritis.
    - Pain in a nonanatomic distribution or that disturbs unpleasant but not pleasant activities may suggest a functional disorder.
  - **D**uration (eg, continuous, variable, specific time of the day only, frequency)
  - **C**haracter or quality (eg, aching, cramping, deep, burning, tingling, numbness, with stiffness)
    - Muscular pain may be described as aching or cramping.
    - Bone pain is often described as deep.
    - Nerve pain may present as burning, tingling, or numbness.
    - Stiffness, especially with clinical evidence of arthritis not associated with trauma, should prompt concern about a rheumatologic process.
  - **A**ssociated factors that relieve or worsen
    - Pain that is worse with sleep or rest and improves with activity may suggest a rheumatologic process.
    - Types of activities that may affect the pain
  - **R**adiating/pattern of pain
- Medical history/review of systems
  - When considering overuse injuries, may assess for repetitive motions, handedness
  - Signs of systemic illness (eg, fever, recent weight loss, sweating, rashes, gastrointestinal symptoms)
  - Signs of spinal disease (eg, retention or incontinence of urine or stool)
  - Recent infectious exposures, including hepatitis B, pharyngitis/strep throat, upper respiratory tract infection
    - Consider transient synovitis of the hip in children <10 years
    - A history of exposure to viral illness might explain myalgia or arthralgia, eg, the prodrome of hepatitis B can cause significant arthralgia.
  - Recent travel or potential infectious exposures (eg, home-processed meats)
  - History of autoimmune disease, or congenital/acquired asplenia
  - Family history of autoimmune diseases, hemoglobinopathies, human leukocyte antigen B27 (HLA-type B27), joint hypermobility, fibromyalgia
    - A sickle cell pain crisis must always be considered in a child of African or Mediterranean origin with a painful extremity.
    - HLA-B27 is associated with Reiter syndrome, psoriatic arthritis, inflammatory bowel disease, and ankylosing spondylitis and may be associated with enthesitis-related arthritis (inflammation at attachments of tendons/ligaments/fascia to bone).
  - Recent medication use
    - A serum sickness–like illness, particularly associated with cefaclor
    - Even a short course of systemic steroids can cause aseptic necrosis of the hip or demineralization of bone.
    - Immunizations, particularly for rubella, may cause joint or extremity pain.
- Growth patterns/growth spurt
- As indicated, consider a full HEADSSS assessment or at a minimum the following:
  - Home situation
  - Educational status
  - Activities (specific activities and changes in activities), exercise patterns
  - Sexual history

PHYSICAL EXAM

- Vital signs
  - Evaluate temperature.
  - Evaluate blood pressure and heart rate.
    - These may be elevated with clinically significant pain, or with endocrine abnormalities.
    - An elevated resting heart rate may be associated with rheumatic fever.
  - Plot previous growth data (especially height, weight, and body mass index).
    - SCFE is more likely in an overweight adolescent.
- Physical examination
  - Conduct a general, if brief, physical examination, even if the history points to extremity pain from minor local trauma.
  - Examine the extremities, especially proximal and distal to the site of the symptom (given the possibility of referred pain), assessing for:
    - Skin color and temperature
      - Color change associated with extremity pain may indicate:
        - Redness—inflammation
        - Intense red with streaking—infection
        - Darkened—bruising or gangrene
        - Pallor—anemia, or systemic illness
    - Vascular status, by palpating pulses and determining distal capillary refill time
    - Muscle strength and distribution pattern (eg, proximal vs distal weakness)
      - Isolated distal weakness is likely to be of neurologic origin, whereas proximal weakness is most likely from muscle disease.
    - Soft-tissue swelling
    - Presence of skeletal deformities
    - Tenderness to palpation
    - Joint disruption or effusions
    - Joint laxity or hyperextensibility
  - Examine the other extremities and joints.
    - Comparing with the opposing limb may be useful when assessing swelling, muscle bulk and tone, and joint mobility.
      - Symmetry of skin folds and limb lengths can be helpful.
    - Examining other limbs may reveal a broader extent of involvement.
    - Observing use of the affected limb (when the patient is unaware) may suggest involvement versus a functional process.
    - If lower extremities are involved, observe and classify gait.
    - Nail pitting may be consistent with psoriasis.
  - Examine for organomegaly.
  - Assess for rashes.
    - Vasculitic rash on extensor surfaces of knuckles, knees, and elbows: Consider dermatomyositis.
    - Palpable purpura: Consider Henoch-Schönlein purpura.
    - Photosensitive rash: Consider systemic lupus erythematosus, dermatomyositis, and parvovirus infection.
  - Pain out of proportion to examination may suggest necrosis or leukemia.

DIFFERENTIAL DIAGNOSIS

- Most visits to a primary care pediatrician for extremity pain involve pain caused by:
  - Minor trauma
  - Overuse syndromes
  - Normal skeletal growth variants
- Limb pain may be related to primary processes related to infection, nutritional derangements, neoplasms, or specific orthopedic disorders.
  - Also may be related to systemic illnesses or to psychosocial issues
- The challenge is to determine when the pain is significant without exposing the child to excessive diagnostic studies, so that referrals can be made in a timely manner.
- The differential diagnosis of extremity pain is extremely broad.
- Most limb pain is benign, requires no intervention, and is self-limited.
- Mild trauma that leads to a fracture may suggest previous underlying bone pathology.
- Consider physical abuse if clinical findings and/or imaging are not consistent with history.

Orthopedic

- Trauma
  - Fracture
    - Myohematoma
    - Myositis ossificans
    - Osteoporosis
    - Pathologic fracture/osteogenesis imperfecta
  - Sprain: a physical disruption of a ligament
    - Less common in children than in adults
    - Consider fractures when physical examination reveals point tenderness or pain on stretching the ligament.
  - Physical abuse

- Overuse injury
  - Chondromalacia patella (patellofemoral syndrome)
  - Little League elbow: painful inflammation of the epicondyles related to repetitive throwing, potentially with diminished range of joint motion
    - Fragments of bone splintered into the joint may cause the joint to catch or lock.
  - Shin splints
    - Occurs most commonly at the beginning of a training season and is exacerbated by running and jumping
      - Although the pain occurs initially after activity, it may occur during or before activity as the syndrome progresses.
      - Tenderness may be felt overt the posteromedial aspect of the tibia, proximal portion of the posterior tibia, or anterior tibia.
  - Stress fractures
    - Localized, gradually increasing, and persistent extremity pain that worsens with weight bearing, exercise, and activity but diminishes with rest
    - Rare in children <12 years of age and most commonly affect the second metatarsal, proximal tibia, or fibula
- Osteochondroses: irregular mineralization of bone resulting from necrosis followed by regeneration of bone tissue
  - Freiberg disease
  - Köhler disease
  - Legg-Calve-Perthes disease
  - Osgood-Schlatter disease
  - Osteochondritis dissecans
  - Sever disease
- Nerve and/or vascular compression syndromes
  - Carpal tunnel syndrome
  - Cervical nerve root entrapment
  - Compartment syndrome
  - Popliteal artery entrapment syndrome
    - Associated with vascular calf pain that radiates to the foot, which begins with activity, sometimes more with walking than with running
    - Consider if normal pedal pulses are lost with simultaneous knee extension and foot plantar flexion.
  - Thoracic outlet syndrome
- Radial head subluxation (nursemaid's elbow)
  - A common injury in toddlers, following sudden, forceful traction of the hand or forearm
  - Often, the child refuses to use the extremity; if verbal, he or she usually localizes the pain to the elbow or occasionally to the wrist.
  - Holds the arm with the elbow flexed, the forearm close to the chest, and the hand in pronation

- SCFE
  - Caused by dislocation of the head of the femur from its neck and shaft at the level of the upper epiphyseal plate
  - Characteristic pain occurs in the affected hip or the medial aspect of the ipsilateral knee.
    - If displacement is sudden, pain is usually severe and associated, with inability to bear weight.
    - Gradual displacement is associated with slowly increasing, dull pain.
  - Examination may reveal diminished abduction and internal rotation of the hip.
  - Typically affects obese children or adolescents
- Anatomic variants (eg, inflexible flat feet, tarsal coalition)
- Growing pains
  - Intermittent, deep extremity pains that affect the lower more often than the upper extremities
  - Pain is nearly always bilateral, lasts <2 hours, and is worse at night, resolving completely in the morning; it rarely involves joints.
  - Onset is described at 3–5 or 8–12 years of age (not most frequently during periods of rapid growth).
  - Most growing pains resolve in 12–24 months, although they may persist into adolescence.
  - The diagnosis is significant for its lack of associated physical signs.
    - Abnormal findings should prompt a search for another cause.

Infectious/post-infectious

- Septic arthritis
- Osteomyelitis
  - A local infection of bone, usually involving 1 of the long bones; incidence is highest in children 3–12 years of age.
  - Infection often occurs by hematogenous seeding, or by direct inoculation after local trauma.
  - Osteomyelitis can produce extremity pain alone or with signs of a systemic infectious disease—fever, irritability, and septic appearance.
  - Most commonly due to *Staphylococcus aureus*
    - In puncture wounds to the foot, consider *Pseudomonas aeruginosa*, especially if injury is through a tennis shoe.
- Cellulitis/abscess
- Transient (toxic) synovitis
  - A self-limited inflammation of the hip joint, most commonly in children <10 years of age
  - The cause is unknown, but the condition often occurs within 2 weeks of upper respiratory infection.
  - Typically, the child refuses to walk because of apparent |pain in the hip, with hip held in flexion, abduction, and external rotation.

- Diskitis, spinal epidural abscess
- Pyogenic or viral myositis
- Meningococcal disease
- Immunization reaction (especially rubella)
- Tuberculosis
- Arthralgia or myalgia associated with streptococcal or viral infection
- Sexually transmitted infection (gonorrhea, syphilis [periostitis])
- Enteric disease (includes trichinosis)
- Histoplasmosis
- Lyme disease

Rheumatologic/immune-mediated

- Dermatomyositis
  - Muscle pain
  - Proximal weakness associated with a vasculitic rash on the extensor surfaces of knuckles, knees, and elbows (Gottron papules)
- Familial Mediterranean fever
- Henoch-Schönlein purpura
  - Palpable purpura and extremity pain
- Hypermobility syndrome/mixed connective-tissue disease
  - Generalized joint laxity and hyperextensibility differentiates benign hypermobility syndrome from a focal ligament injury.
  - Joint laxity allows chronic hyperextension, which can cause pain, typically in weight-bearing joints, that is often worse in the evening.
  - Dancing, gymnastics, and other joint-impacting activities may exacerbate arthralgia.
- Inflammatory bowel disease
- Juvenile idiopathic arthritis
- Kawasaki disease
- Polyarteritis nodosa
- Rheumatic fever
- Reactive arthritis
- Scleroderma
- Serum sickness
- Systemic lupus erythematosus

Genetic/nutrition

- Sickle cell anemia, thalassemia
- Hemophilia
- Hypercholesterolemia
- Hypervitaminosis A
- Vitamin deficiencies (vitamin C, scurvy; vitamin D, rickets)

- Gout
- Enzyme deficiencies (carnitine palmityltransferase deficiency, Fabry disease, McArdle syndrome, phosphofructokinase deficiency)
- Mucolipidosis
- Mucopolysaccharidosis

Neoplasm

- The possibility of a tumor is a common parental concern.
- While rare, neoplasms can cause limb pain.
- The differential diagnosis includes leukemia, benign (osteoblastoma, osteoid osteoma) and malignant neoplasms (eg, sarcomas [chondrosarcoma, Ewing sarcoma, fibrosarcoma, osteogenic sarcoma, rhabdomyosarcoma, synovial cell sarcoma], lymphomas, neuroblastomas, bone tumors, soft-tissue tumors, and spinal cord tumors.
- Osteoid osteoma is a benign prostaglandin-secreting bone tumor that occurs most often in adolescents.
  - Pain, the presenting symptom, is initially dull and increases in intensity to deep and boring (piercing).
    - More intense at night and with weight bearing
    - Usually involves a femur, tibia, or lumbar vertebral body
- Systemic neoplasms in which extremity pain occurs include leukemia and metastatic neuroblastoma.
  - In children with acute lymphocytic leukemia:
    - One-third have bone pain at the time of diagnosis; in one-fourth, joint or bone pain is a significant presenting symptom.
    - Examination may reveal strikingly little to account for the degree of pain.
- Primary malignant bone tumors may cause severe unilateral pain, with swelling and tenderness at the tumor site.
- Metastatic bone tumor may present as extremity pain.
  - Pain is characterized as unrelenting; increasing pain that worsens at night or with rest; and not relieved by analgesics, heat, or massage.
  - Systemic signs may accompany the pain (eg, weight loss, pallor, lymphadenopathy, hepatosplenomegaly, fever).

Other systemic illnesses

- Caffey disease
- Fibromyalgia
- Guillain-Barré syndrome
- Histiocytosis X
- Hypercortisolism
- Hyperparathyroidism
- Hypothyroidism
- Sarcoidosis

Psychosocial

- Behavior disorders
- Psychogenic pain
- Reflex neurovascular dystrophy
- School phobia

LABORATORY EVALUATION

- Laboratory studies are unnecessary for most extremity pain.
- Consider screening tests if there is suspicion of systemic or infectious process, pain persists longer than anticipated, and history and examination do not lead to a definitive diagnosis.
- Screening tests may include:
  - Complete blood count
    - Complete blood count may reveal anemia or may suggest active infectious process.
    - White blood cell (WBC) count and sedimentation rate are often elevated in osteomyelitis.
    - Transient synovitis may cause a slight elevation in the WBC count and the sedimentation rate.
    - With leukemia, the WBC count may vary, with immature WBCs present; or thrombocytopenia may be present.
  - Erythrocyte sedimentation rate and/or C-reactive protein
    - Elevated erythrocyte sedimentation rate raises suspicion of an infectious, inflammatory (or occasionally, neoplastic) disorder.
    - Effectiveness of osteomyelitis treatment can be monitored by a serial sedimentation rate and/or C-reactive protein level.
    - A C-reactive protein <1 mg/dL has been shown to have an 87% negative predictive value for septic arthritis.
- Additional testing may be performed as guided by clinical suspicion, including:
  - Blood cultures
  - If septic arthritis is suspected, synovial fluid analysis and cultures

IMAGING

- When no clear history of trauma is revealed, when symptoms persist, when associated systemic symptoms are present, or with clinical suspicion, imaging may be obtained.
- Radiographs can help to identify:
  - Fractures, acute and/or pathologic
    - Traumatic injury that would ordinarily cause a sprain in an adult is more likely to cause a greenstick or buckle fracture in a child, so a lower threshold for obtaining posttraumatic radiographs in children may therefore be justified.

- Orthopedic conditions, including SCFE
- Bony tumors
- Some metabolic defects
- In Legg-Calve-Perthes disease, radiographs may be normal or show only joint capsule swelling, although subsequent radiographs may show areas of bone resorption, irregular widening of the epiphysis, and dense new bone formation.
- In leukemia, studies of the extremities may show lucent leukemic lines in the subepiphyseal area.
- In osteogenic sarcoma, radiographs may reveal a tumor in the metaphysis.
  - Presence of both radiolucent and radiopaque areas
  - Characteristic sunburst results from extension of calcification into the overlying soft tissue
  - Periosteal elevation may be present, but it is not diagnostic of the disease.
- Bone scans
  - Are a suggested part of the evaluation for a limping child <5 years of age with a nonfocal examination (per the American Academy of Radiology)
  - Should be considered when a stress fracture, osteomyelitis, or cancer is suspected
  - In rare cases of osteomyelitis, a reduction in perfusion caused by pressure from the exudative process may result in a false-negative scan.
  - In Legg-Calve-Perthes disease, the scan may demonstrate diminished blood flow to the femoral head compared with the contralateral hip.
- Magnetic resonance imaging is being used as a replacement for bone scans in the diagnosis of osteomyelitis.
  - ≥2 weeks may be required for radiographic evidence of osteomyelitis to develop.
  - A bone scan is usually, but not always, diagnostic.
  - The combined use of T1, T2, and short-tau inversion-recovery images effectively rules out osteomyelitis with a negative predictive value approaching 100%.
    - Magnetic resonance imaging offers the additional advantages of imaging of soft-tissue and joint disease.

DIAGNOSTIC PROCEDURES

- Diagnostic procedures (eg, biopsies) may be obtained as guided by clinical suspicion.

TREATMENT APPROACH

- Treatment is aimed at the underlying disease entity.
- With chronic extremity pain, serial examinations over the course of weeks may aid in establishing a diagnosis.

SPECIFIC TREATMENT

- Treatment is highly dependent on clinical presentation and diagnosis.
  - Growing pains
    - Treatment involves heat, massage, and analgesics.
  - Little League elbow
    - Treatment consists of resting the arm by avoiding the repetitive movement, and a change in pitching technique may reduce recurrences.
  - Shin splints
    - Treatment of shin splints involves rest, application of ice, and antiinflammatory drugs.
    - For runners, training on a softer surface or with better-quality running shoes may help.
  - Sprains
    - Grade I sprains can be treated with icing and wrapping to minimize swelling.
    - Early range of motion exercises should be encouraged, with a gradual return to activity.
    - The recurrence of pain indicates too rapid a return to a given level of activity.
    - Grade II sprains and grade III sprains should generally be referred to an orthopedist for immobilization.
  - Stress fractures
    - Treatment consists mostly of rest and treatment with nonsteroidal antiinflammatory agents.
    - Casting or splinting is occasionally necessary.
  - Radial head subluxation (nursemaid's elbow)
    - The practitioner can reduce the subluxation by using 1 hand to supinate the patient's forearm quickly while simultaneously exerting traction on the forearm and using the thumb of the other hand to create pressure over the patient's radial head.
    - This maneuver is completed by placing the elbow through full extension and flexion while maintaining pressure over the radial head.
    - Normal use of the extremity usually returns within 30 minutes.
  - SCFE
    - Management involves surgical placement of a pin through the femoral head and the epiphysis to prevent further slippage.
  - Osteochondroses
  - Osteoid osteoma
    - Surgical excision is curative.
  - Transient synovitis
    - Treatment consists of bed rest, usually for <4 days.

WHEN TO REFER

- When a surgical procedure or subspecialist is required for definitive treatment (eg, operative repair of fracture, ligament tear, Ewing sarcoma)
- When a surgical procedure or subspecialist required for diagnostic evaluation (eg, septic arthritis, juvenile idiopathic arthritis, systemic lupus erythematosus)
- When extremity pain occurs in the context of likely systemic illness (eg, Fabry disease, Crohn disease)
- Consider ophthalmology and rheumatology consultation if limb pain occurs in conjunction with uveitis, photophobia, eye injection, or eye pain.

WHEN TO ADMIT

- If a child cannot ambulate, and outpatient or emergency department screening does not confirm a diagnosis
- High clinical suspicion for septic arthritis

COMPLICATIONS

- SCFE
  - Avascular necrosis of the femoral head is a common complication, even with early recognition and treatment.
- Transient synovitis
  - In rare instances, avascular necrosis of the femoral head may be a late complication.

Facial Dysmorphism

DEFINITION

- Congenital malformations are clinically significant abnormalities of form or function that result from localized intrinsic defects in morphogenesis that occur in embryonic or early fetal life.
  - These include clefting of the lip or palate; congenital heart disease, such as tetralogy of Fallot; and multicystic kidney disease.
  - They may result from an unknown cause but increasingly can be traced to mutations in single developmental genes.
  - Malformations usually require surgical intervention.
- Deformations differ from malformations in that they arise as a result of environmental forces acting on normal primordial tissue.
  - For example: A fetus in a uterus where a large fibroid is present may have limited space for normal range of motion for limbs.
    - Limitation of limb motion leads to congenital contractures, arthrogryposis multiplex congenita.
  - Deformations occur later than malformations, usually after the first trimester, and often resolve with minimal therapy.
- A malformation (such as a cleft lip) or a deformation (such as clubfoot deformity) may occur in isolation or as part of a malformation sequence, a syndrome, or an association.
  - When a single malformation causes secondary effects on other structures later in development, a malformation sequence results.
  - In clinical genetics, a syndrome is defined as a group of malformations that occur together and are caused by a clearly identifiable causative agent.
  - Associations have no single underlying cause that explains a recognizable pattern of anomalies that occur together.

EPIDEMIOLOGY

- Prevalence
  - 2–5% of newborns are found during the neonatal period to have ≥1 congenital malformations.
  - 7–8% at 1 year of age, because some malformations (eg, congenital heart disease) may remain clinically silent during the newborn period.
  - In approximately 50% of children with congenital malformations, only a single malformation is identifiable.
    - Multiple malformations are present in the other 50%.
- Causes of multiple malformation syndromes
  - ~7.5% result from single gene mutations.
  - ~6% result from a chromosomal abnormality.
  - ~6% result from teratogens.
  - >50% result from unknown factors.

MECHANISM

- A malformation sequence occurs when a single malformation causes another to develop: for example, the Pierre Robin malformation sequence.
  - Primary malformation, failure of the growth of the mandible during the first weeks of gestation, results in micrognathia (small jaw).
  - Insufficient jaw size forces the normal tongue into an unusual position.
  - The abnormally placed tongue blocks fusion of the palatal shelves that normally come together in the midline, producing a U-shaped cleft of the palate.
  - After delivery, the normal-sized tongue in the abnormal oral cavity can lead to airway obstruction and obstructive apnea, a potentially life-threatening complication.
- Syndromes may be caused by a single gene mutation: for example, Marfan syndrome.
  - A mutation in the *FBN1* gene on chromosome 15 leads to abnormally formed fibrillin, resulting in a characteristic set of abnormalities of the skeletal, cardiovascular, and ophthalmologic systems.
- Syndromes may result from chromosomal abnormality: for example, Down syndrome.
  - An extra copy of chromosome 21 leads to craniofacial dysmorphic features, developmental disabilities, cardiac anomalies, and other abnormalities.
- Syndromes can be caused by a teratogenic agent.
  - A drug, chemical, or environmental toxin that causes damage to the developing embryo or fetus; for example, valproic acid, an anticonvulsant that when used during the first trimester of pregnancy leads to:
    - Spina bifida
    - A characteristic facial appearance
    - Limb defects
    - Other anomalies
- A syndrome can result from unknown factors: for example, Russel-Silver syndrome.
  - Intrauterine growth restriction with failure to thrive, skeletal asymmetry, small and incurved fifth fingers, and learning disabilities.
  - A small number of patients have maternal uniparental disomy of chromosome 7, but 90% of patients have no identifiable cause.
- An association is a group of unconnected anomalies that regularly occur together: for instance, the VACTERL association (vertebral anomalies, anal atresia, cardiac defects, tracheoesophageal fistula, renal anomalies, and limb anomalies)
  - A group of malformations that occur more commonly together than might be expected by chance

F

- No single unifying cause has ever been identified to explain this condition.
- As the cause of an association becomes known, the disorder moves into the category of syndrome.

HISTORY

- Establishing a standardized routine is helpful for the evaluation of the child with dysmorphic features.
  - This routine should include taking the history, including a 3-generational family history, and performing a careful physical examination.
  - Following these steps, specific diagnostic laboratory tests can be ordered to confirm a diagnosis.
- Health care providers should be sensitive about the terminology used to describe the infant.
  - The physician should describe the abnormal features as clearly and concisely as possible.
- In taking the history, the following questions about the pregnancy should be asked:
  - *What was the birth weight?*
    - A lower-than-expected birth weight can be associated with a chromosome anomaly or exposure to a teratogen.
    - Babies who are large for gestational age may have diabetic mothers or an overgrowth syndrome, eg, Beckwith-Wiedemann syndrome.
    - Infants who are accurate for gestational age may have a single gene mutation; a multifactorial condition; or, most likely, no genetic disease at all.
  - *Was the baby full term, or pre- or postmature?*
    - Especially important when evaluating an older child with developmental disabilities
    - Postmaturity is associated with some chromosome anomalies, eg, trisomy 18 and anencephaly.
  - *Was the baby born by vaginal or cesarean delivery? If the latter, what was the indication?*
    - Caesarean delivery may be performed because of fetal distress, a risk factor for developmental disability caused by oxygen deprivation.
    - Babies born from breech presentation are approximately 4 times more likely to have congenital malformations.
  - *How old were the parents at the time of the child's delivery?*
    - Advanced maternal age is associated with an increased risk of nondisjunction leading to trisomies, eg, Down syndrome (trisomy 21).
    - Advanced paternal age may be associated with an increased risk of a new mutation leading to an autosomal-dominant trait, eg, achondroplasia.

- *Did the pregnancy have complications? Does the mother have underlying medical problems? Does she take any medications? Did she smoke cigarettes, drink alcohol, or take any drugs?*
  - Exposure of the embryo to teratogens, medications, or environmental agents known to cause birth defects is a significant cause of congenital malformations.
- *When did the mother feel quickening? Were fetal movements active?*
  - Quickening, which normally occurs between 16 and 20 weeks' gestation, is delayed in hypotonic fetuses, who also have less vigorous movements during fetal life.
  - Persistent hiccups in an infant found to have neonatal seizures suggests prenatal onset of the condition.
- *Was the amount of amniotic fluid normal?*
  - An increased amount of amniotic fluid is associated with intestinal obstruction or a central nervous system anomaly leading to poor swallowing.
  - Decreased fluid may point to a renal or urinary tract abnormality leading to failure to produce urine or chronic amniotic fluid leak.
- A 3-generation pedigree should be constructed, searching for similar and dissimilar abnormalities in first- and second-degree relatives.
  - A history of pregnancy or neonatal losses should be documented.

PHYSICAL EXAM

- In the process of evaluating the child with dysmorphic features, the physical examination is the most important element.
  - Whenever possible, the patient should be examined using a standardized approach.

Growth

- The height (length), weight, and head circumference should be carefully measured and plotted on appropriate growth curves.
- Growth appropriate for age may be consistent with:
  - A single gene disorder
  - A multifactorially inherited condition
  - Most commonly to no genetic disease
- Small size or growth restriction may be secondary to:
  - Chromosomal abnormality
  - Skeletal dysplasia such as achondroplasia
  - Exposure to toxic or teratogenic agents
- Larger-than-expected size suggests an overgrowth syndrome.
  - If in the newborn period, suggests maternal diabetes

- Proportions
  - Do limbs look appropriate for the head and trunk?
    - Short limbs imply presence of a short-limbed bone dysplasia, such as achondroplasia.
    - Trunk and head that are too small for the extremities may suggest a disorder affecting the vertebrae.

Craniofacial features

- Careful examination of the craniofacies is crucial for the diagnosis of many congenital malformation syndromes.
  - In assessing the face, the following should be systematically observed.

Head shape

- In newborns, the examiner may need to allow a few days for the deformation from molding to resolve.
- The head should be described using the following terms:
  - *Normocephaly:* a normal head shape.
  - *Dolichocephaly* or *scaphocephaly:* a long, thin head.
  - *Brachycephaly:* a head that is narrow in the anteroposterior diameter and broad laterally.
  - Plagiocephaly: a head that is asymmetric or lopsided.

Facial features

- A dysmorphic face may be appropriate given the family's physiognomy, or it may indicate a particular syndrome.
- Smith's Recognizable Patterns of Human Malformation aids identification and helps determine whether a particular condition is genetically based.
- Examples of causes of genetic facial malformation
  - Cause: Chromosomal
    - Down syndrome (trisomy 21)
    - Facial dysmorphism: midface hypoplasia, upward obliquity of palpebral fissures, epicanthal folds, flat nasal bridge, anteversion of nares
  - Cause: Autosomal dominant
    - Treacher Collins syndrome
    - Facial dysmorphism: dysplastic ears, maxillary hypoplasia
  - Cause: Autosomal recessive
    - Hurler syndrome
    - Facial dysmorphism: corneal clouding, coarse facies
  - Cause: Teratogenic: intrauterine infection
    - Congenital rubella
    - Facial dysmorphism: cataracts
  - Cause: Drug induced
    - Fetal alcohol syndrome
    - Facial dysmorphism: smooth philtrum, small eyes

- In evaluating the face, the examiner should first note the symmetry; facial asymmetry may be due to:
  - Deformation related to intrauterine or extrauterine positioning
  - Malformation of 1 side of the face: eg, hemifacial microsomia (Goldenhar syndrome or facio-auriculo-vertebral syndrome)
- Evaluate the 4 regions of the face separately.

Forehead

- Extends from the anterior hairline to the eyebrows.
  - Overt prominence: achondroplasia
  - Deficiency: sloping appearance, which occurs in children with primary microcephaly

Midface

- Encompasses the region from the eyebrows to the upper lip and laterally from the outer canthus of each eye to the outer commissure of the lips
- Hypoplasia of the midface is a common component of many syndromes, including Down syndrome and fetal alcohol syndrome.
- In evaluating the midface, carefully measure and plot measurements on appropriate growth curves for:
  - The distance between the eyes: inner and outer canthal distances
  - Pupils: interpupil distance
    - Eyes that are too close together may confirm an impression of hypotelorism, a defect in midline brain formation (holoprosencephaly).
    - Eyes that are too far apart—hypertelorism—are suggestive of such syndromes as Opitz syndrome (ocular hypertelorism, tracheal and esophageal anomalies, and hypospadias).
  - Length of the palpebral fissure
    - Short in fetal alcohol syndrome
    - Excessively long in Kabuki syndrome (short stature, mental retardation, long palpebral fissures with eversion of lateral portion of lower lid)
  - Other features of the eyes
    - The obliquity (slant) of the palpebral fissures may be upward, as in Down syndrome, or downward, as in Treacher Collins syndrome.
    - Epicanthal folds, flaps of skin covering the inner canthus of the eye that are usually associated with flattening of the nasal bridge, may indicate Down syndrome or fetal alcohol syndrome.

- Features of the nose
  - Nasal bridge can be flattened, as in Down syndrome, or prominent, as in velocardiofacial syndrome.
  - Nares may be oriented normally or tipped back (anteversion)
  - Body of the nose may be normal or deficient

Malar region

- Extends on either side from the upper portion of the ear to the midface.
- Ears should be checked for:
  - Size: measured and plotted on growth charts that record length for age
  - Shape: noting abnormal folding or flattening of the helices
  - Position: low set if the top of the ear is below a line drawn from the outer canthus to the occiput
    - May be low set because they are small or microtic or because of a malformation of the mandibular region
  - Orientation: posterior rotation is present when ear appears turned toward the rear of the head.

Mandibular region

- The mandible extends from lower ear to lower ear and includes the lower lip and jaw.
- In most newborns, the chin is often retruded, slightly set back behind the vertical line extending from the forehead to the philtrum.
- If the mandible itself is small, it is described as micrognathic (Pierre Robin malformation sequence).
- An unusually prominent mandible is described as prognathic.

Neck

- Webbing, a feature common in Turner and Noonan syndromes
- Shortening, occasionally seen in:
  - Some skeletal dysplasias
  - Conditions in which anomalies of the cervical spine occur (Klippel-Feil syndrome)
- The position of posterior hairline
- Size of the thyroid gland

Trunk

- Chest should be examined for shape.
  - A shieldlike chest is found in Noonan and Turner syndromes.
- Symmetry
  - Hypoplasia of the pectoralis major and minor muscles, leading to asymmetry (Poland malformation sequence)
- A pectus deformity of the chest, either pectus excavatum or pectus carinatum, is usually an isolated finding.
  - Also a cardinal feature of Marfan syndrome

- Scoliosis is usually an isolated feature
  - Often seen in Marfan syndrome and in several other disorders

Extremities

- Anomalies of the extremities are common in many congenital malformation syndromes.
- All joints should be examined for range of motion.
- The presence of single or multiple joint contractures suggests either:
  - Neuromuscular dysfunction, as in the case of some forms of muscular dystrophy, or
  - External deforming forces that limited motion of the joint in utero
- Radioulnar synostosis, an inability to pronate or supinate the elbow occurs in:
  - Fetal alcohol syndrome
  - In some X chromosome aneuploidy syndromes, such as 48,XXXX and 48,XXXY syndromes
- The hands should be examined.
  - Polydactyly: the presence of extra digits
    - Can occur in isolation as an autosomal-dominant trait in up to 1% of all newborns
    - Can occur as part of a malformation syndrome, such as trisomy 13
  - Oligodactyly: a deficiency in the number of digits
    - Seen in Fanconi syndrome (growth retardation, aplastic anemia, development of leukemia or lymphoma and associated heart, renal, and limb defects including radial aplasia and thumb malformation or aplasia)
    - Generally part of a more severe limb reduction defect or secondary to intrauterine amputation that may occur with amniotic band disruption sequence
  - Syndactyly, a joining of ≥2 digits, is common to several syndromes.
  - Dermatoglyphics are important to note, especially the palmar crease pattern.
    - A transverse palmar crease, indicative of hypotonia during early fetal life (~50% of children with Down syndrome and 10% of individuals in the general population)
    - A characteristic palmar crease pattern is seen in fetal alcohol syndrome.

Genitalia

- Genitalia should be examined for abnormalities in structure.
- In male infants, if the penis appears short, it should be measured and plotted on an appropriate growth chart.
- Ambiguous genitalia can be associated with endocrinologic disorders, such as:
  - Congenital adrenal hyperplasia (female infants have masculinized external genitalia, but male genitals may be unaffected)

- Chromosomal disorders, such as Turner syndrome mosaicism
- Part of a multiple malformation disorder, such as Smith-Lemli-Opitz syndrome
- Hypospadias (occurs in 1 in 300 male newborns) is a common congenital malformation that often occurs as an isolated defect.
  - If it is associated with other anomalies, the possibility of a syndrome is strong.

DIFFERENTIAL DIAGNOSIS

- The differential diagnosis comprises conditions that feature some or all of the clues.
- Once this list has been assembled, a series of laboratory and imaging tests can be performed to move toward a definitive diagnosis.
- In the majority of cases, no specific diagnosis is immediately evident.
  - Some constellations of findings are rare, and finding a match may prove difficult.
  - In many cases, all laboratory tests are normal, and confirmation relies on subjective findings.
- Clinical geneticists have attempted to resolve this difficulty by developing scoring systems.
  - Cross-referenced tables of anomalies that help in developing a differential diagnosis
  - Computerized diagnostic programs
- An accurate diagnosis is important for 3 reasons:
  - It offers the family an explanation of why their child was born with congenital anomalies.
    - This may help allay feelings of guilt, given that parents frequently believe that they are responsible for their child's problem.
  - The natural history of many disorders is well described, and a diagnosis allows:
    - Anticipation of medical problems associated with a particular syndrome and performance of appropriate screening
    - Reassurance that other medical problems are no more likely to occur than they might with children who do not have the diagnosis
  - It permits accurate recurrence risk for future progeny.
    - Genetic counseling
    - Future prenatal diagnostic testing
- The diagnosis enables the clinician to provide the family with:
  - Educational materials
  - The chance to meet other families who have children with the same condition

- The Internet has become an important source for information.
  - Care should be exercised, because information on the Internet is not always subject to editorial control.
    - Some information may be inaccurate or inappropriate.
  - Physicians should try to screen sites before encouraging a family to seek information.
  - 2 good Web sites are:
    - National Organization for Rare Disorders (www.rarediseases.org)
      - A clearinghouse for information about rare diseases and their support groups
    - Genetests (www.genetests.org)
      - Provides information on available clinical and research testing for many diseases

LABORATORY EVALUATION

- Chromosome analysis (karyotype), either metaphase or prophase (high resolution), should be routinely ordered for children with:
  - Multiple congenital anomalies
  - Involvement of 1 major organ system and ≥ 2 dysmorphic features
  - Presence of mental retardation
- Chromosome analysis will identify conditions caused by:
  - Too much chromosomal material, such as trisomies
  - Too little chromosomal material, such as monosomies
- Fluorescent in situ hybridization (FISH) uses DNA technology to identify specific regions of the genome that are missing or duplicated.
  - FISH uses a DNA probe that is complementary to a specific region of the genome.
  - After a fluorescent marker is attached to this probe, it is incubated with chromosomal DNA from the patient.
  - FISH is requested when a syndrome with a known chromosomal defect is suspected, such as:
    - Velocardiofacial syndrome: deletion of 22q11.2
    - Präder-Willi syndrome: deletion of 15q11.2
    - Angelman syndrome: deletion of 15q11.2
    - Beckwith-Wiedemann syndrome: duplication of 11p15.2
- In a growing number of disorders, direct DNA analysis can be performed to identify specific mutations known to cause disease.
  - Uses Web-based resources for the most recent information, because the list of these disorders increases every day
  - Genetests (www.genetests.org), which is updated frequently, provides information about availability of testing for specific conditions.
    - Identifies laboratories performing these tests

F

IMAGING

- Radiologic imaging plays an important role in the evaluation of children with dysmorphic features.
- Individuals found to have multiple external malformations should have a thorough evaluation to detect internal malformations.
- Testing might include ultrasonographic evaluation of:
  - Head
  - Abdomen (possible anomalies in the kidney, bladder, liver and spleen)
- 3-dimensionally reconstructed computed tomography of the head is indicated in craniosynosostosis.
- Skeletal radiographs should be obtained if concern exists about a possible skeletal dysplasia.
- Magnetic resonance imaging may be indicated in children with:
  - Neurologic abnormalities
  - Spinal defect

DIAGNOSTIC PROCEDURES

- The presence of a heart murmur should trigger cardiology consultation.
  - Electrocardiography and echocardiography may be indicated.

TREATMENT APPROACH

- The pediatric health care provider seeing a patient who has dysmorphic facial features must decide whether the patient or family will benefit from a thorough evaluation or referral.
  - The most important task initially is to determine whether features are:
    - Consistent with the individual's genetic background
    - An abnormal phenotype
  - Following systematic diagnosis, the physician should convey the implications to appropriate family members.
    - Including genetic counseling

WHEN TO REFER

- A dysmorphologist should assist with diagnosis and meet with the family in person to explain the condition and all of its ramifications.
- A sufficient amount of time should be allotted for this meeting, because families may have many questions.
  - Each should be answered in a thoughtful and considerate way.
- It is helpful to include social support professionals as participants in these meetings.
  - Genetic counselors, social workers, and psychologists can be helpful in assisting the family in accepting the news and moving on with the next phase of their lives.

Failure to Thrive

DEFINITION

- Abnormal pattern of weight gain in children <2 years
  - Growth pattern irreconcilable with a predetermined standard for age
  - Weight consistently <80% of the median for age
  - Weight on >1 occasion falling below the 3rd percentile for age
  - Weight that has fallen across 2 major percentiles on the National Center for Health Statistics standard growth charts
- Social Security Administration definition
  - A drop in weight to below the 3rd percentile
  - In children <2 years, drop in weight to <75% of the median weight-for-height or age
- When acute malnutrition results in decreased weight-for-age, the condition is referred to as *wasting*.
- If caloric deprivation is prolonged, then it will eventually affect the child's linear growth as well, at which point the child is said to be *stunted*.
- Abnormalities in linear growth not accompanied by wasting (the child who has short stature alone) are not failure to thrive.

MECHANISM

- Infants and children grow in the presence of adequate amounts of 4 fundamental constituents.
  - Oxygen: deprivation at the tissue level will result in poor weight gain.
    - Congestive heart failure
    - Chronic lung disease
    - Anemia
  - Substrate: inadequate calories, protein, or micronutrients
    - Environmental deprivation
    - Malabsorption
    - Inability to metabolize them at the tissue level
  - Hormones: deficiencies can result in failure to thrive
    - Growth hormone
    - Insulin-like growth factors
    - Glucocorticoids
    - Thyroid hormone
    - Other regulators of growth
  - Love
    - Infants or children severely deprived of affection often will not grow despite what appears to be normal caloric intake.

- In the past, patients who had inadequate weight gain have been classified as a minority whose difficulty stems from a readily identifiable organic cause and a majority whose problem resides in a residual nonorganic category.
  - Other researchers have emphasized the overlapping nature of these distinctions and have suggested a third, or mixed, category of failure to thrive.
  - More recent approaches have tended to depart from the organic-nonorganic dichotomy in recognition of the somewhat arbitrary nature of this distinction.
- Energy
  - The largest share of energy consumed, approximately 55–60%, is devoted to maintaining a basal metabolic rate.
  - 5–10% of energy is lost in urine and stool.
  - 5% is accounted for by specific dynamic action.
  - 15% is used for normal physical activity above basal metabolic functions.
  - 15% is directed toward growth.
  - To support all these functions, infants need approximately 100–110 kcal/kg/day.
  - An imbalance between energy needs and energy supplies can arise either from increases in the former or deficiencies in the latter.
- Parenting difficulties may prevent the infant from receiving sufficient calories.
  - Unfamiliarity with proper preparation of infant formula or appropriate breastfeeding techniques
  - Psychosocial dysfunction
  - Maternal depression
  - Frank abuse or neglect
  - Economic deprivation
  - Unsound parental beliefs regarding nutrition
  - Subtle central nervous system abnormalities in the child that make them difficult feeders
- Food refusal in children
  - May begin even in infancy
  - Can result from many causes
    - Pain (from reflux esophagitis)
    - Psychosocial adjustment disorders from emotional deprivation
    - Anorexia from chronic infection or intoxication
    - Structural abnormalities resulting in dysphagia
- Inability to ingest nutrients properly
  - Structural malformations of the naso- or oropharynx
    - Cleft palate
    - Choanal atresia
    - Treacher Collins syndrome

- Muscular weakness
- Cerebral palsy or other central nervous system abnormalities
- Diseases that give rise to excessive dyspnea
- Vomiting
  - May impede growth through caloric deprivation
  - May be caused by
    - Structural abnormalities of the gastrointestinal tract
    - Increased intracranial pressure from any source
    - Chronic acidosis
    - Rumination
    - Gastroesophageal reflux
- The principal organ of nutrient absorption is the small bowel.
  - Malabsorption may result from:
    - Gross structural abnormalities
    - Inflammatory conditions
    - Infectious agents
    - Disorders of organs that elaborate enzymes essential for digestion

HISTORY

- Prompt evaluation of infants and children who do not gain weight as expected is important.
- The physician should begin by asking the parent or parents, guardian or guardians, or principal caregiver or caregivers how they think the baby is doing and what they believe the problem to be.
- Every evaluation of an infant or child who is not gaining weight must begin with a thorough history.
  - Gestational age at birth
  - Any unusual complications of the labor and delivery
  - Presence of malformations or other obvious deformities
- Knowledge of a parent's frame of mind may propel further evaluation toward or away from difficulty in parent-child interaction, including child neglect.
- Feeding history
  - Is the baby bottle-fed or breastfed?
    - How often does the child breastfeed, and for how long?
    - Does the mother feel as though the child is sucking well?
    - Does the baby appear sated after feeding?
  - If bottle-fed, how is the formula prepared and by whom?
  - How many ounces will the baby take in a 24-hour period?
  - Does the infant wet 6–8 diapers a day?
  - For older children, when were solids introduced?
  - Does the parent find the child to be a picky eater or difficult to interest in food?
  - Does the child drink excessive amounts of juice during the day, substituting for more calorically rich nutrients?

- What are meal times like at home?
  - Where does the child eat, and with whom?
  - Are distractions, such as television, game boys, or video games, present during meals?
- Is food being used for discipline or in battles over control?
- A 24-hour dietary recall of a typical day often can help quantify the caloric intake of the patient.
  - If this information proves difficult to elicit, the parents can be sent home with a nutritional diary to fill out prospectively and bring in at the next visit.
- A home visit provides an opportunity to observe the family interaction around feeding in the context in which it normally occurs.
- Vomiting or spitting up
  - Frequency
  - Volume
  - Presence of blood or bile in the emesis
  - Gastric outlet obstructions (pyloric stenosis, antral web) often result in the generation of significant propulsive forces leading to projectile vomiting.
  - Gastroesophageal reflux often results in less dramatic patterns of regurgitation.
  - An obstruction distal to the ligament of Treitz will generally produce bilious vomiting.
    - In infants, this symptom may indicate the presence of a malrotation and midgut volvulus.
- Pattern and frequency of stooling
  - Liquid stools may indicate a small-bowel pathologic condition.
  - Bulky, foul-smelling stools may result from fat malabsorption.
  - Mucus or blood in the stools may indicate an inflammatory condition.
- Additional information should be obtained about the medical history, beginning with the parents' attitudes regarding their decision to have a baby and what their experience with the pregnancy was like.
  - Did the mother gain a reasonable amount of weight?
  - Did she experience any illnesses during her pregnancy?
    - Hypertension or preeclampsia will result in an infant who is small for gestational age.
    - Gestational diabetes may produce an infant with macrosomia who fails to gain weight because of postnatal cardiac complications.
  - Ask about specific toxic exposures in utero.
    - Tobacco use may result in a small baby, but he or she rapidly catches up in weight with peers.
    - Marijuana and alcohol use exert an influence on growth that may be sustained throughout childhood.

- Family history
  - Growth patterns of siblings
  - Occurrence of fetal loss or infant deaths
  - Presence in the family of immune deficiencies, neurologic disorders, or metabolic derangements
  - Any unexplained growth deficiencies in close relatives
  - Recent comprehensive longitudinal studies from England emphasize the extent to which mean parental height and parity overwhelm the influence of traditional markers of socioeconomic deprivation on infant weight gain, such as parental education or occupational status.
- Social history
  - Availability of social supports for the parents
  - Economic or legal circumstances that threaten the stability of the family
  - Nature of the relationship between the parents
  - Presence of affective disorders in the primary caregiver
  - Recent disruptive events in the family's life
- Finally, look for unrealistic expectations regarding feeding patterns, dietary fads, or infant behavior.

PHYSICAL EXAM

- Initial examination begins with observation of how the child relates to the parent or parents and the examiner.
  - Does the child appear listless, easily distractible, or irritable?
  - Can the child be engaged to make eye contact or to play with an age-appropriate toy?
- Repeated anthropometric measurements over time constitute the most important component of the physical evaluation of children who are not gaining weight.
  - Assemble all data available from previous anthropometric measurements of the patient, including weight, height, and head circumference.
  - Premature infants must have their measurements corrected for gestational age
    - Until 18 months of age for head circumference
    - Until 24 months of age for weight
    - Until 40 months of age for height
- The child should be completely undressed, and notations should be made of:
  - Any evidence of wasting
  - Presence and distribution of normal subcutaneous body fat
  - Muscle mass and tone
  - Any dysmorphic features

- Particular attention should be paid to organ systems that may reflect evidence of malnutrition.
  - Mucous membranes, hair, nails, and skin
    - Abnormalities may indicate vitamin, protein, fat, and micronutrient deficiencies.
  - Head, eyes, ears, nose, and throat
    - Open fontanelles may indicate hypothyroidism.
    - Craniotabes are seen in nutritional rickets.
    - Blurred disk margins of increased intracranial pressure are seen in chronic emesis.
    - Submucosal cleft of the hard palate is seen in infant who feeds poorly
- Thyroid
  - Palpated gently
  - Auscultated for evidence of hyperthyroidism
- Lungs and heart
  - Observation, palpation, and particularly auscultation may reveal wheezing, rales, or heart murmurs suggestive of the presence of chronic conditions.
  - These conditions often result in energy expenditures that can outstrip the supply of nutrients available to an infant.
  - Examine the digits for clubbing in the older children.
- Abdominal examination
  - To rule out organomegaly associated with tumor, infection, or storage disease
  - Intestinal distention can be associated with carbohydrate malabsorption.
- Neurologic examination being watchful for
  - Disorders of mentation
  - Cranial nerve abnormalities
  - Generalized weakness
  - Spasticity

DIFFERENTIAL DIAGNOSIS

- Conditions that increase energy needs
  - Chronic heart disease (congenital or acquired)
  - Chronic lung disease (bronchopulmonary dysplasia, cystic fibrosis, pulmonary lymphangiectasis)
  - Chronic anemia (hemaglobinopathies, enzyme deficiencies, membrane abnormalities)
  - Chronic infection (urinary tract infections, respiratory infections, tuberculosis)
  - Endocrine abnormalities (hyperthyroidism)
  - Malignancy (neuroblastoma, ganglioneuroma)
- Conditions that compromise the efficiency of energy utilization
  - Chronic infection
  - Chronic renal disease

F

- Hepatic insufficiency
- Inborn errors of metabolism
- Hormonal abnormalities
- Certain genetic syndromes
- Deficiencies of various micronutrients, including iron, zinc, and carnitine
- Conditions leading to deficiency in energy supply
  - Calories withheld
  - In utero conditions
  - Formula preparation mistakes
  - Breastfeeding difficulties
  - Parent-child psychosocial dysfunction
  - Maternal depression
  - Intentional abuse or neglect
  - Poverty
  - Unsound parental beliefs regarding nutrition
  - Difficult feeders
  - Calories not properly ingested or digested
  - Anorexia (reflux esophagitis, emotional deprivation, chronic infection, dysphagia)
  - Structural abnormalities of the oro- or nasopharynx (cleft palate, choanal atresia, Treacher Collins syndrome, Pierre Robin syndrome, laryngeal web)
  - Structural abnormalities of the gastrointestinal tract (stenosis or atresia of the esophagus or duodenum, tracheoesophageal fistula, vascular ring, strictures, achalasia, malrotation, antral web, pyloric stenosis)
  - Neuromuscular disorders (cerebral palsy, hydrocephalus, myopathies)
  - Conditions leading to excessive dyspnea (congestive heart failure, chronic lung disease)
  - Vomiting and rumination
  - Malabsorption
  - Small bowel (celiac disease, inflammatory bowel disease, disaccharide malabsorption, intestinal lymphangiectasia, jejunal atresia, duplication cysts, chronic parasitic infections)
  - Pancreas (cystic fibrosis, Shwachman-Diamond syndrome, chronic pancreatitis)
  - Liver (cirrhosis, intrahepatic cholestatic syndromes, biliary atresia)

LABORATORY EVALUATION

- If the cause of the failure to thrive is not made clear by history and physical examination, laboratory investigation is unlikely to reveal it.
- In cases in which psychosocial features predominate, most laboratory tests may be unnecessary.

- If the cause of a child's failure to gain weight adequately remains uncertain after careful history and physical examination, a limited number of screening studies may be considered:
  - Complete blood count
  - Blood pH
  - Serum electrolytes
  - Blood urea nitrogen and creatinine
  - Urinalysis and urine culture
  - Stool examination
    - Reducing substances
    - pH
    - Occult blood
    - Ova and parasites
- More extensive testing should be done only when historical or physical examination evidence indicates a specific diagnosis.

TREATMENT APPROACH

- The therapeutic approach to a child failing to gain weight adequately must be tailored to individual needs of the family and the child.
- Therapy should be directed toward the underlying disease or condition where a specific diagnosis has been identified.
- When disturbance in the parent-child interaction is recognized as the cause of the patient's inability to gain weight, the family should be approached nonjudgmentally.
- The severity of the child's condition should dictate the initial approach to treatment.

SPECIFIC TREATMENT

Mild to moderate failure to thrive

- Goals
  - Nutritional rehabilitation
  - Parental education
  - Behavioral intervention
- Infants and children exhibiting mild degrees of malnutrition (>80% of ideal body weight for age)
  - May be managed as outpatients
  - May be managed by primary care physician, with consultation from a nutritionist
    - Occasional consultation may be provided by subspecialist colleagues.
- Patients who have evidence of more severe caloric deprivation require involvement of a multidisciplinary team
  - Primary care physician
  - Nutritionist
  - Mental health or behavioral therapist
  - Social worker

- Hospitalization may be necessary for a subset of these patients whose malnutrition is combined with or results from another significant medical condition.
- Home visitation using professionals may be a successful intervention in select circumstances.
- Child protective services must be alerted about any child thought to be the victim of neglect.
- Refeeding regimen
  - ~10–15% of calories from protein
  - 50–60% from carbohydrate
  - 30–40% from fat
- Attempts to overfeed malnourished infants at the outset of therapy should be avoided.
  - They may exhibit some degree of anorexia initially.
  - Refeeding that is too vigorous may induce malabsorption and diarrhea.
- A typical 3-phase regimen:
- Phase 1
  - Day 1: begin with provision of 100% of daily age-adjusted energy and protein requirements based on the child's weight.
  - If this phase is well tolerated, proceed to Phase 2.
- Phase 2
  - Intake is increased to provide adequate nutrition to achieve catch-up growth.
    - (Age-adjusted energy requirements [kcal/kg/day]) × (ratio of the child's ideal body weight for height)/(the child's actual body weight at presentation) = reasonable estimate of the nutritional requirements for this stage
    - The same calculation can be made for protein requirements.
    - Energy and protein requirements for these phases of infant refeeding usually can be accomplished with the use of a routine infant formula modified to increase its caloric density.
      - Mixing 13 oz of concentrated formula with 10 oz of water rather than 13 oz of water will create a formula that is 24 cal/oz.
    - Alternatively, carbohydrates in the form of glucose polymers or fat in the form of medium-chain triglycerides adds calories while avoiding complications of overhydration.
    - For older children, available caloric supplements will include a wide variety of solid foods.
- Phase 3: consolidation phase of nutritional rehabilitation
  - A varied diet is offered ad libitum.
  - The child gradually approaches ideal body weight.
  - Multivitamin and iron supplementation should be part of every refeeding regimen for undernourished children.

- Initiation of nutritional rehabilitation is an ideal time to educate parents and to address family interactions, psychological vulnerabilities, social needs.
  - Emphasis should be placed on appropriate nutritional information.
  - Concrete suggestions should be offered about how to structure mealtime at home.
    - Minimize distractions.
    - Provide a relaxed social environment that encourages good eating habits.
  - For families in need, access to community resources must be facilitated.
    - Special Supplemental Nutrition Program for Women, Infants, and Children (WIC)
    - Food stamps
  - Pediatricians should be prepared to advocate vigorously for patients in need of supplemental nutrition or special infant formulas when families experience difficulties in obtaining these products.

Severe failure to thrive

- Children who are <60% of ideal body weight for height should be hospitalized.
- The nutritional rehabilitation
  - Will be more prolonged
  - May entail a period of tube feedings in addition to oral supplements
- In cases in which the gastrointestinal tract is temporarily inaccessible, parenteral feedings with central venous access may be necessary.

WHEN TO REFER

- If a diagnosis is made of a chronic disease pertaining to an organ subspecialty discipline such as cardiac, pulmonary, renal, gastrointestinal, or endocrine
- If the psychosocial family dynamic indicates a need for psychiatric intervention for either or both parents
- If nutritional rehabilitation warrants the attention of a nutritionist

WHEN TO ADMIT

- Any child with a weight <60% of ideal body weight should be hospitalized.
  - Care should be provided by a multidisciplinary team.
    - Nutritionists
    - Social workers
    - Pediatricians
    - Pediatric subspecialists, when appropriate

- Other children who should be hospitalized include
  - Any child who, despite aggressive outpatient management, continues to fail to gain weight at an acceptable rate
  - Any child who presents with signs of marasmus or severe protein malnutrition (kwashiorkor)

FOLLOW-UP

- Poor weight gain in infancy should be followed up assiduously.
- Initial weekly visits for infants may be necessary to reassure the parents and practitioner that the therapy undertaken is having the desired effects.
- Children <6 months, when provided with adequate calories, begin to gain weight in a few days.
- Older children may take longer than their younger counterparts before sustained weight gain is established.
- Ongoing developmental, behavioral, and social evaluations must be incorporated into any plan for follow-up.
  - Children who gain weight poorly often have abnormalities in these areas.
  - The lingering effects of calorie, protein, and micronutrient deprivation may manifest as developmental and behavioral abnormalities.
    - Such results are particularly likely in children whose mothers exhibit affective disorders.

COMPLICATIONS

- Most children who fail to gain weight adequately suffer from malnutrition and are therefore at risk for its attendant consequences.

PROGNOSIS

- Caution must be used when predicting outcomes for children who have abnormal weight gain patterns in infancy and childhood.
- A variety of conditions may give rise to this clinical picture.
  - High-quality data on which reasonable predictions might be sustained are lacking.
  - One systematic review of 13 long-term longitudinal studies concluded that growth and neurocognitive outcomes probably do not differ substantially between children with failure to thrive and their unaffected peers.
  - In an extensive review of the literature, the Agency for Healthcare Research and Quality concluded that children with failure to thrive in infancy are likely to suffer immunologic, behavioral, cognitive, and psychomotor developmental deficits that persist despite interventions.
- Such disparate findings suggest that most children in the mild failure to thrive category will
  - Experience brisk nutritional rehabilitation
  - Do well with adequate follow-up
- More severely affected children may require more prolonged or repetitive interventions.
  - Type of intervention depends on the underlying cause
  - These children may suffer residual cognitive, behavioral, and educational consequences.
- All children who exhibit faltering weight gain during infancy and childhood absolutely must receive early comprehensive evaluation and prompt treatment.

Family Screening and Assessments

BACKGROUND

- Because primary care providers develop ongoing relationships with families, they are uniquely poised to discuss and screen for a variety of family stresses that may negatively affect children.
- Family screening and assessment involves identifying parents who face challenges in meeting their child's needs, such as:
  - Depression
  - Smoking
  - Poverty
  - Addiction
  - Violence

Maternal depression

- Prevalence
  - Of the 4 million births annually, depression affects 500,000 women.
    - The most common complication of childbearing
    - 12–42% of maternal depressive symptoms are seen in pediatric primary care settings.
  - Socioeconomic
    - Maternal depressive symptoms are ubiquitous in all social and economic groups.
  - Postpartum blues (mildest)
    - Approximately 70% of women
  - Postpartum depression (moderate)
    - Approximately 15% of women
  - Postpartum psychosis (severe)
    - 1–2 of every 1000 births
  - Women at highest risk
    - Personal or family history of depression
    - Previous episode of postpartum depression
    - Low income
    - Low level of education
    - Poor maternal health status
    - Other stressful life events
- Etiology
  - Probably involves a complex interaction of biochemical, interpersonal, and social factors
- Disease spectrum
  - Postpartum blues
    - Lasts ~10 days
    - Typically does not interfere with a woman's ability to function
  - Postpartum depression
    - More persistent and debilitating than postpartum blues
    - May develop insidiously over the initial 3 postpartum months or occur more acutely

- Can interfere with a mother's ability to care for herself or her child
- Lasts an average of 7 months if left untreated
  - Postpartum psychosis
    - Occurs within the initial 2 weeks of delivery
    - Psychiatric emergency requiring immediate action because of risk of suicide, infanticide
    - Characterized by major disturbances in thinking and behavior, hallucinations, and delusions
  - Maternal depression
    - Term often used to describe chronic or acutely depressed women with dependent children (may include postpartum)
    - Well described in the American Psychiatric Association *Diagnostic and Statistical Manual of Mental Disorders*, 4th edition
    - Signs and symptoms are clinically indistinguishable from those of major depression that occurs in women at other times.
    - Women experience recurrence and relapses.

- Maternal depression: effects on children
  - Infant behaviors in maternal depression
    - Limited play and exploratory behaviors
    - Less responsive to facial expressions
    - More emotionally labile (ie, fussy)
    - Increased drowsiness
    - Less sociable with strangers
    - Difficulties with emotion regulation
  - Maternal-child interactions in maternal depression
    - Decreased reciprocity in interaction of the infant
    - Decreased enjoyment of the infant by mother
    - Lack of patience to soothe the infant
    - Less active interactions with the infant
  - Children's mental and emotional health after maternal depression
    - Hyperactivity
    - Defiance and disrespect
    - Higher rates of depression
    - Increased substance abuse in adolescent years
  - Children's cognitive development with maternal depression
    - Delayed cognitive development
    - Lower scores on the McCarthy Scale of Children's Abilities in infants
    - Poor school performance in later years
  - Preventive health and parenting practices among women with depression
    - Shorter duration of breastfeeding
    - Less play and reading

– Less use of safety items (eg, outlet covers)

– Higher use of acute health services

– Lower rate of up-to-date immunizations

– Fewer optimal parenting practices (eg, reading, playing)

Parental smoking

■ Prevalence

• 43% of children age 2 months to 11 years live in homes with ≥1 smoker.

• 60% of children 3–11 years of age are exposed to environmental tobacco smoke (ETS) (~22 million children).

■ Health risks to children

• Lower respiratory infections

• Middle ear effusions

• Asthma exacerbations

• Sudden infant death syndrome

• Increased risk of cancer as adults

– Lymphoma

– Leukemia

Intimate partner violence

■ Prevalence

• As many as 2 million women will experience intimate partner violence each year.

• >3 million children witness interparental violence.

• Children in this setting are at risk for:

– Developmental delay

– Sleep disorders

– School failure

– Oppositional defiant disorder

– Depression

– Abuse

GOALS

■ Prevent adverse outcomes

■ Maximize each child's potential

• Family well-being is critically important in achieving these goals.

– Identify parents in need of psychosocial services.

– Partner with parents.

– Offer information and resources.

• Use strategies that incorporate theories of behavioral health counseling.

– The 5As (Ask, Advise, Assess, Assist, Arrange) are readily transportable to other family issues.

GENERAL APPROACH

■ A large body of evidence supports family psychological screening.

• The quality of the child's environment, especially the quality of caregiving relationships, influences:

– Development of young children

– Childrens' long-term outcomes

■ How can pediatric providers include family psychosocial screening into pediatric primary care?

• Barriers to discussing family stresses include lack of:

– Time

– Education

– Resources

• Barriers may be community specific, and some may be more difficult to rectify than others.

■ Maternal depression: rationale for screening

• Screening for maternal depression is necessary when viewed in the context of the effects on children.

– Pediatricians are reluctant to discuss maternal mental health in the course of routine pediatric primary care.

– Pediatricians recognize only 25% of mothers with depressive symptoms.

• Mothers at risk for depression may not seek health care from their own primary care physician.

– However, they see their child's pediatrician many times during the postpartum period and beyond.

– Every well-child visit presents the opportunity to ask a mother if she is feeling overwhelmed, stressed, anxious, or depressed.

– Simple steps can be taken that may open windows of communication that will encourage a mother to discuss her feelings.

• Mothers will be open to help if:

– A consistent, trusting relationship exists

– Concerns about maternal emotional needs become an expected component of each pediatric visit

• Treating maternal depression can:

– Have a positive effect on both mothers and their children

– Reduce psychiatric conditions in children

■ Parental smoking: rationale for screening

• The consequences of exposure to tobacco smoke on children pose immediate health risks and long-term health concerns.

• Smoking is a highly addictive behavior, but treatment is effective.

- Exposure to secondhand smoke primarily comes from parental tobacco use.
  - Despite recommendations from Bright Futures, pediatricians infrequently assess and advise parents to quit smoking.
  - Pediatricians can address children's exposure to ETS by asking a few simple questions.
- The AAP issued a policy statement with strong recommendations for pediatricians to:
  - Inform parents about the health hazards of passive smoking
  - Provide guidance on smoking cessation during primary care visits
- Pediatricians should familiarize themselves with treatment options that are available to:
  - Help their adolescent patients who smoke
  - Assist the parents of their youngest patients
- Intimate partner violence: rationale for screening
  - AAP policy statement
    - Pediatricians are in a position to recognize abused women in pediatric settings.
    - Intervening is an active form of child abuse prevention.
  - Barriers to screening
    - Asking mothers about intimate partner violence during a pediatric visit is often difficult, especially when older children are present.
    - Pediatricians may be unprepared to raise questions with mothers.
    - However, this area of inquiry is critical and has been recommended by numerous advisory boards.

SPECIFIC INTERVENTIONS

Maternal depression

- Screening strategies
  - Signs and symptoms of maternal depression
    - Sadness or low mood
    - Feeling down
    - Feeling worthless
    - Loss of interest or pleasure (anhedonia)
    - Anxiety
    - Guilt
    - Loss of energy
    - Anger
    - Increased or decreased sleep
    - Increased or decreased appetite
    - Delusions or paranoia
    - Thoughts of death (their own or their child's)
    - Suicidal ideation

- Note the mother-child interaction.
  - Helps to assess attachment and bonding
  - This assessment is the most rudimentary but is already an inherent component of a primary care visit.
- Ask specific questions:
  - "How are you feeling about being a mother?"
  - "How is your energy level?"
  - "Have you had any periods of sadness? Feeling blue? Crying?"
  - "Are you feeling overly worried about your infant?"
  - "How have you been eating? Sleeping?"
  - "Do you have any worries about your overall mood?"
- Ask about resources mothers have to assist them.
  - Family members
  - Child care
  - Financial assistance
- Ask about other stressors that may have a negative impact on children.
  - Marital problems
  - Substance abuse
  - Housing instability
- Ask about history of depression.
  - Be specific
  - Ask about suicidal ideation.
  - Make appropriate emergency referrals as needed.
- Listen.
  - Mothers will talk about their concerns if they believe you are listening without judging them.

Screening tools

- Edinburgh Postnatal Depression Scale (EPDS)
  - 10-item, 5-minute questionnaire
  - Easy to use
  - Can be scored immediately
  - Sensitivity: 93–100%
  - Specificity: 83–90%
  - EPDS instructions
    - The mother is asked to indicate 1 of 4 possible responses that comes the closest to how she has been feeling in the previous 7 days.
    - All 10 items must be completed.
    - Care should be taken to avoid the possibility of the mother discussing her answers with others.
    - The mother should complete the scale herself, unless she has limited English or has difficulty with reading.

F

- Sample EPDS question:
  - Given that you have recently had a baby, we would like to know how you are feeling. Please check the box next to the answer that comes closest to how you have felt IN THE PAST 7 DAYS, not just how you feel today.
  - Example: I have felt happy:
    - Yes, all the time
    - Yes, most of the time
    - No, not very often
    - Not at all
    - Checking box 2 would mean: "I have felt happy most of the time" during the past week. Please complete the following questions in the same way.
- Patient Health Questionnaire-2
  - 2 questions
  - Answers on a scale of 0–3
    - 0 = Not at all
    - 1 = Several days
    - 2 = More than one-half the days
    - 3 = Nearly every day
  - Score of 3 or more points is considered a positive score.
    - Over the past 2 weeks, how often have you been bothered by any of the following problems?
      - Little interest or pleasure in doing things
      - Feeling down, depressed, or hopeless
- US Preventive Task Force
  - 2 questions are asked of the mother at every primary care visit.
  - *Yes* to either question is considered a positive score.
    - During the past 2 weeks, have you ever felt down, depressed, or hopeless?
    - During the past 2 weeks, have you felt little interest or pleasure in doing things?
- Center for Epidemiologic Studies Depression scale
- Beck Depression Inventory
- Patient Health Questionnaire-9

Using results that reveal depression

- Assure the mother that:
  - She is not alone.
  - Many mothers experience similar feelings.
  - Depression is treatable.
  - Support is available if they need it.
  - You are a partner that can help.
- Encourage her to:
  - Get the help she might need
  - Be the best mother she can be

- Offer to:
  - Help her meet other mothers
  - Provide information about community, print, and online resources
  - Speak to the mother's primary care provider
  - Initiate a referral to a mental health professional, support group, or other therapeutic agency
  - Speak with other family members who might be supportive to the mother
- Intervene if:
  - The mother shows severe impairment, psychosis, or suicidal ideation by initiating an emergency behavioral evaluation by a specialist
  - The child is at any imminent physical risk, strongly consider contacting child protective services
- Be prepared to:
  - Maintain communication with a mother who initially denies her symptoms and is unwilling to seek further treatment
  - Develop a strong therapeutic alliance and close follow-up
  - These strategies can help encourage mothers to address depressive symptoms
  - Schedule frequent office visits to follow up with the mother and her child or children

Parental smoking

- Screening tools for ETS
  - 3-item validated measure of ETS exposure
    - Does the child's mother smoke?
    - Do others smoke?
    - Do others smoke inside?
  - Alternative 5-item screen
    - Does "_____'s" mother currently smoke?
      - In the home?
    - Does "_____'s" father currently smoke?
      - In the home?
    - Is your child exposed to cigarette smoke on a regular basis (any exposure at least 1 time a week) from anyone other than the parents (eg, stepparents, day care providers, grandparents, siblings, friends)

Intimate partner violence

- Screening tools
  - During every pediatric visit, pediatricians can ask mothers a few simple questions, such as:
    - "We all have disagreements at home. What happens when you and your partner disagree?"
    - "Does shouting, pushing, or shoving occur?"
    - "Does anyone get hurt?"

- "Has your partner ever threatened to hurt you or your children?"
- "Do you ever feel afraid of your partner?"
- "Has anyone forced you to have sex in the last few years?"
- The American Medical Association has suggested 3 questions.
  - Are you in a relationship now or have you ever been in a relationship in which you have been harmed or felt afraid of your partner?
  - Has your partner ever hurt any of your children?
  - Are you afraid of your current partner?
- HITS (hurt, insulted, threatened with harm, screamed at)
  - How often does your partner:
    - Physically hurt you?
    - Insult or talk down to you?
    - Threaten you with harm?
    - Scream or curse at you?

- Answers
  - 1 = Never
  - 2 = Rarely
  - 3 = Sometimes
  - 4 = Fairly often
  - 5 = Frequently
- Scoring: A total score >10 is considered positive for partner violence.
- Partner Violence Screen
  - Have you been hit, kicked, punched, or otherwise hurt by someone within the past year? If so, by whom?
  - Do you feel safe in your current relationship?
  - Is there a partner from a previous relationship who is making you feel unsafe?
  - Scoring: A "yes" response on any question is considered positive for partner violence.

F

Fatigue and Weakness

DEFINITION

- *Fatigue* and *weakness* are terms that are difficult to define and often used interchangeably.
  - Ubiquitous symptoms that may or may not be related to medical diagnoses
  - Used commonly in medical and colloquial language
  - Any acute illness or trauma may be accompanied by fatigue.
  - Usually, only prolonged fatigue is noteworthy.
- Adolescents and children often use other terms to describe perceptions of somatic weakness and fatigue.
- Fatigue involves:
  - Extreme and unusual tiredness
  - Decreased physical performance
  - Excessive need for rest
  - Often is accompanied by feelings of:
    - Sleepiness
    - Weariness
    - Irritability
    - Lassitude
    - Boredom
    - Decreased efficiency
- *Weakness* refers to diminished body or muscle strength.
  - True weakness can be identified only by demonstration of abnormal neurologic or muscular function based on:
    - History
    - Physical examination
    - Laboratory studies
- The term *chronic infectious mononucleosis* and *chronic fatigue syndrome* have become popular with both physicians and the media.
  - Attention has led to:
    - Misuse of these terms
    - Mild mass hysteria among young adults and adolescents, convinced they have one of these disorders

EPIDEMIOLOGY

- Age
  - Adolescents are most likely to experience fatigue, lassitude, lack of energy, or mild depression.
- Seasonality
  - Most common in spring among adolescents

MECHANISM

- Fatigue
  - Most commonly associated with recurrent or chronic infection in children

- May be a normal result of any physical or mental work in which energy expenditure exceeds restorative processes
- Temporary fatigue that follows intense exercise involves several complex mechanisms, including:
  - Increased central inhibition mediated by group III and IV muscle afferents
  - Decrease in muscle spindle facilitation and suboptimal cortical output
- At the level of the muscle cell, fatigue results from a reduction in adenosine triphosphate caused by:
  - High utilization rates
  - Depletion of glycogen
- Normal fatigue follows:
  - Such activities as cramming for examinations
  - Lack of food
  - Sleep deprivation
- The degree of fatigue, even when prolonged, is usually appropriate for the amount of physical or mental exertion expended.
- Fatigue may be a pathological state with an organic or psychological foundation.
  - Lassitude associated with somatic illness often has definable physical or laboratory abnormalities.
  - Fatigue has also been shown to have a strong correlation with:
    - Depression
    - Anxiety disorder
- Weakness
  - True weakness in a child is a cause for concern.
  - Results from a derangement of neuromuscular function
    - Cerebral hemispheres
    - Cerebellum
    - Spinal cord
    - Anterior horn cells
    - Peripheral nerves
    - Myoneuronal junction
    - Muscle

HISTORY

- Goals
  - Rule out underlying medical illness.
  - Return the child to a state of well-being.
  - Relieve parental concerns.
- Critical evaluation of history, physical examination, and laboratory tests should enable quick determination of organic causes for fatigue.
- Points to consider
  - Adequate time and concern are needed to evaluate history.

- Symptoms of chronic fatigue cannot be dismissed casually over the telephone or with a quick office visit.
- The problem may seem insignificant, but either the child or parents are worried about the fatigue.
  - Family members may disagree about the significance of the symptoms.
- Patients who come to the primary care physician complaining of fatigue often have emotionally based problems.
  - A careful history, with information from both child and parents (taken separately when appropriate), often helps narrow the differential diagnosis.
  - Discrepancies between the child's and the parents' observations become evident.
  - Emotional stress or some disruption in the patient's life is often part of the history.
  - In most cases, a diagnosis of emotionally related fatigue emerges on the basis of the history alone.
  - Information derived from a long-standing physician-patient relationship helps reduce tensions during the evaluation.
- Fatigue
  - Young children infrequently complain of feeling fatigued.
    - Before adolescence, most children cannot verbalize a feeling of fatigue.
      - Even with chronic organic diseases, most children do not express fatigue verbally.
      - Younger children occasionally express a sense of lassitude and fatigue on questioning.
    - Fatigue is usually exhibited in terms of a child's physical activity and performance in school, sports, and other organized activities.
    - The problem may be manifested by trouble running or keeping up in gym class, clumsiness, or lack of agility.
    - Concerned parents usually report that the child appears fatigued.
      - "He has no energy."
      - "She lies around all the time."
      - "She seems bored and droopy."
      - "He's sleeping a lot of the time."
      - "She has no pep."
      - "He drags around."
      - "I can't get her to do a thing."
    - The younger the child, the more likely that the expressed or observed fatigue has a pathological basis.
  - Chronic fatigue is common among adolescents.
    - Even minor illnesses often precipitate prolonged fatigue in adolescents.
    - Parents often perceive their adolescent children to be fatigued, even when the adolescents do not agree.

PHYSICAL EXAM

- Thorough physical examination may be the only assessment necessary.
- In all age groups
  - Search for sites of chronic latent infection
    - Adenopathy
      - Cervical adenopathy can be a clue to the diagnosis of infectious mononucleosis
    - Enlargement or tenderness of the liver and spleen
    - Abdominal masses
  - Prolonged fever, however low grade, must always be viewed as significant and may suggest:
    - Infection
    - Inflammatory disease
    - Cancer
  - Palpate for an enlarged or tender thyroid gland.
  - Look for mild scleral icterus and petechiae.
  - Examine for pallor from:
    - Anemia
    - Hypothyroidism
  - Examine the oropharynx for hyperpigmentation of gums and buccal mucosa (Addison disease).
  - Assess plotted height and weight.
    - Failure to progress along expected growth parameters may indicate an underlying systemic process.
      - Chronic cardiac disorder
      - Pulmonary disorder
      - Gastrointestinal disorder
      - Renal disorder
    - Poor growth velocity and obesity may indicate underlying endocrinopathy.
      - Hypothyroidism
      - Cushing syndrome
    - In adolescents with unexplained fatigue, poor weight gain may be a manifestation of inflammatory bowel disease.
- A young child's affect and appearance are most revealing.
- Adolescents may be more difficult to evaluate and may:
  - Be slovenly
  - Be uncommunicative
  - Be depressed
  - Be unwilling to express their feelings
  - Appear physically ill

F

DIFFERENTIAL DIAGNOSIS

Fatigue

Infants

- The term fatigue is rarely pertinent in this age group.
- Parents sometimes report that the infant tires easily during feedings or seems droopy.
- Infants with cyanotic or congestive heart disease:
  - Often appear to tire easily
  - Sweat excessively with feedings
- Other serious conditions, including severe anemia and hypothyroidism, may present as listlessness.

Children

- Recurrent or chronic infection is the most common cause.
- Otitis media, sinusitis, and tonsillitis of a recurrent and smoldering nature
  - Often overlooked for systemic effects
  - Fatigue may be prominent.
- Upper respiratory tract allergies
  - Often mistakenly considered insignificant
  - May cause impressive fatigue, irritability, and mild depression
- Toxoplasmosis and cytomegalovirus infections
  - May mimic mononucleosis
  - Produce significant fatigue, but with only minimal cervical adenopathy and fever
  - Fluorescent antibody test positive for toxoplasmosis or cytomegalovirus with negative results of a heterophil antibody test confirms the diagnosis.
- Hepatitis and other viral infections
  - Child may be anicteric (or only slightly icteric), with little or no hepatic tenderness or enlargement.
  - Other common viral infections, especially during convalescence, can cause prolonged fatigue accompanied by depression.
- Endocrine disorders
  - Only hypothyroidism is likely to be associated with fatigue.
    - A child with hypothyroidism whose growth rate has decreased may exhibit increasing fatigue and lassitude, at first subtle, as the only symptoms.
  - Thyrotoxicosis is uncommon in young children but occasionally produces isolated fatigue in adolescents.
- Diabetes mellitus
  - Any metabolic disorder can cause fatigue, but only diabetes mellitus occurs with enough frequency to merit consideration.
  - Fatigue almost always accompanies an initial or uncontrolled diabetic state.

- Inflammatory diseases
  - Rheumatoid arthritis and other rheumatoid-like disorders, such as Lyme arthritis
  - Significant fatigue out of proportion to the child's musculoskeletal symptoms
- Pulmonary disease
  - Cyanotic heart disease
  - Chronic advanced pulmonary disease, as with cystic fibrosis
  - Underlying disease is usually readily evident before fatigue becomes severe.
  - Severe fatigue may be caused by a previously undiagnosed hypoxic disorder.
- Anemia
  - Often thought to be cause of fatigue, but generally not the case
  - Symptoms are usually not seen in children until the hemoglobin level decreases to 6 or 7 g/dL.
    - If erythrocyte counts decrease gradually, even lower hemoglobin levels may ensue without clinically evident symptoms.
    - Younger children especially seem to tolerate markedly low hemoglobin levels with no symptoms.
  - Irritability and attention problems may be present.
- Cancer
  - Leukemia or lymphoma occasionally develops insidiously, with fatigue as the major symptom.
- Emotional disorders
  - Most children experience brief, transient periods of lassitude or fatigue that are usually self-limited.
  - Unexplained chronic fatigue is often found to be emotionally related.
  - Before adolescence, the complaint usually stems from the parents' concern about a child's reduced activity level.
  - A younger child will be noted to:
    - Prefer sedentary activities
    - "Lie around the house a lot"
    - Appear tired
    - Lack energy
    - Shrink from social contacts
  - Observed traits may have been long-standing.
    - A comment from grandparents or a teacher may arouse parental anxiety and precipitate a visit to the primary care physician.
    - The family usually suspects that the child has a serious organic disease.
    - Further evaluation usually reveals that the child is performing very satisfactorily but not up to the family's excessive expectations.

– The child may be withdrawing because of:

- ▪ Failure to compete with an exceptional sibling
- ▪ Real or imagined failure in school

– A child may feel a lack of well-being because of parental discord.

– Lack of parental involvement with a child may lead to lassitude and boredom.

- Stress and anxiety in children often result in either hyperactivity or withdrawal.

  – The more common withdrawal reaction may express itself as chronic fatigue.

  – Protracted and severe periods of withdrawal are more likely to be caused by a pathological process.

- In some children, chronic fatigue may be a sign of true psychiatric depression.

Adolescents

- ▪ Chronic fatigue is encountered most frequently in adolescents.

- ▪ Even minor illnesses often precipitate prolonged fatigue in adolescents.

- ▪ Normal swings of mood and energy are usually of more concern to parents and teachers than to the patient.

  - However, some adolescents initiate visits to their primary care physician because they feel fatigue.

- ▪ Infectious illnesses

  - Infectious mononucleosis

    – Most adults and many infants and children have been infected with the Epstein-Barr virus (EBV).

    – Clinical manifestations in proved cases are extremely variable.

    – Some patients remain symptom free.

    – Symptoms usually resolve in several weeks, but the occasional patient may have an atypical or more prolonged course.

    – The leukocyte count may be normal.

    – Lymphocytosis with atypical lymphocytes will most likely be present.

    – The heterophil antibody screening test (mono test) is diagnostic in most circumstances.

    – Initial clinical findings either persist or are intermittent over months or, in rare cases, years and typically include chronic fatigue.

    – Patients should not be labeled with a diagnosis of chronic infectious mononucleosis syndrome or chronic EBV infection, which used to be and still is a quick fix diagnosis for patients who are chronically fatigued.

  - *Mycoplasma* pneumonia

    – Often low grade and without fever; produces progressive fatigue

- Hepatitis
- Cytomegalovirus infection
- Toxoplasmosis

▪ Addison disease

- Unexplained fatigue and associated weakness
- Anorexia
- Nausea
- Vomiting
- Weight loss

▪ Alcoholism and drug abuse

- Possible cause of chronic fatigue that should not be overlooked in this age group

▪ Emotional disorders

- Fatigue
- Lassitude
- Lack of energy
- Mild depression
- May be sleep deprived, have unhealthy eating habits
- Hypochondriacal symptoms
- Possible fever, usually caused by infection (eg, infectious mononucleosis, influenza)

  – Emotional reaction may be precipitated by a physical illness, particularly infection

- Usually seen during periods of greatest stress

  – May collapse with fatigue after intense and exuberant activity, eg, schoolwork, extracurricular activity, sports, social events

- Burnout and fatigue are common in overachieving high school and college students.

▪ Chronic fatigue syndrome (CFS)

- Initially attributed to infection with EBV
- Symptoms include:

  – Persistent or relapsing severe fatigue
  – Fever
  – Headache
  – Sore throat
  – Tender lymphadenitis
  – Nausea or vomiting
  – Myalgia
  – Arthralgia
  – Abdominal pain

- Neurocognitive symptoms, such as:

  – Inability to concentrate
  – Sleep disturbances
  – Episodic confusion

F

- Memory problems
- Depression
- Anxiety
- Irritability
- Neurocognitive symptoms are the most difficult to evaluate because of individual differences in emotional perception.
- Extensive laboratory evaluations usually produce normal results.
- Centers for Disease Control and Prevention (CDC) criteria for the case definition of CFS (based mainly on observations in adults):
  - New onset of persistent or relapsing fatigue lasting ≥6 months
  - No prior history of such fatigue
  - Exclusion of other clinical conditions that might produce similar symptoms
  - In addition, symptoms must include ≥4 of the following:
    - Muscle pain
    - Tender lymphadenopathy
    - Headaches of new type, pattern, or severity
    - Arthralgia
    - Impaired memory or concentration
    - Pharyngitis
    - Low-grade fever
    - Postexertional malaise lasting >24 hours
    - Sleep disturbances
  - Individuals with >6 months of disabling fatigue but an insufficient number of symptoms to meet criteria have been labeled as having idiopathic chronic fatigue.
  - CDC criteria exclude most past or current major psychiatric disorders but allow some comorbid psychiatric symptoms (eg, anxiety and nonmelancholic depression).
- Autoimmune disease
  - Children with autoimmune disease may initially have fatigue with little else.
  - Mild articular or periarticular inflammation may be missed on examination.
  - Children with the following conditions may have prolonged symptoms, including fatigue, without any physical findings.
    - Inflammatory bowel disease
      - Unexplained fatigue may continue for months as the only major symptom.
      - A loss of sense of well-being
      - Eventually accompanied by fever, abdominal symptoms, abnormal stools
    - Arthritis
    - Arthritis-like illness
    - Cancer (monocytic leukemia, in particular)

- Thyroid disease
  - Enlarged, tender thyroid gland and fatigue may indicate thyroiditis with emerging hypothyroidism.
  - Thyroid is often palpable and full in healthy adolescents.
  - Chronic fatigue from thyroid disease can usually be ruled out quickly with:
    - A thyroid-stimulating hormone test
    - A free thyroxine (free T_4) test
  - Some patients with hypothyroidism also demonstrate mild to moderate anemia.
  - Those who have active thyroiditis may have an elevated sedimentation rate.
- Anemia
  - The diagnosis of pure anemia requires a marked reduction of the hemoglobin level.
  - Erythrocyte indices and a reticulocyte count will characterize the anemia and its probable cause.
  - Anemia accompanied by thrombocytopenia suggests leukemia or aplastic anemia.

Weakness

Infants

- Infants with weakness are often described by parents as being "floppy."
  - In the newborn period, some may assume a frog-leg position.
- Usually indicates hypotonia caused by a neuromuscular disorder.
- Chromosomal anomalies are among the more common causes of hypotonia in infants.
  - Down syndrome
  - Congenital hypothyroidism
  - Infantile form of spinal muscular atrophy (Werdnig-Hoffmann disease)
- Infant botulism
  - Caused by ingesting *Clostridium botulinum* spores in honey
  - Can cause floppy appearance accompanied by:
    - A weak cry caused by muscle weakness
    - Loss of head control
    - Lethargy
    - Inability to feed
    - Constipation

Older children and adolescents

- Myasthenia gravis and Guillain-Barré syndrome (postinfectious polyneuropathy)
  - Perhaps the 2 most common causes of weakness in this age group

- In myasthenia gravis, deep-tendon reflexes may be diminished but are rarely absent.
- Guillain-Barré syndrome is remarkable for bilateral, symmetrically absent tendon stretch reflexes.
■ Other causes of weakness in the older child include:
  - Muscular dystrophies
  - The juvenile form of spinal muscular atrophy
  - Dermatomyositis
  - Polymyositis

LABORATORY EVALUATION

■ Initial laboratory evaluation can include:
  - Complete blood count with erythrocyte indices
  - Thyroid and liver function tests
  - Throat culture
  - Stool examination for blood
  - Cold agglutinin test (simple screen for *Mycoplasma* infection)
  - Erythrocyte sedimentation rate (ESR)
    - The most valuable screening test for inflammatory diseases of all varieties
    - Normal sedimentation rate almost always rules out:
      - Autoimmune disease
      - Inflammatory bowel disease
      - Chronic smoldering infections
      - Disseminated cancer
    - Elevated ESR requires further investigation.
■ Routine urinalysis
  - Almost always reveals diabetes
  - Most patients who have chronic renal failure have abnormal urinalyses, as well as significant anemia.
  - Confirm these diagnoses with:
    - Measurement of blood glucose in diabetes
    - Measurement of creatinine or blood urea nitrogen in renal disease
■ Thyroid disease can usually be ruled out quickly with:
  - A thyroid-stimulating hormone test
  - A free T_4 test
■ Infectious mononucleosis
  - Results of the heterophil antibody test may be negative in many young children and infants and ~10% of older children and adolescents with the disease.
  - Reliability of EBV antibody testing can confirm active infectious mononucleosis.

- EBV antibody titers can usually differentiate long-past infection from recent and active infection.
  - Eliminates EBV infection and infectious mononucleosis as causes for the fatigue
  - Permits a search for other likely neuropsychiatric causes
■ Toxoplasmosis or cytomegalovirus can be confirmed by:
  - Positive results of a fluorescent antibody test
  - Negative results of a heterophil antibody test
■ Adrenocorticotropic hormone stimulation test
  - Definitive diagnostic test for Addison disease
    - Hyperkalemia, hyponatremia, and hypoglycemia are useful diagnostic features.
■ Laboratory studies for muscle weakness may include:
  - Chromosomal studies
  - Muscle enzyme assays

IMAGING

■ Radiography is rarely necessary and should be discouraged.

DIAGNOSTIC PROCEDURES

■ The evaluation of a patient who has weakness may include:
  - Nerve conduction studies
  - Electromyography
  - Edrophonium (Tensilon) challenge
  - Muscle biopsy
  - Lumbar puncture

TREATMENT APPROACH

■ Chronic fatigue, in the absence of other physical symptoms, is usually emotionally based.
■ In most patients, further management requires meaningful communication among primary care physician, patient, and parents.
■ Older children and adolescents benefit from personal, warm attention and a continuous relationship with one physician.

SPECIFIC TREATMENT

■ In younger children, variability in performance and behavior of healthy children must be put into perspective.
■ Appropriate parental expectations must be emphasized.
■ Conversation after the physical examination, with appropriate give and take, should:
  - Reassure children or adolescents about basic health
  - Reiterate common and normal occurrence of fatigue
  - Examine daily routine and stresses
  - Suggest modifications of lifestyle and approach to life's situations

- If emotional fatigue is thought to exist:
  - The patient (especially adolescents) must accept that organic diseases have been ruled out.
  - The patient must be made aware of emotional basis for the fatigue.
  - Reasons for any psychiatric referral must be made clear.

WHEN TO REFER

- Attempting to establish the probable cause of the fatigue is the primary care physician's responsibility.
- Referral to a specialist is appropriate with:
  - Hypotonia in infants
  - Unexplained weight loss
  - Suspected major affective disorder, eg, depression
  - Suspected cancer

WHEN TO ADMIT

- Severe depression or suicidal ideation
- Need for evaluation of neuromuscular disorders, including:
  - Werdnig-Hoffmann disease
  - Guillain-Barré syndrome
  - Myasthenia gravis

PROGNOSIS

- CFS
  - Although few longitudinal data are available, the prognosis for adolescents with CFS is better than that for adults.
  - Symptoms may persist for months or several years, but most adolescents with CFS have a good outcome.
    - Complete recovery in approximately 50%

Fever

DEFINITION

- General definition: an increase in body temperature
- More accurately described as a homeostatic response under control of thermoregulation
  - Distinct from hyperthermia: an increase in body temperature from conditions that overwhelm normal thermoregulation
- Normal core body temperature measured rectally ranges from 97°F to 100°F (36.1°C–37.8°C).
  - May be as low as 95.5°F (35.3°C) or as high as 101°F (38.3°C)
- "Normal" temperature of 98.6°F (37°C) was derived from an 1868 study of >1 million axillary temperatures taken in adults.
  - This value may have no relevance for children, not only because adults were studied but also because axillary and rectal (core) temperatures correlate poorly.
  - Young children appear to have higher core body temperatures than adults, with temperatures slightly higher than 37.8°C occurring frequently in those <2 years.
- Upper limits of the normal range for a rectal temperature
  - 100.4°F (38.0°C) for infants <1 month
  - 100.6°F (38.1°C) in 1-month-olds
  - 100.8°F (38.2°C) in 2-month-olds
- The lowest body temperatures occur between 2AM and 6AM, and the highest occur between 5PM and 7PM.
- A consensus panel has recommended the lower limit of fever be defined as a rectal temperature of 38°C (100.4°F).

EPIDEMIOLOGY

- Newborns
  - Temperature >98.6°F (37°C) occurs in 1% of all newborns.
    - 10% of these children have a bacterial infection.
  - Fever during the first 4 days of life has been associated with a high incidence of bacterial disease.
    - Neonates up to 28 days of age with fever have a significant risk of a bacterial infection (approximately 12% in some studies).
- Infants
  - 5–8% of children in the 3- to 36-month-old age group with undifferentiated febrile illness have a urinary tract infection (UTI).
    - Female infants with temperatures above 39°C (102.2°F) have a UTI incidence of 16–17%.
    - Uncircumcised boys in the first 12 months of life have an 8- to 9-fold higher rate of UTI than circumcised boys.
- Types of bacterial infection
  - Except for neonates <28 days, the rate of serious bacterial infections in febrile patients is lower if they are infected with influenza and respiratory syncytial virus.
  - UTI and occult bacteremias are the most common types of infection.
  - Pneumococcal infection is uncommon; group B *Streptococcus, Escherichia coli*, and other enteric pathogens are more usual.
  - With group B *Streptococcus* infection, the risk of accompanying meningitis is as high as 39%.
  - Since the introduction of pneumococcal vaccine, the disease has decreased 60–80% in children <24 months.
    - Because occult pneumococcal bacteremia and other pneumococcal infections previously made up most of the serious bacterial infections in young children with high fever (>102°F [>39°C]), use of this vaccine has greatly decreased the incidence of serious bacterial infections in children at greatest risk.
    - Given the marked decrease in pneumococcal and *Haemophilus influenzae* type b (Hib) serious bacterial infections, the likelihood of a serious bacterial infection in infants and toddlers with high fever (>102°F [>39°C]) has been reduced.

HISTORY

- Because many evaluations of the febrile child take place over the telephone, the clinician must take a pertinent history, including:
  - Patient age (the younger the child, the more thorough the evaluation)
  - Associated signs and symptoms
  - Exposure to illness in family or community
  - History of recent immunizations
  - History of any recurrent infections (eg, urinary tract infections, streptococcal infections, otitis media)
  - Duration and height of the fever
    - Low-grade fever present for many days (signifying chronic or benign illness) usually does not need to be evaluated as urgently as a temperature of 106°F (41°C) present for a few hours (indicating potentially serious infectious disease).
  - Time of year
    - Winter: respiratory syncytial and influenza virus infections
    - Spring and fall: parainfluenza virus infections (the most common cause of croup)
    - Summer: enterovirus infections

PHYSICAL EXAM

Findings on general physical examination

- Pronounced hypermetabolic state
- Flushed cheeks
- Unusual glitter in the eyes

- Sleepiness and lethargy or exceptional alertness and excited demeanor (particularly 5- to 10-year-olds)
- Pulse increased by about 10–15 beats per 1°C of fever
- Increased respiratory rate
- Hot and dry skin ("burning up with fever")
  - Distal extremities may be cold and pale (vasoconstricted), obscuring an extremely high core body temperature.
- Shivering or sweating (mechanisms by which the body increases or decreases temperature).
  - Excessive sweating may cause dehydration, particularly with poor fluid intake.
- Dry mouth and lips from rapid mouth breathing and dehydration
- Febrile seizure may occur if irritability of the central nervous system increases.

Small infant

- Signs and symptoms may be less obvious.
- Shivering does not occur in the first few months of life.
- Diaphoresis is less frequent than in the older child.
- Irritability, pallor, and anorexia may be the only suggestions of illness; carefully measure temperature if the parent mentions these signs.

Examine the following:

- Respiratory tract
- Tympanic membranes
  - Otitis media
- Pharynx
  - Pharyngitis
- Nose
  - Discharge of sinusitis or viral upper respiratory tract infection
- Lungs
  - Evidence of pneumonia or bronchiolitis
- Eyes
  - Conjunctivitis as a clue to adenovirus, influenza, or respiratory syncytial virus infection, conjunctivitis-otitis syndrome, or Kawasaki disease
- Skin
  - Typical viral exanthems (rubella, roseola, or chickenpox)
  - Erythema marginatum (rheumatic fever)
  - Rose spots (typhoid fever)
- Lymph nodes
  - Generalized lymphadenopathy
    - Viral illnesses (eg, infectious mononucleosis, hepatitis, or cytomegalovirus infection)
    - Leukemia or lymphoma

- Localized enlargement
  - Skin infection
  - Tumor
- Isolated cervical lymphadenopathy
  - Tuberculosis
  - Cat-scratch disease (*Bartonella* infection)
- Musculoskeletal system
  - Localized bone tenderness (osteomyelitis)
  - Restricted range of motion in a warm joint (arthritis)
- Heart
  - Carditis of rheumatic fever
  - Infective endocarditis
- Spine
  - Diskitis
  - Costovertebral angle tenderness should prompt examination of the urine for evidence of UTI.

Factitious fever

- Pulse that is not correlated with the increase in temperature
- Inability to document fever when temperature is measured rectally
- Absence of sweating during defervescence

DIFFERENTIAL DIAGNOSIS

General

- Differentiate fever from hyperthermia, an increased body temperature resulting from conditions that overwhelm the normal process of thermoregulation.
  - Dehydration
  - Excessive muscle activity
  - Heat exposure
- Conditions associated with fever
  - Infection
    - If pulse rate is less than expected for the degree of fever, consider typhoid fever, tularemia, mycoplasma infection, or factitious fever.
  - Autoimmune disease
  - Neoplastic disease
  - Metabolic disease (eg, hyperthyroidism)
  - Chronic inflammatory disease
  - Hematologic disease (eg, sickle cell disease, transfusion reaction)
  - Drug fever and immunization reaction
  - Poisoning (eg, aspirin, atropine)
  - Central nervous system abnormalities
  - Factitious fever

- Although any disease in these categories may cause fever at any age, some diseases are more likely to occur at some ages than at others.

Viral infections

- Use findings of viral infections and their course to distinguish them from bacterial diseases.

- Viral infections tend to be less serious than bacterial infections.
  - Enterovirus
  - Influenza virus
  - Parainfluenza virus
  - Respiratory syncytial virus
  - Adenovirus
  - Rhinovirus
  - Rotavirus

Bacterial infections

- More aggressive and more serious outcomes compared with viral infections

- May be especially devastating in younger children with immature immune systems

- Infection that remains localized in the older child may in the infant and toddler disseminate rapidly to:
  - Blood (bacteremia)
  - Lungs (pneumonia)
  - Meninges (meningitis)
  - Bones (osteomyelitis)
  - Joints (arthritis)

Distinguishing bacterial from viral infections

- In younger children:
  - Difficult to recognize bacterial infection because children cannot verbalize complaints
  - Physical signs and symptoms are more subtle and easily missed.
  - Serious bacterial disease is especially difficult to diagnose in children with no obvious focus of infection.

- Efforts to improve the ability to diagnose a serious bacterial infection focus on 3 areas.
  - History and physical examination
    - Neither height of fever nor degree of toxicity is a reliable predictor by itself of bacteremia or serious bacterial infection.
  - Laboratory data
  - Response to antipyretics
    - The most unhelpful criterion in distinguishing serious bacterial infection from more benign viral infection
    - Children with a serious infection respond to antipyretics no differently from those whose illness is less significant.

- Rochester criteria, a combination of clinical and laboratory criteria to identify infants at low risk for a bacterial infection
  - The infant appears generally well.
  - The infant has been previously healthy.
    - Born at term (≥37 weeks' gestation)
    - Did not receive perinatal antimicrobial therapy
    - Was not treated for unexplained hyperbilirubinemia
    - Had not received and was not receiving antimicrobial agents
    - Had not been previously hospitalized
    - Was not hospitalized longer than the mother
  - No evidence of skin, soft tissue, bone, joint, or ear infection
  - Laboratory values
    - Peripheral blood leukocyte count 5.0–15.0 × 10^9 cells/L (5000–15,000/mm^3)
    - Absolute band form count ≤1.5 × 10^9 cells/L (≤1500 cells/mm^3)
    - ≤10 leukocytes per high-power field (×40) on microscopic examination of a spun urine sediment
    - ≤5 leukocytes per high-power field (×40) on microscopic examination of a stool smear (only for infants with diarrhea)

Seizure

- Most dramatic manifestation of fever in a child

- Generalized tonic or tonic-clonic seizure, usually lasting <15 minutes and occurring within 24 hours of the onset of fever, may begin without warning.

- Most parents are not aware that fever was present.

- The primary care physician may be called immediately after the seizure has occurred or after transport to the emergency department.
  - The child is likely to be postictal and have a rectal temperature of 102°F–104°F (39°C–40°C).
  - Seizure may be the first sign of meningitis or encephalitis.

Psychosocial factors

- A visit or telephone call for minimal fever and little evidence of disease should prompt thorough assessment of the psychosocial factors that may be contributing to parental concern.

- Answers to the following questions and others may clarify the situation.
  - Is the main concern about something else—a hidden agenda?
  - What knowledge about fever and disease does the caregiver have?
  - Has the caregiver had a previous traumatic experience with disease resulting in excessive anxiety?
  - Might the patient be a vulnerable child?

- Is this family dysfunctional, in which minor illness either cannot be dealt with or is used as a means to meet other needs?

Factitious fever

- Infrequent but well-described entity
- Children as young as 8 years have been known to increase the thermometer reading artificially by rubbing the mercury thermometer bulb on the sheets or by exposing it to warm liquids.

LABORATORY EVALUATION

- In newborns (≤4 days old) with fever, a full workup is indicated.
  - Complete blood count
  - Differential count
  - Urine analysis
  - Cultures of blood, urine, and cerebrospinal fluid (CSF)
- In an older infant who appears nontoxic and is at low risk for bacterial infection
  - CSF and blood culture may be avoided if:
    - Good observation and follow-up can be made within 24 hours.
    - Antibiotics are not administered.
  - If antibiotics are to be administered, then full workup, including blood and CSF cultures, should always be performed.
- For children who do not appear toxic:
  - Consider obtaining a leukocyte count.
  - If the count is >15,000 leukocytes/mm³, consider blood culture.
  - Obtaining a leukocyte count and blood culture at the same time is easiest, with the blood sent for culture only if the leukocyte count warrants doing so.
  - Procalcitonin and C-reactive protein blood levels might have better sensitivity and specificity than leukocyte count in predicting serious bacterial infection, but studies vary widely with respect to the best cut-off levels.
- Given the current lower incidence of pneumococcal disease, avoiding blood tests altogether might be more cost-effective and reasonable if the child:
  - Has received ≥3 doses of the Hib and pneumococcal vaccines
  - Does not appear toxic
  - Has no obvious focus of infection
  - Has reliable health care providers and excellent follow-up capabilities
- Urine culture
  - For febrile boys <6 months of age (<12 months if uncircumcised)
  - Girls <12–24 months

- Rapid diagnostic viral testing
  - Available for influenza A and B, respiratory syncytial virus, and enterovirus
  - Sensitivity and specificity vary, but a positive result may help decrease the number of other tests that need to be performed to rule out bacterial infection.

IMAGING

- Chest radiography
  - Generally necessary only if clinical symptoms or signs suggest pneumonia (eg, cough, tachypnea, dyspnea, rales, decreased breath sounds, dullness to percussion)
  - At least 1 study has suggested that as many as 20% of children with a temperature of ≥102.2°F (39°C) and a leukocyte count >20,000 cells/mm³ have pneumonia on the chest radiograph, even in the absence of respiratory symptoms and signs.

DIAGNOSTIC PROCEDURES

- Lumbar puncture
  - The younger the child is, the more difficult it is to diagnose meningitis clinically (eg, meningismus, Kernig sign, Brudzinski sign).
    - Children <12 months: strongly consider lumbar puncture since clinical signs of meningitis may be absent
    - Children 12–18 months of age: Consider lumbar puncture.
    - Children >18 months: Lumbar puncture is not routinely warranted except in the presence of signs and symptoms suggestive of meningitis or other intracranial infection.
  - Antibiotic treatment can mask meningitis; consider lumbar puncture in a child with a febrile seizure who has received antibiotics.
  - Reexamination after a convulsive episode may help determine whether examination of the CSF is needed.

WHEN TO REFER

- Patients with prolonged fever may be referred to rheumatologists.

WHEN TO ADMIT

- If the child appears toxic (eg, lethargic or irritable, noninteractive, poor perfusion)
  - Consider hospitalization *and*
  - Further diagnostic tests to assess for serious bacterial infection

Fever of Unknown Origin

DEFINITION

- Fever of unknown origin (FUO) is defined as ≥2 weeks of daily rectal temperature >38.3°C (101°F) with cause not determined by simple diagnostic tests, including:
  - Complete history
  - Thorough physical examination
- Some experts say that 1 of the 2 weeks of fever should be documented in the hospital.

MECHANISM

- Most cases of FUO eventually are found to be caused by common pediatric illnesses that are either self-limited or treatable.
  - Infectious illness accounts for 40–60% of FUO in children.
    - Although most infections that exhibit as FUO are an atypical or incomplete manifestation of a common infectious disease, several other types of infections should be considered.
  - Autoimmune disease accounts for 7–20% of cases.
  - Cancer is a much less common cause of FUO in children (1.5–6%) than in adults (7–16%).
- Children <6 years are most likely to have FUO resulting from an infection.
- Autoimmune diseases start to become more common after 6 years of age.
  - However, infection remains the most frequent cause of FUO.

HISTORY

- Careful documentation of fever is necessary before diagnosing FUO.
  - "Day of fever" is defined as a 24-hour period in which a temperature >38.3°C (101°F) occurs at least once.
  - Thorough explanation of the range of normal core body temperature for age, with its diurnal variation, may help to exclude patients who are not truly febrile but who instead have a high normal body temperature.
  - Physician should instruct parents in the technique of taking a rectal temperature.
  - Circumstances that may affect body temperature must be recorded.
    - All medications taken
    - Activities in which the child has participated
    - Environmental temperature
- Information must be obtained regarding:
  - Travel
  - Patient residence if outside the US
  - Animal exposure
  - Frequency of exposure to other persons who have common febrile illnesses
  - Previous illness
  - Hospitalizations
  - Medications
  - Family history of disease
  - Race and ethnicity
  - Precise course of the exhibiting symptoms
- Meticulous documentation of dates is especially important.
  - Family should record on a calendar the daily time and degree of the fever, along with associated symptoms.
  - For children >11–12 years of age, a separate interview should be conducted alone with the child to:
    - Obtain the child's perspective on the illness
    - Elicit information about subjects difficult to discuss in presence of parents
      - School
      - Peer relationships
      - Family functioning
      - Sexual identity and activity
- Some inflammatory diseases have recognizable fever patterns (eg, double quotidian fever of systemic juvenile idiopathic arthritis).
  - Fever patterns (ie, remittent, intermittent, sustained) rarely are diagnostic of a specific disease.
  - Determine whether even 1 or 2 days of normal temperature are interspersed between days of fever.
    - Child may have a series of rapidly sequenced brief febrile illnesses, masquerading as a single febrile illness.
- Careful documentation of fever should also help exclude pseudo-FUO, characterized by:
  - Absence of documented, persistent fever
  - Lack of objective, abnormal physical findings
  - History of significant or near-fatal illness
  - Parental fear of malignant or crippling disease
  - Frequent environmental exposure to illness
  - Absence of persistent weight loss
  - Normal erythrocyte sedimentation rate (ESR) and platelet count
  - Many missed school days because of subjective morning symptoms
    - Excessive amount of school missed, given the general degree of illness described
    - School absence for symptoms that are conspicuously absent during the rest of the day: fatigue, abdominal pain, and headache in the morning

- Discordance of fever and pulse rate
- Medical or paramedical family background
- ≥1 of the following:
  - Mild self-limited diseases
  - Behavioral problems
  - Parents who have misconceptions concerning health and disease
- Families under stress
- Child without a true fever if body temperature is measured accurately and consistently
  - Sometimes this must be done under hospital supervision.
- Periodic fever syndromes
  - Some children have shorter-than-normal episodes of fevers that recur in a regular (periodic) fashion with predictable symptoms.
  - Many of these periodic fevers are now known to be genetically based and can be diagnosed by sophisticated genetic testing.

PHYSICAL EXAM

- A full physical examination must be performed.
  - Rectal temperature
  - Respiratory rate
  - Heart rate
  - Blood pressure
- A discrepancy between heart rate and temperature suggests factitious fever.
- A thorough examination of the respiratory tract is indicated.
  - Inspection of the pharynx for hyperemia and exudate
  - Transillumination of the sinuses for sinusitis
  - Search for purulent nasal discharge
  - Auscultation of the chest for localized wheezing
- Inspection of the tympanic membranes for chronic otitis media
- In the older child, examination of the teeth to exclude dental caries and periodontal disease
- A new cardiac murmur may be a clue to rheumatic fever or infective endocarditis.
- Lymphadenopathy, especially if generalized, may suggest a viral infection.
  - Infectious mononucleosis
  - Cytomegalovirus
  - Toxoplasmosis
  - HIV
- Joints must be examined meticulously for:
  - Swelling
  - Restricted range of motion
  - Tenderness

- Skin rashes may suggest:
  - Viral disease
  - Autoimmune disease, such as juvenile idiopathic arthritis
- Absence of sweating and presence of a smooth tongue are consistent with familial dysautonomia.
  - Rare genetic disorder of thermoregulation
- Imperative tests
  - Rectal examination in the older child
    - Pararectal lymphadenopathy may suggest a pelvic infection.
  - Stool guaiac test
    - Positive result may be consistent with inflammatory bowel disease.

DIFFERENTIAL DIAGNOSIS

Bacterial infectious diseases

- Bacterial endocarditis
- Bartonellosis (caused by *Bartonella henselae*)
  - Usually exhibits as classic cat-scratch disease
  - May also appear as atypical cat-scratch disease, producing prolonged fever and hepatosplenic abscesses, lymphadenopathy, or central nervous system disease
  - When exposure to kittens and cats can be documented, serologic testing for *Bartonella* should be obtained.
    - If positive, abdominal ultrasonography should be considered.
- Brucellosis
- Chlamydia
  - Lymphogranuloma venereum
  - Psittacosis
- Leptospirosis
- Liver abscess
- Mastoiditis (chronic)
- Osteomyelitis
  - Particularly of the axial skeleton (intervertebral disk space and vertebral body infections) and the pelvis
- Pelvic abscess
- Perinephric abscess
- Pyelonephritis
- Salmonellosis
- Sinusitis
- Subdiaphragmatic abscess
- Tuberculosis
- Tularemia

F

Viral infectious diseases

- Cytomegalovirus
- Epstein-Barr virus (infectious mononucleosis) is the most common infectious cause of FUO.
- Hepatitis viruses
- HIV and AIDS
  - Assess the child thoroughly for characteristic physical signs and symptoms, as well as known risk factors for HIV.
    - Parental intravenous drug abuse
    - Parental sexual contact with individuals who may be HIV positive
    - HIV-positive mother
    - Hemophilia requiring transfusion of blood products
  - Fever is not usually the sole manifestation of HIV infection.
  - HIV infection should be strongly considered and the appropriate laboratory tests performed if fever has been present for >2 months and is associated with ≥1 of the following:
    - Failure to thrive or weight loss >10% from baseline
    - Hepatomegaly
    - Splenomegaly
    - Generalized lymphadenopathy (lymph nodes measuring ≥0.5 cm in ≥2 sites, with bilateral site involvement counting as 1 site)
    - Parotitis
    - Persistent or recurrent diarrhea
- Rickettsial diseases
  - Q fever
  - Rocky Mountain spotted fever

Fungal infectious diseases

- Blastomycosis (nonpulmonary)
- Histoplasmosis (disseminated)

Parasitic infectious diseases

- Malaria
- Toxoplasmosis
- Visceral larva migrans
- Visceral leishmaniasis

Autoimmune diseases

- Systemic juvenile idiopathic arthritis
  - Fever is almost always associated with this illness.
    - Often precedes the joint manifestations by weeks or months
  - The typical double quotidian fever (2 fever spikes in 24 hours with a normal temperature in between) is a helpful clue to this diagnosis.

- Polyarteritis nodosa
- Systemic lupus erythematosus
- Chronic regional enteritis
  - More common among children >6 years

Cancer

- Diagnosis that provokes the most anxiety
- Malignancies that may present with FUO in children include:
  - Leukemia (the most common malignancy in children)
  - Solid tumors, such as lymphoma, neuroblastoma, hypernephroma, and hepatoma
  - Hodgkin disease
- The reason for fever in these diseases is unclear.
  - May be related to endogenous pyrogen and other cytokines produced by the neoplastic cells

Periodic fever syndromes

- Recurrent fevers that do not satisfy the classic definition of FUO
  - Associated with a well-defined constellation of symptoms each time
- PFAPA (periodic fever, aphthous stomatitis, pharyngitis, and cervical adenopathy) is the most common.
  - Nonhereditary autoinflammatory syndrome
  - Onset before the age of 3 years
  - Associated with a sudden fever to 39°C–40°C (102°F–104°F) lasting 3–5 days
  - Anorexia
  - Mild oral ulcerations with pharyngitis, cervical lymphadenopathy, an increased leukocyte count, and an increased ESR
  - This constellation of symptoms recurs every 3–6 weeks.
  - A single dose of corticosteroids may quickly resolve the symptoms of individual episodes.
- Other periodic fever syndromes include:
  - Cyclic neutropenia
  - Familial Mediterranean fever
  - Hyperimmunoglobulinemia D and periodic fever syndrome
  - Tumor necrosis factor receptor–associated periodic syndrome
- Periodic fever syndromes are found in various populations around the world and are associated with known genetic mutations.
  - The primary care physician should know the patient's race, ethnicity, and country of origin.
    - These factors may provide clues about a specific periodic fever syndrome.

F

Miscellaneous causes

- Central diabetes insipidus
- Drug fever
- Ectodermal dysplasia
- Familial dysautonomia
- Granulomatous colitis
- Infantile cortical hyperostosis
- Münchausen by proxy syndrome
- Nephrogenic diabetes insipidus
- Pancreatitis
- Pseudofever
- Sarcoidosis
- Serum sickness
- Thyrotoxicosis
- Ulcerative colitis

LABORATORY EVALUATION

- If history and physical examination disclose no specific findings and growth is normal, only simple diagnostic tests are indicated.
- Routine blood counts and urinalysis
  - Have not been shown to be particularly useful; however, elimination from the workup is not advocated.
- A purified protein derivative tuberculin skin test should be given to detect tuberculosis.
  - Anergy may occur in active tuberculous infection.
- Blood, urine, and throat cultures
  - Negative cultures exclude infections of these areas.
- Erythrocyte sedimentation rate (ESR), C-reactive protein (CRP) level, and albumin/globulin ratio
  - Most useful laboratory tests
  - Higher probability of serious disease exists, particularly an autoimmune vascular disease or cancer; pursue further evaluation if:
    - ESR is >30 mm/h *or*
    - CRP level is elevated *or*
    - Albumin/globulin ratio is inverted
- The remainder of the evaluation should be individualized based on historical and clinical findings.
- Because infectious causes are the most common, specific serologic tests may be useful.
  - Hepatitis A and B
  - Epstein-Barr virus infection (infectious mononucleosis)
  - Bartonellosis
  - Toxoplasmosis
  - Cytomegalovirus

- Bone marrow examination
  - Occasionally helps in diagnosis of:
    - Tuberculosis
    - Leukemia
    - Metastatic cancer
    - Fungal infections
  - Should be considered only in children with:
    - Clinical or laboratory suggestion of cancer *or*
    - Immunocompromise
- If ESR, CRP level, and albumin/globulin ratio are normal and no signs and symptoms are present that are specific to a particular disease, little can be gained from any of the previously mentioned tests.
- If the child is not deteriorating visibly, a period of observation may be necessary until new findings appear that can give more direction to the investigation.
- It is likely that the parents and patient will be anxious about an undiagnosable problem.
  - The physician must be ready to provide all family members with a clear explanation of the evaluative process, any normal results, and reassurance.

IMAGING

- Radiologic studies may be appropriate in certain individuals but should not be done routinely.
  - Sinuses
  - Gastrointestinal tract
  - Chest
- Radioactive gallium scan
  - To detect occult abscesses and infections
  - Less useful in children than in adults
- Total-body computed tomography
  - May help find tumors
- Abdominal ultrasonography
  - If the abdomen is of primary concern

DIAGNOSTIC PROCEDURES

- Bone marrow aspiration may need to be done to rule out cancer and to culture the bone marrow for bacterial and fungal organisms.

TREATMENT APPROACH

- Fever without a discernible cause is always difficult for clinicians because fever suggests disease.
  - Inability to identify the cause of fever can undermine the physician's credibility and can affect rapport with patients.
  - The longer fever persists, the more concern is raised by the parents.

■ Intensive examination of all of the following is the physician's responsibility and first stage of managing the patient.

- History
- Physical examination
- Particular social environment in which the child and family live

WHEN TO REFER

■ Referrals to the following may occasionally be necessary for additional assistance in determining diagnosis.

- Pediatric infectious disease specialists
- Rheumatologists
- Specialized diagnosticians
- Any combination of these professionals

WHEN TO ADMIT

■ Need for hospitalization depends on:

- Amount of parental anxiety
- Necessity to document fever
- Need to perform diagnostic tests that cannot be done on an outpatient basis

FOLLOW-UP

■ The health care professional must continue to assess these children frequently to:

- Detect new findings early
- Maintain the confidence of the family while the fever continues

PROGNOSIS

■ Children with FUO generally do well, even though fever may last for weeks or months.

F

Foot and Leg Problems

DEFINITION

- Terms used to describe leg and foot disorders
  - *Abduction:* deviation away from the midline of the body
  - *Adduction:* deviation toward the midline of the body
  - *Calcaneus:* foot dorsiflexed, placing the heel below the level of the toes
  - *Cavus:* medial longitudinal arch of the foot elevated
  - *Equinus:* foot plantar flexed, placing the toes below the level of the heel
  - *Pes:* the foot
  - *Planus:* medial longitudinal arch of the foot flattened
  - *Talipes:* congenital deformities of the foot that, if untreated, result in walking on the ankle (talus)
  - *Torsion:* excessive or abnormal twisting along the long axis
    - *Internal torsion:* excessive or abnormal inward twisting
    - *External torsion:* excessive or abnormal outward twisting
  - *Varus:* medial or inward deviation of 1 segment of an extremity relative to the proximal (previous) segment
  - *Valgus:* lateral or outward deviation of 1 segment of an extremity relative to the proximal (previous) segment
  - *Version:* physiologic or normal twisting along the long axis
    - *Inversion:* physiologic or normal twist inward
    - *Eversion:* physiologic or normal twist outward
    - *Anteversion:* physiologic or normal twist forward
    - *Retroversion:* physiologic or normal twist backward
  - *Pronation:* outward rolling of the foot with eversion of the heel and eversion and abduction of the forefoot (*flexible foot, relaxed foot, fatfoot, flatfoot, pes planus*)

EPIDEMIOLOGY

- Clubfoot: both forms (*talipes equinovarus* and *talipes calcaneovalgus*)
  - 1 of every 200 live births
  - Bilateral in 50% of cases
  - Affect boys almost twice as often as girls
  - Incidence in siblings if one has clubfoot is 3–4%.
  - If 1 parent and a child have clubfoot, then subsequent children have a 25% chance of having clubfoot.
- Curly toe
  - Curly toe is quite common in infancy and childhood.
- Polydactyly
  - Common
- Accessory tarsonavicular
  - Fairly common; probably occurs in 1% of the population
  - Bilateral in 50% of patients

- Forefoot adductive deformities (*talipes varus, metatarsus varus,* and *metatarsus adductus*)
  - Combined incidence of these 3 deformities is ~1 per 100 live births (the most frequent musculoskeletal congenital malformation).
  - Metatarsus adductus: the most common
  - Talipes varus: the least common
- Femoral anteversion occurs twice as frequently in girls as in boys.

MECHANISM

- Hallux valgus
  - Many factors cause the problem.
    - Foot structure (which may or may not be hereditary)
    - Narrow stylized shoes that crimp toes
- Hammertoe
  - In infants, usually hereditary
  - In the older child, usually results from faulty shoe wear
- Clubfoot
  - Usually idiopathic
- Claw toe
  - Usually occurs in conjunction with a cavus foot, in neuromuscular diseases
    - Charcot-Marie-Tooth disease
    - Myelomeningocele
- Extra toe
  - Usually, family history
- Syndactyly (webbed toes)
  - May exist as an isolated finding or as part of a more extensive syndrome of congenital anomalies
  - Family history often found
- Metatarsus adductus
  - Crowded intrauterine environment
    - Uterine fibroids
    - Bicornate uterus
    - Multiple gestation
    - Oligohydramnios
- Toe-walking
  - Commonly associated with cerebral palsy if persists beyond 2 years of age
  - Also caused by congenitally short tendocalcaneus

HISTORY

- Pronation (flatfoot)
  - Most infants have flexible flatfeet.
    - Transient, with resolution by 2.5 years of age in 97%

- Family history of pronation may be found in children with flatfoot that persists beyond the usual time of physiologic resolution.
- Symptoms are uncommon but may occur.
  - Aching of the feet and legs
  - Muscle cramps in the calves at night
  - Easy fatigability
  - Reluctance to participate in strenuous activity
- Tarsal coalitions
  - May be found in other family members who are asymptomatic but have no hindfoot motion
- Pes cavus
  - Seen in:
    - Muscular dystrophy
    - Peripheral neuropathies
    - Disease of the spinal cord, brainstem, and cerebral cortex
  - Conditions producing it as a late manifestation
    - Cerebral palsy
    - Meningomyelocele
    - Poliomyelitis
    - Charcot-Marie-Tooth disease
    - Friedreich ataxia
  - Family history should be sought because many conditions producing this deformity are inherited.
- Bowed legs/knock-knees
  - History of uterine crowding during fetal development can be associated with extreme cases.
  - Prior trauma
  - Abnormalities
    - Endocrine
    - Metabolic
    - Bone
- Femoral anteversion
  - In utero and postnatal positioning of the legs and hips

PHYSICAL EXAM

- If a pathologic deformity of the legs or feet is diagnosed, the clinician should look for other congenital anomalies, especially those involving the skeletal system.

Forefoot adductive deformities

- Talipes varus
  - The entire foot is inverted and the forefoot is adducted.
- Metatarsus varus
  - The forefoot is inverted and adducted while the hind foot and heel are in the normal position.
  - The great toe is widely separated from the second toe.
  - The lateral border of the foot is convex.

- Metatarsus adductus
  - The only finding is adduction of the metatarsals at the tarsometatarsal joints.
  - The forefoot is adducted but not inverted.
  - Severity may be graded by the heel bisector method (line bisecting the heel that falls between the second and third toes).
    - Mild if line falls through third toe
    - Moderate if between the third and the fourth toes
    - Severe if between the fourth and fifth toes
  - Flexibility of the forefoot should be assessed.
    - With a flexible foot, the second toe can be easily brought in line with or past the heel bisector.

Clubfoot

- The leg and its appended foot are turned to resemble a club.
  - Plantar flexion (equinus) of the ankle
  - Adduction (varus) of the heel (hindfoot)
  - High arch (cavus) at the midfoot
- 2 varieties
  - Talipes equinovarus (more severe)
    - The heel and forefoot are inverted.
    - The forefoot is adducted.
    - The entire foot is plantar flexed.
  - Talipes calcaneovalgus
    - Eversion of the heel and forefoot
    - Abduction of the forefoot
    - Dorsiflexion of the entire foot
  - Associated neurologic, muscular, or other skeletal anomalies should be sought.
    - Neuromuscular clubfoot is associated with arthrogryposis, meningomyelocele, and congenital constriction band syndrome.

Toe deformities and their presentations

- Hallux valgus
  - The great toe is deviated laterally to overlap the second toe.
  - The first metatarsal bone is deviated medially.
  - Prominence on the medial aspect of the metatarsophalangeal (MTP) joint
  - Bursa forms from the constant irritation and inflammation, forming a painful bunion.
  - May see some degree of pronation (flatfoot)
- Hammertoe
  - Occurs at the proximal interphalangeal joint
- Mallet toe
  - Occurs at the distal interphalangeal joint

F

- Claw toe
  - Involves all joints of the toe—hyperextension of the MTP joints and flexion at both the proximal interphalangeal and distal interphalangeal joints
- Curly toe
  - The fourth or fifth toe is usually flexed downward and twisted underneath the adjacent toe.
- Syndactyly
  - Interconnection between ≥2 toes can vary from thin skin to a bony attachment.
  - Growth differential between the involved toes tends not to be significant.
- Bunionette (tailor bunion)
  - Bunionette occurring at the fifth MTP joint
  - Bursa over the lateral aspect of the fifth MTP joint is prominent, inflamed, and painful.
- Associated neurologic, muscular, or other skeletal anomalies should be sought.
  - Neuromuscular clubfoot is associated with arthrogryposis, meningomyelocele, and congenital constriction band syndrome.

Pronation (flatfoot)

- The Achilles tendon curves inward.
- The medial longitudinal arch of the foot, observed without weight bearing, disappears on standing.
- Look for associated conditions, such as:
  - Obesity
  - Neuromuscular disorders
  - Structural abnormalities above the ankle
- In newborns, bony prominences on the medial and plantar aspects of the foot, with limited plantar flexion and forefoot inversion, indicate vertical talus and accessory tarsonavicular.

Tarsal coalitions

- Usually detected in late childhood or adolescence
- A fibrous/cartilaginous bar connecting the hindfoot bones becomes ossified, producing pain with walking and an inability to invert the foot.
- The foot is held in a pronated position, with eversion of the forefoot.
- Peroneal tendons stand out prominently when attempts are made to invert the foot.
- Calcaneonavicular coalition tends to develop between 9 and 13 years of age.
- Talocalcaneal coalition develops at 13–16 years of age.

Pes cavus

- Weakness or paralysis of the intrinsic muscles of the foot and its dorsiflexors
- Leads to deformity over time; usually seen in late childhood or adulthood

- A high-arched foot characterizes the deformity.
- Takes 1 of 2 forms
  - *Cavovarus*, in which the calcaneus is inverted with tightness of the heel cord
  - *Calcaneocavus*, in which a high arch with normal heel alignment is present

Bowed legs (genu varum)/knock-knees (genu valgum)

- From birth until 18 months, some bowing is normal.
- Continued growth results in a knock-knee pattern of 10–15 degrees, which assumes prominence by age 3–4 years.
- Persists until later childhood or early adolescence, when balancing and straightening occur spontaneously (normal).
- Marked degrees of these conditions require investigation to rule out underlying disease that can result in permanent deformity.

In-toeing (pigeon toe)

- If the child's patellae are rotated inward (kissing knees) while walking, the underlying problem is above the knee.
- If the patellae face straight forward, the underlying problem is below the knee.
- Excessive in-toeing is likely to be caused by benign conditions representing variations of normal development from excessive rotations of the femur, the tibia, or both.
- In-toeing does not usually cause pain or interfere with development or stability of gait.
- Best position to assess rotation of the lower extremities:
  - Child in the prone position
  - Hips fully extended
  - Knees flexed to 90 degrees
  - To measure hip rotation, the lower leg is used as a pointer and the legs are rotated through the axis of the hip joint.
    - Until 1–2 years of age, clinical measurement of hip rotation is limited by the physiological tightness of the hip joint capsule.
    - After 18–24 months, measurement of hip rotation is a close approximation of bony femoral rotation, averaging 50 degrees of internal rotation and 40 degrees of external rotation.

Out-toeing (slew foot)

- To assess tibial rotation: measure the thigh-foot angle, the axis of the foot relative to the axis of the thigh.
  - Normal angle ranges from 0–30 degrees of external rotation; an internal thigh-foot angle indicates internal tibial torsion.
  - By age 2 years, children typically walk with feet turned out relative to the line of progression.
  - Thigh-foot angle of 10–15 degrees is normal in older children.

Femoral anteversion

- Produces kissing knees, in-toeing, and clumsy gait.
  - With the patella in neutral position, the greater trochanter of the femur lies posterior to the lateral, longitudinal midthigh line.
  - External rotation is decreased.
  - Internal rotation of the hip in extension is increased (normally 35–45 degrees for both).
  - External rotation of the hip in flexion is normal.

Femoral retroversion

- Findings are the opposite of those found in anteversion of the femoral neck.

DIFFERENTIAL DIAGNOSIS

- Pronation
  - Foot flattening includes vertical talus, accessory tarsonavicular, and fusion of ≥1 of the tarsal bones (tarsal coalition).
    - Accessory tarsonavicular
      - A normal anatomic variant
      - A secondary center of ossification forms in the medial portion of the tarsonavicular at the attachment of the posterior tibialis tendon.
      - Ossification becomes more prominent or symptomatic during adolescence.
      - Can have repetitive sprains of the fibrous attachment of the ossicle to the navicular
    - Tarsal coalitions
      - Not usually detected until late childhood or adolescence, when they produce pain with walking and inability to invert the foot
      - 2 types have been identified.
        - o Calcaneonavicular coalition, which involves the calcaneus and the navicular bones
        - o Talocalcaneal coalition, in which is the calcaneus is coalesced to the talus
- Toe-walking
  - May be habitual (idiopathic toe-walking)
  - Cerebral palsyis associated with toe-walking that persists beyond 2 years of age.
  - Congenitally short tendocalcaneus causes persistent toe-walking even though the child can toe-heel and heel-toe walk; the condition disappears at 6–8 years of age.
- In-toeing is generally caused by benign conditions.
  - Protective or compensatory shifting of body weight in pronation and knock-knee, both normal developmental stages
    - Most common cause of in-toeing
    - Corrects itself in time

- Developmental bowing
  - Self-correcting
  - May lead to temporary in-toeing
- Internal tibial torsion
- Femoral anteversion
- Metatarsus adductus
- Talipes equinovarus and metatarsus varus
- Spasticity of the internal rotator muscles of the hip (seen in cerebral palsy)
- Anterior maldirection of the acetabulum
- Out-toeing is seen with:
  - Calcaneovalgus
  - Pes planovalgus
  - Flaccid paralysis of the internal rotator muscles of the hip
  - Posterior maldirection of the acetabulum
  - External tibial torsion
- Tibial torsion
  - Pathologic degrees of internal/external tibial torsion due to:
    - Deformities of the feet, ankles, knees, and hips *or*
    - Improperly applied casts, braces, or Denis Browne splints
- Genu varum (bowed legs)
  - When extreme or unilateral, may result from:
    - Rickets
    - Dyschondroplasia
    - Osteogenesis imperfecta
    - Osteochondritis
    - Blount disease (tibia vara)
    - Injury to the medial proximal epiphysis of the tibia
- Genu valgum (knock-knees)
  - Often associated with pronation
  - More apt to be marked in overweight children
  - Injury to the lateral proximal tibial epiphysis can cause unilateral genu valgum.
  - Underlying generalized diseases of the bone can cause marked bilateral genu valgum.

IMAGING

- Clubfoot
  - Radiographic examination is required at the time of diagnosis and periodically during treatment.
    - Delineates the pathologic finding
    - Guides management
- Metatarsus adductus
  - In babies with limited forefoot flexibility, radiographic examination is necessary to rule out talipes varus and metatarsus varus.

F

- In the primary care physician's office, placing the child in a standing position on a copy machine and taking a photocopy of the soles of the feet is an easy way to assess the heel bisector position.
- Allows for tracking of the progression or improvement of the condition over time.
■ Pronation
- Flexible flatfoot (pes planus) does not require any imaging in most cases.
- Radiograph may be necessary if:
  - Pronation persists beyond 2.5 years of age.
  - Symptoms are present.
  - Flexibility is limited.
  - Planovalgus is suspected.
■ Pes cavus
- Radiographic examination may be necessary, especially if surgical management is under consideration.
■ Genu varum (bowed legs), when extreme or unilateral, requires roentgenographic examination to exclude:
- Rickets
- Dyschondroplasia
- Osteogenesis imperfecta
- Osteochondritis
- Blount disease (tibia vara)
- Injury to the medial proximal epiphysis of the tibia
■ In-toeing and out-toeing rarely require imaging studies.

TREATMENT APPROACH

■ Most problems require no treatment or are managed easily without consultations.
■ A few require services of an orthopedist.

SPECIFIC TREATMENT

Talipes varus and metatarsus varus

■ Fixed deformities of the foot that require early treatment
■ Serial casting
- Abduction stretching exercises and out-flare last shoes may be used as an adjunct to cast treatment but should not be relied on as the only therapy.
- Long-leg splints on both legs

Metarsus adductus

■ Requires no treatment because resolves spontaneously, usually within the first year

Hallux valgus

■ Patients should wear shoes with plenty of toe room and no heels.

■ If flatfoot is present, a shoe insert to correct the foot pronation may help prevent progression of the disease.
■ In more severe cases, surgical correction may be needed.

Hammertoe

■ Most cases are mild, cause no pain, and can be left alone.
■ The child should have roomy shoes that allow the toes to stretch.
■ In more severe cases, at an older age, surgical correction may be needed.

Mallet toe

■ Most cases are mild and need no treatment.
■ If a corn develops over the deformity, shaving and padding will help.
■ In more severe cases, surgical correction can be performed.

Curly toe

■ If the condition is severe and causes irritation with shoe wear, surgical transfer of the toe flexor may correct the problem.

Extra toe

■ If the extra toe is not causing problems with walking and shoe wear, no treatment is needed.
■ Can be ablated by suture ligation
■ If an extra little or big toe and sticks out prominently, difficulty with shoe wear is common.
- In these cases, surgical excision will remove the problem.
  - Typically performed after 9–12 months of age

Bunionette

■ If padding does not help relieve the discomfort of a bunionette, surgical correction is needed.

Clubfoot

■ Treatment is with casting immediately on initial diagnosis.
■ 2–4 months of manipulation and casting are usually required.
■ Recurrence is common after correction by manipulation alone, and prolonged casting is usually required.
- Recurrence is most common in the first 2–3 years but may still happen up to age 5–7 years.
■ Surgical correction (tenotomies, muscle transplants, and arthrodeses) may be required in severe cases.
- When conservative management fails *or*
- Because of recurrence when the child is older
■ Recurrence is much less likely after surgical correction.
■ Early initiation of therapy will:
- Increase success rate of manipulative or conservative management
- Decrease the need for surgical intervention

Pronation

- Usually disappears before 2.5 years of age and requires no treatment

- If pronation persists, treatment is not necessary unless symptoms occur.

- Corrective shoes with a long medial counter and a Thomas heel

- Support to the medial longitudinal arch with a flexible felt, rubber, or leather pad placed beneath the inner sole may help.

- Wedges that are 1/8- to 3/16-inch thick applied to the medial aspect of the heel and the lateral aspect of the sole are sometimes helpful.

- Steel arch supports placed in the shoe rarely are required.

- If neuromuscular disorders (eg, tight heel cords) are present, then heel cord–stretching exercises may reduce discomfort.

- Pes planovalgus
  - Orthopedic shoes
  - Surgical correction is required only for accessory tarsonavicular or tarsal coalition if symptoms cannot be relieved through conservative means (~10% of cases)
    - Usually performed in adulthood

Vertical talus

- Usually requires surgical correction early in infancy

Toe-walking

- The only treatment required for either idiopathic or habitual toe-walking is reassurance.

- If it persists beyond 2 years of age, a dorsiflexion-assist ankle-foot orthosis may be of benefit.

Bowed legs/knock-knees

- Simple observation and reassurance are all that are required, because the condition spontaneously corrects 99% of the time.

- When identified, the underlying causes of extreme varus or valgum deformities must be effectively treated to improve angulation.

- Treatment of severe bowing or knocking of the knees caused by underlying disease is determined by the nature of the condition and may include:
  - Wedge osteotomy
  - Epiphyseal stapling

In-toeing/out-toeing

- Most children will simply outgrow their variant.

- Tibial torsion
  - If a child trips on his or her feet and falls frequently, or if parents are unduly concerned about in-toeing, use:
    - Passive stretching exercises (externally rotating the foot at the ankle)

- Corrective shoes
  - Thomas heel
  - Longitudinal arch pad
  - Inner heel
  - Outsole wedges
  - Application of torque heels
- Denis Browne splints should not be used without orthopedic consultation, as they may create abnormal stress on the hip joint.
- In extreme cases, orthopedic treatment
  - Use of a bivalve lower-trunk and leg cast during sleeping hours
  - Rarely, derotation osteotomy of the middle or lower femoral shaft

- Femoral anteversion (in-toeing)
  - A simple measure if parents are concerned is to have the child learn to sit in the tailor, modified lotus, or Indian-style sitting position.
  - Use of Denis Browne splints is contraindicated.
  - Corrective shoes are of no value.

WHEN TO REFER

- Toe anomalies
  - Referral to a podiatrist or orthopedist may be indicated if:
    - The anomaly leads to pain or uncomfortable shoe wear or ambulation.
    - These symptoms do not respond to conservative management.

- Clubfoot
  - Immediate referral to an orthopedist should be made on diagnosis.

- Metatarsus varus
  - Forefoot has limited flexibility.
  - Condition appears to be progressing or is not improving with growth.

- Pronation
  - Limited flexibility or a suspicion of planovalgus
  - Persistence of pronation beyond 2.5 years of age
  - Symptoms are present that are not relieved through conservative management

- Pes cavus
  - Always refer for evaluation by a neurologist, physiatrist, or orthopedist, individually or in collaboration.

- Toe-walking
  - If it persists beyond 2 years of age
  - If the child has an abnormal neurologic history or examination

- Bowed legs and knock-knees
  - Severe, asymmetric, or unilateral genu varum or genu valgus
  - Condition that does not follow the expected physiologic progression with growth
- In-toeing and out-toeing
  - If in-toeing is severe
  - Unsteady gait (especially while running) that causes stumbling
  - Condition that does not follow the expected physiologic progression with growth
- Tibial torsion
  - Extreme rotation (especially when associated with difficulty walking or running)
  - Significant asymmetry
  - Sudden proximal tibial deviation
  - Condition that does not follow the typical pattern of improvement with growth
- Femoral anteversion
  - Extreme rotation (especially when associated with difficulty walking or running)
  - Significant asymmetry
  - If the condition does not follow the typical pattern of improvement of growth by 7 years of age

FOLLOW-UP

- Many foot and leg problems are benign and resolve with time.
  - Close follow-up and monitoring for the resolution of condition is necessary.
  - If the condition does not resolve at the expected time, a referral to a specialist should be made.

PROGNOSIS

- Many common foot and leg problems are benign and resolve with time.

PREVENTION

- The foot takes the shape of the shoe, not vice versa.
  - Improperly fitted or manufactured shoes may be the primary cause of acquired foot deformities and problems.
  - Shoes that do not fit properly can deform an otherwise normal foot, resulting in hammertoe, hallux valgus, bunionettes, corns and, ultimately, the need for surgery.

- Determining the proper fitting for shoes involves no great science.
  - The foot widens while standing and throughout the day, so measurements should:
    - Be made later in the day
    - Be made with the child standing
    - Should apply only to the time the shoes are newly acquired
  - Both feet should be measured, and shoes should be fitted to the larger foot.
  - The counter should hug the heel snugly.
  - Length should allow a fingerbreadth (0.5 inch) between the tip of the great toe and the toe box.
  - The foot should fit snugly into the widest part of the shoe.
  - Width should not crowd the ball of the foot and should allow the toes to extend without wrinkling the upper.
  - While still in the store, the parents should have the child walk in the shoes to ensure comfort.
  - Shoes should not be expected to stretch to fit; if shoes do not fit, then they should not be purchased.
- Shoes in good condition can be handed down from 1 child to another.
- The frequency with which shoes should be changed depends on the:
  - Rate of growth of the feet
  - Quality of the shoes
  - Degree of their use
  - Parents can usually tell when shoes become too small (or rather, when feet become too large) without professional advice.
    - The toes will be felt to press against the toe box.
    - Getting the shoes on or having the child keep them on will be increasingly difficult.
- Lightweight cotton, nylon, or wool socks that adjust to the length and width of the foot for foot comfort

Foreign Bodies of the Ear, Nose, Airway, and Esophagus

DEFINITION

- Foreign bodies of the ear, nose, respiratory, and digestive tracts are a common problem among children, particularly those <5 years.
- Children are at risk as soon as the pincer grasp is achieved around 9 months of age.

EPIDEMIOLOGY

- Prevalence
  - In 1998 foreign-body aspiration and asphyxiation was the fourth leading cause of accidental death in the home among children <5 years.
  - As of 2006 foreign body aspiration and asphyxiation accounted for ~9% of all home accidental deaths of children <5 years.
    - The incidence declines rapidly among those ≥5 years.
  - National Safety Council data from 2005 to 2006 report choking deaths in 133 per 100,000 population in children from birth to 4 years.
  - Increased parental awareness of the risks of leaving small objects within the reach of young children.
    - Consumer education has been important in diminishing this hazard.
  - Development of life-saving techniques (Heimlich maneuver) that can be performed by people who are not health care workers account for a higher survival rate.

ETIOLOGY

Ear and auditory canal

- Foreign bodies of the ear and external auditory canal can include:
  - Food
  - Insects
  - Toys
  - Buttons
  - Crayon pieces
  - Pencil erasers
  - Button-shaped batteries
- Accidental entry of a foreign object through external auditory canal
  - The child or a companion can insert the object during play.
  - Insects can fly or crawl into the ear canal.
- Children who have chronic external otitis or itching may be more likely than healthy children to place objects in their ear canal.
- Earrings can become embedded in the auricle when a chronic infection of the pierced site is followed by overgrowth of granulation tissue.
  - Use of the spring-loaded piercing gun has resulted in numerous cases of embedded earrings.

Nose

- Foreign bodies in the nose fall into 2 categories.
  - Soft
    - Tissue paper
    - Eraser material
    - Clay
  - Hard
    - Bead
    - Pebble
    - Candy
- A foreign object may enter the nose accidentally while the child is attempting to sniff or smell it.
- Chronic rhinitis is the most common underlying factor in children placing objects in the nose.
- Frequency of foreign bodies in the nose increases during the summer and Christmas, when toy sales increase.

Airway

- Infants in particular will place almost anything they can handle into their mouth.
  - A startle may cause inadvertent ingestion or aspiration.
- Lack of complete dentition and lack of attention to chewing may allow large food particles to enter the posterior pharynx.
- Other contributors to foreign body ingestion
  - Incomplete development of mouth and tongue coordination
  - Neuromuscular mechanism for swallowing in young children
- A positive association exists between the occurrence of upper respiratory tract infections and foreign body aspiration.
  - A cold interrupts a smooth breathing-swallowing pattern and leads to an increase in aspiration.
  - More common among younger children, but some estimates indicate that 23% occurred in children >5 years
- Complete airway obstruction is generally caused by globular foods and objects.
  - Hot dogs
  - Nuts
  - Candies
  - Grapes
  - Toys
  - Latex balloons
- Impaction may take place in 3 segments of the airway.
  - Larynx
    - A review found 11 of 91 cases of a foreign body lodged in the larynx.
    - Of these, 5 died and 3 had anoxic encephalopathy.
  - Trachea
  - Bronchial tree

F

Esophagus

- More than one-half of foreign bodies in children involve the esophagus.
  - Coins, food, marbles, buttons, pins, tacks, jewelry, and batteries are a few of the numerous foreign bodies children have ingested.
    - Coins are the most common foreign body in the esophagus in children <10 years in the US.
    - Fish bones are the most common in children ≥10 years.
    - The esophagus has 4 physiologic areas of narrowing.
      - Cricopharyngeal sphincter
      - Aortic arch
      - Region of the left main bronchus
      - Gastroesophageal sphincter
      - These correspond to the 4 most common sites of foreign body obstruction.
        - The cricopharyngeus is the most common.
        - Arch of the aortic region is the most dangerous.
      - If the foreign body is lodged at the lower border of the cricopharyngeus muscle, it will be visualized at the level of the clavicles on the chest radiograph.

RISK FACTORS

- Children at risk
  - Those with developmental delays
  - Children who have undergone esophageal surgery
  - Children with a damaged esophagus from prior caustic ingestions

SIGNS AND SYMPTOMS

Foreign bodies in the ear

- Most common among children between 2 and 4 years of age
- Eliciting a history of placing an object in the ear canal is difficult.
  - Most children are reluctant to admit to this activity.
  - If insertion is not witnessed, the foreign body may go undetected for an extended period.
- Findings depend on:
  - Depth of the foreign object within the external auditory canal
  - Nature and composition of the object
  - Duration in the canal
- Children may complain of or the following may be observed.
  - Ear pain
  - Discomfort
  - Bleeding
  - Discharge
  - Odor
  - Aural fullness
  - Hearing loss
  - Nausea
  - Vomiting
  - Coughing
  - Tearing
  - Dizziness
- Inert substances, such as plastic, that are not obstructing the canal and are not abutting the tympanic membrane may not cause symptoms.
- Insects tend to incite local irritation.
  - Discomfort
  - Erythema
  - Drainage
- Food may cause local inflammation.
  - Often leads to local pain and itching
- Objects that touch the tympanic membrane cause pain, particularly with movement of the drum or swallowing.
- If the entire canal is obstructed, hearing will likely be decreased.
- Button-size alkaline batteries may leak battery alkali and cause a severe local tissue reaction or destruction.
  - Pain, swelling, or discharge may be seen.
  - Expeditious management prevents serious injury to the canal, tympanic membrane, or middle ear.
- When the history indicates a small foreign body that cannot be seen, it may be lodged anteriorly in the tympanic sulcus.
  - Instillation of water to fill the medial half of the external canal may act as a concave lens and allow visualization of the tympanic sulcus.
- Microscopic evaluation will aid in visualization if a patient has a small, narrow, or swollen external ear canal.

Foreign bodies in the nose

- Children will usually not admit to placing foreign bodies in the nose.
- Most common symptom is unilateral nasal discharge that may be foul smelling.
  - Unilateral nasal discharge in a young child should be considered evidence of a foreign body until proved otherwise.
- Epistaxis may be the presenting symptom.
- Anterior nasal cavities should be examined with a nasal speculum and suction.
  - Powerful illumination is important.
- When an alkaline disk battery is lodged in the nose, symptoms may be acute.

■ Tissue damage can occur through 3 mechanisms.
- Electrical burn
- Liquefaction necrosis (from sodium hydroxide)
- Pressure necrosis

Foreign bodies in the airway

■ When an object is aspirated, it initially produces:
- Choking
- Gagging
- Coughing
- Wheezing

■ This may be followed by an asymptomatic interval during which little evidence remains to suggest the presence of a foreign body.

■ Depending on the site of the foreign body in the airway, a patient may exhibit a spectrum of findings from an almost complete lack of symptoms to signs of complete airway obstruction.

■ High index of suspicion and knowledge of possible presentation scenarios are the best insurance against missed or delayed diagnoses.

■ Laryngeal foreign bodies
- Most likely to produce acute and dramatic presentation
- Large objects that completely obstruct the airway cause:
  - Stridor
  - High-pitched wheezing
  - Cough
  - Dysphonia
  - Aphonia
  - Cyanosis
- Small objects that obstruct partially but allow adequate air exchange produce:
  - Cough
  - Stridor
  - Hoarseness
  - Pain or discomfort

■ Tracheal foreign bodies
- Usually associated with cough, some degree of stridor, or wheezing
- May produce an audible slap as the object moves from the carina to the glottis with respiration

■ Bronchial foreign bodies
- Usually cause wheezing or coughing if they are partly obstructing
- Are often misdiagnosed as asthma
- With complete obstruction of a bronchus, initial asymptomatic period is followed by a postobstructive pneumonitis or bronchiectasis.

- Sharp objects, such as pins or tacks, may cause pain or hemoptysis.

Foreign bodies of the esophagus

■ Highest incidence in children 14 months to 6 years

■ History of foreign body ingestion is often not obtained.

■ Most foreign bodies pass through the esophagus undetected.

■ Swallowed or aspirated object can cause a respiratory emergency, no symptom at all, or anything in between.

■ Objects that do not pass freely initially stimulate the larynx and cause gagging and coughing.

■ Subsequent symptoms depend on size, composition, and nature of the foreign body.

■ In young children, the following symptoms are common.
- Poor feeding
- Refusal to eat or drink
- Increased salivation

■ When the esophagus is completely or almost completely obstructed
- Choking
- Vomiting

■ Duration of obstruction can affect clinical presentation.
- Longer time, increased tissue reaction and local inflammation
- In the later stages
  - Pain on swallowing
  - Airway compromise
  - Fever
  - Leukocytosis

DIFFERENTIAL DIAGNOSIS

■ Differential diagnosis of foreign bodies in the nose includes:
- Suppurative rhinitis
- Adenoiditis
- Sinusitis
- Nasal or nasopharyngeal tumors
- Nasal polyps also may cause unilateral nasal discharge.
- In a young child, cystic fibrosis must be ruled out.

IMAGING

■ Foreign bodies in the nose
- Radiography may be helpful if the object is radiopaque or has become calcified.
- Incidental finding of a nasal foreign body on a routine dental radiograph examination has been reported.
- In a review of children who had nasal foreign bodies, 28 of 71 (39%) radiographs demonstrated a foreign body.

F

- US toy manufacturers are required by law to make toy parts radiopaque.
  - Those manufactured outside the US do not have to conform to this regulation.
- Foreign bodies of the airway
  - For objects suspected of being lodged in the laryngeal inlet, high-kilovolt anteroposterior and lateral radiographs of the upper trachea or esophageal inlet should be obtained if the patient's condition permits.
  - Bronchial foreign bodies may be suggested by a dynamic radiographic study.
    - Inspiratory-expiratory films
    - Lateral decubitus films
    - Videofluoroscopy
    - These studies can demonstrate air-trapping in the affected lung.
- Foreign bodies of the esophagus
  - Posteroanterior and lateral chest radiographs, in addition to neck radiographs, are diagnostic if the object is radiopaque.
  - If the foreign body is a coin, it will be oriented in a transverse position because the opening of the esophagus is widest in a transverse position.
  - Contrast studies can be used when a foreign body that does not show on routine radiographs is strongly suspected.

DIAGNOSTIC PROCEDURES

- Direct visualization of the foreign body by endoscopy may be necessary when the foreign body is not visualized by different imaging techniques.

TREATMENT APPROACH

- The severity of the problems caused by the presence of a foreign body depends on site, composition, and duration of time in the body.
- Removal of a foreign body is not usually an emergency except:
  - If the airway is compromised
  - If the object is a battery
- Removal should be attempted only if the following are available.
  - Appropriate sedation or anesthesia
  - Proper instrumentation and illumination
  - Skilled practitioner
  - Attempts to remove the foreign body without these may aggravate the problem and jeopardize the child's well-being.

SPECIFIC TREATMENTS

Foreign bodies in the ear

- Nonurgent situations
  - Nonreactive foreign bodies that do not occlude the external canal completely or impinge on the tympanic membrane do not present an emergency.
- Aural foreign bodies may be removed by:
  - Irrigation
    - Gentle irrigation may be used on nonabsorbable substances.
      - Ensure that the tympanic membrane can be visualized.
      - Make sure it is intact and that there is no evidence of inflammation of the external canal.
    - 18-gauge catheter attached to a 10- to 20-mL syringe
      - The pressure generated is well below the pressure required to burst a tympanic membrane.
    - Flow of fluid should be directed around the retained object.
      - Allow backpressure to force the object out of the canal.
    - Fluids should be warmed to avoid irritation of the labyrinths.
    - Food tends to swell when water is applied, making removal difficult.
  - Suction
    - Frazier tip suction
  - Instrumentation
    - Choice of instrument will depend on the shape and composition of the object.
      - Alligator forceps
      - Right-angle hook
    - Pass instrument beyond the object, hook it from behind, and pull it out gently.
- Urgent situations
  - In older children who are cooperative
    - Local anesthetic injected with a small-gauge needle into the skin lining the external canal may allow complete removal of the foreign body and subsequent examination.
  - In younger children or for those who are uncooperative:
    - General anesthesia may be necessary.
    - This is preferable to traumatic removal if the child cannot cooperate or cannot be restrained adequately.
    - Remove the foreign body immediately when:
      - The tympanic membrane cannot be visualized
      - Evidence exists of inflammation or injury to the external canal

- Expeditious removal is particularly important with an alkaline battery.
  - Tympanic membrane perforations have been reported within only 8 hours of entry.
  - Magnets may be helpful for removing metallic objects, such as batteries or metal beads.
- Insects
  - Kill before removal.
    - Instill water, mineral oil, or topical lidocaine into the external canal.
    - Extract the insect with suction or alligator forceps.

Foreign bodies of the nose

- Remove as quickly as possible, particularly in the case of an alkaline battery.
  - Can cause severe local inflammation, with tissue damage occurring within 1 hour of placement
  - Saline irrigation should be avoided as it can cause further tissue damage.
- Young children are averse to nasal instrumentation, and removing a nasal foreign body requires cooperation or restraint.
  - Sedation or general anesthesia may be needed.
  - Topical application of a vasoconstrictor agent (eg, oxymetazoline, phenylephrine) in conjunction with removal of secretions by a small suction tip aids visualization, particularly when the object is lodged in the middle or posterior nasal cavity.
- An endoscope is recommended for visualization.
- Most items can be removed with a grasping instrument, eg, straight forcep, mosquito clamp.
  - If foreign body is firm and flat or has an edge, then it may be removed by using a nasal bayonet or Hartmann or alligator forceps.
  - A wire loop may be placed beyond a spherical object, which is then removed by pulling loop forward.
- Other methods include suction, irrigation, and adhesives.
  - Soft, friable objects can usually be removed with a Frazier tip suction device.
  - A Fogarty or a small Foley catheter may be used for removal.
    - Place the catheter beyond the foreign body into the posterior portion of the nasal cavity or nasopharynx.
    - Inflate with 2–3 mL of saline solution.
    - Draw the catheter gently forward and out of the nose, expelling the object.
    - Foreign object may be dislodged by pushing it posteriorly into the nasopharynx, which may lead to aspiration of the object.

- Nebulized adrenaline together with nose blowing has been reported to expel nasal foreign bodies successfully.
  - Using pepper to induce a sneeze while the uninvolved nostril is occluded or blowing in the child's mouth while the contralateral nostril is held shut is not suggested.
- Ambu-bag insufflation of the mouth with the patient in Trendelenburg position has been described.
- After removal, local inflammation exhibited by bloody or purulent oozing may be controlled with:
  - Saline nose drops
    - Sterile water should be used in place of saline if the foreign object removed was an alkaline battery.
  - Antibacterial ointment, eg, bacitracin, mupirocin
- A foreign body that has remained in the nose for a long time may become calcified and form a rhinolith.
  - Removal is often difficult and bloody.

Foreign bodies of the airway

- Foreign bodies that completely obstruct the laryngeal inlet create a life-threatening emergency.
  - They should be expelled immediately by using the Heimlich maneuver (abdominal thrusts).
    - For infants <1 year, the AAP recommends 5 back blows in the head-down position followed by 5 chest thrusts in the supine position, in place of the Heimlich maneuver.
    - Blind finger sweeps are dangerous and should be avoided.
  - If the foreign body cannot be expelled, a large-bore needle or angiocatheter (14 gauge) should be inserted into the cricothyroid space to allow ventilation until the patient can be taken to the operating room.
  - Alternatively, emergency tracheotomy may be necessary.
- Partly obstructing laryngeal foreign bodies should be treated in a manner that prevents total obstruction of the airway.
  - Back blows and abdominal thrusts should not be used in these cases.
- Tracheal and bronchial foreign bodies should be removed by a physician specifically trained for the task.
  - Procedure requires controlled endoscopic removal in the operating room.
  - It is not usually an emergency, and adequate preparations can be made.

Foreign bodies of the esophagus

- Usually does not require emergency intervention
- Endoscopic removal under anesthesia by a trained expert remains the method of choice.
- Remove the object as soon as possible after proper evaluation and preparation.
  - If the child has eaten recently, allow an appropriate period pass before general anesthesia is administered.

F

- If the foreign body is corrosive, such as an alkaline button battery, it should be removed as soon as possible to prevent severe inflammation and potential perforation of the esophageal wall.
- Rigid esophagoscopy
  - Optical forceps are passed through the central channel for retrieval of the foreign body.
    - Allows for direct visualization of the esophagus, mucosa, and foreign body
- Flexible endoscopy
  - Once the scope is passed, a variety of flexible graspers, forceps, baskets, and magnets can be passed through the instrument channel for retrieval.
  - Nonendoscopic techniques are not recommended.
    - Using catheters to remove the foreign body can lead to aspiration, airway obstruction, and death.

WHEN TO ADMIT

- Foreign bodies in the airway
  - If prolonged or difficult instrumentation of the airway occurred during removal of the foreign body
  - If postoperative edema develops
- Foreign bodies in the esophagus
  - If the object is sharp and irretrievable by endoscope

WHEN TO REFER

- If airway compromise exists
- Anytime a battery is involved
- If the child cannot be restrained adequately
- If an object cannot be removed
  - Ear
    - If the tympanic membrane cannot be visualized or perforation is suspected
    - If the object is touching the tympanic membrane
    - If the object is spherical or in the canal for >24 hours
    - If hearing loss, nystagmus, vertigo, central nervous system deficits, or deep-seated infection exists
  - Nose
    - If a rhinolith has formed
  - Airway
    - For tracheal and bronchial foreign bodies
  - Esophagus
    - For endoscopic removal if perforation is suspected

FOLLOW-UP

- Foreign bodies of the ear
  - Postextraction care
    - After any foreign body is removed, the external canal and tympanic membrane should be thoroughly inspected.

- If the external auditory canal appears infected or irritated
  - Topical antibiotic otic drops with steroids may be instilled.
  - The affected ear should be protected from water until it has healed completely.

COMPLICATIONS

Foreign bodies of the ear

- Complications can be caused by:
  - The foreign body
  - Traumatic removal
- Laceration or inflammation of the external canal
  - Usually not serious
  - Resolves with instillation of liquid analgesics and antibiotics
- Perforations of the tympanic membrane
  - Carefully inspect to ensure that a flap of the membrane has not folded into the middle ear, leading to a permanent perforation or a cholesteatoma.
  - The middle ear space can become contaminated, and otitis media can develop.

Foreign bodies of the nose

- Complications include:
  - Epistaxis
  - Local infection
  - Inflammation
  - Nasal septal perforation
- Occasionally a scar band, or synechia, may form between the turbinate and septum.
  - Prevent synechia by placing a splint made of Gelfilm or Silastic over the raw, exposed area.
- Obstruction of a sinus ostium by a foreign object may lead to the development of sinusitis.
  - Typically causes pain and tenderness over the affected sinus
  - Clouding and an air-fluid level will be observed on the radiograph.
  - Treatment includes oral antibiotics and nasal decongestant drops.
- Aspiration can be prevented in most cases by prompt and skilled removal.

Foreign bodies of the airway

- Abdominal and chest thrusts may damage intraabdominal contents (eg, liver, spleen) and ribs.
  - Should be used only in cases of complete airway obstruction that would otherwise cause certain death
- Conversion of a partial airway obstruction to a complete obstruction can be prevented by having skilled personnel retrieve the foreign body.

- Pneumonia was the most common complication in 127 cases of foreign body aspiration.
- A bronchial foreign body that remains in place for an extended period may cause air trapping and irreversible bronchiectatic changes distal to the obstruction.
- Prolonged or difficult instrumentation of the airway during removal of a foreign body can lead to laryngeal edema or injury, with obstructive symptoms.
  - May require a period of intubation after surgery
  - Postoperative edema can sometimes be prevented by using steroids during and after surgery.

Foreign bodies of the esophagus

- Perforation of the esophagus can result from:
  - Endoscopic retrieval procedure
  - By the foreign body itself
- Endoscopic removal is particularly dangerous with objects lodged at the level of the aortic arch.

- If an esophageal tear is suspected, a radiographic gastrograffin swallow study will usually confirm or negate the suspicion.
- Retropharyngeal abscess has been reported as the most frequent complication of a sharp esophageal foreign body.
- Foreign bodies that have been in the esophagus for long periods can cause a stricture to develop.
  - A contrast study, computed tomography, or esophagoscopy should be performed to aid in the diagnosis.

PREVENTION

- During anticipatory guidance, parents and caregivers should be instructed not to:
  - Leave small objects or inappropriate food where a young child can reach them
  - Give small objects or inappropriate food to a young infant

F

Fractures and Dislocations

DEFINITION

- A fracture is a break or crack in a bone.
  - Direct fracture: at the site of injury
  - Indirect fracture: at a site different from the applied force
  - Closed fracture: no break in the skin
  - Open fracture: bone fragment is exposed to air.
  - Comminuted fracture: bone has ≥3 fragments.
  - Impacted fracture: bone ends are compressed into each other.
- Salter-Harris classification system
  - Describes injury to the growth plate
    - Fractures that do not cause any direct injury to the growth plate (eg, chip fractures) are not usually included in the Salter-Harris classification system.
  - Type I fracture
    - The epiphysis is separated from the metaphysis without a true break in the bone.
  - Type II fracture
    - The most common growth plate fracture
    - A fragment of metaphyseal bone separates from the epiphysis.
  - Type III fracture
    - Partial growth plate injury through the epiphysis
  - Type IV fracture
    - Extends across the growth plate, injuring both the epiphysis and the metaphysis
  - Type V fracture
    - Growth plate is compressed.
- Dislocation
  - Malposition of bone ends that normally appose each other within a joint

EPIDEMIOLOGY

- Fractures
  - Fractured clavicle
    - Most common fracture in children
    - Incidence can be as high as 3.5% in babies delivered vaginally.
  - Growth plate injuries
    - ~15% of all childhood fractures
- Dislocations
  - In children, far less common than fractures
  - A child's ligaments are quite strong compared with an adult's.
  - With an injury, it is more likely that bone will break or growth plate will separate than that ligament will tear.
  - Developmental dysplasia of the hip (DDH)
    - Formerly known as *congenital hip dislocation*

- The femoral head has a tendency to dislocate in as many as 5 of every 1000 infants.
    - 6–8 times more common in girls than in boys
  - Nursemaid's elbow
    - Common dislocation in pediatrics
    - Usually occurs in children between 1 and 4 years of age

ETIOLOGY

- Stress fractures
  - Result from recurrent trauma to a bone
- Pathologic fractures
  - Can occur without trauma or with minor trauma
- Toddler's fracture
  - Torsion of the foot creates a spiral break in the tibia.
- DDH
  - May be related to left occiput anterior fetal position, which puts pressure on the left hip to dislocate
  - Genetic predisposition
  - Theories suggest that female fetuses are more sensitive to maternal hormones that can induce ligamentous laxity of the hip.
- Nursemaid's elbow
  - Pulling or yanking a child's arm, often by a parent or caretaker
  - Annular ligament of the radial head becomes entrapped in the radiohumeral joint

RISK FACTORS

- Stress fracture
  - Athletic activity
    - Long-distance running is associated with long-bone fractures.
- Pathologic fracture
  - Conditions resulting in weakened bone
    - Osteogenesis imperfecta
    - Tumor
- Fractured clavicle
  - Difficult vaginal delivery
- DDH
  - Positive family history of hip dislocation
  - Breech delivery
  - Cesarean section

SIGNS AND SYMPTOMS

History

- Whenever a fracture or dislocation is suspected, an accurate history is essential.

- Historical details may provide clues about the mechanism of injury.
  - Where any pain is located
  - How, where, and when the injury occurred
  - A fall off of a skateboard or scooter increases suspicion for a forearm fracture.
- Does the parent or child report any loss of function in the affected limb?
  - Does the history show acute or recurrent trauma?

Physical examination

- Key to revealing signs of serious trauma and secondary sites of injury
  - Includes vital signs and neurovascular assessment
- Pulses
  - Should be normal
  - Absence of pulses signifies a serious injury requiring immediate medical attention.
- Sensation
  - Should be intact
  - Absence of sensation signifies a serious injury requiring immediate medical attention.
- Movement
  - Should be present even if limited by discomfort
  - Absence of movement signifies a serious injury requiring immediate medical attention.
- The examiner should look carefully for:
  - Any unnatural or deformed position of joints or limbs
  - Pain on palpation or attempted movement
  - Swelling and discoloration
  - Crepitus, which can sometimes be elicited at a fracture site
  - Any of the above findings should alert the clinician to order imaging studies.
- Clinical appearance of fractures
  - Closed fracture
    - Hidden fracture causes slight pain and swelling but no obvious bone deformity.
    - Radiographs are necessary to confirm diagnosis.
  - Open, or compound, fracture
    - Patient is at risk for infection and injury to adjacent nerves and blood vessels.
    - Immediate medical attention is necessary.

Fractured clavicle

- Can occur at any time during childhood as a result of trauma
  - Diagnosis is often made after the fact, when a callus at the fracture site is noted at a well-baby visit.
- Physical findings
  - Decreased arm motion on the affected side

- Crepitus
- Swelling at the fracture site
- Imaging may be needed to confirm diagnosis.

DDH

- 3 times more common on the left than the right side
- Bilateral in approximately 20% of cases
  - Children <1 year should be examined for hip dislocation at every routine visit with the appropriate tests.
  - Ortolani test (not usually positive beyond 3 or 4 months)
    - With the baby laying supine, the hips and knees are flexed and the knees brought together.
    - The examiner then places a hand on each of the baby's knees, with each middle finger over the greater trochanter and each thumb over the medial thigh.
    - With gentle abduction of the knees, the dislocated femoral head will slip back into the acetabulum with an audible or palpable *clunk.*
    - This motion pushes a dislocated hip back into the hip socket.
    - Notably, a hip *click* (without a *clunk* and without any movement of the femoral head) does not indicate hip dislocation.
  - Barlow test (not usually positive beyond 3 or 4 months)
    - The reverse of the Ortolani test
    - The femoral head can be felt slipping out of the acetabulum when the knees are brought back together.
    - This motion pushes a dislocatable hip out of the hip socket.
  - Telescoping sign
    - The examiner may feel unusual laxity of the hip by pushing up and down on the thigh when hips are flexed and adducted.
  - Older infants should be examined for:
    - Limited hip abduction
    - Asymmetry of the thigh skin folds
    - Limp when cruising or walking
    - Leg length discrepancy
- Galeazzi sign to determine leg-length discrepancy
  - With the infant lying supine, the examiner flexes the infant's thighs and brings the knees together.
  - If one knee is higher than the other, the Galeazzi sign is positive and the possibility of a dislocated hip exists.

Nursemaid's elbow

- Transient subluxation of the proximal radial head
- The child refuses to move the arm and keeps it flexed and pronated.
- History (yanking or pulling of the arm by another person) and characteristic posture of the child's arm confirm the diagnosis.

F

Child abuse

- Fractures and dislocations are commonly suggestive of child abuse.
- Child abuse may be suspected when:
  - Unexplained injury occurs.
  - Inconsistency exists between history and physical findings.
  - Delay between time of injury and time that medical attention is sought is unusually long.
  - Multiple bruises are noted on physical examination.

Toddler's fracture

- Spiral fracture of the tibia in a child <6 years of age
- Trauma to the leg often is minor or unwitnessed; therefore, no history of trauma may be found.
- If the cause of the fracture is unexplained, child abuse may be a consideration.
- Symptoms may be minimal.
  - The child may be brought for medical attention only because of reluctance to bear weight on the affected leg.
  - Physical examination is significant for tenderness over the affected area of the tibia.
  - The examiner should have a high index of suspicion in a child who has a limp or fails to bear weight.

Injury to growth plate

- Growth or epiphyseal plate injuries occur only in childhood.
- They must be treated with care to protect a bone's growth potential.
- Type I fractures
  - Radiographs are often normal.
  - Therefore, diagnosis is based on the clinical picture: tenderness over the area of the growth plate.

DIAGNOSTIC APPROACH

- Careful history to elicit precipitating event
- Physical examination to reveal signs of trauma and secondary injury
- Radiography to detect subtle fractures and to exclude dislocation
- Infants and children should be assessed for DDH annually.
- Pediatric care practitioners are morally and legally responsible for detecting child abuse and reporting all suspected cases.

IMAGING

- Radiography
  - A mainstay in the diagnosis of fractures and dislocations
    - Confirms diagnosis of closed fracture
    - 2 angles are used to delineate subtle fractures.
    - Including the joint above and below the injury can be helpful in excluding dislocation.

- In many cases, a film of the unaffected side for a comparison view is needed.
- Breaks in the bone may be described by their radiographic appearance as:
  - Transverse
  - Oblique
  - Spiral
- Stress fractures are often missed on radiographs.
- Torus or buckle fracture
  - Most commonly occurs after injury to the forearm
  - The radiograph shows a wrinkled appearing break of the distal radius.
- DDH
  - A radiograph in infants >4–6 months of age will confirm or rule out a dysplastic hip.
- Nursemaid's elbow
  - Imaging is unnecessary.
- Child abuse
  - If abuse is suspected, a radiographic bone survey should be performed in younger children.
  - Silent fractures, or multiple fractures in varying stages of healing, may be seen.
- Toddler's fracture
  - Anteroposterior and lateral radiographs of the tibia-fibula confirm the diagnosis.
  - Fracture is sometimes not evident on a radiograph for a few days.
  - Physician should not hesitate to repeat films in a child who has an unexplained limp that does not resolve spontaneously.
- Computed tomography
  - Can be useful when injury to the growth plate is a concern
- Magnetic resonance imaging
  - May be indicated to confirm torus or buckle fracture
- Radionuclide bone scan
  - May be indicated to confirm torus or buckle fracture
- Ultrasonography
  - May be needed to confirm:
    - Fractured clavicle
    - DDH

TREATMENT APPROACH

- Fractures and dislocations should be splinted and immobilized immediately.
  - Most pediatric fractures respond to closed reduction by an orthopedist.
  - Even some compound fractures can be managed nonoperatively.

- Close pediatric and orthopedic follow-up are important.

■ If the growth plate is affected:

- Open reduction in the operating room is performed.

SPECIFIC TREATMENTS

Fractured clavicle

■ If the condition is asymptomatic:

- No treatment is needed.

■ If the fracture causes pain or reduced arm movement:

- Immobilization of the arm on the affected side for 2–3 weeks
- In older children, splinting for 3–4 weeks in a simple sling is required.
- Figure-of-8 bandages are cumbersome and work no better than a sling.

■ Most of the fracture's healing and realignment are spontaneous.

DDH

■ Treatment requires referral to an orthopedist for a harness or casting.

- Treatment is more straightforward the earlier the diagnosis is made.

■ Infants <6 months of age

- A Pavlik harness is worn for up to 5 months.

■ Infants ≥6 months of age, and infants in whom the harness was not successful

- Casting
- Possibly surgery

Nursemaid's elbow

■ Treatment is easily performed by the pediatrician.

- Rapid, forceful supination of the forearm while pressure is placed over the proximal radial head, followed by extension then flexion of the elbow

■ Symptoms usually resolve within 30 minutes.

■ The condition is sometimes recurrent.

- Great care must be taken when holding hands with the affected child, lest the child suddenly tries to pull away.

Child abuse

■ When child abuse is suspected, the child should be hospitalized for protection and for appropriate evaluation and orthopedic care.

■ Child protective services and social services should be involved.

Toddler's fracture

■ Immobilization in a cast for 3–4 weeks.

Long-bone fractures

■ Often corrected with overriding of broken ends to prevent length discrepancies with the uninjured side

Growth plate injuries

■ The growth plate must be protected when treating children's fractures.

- A growth plate injury can result in the loss of growth potential.

■ Type I fracture

- Immobilization by cast for approximately 3 weeks

■ Type II fracture

- Closed reduction of the fracture is usually possible; with proper casting, growth is not disturbed.

■ Type III fracture

- Open repair of the fracture in the operating room is indicated to align articular surfaces and preserve joint function.

■ Type IV fracture

- The fracture must be perfectly realigned to protect growth potential.

WHEN TO ADMIT

■ Whenever child abuse is suspected or if the patient is not medically stable (ie, multiple injuries)

WHEN TO REFER

■ All fractures and dislocations not easily managed in a primary care setting

■ In most cases, consultation with an orthopedic specialist is necessary.

FOLLOW-UP

■ A child in a cast should be comfortable.

■ The child needs reevaluation and possibly requires recasting if:

- Pain is persistent *or*
- Color changes or sensory changes occur to the casted extremity.

PROGNOSIS

■ Fractures heal more quickly in children than in adults.

- Remodeling that occurs in the healing of pediatric fractures often corrects residual bony deformities.

■ Accelerated growth rate of bony fragments during healing (overgrowth) occurs in pediatric long-bone fractures.

■ Type I and II fractures

- Growth is usually not disturbed.

■ Type V fracture

- Prognosis for preserving growth is poor because of a crush injury to the growth plate.

Gastroesophageal Reflux Disease

DEFINITION

- Gastroesophageal reflux (GER) is the passage of gastric contents into the esophagus.
  - Most episodes are brief and unaccompanied by symptoms.
- Gastroesophageal reflux disease (GERD) is symptoms or complications resulting from exposure of the esophagus, the oropharynx, or the airway to gastric refluxate (acid, food, bile).
  - *Regurgitation* occurs when gastric contents enter into the oropharynx.
  - *Vomiting* refers to gastric contents exiting through the mouth.
  - *Rumination* is regurgitation with subsequent reswallowing of the gastric contents.

EPIDEMIOLOGY

- GER
  - Age
    - Infants <1 year frequently have GER.
    - 50% of infants <3 months have recurrent regurgitation and other GER symptoms.
    - 67% of healthy infants 4 months of age have these symptoms; the peak prevalence is between 4 and 6 months of age.
    - The prevalence of GER decreases to 5% among infants 10–12 months of age.
    - By 1 year of age, most infants have stopped having symptoms of GER.
- Barrett syndrome, often called *Barrett esophagus*, is a metaplasia of lining of lower esophagus from squamous epithelium to columnar epithelium that is acquired as a result of long-standing esophagitis.
  - The incidence of Barrett esophagus in children is rare and <1 per 1000 in children undergoing endoscopy.

ETIOLOGY

- The causes of GERD are multifactorial and depend on anatomy, motility, and physiologic factors.
- Anatomy
  - In an infant, the normal obtuse angle of His does not occlude the hiatus when the stomach is distended postprandially and may result in regurgitation.
  - Abnormalities such as malrotation, annular pancreas, or antral web may also result in symptoms of GERD.
- Motility
  - Impaired esophageal motility associated with repair of esophageal atresia or tracheoesophageal fistula or delayed gastric emptying may result in prolonged acid exposure in the esophagus and eventual complications of GERD.

- Impaired buffering of acid in the esophagus by saliva may lead to esophagitis in children with cystic fibrosis or adults with autoimmune disease.
- Lower esophageal sphincter (LES) pressure is an important antireflux barrier.
  - Possibly because of the other factors, LES pressure by itself correlates poorly with GER.
- Physiologic factors
  - In both children and adults, the most common cause of reflux is inappropriate transient LES relaxation with inhibition of esophageal peristalsis.
    - Transient LES relaxations typically occur up to 5 times in the immediate postprandial hour with episodic movement of gastric contents into the distal esophagus.
    - These relaxations are vagally mediated, brief in duration, and probably play a normal role in eliminating gas from the stomach.
    - When the refluxate enters the esophagus, it is buffered by saliva and cleared by normal esophageal peristalsis.
    - In patients with GERD, these relaxations last longer, from 5–35 seconds.
    - During this period, a combination of LES hypotonia and inhibited esophageal peristalsis prolong the contact time of the gastric contents with the esophageal mucosa and contribute to tissue injury.
    - Inappropriate LES relaxation and delayed gastric emptying has been shown to occur in 28–50% of children with GERD.
- Conditions associated with GERD
  - Asthma and chronic cough are associated with GERD.
    - Vagal afferents innervate both the esophagus and the bronchi and acid stimulation of receptors in the esophagus may induce reflex bronchoconstriction.
  - Bronchoconstriction and laryngospasm
    - May be caused by microaspiration of gastric contents into the trachea
  - Increased airway responsiveness in asthmatic patients
    - Esophageal acid exposure per se, even though it has a minimal effect on pulmonary function, is a contributor.
  - No convincing temporal relationship exists between esophageal acidification and apnea or bradycardia in unselected patients.

RISK FACTORS

- GERD occurs in infants who have irritability associated with feeding or food refusal.
- Infants who have symptoms for >90 days are at increased risk of having symptoms of GERD 9–11 years later.
- The significance of heartburn at age 10 years and whether it predisposes one to complications of GERD later in life is not known.

■ Factors in increased risk and severity of GER

- Increasing intraabdominal pressure (crying in infants, coughing, obesity)
- Gastric acid secretion
- Consumption of:
  - Large meals
  - Fatty foods
  - Caffeinated beverages
  - Candy
  - Certain medications (theophylline, morphine, calcium-channel blockers)

SIGNS AND SYMPTOMS

■ Symptoms of GER depend on the age of the patient.

■ Clinical manifestations change with age and the development of language.

- Infants may express discomfort from acid reflux by crying, refusing to eat, or failing to thrive.
- Older children may mention abdominal pain but will not localize the pain to the epigastrium or retrosternal areas.
- Adolescents are more likely to report heartburn symptoms similar to those reported by adults.
- Extraesophageal symptoms, such as pneumonia, cough, hoarse voice, or dental disease, may occur at any age.

Symptoms of GER

■ Gastrointestinal

- Nausea
- Vomiting
- Regurgitation
- Irritability during and after feedings
- Refusal to feed
- Failure to thrive
- Heartburn
- Dysphagia
- Odynophagia
- Hematemesis
- Melena
- Eructation
- Anorexia

■ Respiratory

- Chronic cough
- Reactive airway disease
- Recurrent pneumonia
- Stridor
- Chest pain

- Apnea
- Hoarseness of voice
- Choking
- Gagging

■ Neurobehavioral

- Apnea or apparent life-threatening event (ALTE)
- Seizure-like events
- Sandifer syndrome
- Rumination

History in the child with suspected GER/GERD

■ Little is known about the natural history of children and adolescents with symptoms of GER/GERD.

■ The following information should be obtained.

- Feeding history
  - Amount and frequency (overfeeding)
  - Preparation of formula
  - Source of dietary protein
  - Position and burping
  - Behavior during feedings (choking, gagging, coughing, arching, discomfort, feeding refusal)
- Pattern of vomiting
  - Frequency and amount
  - Painful
  - Forceful
  - Hematemesis
  - Association with fever, lethargy, diarrhea
- Medical history
  - Prematurity
  - Growth and development (mental retardation, cerebral palsy, developmental delay)
  - Surgery
  - Hospitalizations
  - Newborn screen (galactosemia, maple sugar urine disease, congenital heart disease)
  - Recurrent illness (croup or stridor, pneumonia, wheeze, hoarseness, excessive fussiness or crying, hiccups)
  - Apnea
  - Inadequate weight gain
- Psychosocial history
  - Stress
- Family history
  - Significant illness
  - Gastrointestinal disorders (familial pattern to obstructive disorders, celiac disease)
  - Other (metabolic, energy)

- Growth chart
  - Length, weight
  - Head circumference
- Warning signs
  - Bilious vomiting
  - Gastrointestinal bleeding: hematemesis, hematochezia
  - Forceful vomiting
  - Onset of vomiting after 6 months of life
  - Failure to thrive
  - Diarrhea
  - Constipation
  - Fever
  - Lethargy
  - Hepatosplenomegaly
  - Bulging fontanelle
  - Macrocephaly, microcephaly
  - Seizures
  - Abdominal tenderness, distention
  - Genetic disorders (eg, trisomy 21)
  - Other chronic disorders (eg, HIV)

DIFFERENTIAL DIAGNOSIS

Conditions similar to GER

- A variety of conditions have clinical features that resemble GER, including:
  - Eosinophilic esophagitis
  - Food allergy
  - Achalasia
  - Cyclic vomiting syndrome
  - Pill esophagitis
  - Infectious esophagitis
  - Rumination syndrome
- These conditions may be suspected on the basis of characteristic features, diagnostic testing, or a failure of symptoms to respond to standard medical therapy for acid reflux.

Specific conditions

Eosinophilic esophagitis

- Occurs in young children, teenagers, and adults
- Appears to be more common today than 25 years ago
- The majority of patients are male, and most have dysphagia or food impaction.
- Younger children may have symptoms suggestive of GERD such as abdominal pain or food refusal.
- Dysphagia or esophageal food impaction is more commonly noted in older children.

- Partial or complete unresponsiveness to acid-suppression therapy suggests that GERD is not a contributing factor.
- A personal or family history of allergic disease is found in 75% of cases.
- The diagnosis is suspected when white exudate, circular rings, or linear furrowing is seen during upper endoscopy.
- Establishing diagnosis depends on finding >15–20 eosinophils per high-power field on an esophageal mucosal biopsy.

Food allergy

- Milk protein and other food allergies in young infants may mimic symptoms of GER, but they usually resolve with dietary restriction or time.
- A challenge with the suspected allergen may reproduce the symptoms but is usually not necessary for managing the patient.
- Eczema, skin rash, wheezing, concomitant diarrhea, or blood in the stool should alert the clinician to the possibility of allergy.

Achalasia

- A motor disorder characterized by lack of peristalsis in the distal two-thirds of the esophagus, an elevated resting pressure in the distal esophagus, and failure of the LES to relax
- Results in functional obstruction in the lower esophagus and accumulation of food in the esophagus
- Children may have weight loss; regurgitation of undigested food; halitosis; cough, especially when supine; or pneumonia.
- The most common feature on chest radiograph is absence of air in the stomach and an air-fluid level in the esophagus.
- Widening of the mediastinum may be seen in long-standing disease.
- Esophageal manometry is often diagnostic and demonstrates:
  - Aperistalsis in the distal two-thirds of the esophagus
  - Elevated resting LES
  - Failure or incomplete relaxation of the LES
- In young children with achalasia, sphincter relaxation and occasional peristalsis may be present.
- Barium esophagraphy often reveals a symmetrical narrowing in distal esophagus with the appearance of a bird beak.

Cyclic vomiting syndrome

- A functional gastrointestinal disorder characterized by:
  - Bouts of intractable nausea
  - Vomiting lasting for hours
  - Lethargy and pallor
  - Periods of complete symptom relief
- These episodes are intense in severity, but unlike in GER, the patient is completely asymptomatic between episodes.
- A bout may be triggered spontaneously, by stress, or by menstruation.
- No diagnostic test or identifiable neurologic, metabolic, or other gastrointestinal disease exists to explain the condition.

- Differential diagnosis of vomiting
  - Gastrointestinal obstruction
    - Pyloric stenosis
    - Malrotation with intermittent volvulus
    - Intermittent intussusception
    - Intestinal duplication
    - Hirschsprung disease
    - Antral or duodenal web
    - Foreign body
    - Incarcerated hernia
  - Gastrointestinal disorders
    - Achalasia
    - Gastroparesis
    - Gastroenteritis
    - Peptic ulcer disease
    - GER
    - Eosinophilic esophagitis, gastroenteritis
    - Food allergy or intolerance
    - Inflammatory bowel disease
    - Pancreatitis
    - Appendicitis
  - Neurologic disorders
    - Hydrocephalus
    - Subdural hematoma
    - Intracranial hemorrhage
    - Mass lesion
  - Infection
- Sepsis
- Meningitis
- Urinary tract infection
- Pneumonia
- Otitis media
- Hepatitis
- Metabolic or endocrine disorders
  - Galactosemia
  - Hereditary fructose intolerance
  - Urea cycle defects
  - Amino and organic acidemias
  - Congenital adrenal hyperplasia
  - Maple syrup urine disease
- Renal disorders
  - Obstructive uropathy
  - Renal insufficiency

- Toxic agents
  - Lead
  - Iron
  - Vitamin A or D
  - Medications (eg, ipecac, digoxin, theophylline)
- Cardiac disorders
  - Congestive heart failure

Pill esophagitis

- Occurs when a pill is lodged in the esophagus
- Usually causes acute onset of severe midchest or substernal pain and dysphagia
- Minocycline, ibuprofen, iron, and potassium hydroxide are the usual suspects.
- Condition is suspected based on history; endoscopy may not be necessary if symptoms improve with acid-suppression therapy or sucralfate.

Infectious esophagitis

- Most infectious causes of esophagitis present with odynophagia and not dysphagia.
- Herpes simplex virus; cytomegalovirus; and fungal infection, such as candidiasis, may occur in both immunocompetent and immunocompromised hosts.
- Upper endoscopy is beneficial in making the diagnosis both by histopathologic features and by culture.

Rumination syndrome

- Characterized by regurgitation of food into the mouth with subsequent reswallowing of the material
- This syndrome was typically thought to occur in neurologically compromised children but is now recognized as occurring in otherwise healthy children and adolescents.
- Repeated masticatory movements, swallowing air, and tensing abdominal musculature help distinguish rumination from effortless GER.

IMAGING

- Scintigraphy
  - Oral intake of radiolabeled technetium followed by scan of esophagus, stomach, and the lungs to detect radiolabeled colloid that has been refluxed or aspirated
  - Gastric emptying time may be calculated for potential therapeutic intervention.
  - Techniques of performing this test are not standardized, and age-specific normative data are not available.
    - Their role in evaluating GERD in children is unclear at this time.
    - Determining gastric emptying may contribute to management.

- Upper gastrointestinal radiography (barium swallow)
  - Primary role is to rule out anatomic causes of GERD such as malrotation, annular pancreas, and antral web.
  - When compared with esophageal pH, upper gastro-intestinal radiography:
    - Is neither sensitive nor specific for GER (31–86% and 21–83%, respectively)
    - Does not reliably determine the presence or absence of GER

DIAGNOSTIC PROCEDURES

- Esophageal pH monitoring
  - Frequency and duration of acid reflux episodes occurring over 20 hours recorded with:
    - Transnasally placed probe
    - Bravo pH probe clipped to the wall of the distal esophagus that transmits to a recorder using radiofrequency signals
  - Percentage of total time the esophageal pH is <4.0 (called the *reflux index*) is considered the most valid measure of reflux.
    - A reflux index ≥12% in infants <1 year and ≥6% in children >1 year is considered abnormal.
  - Not all patients with GER test positive on this study, but 95% of children with esophagitis (gross and microscopic) have an abnormal reflux index.
  - Only 50% of patients with a positive pH study have esophagitis, and the severity of esophagitis does not correlate with the reflux index.
  - Daily variation in severity raises questions about the diagnostic utility of pH probe testing for a condition that is diagnosed by clinical criteria.
  - Proximal esophageal and pharyngeal pH monitoring have not been proven useful in predicting which patients are at risk for upper airway complications.
  - Esophageal pH monitoring is not necessary to establish a diagnosis of GER.
  - It may be beneficial to relate acid reflux with cough, apnea, bradycardia, or other extraesophageal symptoms or to determine efficacy of therapy when symptoms persist.
  - The volume of acid needed to cause extraesophageal symptoms may be very small, and changes in pH may not be detected by pH probe monitoring.
  - The technique is limited because it detects only acid reflux and will not detect nonacidic, postprandial reflux.
- Multiple intraluminal electrical impedance measurement
  - Measures changes in electrical resistance and conductance in the mucosa when a fluid bolus moves down the esophagus, indicating nonacid and acid reflux
  - The clinical value of this test is not yet determined, but preliminary studies suggest that children with pulmonary symptoms may have increased nonacid reflux.

- In conjunction with pH probe, monitoring study may be useful in evaluating patients who do not respond to acid-suppression therapy.
- Endoscopy and biopsy
  - Endoscopy allows direct visualization of esophageal mucosa to detect erosions, ulceration, and reflux-related complications, such as peptic stricture and Barrett esophagus.
    - Because endoscopy requires sedation and the diagnosis of GERD is established based on clinical evidence, indications for this test are based on suspicion of complications of GERD or the need to rule out other disorders.
  - Biopsies routinely obtained at endoscopy determine presence and severity of esophagitis and may help exclude such conditions as Crohn disease of the esophagus, eosinophilic esophagitis, and infection.

TREATMENT APPROACH

- Management of GER/GERD involves:
  - Lifestyle modifications
  - Acid suppression
  - Promotility agents
  - Surgical therapy
- Children at different ages may respond differently to specific interventions.
- Consideration of issues related to growth, development, and compliance are important in determining the best therapeutic intervention.

SPECIFIC TREATMENTS

Lifestyle changes in infants

- Often the first therapy that should be initiated to treat a child with GER or GERD
- Normalization of feeding volume and frequency is essential.
  - Some infants may be fed an excessive volume.
  - By simply reviewing feeding history and educating the family, GER may resolve.
- Thickening formula with rice cereal or purchasing a commercial formula that becomes denser in the stomach may decrease frequency and volume of regurgitation.
  - 1 tablespoon of rice cereal added to each ounce of formula decreases the number of vomiting episodes without reducing the reflux index.
  - Increasing the hole in the nipple may be necessary, avoiding increasing flow so much so that the infant cannot swallow the volume and begins to cough.
  - May lead to constipation, decreasing gastric emptying, and increasing GER

- Increases calories (~34 cal/oz with addition of 1 tbsp/oz), which may be beneficial for infant with slow or poor weight gain
  - As GER resolves, the infant may gain excessive weight.
- Closely monitor growth during treatment for GER in the first year of life.

■ Intolerance of dietary proteins, such as cow's milk or soy, may lead to symptoms identical to those of GER.
  - Generally seen in formula-fed infants; less common in breastfed babies
  - Diagnostic tests are generally not helpful, but children with GER related to dietary protein often improve with a switch to another formula.
  - 1- to 2-week trial of hypoallergenic formula may answer the question about the role of nutrition in causing GER.
  - In a breastfed infant with GER, symptoms often resolve with time.
    - If intervention is required, some infants will improve if the mother eliminates cow's milk and beef from her diet.
    - Soy is more ubiquitous, and restricting cow's milk, beef, and soy is more limiting for a mother's diet.

■ A change in position may decrease GER in infants
  - The prone position is optimal when the infant is awake.
  - Sleeping in the prone position has been recognized to be associated with a higher risk for sudden infant death syndrome (SIDS) compared with the supine position.
  - Based on the new AAP recommendations, the supine position is recommended during sleep for children <12 months
    - The reduced risk of SIDS outweighs the potential benefits of prone sleeping with respect to GERD.
      ■ In certain unusual situations, prone positioning during sleep may be considered when risk of death from complications of GERD outweighs potential increased risk of SIDS.
      ■ When the prone position is a recommendation in a given case, the family should understand the rationale and be advised to avoid using soft bedding that is known to be a suffocation risk.
  - Use of infant seats may increase frequency and severity of reflux.
  - No evidence has been found for decreasing regurgitation by elevating the head of the crib, but many families report improvement with this intervention.
  - As infants begin to move around in their cribs, maintaining their head higher than their feet may become a challenge.
  - For the thriving infant with GER, feeding and positioning are important interventions that may decrease severity of regurgitation and prevent the need for medical therapy.

Lifestyle changes in children and adolescents

■ Evidence-based data in children and adolescents with GER are limited, but avoiding lying down after meals and elevating the head of the bed may decrease symptoms of GER.

■ Older children should avoid caffeine, chocolate, and spicy foods that exacerbate reflux-related symptoms.

■ Active or passive exposure to nicotine will exacerbate GER, and children with GER should be aware of the additional risks in cigarette smoking.

■ Obesity is a known risk factor for complications of GER, and reducing body weight should be discussed with every relevant child and family.

Drug therapy

■ Several categories of drugs are effective for the management of infants, children, and adolescents with GER/GERD.
  - Histamine-2 receptor antagonists (H_2RAs) and proton-pump inhibitors (PPIs) suppress acid production.
  - Antacids neutralize acid that has been produced.
  - Prokinetic agents enhance gastric emptying and some may increase LES pressure.

■ Each class of drugs has a specific role.
  - Acid suppressants reduce exposure of the esophagus to acid gastric contents and promote healing of the esophageal mucosa.
  - Prokinetic agents have not been shown to be effective in clinical trials but in theory may decrease reflux volume by increasing LES pressure, reducing frequency of transient LES relaxations, and accelerating gastric emptying.
  - Empiric trials of medication are often used in adults to support a clinical diagnosis of GER.
    - While recommended by many experts in pediatric gastroenterology, it has not been validated in children.

■ Antacids
  - Buffer gastric acid and decrease its corrosive effect on esophageal mucosa
  - May relieve symptoms of heartburn, improve esophagitis, and prevent acid-related respiratory symptoms
  - Intensive high-dose antacid therapy with magnesium and aluminum hydroxide was shown to be as effective as cimetidine for treatment of esophagitis in children.
    - However, aluminum-containing antacids may increase aluminum levels, potentially causing osteopenia, anemia, and neurotoxicity.
  - Antacids are generally used for short-term management of intermittent symptoms of GERD.

■ H_2RAs
  - Exert their antisecretory effect by blocking the H_2 receptors on gastric parietal epithelial cells
    - Ranitidine, 1 month–16 years: 5–10 mg/kg/day in 2 divided doses

G

- Famotidine, 1 year–16 years: 1 mg/kg/day in 2 divided doses up to 40 mg twice a day
- Nizatidine, ≥12 years: 150 mg twice a day
- Cimetidine, ≥16 years: 800 mg twice a day or 400 mg 4 times a day
- All are approved by the US Food and Drug Administration (FDA) for use in children; no over-the-counter H_2RAs are labeled for pediatric use.

- Numerous randomized controlled studies in adults have documented efficacy of this class of medication in relieving reflux symptoms and healing esophagitis.
- 2 randomized placebo-controlled studies in children report on the efficacy of cimetidine and nizatidine at improving reflux symptoms and healing of esophagitis with the medication.
- Concern exists about development of tolerance or tachyphylaxis with H_2RAs.
- In adults, antisecretory potency of medications in this class decreases after 3 days compared with PPIs, suggesting benefit for long-term use may not be as good as that with other classes of medications.
- Nevertheless, based on case series and expert opinion, H_2RAs are considered to be efficacious and safe in infants and children with GER.

- **PPIs**
  - The most potent class of acid-suppressive medications
  - Block the final step of acid production by covalently binding and deactivating hydrogen-potassium-adenosine triphosphatase enzyme (pump) in the gastric parietal cell
  - PPIs require acid in the parietal cell canaliculus to be activated and are most effective when taken after a prolonged fast, such as 30 minutes before the first meal of the day
  - When required, an evening dose should be administered 30 minutes before the evening meal.
  - Concomitant administration of H_2RAs may, in theory, reduce the efficacy of PPI therapy by reducing available hydrogen ions needed to activate the PPI.
  - Pharmacokinetic parameters for PPIs in adolescents are similar to those reported in adults; however, children <12 years require doses ranging from 1.5 to 2 times the adult dose on a per-kilogram basis to achieve adequate acid suppression.
    - Dose adjustment is attributed to a higher metabolic capacity in children, particularly those 1–6 years of age.
  - Drugs that are FDA approved for children
    - Esomeprazole, 12–17 years: 20 mg or 40 mg by mouth daily (capsule, oral suspension intravenous solution)
    - Lansoprazole, 1–17 years
      - 1–11 years, ≤30 kg: 15 mg by mouth daily
      - 1–11 years, >30 kg: 30 mg by mouth daily
      - 12–17 years, nonerosive: 15 mg by mouth daily
      - 12–17 years, erosive: 30 mg by mouth daily
      - Capsule, oral suspension, rapidly dissolving tablet, intravenous solution
    - Omeprazole, 1–16 years
      - 2–16 years, <20 kg: 10 mg by mouth daily
      - 2–16 years, ≥20 kg: 20 mg by mouth daily
      - Capsule, oral suspension
  - Not FDA approved for children:
    - Rabeprazole, 18 years (tablet)
    - Pantoprazole, 18 years (capsule, oral suspension, intravenous solution)
    - Zegerid
  - Efficacy data in children are mainly from open-label trials and a few controlled trials.
  - PPIs are most effective in decreasing symptoms of reflux and healing esophagitis in children and adolescents.
  - The benefit of PPIs alone in the treatment of GERD in children with asthma has not been well studied, but studies suggest that this class of medication is effective and is an excellent choice for an empiric trial.
  - Over 10 years of safety data are reported with continuous use of omeprazole in adults, but safety data in children are more limited.
    - A limited number of children receiving omeprazole have been monitored for >8 years, with good safety data, and the safety of lansoprazole in children appears to be similar.

- **Prokinetic agents**
  - Used in the treatment of GERD to accelerate gastric emptying.
  - Studies have not shown a decrease in acid reflux episodes, thereby raising questions that these drugs may not reduce transient LES relaxations that are the most important pathophysiologic mechanism of GER.
  - The only prokinetic agents that are available in the United States are metoclopramide and erythromycin.
  - Metoclopramide has limited efficacy in treating GER and has potentially serious side effects that limit its value in treating children with GER.
    - Dyskinesia and tardive dyskinesia that result from crossing the blood-brain barrier
    - Increased serum prolactin levels
  - Erythromycin is rarely used in children who have only GER unless they have significant delay in gastric emptying.

Surgery for GERD

- Surgical therapy is an option for children who remain symptomatic during long-term medical therapy or have side effects of medication.

- Life-threatening complications, such as aspiration, may lead to recommendation of a fundoplication, but the concern that aspiration may result from swallowing and not from reflux is always present.
- If esophageal clearance is impaired, aspiration related to pharyngeal dysfunction may worsen after fundoplication.
- The rationale for surgery to avoid long-term medical therapy has not been well studied in children.
  - ~30% of adults who undergo fundoplication continue to use acid-suppression therapy after surgery.
- Nissen fundoplication is the standard form of surgery
  - It involves wrapping the fundus of the stomach around the LES to reinforce the antireflux barrier.
- Several modifications to Nissen fundoplication have been added, including the newer laparoscopic approach.
  - Recent studies suggest that children who have laparoscopic fundoplication may have fewer complications but a higher rate of reoperation (14%) when compared with children having an open Nissen fundoplication (8%).

WHEN TO ADMIT

- Failure to thrive
- Aspiration pneumonia

WHEN TO REFER

- Failure of medical therapy
- Side effects of medical therapy
- Failure to thrive

FOLLOW-UP

- Infants with GER should be monitored for weight gain, complications of GER and side effects of medication.

COMPLICATIONS

General

- Symptoms
  - Recurrent vomiting
  - Weight loss or poor weight gain
  - Irritability in infants
  - Regurgitation
  - Heartburn or chest pain
  - Hematemesis
  - Dysphagia or feeding refusal
  - Apnea or ALTE
  - Wheezing or stridor
  - Hoarseness
  - Cough
  - Abnormal neck posturing (Sandifer syndrome)

- Findings
  - Esophagitis
  - Esophageal stricture
  - Barrett esophagus
  - Laryngitis
  - Recurrent pneumonia
  - Hypoproteinemia
  - Anemia

Esophageal complications

- Peptic strictures are a known complication of severe GERD, especially in patients with neurologic impairment or esophageal motility disorders.
- Children with peptic stricture usually have dysphagia but, depending on their age, they may refuse to eat solids.
- Impaction of food may be the initial presentation.
- Peptic strictures are readily seen by barium swallow and are usually located in the distal third of the esophagus.
- Endoscopy is essential to look for Barrett epithelium, the columnar esophageal epithelium seen in Barrett syndrome.
- High-dose acid-suppression therapy and balloon dilation may obviate the need for fundoplication.
- In adults, Barrett epithelium is reported to occur in up to one-half of those with stricture, but Barrett epithelium is relatively rare in children.
- Cases have been reported of children with Barrett epithelium-associated adenocarcinoma and with mid-esophageal strictures, but the prevalence in this population is not well known.
- Patients with Barrett esophagus require at least annual surveillance for dysplasia.
- Fundoplication may not reverse Barrett esophagus, and no consensus exists on optimal therapy.
- Gastrointestinal bleeding associated with hematemesis, melena, guaiac positive stools, or anemia can occur as a complication of GERD resulting from erosive esophagitis.
  - Primarily in children who are neurologically impaired

Respiratory complications

- Chronic cough, stridor, hoarseness
- Laryngopharyngeal reflux in infants
  - Feeding resistance or refusal, growth failure
  - Irritability
  - Abnormal crying
  - Sleeping problems
  - Apnea
  - Recurrent croup
  - Laryngomalacia
  - Excessive salivation

G

- Laryngopharyngeal reflux in children
  - Chronic cough
  - Dysphonia
  - Globus, sore throat
  - Halitosis
  - Nasal obstruction
  - Rhinorrhea, headache
  - Regurgitation, vomiting
  - Abdominal pain
  - Dysphagia
- Characteristic laryngoscopic findings attributed to GERD include airway erythema, edema, nodularity, granuloma, and cobblestoning.
- See table Differential Diagnosis of Hoarseness and Laryngeal Edema.
- Therapy with a PPI is usually recommended because of its acid-suppression capacity, but high doses over a prolonged period are often required because relapse after stopping therapy is common.
- Recurrent pneumonia
  - GERD may cause aspiration pneumonia and chronic pulmonary fibrosis and may occur without esophagitis.
  - Children with neurodevelopmental delay present a special diagnostic problem because oropharyngeal incoordination may result in aspiration without reflux.
  - Performing fundoplication in such a child might potentially impair esophageal clearance and increase the risk of aspiration.
  - A videofluoroscopic swallowing study or fiberendoscopic swallowing evaluation with neurosensory testing may help identify patients at risk for aspiration.

- Asthma
  - Several studies suggest that GERD may contribute to the severity of asthma.
  - Although symptoms of reflux are common in children with asthma and a high proportion of children with persistent asthma have abnormal pH monitoring, the relationship between asthma and GERD remains a challenge.
  - The prevalence rates of GERD-associated asthma are reported to be 25–75%.
  - Approximately 50% of patients with persistent asthma who test positive for GERD by pH monitoring have no or minimal symptoms of GERD.
  - In a clinical trial of asthmatic children age 5–10 years, children with normal pH monitoring were randomized to receive a PPI or no acid-suppression treatment.
  - ~25% of asthmatic children with normal pH probe studies were able to decrease asthma medication, whereas children who were not treated with acid-suppression medication continued therapy at the same dose of asthma medication.
  - Studies have shown improvement of asthma symptoms after medical therapies for GERD that included positional therapy, thickening of formula without medication, cisapride, and an H_2RA.
  - Evidence is insufficient to establish optimal medical therapy for GER in children with asthma.
    - The best test to determine whether association between asthma and GERD exists is an empiric trial with a PPI given twice a day for =3 months.
- Apnea or ALTE
  - An episode occurring in an infant that requires intervention and is characterized by a combination of apnea, cyanosis, pallor, rubor, plethora, limpness, stiffness, choking, or gagging

Differential Diagnosis of Hoarseness and Laryngeal Edema[a]

Signs, Symptoms, or Factors	Laryngopharyngeal Reflux[b]	Infection[c]	Rhinosinusitis (Postnasal Drip)[d]	Allergy[e]	Benign Vocal Fold Lesion[f]
Hoarseness	Fluctuates	Acute	Acute, chronic, or recurrent	Fluctuates	Constant
Throat pain	Common (with cough, clearing of throat)	Yes	Uncommon	No	From secondary muscle tension
Laryngeal findings	Edema, granuloma, erythema, pseudosulcus	Erythema, edema	Secretions (thick discolored), edema	Edema, clear secretions, bluish mucosa	Nodules, polyps, cysts, scars

[a] Adapted from: Ford CN. Evaluation and management of laryngopharyngeal reflux. *JAMA.* 2005;294(12):1534–1540. Copyright © 2005 American Medical Association. All rights reserved.
[b] Aggravating factors are cigarette smoke, obesity, diet, or lifestyle.
[c] Aggravating factors are systemic infection, immunosuppression.
[d] Aggravating factors are laryngopharyngeal reflux, allergy, cigarette smoke.
[e] Aggravating factors are environment and season.
[f] Aggravating factors are cigarette smoke, vocal trauma, laryngopharyngeal reflux.

- ALTEs may be caused by cardiac, central nervous system, and infectious diseases, as well as upper airway obstruction, central apnea, and GERD.

- Despite reports that GER can induce obstructive apnea, subsequent investigations in unselected patients with ALTE have not demonstrated a convincing temporal relationship between ALTE and acid reflux, apnea, or bradycardia.

- The most convincing relationship between GERD and obstructive or mixed apnea has been in infants in whom episodes occurred while the patient was awake, in the supine position, and within 1 hour of a feeding.

- No evidence indicates that clinical characteristics of an ALTE or a combined pH study with polysomnography might predict risk for further episodes or sudden death.

- No randomized studies have evaluated usefulness of esophageal pH study in infants with ALTE.

- The benefit of medical therapy of GERD to prevent subsequent ALTE is not known.

- Thickening feeds, prokinetic agents, and acid-suppression therapy are reasonable therapeutic options.

- Surgical therapy is unproven and should be considered only in infants with ALTE that is unresponsive to acid-suppression therapy known to be associated with GERD.

Other complications

- Sandifer syndrome

  - A rare complication of GERD usually seen in otherwise neurologically normal children.

  - Characterized by stereotypical, repetitive stretching and arching movements thought to be related to esophageal pain

  - These behaviors may be mistaken for atypical seizures or dystonia.

- Additional extraesophageal complications

  - Dental erosions, recurrent sinus disease, rhinopharyngitis, hoarse voice, and otitis media have been attributed to GERD.

  - All of these disorders have multiple causes, including infectious agents, immunoregulatory defects, and anatomic abnormalities.

  - Attributing the cause to GERD may oversimplify what should be a more thorough evaluation to look for other underlying causes.

G

Gastrointestinal Allergy

DEFINITION

- Food allergy is a common but often unsubstantiated diagnosis in pediatric practice.
- An adverse reaction to a food is any untoward reaction, regardless of its cause; it can be classified under 2 general categories.
  - Food allergy or hypersensitivity—an immunologic response
  - Food intolerance—a nonimmunologic response caused by:
    - Underlying congenital or acquired enzyme deficiency in which a specific dietary nutrient cannot be metabolized properly
      - Disaccharidase deficiency
      - Galactosemia
      - Hereditary fructose intolerance
    - Ingestion of a toxin in the food
      - *Staphylococcus*
      - Shellfish
      - Mushrooms
    - Ingestion of a pharmacologic agent
      - Metabisulfite in wine or salad may cause bronchospasm.
      - Wine and monosodium glutamate may cause headache.
      - Caffeine may cause arrhythmia.
- Gastrointestinal (GI) allergic manifestations can be classified as
  - Immunoglobulin (Ig) E–mediated
    - Immediate GI hypersensitivity and oral allergy syndrome
  - Mixed GI allergy syndromes (involving some IgE components and some non–IgE- or T-cell–mediated components)
    - Eosinophilic esophagitis
    - Eosinophilic gastroenteritis
  - Non–IgE-mediated or T-cell–mediated allergic GI disorders
    - Dietary protein enteropathy
    - Protein-induced enterocolitis
    - Proctitis
- In all of these conditions, response of the immune system to a specific protein leads to pathologic inflammatory changes in the GI tract.
- Eosinophilic (or allergic) GI disorders (EGIDs) are characterized by infiltration of the GI tract with eosinophils.
  - Multiple food sensitivities are often identified.
  - Disorders are also usually associated with other systemic allergies.
- EGIDs are subdivided into specific areas of the GI tract.
- There is new focus on EGIDs because of the explosion of research into eosinophilic esophagitis.

EPIDEMIOLOGY

- Cow's milk protein allergy (CMPA)
  - Prevalence
    - 2.5% of newborns have hypersensitivity to cow's milk in the first year of life.
  - Age
    - CMPA rarely develops after 1 year of age.
- Soy protein allergy
  - Prevalence
    - 30–50% of infants with CMPA may also be allergic to soy protein; however, soy protein allergy may occur without concomitant CMPA.
- EGID
  - Previously thought to be rare
  - Prevalence
    - Eosinophilic esophagitis (a subset): 4 in 10,000 persons
    - May be underestimated because all incidence studies are based on referrals
    - Increased incidence appears to result from a combination of a higher index of suspicion and a true increase in pediatric allergy.

ETIOLOGY

Food allergy

- The GI tract contains lymphoid tissue capable of mounting an immunologic response to prevent penetration of antigens across the epithelium.
  - Lymphocytes and plasma cells are present in Peyer patches and the lamina propria of the small and large intestine.
  - IgA-containing plasma cells account for only 2%.
- Aberrations in immunologic mechanisms that trigger GI allergic reactions are unknown.
- This immunologic response can elicit symptoms consistent with a GI disorder, such as
  - Diarrhea
  - Vomiting
  - Dysphagia
  - Constipation
  - GI blood loss
- Foods that account for 90% of allergic reactions in children are:
  - Cow's milk protein
    - ß-Lactoglobulin, the main whey protein, appears to be the most antigenic component.
    - Some infants can be sensitive to casein or whey protein.
  - Eggs
  - Peanut
  - Soy

- Tree nuts
- Fish
- Wheat
- Food allergy can cause:
  - Urticaria or angioedema
  - Anaphylaxis
  - Atopic dermatitis
  - Respiratory symptoms
  - GI disorder
- These allergies are much more common in infants than in older children because infants may be predisposed to protein allergy caused by
  - Enzymatic immaturity
  - Increased gut permeability
  - Relatively low secretory IgA

EGID

- Causes of EGID include:
  - Sensitization to aeroallergens
  - Autoimmune processes
  - Ingested food allergies
  - Predisposition as a result of severe reflux or cutaneous atopy
- Both IgE-dependent and IgE-independent mechanisms are believed to be involved in the pathogenesis of these conditions.
- An allergic basis for this disease in some patients is indicated by presence of:
  - Peripheral eosinophilia
  - Systemic allergies
  - Elevated IgE levels
  - Therapeutic response to steroids

SIGNS AND SYMPTOMS

CMPA

- Systemic manifestations
  - Anaphylaxis
  - Iron-deficiency anemia (caused by GI blood loss)
  - Atopic dermatitis, urticaria
  - Peripheral eosinophilia
  - Poor sleep
- Respiratory manifestations
  - Rhinitis
  - Wheezing
  - Pulmonary hemosiderosis
  - Nasopharyngeal obstruction leading to cor pulmonale

- GI manifestations
  - Vomiting or gastroesophageal reflux
  - Diarrhea, malabsorption, protein-losing enteropathy
  - Enterocolitis
  - Constipation
  - GI bleeding
  - Failure to thrive
- The GI manifestations depend on the site of predominant inflammation in the GI tract.
  - Esophagitis causes recurrent vomiting and reflux.
  - Gastritis causes vomiting, irritability or pain, and occult GI bleeding.
    - Antral gastritis is a common finding, with increased eosinophils and inflammatory cells in the antrum.
  - Enteritis causes diarrhea, malabsorption, or protein-losing enteropathy.
  - Colitis causes rectal bleeding, with blood or mucus in the stool.
  - Some infants can exhibit severe enterocolitis.
  - A significant number of these infants experience straining or discomfort with stools.

Soy protein allergy

- The clinical features of soy protein allergy are similar to those of CMPA, including:
  - Esophagitis
  - Gastritis
  - Enteritis
  - Colitis

Human milk allergy

- Breastfed infants may develop the same symptoms as those who are formula-fed.
  - Allergic colitis
    - Most common symptom
  - Esophagitis
  - Gastritis
  - Enteritis
  - Significant irritability
  - Occult blood or obvious rectal bleeding
  - Commonly asymptomatic

EGID

- Disease manifestations of EGIDs depend on the depth of GI involvement.
- Mucosal disease (more common in children)
  - Dysphagia and heartburn if limited to the esophagus
  - Vomiting if involving the stomach

G

- Protein-losing enteropathy, malabsorption, and diarrhea if involving the small bowel
- Bloody stools if involving the colon
■ Muscular disease (or submucosal)
- Prominent inflammation in the stomach antrum can lead to pyloric obstruction.
■ Serosal disease
- Causes eosinophilic ascites
- Symptoms resemble those of peritonitis.
■ Patients with eosinophilic esophagitis have variable manifestations that may include:
- Feeding disorder
- Abdominal pain
- Vomiting
- Symptoms mimicking gastroesophageal reflux in young children
  - May have normal pH probe studies and fail to respond to antireflux medications
- Symptoms may include dysphagia for solids or food impaction in older children.
■ Other EGIDs have symptoms that vary with the anatomic site of eosinophilia and the depth of eosinophilic infiltration.
- Mucosal form
  - Nausea, vomiting, colicky abdominal pain, diarrhea
  - Occult blood loss, iron deficiency anemia
  - Protein losing enteropathy leading to hypoalbuminemia
  - Failure to thrive/grow
- Muscular (transmural) form
  - Obstructive symptoms, mimicking pyloric stenosis or thickening of the gastric outlet
- Serosal form
  - Eosinophilic ascites
- Approximately 75% of affected patients have peripheral eosinophilia (with all 3 types)
■ If the stomach is involved, patients may have evidence of delayed gastric emptying, including nausea and bloating or vomiting, a symptom suggestive of pyloric obstructive disease.

DIFFERENTIAL DIAGNOSIS

■ CMPA
- Other causes of rectal bleeding
  - Rectal bleeding or guaiac-positive stools are probably the most common symptoms in infants with formula sensitivity.
  - Allergy is the most common cause of rectal bleeding among infants <6 months of age.
- Celiac disease
  - Differentiation is made by the absence of antiendomysial or anti–tissue transglutaminase antibodies in CMPA.

■ EGIDs
- Eosinophilia can be associated with:
  - Parasitic infestations
  - Nutritional deficiencies
  - Inflammatory bowel disease
  - Neoplasms

DIAGNOSTIC APPROACH

■ In patients with specific food allergies, removing specific food allergens from the diet ameliorates symptoms.
- Reintroduction of the allergen leads to recurrence of symptoms.
■ CMPA and soy protein allergy are the most clearly defined allergies in infants.
■ In patients with refractory reflux food allergy or formula sensitivity should always be considered because these 2 conditions may coexist.
■ CMPA
- GI symptoms predominate in many patients.
- In others, anaphylaxis or pulmonary symptoms occur.
- Infants with severe atopic dermatitis should also be evaluated for possible CMPA and other food allergy.
■ EGID has no classic symptoms; it can go undetected for several years.
■ Whether these entities are variants of a similar disease process or distinctly different conditions remains to be solved.
■ The diagnosis of EGID is based on clinical features and laboratory findings; endoscopy is essential to confirm a diagnosis
- Collaboration with a pediatric gastroenterologist is necessary.
- A pediatric allergist can help direct specific testing for allergy.
■ For eosinophilic esophagitis, diagnosis is based on:
- Patient or family history of allergy
- Evaluation to rule out reflux
- Typical eosinophilic infiltration of the esophagus on the biopsy specimen
- Allergy testing

LABORATORY FINDINGS

■ In formula allergy, the infant may not have peripheral eosinophilia.
■ IgE measurement and radioallergosorbent tests (RASTs) to detect IgE antibodies specific for milk and soy proteins
- Usually negative, suggesting that the immunologic mechanism occurs by means of a non-IgE (T-cell–mediated) mechanism.
- A significant number of these patients have a concomitant transient hypogammaglobulinemia or hypoalbuminemia caused by protein-losing enteropathy.

- Treatment of the milk or soy or other food allergy results in normalization of serum proteins.
- An elevated IgE level or positive RAST result with these foods at this age in most cases suggests long-term rather than self-limited sensitivity.

■ EGIDs

- Half of patients have peripheral blood eosinophilia, elevated IgE levels, and an atopic history.
- Hypereosinophilic syndromes are characterized by infiltration of many organs with eosinophils.
- All EGIDs share a common feature of eosinophils infiltrating the GI tract, without involvement of extraintestinal organs.
- Eosinophilic esophagitis is the only EGID for which normal and abnormal eosinophil counts are established.
- Because the mechanism of allergic GI diseases is probably on a spectrum between immediate hypersensitivity and cell-mediated immunity, the value of any single test is variable.
  - Allergy testing can include skin prick tests, RASTs, and patch testing.
  - Peripheral eosinophilia occurs, and an elevated IgE level is a variable finding; absence does not rule out eosinophilic esophagitis or other eosinophilic gastroenteropathies.
- In other EGIDs
  - Laboratory studies may include hypoalbuminemia and low immunoglobulin levels caused by malabsorption and protein-losing enteropathy.
  - If the patient has long-term blood loss, laboratory studies may show iron-deficiency anemia.

IMAGING

■ Eosinophilic esophagitis

- X-ray studies, including esophagraphy, may show thickened folds or a narrowing of the esophagus.

■ Other EGIDs

- X-ray studies, including esophagraphy or upper GI tract study:
  - May show thickened folds caused by edema in the esophagus or stomach
  - May show gastric outlet obstruction
  - Small-bowel follow-through may show nodular small bowel.

DIAGNOSTIC PROCEDURES

■ Biopsy

- The hallmark of GI biopsy results is an increased eosinophil count.

- >20 eosinophils per high-power field on a rectal biopsy specimen is indicative of an allergic cause for colitis; however, any inflammatory lesion of the GI tract appears to attract eosinophils.
- In CMPA, duodenal biopsy specimens reveal patchy changes, ranging from normal mucosa to flat gut lesions.
- Although scattered eosinophils are normal throughout the rest of the GI tract, they are pathologic when seen in esophagus.
  - Esophageal eosinophilia in reflux is mild (<15–20 eosinophils per high-power field) and is usually limited to the distal esophagus.
  - In eosinophilic esophagitis, eosinophilia is severe (>20 eosinophils per high-power field) and can involve most of the length of the esophagus.
- If allergic gastroenteropathy involves the small bowel, the lesions are in a patchy distribution, ranging from areas of normal mucosa to a flat villus lesion.
  - Eosinophilic infiltration may be mild or marked.
  - Gastric abnormalities, found more commonly in the antrum, have been described as being consistent in the mucosal form of the disease.
  - The stomach shows evidence of gastritis, with destruction and regeneration of gastric glands and surface epithelium, and eosinophilic infiltration usually is marked.
- In endoscopy of eosinophilic esophagitis
  - Mucosa may appear normal on gross examination.
  - Suggestive findings are often apparent, especially the classic ringed or furrowed esophagus and white exudates (seen exclusively in eosinophilic esophagitits).
- Biopsy samples of eosinophilic esophagitis help quantify eosinophilic infiltration and inflammation if mucosal disease is present.
- In other EGIDs, findings may be confusing because there is no consensus on histopathologic criteria.
  - The small intestine can reveal both normal mucosa (with or without eosinophilic infiltration) and a flat villus lesion.
  - In the stomach, a gastric antral biopsy specimen is of diagnostic value in the mucosal form of the disease and is usually positive, revealing evidence of gastritis with marked eosinophilic infiltration.

TREATMENT APPROACH

■ Treatment of food allergy includes primary prevention to prevent sensitization to proteins.

■ See Prevention for the AAP recommendations.

SPECIFIC TREATMENTS

Infant formulas

- Once a specific protein allergy is suspected or diagnosed, the infant should initially be fed a hypoallergenic formula.
- The choice of formula depends on the formula used at the time of diagnosis.
- Nonstandard infant formulas
  - Soy protein with L-methionine
    - Bright Beginnings Soy, Good Start Supreme Soy, Isomil Advance, Enfamil Prosobee
  - Partially hydrolyzed whey may help reduce the risk of CMPA but should not be used as treatment of existing allergy symptoms.
    - Good Start Supreme
  - Partially hydrolyzed casein, partially hydrolyzed whey
    - Gentlease
  - Casein hydrolysate (hypoallergenic) if the patient is taking a milk-based or soy-based formula
    - Alimentum, Nutramigen, Pregestimil
  - Amino acid base
    - Neocate, Elecare
- A comparison of partial versus extensive hydrolysates appears in the table Soy vs Partial vs Extensive Hydrolysates vs L-Amino Acid Formulas.
- Allergy may last as little as 3–12 months; therefore, this period is one of trial and error as the patient is gradually retried on the previously proved allergen.
- Approximately 10–15% of infants given casein hydrolysate formula still have a persistent sensitivity, as evidenced by continual guaiac-positive stools or overt GI bleeding.
  - Many respond to the L-amino acid formulas, such as Neocate and Elecare.

- These formulas are expensive and should be used only when persistent sensitivity to all other formulas is well documented.
- Milk or milk products from animals other than cows have been used anecdotally, eg, sheep's or goat's milk.
  - Risk of possible cross-reactivity between cow's milk proteins and sheep's or goat's milk proteins
  - Goat's milk is folate deficient.

Human milk allergy

- Treatment in infants who are sensitive to mother's milk involves persuading mothers to avoid cow's milk products.
- Not all infants will respond to this measure.
  - Accidental maternal ingestion of milk proteins
  - Some other factor
- Preventing many breastfeeding mothers from eliminating foods from their diet, which can cause significant maternal weight loss, can sometimes become extremely difficult.
- Mothers should be told that most infants who show sensitivity to foods the mother is eating do not have severe disease and breastfeeding can be continued unless symptoms are significant.
- Mothers who exclude multiple foods from their diets should consider vitamin and calcium supplementation.
- Use of a hypoallergenic formula may be worth a trial to determine whether the infant's symptoms disappear.

EGID

- If foods test positive on a combination of tests for immediate or delayed hypersensitivity and food challenges, these foods should be eliminated from the diet.
- The most common foods implicated are, in order: milk, egg, soy, corn, and wheat.
  - Several foods may be found to cause symptoms.

Soy vs Partial vs Extensive Hydrolysates vs L-Amino Acid Formulas

Category	Soy	Partially Hydrolyzed[a]	Extensively Hydrolyzed[b]	L-Amino Acid
Decreases protein sensitization	No	Yes	Yes	Yes
Treatment for established CMPA	No	No	Yes	Yes
Type of formula	Routine	Routine	Specialty	Specialty
Cost	Comparable with standard cow's milk	Comparable with standard cow's milk formula	3 to 4 times more costly than standard	Even more expensive then extensively hydrolyzed formula
Palatability	Comparable with standard	Comparable with standard	Less than standard	Less than standard

Abbreviation: CMPA, cow's milk protein allergy.
[a] Partially hydrolyzed whey.
[b] Extensively hydrolyzed casein.

- Dietary elimination of these allergens may alleviate most symptoms.
  - Some patients require complete dietary elimination with an L-amino acid–based formula.
  - An advantage of dietary management is a good rate of cure.
  - Restrictive diets may be difficult for children and may create social and behavioral problems.
  - Exclusive reliance on specialized formulas can be very expensive.
- For patients who cannot follow a restrictive diet, corticosteroid therapy may be required intermittently.
  - Quickly improves symptoms and normalizes tissue on biopsy specimens.
  - Steroids cannot be used on a long-term basis, and esophageal eosinophils and symptoms can recur after discontinuing therapy.
  - Topical steroids, such as swallowed fluticasone propionate, improve symptoms and histologic findings.
    - Eradication of eosinophils in the esophagus is less consistent with topical therapy, and symptoms and baseline histologic values return on discontinuation.
    - Topical treatment is associated with esophageal candidiasis.
- Oral cromolyn sodium (Gastrochrome®) has not been proven helpful.
- Leukotriene receptor antagonists improve symptoms but do not change histologic values.
- Symptomatic strictures resulting in food impactions or severe dysphagia may require endoscopic dilatation.
- Pyloric obstructive disease may require surgery.
- If patients have other symptoms of allergy or atopy, these should be addressed as well.

WHEN TO ADMIT
- Anaphylaxis
- Severe malnutrition

WHEN TO REFER
- Poor weight gain
- Immediate GI response after particular food or foods
- Incomplete response to exclusion or elemental diet
- Multiple food allergies
- Multiple allergic symptoms
- Malabsorption or protein-losing enteropathy
- Gastroesophageal reflux disease recalcitrant to appropriate therapy

COMPLICATIONS
- CMPA
  - Profuse vomiting and or diarrhea can lead to shock, anemia, and methemoglobinemia.
  - Children with enterocolitis may be predisposed to a severe rare form of enterocolitis to solid-food antigens later in life.
    - They may develop severe reactions to food proteins considered to be of low allergenicity.

PROGNOSIS
- CMPA
  - Previously, physicians counseled families that infants with CMPA would outgrow it by 2 years of age.
  - Later studies revealed that allergy may persist in:
    - 72% at age 2 years
    - 44% at age 4 years
    - 32% at age 6 years
  - Other studies are less pessimistic.
    - 44% with persistent symptoms at 1 year
    - 33% at 2 years
    - 23% at 3 years
  - Patients who have longer persistence of symptoms have:
    - Symptoms later after initial introduction of milk
    - Higher frequency of allergic disease
    - Multiple food allergies
- EGID
  - Evidence indicates that EGIDs are lifelong conditions with remissions and exacerbations, often requiring careful dietary manipulation and intermittent steroid therapy.
  - Preliminary data suggest that younger adolescents go through a phase in which they are much better able to tolerate foods to which they were previously sensitive.
  - If the EGID produces significant malabsorption, osteoporosis may occur.
  - Natural history of eosinophilic esophagitis remains unclear.
    - Among adults with initial misdiagnoses of reflux, some develop strictures requiring dilation.
    - The esophagus can be friable, tearing with the mere passage of an endoscope.
    - Possible evolution to Barrett esophagus remains to be studied.

PREVENTION
- AAP 2008 Recommendations for Prevention of Allergy
  - Nutritional interventions are largely limited to infants at high risk of developing allergy (ie, infants with at least 1 first degree relative with allergic disease).

G

- There is "evidence" that compared to intact cow's milk protein formula, exclusive breastfeeding for at least 4 months prevents or delays the occurrence of atopic dermatitis, cow's milk allergy, and wheezing.

- There is "modest evidence" that atopic disease may be delayed or prevented by the use of extensively or partially hydrolyzed formulas compared with intact cow's milk formula, particularly for atopic dermatitis.

- There is "little" or "no current convincing" evidence that the timing (delaying) of introduction of complementary foods beyond 4 to 6 months of age prevents the occurrence of atopic disease.

- There is "no convincing" evidence for the use of soy formula for allergy prevention.

- Current evidence does not support maternal dietary restrictions during pregnancy or lactation.

G

Gastrointestinal Hemorrhage

DEFINITION

- Bleeding at any point along the length of the gastrointestinal (GI) tract, from the mouth to the anus
- Bleeding may be arterial, venous, or both.

MECHANISM

- A large vascular supply to the GI tract accounts for an appreciable fraction of cardiac output, especially after eating meals.
- Most bleeding is slow and involves oozing from the mucosal surface.
- Acute GI bleeding
  - May occur with or without symptoms
  - Can originate in either the upper or the lower GI tract
  - Massive bleeding can result from lesions involving high-pressure arteries or a large, engorged venous plexus.
- Chronic GI bleeding
  - Usually slow and intermittent

HISTORY

- The physician must quickly assess severity to expedite appropriate resuscitative measures.
- The physician must consider the most likely causes.
  - Does the problem require immediate surgery?
  - Does the problem require medical evaluation and management?
- The workup is based on:
  - Patient's age and history
  - Patient's clinical appearance
  - Physician's familiarity with the patient
- A detailed history may help determine the location and duration of the bleeding.
- A family history of polyps, bleeding disorders, or GI diseases is important.
- Presence or absence of abdominal pain
  - If present: location, severity, and quality
- Associated systemic symptoms (eg, with hemolytic-uremic syndrome [HUS] or inflammatory bowel disease [IBD])
- Altered mental status or lethargy
- Suggestion of surgical etiology (eg, Meckel diverticulum, intussusception, volvulus)
- Color of the stool
- Description of emesis
  - Whether a change has occurred in either in the preceding days or weeks
- Vomiting that progresses from bile-stained to bloody
  - Intestinal obstruction (volvulus, intussusception, necrotizing enterocolitis [NEC])
  - Mallory-Weiss tears

- Bloody diarrhea
  - Infectious enteritis
  - Food allergy
  - IBD
  - May precede HUS
- Painless lower GI bleeding
  - If substantial
    - Meckel diverticulum
    - GI vascular anomalies
  - If less severe
    - Polyps
    - Lymphonodular hyperplasia
- Fever
  - Common in infectious or inflammatory disorders
- Arthritis and rash are seen with Henoch-Schönlein purpura (HSP).
- Neonatal history should focus on risk factors for NEC or varices.
  - Umbilical vein catheters
  - Liver disease
  - Birth asphyxia
- Sexual activity or abuse involving anal penetration should alert the clinician to anal and rectal trauma.

PHYSICAL EXAM

- A complete and systematic examination should be performed because clues to the diagnosis may be present in any organ system.
- General appearance and vital signs can be helpful in determining duration of bleeding.
  - Acute GI bleeding may occur with or without signs of shock, depending on the amount of blood loss.
  - Slow, chronic bleeding allows time for physiologic changes.
    - Compensatory tachycardia
    - Orthostasis
    - Decreased pulse pressure
    - Iron-deficiency anemia
    - Fatigue
    - Pallor
- The nose and mouth should be examined for bleeding lesions or burns.
- The abdomen, perineum, and rectum should be thoroughly examined.
  - Abdominal examination to assess:
    - Tenderness
    - Bowel sounds

– Masses

– Hepatosplenomegaly

– Signs of chronic liver disease

■ Telangiectasias

■ Jaundice

■ Hepatosplenomegaly

■ Prominent abdominal venous pattern

- Rectal examination, with special attention to the perianal region

• Skin tags

• Abscesses

• Fissures

• Bleeding points

• Hemorrhoids (uncommon)

• Character and color of stool

• Occult blood on guaiac testing

• Palpation for polyps and pelvic masses

- Digital rectal examination should follow in an attempt to discover:

• Anal fissures

• Rectal polyps

• Hemorrhoids

- Sigmoidoscopy for children who have persistent rectal bleeding to identify polyps or mucosal lesions

• Blood originating from above the reach of the sigmoidoscope indicates the need to proceed with other diagnostic studies.

- Skin

• Eczema

– Possible association with food allergy

• Skin lesions, such as purpura and petechiae

– Bleeding disorders

– HSP

– HUS

DIFFERENTIAL DIAGNOSIS

Newborns

- Usually appears as rectal bleeding or blood suctioned from the stomach during routine postnatal care

- In many instances, no lesion is readily discernible, and bleeding resolves spontaneously and permanently.

- Common causes of GI bleeding in the first 24 hours of life include:

• Maternal blood swallowed during delivery

• Local trauma after nasogastric suctioning

- Premature infants and newborns who have low Apgar scores are at increased risk for gastric ulcerations and erosions that can bleed.

• These lesions rarely are primary.

• Usually result from asphyxia associated with a difficult delivery, a cardiac lesion, or sepsis

- Hemorrhagic disease of the newborn

• Inherited deficits of coagulation factors or delay in administration of postnatal vitamin K occasionally produces GI bleeding.

• More commonly, these disorders show as diffuse bleeding from venipuncture sites.

- NEC usually manifests as lower GI bleeding with bilious vomiting, abdominal distention, and lethargy.

• Symptoms usually occur after the first feeding but may be delayed for a few weeks.

• Most common in premature infants

• Occasionally occurs in stressed full-term infants

• Up to 5% of neonates in intensive care units develop NEC.

• Overall mortality may be as high as 30%.

• Complications include sepsis and shock.

- Intrinsic structural lesions can cause lower GI bleeding.

• Duplication

– A tubular structure lined with normal GI mucosa adjacent to the true intestine can be present anywhere along the GI tract.

– Can cause lower GI bleeding, either acute or chronic, along with abdominal distention and vomiting.

– Unrepaired duplications may lead to obstruction, volvulus, or perforation.

• Volvulus or malrotation

– A volvulus or malrotation of the GI tract should be suspected in any infant who has abdominal pain, bilious vomiting, and melena.

– Because these symptoms and signs are often unreliable, the diagnosis should be considered in any newborn who vomits and has guaiac-positive stools.

• Vascular malformation

– Must be considered in the evaluation for painless rectal bleeding

■ Hemangiomas

■ Other vascular lesions, such as hereditary hemorrhagic telangiectasia (Rendu-Osler-Weber syndrome)

– The most common form is the larger cavernous hemangioma.

■ Either polypoid or diffuse

■ Extends several centimeters through the submucosa of the small or large intestine

- The diffuse type usually involves the large bowel, specifically the rectum.
- Cutaneous vascular malformations are often present but may require scrupulous searching to detect.
- Can occur anywhere along the GI tract
- Produce slow or diffuse lower GI bleeding
- The bleeding is usually painless.
- The color of the blood in the stool varies, depending on the level of the lesion.
- Vascular malformations may be associated with cutaneous hemangiomas or cardiac defects.
- Milk protein allergy or soy protein allergy
  - Can begin as early as the first week of life
  - Exhibits as:
    - Severe diarrhea
    - Gross blood in the stool
    - Abdominal distention
    - Vomiting
  - Older infants may have occult lower GI bleeding and mucus in the stool.
  - The diagnosis is made by clinical response to withdrawal and rechallenge with the offending protein.
- Infectious enteritis
  - Rare in the newborn
  - May appear later in the first month of life
  - In very young infants, bacterial gastroenteritis, especially that caused by *Salmonella*, can cause bloody diarrhea with or without fever.
  - 8–13% of infants may have associated bacteremia.
- Anal fissure
  - Suggested by bright red blood streaks on the surface of the stool
  - Often associated with hard stools
  - The most common cause of rectal bleeding
  - Visual inspection of the anus usually confirms the diagnosis.

Infants and young children

Upper GI bleeding

- Upper GI bleeding in the young child usually is caused by mucosal lesions in the esophagus and the stomach.

Esophageal bleeding

- Often slow and occult (without hematemesis), manifesting with signs of anemia or guaiac-positive stools
  - Acid reflux
    - Newborns who have persistent or severe gastroesophageal reflux can develop esophagitis.
  - Viral infection, or fungal infection particularly with immunocompromise.

- Caustic ingestion severe enough to burn the esophageal mucosa can result in painful swallowing, drooling, oral burns, and hematemesis.
- Esophageal foreign body
  - As infants become more mobile and dexterous, they are at higher risk for foreign body and toxic ingestions.
  - Coins and small toys, when lodged in the esophagus, can cause drooling, vomiting, and chest pain.
  - Persistent or unrecognized esophageal foreign bodies
    - Lead to edema and erosion of the esophagus
    - May cause hematemesis
- Mallory-Weiss tear
  - A rent at the gastroesophageal junction that may result from forceful or prolonged vomiting
  - The emesis becomes streaked with bright-red blood and may develop into coffee-ground emesis if the tear persists.

Gastroesophageal varices

- Variceal bleeding ranges from slow, persistent oozing to acute massive hematemesis.
- Physical examination usually reveals signs of portal hypertension, such as enlarged liver or spleen, or both.
- Most cases result from the cavernous transformation of the extrahepatic portion of the portal vein, which has been associated with:
  - Umbilical vessel catheterization
  - Omphalitis
  - Neonatal conditions associated with hypoxia, prolonged jaundice, or sepsis

Gastritis

- Infectious
- Medications (eg, nonsteroidal antiinflammatory drugs, corticosteroids)

Lower GI bleeding

- The differential diagnosis is broad.
- Polyps
  - Juvenile polyps
    - Most common cause of lower GI bleeding in 3- to 7-year-old children
    - Typically located in the colon
    - Simple, solitary, benign hamartomatous lesions
    - May irritate the GI tract, causing intermittent, painless, bright-red rectal bleeding
    - Many of these polyps autoamputate if left alone and are passed with the stool.
    - Most polyps are located within 25 cm of the anus.

– They are easily identified by:
  ■ Digital examination
  ■ Air-contrast barium enema
  ■ Sigmoidoscopy
– Can be removed with snare electrocautery
- Adenomatous polyps
  – Adenomatous polyps are premalignant tumors.
  – May transform into cancer over an average of 10 years
  – May produce rectal bleeding as early as infancy
  – Managed differently from juvenile polyps
  – Associated with familial polyposis and Gardner syndrome
  – Juvenile polyposis coli (JPC) is suggested by the presence of 5–10 juvenile polyps; ≥10 polyps is considered diagnostic.
    ■ JPC occurs in approximately 10% of patients with colonic polyps.
    ■ Associated with anemia, right-colon polyps, and adenomas

Meckel diverticulum
■ A remnant of the omphalomesenteric duct
■ Found within 2 feet of the ileocecal valve
■ Present in up to 2% of the population
■ The acid secreted by ectopic gastric mucosa, which is usually present in diverticula that bleed, causes peptic ulceration of the ileal mucosa.
  - Typically occurs in children <3 years
  - Causes painless, maroon- or red-colored lower GI bleeding
  - Typically, the bleeding is severe enough to cause the hemoglobin level to decrease to approximately 8 g/dL.

Intussusception
■ Telescoping of an intestinal segment
■ Typically seen in children 6–24 months of age
■ Often idiopathic
■ Usually involves invagination of the distal ileum through the ileocecal valve into the colon
■ Older children with intussusception and those with multiple recurrences may have pathologic lesions that serve as lead points (eg, Meckel diverticulum, polyp, tumor).
■ Classic presentation begins with intermittent, severe, crampy abdominal pain, with vomiting shortly thereafter.
■ As the intussusception progresses, lethargy or paradoxical irritability develops.
■ Guaiac-positive stools
  - Seen as the bowel becomes ischemic
  - May progress to the passage of red bloody mucus, classically referred to as *currant jelly stools*

■ Complications include:
  - Intestinal perforation
  - Peritonitis
  - Significant bleeding

Lymphonodular hyperplasia
■ May cause painless, blood-streaked stools
■ Usually seen in children <6 years
■ May be associated with food allergy
■ Diagnosis is made by endoscopic examination and histologic confirmation.

Infectious enterocolitis
■ Symptoms range from mild diarrhea to fever, abdominal cramping, and watery or mucoid stools (or both forms) with or without blood.
■ *Salmonella, Shigella, Yersinia,* and *Campylobacter* are the most common bacterial causes of bloody diarrhea.
■ Pseudomembranous colitis, caused by *Clostridium difficile,* also causes fever, diarrhea, abdominal cramping, and bloody stools.
■ The child often has a history of recent hospitalization and antimicrobial therapy.
■ Onset of symptoms can be delayed for weeks.
■ A variety of parasites, such as amoebae, can cause bloody diarrhea.

Systemic diseases
■ HSP: purpura with arthritis, hematuria, abdominal cramping, and bloody stool
■ HUS: prodrome of hemorrhagic colitis, followed by thrombocytopenia, hemolytic anemia, and renal disease
  - Most commonly caused by Shigatoxin-producing *Escherichia coli* O157:H7

Other causes
■ Milk protein allergy, anal fissures, and congenital GI structural anomalies can also occur in this age group.

Older children and adolescents
■ Nasopharyngeal bleeding
■ Esophagitis
■ Mallory-Weiss tear
■ Gastroesophageal varices
■ Gastritis
  - Infectious
  - Medications (eg, nonsteroidal antiinflammatory drugs, corticosteroids, tetracycline)
■ Peptic ulcer disease
  - Can occur at any age, but more common in the older child and adolescent
  - Symptoms usually begin with epigastric or periumbilical pain accompanied by nausea.

- GI bleeding is evident in approximately 50% of children as either hematemesis or melena.
- *Helicobacter pylori*
  - Bacteria found in the gastric mucous layer or adherent to the epithelial lining of the stomach causally associated with ulcers
  - Infection is common worldwide.
  - In areas of high prevalence, most children are infected by 10 years of age.
  - Infected children usually are asymptomatic and only occasionally develop disease in childhood.
- Duplication
- Vascular malformation
- Polyps
  - Juvenile (see above)
  - Adenomatous (see above)
- Infectious enterocolitis (see above)
- Inflammatory bowel disease
  - May appear in the adolescent age group as episodes of bloody diarrhea, cramping, and tenesmus
  - The course may be atypical in children, making the diagnosis difficult.
  - The diagnosis is suggested by:
    - Growth failure
    - Weight loss
    - Anemia
    - Evidence of recurrent bouts of GI bleeding
  - Abdominal pain, fever, and weight loss suggest inflammatory bowel disease.
- Systemic diseases (HSP, HUS)
- Vascular malformation (see above)
- Meckel diverticulum
- Hemorrhoids
- Anal fissure

Cirrhosis and chronic liver disease

- Intrahepatic causes of cirrhosis, leading to portal hypertension, that may first show during childhood, include
  - Wilson disease (after 6 years of age)
  - α_1-Antitrypsin deficiency
  - Biliary cirrhosis
  - Metabolic, infectious, or anatomic forms of chronic liver disease
- These chronic liver diseases also may be associated with coagulopathy and thrombocytopenia from the hypersplenism that usually accompanies them.
- If the cause of the portal hypertension is extrahepatic, bleeding may be tolerated remarkably well.

- In patients with cirrhotic liver disease, bleeding may lead to rapid hepatic decompensation.

False bleeding

- Red color in the stool often is assumed to be blood; however, many other substances cause change in stool color.
  - Foods that contain a high concentration of red pigments, such as tomatoes, cranberries, beets, and red fruit juices and gelatin (Jell-O)
  - Red-colored medications, such as acetaminophen and amoxicillin, can be passed in the stools, especially if diarrhea is present.
  - Spinach, licorice, iron, and bismuth (Pepto-Bismol) often lead to dark, black stools, which can be confused with true melena.
- In infants, *Serratia marcescens* can cause red diaper syndrome as a result of the formation of red pigment in soiled diapers stored for >1 day.

Nongastrointestinal sources of bleeding

Infants

- An infant may swallow maternal blood either during delivery or when breastfeeding if the mother has bleeding nipples.
  - The Apt-Downey test is helpful in differentiating maternal blood from infant blood.
    - 1 part of the bloody stool (or gastric aspirate) is mixed with 5 parts of water to lyse the erythrocytes.
    - After the mixture is centrifuged, 1 mL of 0.2 normal sodium hydroxide is added to the supernatant hemoglobin solution.
    - After 2 minutes, fetal hemoglobin, which resists the alkaline reduction, remains pink, whereas maternal hemoglobin turns yellow-brown.
    - Melena contains denatured hemoglobin and therefore cannot be used for the Apt-Downey test.
- Vaginal bleeding in a newborn with estrogen withdrawal may be mistaken for rectal bleeding.

Older children

- Swallowed blood usually is the result of nosebleeds or bleeding mouth lesions.
  - This nasopharyngeal bleeding can mimic hematemesis or melena.
- Pulmonary hemorrhage
  - Rare in children
  - May exhibit acutely as hematemesis
  - May exhibit more chronically as melena and anemia
- In the menstruating teenager, vaginal blood may affect the accuracy of stool guaiac testing.
- The possibility of blood being added to the stool by a caretaker suggests Munchausen syndrome by proxy.

G

LABORATORY EVALUATION

- Laboratory testing should focus on:
  - Determining the amount and duration of the bleeding
  - Assessing for coagulopathy
  - Evaluating for other laboratory abnormalities that may be associated with the underlying disease process
- Initial laboratory studies
  - Complete blood count with reticulocyte count
    - Hemoglobin determination can help assess the degree of blood loss.
    - Acute bleeding may not decrease the hemoglobin level until intravascular equilibration has taken place.
    - The leukocyte count may be elevated in infectious colitis.
  - Coagulation studies
    - Prothrombin time may be elevated as a sign of a bleeding disorder or as result of abnormalities in liver synthetic function.
    - Partial prothrombin time
    - Platelet count
  - Serum chemistries
    - To assess renal function
    - An elevated blood urea nitrogen level may result from increased intestinal absorption of blood with long-standing upper GI bleeding.
  - Liver function tests for suspected liver disease
  - Blood type and screen
    - If patient has significant bleeding or a low hemoglobin level and transfusion may be needed
  - Stool specimen
    - If bloody diarrhea is present
    - For culture, if appropriate
    - For ova and parasites, if appropriate
  - Stool guaiac
    - The most common test
    - Highly sensitive
    - Uses the peroxidase activity of hemoglobin to catalyze a color change on a test card or paper strip
    - Can identify even trace amounts of blood
    - Foods that have peroxidase activity may cause false-positive results if eaten within 3 days of testing.
      - Red meat
      - Liver
      - Processed meats
      - Raw fruits and vegetables, especially melon, turnip, radishes, and horseradish
    - High vitamin C intake interferes with the peroxidase reaction and can cause false-negative results.
    - Outdated guaiac cards and prolonged storage may affect the accuracy of the test.
    - Stool guaiac cards are not accurate for testing emesis for the presence of blood because gastric acid can affect the reaction that causes the color change.
  - Serologic tests
    - *H pylori* IgG antibodies
    - IBD serologies

IMAGING

- Imaging studies are needed in most children with GI bleeding:
  - To locate the source of the bleeding
  - To confirm a suspected diagnosis
- The type of study is chosen on the basis of:
  - The child's age
  - Clinical presentation
  - Possible diagnosis
- Radiography
  - Plain radiographic films:
    - Usually are nonspecific
    - Usually require additional imaging to confirm a diagnosis
  - 2-view (flat and upright) abdominal radiographs will reveal:
    - Signs of obstruction or calcifications
    - Air-fluid levels
    - Dilated bowel loops
  - Some specific radiographic findings include:
    - Pneumatosis intestinalis in NEC
    - Intestinal obstruction with absence of gas in the right colon in intussusception
    - In volvulus/malrotation, the radiograph may show loops of small bowel overriding the liver shadow, with paucity of air in the GI tract distal to the volvulus.
- Barium studies
  - For identification of:
    - Intestinal foreign bodies
    - Polyps
    - Lymphonodular hyperplasia
    - IBD
  - An upper GI series, barium enema, or both are sometimes needed to confirm the diagnosis of volvulus/malrotation.
  - Barium swallow has poor sensitivity in esophagitis.
  - Barium enema or upper GI series with small-bowel follow-through should be the last studies performed.
    - They make use of arteriography, isotope scans, and endoscopy impossible for several days thereafter.

- Confirmation of intussusception, followed by hydrostatic reduction with barium or air enema, is successful in approximately 70–80% of cases, even in those with symptoms for >24 hours.
- Ultrasonography
  - The use of screening ultrasonography has decreased unnecessary enemas for clinically suspected intussusception.
    - Diagnosis can be confirmed by identification of the layering of intestinal mucosa as a bulls-eye or coiled spring lesion.
- Color Doppler ultrasonography
  - Increasingly useful as a diagnostic aid in both intussusception and malrotation
  - Usefulness depends on the skill of the operator.
- Computed tomography
  - Occasionally helpful in defining related anatomic features if the child is hemodynamically stable and either cooperative or sedated
  - Midgut volvulus also may be diagnosed by computed tomography or ultrasonography.
    - Duodenal dilatation
    - Fixed midline bowel
    - Wrapping of the bowel and the superior mesenteric vein around the superior mesenteric artery (whirlpool sign)
- Angiography
  - For severe, life-threatening bleeding
  - Can be both diagnostic and therapeutic, depending on the ability to embolize the bleeding vessels
  - Limited sensitivity in detecting slow or past bleeding, so best performed when bleeding is active
  - Selective arteriography or digital subtraction angiography may aid in demonstrating vascular malformation.
- Arteriography
  - If the bleeding is not immediately life threatening
  - Can demonstrate bleeding that occurs at a rate ≥0.5 mL/min
- Radionuclide scanning
  - For children with persistent, active bleeding who are clinically stable
  - Often can identify the source of an acute, ongoing bleed by pinpointing accumulation of an isotope at the bleeding site
  - Sulfur-colloid isotopic study
    - More sensitive and less invasive than arteriography
    - Can demonstrate active bleeding at rates as low as 0.05–0.1 mL/min
    - Demonstrates active bleeding by using a tracer with a very short half-life

- Isotope is extracted rapidly so that background radioactivity is low.
- In small infants, a large uptake of the isotope by the liver may mask the right upper quadrant.
- The bleeding site may be determined with technetium-99-pertechnetate–labeled red blood cells.
  - Labeled cells may remain in circulation for more than a day and allow repeated imaging to locate the site of intermittent bleeding.
- An isotope-labeled red blood cell infusion has a lower contrast ratio but is better at detecting slower or intermittent bleeds than a sulfur-colloid isotopic scan.
- A Meckel scan uses technetium-99 pertechnetate, which is secreted by ectopic gastric mucosa, to identify the diverticulum.
  - The test is fairly sensitive, but only during active bleeding.
  - A repeat scan is sometimes necessary.
- If the rate of bleeding does not permit enough time to perform these studies, vasopressin or octreotide may be administered parenterally in an attempt to control the bleeding and to stabilize the patient.

DIAGNOSTIC PROCEDURES

- Upper GI fiberoptic endoscopy can establish diagnosis in 75%–90% of patients.
  - Is unlikely to achieve adequate visualization if bleeding is massive and cannot be controlled with saline lavage.
  - Gastric ulceration is diagnosed in newborns by radiography or upper GI endoscopy
- Gastroduodenoscopy to determine source and type of lesion present if bleeding ceases.
- Colonoscopy and biopsy usually confirm diagnosis of inflammatory bowel disease.
- Esophagoscopy and pH probe manometry are used to diagnose gastroesophageal reflux.
- *H pylori* infection is diagnosed by culture of biopsy specimens from the stomach and duodenum.

TREATMENT APPROACH

- The approach to acute massive GI bleeding must be the same as that in any other emergency.
  - Obtain the pertinent historical information.
  - Perform a brief but adequate examination.
  - Stabilize the patient clinically.
  - Arrive at a working diagnosis
  - Institute appropriate therapy or consultations.
- Massive upper GI bleeding may lead to vomiting, aspiration, and airway obstruction requiring stabilization of the airway with endotracheal intubation.

- Administration of oxygen is always indicated.
- Assess adequacy of circulation by evaluating:
  - Peripheral perfusion
  - Quality of pulses
  - Capillary refill time
- In children, the initial response to hypovolemic shock is tachycardia.
- In acute bleeding, adequate blood pressure can be maintained with blood loss of up to 30% without replacement.
- Prompt surgical intervention is required:
  - In vascular compromise of the intestine
  - When the rate of bleeding is excessive and uncontrollable by more conservative methods
- Conservative measures control most acute episodes of GI bleeding relatively easily.
  - Patients who eventually require surgical intervention can usually undergo surgery electively at a later time.

SPECIFIC TREATMENT

Emergency management

Immediate response

- Tachycardia and capillary refill time are essential in determining the nature of the resuscitation required.
- Skin turgor and the color of the mucous membranes should be noted.
- Place a large-bore intravenous catheter if there are signs of shock.
  - Orthostasis or frank hypotension
  - Tachycardia
  - Poorly perfused extremities
  - Pale mucous membranes
- If percutaneous venous access is not obtained within a few minutes, an intraosseous line should be placed.
  - 20 mL/kg of normal saline should be given rapidly to reexpand the vascular volume.
  - Fluid bolus may need to be repeated several times.
  - Additional fluid should be given as needed
  - With >30–40% acute blood loss, packed red blood cells should be given as soon as possible (see Shock).
- A nasogastric tube, preferably of the vented sump type, helps to:
  - Determine the source of bleeding
  - Estimate the volume of ongoing blood loss
- The nasogastric tube should be left in place and attached to:
  - Low-pressure continuous suction, if vented
  - Intermittent suction, if nonvented

- Nasogastric tube placement may aggravate bleeding in a patient with varices.
  - Even in this case, a nasogastric tube may be required to quantitate blood loss adequately.

Controlling bleeding and determining specific diagnosis

- If the nasogastric aspirate contains blood, or if the patient has hematemesis
  - Saline irrigation may be instituted through the nasogastric tube to decrease mucosal blood flow and stop profuse bleeding.
  - The efficacy of lavage in decreasing and controlling gastric bleeding has not been demonstrated conclusively.
    - It allows easier assessment of the rate of bleeding
    - It helps in removing clotted blood.
  - Use saline at room temperature, because irrigation with water can lead to hyponatremia and iced or cold fluid may cause hypothermia.
  - Withdraw after 3–5 minutes.
  - Aspirate returns that do not clear in 15 minutes:
    - Suggest continued GI bleeding
    - Should prompt additional evaluation
- Gastroduodenoscopy if bleeding ceases:
  - To demonstrate the bleeding source
  - To determine the type of lesion present
  - Upper GI fiberoptic endoscopy can establish the diagnosis in 75–90% of patients.
  - Adequate visualization is unlikely if the bleeding is massive and cannot be controlled with saline lavage.
- If the bleeding is not immediately life threatening:
  - Arteriography can demonstrate bleeding that occurs at a rate ≥0.5 mL/min.
  - Sulfur-colloid isotopic study, more sensitive and less invasive than arteriography, can demonstrate active bleeding at rates as low as 0.05–0.1 mL/min.
  - Injection with technetium-99-pertechnetate–labeled red blood cells that may remain in the circulation for more than a day and allow repeated imaging can be used to locate the site of intermittent bleeding.

Mucosal erosion or inflammation

- Antacid therapy, with or without concomitant use of a histamine 2-blocker
- For bleeding ulcers, intravenous therapy with a proton-pump inhibitor:
  - Reduces risk of rebleeding
  - Does not appear to influence overall mortality

Variceal bleeding

- The cause of the lesions must be determined for appropriate treatment of the underlying disease.

- In particular, liver or portal venous disease should be sought.

- Clotting factors and platelets should be replaced as indicated.

- Use of balloon tamponade with a Sengstaken-Blakemore tube is effective in controlling bleeding but has a high incidence of complications.

- Vasoactive drugs and endoscopy have replaced the Sengstaken-Blakemore tube in most cases.
  - Somatostatin and octreotide have been found to be effective in adults and in smaller studies in children.
    - Octreotide decreases splanchnic blood flow, thereby decreasing portal pressure.
    - Octreotide has less effect on systemic blood flow and is associated with fewer side effects than vasopressin.
    - Pediatric studies (with no control groups) have shown octreotide to be 50–63% effective in controlling acute variceal bleeding.
    - Initially, a 50-mcg bolus is infused, preferably through a central or intraosseous line, followed by an infusion of 50 mcg/hour for 5 days.
  - Endoscopy is the preferred intervention for variceal bleeding because it can provide both diagnosis and therapy.
    - Endoscopic injection sclerotherapy (EIS) uses an injection of a sclerosing solution into the varices.
    - Endoscopic variceal band ligation (EVL) uses elastic bands placed around the varices in the distal esophagus.
    - Endoscopy has been found to be 80–100% effective in controlling variceal bleeding.
      - In a randomized controlled trial in 49 children, EVL achieved variceal eradication faster than EIS, with a lower rebleeding rate and fewer complications.
    - Endoscopy should be performed by an experienced gastroenterologist, with general anesthesia and endotracheal intubation available, especially when performed on small children.

- Studies in adults and experience in pediatrics, although limited to date, suggest:
  - Octreotide as the initial treatment for bleeding varices
  - Followed by endoscopic therapy, either EVL or EIS
  - If bleeding continues despite vasoactive and endoscopic therapies, then balloon tamponade can be attempted.

H pylori infection

- Treatment, when indicated, consists of:
  - A 7- to 14-day course of any of a variety of antibiotic regimens
  - A proton-pump inhibitor

Necrotizing enterocolitis

- Neonates remain hospitalized for bowel rest and intravenous antibiotics.

- Occasionally requires surgical intervention

Meckel diverticulum

- Treatment requires surgical excision.

Mallory-Weiss tear

- Although the bleeding is minor and usually resolves spontaneously, a histamine 2-blocker may be needed to prevent continued irritation by stomach acid.

Volvulus malrotation

- Immediate surgical repair is necessary.

WHEN TO REFER

- Upper GI bleeding
- Lower GI bleeding
  - Of moderate amount
  - Persistent or intermittent

WHEN TO ADMIT

- Any nontrivial upper GI bleeding
  - Active bleeding
  - Moderate amount of blood
  - Anemia
  - Abdominal pain
- Significant lower GI bleeding

G

Gastrointestinal Obstruction

DEFINITION

- Gastrointestinal obstruction (GIO) is relatively uncommon during infancy, childhood, and adolescence.
- Obstructions distal to the pylorus are potential surgical emergencies.
  - The younger the patient is, the more ominous the probable cause and the more urgent the required therapy.

ETIOLOGY

- The presence or absence of key symptoms and signs, along with patient age, are important clues to the cause of the obstruction (see table Clinical Findings for Pediatric Gastrointestinal Obstruction):
  - Esophageal atresia
  - Gastric obstruction
  - Hypertrophic pyloric stenosis
  - Duodenal obstruction
  - Volvulus
  - Jejunoileal atresia
  - Intussusception
  - Meconium ileus
  - Meconium plug
  - Congenital aganglionosis
  - Obstipation of prematurity
  - Incarcerated inguinal hernia
  - Imperforate anus

SIGNS AND SYMPTOMS

- The symptoms and signs of a GIO (see table Clinical Findings for Pediatric Gastrointestinal Obstruction) vary but involve the following, either singly or in combination:
  - Vomiting (often bilious)
  - Abdominal pain
  - Abdominal distention
  - Change in bowel habits
  - Fever
  - Abdominal tenderness
  - Palpable abdominal mass

DIFFERENTIAL DIAGNOSIS

Vomiting

- Vomiting usually is *not* caused by GIO.
- Diseases in neonates or infants associated with nonbilious, nonprojectile vomiting include:
  - Gastroesophageal reflux (chalazia) or regurgitation in an infant
    - Benign and self-limited
    - Can be ruled out by 24-hour pH probe study or a nuclear medicine milk reflux scan

- Esophageal obstruction (atresia)
  - Neonate may have copious, frothy bubbles of mucus that cause rattling respirations, coughing, choking, and cyanosis.
  - Respiratory distress caused by tracheal aspiration of saliva retained in the upper esophagus or aspiration through the commonly associated tracheoesophageal fistula proximal or distal to the atresia can be associated with this anomaly.
  - Denoted by esophageal block encountered during attempts to pass an 8- or 10-French transoral soft catheter approximately 17 cm into the stomach
  - With pediatric gastric volvulus, 1 of the 2 most likely neonatal conditions in which a congenital or early-acquired esophageal obstruction is likely to be encountered
- Acute gastric volvulus
  - Often accompanied by severe pain, unlike esophageal atresia
  - Can be associated with signs of shock, chest pain, dysphagia, dyspepsia, and acute respiratory distress
- Complete or incomplete gastric antral web
  - Diagnosis often delayed, made in late infancy
  - Associated with failure to thrive
- Diseases associated with projectile, nonbilious vomiting of early infancy include:
  - Congenital hypertrophic pyloric stenosis
    - Semiurgent medical condition of dehydration and electrolyte disturbances
    - Typically a hyponatremic, hypochloremic, hypokalemic contraction metabolic alkalosis with a possible late paradoxical aciduria
  - Suspected hypertrophic pyloric stenosis in infants
    - Usually does not require an upper GI series to confirm
    - Classic symptoms of upper abdominal peristaltic waves and palpable, olive-sized mass in the mid- to right upper quadrant are diagnostic.
    - Experienced pediatrician or surgeon will be able to palpate the mass in approximately 80–90% of affected patients.
    - Diagnosis may be aided by physical findings of hypoplastic inferior labial frenulum or an abnormal mucosal reflectance of the oral mucosa.
    - Abdominal ultrasound can aid diagnosis where pyloric stenosis is suspected but not palpable.
    - Radiographic confirmation is unnecessary, costly, and potentially hazardous.
- Bilious vomiting in infants, usually nonprojectile, is more ominous and denotes GIO below the level of the ampulla of Vater.
  - Possible intestinal malrotation with a complicating midgut volvulus

Clinical Findings for Pediatric Gastrointestinal Obstruction

Cause	Findings						
	Vomiting	**Pain**	**Stool Pattern**	**Distention**	**Bowel Sounds**	**Tenderness**	**Masses**
Esophageal atresia	Nonbilious (saliva)	No	Normal meconium	No	Absent to normal	No	No
Gastric obstruction	Nonbilious (curdled formula)	Severe with gastric volvulus; none with antral web	Normal meconium	Epigastric	Absent to normal	Severe with volvulus	No
Hypertrophic pyloric stenosis	Nonbilious, projectile	No	Constipation (dehydration)	Epigastric	Hyperactive (epigastric)	No	Yes (olive-sized mass)
Duodenal obstruction	Bilious	Minimal	Small meconium stool	Epigastric	Absent to normal	No	No
Volvulus	Bilious	Severe	Hematochezia	Epigastric to generalized	Hyperactive	Yes (severe)	No
Jejunoileal atresia	Bilious	No	Small, hard, light-colored meconium stool	Generalized	Variable	No	No
Intussusception	Bilious	Yes (crampy)	Currant jelly stool	Generalized	Hyperactive	Yes	Yes (sausage shaped)
Meconium ileus	Bilious	No	Obstipation	Generalized	Variable	No	Yes (doughy beads)
Meconium plug	Bilious	No	Obstipation	Generalized	Variable	No	No
Congenital aganglionosis	Bilious	No	Obstipation, constipation, and intermittent diarrhea	Generalized	Hyperactive	No	Palpable stool
Obstipation of prematurity	Bilious	No	Obstipation	Generalized	Hyperactive	No	No
Incarcerated inguinal hernia	Bilious	Yes	Diarrhea or constipation	Generalized	Hyperactive	Yes	Inguinal or scrotal
Imperforate anus	Bilious	No	Obstipation	Generalized	Hyperactive	No	No

- Can produce GIO with ischemia and subsequent bowel necrosis within a few hours
- Requires immediate radiologic examination for diagnosis
- Premature infant who has an immature pyloric sphincter can have bilious regurgitation without obstruction, especially when it is associated with an ileus related to an underlying septic process.
- Clinical signs of peritonitis preclude radiologic study for diagnosis

- Immediate exploratory laparotomy is necessary.
- Upper gastrointestinal (GI) radiographic series is the diagnostic study of choice in less severely ill neonates, although diagnosis may be made by ultrasound.
- Other causes of bilious vomiting in the neonate and infant include:
  - Duodenal, jejunal, and ileal atresias
  - Duodenal stenosis caused by an annular pancreas or Ladd bands (colonic peritoneal bands crossing the duodenum) associated with malrotation

- Meconium ileus
- Colonic atresia
- Congenital aganglionosis of the colon (Hirschsprung disease)
- Imperforate anus

■ Infant or older toddler who has bilious vomiting can have a GIO produced by:

- Incarcerated hernia
- Intussusception
- Previously unrecognized malrotation with associated volvulus

■ Bilious vomiting in an adolescent can be caused by:

- Incarcerated hernia
- Postoperative adhesion
- Meconium ileus equivalent associated with cystic fibrosis
- Acute inflammation (appendicitis and pelvic inflammatory disease)
- Chronic inflammation (regional ileitis or ulcerative colitis)
- At this age, malrotation is less likely.

■ In less developed countries, obstruction may be caused by:

- Masses of worms, especially *Ascaris lumbricoides*
- Tuberculosis

■ A significant number of all patients with persistent bilious emesis will have an underlying pathological abnormality requiring early diagnosis and definitive surgical treatment.

■ Hematemesis

- Small amounts of blood may be observed in the vomitus of infants who have congenital hypertrophic pyloric stenosis, caused by gastric irritation as a result of repeated emesis.
- In rare cases, hematemesis with larger amounts of blood is associated with GIO:
  - Acute peptic ulcer resulting in obstruction in a newborn (uncommon)
  - In an older, chronically stressed infant or child (more common)
- *Helicobacter pylori* is a potential cause of peptic ulcer disease in children, more so in developing countries.

Abdominal pain

■ Abdominal pain, which may cause inconsolable crying or irritability in an infant, usually accompanies GIO.

- Intussusception
  - The pain is likely to be crampy or intermittent.
  - Results in crying and flexion of the legs to the abdomen, interspersed with periods of decreased distress
  - In ~10% of children who have intussusception, lethargy is the only symptom.

• Complete or partial obstruction of the intestine

- Produces acute intermittent abdominal pain, which becomes constant in a matter of hours
- Caused by intestinal distention, peritoneal inflammation, or both
- Bowel wall edema ensues, increasing the degree of obstruction and causing a progression of changes that place the intussuscepted intestine at further risk for ischemic damage.

• Malignancies in the intestinal tract are rare and usually do not produce intestinal obstruction.

- Intestinal or mesenteric lymphomas may cause GIO in patients >4 years.
  - Commonly present as intussusception
- An immunocompromised child who has a malignancy or AIDS may develop primary or secondary inflammatory lesions that lead to obstruction.

Stools

■ Obstipation in a newborn

- Delay of initial bowel movement in:
  - Premature infants
  - Infants who are small for gestational age
  - Infants of mothers with diabetes
  - Infants with mothers with problems of substance abuse (narcotics such as morphine)
  - Infants with complications of maternal drug therapy (eg, magnesium sulfate for toxemia)
  - Neonatal stress (hypoxemia or sepsis)
- Atresias of the proximal portion of the intestinal tract usually do not cause obstipation, except for those involving the most distal terminal ileum.
- However, meconium passed by these infants usually is sparse and lighter in color, and may be hard and dry.

■ The differential diagnosis of newborn obstipation includes:

- Congenital aganglionosis of the colon
- Meconium ileus (with underlying cystic fibrosis)
- Meconium plug syndrome (30% of these are associated with congenital aganglionosis of the colon or cystic fibrosis)
- Small left colon syndrome
- Colonic atresia
- Imperforate anus
- Rectal atresia (rare)

■ Strictures produce obstipation or constipation in an older infant or child and may result from:

- Neonatal necrotizing enterocolitis
- Intestinal surgery

- Extrinsic compression of the GI tract caused by:
  - Congenital cysts
  - Intestinal duplication
  - Inflammatory masses
  - Malignancies
- Particularly in neonates and infants, diarrhea or alternating diarrhea and constipation can be a sign of:
  - Functional GIO
  - Partial or intermittent GIO
  - Congenital colonic aganglionosis
  - Intussusception (frequently seen with hematochezia or melena)
  - Intermittent volvulus (frequently seen with hematochezia or melena)
- Hematochezia, or grossly bloody stools, in association with GIO symptoms, indicates intestinal vascular compromise.
  - Most common in patients who have an intussusception or volvulus
  - So-called currant jelly stools of intussusception that result from the admixture of blood and mucus, or darker (mahogany to black), melena-type stools from a more proximal intestinal bleeding site
    - A sign of superficial mucosal sloughing
    - Also accompany full-thickness necrosis of the bowel wall
- In infants without grossly bloody stools, occult blood is present in up to 75% of cases of intussusception.
- Hemoccult test should be performed in all infants with altered mental status.

DIAGNOSTIC APPROACH

- The infant with a history of vomiting must be evaluated for signs of dehydration by examining:
  - Anterior fontanelle
  - Rate and intensity of distal pulses
  - Level of consciousness
  - Perfusion of the extremities
  - Condition of the mucous membranes
- Abdominal auscultation should be performed before any other aspect of abdominal examination.
  - Listen to all the abdominal quadrants.
  - High-pitched, *tinkling* bowel sounds heard in rushes are diagnostic of a complete GIO.
  - Bowel sounds often are normal early, and become diminished or absent late in obstruction.
- When GIO is suspected, physical examination of the abdomen includes:
  - Evaluation for distention (see table Clinical Findings for Pediatric Gastrointestinal Obstruction)

- Likely to be prominent if obstruction is distal to the duodenum
- Mild to moderate epigastric distention seen with obstruction caused by:
  - Antral web
  - Hypertrophic pyloric stenosis
  - Duodenal atresia that produces only mild to moderate epigastric distention
- Distal intestinal atresia or other forms of lower GIO produce generalized distention.
- Distention does not aid in the diagnosis of a potential underlying midgut volvulus.
- Palpation
  - Mild tenderness or discomfort is expected if the abdomen is moderately to grossly distended.
    - Pressure applied to gas- or fluid-filled loops of bowel causes pain.
  - Marked tenderness clearly indicates an accompanying peritoneal inflammation.
    - Peritonitis in the setting of GIO
      - Indicates ischemia of the bowel wall with possible necrosis
      - Demands immediate surgical evaluation and treatment
    - Diagnostic radiologic studies that use contrast material are contraindicated.
  - Multiple doughy, compressible, mobile, nontender abdominal masses in a newborn who has GIO
    - Associated with meconium ileus
  - A tender, palpable, immobile mass most likely is cellulitis or abscess related to visceral perforation caused by:
    - Necrotizing enterocolitis in infants
    - Appendicitis in children or adolescents
    - Inflammatory bowel disease in children and adolescents
  - Nontender, mobile mass that produces GIO symptoms
    - Congenital intestinal duplication cysts
    - Mesenteric cysts
  - Sausage-like mass in the right upper quadrant with absence of bowel in the right lower quadrant
    - Pathognomonic of intussusception
    - Called the *Dance sign*
- Rectal examination often can clarify the cause of GIO.
  - In infant suspected of having an incarcerated inguinal hernia:
    - Palpate the peritoneal side of the internal inguinal ring transanally and identify an exiting intraperitoneal structure.

G

- Diagnosis of any suspected colonic or distal GIO
  - Previously unsuspected perirectal or presacral pelvic masses (eg, hydrometrocolpos, appendiceal inflammatory mass, presacral teratoma)
- Abnormal stool (as in the patient who has meconium plug syndrome) or blood (associated with intussusception or inflammatory bowel disease)
- Rarely, intraluminal rectal mass, such as with a low-lying intussusception

LABORATORY FINDINGS

- To ensure readiness of patients for surgery
  - Urinalysis, with catheterization if necessary
  - Complete blood count
  - Blood chemistry studies

IMAGING

- Studies are dictated by the results of the history and physical examination.
- See the table Roentgenographic Findings for Common Causes of Gastrointestinal Obstruction for radiographic diagnostic studies required for a patient who has GIO.

Plain-film radiograph studies

- A plain-film radiograph of the abdomen should be obtained for all patients suspected of having GIO.
  - Presence of even a large number of air-filled loops does not eliminate the need for a contrast study.
  - In a patient with volvulus, contrast study may show a corkscrew appearance projecting forward, away from the posterior abdominal wall.
- Chest radiography can demonstrate the curling of a nasogastric tube or dilated pouch in esophageal atresia.
- In a newborn infant, air localized to the stomach and duodenum (double-bubble sign) is diagnostic of a duodenal obstruction.
  - If no distal intestinal intraluminal air is seen, then GIO usually is caused by an atresia.
  - If even a small amount of air is found distally, then malrotation with possible volvulus must be suspected.
- Calcifications visualized by an abdominal radiograph in a neonate with suspected GIO
  - Evidence of an intrauterine intestinal perforation (meconium peritonitis), which often is associated with intestinal atresia
  - Calcifications may:
    - Be small, single, or multiple
    - Be scattered throughout the entire peritoneal cavity
    - Outline the peritoneal cavity
  - Cystic fibrosis may be the underlying disease.

- Abdominal radiograph of GIO in association with suspected cystic fibrosis (meconium ileus)
  - Gas may be absent in the right iliac fossa because of a meconium cyst.
  - Peculiar hazy pattern described as a *ground glass* or *soap bubble* appearance
    - The pattern is caused by abnormal meconium mixed with air that is inspissated in the bowel lumen.
  - Occasionally, this hard, dense meconium, palpable as multiple abdominal masses, appears on a radiograph as a chain of radiolucencies, known as the *string of beads* sign.
  - Air-fluid levels are rare in meconium ileus.
- Blunt injury to the abdomen, either accidental or intentional, can result in early obstruction from bowel wall edema and from a hematoma in the infant or toddler.
  - A full-thickness bowel wall injury often produces late sequelae such as an intestinal leak with initially normal or equivocal examination resulting in delay in diagnosis.
  - Diagnosis requires a high index of suspicion and, often, thorough and repeated radiologic evaluations.

Upper GI and barium enema

- Use of an upper GI series or a barium enema is necessary to rule out a malrotation or nonrotation of the intestine.
  - Upper GI series can determine the relationship among the duodenum, the jejunum, and the ligament of Treitz.
  - Barium enema can ascertain cecal position.
  - Barium enema of an *unused,* small-caliber distal colon (microcolon) in a normal position makes diagnosis of intestinal atresia or meconium ileus more likely than acute volvulus.
- Meconium ileus and meconium plug syndrome are neonatal GIO conditions that can be diagnosed and frequently can be treated with a water-soluble contrast enema.
  - Procedure is appropriate in a neonate suspected of having meconium ileus, but no evidence of perforation, and who is well hydrated.
  - Inspissated meconium is localized to the distal ileum, and may be freed from the bowel wall for spontaneous expulsion.
  - Technique is limited in application and duration, with subsequent surgical therapy required in as many as 50%.
- Uncomplicated meconium plug syndrome, infrequently associated with cystic fibrosis but occasionally associated with congenital aganglionosis, also is diagnosed and treated successfully with a barium enema.
  - Unlike meconium ileus, the meconium in meconium plug is localized to the distal colon.
  - Contrast enema is contraindicated when there is
    - Evidence of intestinal vascular compromise
    - Evidence of perforation, such as peritonitis, free intraperitoneal air, or intraperitoneal calcification

Roentgenographic Findings for Common Causes of Pediatric Gastrointestinal Obstruction

Cause	Dilated Area	Air or Fluid Levels	Calcium Deposits	Noncalcium Opacities	Further Studies That May Be Indicated
Esophageal atresia	Esophagus and stomach	Yes (gastric)	No	No	Esophageal air instillation
Gastric obstruction	Stomach	Yes	No	No	Gastric barium instillation[a]
Hypertrophic pyloric stenosis	Stomach	Yes	No	No	Ultrasonography
Duodenal obstruction	Stomach, duodenum (double bubble)	Yes	No	No	None
Volvulus	Variable	Variable	No	No	Upper gastrointestinal series or barium enema
Jejunoileal atresia	Stomach and small intestine	Yes	Yes (with prenatal perforation)	No	Barium enema to rule out nonrotation
Intussusception	Stomach and small intestine	Variable	No	Yes (soft-tissue densities)	Ultrasonography, barium/air enema[b], or both
Meconium ileus	Stomach and small intestine	No	Yes (meconium peritonitis)	Yes (ground-glass appearance)	Water-soluble contrast enema[c]
Meconium plug	Stomach to colon	Yes	No	No	Water-soluble contrast enema
Congenital aganglionosis	Stomach to colon	Yes	No	No	Barium enema
Obstipation of prematurity (short left colon syndrome)	Stomach to colon	Yes	No	No	Barium enema
Incarcerated inguinal hernia	Stomach and small intestine	Yes	No	No	None
Imperforate anus	Stomach to colon	Yes	No	No	Complete evaluation of genitourinary tract

[a] Should be performed cautiously to avoid aspiration.
[b] Should be performed cautiously to avoid bowel perforation.
[c] May be therapeutic and diagnostic.

- Colonic dysfunction of prematurity, or *small left colon syndrome* (SLCS)
  - Produces a functional mechanical obstruction
  - Related to:
    - Extreme prematurity
    - Maternal diabetes
    - Prenatal maternal medications for eclampsia (magnesium sulfate)
    - Hypothyroidism
    - Maternal narcotic use
  - A diagnosis of exclusion, because its barium contrast appearance resembles Hirschsprung disease.
- Older infants and toddlers suspected of having GIO produced by intussusception can be diagnosed and often treated successfully with a barium enema.
  - The study is performed with a limited pressure (3 feet) barium column.
  - Intussusception is slowly reduced by the hydrostatic pressure.
  - Because of the potential hazard of a barium perforation, the study should always be performed by an experienced radiologist with a surgical team standing by.

- Procedure can be used in approximately 75% of patients, with successful reduction of the intussusception in 85% to 90%.
- Surgical reduction is required in cases that cannot be reduced radiologically.
- The patient always should be observed for 12–24 hours in the hospital after successful intussusception reduction.

■ Air enema reduction of the intussusception recently has become available.

- Air insufflation of the rectum and colon using an in-line pressure-limiting valve while maintaining fluoroscopic or sonographic observation
- Advantages of this technique
  - Elimination of barium and threat of severe chemical peritonitis if perforation inadvertently occurs
  - Possibly an improved mechanical advantage by using air reduction

Ultrasound

■ May provide prenatal diagnosis of GIO

- In up to 40% of cases, GIO may be suggested by findings such as:
  - Polyhydramnios, inability to identify the stomach
  - Cystic abdominal lesions
  - Dilated loops of bowel

■ Prenatal diagnosis of GIO (eg, atresia, volvulus) eliminates the need for emergent postnatal workup.

■ Color Doppler ultrasound

- May show a distorted relationship of the superior mesenteric vessels in a patient with volvulus

■ Duplication cysts can occur anywhere in the GI tract but are most common in the ileum, followed by the stomach.

- Ultrasound is the most useful imaging modality to diagnose enteric duplication cysts.
- *Rim sign* refers to an echogenic inner rim of mucosa and hypoechoic outer rim of the muscle layer.
- Peristalsis of the cyst wall and septations aid in diagnosis.

■ In meconium peritonitis, sonography may show ascites with echogenic debris, abnormal cystic masses, and thickening and dilatation of the bowel wall.

■ Diagnosis of suspected intussusception can be made effectively by ultrasound or CT.

- Both tests are useful in a patient whose examination is unremarkable and whose history is equivocal.

DIAGNOSTIC PROCEDURES

■ Hypertrophic pyloric stenosis

- Barium study of the upper GI tract may show normal duodenal bulb with a proximal antral chamber between the web and the pylorus, known as the *double duodenal bulb appearance*.

- Esophagogastroduodenoscopy may help identify and potentially divide the web.
- If the web cannot be treated safely during endoscopy, then open gastric antroplasty is effective.

■ Hirschsprung disease

- Initial diagnosis is made based on clinical suspicion because it cannot be verified by noninvasive diagnostic procedures.
  - Barium enema or anorectal manometry reflecting an absent rectosphincteric reflex often is helpful in diagnosis of older children.
  - Either a rectal mucosal or full-thickness rectal wall biopsy specimen is required to confirm the diagnosis in infants.

TREATMENT APPROACH

■ Gastric decompression to prevent continued bowel distention, vomiting, and possibly aspiration

■ Intravenous fluid therapy

- Required immediately to replace intraluminal and intra-peritoneal fluid loss
  - Luminal losses are high in electrolyte content, requiring administration of higher-than-maintenance concentrations of sodium, chloride, and potassium.
  - Solutions such as lactated Ringer's solution are needed to provide appropriate replacement.

■ Emergent or semi-urgent surgery

- Required by almost all children with GIO
- The child must be well prepared for anesthesia and the surgical procedure.
  - This requires correcting fluid and electrolyte, hematologic, and metabolic imbalances before surgery.
  - Such measures should begin before extensive diagnostic imaging studies are undertaken.

■ Nonsurgical therapy for failure to pass meconium caused by

- Hypothyroidism
- Hypercalcemia
- Hypokalemia
- Sepsis
- Congestive heart failure

SPECIFIC TREATMENTS

■ The type of surgical procedure performed and the patient's postoperative course and prognosis depend on the type of lesion causing GIO.

Incarcerated inguinal hernia

■ Important cause of GIO in children and adolescents

- Reduction can be accomplished by
  - Sedation with a tranquilizer, with or without an added narcotic analgesic

– Keeping the patient supine in mild Trendelenburg position

– Applying an ice pack to the inguinal region

- Medications must be used cautiously to prevent excessive sedation, because vomiting and aspiration can occur.

■ Should be reduced gently and repaired later, after GIO and local edema have subsided

- If reduced but left unrepaired, recurrent incarcerations are likely, with potential strangulation and necrosis of the bowel.

Colonic dysfunction of prematurity/small left colon syndrome (SLCS)

■ Surgically, a temporary colostomy is indicated only by

- Failure to respond to careful, small-volume, saline enema therapy

- Signs of peritonitis or intestinal perforation

■ Prognosis for uncomplicated cases is excellent.

Esophageal obstruction

■ Esophageal atresia with associated tracheoesophageal fistula

- A relative emergency that requires either

– Primary repair, *or*

– Staged procedure with initial gastrostomy for gastric decompression and prevention of aspiration

– Subsequent definitive repair, including division of the fistula and anastomosis of the esophageal ends, after treatment of existing underlying pneumonic process

- Gastrostomy and definitive repair occasionally are performed simultaneously.

- Esophageal repair is performed without gastrostomy in selected patients.

- Complications of definitive procedure include esophageal leaks, infection, and strictures.

- As many as 50% of cases have associated anomalies:

– Cardiovascular system

– Imperforate anus

– Duodenal atresia

– Intestinal malrotation

- In uncomplicated atresia and tracheoesophageal fistula, morbidity is low and mortality is negligible.

– Associated cardiovascular anomalies and low birth weight lead to a mortality rate as high as 70%.

– Late complications of atresia and tracheoesophageal fistula include congenital hypertrophic pyloric stenosis and chronic gastroesophageal reflux with reactive airway symptoms.

Gastric obstructions

■ Gastric volvulus

- Usually an acute problem

- Requires

– Immediate surgical gastropexy to prevent ischemia and necrosis

– Temporary gastrostomy tube for fixation and decompression

- If no gastric necrosis is found, then recovery usually is uneventful.

- Gastric necrosis with resulting peritonitis results in high morbidity and mortality.

■ Gastric antral web

- Difficult to diagnose and often requires repeated diagnostic studies, but is not a critical problem

- Surgical therapy consists of simple incision of the web and performance of a modified pyloroplasty.

- Few postoperative complications

■ Hypertrophic pyloric stenosis

- Surgical therapy after adequate correction of associated, potentially life-threatening dehydration and hypochloremic alkalosis

- Procedure is a muscle-splitting pyloromyotomy, leaving the mucosa intact.

– Can be performed laparoscopically or through a right upper quadrant or supraumbilical incision with similar operative times, complications, and costs

– Acute complications are unusual.

- Patient without sequelae resumes postoperative feedings within 8–24 hr, sometimes as early as in the recovery room.

- Chronic complications such as stricture related to intra-operative mucosal perforations and adhesions are rare.

Duodenal obstructions

■ Duodenal atresia, stenosis, and annular pancreas

- Semiurgent problems, as long as they are not accompanied by volvulus

- Volvulus demands immediate abdominal exploration.

- Surgical therapy consists of bypassing obstructed area via

– Duodenoduodenostomy

– Duodenojejunostomy

– Gastrojejunostomy

- Moderate feeding problems necessitating longer hospitalization may be encountered, particularly with gastrojejunostomy.

- Prognosis is good.

- With associated congenital cardiac problems, mortality can be as high as 50%.

■ As many as 10% of cases of duodenal atresia are associated with Down syndrome (trisomy 21).

■ Growth and development of patients who have uncomplicated and isolated duodenal obstructions are normal.

- Duodenal and other intestinal duplication cysts are completely excised if possible.
  - At the least, mucosal lining should be excised, since cysts are associated with a late malignant transformation.

Jejunal and ileal obstructions

- Jejunal and ileal atresia
  - Semiurgent, unless associated with a volvulus
  - Surgical treatment involves:
    - Excision of the atretic bowel
    - Primary anastomosis of the dilated proximal and the narrowed distal segments
    - When multiple atretic segments of bowel, or small-bowel atresias associated with absence of the superior mesenteric artery, are present, overall intestinal length (absorptive surface) may be greatly reduced.
  - Total parenteral nutrition commonly is required after surgery.
  - Overall survival and prognosis are good, unless the atresia is complicated by:
    - Cystic fibrosis
    - Remaining small intestine that is too short for adequate absorption
- Malrotation with a complicating volvulus
  - The most critical diagnosis in any child suspected of having GIO
  - Twisted bowel mesentery may lead to ischemia and bowel necrosis within 4–6 hr after the onset of symptoms.
  - Untreated volvulus has a high acute mortality rate because of associated metabolic imbalance and sepsis.
  - Successful surgical resection of the involved necrotic bowel is associated with high long-term morbidity.
  - Entire embryonically derived midgut may have to be resected, leading to
    - Reduced intestinal absorption of nutrients
    - Short-gut syndrome
- Early diagnosis, rapid correction of fluid and electrolyte imbalances, and surgical reduction of mesenteric torsion with or without resection of potentially necrotic bowel are imperative.
- Proximal and distal segments of involved intestine that appear ischemic but may be viable should be retained.
  - Creation of abdominal enterostomas in lieu of extensive initial intestinal resection
  - Second-look operation performed in 24 hours
- Postoperative complications include:
  - Marked fluid and electrolyte disturbances
  - Local and systemic infections
  - Malnutrition

- Long-term parenteral nutrition, dietary adjustments, and repeated surgical procedures should be expected.
- Survival with reasonable quality of life can be expected if remaining viable small bowel is ≥30 cm.
- Morbidity is lessened when ileocecal valve remains intact.
- Long-term hospitalization and prolonged nutritional support with total parenteral nutrition usually are required.
- Meconium ileus may respond to water-soluble contrast enemas (see Imaging).
  - Evidence of accompanying intestinal perforation or failure of carefully managed water-soluble contrast enema necessitates surgical therapy.
  - Cystic fibrosis, almost always an underlying disease, complicates postoperative respiratory and nutritional status.
  - Administration of solutions such as N-acetyl-cysteine by means of an enterotomy usually cleanses the intestinal lumen.
  - Associated atretic or necrotic intestinal segments are excised.
  - Primary anastomoses are performed.
  - Enterostomas are created for:
    - Postoperative lavage of massively impacted meconium
    - Instances in which viability of the remaining bowel segments is in question.
  - A stoma may be needed to protect an anastomosis.
  - A transabdominal T tube may be left intraluminally to allow decompression and irrigation.
  - Appendix may be used as a conduit.
- Surgical survival is good.
- Morbidity is high; ultimate prognosis is related to severity of other manifestations of cystic fibrosis.

Colonic and rectal obstruction

- Intussusception that is uncomplicated by a lead point, eg, Meckel diverticulum, polyp, or malignancy
  - Hydrostatic air reduction is successful in up to 90% of appropriately selected patients.
  - Recurrences seen in 5–7%.
  - Surgical intervention is required if evidence of compromised bowel is found, eg, in free perforation or peritoneal irritation, and in failures of air–hydrostatic reduction.
    - Successful reduction requires retrograde reflux of contrast media or air into the terminal ileum.
    - Most intussusceptions that are reduced intraoperatively do well postoperatively, with a low (2–5%) recurrence rate.
    - Bowel resection is required when:
      - Intraoperatively recognized pathological lead point is present
      - Ischemic complication is found

- Early diagnosis and treatment of intussusception reduces morbidity and mortality.
- Rectal atresia and imperforate anus require diagnosis, initial therapy, and colostomy within 24 hr.
  - Very low perineal lesions (anterior displaced anus and fourchette fistula) can be treated with initial dilatations only.
  - Definitive therapy is a pull-through procedure and anoplasty.
    - Performed when the infant is 2–3 months of age
  - If lesion is not associated with other congenital anomalies, then survival is good.
    - Clinician should look for other anomalies, particularly those of the genitourinary tract (rectovaginal and rectovesicular fistulas, lower urinary tract obstructions with megacystis, hydroureter, and hydronephrosis).
  - Future stool continence is related directly to severity of the deformity, which is influenced by degree of normal embryologic descent of the colon through the levator muscle.
  - Definitive surgery for high lesions, in which colon descent is limited to a position above the levator muscle, results in daytime stool continence in ~60% of patients.
    - Overall continence rate for high lesions is 10–20%.
  - Repair of low lesions, in which the colon has descended below levator muscle, results in continence rate of at least 80–90%.
- Congenital aganglionosis of the colon (Hirschsprung disease)
  - Colostomy using a segment of proximal ganglionic colon
  - 6 months to 1 year later, excision of affected aganglionic segment and anastomosis of normally innervated (ganglionic) bowel to the anus (the pull-through procedure).
  - Many patients respond preoperatively to regular rectal stimulation and irrigations to evacuate the colon.
  - This measure allows performance of a primary pull-through procedure during the immediate newborn period and up to several months of age and avoidance of a colostomy.
  - Infant morbidity and mortality rates are high when the disease is complicated by enterocolitis; however, patients who have no such complications usually do well, with good anal continence, growth, and development.

Minimally invasive surgery

- Many procedures can be performed laparoscopically:
  - Pyloromyotomy
  - Fundoplication
  - Endorectal pull-throughs
- Obstructions caused by the following processes can be successfully treated with minimally invasive laparoscopic techniques:
  - Adhesions

- Inflammation (inflammatory bowel disease, appendicitis, and Meckel diverticulitis)
- Intussusception
- Procedures such as pyloromyotomy may be performed with a modified open technique, with less expensive and equally acceptable cosmetic results.
- Use of the minimally invasive technique for the Ladd procedure may be less effective than original open procedure.
- As smaller-size instrumentation improves and surgeons gain more experience, the list of procedures that can be performed laparoscopically continues to grow.

Fetal surgery

- Due to the risk to the mother from invasive procedures, in utero treatment or newly developed endoscopic fetal procedures must be considered only when death of the fetus or newborn is certain without such intervention.
- Open or endoscopic fetal surgery is accepted for:
  - Congenital cystic adenomatoid malformation
  - Fetal sacrococcygeal teratoma
  - Congenital diaphragmatic hernia
  - Obstructive uropathy
- None of the prenatal GIO diagnoses or their causes pose an immediate threat to the fetus or the mother.
  - Overall combined mortality rate is <5%.
  - Benefits to the baby do not outweigh the risk to the mother; therefore, these lesions are not appropriate for prenatal interventional therapy.

WHEN TO ADMIT

- All cases of intestinal obstruction

WHEN TO REFER

- All patients with suspected and confirmed intestinal obstruction should be referred to pediatric surgery.

COMPLICATIONS

- Decreased blood supply to the intestines may occur in patients with conditions such as volvulus.
  - Delayed diagnosis of this compromise in blood supply may lead to necrosis of the intestines and intestinal perforation, resulting in peritonitis, sepsis, and severe metabolic derangements.
- Problems related to malabsorption, if large portion of small intestine has been resected.

PROGNOSIS

- Prognosis depends on the underlying condition, rapidity in diagnosis, and surgical intervention.
  - Hypertrophic pyloric stenosis has excellent prognosis as compared to small gut volvulus.

G

Genetic Metabolic Disease Recognition

DEFINITION

- Prompt diagnosis of genetic disease is important.
  - Therapeutic interventions are available for some conditions; early therapy may improve outcomes.
  - Genetic counseling informs parents about recurrence risk and reproductive options.
- >300 diseases caused by inborn errors of metabolism have been identified.
- The primary care physician can expect to see several patients who have these disorders.
  - Often the first clinician to evaluate
  - Familiarity with clinical presentations and knowledge of initial laboratory evaluation are important.
  - Formal diagnosis and treatment is usually done in consultation with a specialist.
- Disease is detected:
  - By population-wide screening of newborns
  - By testing following clinical manifestation of disease
- With advances in understanding cellular processes, some defects can now be recognized.
  - Transport proteins
  - Membrane proteins
  - Organelle assembly
  - Intracellular processing and trafficking
  - Other biological processes that result in biochemical disturbances with clinical expression

EPIDEMIOLOGY

- Prevalence
  - Inborn errors of metabolism individually are rare.
  - Collective incidence is approximately 1 in 1000 live births.
  - Metabolic disease will be origin of symptoms in:
    - ~1 in 5 sick, full-term newborns who have no risk factors for infection
    - 1 in 100 children who have a serious medical problem

MECHANISM

Classification of genetic metabolic disorders

- Many of the clinical examples provided below refer to groups of disorders and do not distinguish specific enzymatic defects.
- All disorders listed below are autosomal-recessive unless otherwise noted.
- Diagnostic suspicion of a metabolic disorder does not require comprehensive knowledge of the various biochemical pathways involved.
  - Typical clinical presentations, specific historical clues, and pertinent findings on clinical examination should lead to their consideration.

- Some laboratory tests routinely obtained in ill children can help determine the presence of metabolic disease.

Metabolites

- Amino acids
  - Amino acid catabolism
    - Phenylketonuria
    - Homocystinuria
    - Tyrosinemia type 1
    - Maple syrup urine disease (MSUD)
    - Nonketotic hyperglycinemia
- Urea cycle disorders
  - Ornithine transcarbamylase deficiency (X-linked)
  - Citrullinemia
  - Arginosuccinic aciduria
  - Carbamoylphosphate synthase deficiency
- Amino acid transport
  - Lysinuric protein intolerance
  - Cystinuria hyperornithinemia-hyperammonemia-homo-citrullinuria syndrome
- Synthesis of creatine and neurotransmitters
  - Creatine deficiency disorders
  - Disorders of γ-aminobutyric acid metabolism and mono-amine synthesis
- Organic acids
  - Organic acid metabolism
    - Propionic acidemia
    - Methylmalonic acidemia
    - Isovaleric acidemia
    - Glutaric acidemia type 1
    - Holocarboxylase synthetase deficiency
- Fatty acids
  - Fatty acid oxidation
    - Short-chain, medium-chain, and very long–chain acyl-coenzyme A (CoA) dehydrogenase deficiency
    - Long-chain 3-hydroxyacyl-CoA hydrogenase deficiency
    - Carnitine uptake defect
    - Carnitine palmitoyl transferase (CPT) deficiencies (CPT 1 and CPT 2)
  - Cholesterol synthesis
    - Mevalonic acidemia
    - Smith-Lemli-Opitz syndrome
    - Conradi-Hünermann-Happle syndrome (X-linked)
- Carbohydrates
  - Carbohydrate intolerances
    - Galactosemia
    - Hereditary fructose intolerance

- Glycogen breakdown (glycogen storage disorders [GSDs])
  - Hepatic forms
    - Glucose-6-phosphatase deficiency (GSD 1)
    - Debrancher enzyme deficiency (GSD 3)
  - Muscle form
    - Muscle glycogen phosphorylase deficiency (GSD 5)
  - Lysosomal form
    - Pompe disease (GSD 2)
- Glucose catabolism (glycolysis) and synthesis (gluconeogenesis)
  - Pyruvate dehydrogenase deficiency
  - Pyruvate carboxylase deficiency
  - Fructose diphosphatase deficiency
- Vitamins, minerals, and cofactors
  - Activation, transport, recycling
    - Biotinidase deficiency
    - Molybdenum cofactor deficiency
    - Biopterin, cobalamin, and copper disorders

Organelles

- Peroxisome
  - Peroxisome biogenesis
    - Zellweger syndrome
    - Neonatal adrenoleukodystrophy
    - Infantile Refsum disease
    - Rhizomelic chondrodysplasia punctata
  - Single peroxisome enzyme or protein deficiencies
    - X-linked adrenoleukodystrophy
    - Adult Refsum disease
    - Hyperoxaluria type 1
- Lysosome
  - Lysosomal storage disorders
    - Mucopolysaccharidoses (MPSs)
      - Hurler-Scheie syndrome (MPS 1)
      - Hunter syndrome (MPS 2, X-linked)
      - Sanfilippo syndrome (MPS 3A-D)
    - Sphingolipidoses
      - Tay-Sachs disease
      - Krabbe disease
      - Metachromatic leukodystrophy
      - Niemann-Pick, Gaucher, Fabry diseases (X-linked)
  - Lysosomal enzyme transport
    - Mucolipidoses (MLs)
    - I-cell disease (ML 2, ML 3)
      - Cystinosis
      - Sialic acid storage disease
- Mitochondria
  - Respiratory chain complexes
    - Leigh syndrome
    - Multiple acyl-CoA dehydrogenase deficiency (glutaric acidemia type 2)
    - Mitochondrial encephalomyopathy, lactic acidosis, and stroke syndrome; mitochondrial encephalomyopathy and ragged red fibers; neuropathy, ataxia, and retinitis pigmentosa (mitochondrial DNA–encoded defects)
- Endoplasmic reticulum, Golgi
  - Intracellular protein processing and trafficking
    - Glycosylation
      - Congenital disorders of glycosylation

HISTORY

Dietary history

- High protein intake precipitates such symptoms as vomiting, lethargy, and coma.
  - Disorders in which protein catabolism is defective
    - Amino acid disorders
    - Organic acid disorders
- An infant who vomits but improves on glucose feeding, and in whom vomiting recurs within a few days of reinstitution of milk feeding, might have a metabolic disease.
- History may reveal onset of illness on weaning from breast milk, which has lower protein content than commercial formulas, or association of illness with high-protein meals.
  - Older patients may avoid protein by limiting protein intake.
- Carbohydrate intolerances
  - Fructose (fruit juices) in hereditary fructose intolerance
  - Lactose (human or cow's milk) in galactosemia

Response to infection, fever, and fasting

- History of unusual lethargy during mild illness or intolerance of fasting is an important clue for diagnosing metabolic disease.
- Infections, fever, and fasting result in an overall catabolic state.
  - Under these conditions, disorders involving impaired glucose production and fatty acid catabolism are exacerbated.
  - Endogenous protein catabolism may precipitate expression of amino acid and organic acid disorders.
- GSD may present within first few months of life at the time when the interval between feedings is lengthened.
- Disorders of fatty acid oxidation classically occur during an episode of intercurrent illness with prolonged fasting.

G

G

■ Immunizations, which may produce mild illness in normal children, can cause metabolic decompensation in children with inborn errors of metabolism.

- Immunization should not be avoided in these children.
- Patients with metabolic disorders should be monitored carefully after immunization.
- Influenza vaccines are recommended yearly.

Adverse reactions to anesthesia and surgery

■ General anesthesia, surgery, and other causes of stress to metabolic systems and can precipitate illness in patients with metabolic disease.

- Patients with homocystinuria are prone to thromboembolism
  - On administration of high-osmolar contrast dyes
  - During surgery
- Some patients with myopathy are at risk of malignant hyperthermia when halothane is administered.

Family history

■ Complete family history for all patients with suspected metabolic disease is essential.

■ Most of these disorders are inherited in autosomal-recessive fashion.

- Factors that increase the likelihood of autosomal-recessive disease
  - Parental consanguinity
    - 2.5-fold increase in risk for autosomal-recessive disorders
    - Consanguinity is practiced in Asia; North Africa; Switzerland; the Middle East; and some parts of China, Japan, Europe, and the United States
    - Intermarriage in the US occurs within some cultural religious groups, including members of the Amish and Latter-Day Saints (Mormon) communities.
  - Similarly affected siblings
  - Early death of a sibling
- Some autosomal-recessive metabolic disorders are found at higher frequency in certain ethnic groups.

■ Consanguinity is less common in the US than in other countries.

- However, increased immigration from Asia, Africa, and Europe necessitates increased awareness.
- Negative family history does not exclude the possibility of a metabolic disorder.

■ Similarly affected male relatives on maternal side is consistent with X-linked disorders.

■ Disorders of mitochondrial genome show an exclusively maternal pattern of inheritance.

PHYSICAL EXAM

■ Metabolic disease affects multiple organ systems and produces a variety of physical findings; however, some general themes exist.

- With disorders that occur along with episodic illness, significant findings may be present or exacerbated only during the acute phase.
- Neurologic abnormalities and vomiting predominate in episodic presentations.
  - Hepatomegaly, cardiomyopathy, and muscle weakness may also be present, as in disorders of fatty acid oxidation.
- Tachypnea and hyperpnea are often overlooked as signs of metabolic acidosis or respiratory alkalosis.
- Other disorders feature characteristic pattern of findings that develop over time.
  - Coarse facial features, corneal clouding, hepatosplenomegaly, macrocephaly, and skeletal changes suggest:
    - MPSs
    - Disorders of glycoprotein degradation
    - MLs
- A constellation of alopecia, chronic dermatitis, ataxia, and seizures is seen with biotinidase deficiency.
- Lens dislocation, long extremities, and vascular occlusion caused by thrombosis are found in homocystinuria.
- Metabolic disease should be suspected when physical examination reveals abnormalities in >1 organ system.

■ Pertinent clinical findings in genetic metabolic disorders

- Neurologic
  - Encephalopathy
  - Stroke-like episode
  - Macrocephaly or microcephaly
  - Developmental delay
  - Ataxia
  - Choreoathetosis
  - Dystonia
  - Peripheral neuropathy
  - Hypotonia or hypertonia
  - Seizures
  - Myoclonus
  - Deafness
  - Brain malformation
  - Cerebral calcification
- Ophthalmalogic
  - Cataracts
  - Lens dislocation
  - Corneal opacity
  - Macular cherry-red spot

- Macular degeneration
- Retinal pigment change
- Optic atrophy
- Respiratory
  - Tachypnea
  - Hyperpnea
- Cardiovascular
  - Cardiomyopathy
  - Pericardial effusion
  - Rhythm disturbance
  - Thrombosis
  - Bleeding diathesis
  - Anemia
- Abdominal
  - Hepatomegaly
  - Cirrhosis
  - Jaundice
  - Splenomegaly
  - Nephrolithiasis
  - Renal Fanconi syndrome
  - Renal cyst
  - Pancreatitis
- Muscular
  - Hypertrophy
  - Myopathy
  - Myalgias
  - Recurrent myoglobinuria
- Skin
  - Eczematous rash
  - Ichthyosis
  - Photosensitivity
  - Angiokeratomas
  - Xanthomas
- Hair
  - Sparse
  - Brittle, dry, coarse
- Skeletal
  - Scoliosis
  - Kyphosis
  - Joint contractures
  - Dysostosis multiplex
  - Epiphyseal calcifications
- Other
  - Dysmorphic features
  - Coarse facial features

DIFFERENTIAL DIAGNOSIS

- Many common pediatric illnesses produce similar signs and symptoms.
  - Unfortunately, metabolic disease is often not considered until other disorders are excluded.
    - Diagnostic delay is particularly common for metabolic disorders with nonacute presentation, especially when slow development is the major initial finding.
    - For best outcomes, metabolic disease should be included in the earliest differential diagnoses.

High-risk scenarios for consideration of metabolic disorders

- Acute illness in a previously normal newborn; consider:
  - Aminoacidopathies
  - Organic acidemias
  - Urea cycle defects
  - Galactosemia
- Neonatalseizure disorder; consider:
  - Pyridoxine-dependent seizures
  - Nonketotic hyperglycinemia
  - Sulfite oxidase deficiency
  - Zellweger syndrome
- Recurrent episodes of illness (lethargy, vomiting, ataxia, encephalopathy, stroke-like episodes, myopathy); consider:
  - Aminoacidopathies
  - Organic acidemias
  - Urea cycle defects
  - Defects in fatty acid metabolism
  - Disorders of carbohydrate metabolism
  - Mitochondrial disorders
- Acute life-threatening event; consider:
  - Fatty acid oxidation defects
- Neurologic regression; consider:
  - Lysosomal storage disorders
  - X-linked adrenoleukodystrophy
- Chronic, progressive symptoms (poor feeding, poor growth, slow development, neurologic and other organ system dysfunction); consider:
  - Aminoacidopathies
  - Organic acidemias
  - Disorders of carbohydrate metabolism
  - Mitochondrial and peroxisomal diseases
- Cardiomyopathy; consider:
  - Pompe disease
  - Mitochondrial disorders
  - Fatty acid oxidation defects
  - Congenital disorders of glycosylation

G

- Hepatopathy, consider:
  - Tyrosinemia type 1
  - Galactosemia
  - Mitochondrial disorders
  - Bile acid defects
- Maternal HELLP syndrome (hemolysis, elevated liver enzymes, low platelets); consider:
  - Fatty acid oxidation disorders

Neonatal presentation

- Sudden deterioration of a full-term normal neonate within first few days of life is a hallmark of metabolic disease.
  - Many infants remain free of symptoms for the first 24 hours of life.
  - When feeding begins, toxic metabolites accumulate, vomiting may occur, and the infant becomes increasingly lethargic.
  - Symptoms that highlight progression of many severe illnesses in neonate with limited repertoire of responses
    - Neurologic abnormalities
    - Respiratory distress
    - Shock
  - The differential diagnosis includes:
    - Sepsis
    - Congenital heart disease
    - Neurologic insults
    - Gastrointestinal obstruction
    - Metabolic disease
  - Clinician should pay particular attention to possibility of metabolic disease:
    - When risk factors for infection are absent *or*
    - When the infant deteriorates despite antibiotic therapy
- Documentation of infection, cardiomyopathy, or brain abnormalities does not exclude underlying metabolic disease.
  - Serious infection occurs in metabolically debilitated patients (eg, untreated infants with galactosemia are at increased risk for *Escherichia coli* sepsis).
  - Cardiomyopathies develop in several categories of metabolic disease, including disorders of fatty acid oxidation.
  - Metabolic crisis may result in diffuse cerebral swelling and stroke.
  - Seizure activity predominates in certain disorders; others are associated with developmental brain abnormalities.
- Some disorders occur within the first 24 hours of life and affected infants may have associated dysmorphic features and congenital abnormalities.
  - Peroxisomal defects
  - Disorders of pyruvate metabolism

- Respiratory chain defects
- Hydrops is an unusual presentation of some lysosomal storage diseases.
- The infant with a metabolic disorder may also present with less fulminant signs during the first few months of life.
  - Poor feeding, recurrent vomiting, and generalized hypotonia
  - Infants who have tyrosinemia type I experience liver dysfunction, and their status can deteriorate rapidly.

Late-onset presentation

- In one-third of patients, disease does not become clinically apparent until childhood or even later.
- Late-onset presentation is more variable than neonatal presentation and frequently involves precipitating factors, such as diet and illness.
- Mutations in responsible genes may encode a protein with more residual activity; patients with neonatal presentations may have none.
- Poor growth, developmental delay, or other underlying chronic abnormalities are often found.
  - However, illness can also occur acutely in a previously well individual.
  - Toddlers with medium-chain acyl-CoA dehydrogenase deficiency typically exhibit the condition acutely.
- Some patients with urea cycle defects have late-onset presentations.
  - May involve neurologic symptoms and include:
    - Encephalopathy
    - Psychiatric symptoms
    - Ataxia
    - Stroke-like episodes
    - Recovery may be slow, with permanent or transient neurologic dysfunction.
  - Nongenetic diagnoses usually considered include:
    - Reye syndrome
    - Ingestion of toxic substances
    - Encephalitis
- In children with recurrent vomiting, lethargy, and dehydration resembling viral illness, each episode is protracted.
  - Improvement often requires parenteral fluids.
  - Patients with methylmalonic academia, isovaleric acidemia, and MSUD can exhibit symptoms later on in this fashion.
- Recurrent crises of fever, vomiting, and diarrhea associated with dysmorphic features are found in mevalonic aciduria.
- Recurrence of similar episodes of illness is characteristic of metabolic disease.
- Abdominal pain, vomiting, and evidence of pancreatitis (eg, increased serum amylase) occur in ~8% of patients with organic acidemia.

- Organic acidemias constitute a high proportion of otherwise unexplained pancreatitis in children.
- Postpartum coma may lead to the diagnosis of an underlying urea cycle defect.

Neuropsychological regression

- Characteristic feature of lysosomal storage disorders
  - Typically, the child demonstrates either normal or slow developmental progress, then fails to reach developmental milestones.
  - Progressive deterioration occurs at variable ages and rates.
  - Certain associated physical findings can narrow the differential diagnosis in this group.

Chronic, progressive symptoms

- Metabolic disease can affect any major organ system chronically and progressively without episodes of acute illness.

LABORATORY EVALUATION

- Routine laboratory investigation can provide useful diagnostic clues.
- In disorders that have episodic symptoms, laboratory values may be abnormal only at the time of acute illness.
- Partial treatment with intravenous fluids, transfusions, or dietary changes can mask abnormalities.
- Drug metabolites can result in false-positive findings.
- Diagnostic results are more likely to be obtained by testing for metabolic disease early in the course of illness.
  - Collect specimens early.
    - Urine, heparinized plasma, spinal fluid
  - Store specimens frozen.
  - Send them later for analysis, if warranted.
- Key laboratory abnormalities are metabolic acidosis; hypoglycemia, with or without ketosis; and hyperammonemia.
- Low uric acid levels often escape attention.
  - Consistently present in molybdenum cofactor deficiency and disorders of purine catabolism
  - May be the result of renal tubular defects
  - Leukopenia and thrombocytopenia have been found in patients with organic acidemias.
    - Patients who have methylmalonic acidemia develop evidence of renal dysfunction.

Initial blood and urine tests for suspected genetic metabolic disorders

- Blood
  - Blood gases, electrolytes: Metabolic acidosis, increased anion gap
    - Disease: Organic acidemias, MSUD, disorders of carbohydrate metabolism, mitochondrial defects
  - Blood gases, electrolytes: Respiratory alkalosis
    - Disease: Urea cycle defects

- Glucose: Low with ketosis
  - Disease: Disorders of carbohydrate metabolism, organic acidemias
- Glucose: Low without ketosis
  - Disease: Fatty acid oxidation defects
- Ammonia: High
  - Disease: Urea cycle defects, organic acidemias, fatty acid oxidation defects
- Lactate, pyruvate: High
  - Disease: Disorders of carbohydrate metabolism, respiratory chain defects
- Uric acid: High
  - Disease: Glycogen storage disorders, fatty acid oxidation defects, organic acidemias
- Uric acid: Low
  - Disease: Molybdenum cofactor deficiency
- Urea nitrogen: Low
  - Disease: Urea cycle disorders
- Liver transaminases: High
  - Disease: Tyrosinemia, galactosemia, hereditary fructose intolerance, fatty acid oxidation defects
- Phosphate: Low
  - Disease: Hereditary fructose intolerance, fructose 1,6 diphosphatase deficiency
- Creatine kinase: High
  - Disease: Fatty acid oxidation disorders, mitochondrial myopathies, muscular dystrophies
- Blood count: Neutropenia, thrombocytopenia
  - Disease: Organic acidemias
- Urine
  - Odor
    - Assess by opening a closed container left at room temperature for 3 hours.
    - Sweaty feet, musty, tomcat urine, maple syrup odor
      - Disease: Organic acidemias, aminoacidopathies
  - Ketones
    - Essential test whenever hypoglycemia is documented
    - Positive
      - Disease: Organic acidemias, MSUD, disorders of carbohydrate metabolism
  - Reducing substances
    - Requires urine glucose determination for interpretation
    - Positive with glucose, galactose, fructose
      - Disease: Galactosemia, hereditary fructose intolerance

G

Specific laboratory tests for genetic metabolic disorders

■ Blood

- Test: Quantitative plasma amino acids
  - Disease: Aminoacidopathies, organic acidemias, disorders of carbohydrate metabolism
- Test: Carnitine levels (total, free, and esterified), acylcarnitine profile
  - Disease: Disorders of fatty acid metabolism
- Test: Very long–chain fatty acids, plasmalogens, phytanic acid
  - Disease: Peroxisomal disorders (leukodystrophies)

■ Urine

- Test: Quantitative amino acids
  - Disease: Specific amino acid transport defects
- Test: Organic acids
  - Disease: Organic acidemias
- Test: Oligosaccharide thin-layer chromatography
  - Disease: Lysosomal disorders of glycoprotein degradation
- Test: Screens (ferric chloride, dinitrophenylhydrazine, sulfite MPS spot)
  - Disease: Aminoacidopathies, organic acidemias, sulfite oxidase–deficiency MPSs (frequent false positives and false negatives)

■ Cerebrospinal fluid

- Test: Amino acids, glucose, neurotransmitters, lactate
  - Disease: Nonketotic hyperglycinemia (requires simultaneous plasma amino acids), disorders of neurotransmitters, mitochondrial disorders

■ Blood, skin, or other tissue

- Test: Enzyme assays
  - Disease: Lysosomal enzymes, definitive diagnosis of most metabolic disorders

■ If the child dies before a definitive diagnosis is made:

- A small piece of muscle and liver should be flash frozen and held at –80°C.
- A skin sample to culture fibroblasts should be obtained by biopsy before death for enzyme studies.
- Heparinized plasma and urine should be frozen for metabolic studies.
- EDTA-anticoagulated blood should be obtained for DNA studies.

DIAGNOSTIC PROCEDURES

■ Skin biopsy for fibroblast cultures for enzyme studies and liver biopsy

TREATMENT APPROACH

■ Treatment of metabolic disease can be divided into 2 categories.
- Short-term therapy
- Long-term management

■ Short-term therapy and long-term management should be provided in consultation with a physician skilled in treating metabolic diseases.

■ Careful monitoring of laboratory parameters and clinical status is required.
- Attention needs to be given to complications that may result from biochemical abnormalities and therapy.

Short-term therapy

■ In treatment of episodes of metabolic decompensation (before or after diagnosis has been established), the ill child is approached as usual.
- Particular attention paid to:
  - Respiratory status
  - Cardiovascular status
  - Fluid status
  - Neurologic status
- Intake of all potentially offending compounds (protein, lactose, fructose) is stopped.
- Further catabolism is inhibited by providing high caloric intake.
  - Caloric supplements should include at least 60 calories/kg per day from glucose to prevent proteolysis.
    - Generally conforms to hourly rate of D10 (with appropriate electrolytes) at twice maintenance or 8–10 mg/kg per min of glucose
- Insulin, starting at a low dose, may be required to maintain euglycemia and promote anabolism.
- Bicarbonate is useful in cases of severe acidosis.
- If a vitamin-responsive disorder is suspected, a trial of vitamin cofactors can be instituted.
  - Hydroxocobalamin
  - Biotin
  - Thiamine
  - Riboflavin
  - Pyridoxine
  - Folate
- Carnitine may be added in organic acidurias to promote excretion of toxic metabolites.
- In disorders of fatty acid oxidation, carnitine should be used judiciously and only to restore normal levels of free carnitine.

■ Patients with hyperammonemia—detoxify and remove ammonia with:

- Intravenous phenylacetate
- Sodium benzoate
- Arginine

■ Situations requiring prompt institution of hemodialysis

- Progressive hyperammonemia unresponsive to medications
- Comatose states that result from hyperammonemia or other toxic metabolites

■ For patients with MSUD, acute crises are best managed with the use of nasogastric branched-chain amino acid–free synthetic feeds.

Long-term management

■ Long-term therapy is disease specific and involves several strategies.

■ To reduce the accumulation of toxic metabolites, intake of offending compounds is limited to the smallest amount needed for growth and development.

- This approach often requires an artificial diet that includes special formulas and caloric supplementation.
- Regular monitoring of amino acids and other laboratory values is required to optimize diet for each individual patient.
- For some disorders, the offending compound is non-essential and can be eliminated entirely.
- When the enzyme defect involves binding of a cofactor (usually a vitamin) or defective synthesis of the cofactor itself, therapy centers on dietary supplementation of the cofactor.
  - Other strategies include stimulation of alternative biochemical pathways to detoxify and remove the offending substance.

■ Tyrosinemia type I

- Treatment with nitisinone blocks formation of succinylacetone, a toxic compound.

■ Cystinosis

- Administration of cysteamine, an aminothiol, reduces lysosomal storage of cystine.

■ In disorders accompanied by fasting intolerance

- Treatment consists of frequent meals.
- May require administration of complex carbohydrates, such as cornstarch, between meals to allow prolonged absorption of glucose and nocturnal nasogastric feeding.

■ Other therapeutic approaches directly provide the missing product.

- Congenital disorders of glycosylation
  - Mannose supplements
- Smith-Lemli-Opitz syndrome
  - Cholesterol

■ None of these interventions constitutes a cure, and most are only partially successful in alleviating clinical symptoms.

■ Chaperone therapy (use of pharmacologic molecules to normalize or stabilize protein structure or function) to optimize residual enzymatic activities has been proposed.

■ Liver and bone marrow transplantations have been performed in several disorders, with mixed results.

■ Enzyme replacement therapies have been developed for some lysosomal storage disorders; others are in the pipeline.

■ Gene therapies and in utero therapies continue to be explored.

■ On a community level, daily care of patients can be extensive.

- The team approach includes education of ancillary caretakers, school systems, and the public.
- There are psychosocial and financial consequences to patient and family.

SPECIFIC TREATMENT

Screening for genetic metabolic disease

■ Newborn screening can accelerate diagnosis.

- Specimens must be analyzed quickly and abnormal results reported promptly.
- A sine qua non of newborn screening is that the prognosis can be improved by prompt institution of therapy.
  - Accumulated experience with screening has demonstrated that the outcome is not always as good as anticipated.
  - For some disorders, a few infants may receive therapy unnecessarily.

■ Certain disorders for which treatment is effective are asymptomatic until it is too late for effective intervention.

- In phenylketonuria (PKU), nonspecific signs (eg, eczema) occasionally appear early in infancy.
  - However, by the time developmental delay is apparent, irreversible damage has occurred.
- For other disorders, symptoms appear early, but diagnosis is often delayed.
  - Galactosemia
  - MSUD
  - Some cases of congenital hypothyroidism (CH)

■ A few single-gene conditions occur only after exposure to environmental agents that are not harmful to most in the doses encountered.

- Screening might result in treatment that ameliorates harmful effects or warns those at risk to avoid exposure.
- <10% of people who develop cancer have inherited alleles at single loci that greatly increase susceptibility to malignant transformation.
  - Retinoblastoma and breast and colon cancer have been studied most thoroughly.
- The benefits of screening the entire population for genetic susceptibilities remain to be established.

- Most single-gene disorders are not treatable, but persons at risk, as well as heterozygous carriers, can be detected by genetic tests (see Prevention).

■ Primary health care clinicians will be increasingly involved with neonatal, carrier, and prenatal screening and presymptomatic testing for adult-onset disorders.

- In some cases, the clinician will:
  – Inform patients about availability of tests
  – Counsel patients about having tests
  – Interpret meaning of test results for patients

False-positive and false-negative findings

■ Few people being screened will be at risk of disease in themselves or their offspring.

■ False-positive findings frequently occur more often than the condition of interest in the population being screened.

- Immunoreactive trypsinogen (IRT) test used in a few states to screen newborns for cystic fibrosis (CF) yields >5 times as many false-positive as true-positive results.

- Because blood phenylalanine concentration may exceed normal levels only minimally during the first few days of life in infants who have PKU, the cutoff for phenylalanine level (and other metabolites) must be set lower than the minimal phenylalanine concentration needed to establish a diagnosis of PKU.

■ On average, by using current methods, >50 false-positive findings are identified for every confirmed case.

■ When DNA tests are performed appropriately for single-gene disorders, false-positive results are seldom encountered.

- For disorders in which a single-gene mutation increases risk of disease but is insufficient to cause it, positive DNA test results do not always mean that disease will occur.

■ False-negative results are a problem with both DNA tests and more traditional tests.

- In DNA tests, they occur when the test does not detect all the different mutations capable of causing disease.

■ Early discharge of healthy newborns before 24 hours of age increases the number of infants who have false-negative and false-positive test results.

- Infants with PKU have near-normal levels of phenylalanine in cord blood; adequate exposure to exogenous protein is required to develop a high phenylalanine level.

- When quantitation of blood galactose is used to screen for galactosemia, infants with galactosemia must have consumed sufficient amounts of galactose-containing human milk or cow's milk formula to accumulate galactose.

- ~10% of infants with CH will have normal thyroxine (T_4) levels when screened early.
  – Most also have normal thyroid-stimulating hormone (TSH) levels.

- When TSH is used as the initial screening test (common in Europe but not in US), ≤25% of infants discharged early may have increased levels.

- In screening for congenital adrenal hyperplasia (CAH), samples collected before 36 hours of age are much more likely to yield false-positive increases in 17-hydroxyprogesterone than are samples collected after 48 hours.

■ The chance of misclassification is higher the earlier an infant is screened.

- Most, but not all, infants who have disorders for which screening usually is provided will be detected when tested after 24 hours of age.

■ It is difficult to guarantee that a screening test will be performed soon after discharge.

- Therefore, no infant should be discharged, even if <24 hours, without first being screened.

■ Raising the threshold value to reduce the number of false-positive results or lowering it to reduce the number of false-negative results for infants screened before 48 hours:

- Increases, respectively, the number of false-negative and false-positive results

- Use of a different value for infants screened early or late requires the laboratory to treat the 2 groups of infants separately.

- The best solution to prevent these errors is not to discharge infants until they are at least 48 hours of age.
  – Some state newborn screening programs require a second screening test at 2 weeks of age.

■ No clinician should ever assume that an infant with symptoms of a disorder for which screening was performed might not have that disorder.

■ Screening tests can give erroneous results because of the presence of other substances that interfere with analysis.

- Donor blood products from recent transfusion can affect DNA tests.

- Certain antibiotics can interfere with the bacterial inhibition assays used in some newborn screening.

■ In absence of rigorous quality-control programs, laboratory error is probably the most common cause of false-positive and false-negative newborn screening test results.

- Misidentification of specimens
- Failure to transmit results properly
- Erroneous assays

Newborn screening

General

■ In the US, newborn screening is mandated by each state.

- For many years, most states screened only for PKU and hypothyroidism.

- Now, the scope includes conditions for which the hope is that early recognition will ameliorate outcome.

- The National Newborn Screening and Genetics Resource Center maintains current information on states screening requirements.
- All states and the District of Columbia routinely screen newborns for:
  - PKU (1 in 14,000 live births)
  - CH (1 in 3300 live births)
  - Galactosemia (approximately 1 in 59,000 live births)
  - Sickle cell anemia (>1 in 400 live births of black infants)
- All states except Florida screen for other hemoglobinopathies.
- Other state screening
  - 46 states screen for MSUD (<1 in 100,000 live births).
  - 45 for homocystinuria (<1 in 100,000 live births)
  - 44 for biotinidase deficiency (~1 in 80,000 live births)
  - 48 for CAH (1 in 20,000 live births)
  - 46 for medium-chain acyl-CoA dehydrogenase deficiency (1 in 15,000 live births)
  - 24 for CF (1 in 3200 white live births)
- Physicians should document screening test results and any follow-up in the child's medical record.
- Practitioners should not place undue faith in a negative result.
  - Screening tests can be falsely negative.
  - Repeat or more definitive testing should be obtained for infants whose findings arouse suspicion.
  - Treatment should not be started on the basis of a single positive screening test result.
  - Consultation with someone experienced in evaluation of metabolic disorders should be initiated.
  - When treatment is indicated, response may vary.
- Some infants may escape screening.
  - The largest group is composed of infants born at home; they should be screened at their first visit for pediatric care.
  - Sick infants transferred from one hospital to another may be missed; if any doubt exists, the receiving hospital should rescreen the baby.

PKU

- Infants with PKU show few signs until they develop mental retardation.
  - PKU may not be appreciated until the second year of life.
  - Disease is irreversible.
- Screening early in infancy, followed by prompt administration of a diet low in phenylalanine, is the only way to improve outcome.
  - Intellectual performance correlates with age at which dietary treatment is started and with success of dietary control.
  - Studies to confirm positive test results should be performed quickly to permit initiation of a low-phenylalanine diet as soon as possible, no later than the third week of life.

- The AAP recommends that every infant in the US be screened before discharge from the nursery.
  - Infants initially screened before 24 hours of age should be rescreened before the third week of life.
  - Premature and sick infants should be screened by the seventh day of life.
- A few states recommend that all infants undergo a second screening between 2 and 4 weeks of age.
- Defects in the synthesis or regeneration of biopterin cofactors for the conversion of phenylalanine to tyrosine also result in positive screening test results and clinical disease.
  - In addition to the predominant phenylalanine hydroxylase deficiency
  - Dietary restriction of phenylalanine is insufficient to prevent mental deterioration and seizures in these infants.
    - Use of biopterin or neurotransmitter precursors offers some hope.
    - Infants with these disorders will be identified by neonatal screening for PKU.
    - They represent <3% of all infants with hyperphenylalaninemia.
    - Tests for these variant forms should be performed in any infant who persistently has high blood phenylalanine levels, even in the moderate range of 10–20 mg/dL, while on a normal diet.

CH

- Causes of CH are multiple and complex.
  - Transplacental passage of maternal antibodies that interfere with fetal thyroid development or thyroid function
  - Maternal antibodies can cause transient hypothyroidism.
  - Mothers receiving antithyroid medication (propylthiouracil) may have babies with transient hypothyroidism.
  - Genetic factors are suggested in families with >1 affected infant.
    - Such findings do not rule out environmental or maternally acquired causes.
  - For unknown reasons, girls are twice as likely as boys to have CH.
  - Birth prevalence is somewhat higher in Hispanic and Native American persons than in white or Asian persons, in whom it is higher than in black persons.
- Infants with the most profound deficiencies of T_4, usually as a result of thyroid agenesis, are more likely to have neonatal symptoms.
  - Persistent jaundice, difficulty feeding, and lethargy are most frequent.
  - Even infants with agenesis may be asymptomatic when examined following an abnormal screening test result.
    - Placental transfer of T_4 and some fetal production of triiodothyronine in the brain may explain this circumstance.

G

- The 10% of infants with CH found by a second screening (in states that screen twice) are less often symptomatic and have lower increases of TSH.
- Even if newborn test results are negative, hypothyroidism may still develop in infancy or childhood.
- The incidence of CH detected by neonatal screening is higher than that detected by clinical diagnosis in the prescreening era, suggesting either:
  - That infants who have milder disease escaped diagnosis *or*
  - That some infants receiving a diagnosis today do not really have CH
    - Thus it is important to ensure that CH persists in equivocal cases.
- In most laboratories in the US, T_4 is measured on the screening specimen.
  - If low, then TSH is measured on the same specimen.
    - If TSH is high and findings are confirmed by another specimen, treatment with T_4 is initiated.
  - Most infants who persistently have low T_4 levels but normal TSH levels will prove on further study to have normal free T_4 concentrations and thyroid-binding globulin deficiency and do not require treatment.
  - A few infants with low T_4 and normal TSH levels have pituitary gland failure, which is encountered much less frequently than thyroid-binding globulin deficiency.
  - Occasionally, an infant with initial low T_4 and normal TSH levels will have a delayed increase in TSH level and symptoms of hypothyroidism.
    - TSH should be retested if symptoms appear.
- Motor and cognitive development of infants with CH at 7.5 years of age correlate with the age at which T_4 treatment is started.
  - Most infants who receive early treatment have IQ scores in the normal range.
    - Many are at the low end compared with matched controls (approximately a 5- to 10-point loss in IQ).
- Patients with CH have persistent deficits in visuospatial abilities, memory, and attention, correlated to severity of early hypothyroidism.

Sickle cell anemia

- States have added sickle cell disease to their newborn screening programs.
- Before screening, ~10% of infants in the US with sickle cell disease died by 10 years of age.
- Effectiveness of screening in reducing morbidity and mortality depends on:
  - Ensuring that infants detected by screening are referred to a continuing source of care to receive prophylactic penicillin
  - Parents learning how to manage situations that increase chance of sickle cell crises

- No specific treatment is available for sickle cell anemia.
- Tests used for screening
  - Hemoglobin electrophoresis, isoelectric focusing, high-performance liquid chromatography
    - Reveals hemoglobinopathies in addition to sickle cell anemia
  - Specific sickle cell anemia DNA testing
    - Does not identify other hemoglobinopathies
  - All forms of sickle cell testing identify infants with sickle cell trait who will remain healthy.
  - Parents of an infant with sickle cell trait may be at risk for having an infant who has sickle cell anemia if both partners are carriers of the sickle cell gene.
  - A screening program will have 40 times more carriers to notify than parents of infants who have sickle cell anemia.
  - The purpose of notifying parents is to offer testing to determine whether they are both carriers and at 25% risk of having affected offspring with each subsequent pregnancy.
  - An infant who has this trait and triggers the investigative process has nothing to gain from it.
    - In most couples that have an infant with the trait, only 1 partner is a carrier.
  - Parents should be informed that newborn screening might provide information about their future risks of having a child with a serious hemoglobinopathy.
    - They should be given the opportunity to request the results.
  - Thalassemias are not directly screened for in the US
    - Will be detected when general hemoglobin electrophoresis is performed

Galactosemia

- In contrast to PKU, serious manifestations of classic galactosemia occur soon after milk feedings are started.
  - Diagnosis can be, and often is, made clinically before screening test results are reported.
  - Prompt administration of a lactose-free diet in newborns will save the lives of patients with this disorder.
  - May not prevent mental retardation or other developmental problems, including a high incidence of ovarian failure
  - The age of starting the galactose-free diet is not significantly associated with the magnitude of problems (developmental delay, physical growth, or speech).
- It is uncertain whether infants whose galactosemia is found by screening would have developed symptoms had they not been started on a lactose-free diet.
  - Some infants discovered by screening have variant forms of galactosemia.
  - Residual amounts of galactosyl-1-phosphate uridylyltransferase (ie, enzyme that is absent in classic cases) are found.

G

- Infants with some of these variants have acute neonatal symptoms, generally milder than in classic cases.
- Some infants exhibit no symptoms.
  - It is unclear whether they are less likely to have long-term manifestations, such as developmental delay.

■ Much remains to be learned about the pathogenesis of galactosemia and development of effective therapy.
- The value of neonatal screening for galactosemia is questionable, although classic galactosemia will result in death if untreated.

■ The principal goal is to ensure prompt intervention in individuals who have early onset of symptoms and whose lives are threatened.
- These infants can be diagnosed clinically.

MSUD

■ Infants with the classic form of MSUD usually show signs within 2 weeks of birth.
- The course can be fulminant and rapidly fatal.
- Early treatment can prevent or ameliorate acute symptoms.

■ Patients require a special diet low in branched-chain amino acids.
- If the diet is started early, long-term outcome can be good.

■ One problem with routine screening is the inherent delay in obtaining results.
- A specimen collected on day 2 may not be reported until day 10.
  - By that time, most infants with classic MSUD will be severely ill or dead.
  - Starting the special diet will usually save infants who are still alive at this point, but survivors often have mental retardation and neurologic problems.
- Confirmation of MSUD in sick infants can sometimes be hastened by contacting the laboratory responsible for performing newborn screening.
  - In many instances, the laboratory will process the specimen more quickly when it receives a special request.
  - Infants known to be at risk because of a previously affected family member or North American Mennonite descent:
    ■ Should undergo definitive testing (quantitative plasma amino acids) on the second day of life
    ■ Immediately begin a special diet to ensure the best possible outcome

■ Lapse into coma is associated with a decrease of up to 40 IQ points.

■ The enzyme defect in MSUD is complex, and many different mutations have been characterized.
- Exception: a North American Mennonite community, in which a single mutation accounts for a high prevalence of the condition

■ Many patients are compound heterozygotes.
- As a result of screening and immediate institution of the special diet, establishing the genotype-phenotype relationship has been difficult.
- Some infants started on the diet may have forms of the disorder that would have appeared only later in infancy or childhood with:
  - Episodes of ataxia
  - Failure to thrive
  - Mild ketoacidosis, particularly after infection or high-protein ingestion

CAH

■ In 21-hydroxylase deficiency and 11-hydroxylase deficiency, cortisol production is impaired.
- 21-hydroxylase deficiency accounts for >90% of patients with CAH.
- 11-hydroxylase deficiency accounts for ~5% of cases.
- As a result of the deficiency, feedback inhibition of adrenocorticotropic hormone is lacking.
- Cortisol precursors, including those that have androgenic activity, are overproduced.

■ In girls, ambiguous genitalia should permit clinical diagnosis in the neonatal period.
- Because the diagnosis is not always made, screening might increase recognition of girls, permitting them to be raised as girls.
- The diagnosis is much more difficult to establish in newborn boys.

■ Approximately two-thirds of infants who have 21-hydroxylase deficiency lose salt.
- They may experience severe dehydration and vascular collapse accompanied by hyponatremia during the first 3 weeks of life.
- Unscreened boys who have salt-losing CAH receive a diagnosis at a median age of 26 days vs 12 days for screened boys.

■ Boys who have simple virilizing CAH are detected only by screening.

■ Several different mutations in the gene for 21-hydroxylase have been found.
- The presence of salt losing depends on the particular mutation, but a complete genotype-phenotype correlation has not been established.

Biotinidase deficiency

■ Biotin is a cofactor of several carboxylases.

■ Availability through recycling is reduced in inherited deficiencies of biotinidase.

G

- Manifestations and age at onset of biotinidase deficiency vary, possibly because of differences in degree of enzyme deficiency and amount of biotin available to the infant.
  - Symptoms usually appear between 2 weeks and 3 years.
    - Ataxia
    - Alopecia
    - Hearing loss
    - Decreased vision
    - Optic atrophy
    - Seizures
  - Not yet known whether some infants who have the disorder remain free of symptoms
    - It is possible that not all infants discovered by screening will develop symptoms.
      - Infants found by screening have higher levels of residual biotinidase than those diagnosed clinically.
      - Treatment with supplemental biotin is simple and inexpensive.
  - Biotin reverses some symptoms after they appear.
    - Not always true for hearing and visual impairments and developmental delay
    - Unclear whether clinical diagnosis will always be made expeditiously
  - Infants treated as a result of screening have so far remained free of symptoms.

CF

- IRT is increased in the blood of most newborns with CF.
- 24 states currently perform this test.
  - Those that mandate 2 screenings use this method alone.
    - Other states follow IRT with second-tier DNA testing for common CF transmembrane conductance regulator mutations.
  - Some states screen only for the *F508* delmutation, which is present in 70% of CF alleles worldwide.
    - Other states require a broader panel, which is enriched for mutations seen in black and Hispanic persons.
    - Decreases the rate of false-positive findings identified by IRT screening alone
    - May miss up to 10% of patients with CF who do not carry a common mutation on either allele
- Neonates with CF and meconium ileus usually have false-negative results.
- The Centers for Disease Control and Prevention issued a report concluding that screening newborns for CF was justified.
  - Long-term nutritional outcome is improved in children identified by screening compared with those identified clinically.
  - Newborn screening may improve childhood survival.

- No treatment is yet available that prevents the clinical manifestations.

Homocystinuria

- Vitamin B_6–dependent forms of homocystinuria
  - Treated easily and effectively
  - Account for ~50% of cases
- Newborn screening will not detect all affected infants.
- The detection rate after the first week of life by tests that measure blood or urine homocystine will be higher than that of neonatal screening, which detects hypermethioninemia.
  - Hard to justify newborn screening by bacterial inhibition assay
  - Some experts have suggested lowering the blood methionine cutoff to 1 mg/dL to decrease the false-negative rate.
    - Argument has been obviated by institution of tandem mass spectrometry (MS/MS) for newborn screening.
    - Results are quantitative, and MS/MS is currently being used to some extent in all but 6 states.

Medium-chain acyl-CoA dehydrogenase deficiency

- Medium-chain acyl-CoA dehydrogenase deficiency has an incidence of 1 in 10,000 to 14,000 in the white population.
  - 25–50% initial decompensation fatality rate
  - Easily treated by:
    - Avoiding fasting and catabolism
    - Instituting carnitine supplementation and intravenous glucose early in course of intercurrent illness
- Unscreened infants are usually discovered at between 6 and 18 months of age after decreased caloric intake usually associated with intercurrent illness.
  - The child develops hypoketotic hypoglycemia, followed by hepatic encephalopathy and ultimately death if untreated.
    - The whole progression can occur during the 12 hours of nighttime sleep.
    - Accounted for small percentage of deaths caused by sudden infant death syndrome in the prescreening era

Glucose-6-phosphate dehydrogenase deficiency

- A significant number of different alleles result in this X-linked genetic susceptibility.
- The usual manifestations are hemolytic anemia accompanied by jaundice and hemoglobinuria.
- ~10% of black boys inherit the mild A form.
  - Except for some sulfur compounds (eg, sulfamethoxazole), drugs that trigger reactions are seldom used in the US (eg, primaquine).
    - Some individuals may develop hemolysis after heavy exposure to naphthalene (mothballs).

- In the more severe Mediterranean variant (only occasionally in the A variant), hemolytic anemia (favism) is encountered after ingestion of fava beans.
  - A staple in many Mediterranean diets
  - Initiation of a newborn screening program for glucose-6-phosphate dehydrogenase deficiency in Sardinia, together with more education about the deficiency, was associated with a marked decline in occurrence of favism and need for blood transfusions.

α_1-Antitrypsin (α_1-AT) deficiency

- α_1-AT deficiency is usually the result of inheriting Z alleles from both parents.
- Individuals with severe α_1-AT are at increased risk of chronic obstructive pulmonary disease (COPD).
  - In population-based surveys, many people who have severe deficiency remain asymptomatic throughout life.
  - Smokers who have the deficiency are likely to encounter pulmonary problems between 20 and 40 years of age, ~15 years earlier than nonsmokers.
  - Not all nonsmokers who have α_1-AT deficiency get COPD (accounts for ~1% of all COPD).
  - Presymptomatic screening might alert individuals who have α_1-AT deficiency to the especially harmful consequences of smoking.
- Treatment of α_1-AT–deficient adults with emphysema with human α_1-AT increased serum and lung α_1-AT levels but did not improve their pulmonary function.
  - Whether treatment would prevent COPD remains to be established.
- Screening of newborns or young children is of questionable value because adolescents who have α_1-AT deficiency have normal pulmonary function.
- ~10% of infants who have α_1-AT deficiency develop cholestasis.
  - 2–3% later develop cirrhosis.
  - No specific treatment or known means of preventing liver manifestations is available.
  - Human milk may be protective.
  - Newborn screening would not be expected to alter prognosis.
- α_1-AT deficiency should be included in the differential diagnosis of persistent jaundice in young infants.
- Screening adolescents or young adults might be of benefit.

New techniques for newborn screening

General

- Enzyme replacement therapy has been developed to treat infant-onset Pompe disease.
  - For the best outcome, treatment should be initiated before 6 months of age.

- A dried-blood spot filter paper assay has been developed.
  - Many experts are advocating for adding this condition to the newborn screening panel.
- Treatment is variably effective.
  - In some patients, it affords complete resolution of heart and muscle disease.
  - In others, it converts a fatal disorder to a severe chronic illness, resulting in numerous hospitalizations and slow deterioration.
- Cord blood stem cell transplantation can cure Krabbe disease if undertaken in the first month of life.
  - One state has already added this condition to its newborn screening panel.
- New tests are being developed to screen for severe combined immunodeficiency and adrenoleukodystrophy.
  - Much research and interest exists in this area.

MS/MS

- MS/MS can quantitate accurately multiple amino acids, organic acids, and metabolites of fatty acid oxidation from dried blood on filter paper.
- The advent of this technique has:
  - Broadened the scope of newborn screening
  - Dramatically decreased (by 2 orders of magnitude) some false-positive rates
  - Decreased the false-negative rates for homocystinuria
- MS/MS is used to screen for:
  - PKU
  - MSUD
  - Homocystinuria
  - Tyrosinemia
  - Citrullinemia, by detecting increased citrulline
  - Argininosuccinic acidemia, by detecting increased citrulline
- MS/MS cannot detect ornithine transcarbamylase or carbamoylphosphate synthetase deficiencies.
  - Cannot reliably detect a low citrulline level
- MS/MS can detect a broad array of organic acids and metabolites of fatty acid oxidation.
- For many disorders that can be identified by MS/MS, no fully effective treatment exists.
  - Early intervention may not affect outcome.
  - Undiagnosed infant deaths would decrease.
  - Availability of prenatal diagnosis in subsequent pregnancies for at-risk families would increase.
- The American College of Medical Genetics and March of Dimes concurred on a core panel of disorders and secondary target conditions that can be detected by MS/MS.

G

Genetic susceptibilities

■ In a few genetic conditions, disease is likely to appear only in certain environments.

● Screening of infants or young children provides warning that certain exposures will be harmful and should be avoided.

– If harmful exposures occur, awareness of the genetic susceptibility might speed appropriate management.

● In the US, no state currently screens newborns for such genetic susceptibilities.

– May reflect a lack of confidence in the ability of the health care system or parents to ensure that the harmful exposures will be avoided

● Screening workers or prospective employees for genetic susceptibilities to agents that may be encountered is of interest to some employers.

Carrier screening

■ Carrier screening is undertaken for severe untreatable inherited disorders to provide persons identified as carriers with options for preventing conception or birth of affected children.

● Tay-Sachs disease

– Carrier screening has resulted in a significant decrease in disease in many Jewish communities.

● Thalassemia

– Carrier screening in Sardinia and elsewhere in the Mediterranean Basin has lowered incidence.

● Sickle cell anemia

– Most American couples found by carrier screening to be at risk of having a child with sickle cell anemia decide not to terminate the pregnancy.

– With nondirective counseling, they may not view the disorder as severe.

■ School-based screening programs for sickle cell and Tay-Sachs disease carriers probably recruit a much higher proportion of the at-risk population than do community programs or office or clinic screening programs.

● However, may lead to stigmatization of students identified as carriers

● Unclear that adolescents identified as carriers will retain this information or act on it when they consider having children

■ If prenatal diagnosis of a condition is available and abortion of an affected fetus is acceptable, then less reason exists to offer screening before pregnancy.

● Couples might be screened before the woman becomes pregnant or early in pregnancy.

■ Since 2001, the American College of Obstetricians and Gynecologists has recommended offering carrier testing for CF for all pregnant white women.

● In 2005 it altered its recommended panel of 25 mutations.

● Uptake of screening approached 25% of pregnancies in 2004.

■ Screening young women to determine whether they are carriers of X-linked disorders is technically feasible with DNA analysis.

● Fragile X syndrome

● Hemophilia

● Duchenne muscular dystrophy

● Because of new mutations, not all births of infants with these disorders might potentially be avoided.

● Such testing is not routinely offered at this time.

Prenatal screening

■ Practitioners who provide care to young persons do not usually have primary responsibility for managing pregnancies.

● However, they often will have prior contact with the mother and father.

– Can contribute to the parents' understanding of the indications for screening in pregnancy

– May also be contacted by obstetricians to assist in counseling or in anticipation of high-risk newborns

■ Neural tube defects

■ Folate supplementation of bread products was initiated in January 1998.

■ Maternal serum screening of α-fetoprotein (AFP) between the 15th and 21st weeks of pregnancy

● Maternal serum AFP test can detecting 90% of fetuses that have anencephaly and ~80% of those that have open spina bifida.

● For every true-positive result, there will be ~30 false-positive results.

● Normal maternal serum AFP concentration is highly dependent on gestational age.

● In women with high maternal serum AFP, sonographic examination is needed to determine the accuracy of estimated gestational age.

– If sonography confirms gestational age, amniotic fluid is obtained by amniocentesis.

– If amniotic fluid AFP is high, the likelihood of an open neural tube defect is >90%.

● Further assurance that a defect is present is obtained by performing acetylcholinesterase determinations and high-detail (level 2) ultrasonography.

– Although high-level ultrasonography performed by expert sonographers detects most fetuses with open spina bifida, it should not replace AFP screening.

- Down syndrome
  - Prenatal diagnosis for Down syndrome is rapidly evolving.
    - Definitive testing requires chorionic villi sampling or amniocentesis.
      - Routinely offered to women >35 years of age
      - Costly and invasive
    - Biochemical marker screening tests are now available for:
      - Younger women
      - Women >35 years for whom risks of amniocentesis or chorionic villi sampling are unacceptable
    - Second-trimester triple screening detects approximately 60% of fetuses with Down syndrome.
      - Free ß-human chorionic gonadotropin
      - Maternal serum AFP
      - Estriol
    - Addition of inhibin A to form quadruple screening increases sensitivity to ~70%, with a 5% false-negative rate.
  - New first-trimester screening can detect 70% of fetuses with Down syndrome.
    - Includes testing for pregnancy-associated plasma protein A and free ß-human chorionic gonadotropin
    - When coupled with first-trimester nuchal translucency testing by ultrasonography, sensitivity increases to 86%, with only a 5% false-negative rate.
    - Technically challenging and not yet widely available
    - Sequential screening can detect ≤95% of affected pregnancies, with only an overall false-positive rate of 5%.
    - First-trimester screening, followed by second-trimester quadruple screening for persons not at high risk by first-trimester screening
  - First-trimester screening for Down syndrome does not obviate the need for second-trimester screening for neural tube defects.

WHEN TO REFER

- All patients suspected of having genetic metabolic disease should be referred to a physician who has expertise in this area.

WHEN TO ADMIT

- All infants whose respiratory, cardiac, hematologic, and neurologic status is unstable
- Patients in coma
- Patients with metabolic acidosis or respiratory alkalosis
- Patients with hypoglycemia and also elevated ammonia level
- Patients with significant electrolyte abnormalities
- Patients with significantly abnormal liver enzymes and liver function tests

PREVENTION

- Carrier testing before pregnancy provides couples the option of preventing conception of children who will have severe, untreatable, inherited disorders by:
  - Adoption
  - Artificial insemination of donor sperm
  - Ovum donation or surrogacy in the case of X-linked disorders
- Carrier testing early in pregnancy by chorionic villi sampling or amniocentesis provides couples the option of preventing the birth of an affected child.
  - By selective abortion
- Prenatal cytogenetic and biochemical testing can avoid the birth of children who have aneuploidy or neural tube defects, respectively.

G

Giardiasis

DEFINITION

- Gastrointestinal (GI) symptoms of waterborne disease caused by *Giardia intestinalis* (also known as *Giardia lamblia* and *iardia duodenalis*), an extracellular parasite that has no intermediate development outside of the intestinal lumen

EPIDEMIOLOGY

- *G intestinalis* is holoendemic in the US.
  - One of the most commonly identified pathogens in waterborne diarrheal disease
- Geographic distribution
  - Prevalence high in:
    - Mountainous regions
    - Child care centers
    - Major metropolitan areas
    - Among campers
    - Among international tourists
- Age
  - Children <5 years most commonly affected in the US.
    - With intensive exposure to stool, as in child care centers caring for infants in diapers, giardiasis quickly may become hyperendemic.
- Seasonality
  - Infection rates peak in late summer and early fall.

ETIOLOGY

- Many large common-source outbreaks have been traced to contaminated drinking water.
  - Municipal drinking water supplies that have sewage contamination, defective or deficient filtration facilities, and reliance on chlorination as the principal method of water disinfection
  - Use of surface water for drinking in mountainous regions
  - Although zoonotic infections have been documented, recent molecular epidemiologic studies suggest it is rare.
- *G intestinalis* exists in 2 forms.
  - Motile, flagellated trophozoite that causes disease
  - Dormant cyst that transmits infection
- Because cysts may be shed in abundance in the stool, *G intestinalis* may be transmitted by the fecal-oral route.
  - Main route of spread in families, institutions, and child care centers
- Foodborne giardiasis has been reported.
  - Food probably contaminated during preparation

RISK FACTORS

- HIV infection
- Intensive exposure to stool
- Poor sanitation
- Poor hygiene

SIGNS AND SYMPTOMS

- Incubation period of giardiasis is 7–14 days.
- Most infected patients remain asymptomatic; however, they shed cysts in their feces and are infectious.
- Children are more likely than adults to have symptomatic disease.
- Principal GI symptoms last 7–10 days or longer.
  - Most common
    - Diarrhea
    - Abdominal cramps
    - Nausea
  - Less common
    - Vomiting
    - Malodorous stools
    - Flatulence
    - Bloating
    - Anorexia
    - Constipation
  - Because of the disaccharidase deficiency that accompanies severe infections, some patients report milk intolerance, which may last for weeks.
- Giardiasis must be considered in the differential diagnosis of failure to thrive since some patients, particularly children, develop:
  - Chronic diarrhea
  - Frank malabsorption
  - Weight loss
  - Malnutrition
  - Growth retardation
- Malabsorption leading to iron-deficiency anemia also has been reported.
- Constitutional symptoms are not prominent, but up to 25% of patients experience:
  - Fatigue
  - Headache
  - Low-grade fever
- Extra intestinal syndromes (rare)
  - Urticaria
  - Erythema multiforme
  - Arthralgia
- Because the colon and rectum are not involved, tenesmus should suggest another diagnosis.
- Blood almost never is found in the stool.
- Presence of mucus is unusual.

- Physical examination
  - Generally unremarkable unless secondary malnutrition has developed

DIFFERENTIAL DIAGNOSIS

- Sprue
- Food allergy
- Psychogenic abdominal pain
- A wide variety of GI disturbances

DIAGNOSTIC APPROACH

- Confirm GI symptoms.
- Order laboratory workup for detection of parasites in stool.

LABORATORY FINDINGS

- Heat-stable antigen-detection in stool or detection of parasites by fluorescence is used more commonly now than microscopic examination of stool.
  - Tests often combined for simultaneous detection of *Cryptosporidium* species
  - These tests compare well with standard microscopic procedures.
    - In most cases, more sensitive
    - Multiple samples may be needed for optimal detection.
- Serologic tests are valuable in epidemiologic studies.
  - Of little use diagnostically
- Other blood tests
  - Sedimentation rate is normal.
  - No eosinophilia is found because the parasite is noninvasive.
- Biochemical evidence of malabsorption may be found, including:
  - Disaccharidase deficiency
  - Abnormal absorption of D-xylose and fat
  - Deficiency of folic acid

IMAGING

- Upper GI x-rays may reveal:
  - Mild dilation of the small bowel
  - Edema of the mucosa
  - Segmentation of barium
  - Either increased or decreased transit times
  - However, these changes are nonspecific.

DIAGNOSTIC PROCEDURES

- Direct duodenal aspiration or EnteroTest
  - Analysis of duodenal contents provides the optimum yield in patients requiring additional measures to have the pathogen detected.

- Small-bowel biopsy
  - In rare patients with chronic symptoms in whom the diagnosis must be excluded
    - Several sections of the biopsy specimen stained may be needed.
    - *Giardia* organisms are detected more easily in Giemsa-stained mucosal impression smears than in stool samples.
  - Biochemical evidence of malabsorption may be found, including:
    - Disaccharidase deficiency
    - Abnormal absorption of D-xylose and fat
    - Deficiency of folic acid

TREATMENT APPROACH

- Treat with an antiparasitic agent when infection is recognized, even if the patient is asymptomatic.
  - Carriers of the parasite are potential transmitters of disease and may have subclinical malabsorption.
  - Physicians may elect not to treat asymptomatic patients if reexposure to *G intestinalis* seems unavoidable in some hyperendemic settings.

SPECIFIC TREATMENTS

Metronidazole

- Used widely in adults and children
  - Giardiasis is not an approved indication for metronidazo-lein the US.
- Acceptable cure rate
  - Well tolerated (except for the mild metallic aftertaste)
    - Can be formulated as a suspension
  - Low incidence of serious side effects
    - Alcohol ingestion, including in concurrent medications, should be avoided with metronidazole because of disulfiram-like reactions.

Tinidazole

- Tinidazole is an itroimidazole similar to metronidazole
  - Had been used extensively in a single-dose regimen outside of the US
- FDA-approved for the treatment of giardiasis
  - Including in children ≥3 years
- Can be formulated as a suspension

Furazolidone

- Efficacy of furazolidone in children has been as high as 92%.
  - Comparable if not superior to cure rates seen with alternative agents
- Pleasant taste
- Available in a pediatric suspension

G

- Side effects have been minimal in children.
  - Mild GI distress
  - Hypersensitivity reactions
  - Hemolysis in individuals who have glucose-6-phosphate dehydrogenase deficiency
  - Brown discoloration of urine
  - Disulfiram-like reactions
- Contraindicated with monoamine oxidase inhibitors

Nitazoxanide

- Nitazoxanide is a recently FDA-approved antiparasitic agent with specific indications for the treatment of cryptosporidiosis and giardiasis in children
- Cure rates in small, randomized trials are similar to those with standard agents for giardiasis.
- Side effect rates seem similar to those with placebo.
  - Yellow sclera noted rarely
    - Clears with discontinuation of the drug
- More costly than other agents

Albendazole

- Albendazole is reported to be as effective as metronidazole in a study of children 5–10 years of age
- Active against a broad range of intestinal parasites, including helminths

Paromomycin

- Paromomycin is a nonabsorbable aminoglycoside
- Has been used to treat giardiasis in pregnancy
  - Data regarding its efficacy are limited.

Quinacrine

- Quinacrine was previously commonly used as therapy.
- Not commercially available in the US but can be obtained if needed (www.medicalletter.com).

Drug resistance

- No well-documented evidence exists for actual drug resistance in *Giardia* on an individual clinical case level.
- In vitro sensitivity has shown variations but is assay- and inoculum-dependent.
- For cases of severe or recalcitrant infections, prolonged or combination therapy may be necessary.

PROGNOSIS

- Relapse is possible after any of the treatment regimens.
- Re-treatment with the same agent or an alternative drug is often successful.

PREVENTION

- Because giardiasis is so prevalent, total prevention of transmission is virtually impossible.
  - Good hand washing is essential to limit spread by the fecal-oral route.
    - Especially important when infants in diapers are affected
- When an outbreak is suspected in child care centers that have infants in diapers, the local health department should be contacted.
  - Epidemiologic investigation should be undertaken to identify and treat all symptomatic children, child care workers, and family members infected with *Giardia.*
- Prevention of waterborne giardiasis is contingent on adequate water purification, including filtration, sedimentation, and flocculation in addition to chlorination.
  - Tourists in endemic areas should avoid drinking tap water.
  - Campers should not rely on chlorination tablets, which are ineffective against *Giardia* cysts.
  - Boiling for ≥2 minutes, even at high altitudes, and filtration (pore size ≤1 μm or with a filter rated for cyst removal) are satisfactory means for preparing drinking water free of *G intestinalis.*

Gluten-Sensitive Enteropathy (Celiac Sprue)

DEFINITION

- Gluten-sensitive enteropathy (GSE) is a condition characterized by clinical features of malabsorption and pathologic changes in the jejunal mucosa.
  - Both improve when gluten is removed from the diet and recur when it is reintroduced.
- Also known as *celiac sprue*
- Second-most common cause of malabsorption in children (cystic fibrosis is the most common cause)

EPIDEMIOLOGY

- Race/ethnicity
  - Has been identified in most ethnicities, including European, Hispanic, Indian, Chinese, Sudanese, African-Caribbean, and Middle Eastern persons
  - Prevalence in US is 1 in 133 persons.
  - Worldwide prevalence estimated to be 1 in 266 persons.
- Age
  - Average age at diagnosis is <24 months.
  - The diagnosis occurs sooner in infants who are fed cereal at an early age.
  - Incidence declines markedly after age 2 years.
    - Diagnosing GSE in a teenager is even less common.

ETIOLOGY

- GSE affects the mucosa of the small intestine, sparing the submucosa, muscularis, and serosa.
  - Mucosal lesions of the small intestine vary in severity and extent.
  - Lesions in the jejunum are generally more severe than those in the ileum.
- In active GSE, surface epithelial-cell damage occurs.
  - Compensatory crypt hypertrophy occurs, resulting in villus flattening.
  - Surface epithelial cells become more cuboidal.
  - Many intraepithelial lymphocytes are noted, and the lamina propria shows a marked increase in plasma cells and lymphocytes.
- GSE is a genetic disease, although the mode of inheritance is unknown.
  - Incidence in first-degree relatives is between 1 in 18–22; for second-degree relatives, the incidence is 1 in 24–39.
  - The presence of *HLA-DQ2* or *-DQ8* is necessary to develop GSE.
  - The *HLA-DQ2* allele combination is found in 90–95% of patients with GSE (however, 20–30% of the normal population also has this combination).
  - Remaining 5–10% of patients are *HLA-DQ8* positive.

- 2 possible mechanisms explain the cause of GSE.
  - Lack of a specific dipeptidase results in accumulation of toxic gluten peptides that initiate an inflammatory response.
  - May be mediated through immunologic aberrations associated with genetically determined cell-surface markers
- Various immunologic abnormalities have been described.
  - Increased levels of serum immunoglobulin (Ig)A and lower levels of serum IgM
  - Intestinal mucosal immunoglobulin synthesis, notably IgA and IgM, is markedly increased in active GSE.
    - 50% of the increased IgA is associated with specific anti-gluten antibody.
  - In vitro duodenal mucosa and peripheral lymphocyte transformation in response to gluten has been described.

RISK FACTORS

- Diseases associated with increased incidence of GSE
  - Type 1 diabetes
  - IgA deficiency
  - Down syndrome
  - Turner syndrome
  - Williams syndrome
  - Autoimmune thyroiditis

SIGNS AND SYMPTOMS

- Symptoms of an advanced case of GSE
  - Irritability
  - Anorexia
  - Chronic diarrhea
  - Failure to thrive
  - A potbelly
  - Muscle wasting, especially of the buttocks and proximal limbs
- Other manifestations
  - Growth failure (without gastrointestinal symptoms)
  - Anemia
  - Iron deficiency
  - Folate deficiency
  - Vitamin-B_{12} deficiency (rare)
  - Rickets, osteoporosis, bone pain, pathologic fractures
  - Bleeding disorders
  - Edema
  - Constipation
  - Vomiting
  - Recurrent abdominal pain
  - Rectal prolapse
  - Clubbing of the fingernails

■ Celiac crisis (life-threatening condition)

- Massive diarrhea
- Severe electrolyte imbalance
- Dehydration
- Shock

DIFFERENTIAL DIAGNOSIS

■ Common causes of flat villus lesions include:

- Food sensitivity
- Cow's milk protein allergy
- Soy protein allergy
- Eosinophilic gastroenteritis
- Infection: viruses (rotavirus), bacteria (*Escherichia coli*), parasites (*Giardia lamblia*), or fungi (*Candida albicans*)
- Malnutrition (kwashiorkor, not marasmus)
- Tropical sprue
- Immunodeficiency disorders (most notably AIDS)
- Familial enteropathy
- Lymphoma
- Crohn disease
- Whipple disease

■ A sweat test should be performed to exclude cystic fibrosis.

- Most common cause of malabsorption in childhood
- May coexist with GSE

DIAGNOSTIC APPROACH

■ For definitive diagnosis of GSE, the clinician must see:

- Demonstration of clinical malabsorption and abnormal intestinal lesions
- Clinical and histologic response to gluten withdrawal
- Subsequent gluten challenge that may exacerbate clinical symptoms but that always produces abnormal intestinal histologic findings

■ Diagnosis must be made with certainty because:

- GSE means lifelong gluten restriction.
- Untreated patients have higher risk of gastrointestinal cancer in late adulthood.

LABORATORY FINDINGS

■ Serologic markers for diagnosis and screening

- Anti–tissue transglutaminase (tTG) antibodies
  - First step in screening
- IgA endomysial antibodies
  - Most specific
  - Used as a confirmatory test when findings of tTG antibody testing are equivocal

- Anti-gliadin antibodies
  - Less specific and less sensitive than endomysial antibodies
  - Not suggested for screening
- False-positive endomysial and tTG antibody tests are unusual.
- When IgA is low or absent, consider measuring serum tTG-IgG and endomysial antibody-IgG levels.
- 10–15% of patients with GSE may have negative markers.
  - Thus a negative serologic test result does not exclude diagnosis.

■ Genetic markers *HLA-DQ2* and *-DQ8*

- If negative, this excludes GSE.
- Markers are present in people without GSE.

■ Hematology and electrolytes

- Anemia
- Hypoprothrombinemia
- Abnormal serum albumin and globulin levels
- Electrolyte disturbances, especially hypokalemia
- Calcium, phosphorus, and alkaline phosphatase levels may be abnormal in patients with rickets.

IMAGING

■ Radiographic findings in GSE are nonspecific.

- May see distended small intestine and segmented barium on a small-bowel follow-through

DIAGNOSTIC PROCEDURES

■ Biopsy of the small intestine is the best way to diagnose GSE.

- Should be performed to confirm diagnosis when serologic markers are positive
- Are routinely obtained by fiberoptic endoscopy, permitting visualization of the duodenum
- Scalloping of the small intestinal valvulae of Kerckring has been described as pathognomonic for GSE.
  - In young infants, edema of the duodenal mucosa is more common.

■ Repeat biopsy and rechallenge

- Not necessary if a child >2 years old has become asymptomatic on a gluten-free diet.
- Children <2 years old should undergo another biopsy to demonstrate healing then undergo rechallenge and another biopsy.
  - The same approach is suggested in children with an indeterminate diagnosis.

TREATMENT APPROACH

- Treatment of GSE is a gluten-free diet (GFD).
  - Remove gluten from the diet, including wheat, rye, and barley.
    - Oats do not contain gluten but may be cross-contaminated with gluten during manufacturing.
  - A lactose-free diet is advocated during the initial 4–6 weeks to alleviate diarrhea.
    - Lactose may be gradually reintroduced, provided that there is no concurrent infection, severe electrolyte imbalance, dehydration, or celiac crisis.
  - Nutrition counseling by a qualified dietician is an important component of treatment.
- Replacement iron, folic acid, vitamin K, vitamin D, and calcium should be initiated when appropriate.
- Compliance with GFD can be tracked by assessing serologic markers.
  - An increase in tTG antibody will be observed if the patient is noncompliant.
  - Weeks may be required for symptoms to disappear completely; subjective improvement occurs within the first few days.

WHEN TO ADMIT

- Failure to thrive and intractable diarrhea
- Dehydration and electrolyte abnormailities
- Celiac crisis

WHEN TO REFER

- Referral to a gastroenterologist is based on
  - Clinical suspicion
  - Presence of positive serologic markers
  - First-degree relatives with GSE
  - Syndromic presentations
  - Existence of other autoimmune disorders

FOLLOW-UP

- After GFD, monitoring serum tTG or endomysial antibodies (or both) is the preferred method for children >2 years.

COMPLICATIONS

- Celiac crisis
  - Triggers include:
    - Severe malnutrition
    - An infectious process
    - Poor compliance with GFD
    - Bacterial overgrowth caused by dysmotility
    - Hypoproteinemia
  - Patient needs to be admitted to the intensive care unit for further stabilization of electrolytes and fluids.
  - Once fluids have stabilized, start parenteral nutrition with total gut rest.
  - Slowly, introduction of a GFD with oral supplementation of iron, folic acid, vitamin D, and calcium should be attempted.
  - These patients might require prolonged total parenteral nutrition.

PROGNOSIS

- GSE means lifelong gluten restriction.
- Untreated patients risk developing gastrointestinal cancer in late adulthood.
- Refractory GSE occurs in 7–30% of patients.
  - Patients resistant to a GFD require therapy with immunomodulators.

G

Headache

DEFINITION

- Headaches are classified as primary or secondary.
- Primary headaches are directly attributed to a neurologic basis and include:
  - Migraine
  - Tension-type headaches (TTHs)
  - Cluster headaches
  - Other primary neuralgias
- Secondary headaches are attributed to a specific nonneurologic cause.
  - Infectious
  - Vascular
  - Traumatic
  - Toxic
    - Including medications and overuse of medications
  - Mass lesion

EPIDEMIOLOGY

- Prevalence
  - Headaches, particularly migraine, are being increasingly recognized as a significant health problem for children and adolescents.
    - Up to 75% of children report having a significant headache by the time they are 15 years of age.
    - Up to 28% of adolescents have had a migraine.
  - 10.6% of children between 5 and 15 years of age had significant headaches consistent with migraine.
  - There is an increasing 1-year prevalence in children between the ages of 10 and 19 years.
- Age and sex
  - In a meta-analysis of pediatric headache:
    - 1.2–3.2% of children between 3 and 7 years of age had migraine, with a slight male predominance.
    - Incidence of migraine increased to 4–11% between 7 and 11 years of age, with equal male and female occurrence.
    - Incidence of migraine increased to 18–23% between 11 and 15 years of age, with female predominance.
    - In the 15- to 19-year-old range, using the International Classification of Headache Disorders I (ICHD-I) criteria:
      - 28% of these adolescents had migraine.
      - Female predominance
      - Migraine without aura was more common than migraine with aura.
      - Mixed headaches were seen in 6.3% of the patients, with some TTHs in addition to migraines.
  - 81% of adolescents with migraine had a positive family history.
    - Nearly one-quarter of female adolescents reported a relationship between headaches and menstruation.
    - Status migrainosus was noted in 14.8% of girls and 4.7% of boys.
- TTHs have been less well studied than migraine.
  - Estimates of prevalence in children range from 1–73%.
- Impact of headaches
  - 1989 National Health Interview Survey found that within a 2-week period, 975,000 children had a migraine, resulting in 164,454 missed school days.

MECHANISM

- Migraine has a genetic component.
  - Studies have shown a degree of inheritance as high as 90% in first- or second-degree relatives.
- TTHs are generally considered mild recurrent headaches, previously called *muscle contraction headache, idiopathic headache,* and *tension headache.*

HISTORY

- The first step in evaluating a child with headache is to rule out secondary causes.
  - Detailed headache history
    - Length of time the child has had headaches
    - Severity
    - Quality
    - Location
    - Frequency
    - The effect on the child's quality of life and disability
    - Factors that exacerbate and relieve the headaches.
    - Any aura before headaches
  - Detailed review of systems
  - Medical history
  - A psychosocial and family history to identify stressors that may be contributory

PHYSICAL EXAM

- Conducting a physical examination is important, with an emphasis on the neurologic examination.
  - Include a thorough search for potential sources of secondary headache.
    - Increased intracranial pressure
    - Sinusitis
    - Dental disease
    - Abnormalities of the cervical spine
    - Temporomandibular joint disorders

DIFFERENTIAL DIAGNOSIS

- After the detailed history and medical examination, it should be possible to determine whether the patient has a primary or secondary headache.

Secondary headache causes

- Head or neck trauma
- Cranial or cervical vascular disorder
- Nonvascular intracranial disorder
  - High-pressure headaches
  - Low-pressure headaches
- Substance use/abuse or withdrawal
  - Includes medication overuse headaches
- Infection
  - Meningitis
  - Encephalitis
  - Brain abscess
- Disorders of homeostasis or facial pain extending from
  - Cranium
  - Neck
  - Eyes
  - Ears
  - Nose
  - Sinuses
  - Teeth
  - Mouth
- Psychiatric disorders

Primary headache disorders

- Migraine
  - Migraine without aura, previously called *common migraine* or *hemicrania simplex*
    - Recurrent headache disorder
    - Attacks last 4–72 hours.
    - Typical characteristics
      - Unilateral location
      - Pulsating quality
      - Moderate or severe intensity
      - Aggravation by routine physical activity
      - Association with nausea, photophobia, phonophobia
  - Migraine with aura
    - Aura consists of visual, sensory, or speech symptoms.
    - Gradual development
    - Duration ≤1 hour
    - Complete reversibility
    - In addition to the aura, the headache will have symptoms of migraine without aura.
  - Childhood periodic syndromes
  - Retinal migraine
- Complications of migraine
  - Chronic migraine
    - Frequent headaches (≥15 times per month for the previous 3 months)
    - Presence of migraine features
    - Cannot be attributed to a secondary cause
  - Status migrainosus
  - Probable migraine
- TTHs
  - Generally considered mild recurrent headaches
  - Many features are the opposite of those of migraine.
  - TTHs can be subdivided based on frequency.
- Infrequent, episodic
- Frequent, episodic
- Chronic
- The headaches themselves are usually described as:
  - Mild and moderate in severity
  - Diffuse in location
  - Having a pressing quality
  - No secondary causes are identified.
- Cluster headache
  - Trigeminal autonomic cephalagias
- Other primary headaches

IMAGING

- If abnormalities on the neurologic examination cannot be explained by medical history, then neuroimaging may be required to identify a medically or surgically treatable cause of the headaches.

TREATMENT APPROACH

- In patients with secondary headaches, the treatment goal is to address the underlying cause.
  - Headaches should resolve once the underlying cause is addressed.
- Treatment of primary headache disorders in children must be 3-fold.
  - Acute therapy
  - Preventive therapy
  - Biobehavioral therapy
- Clear goals of treatment must be discussed with the patient and parents.

SPECIFIC TREATMENT

Short-term therapy

- Short-term therapy is designed to ameliorate the episodic headache.
- The goal of this treatment is a quick return to normal activity without relapse.
- For headache in children, medications include:
  - Nonsteroidal antiinflammatory drugs (NSAIDs)
    - Ibuprofen, naproxen sodium
      - Ibuprofen has become a mainstay for the acute treatment of childhood headaches and migraines.
      - Good tolerability
      - Effective in clinical trials
      - Proper use of ibuprofen requires:
        - o Identification by the child of onset of the headache
        - o Initiation of rapid treatment
        - o Proper dosing based on weight
        - o Avoidance of overuse; limited to ≤3 times per week
    - Aspirin for older children
    - General pain relievers, eg, acetaminophen
- Most prescriptive nonspecific medications have either not been evaluated in children or have not been proven effective.
- Many prescriptive medications contain sedatives or narcotics that may treat the pain but do not allow the child to return to normal functioning.
- When NSAIDs are ineffective or not completely effective, migraine-specific therapy is often required.
- Triptans
  - Triptans are 5-HT$_{1B-1D}$ agonist migraine-specific medications.
  - Currently, 7 triptans have been approved for use in the US in adults.
    - Not approved for use in childhood migraine
    - Several studies in children, however, have shown their effectiveness.
  - Sumatriptan, zolmitriptan, rizatriptan
    - Two treatment methods may be used when prescribing triptans: rescue therapy or stepwise treatment within an attack.
    - The child starts with an NSAID at an appropriate dose at the onset of the headache.
      - If this medication is not working, then a triptan is used as rescue therapy.

- The stratified care model requires the patient to determine the headache severity at the onset.
  - For a mild or moderate headache, the patient takes an NSAID.
  - For a severe headache, the patient takes a prescribed triptan.
  - In this way, patients stratify their headaches and the subsequent treatment.
  - This method has not been successful in children because they often have difficulty recognizing the headache severity at its onset.
- Dihydroergotamine (DHE)
  - Ergot alkaloids have a long history of usefulness in migraines.
  - Frequently used in the emergency management of childhood headaches
  - Limited reports have shown usefulness of intravenous DHE in an inpatient setting.
    - Breaks status migrainosus or prolonged migraines in children
    - The effect may be enhanced if patients are premedicated with dopamine antagonists.
- Dopamine antagonists (prochlorperazine, metoclopramide)
  - Initially used for nausea and vomiting effects of migraine headaches
  - The dopaminergic model of migraine was developed, and these medications have been reanalyzed for usefulness in short-term therapy of the headaches themselves.
  - Dopamine antagonists should be given intravenously.
  - Their utility is limited by extrapyramidal side effects.
  - It is suggested that prochlorperazine can be used to break an acute episode of status migrainosus.
    - Best given with rehydrating fluids in the emergency department setting

Prophylactic treatment

- The second component of effective headache treatment
- Should be instituted when the headache or migraine becomes frequent or disabling
- Goals
  - Minimize the effect of the headache
  - Reduce the number of headaches
- A clear diminishment in severity and headache features may be observed.
- Having >2–3 headaches per month typically warrants treatment.

- For all prophylactic medications, titrate doses slowly to an effective level.
  - Requires understanding by the patient and family that this may be a lengthy process (weeks, months)
  - Failure to respond may be due to:
    - Inadequate time of treatment
    - Inadequate dosing
- Prophylactic medications can be grouped into:
  - Antiepileptics
  - Only divalproate sodium and topiramate are currently approved for the prevention of migraines in adults; they are not approved for children.
    - Divalproate sodium
      - 15–20 mg/kg/day
  - Topiramate
    - 2–4 mg/kg/day
    - Taper up to this dose slowly, in quarter steps, over 8–10 weeks.
  - Gabapentin
  - Levetiracetam
  - Zonisamide
  - Antidepressants
    - The most widely used tricyclic antidepressant for headache prevention is amitriptyline.
    - Has been used for many decades for its antidepressive properties
    - First recognized in the 1970s as an effective migraine therapy
    - Most studies in children with amitriptyline have been open-label studies; there are no placebo-controlled studies.
      - Amitriptyline was found to be effective in 50–60% of children in a cross-over study comparing amitriptyline with propranolol and cyproheptadine.
      - In an open-label study, amitriptyline resulted in a perceived improvement in >80% of the children.
    - Titrate slowly to the full dose over 8–10 weeks to minimize side effects, particularly somnolence.
  - Nortriptyline has been used instead of amitriptyline.
    - Potential for increased arrhythmias
    - Regular electrocardiographic evaluation may be required if nortriptyline is chosen.
  - Serotonin selective reuptake inhibitors have been studied for the treatment of headaches in adults; it has not yet been studied in children.
    - Effectiveness is not as notable as that of tricyclic antidepressants.
    - Suggests that a more global decrease in neurotransmitter reuptake inhibition is needed to treat childhood headache disorders

- Antiserotonergic medications
- Cyproheptadine has long been used for preventing childhood headaches.
  - Antihistamine with antiserotonergic effects
  - May have some calcium channel–blocking properties
  - Tends to be well tolerated
  - Increased weight gain is the most significant side effect.
    - Because weight gain is substantial, use of this medication tends to be limited to younger children.
- Antihypertensive medications
- ß-Blockers have a long history of use for preventing childhood headaches.
  - Propranolol was found to provide mixed responsiveness when used for childhood headaches.
  - Even with their long history, ß-blockers have limited usefulness in children.
    - They cause a decrease in blood pressure.
    - There is a risk for exercise-induced asthma.
    - They can result in depressive effects.
- Calcium-channel blockers have been extensively studied in adults for headache prevention.
  - Flunarizine has been demonstrated to be an effective migraine preventive agent.
    - Available in Europe but not in the US.
  - Baseline headache frequency was significantly reduced in flunarizine-treated children.
    - These data cannot be extrapolated to other calcium-channel blockers.

Biobehavioral therapy

- Third component of effective headache treatment
- Essential for children to maintain a lifetime response to the treatment and management of their headaches
- Biobehavioral therapy can be divided into 3 components.
  - Treatment adherence
    - A clear understanding by the patient and parent about the importance of the treatment is essential.
    - Psychological or biobehavioral intervention may be useful in assisting with adherence by identifying roadblocks to the medical plan and helping to overcome these barriers.
  - Lifestyle management
    - In many instances, unhealthy lifestyle habits serve as a trigger for childhood headaches.
      - Inadequate nutrition
      - Skipping meals
      - Altered sleep patterns

H

- Maintaining healthy lifestyle habits includes:
  - Adequate fluid hydration, with limited use of caffeine
  - Regular exercise
  - Adequate nutrition through regular meals and a balanced diet
  - Adequate sleep
  - The patient and parents must understand that these objectives are lifetime goals that can control the effect of migraines and minimize the use of medication.
  - Lifestyle changes may result in an overall long-term improvement in quality of life and may reverse any progressive nature of the disease.
- Biofeedback-assisted relaxation therapy
  - May be a useful addition
  - For children, single-session biofeedback-assisted relaxation therapy has been demonstrated to be learned quickly and efficiently.

WHEN TO REFER

- Headaches that do not respond routinely to acute treatment
- Headaches that are increasing in frequency, severity, or duration
- Headaches in which the features acutely change
- Side effects of medications that limit increasing the medication to an effective dose
- Psychological factors that interfere with management
- Disability that impairs functioning

WHEN TO ADMIT

- Admission or emergency department treatment should be considered when:
  - Home therapies are ineffective for acute treatment.
  - Headache has continued for >24 hours.
  - Headache pain becomes intolerable.

FOLLOW-UP

- Important to assess regularly the morbidity of headaches and effectiveness of treatment
- Regular measurement of both disability and quality of life are helpful in assessing treatment strategies and improvement in outcomes.

- Disability
  - Pediatric Migraine Disability Assessment (PedMIDAS) uses a patient-based disability scale.
- Quality of Life
  - Pediatric Quality of Life Inventory version 4.0 (PedsQL 4.0) uses both parent and child input.
    - Evaluates functioning in health, emotional, social, and school domains
    - Headaches have been found to substantially affect emotional development and school functioning.

COMPLICATIONS

- Avoiding overuse of medication is critical in short-term therapy.
- Overuse can cause analgesic rebound headaches.
  - Transformed migraines
  - Chronic daily headaches
- Overuse of medication is characterized by inadequate treatment of headache.
  - Low-dose or delayed treatment
    - Increase in analgesic use over time, with decreased effectiveness
  - When rebound headaches are identified, a recovery period free of analgesic use is required.
- Allodynia
  - A painful or heightened sensation beyond the location of the headache
  - Once allodynia has been established, patients have decreased response to medication.
  - For these patients, stress the need for early treatment.

PROGNOSIS

- Primary headaches can have a significant effect on a child's life.

Head Injuries

DEFINITION

- *Traumatic brain injury* (TBI) is a leading cause of death and disability in the US.
- *Primary brain injury* refers to the neural injury caused by the traumatic insult itself and exhibits in the form of:
  - Contusions
  - Intracranial bleeding
  - Fractures
  - Diffuse axonal injuries
- *Secondary brain injury* refers to the subsequent injury to neural tissue after trauma has occurred.
- *Concussion* is any head injury associated with alteration in mental status.
- *Cerebral contusions* are bruises of the cerebral cortex that can occur as a result of:
  - Direct injury (coup injury)
  - Injury at the opposite point where the relatively mobile brain strikes the bone on the other side (contrecoup injury)
- *Growing fractures* occur as a result of leptomeningeal cyst formation and frequently require neurosurgical closure.
- *Diffuse axonal injury* refers to damage at the gray-white matter junction, seen after an acceleration-deceleration mechanism.

EPIDEMIOLOGY

- Incidence
  - 1.6 million head injuries occur every year.
  - 250,000 require hospitalization.
  - 60,000 deaths are caused by head injuries occur every year.
- Prevalence
  - 70,000–90,000 patients are left with permanent neurologic sequelae.
- Cost
  - $100 billion per year
  - In 2000 injuries to children <14 years old were projected to have a total lifetime economic costs >$50 billion in medical expenses and lost productivity.
- Age
  - Among children age 0–14 years, TBI results annually in:
    - ~2685 deaths
    - 37,000 hospitalizations
    - 435,000 emergency department (ED) visits
  - ~50% of patients hospitalized with head injury are <20 years of age.
  - >75% of trauma deaths in children are due to brain injury.
  - Skull fractures occur in approximately 2 per 1000 infants and 0.5 to 1 per 1000 older children and adolescents.
- Sex
  - Boys are injured twice as often as girls.

ETIOLOGY

- The brain is covered by 3 layers of meningeal tissue (pia mater, arachnoid mater, and dura mater), followed by the skull bones (calvarium) and scalp, which has a strong layer of tissue (galea aponeurotica).
- The brain does not adhere to the skull, but is able to move freely within it, cushioned by cerebrospinal fluid.
- Causes of primary brain injury vary with age.
  - In infants
    - Falls
    - Child abuse
  - In preschool and school-age children
    - Vehicular accidents
  - In adolescents
    - Sports injuries
    - Assault
  - For all ages
    - Falls are the most common cause of head trauma.
    - Vehicular accidents are the leading cause of serious injury.
      - In most cases, the child is a pedestrian.
- Secondary brain injury results from numerous causes, including:
  - Hypoxia
  - Hypoperfusion
  - Excitotoxic damage
  - Free radical damage
  - Metabolic derangements
- Damage caused by secondary brain injury can be more devastating than that from the primary insult itself.
- The most important cause for secondary brain injury is brain ischemia resulting from inadequate cerebral blood flow.
  - Adequate cerebral blood flow depends on the cerebral perfusion pressure, which is the difference between mean arterial pressure and intracranial pressure (ICP).
  - Normally the cerebral perfusion pressure fluctuates inside a narrow range, the result of cerebral autoregulation.
  - When this control mechanism is lost because of brain injury and secondary brain tissue damage, an increase in intracranial volume (mainly the result of intracranial hemorrhage or cerebral edema) will lead to a disproportionate increase in ICP.
  - This increase further accentuates neuronal damage by reducing cerebral blood flow.
  - An increase in ICP leads to cerebral herniation syndromes.
  - These syndromes are characterized by:
    - Worsening of sensorium
    - Pupillary changes

– The Cushing triad

- Bradycardia

- Irregular respirations

- Hypertension

RISK FACTORS

■ Most children hit by a vehicle are not supervised by an adult at the time of the accident.

SIGNS AND SYMPTOMS

History

■ The possibility of child abuse must be kept in mind.

- Suggested when the given history is not proportional to the severity of injury

  – For instance, children rarely experience a serious injury when they fall out of bed.

■ Indicators of severe head trauma include:

- Loss of consciousness

- Seizures

- Amnesia for the circumstances surrounding the injury

- Focal neurologic deficits

■ Vomiting and headache are common symptoms after head trauma.

- If not persistent or severe, they are not suggestive of any specific pathologic finding.

■ Persistent clouding of consciousness is the most reliable sign of a significant brain injury.

■ The duration of posttraumatic amnesia, defined as an inability to generate new memories after head injury, correlates positively with the severity of the injury.

Physical examination

■ A detailed neurologic evaluation should be performed only when adequacy of the airway, breathing, and circulation are ensured.

■ Should begin with assessment of mental status and assignment of a Glasgow Coma Scale (GCS) score

■ Neurologic examination begins with assessment of the cranial nerves.

■ Particular attention needs to be given to:

- Pupillary responses and symmetry

- Funduscopic examination (to rule out papilledema or hemorrhage)

  – Retinal hemorrhage suggests child abuse.

- Eye movements (to assess for dysconjugate gaze)

- Asymmetries of facial sensation or movement

- Tongue movement

- Gag reflex

■ As a sensory screening examination, symmetrical responses to pain in all 4 limbs should be determined.

■ The motor examination should assess:

- Symmetry of muscle tone and movement and of the deep-tendon reflexes and plantar responses

- The alert, cooperative child's ability to manipulate small objects

- The child's gait and station

■ General physical examination should focus on:

- Presence of injury to other body systems

- Seeking evidence of physical neglect or abuse

■ The GCS (see table Glasgow Coma Scale), or a modified GCS for children and infants, can be used to evaluate mental status, assess prognosis, and follow the patient's progress.

- The scale is based on the patient's response in 3 areas.

  – Motor response

  – Verbal response

  – Eye-opening response

- Severe head injury may be defined as that resulting in a GCS score <9.

- Moderate head injury is associated with a score of 9 to 12.

- A score of 13–15 indicates a mild head injury.

■ Pontine and midbrain function may be assessed by examining oculovestibular reflexes.

- In the unconscious patient, the head should be rotated briskly from side to side after confirming there is no cervical spine injury.

- Normally, when the head moves to the right, the eyes move to the left, and vice versa.

- Loss of these reflex eye movements in a comatose patient suggests an injury to the midbrain or pons.

- If the tympanic membranes are intact, then ice water caloric responses should be elicited.

  – With the patient's head elevated to 30 degrees, 120 mL of ice water is infused alternately into each ear canal.

  – The eyes should turn toward the irrigated ear.

  – If they do not, then a brainstem injury is likely.

- To assess pontine function, the quality and symmetry of the grimace evoked by painful stimulation of the face should be observed.

  – In patients who do not respond to this stimulation, or in those who do so minimally, corneal reflex should be tested.

  – Failure to react by blinking is consistent with pontine injury or deep coma.

■ Medullary function is evaluated by assessing the patient's gag reflex and tongue movement.

- Examination of the patient's craniospinal axis should be performed in concert with the neurologic assessment, assessing for signs of trauma.

Glasgow Coma Scale [a,b]

Eye-Opening Response		
Score	**>1 Year**	**<1 Year**
4	Spontaneous	Spontaneous
3	To verbal command	To shout
2	To pain	To pain
1	None	None
Motor Response		
Score	**>1 Year**	**<1 Year**
6	Obeys commands	Displays spontaneous response
5	Localizes pain	Localizes pain
4	Withdraws from pain	Withdraws from pain
3	Displays abnormal flexion to pain (decorticate rigidity)	Displays abnormal flexion to pain (decorticate rigidity)
2	Displays abnormal extension to pain (decerebrate rigidity)	Displays abnormal extension to pain (decerebrate rigidity)
1	None	None

Verbal Response			
Score	**>5 Years**	**2–5 Years**	**0–23 Months**
5	Is oriented and converses	Uses appropriate words and phrases	Babbles, coos appropriately
4	Conversation is confused	Uses inappropriate words	Cries, but is consolable
3	Words are inappropriate	Cries or screams persistently to pain	Cries or screams persistently to pain
2	Sounds are incomprehensible	Grunts or moans to pain	Grunts or moans to pain
1	None	None	None

[a] Modified from: Teasdale G, Jennett B. Assessment of coma and impaired consciousness: a practical scale. *Lancet.* 1974;304(7872):81–84. Copyright © Elsevier 1974.
[b] Glasgow Coma Scale score equals sum of best eye opening, motor, and verbal responses. Range is 3–15. Usual definitions of severity of head injury: severe, ≤9; moderate, 9–12; mild, 13–15.

- Swelling and bony depression of the skull suggests an underlying fracture.
- Signs of basilar skull fracture include:
  - Ecchymoses behind the ear (the Battle sign)
  - Ecchymoses around the orbits (raccoon sign)
  - Cerebrospinal fluid rhinorrhea
  - Otorrhea
  - Hemotympanum
- Basilar fractures or scalp lacerations overlying fractures serve as portals of entry for bacteria into the subarachnoid space and may cause meningitis .

DIFFERENTIAL DIAGNOSIS

■ Concussion
- Mild head injury with a GCS score of 13–15 and no focal neurologic findings

- Most concussion patients can be discharged home after a period of evaluation and observation.
- Thorough evaluation is important, and the physician should advise parents regarding the child's return to sports.
- Guidelines for assessment and management of concussion from the American Academy of Neurology are presented in table Classification of Concussion.

■ Skull fractures
- The most common bone to fracture is the parietal bone.

■ Parenchymal injuries
- Clinical manifestations vary, but patients often exhibit:
  - Alteration in consciousness
  - Focal seizures
  - Focal neurologic findings (eg, cortical blindness in cases of occipital lobe injury)

Classification of Concussion[a,b]

Grade	Definition	Management
1	• Transient confusion • No loss of consciousness, mental status abnormalities for <15 min	• Return to sports activities same day only if all symptoms resolve within 15 min • If a second grade-1 concussion occurs, no sports activity until asymptomatic for 1 week
2	• Transient confusion • No loss of consciousness, mental status abnormalities for >15 min	• No sports activity until asymptomatic for 1 week • If a grade-2 concussion occurs on the same day as a previous grade-1 concussion, no sports activity for 2 weeks
3	• Concussion involving any loss of consciousness	• No sports activity until asymptomatic for 1 week if loss of consciousness was brief (seconds) • No sports activity until asymptomatic for 2 weeks if loss of consciousness was prolonged (minutes or longer) • Second grade-3 concussion — No sports activity until asymptomatic for 1 month • Any abnormality on CT or MRI — No sports activity for remainder of season — Patient should be discouraged from any future return to contact sports

Abbreviations: CT, computed tomography; MRI, magnetic resonance imaging.

[a] Modified from: Quality Standards Subcommittee, American Academy of Neurology. Practice parameter: the management of concussion in sports (summary statement). *Neurology.* 1977;48:581–585.

[b] Concussion symptoms: early (minutes and hours)—headache, dizziness or vertigo, lack of awareness of surroundings, nausea or vomiting. Late (days to weeks)—persistent low-grade headache, light-headedness, poor attention and concentration, memory dysfunction, easy fatigability, irritability and low frustration tolerance, intolerance to bright lights or difficulty focusing vision, intolerance of loud noises, sometimes ringing in the ears, anxiety or depressed mood, sleep disturbance.

■ Diffuse axonal injury
- Often seen after an acceleration-deceleration mechanism (whiplash injury)
- Damage is at the gray-white matter junction.
- Most children will experience changes in sensorium.
- Some studies have reported that 82% will develop coma.

■ Intracranial hematoma
- Hematomas can occur anywhere in the intracranial space.
- Differences between the 2 most common types—epidural and subdural—are described in table Differences Between Epideral and Subdural Hematomas.

IMAGING
■ Cervical spine films to rule out fracture or subluxation
- Most ED physicians do not obtain cervical spine radiographs if:
  - Mental status and neurologic examinations are normal.
  - No tenderness of the spine is present.
  - The child moves his or her head around without difficulty, especially if >5 years of age.
  - The younger the child is, the lower the threshold for obtaining cervical spine films.

■ Noncontrast computed tomography (CT) of the brain with bone windows
- CT is the imaging study of choice in acute trauma.
  - Easier to obtain than magnetic resonance imaging (MRI)
  - May not require sedation
- CT identifies the relationship between bone fragments and intracranial contents.
- CT reveals extraaxial fluid collections such as epidural and subdural hematomas.
- CT often detects parenchymal brain injury.
- Has supplanted the use of skull radiographs
- All high-risk head injury patients require cranial CT.

■ Disadvantages of CT
- Exposure to radiation
  - Lifetime attributable cancer mortality risk for a child after a typical head CT is estimated at 1 per 5000.
  - Cranial CT should be used selectively in the ED evaluation of children with minor blunt head trauma.
- Transport of the child away from supervision in the ED
- Potential need for pharmacologic sedation
- Additional health care costs
- Increased time for completing the ED evaluation

Differences Between Epidural and Subdural Hematomas

Characteristic	Epidural Hematoma	Subdural Hematoma
Mechanism	Direct trauma that leads to bleeding from middle meningeal artery or shearing of epidural veins	• Shaking (acceleration-deceleration) injury leading to tearing of bridging veins in the subdural space. • In young children, this may result from child abuse.
Clinical manifestations	• Lucid interval—symptom-free interval between time of injury and time of manifestation can be seen • Patients run the gamut from asymptomatic to those who exhibit focal seizures and coma	• Lucid interval unlikely. • Many children have coma, seizures, or evidence of chronic changes (tense anterior fontanelle, macrocephaly).
Investigations	CT is diagnostic for a lenticular lesion with an overlying fracture	• CT reveals blood collection as a hyperdense crescentic collection along the cerebral hemisphere. • In cases of child abuse, hemorrhage of different ages can be seen with changes suggestive of hydrocephalus.
Management	Craniotomy with drainage of hematoma and repair of the ruptured blood vessel	Management will vary depending on extent of bleeding, and in some cases, ICP monitoring with expectant observation may be the only therapy; intracranial evacuation of blood clot may be the therapy of choice for some cases.
Prognosis	Excellent after initial insult is adequately treated	Poor, with high mortality and high morbidity (sequelae).

Abbreviations: CT, computed tomography; ICP, intracranial pressure.

■ MRI may be useful in later assessments because it is more sensitive than CT at detecting intrinsic brain injuries, such as diffuse axonal injury.

TREATMENT APPROACH

Emergency care

■ The basic ABCs of resuscitation (airway, breathing, and circulation) should be addressed first.

■ Maintaining normal oxygenation is imperative.

• Ischemia, increased ICP, and uncontrolled seizures may cause further brain injury.

• Correction of anoxia and poor cerebral perfusion is more important than detection of an intracranial hematoma.

■ Coexisting cervical spine injury should be assumed until proved otherwise.

• The neck should not be moved until cervical spine films can rule out a fracture or dislocation, which may result in spinal cord trauma if movement occurs.

• The preferred initial radiographs are cross-table lateral, anteroposterior, and odontoid views.

■ In the severely injured patient, the airway requires intubation to ensure adequate ventilation to reduce the chance of developing increased ICP.

• When possible, an anesthesiologist should perform the intubation.

• Rapid sequence intubation is indicated for most patients with head injuries to ensure that they are comfortable and that intubation can be safely achieved.

• This task is usually accomplished with a combination of:

– Sedative to induce anesthesia (thiopental, etomidate, fentanyl, or midazolam)

– Atropine to reduce secretions and prevent vagal reflexes

– Neuromuscular blocking agent to produce paralysis (rocuronium or succinylcholine)

• Close attention to blood pressure is necessary because sedatives may cause hypotension.

• Cricoid pressure may be applied to reduce the risk of aspiration.

• Prolonged hyperventilation is no longer suggested for patients with acute severe head injury.

SPECIFIC TREATMENTS

Secondary brain damage

■ Once TBI has been detected and the patient resuscitated, subsequent management is directed at preventing secondary insults.

- The most important causes of secondary brain damage are:
  - Hypoxia
  - Systemic hypotension
  - Increased ICP (intracranial hypertension)
- Vital signs should be frequently assessed to ensure adequacy of circulation.
- Shock leads to further brain injury despite adequate airway management and oxygenation.
- Vigorous fluid therapy to restore adequate circulating blood volume and sufficient cerebral perfusion is essential.
- Isotonic solutions or blood products
  - Preferred because hypotonic solutions may promote movement of free water into damaged brain tissue, increasing the potential for cerebral edema
  - Some authorities argue for the use of hypertonic solutions in acute severe brain trauma, although this approach is not widely used.
- If the patient is in shock, then a source of bleeding should be sought.
- Patients rarely sequester sufficient blood volume in the head to produce shock
  - Notable exceptions: the infant with an expansible skull, the presence of a large subgaleal hematoma
- Additional measures directed at reducing secondary brain injury
  - Elevation of the patient's head 30 degrees
  - Maintenance of the head in a midline position to maximize venous outflow from the cranial vault
- ICP should be monitored and decreased if necessary.
  - Placement of an intracranial ventricular catheter is the most accurate and reliable method for monitoring ICP.
  - Intracranial hypertension is defined as an ICP of >20 mm Hg.
  - Cushing response (hypertension and bradycardia) implies increased ICP.
  - This response and unilateral pupillary dilation (a sign of impending catastrophic temporal lobe herniation) should prompt administration of mannitol.
  - Reduction of cerebral metabolism by initiating barbiturate coma may improve outcomes and should be considered when pediatric neurosurgeons and pediatric intensive care units are available.
  - The role of therapeutic hypothermia in the treatment of children with severe TBI is still unclear.
  - Corticosteroids do not improve outcome when used in acute-phase management of TBI.
- Antipyretics should be administered to reduce fever.
  - Hyperthermia may increase cerebral metabolic demands, further taxing delivery of nutrients to the injured brain.

- Seizures greatly increase metabolic demands of the brain and should be treated promptly with intravenous diazepam or lorazepam, followed by intravenous phenytoin.
- Intravenous phenytoin should be provided if the patient is pharmacologically paralyzed because it results in an inability to detect seizure activity.
- Intravenous phenytoin is advisable before transfer to another medical center.

Types of TBI

- Concussion
  - Most patients can be discharged home after a period of evaluation and observation.
  - Physician should advise parents regarding the child's return to sports (table Classification of Concussion).
- Skull fractures
  - Linear skull fractures often require no intervention.
    - Admit the child for a period of observation.
  - Depressed skull fractures are often associated with underlying brain abnormalities and may require surgical interventions.
  - Basilar skull fractures are often associated with cerebrospinal fluid leakage and cranial nerve damage.
    - Require pediatric neurosurgical intervention
    - Should be managed at tertiary-care pediatric trauma centers
- Diffuse axonal injury
  - Most patients with will need hospitalization along with ICP monitoring in the intensive care unit.

Care of the less severely injured patient

- Intermediate-risk patients might be managed in 1 of 2 ways.
  - 4- to 5-hour period of observation and reevaluation
  - Head CT
- Low-risk patients may be observed in the ED or at home with reliable caretakers.
- Management of closed head trauma
  - In 1999, the AAP published guidelines for the management of closed head trauma in previously healthy children 2–20 years of age.
  - This consensus statement used historical features of loss of consciousness and presence of symptoms as an indication for CT of the head.
  - For children without a loss of consciousness, a complete history and a physical examination should be performed.
    - The caregiver should observe the patient for any deterioration in mental status.
  - For patients who have a history of a brief loss of consciousness, along with amnesia, headache, or vomiting at the time of evaluation, the prevalence of intracranial injury may be as high as 7%.

- Many of these brain injuries have little clinical consequence.
  - A minority of these children may require neurosurgical intervention.
  - In symptomatic children with a brief loss of consciousness, CT of the head may be useful.
  - With a brief loss of consciousness in an otherwise asymptomatic patient, observation for neurologic deterioration may be an acceptable alternative to head CT.
- The following 5 clinical findings have been found to identify 99% of all children with TBI on CT and 100% of those who required neurosurgery.
  - Abnormal mental status
  - Clinical signs of skull fracture
  - Scalp hematoma
  - History of headache
  - Vomiting
- A clinical decision rule excludes TBI in need of neurosurgical intervention (negative predictive value of 100%) when none of these 5 clinical variables is present.
- Use of this rule will reduce unnecessary exposure to radiation from CT by 25%.
- Discharge home
  - Patients with mild head injury can be discharged home with appropriate instructions so long as they:
    - Promptly recover their neurologic function
    - Are not suspected of being abused
    - Have reliable caregivers
  - Children with normal neurologic examinations and negative CT rarely have neurologic deterioration after discharge from the ED.
  - Parents are often instructed to observe the child carefully for at least 24 hours, periodically awakening the child from sleep.
  - Caregivers should return immediately to the ED if their child:
    - Cannot be awakened
    - Demonstrates decreasing mental status while awake
    - Develops seizures, focal weakness, increasing headache, progressive instability, or vomiting to the point of dehydration
  - Linear skull fractures do not require admission to the hospital if the child is asymptomatic; they do require close observation because of the significant force required to fracture the skull.
  - After hospital or ED discharge, office follow-up is suggested at 2 weeks.
  - Recovery can be reviewed and further anticipatory guidance provided to the family regarding relevant neurologic sequelae.

- Children <2 years who have diastatic fractures (fractures that involve normal suture lines) should be evaluated again in 6–8 weeks to check for a growing fracture .

WHEN TO ADMIT

- Persistent alteration in mental state
- Focal neurologic deficits
- Seizures
- Persistent vomiting that precludes adequate hydration
- Severe headache
- Suspicion of abuse
- Unreliable caregivers or observers at home
- Any injury requiring neurosurgical intervention
- CT indicating intracranial bleeding or brain injury

Admission of the less severely injured patient

- The decision to admit a child with mild to moderate head trauma must be individualized.
- Controversy exists regarding the use of clinical signs and symptoms to identify children at risk for TBI after blunt trauma.
- Guidelines have been proposed in the approach of children with blunt injury.
- These children have been traditionally divided into 2 groups.
  - Age ≤2 years
    - A multidisciplinary panel suggested stratifying patients into risk categories based on clinical features (eg, history and physical examination, mechanism of injury, presence or absence of skull fracture).
  - Between 2 and 20 years of age
- Patient characteristics
  - High-risk patients have any of the following.
    - Depressed mental status
    - Focal neurologic findings
    - Signs of depressed or basilar skull fracture
    - Seizure
    - Irritability
    - Acute skull fracture
    - Bulging fontanelle
    - >5 episodes of vomiting or vomiting for >6 hours
    - Loss of consciousness that lasts >1 minute
  - Intermediate-risk patients have any of the following characteristics.
    - Vomiting 3–4 times
    - Loss of consciousness that lasts for <1 minute
    - History of lethargy or irritability, now resolved
    - Caretakers concerned about current behavior
    - Higher force mechanism
    - Hematoma (especially large or nonfrontal in location)

– Unwitnessed trauma

– Fall onto a hard surface

– Vague or no history of trauma with evidence of trauma

– Nonacute skull fracture older than 24–48 hours

– Patients in this category might be managed in 1 of 2 ways.

  ■ 4- to 5-hour period of observation

  ■ Reevaluation or a head CT

• Low-risk patients have:

– Low-energy mechanism (eg, a fall of <3 feet)

– No signs or symptoms

– >2 hours since the injury

– As the patient's age increases, the risk decreases.

WHEN TO REFER

■ Deteriorating mental status

■ Coma or persistent alteration in mental status

■ A GCS score <9

■ Subdural, epidural, or intraparenchymal hematoma

■ Focal abnormalities on neurologic examination

■ Seizures after the first week or recurrent seizures

■ Shock

■ Signs of Cushing response (bradycardia and hypertension)

■ Suspicion of child abuse (refer to appropriate local governmental agency)

■ Cervical spine injury

■ Basilar skull fracture

■ Depressed skull fracture

■ Increasingly severe headaches

■ Facial laceration or suspicion of significant trauma at other locations

PROGNOSIS

■ Children who experienced mild head trauma (GCS score of 13–15) are indistinguishable from their peers 1 year after their injuries.

• Significant neurologic dysfunction may be seen immediately after the child's injury and may persist for as long as 8 weeks.

• Symptoms include:

– Irritability

– Sleep disturbance

– Clinging behavior

– Hyperactivity

– Headache

• Anticipatory guidance for parents regarding the transient nature of these symptoms in mild head injuries is important.

■ Children who have moderate head injury (GCS score of 9–12) and severe head injury (a score of 3–8) may suffer from multiple physical, cognitive, and psychological disabilities.

• Prognosis is generally more favorable for head-injured children than adults.

• Children with an initial GCS score >6 have an 80% chance of achieving functional independence.

• Intellectual recovery continues for as long as 2 years after head injury in children.

• Long-term rehabilitative services are needed.

• Formal psychological assessment for staging school reentry and for ongoing adjustment of the child's academic curriculum should be obtained.

■ 5% of patients will experience seizures within the first week after their head injury.

• Occurrence of these early-onset seizures does not accurately predict development of later posttraumatic epilepsy.

• The risk of subsequently developing epilepsy is significantly increased if seizures are present beyond the first week after head injury, particularly with severe head trauma, intraparenchymal hematoma, or depressed skull fracture.

• With these risk factors, approximately one-third of patients will develop posttraumatic epilepsy.

• Electroencephalographic studies do not accurately predict subsequent development of epilepsy; use of prophylactic anticonvulsant medications does not appear to reduce risk.

• Anticonvulsants are generally not used in mild brain injury but are indicated for children with severe brain injury to prevent increased ICP caused by seizures per se.

PREVENTION

■ Education regarding prevention of head injury is essential.

• Anticipatory guidance can dramatically reduce the morbidity and mortality that result from head injury and includes:

– Appropriate supervision of children

  ■ High-risk activities

– Protective equipment

  ■ Car seats for infants

  ■ Bicycle helmets for older children

Hearing Loss

DEFINITION

- Pediatricians must recognize the signs, symptoms, and risk factors for hearing loss and become aware of appropriate referral paths.
  - Pediatricians are usually the first health care practitioners approached by parents who have concerns about their child's hearing.
  - Parents become concerned about the child's hearing at ~6 months of age when the hearing loss is severe.
  - Milder degrees of hearing loss typically do not generate concern until the child reaches school age.
  - Patterns of hearing loss that are termed *mild* or *minimal* are far from benign and cause academic, communicative, social, and emotional difficulty for school-age children.

EPIDEMIOLOGY

- Advent of vaccines for rubella and meningitis
  - Virtually eliminated hearing loss caused by congenital rubella
  - Dramatically reduced hearing loss resulting from meningitis
- Prevalence
  - Severe to profound hearing loss is not as common as it once was.
    - The incidence of severe bilateral hearing loss in newborns is 1 per 1000.
  - Milder degrees of hearing loss are more prevalent.
    - The incidence of very mild or minimal losses approach 1 per 20.
  - In the neonatal intensive care unit, hearing loss is seen in ~20 to 40 per 1000 babies.
  - In the course of a typical practice a pediatrician will encounter approximately a dozen children with severe to profound hearing loss.
- Impact
  - ~35% of children with minimal hearing loss fail ≥1 grade in school, compared with an overall failure rate of ~3%.

MECHANISM

- Newborn hearing screening is widespread, however such screening programs are designed to identify moderate degrees of hearing loss and greater.
- A child who passed a hearing screening as a newborn may still have hearing loss.
- Hearing loss from otitis media is the most common type of loss encountered by pediatricians.

HISTORY

- Approximately 35–50% of children with hearing loss have no known risk factors.
- Complete history and observation accompanied by hearing screening are essential.

- Significant speech and language delays, because of their association with severe to profound hearing loss, provide a high level of suspicion.
- A history of any of the following should also prompt screening for hearing loss.
  - Behavioral problems
  - Social difficulties
  - Academic difficulties
- Parents' comments and potential explanations for mild-to-moderate hearing loss.
  - "He can hear me when he wants to hear me. Sometimes he just ignores me."
    - With mild hearing loss, little or no difficulty listening in quiet settings
    - More difficulty when background noise is present
  - "When I call her, she has to look around for me. She never seems to know where I am in the house."
    - With unilateral hearing loss, difficulty localizing a sound source
  - "When we are in crowds, I have to call his name several times before he responds."
    - Difficulty hearing in the presence of background noise
  - "My child is exhausted when she comes home from school."
    - Fatigue from the effort exerted to listen throughout the day
  - "His speech is very difficult to understand. I don't think it's his hearing, because he always responds when I call him."
    - Children with high-frequency hearing loss may have poor speech production.
      - They cannot hear high-frequency speech sounds (consonants).
      - They can hear low- and mid-frequency sounds.
  - "My child is doing poorly in school, but I know she understands the material because we go over her homework at night."
    - Difficulty hearing in school settings because of background noise
    - No hearing difficulty apparent when working at home in a one-on-one situation

DIFFERENTIAL DIAGNOSIS

- Most congenital hearing loss is hereditary.
  - However, a negative family history is common.
  - 80% of inherited hearing loss results from autosomal recessive transmission.
  - 18% results from autosomal dominant transmission.
  - Approximately 2% results from X-linked recessive transmission.
  - Children with dominantly inherited hearing loss may have families who demonstrate incomplete penetrance.

- Evidence of the gene expression can be highly variable.
- Most children with inherited hearing loss are nonsyndromic.
- Several syndromes are associated with sensory hearing loss.
  - Alport syndrome
  - Neurofibromatosis
  - Usher syndrome
  - Waardenburg syndrome
- Children with Down syndrome are at high risk for conductive hearing loss and have a higher-than-average risk for sensory loss.
- Infants in the neonatal intensive care unit are at increased risk for:
  - Neural conduction dysfunction
  - Auditory brainstem dysfunction
  - Auditory neuropathy/dyssynchrony
    - A recently identified disorder characterized by a unique constellation of behavioral and physiologic auditory test results
    - Ranges from normal hearing to profound hearing loss and poor speech perception
    - Children with family history of childhood hearing loss or with hyperbilirubinemia are at particular risk.
- Audiologic and medical monitoring of infants at risk are recommended.

DIAGNOSTIC PROCEDURES

- If an infant or child fails a hearing, speech, or language screening measure in the pediatrician's office, referral for a full audiologic evaluation is recommended.
- A recent study suggested that more than one-half of children who failed screenings in primary care practices did not receive rescreening or referral for further testing.
- Audiologists with pediatric experience can define degree of hearing loss.
  - Distinguish among conductive, sensory, and neural types of loss in children of all chronologic ages and developmental levels
- Evaluation of hearing in infants and young children consists of a combination of physiological and behavioral measures.
  - For infants <6 months, testing is typically limited to physiologic measures because behavioral responses are not yet reliable enough to define the extent of loss.
  - See Auditory Screening.

TREATMENT APPROACH

- Early identification of hearing loss is of little value without timely intervention.
- Many children have conductive and sensorineural hearing losses not amenable to medical treatment; they may benefit from amplification.

SPECIFIC TREATMENT

Hearing aids

- Traditional hearing aids are designed to:
  - Pick up sounds
  - Convert them to electrical signals
  - Amplify, filter, and convert signals back to acoustic signals for a receiver
  - In noisy settings, frequency-modulated systems can be used alone or in combination with hearing aids.
    - For instance, a microphone worn by a teacher to amplify only the teacher's voice while minimizing interfering background noise

Cochlear implants

- An alternative to traditional hearing aids
- The device is surgically implanted in the cochlea.
  - Electrodes stimulate the auditory nerve with electrical current.
- Cochlear implants do not restore normal hearing.
- Children vary markedly in the benefits they derive from the implant.
  - Most experience at least an awareness of sound.
  - Some reach a high level of speech recognition and can develop normal speech and language skills.

WHEN TO REFER

- Family history of permanent hearing loss
- Postnatal infections associated with sensorineural hearing loss (eg, meningitis)
- History of in utero infections
  - Syphilis
  - Toxoplasmosis
  - Rubella
  - Cytomegalovirus
  - Herpes
- Neonatal indicators associated with progressive or late-onset hearing loss
  - Hyperbilirubinemia requiring exchange transfusion
  - Persistent pulmonary hypertension of the newborn associated with mechanical ventilation
  - Use of extracorporeal membrane oxygenation
- Syndromes associated with hearing loss
  - Alport syndrome
  - Down syndrome
  - Neurofibromatosis
  - Usher syndrome
  - Waardenburg syndrome

- Neurodegenerative disorders
  - Charcot-Marie-Tooth disease
  - Friedreich ataxia
- Head trauma
- The child does not pass a hearing screen in the pediatrician's office.
- The patient or caregiver is concerned about hearing, speech, or language development.

FOLLOW-UP

- For infants with permanent hearing loss:
  - Communicate with the state's coordinator for early hearing detection and intervention to ensure that the child and family are enrolled in appropriate services.
  - Be sure that the child has received a thorough medical evaluation (including genetics consultation) to determine the cause of the hearing loss.

- There is a high incidence of vision problems in children with hearing loss.
  - Referral for ophthalmologic evaluation may be warranted.
- Approximately 30–40% of children with hearing loss have additional disabilities.
  - Periodic developmental screening and surveillance is an integral part of their management.

COMPLICATIONS

- Children with hearing loss are especially vulnerable to the effects of otitis media with effusion because additional hearing loss can negatively affect the audibility of speech through hearing aids.
- Closely monitor and manage children who have persistent otitis media with effusion.

H

Hearing Screening

BACKGROUND

- Hearing loss is the most common congenital abnormality in newborns.
- Routine screening for hearing loss is a justifiable procedure, based on its prevalence and potential for treatment.
  - 1 to 6 in 1000 babies without risk factors are born with hearing loss >40 dB.
  - ~13.3 per 1000 babies with high-risk factors are born with hearing loss >40 dB.
  - ~15% of all children in the US have a hearing loss with thresholds ≥16 dB.
- Hearing loss may be progressive or acquired.
  - 20–30% of hearing loss up to age 18 is acquired or progressive.
  - 75% of children have ≥1 episode of otitis media by their third birthday.
  - The principal cause of hearing loss in preschool children is otitis media.
  - Many conditions place children at risk for late-onset or progressive hearing loss.
    - Neurofibromatosis
    - Osteopetrosis
    - Usher syndrome
    - Other syndromes (Waardenburg, Alport, Pendred, Jervell, and Lange–Nielson)
    - Neurodegenerative disorders, eg, Hunter syndrome
    - Sensory motor neuropathies, eg, Friedreich ataxia and Charcot–Marie–Tooth syndrome
    - Postnatal infections associated with sensorineural hearing loss (confirmed bacterial and viral meningitis)
    - Head trauma, especially basal skull or temporal bone fracture requiring hospitalization
    - Chemotherapy
- Hearing loss may cause:
  - Speech and language delay
  - Difficulty in social and educational environments
- Profound consequences
  - ~37% of children with mild hearing loss will fail ≥1 grade in school.
  - Late-identified children with bilateral permanent hearing loss leave school at age 18 with a sixth-grade reading level and a language-age equivalent of 12 years.

GOALS

General

- To identify children with moderate to severe hearing loss as early as possible to prevent detrimental effects on language and speech development

- Joint Committee on Infant Hearing–endorsed goals
  - Test children by 1 month of age.
  - Identify those with hearing loss by 3 months of age.
  - Treat hearing-impaired children by 6 months of age.
- All 50 states and the District of Columbia have mandatory universal newborn hearing screening programs to detect moderate to severe hearing loss.

Goals of screening, by age group

- Neonatal/early infancy
  - Primary goal is to identify congenital or in utero acquired hearing loss and to ensure speech development.
  - If risk factors for delayed-onset or progressive hearing loss are present, the child should receive audiologic monitoring every 6 months for the first 3 years.
  - All infants should receive ongoing surveillance of communicative development during well-child visits, beginning at 2 months of age.
  - Objective physiological measures used together
    - Otoacoustic emissions
    - Auditory brainstem response (ABR) measures
  - Best time frame: approximately 3–4 days after birth or before hospital discharge
  - The Joint Committee on Infant Hearing recommends different protocols for neonatal intensive care unit and well-baby nurseries.
    - Screening of neonatal intensive care unit babies admitted for >5 days should always include ABR testing.
    - Any baby readmitted within first month of life who has risk factors for hearing loss should have repeat hearing screening before discharge.
  - Despite the sensitivity of a 2-step screening protocol, some infants with hearing loss will still be missed.
    - Acquired or progressive hearing loss will be unidentified in the neonatal population.
    - The main factor for effectiveness of hearing screening is appropriate follow-up.
- Toddler and preschool (2–5 years)
  - The primary goal is detection of remediable otopathologic abnormalities, or of progressive or acquired hearing loss.
  - Screening assumes that the more severe sensorineural hearing losses will have been identified by 2 years.
  - The screening protocol includes identification of:
    - Otopathologic abnormalities (especially otitis media with effusion)
    - Mild conductive hearing loss
    - Sensorineural hearing impairment

- School age
  - Primary goal: identical to that of toddler-preschool period, with addition of the maintenance of educationally optimal hearing
  - Typically screened in school by trained professionals; referred to physician only if they fail screening
  - Children are screened:
    - On initial entry
    - Annually through third grade
    - In seventh and eleventh grades
    - As needed, requested, or mandated by regulation
  - At-risk children should be routinely monitored for hearing loss.
  - During this period, central auditory processing disorders become apparent.
  - Elicitation of parental/caregiver concern about child's hearing and speech/language development is key.

GENERAL APPROACH

- Early identification and intervention are critical for:
  - Overall communicative development
  - Cognitive development
  - Educational development
  - Emotional/behavioral development
- Early intervention methods include:
  - Audiologic management
  - Otologic treatment
  - Amplification
  - Parental counseling
  - Special education
- Infants: auditory screening using a physiologic measure should be completed no later than 1 month of age.
  - Infants who do not pass initial and subsequent screening should have audiologic and medical evaluations no later than 3 months of age.
  - Infants with confirmed permanent hearing loss should receive early intervention services as soon as possible, but no later than 6 months of age.
    - A simplified, single point of entry into the intervention system is optimal.
- The intervention should be family centered, with infant and family rights and privacy guaranteed.
  - Informed choice
  - Shared decision making
  - Parental consent
  - Families should have access to information about all intervention and treatment options and counseling regarding hearing loss.

- Immediate access to high-quality technology, including hearing aids, cochlear implants, and other assistive devices when appropriate.
- Continued assessment of communication development should be provided to all children with or without risk indicators for hearing loss.
- Appropriate interdisciplinary intervention programs:
  - Should be provided by professionals knowledgeable about childhood hearing loss
  - Should recognize and build on strengths, informed choices, traditions, and cultural beliefs of the families
- Information systems should be designed and implemented to interface with electronic health records.
- Routinely refer children who fail their hearing screenings to a licensed audiologist for appropriate follow-up and management.

SPECIFIC INTERVENTIONS

- Initial follow-up evaluation for infant or child who fails hearing screen or is at risk for acquired or progressive hearing loss
  - Comprehensive audiologic evaluation by licensed audiologist
  - ≥1 ABR test, as part of assessment of children <3 years, before permanent hearing loss can be confirmed
  - If hearing loss or middle-ear dysfunction is confirmed, refer for otologic and medical consultation to:
    - Determine the cause of the hearing loss
    - Identify related physical conditions (present in 40%)
    - Provide recommendations for medical treatment and other referrals, if appropriate
- Comprehensive evaluations should include:
  - Complete patient and family history to identify risk factors
  - Tests to identify any anatomic malformations
    - Physical examination
    - Possible laboratory and radiologic tests
  - Monitoring of developmental milestones
  - Referral for genetic evaluation and counseling by medical geneticist
  - Referral to an ophthalmologist to test for visual acuity
  - Other specialty referrals, such as a speech and language evaluation, once etiology and developmental concerns have been identified
- Audiologic intervention depends on type and degree of hearing loss.
  - For conductive hearing loss, medical and surgical options are often available.
  - For atresia or similar anatomic condition that precludes medical or surgical treatment, bone-conduction or bone-anchored hearing aid, with fit by an audiologist

- For sensorineural hearing loss, amplification or assistive listening devices are typically recommended.
  - Children as young as 4 weeks may be fitted with hearing aids following appropriate physiological tests.
  - If diagnosed with permanent hearing loss, children should be fitted with hearing aids within 1 month.
- Cochlear implantation is often considered for severe to profound hearing loss in children as young as 12 months; criteria for use by age:
  - 12–24 months
    - Profound sensorineural hearing loss in both ears
    - Lack of progress in development of auditory skills with appropriate binaural hearing aids
    - High motivation and realistic expectations from the family
    - Other medical conditions, if present, do not interfere with implant procedure.
  - 25 months to 17 years 11 months
    - Severe to profound sensorineural hearing loss in both ears
    - Little or no benefit from hearing aids (speech scores ≤30% in best-aided condition)
    - Lack of progress in development of auditory skills
    - High motivation and realistic expectations from family
    - No medical contraindications
- Speech and language assessment and therapy are essential to development and intelligible speech by entry into kindergarten.
- Financial concerns should not limit a child's access to intervention services.
  - The Individuals with Disabilities Education Act (IDEA) ensures that children who have hearing loss receive appropriate, family-centered, multidisciplinary intervention services at no charge from birth through the school years.
  - Options available to cover cost of amplification due to permanent hearing loss
    - Private insurance
    - Medicaid
    - Services provided by IDEA/school education resources

Heart Failure

DEFINITION

- Congestive heart failure (CHF) is an inability to perfuse the body tissues adequately.

EPIDEMIOLOGY

- Age
  - CHF can occur in infants or children of any age, but up to 90% of cases occur during the first year of life, most during the neonatal period.

ETIOLOGY

- For a particular left ventricular (LV) preload, cardiac output or stroke volume increases progressively from fetal to neonatal to adult stages of life.
- Mechanisms are not entirely clear, but properties of contractile proteins, ion channels, and cell surface receptors are expressed differently at each developmental stage.
- These changes in protein expression affect contractility of the LV myocardium at different developmental stages.
- Animal studies suggest that neonates operate closer to maximal inotropic potential than adults, and neonates may have less reserve to handle excess ventricular preload and are more likely than adults to experience episodes of CHF.
- The age at onset of heart failure (HF) in children, especially in infants, is important in determining cause.

SIGNS AND SYMPTOMS

- Feeding
  - Helps quantify nutritional intake and compare it with weight gain
  - Children with CHF often have greater nutritional needs because of increased metabolic demands.
    - Often require ≥150 kcal/kg daily to gain adequate weight
  - Frequently, infants with CHF do not feed vigorously and may feed only in short, interrupted periods.
  - For older children, CHF over long intervals results in malnutrition.
  - Weight is usually the initial anthropometric measurement to be affected, followed by height and then head circumference.
- Activity level
  - Children with CHF usually change their activity level, becoming less active or more irritable and anxious.
- Tachycardia
  - Children with CHF may have persistent sinus tachycardia, with heart rates far higher than the normal range for their age.
- Tachypnea
  - Higher respiratory rates during sleep are often found in children with CHF.

- Rales
  - Clinically evident rales are less likely to be found in infants and young children with CHF.
  - In a young child, rales may suggest active pulmonary disease.
- Jugular venous distention
  - Found in many older patients with HF, but not seen as frequently in infants and children, largely because observing their jugular veins is difficult
- Hepatomegaly
  - The liver is frequently enlarged in infants and children with CHF.
  - Measuring the total liver span by percussion is more useful than determining how far the liver edge extends below the right costal margin.
  - The left lobe of the liver is frequently enlarged in CHF, and thus a palpable liver edge that crosses the midline is suggestive of CHF.
- Third heart sound gallop
  - Frequently observed in children of all ages with CHF
  - An S_3 gallop may not indicate CHF in a neonate.
- Pulses and perfusion
  - Diminished strength of the peripheral pulses and perfusion are common signs.
  - Simultaneously palpating upper and lower extremity pulses may reveal differences in intensity or timing of the pulses, indicating:
    - Coarctation of the aorta
    - Interrupted aortic arch
    - Another lesion interfering with arterial blood flow
- Arrhythmias and sudden death
  - Arrhythmias can be both a cause and a result of HF in children and young adults.
  - Ventricular dysfunction resulting from dilated cardiomyopathy may be associated with high-grade ectopy.
  - This may increase the risk of death associated with HF.
  - Unexplained syncope or palpitations in children with HF or cardiomyopathy should prompt evaluation for arrhythmias.
  - Syncope may be an important predictor of sudden death in these children.

DIFFERENTIAL DIAGNOSIS

- The transition from fetal circulation to postnatal circulation requires precise steps, any of which may be compromised and lead to HF.

Prenatal period

- Infections, such as those caused by parvovirus, can lead to CHF with or without myocarditis.
- Abnormalities of heart rhythm

- Fetuses tolerate prolonged supraventricular tachycardia poorly, and the mother must often be treated with antiarrhythmic medications to control the condition in the fetus.
- Fetuses with chronic or severe CHF have a greater likelihood of developing hydrops fetalis and dying.

First day of life

- Persistent fetal circulation or persistent pulmonary hypertension is the leading cause of CHF.
  - Associated with meconium aspiration and neonatal acidosis
  - In persistent pulmonary hypertension, CHF may not be clinically apparent.
  - When recognized early, careful use of fluids, inotropes, and oxygen can be beneficial.
- Neonatal sepsis
  - Prolonged rupture of membranes, maternal infection, and associated findings are risk factors.
  - Usually accompanied by the classic signs or symptoms
  - Treating sepsis with antibiotics and judicious use of fluids in conjunction with anticongestive therapy is often effective.
- Hematologic or metabolic disorders
  - Hematocrit that is too high or too low is a risk for HF.
  - Polycythemia resulting in sludging and hyperviscosity, most common in infants of mothers with diabetes
  - Partial exchange transfusion will often lead to a rapid improvement in signs of HF.
- Severe anemia
  - Determining whether reduced erythrocyte count has an acute or a chronic cause is important.
  - Acute blood loss, as from abruptio placentae, can be managed with blood transfusion and by otherwise increasing intravascular fluid volume.
  - Chronic anemia, such as that caused by Rh sensitization, may produce low erythrocyte count and a low hematocrit.
  - Intravascular volume may be high, and transfusion may worsen HF.
  - Such patients may benefit from double-volume exchange transfusion.
- Metabolic causes of cardiomyopathy include hypoglycemia and hypocalcemia.
  - The neonatal myocardium uses glucose for energy metabolism, diminishing fat reserves.
  - A newborn with a low blood glucose level and signs or symptoms of CHF will often improve when the blood glucose level is normalized.
  - Hypocalcemia is another metabolic cause; normalization of calcium, a potent inotrope, can reduce signs or symptoms of CHF.
  - Hypoglycemia and hypocalcemia are often seen together in infants of mothers with diabetes.

- Rare congenital heart defects, such as absent pulmonary valve syndrome, free tricuspid orifice, or severe anomaly of the tricuspid valve associated with severe pulmonary stenosis
- Heart rate abnormalities
  - A newborn can tolerate supraventricular tachycardia of 250–300 beats/min for only 12–36 hours before developing signs and symptoms of CHF.
  - Sinus rhythm should be established immediately in symptomatic neonates with supraventricular tachycardia and CHF.
  - If vagal maneuvers or intravenous administration of adenosine do not result in normal sinus rhythm and a pacemaker is unavailable, then cardioversion should be attempted, followed by treatment with drugs.
  - Slow heart rates may lead to CHF.
    - Heart rates <60 beats/min result in symptomatic CHF.

Days 1–2 of life

- Obstructed total anomalous pulmonary venous return
  - Persistent or progressive tachypnea and hypoxia and
  - Chest radiographs showing a snowman or snowball pattern, with vessels radiating from a small cardiac silhouette
  - Echocardiography can confirm the diagnosis.
  - Early identification is essential because surgery is the only effective intervention.

Days 2–3 of life

- Ductus arteriosus–dependent lesions, including the following:
  - Right-sided obstructive lesions, such as pulmonary atresia, maximal tetralogy of Fallot, or tricuspid atresia
  - Transposition of the great arteries (the most common type of cyanotic heart disease)
  - Left-sided obstructive lesions, such as hypoplastic left-heart syndrome, critical aortic stenosis, or complex coarctation of the aorta
- CHF is less likely when any of these conditions is accompanied by a patent ductus arteriosus but may develop after the ductus arteriosus has closed, especially in cases of left-sided obstructive lesions.
- If diagnosed in time, these patients can often be stabilized by infusions of prostaglandin E_1 to maintain patency of the ductus arteriosus.

Days 3–7 of life

- Endocrine disorders, including congenital adrenal hypoplasia, hyperthyroidism
- Renal disorders, such as renal vein thrombus, renal artery stenosis, and hypertension or oliguria of any cause

Weeks 1–2 of life

- Complex coarctation of the aorta
- Similar lesions, such as an interrupted aortic arch, also may present at this age.

- Typically, ductus arteriosus closes by 3 days of life in children without these conditions.
- In complex coarctation of the aorta, the ductus remains open for up to 1 or 2 weeks.
- A child with coarctation of the aorta and CHF at 1–2 weeks of age may have no pulse differential between the upper and lower extremities if cardiac output is low.
- Any suspected complex coarctation or interrupted aortic arch should be investigated by echocardiography.
- When diagnosed early, the child can often be stabilized quickly with anticongestive therapy and prostaglandin E_1.

Months 1–2 of life

- Left-to-right shunt lesions
  - For example, ventricular septal defect where pulmonary artery resistance has decreased over the first few postnatal weeks, resulting in increased left-to-right shunting
  - Others include atrial-level shunts (eg, atrial septal defect); common atria; ventricular-level left-to-right shunts (eg, complete atrioventricular canal defects, ventricular septal defects, single ventricle); and great vessel-level shunts, such as patent ductus arteriosus.
  - The timing of presentation often suggests existence of a left-to-right shunt.
  - Whether CHF in this circumstance is easily treated is unclear.
    - In the past, hypertransfusion therapy to reduce shunting was found to be useful.
      - This therapy is not commonly used.

Months 6–12 of life

- Metabolic, genetic, infectious, and inflammatory cardiomyopathies
- Children with metabolic or genetic cardiomyopathy seem asymptomatic to the family for the first 6 months of life.
- Children may exhibit growth failure and hypotonia.
- Such disorders as glycogen storage diseases also present in this way.
- Infectious and inflammatory diseases, such as HIV, enterovirus infections, and Kawasaki disease, can cause myocarditis at this age.

Years 1–18 of life

- Most common in children with comorbid severe or chronic illnesses
- Beyond the first year of life, CHF is unusual.
- Older children with congenital heart disease, other than those who have had corrective surgery, rarely develop CHF.
- Leading indications for pediatric heart transplantations, which indicate a failure of the medical management of CHF, are congenital heart disease during the first year of life and cardiomyopathies thereafter.

DIAGNOSTIC APPROACH

- A thoroughly obtained clinical history often provides clues to the cause of CHF.
- Classification systems for adults are not particularly useful in infants and children because of:
  - Variation in normal respiratory rates
  - Different developmental stages, reflecting different exercise capabilities
  - Different causes for HF across age groups

Ross scoring system of HF in infants

- Volume per feeding (oz)
  - 0 points: >3.5
  - 1 point: 2.5–3.5
  - 2 points: <2.5
- Time per feeding (min)
  - 0 points: <40
  - 1 point: ≥40
- Respiratory rate (breaths/min)
  - 0 points: <50
  - 1 point: 50–60
  - 2 points: >60
- Respiratory pattern
  - 0 points: normal
  - 1 point: abnormal
- Peripheral perfusion
  - 0 points: normal
  - 1 point: decreased
- S_3 or diastolic rumble
  - 0 points: absent
  - 1 point: present
- Liver edge from costal margin, cm
  - 0 points: <2
  - 1 point: 2–3
  - 2 points: >3
- Totals
  - No CHF: 0–2 points
  - Mild CHF: 3–6 points
  - Moderate CHF: 7–9 points
  - Severe CHF: 10–12 points

Pediatric clinical HF score

- Diaphoresis
  - 0 points: head only
  - 1 point: head and body during exercise
  - 2 points: head and body at rest

H

- Tachypnea
  - 0 points: rare
  - 1 point: several times
  - 2 points: frequent
- Breathing
  - 0 points: normal
  - 1 point: retractions
  - 2 points: dyspnea
- Respiratory rate (breaths/min)
  - 0–1 year
    - 0 points: <50
    - 1 point: 50–60
    - 2 points: >60
  - 1–6 years
    - 0 points: <35
    - 1 point: 35–45
    - 2 points: >45
  - 7–10 years
    - 0 points: <25
    - 1 point: 25–35
    - 2 points: >35
  - 11–14 years
    - 0 points: <18
    - 1 point: 18–28
    - 2 points: >28
- Heart rate (beats/min)
  - 0–1 year
    - 0 points: <160
    - 1 point: 160–170
    - 2 points: >170
  - 1–6 years
    - 0 points: <105
    - 1 point: 105–115
    - 2 points: >115
  - 7–10 years
    - 0 points: <90
    - 1 point: 90–100
    - 2 points: >100
  - 11–14 years
    - 0 points: <80
    - 1 point: 80–90
    - 2 points: >90
- Liver edge from costal margin, cm
  - 0 points: <2
  - 1 point: 2–3
  - 2 points: >3

CLASSIFICATION

- The Ross classification of HF in infants has been validated to address pediatric differences from adult classification systems.
  - Class I: no limitations or symptoms
  - Class II
    - Mild tachypnea or diaphoresis with feeding in infants
    - Dyspnea on exertion in older children
    - No growth failure
  - Class III
    - Marked tachypnea or diaphoresis with feeding or exertion
    - Prolonged feeding times
    - Growth failure from CHF
  - Class IV: symptoms at rest, with tachypnea, retractions, grunting, or diaphoresis
- Proposed HF staging for infants and children by the International Society for Heart and Lung Transplantation
  - Modified from the American College of Cardiology/American Heart Association guidelines and complementing the Ross classification system
  - Stage A: patients with increased risk of HF but normal cardiac function and no evidence of cardiac chamber volume overload
    - Examples: previous exposure to cardiotoxic agents, family history of heritable cardiomyopathy, univentricular heart, congenitally corrected transposition of the great arteries
  - Stage B: patients with abnormal cardiac morphology or cardiac function, with no symptoms of HF, past or present
    - Examples: aortic insufficiency with LV enlargement, history of anthracycline use with decreased LV systolic function
  - Stage C: patients with underlying structural or functional heart diseases and past or current symptoms of HF
  - Stage D: patients with end-stage HF requiring continuous infusion of inotropic agents, mechanical circulatory support, cardiac transplantation, or hospice care

TREATMENT APPROACH

- The 4 classes of drugs used most frequently in the management of CHF in children are:
  - Diuretics
  - Inotropes
  - Agents to reduce afterload
  - ß-Adrenergic antagonists

- Each class targets a different pathophysiologic feature of CHF, and they are often used in combination.
- A pediatric cardiologist should direct the treatment of CHF in children.

SPECIFIC TREATMENTS

Current consensus recommendations for management of pediatric HF

- All recommendations presented are class I (conditions for which general agreement exists that a given therapy is useful and effective).
- Recommendation 1
  - The underlying cause of new-onset ventricular dysfunction (HF stages B, C, or D) should be evaluated thoroughly in all patients.
    - The evaluation may include metabolic and genetic evaluation in selected cases, as indicated by the available history and physical findings.
    - Invasive assessment, including myocardial biopsy, may be considered in selected cases.
    - In infants, particular care should be given to the exclusion of coronary artery anomalies and other anatomic causes.
- Recommendation 2
  - Screening of first-degree relatives should be considered in patients with new-onset ventricular dysfunction caused by dilated cardiomyopathy (HF stages B, C, or D).
- Recommendation 3
  - Patients with fluid retention associated with ventricular dysfunction (HF stage C) should be treated with diuretics to achieve a euvolemic state using clinical criteria of fluid status and cardiac output.
- Recommendation 4
  - Digoxin should be used in patients with ventricular dysfunction and symptoms of HF (HF stage C) to relieve symptoms. Lower doses of digoxin are preferred for this purpose.
- Recommendation 5
  - For the treatment of moderate or severe LV dysfunction with or without symptoms (HF stages B and C), angiotensin-converting enzyme (ACE) inhibitors should be routinely used unless a specific contraindication exists.
    - These medications should be started at low doses and titrated up to a maximal tolerated safe dose.
    - Uptitration may require a reduction in the dose of diuretics.
- Recommendation 6
  - In all cases of HF associated with structural heart disease (HF stages B, C, or D), surgical repair of significant lesions should be considered because the long-term outlook may be more favorable than with medical management alone.

- Recommendation 7
  - Clinical management of diastolic dysfunction should address symptoms and attempt to address the underlying cause of the diastolic dysfunction, if known.
    - This management should include a careful evaluation for pericardial disease and coronary insufficiency with attendant myocardial ischemia.
    - Systemic hypertension, if present, should be aggressively controlled.
- Recommendation 8
  - Fluid management to control symptoms remains a cornerstone in the management of symptomatic diastolic dysfunction (HF stage C).
    - Diuretics can help control symptoms but must be used cautiously because cardiac output depends on increased filling pressures.
    - Renal function should be followed closely, with care taken not to administer too much.
    - Sodium and fluid restriction may be helpful in controlling symptoms.
- Recommendation 9
  - Atrial arrhythmias are not infrequent in patients with diastolic dysfunction caused by atrial enlargement. However, atrial contribution to ventricular filling is particularly important for this group of patients (HF stages B and C).
    - Therefore, efforts should be made to maintain sinus rhythm by use of antiarrhythmic therapy and pacemakers.
- Recommendation 10
  - Patients with diastolic dysfunction refractory to optimal medical or surgical management should be evaluated for heart transplantation because such patients are at high risk for pulmonary hypertension and sudden death (HF stage C).
- Recommendation 11
  - Institution of mechanical cardiac support should be considered in patients without structural congenital heart disease, those who present with acute low cardiac output, or those who have intractable arrhythmias during a presumably temporary condition that is refractory to medical therapy (HF stage D), such as myocarditis, septic shock, or acute rejection after heart transplantation.
- Recommendation 12
  - Institution of mechanical cardiac support should be considered in patients with or without structural congenital heart disease and who have acute decompensation of end-stage HF, primarily as a bridge to heart transplantation (HF stage D).

H

■ Recommendation 13

- In patients with significant arrhythmias in the setting of HF associated with structural heart disease (HF stages B, C, or D), surgical repair of important uncorrected or residual defects should be considered because this is likely to be essential in achieving adequate rhythm control.

■ Recommendation 14

- In patients with significant arrhythmias in the setting of HF associated with structural heart disease (HF stages B, C, or D), improving or optimizing the medical treatment for HF and correcting aggravating factors, such as electrolyte abnormalities, should be considered because this is likely to be a key determinant of the successful control of arrhythmias.

■ Recommendation 15

- In patients with significant arrhythmias in the setting of HF associated with structural heart disease (HF stages B, C, or D), maintenance of atrioventricular synchrony is of great importance in optimizing hemodynamics, and management of intraatrial arrhythmias should be oriented toward restoration of sinus rhythm rather than toward ventricular rate control alone.

Pharmacotherapy

■ Symptomatic LV dysfunction or CHF in children can be caused by many different pathophysiologic mechanisms.

■ The basis for using these agents is extrapolated from adults, and generally they are used for the palliative relief of symptoms in children.

■ Treatments directed at prevention or cure of CHF in children have not been evaluated.

■ Diuretics

- Increased preload is 1 common mechanism.
- Overall systolic performance of the ventricle is reduced.
- Preload reduction with diuretic therapy is often beneficial.

■ Inotropes

- Depressed contractility of unhealthy LV myocytes and inotropic support frequently bring early symptom relief.
- However, determining the cause of HF in a child becomes critical because many children with unexplained HF have mitochondrial defects that impair their ability to respond to inotropic support.
- Aggressive use of inotropic support in such patients may hasten their deaths.
- Digoxin, an inotrope administered orally or intravenously, will raise a child to a higher inotropic state and, in the process, lead to a reduction in preload.
- Frequently, digoxin is used in combination with a diuretic.
- Some studies suggest synergy between digoxin and diuretics that potentiates primary ventricular function and reduces preload more than either agent alone.

- Combination therapy can also reduce the chance of individual agent toxicity.
- ß-Adrenergic agonists, such as dopamine and dobutamine, are also inotropic and are useful for treating children with HF, especially those in a decompensated state.
- Newer inotropic agents are being investigated.
  - Calcium-sensitizing agents, in particular, improve cardiac output with minimal increases in heart rate, a common side effect of ß-adrenergic agonists.

■ Agents that reduce afterload

- LV afterload reduction in a child with symptomatic LV dysfunction will improve function and reduce symptoms.
- ACE inhibitors, such as captopril and enalapril, are used most frequently.
  - They are vasodilators, but they affect neurohormonal mechanisms.
  - In adults with asymptomatic LV dysfunction or CHF, ACE inhibitors have been associated with slowing progression from asymptomatic LV dysfunction to CHF and reducing mortality from HF.
  - These benefits are believed to be caused by combination of vasodilatory and neurohormonal activation.
  - The vasodilatory effects of ACE inhibitors will often move a child to a more favorable preload state and reduce afterload, thus improving LV contractility.

■ ß-Adrenergic antagonists

- ß-Adrenergic antagonists reverse adrenergically mediated intrinsic myocardial dysfunction and remodeling.
- Atenolol and carvedilol
- In adults with CHF, ß-antagonists improve symptoms, ventricular function, and survival.
- Small studies suggest that ß-antagonists improve ventricular function in children with CHF.
- These agents have not yet been used extensively, and further evaluation of this class of drugs is under way.

■ Newer agents for management of CHF

- Angiotensin-receptor blockers
- Endothelin-receptor antagonists
- Phosphodiesterase inhibitors
- Aldosterone antagonists
- Calcium-sensitizing agents
- Tumor necrosis factor a inhibitors
- Neural endopeptidase inhibitors
- Vasopressin antagonists

Arrhythmias

■ Arrhythmias are a major cause of morbidity and mortality in children with HF, especially in the later stages of disease.

- Short-term treatment with intravenous antiarrhythmic agents and cardioversion or defibrillation should be considered for all children with hemodynamic instability.
- Long-term suppressive therapy or radiofrequency surgical ablation therapy may be required for long-term management of recurring arrhythmias.
- In adults with HF and arrhythmias, implantable cardiac defibrillators have greatly improved survival.
- These devices have not been used extensively in young children, and only a few small studies have assessed their use.
- However, technologic advances suggest the potential for decreased complications and infections; thus, they hold promise for use in younger children.

Nutritional management

- A systematic approach to overcoming failure to thrive has been suggested, starting with dietary intervention.
  - Counseling and educating patient and parents to optimize feeding to increase mean caloric intake and weight
- The high energy cost of eating might prevent a child from consuming larger quantities of food; fortified formula and breast milk have improved weight gain.
  - Monitor the patient closely, because high-energy formula can induce thermogenesis and increase metabolic inefficiency.
  - Breastfeeding is less stressful than bottle feeding for infants with congenital heart disease.
- Gastrostomy placement and parenteral feeding may be important considerations in severely malnourished infants, in part because they do not incur the energy costs of feeding.
- Mortality and morbidity associated with cardiac surgery increase in underweight infants.
- Conversely, some findings show that energy expenditures decrease and return to normal after surgery.
- Therefore, if an infant fails to thrive after all aggressive feeding and nutrition measures have been tried, surgery may be advisable even if the infant is not at an ideal weight.
- Other nutritional considerations
  - Managing electrolyte abnormalities that may occur from diuretic use
  - Balancing fluid intake with fluid overload in children with HF

Surgery

- Children with cardiomyopathy or HF after repair of a congenital cardiac defect may be candidates for heart transplantation.
- Aggressive pretransplantation evaluation is required, given the potential for long-term complications.
- Newer surgical techniques for congenital cardiac defects include techniques to correct failed procedures or revise older, less effective surgical procedures.
- As children with congenital heart disease live longer, revision procedures in young adulthood may become important in long-term management.
- For children at risk of sudden death from arrhythmias, implantable cardioverter defibrillators may be considered, although not well studied or used extensively in children.
- Difficulties include large size of the device and leads, difficult surgical access due to previous cardiac surgeries, and difficulties with programming devices as a result of inconsistent rate patterns.

WHEN TO ADMIT

- All pediatric patients with HF must be admitted for evaluation and management and monitoring of the progress.

WHEN TO REFER

- All pediatric patients with HF must be managed in consultation with pediatric cardiologists.

FOLLOW-UP

- All pediatric patients with HF must be closely monitored for growth and development.

PROGNOSIS

- Prognosis depends on the underlying cardiac cause leading to HF as well as on early and appropriate management.

PREVENTION

- All patients with congenital heart disease, with or without repair, must be monitored closely for symptoms.
  - Educate patients and parents on the early identification of HF symptoms.

H

Heart Murmurs

DEFINITION

- A heart murmur results from turbulent blood flow.

EPIDEMIOLOGY

- Heart murmur is a common finding during the physical examination of children.
- Few children have structural cardiac disease.

MECHANISM

Cardiac cycle and associated heart sounds

- When determining the significance of a heart murmur, the pediatric primary care physician needs to understand:
  - Events of the cardiac cycle
  - Associated heart sounds
- Heart sounds as auscultated during physical examination are directly related to the hemodynamic events of systole and diastole.
- The first heart sound (S1) is related to the closure of the mitral and tricuspid valves at the very end of diastole.
  - The ventricles are completely filled.
  - The ventricles then undergo a period of isovolumic contraction.
  - The aortic and pulmonary valves begin opening.
  - Rapid systolic ejection phase begins.
  - This phase is followed by a phase of reduced ejection later in systole.
- The second heart sound (S2) is created by closure of the aortic and pulmonary valves at the very end of systole.
  - Physiologic splitting of S2 is particularly important in the diagnosis of cardiac disease.
  - The first component of S2 is created by closure of the aortic valve (A2).
  - The second component of S2 is created by closure of the pulmonary valve (P2).
  - During inspiration, P2 occurs after A2, generating an audibly split S2 (A2-P2).
  - During exhalation, closure of the aortic and pulmonary valves is nearly coincident, creating a single S2.
  - Splitting of S2 can be difficult to hear in infants or children with accelerated heart rates.
  - Normal splitting pattern helps distinguish an abnormality from normalcy.
    - Wide splitting of S2 is associated with prolonged ejection from the right ventricle, as occurs with such conditions as an atrial septal defect (ASD), in which S2 is widely split and fixed.
    - A narrowly split S2 is associated with pulmonary hypertension, in which closure of P2 is early, or aortic stenosis, when closure of A2 is delayed.

- Failure of S2 to split at all can be the result of simultaneous closure of the aortic and pulmonary valves during all phases of the respiratory cycle.
  - This is found with conditions that result in high pulmonary artery pressure.
- A single S2 can also be associated with certain congenital cardiac anomalies, such as:
  - Truncus arteriosus
  - Tetralogy of Fallot
  - Cardiac surgical palliations
  - Bidirectional Glenn shunt
  - Fontan completion
- Third and fourth heart sounds may also be heard during physical examination.
  - The third heart sound (S3) is heard early in diastole, during the initial phase of passive rapid ventricular filling.
  - It is a low-frequency sound that can be best heard at the left lower sternal border or at the apex.
  - An apical S3 can frequently be heard in normal children, as well as in competitive athletes.
- The fourth heart sound (S4) is always pathologic.
  - S4 is also a low-frequency sound, but is heard late in diastole, just before S1.
  - It results from rapid filling of the ventricle caused by atrial contraction.
  - An S4 gallop is associated with decreased ventricular compliance (as is seen in cardiomyopathy) and congestive heart failure.
  - Auscultation of an S4 gallop warrants immediate evaluation by a pediatric cardiologist.
- Clicks may be audible during the cardiac cycle.
  - Ejection clicks are heard in systole.
  - The timing of the click in the cardiac cycle helps elucidate the cause.
  - An early systolic click, heard just after S1, is associated with:
    - Semilunar valve stenosis (aortic stenosis or pulmonary stenosis)
    - Dilation of the great arteries (the aorta or pulmonary artery)
  - Aortic valve clicks, best heard at the apex or right upper sternal border, do not vary in intensity with respiration.
  - Pulmonary valve clicks increase in intensity with exhalation and are best heard along the left sternal border.
  - A midsystolic apical click is heard with mitral valve prolapse and may be accompanied by a late systolic murmur.

Cardiac anatomy

- The physician must understand the anatomy of the heart and its position in the chest.
- Location of the heart murmur on the chest wall serves as an important tool in deciding whether the murmur is innocent or abnormal.

HISTORY

- A complete and accurate history is the most important aspect of evaluating a cardiac murmur in children.
- Certain aspects of the patient's history may raise or lower the index of suspicion regarding the cause of a heart murmur.
- History should include the patient's chief symptoms and:
  - Medical history
  - Birth history
  - Family history
- Patient history
  - Poor weight gain
  - Difficulty feeding
  - Frequent respiratory difficulties
  - Respiratory distress
  - Cyanosis
  - Exercise intolerance
  - Chest pain with exercise
  - Unexplained syncope (especially syncope resulting in injury)
  - Concurrent syndromic disorder or genetic disease
  - Concurrent metabolic disorder or storage disease
  - Sickle cell anemia or blood dyscrasias resulting in anemia
  - History of cardiotoxic chemotherapy
  - Concurrent HIV disease
  - Hypertension
- Birth history
  - Maternal diabetes
  - Maternal TORCH (toxoplasmosis, other agents, rubella, cytomegalovirus, herpes simplex) infections during pregnancy
  - Multiple gestation pregnancy
  - In vitro fertilization pregnancy
  - Maternal drug use (either legal or illicit), known teratogens
  - Abnormal amniocentesis
  - Abnormal fetal ultrasonogram
  - Maternal history of congenital heart disease
- Family history
  - Congenital heart disease
  - Sudden cardiac death
  - Unexplained death in young people
  - Cardiac disease in the young
  - Stroke or myocardial infarction in men <55 years or women <65 years
  - Seizure disorders
  - Congenital deafness

PHYSICAL EXAM

Patient evaluation

- Evaluation of a cardiac murmur involves more than auscultation of the heart.
- Complete physical examination is needed to put the murmur in perspective.
- Pertinent aspects of physical examination include:
  - Vital signs
    - Temperature, heart rate, respiratory rate, length/height, weight
    - Blood pressures in the right arm, left arm, leg
    - Pulse oximetry on room air (right hand and either foot if infant)
  - General
    - Cyanosis, pallor, dysmorphic features, overall distress
    - Breathing pattern: retractions, grunting, nasal flaring
  - Head and neck
    - Jugular venous distention
    - Thyromegaly, thyroid nodules
  - Chest
    - Chest wall deformity, asymmetry, surgical scars
    - Lung aeration
    - Rales, rhonchi, wheezes, stridor
  - Cardiac
    - Inspection
    - Palpation
    - Auscultation
  - Abdominal
    - Liver span
    - Tenderness
    - Distention, ascites
  - Extremities
    - Perfusion: capillary refill, temperature, quality of pulses
    - Clubbing, cyanosis, edema
    - Arachnodactyly, joint laxity (Marfan syndrome)
    - Increased arm span/upper to lower body ratio (Marfan syndrome)

Cardiac evaluation

- Includes:
  - Inspection
  - Palpation
  - Auscultation
- Inspection
  - Begin with:
    - General appearance
    - Nutritional status

H

– Genetic abnormalities

– Color

– Comfort

• Then inspect the chest wall for abnormalities, including:

– Deformities, such as pectus excavatum

– Asymmetry

– Surgical scars

■ Palpation

• Begin with the extremities.

• Evaluation of overall perfusion includes assessment of:

– Pulses

– Capillary refill

– Temperature of extremities

• The precordium is then palpated to detect the point of maximal impulse (PMI) of the left and right ventricles and to detect thrills.

– PMI for the left ventricle is palpated in the left fourth or fifth intercostal space in the midclavicular line.

– PMI for the right ventricle is appreciated in the fourth to fifth intercostal space along the left lower sternal border.

• Displacement of the PMI suggests an underlying abnormality.

• Thrills can be palpated:

– In the suprasternal notch (suggesting aortic valve disease or coarctation of the aorta)

– Along left upper sternal border (suggesting pulmonary valve disease)

– Along right upper sternal border (suggesting aortic valve disease)

– Along left lower sternal border, in association with ventricular septal defects (VSDs)

■ Auscultation

• A systematic approach to auscultation of the heart ensures that each major anatomic area of the heart is heard in systole and diastole.

• The major areas of auscultation on the precordium

– Apex

– Left lower sternal border

– Left mid or upper sternal border

– Right upper sternal border

• These areas correspond to each atrioventricular and semilunar valve, as well as the outflow tracts of the right and left ventricles.

• The clinician should also auscultate:

– Left and right infraclavicular areas

– Axillae

– Back

• Auscultation for a continuous sound (bruit) should be performed over the liver and fontanelle.

– A bruit suggests an arteriovenous malformation.

• The patient should be examined in the following positions.

– Supine

– Sitting

– Left lateral decubitus

• Other postural maneuvers that may be useful:

– Squatting

– Standing

– While performing a Valsalva maneuver

• Auscultation includes an assessment of S1 and S2, including the nature of the splitting of S2.

• Consideration of any S3 and S4, murmurs, clicks, and rubs completes the auscultation.

Evaluation of heart murmur

■ Random fluctuations in velocity and pressure during blood flow results in vibration of the surrounding tissue, which is auscultated as a murmur.

■ A complete description of a heart murmur includes:

• Intensity

• Timing

• Location

• Radiation

• Quality

Intensity

■ Graded on a scale of I to VI for murmurs in systole

• Grade 1: Barely audible

• Grade II: Soft, but easily audible

• Grade III: Moderately loud without a thrill

• Grade IV: Moderately loud with a thrill

• Grade V: Loud with a thrill, heard with stethoscope barely on the chest

• Grade VI: Loud with a thrill, heard with stethoscope off the chest

■ Some cardiologists use a scale of I to IV for murmurs in diastole.

• Grade I: Barely audible

• Grade II: Soft, but immediately heard

• Grade III: Easily heard

• Grade IV: Very loud

■ The intensity of a murmur does not necessarily reflect the severity of abnormality.

■ A small VSD may have a very loud murmur.

■ Critical aortic stenosis may have a very soft murmur if cardiac output is low.

Timing

- The point in the cardiac cycle at which the murmur is heard
- Murmurs are described as being:
  - Systolic
  - Diastolic
  - Continuous
- Systolic murmurs occur during anatomic systole, the time beginning with atrioventricular valve closure (S1) and ending with semilunar valve closure (S2).
- Systolic murmurs are further divided into:
  - Ejection (crescendo-decrescendo) murmurs
    - Begin shortly after S1, peak in intensity
    - End at or before S2
    - May be innocent or abnormal
    - Most innocent murmurs are grade I to III systolic ejection murmurs.
    - Abnormal murmurs result from:
      - Obstructed blood flow across a semilunar valve (aortic or pulmonary stenosis)
      - Excessive volume crossing a normal semilunar valve (ASD)
    - Abnormal murmurs may be of any grade of intensity.
  - Holosystolic (pansystolic, S1 coincident) murmurs
    - Start with S1
    - Continue to S2 at the same level of intensity
    - Sometimes obscure S2 during auscultation
    - Result from movement of blood from a higher-pressure chamber to a lower-pressure chamber, such as with a VSD or mitral regurgitation
  - Late systolic murmurs
    - Associated with mitral valve prolapse and resultant mitral regurgitation
    - Classically preceded by a midsystolic click
- Diastolic murmurs occur during anatomic diastole.
  - The time beginning with semilunar valve closure (S2) and ending with atrioventricular valve closure (S1)
  - Diastolic murmurs are divided into early, mid, and late diastolic murmurs.
  - All are abnormal by definition.
  - Early diastolic murmurs begin immediately after S2 and are decrescendo in nature, becoming less audible as the ventricle fills.
  - Aortic insufficiency and pulmonary insufficiency are heard in early diastole.
  - Mid-diastolic murmurs occur clearly after S2 during the rapid filling phase of the ventricle.
  - Mitral stenosis and tricuspid stenosis murmurs are heard in mid-diastole.
  - Late diastolic (presystolic) murmurs occur near the end of diastole during the phase of atrial contraction.
  - Severe mitral stenosis or tricuspid stenosis murmurs increase in late diastole.
- Continuous murmurs
  - Begin in systole
  - Continue throughout systole
  - End some time during diastole
  - Vascular in origin
  - Caused by:
    - Aortopulmonary (eg, patent ductus arteriosus)
    - Arteriovenous (eg, arteriovenous fistula)
    - Connections
    - Turbulent flow in arteries (eg, coarctation of the aorta)
    - Turbulent flow in veins (eg, venous hum)
  - These murmurs are abnormal, except for the innocent venous hum (see table Common Innocent Murmurs).
  - Continuous murmurs sound fairly uniform until they soften in late diastole.
  - They result from such lesions as:
    - A patent ductus arteriosus
    - An arteriovenous malformation
    - A surgical shunt
  - A to-and-fro murmur describes an ejection murmur heard in systole, coupled to a decrescendo murmur early in diastole.
    - To-and-fro murmurs are not true continuous murmurs.
    - Combined aortic stenosis and aortic insufficiency or pulmonary stenosis and pulmonary insufficiency produce to-and-fro murmurs.

Location and radiation

- Refer to the area where the murmur is best heard and where it radiates
- Useful in differential diagnosis

Quality

- Refers to the pitch and nature of a murmur
- Pitch is generally described as either high or low.
  - High-pitched murmurs occur when the pressure differential involved is large.
    - Aortic insufficiency is a high-pitched murmur.
  - Low-pitched murmurs occur when a lower pressure differential is involved.
    - Pulmonary insufficiency causes a low-pitched murmur.
- Systolic murmurs are described as ejection, regurgitant, harsh, blowing, musical, or vibratory.
- Diastolic murmurs are described as blowing, rumbling, crescendo, or decrescendo.

Common Innocent Murmurs

Murmur	Intensity	Timing	Location	Quality
Still	I–III or VI	Early-mid systolic	LM-LLSB or apex	Vibratory, musical
Pulmonary	I–III or VI	Early-mid systolic	LUSB	Low-pitched, ejection flow
Venous hum	I–III or VI	Continuous	Right or left infra- or supraclavicular	Low-pitched, disappears with head turn, supine position, jugular compression

Abbreviations: LM-LLSB, left mid to left lower sternal border; LUSB, left upper sternal border.

DIFFERENTIAL DIAGNOSIS

- The challenge for the primary care physician lies in distinguishing innocent murmurs from those that indicate a cardiac abnormality.
- Location helps narrow the differential diagnosis of the murmur.
- Radiation of the murmur can also aid in forming the differential diagnosis.
  - Murmurs that radiate to the neck tend to be of aortic or left ventricular outflow tract origin.
  - A murmur heard best at the left upper sternal border with radiation to the axillae and back is more likely to be pulmonary in origin.
- Postural maneuvers are useful in distinguishing among different types of murmurs.
  - Innocent murmurs tend to become louder when the patient moves from an upright to a supine position.
  - Placing the patient in the left lateral decubitus position increases the murmur of mitral stenosis.
  - Valsalva maneuver, by decreasing venous return:
    - Makes the murmur of aortic stenosis softer
    - Makes the murmur of hypertrophic obstructive cardiomyopathy louder
    - Decreases the murmurs associated with a VSD and mitral regurgitation
    - Can nearly eliminate innocent still murmurs (see table Common Innocent Murmurs)
  - Squatting increases venous return and makes the murmur of hypertrophic obstructive cardiomyopathy softer.
  - Standing up after squatting can accentuate the murmur or click of mitral valve prolapse by moving the murmur and click closer to the S1.
  - Turning the head can eliminate the innocent continuous murmur of a venous hum.

LABORATORY EVALUATION

- Patients with cyanotic heart diseases are polycythemic, with very high hemoglobin level and hematocrit.

IMAGING

- Chest radiograph may be done to determine the size of heart, the status of pulmonary vasculature, and evidence of congestive cardiac failure.

DIAGNOSTIC PROCEDURES

- Electrocardiography and echocardiography are usually done to define the lesion of organic heart disease that is causing the murmur.

TREATMENT APPROACH

- It is important to differentiate innocent murmur from abnormal murmur.
  - Once innocent murmur is established, reassurance is the mainstay of management.

SPECIFIC TREATMENT

- The specific management of cardiac murmur depends on the underlying cardiac lesion.

WHEN TO REFER

- Patient, maternal, or family history that raises the index of suspicion for heart disease
- All diastolic murmurs require referral to a pediatric cardiologist.
- Continuous murmurs, except venous hum
- All systolic murmurs grade IV or higher
- All systolic murmurs not clearly fitting the pattern of innocent murmur
- A thrill is an abnormal finding and warrants referral to a pediatric cardiologist.
- Cyanosis, clubbing
- Higher blood pressure in 1 or both arms than in a leg
- Congestive heart failure—rales, respiratory distress, hepatomegaly, edema
- Abnormal electrocardiogram
- Symptoms that suggest reactive airway disease that do not improve with appropriate medical therapy

H

Hematuria

DEFINITION

- Urine that contains blood or erythrocytes
- Microscopic
  - >5 erythrocytes per high-power field seen on microscopy of centrifuged urine
- Macroscopic (or gross)
  - Red or brown (cola-colored) urine with erythrocytes seen on microscopy

EPIDEMIOLOGY

- Prevalence
  - The rate of macroscopic hematuria in children presenting to a pediatric emergency department was 1.3 per 1000 visits in 1 study.
  - Studies of routine screenings for microscopic hematuria suggest rates of up to 32 per 1000 girls and 14 per 1000 boys.
- Thin basement membrane nephropathy (one of the common causes of microscopic hematuria)
  - Prevalence
    - Estimated at 1–10% of the population
  - Sex
    - More common in females than in males
  - Age
    - Has been diagnosed in children as young as 1 year

MECHANISM

- Infection of the upper or lower urinary tract is the most common cause of hematuria overall.
- Macroscopic hematuria may originate from any component of the genitourinary tract; possible causes include:
  - Infection
  - Glomerular, interstitial, and tubular diseases
  - Bleeding from trauma, stones, or coagulopathy
- Microscopic hematuria may be caused by:
  - Infection
  - Nephrolithiasis (hypercalciuria)
  - Glomerulonephritis
- The most common causes of asymptomatic isolated microscopic hematuria are:
  - Thin basement membrane nephropathy (TBMN)
  - Idiopathic hypercalciuria
  - Immunoglobulin A (IgA) nephropathy
  - Sickle cell diseaseor trait
- The most common glomerulonephritis is postinfectious.
  - Prodromal infection 1–6 weeks before the onset of hematuria
  - Often a streptococcal skin or throat infection

- Viral infections, such as:
  - Varicella
  - Cytomegalovirus
  - Epstein-Barr virus
  - Hepatitis B virus and hepatitis C virus
- Parasitic infections, such as toxoplasmosis
- Other causes of acute postinfectious glomerulonephritis include:
  - Ventriculoperitoneal shunt infections (shunt nephritis)
  - Acute or subacute endocarditis
- Henoch-Schönlein purpura
  - Can produce glomerulonephritis with hematuria

HISTORY

- Hematuria may manifest as:
  - Dramatic change in the color of a child's urine
  - Blood on a diaper or underwear
  - Finding on urinalysis
    - Routine screening urinalysis is recommended by the AAP at 5 years of age and again at 11–21 years of age.
- Hematuria of glomerular origin:
  - Presents with tea- or cola-colored urine
  - Is marked by the presence of erythrocyte casts
  - Is typically painless

Macroscopic hematuria

- Obtain a detailed description of the urine (see Figure 31 on page F12).
  - Renal or glomerular causes of hematuria result in tea- or cola-colored urine.
  - Hematuria of lower tract origin causes red or pink urine.
  - Highly turbid urine may indicate the presence of cells.
    - Suggests glomerular disease or infection
- Blood clots suggest urinary tract bleeding.
  - Timing of the bleeding may be helpful.
  - If bleeding occurs only with the onset of micturition, the source of the bleeding is likely to be in the lower tract.
- Laboratory and radiologic evaluation is dictated by associated signs and symptoms from a detailed history and physical examination.
  - Important historical elements include associated urinary symptoms, such as:
    - Dysuria
    - Frequency
    - Urgency
    - Enuresis
  - A decrease in urine output should prompt particular concern and rapid evaluation and treatment.

- A review of systems should include associated symptoms.
  - Abdominal pain or colic
  - Upper respiratory infection symptoms
  - Swelling of extremities
  - Blurry vision or headaches suggestive of hypertension
- Ask patient or parents about:
  - Prior episodes of hematuria
  - Preceding infections
    - Documented group A streptococcal throat infection
    - History of sore throat or skin infection
  - History of trauma
  - Other illnesses, such as the presence of sickle cell trait or sickle cell disease
- Systemic illnesses may be suggested by history of:
  - Fever
  - Malaise
  - Weight loss
  - Alopecia
  - Rash
  - Joint pains, such as may be seen in rheumatologic disease
- Important points of family history include:
  - Other family members with hematuria or kidney or rheumatologic disease
  - Any history of deafness, which may occur with Alport syndrome

Microscopic hematuria

- Figure 32 on page F12 shows a proposed algorithm for the evaluation of microscopic hematuria.
- Recent history of throat or skin infections
- Family history of hematuria, deafness, or kidney disease

PHYSICAL EXAM

- Growth parameters
- Measurement of blood pressure
- Evaluation of abdominal or costovertebral angle tenderness
- Search for evidence of local trauma to the genitourinary tract.
- Inspection and palpation for periorbital, genital, or extremity edema

DIFFERENTIAL DIAGNOSIS

- Macroscopic hematuria:
  - Is a common sign of glomerular and urologic disease
  - Rarely is a cause of anemia
- Blood on a diaper or underwear
  - Most commonly occurs with trauma to or manipulation of the genital area

- In boys, localized irritation of the meatus is the most frequent cause.
- Responds to treatment with petroleum jelly and reassurance to the parent without further evaluation
  - Other causes include:
    - Sexual abuse
    - Urinary tract infection with *Serratia marcescens*
- Hematuria in association with edema and hypertension suggests glomerulonephritis.
- Hematuria arising from the urinary tract is usually red-pink, with or without clots.
- TBMN
  - Also known as *thin basement membrane disease, hereditary hematuria, benign familial hematuria,* or *benign hereditary nephritis*
  - One of the most common causes of persistent microhematuria
  - 5–22% of affected individuals will have an episode of macroscopic hematuria associated with an infection or exercise.
  - Persistent microhematuria distinguishes TBMN from other acute renal causes of hematuria, such as postinfectious glomerulonephritis.
  - Characterized by:
    - Painless microscopic hematuria with minimal proteinuria
    - Normal renal function
  - Renal biopsy reveals uniform thinning of the glomerular basement membrane.
  - Transmitted in an autosomal dominant fashion.
  - Diagnosis is suggested by:
    - Family history of microscopic hematuria without symptomatic renal disease
    - Asymptomatic parent testing positive for hematuria TBMN
  - No evidence has been found to support treatment of TBMN, which is typically nonprogressive.
  - Affected children should be monitored for hypertension, proteinuria, and renal insufficiency.
    - May point to the diagnosis of:
      - IgA nephropathy
      - Alport syndrome
      - Nephrolithiasis
      - Glomerulonephritis
      - Each has been reported in association with TBMN.
- Hypercalciuria
  - A common cause of microscopic hematuria
  - Defined as:
    - Urine calcium-to-creatinine ratio >0.21

— >4 mg/kg per day of excreted calcium on a 24-hour urine collection

- Children with hematuria and underlying hypercalciuria are at risk for nephrolithiasis.
  - The risk appears to be greater:
    - In older children
    - In children with macroscopic rather than microscopic hematuria
    - When there is a family history of stone formation
- Henoch-Schönlein purpura
  - Common systemic vasculitis in children
  - Usually associated with:
    - Crampy abdominal pain
    - Arthralgia
    - Palpable purpura
  - Can produce glomerulonephritis with hematuria

LABORATORY EVALUATION

- Most children with isolated microscopic hematuria do not have a serious or treatable cause for the hematuria and do not require an extensive workup.
- Begin with urinalysis with microscopic examination of fresh-spun urine sample to confirm the presence of erythrocytes.
  - Dysmorphic erythrocytes and erythrocyte casts are pathognomonic of hematuria of glomerular origin.
- Urine dipstick positive for blood and <5 erythrocytes found on microscopy
  - The diagnosis is hemoglobinuria or myoglobinuria rather than hematuria.
- Several drugs and foods can discolor urine to give it the appearance of hematuria (urinalysis will be negative for blood).
  - Rifampin
  - Ibuprofen
  - Nitrofurantoin
  - Beets
  - Blackberries
- Nephrolithiasis may be suggested by the presence in urine of:
  - Calcium
  - Uric acid
  - Cystine crystals
- Infectious causes of hematuria are indicated by:
  - Leukocyte casts
  - Leukocyte esterase
  - Nitrate positivity on urine dipstick
- Further evaluation is determined by the most likely cause of the blood in the urine.

- If microscopy is not immediately available, a reasonable panel of tests would include:
  - Serum electrolytes
  - Blood urea nitrogen
  - Creatinine
  - Calcium and phosphorus
  - Liver function tests
  - Antinuclear antibody test
  - Complement studies (C3, C4, and total complement)
  - Complete blood count with differential
  - Streptozyme (deoxyribonuclease B) and streptolysin O antibody titers
- Patients with a history of sore throat should undergo:
  - Throat culture
  - Rapid testing for group A ß-hemolytic streptococci
- Urine culture should be performed on:
  - All patients with urinary symptoms
  - Infants with unexplained fever or sepsis
- Proteinuria on urinalysis should be further evaluated with a morning void for protein-to-creatinine ratio.
- Asymptomatic, normotensive child with isolated microhematuria
  - Repeating urinalysis ≥1 times before further evaluation often is prudent.
- Persistent microhematuria may represent an early presentation of a progressive glomerular disease, such as:
  - IgA nephropathy
  - Alport syndrome
- Periodic urinalysis should be done to monitor for the development of significant proteinuria.

IMAGING

- Every child with macroscopic hematuria should have renal ultrasonography to rule out:
  - Nephrolithiasis
  - Tumor
  - Urologic abnormalities
    - Cystic disease
    - Obstructive uropathy
    - Parenchymal renal disease

DIAGNOSTIC PROCEDURES

- Renal biopsy may be performed for:
  - Family history of hematuria
  - History or laboratory evaluation suggestive of rheumatologic disease, such as systemic lupus erythematosus

H

- Renal biopsy is absolutely indicated in cases of hematuria with:
  - Nephrotic syndrome
  - Recurrent hematuria
  - Azotemia
  - Renal insufficiency

TREATMENT APPROACH

- Management of glomerular disease depends on the cause of the glomerulonephritis.
- Poststreptococcal glomerulonephritis
  - Low C3 levels and elevated streptolysin O antibody titers are characteristic.
  - Typically self-limited
  - Good prognosis for long-term renal function
- Microhematuria without any other signs and symptoms:
  - Often is benign
  - Resolves spontaneously in many cases (transient hematuria)
- School-aged children with microscopic hematuria may be observed for ≥2 years before more extensive testing is undertaken.
- Patients with glomerulonephritis need to be monitored for hypertension and, if present, need to be treated with antihypertensive medications.

SPECIFIC TREATMENT

- Treat urinary tract infections with an appropriate antimicrobial regimen
- Skin or throat streptococcal infections should be treated with penicillin.

WHEN TO REFER

- Hematuria associated with pain
- Persistent microscopic hematuria with:
  - Associated proteinuria
  - Hypertension
  - Hearing loss
  - Family history of renal disease or deafness
- Glomerulonephritis
  - Some types require management by a nephrologist.
- Urologic evaluation, which may include direct visualization by cystoscopy, may be required for:
  - Trauma
  - Tumors
  - Cystic disease
  - Congenital obstruction
  - Hemorrhagic cystitis
  - Lower urinary tract bleeding
  - Nephrolithiasis
- Children with nephrolithiasis benefit from both nephrologic and urologic evaluation.
- A family history of deafness or kidney disease and the presence of hypertension, proteinuria, or edema
- Significant proteinuria
- Occurrence of macroscopic hematuria

WHEN TO ADMIT

- Admission for intravenous hydration may be required for:
  - Patients withsickle cell disease or sickle cell trait and macroscopic hematuria from papillary necrosis
- Severe abdominal pain or flank pain
- Congestive heart failure or fluid overload indicative of oliguria or anuria
- Hypertension
- Renal insufficiency
- Anasarca (generalized edema)
- Oliguria
- Decreased urine output
- Azotemia
- Acute hypertension
  - Requires aggressive management with:
    - Fluid and salt restriction
    - Antihypertensive medications
- Further evaluation of glomerular hematuria may be continued as an outpatient or inpatient.

FOLLOW-UP

- Monitor growth (height).
- Monitor patients for hypertension.
- Hematuria should be monitored by periodic urine analysis.
- Kidney function (serum blood urea nitrogen, creatinine) may need to be monitored as appropriate.

COMPLICATIONS

- Some renal disorders associated with hematuria may lead to:
  - Hypertension
  - Progressive kidney disease leading to renal failure

PROGNOSIS

- Proteinuria is a more important prognostic finding than macroscopic hematuria.
- Proteinuria and hypertension are poor prognostic indicators.

Hemoglobinopathies and Sickle Cell Disease

DEFINITION

- The normal hemoglobins (Hb) are Hb A (96% of the total content), Hb F (1%), and Hb A_2 (3%).
- Hemoglobin synthesis is directed by controlling genes that are switched on and off at certain stages of human life, resulting in different globin-chain synthesis at different times.
- Inherited Hb disorders due to single-gene defects
  - Thalassemias: structurally normal but decreased amounts of globin chains
    - α-Thalassemias
    - ß-Thalassemias
  - Structural Hb abnormalities: abnormal globin chains
    - Sickling disorders
    - Sickle cell trait
      - Benign carrier state
    - Rare structural hemoglobinopathies

EPIDEMIOLOGY

- Inherited Hb disorders comprise most common single-gene defects in humans.
- In the US and other developed countries, hemoglobinopathies remain a concern, particularly among certain ethnic groups.
- Incidence
  - Approximately 400,000 births per year of infants with serious hemoglobinopathies
- Prevalence
  - Worldwide frequency of carrier state estimated at 270 million
    - Prevalence is increasing worldwide.
  - Sickle cell trait
    - Varies from 6.7–10.1% in blacks
  - ß-Thalassemia prevalence
    - Mediterranean region
    - Africa
    - Middle East
    - Indian subcontinent
    - Burma
    - Southeast Asia (including the Malay Peninsula)
    - Southern China
    - Indonesia
- α-Thalassemia retardation (ATR)
  - Occurs in racial groups in which α-thalassemia is otherwise rare
- Hb Bart disease accounts for 90% of all hydrops fetalis in Southeast Asia.
- Hb E is common in Southeast Asia and in certain areas of the Indian subcontinent.

ETIOLOGY

- Thalassemias are caused by mutations in the globin gene cluster, resulting in a genetic decrease in globin chain synthesis.
  - In theory, as many types of thalassemias exist as types of globin chains.
  - Practically, the most clinically relevant thalassemias are α- and ß-thalassemia.
  - α-Thalassemia
    - Characterized by decreased α-chain synthesis
    - The most common defect is deletional, although nondeletional defects have been described.
    - The a gene is duplicated, and 2 α-globin genes per haploid genome are present.
    - See Classification for types of α-thalassemias.
  - ATR
    - The pattern of inheritance is different from that seen in α-thalassemia.
    - Occurs in association with a deletion on chromosome 16 (ATR-16) and in association with the ATR-X syndrome, which results from mutations of the *XH2* gene, located on the long arm of the X chromosome (Xq13.3)
  - ß-Thalassemia
    - Caused by a decrease in production of ß-globin chains as a result of mutations in the ß-globin gene
    - Mutations cause variable impairments of globin synthesis.
    - More severe forms result from homozygosity or compound heterozygosity for the mutant ß-globin allele.
      - Result in thalassemia major or thalassemia intermedia
- Structural hemoglobinopathies
  - Usually result from a point mutation in the α- or ß-globin gene that causes a functional abnormality, effects of which depend on where the missense mutation occurs
  - Sickling disorders
    - Sickling disorders depend on gene interactions.
    - SS (known as sickle cell anemia)
      - Homozygosity for the mutant Hb S
      - Results in no normal ß alleles and no Hb A
    - SC
      - Double heterozygosity for 2 ß-chain mutants (Hb S and Hb C)
      - Results in no normal ß alleles and no Hb A
    - Sickle ß-thalassemia
      - Double heterozygosity for Hb S and ß-thalassemia

- One ß gene directs the synthesis of Hb S, and the other is either:
  - Completely suppressed, and patient has no Hb A (S ß$^+$-thalassemia) *or*
  - Incompletely suppressed, and patient produces a small amount of Hb A (S ß$^+$-thalassemia)
  - Hb A$_2$ is increased.
- SO Arab and SD
  - Double heterozygosity for Hb S and Hb O or D, respectively
- Rare structural hemoglobinopathies (prototypes)
  - Hb Zurich
    - Unstable hemoglobin: usually results from amino acid substitutions near the heme pocket
  - Hb Bethesda
    - Hemoglobin with high oxygen affinity: amino acid substitution near the α$_1$-ß$_2$ interface
  - Hb Kansas
    - Hemoglobin with low oxygen affinity: amino acid substitution near the α$_1$-ß$_2$ interface
  - Hb M
    - Amino acid substitution near the heme pocket, close to the site of the iron molecule
  - Hb C, D, and E
    - Structural variant hemoglobins synthesized at a lower rate than normal ß chains
    - Heterozygous Hb C (AC) results in mild target cells but no anemia.
    - Homozygous C (CC) produces mild hemolytic anemia, marked red blood cell (RBC) morphologic changes (target cells, hemoglobin crystals, and microsphero-cytes), and mild splenomegaly.
    - Heterozygous E (AE) causes mild thalassemic pheno-type with mild microcytosis and hypochromia.
    - Homozygous E (EE) results in moderate thalassemic phenotype, with hypochromia, microcytosis, and mild anemia.
    - Combined E- and ß-thalassemia inheritance results in a transfusion-dependent thalassemic phenotype.

SIGNS AND SYMPTOMS

- α-Thalassemia
  - Silent carrier
    - No anemia
  - α-Thalassemia-1
    - Mild anemia
  - Hb H disease
    - Moderate anemia
  - Hb Bart disease
    - Severe anemia
  - ATR-X syndrome: α-thalassemia seen in nontropical populations
    - Severe intellectual disability
    - Minor facial anomalies
    - Genital anomalies
    - Mild form of Hb H disease
- ß-Thalassemia
  - Clinical presentation is variable.
  - Thalassemia major
    - Symptoms at approximately 6 months with anemia that can be severe and symptomatic
    - Growth failure
    - Cardiac dysfunction
    - Pallor
    - Jaundice
    - Hepatosplenomegaly
    - The patient's body becomes loaded with iron, even when transfusions are sparingly provided.
      - Liver effects (leading to cirrhosis)
      - Pituitary effects (leading to hypogonadism and growth failure)
      - Heart effects (leading to arrhythmia and cardiomyopathy)
      - Bone effects (leading to pathologic fractures)
  - Thalassemia intermedia
    - Patients exhibit symptoms later in life.
    - Anemia is well compensated.
      - May be exacerbated by infection, folate deficiency, or increasing hypersplenism
- Sickling disorders
  - Pallor
  - Jaundice
  - Increased fatigue
  - Gallstones
  - Poor growth
  - Aplastic crises occur:
    - After viral infections
    - In situations in which transient marrow suppression results in a life-threatening decrease in hemoglobin
  - Episodic, variable, and unpredictable musculoskeletal pain
    - Disabling if frequent and severe
    - Usually uncomplicated and not life threatening
  - Acute bone pain or infarction
    - Common at all ages

- Dactylitis (foot and hand swelling) is classic early childhood symptom.
- Splenic sequestration crisis may occur.
  - Sudden pooling of blood in the spleen with hypovolemic shock
  - Life-threatening and recurrent syndrome of early childhood
- Strokes, although uncommon, are a recurrent and serious problem.
- Variety of cerebrovascular catastrophes, such as hemorrhage and thrombosis, can occur.
- Acute chest syndrome is common.
  - Pulmonary infarction or pneumonia (or both)
- Large volumes of dilute urine even in young children
  - Need copious fluid intake to avoid dehydration
- Hematuria
- Priapism
- Trophic leg ulcers
- Blindness
- Sickle cell trait
  - Most people have no clinical symptoms.
  - Can cause hematuria and a loss of urine-concentration capacity
  - Symptoms from intravascular sickling have been reported with:
    - Strenuous exercise at high altitudes
    - Flying at high altitudes in unpressurized aircraft
- High oxygen–affinity hemoglobins
  - High arterial oxygen saturation
    - Markedly left-shifted oxygen-dissociation curve
  - Presence of familial erythrocytosis (polycythemia)
- Hb M
  - History of cyanosis since birth, with a normal oxygen saturation
- Low oxygen–affinity hemoglobins
  - Right-shifted oxygen-dissociation curve

DIAGNOSTIC APPROACH

- Prenatal diagnosis
  - Specific tests, such as:
    - Globin chain synthesis ratios
    - DNA analysis by sampling of fetal blood or chorionic villus
    - Restriction fragment polymorphism
- α-Thalassemias
  - Confirmation of decreased a chains by globin-chain synthesis measured in reticulocytes
    - Expensive and hard to do

- Sickling disorders
  - Clinical history and physical findings are the first steps to diagnosis.

LABORATORY FINDINGS

Thalassemias

- α-Thalassemias
  - Routine complete blood count shows hypochromia (mean cell Hb <27 pg).
  - Microcytosis (mean cell volume <80 fL)
  - Mild anemia with normal Hb A_2
  - Abnormal Hb tetramers are demonstrated by:
    - Presence of RBC inclusions on cresyl blue stain
    - Hemoglobin electrophoresis
    - Rapid movement (faster than Hb A)
      - Require special attention during electrophoresis testing
  - Hb Bart (γ-tetramers) are found in the first few weeks of life, and Hb H can be found in older patients.
  - Silent carrier: normal RBC count
  - Hb H disease: fragmented cells with hypochromia and microcytosis
- ß-Thalassemia: thalassemia major
  - RBCs may be destroyed within the marrow, leading to ineffective erythropoiesis.
    - Hallmark of ß-thalassemia
  - Decreased hemoglobin content per cell
  - Hypochromia
  - Microcytosis

Structural hemoglobinopathies

- Sickling disorders
  - Morphologic sickling can be assessed by blood smears.
  - Presence of Hb S is evaluated by the solubility test.
    - Inexpensive and sensitive to the carrier state
  - Hemoglobin electrophoresis confirms the exact phenotype.
- Unstable hemoglobins
  - Hemolytic anemia
  - Detection of Heinz bodies by staining and heat precipitation test
  - Hemoglobin electrophoresis is not always useful because of the tendency of hemoglobin to rapidly denature.
- High oxygen–affinity hemoglobins
  - High RBC mass
- Low oxygen–affinity hemoglobins
  - Hemoglobin level and RBC mass are normal.
- Hb M
  - Brown discoloration of freshly drawn blood
    - Does not change with aeration

H

- Spectrophotometry confirms presence of methemoglobin.
- Electrophoresis demonstrates abnormal hemoglobin.

DIAGNOSTIC PROCEDURES

- Hemoglobin electrophoresis may be diagnostic in many hemoglobinopathies and thalassemias.

CLASSIFICATION

- Classification of a thalassemias, by phenotype (number of a genes; genotype)
  - Normal (4; αα/αα)
  - Silent carrier (3; –α/αα)
  - 2-gene deletion (α-thalassemia-1) (2; ––/αα or –α/–α)
  - Hb H disease (1; ––/–α)
  - Hb Bart disease (hydrops fetalis) (0; ––/––)

TREATMENT APPROACH

- Blood transfusion
  - Continues to be the mainstay of care of patients with hemoglobinopathies
  - Transfusion safety is an important consideration, particularly prevention of transfusion-transmitted infections.
    - Donors should be screened forhepatitis B and C, HIV, syphilis, and malaria.
    - Donor screening may sometimes be ineffective.
      - Insensitive tests
      - Expired kits and reagents
      - Improper procedures
- Iron chelation
  - Deferrioxamine
    - Daily 8-hour subcutaneous infusion via small portable pumps
    - Well tolerated and extremely effective
  - Oral deferasirox
    - Similar efficacy as deferrioxamine in preclinical trials, and much less cumbersome for patients
    - Starting dose is 20 mg/kg once daily as a dispersion in water or orange or apple juice.
    - Highest recommended dose is 30 mg/kg per day.
  - Toxicities
    - Increase over baseline of creatinine and proteinuria
    - Pediatric patients with sickle cell disease have low creatinine concentration.
      - Increases of 30% over baseline should prompt dose decreases for such patients.
    - Chemical hepatitis or aminotransferase elevation over baseline
      - Usually respond to dose decreases to 10 mg/kg per day

- Treatment effectiveness is measured by monitoring serum ferritin level.
  - Although not the most accurate measure of total body iron stores
  - Levels <2500 mg/dL are associated with improved cardiac disease–free survival.
  - Chelation should be interrupted for serum ferritin levels ≤500 ng/mL because of increased drug toxicity at low ferritin levels.
  - Magnetic susceptometry provides a noninvasive method for measuring hepatic iron stores.
    - This test is available in only a few centers worldwide.
- Stem cell transplantation
  - Improved techniques that use human leukocyte antigen (HLA)–matched sibling donors may result in cures for the hemoglobinopathies.
  - Interest exists in nonmyeloablative or reduced-intensity myeloablative stem cell transplantation.
    - Has reduced morbidity but leads to a chimerism in the recipient
    - This procedure is still investigational.
- Advances in genomics and other technologies
  - Have promise to improve treatment of patients with hemoglobinopathies

SPECIFIC TREATMENTS

ß-Thalassemia

- Blood transfusions are provided to:
  - Correct anemia
  - Suppress erythropoiesis
  - Prevent growth failure
  - Inhibit increased gastrointestinal absorption of iron
- Splenectomy
  - Usually performed if transfusion requirements increase because of hypersplenism
- Folic acid supplementation
  - May be considered to meet its increased requirement
- Iron chelation
- Hematopoietic stem cell transplantation
  - May be performed when chronic transfusions and chelation are not possible
    - If successful, reverses need for transfusions or chelation therapy
    - Carries risk of serious adverse effects
      - Graft failure
      - Rejection
      - Graft-versus-host disease
      - Death

- Does not reverse preexisting and established growth failure, endocrinopathies, and gonadal dysfunction
- Must also consider availability of supportive care after transplantation
- Using either related or unrelated HLA-matched donors results in excellent outcomes in low-risk patients without extensive organ damage.

Structural hemoglobinopathies

Sickling disorders

- Give symptomatic and supportive care of complications.
  - Treat pain episodes with analgesics (often narcotics) and local heat packs.
  - Ensure adequate hydration.
  - Adjust acid-base balance.
  - Prevent hypoxia.
  - Avoid exposure to cold.
  - Treat febrile episodes early and aggressively with antibiotics.
- Judicious use of blood transfusions will help:
  - Prevent strokes
  - Correct severe anemia (Hb level <5 g/dL, usually with aplastic crisis or splenic sequestration)
- Management is optimized by early diagnosis with screening of newborns.
- Routine daily prophylactic penicillin and pneumococcal vaccine
  - To prevent high childhood mortality from infections
- Agents that stimulate fetal hemoglobin production (eg, hydroxyurea) may be administered.
- Peripheral or cord blood stem cell transplantation from an HLA-identical sibling
  - High-risk procedure
  - Can be curative
  - Used for certain individuals with markers for adverse outcome (eg, stroke in a young child)
- Future directions
  - Antisickling agents, such as membrane-active drugs
  - Gene therapy

Rare structural hemoglobinopathies

- Unstable hemoglobin
  - Avoid oxidant drugs.
  - Provide transfusions as clinically indicated.
  - Remove the spleen if anemia is severe.
- High oxygen–affinity hemoglobins
  - Maintain hematocrit at 70% by phlebotomy to prevent high viscosity.

- Low oxygen–affinity hemoglobins
  - No specific management is necessary or effective.
  - Cyanosis is relatively well tolerated if strenuous activities are avoided.
- Hb M
  - No management is needed; the amount of Hb M is insufficient to cause physiologic derangements.

WHEN TO ADMIT

- Anemic crisis (Hb level <5 g/dL)
- Sudden splenic enlargement
- Pain not responding to home care and narcotics
- Difficulty in breathing, chest pain
- High fever spikes (>38°C core)
- Any central nervous system symptoms

WHEN TO REFER

- Initial and routine annual or biannual evaluation
- Serious complications, such as stroke, splenic sequestration, recurrent acute chest syndrome
- Care during pregnancy

FOLLOW-UP

- Patients with thalassemia major require regular transfusions for survival.
- Monitoring for chelation regimens
  - Annual audiologic and ophthalmologic examinations
  - Annual echocardiographic examinations

COMPLICATIONS

- Beginning in early childhood, risk of severe bacterial infections is lifelong.
  - Common cause of death
- Transfusion-transmitted infections remain a risk.
- Hb Bart disease
  - Invariably results in death in utero or shortly after birth due to severe anemia
  - Associated with life-threatening complications to the mother
    - Placentomegaly
    - Hypertension and preeclampsia
    - Disseminated intravascular coagulation
    - Hemorrhage

H

- Hb H disease
  - A serious decrease in hemoglobin can occur with infections or with ingestion of substances that induce oxidant stress.
  - Hydrops fetalis syndrome
    - Devastating complication associated with nondeletional forms of Hb H disease
    - Associated with similar fetal and maternal complications as Hb Bart hydrops fetalis, including death in utero

PROGNOSIS

- Sickling disorders
  - Disease is extremely variable in severity.
  - Factors that affect disease severity include:
    - Presence of genetic markers, such as the ß-gene haplotype
    - Coinheritance of α-thalassemia (beneficial)
    - Amount/distribution of Hb F (higher levels are beneficial)
- Hb Bart disease
  - Invariably results in death in utero or shortly after birth due to severe anemia

PREVENTION

- Simple awareness of genetic diseases and education and counseling of families at risk
  - Low-tech but crucial in avoiding burden of these diseases to individuals and society
- The primary reason to screen patients for hemoglobinopathy is to identify risk of producing offspring with clinically important disease, such as:
  - ß-Thalassemia major
  - Sickle cell disease
  - Severe α-thalassemia (hydrops fetalis)
- Screening of parents
  - Complete blood count while paying attention to RBC indices
    - Thalassemias are usually associated with:
      - Low mean cell volume (microcytosis)
      - Normal or near-normal mean cell hemoglobin concentration
      - Hemoglobin concentration may be decreased or normal with a high RBC count.
    - Once iron deficiency is ruled out and hemoglobinopathy is suspected
      - Perform hemoglobin electrophoresis evaluation for levels of Hb A2 and F and presence of an abnormal hemoglobin, such as Hb C, Hb S, or Hb E.
- Premarital screening and genetic counseling
  - Easy and inexpensive
  - Good ways to provide reproductive options for couples at risk for children with hemoglobinopathies
  - Nondirective genetic counseling should be provided and targeted to populations with a high prevalence of the hemoglobinopathy traits.
- Prenatal diagnosis
  - Specific tests, such as globin-chain synthesis ratios or DNA analysis by sampling fetal blood or chorionic villus
  - Chorionic villus sampling
    - Challenges include technical difficulties of the various methods used, as well as expense.
    - Women with at-risk pregnancies must be assessed for prenatal diagnosis, ideally in the first trimester (8–14 weeks' gestation).
    - Choice of therapeutic abortion for involved pregnancies can be difficult, depending on cultural and religious beliefs.
    - Research studies report a higher acceptance of prenatal diagnosis if another child is affected.
  - Preconception diagnosis and implantation of normal embryos after in vitro fertilization
    - Extremely expensive alternative
    - Currently available in the West
  - In utero therapy that uses stem cell transplantation
    - Would help at-risk couples that do not opt for termination
    - Currently in early trials

Hemolytic-Uremic Syndrome

DEFINITION

- Hemolytic-uremic syndrome (HUS) is a systemic thrombotic microangiopathy with multiple causes.
- It is characterized by the classic triad of microangiopathic hemolytic anemia, thrombocytopenia, and acute kidney failure.
- The end result is endothelial lesions leading to thrombosis of the microcirculation in many organ systems (see table Hemolytic-Uremic Syndrome Clinical Entities).
- HUS is divided into 2 types, depending on whether the patient has had diarrhea.
  - Presence of diarrhea is designated *D+ HUS*.
    - Most common type
    - Caused by toxins from a group of Enterobacteriae, enterohemorrhagic *Escherichia coli* (EHEC)
  - Absence of diarrhea is designated *D– HUS*.
    - Only 10% of cases are classified as D– HUS.

EPIDEMIOLOGY

- Geographic distribution
  - Shigatoxin (ST)-associated HUS is prevalent in areas of the world with high incidence of gastrointestinal infections by ST-producing EHEC (STEC).
  - In Argentina, ST-associated HUS is approximately 10 times more frequent than in other locations with high incidence, such as Canada, some Western European countries, and California and Utah.
  - In countries with a high incidence of ST-associated HUS, the prevalence of atypical forms is <10%.
- Incidence
  - The incidence of atypical genetic HUS is low.

ETIOLOGY

- Clinically, HUS caused by genetic mutations tends to be more severe than HUS caused by STEC.
  - Tends to recur and have persistent activity
  - The long-term course is more severe, leading more frequently to chronic renal disease.
- Multiple genetic mutations have been found in patients with atypical HUS.
  - Mutations in the complement system activation can cause atypical HUS.
- Another pathogenetic mechanism for atypical HUS depends on lack of the activity of ADAMTS-13 (a disintegrin and metalloproteinase with thrombospondin-1–like domains).

RISK FACTORS

- Antimotility agents, although useful for symptomatic relief of diarrhea, have been shown to increase the risk of toxic mega-colon in patients with HUS and are contraindicated.
- Use of some antibiotics to treat *E coli* bowel infection has been found to increase the risk of HUS by promoting release of ST from the bacteria.
- Patients with factor H and factor I mutations have posttransplantation recurrence rates for HUS of 30–100%.
- ADAMTS-13 deficiency HUS can recur after transplantation.

Hemolytic-Uremic Syndrome Clinical Entities

Classification	Cause	Clinical Manifestation
Infectious	Bacterial cytotoxin (*Escherichia coli*, *Shigella*, *Salmonella*) pneumococcal, viral	Epidemic/classical/D+ enteropathic
Idiopathic	• Endothelial dysfunction? • Other regulatory C proteins?	• Hereditary (autosomal dominant, autosomal recessive) • Sporadic, atypical
Genetic	• Factor H, factor I deficiency • MCP (CD46) • vWF protease ADAMTS 13	• Recurrent • Recurrent except posttransplant • Recurrent
Immunologic	• vWF protease antibodies • Factor H autoantibodies	TTP
Other	Cancer, pregnancy, malignant hypertension, transplant rejection glomerulonephritis	
Toxic related	Cyclosporine, tacrolimus, sirolimus, mitomycin, radiation	

Abbreviations: ADAMTS, a disintegrin and metalloproteinase with thrombospondin; MCP, membrane cofactor protein; TTP, thrombotic thrombocytopenic purpura; vWF, von Willebrand factor.

SIGNS AND SYMPTOMS

- In the classical form, most patients have:
  - Diarrhea (bloody in two-thirds of cases)
  - Vomiting
  - Fever
- Several days later
  - Sudden onset of pallor
  - Severe malaise
  - Decrease in urine output
  - Edema
- During the acute phase, approximately one-third of patients may have symptoms of central nervous system involvement, including:
  - Change in sensorium (excitement or somnolence)
  - Convulsions
  - Possibly severe coma
- Intestinal (generally colonic) necrosis can be severe enough to require surgical intervention.
- Hypertension in approximately one-half of children with HUS
  - May have either short-term or persistent patterns
  - Short-term hypertension is caused by volume expansion and improves with salt restriction or dialysis.
  - Persistent hypertension is generally associated with renal ischemia in the presence of severe lesions.
- Hyperglycemia caused by pancreatic insufficiency, cardiac involvement, and hepatic failure are rare.

DIFFERENTIAL DIAGNOSIS

- Differential diagnosis of HUS is wide and includes:
  - Thrombotic thrombocytopenic purpura
  - Malignant hypertension
  - Vasculitis
  - Disseminated intravascular coagulation
  - Sepsis
  - Reye syndrome
  - Intussusception
  - Renal vein thrombosis
- The best differential sign of HUS is microangiopathic anemia with schistocytes in the peripheral smear.

DIAGNOSTIC APPROACH

- Both the clinical outcome and short-term and long-term treatment of HUS vary greatly depending on the cause; thus, finding the causes and acting accordingly is important.

LABORATORY FINDINGS

- Laboratory studies reveal:
  - Low hemoglobin
  - Fragmented erythrocytes (schistocytes)
  - Thrombocytopenia, indicating acute microangiopathic anemia
- Urine sample (if one can be obtained) shows signs of:
  - Glomerular involvement (hematuria with erythrocyte casts)
  - Proteinuria
- Decrease in the glomerular filtration rate is indicated by elevated levels of:
  - Serum creatinine
  - Blood urea nitrogen

IMAGING

- Renal ultrasonography shows symmetrical enlargement of both kidneys compared with patients with renal vein thrombosis, in which the kidneys are generally enlarged unilaterally.

TREATMENT APPROACH

- Treatment for HUS remains almost entirely supportive (see table Treatment Strategies for Hemolytic-Uremic Syndrome).
- The advent of dialysis and improvements in management of acid-base, electrolyte, and volume disorders in children has significantly improved outcomes.
- The prudent use of intensive care, nephrology, and genetic counseling can make a difference in the outcome of HUS.

SPECIFIC TREATMENTS

Supportive care

- Antimotility agents, although useful for symptomatic relief of diarrhea, have been shown to increase the risk of toxic megacolon in patients with HUS and are contraindicated.
  - This problem should be explained to both patient and parents, providing clear reasons why the diarrhea is not being treated.
- Use of some antibiotics to treat *E coli* bowel infection has been found to increase the risk of HUS by promoting the release of ST from the bacteria.
- HUS associated with diarrhea seems to respond to plasma exchange.
  - In patients with severe and progressive acute kidney failure and heart failure, plasma exchange might be considered.
  - Plasma exchange is started within 24 hours of presentation, using ≥1 volume (40 mL/kg) exchange as needed.
  - In HUS caused by *Streptococcus pneumoniae,* plasma therapy is contraindicated because adult plasma contains antibodies to the Thomsen-Friedenreich antigen and may worsen the disease process.

H

Treatment Strategies for Hemolytic-Uremic Syndrome[a]

	Antibiotics	Antimotility Agents	Plasma Exchange or Plasma Infusion	Kidney Transplant
Escherichia coli associated	Contraindicated	Contraindicated	Not effective	Recommended
Streptococcus pneumoniae	Not known	Not known	Contraindicated	Recommended
Factor H mutation	Not known	Not known	• Variably effective • Recommended	Contraindicated
Factor I mutation	Not known	Not known	• Variably effective • Recommended	Contraindicated
MCP mutation	Not known	Not known	Not effective	Recommended
ADAMTS 13 mutation	Unrelated	Unrelated	Recommended	Risk of recurrence

Abbreviations: ADAMTS, a disintegrin and metalloproteinase with thrombospondin; MCP, membrane cofactor protein.
[a] Supportive care is appropriate in all types as needed.

- Angiotensin-converting enzyme inhibitors are recommended in patients with persistent proteinuria.
  - Women should be advised that these agents are teratogenic, and care should be taken to prevent pregnancy.

Kidney transplantation after HUS

- Should be considered for patients (approximately 10–15%) who progress to terminal renal failure after HUS associated with diarrhea
- Depending on the availability of a graft, they may:
  - Require dialysis
  - Get a preemptive transplantation
- These children are excellent candidates because of:
  - The likelihood of recurrence of HUS is low.
  - Patient and graft survival rates are similar or superior to those in children who have received transplants for other renal diseases.
- For patients who are on dialysis as a result of genetic HUS and who then receive a kidney transplant:
  - Overall 1-year graft survival is <30% (vs the expected 95%) because of a 50% recurrence rate of HUS.
  - Results vary depending on the genetic defect.
- Patients with factor H mutations have posttransplantation recurrence rates of 30–100%.
  - In part because factor H is made chiefly in the liver
  - Combined kidney and liver transplants have had mixed success and are not recommended.
- Factor I mutation patients have a similar circumstance and outcome and are not recommended for kidney transplantation.
- ADAMTS-13 deficiency HUS can recur after transplantation.

- Outcomes in the 4 patients with MCP mutations (CD46) who have received transplants were very good.
  - MCP is a protein that is highly expressed in the kidney; thus, kidney transplantation appears to be a good alternative to long-term dialysis.

WHEN TO ADMIT

- All patients with HUS must be admitted.

WHEN TO REFER

- All patients with HUS should be referred to a nephrologist and other subspecialist as indicated.

FOLLOW-UP

- Growth and blood pressure should be closely monitored.
- Regularly test the glomerular filtration rate.
- Proteinuria may remain after all these signs normalize.
  - Persistence for >6 months after the acute stage is a sign of risk for hyperfiltration caused by reduced renal mass, leading to progressive kidney fibrosis.

COMPLICATIONS

- HUS is the most frequent cause of acute kidney injury in children.
- These patients have a hypercatabolic state and may develop several conditions requiring aggressive dialysis.
  - Hypervolemia leading to hypertension, cardiac failure, pulmonary edema, and encephalopathy
  - Hyperkalemia producing cardiac arrhythmias
  - Severe metabolic acidosis
  - Hyponatremia (10% may exhibit hypernatremia), which may be associated with volume contraction caused by the preceding diarrhea or may be dilutional caused by oliguria.

H

PROGNOSIS

- The mortality rate has plummeted over the past 40 years from 40–50% to 3–5%.

- In STEC HUS, >95% of children recover from the acute phase of the illness.

- Mortality is associated with intercurrent infection or severe neurologic, intestinal, or myocardial complications associated with the more severe patterns of the systemic acute disease.

- With current management of fluid and electrolyte disorders and hypertension, no patient should die of complications related to acute kidney injury.

- Long-term renal course depends on intensity of the acute injury and initial destruction of the nephron mass.

- During the acute phase, signs associated with an increased risk of residual kidney lesion and progression to chronic renal insufficiency include:

  - Presence and length of the anuria
  - Need for and duration of dialysis
  - Presence of persistent hypertension
  - Magnitude of extrarenal involvement (central nervous system, intestine)

- Large groups of patients followed for >3 years after recovery of the acute period have shown that:

  - ~65% may have normal function, normal blood pressure, and no proteinuria .
  - 15% may have persistent proteinuria with or without hypertension but normal creatinine clearance.
  - 20% will have chronic renal failure of different degrees.

PREVENTION

- Properly cooking meats and good hygiene will prevent infections with organisms associated with HUS and thus prevent D+ HUS.

Hemophilia and Other Hereditary Bleeding Disorders

DEFINITION

- Hemophilia A (classic hemophilia)
  - Due to congenital factor VIII deficiency
- Hemophilia B (Christmas disease)
  - Due to congenital factor IX deficiency
- von Willebrand disease (vWD)
  - Most common hereditary coagulation disorder, usually asymptomatic
- Coagulant deficiencies
  - Congenital lack or dysfunction of any of the factors needed for coagulation
    - Factor XI deficiency
    - Afibrinogenemia
    - Dysfibrinogenemia

EPIDEMIOLOGY

- Prevalence
  - Hemophilia is seen in ~1 in 5000 male patients.
    - 80–85% have hemophilia A.
    - 10–15% have hemophilia B.
  - vWD is found in 1% of the population.

RISK FACTORS

- Family history of hemophilia in approximately two-thirds of cases

SIGNS AND SYMPTOMS

- Severe disease is characterized by hemarthroses and hematoma formation with minimal or no apparent trauma.
- Mild disease results in bleeding only with trauma.
- Recurrent bleeding into joints is the most frequent clinical problem for patients with hemophilia.
  - Knees, ankles, and elbows are involved most often.
  - Many have 1 particular target joint.
  - Synovial thickening and vascular friability may develop.
    - Results in vicious cycle with increased susceptibility to bleeding
  - Synovitis accompanied by chronic effusion often develops and may progress to joint destruction (hemophilic arthropathy) and severe disability.
- vWD
  - Bleeding after surgery and trauma
  - Mucosal bleeding; most frequently exhibits as epistaxis
  - Menorrhagia
  - Gastrointestinal bleeding
  - Hemarthrosis and deep hematomas may be seen in severe (type III) vWD.

DIAGNOSTIC APPROACH

- Bleeding disorders are suspected on the basis of family and personal history.
- Laboratory tests will identify the specific deficiency.
  - Hemophilia
    - Severe hemophilia is defined by a factor VIII or IX level <1%.
    - Levels >5% are associated with mild disease.
    - Intermediate levels are associated with moderate disease.
- Most useful screening tests
  - Partial thromboplastin time or activated partial thromboplastin time (aPTT)
  - Prothrombin time (PT)
    - PT alone is not adequate for screening for coagulation disorders because it misses the most common congenital deficiencies.
  - Falsely prolonged clotting tests may result from an insufficient amount of blood in the specimen tube due to difficulty accessing the vein.
  - Tests are sensitive to clotting factor levels <30–40% of normal.

LABORATORY FINDINGS

- Prolonged partial thromboplastin time or aPTT and PT
  - Prolonged aPTT or PT must be followed by individual clotting factor assays.
  - If both test results indicate prolonged times:
    - Abnormal liver function or vitamin K deficiency with multiple reduced factors should be considered.
- Factor XIII deficiency will not be detected with aPTT or PT.
- Individual clotting factor assays
- Thrombin time
  - Measure to look for abnormalities of fibrinogen or possible interference by heparin.
  - If results are abnormal, measure reptilase time (which is not sensitive to heparin).
- Bleeding time
  - Useful screening test for vWD, and acquired and congenital abnormalities of platelet function)
  - Difficult to standardize
  - Assessment in an uncooperative child is difficult.
  - Replaced in many centers by Platelet Function Analyzer-100, which is more sensitive and reproducible.
- vWD
  - Several components of the vWF–factor VIII complex and function can be determined.
    - Factor VIII activity
    - vWF activity (ristocetin cofactor)

- – vWF antigen
- – Pattern of multimers
- Many variants of vWD
  - – Type I
    - All components are similarly reduced.
    - Multimer pattern is normal.
  - – Type II
    - Decrease or absence of the larger multimers
    - Type IIB exhibits increased binding to platelets.
  - – Type III
    - Very low or absent levels of all components
- Usually, decreased levels of factor VIII
- aPTT may be normal if the factor VIII level is >30–40%.
  - – Results may be variable; if normal, the test should be repeated if the index of suspicion is high.
- vWF levels of 35–50% may exist both in patients with vWD and normal individuals with blood type O, making definitive diagnosis difficult.

TREATMENT APPROACH

General management principles

- Ideal management of hemophilia is in a comprehensive center where all needs can be met, including:
  - Medical
  - Orthopedic
  - Physical rehabilitation
  - Dental
  - Psychosocial
- All elective surgical procedures must be performed in a center that has:
  - Experienced personnel
  - Immediate availability of blood clotting factor assays
  - Ready supply of clotting concentrates
  - Factor inhibitor testing prior to procedures
- Factor replacement
  - Should always be given promptly when bleeding is suspected
  - Should be given before radiographic examination or other diagnostic studies
- A patient with severe injury or life-threatening bleeding needs:
  - An immediate dose of the appropriate clotting factor to increase its level to 100%
  - Subsequent transfer to a hemophilia center
- A patient with any significant injury:
  - Must be treated promptly, even without apparent evidence of active bleeding (bleeding is often delayed)

- A small, superficial laceration
  - If not bleeding or in need of cleaning, may be managed with a simple pressure dressing
  - If bleeding occurs or if suturing is required, appropriate clotting factor must be administered immediately.
- Treatment must be given before all surgical procedures, arterial puncture, and lumbar puncture.

Specific scenarios

- Casts
  - Should not be applied without previous administration of factor
  - Factor administration should be continued for several days after casting.
  - The involved area should be monitored closely for evidence of nerve or vascular compression.
- Hemarthrosis
  - Treat as soon as pain, tingling, or limping begins, even if there is no evidence of swelling.
  - If marked swelling is present, joint should be aspirated and immobilized after factor replacement.
- Early synovitis
  - Manage by providing factor VIII or IX prophylactically for several weeks, often with a short course of corticosteroids.
  - Synovectomy may be effective if medical management fails.
    - – Accomplished by arthroscopy, even in young children
    - – Intensive physical therapy is required with the procedure.
  - Radiosynovectomy
    - – A simpler procedure, requiring less factor replacement and physical therapy
    - – Has been performed in young children, with good joint outcomes
    - – Some concern exists about inducing cancer and interfering with growth.
- Pain
  - Manage with acetaminophen whenever possible.
  - Codeine and other oral narcotics can be provided if necessary.
  - Aspirin must be avoided.
  - Nonacetylated salicylates (eg, choline magnesium trisalicylate [Trilisate]) can be used.
  - Nonsteroidal antiinflammatory drugs (eg, ibuprofen) can be given cautiously if the patient is not receiving zidovudine.
- Treatment for mild hemophilia
  - Desmopressin may be effective if the baseline factor VIII level is >5%, depending on the level desired.
    - – Overhydration must be prevented because water retention and hyponatremia may occur, particularly in young children and with repeated doses.

- A concentrated intranasal preparation (Stimate) is available and has been used in children ≥6 years of age.
- A stimulation test with response assessment should be performed in each patient with both intravenous and nasal preparations before they are used for the first time.
- Desmopressin is ineffective in factor IX deficiency.

■ Treatment for inhibitor antibodies

- Up to 50% of patients with severe hemophilia A and 3% with hemophilia B develop antibodies that inhibit factor VIII or factor IX.
  - Usually early in treatment
  - Many of these antibodies are present in low titer and may subsequently disappear.
- Management (by experienced practitioners) may include:
  - Large doses of factor VIII or factors that bypass factor VIII in the coagulation cascade
    ■ Prothrombin complex
    ■ Activated prothrombin complex
    ■ Recombinant factor VIIa
  - Induction of immune tolerance by continuous exposure to high doses of factor over months usually is effective in controlling inhibitor, with or without concomitant immunosuppression.
  - Suspect inhibitor antibodies if response to appropriate therapy is inadequate.
  - Assess for inhibitor antibodies in all patients and before all elective surgery.
    ■ Bethesda inhibitor assay determines presence and strength of inhibitors.
  - Patients with hemophilia B and inhibitor antibodies
    ■ May develop anaphylaxis or nephrotic syndrome when given factor IX
    ■ Recombinant factor VIIa has been effective.

■ vWD

- Most patients with type I vWD will respond to desmopressin; this approach can be used for most bleeding episodes.
- Most patients with type IIA and all with type III do not respond to desmopressin.
  - Contraindicated in type IIB disease; may cause platelet aggregation and disseminated intravascular coagulation (DIC)
- Patients who have severe bleeding or do not respond to desmopressin should be treated with Humate P, a concentrate containing both factor VIII and vWF.
- Mild epistaxis can often be controlled with ε-aminocaproic acid or tranexamic acid.
  - Should be used as adjunctive therapy for mucosal bleeding other than hematuria

■ Deficiencies can be treated with fresh-frozen plasma.

- Used for patients with factor V or XI deficiency
- Used in an emergency for patients who are bleeding but whose deficiency has not yet been identified
- Concentrates are preferable for treating factor VII deficiency because of their short half-life, and because all are virus depleted.

■ Prothrombin complex products contain factor VII, II and X (but content of each factor varies in different lots).

- May induce thrombosis or DIC
- Must be used cautiously, particularly in patients with liver disease

SPECIFIC TREATMENTS

Treatment of bleeding episodes in hemophilia, by type of bleeding

■ Hematoma, simple

- Increase factor VIII or IX to 20–40%.
- Treat only once.

■ Hemarthrosis, mild muscle hematoma

- Increase factor VIII or IX to 30–40%.
- Treat once as soon as symptoms begin; if severe, repeat daily until better.
- Ancillary treatment
  - Aspirate joint after treatment if swelling is marked.
  - Do not use ε-aminocaproic acid.

■ Severe muscle hematoma

- Increase factor VIII or IX to 50–100%.
- Treat for 3–7 days.

■ Mouth bleeding, epistaxis, dental extractions

- Increase factor VIII or IX to 80–100%.
- Treat once.
- Ancillary treatment: Start ε-aminocaproic acid, 75–100 mg/kg every 6 hr, or tranexamic acid, 25 mg/kg every 6–8 hr by mouth for 3–7 days (until clot is gone).

■ Gastrointestinal bleeding

- Increase factor VIII or IX to 100%.
- Treat for 3–7 days.
- Ancillary treatment, ε-aminocaproic acid or tranexamic acid

■ Hematuria

- Factor VIII or IX (in mild cases, may not be needed)
- Treat for 3–7 days.
- Ancillary treatment
  - Bed rest
  - Hydration
  - Prednisone, 2 mg/kg daily (in selected patients)
  - Do not use ε-aminocaproic acid.

- Life-threatening, central nervous system, airway obstruction, retroperitoneal
  - Increase factor VIII or IX to 100%; do not allow decrease to <50%.
  - Treat for 7–14 days.
  - Monitor levels.
- Surgery
  - Factor VIII or IX should be at 100%; do not allow decrease to <50%.
  - Treat for 7–14 days.
  - Monitor levels.
- Prophylaxis
  - Factor VIII or IX, 20–40 U/kg
  - Treat 3 times per week for factor VIII, 2 times per week for factor IX.

Treating with factor VIII or IX

- Whole vials with the calculated/desired dose or a higher level should be given because products are too expensive to waste.
- Continuous infusion can be used for patients undergoing surgery or those who are bleeding extensively.
- Factor VIII: 1 U/kg increases plasma level by 2%; biological half-life = 10–12 hours
- Factor IX: 1 U/kg increases level by 1%; 1 U/kg of recombinant factor IX increases level by 0.8%; biological half-life = 20–24 hours
- Slightly lower levels of factor IX than of factor VIII are effective.
- Initial dose = 50 U/kg of factor VIII and 80–100 U/kg of factor IX
  - Repeat half the factor VIII dose in 8–12 hours.
  - Repeat half the factor IX dose in 12–24 hours.
  - Alternatively, provide continuous infusion of 3–4 U/kg per hour of either factor after initial bolus dose.

Product: content, dose, and indications

- Fresh-frozen plasma
  - Whole plasma
  - 5–15 mL/kg; 1 U of each of the coagulation factors/mL; 220 or 600 mL/bag
  - Multiple factor deficiency; DIC; reversal of warfarin effect; hemolytic-uremic syndrome or thrombotic thrombocytopenic purpura; unknown coagulation defect; when no specific concentrate exists
- Cryoprecipitate (not virus inactivated)
  - Factor VIII, vWF, factor XIII, fibrinogen, fibronectin
  - 1 U/kg increases factor VIII 2%; 75–100 U factor VIII and vWF/ bag; volume approximately 20 mL; not assayed
  - Factor XIII deficiency, hypofibrinogenemia

- Factor VIII
  - Factor VIII
  - 1 U/kg increases factor VIII 2%; preassayed; up to 100 U/mL
  - Hemophilia A
- Humate P
  - Factor VIII, vWF
  - Preassayed; factor VIII 20-40 U/mL; vWF 50-100 U/mL
  - Severe vWD; mild to moderate vWD if desmopressin is ineffective or inadequate
- Factor IX
  - Factor IX
  - 1 U/kg (1.2–1.4 U/kg of recombinant) increases factor IX by 1%; preassayed; up to 100 U/mL
  - Hemophilia B
- Prothrombin complex
  - Factor II, VII, IX, X
  - Preassayed for factor IX; content of other factors varies among products
  - Hemophilia B when purified factor IX cannot be used; mild bleeding in hemophilia A with inhibitor; congenital deficiency of factor II or X
  - Danger of thrombosis (including myocardial infarction and DIC) in presence of liver disease, prolonged use
- Activated prothrombin complex
  - Factor II, VII, IX, X; factor VIII–bypassing activity
  - Preassayed for ability to shorten aPTT of plasma with high-titer factor VIII inhibitor
  - Hemophilia A or B with inhibitor
  - Cannot evaluate response by measuring factor VIII activity
  - Risk of DIC and thrombosis
- Novoseven
  - Recombinant factor VIIa
  - Preassayed
  - Hemophilia A or B with inhibitor; factor VII deficiency
  - Risk of thrombosis

WHEN TO ADMIT

- Significant trauma is present.
- Bleeding is present in a potentially life-threatening area.
- Severe abdominal pain exists.
- Any surgical procedure must be performed.

WHEN TO REFER

- All children with hemophilia should be seen at least once a year at a comprehensive hemophilia center if possible.
- All elective surgery should be performed at a hemophilia center.

- All patients with significant trauma or potentially life-threatening bleeding should be given an initial loading dose of factor (to 100%) and transferred to a hemophilia center.
- All patients with inhibitors should be managed at a hemophilia center.
- Children with vWD should have an initial evaluation by a specialized coagulation laboratory.

FOLLOW-UP

- If a child has reasonably easy venous access and family dynamics permit it:
  - Parents can be taught to administer treatment to children as young as 3 years.
  - 9- or 10-year-olds can be taught to self-administer factor concentrates.
  - Benefits
    - Much earlier treatment of bleeding episodes
    - Satisfaction of self-sufficiency
    - Prevention of frustration of having to get to a treatment center or emergency department
  - Indwelling venous access devices are simpler, although infections and thrombosis have been problems.
  - Home intravenous therapy is a convenient way to administer prophylaxis or immune tolerance induction.

COMPLICATIONS

- Synovitis accompanied by chronic effusion often develops and may progress to joint destruction (hemophilic arthropathy) and severe crippling.

PREVENTION

- Routine immunizations
  - Must include hepatitis B and hepatitis A vaccines
  - Should be given subcutaneously with a 25-gauge needle; pressure should be maintained for 5–10 minutes
  - Intramuscular injections should be minimized.
- Using appropriate caution while allowing development of independence is a difficult balance.
  - Psychosocial problems can be associated with a serious chronic illness and frequent pain and limitation of normal activities.
  - Family education about the disease is essential.
  - Support groups are beneficial.
- Synovitis leading to joint destruction is minimized by prompt, adequate treatment or prevention of bleeding.
- Prophylaxis for patients with severe hemophilia
  - Prophylactic factor concentrate treatment administered several times a week
    - Prevents hemarthrosis and joint damage
    - Normalizes living
    - More expensive than episodic treatment for bleeding, but saves cost by preventing orthopedic complications
    - Results in psychological benefits

H

Hemoptysis

DEFINITION

- Hemoptysis is spitting or coughing of blood that originates within the thorax.
- Presentation ranges from flecks of blood in the sputum to massive, potentially life-threatening bleeding that can lead to respiratory distress or death.
- Most commonly associated with previously diagnosed congenital heart disease or cystic fibrosis (CF), but also with infectious respiratory illnesses and, rarely, neoplasms
- May be seen in infants with a variety of congenital defects
  - Arteriovenous malformations
  - Extralobar sequestration
  - Hereditary hemorrhagic telangiectasia (Rendu-Osler-Weber syndrome)
- Diffuse pulmonary hemorrhage is not uncommon in infants of very low birth weight.

EPIDEMIOLOGY

- Rare in children

MECHANISM

- Hemoptysis can result from:
  - Disruption of either arm of the dual pulmonary vascular system
  - Damage to the alveolar endothelial junction
- Localized hemoptysis usually is the result of bleeding from the high-pressure bronchial circulation in inflamed airways.
- The low-pressure pulmonary circulation rarely is to blame for hemoptysis, except in necrotic infarcts and pulmonary arterial aneurysms in tubercular cavities.
  - Both of these conditions are extremely rare in children.
- Increased cardiac output to the bronchial circulation may contribute to hemoptysis and can be caused by:
  - Inflammation in the lungs
    - With chronic inflammation (eg, bronchiectasis), broncho-pulmonary anastomoses are increased, thereby increasing the potential for erosion of vessels in the presence of superimposed infection.
  - Pulmonary vascular obstruction
  - Neoplasia

HISTORY

- 4 important considerations should be kept in mind in evaluating children with hemoptysis.
  - Whether the bleeding requires an emergency resuscitative effort
  - Whether what appears to be hemoptysis is bleeding from the upper airway or gastrointestinal tract
    - The source of the bleeding should be established.
- Children with lower respiratory tract infection but no chronic disease usually:
  - Have mild, self-limited bleeding
  - Require no specific treatment other than management of the underlying acute illness
- Management of hemoptysis that arises from a localized site differs from that which causes a diffuse alveolar hemorrhage, which may be the presenting sign of an underlying immunologic disorder.
- A detailed history of both pulmonary and nonpulmonary symptoms often permits a tentative diagnosis.
- The presumptive diagnosis can then be proven or disproven by findings of specific laboratory tests and procedures.
- Aspects of the history that help focus the evaluation include:
  - Recent trauma
  - Easy bruising
  - Changes in urine color
  - Weight loss
  - Arthralgias
  - Previous heart disease or surgery
  - Medication use
  - Substance abuse
  - Family history of bleeding disorders
  - Surgical procedures
  - Pica
  - Fever
  - Pleuritic chest pain
  - Menstrual irregularities
  - Asthma not responsive to appropriate medical therapy
  - Travel to or from developing countries and areas that raise sheep may necessitate evaluation for mycobacterial, mycotic, or parasitic lung infections.
- Recurrent pneumonitis, sinus infections, and chronic sputum production may be indicative of:
  - Bronchiectasis from CF
  - Foreign body aspiration
  - Ciliary dyskinesias
  - Immunodeficiency disorders
  - Other chronic lung diseases

PHYSICAL EXAM

- Physical examination begins with the vital signs to determine the speed at which the examination should be conducted.
- Thorough inspection of the nasal passages and oropharynx is done to rule out a nonpulmonary cause of the hemoptysis.

- As the examination proceeds caudally, certain findings on inspection and auscultation may suggest a specific diagnosis.
  - Cutaneous telangiectases and a murmur or bruit over the lung fields suggest hereditary hemorrhagic telangiectasia (Rendu-Osler-Weber syndrome).
  - Clubbing with or without adventitial breath sounds suggests bronchiectasis.
  - A saddle nose and stridor suggestive of subglottic stenosis are often seen in patients with Wegener granulomatosis.
  - A pleuritic rub, acute pleuritic chest pain, and history of oral contraceptive use or recent abortion suggest a pulmonary embolic event or other pleural-based lesion.
  - Localized homophonous wheezing over a major airway or decreased breath sounds, with or without a cough, suggests an intraluminal obstruction, such as an aspirated foreign body.
- Evidence of trauma to the thorax may be subtle.
  - 30% of children who experience major trauma to other organ systems will be found to have thoracic trauma as well.
- Examination of the heart may provide evidence of pulmonary hypertension or a new murmur.
- Lymphadenopathy and hepatosplenomegaly raise the possibility of a lymphoproliferative disease with an associated bleeding diathesis.

DIFFERENTIAL DIAGNOSIS

No preexisting medical condition

- For a child or adolescent without a preexisting medical condition who has a first episode of hemoptysis, the most common causes are:
  - Acute infectious pneumonia
  - Foreign body aspiration
- Classically, a child with pneumococcal pneumonia and hemoptysis who is old enough to expectorate:
  - Is febrile
  - Appears ill
  - Has a cough that is productive of rusty sputum
- Certain other bacterial and viral lower respiratory tract infections can cause hemoptysis.
  - In these cases, hemoptysis usually:
    - Occurs early in the course of the illness
    - Is self-limited
    - Consists of only blood-tinged sputum
  - Globally, the most common causes of hemoptysis in children probably are:
    - Tuberculosis
    - Echinococcus
    - Paragonimiasis

- Foreign body aspiration
  - In many cases of aspiration, the initial choking episode is not observed or not remembered.
  - A bout of paroxysmal coughing may occur after the initial event, but as cough receptors in the bronchi or trachea adapt, coughing will stop.
  - Over time, and depending on the location and composition of the foreign object, subsequent inflammation will develop.
    - May result in airway obstruction, with wheezing or recurrent pneumonitis
  - If neovascularization of granulation tissue in the airways occurs, or if bronchiectasis develops, hemoptysis can occur weeks to months after the initial event.
  - Only 40% of children with foreign body aspiration exhibit the classic triad of wheezing, cough, and decreased breath sounds distal to the site of obstruction.
- Pulmonary tuberculosis, usually with systemic manifestations of anorexia and weight loss
  - Purified protein derivative test may be negative.
- Autoimmune disorder or other immunologic abnormality, although rare as a presenting symptom
  - More common in girls
  - Rarely produces hemoptysis alone
  - More commonly characterized by systemic manifestations, including (in addition to the hemoptysis):
    - Fever
    - Weight loss
    - Malaise
    - Anorexia
    - Amenorrhea
    - Rashes
    - Hypertension
- Diffuse pulmonary hemorrhage
  - May be divided into 4 categories, all rare
    - Hemorrhage associated with antiglomerular basement membrane antibodies in serum or tissue (eg, Goodpasture syndrome)
    - Hemorrhage associated with an autoimmune-mediated disease (eg, systemic lupus erythematosus)
    - No immunologic abnormalities, but an association with antibodies
    - Idiopathic pulmonary hemosiderosis (IPH)
      - No evidence of immune-mediated mechanism is found.
      - IPH is diagnosed in most children before the age of 7 years or after the age of 16 years.
      - Symptoms include respiratory distress, bilateral alveolar infiltrates, and iron-deficiency anemia.

- Heiner syndrome (pulmonary hemosiderosis associated with cow's milk allergy) manifests as hemoptysis with:
  - Failure to thrive
  - Vomiting
  - Gastrointestinal bleeding
  - Upper respiratory tract congestion
- Congenital malformations
  - Symptoms depend on the nature of the lesion.
  - May be associated with massive hemoptysis or respiratory distress in newborns
- Primary pulmonary neoplasms
  - Extremely rare in children, especially immunocompetent children
  - <5% of tumors reported in the literature have been associated with hemoptysis.
  - The most common presentations of primary pulmonary neoplasms in children are:
    - Fever
    - Cough
    - Pleural pain
- Other rare causes of hemoptysis without preexisting medical problems
  - Pulmonary embolism
    - Pleuritic pain, cough, and dyspnea
    - Probably associated with oral contraceptive use, recent abortion, or trauma to lower extremities
  - Parasitic lung infections (rare in the US)
    - Travel to endemic areas or sheep-raising areas
    - Peripheral eosinophilia
  - Arteriovenous malformations
    - Recurrent epistaxis
    - Positive family history for hereditary hemorrhagic telangiectasia (Rendu-Osler-Weber syndrome)
    - Cutaneous telangiectasia
  - Catamenial hemoptysis
    - Occurs with onset of menses
  - Factitious hemoptysis, a form of Munchausen syndrome
    - A consideration in adolescents with unusual or perplexing symptoms and normal findings
    - Has been reported in children who had undergone numerous invasive procedures and were biting their oral mucosa to simulate hemoptysis

Preexisting medical conditions

- CF
  - The most common chronic disease associated with hemoptysis

- Hemoptysis usually begins in the second or third decade of life and ranges from the production of blood-tinged sputum with excessive coughing to massive bleeding.
- Massive hemoptysis has an annual incidence of 1% among patients with CF and carries a high mortality rate.
- Bronchiectasis
  - The number of children with bronchiectasis has decreased because of the decline of tuberculosis and the use of effective vaccines against measles and pertussis.
  - Children with immunodeficiencies, recurrent aspiration, and ciliary dyskinesias may develop bronchiectasis.
  - Most have a history of a chronic productive cough with purulent sputum and changes on the lung examination preceding the onset of hemoptysis.
- Congenital heart diseaseis becoming a less common cause of hemoptysis because of advances in corrective cardiac surgery.
  - Seen with Eisenmenger complex and pulmonary venous congestion
- Primary or secondary pulmonary hypertension can lead to hemoptysis as a result of thromboembolic events.
- Right-ventricular outflow obstruction with increased bronchial arterial circulation
  - Hemoptysis is due to hemorrhage from enlarged and tortuous bronchial arteries.
- Pulmonary vascular obstructive disease
  - Hemoptysis occurs because of pulmonary hypertension as well as thrombosis.
  - These vascular changes take years to develop and are usually first observed in adolescents.
- Less common causes in children with a preexisting medical problem
  - Sickle cell anemia
    - Acute chest syndrome or pulmonary infarction
  - Aspergillosis in association with CF or asthma
    - Peripheral eosinophilia and fungi seen on Gram stain of sputum

LABORATORY EVALUATION

- Laboratory tests should be depend on findings at history and physical examination.
- Arterial blood gas measurement if the patient has a compromised airway
  - May aid decisions about need for intensive care
- Urinalysis or specific serologic markers
  - To determine whether the child has an immunologic disease involving the basement membranes of both the kidneys and the lungs
- Complete blood count with eosinophil count
  - To differentiate bacterial from parasitic pneumonia

- Clotting studies
  - Routinely ordered, but invariably normal
  - Bleeding disorders generally do not cause spontaneous hemoptysis.
- Skin tests
  - Should always be performed for suspected mycobacteria
  - Other skin tests, or serologic testing for fungi or other infectious agents, should be guided by clinical acumen.
- Pulmonary fluid culture
  - If sputum is produced or bronchoscopy is performed, it should be cultured and examined for:
    - Bacteria
    - Fungi
    - Ova
    - Parasites
    - Mycobacteria
  - Should be stained for the presence of hemosiderin-laden macrophages
- If warranted, early-morning gastric aspirates can be cultured and stained for microorganisms and macrophages.

IMAGING

- The history and physical examination should produce a tentative diagnosis that guides what imaging studies or procedures are needed to reach a definitive diagnosis.
- Chest radiography should be done if the child is stable.
  - Any abnormality on a chest film should be considered as a potential source for the hemoptysis.
  - A normal radiograph does not exclude the thorax as the source of bleeding.
  - In approximately one-third of children with hemoptysis, initial chest radiographic examination reveals no abnormality.
  - Significant findings on chest film include:
    - Hilar adenopathy
    - Air-fluid level in an abscess
    - Mass
    - Cavitary lesion
    - Mediastinal widening
    - Alveolar infiltrates
      - A common finding in children with autoimmune diseases that involve the lungs
    - Thickening of the bronchial walls with ring shadows and tramlines suggests bronchiectasis.
  - If a foreign body is suspected, views that may help localize the foreign body include:
    - Inspiratory and expiratory films
    - Left and right lateral decubitus films
    - Fluoroscopy

- If a foreign body is causing airway obstruction, then the side of the thorax that does not deflate normally on expiration or when dependent is the side with the foreign body.
  - Chest radiography may reveal nothing abnormal if:
    - The foreign body is embedded in the mucosa of the airway.
    - Obstruction is partial.
  - The chest radiograph is normal in 25% of children with bronchial foreign bodies and >50% of children with tracheal foreign bodies.
    - Because only 10% of aspirated foreign bodies are radiopaque, a normal chest radiograph does not preclude aspiration.
- Additional imaging studies depend on the presumptive diagnosis.
  - Computed tomography (CT)
    - If the chest radiographic examination is normal or does not add any information to that obtained from the history and physical examination, CT can:
      - Identify airway abnormalities
      - Elucidate abnormalities seen on chest radiographs
      - Define mediastinal structures
      - Detect parenchymal disease
      - Help categorize congenital pulmonary malformations and pulmonary vasculitis syndromes
      - Provide a road map for subsequent bronchoscopy
    - High-resolution CT has replaced bronchography for diagnosing bronchiectasis.
  - Magnetic resonance imaging (MRI) is appropriate for:
    - Evaluating possible congenital vascular malformation
    - Differentiation of structures within the mediastinum and hilum
    - The advantages of MRI do not outweigh its disadvantages, especially if excessive respiratory motion is present or the child's condition is unstable.

DIAGNOSTIC PROCEDURES

- Indications for bronchoscopy include:
  - A diagnosis that is in question
  - Massive hemoptysis
  - Incomplete response to therapy
- Timing and need for bronchoscopy, either rigid or flexible, depend on:
  - Stability of the child's condition
  - Suspected cause of the hemoptysis

H

- Not every child with hemoptysis needs bronchoscopy.
  - Hemoptysis rarely is the primary indication.
  - If hemoptysis resolves rapidly and completely after medical therapy, bronchoscopy is not needed.
- No studies have compared the use of fiberoptic versus rigid bronchoscopy for evaluating hemoptysis in either adults or children.
  - Fiberoptic bronchoscopy may be used for initial evaluation.
  - If an anatomic lesion or foreign body is discovered, rigid bronchoscopy will be needed.
  - Both instruments can be used to:
    - Administer therapeutic agents to the airways
    - Sample bronchial fluids
    - Take biopsy samples
  - With the rigid bronchoscope, the bronchoscopist has complete airway control and can:
    - Suction through a larger channel
    - Sample suspicious lesions
    - Insert packing material to tamponade the bleeding
    - Remove foreign bodies from the airway (preferred instrument for this purpose)
  - With the fiberoptic bronchoscope:
    - General anesthesia is not required.
    - The scope usually is passed transnasally (so that upper airways can also be examined).
    - The scope can be easily maneuvered into the upper lobes and more distal airways.

TREATMENT APPROACH

- Treatment for hemoptysis is typically directed at the underlying disease process.

SPECIFIC TREATMENT

- CF
  - Mild hemoptysis can be treated with conservative medical therapy, which includes:
    - Bed rest
    - Intravenous or oral antibiotics
    - Withholding of chest physiotherapy
    - Administration of vitamin K
  - Massive or recurrent hemoptysis in CF and other diseases is now treated with bronchial artery embolization.
    - Despite a moderately high rate of recurrent bleeding, embolization can relieve symptoms for a significant period.
- Bronchiectasis
  - Management is similar to that for CF.

- Treatment of acute exacerbations of IPH includes:
  - High-dose oral or intravenous corticosteroids
  - Supportive care for acute bleeding into the lungs
  - Controversy exists regarding the need for long-term immunosuppressive therapy.
    - Most clinicians caring for children with IPH use azathioprine, chloroquine, or cyclophosphamide to help maintain normal lung function and prevent further episodes of hemoptysis.
- Heiner syndrome
  - Although the mechanism whereby milk causes multisystem damage is unclear, elimination of milk from the diet results in dramatic improvement.

WHEN TO REFER

- If evidence for aspiration is definitive, the child should be referred to a pediatric surgeon or otolaryngologist experienced in retrieving foreign bodies for rigid bronchoscopy.
- If the diagnosis is uncertain, the child should be referred to a pediatric pulmonologist or other clinician skilled in the use of the fiberoptic/rigid bronchoscope to determine whether foreign body is present.
- Before bronchial artery embolization, the child should be evaluated by a team consisting of a pulmonologist, thoracic surgeon, and interventional radiologist.

WHEN TO ADMIT

- Evidence of hemodynamic instability
- Mental status changes
- High suspicion of tuberculosis
- Known heart disease
- Chronic lung disease (eg, CF, ciliary dyskinesias, immunodeficiencies)
- High suspicion of pulmonary neoplasm
- Sickle cell anemia, vasoocclusive crisis, or acute chest syndrome
- Inability to protect airway
- Risk of pulmonary embolism
- Lung abscess
- Children <1 year of age
- Foreign body aspiration
- Pulmonary hypertension

FOLLOW-UP

- Children with mild hemoptysis who are not hospitalized need close outpatient follow-up.

PROGNOSIS

- Prognosis depends on the underlying cause of hemoptysis.

Henoch-Schönlein Purpura

DEFINITION

- Henoch-Schönlein purpura (HSP) is the most common form of vasculitis in children.
- A small-vessel vasculitis mediated by immunoglobulin (Ig) A–containing immune complexes and characterized by non-thrombocytopenic purpura, abdominal pain, arthralgias, and renal disease
- Diagnostic criteria published in 1990 by the American College of Rheumatology state that if ≥2 of the following are present, sensitivity and specificity for HSP are >87%.
  - Palpable purpura
  - Initial presentation at ≤20 years
  - Bowel angina
  - Typical biopsy findings

EPIDEMIOLOGY

- Incidence
  - Annual incidence in the United Kingdom: ~20.4 per 100,000 children
- Age
  - HSP mainly affects young children.
  - Peak incidence at 4–6 years of age
- Sex
  - 1.5:1 male-to-female ratio
- Geographic distribution
  - HSP is more common in Europe and Asia than in the US.
- Seasonality
  - More prevalent during the winter and spring

RISK FACTORS

- In ≥30% of cases, an upper respiratory infection precedes the onset of symptoms.
- Other conditions that can precipitate HSP
  - Infections
  - Drug allergies
  - Insect bites
  - Vaccines
- Cases have been reported in children with C2 and C4 complement deficiencies.

SIGNS AND SYMPTOMS

- Cutaneous manifestations
  - 50% of patients have a macular-petechial rash.
    - Symmetric
    - Sometimes purpuric
    - Localized predominantly in the extensor surface of the lower extremities, forearms, and buttocks; tends to spare the trunk
  - Lesions tend to fade with time, but new lesions appear for up to 3 months after initial presentation.
  - Nonpitting edema of the scalp, hands, and feet in 30–70%
- Joint manifestations in 60–80% patients
  - Knees, ankles, wrists, and fingers are most commonly affected.
  - Joints are usually tender and swollen.
  - Symptoms resolve without residual deformity.
- Gastrointestinal manifestations in 50–70%
  - Higher incidence in patients with renal involvement
  - Intermittent colicky abdominal pain, vomiting, or gastro-intestinal bleeding are most common.
  - Up to 5% develop intestinal infarction, perforation, or intussusception.
- Renal involvement in 20–50%
  - Responsible for long-term morbidity in affected patients
  - HSP nephritis usually coincides with or follows cutaneous manifestations.
  - Nephritis usually presents within 4 weeks of onset of joint or gastrointestinal manifestations.
  - Spectrum of renal involvement is broad and may include:
    - Microscopic hematuria (transient or persistent)
    - Macroscopic hematuria (initial or recurrent)
    - Proteinuria
    - Nephritic syndrome
    - Nephritic-nephrotic syndrome
- Testicular swelling and tenderness in up to 35% of male patients
  - If present, a thorough evaluation is necessary to rule out testicular torsion.
- Pulmonary hemorrhage and central nervous system involvement have been described.

DIFFERENTIAL DIAGNOSIS

- In a child with acute purpuric and petechial eruptions, clinicians must ensure that the differential diagnosis is kept broad.
- Possible diagnoses include, but are not limited to:
  - Acute bacterial infections (invasive meningococcal disease)
  - Rocky Mountain spotted fever
  - Toxic shock
  - Enteroviral infections
  - Endocarditis
  - Idiopathic thrombocytopenic purpura
  - Parvovirus B19
  - Kawasaki disease
  - Acute hepatitis A

- Differential diagnosis for hematuria is wide and can range from very benign to life threatening.
  - Normal activities, such as bike riding or snowboarding, can cause benign hematuria.
  - Important distinction is whether proteinuria is also present with hematuria.
  - Patients without protein in the urine are more likely to have:
    - Kidney cysts
    - Hypercalciuria
    - Kidney stones
    - Thin basement membrane syndrome
  - When proteinuria is also found, the following should be considered:
    - Poststreptococcal acute glomerulonephritis
    - IgA nephropathy
    - Systemic lupus erythematosus
    - Alport syndrome

DIAGNOSTIC APPROACH

- Diagnosis of HSP is based on clinical findings.
- Hematuria is defined as >5–10 erythrocytes per high-power field from a freshly voided centrifuged midstream urine sample.
  - Hematuria should persist for ≥1 month to merit a workup.

LABORATORY FINDINGS

- In general, complete blood count, platelet count, coagulation studies, and complement levels are normal.
- Serum albumin and renal function are usually normal.
  - Vary according to the degree of renal involvement
- IgA levels may be transiently elevated in 50% of patients with HSP.
- Urinalyses obtained at various times in the disease process may reveal:
  - Hematuria
  - Proteinuria

DIAGNOSTIC PROCEDURES

- Renal biopsy is not indicated in all patients with a diagnosis of HSP.
  - It should be considered in patients with:
    - Significant proteinuria for ≥1 month
    - Renal insufficiency
    - Hypertension
    - Nephrotic syndrome

TREATMENT APPROACH

- Once the diagnosis of HSP is established, supportive care is the most important first step.
- Partnership between primary care physician and nephrologist ensures a balance of safety and efficacy.
- Careful attention to the following will be the cornerstone of treatment for most patients.
  - Nutrition
  - Volume status
  - Vital signs
  - Laboratory data (complete blood count, kidney function, electrolytes)
- Specific therapy for HSP remains controversial.
- Children who do not show any urinary abnormalities within 6 months of diagnosis do not develop chronic kidney disease (CKD).
  - Therefore, steroids or other immunosuppressants are not advised for this group.
- Children who show only isolated hematuria or proteinuria have a very low risk of CKD (1.6%).
  - This group should receive supportive care only and not more aggressive treatment.
- Patients who have nephritic or nephrotic syndrome have a much higher risk of CKD (10–19.5%).
  - This group merits serious consideration for aggressive therapy.
  - Girls are especially at risk of CKD (2.5 times higher than their male counterparts) and will likely benefit most of all from therapy.

SPECIFIC TREATMENTS

Steroids

- Long-term follow-up of 219 patients (83 children <16 years and 136 adults) with biopsy-proven HSP found that:
  - 60% of children and 72% of adults had been treated with steroids.
  - 14% of children and 22% of adults had received immunosuppressants.
  - Use of steroids or immunosuppressants failed to show any protective influence over supportive care.
  - 7% of these children ended up receiving dialysis after a mean follow-up of 6.7 years.
  - Girls were at higher risk of eventual dialysis.
- Use of steroids in patients with HSP should be decided on individual bases; cases considered for steroid treatment should be referred to nephrologists.

- Steroids for extrarenal manifestations may be of use.
  - Randomized, double-blind, placebo-controlled trial of early steroid therapy that followed patients for 6 months
  - Of the 171 patients who were included, 84 were treated with prednisone and 87 received placebo.
  - Endpoints were renal involvement at 1, 3, and 6 months and healing of extrarenal symptoms.
  - Use of prednisone (1 mg/kg/day for 2 weeks, with weaning over the subsequent 2 weeks) was effective in reducing the intensity of abdominal pain and joint pain (4.6 vs 7.3; $P = 0.030$).
  - Prednisone did not prevent development of renal symptoms, but it was effective in treating them.
  - Renal symptoms resolved in 61% of prednisone recipients and 34% of placebo recipients.
  - Conclusion: general use of prednisone in HSP is not supported, but patients with disturbing symptoms may benefit from early treatment.
    - Prednisone reduces extrarenal symptoms and is effective in altering, but not preventing, the course of renal involvement.

Fish oil, enalapril, and angiotensin-converting enzyme (ACE) inhibitors

- Fish oil and enalapril for hypertension, hematuria, and proteinuria
  - Children in a study were given 1000 mg fish oil twice daily and enalapril 2.5–10 mg/day.
  - Enalapril was subsequently stopped in all patients within 1 year.
  - 6-month follow-up off ACE inhibition but on fish oil
    - Renal function remained the same (mean creatinine level, 0.6 mg/dL) before and after treatment.
    - Hypertension (135/82 vs 100/54; $P <0.05$) remained better controlled.
    - Proteinuria (1041 mg/day vs 104 mg/day; $P <0.05$) remained minimal.
  - Conclusion: this case series was very small, but fish oil is a benign treatment that may provide other added benefits, such as reduction of hypertriglyceridemia.
  - Fish oils (omega-3-acid ethyl esters) have been shown to be promising in IgA nephropathy, which many researchers believe is part of the spectrum of disease related to HSP.
  - Antiinflammatory and immune-modulating effects of fish oil have been demonstrated in other studies.
- ACE inhibitors are also indicated for control of hypertension, especially for patients with proteinuria.
  - ACE inhibitors are contraindicated during pregnancy.

- Cyclosporine and prednisone, plasmapheresis, tonsillectomy, dapsone, and cyclophosphamide have been tried, with varying degrees of success.
  - These approaches have the possibility of toxicity and lack verification.

WHEN TO ADMIT

- Toxic appearance (febrile, lethargic, hypotensive, or hypertensive, with altered mental status or "not acting themselves")
- Abdominal pain may indicate acute appendicitis, intussusception, small-bowel obstruction or infarction, or pain caused by HSP.
  - Obtaining a surgical consultation is advisable if abdominal pain is particularly severe or out of proportion to findings on physical examination.
- A significant reduction in urine output for age and weight or inability to keep fluids down
- Any alteration from normal in the patient's kidney function (blood urea nitrogen or creatinine)
- Given that the presenting rash with HSP may be the manifestation of many other very severe diseases, a short admit in all but the most healthy looking patients may be prudent.
- Any child not able to communicate (infants or mentally handicapped patients) should be admitted for close observation.

WHEN TO REFER

- Significant and persistent signs of kidney inflammation (nephritic or nephrotic syndrome)
- Acute kidney injury (elevation in blood, urea, nitrogen or creatinine levels) should be referred to a nephrologist.

FOLLOW-UP

- Patients must be monitored for changes in renal function and for hypertension.

COMPLICATIONS

- 2–5% of patients with renal involvement progress to end-stage renal disease.

PROGNOSIS

- HSP nephritis
  - When mild, tends to resolve without any particular intervention
  - 2–5% of patients with renal involvement progress to end-stage renal disease.
- Predictors of poor renal prognosis
  - Abnormal creatinine clearance at 3 years after onset
  - Ultrastructural abnormalities in the renal biopsy

Hepatitis

DEFINITION

- *Hepatitis* describes inflammation of the liver and does not imply a cause.
  - Hepatitis in the pediatric age group may be viral, autoimmune, metabolic, or drug related.
- *Fulminant hepatic failure* is hepatic encephalopathy within 8 weeks of onset of illness.
  - Definition is problematic in children because:
    - It is difficult to detect encephalopathy in infants and young children.
    - Encephalopathy may arise late or not at all.
  - In children, fulminant hepatic failure can be defined as lack of preexisting liver disease and severe impairment of hepatic function evidenced by prothrombin time >4 seconds over control values and unresponsive to large doses of vitamin K.

EPIDEMIOLOGY

Viral hepatitis

- Incidence
  - >16,000 cases of viral hepatitis are reported annually to the Centers for Disease Control and Prevention.
  - Additional unrecognized anicteric cases occur, especially in the pediatric population, in which the anicteric/icteric case ratio is thought to approach 10:1.

Hepatitis A virus (HAV)

- HAV is a 27-nm RNA virus that is a member of the picornavirus group.
- Prevalence
  - Antibody to hepatitis A is present in 33% of the US adult population.
- Transmission is predominantly by the fecal-oral route.
  - Saliva and urine are potentially important vehicles, particularly among siblings.
  - Other identified causes for the acquisition of type-A infection include:
    - Contaminated shellfish
    - Polluted water
    - Travel to endemic areas
  - Parenteral transmission is possible but uncommon.
- Children with acute HAV may be completely asymptomatic, but infectious.
- Incubation period is 15–40 days.

Hepatitis B virus (HBV)

- HBV is a common, highly infectious virus of the Hepadnaviridae family.
- Age
  - In highly endemic areas, acquired at a very young age
  - Age at acquisition is the major determinant of chronicity.

- In low-prevalence countries, HBV infection occurs more often in adolescents and occurs sporadically.
- Prevalence
  - Approximately 90% of children who acquire HBV as neonates will develop chronic hepatitis.
    - Only 20% of children and 10% of adults follow the same course.
- Transmission
  - More likely (up to 90%) if mother is hepatitis B e antigen (HBeAg) positive
  - Less likely (20%) if mother is HBeAg negative
  - Occurs through contact with:
    - Blood
    - Vaginal and menstrual fluids
    - Semen
  - The virus is stable on environmental surfaces for at least 7 days.
  - Horizontal transmission
    - Most frequent route in hyperendemic areas (Asia, Africa, Southern Europe, Latin America) perinatally or in early childhood
    - Uncommon in early childhood from infectious siblings and among institutionalized patients
  - Improperly sterilized syringes and nosocomial transmission are also means of acquisition in some parts of Africa and Asia.
  - Fulminant hepatitis has been reported if the mother is HBeAg negative.
    - The mechanism is not clear.
    - Thought to be the result of selection of more potent mutant viruses
  - Maternal antibody to HBeAg does not prevent perinatal transmission.
  - Risk of infection to infant seems to be markedly increased (65–100%) if the mother has had clinical hepatitis in the third trimester.
  - Principal route of infection with HBV is at birth by microtransfusions or swallowing blood and genital secretions.
- Incubation period is 50–180 days.

Hepatitis C virus (HCV)

- HCV, recognized in 1989, is a single-stranded RNA virus of the Flaviviridae family.
- Prevalence
  - Seroprevalence of HCV in the US is estimated at 1.8%.
  - In children, the seroprevalence rate for those without known risk factors is:
    - 0.2% for those <12 years of age
    - 0.4% for those 12–19 years of age

- Responsible for the majority of posttransfusion non-A, non-B hepatitis
  - Before screening of donor blood in 1990, most children were infected by parenteral exposure to contaminated blood and blood products.
  - Since screening, risk of HCV infection has been reduced to 0.004–0.0004% per unit transfused.
- The major cause of new pediatric HCV infection is perinatal transmission.
  - Overall risk of transmission is 6% from HCV antibody–positive mothers.
  - Risk is minimal when the mother is HCV RNA negative but higher when mothers are coinfected with HIV.
    - A recent European multicenter study showed no increase in transmission of HCV from HCV-HIV–coinfected mothers to their infants.
    - A possible explanation is that effective highly active antiretroviral therapy of coinfected women led to reduced immunosuppression and reduced maternal viral load.
    - This study also found doubling of the risk of HCV infection in female offspring.
- Horizontal transmission from parent to child, sibling to sibling, and via sexual transmission is extremely low.
- Incubation period is 20 to 90 days.

Hepatitis D virus (HDV)

- HDV, discovered in 1977, is a defective virus that requires replication of HBV for its own replication.
- Its epidemiologic mechanism is parallel to that for HBV infection.
- Prevalence
  - Significantly decreased with better control of HBV infection
- Replication occurs in the liver.
- Pathologic effects are limited to liver.
- Hepatitis D antigen can be found in both liver and serum of individuals with the disease.
- Infection may occur as a coinfection with chronic HBV or as acute superinfection of HBV.
  - In both cases, it causes a more severe illness, with significant morbidity and mortality.
- HDV may be transmitted perinatally with HBV.

Hepatitis E virus (HEV)

- HEV is a 27- to 34-nm single-stranded RNA virus.
- Only imported cases have been identified in the US.
  - Cause of epidemic, enteric transmitted hepatitis in India, Pakistan, Nepal, Russia, China, Algeria, Central Africa, Peru, and Mexico

- Illness usually occurs in areas where the water supply is contaminated by feces.

Hepatitis G virus (HGV)

- HGV, identified in 1995, is an RNA virus of the Flaviviridae family and a distant relative of HCV.
- Prevalence
  - Estimated to be 13.8% among US children, based on a small study of blood bank samples
- Mainly transmitted parenterally through blood, blood products, and intravenous drug use
- Infection may be self-limited, resulting in the production of neutralizing antibody to the E2 envelope protein, or may result in a carrier state.
- Virus does not replicate in the liver and does not appear to alter the course and severity in persons coinfected with HCV, but it may be protective in HIV infection.

TT virus (TTV)

- TTV is a DNA virus discovered in 1997 in the sera of 3 of 5 patients with biopsy-proven hepatitis and elevated serum alanine aminotransferase levels.
- Prevalence (North America)
  - 10% in volunteer blood donors
  - 13% of commercial blood donors
  - 17% of intravenous drug users
- The role of TTV in the pathogenesis of acute and chronic liver disease is undetermined.

Autoimmune hepatitis (AIH)

- Approximately two-thirds of affected children are girls.
- 2 types
  - Type 1
    - More common
    - Usual onset in adolescence, early adulthood
  - Type 2
    - Less common
    - Usual onset in childhood, before adolescence

Metabolic liver disease

- α_1-Antitrypsin (α_1-AT) deficiency is the most common genetic cause of liver disease in children.
  - 1 in 1,600–2,000 live births
- Nonalcoholic steatohepatitis (NASH) generally occurs in prepubertal children (slightly more often in boys than girls), in association with:
  - Obesity (body mass index >30 kg/m^2)
  - Insulin resistance
  - Hypertriglyceridemia

ETIOLOGY

- Causes of hepatitis vary with:
  - Age
  - Geographic location
  - Presence or absence of underlying illness

Types of pediatric hepatitis

- Viral
  - Specific hepatitis viruses (eg, HAV, HBV, HCV)
  - Other viruses (eg, Epstein-Barr virus, cytomegalovirus, herpes simplex virus, coxsackievirus)
- AIH
  - A chronic necroinflammatory hepatitis characterized by:
    - Mononuclear cell infiltration of the portal tracts
    - Hypergammaglobulinemia
    - Non–liver-specific autoantibodies
      - Type 1: positive for antinuclear antibody (ANA) and anti–smooth-muscle antibody (SMA)
      - Type 2: positive for anti–liver-kidney microsomal antibodies (LKM)
- Metabolic
  - α_1-AT deficiency
    - The most common genetic cause of liver disease in children
    - Results from the retention of the mutant α_1-AT inside the endoplasmic reticulum of liver cells
    - May predispose certain individuals with homozygous phenotype ZZ to significant liver injury
  - Wilson disease results from a mutation in the *ATP7B* gene, which encodes a copper-binding membrane protein regulating the transport of copper across cell membranes.
    - >200 mutations that may produce disease in humans have been identified.
    - Accumulation of copper in hepatocytes and other organs results in a constellation of clinical symptoms, including:
      - Hepatitis
      - Neuropsychiatric disease
      - Kayser-Fleischer rings in the Descemet membrane of the cornea
  - Tyrosinemia
    - Deficiency in fumarylacetoacetate hydrolase leads to an accumulation of intermediary toxic metabolites, such as maleylacetoacetate and fumarylacetoacetate.
    - Metabolites are thought to cause hepatorenal damage and eventual hepatocellular carcinoma.
  - Hereditary fructose intolerance (HFI)
    - Absence of the enzyme aldolase-B
    - Results in the build up of fructose-1-phosphate, which inhibits gluconeogenesis and glycolysis

- Progressive familial intrahepatic cholestasis (PFIC) type 1, or Byler disease
  - Caused by a mutation in the gene *FIC 1,* which codes for a P-type adenosine triphosphatase involved in amino-phospholipid transport
    - Mechanism by which cholestatic injury occurs in this condition is to be determined.
  - PFIC type 2 is caused by a mutation in the gene encoding for the main adenosine triphosphate–dependent bile acid pump on the canalicular membrane.
  - PFIC type 3 is caused by a mutation in the gene encoding the *MDR* protein, which is a phospholipid flippase also located on the canalicular membrane.
  - PFIC types 1 and 2 cause cholestatic liver disease in infancy.
- Inborn errors of bile acid metabolism lead to severe cholestatic liver disease, necessitating early recognition and treatment.
- Alagille syndrome, or paucity of the intrahepatic bile ducts
  - Caused by a mutation in the human *jagged 1* gene
  - Approximately 50% of patients inherit the disease in an autosomal dominant manner.
  - Others have spontaneous mutations.
  - Multiple mutations have been identified, but genotype-phenotype correlations are more difficult to determine.
- NASH is associated with obesity, but most obese children do not have NASH.
  - Other factors, unidentified as yet, must be involved.

Fulminant hepatic failure

- Acetaminophen toxicity is the most common cause of fulminant hepatic failure in the US.
- In infancy, metabolic disorders may cause fulminant hepatic failure.
  - Galactosemia
  - HFI
  - Tyrosinemia
  - Neonatal hemochromatosis
- See the table Diagnostic Investigations for Liver Disease for appropriate investigations.
- In older children, the following should be considered in the etiology of fulminant hepatic failure.
  - Wilson disease
  - Autoimmune hepatitis, particularly type 2
  - Medications
  - Toxins

Diagnostic Investigations for Liver Diseases

Disease	Investigation	Interpretation
α_1-AT deficiency	Serologic Pi type	• MM (normal) • ZZ (α_1-AT deficiency)
	Serum α_1-AT	<50 mg/dL
	Liver biopsy	PAS-positive diastase resistant granules in the hepatocytes endoplasmic reticulum
Tyrosinemia	Urinary succinyl acetone	Elevated
	α-fetoprotein	• Increased (indicative of immature hepatocytes) • May be increased in many types of neonatal hepatitis but significantly raised in tyrosinemia
PFIC 1, 2, 3	Serum bile acids	Increased
PFIC 1, 2	GGT	Low
PFIC 3	GGT	High
Bile acid metabolic disorder	Fast atom bombardment mass spectroscopy of urine	Typical profiles
	Serum bile acids	Low
	GGT	Low
Hereditary fructose intolerance	Urine reducing substances	Positive when ingesting fructose
	Gene testing	22 Mutations for HFI, 70% of patients have two mutations in exon 5 (*A149P, A174D*)
Cystic fibrosis	Sweat chloride test	Sweat chloride >60 mEq/L
Autoimmune hepatitis		ANA; anti-SMA or anti-LKM
Neonatal hemochromatosis	Serum transferrin	Low (reflects low functioning liver cell mass)
	Serum ferritin	Markedly increased (nonspecific)
	MRI	Siderosis of pancreas, myocardium
	Buccal biopsy	Siderosis of salivary glands
Niemann-Pick type C	Liver biopsy (electron microscopy)	Whirled inclusions of sphingomyelin in lysosomes
	Skin fibroblast culture	Measurement of sphingomyelinase activity

Abbreviations: α_1-AT, α_1-antitrypsin; ANA, antinuclear antibody; anti-LKM, anti–liver-kidney microsomal antibodies; anti-SMA, anti–smooth-muscle antibody; GGT, γ-glutamyl transferase; HFI, hereditary fructose intolerance; MRI, magnetic resonance imaging; PAS, periodic acid–Schiff; PFIC, progressive familial intrahepatic cholestasis.

SIGNS AND SYMPTOMS

- Evaluation of a child with hepatitis depends primarily on:
  - Age of the child
  - Nature of the symptoms
- Common presentations include:
  - Jaundice
  - Incidental finding of elevated liver enzymes during routine workup
  - Fulminant hepatic failure
- Clinical syndromes of viral hepatitis vary from asymptomatic to fulminant hepatic failure, depending on the virus and host factors.
  - Acute viral hepatitis may also progress to chronic liver disease, particularly with HBV and HCV.
  - See table Clinical Features of Acute Viral Hepatitis.

Jaundice in newborns and infants

- Infants with jaundice and elevated liver enzymes may:
  - Be otherwise well
  - Have failure to thrive
  - Display signs of liver decompensation
- The primary care physician must determine:
  - Family history of jaundice, liver, or metabolic disease
  - Maternal exposure to drugs and toxins
  - Maternal serologic status for hepatitis A, B, and C
- Maternal illnesses during pregnancy suggesting the presence of an in utero infection should be noted, particularly if the infant is malnourished.
- A complete dietary history to determine fructose ingestion in the infant (either through food or medication) is required if HFI is suspected.
- Examination may reveal hepatosplenomegaly, icterus, and little else.

Child with jaundice

- HAV infection is heralded by an abrupt onset associated with:
  - Fever
  - Malaise
  - Anorexia
  - Nausea
  - Vomiting
  - Upper abdominal discomfort
  - Darkening of the urine and enlargement and tenderness of the liver
  - Jaundice (infrequent in young children)
  - Disease is rarely fulminant.
    - A small percentage of patients with HAV may have a relapsing or protracted course.

- HBV
  - Onset is usually insidious.
  - Extrahepatic manifestations, such as skin rash and arthralgia, are common and may be prodromal.
  - Younger children may be asymptomatic.
  - Duration of illness is usually 4–6 weeks.
  - >80–90% of children recover without sequelae.
  - Fulminant hepatitis is seen in infants born to HBeAg-positive mothers with low levels of HBV DNA.
  - Liver cirrhosis is encountered in 3–5% of children with chronic HBV.
- Acute HCV infection is asymptomatic in most children.
  - Both acute liver failure and cirrhosis have been reported in infancy.
  - 2 characteristic clinical features of HCV infection are:
    - Fluctuation in the serum aminotransferase concentrations
    - Progression to chronicity in 50–90% of patients
  - Most patients remain asymptomatic without stigmata of chronic liver disease.
  - Liver histologic test shows mild to moderate hepatitis.
- Acute HDV infection in a child who is a chronic HBV carrier may produce a severe episode of hepatitis with fulminant hepatic failure or chronic hepatitis.
- HEV is similar clinically to HAV.
  - Its most unusual clinical feature is a high mortality rate in pregnant women (approximately 10%).
- The mode of presentation of AIH is highly variable.
  - Hepatomegaly, splenomegaly, and jaundice are common.
  - AIH is strongly associated with ulcerative colitis and may precede or follow the colitis.
  - Associated extrahepatic manifestations include:
    - Nephrotic syndrome
    - Autoimmune thyroiditis
    - Behçet disease
    - Crohn disease
    - Insulin-dependent diabetes
    - Urticaria pigmentosa
    - Vitiligo
    - Hypoparathyroidism
    - Addison disease
  - Fibrosis may be seen to a variable degree.
  - True cirrhosis may be present.

Clinical Features of Acute Viral Hepatitis[a]

		HAV	HBV	HCV
Characteristics	Age distribution	Children and young adults	All age groups	All age groups
	Route of infection	Predominantly fecal-oral route	Parenteral	Parenteral
	Incubation period (days)	15–40	50–180	20–90
	Onset	Acute	Insidious	Insidious
	Duration of clinical illness	Weeks	Weeks to months	Weeks to months
Virus Present	Feces	Late incubation, acute	May be present	Absent
	Blood	Late incubation, acute	Late incubation, acute, may persist for months	Present chronically
Signs and Symptoms	Fever	High, common early	Moderate, less common	Moderate, less common
	Nausea and vomiting	Common	Less common	Less common
	Anorexia	Severe	Mild to moderate	Mild to moderate
	Arthralgia or arthritis	Rare	Common	?
	Rash or urticaria	Rare	Common	?
Laboratory Findings	Aminotransferase elevation	1–3 weeks	Months	Fluctuates for months
	Bilirubin elevation	Weeks	May be months	Unusual
	HBsAg	Absent	Present	Absent
	Severity	Usually mild	Often severe	Usually mild
	Progression to chronic hepatitis	Rare	More common	High rate
	Immunity	Homologous, lifelong	Homologous, lifelong	Unusual
	Prevention	Immune serum globulin	Hyperimmune globulin; vaccine	Screen donor blood

Abbreviations: HAV, hepatitis A virus; HBsAg, hepatitis B surface antigen; HBV, hepatitis B virus; HCV, hepatitis C virus.

[a] Modified from: Krugman S, Katz SL. *Infectious Diseases of Children*, 8th ed. St Louis, MO: Mosby; 1985. Copyright © Elsevier 1975. deBelle RC, Lester R. Current concepts of acute and chronic viral hepatitis. *Pediatr Clin North Am.*1975;22(4):943–961. Copyright © Elsevier 1975.

■ Metabolic diseases
  • NASH is seen in children with a significant number of risk factors, including:
    – Obesity (body mass index >30 kg/m^2)
      ■ Many children are obese, but only a minority have NASH.
    – Diabetes
    – Insulin resistance
    – Hypertriglyceridemia
  • HFI in the older child with an aversion to fructose-containing products who, after inadvertent ingestion, develops:
    – Vomiting
    – Elevation of serum aminotransferases
■ To evaluate for drug or toxin-induced hepatitis, a complete medical history should be obtained for:
  • Prescribed medications
  • Herbal teas

- Poisons
- Wild mushrooms

DIFFERENTIAL DIAGNOSIS

Viral

- Specific hepatitis viruses
  - Such as HAV, HBV, HCV
- Other viruses
  - Such as Epstein-Barr virus, cytomegalovirus, herpes simplex virus, coxsackievirus

Autoimmune

- Type 1
- Type 2

Metabolic

- α_1-AT deficiency
- Wilson disease
- HFI
- Tyrosinemia
- Galactosemia
- Progressive familial intrahepatic cholestasis
  - 3 types
- Alagille syndrome
- NASH

Drugs

- Anesthetics
- Anticonvulsants
- Antihypertensives
- Chemotherapeutics
- Diuretics
- Laxatives
- Many others

Fulminant hepatic failure

- Acetaminophen toxicity is the most common cause of fulminant hepatic failure in the US.
- In infancy, metabolic disorders may cause fulminant failure
  - Galactosemia
  - HFI
  - Tyrosinemia
  - Neonatal hemochromatosis
- See the table Diagnostic Investigations for Liver Disease for appropriate investigations.
- In children beyond infancy, the following should be considered in the etiology of fulminant hepatic failure.
  - Wilson disease
  - AIH, particularly type 2

- Medications
- Toxins

Newborns and infants

- Other conditions that should be considered in an infant with jaundice include:
  - α_1-AT deficiency
  - Cystic fibrosis
  - Defects in amino acid synthesis
  - Organic acid synthesis and fatty acid oxidation
  - Glycogen storage disease
  - Niemann-Pick type C disease
- The association of renal Fanconi syndrome and clotting abnormalities that are unresponsive to vitamin K therapy suggests tyrosinemia.
- Neonatal hemochromatosis may present with hepatitis but often occurs with acute liver failure.
- Patients with Alagille syndrome may have jaundice and hepatitis in the first 2 years of life.
  - The diagnosis is a clinical one based on the association of bile duct paucity together with ≥3 of the following.
    - Typical facies
    - Posterior embryotoxon (ophthalmologic examination)
    - Butterfly vertebrae (on chest radiograph)
    - Consistent cardiac disease (eg, pulmonary stenosis)
    - Renal disease
  - Other features include:
    - Markedly elevated γ-glutamyl transferase (GGT) level (eg, 800 IU/L)
    - Hypercholesterolemia
    - Growth retardation
    - Intracranial bleeding
- Tyrosinemia
  - The usual presentation in infants is acute liver failure with pronounced coagulopathy.
- Galactosemia exhibits in the neonatal period with:
  - Cholestatic jaundice
  - Hypoglycemia
  - Hepatitis
- HFI manifests as:
  - Metabolic acidosis
  - Hypoglycemia
  - Liver failure

Children

- Viral hepatitis, particularly HAV, HBV, HCV, and Epstein-Barr virus, should be actively sought in this age group.
- HBV should be considered in the differential diagnosis of serum sickness–like illness.

- Wilson disease should be considered in assessment of pediatric liver disease, because of its variable presentation and availability of effective therapy.
  - Kayser-Fleischer rings and neurologic findings may be absent.
  - Ceruloplasmin may be normal in young children.
- AIH
  - Type 1 is characterized by the presence of ANA and anti-SMA.
  - Type 2 is characterized by the presence of anti-LKM.
- NASH
  - Fat in the liver associated with inflammation
  - Consider in prepubertal children with obesity

DIAGNOSTIC APPROACH

- Complete clinical history and thorough physical examination are important in making a timely diagnosis and preventing unnecessary investigations.

LABORATORY FINDINGS

Jaundice in newborns and infants

- Investigations in the infant in whom a cause of hepatitis is not obvious should include serologic testing for viruses and general investigations, such as:
  - Blood ammonia
  - Serum glucose
  - Blood gases with pH
  - Blood lactate
  - Urine metabolic screen and reducing substances
  - Erythrocyte galactose-1-phosphate uridyl transferase tests
  - Thyroid function tests
  - Serum and urine bile acid tests
  - More sophisticated tests are required for many metabolic and inherited disorders.

Child with jaundice

HAV

- Presence of IgM-class anti–hepatitis A coinciding with clinical symptoms confirms diagnosis of acute HAV.
- HAV RNA can be detected in serum and stool as early as 2–3 weeks before acute illness.
- HAV RNA can be detected in serum and stool up to 1 week after the onset of illness.
- Recovery in the stool decreases as jaundice becomes evident.
- HAV IgM antibody is short lived.
- HAV IgG antibody is present at least 10 years after infection.
  - Probably confers lifelong immunity to the virus
- Bilirubin level increases in both direct and indirect fractions but does not generally exceed 15 mg/dL.

- Generally, aminotransferase level elevation does not last >3 weeks.
- Clinical and laboratory abnormalities do not generally persist beyond 4 weeks.

HBV

- Its double-stranded overlapping DNA codes for:
  - Surface antigen (HBsAg)
  - Core antigen (HBcAg)
  - HBeAg
  - DNA polymerase
- HBsAg has been found in all body secretions and excretions from infected persons.
- Presence of HBsAg in the serum implies HBV infection.
- First marker to appear; detected 2 weeks to 6 months after exposure
- Children with HBV infection are initially HBsAg and HBeAg positive.
- HBeAg reflects active viral replication and infectivity.
- During this immunotolerant stage, which may persist for years, viral replication and serum HBV DNA levels are very high.
  - Serum aminotransferase levels fluctuate and may be in the upper limit of normal range.
  - HBV aminotransferase elevation usually peaks approximately 1 month after the onset of illness.
- During childhood, conversion from HBeAg to anti-HBeAg may occur spontaneously, at a rate of 3% per year, although rates vary with the mode of acquisition.
- Seroconversion to anti-HBeAg is often preceded by a transient elevation in serum aminotransferases.
- After anti-HBeAg seroconversion, HBV DNA levels remain low or undetectable.
- Most children remain HBsAg positive, and this chronic carrier state is not generally associated with overt disease.
- Annual HBsAg clearance rate in chronic carriers is low (1–2%) and may be associated with persistence of HBV DNA.
- HBV DNA is detectable in serum very early in the infection, but its measurement is limited by the sensitivity of the techniques used.
  - Target amplification techniques, such as polymerase chain reaction (PCR), have a lower limit of detection of 100–400 copies/mL.
  - Signal amplification techniques such DNA hybridization assays and branched chain DNA assays are less sensitive.
  - Interassay variation is significant.
- Viral load from different assays cannot be compared directly.
- To standardize measurements, an international unit has been recently adopted, and most laboratories will report with the new unit in the near future.
- Anti-HBsAg confers immunity and indicates resolving or past infection.

H

- Anti-HBsAg is also seen after vaccination because the vaccine contains recombinant HBsAg.
- Presence of anti-HBcAg, which appears 3–5 weeks after HBsAg, implies exposure to the native HBV and can indicate ongoing or past infection, but does not appear after vaccination.

HCV

- Presence of antibodies to HCV implies exposure to native HCV virus but does not confer protective immunity.
- Most laboratories currently use third-generation enzyme-linked immunosorbent assay (ELISA) with >99% sensitivity and specificity.
- Recombinant immunoblot assay can be used when HCV infection is suspected but ELISA is negative or inconclusive.
- Both of these tests become positive weeks after exposure to the virus.
- Highly sensitive PCR assay becomes positive within days after exposure to the virus.
- Assays for viral detection may be quantitative or qualitative.
  - Quantitation is an important component of guiding therapy.
  - Quantitative assays are used more often.
- As with HBV infection, an international unit is being adopted to overcome variability between laboratories and commercially available assays.
- Vertically acquired infection is confirmed by:
  - Persistence of anti-HCV antibody beyond 18 months of age
  - Presence of HCV RNA in serum after the first 3 months of life
- PCR testing before this period is unreliable.

HDV

- A test for anti-HDV is commercially available.
- Evaluation for acute HDV is appropriate in a child with fulminant hepatic failure and HBV.

HEV

- Evaluation for acute HEV infection is appropriate in a child from a developing country with acute hepatitis.
- Cholestasis may be more common than with HAV.
- Elevation of serum aminotransferase levels is modest.
- Real-time PCR has recently been developed.

HGV and TTV

- Evaluation for HGV and TTV is not indicated outside of epidemiologic studies.
  - No clear evidence that they are pathogens
- Diagnosed by detection of HGV RNA and TTV DNA by PCR methods

AIH

- AIH should be excluded with serologic testing in all children with signs of acute or chronic liver disease and liver failure.
  - Routine investigations reveal hypergammaglobulinemia and increased ANA, SMA, or LKM antibody titers.
  - In 1999 the International Auto-Immune Hepatitis Group modified a scoring system to diagnose AIH in adults.
    - Useful in children, particularly when a GGT ratio was used instead of alanine aminotransferase/alkaline phosphatase ratio
  - Histologically, portal tracts are infiltrated by lymphocytes and plasma cells.
  - Inflammatory cells often infiltrate the parenchyma, accompanied by necrosis of cells at the periphery of the hepatic lobule (piecemeal necrosis).

Metabolic diseases

- No single test is available to diagnose Wilson disease.
  - The combination of ≥2 of the following is highly suggestive.
    - Decreased serum ceruloplasmin level (<20 mg/dL)
    - Elevated urinary copper excretion (>100 mcg/24 hours)
    - Elevated liver copper concentration (>250 mcg/g of dry weight)
    - Kayser-Fleischer rings
  - Genetic testing is available in some centers.

Drug or toxin-induced hepatitis

- Serum acetaminophen should be measured and appropriate therapy instituted immediately.
- Urine toxicologic screen should be performed when the index of suspicion is high.

Abnormal liver enzyme levels

- Systemic disorders may increased aminotransferase levels.
- Elevated levels of aminotransferases have been found in 32% of children with celiac disease .
  - Celiac screen should be performed in all children with unexplained elevation of serum aminotransferase levels after hepatologic causes have been excluded.

PFIC

- Types 1 and 2 and inborn errors of bile acid synthesis should be suspected in any child with:
  - Elevated serum bile acid levels
  - Low GGT level
  - Elevated aminotransferase levels
- Type 3 has a similar clinical picture, except that the GGT level is elevated and presentation may be delayed.

IMAGING

- Ultrasonography
  - In NASH, fatty liver can be identified on sonography by uniform or patchy increased echogenicity.

DIAGNOSTIC PROCEDURES

- Liver biopsy is required:
  - When chronic liver disease is suspected and cannot be diagnosed
  - To determine the degree of inflammation and fibrosis, which may influence treatment
  - Needle biopsy is usually adequate.
  - Risks are low when clotting function is normal, ultrasonographic guidance is used, and the biopsy is performed by an experienced physician.
  - The biopsy sample should be sent for histologic testing with additional stains (eg, copper, iron) if necessary.
  - A small sample should be preserved in glutaraldehyde for electron microscopy if metabolic liver disease is suspected.
  - If Wilson disease is suspected, hepatic copper should be quantified.
    - Obtaining a second biopsy core is usually necessary for this purpose.

SPECIFIC TREATMENTS

HAV

- Vaccines
  - 2 inactivated vaccines against HAV are licensed in the US for children age 1–18 years and adults.
- Twinrix, the HAB-HBV combination vaccine, is licensed for >18 years of age.
- Vaccine is given in a 2- or 3-dose schedule depending on the formulation (see table Recommended Doses and Schedules for Inactivated Hepatitis A Vaccines).
- Children with underlying liver disease should receive the HAV vaccination.
- Either pediatric formulation induces seroconversion rates >90% after the initial dose and 100% after the second dose.
- Indications for HAV vaccination
  - All children at 1 year of age
  - Catch-up immunization of unimmunized children 2–18 years of age
    - Especially with increase in incidence among children and adolescents
  - Travelers to endemic areas
  - Patients with chronic liver disease
  - Men who have sex with men
  - Users of injection and illicit drugs
  - Patients at high risk of exposure secondary to occupation
- No particular diet or restriction of activity appears to affect course or outcome of acute viral hepatitis.
- Return to school 1 week after onset of illness, provided that the child feels well, is recommended.
- Household contacts are already likely to be infected by the time of diagnosis.
  - Infection-control measures should be instituted, including:
    - Scrupulous hand washing
    - Use of disposable eating utensils until jaundice clears

Recommended Doses and Schedules for Inactivated Hepatitis A Vaccines[a]

Age (yr)	Vaccine[b]	Hepatitis A Antigen Dose	Volume per Dose (mL)	Number of Doses	Schedule
1-18	Havrix	720 ELU	0.5	2	Initial and 6–12 mo later
1-18	Vaqta	25 U[c]	0.5	2	Initial and 6–18 mo later
≥19	Havrix	1440 ELU	1.0	2	Initial and 6–12 mo later
≥19	Vaqta	50 U[c]	1.0	2	Initial and 6–18 mo later
≥18	Twinrix[d]	720 ELU	1.0	3 or 4	Initial and 1 and 6 mo later OR Initial, 7 and 21–30 days followed by a dose at 12 mo

Abbreviation: ELU, enzyme-linked immunosorbent assay units.

[a] From: American Academy of Pediatrics. Hepatitis A. In: Pickering LK, Baker CJ, Kimberlin DW, Long SS, eds. *Red Book: 2009 Report of the Committee on Infectious Diseases*. 28th ed. Elk Grove Village, IL: American Academy of Pediatrics; 2009:332.

[b] Havrix and Twinrix are manufactured by GlaxoSmithKline Biologicals; Vaqta is manufactured and distributed by Merck & Co, Inc.

[c] Antigen units (each unit is equivalent to approximately 1 mcg of viral protein).

[d] A combination of hepatitis B (Engerix-B, 20 mcg) and hepatitis A (Havrix, 720 ELU) vaccine (Twinrix) is licensed for use in people 18 years of age and older in a 3-dose schedule. Havrix 360 ELU in single-dose vials is licensed in the US but no longer available.

- Pooled serum Ig given within 2 weeks postexposure is effective in preventing symptomatic infection, as is immunization within an 8-day window period.
- Ig should be given to household contacts; institutional contacts, and persons exposed in common source outbreaks.
- Neonates born of infected mothers do not need special care if the mother is not jaundiced.
- Children traveling to endemic areas should be immunized prophylactically.
  - Vaccination is preferable.
    - If travel is imminent (in <1 month), then IgG may be substituted.

HBV

- History of vaccination in the US
  - In 1991 universal newborn infant HCV immunization
  - In 1995 routine vaccination of all adolescents age 11–12 years
  - In 1999 inclusion of children <18 years who had not been vaccinated previously
  - These efforts resulted in a significant reduction of HBV in children.
  - The rate of acute HBV infection in children and adolescents decreased by 89% during 1990–2002.
- Racial disparities in hepatitis B incidence have narrowed.
- A recent study showed that 40% of homeless inner-city children age 13–18 years had no record of HBV vaccination.
  - HBV vaccine must be administered on any chance encounter with such children.
- Persons who should receive HBV immunization:
  - All infants (infants of HBsAg-positive mothers require postexposure immunoprophylaxis with HBIg and vaccine)
  - Infants and children at risk of acquisition of HBV by person-to-person (horizontal) transmission should be immunized by 6–9 months of age.
  - Adolescents (special efforts should be made to vaccinate adolescents at high risk for HBV infection)
  - Users of intravenous drugs
  - Sexually active heterosexual persons with >1 sex partner in the previous 6 months or those with a sexually transmitted infection
  - Men who have sex with men
  - Health care workers at risk of exposure to blood or body fluids
  - Residents and staff of institutions for developmentally disabled persons
  - Staff of nonresidential child care and school programs for developmentally disabled persons, if attended by a known HBV carrier
  - Patients on hemodialysis
  - Patients with bleeding disorders who receive certain blood products

- Household contacts and sexual partners of HBV carriers
- Members of households with adoptees from countries where HBV infection is endemic and who are HBsAg positive
- International travelers who will reside for >6 months in an area of high endemic HBV and who otherwise will be at risk
- Inmates of long-term correctional facilities
- Detailed recommendations regarding doses and postexposure prophylaxis are provided in the tables Recommended Doses of Hepatitis B Vaccines and Guide to Postexposure Immunoprophylaxis of Unimmunized People to Prevent Hepatitis B Virus Infection.
- A neonate born to an HBsAg-positive mother or a mother who has had hepatitis B during pregnancy should be given:
  - 0.5 mL of HBIg intramuscularly within the first 12 hours of life *and*
  - 0.5 mL of HBV vaccine intramuscularly before hospital discharge but definitely within the first week of life *and*
  - 0.5 mL of HBV vaccine intramuscularly at 1 and 6 months
- Data linking breastfeeding to the acquisition of viremia are equivocal.
  - HBsAg-positive mothers whose infants have received immunoprophylaxis may breastfeed without risk of transmitting HBV.
- HBV immunization also protects against HDV infection.
- 2 treatments for HBV in children have been approved.
  - Interferon-α
    - May be given to children ≥1 year of age
    - Results in HBeAg seroconversion in 25–50% of children with chronic HBV
    - Effect on HBsAg clearance is poor, but serum aminotransferase levels and liver histologic results improve.
  - Lamivudine (3 mg/kg daily up to 100 mg/day)
    - May be given to children ≥3 years of age
    - Has been shown to produce HBeAg seroconversion in 22% of children versus 13% of placebo controls
    - Response is greatest in patients with an elevated alanine aminotransferase level.
    - Resistance rates in the first year of therapy were 19%.
  - Adefovir dipivoxil
    - Latest drug to be approved by the US Food and Drug Administration for HBV infection in adults
    - Currently being evaluated in pediatric trials
- Seroconversion may not be permanent; seroreversion may occur, particularly in the first year after therapy.
  - Newer nucleoside analogues and other families of drugs are available for treating HBV infection; resistance to each has developed after monotherapy.
  - The decision to treat should be made in conjunction with a pediatric hepatologist.

Recommended Doses of Hepatitis B Vaccines[a]

Patients	Vaccine[b]		Combination Vaccine
	Recombivax HB[c] dose, µg (mL)	Engerix-B[d] dose, µg (mL)	Twinrix[e]
Infants of HBsAg-negative mothers and children and adolescents <20 yr of age	5 (0.5)	10 (0.5)	Not applicable
Infants of HBsAg-positive mothers (HBIg [0.5 mL] also is recommended)	5 (0.5)	10 (0.5)	Not applicable
Adults ≥20 yr of age	10 (1.0)	20 (1.0)	20 (1.0)
Adults undergoing dialysis and other immunosuppressed adults	40 (1.0)[f]	40 (2.0)[g]	Not applicable

Abbreviations: HBsAg, hepatitis B surface antigen; HBIG, hepatitis B immune globulin.

[a] Modified from: American Academy of Pediatrics. Hepatitis B. In: Pickering LK, Baker CJ, Kimberlin DW, Long SS, eds. *Red Book: 2009 Report of the Committee on Infectious Diseases*. 28th ed. Elk Grove Village, IL: American Academy of Pediatrics; 2009:344.

[b] Both vaccines are administered in a 3-dose schedule; 4 doses may be administered if a birth dose is given and a combination vaccine is used to complete the series. Only single-antigen hepatitis B vaccine can be used for the birth dose. Single-antigen or combination vaccine containing hepatitis B vaccine may be used to complete the series.

[c] Available from Merck & Co Inc.
- A 2-dose schedule, administered at 0 months and then 4 to 6 months later, is licensed for adolescents 11 through 15 years of age using the adult formulation of Recombivax HB (10 µg).
- A combination of hepatitis B (Recombivax, 5 µg) and *Haemophilus influenzae* type b (PRP-OMP) vaccine is recommended for use at 2, 4, and 12 through 15 months of age (Comvax). This vaccine should not be administered at birth, before 6 weeks of age, or after 71 months of age.

[d] Available from GlaxoSmithKline Biologicals. The US Food and Drug Administration also has licensed this vaccine for use in an optional 4-dose schedule at 0, 1, 2, and 12 months for all age groups. A 0-, 12-, and 24-month schedule is licensed for children 5 through 16 years of age, and a 0-, 1-, and 6-month schedule is licensed for adolescents 11 through 16 years of age.
- A combination of diphtheria and tetanus toxoids and acellular pertussis (DTaP), inactivated poliovirus (IPV), and hepatitis B (Engerix-B 10 µg) is recommended for use at 2, 4, and 6 months of age (Pediarix). This vaccine should not be administered at birth, before 6 weeks of age, or at 7 years of age or older.

[e] A combination of hepatitis B (Engerix-B, 20 µg) and hepatitis A (Havrix, 720 enzyme-linked immunosorbent assay units [ELU]) vaccine (Twinrix) is licensed for use in people 18 years of age and older in a 3-dose schedule administered at 0 mo, 1 mo, and 6 or more months later. Alternately, a 4-dose schedule at days 0, 7, and 21 to 30 followed by a booster dose at 12 months may be used.

[f] Special formulation for adult dialysis patients given at 0, 1, 2, and 6 months.

[g] Two 1.0-mL doses given in 1 or 2 injections in a 4-dose schedule at 0, 1, 2, and 6 months of age.

HCV

- No vaccine is available for prevention of HCV.
- Natural infection does not protect from reinfection with the same or different genotypes.
- The most important strategies for controlling hepatitis C include:
  - Screening donor blood for anti-HCV
  - Identifying and educating of persons at risk
  - Establishing risk-minimization programs for intravenous drug users
- Screening should include:
  - Injection drug users
  - Patients receiving hemodialysis
  - Recipients of ≥1 unit of blood or blood products before 1992
  - Children with clinical non-A, non-B hepatitis
  - Children >18 months of age born to mothers infected with HCV
  - International adoptees born to high-risk mothers
- Patients with HCV infection should:
  - Avoid hepatotoxic medications and alcohol
  - Receive vaccination against HAV and HBV infections to prevent additional liver damage
- The American Association for the Study of Liver Diseases presents arguments for and against treatment of HCV infection in children.
  - On the basis of treatment trials in children, the US Food and Drug Administration has approved treatment of children with HCV age 3–17 years with a combination regimen of:
    - Interferon-α (subcutaneously 3 times per week)
    - Oral ribavirin
  - Side effects are better tolerated in children but require close monitoring.

Guide to Postexposure Immunoprophylaxis of Unimmunized People to Prevent Hepatitis B Virus Infection[a]

Type of Exposure	Immunoprophylaxis[b]
Household contact of HBsAg-positive person	Administer hepatitis B vaccine series
Discrete exposure to an HBsAg-positive source[c]:	
• Percutaneous (eg, bite, needlestick) or mucosal exposure to HBsAg-positive blood or body fluids that contain blood	Administer hepatitis B vaccine + HBIG; complete vaccine series
• Sexual contact or needle sharing with an HBsAg-positive person	Administer hepatitis B vaccine + HBIG; complete vaccine series
• Victim of sexual assault/abuse by a perpetrator who is HBsAg positive	Administer hepatitis B vaccine + HBIG; complete vaccine series
Discrete exposure to a source with unknown HBsAg status:	
• Percutaneous (eg, bite, needlestick) or mucosal exposure to blood or body fluids that contain blood with unknown HBsAg status	Administer hepatitis B vaccine series
• Victim of sexual assault/abuse by a perpetrator with unknown HBsAg status	Administer hepatitis B vaccine series

Abbreviations: HBsAg, hepatitis B surface antigen; HBIG, hepatitis B immune globulin.

[a] Modified from: American Academy of Pediatrics. Hepatitis B. In: Pickering LK, Baker CJ, Long SS, et al, eds. *Red Book: 2009 Report of the Committee on Infectious Diseases.* 28th ed. Elk Grove Village, IL: American Academy of Pediatrics; 2009: 353.

[b] Immunoprophylaxis should be administered as soon as possible, preferably within 24 hours after exposure. Studies are limited on the maximum interval after exposure during which postexposure prophylaxis is effective, but the interval is unlikely to exceed 7 days for percutaneous exposures and 14 days for sexual exposures.

[c] If person previously was immunized with hepatitis B vaccine series, administer hepatitis B vaccine booster dose.

- Therapy should be supervised by persons who are experienced in treating children.
- Recently, a trial has evaluated pegylated interferon and ribavirin in children.
  - Sustained viral response was documented in 22 (47.8%) of 46 patients with genotype 1.
  - A multicenter, placebo-controlled trial of pegylated interferon with or without ribavirin is currently under way.

HEV

- Treatment of HEV infection is supportive.
- Development of recombinant peptide vaccines is under way.

AIH

- Prednisone can suppress activity in AIH.
  - Has side effects on growth
- Azathioprine, an immunosuppressive, is frequently added.
  - Allows a reduction in dose of or complete weaning from prednisone
- Cyclosporine or tacrolimus may be effective in patients who are refractory to azathioprine and steroids.
- Prednisone is initiated at a steady dose.
  - On improvement, prednisone dose may be tapered at weekly intervals to a dose that maintains remission.
- Azathioprine may be added after symptoms improve.
  - Monitor for azathioprine toxicity (eg, hematopoietic toxicity), particularly in patients with thiopurine *S*-methyltransferase deficiency.

- Remission is defined as:
  - Absence of clinical symptoms
  - Aminotransferase level no more than 2 times normal
  - Decreasing serum GGT level
  - Resolution of aggressive histologic appearance on a liver biopsy specimen
- Duration of therapy once remission is achieved is controversial.
  - Clinical remission generally occurs within 3–6 months.
  - Biochemical remission occurs within 6–12 months.
  - Histologic remission occurs within 12–24 months.
- Once remission is achieved, steroids may be tapered gradually over 2–3 months.
- Long-term treatment with a low-dose steroid is often required.
- During steroid taper, monitor at 2- to 4-week intervals for ~3 months for early evidence of recurrence.
  - If disease does not recur within this time, the frequency of observation can be decreased.
  - ≥80% of children appear to achieve initial remission.
  - Although relapses are common, long-term control usually is achieved with continuous immunosuppressive therapy.
- The child with AIH and fulminant hepatic failure poses a difficult therapeutic problem.
  - Prednisone and azathioprine have been used in this situation with success.

- Liver transplantation may be necessary for survival.
- Most children are likely to have prolonged survival on minimal long-term immunosuppression.

Drug-induced hepatitis

■ Profound effects of acetaminophen toxicity can be treated with intravenous *N*-acetylcysteine.

■ In all other cases of suspected drug-induced hepatitis, supportive care is recommended along with discontinuation of the suspected drug.

Metabolic liver disease

■ Aim of therapy in Wilson disease is copper chelation in a controlled manner.

- First-line therapy is penicillamine in the majority of cases.
  - Requires close monitoring for significant side effects, including allergies and renal disease
- Triethylene tetramine hydrochloride (trientine) has been effective in the same dose as penicillamine.
  - Also associated with significant side effects
- Tetrathiomolybdate can be used when significant neurologic disease exists.
  - Toxicity needs to be monitored carefully.
- Zinc may be used as initial therapy in patients without clinical disease diagnosed incidentally on family screening.

■ No specific therapy is available for α_1-AT deficiency.

- Liver transplantation should be considered for end-stage liver disease.

■ Dietary restriction of galactose is the treatment of choice for galactosemia.

■ Tyrosinemia may be treated with a phenylalanine and a tyrosine-restricted diet, together with 2-nitro 4-trifluorom-ethyl-benzoyl-1-1,3-cyclohexanedione (NTBC).

- NTBC is an inhibitor of an early enzyme in the tyrosine degradation pathway that is thought to prevent the accumulation of toxic products, resulting in clinical improvement in most patients.
- Although costly, NTBC has been proposed as an alternative to liver transplantation.
- Whether it will decrease the risk of hepatocellular carcinoma is not yet determined.

■ Bile acid–replacement therapy is the treatment of choice for inborn errors of bile acid synthesis.

■ Ursodeoxycholic acid may be used in the treatment of liver disease secondary to cystic fibrosis, although no data exist to support its use.

Fulminant hepatic failure

■ Needs to be managed in a setting with liver transplantation expertise

■ Requirements of liver support must be balanced with management of fluids, nutrition, and encephalopathy.

■ Transferring a child with severe hepatitis early before the need for intensive care management is preferable.

Liver transplantation

■ Has improved mortality and morbidity of children who have severe liver disease

■ Indications include:

- Liver failure
- Growth failure
- Intractable itch from cholestasis

■ Pretransplant management involves aggressive nutritional therapy and prevention of complications, such as bacterial peritonitis and variceal hemorrhage.

■ Transplantation for chronic liver failure secondary to HBV infection is complicated by almost 100% recurrence of infection.

- HBIg followed by lamivudine improves the outcome.

■ Recurrence of HCV infection after transplantation is ~90%, but transplantation is recommended because recurrent disease is usually mild.

■ Recurrence is related to donor risk factors, recipient risk factors, and viral and clinical factors.

■ Liver transplantation for all causes results in 5-year survival rates in children approaching 70–80%.

■ Focus is directed toward improving morbidity related to immunosuppressive medications and quality-of-life issues.

WHEN TO ADMIT

■ Children with fulminant liver failure of any cause should be promptly hospitalized at a pediatric liver transplantation center.

- Fulminant hepatic failure is defined as lack of a preexisting liver disease and severe impairment of hepatic function, as evidenced by prolonged prothrombin time (>4 seconds over control value) that is unresponsive to large doses of vitamin K.

■ Hospitalization is generally unnecessary for the patient with acute HAV.

- An infant or young child should be hospitalized if coagulopathy or other evidence of liver decompensation is present.

■ Prolonged prothrombin time (>4 seconds over control value) in a child with severe hepatitis of any cause

■ Acute encephalopathy in a child with severe hepatitis of any cause

■ Dehydration requiring intravenous fluid resuscitation in a child with severe hepatitis

■ Gastrointestinal bleeding in a child with acute or chronic hepatitis

H

WHEN TO REFER

- Children with uncomplicated HAV can usually be managed by a general pediatrician.
  - Chronic hepatitis B, D, or C should be referred to a pediatric gastroenterologist or infectious disease specialist.
- Children with metabolic liver disease, drug-induced hepatitis, or AIH should be referred to a pediatric specialist in metabolic disease or gastroenterology.
- HBsAg-positive serologic test in children ≥1 year of age
- Anti–HCV-positive serologic test in children ≥3 years of age
- Any diagnosis of drug-induced hepatitis (unexplained elevation of serum aminotransferase levels or bilirubin level in a child who is taking or has recently taken any medication)
- Any diagnosis of metabolic liver disease (unexplained elevation of serum aminotransferase levels or bilirubin level in a child) and a positive screening test, such as low ceruloplasmin level, low galactose-1-phosphate uridyl transferase level, and positive urine-reducing substances

FOLLOW-UP

- HBV
  - Although the best methods and frequency of surveillance have not been determined, careful follow-up includes:
    - Serial serum α-fetoprotein measurement
    - Ultrasonography of the liver

COMPLICATIONS

- HBV
  - Long-term effects of acquiring HBV in infancy include cirrhosis and hepatocellular carcinoma.
  - Many cases of HBV-related liver cancer have been described in children.
  - Most cases of HBV-related hepatocellular carcinoma occur in adults.

- Recent studies suggest that perinatal transmission is important in hepatocarcinogenesis, perhaps related to the high dose of HBV DNA with subsequent tolerance and persistent necroinflammatory activity.
- HCV
  - Fibrosis increases with duration of infection, but in an unpredictable manner.
  - Patients with chronic HCV infection who become infected with HAV are at substantial risk of fulminant hepatic failure.
  - Chronic HCV infection predisposes patients to cirrhosis and hepatocellular carcinoma over 20 years in those with adult-acquired infection.
  - The natural history of perinatally acquired HCV infection is still under evaluation.

PREVENTION

- HAV vaccination routinely after 1 year of age and in all adolescents
- HBV
  - Aggressive immunization programs have substantially lowered risks.
- HCV
  - Maternal-fetal transmission has been linked to in utero monitoring and prolonged rupture of membranes.
    - HCV does not appear to be prevented by cesarean section.
  - Although HCV RNA has been detected in breast milk, current evidence suggests that breastfeeding is not contraindicated.
    - In developed countries, mothers should consider abstaining from breastfeeding if nipples are cracked and bleeding.

Hepatomegaly

DEFINITION

- *Hepatomegaly* denotes an enlarged liver.

MECHANISM

- Hepatomegaly results from an increase in either the number of cells or the size of structures within the liver.
- This may result from broad categories of disorders.
  - Inflammatory/infectious
  - Neoplastic/infiltrative
  - Storage disorders
  - Vascular congestion
  - Biliary obstruction

HISTORY

- Describe the hepatomegaly.
  - Timing of onset
  - Associated signs/symptoms
- Review of systems
  - Pulmonary manifestations (dyspnea, hyperinflation, tracheal deviation)
  - Cardiac manifestations (cough, chest pain)
  - Gastrointestinal symptoms (hematemesis)
  - Neuropsychiatric symptoms
  - Assess for trauma.
  - Assess the likelihood of hypercoagulability.
  - Assess exposure to toxins and medications.
- Medical history
  - Asthma
  - Cardiac disease
  - Infectious exposures
  - Medication history
- Perinatal history
  - Jaundice
- Family history
  - Inflammatory conditions (systemic lupus erythematosus, sarcoidosis)
  - Cancer
  - Metabolic conditions/storage disorders (Wilson disease, glycogen storage disease)

PHYSICAL EXAM

- Vital signs
  - Temperature
  - Heart rate, blood pressure, respiratory rate

- Physical examination
  - Liver
    - Determine size and span.
      - Determine the upper margin by percussion.
      - Determine the lower margin by either percussion or palpation; palpate upwards from iliac.
      - The upper edge of liver dullness is usually at the level of the fifth rib in the right midclavicular line.
      - Normal span ranges from 5.9 cm in the first week of life to 6.5–8 cm by 15 years of age.
      - Estimation of liver span is more strongly correlated with hepatomegaly than is projection below the costal margin.
    - Determine characteristics.
      - Firm and tender suggests an acute inflammatory disorder.
      - A hard liver may be neoplastic.
      - Smooth and exquisitely tender liver may result from vascular distention.
    - Auscultate for bruits.
  - Spleen
    - An enlarged spleen with a palpable liver usually suggests significant disease.
  - Assess other systems.
    - Ocular: Look for Kayser-Fleischer rings.
    - Respiratory: Examine for evidence of hyperinflation.
    - Cardiovascular
      - Examine for evidence of congestive heart failure.
      - Examine for evidence of cardiac tamponade (eg, pulsus paradoxus).
    - Skin: Assess for jaundice and evidence of trauma.

DIFFERENTIAL DIAGNOSIS

- The differential diagnosis includes inflammatory/infectious causes, neoplastic/infiltrative disorders, storage disorders, vascular congestion, and biliary obstruction.
  - Inflammatory/infectious causes
    - Hepatitis
      - Viral
      - Bacterial (eg, abscess, sepsis)
      - Toxic (eg, drugs, including acetaminophen)
      - Neonatal
      - Autoimmune (eg, systemic lupus erythematosus, sarcoidosis)
    - Trauma

- Neoplastic/infiltrative disorders
  - Primary tumors
    - Hepatoblastoma
    - Hepatocellular carcinoma
    - Hemangioma
    - Focal nodular hyperplasia
  - Metastases
- Storage disorders
  - Fat accumulation
    - Obesity
    - Malnutrition
    - Reye syndrome
    - Cystic fibrosis
    - Diabetes mellitus, type 2
    - Lipid infusion
    - Metabolic liver disease
    - Lipidoses (eg, Niemann-Pick, Gaucher, Wolman diseases)
  - Glycogen excess
    - Glycogen storage diseases
    - Infant of mother who has diabetes
    - Beckwith-Wiedemann syndrome
    - Total parenteral nutrition
  - Copper accumulation
    - Indian childhood cirrhosis
    - Wilson disease
  - α_1-Antitrypsin deficiency
    - Icterus and acholic stools in first week of life are characteristic.
    - Signs of chronic liver disease in older children
  - Hypervitaminosis A
- Vascular congestion
  - Suprahepatic
    - Congestive heart failure
    - Cardiac tamponade
    - Constrictive pericarditis
  - Intrahepatic
    - Hepatic vein thrombosis (Budd-Chiari syndrome)
    - Hepatic vein web
  - Vascular malformations
    - Cavernous hemangioma
    - Capillary hemangioma
    - Hemangioendothelioma

- Biliary obstruction
  - Congenital biliary atresia
  - Congenital hepatic fibrosis
  - Caroli disease
- Displaced or prominent liver edge, without true hepatomegaly
  - Downward displacement of the right hemidiaphragm
    - Hyperinflated lung (eg, asthma, bronchiolitis, pneumonitis)
    - Tension pneumothorax
    - Congenital diaphragmatic hernia
    - Thoracic tumors
  - Subdiaphragmatic lesions (eg, abscess)
  - Aberrant lobe of liver

LABORATORY EVALUATION

- Evaluation is directed toward the suspected cause; thus, laboratory work is not always indicated.
- Possible tests include:
  - Toxin screens, including acetaminophen, aspirin
  - Complete blood count, peripheral blood smear
    - Hemolytic anemia may indicate Wilson disease
  - Liver enzymes (aspartate aminotransferase, alanine aminotransferase)
  - Liver function studies (prothrombin time, international normalized ration, partial thromboplastin time, albumin, protein; ammonia if mental status changes)
  - Fractionated bilirubin
  - Hepatitis panel
  - Blood cultures
  - Vitamin A level
  - Copper studies
  - Tumor markers

IMAGING

- Imaging studies are determined by clinical suspicion.
- Imaging can help to assess liver size.
  - Radiography
  - Ultrasonography
    - May help to identify liver masses, abscesses
  - Computed tomography, magnetic resonance imaging, sulfur colloid scintigraphy
    - Define masses detected on ultrasonography
  - Hepatic angiography
    - May be indicated to evaluate suspected vascular tumors

DIAGNOSTIC PROCEDURES

- Percutaneous liver biopsy
  - Can be used to confirm some metabolic and genetic disorders
  - Idiopathic neonatal hepatitis
    - Marked infiltration with inflammatory cells
    - Giant-cell transformation
  - Biliary atresia
    - Bile duct proliferation
    - Giant-cell transformation
  - Congenital hepatic fibrosis
    - Diffuse periportal and perilobular fibrosis on histologic analysis
- Percutaneous liver aspiration
  - Often performed under ultrasonography or computed tomographic guidance
  - Confirms liver abscess and allows sampling of organisms for culture

TREATMENT APPROACH

- Treatment is aimed at the underlying disease entity.

SPECIFIC TREATMENT

Inflammatory disease

- Inflammatory hepatitis
  - Supportive care
- Bacterial infection
  - Appropriate antimicrobial agents

Liver tumors

- Surgical excision
- Chemotherapy may be a helpful adjunct in reducing tumor size either pre- or postoperatively.

Biliary atresia

- Extrahepatic
  - Surgery
- Intrahepatic
  - Hepatoportoenterostomy procedure of Kasai

Other disorders

- Metabolic or genetic disorders
  - Dietary modifications
  - Gaucher disease: imiglucerase, a new synthetic enzyme
  - Wilson disease: D-penicillamine chelation therapy, with zinc acetate for maintenance therapy
  - Glycogen storage disorders
    - Frequent small feedings of a high-protein, complex-carbohydrate diet
    - Continuous nighttime feeding via gastrostomy tubes
- Indian childhood cirrhosis
  - Chelation therapy with D-penicillamine reduces mortality significantly if administered early in the disease course.

WHEN TO REFER

- Refer for hepatomegaly when there is:
  - Concomitant splenomegaly
  - Liver with hard consistency
  - Distended abdominal veins
  - Audible bruit over the liver
  - Suspicion of cancer

WHEN TO ADMIT

- Impending liver failure
- Not clinically stable because of underlying conditions (eg, large pneumothorax, cardiac tamponade, congestive heart failure, hepatitis)
- For intravenous antibiotics

PROGNOSIS

- Biliary atresia
  - Even with treatment, many patients develop cirrhosis and portal hypertension.
- Indian childhood cirrhosis
  - Rapid evolution to cirrhosis and hepatic failure if left untreated

Herpes Infections

DEFINITION

- Herpesvirus hominis, or herpes simplex virus (HSV)
  - DNA virus with a protein coat
  - One of the most common agents infecting humans
  - Although 85–95% of primary infections may be inapparent, in certain circumstances, the disease can be fatal.
  - Can be divided definitively into 2 immunologic types that correlate with clinical manifestations
    - Herpesvirus type 1 (HSV-1): tends to be associated with disease above the waist
    - Herpesvirus type 2 (HSV-2): associated with disease below the waist, with sexually related transmission, or with disease acquired neonatally

EPIDEMIOLOGY

- Prevalence
  - Since the late 1970s, the prevalence of HSV-2 infection has increased dramatically.
  - In lower socioeconomic groups where crowding probably plays an important epidemiologic role
    - 80–100% of adults demonstrate antibodies to HSV-1.
    - 30–40% or more may be positive for HSV-2.
  - Of persons in higher socioeconomic groups:
    - 21% demonstrate antibodies to HSV-2, compared with 34% of those below the poverty level.
- Age
  - Studies have shown
    - Sharp rise in the prevalence of antibodies to HSV-1 between 1 and 4 years of age
    - Slower increase in antibody acquisition between 5 and 14 years of age
  - From adolescence into early adulthood, coincident with the beginning of sexual activity, the presence of antibodies to HSV-2 increases significantly.
    - HSV-2 antibody is now detectable in at least 1 of 5 persons 12 years or older nationwide.
- Neonatal herpes
  - Incidence
    - Varies between 1 in 3200 and 1 in 15,000 deliveries
    - An estimated 1500 to 2200 infants per year in the US are infected with HSV.
  - Prevalence
    - Between 10% and 60% of healthy American women have HSV-2.
    - As many as 50–60% of women from lower socioeconomic groups in the US have antibodies to HSV-2.
    - Postnatal transmission from a caregiver accounts for approximately 10% of cases.

ETIOLOGY

- HSV-1 transmission
  - Presumed to occur via person-to-person respiratory spread
    - Probably involves close contact, such as kissing an infected person
    - Can occur regardless of whether the source is symptomatic with an apparent vesicular lesion at the time
  - After healing and recovering from the initial infection, the host is not rid of the organism.
    - Organism is presumed to remain in a latent phase in the ganglion cells or nerves innervating the region of localized infection.
- Neonatal herpes infections
  - Most are caused by HSV-2.
  - Antibodies to HSV-1 are associated in 25% of cases.
  - Transplacental transmission of HSV can occur and may induce spontaneous abortion or, rarely, congenital defects in newborns.
  - Pediatricians are more often faced with postnatal herpetic disease contracted by the newborn during the second stage of labor while moving through an infected birth canal.

RISK FACTORS

- HSV-1
  - Sports that involve close skin contact
    - Wrestlers may acquire herpes gladiatorum as a result of viral shedding from an infected opponent.
    - Herpes rugbeiorum, or scrum pox, may result from close skin contact between rugby players.
  - 5–10% of cases of genital herpes associated with HSV-1 are believed to result from orogenital sex.
- HSV-2
  - Sexual activity
  - Frequency of infection is high and underestimated by clinical history in the adolescent population.
- Recurrent infection
  - May be induced by various stimuli, including:
    - Sunlight
    - Fever
    - Physical or emotional trauma
    - Menses
- Neonatal
  - Greatest risk occurs when the mother has contracted primary herpes 2–4 weeks before delivery.
    - Disease may be transmitted to the infant in recurrent cases with or without a clinically detectable herpetic lesion.

- Risk for a child born vaginally to a mother with primary genital herpes is 33–50%.
  - <5% if the mother is shedding virus as a result of reactivated infection
  - Distinguishing primary versus recurrent infection may be impossible because both may be asymptomatic.
    - Approximately 75% of infants with HSV infection are born to women without history, physical, or symptomatic evidence of infection.
- Risk factors for neonatal disease include:
  - History of a first HSV infection during the third trimester
  - Invasive monitoring of the fetus
  - Delivery <38 weeks
  - Maternal age <21 years

SIGNS AND SYMPTOMS

- General
  - Incubation period of 2–12 days
  - Primary infection, if apparent, is usually heralded by:
    - Classic herpetic enanthem or exanthem
    - Lesions are painful vesicles, usually several millimeters in diameter, on an erythematous base.
  - Constitutional symptoms
    - Malaise
    - Fever
    - Anorexia
    - Irritability
  - Recurrent episodes
    - Demonstrate a similar vesicular eruption in the same general anatomic area as the primary eruption, but without concomitant constitutional symptoms
- HSV-1
  - Acute gingivostomatitis
    - The most common form of HSV-1 seen in children
    - Peak incidence between 1 and 4 years of age
    - Characterized by abrupt onset of fever, irritability, poor feeding
    - 1–2 days later:
      - Very tender, red, friable mucous membranes surrounding 2- to 3-mm white ulcerations
      - Severe halitosis
    - Vesicular stage is rarely seen.
    - Large, tender anterior cervical and submandibular lymphadenopathy is common.
    - Duration of illness from 5–14 days
    - Severity ranges from mild to so severe that oral intake becomes negligible, and hospitalization for intravenous hydration may be required.

- Herpes labialis (cold sores):
  - Crust and heal without scarring in 7–10 days
  - May be found on either the upper or lower lip
  - Recurrence at the same site is extremely common.
- Traumatic herpes
  - The result of inoculation at the site of local trauma
  - Includes herpetic whitlow, an extremely painful syndrome involving herpetic infection of a digit
    - Although the sore may resemble a bacterial paronychia, it should not be incised.
    - This condition is common in thumb-suckers who have oral herpes.
- Ocular herpes
  - One of the most common causes of corneal blindness in the US
  - Primary infection usually involves acute keratoconjunctivitis with intense swelling of the lids, but without exudate.
  - Frequently, typical herpetic vesicles are found on the skin surrounding the involved eye.
  - Recurrent disease
    - Can be even more severe
    - May involve superficial or deep epithelial ulceration, stromal damage, or uveitis
  - Should always be referred to an ophthalmologist for care
  - The use of topical steroid preparations in a probable case of ocular herpes can have devastating consequences.
- Viral encephalitis
  - Estimated 250–500 cases reported per year
  - Characterized by fever and personality change
  - Often involves seizures
  - Rapidly progressive encephalopathy culminates in death in 1–2 weeks in >70% of untreated cases.
  - Infection most often localizes to a single lobe.
  - Definitive diagnosis in the past was most often made by biopsy, demonstrating the typical morphologic picture of herpes microscopically.
- HSV-2
  - Usually exhibited by typical herpetic vesicles on
    - Penile shaft, prepuce, or glans penis in the male patient
    - The labia minora or majora, mons, or nearby skin or within the vagina in the female patient
  - Primary infection is accompanied by:
    - Significant local pain, burning, or paresthesia
    - Constitutional symptoms offever and malaise, dysuria, and inguinal lymphadenopathy
  - Recurrent bouts are less severe than initial occurrences.

- Neonatal
  - Must always be included in the differential diagnosis when the newborn or infant has a skin rash ranging from vesiculopapular to vesiculoulcerative

DIFFERENTIAL DIAGNOSIS

- HSV-1
  - Coxsackievirus A herpangina
    - Most common ulcerative enanthem to be considered
    - Results in lesions very similar in appearance to herpes
    - Is located in the posterior oral cavity, unlike the anterior localization of herpetic lesions
  - Other infections include:
    - Varicella
    - Cytomegalovirus
    - Syphilis
  - Autoimmune diseases, such as:
    - Behçet syndrome
    - Reiter syndrome
    - Inflammatory bowel disease
  - Systemic lupus erythematosus and cyclic neutropenia
    - Might be considered in a broader differential diagnosis
    - Cultures for herpes can confirm the final diagnosis if necessary.

LABORATORY FINDINGS

- HSV-1
  - Clinical diagnosis rarely requires laboratory confirmation.
- HSV-2
  - Viral culture
    - In general, the most sensitive method of diagnosis
    - Requires several days for definitive result, depending on the size of the inoculum
    - Vesicles, stool, urine, and mucosal surfaces may be used as sites to obtain culture sample.
  - Direct detection methods, including fluorescent antibody and immunoperoxidase assays
    - Can be used when lesions are available for scraping
    - Test results are rapid but have lower sensitivity; viral culture is still required for confirmation of a negative finding.
  - Tzanck test and Papanicolaou stains
    - Neither is sufficiently specific nor sensitive to serve as a screen for HSV.

- Polymerase chain reaction
  - Highly specific and sensitive
  - Can discriminate between HSV-1 and HSV-2 in cerebral spinal fluid
  - The diagnostic method of choice in HSV encephalitis
- Several point-of-care tests are available using glycoprotein-based assays for HSV-2 antibodies, with sensitivities of 80–98% and specificities >95%.

TREATMENT APPROACH

- No universal cure exists for herpesvirus infections
- Neonatal herpes involving the central nervous system (CNS)
  - By the 1980s, acyclovir had become the treatment of choice.
    - More recent work demonstrates some improved mortality with prolonged high-dose (60 mg/kg/day divided every 8 hours) intravenous acyclovir.
    - Unfortunately, no significant decrease in long-term developmental results among survivors has been demonstrated, allowing morbidity to remain unacceptably high.
    - Due at least in part to the fact that <10% of typical herpetic lesions appear in the first 24 hours of life
      - Early identification of affected infants is difficult; thus, initiation of appropriate therapy is frequently delayed.

SPECIFIC TREATMENTS

Genital herpes

- First clinical episode
  - Oral antiviral therapy shortens the duration of symptoms and viral shedding.
  - Definitely indicated for at least a 10-day course
  - If begun within 1 day of the onset of the first lesion, then episodic therapy may limit the duration and severity of recurrences as well.
    - Acyclovir 400 mg orally 3 times a day for 7–10 days *or*
    - Acyclovir 200 mg orally 5 times a day for 7–10 days *or*
    - Famciclovir 250 mg orally 3 times a day for 7–10 days *or*
    - Valacyclovir 1 g orally twice a day for 7–10 days
    - Treatment may be extended if healing is incomplete after 10 days of therapy.
- Episodic therapy for recurrent genital herpes
  - Acyclovir 400 mg orally 3 times a day for 5 days *or*
  - Acyclovir 800 mg orally 3 times a day for 2 days *or*
  - Acyclovir 800 mg orally twice a day for 5 days *or*
  - Famciclovir 125 mg orally twice a day for 5 days *or*
  - Valacyclovir 500 mg orally twice a day for 3 days *or*
  - Valacyclovir 1.0 g orally once a day for 5 days

- Suppressive therapy for recurrent genital herpes
  - The same medications have been shown to decrease recurrences by 70–80% when used as long-term suppressive therapy in patients with particularly severe or frequent recurrences.
  - The cost of such therapy may limit its usefulness.
    - Acyclovir 400 mg orally twice a day *or*
    - Famciclovir 250 mg orally twice a day *or*
    - Valacyclovir 500 mg orally once a day *or*
    - Valacyclovir 1.0 g orally once a day
- Therapy for immunosuppressed individuals
  - May warrant hospitalization and the use of intravenous acyclovir

Other herpetic syndromes

- Herpetic gingivostomatitis
  - Oral acyclovir
    - Can shorten the duration in children by 6 days if begun within the first 72 hours of illness
    - Potential for significant cost savings because of the frequent need of intravenous hydration among children with this syndrome
    - Only modest efficacy has been shown with treatment of episodic oral herpes.
    - Topical antiviral therapy for recurrences has been demonstrated to decrease the duration of symptoms by ≤1 day.
- Keratitis
  - Topical antivirals treat superficial keratitis effectively.
  - Oral acyclovir may be beneficial in situations of recurrent ocular lesions.
- Herpes encephalitis
  - Intravenous acyclovir remains the mainstay of treatment.
  - Acyclovir has significantly decreased mortality from this condition but has only modestly affected morbidity.
  - Therapy must be initiated promptly to ensure the most favorable outcome.
    - Early treatment has improved the prognosis of this disastrous condition among children but is most effective when begun before the onset of loss of consciousness.
  - For neonates <3 months
    - Treatment should be continued for 21 days.
  - For children ≥3 months
    - Treatment should last 14–21 days.

WHEN TO ADMIT

- Infants with suggested or confirmed neonatal herpes:
  - Must be carefully monitored and treated with intravenous acyclovir
- All individuals thought to have herpes encephalitis:
  - Must be hospitalized and treated expectantly with intravenous acyclovir
- Immunosuppressed individuals with herpes infections:
  - May require intravenous antiviral therapy and will require hospitalization

WHEN TO REFER

- All infants who are thought to have neonatal herpes
  - Should be considered potentially critically ill
  - Would benefit from subspecialty involvement to include critical care or neonatologic and infectious disease, among others
- Regardless of age, patients who have known or suggested immunosuppression who contract herpes
  - May benefit from subspecialty consultation
- Ocular herpes should always be referred to an ophthalmologist.
  - Children in whom ocular steroid therapy is considered may benefit from ophthalmologic consultation to rule out possible ocular herpes infection.

COMPLICATIONS

- HSV-1
  - Certain human hosts are at more serious risk than others for contracting or developing severe disease.
  - Individuals who may be more likely to show serious disseminated disease are those who:
    - Have deficiencies in cell-mediated immunity
    - Are undergoing immunosuppressive therapy for cancer or transplantation
    - Are extremely malnourished
  - The inoculation of herpes into eczematous skin:
    - Can result in eczema herpeticum, which can vary in severity from mild to fatal
    - Constitutional symptoms are the rule, and temperatures of 39.4°C to 40.6°C may last for ≥1 week.
    - Wide areas of skin can become denuded.
    - Enormous fluid, protein, and electrolyte losses are potentially life threatening.
    - Secondary bacterial infection may complicate the condition.
    - Recurrences that are milder than the initial infection occur commonly on areas of the skin affected with chronic eczema.

H

PROGNOSIS

- Prognosis for the many syndromes of HSV has improved greatly with currently available therapies.
- Neonatal herpes
  - The National Institute of Allergy and Infectious Diseases Collaborative Antiviral Study Group classifies cases of neonatal HSV infection into 3 categories according to clinical manifestations.
    - Infants with disseminated disease involving visceral organs with or without CNS involvement
      - Most likely to die (>80% without treatment and 31% with high dose treatment)
      - Infants with HSV-1 disseminated infection have poorer outcomes than those with HSV-2 infection.
      - Hepatoadrenal necrosis is virtually always found.
      - Microcephaly, hydrocephalus, mental retardation, or seizures occur in many survivors.
    - Infants with CNS abnormalities without involvement of viscera
      - Without antiviral therapy, mortality exceeds 50% and morbidity exceeds 90%.
      - With appropriate antiviral therapy, mortality has decreased to 6%, but morbidity remains high.
    - Infants whose skin, eyes, or mouth (SEM) are involved but not the CNS or viscera.
      - Infants who had SEM involvement before antiviral drugs became available
        - Were not expected to die
        - Only 20–30% were left neurologically impaired.
        - However, many who appeared to have SEM involvement went on to develop disseminated or CNS involvement and to suffer disastrous consequences.
        - Classically, >50% of all neonatal HSV infections exhibited as disseminated disease, with only a minority classified as SEM involved.
      - As a result of earlier diagnosis and treatment:
        - 34% now have SEM involvement.
        - 32% have disseminated disease.
        - 34% have CNS disease.

PREVENTION

- Neonatal herpes
  - Stringent prenatal screening programs
    - Previously recommended to prevent HSV infection in offspring of women with recurrent genital herpes
    - Proved costly, impractical to administer, and medically ineffective
  - Current guidelines for managing labor in women with a history of genital herpes
    - History of genital HSV alone is not an indication for cesarean delivery.
    - Expeditious cesarean delivery is recommended if active genital lesions are present at the time of delivery and duration since rupture of membranes is <4–6 hours
    - Some advocate cesarean delivery if the canal is visibly infected, even when the rupture of membranes has been more prolonged.
    - Several studies demonstrated varied results on the rate of cesarean delivery caused by genital HSV at delivery, but they were underpowered to show an effect on HSV in the infants.
    - Scalp electrodes should be avoided when the mother is suspected of having active genital HSV infection.
  - Daily oral acyclovir has been shown to:
    - Suppress subclinical shedding of HSV-2 in the genital tract
    - Prevent clinical recurrences in pregnant women at delivery
  - Joint guidelines to decrease the likelihood of postpartum herpes infection in the infant (AAP and American College of Obstetricians and Gynecologists):
    - Specify isolation criteria to protect healthy infants from their HSV-infected mothers, other infected infants, or infected staff.

Hirsutism, Hypertrichosis, and Precocious Sexual Hair Development

DEFINITION

- Hirsutism: excessive body hair growth in the sex hormone–dependent areas
  - Represents androgen overproduction or enhanced androgen metabolism in the skin
- Hypertrichosis: generalized increase in fine body hair with no preferential sites
  - Usually not associated with pathologic sex hormone production
- Virilization, or masculinization, results from androgen overproduction manifested by:
  - Phallic or clitoral enlargement
  - Masculine body habitus
  - Temporal hair loss
  - Voice changes
  - Breast atrophy
  - Menstrual disorders
- Gonadarche: the maturation of the hypothalamic-pituitary-gonadal axis
- Adrenarche: the activation of the hypothalamic-pituitary-adrenal axis
- Precocious puberty
  - True (central) precocious puberty: early maturation of the hypothalamic-pituitary-gonadal axis
  - Peripheral precocious puberty: early production of sex steroids independent of an activated hypothalamic-pituitary-gonadal axis
    - In boys: from either the testes or the adrenals
    - In girls: from the ovaries, the adrenals, or both
- Adrenal hyperplasia: the histologic change that occurs in the adrenal glands as a result of a deficiency of 1 of the several enzymes necessary for normal steroid biosynthesis

MECHANISM

Excessive androgen exposure

- Prenatal exposure
  - In female infants, exposure to significant androgens during the first trimester (as in the congenital adrenal hyperplasia syndromes) causes genital ambiguity, including varying degrees of clitoral enlargement and labial fusion.
  - Exposure to excessive androgens after the first trimester results in clitoral enlargement, but not labial fusion.
  - Male infants exposed to excessive androgens in utero are not born with abnormal genitalia.
- Postnatal exposure
  - In the growing child, excessive androgens contribute to:
    - Increased growth velocity
    - Rapid epiphyseal maturation
    - Excessive bone age advancement
    - Short adult stature
- If the condition causing androgen overproduction is undiagnosed or inadequately treated, the child will:
  - Develop early sexual hair growth
  - Continue to virilize

Gonadarche

- Activation of the pulsatile release of gonadotropin-releasing hormone (GnRH) from the hypothalamus results in:
  - Increased amplitude and frequency of pituitary gonadotropin secretion
  - Gonadal maturation
- Pituitary luteinizing hormone stimulates ovarian androgen synthesis, occurring mainly in theca cells, stroma cells, and the corpus luteum.
- Levels of the major androgens (Δ-4-androstenedione and testosterone) secreted by the ovaries gradually increase during gonadarche.
  - These androgens contribute to the development of:
    - Pubic hair
    - Axillary hair and odor
    - Acne
- The ovary converts androgens to estrogen in the granulosa cell layer via stimulation from pituitary follicle-stimulating hormone.
  - Estrogens contribute to:
    - Breast development
    - Uterine enlargement
    - Vaginal discharge
    - Menarche
  - Puberty is characterized by an increase in growth velocity (pubertal growth spurt) that results from an increase in growth hormone secretion.

Peripheral precocious puberty

- Ovarian tumors producing androgens can cause early sexual hair growth, hirsutism, virilization, or polycystic ovary syndrome (PCOS).

Cortisol

- The most important of the glucocorticoids made by the adrenal gland
- Its synthesis is regulated primarily by a sensitive negative feedback system with pituitary adrenocorticotropic hormone (ACTH).
- Any condition that causes a decrease in cortisol biosynthesis results in a compensatory increase in ACTH.
- In enzymatic defects of cortisol biosynthesis, cortisol levels decrease.

- The compensatory increase in ACTH stimulates adrenal steroidogenesis, with the resultant accumulation of steroids proximal to the enzymatic defect.
  - These precursor steroids are then shunted to the androgen pathways, with resultant hyperandrogenism.
- 3 alleles are associated with the 21-hydroxylase locus.
  - Individuals may be:
    - Unaffected heterozygote carriers *or*
    - Affected, with classical or nonclassical disease
- Deficiency of the 11-ß-hydroxylase enzyme is characterized by sexual ambiguity in affected girls.
  - Inadequate therapy can result in early virilization.
  - The accumulation of deoxycorticosterone, a weak mineralocorticoid, eventually leads to low renin hypertension.
  - Milder forms of 11-ß-hydroxylase deficiency have been described and exhibit very similarly to the late-onset form of 21-hydroxylase deficiency.

PCOS

- The precise cause of chronic ovarian hyperandrogenism is not known.
- Several factors have been implicated.
  - Altered gonadotropin secretion
  - Hyperinsulinism
  - Insulin-like growth factor-1 and alterations of insulin-like growth factor-1–binding proteins
  - Hyperprolactinemia
  - Thyroid disease
  - Adrenal hyperandrogenism
- Evidence demonstrates a link between PCOS and inappropriate gonadotropin secretion, hyperinsulinemia, and impaired glucose tolerance (IGT) independent of weight.

Adrenal hyperandrogenism

- The adrenal glands produce:
  - Glucocorticoids (cortisol)
  - Mineralocorticoids (aldosterone and desoxycorticosterone)
  - Androgens (dehydroepiandrosterone, Δ-4-androstenedione, and testosterone)
- Glucocorticoid and androgen production are stimulated primarily by pituitary ACTH.
- Exogenous glucocorticoids, by suppressing ACTH, suppress glucocorticoid and androgen production.
- The mineralocorticoids are regulated primarily by the renin-angiotensin enzyme system, which is stimulated and suppressed by low- and high-salt diets, respectively.

HISTORY

- A family history should be obtained.
  - Families of patients with premature adrenarche and PCOS may have a history of cardiovascular disease, atherosclerosis, obesity, or diabetes.
  - A family history of early fetal demise suggests the presence of adrenal hyperplasia.
- Increase in growth velocity with crossing percentile channels suggests:
  - Precocious puberty
    - Sexual hair growth with early breast development is consistent with either central (true) or peripheral precocious puberty.
  - Tumor
  - Adrenal hyperplasia
- Abdominal symptoms (cramps, pain, mass, distention) suggest ovarian androgen-producing tumors.

PHYSICAL EXAM

- The rapid development of sexual hair associated with signs of virilization (eg, severe acne, voice changes, change in body habitus, clitoral or phallic enlargement, rapid growth) suggests marked hyperandrogenism.
  - Severe adrenal enzyme deficiencies
  - Adrenal or ovarian tumor
- Labial fusion indicates exposure to hyperandrogenism during fetal life, which occurs in the congenital adrenal hyperplasia syndromes.
- The presence of sexual hair growth with early breast development is consistent with either central or peripheral precocious puberty.
- Hypertension on physical examination may be caused by:
  - 11-hydroxylase deficiency
  - Adrenal tumor
  - Obesity
- Virilization indicates severe hyperandrogenism.
- Central precocious puberty
  - Clinically, girls have early development of pubic hair, axillary hair and odor, acne, and breast development.
  - Most commonly, breast development occurs initially, but sexual hair growth may precede breast development.
  - In boys, the increase in gonadotropins causes testicular growth and full physical pubertal development.
- Peripheral precocious puberty caused by ovarian androgen-producing tumors
  - The concurrent secretion of estrogen can result in premature breast development, vaginal discharge, or irregular uterine bleeding.
  - Patients may have excessive weight gain, acceleration of linear growth, and advanced bone age.

- PCOS may manifest, in addition to hirsutism, with:
  - Obesity
  - Acne
  - Hyperpigmentation in the intertriginal skin sites, known as *acanthosis nigricans*
  - Male pattern baldness
- Adrenal hyperandrogenism
  - Premature adrenarche
    - Adrenarche in girls before the age of 8 years and in boys before the age of 9 years
    - These children display early sexual hair growth, usually limited to the axillary and pubic areas.
    - The presence of facial, abdominal, or back hair is not consistent with this syndrome.
    - Affected children may develop mildly oily skin and minimal acne, especially on the nose and forehead.
    - Axillary odor is common and generally requires deodorant.
    - Children with premature adrenarche are never virilized; the presence of virilization suggests either a tumor or an enzymatic defect of steroidogenesis.
    - The child's growth velocity may increase slightly.
    - Bone-age maturation may advance but generally stays within 2 years of the chronologic age.
    - Androgen levels are in the range typical of the early Tanner II–III stages of puberty.
  - Enzymatic effects of steroidogenesis
    - Specific symptoms depend on which class of steroids is deficient or overproduced.
    - 21-hydroxylase deficiency
      - Severe salt-wasting form
        - Prenatal exposure of the genetic female external genitalia to the high androgens in the first trimester causes genital ambiguity.
        - Boys with similar exposure do not have genital abnormalities.
        - Children of either sex will develop salt-wasting symptoms, generally within the first 3 months of life.
      - Simple virilizing form
        - The genetic female child is born with genital ambiguity.
        - The genetic male child appears normal.
      - In either form of 21-hydroxylase deficiency, delay in diagnosis or inadequate treatment results in postnatal virilization.
        - Progressive clitoral and phallic enlargement
        - Early development of axillary and pubic hair, axillary odor, and acne
        - Increased growth velocity

- Advanced bone age
- Precocious puberty
- Short adult stature
  - Young women inadequately treated will develop PCOS along with its associated menstrual irregularities and infertility.
- Variable signs and symptoms of hyperandrogenism are common to both types of the disorder.
  - Hirsutism
  - Acne
  - Virilization of the external genitalia or the body
  - Short stature
  - Menstrual irregularities
- The nonclassical late-onset form of 21-hydroxylase deficiency has clinical variability.
  - Symptoms of hyperandrogenism can develop at any age.
  - Affected girls do not have genital ambiguity.
  - The spectrum of symptoms includes:
    - Premature pubic and axillary hair growth
    - Premature axillary odor
    - Acne
    - Increased growth velocity and advanced bone age
    - Hirsutism
    - Male-pattern baldness in young women
    - PCOS
- 11-ß-hydroxylase enzyme deficiency
  - Characterized by sexual ambiguity in affected girls
  - As with 21-hydroxylase deficiency, inadequate therapy can result in early virilization.
- Idiopathic hirsutism or acne
  - Girls who have these signs have no other signs of androgen excess and normal circulating androgen concentrations.
  - Menses and reproductive function are normal.
  - Hirsutism and acne in these women have been attributed to "increased peripheral metabolism" of androgens.

DIFFERENTIAL DIAGNOSIS

Central (true) precocious puberty

- In most cases, not caused by a specific identifiable lesion
  - A hypothalamic or pituitary lesion may be the cause of early puberty, especially in a child <6 years.
- May be associated with:
  - Astrocytoma
  - Craniopharyngioma
  - Ependymoma
  - Germinoma
  - Glioma

- Hypothalamic hamartoma
- Virtually any central nervous system (CNS) insult
  - Trauma
  - Surgery
  - Inflammation
  - Neurologic or mental deficits
- Prolonged exposure to sex steroids

Peripheral precocious puberty

- Ovarian androgen-producing tumors
  - Symptoms can mimic true precocious puberty in the young child.
  - Rapid pubertal progression suggests the presence of a tumor, but not all ovarian tumors affect pubertal progression.
  - A markedly elevated estradiol, androstenedione, or testosterone level is consistent with an ovarian lesion.
  - In contrast to central precocious puberty, peripheral precocious puberty resulting from an ovarian tumor occurs independently of the hypothalamic-pituitary axis.
- Androgen-producing cells can occur in association with:
  - Embryonal carcinoma
  - Dysgerminoma
  - Choriocarcinoma
  - Gonadoblastoma
  - Granulosa-theca cell tumor
  - Sertoli-Leydig cell tumor
  - Arrhenoblastoma
  - These tumors can occur in phenotypic girls who have an abnormal karyotype containing components of the Y chromosome.

PCOS

- Ovarian hyperandrogenism can occur in certain insulin-resistant syndromes.
  - Leprechaunism (associated with severe congenital growth retardation)
  - Kahn type B insulin resistance syndrome caused by the presence of circulating antibodies for the insulin receptor

Testicular androgen production

- Central (true) precocious puberty
  - CNS disease in boys
  - Rarely, associated with severe chronic hypothyroidism

Testicular tumors

- Leydig cell tumors and seminomas can produce testosterone.
- However, many testicular tumors can cause testicular enlargement without symptoms of hyperandrogenism (eg, embryonal carcinoma, endodermal sinus tumor, and teratoma).
- Boys with cryptorchidism and delayed orchiopexy after the age of 6 years are at increased risk.

- Dysgenetic gonads associated with androgen insensitivity, persistent müllerian syndrome, true hermaphroditism, and Klinefelter syndrome have a higher incidence of germ cell tumors as well.

Chorionic gonadotropin-secreting tumors

- Teratomas, embryonal tumors, hepatoblastomas, and CNS germinomas can produce human chorionic gonadotropin, which has been implicated in peripheral precocious puberty among male patients.

Adrenal hyperandrogenism

- Premature adrenarche may be associated with:
  - Functional ovarian hyperandrogenism
  - ACTH-stimulated androgens >2 standard deviations above the mean for normal Tanner II–III pubertal girls
  - Association among acanthosis nigricans, hyperinsulinism stemming from insulin resistance, and hyperandrogenism in adolescent and adult women with PCOS
  - Marked insulin resistance is associated with more severe hyperandrogenism, with an exaggerated increase Δ5 steroids in response to ACTH stimulation.
  - Hyperinsulinism, possibly exacerbated by obesity
  - Minority children are known to be at increased risk for the complications of hyperinsulinism.

Drug-related hirsutism and hypertrichosis

- Hirsutism may result from use of:
  - Anabolic steroids
  - Danazol (Danocrine)
  - Metoclopramide (Reglan)
  - Methyldopa (Aldomet)
  - Phenothiazines
  - Progestins
  - Reserpine (Serpasil)
  - Testosterone
- Hypertrichosis may be caused by:
  - Cyclosporine (Sandimmune)
  - Diazoxide (Hyperstat)
  - Hydrocortisone
  - Minoxidil (Rogaine)
  - Penicillamine (Cuprimine)
  - Phenytoin (Dilantin)
  - Psoralens (Oxsoralen)
  - Streptomycin
- Idiopathic hirsutism or acne
  - Girls with these signs have no other signs of androgen excess and normal circulating androgen concentrations.
  - Menses and reproductive function are normal.
  - Hirsutism and acne in these women have been attributed to "increased peripheral metabolism" of androgens.

LABORATORY EVALUATION

- For a summary laboratory findings and recommended additional testing for hirsutism, see the table Causes of Hirsutism, Associated Laboratory Findings, and Recommended Additional Testing.

Precocious puberty

- GnRH stimulation test to distinguish central from peripheral sexual precocity
- ACTH stimulation test
  - If ACTH testing is consistent with an enzymatic defect in the virilized patient, the nonmalignant nature of the condition should be confirmed by suppression of hyperandrogenism with dexamethasone.
- The presence of virilization or high levels of testosterone (>150 ng/dL) or of dehydroepiandrosterone sulfate (>750 mcg/dL) suggests an ovarian or adrenal tumor.

Karyotype

- If an ovarian tumor is suspected

Central (true) precocious puberty

- Pubertal gonadotropin response to a GnRH stimulation test confirms diagnosis.

Ovarian androgen-producing tumors

- A GnRH stimulation test can distinguish these tumors from central precocious puberty.

- The gonadotropin response is suppressed in peripheral precocious puberty.

PCOS

- Compared with age-matched controls, women with PCOS have an 11-fold increase in the prevalence of metabolic syndrome.
- The risk of metabolic syndrome is high even at a young age, highlighting the importance of early and regular screening.
- 33% of adolescent girls with PCOS have abnormal oral glucose tolerance tests indicating IGT or type 2 diabetes mellitus.
- Insulin resistance can be confirmed by fasting hyperinsulinism and a reduced fasting glucose/insulin ratio or an increased homeostatic model assessment.
- Glucose tolerance test is the most reliable screening test for these conditions in girls with PCOS and can detect IGT or type 2 diabetes mellitus.
- Hormonal evidence of PCOS
  - Luteinizing hormone/follicle-stimulating hormone ratio >2
  - Generous levels of Δ-4-androstenedione
  - Increased total and free testosterone with a reduced level of sex hormone–binding globulin
  - Variable levels of estradiol
- Total testosterone level >150 ng/dL suggests the presence of a tumor.

Causes of Hirsutism, Associated Laboratory Findings, and Recommended Additional Testing

Diagnosis	Testosterone	17-OHP	LH/FSH Ratio	Prolactin	DHEAS	Cortisol	Additional Testing
Congenital adrenal hyperplasia	Normal to increased	Increased	Normal	Normal	Normal to increased	Normal to decreased	ACTH stimulation may be necessary to make the diagnosis
Polycystic ovary syndrome	Normal to increased	Normal	Normal to increased LH and decreased to normal FSH	Normal to increased	Normal to increased	Normal	Primarily a clinical diagnosis; consider laboratory testing and ultrasonography of ovaries to rule out other disorders or tumors; consider screening for the metabolic syndrome with lipids, glucose, oral glucose tolerance test
	Increased free testosterone						
	Decreased SHBG						
Ovarian tumor	Increased	Normal	Suppressed/30 suppressed	Normal	Normal	Normal	Ultrasonography or CT to image tumors

Abbreviations: ACTH, adrenocorticotropic hormone; CT, computed tomography; DHEAS, dehydroepiandrosterone; FSH, follicle-stimulating hormone; LH, luteinizing hormone; OHP, hydroxyprogesterone; SHBG, sex hormone–binding globulin.

Testicular androgen production

- In central (true) precocious puberty, levels of testosterone increase and a pubertal pattern of gonadotropin release can be detected with a GnRH stimulation test.
- In familial gonadotropin-independent puberty, boys who clinically have precocious puberty have high testosterone levels and low GnRH-stimulated gonadotropin levels.

Adrenal hyperandrogenism

- Disorders of adrenal hyperandrogenism caused by enzymatic defects of steroidogenesis (congenital adrenal hyperplasia) respond to stimulation and suppression tests.
- Functional adrenal tumors
  - Characterized by their ability to produce steroids independently of pituitary ACTH or the renin-angiotensin enzyme system
  - As a rule, do not respond to the dynamic tests known to affect adrenal steroidogenesis
- Premature adrenarche
  - The increase in adrenal androgen production can be detected at approximately 6 years.
  - As puberty progresses, an ACTH stimulation test detects the gradual increase in androgen levels.
- 3 autosomal-recessive disorders of adrenal steroidogenesis cause cortisol deficiency and hyperandrogenism.
  - 21-Hydroxylase deficiency
    - Molecular genetic studies have identified the responsible gene: *CYP21A2.*
    - Currently, an affected fetus can be identified by chorionic villus sampling between the 8th and 11th week of gestation.
    - 21-Hydroxylase deficiency is confirmed by an elevated 17-hydroxyprogesterone level.
    - A nonclassical late-onset form of 21-hydroxylase deficiency has clinical variability and symptoms of hyperandrogenism can develop at any age.
      - Because the hyperandrogenism in this form of 21-hydroxylase deficiency is not as severe as the classical form, the basal unstimulated 17-hydroxyprogesterone level may not be elevated.
      - The diagnosis is confirmed by an exaggerated 17-hydroxyprogesterone response to ACTH stimulation.
  - 11-ß-Hydroxylase deficiency
    - The diagnosis is made by an elevated 11-deoxycortisol that is stimulated by ACTH and suppressed by dexamethasone.
  - 3-ß-Hydroxysteroid dehydrogenase deficiency
    - The diagnosis is confirmed by finding elevated precursor steroids either in the basal state or in response to a bolus dose of ACTH.

IMAGING

- Central (true) precocious puberty
  - Evaluation should include magnetic resonance imaging with gadolinium contrast of the hypothalamic-pituitary area.
  - A bone-age radiograph can help identify the child who is at risk for short stature.
  - Early production of sex steroids can cause rapid epiphyseal maturation and result in short stature.
- Peripheral precocious puberty
  - Ovarian androgen-producing tumors
    - Pelvic ultrasonography can be useful in identifying cystic or solid ovarian lesions.
- PCOS
  - The ovaries in PCOS have subcapsular cysts that may be detected by ultrasonography.
  - The absence of cysts on ultrasonography does not exclude PCOS.
  - Hormonal evidence of PCOS can be discerned before morphologic changes can be seen on ultrasonography.
  - Ultrasonography should be performed if an ovarian lesion is suspected.

TREATMENT APPROACH

- For mild hirsutism, local measures, such as shaving, bleaching, depilatories, and electrolysis
- Weight loss
  - Obese patients should be encouraged to lose weight.
- Very few pharmacologic agents are approved by the US Food and Drug Administration for hirsutism.
  - Response to these agents is slow.
  - They often are used with local cosmetic options.

SPECIFIC TREATMENT

PCOS

- Oral contraceptives
  - Decrease circulating androgens in patients with PCOS
  - Synergize with the effects of antiandrogens, such as spironolactone
- Metformin
  - Adolescents with PCOS are severely insulin resistant compared with a control group matched for body composition and abdominal obesity.
  - The use of metformin in girls with PCOS has been reported to:
    - Improve insulin sensitivity
    - Reduce ACTH-stimulated androgens

- Metformin has been reported to prevent development of PCOS symptoms in prepubertal and adolescent girls with premature pubarche and a history of low birth weight.

Central (true) precocious puberty

- Long-acting preparations of GnRH (GnRH analogue)
  - For children whose parents are particularly concerned about the psychosocial issues surrounding early sexual development or the risk for short stature
  - GnRH analogues are effective in halting pubertal progression in girls and boys and preventing menses in girls.
  - Reduction in growth hormone secretion causes the child's growth velocity to decline.
  - The reduction in sex steroids either halts or reduces the rate of bone-age maturation.
  - The net result is an improvement in predicted height and, ultimately, adult stature.

Peripheral precocious puberty

- Ovarian androgen-producing tumors
  - Because dysgenetic gonads, in which differentiation into testis or ovary is either absent or incomplete, are at risk for malignant deterioration, prophylactic gonadectomy is recommended in these girls.

Enzymatic effects of steroidogenesis

- The goal of early diagnosis and treatment is to prevent genital ambiguity in the affected female fetus.
  - Prenatal treatment with dexamethasone should be instituted by 6–7 weeks of gestation (before prenatal diagnosis is possible) to be effective in preventing virilization in female fetuses with congenital adrenal hyperplasia.
  - Preventive therapy is controversial because many unaffected fetuses would be treated prenatally with dexamethasone.

21-Hydroxylase deficiency

- Treatment includes glucocorticoid replacement therapy as hydrocortisone at a dose of 10–25 mg/m² daily to maintain:
  - Normal growth and development
  - Normal rate of bone-age advancement
- Salt-wasting variant
  - Treated with the salt-retaining steroid 9-α fludrocortisone acetate
    - Sometimes useful with elevated plasma renin activity

11-ß-Hydroxylase and 3-ß-hydroxysteroid dehydrogenase deficiency

- Treatment is similar to that for 21-hydroxylase deficiency, with glucocorticoid replacement.

WHEN TO REFER

- Pubic hair, axillary hair, or axillary odor before 8 years of age in girls and 9 years of age in boys

- Breast development, vaginal discharge, or menses in girls before 8 years of age
- Increased facial or body hair (chest, abdomen, back) in girls with or without menstrual irregularities
- Signs of virilization in girls (clitoromegaly, masculine body habitus, voice changes) or in boys (phallic enlargement, change in body habitus, voice change) before the age of 9 years
- Rapid virilization (<1 year) in a pubertal boy

WHEN TO ADMIT

- Severe hypertension with precocious sexual development
  - 11-hydroxylase deficiency
  - Adrenal tumor
- Severe anemia secondary to vaginal bleeding
  - Ovarian cyst
  - Dysfunctional uterine bleeding
- Any suspicion of sexual abuse
- Severe headaches, visual loss, change in mental status
  - Increased intracranial pressure associated with CNS lesion
- Hypotension or shock
  - Addison disease secondary to ACTH deficiency
  - Pituitary apoplexy secondary to a bleed into a pituitary lesion
- Marked hyperglycemia requiring insulin
  - Type 2 diabetes mellitus
  - PCOS
- Severe abdominal pain (torsion of ovarian cyst)

FOLLOW-UP

- Children with hirsutism, hypertrichosis, and precocious sexual hair development need to be followed carefully to monitor the response to the therapy or progression of pubertal changes, because this may lead to short stature.

COMPLICATIONS

- Girls with precocious pubarche who had low birth weight are at high risk for a variant of PCOS even if they are not obese.
  - Hyperinsulinemic hyperandrogenism
  - Dyslipidemia
  - Dysadipocytokinemia
  - Central fat excess
  - Deficit of lean body mass

PROGNOSIS

- Prognosis for children with hirsutism, hypertrichosis, and precocious sexual hair development depends on the underlying conditions leading to these physical findings, early appropriate evaluation, and appropriate treatment.

H

HIV Infection and AIDS

DEFINITION

- Acquired immunodeficiency syndrome (AIDS) results from progressive immune dysfunction after infection with the human immunodeficiency virus (HIV).
- 2 separate HIV viruses have been identified.
  - HIV-1 is the predominant virus responsible for disease in the US and rest of the world.
  - HIV-2 is primarily detected in patients in West Africa.
- Clinical manifestations of HIV infection range from asymptomatic infection to debilitating disease and death.

EPIDEMIOLOGY

- Prevalence
  - In 2006 approximately 10,000 children <13 years were living with AIDS in the US.
  - Acquisition of HIV through adult behaviors is increasing.
    - AIDS in young adults reflects acquisition of HIV during adolescence.
- Transmission
  - Perinatal transmission is the most common mode of acquisition of HIV infection among children in the US.
  - Before the availability of antiretroviral chemotherapy to prevent perinatal HIV transmission, intrapartum transmission was the most common mode of transmission.
  - Before widespread use of antiretroviral prophylaxis, as many as 1800 HIV-infected children were born in the US annually.
    - Now, <50 infants are diagnosed with HIV in the US each year.
  - Not all infants born to HIV-infected women acquire HIV infection.
    - Estimated perinatal transmission rates from untreated women to infants range from 13–30%.
- Geographic distribution
  - The great burden of pediatric HIV infection is in resource-poor countries of Africa and Asia.

ETIOLOGY

- Prepubertal children most commonly acquire HIV infection through maternal-infant transmission.
  - Rarely, they may be infected through:
    - Receipt of infected blood or blood products
    - Sexual abuse
- Perinatal HIV transmission can occur by 3 mechanisms.
  - Transplacental infection in utero
  - Intrapartum infection during labor and delivery
  - Postpartum infection through mother's milk

- Perinatal HIV infection occurs during the development and maturation of the immune system.
  - This distinguishes pediatric HIV infection from adult infection and has profound effects on the:
    - Clinical course
    - Nature
    - Timing of opportunistic infections and immune responses to immunizations
- A substantial number of adolescents contract HIV through adult behaviors.
  - Unprotected sexual activities
  - Intravenous drug use
- HIV transmission through sexual contact occurs in:
  - Children who are sexually abused
  - Sexually active adolescents

RISK FACTORS

- High maternal plasma HIV levels correlate with increased risk of transmission.
- Women with advanced HIV disease or recently acquired infection are more likely to transmit HIV to newborns.
- Receipt of blood
  - Routine testing of blood donors for HIV antibody began in March 1985.
  - Children who received blood or blood products before this time were at risk.
  - Children with hemophilia were at particularly high risk because they received pooled factors from hundreds to thousands of donors.
  - Risk of HIV infection from blood or blood products is now estimated to be 1 in 2 million from a single unit of blood.
- Behaviors that place adolescents at high risk of HIV infection are:
  - Initiation of sexual activity at a young age
  - Unprotected sexual intercourse
- Risk factors are associated with HIV infection in women of childbearing age include:
  - Illicit drug use
  - Sexual contact with persons at high risk

SIGNS AND SYMPTOMS

Diagnosis of HIV/AIDS

- Clinical manifestations range from asymptomatic infection to debilitating disease and death.
- In children, the time from infection to onset of clinical symptoms may be shorter:
  - For those who have perinatally acquired infection than for those infected through blood or blood products
  - Than for adults

- Frequently asymptomatic
  - Infected infants in the neonatal period
    - Most with untreated perinatal HIV infection develop symptoms by 2 years of age.
  - Other children may have no or few symptoms for many years.
- Early clinical signs and symptoms of HIV infection are nonspecific but generally indicate a systemic illness.
  - Children may exhibit:
    - Failure to thrive
    - Developmental delay
    - Persistent oral candidiasis
    - Lymphadenopathy
    - Hepatosplenomegaly
    - Chronic diarrhea
    - Recurrent bacterial infections
    - Recurrent herpesvirus infections
- Delayed acquisition of developmental milestones and loss of previously acquired milestones are common manifestations.
  - Growth failure is common early in the course of disease.
  - Frequent measurements of weight and height are important in:
    - Detecting growth disturbances early
    - Monitoring response to interventions

Diagnosing illness in HIV-infected children

- Most HIV-infected children with fever and normal clinical examination have self-limited febrile illnesses similar to those of non-HIV-infected children.
  - Fever may indicate a serious infection.
  - Persistent fever can be a diagnostic challenge; identifiable and treatable causes include mycobacterial infection and drug-induced fever.
  - Detailed clinical history and thorough physical examination is essential in the initial assessment.
  - Close attention should be paid to general appearance and potential areas of focal inflammation, such as:
    - Skin
    - Ears
    - Sinuses
    - Lungs
    - Gastrointestinal tract
  - Bacteremia with *Streptococcus pneumoniae* and *Salmonella* can occur in the absence of physical findings.
- Additional diagnostic studies should be obtained on the basis:
  - Child's age
  - Clinical appearance
  - Degree of immunosuppression
  - Signs and symptoms at the time that the patient seeks care

- Primary HIV infection in adolescents and adults is frequently accompanied by a mononucleosis-like illness characterized by:
  - Fever
  - Sore throat
  - Lethargy
  - Lymphadenopathy (seroconversion syndrome)
- See Complications for more information on secondary and opportunistic infections.

DIAGNOSTIC APPROACH

- The most important factor in identifying HIV-infected women and children is consideration of the diagnosis.
  - Absence of identifiable risk factors does not exclude HIV infection.

LABORATORY FINDINGS

- The number of copies of HIV RNA in plasma can be quantified.
  - Given that HIV is an obligate intracellular parasite, virus in the plasma is a replicating virus looking for a new host cell.
  - Plasma HIV RNA levels are useful in:
    - Predicting the rate of disease progression
    - Modifying antiretroviral therapy
    - Understanding viral dynamics
  - In children with perinatally acquired HIV, HIV RNA levels peak in the first few months of life and decline slowly over several years.
  - Steady-state HIV RNA levels in children are not achieved until 2–6 years of age.
  - HIV RNA levels in adults decrease rapidly to steady-state levels within several months after primary infection.
  - Despite this decrease in HIV RNA level, intense viral replication continues.
- Infection with HIV leads to a progressive decrease in CD4+ T lymphocytes.
  - Qualitative changes in function of CD4+ T lymphocytes occur before the decrease in number.
  - CD4+ T lymphocytes are crucial to B-lymphocyte function; thus, humoral immunity (antibody production) can be significantly impaired in HIV-infected children.
    - Results in poor antibody responses to encapsulated bacteria and immunizations, despite increase in total immunoglobulins
- Detection of HIV DNA or RNA by polymerase chain reaction (PCR) is the preferred method for diagnosing HIV infection in infants.
  - PCR amplifies HIV DNA or RNA sequences and is extremely sensitive in detecting small amounts of virus.

H

- Almost all HIV-infected infants have a positive HIV PCR result by 1 month of age; 40% can be identified in the first 2 days of life.
- False-positive results occur on rare occasions because of laboratory contamination.
- Positive results should be confirmed by PCR testing of a second blood specimen.
- Early detection of HIV infection allows for initiation of combination antiretroviral therapy in infancy.
  - HIV-exposed infants should be tested by 48 hours of age.
    - A positive PCR result at 48 hours of age suggests intrauterine infection.
- If negative, PCR testing should be repeated at 14 day.
  - >90% of infected infants will have a positive PCR result by 2 weeks of age.
- Infants negative for HIV by PCR at 48 hours and at 14 days:
  - Should be tested at 1–2 months of age
  - Again at 3–6 months of age if previously negative
- HIV infection is diagnosed by 2 positive HIV PCR tests performed on separate blood samples.
- 2 negative PCR results, one performed at 1–2 months of age and the other at 4–6 months of age, make the diagnosis of HIV infection extremely unlikely.
- The Centers for Disease Control and Prevention (CDC) is considering a modification of this schedule for diagnosis.

- The HIV enzyme immunosorbent assay (ELISA) detects antibody to HIV and is appropriate for screening children >18 months of age.
  - HIV ELISA has high sensitivity but lacks specificity.
  - Positive ELISA reactions for HIV are confirmed by Western blot analysis, which detects antibodies to several HIV proteins and is highly specific.
    - False-negative results may occur shortly after primary infection because antibodies to HIV do not achieve detectable levels until 2–3 months after infection.
  - Serologic methods should not be used to confirm HIV infection in children <18 months.
    - Transplacentally derived maternal antibodies result in a positive HIV ELISA with HIV-seropositive mothers, even if the child is not infected.
  - Maternal antibodies can persist for 18 months.
- Laboratory abnormalities often include:
- Anemia
- Thrombocytopenia
- Increased immunoglobulin levels
- Laboratory tests to be considered include:
- Complete blood count with differential, large-volume blood culture
- Urinalysis and urine culture
- Lumbar puncture

- Because HIV antibodies take several months to achieve detectable levels, nucleic acid–based assays (PCR) should be used to diagnose symptomatic primary HIV infection.

IMAGING

- Radiography
  - *Pneumocystic (carinii) jiroveci* pneumonia (PCP) is most commonly characterized by diffuse alveolar infiltrates.
  - Early in the course of PCP in older children, the radiograph may be normal or show minimal changes despite significant cough and even hypoxia.
  - In bilateral lymphoid interstitial pneumonitis (LIP), reticulonodular densities are seen, resembling miliary tuberculosis.
- Computed tomography
  - Characteristic central nervous system findings include cerebral atrophy and basal ganglia calcifications.
  - Initial diagnostic studies often include brain imaging.

DIAGNOSTIC PROCEDURES

- HIV-infected children with pulmonary disease who fail to respond to empirical antibiotic therapy, those who are severely ill, and those who are suspected of having PCP should undergo an invasive diagnostic procedure, such as:
  - Bronchoscopy with bronchoalveolar lavage
  - Lung biopsy
- Persistent diarrhea
  - Endoscopy should be considered in refractory cases.
- Initial diagnostic studies of bacterial and viral pathogens may include analysis of cerebrospinal fluid.

CLASSIFICATION

- CDC immunologic categories based on age-specific CD4+ T lymphocyte count and percentage of total lymphocytes
  - No evidence of suppression
    - <1 year: ≥1500 mcL, ≥25%
    - 1–5 years: ≥1000 mcL, ≥25%
    - 6–12 years: ≥500 mcL, 25%
  - Evidence of moderate suppression
    - <1 year: 750–1499 mcL, 15–24%
    - 1–5 years: 500–999 mcL, 15–24%
    - 6–12 years: 200–499 mcL, 15–24%
  - Severe suppression
    - <1 year: <750 mcL, <15%
    - 1–5 years: <500 mcL, <15%
    - 6–12 years: <200 mcL, <15%

- CDC clinical categories of HIV classification in children
  - N: No signs or symptoms
    - N1: No evidence of suppression
    - N2: Evidence of moderate suppression
    - N3: Severe suppression
  - A: Mild signs or symptoms
    - A1: No evidence of suppression
    - A2: Evidence of moderate suppression
    - A3: Severe suppression
  - B: Moderate signs or symptoms
    - B1: No evidence of suppression
    - B2: Evidence of moderate suppression
    - B3: Severe suppression
  - C: Severe signs or symptoms
    - C1: No evidence of suppression
    - C2: Evidence of moderate suppression
    - C3: Severe suppression

TREATMENT APPROACH

- Care of HIV-infected children is complex and requires a multidisciplinary team including:
  - Pediatricians
  - Experts in antiretroviral therapy
  - Nutritionists
  - Physical therapists
  - Pharmacists
  - Psychologists
  - Social workers
  - Outreach workers
- A cure remains elusive.
- Effective antiretroviral therapy, with suppression of viral replication and nutritional supplementation, is important to maintaining growth.
  - Supplementation with high-calorie foods or formulas often results in increased body fat rather than lean body weight.
- Effective antiretroviral therapy can minimize or reverse the neurocognitive effects of HIV infection.
- Management of antiretroviral therapy should be directed by a specialist who has knowledge of:
  - Mechanisms of action of antiretroviral agents
  - Potential toxicities
  - Drug interactions
  - Cross-resistance patterns
- Currently available antiretroviral therapy works by interfering with the functions of these enzymes:
  - Nucleoside and nonnucleoside reverse transcriptase inhibitors

- Protease inhibitors
- Entry inhibitors
- Integrase inhibitors

- Most children acquire HIV infection during or near the time of birth, and antiretroviral therapy should be initiated in infancy.
  - Risks of drug toxicity and acquisition of drug-resistant virus are increased.
  - Decisions to initiate early therapy require balancing the benefits and risks.
  - Combination antiretroviral therapy is recommended for all infants in whom HIV infection is diagnosed in the first year of life, regardless of clinical, immunologic, or virologic status.
- For children in whom infection is diagnosed after 12 months of age, the decision to start treatment should be based on:
  - Clinical symptoms
  - Plasma HIV RNA level
  - CD4+ T lymphocyte count
- Combination therapy with reverse transcriptase and protease inhibitors block HIV replication and can result in:
  - Dramatic decline in virus production
  - Undetectable plasma HIV RNA levels

SPECIFIC TREATMENTS

Antiretroviral therapy

- The choice of antiretroviral regimen for children is based on several factors, including:
  - Availability of pediatric formulations
  - Potential drug interactions
  - Frequency of drug dosing
  - Potential interactions with other medications
- Before therapy begins, the child's clinical, virologic, immunologic, and nutritional status should be documented.
  - Neuropsychometric testing should be performed in children with deficits.
  - Baseline laboratory studies should include:
    - Complete blood count with differential
    - Liver function tests
    - CD4+ T lymphocyte count
    - Plasma HIV RNA level
- Combination antiretroviral therapy consists of a protease inhibitor or nonnucleoside reverse transcriptase inhibitor in combination with ≥2 nucleoside reverse transcriptase inhibitors.
  - Protease inhibitors that may be used in children include:
    - Lopinavir/ritonavir (preferred)
    - Nelfinavir
    - Ritonavir (alone)

– Amprenavir

– Indinavir

- Preferred combinations of nucleoside reverse transcriptase inhibitors are:
  – Zidovudine plus either lamivudine or emtricitabine
  – Zidovudine plus didanosine
  – Didanosine plus either lamivudine or emtricitabine
- Alternative combinations that have been less well studied in children are:
  – Abacavir plus zidovudine
  – Abacavir plus either lamivudine or emtricitabine
  – Stavudine plus either lamivudine or emtricitabine
- Stavudine and didanosine should not be used or should be used with substantial caution because of potential synergistic toxicities.
- Several combinations are not recommended because of antagonism (stavudine-zidovudine) or because of overlapping toxicities.
- Nonnucleoside reverse transcriptase inhibitors (nevirapine, delavirdine, and efavirenz) can be used in combination with nucleoside reverse transcriptase inhibitors.
- Protease inhibitors with insufficient data in children to recommend at this time
  – Atazanavir
  – Darunavir
  – Fosamprenavir
  – Tipranavir
  – Saquinavir
- Plasma HIV RNA levels should be measured 4 weeks after the child has started therapy to assess response.

Side effects

- Common side effects of nucleoside reverse transcriptase inhibitors are:
  - Anemiaand neutropenia with zidovudine
  - Pancreatitis with didanosine
  - Peripheral neuropathy with didanosine and stavudine
  - Influenza-like hypersensitivity reaction with abacavir
    – Rechallenge with abacavir can be fatal.
- Common side effects of the nonnucleoside reverse transcriptase inhibitors nevirapine, delavirdine, and efavirenzare:
  - Rashes
  - Hepatitis
- Side effects of efavirenz
  - Bad dreams
  - Hallucinations
  - Confusion
  - Impaired concentration

- Side effects of protease inhibitors are gastrointestinal symptoms.
- Long-term complications of combination antiretroviral therapy include:
  - Lipoatrophy
  - Lipodystrophy
  - Hypercholesterolemia
  - Bone demineralization

Compliance

- Compliance to complex drug regimens is hindered by:
  - Large number or volume of medications
  - Poor palatability
  - Varied dosing schedules
  - Different effects of food on drug bioavailability
- Mixing drugs with foods, such as peanut butter or ice cream, may improve compliance in children.
- Behavioral therapy, begun before combination therapy is initiated, can be helpful in:
  - Designing a routine medication schedule
  - Teaching parents and caregivers methods to improve compliance
  - Teaching the child techniques for swallowing unsavory medications
- Gastric tubes may be necessary to ensure medication compliance in children who are not adherent because of medication taste or volume.
- Strict adherence to the treatment regimen is essential for the prevention of drug resistance.
  - Because of cross-resistance, resistance to 1 drug can limit effectiveness of other drugs of the same class.
  - Viral sequences obtained from plasma samples can be tested for:
    – Drug resistance mutations
    – Susceptibility profiles

Drug interactions

- HIV protease inhibitors, as well as the nonnucleoside reverse transcriptase inhibitors, are metabolized in the liver by a cytochrome P450 enzyme.
  - Protease inhibitors can inhibit this enzyme and interfere with the metabolism of many other drugs.
  - Protease inhibitors can act as potent inhibitors of 2 other P450 enzymes active in the metabolism of analgesics: ß-blockers and phenytoin.
  - Ritonavir can stimulate glucuronidation, thus decreasing concentration of drugs metabolized by this pathway, including sedatives (such as lorazepam) and the narcotics morphine and codeine.

- Many drugs that have altered metabolism because of protease inhibitors are used in pediatric emergencies, including narcotic analgesics, anticonvulsants, antiarrhythmics, calcium-channel blockers, and corticosteroids.
  - These drugs should be used with caution in children receiving protease inhibitors.
  - Drugs that have narrow therapeutic margins require careful monitoring for adverse effects and measurement of drug concentrations.
- Drugs contraindicated for use with protease inhibitors include:
  - Meperidine
  - Midazolam
  - Astemizole
  - Terfenadine
  - Cisapride
  - Rifampin
- Other medications frequently prescribed for HIV-infected children are inhibitors of cytochrome P450 enzymes, including:
  - Ketoconazole
  - Itraconazole
  - Clarithromycin
  - Erythromycin
- Dose reduction of protease inhibitor may be required because inhibition of cytochrome P450 enzymes by these medications may lead to increase in the plasma concentration of protease inhibitors.
- Inducers of the cytochrome P450 enzyme system are frequently prescribed for HIV-infected children, including:
  - Antimycobacterial drugs (rifampin, rifabutin)
  - Anticonvulsants (phenobarbital, phenytoin, carbamazepine)
  - Glucocorticoids (dexamethasone)
- Increased metabolism of protease inhibitors may result in subtherapeutic levels, with the potential emergence of drug resistance.

PCP

- Before widespread prophylaxis for PCP and early antiretroviral therapy, a subset of HIV-infected children had rapidly progressive disease and died within the first year of life, frequently of PCP.
- Empirical antibiotic therapy depends on the results of clinical assessment and laboratory tests, and likelihood of adequate monitoring.
  - A third-generation cephalosporin, such as ceftriaxone or cefotaxime, can be used against both gram-positive and gram-negative bacteria.
- PCP should be treated early, usually with co-trimoxazole and corticosteroids.

Varicella and herpes zoster

- HIV-infected children who are susceptible to varicella (no prior natural infection or age-appropriate varicella immunization) should receive:
  - Varicella-zoster immunoglobulin preparation within 96 hours of exposure to varicella *or*
  - Intravenous immunoglobulin, if varicella-zoster immunoglobulin is not available
- Disseminated infection can occur with herpes zoster, and oral or parenteral therapy with acyclovir is warranted.

WHEN TO ADMIT

- Ill-appearing children should be hospitalized.

WHEN TO REFER

- HIV-infected children should be managed by physicians who have knowledge and experience in taking care of children with HIV infection.

FOLLOW-UP

- Frequency of medical follow-up visits depends on many factors, including:
  - Child's clinical status
  - Expected compliance with therapy
- Follow-up should include measurements of HIV RNA levels and CD4+ T lymphocyte counts every 3 months.
- Child care or school attendance
  - Risk of HIV transmission appears to be negligible, and HIV-infected children should not be restricted from attending child care or school.
    - Special consideration may be warranted for those with unusual risk factors for transmission, such as frequent biting or scratching, severe dermatitis, or bleeding disorders.
- Supportive care
  - Many parents and guardians are not willing to tell the child that he or she is infected with HIV.
    - Most children are made aware of their illness through frequent medical visits and medications.
    - The primary care physician's relationship with the patient provides the best position to promote and assist with disclosure.
    - Appropriate disclosure tailored to the child's cognitive level is helpful in alleviating guilt and allowing discussion among the child, caregivers, and health care professionals.
    - Uninfected siblings of HIV-infected children are emotionally affected by the diagnosis and should be included in support groups and counseling.

H

- The primary care physician plays a critical role in providing advice and support as the child nears death, helping the family interpret the complexities of critical care and assisting decisions on the appropriateness of heroic interventions.
  - The physician may be able to assist in family care for the dying child at home if critical care is deemed futile.
  - After the child's death, the physician should continue to support the family through the grief process.
  - Because many pediatricians invest much time and emotional energy in caring for an HIV-infected child, many take the opportunity to express sympathy by attending the funeral.

COMPLICATIONS

- HIV infection and secondary opportunistic infections can involve all organ systems.
- Bacterial and viral pathogens causing meningitis and encephalitis are similar to those in nonimmunocompromised children.
  - Common pathogens include:
    - *Cryptococcus neoformans*
    - *Toxoplasma gondii*
    - Cytomegalovirus
- Pulmonary disease
  - PCP
    - Was frequently found before routine prophylaxis of HIV-exposed infants
    - Typically appears at 3–6 months of age
    - Characterized by:
      - Tachypnea
      - Cough
      - Hypoxemia
      - Diffuse alveolar infiltrates on chest radiograph
  - Common respiratory pathogens seen in children with HIV include:
    - Respiratory syncytial virus
    - Parainfluenza virus
    - Influenza virus
    - Adenovirus
  - Pneumococcus is the most common bacterial cause of pneumonia in HIV-infected children.
  - LIP is a chronic lung disease resulting from lymphoid hyperplasia in the lungs.
    - Children may be asymptomatic or may have chronic cough and wheezing.
    - Children are typically older than those with PCP.
    - Children with LIP frequently have generalized lymphadenopathy and parotid enlargement.

- Infectious causes of diarrhea in HIV-infected children include pathogens of healthy children and numerous opportunistic pathogens.
  - Common parasitic pathogens causing persistent diarrhea include:
    - *Giardia lamblia*
    - *Entamoeba histolytica*
    - *Cryptosporidium* species
    - *Isospora belli*
  - Cytomegalovirus may cause colitis in advanced immunosuppression.
  - Persistent diarrhea can significantly compromise quality of life and nutritional status.
- Central nervous system disease
  - Microcephaly
  - Developmental delay
  - Spasticity
  - Abnormal reflexes
  - Gait abnormalities
  - Central nervous system lymphomas (rare)
- Hematologic abnormalities
  - Leukopenia
  - Anemia
  - Thrombocytopenia (may be the presenting illness)
- Dermatologic conditions include:
  - Recurrent herpes simplex
  - Varicella-zoster virus infections
  - Severe molluscum contagiosum
  - Chronic fungal infections
  - Atopic dermatitis
  - Drug-induced eruptions, particularly with co-trimoxazole
- Drug-induced bone marrow suppression can follow therapy with:
  - Zidovudine
  - Co-trimoxazole
  - Ganciclovir
- Hepatomegaly and increases in hepatic aminotransferase levels are commonly seen, often in the absence of clinically apparent liver disease.
- HIV cardiomyopathy may lead to congestive heart failure.
- HIV nephropathy is a common cause of proteinuria and can progress to nephrotic syndrome.
- HIV-infected children in whom virus replication is not controlled by antiretroviral therapy are frequently stunted in growth.
  - Severe wasting may be seen in advanced disease.
- Cancers are not as common in HIV-infected children, but lymphomas and leiomyosarcomas can occur.

PROGNOSIS

■ High plasma HIV levels and low CD4+ T lymphocyte counts are predictive of poor prognosis.

PREVENTION

Preventing perinatal HIV transmission

■ Antiretroviral therapy administered to women during pregnancy and delivery and to infants during the first 6 weeks of life greatly reduces the rate of perinatal HIV transmission.

■ Although the total number of perinatal infections has decreased, the proportion caused by intrauterine transmission has increased.

  • This supports a greater role for antiretroviral therapy and mode of delivery on influencing intrapartum transmission.

■ Administration of zidovudine to women during pregnancy and labor and to infants for the first 6 weeks of life has been shown to reduce perinatal HIV transmission by two-thirds (from 26% to 8%).

  • This regimen is the standard of care for HIV-infected pregnant women and their newborns.

■ Early identification of HIV-infected pregnant women allows for:

  • Appropriate care of the mother

  • Avoidance of ongoing HIV exposure of the infant through human milk

  • Early institution of PCP prophylaxis for the infant at 4–6 weeks of age

■ Prevention of maternal-infant HIV transmission

  • Identification of HIV-infected women before or during pregnancy is critical.

  • Prenatal HIV counseling and testing should be provided to all pregnant women.

  • Initial HIV antibody testing should be performed early in pregnancy and repeated in the third trimester for women at risk.

Immunization

■ Immunizations are generally safe for HIV-infected children.

■ Immune suppression caused by HIV results in less assurance of protection after immunization than in HIV-uninfected children.

■ The small risk of serious complications from live viral vaccines has led to special recommendations for HIV-infected children.

■ RotaTeq should not be administered to immunocompromised children.

  • HIV-exposed infants with testing that does not support HIV infection may receive an initial dose of RotaTeq before documentation that infant is not infected (negative PCR after 4 months of age).

■ Toxoids, subunit vaccines, inactivated vaccines, and recombinant vaccines are not associated with increased risks of complications in HIV-infected children, including:

  • Diphtheria and tetanus toxoids

  • Acellular pertussis vaccines

  • Inactivated poliovirus vaccine

  • *Haemophilus influenzae* type b

  • Pneumococcal conjugate vaccines

  • Inactivated influenza vaccine

  • Hepatitis A and B vaccines

■ These vaccines should be administered to HIV-infected children according to routine immunization schedule.

  • Because of an increased risk of invasive infection with *S pneumoniae,* immunization of HIV-infected children with pneumococcal conjugate vaccine is particularly important.

  • HIV-infected children may develop lower antibody titers than healthy children after immunization and are more likely to lose protective antibody earlier.

■ Live viral vaccines may result in infection and disease resulting from vaccine virus in severely immunocompromised HIV-infected children, although the risk is quite small. Examples include:

  • Varicella vaccine

  • Measles, mumps, and rubella vaccines

■ After a single reported death, advisory groups in the US have recommended withholding measles vaccine from HIV-infected children with severe immunosuppression, defined as CD4+ T lymphocyte count <15%.

  • Measles-mumps-rubella vaccine should be administered to HIV-infected children at 12 months unless severely immunocompromised (CD4+ <15%).

  • Immune response to measles vaccine in HIV-infected children may be poor, and vaccinated children may remain susceptible.

  • Serious complications after mumps or rubella immunization have not been reported.

■ Live varicella virus vaccine is also recommended for HIV-infected children on the basis of their degree of immunosuppression and symptoms.

  • The AAP Committee on Infectious Diseases recommends varicella vaccine for asymptomatic and mildly symptomatic HIV-infected children who have CD4+ T lymphocyte percentages ≥15%.

  • Serious adverse events after administration of varicella vaccine to HIV-infected children are rare.

Antimicrobial prophylaxis

■ PCP prophylaxis should be administered to HIV-exposed infants beginning at 6 weeks of age, even if HIV infection is not confirmed.

  • Continue until 12 months of age or until HIV has been excluded.

- PCP prophylaxis is administered:
  - For children 1–5 years of age if CD4$^+$ T lymphocyte count is <500 cells/mL
  - For children 6–12 years of age if it is <200 cells/mL
- Lifelong PCP prophylaxis is recommended for children who have a history of PCP, despite immune reconstitution.
- Recommended regimen isco-trimoxazole taken orally 3 days a week.
- Alternative regimens include dapsone or pentamidine.

■ HIV-infected children who have recurrent oral candidiasis may benefit from antifungal prophylaxis.
  - Oral nystatin
  - Clotrimazole
  - Fluconazole

■ *Mycobacterium avium-intracellulare* in children with CD4$^+$ T lymphocyte counts <100 cells/mL
  - Weekly oral azithromycin for prophylaxis
  - Daily rifabutin for infection

■ Immunoglobulin should be provided to susceptible (no age-appropriate measles immunization) HIV-infected children within 6 days of exposure to measles.
  - Measles immunization should be delayed 6 months after receipt of immunoglobulin.

Postexposure prophylaxis after community needlestick injuries

■ Parents, caretakers, and physicians often are most concerned about transmission of HIV after accidental injury from a discarded needle.

■ No consensus or recommendation is available to guide management in such circumstances.

■ Risk of HIV transmission after occupational exposure to HIV-infected blood is 0.3%.

■ Most experts agree that risk after community needlestick injury is lower than risk after occupational exposure.

■ Factors to be considered in the use of antiretroviral agents for postexposure prophylaxis include:
  - Potential risk of HIV transmission
  - Drug toxicities
  - Ability and willingness of the family to adhere to therapy

■ Regimens for occupational postexposure prophylaxis may be followed.

■ Pediatricians caring for adolescents must ensure they have knowledge of risks of acquiring HIV and other sexually transmitted infections through unprotected sex.

H

Hoarseness

DEFINITION

- Hoarseness is a symptom of vocal dysfunction that describes a breathy, harsh, coarse, strained, or raspy voice.
- In children, "hoarseness" can be used to describe both the quality of voice and the quality of cry.
- Hoarseness results from a pathologic change in the vibratory nature of the vocal folds.
- Although sometimes occurring concurrently, hoarseness should be discerned from stridor, a sign of turbulent airflow caused by obstructive lesions in the airway.
- Causes vary by age group and can be attributed to infectious, anatomic, traumatic, inflammatory, neoplastic, neurologic, and iatrogenic sources.

EPIDEMIOLOGY

- Prevalence
  - Described as 6–38% in childhood

MECHANISM

Congenital causes of hoarseness

- Laryngeal anomalies
  - Laryngomalacia
  - Glottic webs
  - Subglottic stenosis
  - Laryngeal cleft
- Cystic lesions
  - Laryngocele
  - Saccular cyst
  - Thyroglossal duct cyst
- Angiomas
  - Lymphatic malformation
  - Hemangioma
  - Arteriovenous malformation
- Cri du chat syndrome

Neurogenic (congenital and acquired)

- Supranuclear (eg, hydrocephalus)
- Nuclear (eg, Arnold-Chiari malformation, Guillain-Barré syndrome)
- Peripheral (eg, myasthenia gravis, cardiovascular anomalies, recurrent laryngeal nerve trauma)
- Psychogenic hoarseness

Vocal cord abuse

- Vocal cord nodules
- Vocal cord polyps

Neoplasia

- Papilloma
- Squamous cell carcinoma

Physical voice change of puberty

- Inflammatory
  - Infectious
    - Simple laryngitis
    - Diphtheria
    - Laryngotracheitis
    - Supraglottitis (epiglottitis)
  - Noninfectious
    - Laryngopharyngeal reflux (LPR)
    - Chronic laryngitis
    - Allergic laryngitis
    - Angioedema
    - Rheumatoid arthritis
    - Relapsing polychondritis
    - Smoking
- Traumatic
  - General
    - Hematoma
    - Laryngeal cartilage fracture
    - Impacted foreign body
  - Postintubation
    - Arytenoid dislocation
    - Cord avulsion
    - Granuloma
    - Acquired glottic web
    - Subglottic stenosis
  - Recurrent laryngeal nerve injury
    - Thyroidectomy
    - Tracheotomy
    - Cardiac surgery
    - Tracheoesophageal fistula repair
    - Tracheal resection
    - Penetrating neck wound

HISTORY

- A thorough history is an essential.
- Age is a critical factor in the development of an appropriate differential diagnosis.
  - Neurologic and congenital fixed anatomic lesions typically occur at birth.
  - Inflammatory, neoplastic, traumatic, or iatrogenic causes occur later.
- Information on quality of the voice with speech or crying, exacerbating or alleviating factors, and associated symptoms
- The onset and course of dysphonia should be considered.
  - Intermittent dysphonia may be related to infectious or inflammatory causes, such as laryngitis.

- Persistent dysphonia may suggest a fixed anatomic lesion.
- Progressive, unremitting hoarseness may suggest an enlarging neoplasm.

■ Underlying reflux may be present in patients with such symptoms as:

- Regurgitation or vomiting
- Feeding difficulties
- Throat clearing
- Foreign body sensation
- Cough

■ Stridor that accompanies hoarseness should be investigated and treated in an expeditious fashion.

- Turbulent airflow resulting from airway obstruction may be life threatening.

PHYSICAL EXAM

■ Thorough physical examination should include a complete head and neck examination with inspection of cranial nerve function for craniofacial anomalies.

- Cutaneous head and neck hemangiomas may suggest a potential laryngeal hemangioma.
- Signs of aspiration during deglutition may be suggestive of sensorimotor causes of dysphonia, such as vocal cord paralysis.

DIFFERENTIAL DIAGNOSIS

■ Forming a differential diagnosis for the hoarse child depends on:

- Quality of hoarseness
- Progression of symptoms
- Related infection
- History of surgery or trauma
- Associated respiratory distress

Causes, by patient age

■ The age of the patient at the onset of hoarseness is a useful way to organize the potential causes.

- 0–6 months
  - Traumatic intubation
  - Iatrogenic: surgical
  - Neurogenic: central or peripheral
  - Neoplastic: hemangioma
  - Congenital: web, cleft, cyst
- 6 months to 5 years
  - Traumatic: foreign bodies, intubation
  - Infection: upper respiratory infection (URI)
  - Neoplastic: papillomas
  - Behavioral, traumatic: nodules
  - Inflammatory: allergy, LPR

- 5–13 years
  - Behavioral, traumatic: nodules
  - Infectious: URI
  - Inflammatory: allergy, LPR
  - Neoplastic
- 13–18 years
  - Infectious: URI
  - Inflammatory: allergy, LPR
  - Behavioral, traumatic:
    - Male: mutational or transitional voice
    - Female: nodules
  - Functional: muscle tension dysphonia

Neonate and infant

■ Hoarseness at birth or shortly thereafter is most often attributable to causes that are:

- Congenital
- Traumatic or iatrogenic
- Neoplastic
- Inflammatory

■ In this age group, "hoarseness" often refers to a weak or breathy cry.

■ Neonatal vocal cord paralysis is a well-known cause of hoarseness and stridor.

- Bilateral vocal cord paralysis is usually congenital and frequently causes respiratory distress and stridor.
  - Central nervous system disease, such as the Arnold-Chiari malformation, must be ruled out.
- Unilateral vocal cord paralysis is more likely to exhibit initially as hoarseness or dysphagia.
- A weak or breathy cry after thoracic or cervical surgery may indicate recurrent laryngeal nerve injury as a source of iatrogenic vocal cord paralysis.
- Traumatic intubation can cause arytenoid cartilage dislocation, with subsequent vocal cord immobility and hoarseness.

■ Congenital laryngeal webs result from of failure of larynx to canalize fully during embryologic development.

- Webs may occur exclusively with hoarseness, but they may be associated with aphonia, stridor, and respiratory distress.
- Webs vary from thin slips of tissue between the anterior of the vocal cords to complete laryngeal atresia (congenital high airway obstruction syndrome).

■ Laryngeal saccular cysts are characterized by symptoms of airway obstruction and dysphagia.

- Saccular cysts are filled with mucinous fluid and arise as a result of an abnormal dilation of the saccule of the larynx secondary to secretory outflow obstruction.

- Posterior laryngeal clefts are an uncommon anomaly resulting in an abnormal opening in the posterior larynx.
  - Clefts can involve the posterior laryngeal commissure or may extend through the cricoid inferiorly through the tracheoesophageal septum.
  - Symptoms depend on extent of the cleft and at birth, typically include aspiration, stridor, respiratory distress, and weak cry.
- Subglottic hemangiomas classically occur at 1–6 months of age, with varying degrees of respiratory distress, stridor, cough, dysphagia, and hoarseness.
  - Natural history of hemangiomas is that of proliferation followed by involution.
  - Subglottic hemangiomas can be unilateral, bilateral, or circumferential.
  - More common in girls than in boys
  - Cutaneous hemangiomas of the head and neck are found concurrently in ~50%.
  - A relationship may exist between pediatric and adult laryngeal disease and reflux.
  - *Gastroesophageal reflux* (GER) refers to the backflow of stomach contents into the esophagus.
  - *LPR* refers to backflow of stomach contents into the laryngopharynx.
  - GER commonly produces emesis, dysphagia, sleep disturbance, and failure to thrive.
  - The association among GER; LPR; and neonatal laryngeal disorders, such as hoarseness, posterior laryngitis, and silent aspiration, remains complicated and controversial (see Dysphagia and Gastroesophageal reflux disease).

Older children

- Subject to many of the same sources of hoarseness as adults
- Leading causes include infectious, inflammatory, traumatic, and neoplastic conditions, such as laryngitis, LPR, vocal nodules, and respiratory papillomata.
- Infectious disorders, such as infective laryngitis, supraglottitis, and laryngotracheobronchitis, rarely present a diagnostic challenge.
- Concern over the airway should always take precedence; a hoarse voice may be an early indicator of impending airway compromise by epiglottitis.
- The role of LPR in children is debated; however, infrequent reflux events have been shown to cause hoarseness in adults.
  - LPR has been found in association with pediatric conditions, such as vocal fold nodules, posterior laryngitis, false vocal cord edema, vocal cord granulomas, functional voice disorders, and hoarseness.
  - Animal studies have shown that subglottic stenosis results when gastric acid is applied to the subglottic mucosa of dogs.

- Vocal nodules arise from phonotrauma or voice abuse more frequently in boys than in girls.
  - Symptoms may fluctuate on the basis of aggravation by vocal abuse and respiratory tract infections.
  - Symptoms may worsen suddenly when polyps swell from internal hemorrhage from vocal trauma.
  - Children with vocal nodules may share symptoms with other family members with similar traits.
- Airway trauma is a potential cause of hoarseness.
  - Sources include blunt or penetrating injuries and intubation trauma.
- Progressive and unrelenting hoarseness suggests a possible neoplastic cause.
  - 98% of pediatric laryngeal neoplasms are benign; recurrent respiratory papillomatosis (RRP) is by far the most common lesion.
  - RRP may be found on other upper aerodigestive tract mucosal surfaces and have a characteristic "cluster of grapes" appearance.
  - RRP may be indistinguishable from the rare laryngeal squamous cell carcinoma of childhood.

Adolescents

- Hoarseness may be of behavioral or psychogenic etiology.
- Mutational voice disorder occurs in male adolescents, resulting in hoarseness and high pitch during the stress of physiologic pubertal voice change.
- Paradoxical vocal fold dysfunction (seen more frequently in girls) is psychogenic in origin and often misdiagnosed as asthma.

IMAGING

- Diagnostic imaging is of prime importance when central nervous system disease, external compression, cancer, or external trauma is suspected.
- Chest and neck plain-film radiography may demonstrate mediastinal masses, cardiovascular anomalies, or abnormalities in the air column suggesting possible infectious or obstructive diseases.
- Computed tomography (CT) and virtual bronchoscopy are excellent methods for:
  - Specifically defining the caliber of the airway
  - Delineating the site and extent of pathologic changes in airway caliber
  - Indications for laryngeal or neck CT include congenital cysts, solid neoplasms, and external trauma.
- Magnetic resonance imaging is helpful:
  - When central nervous system disease is suspected
  - In evaluating possible airway hemangiomas
  - In identifying vascular malformations

H

- Barium esophagraphy has variable sensitivity and specificity for the diagnosis of LPR.
  - Useful mainly for detecting anatomic abnormalities, such as hiatal hernia

DIAGNOSTIC PROCEDURES

Laryngoscopy

- Flexible nasopharyngolaryngoscopy, indirect mirror laryngoscopy, and rigid videostroboscopy are all methods for visualizing the larynx that can provide useful clues.
- Indirect laryngoscopy using a mirror
  - Can be performed on cooperative children
  - Can visualize gross disease and inflammatory changes in the larynx
  - This technique has largely been replaced.
- Flexible fiberoptic nasopharyngolaryngoscopy
  - Provides clear views of laryngeal anatomy and function
  - Can be performed on virtually all age groups, although toddlers and developmentally delayed patients pose the greatest challenge to the examiner
  - Topical anesthesia and topical decongestants can facilitate examination.
  - The flexible endoscope is gently passed though the nose or mouth.
  - Examination in a nonmonitored setting is not advisable if the patient has a tenuous airway or severe congenital cardiac anomalies.
- Videostroboscopy
  - A rigid, angled telescope placed gently into the oropharynx is used for dynamic examination of laryngeal anatomy and function.
  - The examination requires a cooperative child.
  - Uses rapidly pulsed light to examine vibratory characteristics of the vocal fold mucosa
  - Recorded on video to allow repeated assessments viewed at different speeds to enhance visualization of the vibratory quality of the laryngeal mucosa
  - Vocal nodules or other lesions on surface of the vocal fold will dampen the mucosal wave.

Reflux testing

- In the absence of identifiable disease in the hoarse child, investigation into LPR may be warranted.
- Several diagnostic modalities exist for the workup of LPR, including:
  - pH monitoring
  - Impedance testing
  - Nuclear medicine scintiscan
  - Barium esophagoscopy (see Imaging)
  - Direct laryngoscopy with or without biopsy

- Ambulatory 24-hour single-electrode pH monitoring is the gold standard for the diagnosis of GER.
- Double-electrode pH probe, with distal esophageal and pharyngeal electrodes, however, is thought to be the best method for diagnosing LPR and the otolaryngologic manifestations of GER.
- Although pH-monitoring studies remain the gold standard for diagnosis of GER and LPR, they do not detect episodes of nonacidic reflux.
- Multichannel intraluminal impedance monitoring and nuclear medicine scintigraphy
  - Measures both acidic and nonacidic episodes of reflux, which may play a role in apnea, apparent life-threatening events, aspiration, and sleep disturbance.
  - Nuclear medicine scintiscans have specificity of 83–100% but have been shown to be only 15–59% sensitive and lack a standardized technique, making comparisons between studies of limited use.
  - Impedance monitoring evaluates the pH-independent change in intraluminal electrical resistance that occurs with the movement (anterograde or retrograde) of a bolus of food, liquid, or gas within the esophagus.
    - This technique may be a reliable tool for evaluating the association between GER-related symptoms and nonacidic reflux events.
    - It may ultimately replace pH monitoring as the standard tool for detecting LPR in infants and children.
- Laryngoscopy with biopsy
  - May be the most specific test for LPR
  - At least 1 study has failed to show a correlation between laryngoscopy and upper pH probe findings with significant laryngeal histopathologic inflammatory findings.

TREATMENT APPROACH

- Most pediatric hoarseness results from benign, reversible, and self-limited disease.
- Some causes of hoarseness are progressive, malignant, and potentially life threatening.
- Thorough evaluation, precise diagnosis, and appropriate intervention are therefore essential.

SPECIFIC TREATMENT

Congenital lesions

- Management of hoarse voice resulting from unilateral or bilateral vocal cord paralysis is usually secondary to stabilization of the airway and management of dysphagia and aspiration.
- Tracheotomy is sometimes required in patients with bilateral vocal cord paralysis.

- Conservative management has been advocated in selected patients.
  - Patients with congenital or acquired unilateral vocal cord paralysis frequently experience spontaneous resolution of paralysis or compensatory movement of the unaffected cord over time.
  - Recovery has been noted up to 11 years after paralysis.
- In cases of persistent unilateral cord paralysis with persistent hoarseness, the treatment of choice remains speech therapy.
  - Successful surgical vocal cord medialization techniques have been reported.
- Laryngeal webs are managed surgically, endoscopically, or via more extensive open laryngotracheal reconstruction techniques.
  - The type of operation depends primarily on location and extent of lesion.
  - Thin webs are more amenable to endoscopic management.
- Saccular cysts of the larynx
  - Often managed endoscopically via aspiration and marsupialization using sharp dissection or with a carbon dioxide (CO_2) laser.
  - Cyst recurrence is well documented following endoscopic management.
  - Open resection of the cyst may be necessary.
- Posterior laryngeal clefts vary greatly in extent and symptoms.
  - Extensive or symptomatic clefts must be repaired as early as possible.
  - Endoscopic repair is possible in small clefts limited to larynx and upper trachea.
  - More extensive open techniques are used for larger clefts.
  - Tracheotomy may be placed in cases in which staged reconstruction is necessary.
  - A gastrostomy tube is often necessary to limit aspiration and protect the operative site.

Neoplasia

- Subglottic hemangioma is a complicated airway anomaly without universally accepted treatment.
  - Numerous management options exist, including:
    - Close observation
    - Systemic or intralesional steroids
    - Laser ablation
    - Open surgical excision
    - Tracheotomy
- RRP is an airway tumor with a large number of accepted primary and adjuvant therapeutic modalities.
  - CO_2 laser excision remains a popular method for removing laryngeal papilloma, although it is associated with potentially severe sequelae, such as:
    - Airway fire
    - Scarring

- Chronic laryngeal edema with airway compromise
- Vocal fold scarring
- Poor voice
  - Pulsed dye laser therapy was introduced as a less traumatic alternative that can be used safely and effectively under local anesthesia in older patients.
  - Powered instrumentation, such as the microdebrider, is successfully used for excision of RRP.
  - Adjuvant therapies have been used with varying degrees of efficacy and safety, such as:
    - Intralesional cidofovir
    - Interferon-α
    - Indole-3-carbinol
    - Heat-shock protein E7

Inflammation and infection

- Acceptable for the management of GER and LPR in infants and children
  - Behavioral and lifestyle modifications
  - Pharmacotherapy using:
    - Histamine-2 antagonists
    - Proton-pump inhibitors
    - Prokinetic agents
    - Antacids
  - Surgical therapy with fundoplication
- Viral laryngitis and laryngotracheobronchitis are generally treated conservatively.
  - May require airway protection or intravenous steroids in severe cases
- Bacterial infections, such as epiglottitis and membranous laryngotracheobronchitis, necessitate:
  - Early airway protection
  - Intravenous antibiotics directed against *Staphylococcus aureus* and *Haemophilus influenzae*, unless culture results direct differently

Trauma

- Management of vocal fold nodules resulting from phonotrauma
  - Behavioral modification
  - Speech therapy aimed at maximizing vocal hygiene
  - Surgical excision, rarely, because failure to correct underlying voice misuse is likely to result in recurrence
- Arytenoid dislocation resulting from intubation trauma can be adequately treated if recognized and reduced early under anesthesia with microlaryngoscopy.
- Blunt laryngeal trauma
  - Close observation
  - Possibly systemic corticosteroids

- Tracheotomy in cases of severe laryngeal injury and edema
- In adolescents with laryngeal fracture, open reduction and fixation may be required.

WHEN TO REFER

- Recognized cardiac, esophageal, or neurologic disease
- Progressive hoarseness
- Presence of cutaneous hemangioma

- Hoarseness after external trauma or uneventful intubation
- Poor speech intelligibility or psychosocial sequelae
- Hoarseness that has been present since birth

WHEN TO ADMIT

- Presence of respiratory distress, stridor, tachypnea, or tachycardia
- Hoarseness following external trauma

H

Human Herpesvirus-6 and Human Herpesvirus-7 Infections

DEFINITION

- Human herpesvirus (HHV)-6, formerly called *human B-lymphotrophic virus,* and HHV-7 are classified as herpesviruses on the basis of their physical and genetic similarities to others of the group.
  - Herpes simplex virus type 1
  - Herpes simplex virus type 2
  - Cytomegalovirus
  - Epstein-Barr virus
  - Varicella-zoster virus
  - Newly discovered virus associated with Kaposi sarcoma, HHV-8
- HHV-6 and HHV-7 can be distinguished from other herpesviruses by DNA hybridization or by reactions with virus-specific monoclonal antibodies.
- HHV-6 exists in 2 forms.
  - Variant A
    - The range of illnesses, if any, caused by HHV-6A is unknown.
  - Variant B
    - Typically associated with childhood illnesses, such as roseola, and some adult infections.
- HHV-6 and HHV-7 are 2 of the known causative agents of roseola.
  - Classic childhood exanthem, also known as:
    - Roseola infantum
    - Exanthem subitum
    - 3-day fever
    - Sixth disease
    - Pseudorubella
- The spectrum of disease associated with these agents is now understood to be far broader than the benign illness of roseola.

EPIDEMIOLOGY

HHV-6 and HHV-7

- Prevalence
  - The rate of subclinical disease is high.
  - Three-quarters of children are infected with HHV-6 by age 2 years.
  - Most infections are symptomatic.
- Age
  - Recognition of infection is unusual at other ages.
  - Rare cases in adults and neonates have been reported.
- Most HHV-6 and HHV-7 infections are sporadic.
  - Family and institutional epidemics are occasionally noted.
- Serologic surveys show that:
  - Virtually all full-term infants have passively acquired maternal antibody to both HHV-6 and HHV-7 at birth.

- The prevalence of antibody decreases and reaches a low point by 6 months of age.
- Nearly 90% of children have detectable antibody to HHV-6 by 1 year of age.
- Adults from countries around the world show HHV-6 antibody detection rates of 88–90%.
  - Prevalence of antibody to HHV-7 increases with age.
  - 60% of young adolescents have detectable titers.
- For both viruses, these levels persist unchanged through young adulthood and decrease slightly thereafter.
- Primary HHV-6 infection is clearly a major cause of morbidity in infancy and early childhood.
  - 77% of infants from birth through age 24 months acquired primary HHV-6 infection.
  - >90% of episodes were symptomatic.
  - 39% visited a physician for the illness.
- Febrile HHV-6 infection is more significant than previously realized.
  - Primary HHV-6 infection exhibiting as an acute febrile illness was documented in:
    - Approximately 10% of children <3 years of age
    - 20% of children 6–12 months of age
  - HHV-6 infection was the cause of one-third of febrile seizures in children <2 years.
    - 13% were hospitalized after seeking care at an emergency department.
- Most HHV-7 infections seem to be asymptomatic because the rate of seropositivity is high.
  - Detectable viremia with clinical illness occurs in only 1% of children <10 years of age.
- The contribution of HHV-7 infection to emergency department use, hospitalization, or physician visits is unclear.
  - 1% of children <10 years of age have demonstrated HHV-7 viremia.
    - 86% had fever.
    - 40% had seizures.
    - 20% were hospitalized.
- Seizures
  - Not a prominent manifestation of HHV-6 infection, and occur no more frequently than with other febrile illnesses
  - HHV-6 infection is a major factor, accounting for up to one-half of such incidents in children <2 years of age seeking care at an emergency department.
  - HHV-6 DNA can be identified in cerebrospinal fluid (CSF) of up to 70% of children during primary infection and of 28% of previously infected children.

H

Roseola

- Prevalence
  - Primary infection with HHV-7 accounts for approximately 10% of first and most second cases of roseola.
  - HHV-7 infection occurs somewhat later than HHV-6, at a mean age >12 months.
  - Approximately 15% of clinical cases of roseola cannot be attributed to either virus.
- Age
  - 30% of children will experience the clinical roseola between 6 months and 2 years of age.
  - The first episode usually occurs when the child is 7–9 months of age.
  - 60% will be diagnosed by 3 years of age.
  - Nonroseola illness is probably more common.
- Seasonality
  - Cases of roseola are seen year round.
- Geography
  - In Japan, roseola is diagnosed in 60% of children in the first 3 years of life.

ETIOLOGY

- HHV-6 and HHV-7 are 2 of the known causative agents of roseola.
  - A child's first episode of roseola is usually caused by HHV-6B.
- The incubation period for HHV-6 and HHV-7 infection is 5–15 days.
  - Modes of transmission and period of communicability are unclear.
    - Saliva is thought to be the most likely mode of transmission.
    - HHV-6 and HHV-7 can be isolated from saliva of 70–80% of healthy persons >1 year of age.
  - HHV-6 is most frequently isolated from peripheral blood mononuclear cells.
  - In an extensive study of 3-generation families, DNA restriction analysis of HHV-7 isolates showed similar patterns within households.
  - Most patients have no known exposure.
  - Despite direct evidence of intrauterine or perinatal transmission of HHV-6, no consistently recognized sequelae attributed to such infection exist.
- HHV-6 and HHV-7 exist in many healthy persons, including those who have virus-specific antibody.
  - HHV-6 has been isolated from saliva, plasma, and many cell lines.
  - HHV-7 is isolated most often from the saliva in healthy persons.

- As with other herpesviruses, latent or persistent asymptomatic viral infection occurs after the primary infection.
  - The site of latency is not clear, but during reactivation these viruses may appear in:
    - Oral or genital secretions
    - Mononuclear leukocytes
    - Human milk
    - CSF
  - HHV-6 infection may reactivate during:
    - Primary HHV-7 infection
    - Acute febrile illnesses
    - Periods of immunodeficiency, such as treatment with steroids
  - Reactivation characteristics of HHV-7 are unknown.
- Both viruses interfere with the function of certain classes of T lymphocytes.
  - Evidence is emerging that HHV-6, and perhaps HHV-7, act as cofactors in the course of HIV infection.
  - Role of these viruses is under investigation in:
    - Lymphoreticular cancer
    - Chronic fatigue syndrome
    - Other conditions, such as multiple sclerosis

RISK FACTORS

- Poverty and larger family size may be risk factors for early acquisition of HHV-6.

SIGNS AND SYMPTOMS

- Clinical characteristics of HHV-6 and HHV-7 infections in normal children are shown in the table Clinical Characteristics of Human Herpesvirus (HHV)-6 and HHV-7 Infections in Normal Children.

Roseola

- The first recognized clinical manifestation of primary HHV-6, and perhaps HHV-7, infection
- Recognition is based almost entirely on the observation of a classic clinical course.
- Fever with temperature as high as 102.2°F to 105.8°F (39°C–41°C) suddenly develops in a previously well infant.
- Except for irritability, the child does not seem as sick as the temperature indicates.
- Physical findings are few.
  - Painless posterior auricular, suboccipital, or cervical lymphadenopathy
  - Slight eyelid edema, giving the child a sleepy-eyed or droopy appearance
  - Nagayama spots, erythematous macules appearing on the soft palate and near the uvula, are observed regularly after 1–2 days.

Clinical Characteristics of Human Herpesvirus (HHV)-6 and HHV-7 Infections in Normal Children

Signs and Symptoms	Roseola (1945)	Febrile HHV-6 (1994)	Primary HHV-6 (2005)	Febrile HHV-7 (1997, 1998)	Viremic HHV-7 (2006)
Fever	100%	98–100%	58%	100%	87%
Rash at presentation	100%	6–4%	31%	13–86%	0%
Pruritus	1.2%	NR	NR	NR	NR
Desquamation	10%	0%	NR	NR	NR
Pigmentation	0%	7%	NR	NR	NR
Lymphadenopathy	97.5%	NR	NR	NR	NR
Cervical	45%	31%	NR	NR	NR
Erythematous tympanic membranes	92.5%	P	NR	NR	NR
Constipation	40%	NR	NR	NR	NR
Upper respiratory tract symptoms	25%	41%	66%	7%	13%
Nonspecific prodromal symptoms	NR	14%	NR	NR	33%
Diarrhea	15%	33–68%	26%	38%	7%
Meningismus	5%	NR	NR	NR	NR
Convulsions	3.7%	8%	0%	7-75%	40%
Bulging fontanelle	NR	26%	NR	NR	NR
Irritability	92%	P	70%	88%	NR
Edematous eyelids	NR	30%	NR	NR	NR
Nagayama spots[a]	87%	65%	NR	NR	NR
Anorexia	80%	NR	NR	NR	NR
Abdominal pain	25%	NR	NR	NR	NR
Cough	11.2%	P, 50%	34%	NR	NR
Headache	5%	NR	NR	NR	NR
Earache or otitis media	2.5%	30%	NR	NR	7%
Aching joints	2.5%	NR	NR	NR	NR
Vomiting	NR	NR	8%	NR	7%
Asymptomatic	NA	NA	6%	NA	0%
Roseola	100%	17–98%	24%	NR	0%

Abbreviations: NA, not applicable to the study design; NR, not reported; P, reported as present with no numerical value.
[a] Erythematous streaks or spots on the soft palate and uvula.

H

- Rarely, mild coryza, otitis media, or a bulging fontanelle
  - After a 2- to 5-day course, fever resolves dramatically while rash simultaneously appears.
  - With defervescence, the child seems to have recovered, despite the rash.
  - Typical exanthem occurs as macular or maculopapular blanching patches surrounded by a lighter halo.
  - Eruption usually begins on the neck and spreads to trunk and extremities, sparing the face.
  - Rash fades within 4 hours to 4 days and may be missed if it is faint or occurs at night.
- Roseola may also occur in a young infant as an afebrile exanthem.

Mononucleosis-like disease

- HHV-6 infection in adults rarely causes a roseola-like illness.
- Both severe and mild infectious mononucleosis–like disease have been reported in adults with HHV-6 infection.
- Disease lasts several weeks and is associated with:
  - Slight fatigue
  - Headache
  - Sore throat
  - Cervical lymphadenopathy
  - Transient increase in liver enzymes
- Infectious mononucleosis–like illness associated with HHV-6 has been noted in infants.
- HHV-7 has been isolated from a child with a clinical picture of chronic Epstein-Barr virus infection, characterized by:
  - Pancytopenia
  - Fever
  - Hepatosplenomegaly

Seizures

- May be single or recurrent, prolonged, and partial or focal
- May be associated with postictal paralysis or acute resolving hemiplegia
- CSF findings are normal or negative.
- Febrile seizures are noted in symptomatic primary or reactivated infection caused by HHV-7.
  - Some indications suggest that febrile seizures may be more common (and possibly more complicated) with primary HHV-7 than with HHV-6 infection.

Other central nervous system involvement

- Severe meningoencephalitis with neurologic sequelae or death in infants and adults and fatal encephalitis has been attributed to HHV-6B in adult recipients of bone marrow transplants.
- Unclear significance of HHV-6 in relation to:
  - Recurrent seizures
  - Chronic fatigue
  - Multiple sclerosis
  - Other neurologic conditions
- HHV-7 infection has also been described in association with:
  - Encephalopathy
  - Hemiplegia
  - Atypical febrile seizures
- Neurologic conditions associated with HHV-6 and HHV-7 infections are rare.
  - May be severe, requiring intensive care
  - HHV-6 or HHV-7 (or both) infection should be sought to differentiate it from encephalitis associated with vaccines.

Hepatitis

- Mild hepatitis associated with HHV-6 infection is recognized in adults and children.
- A few cases of fulminant or fatal hepatitis have been reported, usually with an associated encephalopathy.
- HHV-6 infection also has been implicated in mild chronic hepatitis in childhood.
- A single case of hepatitis has been reported in relation to HHV-7 infection.

Infection in immunocomprised patients

- Syndrome with fever and rash resembling graft-versus-host disease is recognized in children after they receive bone marrow transplants.
- HHV-6 infection may reactivate during periods of immunosuppression.
- The role of HHV-6 in HIV infection is unclear.
  - Some evidence suggests that HHV-6 may potentiate progression of HIV infection, especially in infants who have acquired HIV vertically.
  - HHV-7 competes with HIV for CD4 receptors on T cells.
    - Virus may interfere with the progression of HIV infection.
- Adult recipients of bone marrow transplants have exhibited the following findings associated with HHV-6 infection.
  - Severe interstitial pneumonitis
  - Disseminated infection
  - Recurrent aseptic meningitis
  - Encephalitis

DIFFERENTIAL DIAGNOSIS

- Roseola is often confused with other exanthematous diseases.
  - Rubella
    - Rash and fever are concurrent.
    - Enlarged lymph nodes are often tender.
  - Rubeola
- Coryza, respiratory symptoms, and Koplik spots distinguish rubeola.

H

- Enterovirus exanthems
  - Usually occur in epidemics
  - Involve both older and younger children
  - Are more common in the late summer and fall
- Erythema infectiosum, or fifth disease
  - Affects the school-aged child
  - Involves the face most prominently
- Scarlet fever
  - More confluent rash
  - Associated with marked pharyngitis
- Drug eruptions (especially those resulting from sulfa-containing preparations)
  - Not regularly preceded by fever
  - Tend to be diffuse
- HHV-8 (causative agent of Kaposi sarcoma)
  - In Egypt, primary infection in childhood with HHV-8 was associated with a mild febrile exanthem indistinguishable from HHV-6– or HHV-7–related roseola.
  - Epidemiologic and clinical characteristics of HHV-8 infection in children in the US are unknown.
- HHV-6 has been isolated from patients who have many other conditions.
  - Because HHV-6 is reactivated by many acute illnesses, attributing causality to the virus is difficult in most cases.
  - Reported associations include:
    - Chronic bone marrow suppression in an immunocompetent adult
    - Idiopathic thrombocytopenic purpura
    - Thrombocytopenia during primary HHV-6 infection
    - Gianotti-Crosti syndrome
    - Hemophagocytic syndrome
    - Fatal disseminated disease in an immunocompetent infant
    - Lymphoproliferative disorders
    - Certain lymphoreticular cancers
- The role of HHV-7 in other diseases is less clear than its association with roseola.
  - Several studies have suggested reactivation of HHV-7 during relapses of adult pityriasis rosea.

DIAGNOSTIC APPROACH

- Roseola is the only manifestation of HHV-6 or HHV-7 infection that is clinically easily recognized.
- Presence of virus may be irrelevant to the disease or condition being investigated.
- Because roseola is an inconsequential illness, confirmation of the diagnosis is rarely needed.

- Signs and symptoms of all other conditions associated with these viruses are too nonspecific to allow definitive diagnosis at the bedside.
- Except in certain situations of infection in immunocompromised hosts and complicated disease in normal hosts, there is no clinical need to confirm infection with HHV-6 or HHV-7 serologically or virologically.
  - Identification of HHV-6 or HHV-7 in febrile infants does not obviate the need to evaluate for serious bacterial infection.
  - Approximately 10% of young infants have concurrent viral and bacterial infections, usually bacteriuria.
- Confirming HHV-6 or HHV-7 infection in children with complex neurologic syndromes may help rule out vaccine administration as the cause.
- Newly developed diagnostic methods to differentiate latent from actively replicating virus may eventually help both diagnosis and pathogenesis of disease associated with HHV-6 and HHV-7.

LABORATORY FINDINGS

- Roseola
  - Leukopenia as low as 2000 leukocytes/mm^3 by the third day of fever is the only helpful laboratory finding.
  - Relative lymphocytosis or monocytosis is typical.
  - Results of urinalysis are normal.
- Neither antibody detection methods nor virus isolation techniques are standardized for HHV-6 or HHV-7.
  - These assays are not available commercially.
  - Presence of maternal antibody in the young infant and reactivation of herpesviruses during other infections confound interpretation of the results.
  - Although polymerase chain reaction identification of virus in body fluids is available as a research tool, the clinical use of this test is questionable.
  - HHV-6 can be detected in high titers in saliva specimens of infants for up to 12 months after primary infection.

IMAGING

- Chest radiograph in roseola is normal.

DIAGNOSTIC PROCEDURES

- CSF examination in roseola is normal.

TREATMENT APPROACH

- Management of roseola is based entirely on symptoms.

SPECIFIC TREATMENTS

- Roseola
  - Acetaminophen is effective in controlling fever.
  - Reassuring parents that the rash is a sign of recovery comforts them and prevents unnecessary office visits.
- Both HHV-6 and HHV-7 have antiviral agent profiles similar to cytomegalovirus, with limited susceptibility to acyclovir.
  - In vitro studies show that either foscarnet or gancicloviris somewhat effective.
    - No clinical trials have been conducted with these drugs.
  - Because infection with either of these agents is self-limited in the immunocompetent child, antiviral therapy is reserved only for life-threatening infection.
- Infection in immunocomprised patients
  - Some patients have recovered after treatment with foscarnet.

WHEN TO ADMIT

- Hospitalization is usually indicated only when an alternate disease process is suspected, such as:
  - Meningitis
  - Encephalitis
  - Recurrent seizures
- Immunocompromised patients may have severe infection with HHV-6 or HHV-7.
  - Typically hospitalized for their severe clinical presentation, for example:
    - Pneumonitis
    - Encephalitis
    - Suspected graft-versus-host disease

WHEN TO REFER

- Primary HHV-6 or HHV-7 infections almost never are clinically recognized until the disease is over.
- Referral is rarely needed, except to rule out an alternative diagnosis, such as:
  - Seizure disorder
  - Treatable encephalopathy
  - Encephalitis
- Severe clinical symptoms in immunocompromised patients should always be managed by an infectious disease consultant.

COMPLICATIONS

- Long-term sequelae are unusual in the normal child with primary HHV-6 or HHV-7 infection.
- Neurologic damage is occasionally noted in children after complicated seizures associated with either virus.

PROGNOSIS

- Even with recurrent seizures during the same illness, complete recovery is the rule.
- The significance of HHV-6 in relation to recurrent seizures is not clear.
  - One study detected no increase in the risk of recurrent seizures in the first year after febrile seizure associated with primary HHV-6 versus first febrile seizures of other causes.
  - Others have noted an increased incidence of subsequent diagnoses of epilepsy.

PREVENTION

- Breastfeeding may delay acquisition of HHV-7 and HHV6.

Hydrocephalus

DEFINITION

- Hydrocephalus is the accumulation of cerebrospinal fluid (CSF) in the cerebral ventricles.
- All hydrocephalus may be considered an obstruction of CSF flow.
  - *Obstructive hydrocephalus* refers to a blockage between the ventricular system and the spinal subarachnoid space.

EPIDEMIOLOGY

- Hydrocephalus is the most common surgically treatable neurologic disorder in children.
- Congenital hydrocephalus occurs in 3 in 1000 live births.
  - The overall incidence of pediatric hydrocephalus is greater when including forms acquired through:
    - Infection
    - Trauma or hemorrhage
    - Tumors
- X-linked hydrocephalus occurs in 1 in 30,000 male births.
  - Represents <2% of all hydrocephalus
- The incidence of subclinical arrested hydrocephalus, which may result in symptoms later in childhood or in adult life, is unknown.
- Hydrocephalus is a principal diagnosis in approximately 27,870 admissions per year.
- Hydrocephalus results in 36,000 operations per year in the US, with a medical cost >$1 billion.

ETIOLOGY

- Disturbance in CSF circulation and absorption (and, rarely, production) results in an accumulation of CSF in the ventricles of the brain.
- Ill effects of hydrocephalus are probably caused by:
  - Decreased blood flow as a result of increased intracranial pressure (ICP)
  - Stretching and compressing of neural fiber and blood vessels that is a consequence of ventricular expansion
  - Although an obstruction can occur in the posterior fossa with blocked fourth-ventricle outflow, it most often results from obstruction of the aqueduct of Sylvius between the third and fourth ventricles.
- X-linked hydrocephalus
  - Defect in chromosomal region Xq28

RISK FACTORS

- Congenital defects
  - Spina bifida with myelomeningocele
    - 80–90% of patients with myelomeningocele require shunting for hydrocephalus.
  - Dandy Walker syndrome

- Holoprosencephaly
- Aqueductal stenosis
- Premature birth
  - Intraventricular hemorrhage (IVH)
    - 20% of premature infants in the US have IVH.
      - 20–75% of them will further develop posthemorrhagic hydrocephalus.
    - Hydrocephalus risk increases with IVH severity or grade.
- Infection
  - Cytomegalovirus
  - Toxoplasmosis
  - Meningitis
- Tumors of the midbrain
- Trauma

SIGNS AND SYMPTOMS

- Premature infants
  - Symptoms
    - Attacks of apnea or bradycardia
  - Signs
    - Tense and nonpulsatile anterior fontanelle
    - Distended scalp veins
    - Abnormal head contour with prominent forehead
    - Rapid (>1 cm/wk) skull circumference increase
- Full-term infants
  - Symptoms
    - Irritability
    - Vomiting
    - Drowsiness
  - Signs
    - Full or tense anterior fontanelle
    - Distended scalp veins
    - Frontal bossing
    - Widening of cranial sutures
    - Cracked pot sign on percussion
    - Macrocephaly
    - Poor head control
    - Sixth cranial nerve palsy
    - Setting sun sign (appearance of sclera above iris)
    - Impairment of upward gaze
- Older children
  - Symptoms
    - Steady or progressive headache
    - Vomiting
    - Blurred vision, diplopia

- Lethargy
- Personality and behavior changes
- Developmental delay
- Signs
  - Papilledema
  - Spasticity, more so in lower limbs
  - Sixth cranial nerve palsy
  - Neuroendocrinopathies
  - Clasped thumbs in approximately half of all cases

DIFFERENTIAL DIAGNOSIS

- Enlarging head circumference
  - Benign familial macrocrania
  - Arachnoid cyst
  - Subdural hygroma or hematoma
  - Intracranial-space–occupying lesion
  - Hydranencephaly
- Increased ICP
  - Subdural hematoma
  - Intracranial-space–occupying tumor or lesion
  - Infection
    - Meningitis
    - Brain abscess
- Neurologic deficit
  - Intracranial-space-occupying lesion
  - Cerebrovascular disease
  - Developmental/neural migration disorder

DIAGNOSTIC APPROACH

- The diagnosis is suspected in:
  - Infants with abnormally rapid head growth
  - Children of any age with symptoms of high ICP or focal neurologic deficit
- It is critical to recognize:
  - Congenital hydrocephalus
  - New-onset acquired hydrocephalus
  - Treatment failure in preexisting hydrocephalus
- Symptoms depend on:
  - Rate of progression
  - Child's age
    - In utero
    - At birth
    - Infancy
    - Early childhood
- The diagnosis of hydrocephalus is verified by brain imaging.
  - Images reveal a dilated ventricular system.

IMAGING

- Computed tomography (CT)
  - Most common form of imaging for establishing hydrocephalus
  - Axial anatomy or size of dilated ventricles
    - Diagnosis and follow-up
  - Periventricular edema
    - Acute hydrocephalus
  - Decreased sulcal or subarachnoid space
  - Confirms ventricular shunt catheter placement
    - Better than magnetic resonance imaging (MRI) for this purpose
  - Guidance during lumbar puncture
- Ultrasonography
  - Used in prenatal examination and in infants
  - Dilatation of lateral and third ventricles
  - Intracerebral blood
    - Neonate with open fontanelle
- MRI
  - Provides much more detail than CT on:
    - Etiology
    - Comorbidity
  - Scans can be obtained antenatally.
  - Guidance during lumbar puncture
  - Axial, sagittal, coronal imaging, and high gray matter resolution
    - Bowing or thinning of corpus callosum
    - Aqueductal stenosis, obstructive masses
    - Posterior fossa abnormalities
  - Cine phase-contrast CSF flow studies to assess:
    - Blockage at aqueduct
    - Fourth ventricular outflow
    - Fenestrations
- Radiography
  - Skull
    - Splaying of sutures
    - Increased gyral marking
    - Erosion of dorsum sellae
  - Shunt series
    - Anteroposterior and lateral view of the head, neck, chest, and abdomen
    - Diagnostic for mechanical shunt failure
    - May reveal a complex set of new and old shunt system components

DIAGNOSTIC PROCEDURES

- Spinal tap
  - Can diagnose increased pressure in communicating hydrocephalus
  - Palliation
- Radioactive tracer and dye studies
  - Lumbar injection
    - Assess lumbar shunt patency of CSF clearance rate
  - Shuntography
    - Injection into shunt to assess patency and flow or cerebral communication
    - Diagnostic for shunt obstruction

CLASSIFICATION

- Classification of hydrocephalus
  - Site of obstruction
    - Obstructive: aqueduct of Sylvius, fourth ventricle outlet
    - Communicating: basal cisterns
    - Multiloculated: atrium, foramen of Monroe, aqueduct, and other
  - Progression
    - Acute: may be caused by hemorrhage, infection, progresses to coma in hours
    - Chronic: congenital, partial obstruction, progresses over months to years, gradual cognitive and ambulatory decline
  - Course
    - Recurrent: with shunt failure; may be acute or chronic in onset
    - Arrested: often congenital without symptoms; symptoms of chronic hydrocephalus can develop later
    - Compensated: similar to arrested but with apparent mechanisms of compensation; treated
  - Location
    - Internal: in ventricular system only
    - External: with accumulation over hemispheres (subdural hematoma, benign macrocrania)
  - Etiology
    - Congenital
    - Acquired
  - Pressure
    - High: acute, brain noncompliant, decreased blood flow, shunt reversible if no permanent ischemia
    - Normal: usually chronic hydrocephalus, brain compliance abnormal with labile pressures
    - Low: very compliant brain, ventricles remain large unless drained at very low pressure, coma may persist without aggressive drainage

- Age of onset
  - Fetal: genetic, congenital, development affected; normal ventricular size unlikely
  - Neonatal: congenital or acquired IVH, infection, tumor, other; comorbidity likely
  - Child: acquired via tumor or other
  - Adult: acquired, idiopathic

TREATMENT APPROACH

- Prompt recognition and treatment of hydrocephalus and treatment failure is important for a favorable outcome.
  - Delay in surgical treatment is a risk factor for a poor outcome in hydrocephalic children.
- Surgical treatment with valved silicone shunts
  - CSF diversion from a cerebral ventricle or lumbar canal to a body cavity
    - Usually the peritoneal cavity
  - Treatment with implanted shunts is life saving.
    - Most children live with hydrocephalus as a chronic surgically arrested disease.
    - Patients have the potential to live full lives into adulthood.
- Endoscopic third ventriculostomy (ETV)
  - Allows fluid to escape without a shunt in obstructive hydrocephalus
- Medical management
  - Usually only a means of palliation before more definitive surgical treatment
  - Acetazolamide slows CSF production.
- Invasive nonsurgical techniques
  - Serial lumbar or ventricular puncture via the fontanelle
    - Performed in emergencies or until a premature infant can tolerate surgery

SPECIFIC TREATMENTS

CSF shunting

- Ventricular catheter
  - Soft, flexible, perforated, straight silicon tube inserted through a 1-cm burr hole in the frontal or occipital cranium
    - Usually on the nondominant side
    - Stabilized at the burr hole with an angle flange or a tapping reservoir
  - The preferred site for the catheter tip is in the anterior horn of a lateral ventricle away from potentially obstructing choroid plexus.

H

- Catheter insertion is most often blind and based on external cranial landmarks.
  - Attempts to visualize catheter tip location with an endoscope during surgery have not resulted in better placement or survival.
- Proximal obstructions are common as a result of tissue growth.
  - Vascular choroid plexus
- Premature infants
  - Implanted ventricular catheter, either externalized or leading to a subgaleal reservoir or space, may be used to obtain more consistent drainage before permanent shunting is considered.

- Valve
  - 2 purposes
    - Allows 1-way flow
    - Regulates the amount of drainage
  - Types of valves
    - Differential-pressure valve
      - Opens when pressure on the cranial side is greater than the distal side
    - High-pressure valve
      - Pressure differential may need to be >140–150 mm Hg.
    - Medium- or low-pressure valve
      - Less of a gradient is needed, and more fluid will be drained.
    - Flow-controlled, antisiphon, or gravity-controlled valve
      - Regulates flow to reduce drainage, especially when standing
      - Overdrainage is common after chronic shunting and can result in slit ventricles or subdural hematomas.
    - Adjustable valve
      - Provides for noninvasive CSF drainage adjustment with growth or if hydrocephalus becomes internally compensated
      - Overdrainage or underdrainage symptoms may be treated with adjustments alone.
- Distal catheter
  - Extends from the valve to the drainage cavity
    - Ventriculoperitoneal
      - Can be placed through an incision ≤1 cm
      - Advantages include extra catheter length insertion to allow for growth and less risk of infection problems compared with vascular shunts.

  - Ventriculoatrial
    - Vascular insertion into the right atrium via the subclavian or internal jugular vein
    - Advantages include less siphoning and possible placement when the abdominal cavity must be avoided.
  - Lumboperitoneal
  - Distal end into pleural cavity
    - Pleural catheters are placed only in adults because CSF drainage of the large infant cranium would too easily overwhelm the pleural space.
  - Distal end into gallbladder
- Complex or loculated hydrocephalus
  - ≥2 proximal catheters may be connected to drain multiple ventricles or cysts.
- Old ventricular catheters may be retained.
  - Pulling catheters out results in some bleeding risk (although they must be removed if a central infection develops).

- The catheter or valve may have a reservoir where fluid can be tapped or pumped.
  - A reservoir that remains depressed (dimpled) after compression is a likely sign of proximal obstruction.
  - This system may be tapped under sterile conditions in the outpatient or emergency department setting to check for patency, pressure, or infection.

ETV

- Used in obstructive hydrocephalus and some cases of communicating hydrocephalus
  - Under endoscopic visualization, fluid trapped in the lateral and third ventricles is released into the basal cisterns through a fenestration made in the floor of the third ventricle, just anterior to the basilar artery.
  - Performed through a right frontal burr hole similar to that used for shunt catheter placement.
  - Advantages
    - Preventing overdrainage
    - Avoiding implanted hardware
- Outcomes
  - Successful in approximately 70% of cases
    - Success does not always decrease ventricular size, as seen with shunting.
  - Failure must often be judged clinically as a return of symptoms.
    - If fenestration is closed (seen in cine phase-contrast CSF-flow MRI or on direct endoscopic inspection), it may be reopened.
    - A shunt may be placed secondarily in other cases.
  - ETV success in communicating hydrocephalus is still not well established.

Serial lumbar or ventricular puncture via the fontanelle

- Indications
  - Emergencies
  - Premature infant not yet able to tolerate surgery (if weight >2 kg)
    - Taps may be performed serially for up to 3–4 weeks in a premature infant with IVH if it is unclear that there will be progressive hydrocephalus requiring a shunt.
- Methods
  - Lumbar puncture
    - Using CT or MRI after confirmation that the hydrocephalus is communicating
    - Lumbar puncture in obstructive hydrocephalus cannot decompress cranial CSF and can cause downward tonsillar herniation.
  - Ventricular puncture
    - Performed at the lateral corner of an open fontanel in infants with obstructive hydrocephalus or when lumbar puncture is not successful

Specific clinical situations

- Myelomeningocele
  - Shunt may be placed at the time of myelomeningocele closure or, if possible, in subsequent days or weeks to reduce infection risk.
  - ETV
    - Controversial in myelomeningocele
    - May be considered an option even in later years in the event of shunt failure
- IVH of prematurity
  - Shunting is usually preceded by several weeks of palliative treatment.
    - Delay allows for infant growth (preferably to >2 kg) and for determining progressive hydrocephalus.
    - Ventricular size may stabilize over weeks.
  - Palliative procedures
    - Lumbar punctures (taking approximately 10 mL/kg)
    - Fontanelle tap
    - Surgical placement of a ventricular catheter for external or subgaleal drainage
- Posterior fossa tumors
  - Tumor resection
    - Allows CSF flow reestablishment
    - Eliminates the need for shunting in most cases
  - ETV or shunt implantation
    - Children with persisting hydrocephalus are excellent candidates for ETV or standard shunt implantation.

- Dandy Walker syndrome
  - Historically treated with cyst resection or fenestration
    - Frequent treatment failure
  - Shunting of the cyst or the ventricles
    - In the presence of aqueductal stenosis, both the ventricles and the cyst may be shunted simultaneously.
  - ETV
    - May be effective
- Postinfectious hydrocephalus
  - Medical treatment
  - External ventricular drain if needed until the infection clears
  - A permanent ventriculoperitoneal shunt may be placed later.
  - ETV
    - Has been attempted in the hopes of avoiding an implanted shunt
    - Alone or in combination with choroid plexus coagulation
    - Viral infections may especially result in minimal leptomeningeal fibrosis with a simultaneous aqueductal stenosis that an ETV may manage.
    - Extensive cistern scarring may limit potential ETV efficacy in many cases.
- Multiloculated hydrocephalus
  - Loculations present a complex drainage problem, sometimes requiring multiple catheters.
  - Open or endoscopic cyst fenestration facilitates fluid communication.
    - Allows simplified drainage through a single shunt catheter
- Aqueductal stenosis
  - ETV
    - Preferred treatment
    - Samples of tectum, posterior third-ventricle, or pineal region tumors can be obtained for biopsy during the same endoscopic procedure.
  - Shunt implantation
    - Still commonly performed

WHEN TO ADMIT

- All newly diagnosed cases of hydrocephalus should be admitted.
- All patients who develop shunt complications, such as shunt malfunction or shunt infection, should be admitted.

H

WHEN TO REFER

- All patients with suspected hydrocephalus should be referred to pediatric neurosurgeons immediately.
- All patients with shunt complications should be referred to pediatric neurosurgeons.

FOLLOW-UP

- Postoperative follow-up schedule
  - 2 weeks after surgery
  - Every 3 months for the first year
  - Every 6 months in the second year
  - Yearly thereafter
- Clinical assessment
  - Developmental milestones
  - Head circumference
  - Symptoms and signs of:
    - Increased intracranial tension
    - Infection
    - Other complications

COMPLICATIONS

Shunt-related complications

- Intracerebral hemorrhage
  - Any probe insertion into the brain may result in bleeding.
    - Occurs in <2% of cases
    - Risk is greater in removing an old ventricular catheter that is obstructed by an ingrowing choroid plexus than in inserting a new one.
  - Minor bleeding may resolve on its own.
    - The greatest concern is increased risk of shunt obstruction.
  - Surgical evacuation
    - Very rarely necessary for bleeding
- Infection
  - Full treatment usually requires:
    - Removing the shunt
    - Placing a temporary external drain if needed
    - Initiating antibiotic treatment
    - Reinserting the shunt after documenting negative CSF cultures
  - Perioperative prophylactic antibiotics
    - Reduce shunt infection risk by 50%.
    - Antibiotic-impregnated shunts may reduce infection rate by 1–2%.

- Risk increases with presence of an inner lumen.
  - Infection rate is 5–10%.
  - Most infections occur in the first 6 months.
  - Indolent infections have been reported after years.
- Usually involves skin flora
  - *Staphylococcus epidermidis*
  - *Propionibacterium acnes*
  - *Staphylococcus aureus*
- Signs and symptoms
  - Signs of systemic or local infection
  - Symptoms ofmeningitis
  - Shunt dysfunction may be a sign of an indolent shunt infection.
  - Chronic infection may be difficult to diagnose; little cellular response
- Shunt obstruction
  - Proximal
    - Choroid plexus ingrowth into the proximal ventricular catheter
  - Distal
    - Scar tissue or thrombus developing in vascular shunts
  - Total or partial/intermittent
    - Hydrocephalic symptoms that recur with ventricular expansion
    - Can be sufficient to indicate surgical exploration
- Mechanical failure
  - Breaks
    - Although shunts may last decades, they become more brittle over time.
    - Calcified scar can evolve around the catheter
    - The valve may become incompetent.
    - A break at a tethering point, such as a valve or connector, is common.
  - Kinks
  - Migration
    - Short shunt caused by growth or migration into the preperitoneal space
  - Displacement
- Overdrainage
  - In CSF shunting, too much drainage (acutely or chronically) can be as problematic as too little.
  - Slit ventricles
    - Ventricles become abnormally small.
    - May result in frequent shunt blockages and episodic headaches

- Subdural hygroma
  - Develops in children with severe cortical thinning
- Chronic subdural hematoma
  - Because the brain has limited elasticity and can reexpand after severe hydrocephalus, cortical walls collapse and a subdural hematoma can develop if bridging vessels are injured.
- Management
  - ICP monitoring
  - Shunt revision to reduce CSF drainage, unless an adjustable valve is in place
  - Implantation of antisiphon or gravity devices
- Complications of shunt implantation
  - Infection
  - Nonphysiologic overdrainage
  - Fever
    - Incidence of all complications combined ranges from 6–20%.
    - Most complications are reversible.
- Complications specific to ventriculocardiac shunts
  - Thrombosis around the distal tube
  - Cor pulmonale
  - Shunt nephritis
  - Septicemia and pyemic abscesses
- Complications specific to ventriculopleural shunts
  - Hydrothorax
    - Characterized by respiratory distress
  - Pyothorax
- Complications specific to ventriculoperitoneal shunts
  - Bowel perforation: rare with current catheter materials
  - Pseudocyst: sterile or infected and presenting as obstruction or abdominal swelling
  - Ascites: malabsorption of CSF; sterile or infected
  - Hernia: at shunt insertion incisions

Complications of ETV

- Injury to the hypothalamus and basilar artery
- Undertreatment/treatment failure
  - Ventricles remain large.
  - Failure may be sudden and catastrophic or gradual and insidious.
  - Success is based on clinical resolution alone.
  - Treatment failure or underdrainage may be missed if it occurs gradually.

PROGNOSIS

- A child with isolated hydrocephalus that is well treated and monitored has the potential for a fully functional life.
- Many factors play a role in overall outcome.
  - Concomitant medical conditions
  - Degree of neurologic compromise at the time of surgical treatment
  - Nature and cause of hydrocephalus
  - Complications greatly affect the long-term outcome.
- Survival
  - Overall shunt mortality rate
    - <5% after 10 years
  - Congenital hydrocephalus
    - 5-year survival rate approximately 90%
  - Posthemorrhagic hydrocephalus
    - Grades I and II: mortality rate, 9%
    - Grades III and IV: mortality rate, 49%
- Functional assessment
  - Intellect/IQ in long-term studies
    - Varies widely with each specific cause
    - >90 in 32%
    - 70–90 in 28%
    - 50–70 in 19%
    - <50 in 21%
    - 60% of patients can be integrated into the normal school system.
  - Degree of intellectual impairment
    - Relates more to the degree of severity of underlying CNS anomalies and defects in the neocortex cytoarchitecture
    - Relates less to severity of hydrocephalus
  - Motor deficit: 80%
  - Visual or auditory deficit: 25%
  - Epilepsy: 30%

Hyperhidrosis

DEFINITION

- Hyperhidrosis is excessive localized sweating.

EPIDEMIOLOGY

- Age
  - Axillary hyperhidrosis usually becomes more of a problem in adolescence.

MECHANISM

- Researchers postulate that emotions and temperature of blood perfusing the hypothalamus stimulate the secretion of hormones that regulate the autonomic nervous system's control of perspiration.
- Eccrine sweat glands
  - Control thermoregulation
  - Most numerous on the palms, soles, and axillae
- Axillary hyperhidrosis
  - Probably stimulated by both heat and emotion
  - Apocrine glands are stimulated at puberty by androgenic hormones.
- Palmar and plantar hyperhidrosis
  - Caused by eccrine sweat production
  - May occur at any age
  - Thought to be stimulated by anxiety

HISTORY

- The child or the family reports:
  - Odiferous sweating
  - Sweating so intense that it interferes with:
    - Hand functions
    - Foot functions
  - Axillary hyperhidrosis in adolescence may cause embarrassment.
    - Sweat ring on clothing
    - Odor associated with bacterial degradation of apocrine sweat

DIFFERENTIAL DIAGNOSIS

- Excessive generalized sweating may be caused by a systemic disorder.
  - Infection
  - Hypoglycemia
  - Drug withdrawal
  - Thyrotoxicosis
  - Pheochromocytoma
  - Riley-Day syndrome

TREATMENT APPROACH

- Topical and systemic agents
  - Anticholinergic agents
  - Prescription 20% aluminum chloride
  - Tap water iontophoresis
- For bromhidrosis (malodorous hyperhidrosis) of the soles
  - Frequent cleansing with drying deodorant soaps
  - Topical antibiotics
  - Going barefoot whenever possible
- For combined axillary hyperhidrosis and bromhidrosis
  - Frequent clothing changes
  - Topical antibiotics and deodorant powders
- For sweating caused by emotional stress
  - Propranolol and anxiolytics

SPECIFIC TREATMENT

Pharmacologic treatment

- Systemic anticholinergic agents
  - May block acetylcholine, the sympathetic innervation terminal neurotransmitter to eccrine glands
  - Side effects preclude long-term use.
- Prescription 20% aluminum chloride
  - Application every other day for palmar sweating or plantar hyperhidrosis
  - Prescription 20% solution of aluminum chloride in anhydrous ethanol applied to the axillary vault
    - May cause an irritant contact dermatitis
    - Hydrocortisone 1% cream for relief of inflammation
- Propranolol and anxiolytics are options to reduce emotional stress
- Botulinum A toxin
  - Approved for axillary sweat gland chemodenervation
  - Palmar and plantar hyperhidrosis
    - Subepidermal injections inhibit sweat production
    - Purportedly blocks presynaptic acetylcholine release
    - Effective for up to 12 months
    - Has been used in patients as young as 14 years
    - Temporarily or, rarely, causes permanent muscle and nerve injury from the injections

Other measures

- In extreme cases
  - Excision of local axillary skin
  - Removal of glands by curettage or liposuction
    - Ganglion sympathectomy cannot be recommended for most patients who have axillary hyperhidrosis, because of attendant complications.

WHEN TO REFER

- Hyperhidrosis that interferes with appropriate bodily function (eg, hand so slippery wet that the child cannot hold a pencil)
- Generalized excessive sweating
- Socially isolating hyperhidrosis as a result of odor or excessive drenching of clothing

H

Hypertension

DEFINITION

- In children and adolescents, hypertension is defined as elevated blood pressure (BP) that persists on repeated measurement at the 95th percentile or greater for age, height, and sex in a healthy population.
  - High-normal or prehypertensive BP is defined as BP ≥90th percentile but <95th percentile (normal systolic and diastolic BPs are <90th percentile).
  - Severe hypertension (with the risk of end-organ injury) is defined as BP >99th percentile.
  - Body size is the single most important determinant of BP in children and adolescents.
  - Using accurate height percentiles is critical for correctly estimating BP percentiles (see Figure 33 on page F13).
- 2 categories of hypertension
  - Primary or essential
  - Secondary

EPIDEMIOLOGY

- Prevalence
  - Recent studies have shown:
    - Mean BP has increased among children and adolescents in the last decade.
    - Elevated BP in childhood often continues into adulthood, predicting hypertension in young adulthood.
    - Essential hypertension is familial in nature.
  - Chronic hypertension is becoming increasingly common in adolescents.
    - Increase in this population of being overweight and obese
    - Obesity rates have more than doubled for children age 2–5 years and 12–19 over the past 3 decades.
    - The obesity rate has more than tripled among children age 6–11 years.
    - Presently in the US, 9 million children >6 years of age are considered obese, with a body mass index (BMI) >95th percentile.
  - Metabolic syndrome
    - Although no standardized definition of metabolic syndrome currently exists, it is increasingly recognized as a significant complication of childhood obesity.
    - National samples indicate that roughly 10% of all 12- to 19-year-olds in the US presently have symptoms of metabolic syndrome.
- Age
  - Essential hypertension
    - The most common type of hypertension in adults
    - Relatively uncommon in (younger) children, but seen more frequently, especially in adolescents

- Secondary hypertension
  - More common in children than in adults
  - Reported in 2–3% of premature infants
- Ethnicity
  - In the US, the distribution of BP in adults differs among racial and ethnic groups.
  - Non-Hispanic black adults have increased prevalence and incidence of hypertension.
  - The age at which differences in BP become apparent across racial and ethnic groups is unclear.
  - Studies repeatedly show that BP levels are higher among black children than among white children.
  - BP levels are significantly higher for black girls than for white girls; the situation for boys is less certain.
  - Mexican-American children have a higher mean-adjusted BP than do non-Hispanic white children.
  - In many instances, a higher BMI explains the difference in BP between different ethnic groups.
  - Increase in BMI in children in the US has accounted for some of the increase in BP.
    - Other factors also probably contribute.

MECHANISM

General

- BP is a product of cardiac output and systemic resistance affected by changes in:
  - Heart rate
  - Stroke volume
  - Blood volume
  - Peripheral resistance
  - Effect of various hormones on vascular bed

Renin-angiotensin system and hypertension

- Angiotensin II
  - Potent vasoconstrictor
  - Major end product of the renin-angiotensin system
  - Exerts the major hormonal control of BP
  - Provides feedback that inhibits renin release
  - Increases intravascular volume
  - Is closely related to renal blood flow
- Renin
  - Enzyme that stimulates production of angiotensin II
  - Release is stimulated by:
    - Volume depletion
    - Hypotension
    - Salt depletion

- Release is inhibited by:
  - Volume expansion
  - Salt loading
  - Elevated electrolyte levels

Other hormonal systems

- Other hormonal systems also affect renin release, such as:
  - Circulating catecholamines
  - Glucagon
  - Adrenocorticotropic hormones
  - Parathyroid hormones

Drugs

- Stimulators of renin release
  - Vasodilators
  - Diuretics
- Inhibitors of renin release
  - Mineralocorticoids
  - ß-Blockers
- Sympathomimetics
  - Cocaine
  - Amphetamines
  - Phenylephrine
  - Nonsteroidal antiinflammatory drugs
  - Erythropoietin
  - Cyclosporins

Age

- BP tends to increase with age throughout the first 2 decades of life.
  - Systolic
    - Average on the first day of life is 70 mm Hg.
  - Increases steadily for the first 2 months
  - Tends to remain stable until 1 year of age, when it increases until adulthood
  - Diastolic
    - Increases slowly for the first week, then declines until 3 months of age
  - Then increases gradually until 1 year of age, when it reaches the level found in the first week
  - Remains steady for the first 5–6 years, after which it increases, along with the systolic BP
  - Children tend to maintain the same BP percentile rank relative to their peers as they grow, a pattern that continues through adolescence, supporting the idea that essential hypertension begins in childhood.

Genetics

- Children from families with a history of hypertension tend to have higher BPs.
- Supports the generally accepted conclusion that genetics influence BP
- Other cardiovascular risk factors among parents correlate with those of their children, including:
  - Disorders of lipid and glucose metabolism
  - Hyperuricemia
  - Poor nutrition
  - Passive smoking
  - Physical inactivity

HISTORY

- Medical history should include questions regarding:
  - All cardiovascular risk factors
  - Symptoms suggestive of secondary hypertension
  - Possible target organ damage
- Particular attention needs to be paid to any history suggesting:
  - Recent onset of renal disease
  - Chronic urinary tract infections
  - Exogenous steroids
  - Oral contraceptives
  - Illicit drugs
  - Tobacco
  - Alcohol
- A systems review that includes the following details:
  - Diet
  - Salt intake
  - Exercise
- In adolescents, use of the following should be explored:
  - Exogenous steroids
  - Oral contraceptives
  - Illicit drugs
  - Tobacco
  - Alcohol
- The following may be helpful in directing further evaluations.
  - A history of prematurity
  - Patent ductus arteriosus
  - Bronchopulmonary dysplasia
  - A positive family history, including age of onset, of:
    - Essential hypertension
    - Systemic disease
    - Endocrinopathy

H

PHYSICAL EXAM

BP measurement

- Figure 34 on page F14 is an algorithm for diagnosing and managing patients with hypertension.
- Systolic BP: defined as the pressure at the onset of the first Korotkoff (K1) sound
- Diastolic BP: pressure at the fifth Korotkoff (K5) sound or at the disappearance or muffling of the Korotkoff sounds
  - In some children, Korotkoff sounds can continue to be heard until 0 mm Hg, generally excluding a diagnosis of diastolic hypertension.
- Height and weight are related independently to BP at all ages (see tables Blood Pressure Levels for Boys by Age and Height Percentiles and Blood Pressure Levels for Girls by Age and Height Percentiles).
- Measure BP in all children >3 years seen in a medical setting.
- Appropriate techniques are important to avoid false-positive readings.
  - Infants should be supine.
  - Children and adolescents should be seated.
    - Child should be quiet for 5 minutes before measurement.
    - Back should be supported and feet on the floor.
    - Right arm should be supported, with antecubital fossa at heart level.
    - Child should not have recently ingested stimulant drugs or food.
  - Appropriately sized cuff
    - Width of cuff must be ≥40% of the mid-arm circumference, as measured midway between the olecranon and the acromion.
    - Cuff should be long enough to cover ≥80% of the circumference of the arm.
    - Cuff should be inflated to ≥30 mm Hg above the expected systolic BP.
    - Inflating too high in young children or infants may cause agitation.
    - Stethoscope or Doppler crystal should be placed lightly over the brachial artery in the antecubital fossa.
    - Arm should be at the level of the heart.
  - Measure in all 4 extremities:
    - Average of at least 2 separate measurements
    - Average 2 systolic and 2 diastolic readings
    - Best to average measurements obtained during several visits
  - Assess radial; brachial; and, most important, femoral pulses.
- Automated BP devices
  - In general, auscultation is recommended method of measuring BP in children.

- Advantages
  - Relative simplicity
  - Ability to minimize observer bias and terminal digit preferences
  - Can provide serial noninvasive BP in newborns and infants, in whom auscultation is difficult
  - Good in the intensive care unit, where frequent BP measurements are needed
  - Automated measurements appear to correlate well with intraarterial readings.
- Reliability in the physician's office is less clear.
  - Devices require frequent calibration.
  - Reference standards have not been established.
- Ambulatory monitoring
  - Recently, has been used to help establish the diagnosis of hypertension and track diurnal variations of BP in older children
  - A monitor is worn on the arm for 24 hours.
  - BP is measured periodically and values stored for later analysis.
  - Specifically helpful in evaluating:
    - White-coat hypertension
    - Risk for hypertensive end-organ injury
    - Apparent drug resistance
    - Hypotensive symptoms that may occur with the use of antihypertensive drugs
  - Can be used to evaluate BP patterns in such conditions as:
    - Episodic hypertension
    - Chronic kidney disease
    - Diabetes
    - Autonomic dysfunction
  - Ambulatory BP monitoring of children and adolescents should be used and interpreted only by those experienced in pediatric hypertension.

Complete physical

- Calculation of BMI
  - Weight in kilograms divided by the square of height in meters
- Auscultation for carotid, abdominal, and femoral bruits
- Palpation of the thyroid gland
- Thorough examination of the heart and lungs
- Examination of the abdomen for:
  - Enlarged kidneys
  - Masses
  - Abnormal aortic pulsation
- Palpation of the legs for edema and pulses
- Examination of the optic fundi

Blood Pressure Levels for Boys by Age and Height Percentiles[a]

BP Age Percentile (Year)[b]		Systolic BP (mm Hg)							Diastolic BP (mm Hg)						
		Percentile of Height							Percentile of Height						
		5th	10th	25th	50th	75th	90th	95th	5th	10th	25th	50th	75th	90th	95th
1	50th	80	81	83	85	87	88	89	34	35	36	37	38	39	39
	90th	94	95	97	99	100	102	103	49	50	51	52	53	53	54
	95th	98	99	101	103	104	106	106	54	54	55	56	57	58	58
	99th	105	106	108	110	112	113	114	61	62	63	64	65	66	66
2	50th	84	85	87	88	90	92	92	39	40	41	42	43	44	44
	90th	97	99	100	102	104	105	106	54	55	56	57	58	58	59
	95th	101	102	104	106	108	109	110	59	59	60	61	62	63	63
	99th	109	110	111	113	115	117	117	66	67	68	69	70	71	71
3	50th	86	87	89	91	93	94	95	44	44	45	46	47	48	48
	90th	100	101	103	105	107	108	109	59	59	60	61	62	63	63
	95th	104	105	107	109	110	112	113	63	63	64	65	66	67	67
	99th	111	112	114	116	118	119	120	71	71	72	73	74	75	75
4	50th	88	89	91	93	95	96	97	47	48	49	50	51	51	52
	90th	102	103	105	107	109	110	111	62	63	64	65	66	66	67
	95th	106	107	109	111	112	114	115	66	67	68	69	70	71	71
	99th	113	114	116	118	120	121	122	74	75	76	77	78	78	79
5	50th	90	91	93	95	96	98	98	50	51	52	53	54	55	55
	90th	104	105	106	108	110	111	112	65	66	67	68	69	69	70
	95th	108	109	110	112	114	115	116	69	70	71	72	73	74	74
	99th	115	116	118	120	121	123	123	77	78	79	80	81	81	82
6	50th	91	92	94	96	98	99	100	53	53	54	55	56	57	57
	90th	105	106	108	110	111	113	113	68	68	69	70	71	72	72
	95th	109	110	112	114	115	117	117	72	72	73	74	75	76	76
	99th	116	117	119	121	123	124	125	80	80	81	82	83	84	84
7	50th	92	94	95	97	99	100	101	55	55	56	57	58	59	59
	90th	106	107	109	111	113	114	115	70	70	71	72	73	74	74
	95th	110	111	113	115	117	118	119	74	74	75	76	77	78	78
	99th	117	118	120	122	124	125	126	82	82	83	84	85	86	86
8	50th	94	95	97	99	100	102	102	56	57	58	59	60	60	61
	90th	107	109	110	112	114	115	116	71	72	72	73	74	75	76
	95th	111	112	114	116	118	119	120	75	76	77	78	79	79	80
	99th	119	120	122	123	125	127	127	83	84	85	86	87	87	88
9	50th	95	96	98	100	102	103	104	57	58	59	60	61	61	62
	90th	109	110	112	114	115	117	118	72	73	74	75	76	76	77
	95th	113	114	116	118	119	121	121	76	77	78	79	80	81	81
	99th	120	121	123	125	127	128	129	84	85	86	87	88	88	89

H

Blood Pressure Levels for Boys by Age and Height Percentile[a], *continued*

BP Age Percentile (Year)[b]		Systolic BP (mm Hg)							Diastolic BP (mm Hg)						
		Percentile of Height							Percentile of Height						
		5th	10th	25th	50th	75th	90th	95th	5th	10th	25th	50th	75th	90th	95th
10	50th	97	98	100	102	103	105	106	58	59	60	61	61	62	63
	90th	111	112	114	115	117	119	119	73	73	74	75	76	77	78
	95th	115	116	117	119	121	122	123	77	78	79	80	81	81	82
	99th	122	123	125	127	128	130	130	85	86	86	88	88	89	90
11	50th	99	100	102	104	105	107	107	59	59	60	61	62	63	63
	90th	113	114	115	117	119	120	121	74	74	75	76	77	78	78
	95th	117	118	119	121	123	124	125	78	78	79	80	81	82	82
	99th	124	125	127	129	130	132	132	86	86	87	88	89	90	90
12	50th	101	102	104	106	108	109	110	59	60	61	62	63	63	64
	90th	115	116	118	120	121	123	123	74	75	75	76	77	78	79
	95th	119	120	122	123	125	127	127	78	79	80	81	82	82	83
	99th	126	127	129	131	133	134	135	86	87	88	89	90	90	91
13	50th	104	105	106	108	110	111	112	60	60	61	62	63	64	64
	90th	117	118	120	122	124	125	126	75	75	76	77	78	79	79
	95th	121	122	124	126	128	129	130	79	79	80	81	82	83	83
	99th	128	130	131	133	135	136	137	87	87	88	89	90	91	91
14	50th	106	107	109	111	113	114	115	60	61	62	63	64	65	65
	90th	120	121	123	125	126	128	128	75	76	77	78	79	79	80
	95th	124	125	127	128	130	132	132	80	80	81	82	83	84	84
	99th	131	132	134	136	138	139	140	87	88	89	90	91	92	92
15	50th	109	110	112	113	115	117	117	61	62	63	64	65	66	66
	90th	122	124	125	127	129	130	131	76	77	78	79	80	80	81
	95th	126	127	129	131	133	134	135	81	81	82	83	84	85	85
	99th	134	135	136	138	140	142	142	88	89	90	91	92	93	93
16	50th	111	112	114	116	118	119	120	63	63	64	65	66	67	67
	90th	125	126	128	130	131	133	134	78	78	79	80	81	82	82
	95th	129	130	132	134	135	137	137	82	83	83	84	85	86	87
	99th	136	137	139	141	143	144	145	90	90	91	92	93	94	94
17	50th	114	115	116	118	120	121	122	65	66	66	67	68	69	70
	90th	127	128	130	132	134	135	136	80	80	81	82	83	84	84
	95th	131	132	134	136	138	139	140	84	85	86	87	87	88	89
	99th	139	140	141	143	145	146	147	92	93	93	94	95	96	97

Abbreviation: BP, blood pressure.

[a] From: National High Blood Pressure Education Program Working Group on High Blood Pressure in Children and Adolescents. The fourth report on the diagnosis, evaluation, and treatment of high blood pressure in children and adolescents. *Pediatrics.* 2004;114(2):555–576.

[b] The 90th percentile is 1.28 3D, 95th percentile is 1.645 SD, and 99th percentile is 2.326 SD over the mean.

Blood Pressure Levels for Girls by Age and Height Percentile[a]

BP Age Percentile (Year)[b]		Systolic BP (mm Hg) Percentile of Height							Diastolic BP (mm Hg) Percentile of Height						
		5th	10th	25th	50th	75th	90th	95th	5th	10th	25th	50th	75th	90th	95th
1	50th	83	84	85	86	88	89	90	38	39	39	40	41	41	42
	90th	97	97	98	100	101	102	103	52	53	53	54	55	55	56
	95th	100	101	102	104	105	106	107	56	57	57	58	59	59	60
	99th	108	108	109	111	112	113	114	64	64	65	65	66	67	67
2	50th	85	85	87	88	89	91	91	43	44	44	45	46	46	47
	90th	98	99	100	101	103	104	105	57	58	58	59	60	61	61
	95th	102	103	104	105	107	108	109	61	62	62	63	64	65	65
	99th	109	110	111	112	114	115	116	69	69	70	70	71	72	72
3	50th	86	87	88	89	91	92	93	47	48	48	49	50	50	51
	90th	100	100	102	103	104	106	106	61	62	62	63	64	64	65
	95th	104	104	105	107	108	109	110	65	66	66	67	68	68	69
	99th	111	111	113	114	115	116	117	73	73	74	74	75	76	76
4	50th	88	88	90	91	92	94	94	50	50	51	52	52	53	54
	90th	101	102	103	104	106	107	108	64	64	65	66	67	67	68
	95th	105	106	107	108	110	111	112	68	68	69	70	71	71	72
	99th	112	113	114	115	117	118	119	76	76	76	77	78	79	79
5	50th	89	90	91	93	94	95	96	52	53	53	54	55	55	56
	90th	103	103	105	106	107	109	109	66	67	67	68	69	69	70
	95th	107	107	108	110	111	112	113	70	71	71	72	73	73	74
	99th	114	114	116	117	118	120	120	78	78	79	79	80	81	81
6	50th	91	92	93	94	96	97	98	54	54	55	56	56	57	58
	90th	104	105	106	108	109	110	111	68	68	69	70	70	71	72
	95th	108	109	110	111	113	114	115	72	72	73	74	74	75	76
	99th	115	116	117	119	120	121	122	80	80	80	81	82	83	83
7	50th	93	93	95	96	97	99	99	55	56	56	57	58	58	59
	90th	106	107	108	109	111	112	113	69	70	70	71	72	72	73
	95th	110	111	112	113	115	116	116	73	74	74	75	76	76	77
	99th	117	118	119	120	122	123	124	81	81	82	82	83	84	84
8	50th	95	95	96	98	99	100	101	57	57	57	58	59	60	60
	90th	108	109	110	111	113	114	114	71	71	71	72	73	74	74
	95th	112	112	114	115	116	118	118	75	75	75	76	77	78	78
	99th	119	120	121	122	123	125	125	82	82	83	83	84	85	86
9	50th	96	97	98	100	101	102	103	58	58	58	59	60	61	61
	90th	110	110	112	113	114	116	116	72	72	72	73	74	75	75
	95th	114	114	115	117	118	119	120	76	76	76	77	78	79	79
	99th	121	121	123	124	125	127	127	83	83	84	84	85	86	87

Blood Pressure Levels for Girls by Age and Height Percentile[a], *continued*

BP Age Percentile (Year)[b]		Systolic BP (mm Hg)							Diastolic BP (mm Hg)						
		Percentile of Height							Percentile of Height						
		5th	10th	25th	50th	75th	90th	95th	5th	10th	25th	50th	75th	90th	95th
10	50th	98	99	100	102	103	104	105	59	59	59	60	61	62	62
	90th	112	112	114	115	116	118	118	73	73	73	74	75	76	76
	95th	116	116	117	119	120	121	122	77	77	77	78	79	80	80
	99th	123	123	125	126	127	129	129	84	84	85	86	86	87	88
11	50th	100	101	102	103	105	106	107	60	60	60	61	62	63	63
	90th	114	114	116	117	118	119	120	74	74	74	75	76	77	77
	95th	118	118	119	121	122	123	124	78	78	78	79	80	81	81
	99th	125	125	126	128	129	130	131	85	85	86	87	87	88	89
12	50th	102	103	104	105	107	108	109	61	61	61	62	63	64	64
	90th	116	116	117	119	120	121	122	75	75	75	76	77	78	78
	95th	119	120	121	123	124	125	126	79	79	79	80	81	82	82
	99th	127	127	128	130	131	132	133	86	86	87	88	88	89	90
13	50th	104	105	106	107	109	110	110	62	62	62	63	64	65	65
	90th	117	118	119	121	122	123	124	76	76	76	77	78	79	79
	95th	121	122	123	124	126	127	128	80	80	80	81	82	83	83
	99th	128	129	130	132	133	134	135	87	87	88	89	89	90	91
14	50th	106	106	107	109	110	111	112	63	63	63	64	65	66	66
	90th	119	120	121	122	124	125	125	77	77	77	78	79	80	80
	95th	123	123	125	126	127	129	129	81	81	81	82	83	84	84
	99th	130	131	132	133	135	136	136	88	88	89	90	90	91	92
15	50th	107	108	109	110	111	113	113	64	64	64	65	66	67	67
	90th	120	121	122	123	125	126	127	78	78	78	79	80	81	81
	95th	124	125	126	127	129	130	131	82	82	82	83	84	85	85
	99th	131	132	133	134	136	137	138	89	89	90	91	91	92	93
16	50th	108	108	110	111	112	114	114	64	64	65	66	66	67	68
	90th	121	122	123	124	126	127	128	78	78	79	80	81	81	82
	95th	125	126	127	128	130	131	132	82	82	83	84	85	85	86
	99th	132	133	134	135	137	138	139	90	90	90	91	92	93	93
17	50th	108	109	110	111	113	114	115	64	65	65	66	67	67	68
	90th	122	122	123	125	126	127	128	78	79	79	80	81	81	82
	95th	125	126	127	129	130	131	132	82	83	83	84	85	85	86
	99th	133	133	134	136	137	138	139	90	90	91	91	92	93	93

Abbreviation: BP, blood pressure.

[a] From: National High Blood Pressure Education Program Working Group on High Blood Pressure in Children and Adolescents. The fourth report on the diagnosis, evaluation, and treatment of high blood pressure in children and adolescents. *Pediatrics.* 2004;114(2):555–576.

[b] The 90th percentile is 1.28 3D, 95th percentile is 1.645 SD, and 99th percentile is 2.326 SD over the mean.

- Neurologic assessment
- Hypertensive neonates often have evidence of:
  - Congestive heart failure
  - Respiratory distress
  - Feeding difficulties
  - Irritability
  - Lethargy
  - Coma

DIFFERENTIAL DIAGNOSIS

General

- Primary hypertension is often seen in patients with:
  - Obesity
  - Positive family history of hypertension or cardiovascular disease

Causes of hypertension in neonates and infants

- Renal parenchymal disease (60–80% of cases)
- Renal artery thrombosis after umbilical artery catheterization
- Coarctation of the aorta
- Congenital structural disease
- Renal artery stenosis
- Bronchopulmonary dysplasia
- Extracorporeal membrane oxygenation

Causes of hypertension in children and adolescents

- In the majority of children, hypertension is secondary to renal or renovascular causes.
  - Renal parenchymal disease
    - The most frequent cause of hypertension in childhood
    - Accounts for 60–80% of cases
    - Hypertension is evident at the initial diagnosis in almost 80% of all cases.
    - Of those who are normotensive at first, nearly one-half will experience hypertension during the course of their illness.
  - Renal artery stenosis, caused by:
    - Fibromuscular dysplasia
    - Takayasu arteritis
    - Williams syndrome
    - Neurofibromatosis
  - Children with renal artery stenosis may have marked symptoms caused by end-organ damage.
    - Congestive heart failure
    - Left ventricular hypertrophy
    - Retinal changes
    - Renal impairment

- Acute poststreptococcal glomerulonephritis
  - Hypertension is evident at the initial diagnosis in almost 80% of all cases.
  - Of those who are normotensive at first, nearly one-half will experience hypertension during the course of their illness.
- Membranoproliferative glomerulonephritis
- Diffuse proliferative glomerulonephritis
- Immunoglobulin A nephropathy
- Hemolytic-uremic syndrome
- Nephrotic syndrome
  - Rarely leads to severe hypertension, unless it is a manifestation of more serious renal disease
- Reflux nephropathy (prevalence of 5–30%)
- Polycystic kidney disease
- Wilms tumor
- Ingestion or abuse of glucocorticoids or other steroids
- Oral contraceptive use

- Coarctation of the aorta
  - The most common nonrenal cause of hypertension in childhood
  - Accounts for 5–15% of cases
  - Hypertension can also occur immediately after repair of coarctation of the aorta and for years thereafter.
  - Risk for postoperative hypertension appears to be lower if the lesion is repaired before 5 years of age.
- Endocrine disorders
  - Mineralocorticoid excess
  - Hyperthyroidism
  - Pheochromocytoma
  - Hypercalcemia
  - Systemic lupus erythematosus
  - Adrenal cortical hyperplasia
- Nervous system disorders
  - Neurogenic tumors
  - Increased intracranial pressure
- Drug-related
  - Ingestion or abuse of glucocorticoids or other steroids
  - Oral contraceptive use
- Immobilization-induced essential hypertension
- Metabolic syndrome is a constellation of risk factors, including:
  - Elevated systolic or diastolic BP
  - Elevated plasma triglyceride level
  - Low high-density lipoprotein cholesterol level
  - Insulin resistance

- A large waist circumference
- Associated with increased risk of type 2 diabetes and with other cardiovascular risk factors
  - A child might have metabolic syndrome if ≥3 risk factors are present.

LABORATORY EVALUATION

- General laboratory screening for possible renal dysfunction, including:
  - Urinalysis
  - Complete blood count
  - Serum urea nitrogen
  - Creatinine
  - Serum electrolytes (including glucose)
  - Urine culture (possibly)
- Positive family history of essential hypertension:
  - Lipid profile, including
    - High-density lipoprotein cholesterol
    - Low-density lipoprotein cholesterol
    - Triglycerides (to assess cardiovascular risk)
- If BP remains elevated after initial treatment, more intensive investigations should include:
  - Screening for mineralocorticoid disease
    - Plasma renin level
    - Plasma renin activity
  - If hyperthyroidism or pheochromocytoma is suspected
    - Thyroid function
    - Serum catecholamines

IMAGING

- If a renal cause is suspected
  - Imaging of the genitourinary system
- Renovascular evaluation generally includes:
  - Standard intraarterial angiography
  - Digital-subtraction angiography
  - Scintigraphy (with or without angiotensin-converting enzyme inhibition)
- Echocardiography
  - May identify coarctation of the aorta
  - Will provide information about left ventricular mass
    - Left ventricular hypertrophy is the most prominent evidence of target-organ damage
    - At diagnosis and for regular follow-up of children with established hypertension

DIAGNOSTIC PROCEDURES

- Cardiac evaluation
  - Important part of the examination

- Determine whether elevated BP will respond to salt restriction and whether it is sensitive to stress.
  - Isometric handgrip exercises
  - Serial subtractions from 100
  - If diastolic BP increases by 20 mm Hg or more and the systolic by 30 mm Hg or more, then the patient is a stress reactor.
  - BP may respond to behavioral modification techniques, diet, and exercise.
- Formal stress testing
  - To assess normal and abnormal BP responses to exercise
  - May be especially helpful in young athletes

TREATMENT APPROACH

- Mild to moderate hypertension in childhood is generally not associated with marked symptoms.
  - BP elevation at this level almost certainly warrants:
    - Close attention
    - Lifestyle modifications
    - Possible therapy
- For children with chronic primary hypertension but no hypertensive target-organ damage:
  - The goal should be to reduce BP to below the 95th percentile for sex, age, and height.
- For children with chronic renal disease, diabetes, or hypertensive target-organ damage:
  - The goal should be to reduce BP to below the 90th percentile for sex, age, and height.
- Justification for treating children who have marked hypertension comes from the results of adult trials.
  - Reduction of BP reduces the risk of target-organ damage.
  - Definitive therapy can decrease later morbidity.

SPECIFIC TREATMENT

Therapeutic lifestyle changes

- Low-salt or no-added-salt diet
- Increased intake of:
  - Fresh vegetables
  - Fruits
  - Fiber
  - Low-fat dairy products
- Weight loss
  - Weight loss is often associated with reduction in both systolic and diastolic pressures.
  - BP tracking and weight-reduction studies support the potential for controlling BP in children through weight reduction.
  - Maintaining normal weight in childhood reduces the likelihood of high BP in adulthood.

- Studies of overweight adolescents with high BP have repeatedly shown that weight loss is associated with a decrease in BP.
- Weight loss also is associated with:
  - Decreased sensitivity to salt
  - Decreased dyslipidemia and insulin resistance
- Focus on health reasons for weight loss instead of appearance.
- Exercise
  - Adjunct to weight loss
  - Often reduces BP even more than weight loss alone
  - Increasing regular physical activity and decreasing sedentary activities are important in preventing hypertension.

Pharmacologic therapy

- Indicated in children and adolescents who:
  - Do not respond to lifestyle modifications
  - Have such conditions as:
    - Systemic hypertension
    - Secondary hypertension
- All classes of antihypertensive drugs lower BP in children.
  - Choice of therapy remains with the treating physician (see table Antihypertensive Drugs Commonly Used to Manage Chronic Hypertension in Children).
- Basic strategy
  - Start with a single drug and assess response.
  - Add additional drugs one at a time, always attempting to target a different organ system.
- Drug of first choice
  - Angiotensin-converting enzyme inhibitor or a calcium-channel blocker
- ß-Blockers
  - Tend to produce more side effects
  - Can be problematic for patients with:
    - Reactive airway disease
    - Diabetes
- α-Agonists
  - Generally considered to be second-line drugs
- Diuretics
  - Now used less often for initial therapy of chronic hypertension

WHEN TO REFER

- Stage 1 hypertension: average systolic or diastolic BP between the 95th and the 99th percentile plus 5 mm Hg
- Stage 2 hypertension: persistent BP >99th percentile plus 5 mm Hg
- Specific conditions requiring referral:
- Abnormal BP by 2 to 3 measurements over 1 month
  - Symptomatic essential hypertension
  - Secondary hypertension
  - Hypertension with diabetes
  - Evidence of target-organ damage (left ventricular hypertrophy)

WHEN TO ADMIT

- Hypertensive emergencies associated with manifestations in other organs
- Hypertensive urgencies (severe BP elevation without other organ involvement)
- Specific conditions requiring admission
  - Hypertensive encephalopathy
  - Acute glomerular diseases
  - Poststreptococcal glomerulonephritis
  - Hemolytic-uremic syndrome
  - Renal artery stenosis
  - Fibromuscular dysplasia
  - Previous umbilical artery catheter
  - Neurofibromatosis
  - Pheochromocytoma
  - Coarctation of aorta
  - Noncompliance with current antihypertensive medication
  - Cocaine toxicity
  - Dialysis patients with excessive volume expansion

H

Antihypertensive Drugs Commonly Used to Manage Chronic Hypertension in Children

Drug		Initial Dose (mg/kg daily)	Maximal Dose (mg/kg daily)	Interval (times/day)
ACE inhibitors	Benazepril	0.2–10	0.6–40	4
	Captopril	0.3–0.5	6	3
	Enalapril	0.08–5	0.6–40	2–4
	Fosinopril	5–10	40	4
	Lisinopril	0.07–5	0.6–40	4
	Quinapril	5–10	80	4
Angiotensin-receptor blockers	Irbesartan			
	6-12 yr	75–150	—	4
	>13 yr	150–300	—	4
	Losartan	0.7–50	1.4–100	4
α- and ß-Blockers	Labetalol	1–3	10–1200	2
	Atenolol	0.5–1	2–100	2–4
	Bisoprolol/HCTZ	2.5/6.25	10/6.25	4
	Metoprolol	1–2	6–200	2
	Propranolol	1–2	4-640	2–3
Calcium-channel blockers	Amlodipine (>6 yr)	2.5–5	—	4
	Felodipine	2.5	10	4
	Isradipine	0.15–0.2	0.8–20	3–4
	Extended-release nifedipine	0.25–0.5	3–120	2–4
Central a-agonist	Clonidine (>12 y)	0.2	2.4	2
	Diuretics			
	HCTZ	1	3–50	4
	Chlorthalidone	0.3	2–50	4
	Furosemide	0.5–2	6	2–4
	Spironolactone	1	3.3–100	2–4
	Triamterene	1–2	3–300	2
	Amiloride	0.4–0.625	20	4
Peripheral α-Agonists	Doxazosin	1	4	4
	Prazosin	0.05–0.1	0.5	3
	Terazosin	1	20	4
Vasodilators	Hydralazine	0.75	7.5-200	4
	Minoxidil			
	<12 yr	0.2	50	3–4
	>12 yr	5	100	3–4

Abbreviations: ACE, angiotensin-converting enzyme; HCTZ, hydrochlorothiazide.

Hypertensive Emergencies

DEFINITION

- Hypertension
  - Systolic or diastolic blood pressure (BP) >95th percentile for sex, age, and height
  - Risk increases with body mass index (BMI).
  - Full clinical manifestations represent potential life-threatening events.
- Hypertensive emergency is associated with acute end-organ dysfunction discovered in the history, physical examination, or laboratory studies and not from BP.
- Malignant hypertension
  - Characterized by marked increases in systolic and diastolic BP
    - ≥160 mm Hg systolic and ≥105 mm Hg diastolic for children <10 years
    - ≥170 mm Hg systolic and ≥110 mm Hg diastolic for children ≥10 years
  - Often associated with spasm and tortuosity of the retinal arteries, papilledema, and hemorrhages and exudates on funduscopic examination

EPIDEMIOLOGY

- Approximately 30% of children with BMI exceeding the 95th percentile have hypertension.
- Acute hypertensive emergencies are relatively infrequent in the pediatric population.

RISK FACTORS

- BMI that exceeds the 95th percentile

SIGNS AND SYMPTOMS

- Key features in history
  - Duration and onset of hypertension
  - Degree of compliance with any drug therapy
  - Possibility of renal disease
    - Urinary tract infections
    - Failure to thrive
    - Hematuria
    - Edema
    - Umbilical artery catheterization
    - Any joint pain
    - Palpitations
    - Weight loss
    - Flushing
    - Weakness
    - Headaches (including characterization)
    - Nausea
    - Vomiting

- White-coat hypertension
  - Patient with BP levels that exceed 95th percentile in a physician's office or clinic but who is normotensive outside a clinical setting
  - Ambulatory BP monitoring is usually required to make this diagnosis.
- Hypertensive encephalopathy (example of hypertensive emergency)
  - Often seen in malignant hypertension
  - Combination of signs and symptoms that can vary
    - Nausea
    - Vomiting
    - Headaches
    - Altered mental status
    - Visual disturbances
    - Seizures
    - Stroke

DIAGNOSTIC APPROACH

- In severe hypertension, evaluation should progress only after the ABCs (airway, breathing, and circulation) of resuscitation have been accomplished.
  - After BP has been taken several times, immediately perform a focused physical examination, checking for evidence of neurologic dysfunction andcongestive heart failure.
  - Funduscopy should be performed to assess for hemorrhage, papilledema, or infarcts.
  - Any discrepancy in upper- and lower-extremity BP measurements should be noted.
  - Presence of abdominal bruit suggests a renovascular cause of hypertension.
- Brief but thorough history and physical examination should be performed to classify the severity.
  - Some key features in the history
    - Duration and onset of hypertension
    - Degree of compliance with any drug therapy
    - Possibility of renal disease
    - Be alert to any history of:
      - Urinary tract infections
      - Failure to thrive
      - Hematuria
      - Edema
      - Umbilical artery catheterization
    - Inquire about any history of:
      - Joint pain
      - Palpitations
      - Weight loss
      - Flushing

- Weakness
- Drug ingestion
- Headaches (including characterization)
- Nausea
- Vomiting
- During initial physical assessment, measure BP in both upper extremities and in ≥1 lower extremity.
  - Using the proper-size cuff is important.
    - Cuff should have an inflatable bladder width ≥40% of arm circumference at a point midway between the olecranon and the acromion; the cuff bladder length should cover 80–100% of arm circumference.
    - If the cuff is too small, the next largest cuff should be used, even if it appears large.
- When newly diagnosed hypertension is seen in a child, the physician should ask:
  - Is the hypertension primary or secondary?
  - Does evidence exist of target organ injury?
  - Are there risk factors that would worsen the prognosis if hypertension is not treated or unsuccessfully treated?
- Perform laboratory tests and electrocardiography.

LABORATORY FINDINGS

- Initial laboratory studies should include:
  - Complete blood count
  - Electrolytes
  - Blood urea nitrogen
  - Serum creatinine
  - Serum calcium
  - Urinalysis
  - Chest radiography
  - Electrocardiography
- Laboratory and radiologic workup can be divided into 3 categories.
  - Tests for diagnosis of primary or secondary hypertension
    - Urinalysis
    - Urine culture
    - Urinary catecholamines
    - Complete blood count with platelet count and blood smear
    - Serum electrolytes, calcium, phosphorus
    - Serum blood urea nitrogen, creatinine
    - Serum C3 complement, antistreptolysin O titer, antinuclear antibody
    - Plasma renin
  - Tests for target organ injury
  - Tests for associated risk factors

IMAGING

- Imaging tests for diagnosis of primary or secondary hypertension
  - Chest radiography
  - Intravenous pyelography
  - Voiding cystourethrography
  - Cardiac catheterization
  - Renal ultrasonography
  - Renal scan
  - Renal arteriography

TREATMENT APPROACH

- Symptomatic hypertensive emergencies should be treated without delay to avoid further damage to vital organs.
  - BP should be decreased by no more than 25% in the first 2 hours.
  - Vascular access should be established immediately.
  - Patient should undergo cardiac and continuous BP monitoring, preferably by intraarterial catheter.
  - Urine output should be monitored from the outset.
  - Any serious complications must be managed before or as hypertension is being treated (eg, anticonvulsants should be administered to a seizing patient along with hypertensive medications).
- Medication choice for hypertensive emergencies depends on several factors.
  - Patient's clinical condition
  - Presumed cause
  - Whether a change occurred in cardiac output or total peripheral resistance
  - Whether end-organ involvement is present
  - The goal is to lower BP promptly but gradually.
    - A sudden decrease can lead to neurologic complications (eg, intracranial bleeding).
    - The aim should be to decrease pressure by ≤25% over the first 8 hours, then gradually normalize BP over 26–48 hours.
- Treatment of hypertensive urgency
  - *Hypertensive urgency* is defined as severe hypertension without evidence of end-organ involvement.
  - Oral antihypertensive agents are generally sufficient, although parenteral therapy is sometimes indicated.
  - Theories suggest:
    - One-third of total planned BP reduction during the first 6 hours
    - Another third during next 24–36 hours
    - Final third during next 24–96 hours or longer
  - 4–6 hours of observation should follow administration of antihypertensive in the emergency department to identify untoward effects, such as orthostasis.

- Patients should be discharged with the same medications as used in the emergency department to treat the hypertension.
- Treatment for malignant hypertension
  - Treatment is urgent, because one-third of severely hypertensive children develop neurologic abnormalities that may be sudden in onset and leave permanent neurologic deficits.
    - Cortical blindness
    - Infarction of the optic nerve
    - Hemiplegias
  - Patients are usually admitted to the intensive care unit for continuous cardiac monitoring and frequent assessment of neurologic status and urine output.
  - An intravenous line is placed to permit administration of fluids and medications.
  - The initial goal of therapy is to reduce mean arterial pressure by approximately 25% over the first 24 hours.
  - An intraarterial line is helpful for continuous titration of BP.
  - Sodium and volume depletion may be severe; volume expansion with isotonic sodium chloride must be considered.
  - Drugs are chosen on the basis of:
    - Rapidity of action
    - Ease of use
    - Special situations
    - Convention
- For asymptomatic patients with BP moderately increased (>5 mm Hg above 99th percentile, as defined in the National Heart, Lung, and Blood Institute report), there are 2 options.
  - Arrange for a future outpatient workup, and a low-dose thiazide diuretic or ß-blocker may be initiated.
  - Alternatively, the patient may be admitted to begin evaluation and therapy while under hospital observation.

SPECIFIC TREATMENTS

Hypertensive emergency

- Nitroprusside
  - 0.5 mcg/kg per min, IV infusion
  - Onset: instantaneous
  - Second dose: 30–60 min later
  - Duration of action: only during infusion
  - Side effects
    - Headache
    - Chest and abdominal pain
  - Disadvantages
    - Requires close observation; may be inappropriate in the emergency department
    - Requires 10 minutes to prepare and is photosensitive
    - Potential exists for cyanide accumulation.

- Diazoxide
  - 3–5 mg/kg (max 150 mg/dose), rapid IV push
  - Onset: in minutes
  - Second dose: 15–30 min later
  - Duration of action: 4–12 hours
  - Side effects
    - Hyperglycemia
    - Hyperuricemia
    - Tachycardia
  - Causes marked salt and water retention, and in patients with edema, should be followed with adiureticagent
- Hydralazine
  - 0.1–0.5 mg/kg (max 20 mg), IV infusion over 15–30 min
  - Onset: 30 min
  - Second dose: 10 min later
  - Duration of action: 4–12 hours
  - Side effects
    - Tachycardia
    - Headache
    - Flushing
    - Vomiting
    - May require the introduction of a ß-blocker
- Labetalol
  - 0.25 mg/kg (max 3–4 mg/kg), IV infusion while supine
  - Onset: 5 min
  - Second dose: 10 min later
  - Duration of action: up to 24 hours
  - Side effects
    - Gastrointestinal upset
    - Scalp tingling
    - Headache
    - Sedation
  - Effective in management of severe hypertension from pheochromocytoma and coarctation of the aorta
  - Reasonable alternative for hypertensive crises in patients with end-stage renal disease
- Nifedipine
  - 0.25–0.5 mg/kg (max 20 mg), bite and swallow or sublingual
  - Onset: 15–30 min
  - Second dose: 30–60 min later
  - Duration of action: 6 hours
  - Side effects
    - Dizziness
    - Facial flushing
    - Nausea

H

- Use depends on the patient's state of consciousness.
- Contraindicated in the presence of intracerebral bleeding
- Phentolamine
  - 0.1 mg/kg per dose, IV
  - Onset: instantaneous
  - Second dose: 30 min later
  - Duration of action: 30–60 min
  - Side effects
    - Tachycardia
    - Abdominal pain
  - Used almost exclusively for treatment of catecholamine crisis (pheochromocytoma or ingestion of sympathomimetic agents, such as cocaine)
  - Carries high risk of hypotension after primary lesion (eg, pheochromocytoma) is excised

Hypertensive urgency
- Nifedipine
  - 0.25–0.5 mg/kg, bite and swallow or sublingual
  - Onset: 15–30 min
  - Duration: 6 hours
- Captopril
  - Age <6 mo: 0.05–0.5 mg/kg, by mouth
  - Age ≥6 mo: 0.3–2.0 mg/kg, by mouth
  - Onset: 15–30 min
  - Duration: 8–12 hours
- Minoxidil
  - 2.5–5.0 mg, by mouth
  - Onset: 2 hours
  - Duration: 12 hours
- Other antihypertensive agents
  - Enalapril
    - Maximum serum concentration approximately 1 hour after administration, and 4–6 hours for its metabolite, enalaprilat
  - Amlodipine is a safe and effective drug in children with chronic renal disease.
  - Intravenous nicardipine is safe and effective in lowering the BP in children with severe hypertension.

WHEN TO ADMIT
- All hypertensive emergencies
- Most cases of hypertensive urgency

WHEN TO REFER
- Consultation with a pediatric nephrologist
  - Diagnostic evaluation of cause of hypertension
  - Short- and long-term management suggestions

- Consultation with a pediatric cardiologist or pediatric neurologist
  - If end-organ cardiac or central nervous system injury is suspected
  - If the relationship between end-organ dysfunction and hypertension is unclear

FOLLOW-UP
- All patients with hypertensive urgency or emergency should be followed by primary physicians as well as nephrologists to monitor blood pressure and adjust medications.

COMPLICATIONS
- Seizure disorders
- Cranial nerve palsies
- Stroke, hemiplegia
- Blindness
- Cardiomyopathy
- Progressive renal damage

PROGNOSIS
- Immediate prognosis for a hypertensive emergency depends on:
  - Rapidity of recognition of the problem
  - Achievement of appropriate BP reduction thereafter
- Although initial neurologic and visual disturbances may improve or resolve, risks remain for residual abnormalities.
  - Seizure disorders
  - Cranial nerve palsies
  - Hemiplegia
  - Blindness
- Renal function often deteriorates acutely in patients who have chronic renal diseases after hypertensive emergency or urgency.
  - With sustained BP control, renal function may improve over weeks or longer.
- Long-term prognosis of hypertension depends, to some extent, on underlying cause as well as success in management.
  - Some causes (eg, acute poststreptococcal glomerulonephritis) may resolve on their own.
  - Such causes as isolated vascular abnormalities are amenable to correction.
  - Hypertension associated with chronic glomerulonephritis may be controlled by continued antihypertensive therapy, but failure to comply with medication regimens remains a problem.
  - Development of end-organ damage (eg, hypertensive cardiomyopathy, stroke) is directly related to adequacy of long-term BP control.

Hyperthyroidism

DEFINITION

- Hyperthyroidism is the result of excessive activity of the thyroid gland.
- The clinical manifestation of excessive circulating thyroid hormone is called *thyrotoxicosis*.
  - With a few exceptions, thyrotoxicosis in children is the result of Graves disease.

EPIDEMIOLOGY

- Graves disease
  - Age
    - Occurs most frequently in early adolescence
    - Is rare in infancy
    - Occurs infrequently in childhood
  - Sex
    - Prevalence is 6–8 times greater in girls than boys.

ETIOLOGY

- Graves disease
  - An autoimmune disorder
  - Occurs in patients who have a genetic predisposition, which is linked to certain human leukocyte antigen haplotypes
  - Results from the interaction between environmental influences and genes, some of which are thyroid specific loci and others that are susceptibility or immuno-regulatory genes
  - Hyperfunction of the thyroid gland
    - Caused by autoantibodies directed against the receptor for thyrotropin
    - These antibodies, called thyrotropin receptor antibodies (TRAbs), are characterized by an overall predominant stimulatory effect on thyroid cells leading to excessive production and release of thyroxine (T_4).
    - Included among the TRAbs are:
      - Thyroid-stimulating immunoglobulins (TSIs) that mimic thyrotropin in their stimulatory action on the production of T_4
      - Thyrotropin-binding inhibitory immunoglobulins that prevent thyrotropin from binding at its receptor and do not stimulate thyroid cells
      - Thyrotropin-blocking antibodies
    - Other antibodies detected in patients include
      - Thyroid growth-stimulating antibodies, which contribute to goiter formation
      - Antithyroglobulin and antiperoxidase antibodies that also are found in Hashimoto thyroiditis

- Eye findings
  - Due to a combination of hyperactivity of the sympathetic system and of mucopolysaccharide accumulation and infiltration of the orbital fat and ocular muscle cells:
    - TRAbs are thought to be the cause of ophthalmopathy because orbital fibroblasts express thyrotropin receptors.
    - In children, mucopolysaccharide accumulation in skin and subcutaneous tissue, as with pretibial myxedema, is infrequent.
- Other causes of thyrotoxicosis include:
  - Early phase of autoimmune hypothyroidism (Hashimoto thyroiditis) before thyroid function is diminished
  - Hyperfunctioning thyroid nodule
  - Pituitary resistance to T_4 that results in excess secretion of thyrotropin
  - Factitious hyperthyroidism caused by administration of exogenous thyroid hormone

RISK FACTORS

- Graves disease
  - Patients frequently have a family history of thyroid disorder.
  - Can occur in conjunction with:
    - Other endocrine autoimmune diseases, such as type 1 diabetes mellitus, hypoparathyroidism, and Addison disease
    - Other autoimmune diseases, such as myasthenia gravis, periodic paralysis, and vitiligo

SIGNS AND SYMPTOMS

- Graves disease often remains undiagnosed for a long time in children because they can continue normal activities without symptoms that are overtly suggestive of hyperthyroidism.
- Clinical signs and symptoms in children who have Graves disease include:
  - Goiter
  - Prominence of eyes
  - Exophthalmos
  - Tachycardia
  - Nervousness
  - Increased appetite
  - Weight loss
  - Emotional lability
  - Heat intolerance
  - Frequent and loose stools

- Early nonspecific findings include behavioral findings that largely reflect hyperactivity of the sympathetic nervous system.
  - Nervousness
  - Sleeplessness
  - Emotional lability
  - Decreased school performance
  - Deteriorating handwriting
- More prominent cardiovascular signs include
  - Tachycardia
  - A widened pulse pressure
  - An overactive precordium
- Neuromuscular signs and symptoms include:
  - Tremor
  - A shortened deep-tendon reflex relaxation phase
  - Fatigability
  - Proximal muscle weakness
- Despite increased appetite, the child loses weight.
- Symptoms that appear later
  - Increased perspiration
  - Warmth
  - Heat intolerance
  - Smoothness of skin
- With long-standing disease
  - Tall stature may accompany advanced skeletal maturation in childhood.
  - Curtailment of final height as a result of early closure of the epiphyses does not occur.
- Goiter
  - Size when first examined varies, and its presence frequently goes unnoticed.
- Thyroid gland
  - Usually seen as diffusely enlarged
    - May be difficult to discern in overweight or obese youngsters
  - Is soft and has a clearly delineated border
  - Neck exam should include
    - Palpation for the presence of a thrill
    - Auscultation for the presence of a bruit
  - Measurement of the size of the lobes and the isthmus is essential in monitoring disease course.
- Eye findings are variable.
  - Severe ophthalmopathy is far less common among children than adults.
  - If present, it is more likely to resolve completely.

- Findings include:
  - Prominence of the eyes (proptosis or exophthalmos)
  - A conspicuous stare (caused by lid retraction and a widened palpebral fissure [see Figure 35 on page F15])
  - Lag of the upper lid on downward gaze

DIFFERENTIAL DIAGNOSIS

- Hashimoto thyroiditis
  - Rarely, children with this disease are:
    - Thyrotoxic
    - Have a high titer of TSI autoantibodies in addition to antithyroid antibodies
  - The condition has been called *hashitoxicosis*.
  - May be differentiated from routine Graves disease in that the hyperthyroidism is usually a transient phase before progression to permanent hypothyroidism
- Other causes of hyperthyroxinemia are rare, including:
  - Generalized resistance to thyroid hormone that is found in association with attention-deficit/hyperactivity disorder
  - Factitious hyperthyroidism from excessive administration of thyroid hormone
  - Thyrotropin-secreting pituitary adenomas
  - Binding-protein changes characterized by normal free T_4 and thyrotropin levels
  - Autonomous thyroid adenomas
    - Can be seen in association with the McCune-Albright syndrome (precocious puberty, café-au-lait pigmentation, and polyostotic fibrous dysplasia)

DIAGNOSTIC APPROACH

- Diagnosis of Graves disease rests on demonstrating:
  - Elevated levels of T_4
  - Depression of thyrotropin levels to below the lower limit of detectability
- A comparison of the patient's levels and age-appropriate normal values of T_4 must be performed before a diagnosis of hyperthyroidism can be made.

LABORATORY FINDINGS

- Measurement of serum free T_4
  - Should be included in initial assessment
  - In patients with binding protein increases, total T_4 may be high, yet free T_4 and thyrotropin will be normal, thereby ruling out hyperthyroidism.
    - Particularly relevant to women taking oral contraceptives, in whom the estrogen increases the binding protein levels, total T_4, total triiodothyronine (T_3), and thyrotropin concentrations

- Measurement of T_3
  - May help confirm the diagnosis of T_3 toxicosis, but rarely necessary
- In thyrotoxicosis, the response of thyrotropin to thyroid-releasing hormone is blunted severely or absent.
  - Thyroid-releasing hormone stimulation test
    - Necessary only when Graves disease is thought to exist but the diagnosis is unclear
    - In equivocal situations, measurement of TRAbs, which are present in 95% of patients who have Graves disease, may help to confirm the diagnosis.
- TSI
  - In pregnant patients, high levels are predictive of neonatal Graves disease.

DIAGNOSTIC PROCEDURES

- Measurement of thyroid gland uptake of radioiodine (^{123}I) or technetium (^{99m}Tc)
  - Useful only to distinguish painless thyroiditis from Graves disease
    - Patients who have thyroiditis (hashitoxicosis) have a low uptake.
    - Patients who have Graves disease have a high uptake.
  - Generally not necessary at the time of diagnosis
  - Required if radioablative therapy is performed

TREATMENT APPROACH

- Graves disease
  - Optimal long-term therapy continues to be the subject of research and some controversy.
    - Some physicians prefer to titrate the dose of antithyroid medication to maintain the patient in a euthyroid state.
    - Others administer antithyroid medication until the patient becomes hypothyroid and supplement thereafter with thyroid hormone.
    - These varying approaches have no effect on rates of relapse.
  - Therapy with antithyroid medication
    - Usually maintained for a minimum of 12–18 months
    - During this time, monitoring the size of the thyroid gland and the TRAb levels can be useful.
    - Shrinkage of the thyroid gland and decreasing TRAb titers predict a greater likelihood of remission after discontinuation of therapy.
    - Thereafter, treatment can be stopped, and 20–40% of patients remain in remission.

- If a relapse occurs on discontinuation
  - Therapeutic choices include either resumption of antithyroid medication or definitive therapy consisting of radioiodine or surgery.
  - The choice depends on factors that affect the chances of success of each form of therapy, such as compliance, patient preference, and surgical expertise.

SPECIFIC TREATMENTS

Antithyroid medications

- Thioamides
  - Aim of treatment is to reduce thyroid hormone production and block its effect on tissue peripherally.
  - Either methimazole or propylthiouracil (PTU) is usually used first.
    - Equally effective in inhibiting thyroid hormone production
    - However, PTU also blocks the peripheral conversion of T_4 to T_3.
    - The half-life is 3–4 hours for PTU and 6–13 hours for methimazole.
    - Both drugs cross the placenta.
      - PTU does so less than methimazole and therefore is the preferred drug during pregnancy.
    - Both drugs are present in small quantities in breast milk.
      - Breastfeeding may be continued.
    - Methimazole induces euthyroidism somewhat faster than does PTU and does so within weeks to a few months, depending on the size of the thyroid gland.
  - PTU
    - Starting doses range from 5–10 mg/kg body weight, with a maximum of 300 mg/day, given in 3–4 divided doses.
  - Methimazole
    - Dose is approximately 0.5–1 mg/kg, with a maximum of 30 mg/day, given in 2–3 divided doses.
  - Once thyroid hormone secretion is depressed, maintenance doses may be given in 2 or 3 daily doses for PTU and 1 or 2 daily doses for methimazole.
  - Potential side effects
    - Minor reactions that subside spontaneously include a purpuric and papular rash, urticaria, joint pain, stiffness, hair loss, nausea, or headaches.
    - Serious reaction—agranulocytosis
      - An idiosyncratic reaction that occurs in 1:500 to 1:1000 cases
      - Usually occurs within the first few months of therapy after either form of antithyroid medication
      - Leukocyte count monitoring is not useful in anticipating agranulocytosis because its onset is sudden.

- Patients thus need to be told about the significance of a sore throat, mouth sores, and fever as potentially heralding agranulocytosis.
    - Supportive treatment, such as antibiotic therapy, and discontinuation of thioamide therapy are necessary.
    - Spontaneously reverses
    - Resumption of therapy with a different thioamide does not usually cause recurrence.
  - Such reactions as drug fever, nephritis, hepatitis, or lupus-like reactions are rare.
- Adjuvant ß-adrenergic blockade
  - In addition to antithyroid medication
  - May be accomplished with propranolol to control the sympathetic hyperactivity of severe Graves disease
    - Therapy is necessary but only transiently.
  - May be contraindicated in patients who have cardiac failure or asthma
- Iodide
  - Has a minor short-term role as adjuvant therapy
    - In patients who develop toxicity to either PTU or methimazole
    - As adjunctive therapy immediately before thyroidectomy and for treatment of severe thyrotoxicosis
  - In practice, it is seldom used.
  - Works by transient inhibitory effect on iodine organification, leading to a decrease in T_4 and T_3

Definitive therapy

- Surgery
  - Resolves symptoms faster than radioiodine therapy
  - Permanent hypothyroidism after surgery is frequent.
  - Potential for surgical complications from injury to adjacent structures (recurrent laryngeal nerve damage and hypoparathyroidism) dictates that referral be made to an experienced surgeon.
- Radioiodine therapy
  - Easy to administer
  - Safer than surgery and equally efficacious
  - Is being used more extensively in the pediatric population
    - Fears regarding thyroid carcinoma, leukemia, radiation, and genetic damage after treatment have been alleviated.
  - Radioactive iodine concentrates in the thyroid gland and induces cell death over time.
    - On average, three-quarters of patients are cured after 1 dose of radioiodine.
    - A small proportion may require a second dose months after the first dose.

- Pregnancy is a contraindication to radioiodine therapy.
  - The iodine crosses the placenta and destroys the fetal thyroid.

Ophthalmopathy

- Most affected children can be treated with topical ophthalmic lubrication.
- Severe ophthalmopathy
  - Management can be either medical or surgical (orbital decompression, eye muscle or lid surgery).
  - Medical management includes high-dose glucocorticoids or orbital radiotherapy, either alone or in combination.

WHEN TO ADMIT

- Routine diagnosis and therapy of hyperthyroidism do not require hospitalization.
- Some severe complications of the disorder or its therapy (ocular, cardiovascular, infectious) may be managed by appropriate subspecialists and with hospitalization.

WHEN TO REFER

- New diagnosis of hyperthyroidism
- Surgical management

FOLLOW-UP

- Graves disease
  - Continued patient monitoring with thyroid function tests is indicated to detect any subclinical relapse.

COMPLICATIONS

- Thyrotoxic crisis
  - An exceptional but severe complication
  - Diagnosis rests on finding uncontrolled hyperthyroidism.
  - Characterized by a constellation of findings, including
    - Cardiac failure
    - Tachycardia
    - Hyperthermia
    - Central nervous system abnormalities, such as confusion, apathy, or coma
  - Infection (even relatively minor) and trauma can be precipitating factors.
  - Therapy must be expeditious and aggressive; should include
    - Antithyroid medication
    - Iodide
    - ß-Blockade
    - Antipyresis
    - Medications to prevent cardiac failure

- Neonatal thyrotoxicosis
  - Rare
  - Due to the transplacental passage of thyroid-directed immunoglobulins from the mother
    - May occur even if the mother no longer has active thyroid disease
    - Stimulatory and blocking maternal thyroid antibodies may disappear at different rates, making the course of neonatal Graves disease difficult to predict.
  - Onset may be immediate or delayed for weeks.
  - Duration may be brief or prolonged, lasting up to 6 months.
  - Notably, transient neonatal hypothyroidism may result from the transfer of maternal thyrotropin-binding inhibitory immunoglobulins.
    - May also be caused by suppression of the hypothalamic-pituitary-thyroid axis by placentally transferred maternal T_4 from mothers with hyperthyroidism
  - Clinical signs and symptoms include
    - Microcephaly
    - Frontal bossing
    - Tachycardia
    - Hypertension
    - Irritability
    - Failure to thrive
    - Flushing
    - Exophthalmos
    - Goiter
  - Can also occur:
    - Vomiting
    - Diarrhea
    - Hepatosplenomegaly
    - Jaundice
    - Thrombocytopenia
  - Cardiac failure and arrhythmias
    - Account for a mortality rate that approaches 25% when the disease is severe and treated inadequately
  - Long-term complications
    - Severe
    - Include hypothyroidism, premature craniosynostosis, and intellectual deficits
  - Adjunctive therapy
    - May be necessary until the disease resolves spontaneously, usually within 1–3 months as the maternal antibodies are degraded
    - In severely hyperactive neonates, propranolol, 2 mg/kg/day, and digital is for cardiac failure may be required.
    - Glucocorticoid therapy may also be beneficial.

PROGNOSIS

- Graves disease
  - No reliable factors predict the natural course in a given patient, aside possibly from goiter size and severity of disease at onset.
  - The clinical course ranges from progression to overt hypothyroidism on the one hand to progression to thyrotoxic crisis on the other.

H

Hypoglycemia

DEFINITION

- Hypoglycemia is serum or plasma glucose concentration <40 mg/dL or whole blood glucose concentration <35 mg/dL.
- The safe plasma glucose is uncertain; some authorities advocate maintaining the plasma glucose level >60 mg/dL in neonates and older children to prevent permanent brain damage.

EPIDEMIOLOGY

- Prevalence
  - Symptomatic hypoglycemia in newborns varies from 1.3 to 3 per 1000 live births.
  - Early feeding decreases the incidence of hypoglycemia.
- Age
  - Hyperinsulinism has 2 peak times of onset.
    - During the first year of life
    - After the 3 years of age
  - Ketotic hypoglycemia is the most likely cause of hypoglycemia with onset after 1 year of age.
  - Hypoglycemia is rare after the age of 5 years.

ETIOLOGY

- Inadequate fasting blood glucose concentration may be due to:
  - Insufficient amounts of endogenous nonglucose precursors
    - Alanine
    - Lactate
    - Glycerol
  - Ineffective hepatic enzyme pathways for gluconeogenesis and glycogenolysis
  - Abnormal hormonal activities for the mobilization of substrates and the regulation of these processes
    - Insulin
    - Growth hormone (GH)
    - Cortisol
    - Glucagon
    - Epinephrine
- Causes
  - Hyperinsulinism
    - Islet cell dysplasia (functional ß-cell secretory disorder)
    - Islet cell adenoma
    - Adenomatosis
    - Beckwith-Wiedemann syndrome
  - Hereditary defects in carbohydrate metabolism
    - Glycogen storage diseases (GSD)
    - Glucose-6-phosphatase deficiency types Ia and Ib
    - Amylo-1,6-glucosidase deficiency type III
    - Defects of liver phosphorylase enzyme system
  - Enzyme deficiencies of gluconeogenesis
    - Fructose-1,6-diphosphatase (FDPase)
    - Phosphoenolpyruvate carboxykinase
    - Pyruvate carboxylase
  - Other enzyme defects
    - Galactose-1-phosphate uridyltransferase (galactosemia)
    - Fructose-1-phosphate aldolase (hereditary fructose intolerance [HFI])
    - Glycogen synthetase
  - Hereditary defects in amino acid and organic acid metabolism
    - Systemic carnitine deficiency
    - Carnitine palmitoyl transferase deficiency
    - Long- and medium-chain acyl-coenzyme A dehydrogenase deficiencies
  - Hormone deficiencies
    - Congenital hypopituitarism or hypothalamic abnormality
    - Growth hormone
    - Cortisol
    - Adrenocorticotropic hormone (ACTH)
    - ACTH unresponsiveness
    - Glucagon
    - Thyroid hormone
    - Catecholamine
  - Ketotic hypoglycemia
    - Nonpancreatic tumors
    - Mesenchymal tumors
    - Epithelial tumors
    - Hepatoma
    - Adrenocortical carcinoma
    - Wilms tumor
    - Neuroblastoma
  - Poisoning or toxins
    - Salicylate
    - Alcohol
    - Propranolol
    - Oral hypoglycemic agents (eg, sulfonylureas)
    - Insulin
    - Unripe ackees (hypoglycin) (Jamaican vomiting sickness)
    - Pentamidine
  - Liver disease
    - Hepatitis, cirrhosis
    - Reye syndrome
  - Other
    - Malnutrition
    - Malabsorption

– Chronic diarrhea

– Cyanotic congenital heart disease

– Postsurgery

RISK FACTORS

- Prematurity
- Hypothermia
- Hypoxia
- Maternal diabetes
- Maternal glucose infusion in labor
- Intrauterine growth retardation

SIGNS AND SYMPTOMS

- The physician should inquire about:
  - Frequency of hypoglycemic episodes
  - Possibility of drug ingestion
  - Malicious administration of drugs
  - Temporal relationship of symptoms to food intake
    - In hereditary defects of amino acid and organic acid metabolism, hypoglycemic symptoms may occur shortly after the ingestion of protein.
    - Symptoms that occur after ingestion of lactose suggest galactosemia.
    - Those that occur after sucrose ingestion suggest HFI.
    - Fasting hypoglycemia is characteristic of ketotic hypoglycemia, hormonal deficiencies, hyperinsulinism, GSD, and FDPase deficiency.
- Clinical findings after 1 month of age
  - Incoordination of eye movements
  - Strabismus
  - Excessive irritability
  - Motor incoordination
  - Convulsions
- In the older child
  - Pallor
  - Tachycardia
  - Sweating
  - Limpness
  - Inattention
  - Staring
  - Listlessness
  - Hunger
  - Abdominal pain
  - Ataxia
  - Stupor
  - Coma
  - Convulsions

DIFFERENTIAL DIAGNOSIS

Hyperinsulinism

- The most common cause of persistent or recurrent hypoglycemia in the first year of life.
  - Islet cell dysplasia (functional ß-cell secretory disorder)
    - Most children who have hypoglycemia caused by persistent hyperinsulinism (previously called *nesidioblastosis*, *islet cell dysplasia*, or *congenital hyperinsulinism*) have symptoms beginning during the first year of life.
  - Islet cell adenoma
    - Uncommon in children
    - Although hypoglycemia caused by varying histologic types of insulinoma may have its onset in the newborn period, symptoms begin after the age of 4 years in 85% of patients.
  - Adenomatosis
  - Beckwith-Wiedemann syndrome (omphalocele, macroglossia, and gigantism)
    - Hypoglycemia occurs in many affected infants and resolves at several months of age.
    - Some have hemihypertrophy.
    - Increased incidence of adrenal, liver, and kidney (Wilms) tumors
  - More commonly, hyperinsulinism is transient and associated with diabetic mothers.

Inborn errors of metabolism

- Carbohydrate enzyme defects
  - GSD
  - Glucose-6-phosphatase deficiency types Ia and Ib
    - Growth retardation
    - Cherubic facies
    - Protuberant abdomen
    - Large smooth liver
    - Enlarged kidneys
    - Normal intelligence
    - Fasting hypoglycemia of only a few hours' duration
    - Ketosis, lactic acidemia, hyperlipidemia, hyperuricemia
    - Bleeding diathesis
    - In type Ib, also have neutropenia and increased frequency of infections.
    - Death may result if hypoglycemia and lactic acidemia are not treated adequately and promptly with intravenous glucose and sodium bicarbonate.
- Reye syndrome
  - Watch for an underlying metabolic defect in young children or in a child with recurrence of Reye syndrome–like symptoms.

- Galactosemia
  - In a lactose-fed infant, characterized by:
    - Failure to thrive
    - Jaundice
    - Vomiting
    - Susceptibility to infection
    - Hepatomegaly
    - Edema
    - Ascites
    - Tendency to bleed
    - Cataracts
    - Proteinuria
    - Aminoaciduria
    - Galactosuria
  - If galactose-containing feedings are not eliminated:
    - Intellectual disability
    - Progressive liver failure
    - Possibly death
  - Symptomatic hypoglycemia is not a common finding.
- HFI (after fructose ingestion)
  - Aversion to sweets
  - Vomiting
  - Profound hypoglycemia
  - Convulsions
  - If ingestion of fructose continues:
    - Failure to thrive
    - Prolonged vomiting
    - Jaundice
    - Hepatosplenomegaly
    - Hemorrhage
    - Abnormal liver function
    - Fructosuria
    - Hepatic failure and death
- Fructose-1,6-diphosphatase deficiency
  - Episodic hyperventilation
  - Fasting hypoglycemia
  - Lactic acidosis, ketosis
  - Hyperuricemia
  - Hepatomegaly
  - Refusal to eat and vomiting precipitates the attacks.
  - Life threatening in neonates and young children
- Amino acid and organic acid metabolism defects
  - Symptoms usually begin in neonatal period, but they may occur later.
  - Amino acid analysis and gas chromatography of blood and urine are often helpful.

- Diagnosis and treatment depend on:
  - Detection of characteristic metabolites in blood and urine
  - Assays of specific enzyme activities in skin fibroblasts or leukocytes
- Medium-chain acyl CoA dehydrogenase (MCAD deficiency) (defect of fatty acid oxidation)
  - Nonketotic hypoglycemia (similar to Reye syndrome)
  - Acute life-threatening event
  - Sudden death
    - An association has been made between infants with known MCAD deficiency and history of a sibling dying of sudden infant death syndrome.
  - Initial screening is best performed with:
    - Analysis of urine organic acids
    - Plasma acylcarnitine profile
    - Measurement of serum carnitine

Hormone deficiencies

- Hypopituarism
  - Severe hypoglycemia during the first few days of life
  - Occasionally, hypoglycemia first appearing later in infancy or childhood
  - A few patients' symptoms
    - Midline deformities, including hypotelorism
    - Abnormality of the frontonasal process
    - Cleft lip or palate
  - Septo-optic dysplasia (optic nerve hypoplasia and absence of the septum pellucidum) is present in some; it may be accompanied by nystagmus.
  - Some male patients have a small penis (microphallus) or genitalia.
  - Children with hypopituitarism are often overweight.
- Cortisol deficiency may be caused by:
  - Addison disease
  - Congenital adrenal hyperplasia
  - ACTH deficiency
  - ACTH unresponsiveness

Ketotic hypoglycemia

- Most common cause of hypoglycemia after 1 year of age
- Combination of ketonuria, hypoglycemia, and central nervous system symptoms
  - Unresponsiveness
  - Pallor
  - Vomiting
  - Coma and convulsions

- Symptoms occurring in the early morning hours associated with an upper respiratory tract infection or prolonged fast, typical of ketotic hypoglycemia for which no cause is known
- Onset is between 9 months and 5.5 years of age, with peak incidence at 2 years.
- Hypoglycemic episode frequency
  - At intervals of a few months to ≥1 year
  - Subsequent decrease in frequency and tendency to disappear usually by 7–8 years of age
- GH, glucagon, cortisol, ß-hydroxybutyrate, and free fatty acid levels in the blood are elevated.
- Urinary ketones are present.
- Blood glucose levels fail to increase after administration of glucagon.
- Symptoms that mimic those noted in ketotic hypoglycemia may occur in children with:
  - GH deficiency
  - ACTH unresponsiveness
  - FDPase deficiency
  - Glycogen synthetase deficiency
  - Reye syndrome

DIAGNOSTIC APPROACH

- When hypoglycemia is suspected, a diagnostic blood sample is generally taken before correcting blood glucose level.
  - Glucose and insulin (priority to do at least these)
  - GH
  - Cortisol
  - Ketone bodies
  - Lactic acid
  - Amino acids
  - Urinary ketones
    - If present, urine should be tested further for presence of amino acids and organic acids.
  - Specific tests for urinary glucose and non–glucose-reducing substances
- For diagnostic purposes, glucagon administration can be useful.
  - Robust glycemic response to glucagon strongly suggests hyperinsulinism.
- Blood glucose level
  - May be approximated quickly at bedside using a visual test strip or glucose meter
  - Can be confirmed later by appropriate chemical laboratory test
- Things to ask about during history
  - History of other affected family members or occurrence of unexplained infant deaths among close relatives
    - Suggest an inherited metabolic disorder

- The frequency of hypoglycemic episodes
- Possibility of drug ingestion
- To establish diagnosis of ketotic hypoglycemia
  - Document hypoglycemic blood glucose levels at the time of symptoms with a diagnostic blood sample.
  - After the child has had several days to recover from acute episode and is eating well, administration of a provocative low-calorie, high-fat ketogenic diet has been useful in establishing diagnosis if a blood sample is unobtainable.
  - The child must be observed carefully for hypoglycemia during the test period.

LABORATORY FINDINGS

- Hyperinsulinism
  - Low fasting plasma levels of ß-hydroxybutyrate and free fatty acids
  - Inappropriate insulin secretion
    - Insulin levels are disproportionately high relative to blood glucose values, particularly during hypoglycemia.
  - A high rate of glucose infusion (>12 mg/kg/min) is often necessary to maintain euglycemia.
  - Immunoreactive insulin
  - Leucine tolerance test
- Inborn errors of metabolism
  - Studies should be performed in a pediatric metabolic center when the child's condition is stable and the blood glucose level is normal.
  - Judgment must be exercised in choosing proper diagnostic test to delineate the underlying abnormality.
  - Presence of specific hepatic enzyme deficiencies may be determined by the use of other tolerance tests.
  - Tolerance tests are performed after variable period of fasting and only with a primary care physician in attendance, who is prepared to interrupt by administering intravenous glucose should signs of hypoglycemia occur.
  - Definitive diagnosis of inherited disorders of carbohydrate metabolism, except galactosemia, depends on assay of specific hepatic enzyme activities.
  - Test results for various hepatic enzyme effects (tolerance tests done after variable fasting period)
    - GSD-I
      - Fasting: glucose decreased, lactic acid increased
      - After glucose: glucose increased, lactic acid decreased
      - After glucagon: glucose same, lactic acid increased
      - After galactose: glucose same, lactic acid increased
      - After fructose: glucose same, lactic acid increased
    - GSD-III
      - Fasting: glucose decreased or normal, lactic acid normal
      - After glucose: glucose increased, lactic acid increased

- After glucagon: glucose increased (2 hours after fasting), lactic acid same
- After galactose: glucose increased, lactic acid increased
- After fructose: glucose increased, lactic acid increased
  - GSD family
    - Fasting: glucose decreased or normal, lactic acid normal
    - After glucose: glucose increased, lactic acid increased
    - After glucagon: glucose increased or same, lactic acid same
    - After galactose: glucose increased, lactic acid increased
    - After fructose: glucose increased, lactic acid increased
  - FDPase
    - Fasting: glucose decreased, lactic acid increased
    - After glucose: glucose increased, lactic acid decreased
    - After glucagon: glucose increased or same (variable; dependent on duration of fast), lactic acid may increase or decrease
    - After galactose: glucose increased, lactic acid same
    - After fructose: glucose decreased, lactic acid increased
  - HFI
    - Fasting: glucose normal, lactic acid normal
    - After glucose: glucose increased, lactic acid same
    - After glucagon: glucose increased (no increase at time of fructose-induced hypoglycemia), lactic acid same
    - After galactose: glucose increased, lactic acid same
    - After fructose: glucose decreased, lactic acid increased
- GH or cortisol deficiencies
  - Low blood values of either in the presence of hypoglycemia raise suspicion of deficiencies of these hormones and need for further studies.
- C-peptide, insulin, and insulin antibodies in blood may identify patient with exogenous source of insulin.
  - C-peptide levels are suppressed.
  - Insulin antibodies may be present.

IMAGING

- Magnetic resonance imaging and computed tomography of the brain may be of diagnostic help if hypopituitarism or GH deficiency is suspected.

TREATMENT APPROACH

- Correction of hypoglycemia
  - Administering 2–4 mL/kg of 10–25% glucose intravenously
  - Intravenous fluids containing appropriate electrolytes and glucose are given at a rate sufficient to maintain plasma or serum glucose levels above 50–60 mg/dL.

- It is important to follow up with sufficiently frequent blood glucose monitoring to determine the adequacy of the continuous glucose infusion.
- Blood glucose level should be monitored initially every 30–60 minutes at the bedside until stable then every 2–4 hours; rate of glucose administered should be adjusted accordingly.
- Overcorrection with subsequent hyperglycemia may complicate fluid management by causing an osmotic diuresis.
- Significant hypoglycemia should be evaluated on an inpatient basis to allow close monitoring.
  - During transport to the hospital, personnel experienced in intravenous techniques and rapid bedside blood glucose measurements must ensure continuous infusion of adequate amounts of glucose.
  - Previously obtained diagnostic blood samples should be sent with the patient to the hospital, preferably on ice.

SPECIFIC TREATMENTS

Hyperinsulinism

- Diazoxide
  - Normal glucose level is restored, use of the drug is continued, and the patient is assessed periodically until 5–7 years of age.
  - Clinical improvement may occur with increasing age, while abnormalities of glucose regulation may remain.
  - Parents should be instructed to monitor urinary glucose and ketones due to possible side effects.
    - Hyperglycemia
    - Ketosis
    - Hyperosmolar nonketotic coma
  - Hyperinsulinism caused by SUR mutations may not respond to diazoxide.
- If hypoglycemia persists or recurs despite diazoxide therapy, then octreotide (a long-acting analogue of somatostatin) may be used.
  - Tachyphylaxis has prevented long-term use in all but a small number of severely affected children.
- Surgery
  - If medical therapy fails
  - Preoperative catheterization and intraoperative histologic studies may allow partial pancreatectomy in approximately 40% of infants with focal abnormalities, reducing the postoperative incidence of diabetes.

Carbohydrate enzyme defects

- Continuous nocturnal glucose-containing gastric feedings
- During the day, frequent feedings, at least every 3–4 hours
- Foods rich in fructose and galactose should be avoided.
- Daily oral administration of uncooked cornstarch suspension is beneficial in older children but less so in infants.

Galactosemia

- Give galactose-free diet immediately.
- Maintain carefully while awaiting results of erythrocyte enzyme studies.
- Continue if diagnosis is confirmed.
- Long-term management consists of avoidance of lactose- and galactose-containing foods.

HFI

- Reverse acute episodes of hypoglycemia by intravenous administration of glucose.
- Long-term treatment consists of:
  - Strict elimination of dietary fructose
  - Elimination of fructose in cough syrups and other drugs

FDPase deficiency

- Treatment of acute attacks
  - Correction of hypoglycemia and acidosis by intravenous infusion of glucose and sodium bicarbonate
- Long-term management
  - Emphasizes avoidance of fasting and provision of a fructose-free, high-carbohydrate diet

Ketotic hypoglycemia

- Reverse acute hypoglycemic attacks by intravenous administration of glucose
- A liberal carbohydrate diet, including a bedtime snack, should be followed.
- Avoid prolonged overnight fasting, particularly during weekends or holidays and periods of illness.
  - Parents should test the child's urine for ketones during illness or periods of fasting.
  - Carbohydrate-containing foods, given promptly when acetonuria develops, are usually successful in aborting attacks.

WHEN TO ADMIT

- A child with documented hypoglycemia not caused by insulin therapy should be hospitalized for careful monitoring and diagnostic testing.
- Surgery
  - If hypoglycemia is diagnosed in an infant <3 months, surgical intervention may be necessary.
  - Surgical exploration is usually performed in severely affected neonates who are unresponsive to glucose and somatostatin therapy.

WHEN TO REFER

- A child with documented hypoglycemia not caused by insulin therapy should be referred to an endocrinologist.

FOLLOW-UP

- Patients with hypoglycemia should be monitored by parents frequently and followed by primary care physician and endocrinologists frequently.

COMPLICATIONS

- Severe and prolonged hypoglycemia can cause permanent brain damage.

PROGNOSIS

- Prognosis for hypoglycemia depends on the underlying cause, severity of hypoglycemia, and rapidity of therapy.

H

Hypospadias, Epispadias, and Cryptorchism

DEFINITION

- An external genital deformity in the newborn boy is usually obvious immediately.
  - Hypospadias: the urethral meatus opens on the ventral surface of the penis.
  - Epispadias: the meatus is formed on the dorsum of the penis at various points along the glans and shaft and, on rare occasions, so far back as to be beneath the symphysis pubis.
  - Circumcision should be delayed in infants with hypospadias and epispadias and should not be performed until a pediatric endocrinologist and a pediatric urologist perform a thorough evaluation.
  - Cryptorchism: undescended testes
    - The testes are generally descended in a full-term infant (depending on the birth weight).
    - Frequently, each testis is of somewhat different size.
    - Testes descend from within the abdomen to the scrotum usually by about week 36 of fetal life.
- Retracted penis may seem to disappear (even though it is 4 cm long) in a suprapubic pad of fat; parents should be assured kindly that the condition will correct itself in time.
- Micropenis is a rare dysmorphic abnormality in which the penis has a stretched length <2 standard deviations below the mean, or is <2.5 cm in length.
  - Circumcision should be delayed in these infants and should not be done until a pediatric endocrinologist and a pediatric urologist perform a thorough evaluation.

EPIDEMIOLOGY

- Prevalence
  - Hypospadias is the most common penile abnormality, occurring in 3 per 1000 newborn boys.
    - Some evidence suggests increasing incidence due to various genetic and environmental factors.
  - Epispadias occurs less frequently: 1 per 117,000 live male births.
  - Cryptorchism
    - 2.2–3.8% in male neonates weighing ≥2500 g at birth
    - 20–30% in the premature infant

ETIOLOGY

- Cryptorchism
  - The testes are in the inguinal canal or abdomen in 50% of those boys with nonpalpable testes.
  - The testes are absent in the remaining 50% because of intrauterine torsion and infarct.
  - Rate of spontaneous descent is lower for full-term infants (50–70%); occurs earlier (usually by age 1–3 months) than for premature infants.

- In a premature infant, the rate of spontaneous descent is as high as 80–90% and may occur later in the first year of life.
- If spontaneous descent does not happen by the first birthday, concern is warranted.
- Cryptorchism affects child's potential for developing testicular cancer, for reproduction capacity, and for sexual function.
  - Testicular cellular damage is increasingly likely with each passing year.
  - Damage is probably not reversible after the age of 4 or 5 years.

RISK FACTORS

- Hypospadias
  - Endocrine disruptors, such as maternal use of progestins, appear to increase risk.

SIGNS AND SYMPTOMS

- Hypospadias
  - The urethral meatus opens on the ventral surface of the penis, located most often on the distal half of the shaft, including the glans penis (60%).
    - May be located at any proximal point along the shaft or scrotum (25%) or the perineum (15%)
    - The prepuce is incompletely formed, covering only the dorsal surface of the glans penis.
    - Associated unilateral or bilateral cryptorchidism in ~10%
- Epispadias
  - Deformity is more proximal than hypospadias.
    - May be associated with complete urinary incontinence because of involvement of bladder neck area and distortion of the normal architecture of the pubic bones
- Cryptorchism
  - In 10% of boys with undescended testes, testes are nonpalpable.
  - On examination, be sure that the testis truly is undescended.
  - Occasionally, an overactive cremasteric reflex may make palpation difficult.
  - Moving the infant or the older child into the tailor position (sitting cross-legged) or a kneeling position can help overcome this difficulty.
  - The examiner must feel from above downward, milking the testis from the inguinal canal into the scrotum.
  - Older patients can help this process by coughing or straining.
  - Cold hands and abrupt palpation can invoke the cremasteric reflex.

- If 1 or the other testis is not palpable, the examiner should search beyond the scrotum and the inguinal canal to the femoral triangle and the inner thigh.
- Undescended testes are associated with inguinal hernia and possibly hydrocele, which can make palpation of the testes more difficult.
- If the testis is impalpable and a hernia is present, the testis usually lies just inside the internal inguinal ring.

■ If undescended, the testes may have stopped descent at some point within the inguinal canal or may still be in the abdomen.

■ If a testis has not reached the inguinal canal, the likelihood is greater that it is abnormal.

■ The lower the testis lies in the inguinal canal, the more likely that it is normal.

■ Some testes that appear descended at birth may ascend later in childhood.

- Testicular ascent may account for between 2% and 20% of all orchiopexies.

DIAGNOSTIC APPROACH

■ Hypospadias

- Severity of the deformity and position of the meatus on the penile undershaft greatly influence surgical decisions.
- Any combination of hypospadias and cryptorchidism should be investigated for possible sex development anomaly.

IMAGING

■ Hypospadias

- Many parents request sonography to be assured that the upper tract is normal.

■ Cryptorchism

- Sonography has proved helpful only with inguinal undescended testis.
- Computed tomography exposes the child to radiation, requires sedation, and has many false-positive and false-negative results.
- Radiation should be avoided.

DIAGNOSTIC PROCEDURES

■ Cryptorchism

- Patients with nonpalpable testes may need endocrine or genetic evaluation.

TREATMENT APPROACH

■ Hypospadias

- Circumcision should not be performed in the presence of hypospadias, however mild.
- None of the tissue that might be needed for repair should be sacrificed.

- If hypospadias is mild and situated at or close to the corona with relatively little deformity, repair is quite straightforward.

■ Cryptorchism

- A testis that retracts because of an overactive cremasteric reflex should not be repaired.
- The truly undescended testis needs repair to:
  - Improve chances of fertility
  - Provide accessible examination (particularly in the event of malignant change)
  - Diminish possibility of testicular torsion
  - Prevent the emotional trauma of an empty scrotum
- Risk of cancer in an undescended testis is 4–10 times that of the normal scrotal testis.
  - Risk is 2 times greater in bilateral undescended testes than in unilateral undescended testis.
- If 1 or both testes truly are ectopic or hidden, the management plan raises questions.
  - How long should one wait for descent before surgical intervention?
  - Does a best time exist emotionally?
  - Is worry about infertility warranted?
  - Can repair help in this regard?
- Orchiopexy does not change the incidence of cancer in undescended testis.
- However, the timing of orchiopexy makes a difference in the outcome of fertility.
- If the testis is not descended by 12 months of age, surgery is indicated.

SPECIFIC TREATMENTS

Hypospadias

■ Same-day surgery

- Occasionally, an associated meatal stenosis can be corrected easily at the time of the hypospadias repair.

■ Chordee, downward curving of the penis as a result of abnormal ventral fibrous bands, is often present and must be addressed at the time of surgery.

- Multiple-stage repairs may be required when chordee is very severe and little dorsal foreskin exists.

■ Currently, most hypospadias defects can be corrected with a single procedure.

■ Frequency of an associated anomaly of the upper urinary tract is low.

■ Even if the defect is severe, a single-stage repair can often be performed.

H

- The pediatric urologist should advise the parents on the right time for surgery and the approach to use.
  - Little research has been conducted on the optimal timing of hypospadias surgery.
  - Many pediatric urologists recommend the surgery as early as age 6 months.
  - In theory, performing the surgery between 6 and 15 months of age avoids any of the sensitive phases of psychosocial development.
- The pediatrician cannot relinquish responsibility for providing concomitant care.
  - Interpretation of events
  - Provision of appropriate counseling to parents and the older child, in a highly charged emotional circumstance
    - Especially important if sexual function is threatened or if sexual identity is of concern
- In the presence of hypospadias alone, little likelihood exists of significant hormonal disturbance, aside from a rare defect in androgen responsiveness.

Epispadias

- Circumcision is to be avoided.

Cryptorchism

- If parents decline surgery or are reluctant, the potential for descent with a therapeutic trial of human chorionic gonadotropin (hCG) can be explored.
  - hCG 1500 U/m² body surface area intramuscularly twice a week for 4 weeks
  - Treating with hCG over a longer period has disadvantages; it can:
    - Hasten onset of puberty
    - Cause testicular damage and sterility
  - Overall success of hCG therapy depends on the initial location of the testis.
    - Greater success reported with lower positioned testes
    - Randomized controlled trials report success rates of 8–43%.
    - Luteinizing hormone–releasing hormone and hCG treatment are equally effective in treating cryptorchism.
- If hormonal treatment fails, surgery is the only other treatment that can be offered:
  - If the testis does not descend
  - If the testis descends but retracts after the hCG trial
- The optimal time for surgical correction of cryptorchism is approximately 12 months of age.
- If surgical correction is delayed until adolescence (eg, because of delayed diagnosis), then possibility of the testis generating viable sperm is significantly decreased.
  - Bringing the testis down at this time does not diminish the potential for cancer, but it increases the likelihood of early detection.

- If the patient with cryptorchism has an associated inguinal hernia (with or without a hydrocele):
  - Herniorrhaphy, along with orchiopexy, should be performed immediately.
  - Elective herniorrhaphy is preferable to a procedure performed in the setting of incarceration and possible strangulation.
- Surgery may be done on an ambulatory basis when the testis is palpated in the inguinal canal.
  - If the testis cannot be felt, a more extensive procedure with an abdominal incision probably is necessary.
    - Unless preliminary laparoscopy reveals the testis to be absent
  - Complete laparoscopic orchiopexy is being performed in specialized centers.
  - In either case, a demonstrably abnormal testis should be removed and replaced with a prosthesis.
- The role of the pediatrician in the care of the patient and his family is important.
  - Emotional support
  - Discussion about child's and parents' fears and concerns in preparation for and after surgery

WHEN TO ADMIT

- Surgical repair of hypospadias
- Surgical repair of epispadias
- Orchiopexy for intraabdominal testis or testes

WHEN TO REFER

- Refer to urology:
  - All cases of hypospadias
  - All cases of epispadias
  - Patients with undescended testis or testes at approximately 1 year of age
- Refer to endocrinology:
  - Hormonal treatment of undescended testes
  - Hypospadias with genital abnormalities

FOLLOW-UP

- Because the incidence of cancer is high in undescended testes/testis, even after orchiopexy, individuals who have undergone orchiopexy should be followed carefully.

PROGNOSIS

- Cryptorchism
  - For persons who respond to administration of hCG, the outlook for full sexual maturity is excellent.
  - If the testes lie within the abdomen and are not palpable in the inguinal canal, then hCG:
    - Will not bring them down into the scrotum
    - May bring them into the inguinal canal, where they are accessible to palpation and long-term observation
    - Avoids immediate surgery
    - If the testes descend into the scrotum, avoids surgery altogether

PREVENTION

- Because the incidence of cancer is high in undescended testes, even after orchiopexy, individuals who have undergone orchiopexy should be taught self-examination of the testes and instructed to seek medical attention if any abnormality is detected.

H

Hypothyroidism

DEFINITION

- Clinical state in which production (or incipient failure of production) of thyroid hormones is insufficient to the extent that it leads to clinical manifestations
- Primary hypothyroidism: insufficient thyroid hormone from failure of thyroid gland
- Secondary hypothyroidism: insufficient production of thyrotropin from pituitary abnormalities
- Tertiary hypothyroidism: insufficient production of thyrotropin from hypothalamic abnormalities

EPIDEMIOLOGY

- Congenital hypothyroidism
  - Age
    - Present at birth
  - Prevalence
    - Approximately 1 infant of every 4000 live births in iodine-sufficient regions of the world
    - Prevalence is greater in iodine-deficient regions.
- Acquired juvenile hypothyroidism
  - Age
    - Occurs outside the newborn period
  - Prevalence in US population
    - Approximately 2% of children 12–19 years of age

ETIOLOGY

Congenital hypothyroidism

- In most cases of permanent congenital hypothyroidism, the underlying mechanism of condition is unknown.
- Approximately 90% of patients with congenital hypothyroidism have:
  - No thyroid tissue (athyreosis)
  - Ectopic thyroid gland
  - Hypoplastic thyroid gland found in the normal anterior cervical location
- Genetic causes
  - Mutations in genes explain only a small portion of cases.
  - Several inborn errors of thyroid hormone synthesis are inherited as autosomal-recessive traits.
  - Rarely, congenital secondary (pituitary) hypothyroidism is caused by mutations in genes that code for pituitary transcription factors.
- Familial abnormalities of thyroid hormone synthesis and metabolism (familial dyshormonogenesis)
- Maternal disease
  - Evidence of maternal autoimmunity has been found in some cases.
    - The etiologic role of autoimmunity is controversial.

- Therapeutic doses of iodine-131 after the 11th week of gestation
- Transient hypothyroidism
  - Transient hypothyroidism can persist for several weeks or months.
  - Thyrotropin receptor–blocking antibodies produced by a mother who has autoimmune thyroid disease cross the placenta and block fetal thyroid function (2% of cases).
  - Drugs prescribed for mother cross the placenta and block fetal thyroid gland.
    - Propylthiouracil
    - Methimazole
    - Iodides
- Endemic goiter and cretinism
- Hypothalamic-pituitary hypothyroidism
  - Pituitary agenesis or aplasia
  - Thyrotropin deficiency: isolated
  - Hypothalamic hormone deficiency
    - Isolated thyrotropin deficiency
    - Multiple tropic hormone deficiencies
    - Septo-optic dysplasia
    - Anencephaly
  - Hypothalamic-pituitary lesions

Juvenile hypothyroidism

- Autoimmune thyroiditis
  - Most common cause of hypothyroidism in children beyond the neonatal period
  - In rare instances, disease may begin as early as 6 months of age.
  - Progresses rapidly during infancy with few symptoms and signs of hypothyroidism
  - Similar to other autoimmune conditions, believed to be the result of interplay between:
    - Unknown environmental factors
    - Genetic predisposition
  - Associated with certain human leukocyte antigen types
- Atrophic thyroiditis of infancy
- Chronic lymphocytic thyroiditis of childhood
- Atrophic thyroiditis of childhood and adolescence
- Hashimoto thyroiditis (struma lymphomatosa)
- Congenital thyroid dysgenesis
  - Ectopic thyroid
  - Hypoplastic thyroid
- Congenital defects in thyroid hormone synthesis or metabolism

- Iatrogenic thyroid ablation
  - Surgical
  - Radioactive iodine-131
- Ingestion of goitrogens
- Endemic goiter
- Hypothalamic-pituitary disease
  - Occasionally, patients who have hypothalamic or pituitary disease may be seen initially with hypothyroidism.
  - These children usually have other clinical features to suggest abnormality of the hypothalamus or pituitary.

SIGNS AND SYMPTOMS

- Hypothyroidism can affect many different organ systems to varying degrees.
- Many of the symptoms and signs of hypothyroidism are different during infancy compared with childhood.

Congenital hypothyroidism

- During the first month of life, affected infants may have no clinical symptoms or signs of hypothyroidism.
- In infants with no functioning thyroid tissue, clinical signs and symptoms rarely present at birth.
  - Almost always present by 6 weeks of age
- Decreased stooling (<1 stool per day)
- Prolonged hyperbilirubinemia (bilirubin level >10 mg/dL after 3 days of age)
- Respiratory distress in a term infant
- Birth weight >4000 g
- Feeding problems
- Sleepiness
- Hoarse cry
- Facial edema
- Large posterior fontanelle (>0.5 cm)
- Rectal temperature <95°F (35°C)
- Umbilical hernia
- Macroglossia
- Bradycardia (pulse <100 beats/min)
- Lethargy
- Cutaneous mottling, vasomotor instability
- Hirsute forehead
- Milder forms of congenital hypothyroidism may be missed by newborn screening programs.
  - Symptoms do not appear until childhood.
  - Children with these milder symptoms usually have:
    - Familial goitrous hypothyroidism (dyshormonogenesis)
    - Thyroid dysgenesis: ectopic thyroid gland located somewhere between the foramen cecum of tongue and anterior mediastinum

Acquired juvenile hypothyroidism

- Clinical symptoms and signs of older children with hypothyroidism may be nonspecific and insidious in development.
- If disease has been present for >6 months, growth deceleration should be evident.
  - Normal thyroid hormone secretion is essential for normal linear growth.
- Most patients who have juvenile hypothyroidism:
  - Have either thyromegaly or deceleration of growth
  - Are usually short in stature
  - Deceleration of linear growth should be identified by the primary care physician who routinely measures height of the patient.
- Frank obesity is uncommon.
  - Reduction in physical activity, if it occurs, is usually less than reduction in caloric intake.
- Growth retardation (<4 cm/yr)
- Delayed dental development and tooth eruption
- Onset of puberty: usually delayed; rarely precocious
- Menstrual disorders
- Galactorrhea
- Constipation
- Cold intolerance
- Weight gain
- Fatigue
- Delayed bone maturation
- Short stature
- Myopathy and muscular hypertrophy
- Increased skin pigmentation
- Physical and mental torpor
- Pale, gray, cool, mottled, thickened, coarse skin
- Coarse, dry brittle hair
- Bradycardia
- Delayed deep-tendon reflexes

DIFFERENTIAL DIAGNOSIS

- The range of nonspecific symptoms and physical findings associated with hypothyroidism may result in other diagnoses being considered initially.
- In newborns
  - Liver abnormalities, suspected because of prolonged jaundice
- In older children
  - Chronic fatigue in children with depression
  - Delayed growth in children with simple delayed puberty
  - Weight gain in children with exogenous obesity

H

DIAGNOSTIC APPROACH

- Most newborns with congenital hypothyroidism will not be discovered on the basis of clinical suspicion.
  - Infants are identified via a newborn hypothyroidism detection program using a dried blood spot collected in the first day or two of life.
    - Analyzed at a central laboratory
  - In most programs, thyrotropin levels are determined:
    - For all infants
    - For infants whose total thyroxine (T_4) level falls below a threshold value
  - Infants identified in these programs must have confirmatory laboratory measurements of free T_4 and thyrotropin performed as soon as possible.
- Thyroid function tests: The most useful tests are usually:
  - Serum thyrotropin
  - Free T_4
    - Has widely supplanted the determination of total T_4
      - Total T_4 values are significantly influenced by circulating protein concentrations.
      - Less clinically useful
  - Tests other than serum T_4 and thyrotropin determinations are not usually required in children with suspected hypothyroidism.
- Varying clinical manifestations of disease make diagnosing congenital hypothyroidism on clinical grounds difficult (see Figure 36 on page F15).
  - Some infants may have clinical features suggestive of hypothyroidism but normal thyroid study results.
  - Others may have minimal clinical features, such as:
    - Mild periorbitaledema
    - Enlarged posterior fontanelle
    - Decreased stooling
    - Abdominal distention
  - Children with advanced hypothyroidism and myxedema are usually:
    - Chubby
    - Have periorbital edema
- Physical examination
  - Inspection and palpation of the anterior cervical area enables the examiner to identify an enlarged thyroid gland, even in a neonate.
  - Easiest method for examining thyroid gland of an infant
    - Place the infant in the supine position with the neck hyperextended over the edge of examining table.
    - Feel for the isthmus of the thyroid, just below the hyoid bone.
  - After identifying the isthmus, palpate laterally to delineate the lobes.
  - Lobes are difficult to define in a healthy infant.
  - Thyroid examination of older child is easier.
    - The thyroid rises during swallowing.
    - Having the patient swallow water will facilitate identification and delineation of both thyroid lobes as distinct from adjacent tissue.

LABORATORY FINDINGS

- Identification of primary hypothyroidism
  - The combination of a low serum T_4 value and elevated thyrotropin value is diagnostic.
  - A normal free T_4 level and elevated thyrotropin level indicates mild hypothyroidism.
  - Elevation of the serum thyrotropin value is the most sensitive test.
  - Free T_4 determination by direct dialysis is the most accurate method.
    - Least likely to give false-positive or false-negative results from interfering drugs or other substances in serum
- Hypothalamic or pituitary hypothyroidism
  - Low free T_4 and thyrotropin levels are strongly suggestive and should prompt further evaluation.
- Thyroid binding–protein deficiency
  - A benign condition
  - Male patients with normal free T_4 and thyrotropin levels but low total T_4 levels
- Occasionally, a child or infant with coexisting and severe illness may have nonthyroidal illness syndrome (euthyroid sick syndrome), in which:
  - The free T_4 level may be low.
  - Low serum triiodothyronine
  - Normal thyrotropin
  - Borderline or frankly elevated reverse triiodothyronine levels
- Autoimmune thyroiditis
  - Elevated serum thyroid peroxidase or thyroglobulin antibodies confirms a presumptive diagnosis.

IMAGING

- Congenital hypothyroidism
  - Some experts suggest use of radioisotopic studies for all infants with suspected; others do not.
  - Thyroid scan is listed as optional in the most recent AAP policy.

- If thyroid scan is performed:
  - Iodine-123 or technetium-99m should be used.
  - Do not use iodine-131, which exposes neonatal thyroid to higher radiation doses.
- Thyroid scan will distinguish sporadic disease, such as thyroid dysgenesis, from familial goitrous thyroid dyshormonogenesis.
  - Important distinction for genetic counseling
  - With dysgenesis, the scan will be consistent with agenesis and atopic thyroid tissue.
  - In familial dyshormonogenesis, a normally sized or enlarged thyroid gland will be found in the normal anterior cervical location of neck.
- Acquired juvenile hypothyroidism
  - Radioisotopic studies are rarely needed.
  - Thyroid uptake studies are indicated when the patient has:
    - Diffuse thyromegaly
    - Biochemical evidence of hypothyroidism not caused by autoimmune thyroiditis or goitrogen ingestion
- Assessment of skeletal maturation can provide additional data regarding the duration of hypothyroidism.
  - Not essential
  - Bone age determination consistent with that of a healthy newborn suggests:
    - Recently acquired, mild congenital hypothyroidism
  - Indications that the fetus was affected by hypothyroidism during third trimester are:
    - Absence of ossification centers at the knee
    - Presence of only 2 ossification centers in the foot

TREATMENT APPROACH

- The treatment of choice for hypothyroidism in infancy and childhood is daily administration of oral L-thyroxine.
  - Dosage
    - Full term: 50 mcg/day; 10–15 mcg/kg per day
    - <6 months: 25–50 mcg/day; 8–10 mcg/kg per day
    - 6–12 months: 50–75 mcg/day; 6–8 mcg/kg per day
    - 1–5 years: 75–100 mcg/day; 5–6 mcg/kg per day
    - 6–12 years: 100–125 mcg/day; 4–5 mcg/kg per day
    - >12 years: 100–200 mcg/day; 2–3 mcg/kg per day
- Transient hypothyroidism can persist for several weeks or months.
  - The infant requires thyroxine therapy until the antibodies disappear.

- The following may interfere with absorption of L-thyroxine and should be avoided when possible.
  - Soy formula
  - Iron
  - Calcium
  - High-fiber foods
- Iodine-containing medications should not be applied to the skin or mucous membranes of neonates for more than a few days.
  - Easily absorbed
  - Block the infant's thyroid gland

SPECIFIC TREATMENTS

Congenital hypothyroidism

- The initial dose of L-thyroxine in a term infant is 50 mcg/day for the first 1–2 weeks.
  - Should be started promptly at initial visit when:
    - Screening test results are abnormal.
    - Serum samples have been sent for confirmatory tests.
    - A scan is abnormal.
  - Clinical studies have indicated that rapid normalization of serum free T_4 and thyroid-stimulating hormone levels with initial L-thyroxine dosing of 50 mcg/day is associated with better long-term development outcomes than using 37.5 mcg/day initially.
  - Infants with hypothalamic or pituitary hypothyroidism generally have milder hypothyroidism.
    - Should be given 25 mcg/day
- At the end of the second to fourth week, determine that the amount of L-thyroxine is adequate but not excessive by measuring:
  - Serum T_4
  - Thyrotropin
- After 1 or 2 weeks
  - 50-mcg/day dose may need to be reduced to 37.5 g/day (or, infrequently, to 25 mcg/day) if:
    - Clinical symptoms of hyperthyroidism develop.
    - The serum T_4 value exceeds 16 mcg/dL.
- In athyreotic infants who have low T_4 values, usually 50 mcg/day is adequate.
- Therapy should be adjusted to maintain serum T_4 levels during infancy in the upper half of the age-adjusted normal range.
  - Optimizes developmental outcome
- Occasionally, the thyrotropin value will not return to normal, even if the T_4 dose is excessive and causes clinical thyrotoxicosis.
  - These infants may have an abnormality in the feedback set point of thyrotropin secretion.

- Goal of therapy should be to maintain:
  - Normal serum T_4 values
  - Clinical euthyroidism
- Discontinuing L-thyroxine therapy some time after 3 years of age is a way of testing for transient congenital hypothyroidism.
  - Serum T_4 and thyrotropin levels are determined 2–4 weeks later.
- A trial of no therapy is not necessary for patients documented to have:
  - Thyroid aplasia
  - Ectopic thyroid dysgenesis
  - Elevated thyrotropin values after the initial period of therapy

Acquired juvenile hypothyroidism

- Older children with hypothyroidism do not share the same urgent need to achieve a euthyroid state.
- Patients who have had a recent onset of mild hypothyroidism may be given a full replacement dose of L-thyroxine.
  - Children ≥3 years of age with chronic hypothyroidism and clinical symptoms should:
    - Be given a low dose
    - Have the dose gradually increased every 2–4 weeks to the full replacement
- Rapid correction of hypothyroid state can often be associated with undesirable behavioral side effects.
  - These children act thyrotoxic despite biochemical euthyroidism.
    - Often restless
    - Have a short attention span
    - Emotionally labile
  - A gradual increase in dose seems to minimize problems in adjustment.

WHEN TO ADMIT

- Myxedema coma
- Parental noncompliance with treatment of a young infant at increased risk for permanent impairment of central nervous system function if thyroid function test results are not maintained in the normal range

WHEN TO REFER

- Severe congenital hypothyroidism
- Cause of hypothyroidism not established on initial evaluation
- Initial therapy does not normalize thyroid function test results within normal range for age.
  - Often not necessarily the normal range provided by the laboratory

- The physician must know the normal range of thyroid function test results for age for patient management during the first 2 decades of life.
- Acquired hypothyroidism that is atypical or complex
  - Disease occurs in infancy or early childhood.
  - Disease is associated with other endocrine or nonendocrine autoimmune diseases.
- When the diagnosis is hypothalamic or pituitary hypothyroidism based on a low free T_4 level (by a method validated in infants and children) and a normal or low thyrotropin level
  - This form of hypothyroidism is rarely an isolated disease.
  - Expected to be associated with other hypothalamic-pituitary abnormalities
  - If isolated, genetic evaluation is needed to define cause and potential for recurrence in a family.

FOLLOW-UP

- Congenital hypothyroidism
  - AAP policy for monitoring free T_4 and thyrotropin values
    - Age <6 months: every 1–2 months
    - Age 6 months to 3 years: every 3–4 months
    - Age 3 years to completion of growth: every 6–12 months
- Acquired juvenile hypothyroidism
  - Once the patient is receiving a full replacement dose with normal values, adequacy of L-thyroxine therapy is monitored by free T_4 and thyrotropin determinations every 6–12 months.
    - An elevated thyrotropin level with or without low T_4 value indicates either inadequate therapy or poor compliance; the latter is characterized by variable serum T_4 and thyrotropin values.
    - Levels may be normal on one occasion and discordant (normal or elevated T_4 value with elevated thyrotropin value) on subsequent determinations, despite no change in therapy.

COMPLICATIONS

- Congenital hypothyroidism
  - Delays in diagnosis and institution of adequate therapy are usually associated with increased risk of intellectual disability.
  - Infants with prolonged fetal hypothyroidism have increased risk for impaired intellectual function.
    - Due to maternal hypothyroidism during first trimester or other factors that blocked fetal thyroid function throughout pregnancy
  - Infants born with delayed skeletal maturation and low T_4 values are most likely to have neurocognitive problems.

- Mild sensorineural hearing impairment may be fairly common.
  - Should be screened to allow for early intervention
- Acquired juvenile hypothyroidism
  - Adolescents with chronic hypothyroidism and severe growth retardation may never achieve full growth potential.
    - In many cases, linear growth response to therapy is not accelerated.
      - Height percentile achieved as an adult is lower than that predicted by patient's growth before development of hypothyroidism.

PROGNOSIS

- Congenital hypothyroidism
  - Infants treated adequately since the first month of age have an excellent prognosis for normal intellectual function and linear growth.
- Acquired juvenile hypothyroidism
  - No permanent intellectual impairment is found among patients with juvenile hypothyroidism.
  - Early diagnosis will prevent:
    - Development of long-standing hypothyroidism
    - Cessation of linear growth
    - Risk of a decrease in final adult height

H

Hypotonia

DEFINITION

- Hypotonia indicates diminished resistance to passive movement.

EPIDEMIOLOGY

- Neonatal hypotonia is most commonly central in origin.
- Hypotonia in general is less likely to be associated with an underlying motor unit disorder.
- Infantile spinal muscular atrophy (Werdnig-Hoffmann disease) is the most common anterior horn cell disease in the US.

MECHANISM

- Hypotonia may result from pathology anywhere from the central nervous system (CNS) to the muscle.
- Consider:
  - Brain disorders or dysgenesis
  - Spinal cord injury
  - Anterior horn cell disorders
  - Peripheral nerve disorders
  - Neuromuscular junction disorders
  - Myopathies

HISTORY

- Determine onset of hypotonia.
  - Review birth and perinatal history, including:
    - Maternal history, birth records
      - Breech presentation is common in infants with a subsequently diagnosed motor unit disorder.
    - Perinatal drug administration
    - If premature, factors surrounding prematurity
    - Newborn screening results
  - If the child is the parents' first, they may be less likely to recognize an abnormality.
- Determine the character of hypotonia.
  - Is hypotonia improving or worsening?
  - Is weakness intermittent or constant?
  - What is the predominant distribution of weakness: proximal, distal, or global?
  - Photographs or videos can be used to document findings outside the office setting.
- Medical history
  - Previous infections
  - History of trauma
  - Results of imaging studies
  - Medication history
- Review of systems, including:
  - Feeding difficulties
  - Recent history of constipation

- Family history
  - Construct a pedigree, noting genetic conditions and individuals with weakness or stiffness.
- Developmental history
  - Include a chronology of developmental milestones.
  - Assess the child's current function and behavior.

PHYSICAL EXAM

- It may be difficult to quantify hypotonia.
  - No readily administered, accurate test exists.
  - Tone may vary greatly during the day, or even during the examination.
  - Difficult to determine true strength of infants and young children
- Examining other family members may help to make the diagnosis.
  - For example, myotonia in the mother of an infant with suspected myotonic dystrophy
- Observation
  - Infants and toddlers
    - Apparent mental status (does the infant appear obtunded?)
    - Sound of cry (eg, cri du chat)
    - Facial expressions (including assessing for ptosis)
    - Head control, ability to sit
    - Respirations (normal or paradoxical)
    - Mobility (rolling over, crawling, walking)
    - Ability to stand
    - Strength of kicking and pushing movements
    - Bulkiness of musculature
    - Functional testing
  - Children and adolescents
    - Posture
    - Gower sign
    - Mobility
- Perform a full neurologic examination, including:
  - Cranial nerve testing
    - Facial and extraocular muscles
      - If weak, the child may sleep with eyelids partly open.
      - Facial muscle weakness may be consistent with congenital myopathies and fascioscapulohumeral muscular dystrophy.
    - Tongue (looking for fasciculations or atrophy)
      - Assess with the tongue not protruded.
      - The child should not be crying.

- Strength assessment
  - Manual muscle group testing
    - Generally cannot be accomplished reliably in children <5 years
    - Note whether there is slowed muscle relaxation after contraction (myotonia).
- Tone assessment
  - In infants, an inability to be held upright and suspended in air without slipping through may indicate poor proximal tone.
  - Decreased tone may be difficult to distinguish from diminished strength.
- Reflexes
  - Deep-tendon reflexes
    - Present or hyperreflexic with central (upper motor neuron) lesions
    - Reduced or absent in peripheral (lower motor neuron) lesions/motor unit disorders
  - Extensor plantar responses
- Gait
- Hearing assessment
■ Examine the skin.
- Level of jaundice in infants
- Signs of trauma (including shaken baby syndrome)
■ Examine carefully for clinical findings consistent with genetic conditions.
- Down syndrome
- Präder-Willi syndrome
- High-arched palate and dental malocclusion are observed in some congenital myopathies (eg, nemaline myopathy).
- An enlarged heart andcongestive heart failure may be observed with glycogen storage disease.
■ Skeletal features
- Joint abnormalities are common.
- Scoliosis is common.

DIFFERENTIAL DIAGNOSIS

■ Focus on diagnosis of the underlying condition.
- The clinician should conduct a thorough search for systemic disorders
- In many instances, a specific diagnosis cannot be made.
■ Central hypotonia (brain disorders or dysgenesis)
- Hypoxic ischemic encephalopathy
- Intracranial hemorrhage
- Infection

- Metabolic disorders
  - Hyperkalemic periodic paralysis (rare autosomal-dominant disorder with onset usually in infancy or early childhood)
- Trauma (including shaken baby syndrome)
- Hypoglycemia
- Hypothyroidism
- Hyperbilirubinemia
- Chromosomal abnormalities (Down syndrome, Präder-Willi syndrome, cri du chat syndrome)
■ Spinal cord injury
- May be a complication of breech deliveries
■ Anterior horn cell disorders
- Infantile progressive spinal muscular atrophy
  - Locus 5q; autosomal recessive; mutation in telomeric copy of SMN gene
  - Striking paucity of spontaneous movement
  - Weakness and muscle wasting are proximal more than distal; more pronounced in legs than in arms
  - Paradoxical respiration (chest wall moves inward during inspiration instead of expanding)
  - Tongue fasciculations
- Poliovirus infection
- Glycogen storage disease type 2 (Pompe disease)
  - Glycogen deposits may form in anterior horn cells.
■ Peripheral nerve disorders
- Rare in infancy and very early childhood
- Most frequently caused by hereditary sensorimotor neuropathies
- Hereditary sensorimotor neuropathies (Charcot-Marie-Tooth disease and variants)
  - Gait abnormalities; with Achilles deep tendon reflexes diminished or absent
- Demyelinating neuropathy (eg, leukodystrophies)
  - Severe weakness, hypotonia, and areflexia
■ Neuromuscular junction disorders
- Passively acquired autoimmune myasthenia gravis (transient neonatal myasthenia)
  - Few patients are symptomatic, and symptoms are usually mild.
  - Weakness is unlikely to develop if it is not present by 1 week of age.
  - Perinatal transmission of antibodies from seropositive mother
- Acquired autoimmune myasthenia gravis (juvenile myasthenia)
- Nonautoimmune myasthenic syndromes (congenital myasthenia gravis)

H

H

- Infantile botulism
  - Rapid onset, usually around age 3 months
  - Constipation; followed by weakness, hypotonia, poor feeding, and diminished activity
- Medications (eg, magnesium, aminoglycosides)
- Myopathies
  - Diverse group of genetic, inflammatory, and metabolic disorders; may exhibit multisystem (muscle, brain, heart) involvement
  - Congenital myopathies (frequently hereditary)
    - Early in life, children will have varying degrees of hypotonia, weakness, and respiratory/feeding difficulties
  - Myotonic dystrophy (locus 19q13; autosomal dominant; trinucleotide repeat disorder)
    - Myotonia will not be present either clinically or electrically until patients are older than 5 years.
    - If suspected in neonatal period, examine mother for characteristic features of the disease
  - Muscular dystrophies
    - Duchenne muscular dystrophy (common)
      - As this condition is progressive, patients do not have hypotonia in infancy
    - Merosin-deficient type
      - Associated with intellectual disability, seizures, white matter abnormalities
    - Fukuyama-type congenital muscular dystrophy (Japan)
      - Associated with severe CNS abnormalities
    - Facioscapulohumeral muscular dystrophy
      - Linked to high-frequency hearing loss
  - Glycogen storage disease
    - May be associated with weakness, marked cardiomegaly/congestive heart failure, hepatosplenomegaly
  - Mitochondrial disease
    - May exhibit CNS and muscle involvement; may have increased serum lactic acid levels
- Benign conditions
  - Benign congenital hypotonia
    - Diagnosis of exclusion
    - Hypotonia with early onset, usually without weakness or developmental delay
    - Frequently associated with joint hyperlaxity, which may lead to dislocations when adult
- Other conditions that may mimic hypotonia
  - Ehlers-Danlos syndrome
    - Hyperlaxity of joints simulates hypotonicity.
  - Inflammatory myopathies (dermatomyositis)
    - Rare in very young children
    - Produce weakness, not hypotonia

LABORATORY EVALUATION

- Laboratory studies may be selected on the basis of the likely cause of hypotonia.
- Central hypotonia
  - If considering infection, consider complete blood count and viral, urine, blood, and cerebrospinal fluid cultures.
  - Consider fractionated bilirubin in a severely jaundiced infant.
  - Consider serum glucose measurement.
  - Consider electrolyte measurement if hyperkalemic periodic paralysis is suspected.
  - Serum thyroid studies
    - Consider if diagnosis is not obvious on physical examination.
    - Neonatal screening generally includes a test for hypothyroidism.
    - Hyperthyroidism or hypothyroidism may be associated with acquired autoimmune myasthenia gravis.
  - Consider genetic studies (see below).
- Anterior horn cell disorders
  - Consider tests for glycogen storage disease type 2 (Pompe disease).
  - Consider stool culture for poliovirus.
  - Consider genetic studies (see below).
- Peripheral nerve disorders
  - Consider genetic studies (see below).
- Neuromuscular junction disorders
  - Acetylcholine receptor antibody test
    - Can be used to confirm diagnosis of acquired autoimmune myasthenia gravis, after edrophonium test
    - May not be positive in milder cases
    - Less useful in children than in older individuals
    - Negative in patients with nonautoimmune myasthenic syndromes (such as congenital myasthenia gravis)
  - Botulism studies
    - Stool analysis: *Clostridium botulinum* or botulinum toxin confirms the diagnosis.
    - Cell culture: Isolation of *C botulinum* confirms the diagnosis.
  - Consider magnesium levels and therapeutic drug monitoring (aminoglycosides).
- Myopathies
  - Serum creatine kinase levels
    - Markedly elevated in:
      - Duchenne muscular dystrophy
      - Becker muscular dystrophy
      - Congenital muscular dystrophies

- Not always increased in congenital myopathies
- Generally normal or only minimally increased in spinal muscular atrophy
- Serum lactic acid
  - May be elevated in mitochondrial disorders
- In setting of hepatomegaly (as can be seen in glycogen storage disease)
  - Consider liver enzymes (aspartate aminotransferase, alanine aminotransferase), liver function tests (prothrombin time, international normalized ratio, partial thromboplastin time, albumin, protein), and ammonia level.
- Genetic studies
  - May confirm genetic disorder suspected on clinical grounds, sparing patient from painful studies when conclusive
  - Consider karyotype and specific studies for:
    - Infantile progressive spinal muscular atrophy
    - Myotonic dystrophy
    - Some hereditary sensorimotor neuropathies (demyelinating and X-linked)
    - Some mitochondrial myopathies
    - Duchenne muscular dystrophy
    - Becker muscular dystrophy
    - Hypomyelinating neuropathy
    - Facioscapulohumeral muscular dystrophy
    - Myasthenic syndromes
    - Cri du chat syndrome
    - Präder-Willi syndrome

IMAGING

- Imaging may be used to examine the CNS or musculature.
- Imaging modalities include:
  - Magnetic resonance imaging or computed tomography
    - Brain scan may reveal a lesion.
    - May be used to assess muscle mass
    - Indicated if muscle biopsy is contemplated in a patient with very small muscles
  - Ultrasonography
    - May be used to assess muscle mass
    - Indicated if muscle biopsy is contemplated in a patient with very small muscles
  - Chest radiograph
    - May be used to assess thymic size in acquired autoimmune myasthenia gravis
- May consider additional focused studies depending on clinical picture (eg, echocardiography in case of cardiomyopathy)

DIAGNOSTIC PROCEDURES

- Procedures may be selected on the basis of the likely cause of hypotonia.
- Sometimes the diagnostic yield of procedures may be higher for other family members.
- Electromyographic studies may be abnormal for neuropathies or myopathies, with differing characteristic findings.
- Peripheral nerve disorders
  - Nerve conduction studies
    - May help to distinguish between axonal and demyelination neuropathies
    - Nerve conduction is extremely abnormal in hypomyelinating neuropathy.
  - Nerve biopsy is diagnostic for hypomyelinating neuropathy.
- Neuromuscular junction disorders
  - Edrophonium test
    - Diagnostic for myasthenia gravis
    - Specialized test that must be performed by a clinician who can interpret the results
  - Repetitive stimulation studies
    - Helpful in diagnosing disorders of the myoneural junction (eg, infantile botulism)
    - Can be quite painful
- Myopathies
  - Muscle biopsy

TREATMENT APPROACH

- Treatment varies according to the underlying condition.

SPECIFIC TREATMENT

- For most causes of hypotonia, treatment is supportive.
- A multidisciplinary team may coordinate interventions.
- For infantile progressive spinal muscular atrophy, consider:
  - Physical therapy
  - Respiratory therapy
  - Nutritional support as needed
  - Genetic counseling
  - Scoliosis treatments (eg, body jacket, molded back support, surgery)
  - Motorized wheelchair for children with type II at approximately 2–3 years of age
- For children with peripheral nerve disorders, consider:
  - Bracing for children with foot drop
- For children with neuromuscular junction disorders
  - Hospitalization, with respiratory and nutritional support as needed

H

- Passively acquired autoimmune myasthenia gravis (transient neonatal myasthenia)
  - Give pyridostigmine until asymptomatic, then taper over 1–2 weeks
- Acquired autoimmune myasthenia gravis (juvenile myasthenia)
  - Consider anticholinesterase drugs, immunosuppressive treatment, intravenous γ-globulin, corticosteroids, or thymectomy.
- Nonautoimmune myasthenic syndromes (congenital myasthenia gravis)
  - Consider anticholinesterase inhibitors, corticosteroids, or diaminopyridine (experimental).
- Infantile botulism
  - Antibotulism immune globulinmay be therapeutic.
- For children with myopathies
  - Infantile form of myotonic dystrophy–type hypotonia
    - Assisted ventilation as indicated
    - Consider gastrostomy tube feedings.
  - Glycogen storage disease
    - Consider enzyme replacement therapy.
      - Without therapy, prognosis is dismal.

WHEN TO REFER

- New onset of neurologic signs
- Persistent lack of normal motor development
- Regression of motor development
- Sudden or precipitous worsening of tone or strength
- Swallowing dysfunction

WHEN TO ADMIT

- Inability to maintain adequate oxygenation
- Mental status changes
- Not clinically stable

PROGNOSIS

- Benign congenital hypotonia
  - By 5 years, many affected children are indistinguishable from other children their age.
- Infantile progressive spinal muscular atrophy
  - Type I: Progressive, with death at age <2 years
  - Type II: Life expectancy into the 20s or later
  - Type III: Normal life expectancy
    - Tremulousness of outstretched fingers (minipolymyoclonus) is associated with a protracted course.
- Myopathies
  - Infantile form of myotonic dystrophy–type hypotonia
    - A neonate who survives will gain strength and tone and will eventually walk.
  - Myotonic dystrophy
    - Severity correlates with the number of trinucleotide repeats.
  - Glycogen storage disease
    - Prognosis is dismal without enzyme replacement therapy.

PREVENTION

- Genetic counseling
- Prenatal diagnosis

Identification and Early Intervention for Development Delays

BACKGROUND

- Every effort should be made to connect a child found to be developmentally delayed to the early intervention system quickly.
- Amendments to the Education of the Handicapped Act (PL 99-457 Part H), enacted by Congress in 1986 and subsequently incorporated into the Individuals with Disabilities Education Act (IDEA) of 1989
  - Requires participating states to develop a system of early intervention services for young children (birth to 3 years) and their families
  - Key components of the legislation
    - Definition of developmental delay
    - Comprehensive system of identifying and referring children ("Child Find")
    - Procedural safeguards to ensure protection of confidentiality and rights of families to due process
    - Requirement of comprehensive, multidisciplinary evaluation to determine the needs of children and families
  - A lead agency in each state is designated to administer, supervise, and monitor early intervention programs and activities.
    - Most states have assigned these roles to the department of education or the department of health.
- Although children may outgrow various problems, a physician should always investigate the parents' concerns thoroughly before reassuring them.
  - Without careful screening and monitoring, only children who have more severe delays are likely to be identified.
  - Evidence suggests that early intervention may make a critical difference in:
    - Development
    - Behavior
    - School success
  - The primary care physician (PCP) is ideally situated to provide ongoing support to families who must navigate the early intervention system.

GOALS

- After evaluation, family members and professionals work together for a child with delays to:
  - Develop an individualized family service plan that describes
    - Services
    - Supports
    - Coordination of services to be provided for the child and family

GENERAL APPROACH

- Screen and refer.
- Monitor progress and guide parents.
- Help overcome barriers to care.

SPECIFIC INTERVENTIONS

Providing early intervention

- Identify and serve children who have developmental delays.
  - May be interpreted narrowly or broadly, depending on the physician's training, interest, level of comfort
  - Screen:
    - For developmental delays by routinely asking the parents during health maintenance visits about their concerns
    - Using appropriate, validated screening instruments
    - Developmental surveillance questions and developmental milestones outlined in the Bright Futures guidelines are effective tools.
    - Routine vision screening and auditory screening are components of health maintenance.
  - Refer:
    - Children whose development is questionable or delayed for evaluation and services
    - Interpret medical information for early intervention providers.
    - Monitor the outcomes of intervention.
- Provide a family orientation.
  - Help parents understand the child's strengths and weaknesses.
  - Support the child's future independent functioning.
  - Any factor affecting a child's functioning affects parents and family, regardless of the cause.
  - Parents need and value the support of their PCP in dealing with the possibility or reality of developmental delay in their child.

Monitoring early intervention

- Areas the PCP should monitor in children with developmental delay
  - Developmental diagnosis
  - Current parental concerns
  - Current intervention
  - Progress reported by parent, with or without a preschool or school report
  - Observed functioning
    - Changes in the child's functioning may require a change in type of intervention.
  - Newly identified needs of child or family
  - Plan for evaluation, coordination, and service provision
  - Ongoing follow-up
    - Ongoing contact with the child enables the PCP to determine that some delays have resolved and to identify others that have emerged.
    - Sharing this information with parents helps them obtain and understand modifications in the child's intervention program.

- Parental expectations
  - Parents often expect that the intervention will correct the developmental delay, although this is not universally true.
  - After dealing with the stress of identifying the delay, parents often need the period of optimism that starting intervention provides.
    - However, some developmental problems will persist and will require different kinds of intervention at different ages.
    - The PCP must be aware of and help parents understand this issue.
- Autism spectrum disorder
  - Increased publicity about early diagnosis has resulted in parents turning to their PCPs for advice.
  - Many biomedical and psychosocial interventions are promoted by various advocacy or professional groups.
    - Only a few have been scientifically studied.
    - For parents seeking guidance, the AAP Committee on Children With Disabilities statement on complementary and alternative medicine is a useful resource.

Barriers to care

- Reluctance to identify developmental delays
  - Parents must be confronted with the possibility.
  - Some parents wait for the PCP to voice the concerns they have begun to feel.
    - They interpret the physician's silence as an indication that no problem exists.
  - The PCP creates a comfortable atmosphere for discussing concerns by:
    - Routinely questioning parents about development and behavior at all contacts
    - Observing the child's development along with the parent
- Questions about the efficacy of early intervention
  - A PCP who is convinced that early intervention will help a child and family is more likely to identify children who need this service.
  - The efficacy of early intervention in improving children's developmental outcomes is documented in well-designed studies.
    - Higher IQ
    - Intervention-related advantages in cognitive and receptive language
    - Stronger school achievement
    - Fewer failing grades at age 12 years
    - Less grade retention and special education placement at age 15 years
  - The best developmental outcomes have been associated with early intervention programs that are:
    - Comprehensive

- Involve both the family and the child
- Focus on strengthening the parent-child relationship
- The 2 groups that appear to benefit most:
  - Children who have biological risk factors and are growing up in adverse circumstances
  - All children who have mild degrees of developmental delay
- Concerns about overidentifying delays, upsetting the family, and subjecting the child to unnecessary evaluations
  - Sensitive exploration of possible delays harms neither the parents nor the child.
    - Avoiding the issue may be detrimental.
  - Evaluation is a way of:
    - Gaining a better understanding of the child
    - Educating the parent
    - Supporting the parent in observing and interpreting the child's behavior
    - Helping the parent explore new ways of interacting with the child
  - Diagnosis of developmental delay is often required to enter the developmental services system.
- Time pressures
  - No other professional whose opinions carry the same authority is involved in the lives of children as their PCP.
  - Several strategies may enable a busy PCP to address developmental issues.
    - Use of short questionnaires for parents who are literate, such as the Child Development Review.
    - Train an office nurse or another staff member to perform developmental screening.
    - Schedule a separate appointment for developmental screening by the PCP when developmental concerns are identified on regular visits.
  - Some early intervention systems and most payors will reimburse participating PCPs for performing developmental screenings.
- Lack of familiarity with resources
  - PCPs must learn how to connect patients and families to the early intervention system so that children may obtain services to which they are entitled.
  - Literature for patients can be obtained from state or county health departments that describe early intervention programs.
    - Such literature should be available in the PCP's office.
  - Most medical school–affiliated pediatric departments have specialists in developmental disabilities.
    - These specialists are a useful resource for evaluation and referral to publicly funded services.

Immune Thrombocytopenia Purpura

DEFINITION

- Immune thrombocytopenia purpura (ITP) of childhood is an acquired immune-mediated, and usually self-limiting, condition of low platelet counts.

EPIDEMIOLOGY

- Incidence
  - Estimated to be between 4 and 8 cases per 100,000 children annually
    - The rate is probably higher because of subclinical cases.
- Age
  - Most common in children 2–10 years of age
  - Peak incidence at 2–4 years of age
- Sex
  - In children, both sexes are equally affected.
  - Female predominance over male (2.3:1) is seen during adolescence and adulthood.

ETIOLOGY

- ITP is caused by antibodies (mostly IgG) directed against antigens normally present on platelet membranes.
- The antibody-coated platelets are then recognized and destroyed by reticuloendothelial cells found mostly in the spleen.

RISK FACTORS

- History of a preceding infection, subsequently resolved
  - Elicited in the majority of patients
  - >70% of cases occur after viral infections.
- In some cases, ITP is seen after measles-mumps-rubella immunization.
  - The best estimate of absolute risk is 1 in 24,000 doses.
  - Usually occurs within 6 weeks of vaccination
  - This risk is considerably less than that of ITP that occurs after natural infections with measles, mumps, or rubella.

SIGNS AND SYMPTOMS

- Typically, there is sudden onset of petechiae, purpura, and ecchymoses in the absence of other signs of illness.
- Mucosal (nose, mouth, and gingival surfaces) bleeding may be present.
- Usually, there are no significant abnormalities on history and physical examination.
  - No other systemic symptoms, such as fever, weight loss, bone pain, or joint pain
  - No significant enlargement of lymph nodes, liver, or spleen
  - If any of these symptoms or physical findings is present, the case is not typical of ITP.
    - Other diagnoses should be considered.

DIFFERENTIAL DIAGNOSIS

- Such infections as Epstein-Barr virus, hepatitis C, and HIV can be ruled out by:
  - History
  - Physical examination
  - Liver enzymes/function tests and viral studies if needed
- Such drugs such as heparin and sulfonamides can be ruled out by history.
- Other autoimmune diseases, such as systemic lupus erythematosus:
  - May be difficult to diagnose
  - Are more likely to affect teenagers and adults than younger children
- Acute leukemia or bone marrow failure
  - Children with leukemia usually have other symptoms and abnormal physical findings not seen in ITP.
    - Hepatosplenomegaly
    - Lymphadenopathy
    - Leukocytosis (leukocyte count >10,000 cells/µL)
    - Significant anemia (hemoglobin level <10 g/dL)
- Acquired aplastic anemia
  - Low platelet count is usually associated with other significant changes in peripheral blood, such as:
    - Macrocytic anemia
    - Leukopenia
    - Neutropenia
- Inherited thrombocytopenia
  - Although thrombocytopenia in most children is either autoimmune or drug related, keeping this category in mind is important.
  - Eliciting a family history of thrombocytopenia, especially parent-child or maternal uncle–nephew, may be important.
  - Diagnostic features on peripheral smear that may point to inherited thrombocytopenia
    - Abnormal size of platelets (either small or giant)
    - Absence of platelet α-granules (gray platelets)
    - Döhle-like bodies
    - Microcytosis
  - Clinical features that suggest inherited thrombocytopenia
    - Bleeding out of proportion to the platelet count
    - Onset of thrombocytopenia early in life
  - Associated features, such as:
    - Absent radii
    - Intellectual disability
    - Renal failure
    - High-frequency hearing loss
    - Cataracts
    - History of a stable level of thrombocytopenia for years

DIAGNOSTIC APPROACH

- ITP is a diagnosis of exclusion after considering the likelihood of other causes of isolated thrombocytopenia.
- For patient with mucocutaneous signs of bleeding who is otherwise healthy, a reasonable workup includes:
  - Complete blood count
  - Peripheral blood smear
  - Reticulocyte count
  - Blood typing

LABORATORY FINDINGS

- Complete blood count
  - Thrombocytopenia is usually the only laboratory abnormality.
  - Platelet count is usually <20,000 cells/μL.
- Peripheral blood smear
  - Will reveal morphologically normal leukocytes and erythrocytes
  - Large, freshly produced platelets are usually seen.
    - These young reticulated platelets contain messenger RNA and are metabolically active.
    - May explain why patients with ITP do not bleed as severely as patients with bone marrow failure, who have similarly low platelet counts
  - If other abnormalities are seen, obtaining additional tests may be indicated, such as:
    - Viral antibodies (HIV, cytomegalovirus, Epstein-Barr virus, varicella, rubeola, mumps, or parvovirus, depending on the clinical picture)
    - Tests for rheumatologic and other hematologic conditions (eg, leukemia, bone marrow failure)
- Reticulocyte count
  - Helpful when diagnosis of ITP is not straightforward (ie, in cases in which associated mild anemia exists, which is not rare)
- Blood typing
  - For determination of Rh status, which determines whether a patient is treatable with anti-D antibodies.
- Both reticulocyte count and blood typing are not strictly needed for evaluation.
  - However, drawing blood to keep aside for reticulocyte count and blood typing is preferable to performing multiple traumatic blood draws on a thrombocytopenic child.
- Platelet antibodies tests
  - Although ITP is caused by platelet antibodies, these tests are sensitive but not specific.
  - Not indicated for the diagnosis of acute ITP in children
- Assessment of bleeding time
  - Bleeding time is prolonged in ITP, but this test is unnecessary, traumatic, and inaccurate in children.

- Tests for prothrombin time and activated partial thromboplastin time are unnecessary.
  - Results are typically normal in these patients.

DIAGNOSTIC PROCEDURES

- Bone marrow biopsy
  - Performed in the past by many pediatric hematologists to rule out acute lymphocytic leukemia for fear of partially treating and thus masking a leukemic process.
  - Now, typically performed when patients have clinical or laboratory features atypical of ITP at presentation that suggest an alternate diagnosis, such as acute leukemia or a bone marrow failure syndrome
  - Also indicated for patients in whom ITP is initially diagnosed but who do not respond to treatment
    - Timing of bone marrow evaluation is an individualized decision.
    - Most likely time is between 7–14 days after treatment is begun, but response is poor
  - May be considered:
    - In patients who have an atypical clinical course
    - In patients in whom splenectomy is contemplated for additional confirmation of diagnosis
    - To rule out a malignant process
  - Bone marrow in ITP
    - Is cellular, with normal erythroid and myeloid precursors
    - Usually shows increased numbers of megakaryocytes

TREATMENT APPROACH

- Most cases in children can be managed on an outpatient basis.
- Consensus is that treatment is indicated for the patient with overt bleeding.
  - Treatment and management recommendations for patients who have different clinical manifestations remain a subject of debate.
  - Current therapy recommendations are not evidence based, but rather are based on expert consensus opinions.
- American Society of Hematology guidelines
  - Children with ITP and platelet counts >30,000 cells/μL
    - These patients require no treatment if they have few or no symptoms, as is usually the case.
  - Patients with platelet counts between 10,000 and 30,000 cells/μL
    - Treatment recommendations are based on the presence and severity of associated bleeding symptoms or the risk of bleeding
    - Severity of symptoms depends on the degree of thrombocytopenia.
    - The lower the platelet count, the more likely the patient is to receive treatment, even in the presence of relatively mild symptoms.

- Children who should be treated
  - Those with platelet counts <10,000 cells/μL and only minor purpura
  - Those with any concomitant or preexisting bleeding disorder
  - Those with extensive purpura of the mucosal membranes may have a higher bleeding risk and should be treated more often than not.
- Other important factors in treatment decision include:
  - Child's age
  - Child's degree of activity
  - Social variables, such as reliability of caregivers and ease of access to emergency medical care, always play a role in the decision to treat or not to treat.
- When therapy is indicated, the primary treatment options for the newly diagnosed patient are:
  - Corticosteroids
  - Intravenous immunoglobulin (IVIG)
  - Intravenous anti-D Ig
- Platelet transfusions
  - Ineffective because the transfused platelets are rapidly destroyed
- General useful advice to families with an affected child includes
  - Avoid activities that are associated with increased likelihood of trauma, such as contact sports.
  - Make sure the child uses a helmet when riding a bicycle.
  - Avoid medications that interfere with platelet function, such as aspirin and nonsteroidal antiinflammatory drugs.

SPECIFIC TREATMENTS

Corticosteroids

- Used for many years in all age groups
- Reduce the risk of symptoms by different mechanisms, most likely by reducing reticuloendothelial system phagocytosis of antibody-coated platelets
- Most pediatric hematologists use prednisone for 2–3 weeks.
  - Shorter courses at higher doses are also effective.
  - Intravenous or oral methylprednisolone up to 3–7 days and dexamethasone for 4 days every 4 weeks have been given.
- Most patients respond to steroids.
  - Response is faster with higher doses (seen after 72 hours of starting treatment).
  - Platelets usually decrease after steroids are discontinued if the titer of platelet antibodies remains elevated.
- A second course of treatment may be necessary:
  - If bleeding develops
  - If the platelet count decreases to <10,000 cells/μL

- Side effects of brief courses of corticosteroids include:
  - Behavioral changes
  - Sleep disturbance
  - Increased appetite
  - Hyperglycemia
  - Weight gain
  - Side effects are more pronounced at higher doses.

IVIG

- Compared with patients receiving steroids
  - Rapid improvement in platelet count is seen, usually within 24 hours.
- Probably interferes with Fc receptor activity, resulting in prolonged survival of antibody-coated platelets
  - Other mechanisms of action include:
    - Regulatory properties of anti-idiotypic antibodies in IVIG
    - IVIG effects on cytokine synthesis and on receptors for cytokines and complement
  - 1 intriguing proposal for mechanism of action
    - Concentration-dependent elimination of IgG can be found from the plasma, and IVIG administration causes acceleration of the rate of IgG catabolism.
    - Such a process would eliminate individual IgG molecules in direct proportion to their relative concentration in plasma.
    - Thus elimination of antiplatelet antibodies is accelerated.
- Far more expensive than steroid therapy
- Side effects
  - Chills
  - Fever
  - Headache
  - Nausea and vomiting
  - Tend to be more pronounced in older patients
  - Neutropenia (absolute neutrophil count <1500 cells/μL) develops in approximately 30% of patients.

Anti-Rho (D) Ig

- Binds to the D-antigen in Rh-positive individuals; the antibody-coated red cells block the Fc receptor of reticuloendothelial cells
  - Results in rapid increase in platelet count, usually in 1–2 days
- A single dose of 50 μg/kg is most commonly used.
  - Many physicians start with a 75-μg/kg dose.
    - Achieves a more rapid increase in platelet count that is similar to that seen with IVIG therapy

■ An average decrease in the hemoglobin level of approximately 1.3 g is seen as a result of the mild hemolysis of the patient's Rho (D)-positive red cells.

- Should be used with caution in children with preexisting anemia
- Should probably be given only to children with a hemoglobin level >10 g/dL

WHEN TO ADMIT

■ Significant bleeding

■ Severe anemia

■ Significant concern for possible traumatic injury

■ Any neurologic change in the setting of thrombocytopenia

WHEN TO REFER

■ History of fever or bone pain

■ Hepatomegaly, splenomegaly, significant lymphadenopathy

■ Family history of thrombocytopenia

■ Platelet count <20,000/µL

■ Abnormal leukocyte count on peripheral smear or associated anemia

■ Lack of response to initial therapy

FOLLOW-UP

■ Patients should have blood counts done once or twice weekly.

■ Blood counts should be done less frequently when the platelet count is:

- Stable
- >30,000 cells/µL
- Increasing with time

COMPLICATIONS

Intracranial hemorrhage

■ Approximately 15–20% of pediatric patients will develop moderate or major hemorrhagic problems.

■ Intracranial hemorrhage (ICH) is rare; it occurs in 0.1–1% of acute ITP.

■ The most serious complication and most likely cause of death in ITP

■ Recognizing which patients are more likely to develop ICH is difficult.

- A literature review of 62 reported pediatric and adolescent cases of ICH in the setting of ITP showed:
  - Median time from the diagnosis of ITP to ICH was 32 days (range, 0 days to 8 years).
  - 72% of cases occurred within 6 months of diagnosis.
  - Platelet count was <10,000 cells/µL in 71.4% of the cases.
  - Treatment before the ICH was primarily steroids but also included IVIG, splenectomy, and others.

- A significant number of patients developed ICH despite having already initiated steroid treatment.

- Many patients have other risk factors, including:
  - Preceding head injury
  - Other preceding mucocutaneous bleeding
  - Prior aspirin treatment
  - Arteriovenous malformations

■ Management is an emergency that requires:

- Immediate imaging (computed tomography) to determine the location and extent of the bleeding
- Immediate consultation with:
  - Pediatric intensivist
  - Hematologist
  - Neurosurgeon
  - General surgeon

■ Treatment includes:

- Administration of IVIG, steroids, continuous platelet transfusions to rapidly increase the platelet count
- Surgical intervention, if needed, including:
  - Craniotomy (especially with posterior fossa hemorrhages that are more likely to cause herniation or brainstem compression)
  - Splenectomy

Immune thrombocytopenia in the neonate

■ Most neonatal thrombocytopenia is not immune in nature but is caused by:

- Sepsis
- Congenital infections
- Drugs
- Asphyxia
- Necrotizing enterocolitis

■ 2 conditions occur when immune thrombocytopenia is seen in neonates.

- Neonatal alloimmune thrombocytopenia (NAIT)
  - A condition in which the mother develops antiplatelet antibodies directed against specific antigens found on fetal platelets but lacking on hers
  - Associated 20% risk of ICH
  - Treatment usually involves administration of maternal washed platelets and IVIG.
  - Importance of detection and accurate diagnosis of NAIT is in the ability to prevent complications in future pregnancies by:
    ■ Treating the mother with IVIG and steroids
    ■ Performing in utero blood sampling and intervening in case of thrombocytopenia
  - Hematologist and high-risk fetal-maternal specialist should be involved in management.

- Another less serious condition is that resulting from passive transfer of maternal platelet autoantibodies in a mother with ITP.
  - Only 4% of babies born to mothers with ITP have platelet counts <20,000 cells/µL.
  - The risk of ICH is low (<1%), and no proof exists that cesarean delivery alters that risk.
- Usually resolves within a few weeks as the antibodies are used up
  - Physicians may choose to treat the babies with IVIG in case the platelet count decreases to <30,000 cells/µL.
  - Maternal ITP is not a contraindication to breastfeeding.

Chronic ITP

- Defined as persistence of thrombocytopenia lasting for >6 months from the time of diagnosis
  - ~10% of patients with typical ITP develop chronic thrombocytopenia.
  - In a prospective Dutch study, variables that predicted the development of chronic disease included:
    - Platelet count >10,000 cells/µL at the onset
    - Absence of infection shortly before the onset of the disease
    - The 232I/T Fc gamma receptor IIB genotype
- Given sufficient time (even years), a significant proportion of such patients will improve or remit.
  - Management should focus on:
    - Minimizing the individual's risk for bleeding
    - Maintaining a safe platelet count, knowing that many patients will require no treatment
- If treatment is needed
  - Periodic short courses of steroids may be given.
  - In case of long-term need for steroids
    - Alternate-day dosing may be effective in preventing bleeding while reducing side effects.
  - IVIG oranti-Rho (D) Ig has also been used, but these measures are only temporary.
  - Splenectomy
    - Effective in improving the platelet count and reducing the associated risk of bleeding in 60–90% of children
    - However, anticipated improvement in hemostasis and platelet count must be balanced with consideration of the small but real risk of overwhelming postsplenectomy sepsis, which may be life threatening.
      - Usually delayed until the child is >5 years because the risk of overwhelming sepsis decreases with age.
    - No universally accepted standards for timing of splenectomy exist.
      - American Society of Hematology guidelines recommend waiting until ≥12 months after diagnosis, if possible.

- Platelet counts in splenectomized patients
  - Generally monitored for an indefinite period
  - Any drop in platelet counts or increase in symptoms should prompt assessment for the presence of an accessory spleen.
- If not previously done, recommendations are to perform a bone marrow biopsy on patients who are being considered for splenectomy.
- Presplenectomy immunizations and subsequent penicillin prophylaxis are necessary.
- Rituximab for refractory chronic ITP
  - A chimeric murine-human anti-CD20 monoclonal antibody
  - Acts by destroying B-lymphocytes by activating complement-dependent and an antibody-dependent cellular toxicity
    - Therefore, mechanism of action is a slow but effective decrease in production of antibodies.
  - In a study of 24 patients 2–19 years of age who received 375 mg/m^2 of rituximab in 4 weekly doses
    - 63% achieved complete remission for 4–30 months (platelet count of >150,000 cells/µL):
  - Although long-term remissions have been documented, use of rituximab in ITP is relatively recent.
  - Long-term follow-up may be needed for accurate prognostication.
  - Use may be associated with:
    - Infusion-related reactions
    - Development of transient hypogammaglobulinemia

PROGNOSIS

- Treatment does not alter the course (ie, the incidence of patients who go on to develop chronic ITP).
  - However, it does shorten the duration of thrombocytopenia in some patients.
- For typical cases of childhood ITP
  - 80% of patients will have platelet counts return to normal within 2 months of presentation, with or without therapy.
  - Another 10% will recover normal platelet levels in the next few months.
  - ~10% will go on to have chronic thrombocytopenia (>6 months' duration).
- Approximately 25% of children will have a relapse after initial treatment.
  - 10% have chronic ITP.
  - 10% have recurrence but resolution within 6 months.
  - 5% have episodes of ITP recurrences and remissions throughout their lives.

Immunization

BACKGROUND

- Vaccination was one of the most important achievements in public health in the 20th century.
- Current US disease levels are 92–100% lower than prevaccination-era disease levels.
- However, many children in the US, as well as other countries, still die from vaccine-preventable diseases.

GOALS

- Routine childhood vaccination is one of the few health care interventions that saves both lives and dollars.
- Routine vaccination saves from $29 (for measles-mumps-rubella [MMR] vaccination) to $2 (for hepatitis B vaccination) for every dollar spent.
- The primary reason for the record low disease incidence is record high immunization coverage levels.
- The process of vaccinating children is becoming increasingly complicated as the number of vaccines and vaccine combination choices increases.
- The current US recommended childhood and adolescent immunization schedule is updated annually or biannually.

GENERAL APPROACH

Live vaccines

- Live vaccines include:
  - MMR
  - Varicella
  - Rotavirus
  - Live attenuated influenza intranasal vaccine (LAIV)
  - Yellow fever
  - Vaccinia
  - Oral poliovirus vaccine (OPV)
  - Bacille Calmette-Guérin (BCG)
  - Oral typhoid vaccine
- Live vaccines replicate in the body.
- Live injected vaccines usually induce immunity through a single dose.
  - Unlike inactivated vaccines, live vaccines are susceptible to vaccine failure caused by circulating antibodies, including residual maternal antibodies in infants.

Inactivated vaccines

- Inactivated vaccines include:
  - Inactivated polio vaccine (IPV)
  - Hepatitis A
  - Rabies
  - Acellular pertussis
  - Hepatitis B
  - Human papillomavirus (HPV)
  - Split virus influenza

- Typhoid Vi
- Toxoid agents
  - Diphtheria
  - Tetanus
- Polysaccharides, unconjugated
  - Pneumococcal
  - Meningococcal
- Polysaccharides, conjugated
  - *Haemophilus influenzae* type B (Hib)
  - Pneumococcal
  - Meningococcal
- Inactivated vaccines
  - Do not contain infectious particles that can replicate in the body
  - Generally require several doses to immunize patients completely

Timing of administration
Routine schedule

- The routine vaccination schedule is harmonized among:
  - The American Academy of Pediatrics (AAP)
  - The American Academy of Family Physicians (AAFP)
  - The Centers for Disease Control and Prevention (CDC) Advisory Committee on Immunization Practices (ACIP)
- The harmonized schedule allows for office preferences by indicating acceptable ranges for routine on-time vaccination scheduling.
- The ranges were created so that offices might accommodate routine vaccination into their well-child care schedule.
- To ensure timely vaccinations, vaccinating early within the acceptable age range is important.
- Intervals between different vaccines not administered simultaneously
  - Using all routine vaccines simultaneously is safe and effective, provided that vaccines are not combined within a single syringe.
  - No contraindications exist to giving any 2 different routine childhood vaccines at the same visit.
  - Vaccines that are not administered simultaneously may be given without regard to intervals, with 1 or 2 exceptions:
    - Live vaccines not given orally (ie, MMR, varicella, LAIV) that are not administered simultaneously should be separated by at least 4 weeks.
    - The 4-week separation rule is intended to reduce theoretical risk of interference from the first vaccine on the subsequent vaccine.
      - If, for example, varicella vaccine is given only 1 week after an MMR, then the varicella vaccine should be repeated or serologic testing should be used to confirm seroconversion.

– AAP guidelines specify that if the adolescent formulation (tetanus toxoid, reduced diphtheria toxoid, and acellular pertussis [Tdap], adsorbed) is not given at the same visit as meningococcal conjugate vaccine, then the 2 should be separated by at least 4 weeks.

  ■ ACIP guidelines do not make this stipulation.

• Combination vaccines:

– Reduce the number of injections

– Are preferred by ACIP, AAFP, and AAP when available

– Are preferred by providers, parents and, no doubt, children

– As a consequence of the increasing number of diseases that can be prevented through vaccination, the number of required injections increased dramatically.

– The number of combination vaccines available also increased.

• All vaccines for which the child is eligible should be offered whenever possible.

– Keeps the child on schedule

– Eliminates an additional, unnecessary office visit

Minimal age and intervals between different doses of a multidose vaccine

■ Vaccine doses that are given too early in life or too soon after a previous dose may be less effective.

• The table Recommended and Minimum Ages and Intervals Between Vaccine Doses shows the earliest acceptable ages of administration of the routinely recommended childhood vaccines and minimal spacing between their doses.

■ Does a vaccine dose given at an interval shorter than the minimal interval count?

• State requirements for school entry vary, but ACIP considers a vaccination valid if the vaccine dose was given within 4 days of the minimal interval.

■ Vaccine doses are considered invalid if an incorrect amount was used.

• Steps should be taken to prevent these errors from occurring.

• The clinician should remember that vaccination is a safe procedure, even if the child is given more than the recommended number of doses.

■ Overvaccination

• With live vaccines, overvaccination is without consequence, because the extra vaccine virus will not infect an already immune person.

• With inactivated vaccines, an increase in local reactions may occur if antibody levels are high.

■ Prolonged intervals between doses of a multidose vaccination series do not diminish vaccine effectiveness once the series has been completed.

■ Series never need to be restarted because of prolonged intervals (with the exception of oral typhoid vaccine).

■ Late-start or interrupted schedule

• Some children start routine vaccination late.

• The recommended schedule for such children is derived from the minimal intervals for the routine vaccinations.

• A catch-up schedule is published annually with the routine schedule.

• For a new patient whose vaccination status is unknown:

– If available, obtain a copy of the record or a report from the previous provider.

– If records are unavailable, the child should be presumed to be unvaccinated, and the vaccination series should be given using the accelerated schedule.

– Serologic testing can be considered for some antigens (eg, MMR, hepatitis B).

Intervals between live injected vaccines and antibody-containing blood products

■ Live injected vaccines (eg, MMR and varicella vaccines)

• Must replicate in the body to induce immunity

• May be compromised by circulating antibodies against the vaccine virus

■ Live vaccines not administered by injection are thought to be unaffected by circulating antibodies.

• LAIV

• Oral typhoid

• OPV

■ Inactivated vaccines

• Are not affected significantly by circulating antibodies

• Relative timing of the administration of immune globulin–containing products need not be considered.

■ MMR and varicella vaccine doses given >14 days before administration of immune globulin–containing products have time to replicate and are effective.

■ When live injected vaccines are given after antibody-containing blood products, the situation is more complex.

• The specific immune globulin–containing product and its dose dictate the waiting period necessary before a live injected vaccine is given.

• MMR and varicella vaccination should be delayed from 3–11 months, depending on the specific immune globulin preparation administered.

• Waiting period details can be found in the AAP *Red Book* and on the CDC Web site.

Vaccinations administered outside the US

■ Determining the immunization status of children who have been partially or completely vaccinated in another country can be difficult.

• Immunization status must be determined for all children.

• Attention must be paid to the rest of the family in the case of recent immigration.

Recommended and Minimum Ages and Intervals Between Vaccine Doses[a]

Vaccine and Dose Number	Recommended Age for This Dose	Minimum Age for This Dose	Recommended Interval to the Next Dose	Minimum Interval to the Next Dose
Hepatitis B (Hep B)-1[b]	Birth	Birth	1–4 months	4 weeks
Hep B-2	1–2 months	4 weeks	2–17 months	8 weeks
Hep B-3[c]	6–18 months	24 weeks	—	—
Diphtheria-tetanus-acellular pertussis (DTaP)-1[b]	2 months	6 weeks	2 months	4 weeks
DTaP-2	4 months	10 weeks	2 months	4 weeks
DTaP-3	6 months	14 weeks	6–12 months[d]	6 months[d,e]
DTaP-4	15–18 months	12 months	3 years	6 months[d]
DTaP-5	4–6 years	4 years	—	—
Haemophilus influenzae type b (Hib)-1[b,f]	2 months	6 weeks	2 months	4 weeks
Hib-2	4 months	10 weeks	2 months	4 weeks
Hib-3[g]	6 months	14 weeks	6–9 months[d]	8 weeks
Hib-4	12–15 months	12 months	—	—
Inactivated poliovirus (IPV)-1[b]	2 months	6 weeks	2 months	4 weeks
IPV-2	4 months	10 weeks	2–14 months	4 weeks
IPV-3	6–18 months	14 weeks	3–5 years	6 months
IPV-4	4–6 years	4 years	—	—
Pneumococcal conjugate (PCV)-1[f]	2 months	6 weeks	2 months	4 weeks
PCV-2	4 months	10 weeks	2 months	4 weeks
PCV-3	6 months	14 weeks	6 months	8 weeks
PCV-4	12–15 months	12 months	—	—
Measles-mumps-rubella (MMR)-1[h]	12–15 months[i]	12 months	3–5 years	4 weeks
MMR-2[h]	4–6 years	13 months	—	—
Varicella (Var)-1[h]	12–15 months	12 months	3–5 years	12 weeks[i]
Var-2[h]	4–6 years	15 months	—	—
Hepatitis A (HepA)-1[b]	12–23 months	12 months	6–18 months[d]	6 months[d]
HepA-2	18–41 months	18 months	—	—
Influenza, Inactivated (TIV)[j]	6-59 months	6 months[k]	1 month	4 weeks
Influenza, Live attenuated (LAIV)[j]	—	2 years	1 month	4 weeks
Meningococcal Conjugate (MCV)	11–12 years	2 years	—	—
Meningococcal Polysaccharide (MPSV)-1	—	2 years	5 years[l]	5 years[l]
MPSV-2[m]	—	7 years	—	—
Tetanus-diphtheria (Td)	11–12 years	7 years	10 years	5 years
Tetanus-diphtheria-acellular pertussis (Tdap)[n]	≥11 years	10 years	—	—
Pneumococcal polysaccharide (PPSV)-1	—	2 years	5 years	5 years
PPSV-2[o]	—	7 years	—	—

continued

Recommended and Minimum Ages and Intervals Between Vaccine Doses[a], *continued*

Vaccine and Dose Number	Recommended Age for this Dose	Minimum Age for this Dose	Recommended Interval to the Next Dose	Minimum Interval to the Next Dose
Human papillomavirus (HPV)-1[p]	11–12 years	9 years	2 months	4 weeks
HPV-2	11–12 years (+2 months)	109 months	4 months	12 months
HPV-3[q]	11–12 years (+6 months)	114 months	—	—
Rotavirus (RV)-1[r]	2 months	6 weeks	2 months	4 weeks
RV-2	4 months	10 weeks	2 months	4 weeks
RV-3[s]	6 months	14 weeks	—	—
Zoster[t]	60 years	60 years	—	—

Abbreviations: DTaP, diphtheria and tetanus toxoids and acellular pertussis vaccine; MMR, measles, mumps, and rubella; TIV, trivalent (inactivated) influenza vaccine; LAIV, live, attenuated (intranasal) influenza vaccine; Td, tetanus and reduced diphtheria toxoids; Tdap, tetanus toxoid, reduced diphtheria toxoid, and reduced acellular pertussis vaccine.

[a] Use of licensed combination vaccines is preferred over separate injections of their equivalent component vaccines. (CDC. Combination vaccines for childhood immunization: recommendations of the Advisory Committee on Immunization Practices [ACIP], the American Academy of Pediatrics [AAP], and the American Academy of Family Physicians [AAFP]. *MMWR.* 1999;48[No. RR-5]). When administering combination vaccines, the minimum age for administration is the oldest age for any of the individual components; the minimum interval between doses is equal to the greatest interval of any of the individual components.

[b] Combination vaccines containing the Hepatitis B component are available (HepB-Hib, DTaP-HepB-IPV, HepA-HepB). These vaccines should not be administered to infants younger than 6 weeks of age because of the other components (i.e., Hib, DTaP, IPV, and HepA).

[c] HepB-3 should be administered at least 8 weeks after HepB-2 and at least 16 weeks after HepB-1, and it should not be administered before age 24 weeks.

[d] Calendar months.

[e] The minimum recommended interval between DTaP-3 and DTaP-4 is 6 months. However, DTaP-4 need not be repeated if administered at least 4 months after DTaP-3.

[f] For Hib and PCV, children receiving the first dose of vaccine at age 7 months of age or older require fewer doses to complete the series (CDC. Recommended childhood and adolescent immunization schedule – United States, 2006. *MMWR.* 2005;54 [Nos. 51 & 52]:Q1-Q4).

[g] If PRP-OMP (Pedvax-Hib®, Merck Vaccine Division), was administered at 2 and 4 months of age a dose at 6 months of age is not required.

[h] Combination measles-mumps-rubella-varicella (MMRV) vaccine can be used for children 12 months through 12 years of age. Also see footnote i.

[i] The minimum interval from Var-1 to Var-2 for persons beginning the series at 13 years or older is 4 weeks.

[j] One dose of influenza vaccine per season is recommended for most people. Children younger than 9 years of age who are receiving influenza vaccine for the first time, or received only 1 dose the previous season (if it was their first vaccination season) should receive 2 doses this season.

[k] The minimum age for inactivated influenza vaccine varies by vaccine manufacturer. Only Fluzone (manufactured by sanofi pasteur) is approved for children 6–35 months of age. The minimum age for Fluvirin (manufactured by Novartis) is 4 years. For Fluarix and FluLaval (manufactured by GlaxoSmithKline) and Afluria (manufactured by CSL Ltd), the minimum age is 18 years.

[l] Some experts recommend a second dose of MPSV-3 years after the first dose for people at increased risk for meningococcal disease.

[m] A second dose of meningococcal vaccine is recommended for people previously vaccinated with MPSV who remain at high risk for meningococcal disease. MCV is preferred when revaccinating persons aged 2-55 years, but a second dose of MPSV is acceptable. (CDC. Prevention and Control of Meningococcal Disease Recommendations of the Advisory Committee on Immunization Practices [ACIP]. *MMWR.* 2005;54: No. RR-7.)

[n] Only one dose of Tdap is recommended. Subsequent doses should be administered as Td. If vaccination to prevent tetanus and/or diphtheria disease is required for children 7 through 9 years of age, Td should be administered (minimum age for Td is 7 years). For one brand of Tdap the minimum age is 11 years. The preferred interval between Tdap and a previous dose of Td is 5 years. In persons who have received a primary series of tetanus-toxoid containing vaccine, for management of a tetanus-prone wound, the minimum interval after a previous dose of any tetanus-containing vaccine is 5 years.

[o] A second dose of PPSV is recommended for persons at highest risk for serious pneumococcal infection and those who are likely to have a rapid decline in pneumococcal antibody concentration. Revaccination 3 years after the previous dose can be considered for children at highest risk for severe pneumococcal infection who would be younger than 10 years of age at the time of revaccination. (CDC. Prevention of pneumococcal disease: recommendations of the Advisory Committee on Immunization Practices [ACIP]. *MMWR.* 1997;46[No. RR-8]).

[p] HPV is approved only for females 9-26 years of age.

[q] HPV-3 should be administered at least 12 weeks after HPV-2 and at least 24 weeks after HPV-1, and it should not be administered before 114 months of age.

[r] The first dose of RV must be administered at 6-14 weeks of age. The vaccine series should not be started after a child has reached 15 weeks of age. RV may be administered on the day a child reaches his or her 8 month birthday but not later, regardless of the number of doses administered previously.

[s] If Rotarix (RV1) is administered as age appropriate, a third dose is not necessary.

[t] Herpes zoster vaccine is approved as a single dose for persons 60 years and older with a history of varicella.

Adapted from: Advisory Committee on Immuniztion Practices (ACIP) General Recommendations on Immunization. *MMWR.* 2006;55(No. RR-15):1–48. Source: Centers for Disease Control and Prevention. Recommended and Minimum Ages and Intervals Between Vaccine Doses. Available at: www.cdc.gov/vaccines/pubs/pinkbook/downloads/appendices/A/age-interval-table.pdf.

- Vaccines, their abbreviations, and vaccination age criteria often differ among countries.
  - The first assumption to make is that the vaccines administered in other countries were as potent as those available in the US.
  - Then, it is necessary to determine which vaccines were administered and in what doses.
    - Determining which vaccines were administered can be difficult, because the standard abbreviations recorded in handheld vaccination records may be different from those used in the US.
    - Translation of foreign-language terms can be facilitated with materials from the CDC.
  - Assistance with specific questions can be obtained from:
    - Your state immunization program
    - The CDC National Center for Immunization and Respiratory Diseases
      - Telephone: 800/232-4636
      - E-mail: nipinfo@cdc.gov
  - Once the vaccine types are determined, the table Recommended Immunization Schedule for Children and Adolescents Who Start Late or Who Are More Than 1 Month Behind can be used to determine:
    - Which doses are valid
    - Which, if any, need to be repeated
  - Doses given earlier than the minimal age or interval generally should be repeated.

Contraindications and precautions

- The CDC's detailed *Guide to Contraindications to Vaccinations*
- *Summary of Recommendations for Childhood and Adolescent Immunization*
- Anaphylactic-type allergy to a vaccine or a vaccine component
  - Includes even mild urticarial reactions
  - Contraindication to further vaccination with the vaccine in question
- Encephalopathy after a previous dose of a pertussis-containing vaccine
  - Contraindication to further vaccination with a pertussis-containing vaccine (eg, diphtheria-tetanus-acellular pertussis [DTaP], Tdap).
- Minor, acute illness
  - Some children are ill at the time of a well-child visit or are in need of a vaccination at an illness visit.
  - In these situations, the clinician must decide whether to recommend vaccination on the basis of 2 questions.
    - Will vaccination be safe for this ill child?

- If the child is not vaccinated at this visit, will he or she be brought back for vaccination?
  - Past appointment-keeping behavior may help in the judgment.
  - Vaccinating the ill child is best, especially if he or she has missed previous preventive care visits.
- Minor illnesses are not valid contraindications to vaccination.
  - Upper respiratory tract infections
  - Otitis media
  - Diarrheal illnesses, whether the individual is febrile or not
- A second, more difficult, consideration is whether minor vaccine side effects, such as fever, will cause diagnostic confusion during the follow-up period for the illness.
  - Particularly likely to be a problem when the patient is a very young infant

Immunocompromised children

- Immunocompromised children and their close contacts require individual attention.
  - Live vaccines
    - In general, live vaccines cannot be used in immunocompromised individuals.
    - Potential for severe or fatal reactions from uncontrolled replication of the vaccine virus
    - Live vaccines should not be given in cases of:
      - Congenital immunodeficiency
      - Leukemia
      - Lymphoma
      - Generalized cancer
      - Treatments that cause immunosuppression (eg, alkylating agents, antimetabolites, and radiation therapy)
      - Persons receiving daily, large doses of corticosteroids (the equivalent of 2 mg/kg of prednisone per day) for ≥14 days
      - Live vaccines should be deferred for at least 30 days after cessation of therapy or reduction in dose.
    - Live vaccine use is not contraindicated:
      - If the corticosteroid is aerosolized (as in asthma inhalers) or a topical agent
      - If it is given on an alternate-day, short course (<14 days)
      - If the child is on a physiologic replacement schedule
  - Inactivated vaccines
    - Cannot replicate and are safe for use in immunocompromised children
    - Immunocompromised children may have a diminished immune response to inactivated vaccines.

Recommended Immunization Schedule for Children and Adolescents Who Start Late or Who Are More Than 1 Month Behind[a]

Catch-up schedule for children aged 4 months through 6 years

Vaccine	Minimum Age for Dose 1	Minimum Interval Between Doses			
		Dose 1 to Dose 2	Dose 2 to Dose 3	Dose 3 to Dose 4	Dose 4 to Dose 5
Hepatitis B[b]	Birth	4 weeks	8 weeks (and at least 16 wks after 1st dose)	—	—
Rotavirus[c]	6 weeks	4 weeks	4 weeks[c]	—	—
Diphtheria, tetanus, pertussis[d]	6 weeks	4 weeks	4 weeks	6 months	6 months[d]
Haemophilus influenza type b[e]	6 weeks	• 4 weeks (if 1st dose is given at age <12 mo) • 8 weeks as the final dose (if 1st dose is given at age 12-14 mo) • No further doses needed (if 1st dose is given at age ≥15 mo)	• 4 weeks[e] (if current age is <12 mo) • 8 weeks as the final dose[e] (if current age is ≥12 mo and 1st dose is given at age <12 and 2nd dose is given at age <15 mo) • No further doses needed (if previous dose is given at age ≥15 mo)	8 weeks as final dose (this dose is only necessary for children aged 12 mo through 59 mo who received 3 doses before age 12 mo)	—
Pneumococcal[f]	6 weeks	• 4 weeks (if 1st dose is given at age <12 mo) • 8 weeks as final dose for healthy children (if 1st dose is given at age ≥12 mo or current age is 24–59 mo) • No further doses needed for healthy children (if 1st dose is given at age ≥24 mo	• 4 weeks (if current age is <12 mo) • 8 weeks as final dose for healthy children (if current age is ≥12 mo) • No further doses needed for healthy children (if previous dose is given at age ≥24 mo	8 weeks as final dose (this dose is only necessary for children aged 12 mo through 59 mo who received 3 doses before age 12 mo or high-risk children who received 3 doses at any age)	—
Inactivated poliovirus[g]	6 weeks	4 weeks	4 weeks	6 months	—
Measles, mumps, rubella[h]	12 months	4 weeks	—	—	—
Varicella[i]	12 months	3 months	—	—	—
Hepatitis A[j]	12 months	6 months	—	—	—

Recommended Immunization Schedule for Children and Adolescents Who Start Late or Who Are More Than 1 Month Behind[a], *continued*

Catch-Up Schedule for Children Aged 7 through 18 Years

Vaccine	Minimum Age for Dose 1	Minimum Interval Between Doses			
		Dose 1 to Dose 2	Dose 2 to Dose 3	Dose 3 to Dose 4	Dose 4 to Dose 5
Tetanus, diphtheria/ Tetanus, diphtheria, pertussis[k]	7 years[k]	4 weeks	• 4 weeks (if 1st dose is given <12 months) • 6 months (if 1st dose is given at ≥12 months)	6 months (if 1st dose is given at age <12 months)	—
Human papillomavirus[l]	9 years	Routine dosing intervals are recommended[l]			
Hepatitis A[j]	12 months	6 months	—	—	—
Hepatitis B[b]	Birth	4 weeks	8 weeks (and at least 16 weeks after 1st dose)	—	—
Inactivated poliovirus[g]	6 weeks	4 weeks	4 weeks	6 months	—
Measles, mumps, rubella[h]	12 months	4 weeks	—	—	—
Varicella[i]	12 months	• 3 mo (if 1st dose is given at ≤13 years) • 4 weeks (if 1st dose is given at ≥13 years)	—	—	—

[a] This table provides catch-up schedules and minimum intervals between doses for children whose vaccinations have been delayed. A vaccine series does not need to be restarted, regardless of the time that has elapsed between doses. Use the section appropriate for the child's age.

[b] Hepatitis B vaccine (HepB).
• Administer the 3-dose series to those not previously vaccinated.
• A 2-dose series (separated by at least 4 months) of adult formulation Recombivax HB is licensed for children aged 11 through 15 years.

[c] Rotavirus vaccine (RV).
• The maximum age for the first dose is 14 weeks 6 days. Vaccination should not be initiated for infants aged 15 weeks 0 days or older.
• The maximum age for the final dose in the series is 8 months 0 days.
• If Rotarix was administered for the first and second doses, a third dose is not indicated.

[d] Diphtheria and tetanus toxoids and acellular pertussis vaccine (DTaP).
• The fifth dose is not necessary if the fourth dose was administered at age 4 years or older.

[e] *Haemophilus influenzae* type b conjugate vaccine (Hib).
• Hib vaccine is not generally recommended for persons aged 5 years or older. No efficacy data are available on which to base a recommendation concerning use of Hib vaccine for older children and adults. However, studies suggest good immunogenicity in persons who have sickle cell disease, leukemia, or HIV infection, or who have had a splenectomy; administering 1 dose of Hib vaccine to these persons who have not previously received Hib vaccine is not contraindicated.
• If the first 2 doses were PRP-OMP (PedvaxHIB or Comvax), and administered at age 11 months or younger, the third (and final) dose should be administered at age 12 through 15 months and at least 8 weeks after the second dose.
• If the first dose was administered at age 7 through 11 months, administer the second dose at least 4 weeks later and a final dose at age 12 through 15 months.

[f] Pneumococcal vaccine.
• Administer 1 dose of pneumococcal conjugate vaccine (PCV) to all healthy children aged 24 through 59 months who have not received at least 1 dose of PCV on or after age 12 months.
• For children aged 24 through 59 months with underlying medical conditions, administer 1 dose of PCV if 3 doses were received previously or administer 2 doses of PCV at least 8 weeks apart if fewer than 3 doses were received previously.
• Administer pneumococcal polysaccharide vaccine (PPSV) to children aged 2 years or older with certain underlying medical conditions, including a cochlear implant, at least 8 weeks after the last dose of PCV.

[g] Inactivated poliovirus vaccine (IPV).
• The final dose in the series should be administered on or after the fourth birthday and at least 6 months following the previous dose.
• A fourth dose is not necessary if the third dose was administered at age 4 years or older and at least 6 months following the previous dose.
• In the first 6 months of life, minimum age and minimum intervals are only recommended if the person is at risk for imminent exposure to circulating poliovirus (ie, travel to a polio-endemic region or during an outbreak).

Recommended Immunization Schedule for Children and Adolescents Who Start Late or Who Are More Than 1 Month Behind[a], *continued*

[h] Measles, mumps, and rubella vaccine (MMR).
- Administer the second dose routinely at age 4 through 6 years. However, the second dose may be administered before age 4, provided at least 28 days have elapsed since the first dose.
- If not previously vaccinated, administer 2 doses with at least 28 days between doses.

[i] Varicella vaccine.
- Administer the second dose routinely at age 4 through 6 years. However, the second dose may be administered before age 4, provided at least 3 months have elapsed since the first dose.
- For persons aged 12 months through 12 years, the minimum interval between doses is 3 months. However, if the second dose was administered at least 28 days after the first dose, it can be accepted as valid.
- For persons aged 13 years and older, the minimum interval between doses is 28 days.

[j] Hepatitis A vaccine (HepA).
- HepA is recommended for children older than 23 months who live in areas where vaccination programs target older children, who are at increased risk for infection, or for whom immunity against hepatitis A is desired.

[k] Tetanus and diphtheria toxoids vaccine (Td) and tetanus and diphtheria toxoids and acellular pertussis vaccine (Tdap).
- Doses of DTaP are counted as part of the Td/Tdap series
- Tdap should be substituted for a single dose of Td in the catch-up series or as a booster for children aged 10 through 18 years; use Td for other doses.

[l] Human papillomavirus vaccine (HPV).
- Administer the series to females at age 13 through 18 years if not previously vaccinated.
- Use recommended routine dosing intervals for series catch-up (ie, the second and third doses should be administered at 1 to 2 and 6 months after the first dose). The minimum interval between the first and second doses is 4 weeks. The minimum interval between the second and third doses is 12 weeks, and the third dose should be administered at least 24 weeks after the first dose.

Information about reporting reactions after immunization is available online at http://www.vaers.hhs.gov or by telephone, 800-822-7967. Suspected cases of vaccine-preventable diseases should be reported to the state or local health department. Additional information, including precautions and contraindications for immunization, is available from the National Center for Immunization and Respiratory Diseases at http://www.cdc.gov/vaccines or telephone, 800-CDC-INFO (800-232-4636).

Department of Health and Human Services • Centers for Disease Control and Prevention

- For vaccination of bone marrow transplant recipients, the clinician should consult the *Red Book* or the CDC guidelines.
- Persons without evidence of severe immunosuppression—even if infected with HIV—should receive MMR and varicella vaccines.
  - Children with symptomatic HIV infection should not receive either of these vaccines.
- Immunocompromised people with limited humoral immunodeficiency (eg, hypogammaglobulinemia, immunoglobulin A deficiency) may be routinely vaccinated with varicella vaccine.
- Persons living with an immunocompromised household contact should be vaccinated as indicated.
- MMR and varicella vaccines, which are live vaccines contraindicated for use in immunocompromised people themselves, should be given to susceptible contacts of immunocompromised people.
- OPV, which is used in countries other than the US, should not be given to people who are immunocompromised or who are close contacts of immunocompromised persons.

Pregnancy
- Pregnant women generally should not receive live vaccines because of the theoretical risk of fetal damage.
- Women should avoid pregnancy for 4 weeks after receiving the MMR, MMR with varicella (MMRV), or varicella vaccine.
- Pregnant women generally may receive inactivated vaccines and toxoids.

- Detailed guidelines for vaccinating pregnant women can be found at the CDC Web site.
- Prematurity
  - Preterm infants should be vaccinated using the routine schedule on the basis of their chronologic age (ie, time since birth, regardless of gestational age) and the standard doses of vaccine.
    - To maximize hepatitis B vaccine efficacy, infants weighing <2000 g and whose mothers are documented to be hepatitis B surface antigen (HBsAg) negative should not receive hepatitis B vaccine until they reach a body weight of 2000 g or chronologic age of 1 month.
  - Premature infants whose mothers' HBsAg status is positive should receive the vaccine and hepatitis B immune globulin (HBIg).
  - If the mother's HBsAg is unknown, the hepatitis B vaccine and HBIg should be given within 12 hours of birth, regardless of birth weight.
    - The birth dose should not be counted as part of the vaccine series.

Vaccine safety
- Vaccine safety concerns have been based on:
  - Data (eg, RotaShield and intussusception)
  - A biologically plausible but unsubstantiated association (eg, thimerosal in the birth dose of hepatitis B vaccine and autism)
  - Speculation (MMR vaccine and autism)

- New concerns are likely to arise.
  - Reliable sources of vaccine safety information that are regularly updated include:
    - Immunization Action Coalition
    - National Network for Immunization Information
    - Vaccine Education Center
    - Institute for Vaccine Safety

SPECIFIC INTERVENTIONS

Universal childhood vaccines

DTaP vaccine

- Recommended form of the oldest combination vaccine, DTP
  - Combination of diphtheria toxoid, tetanus toxoid, and acellular pertussis vaccine
- Vaccination against tetanus and diphtheria has been highly successful.
- DTaP is licensed for all preschool doses.
- Two-thirds of reported cases of pertussis occur in older children and adults, who represent a reservoir for the bacteria and a continuing source of infection for young children.
- Storage
  - DTaP, DTP, or DTP-Hib vaccines should arrive at the office unfrozen.
  - The vaccine should be refrigerated on arrival at a temperature of 2°C to 8°C.
  - The vaccine should not be frozen.
  - Shelf life is up to 1 year.
  - The vials must be shaken vigorously before withdrawing the individual doses.
- Administration
  - The vaccine is administered intramuscularly using a dose of 0.5 mL.
  - The ACIP has stated that, although completing the pertussis vaccination series using vaccine from a single manufacturer is preferred, when this is not feasible, any available licensed pertussis vaccine may be used.
    - Revaccinating individuals with the same manufacturer's product is not necessary to complete the vaccination series; the series can be finished with any of the pediatric acellular vaccines.
- Adverse reactions to diphtheria and tetanus toxoids include:
  - Local reactions, such as redness and induration
  - Nodule at the injection site
  - Arthus-type hypersensitivity reactions
  - Mild adverse reactions to DTaP include:
    - Local reactions of redness, swelling, induration, and tenderness
    - Systemic reactions of drowsiness, vomiting, crying, and low-grade fever

- Moderate-to-severe reactions include:
  - High fevers, with temperature ≥40.5°C (105°F)
  - Persistent and inconsolable crying of >3 hours' duration
  - Hypotonic-hyporesponsive episodes
  - Febrile seizures
- All of these reactions occur much less frequently with DTaP than with DTP, and all are believed to occur without permanent sequelae.
- Contraindications and precautions
  - Contraindication to DTaP vaccination include:
    - A history of severe (anaphylactic) allergic reaction after a prior dose of DTaP vaccine or a vaccine component
    - Encephalopathy within 7 days of a previous dose
  - Precautions to DTaP include:
    - A convulsion within 3 days of a previous dose
    - Persistent, severe, inconsolable screaming or crying for ≥3 hours within 48 hours of a previous dose
    - Collapse or shock like state within 48 hours of a previous dose
    - A temperature of 40.5°C (105°F) that is unexplained by another cause within 48 hours of a previous dose
  - Vaccination should be deferred in the event of a moderate to severe acute illness until the illness subsides.

Hepatitis A virus vaccine

- Recommended for all children between 12 and 23 months of age, with optional catch-up vaccination through the preschool years
- Recommended for persons at increased risk of hepatitis A virus infection, ie, those who:
  - Travel or work in countries of high to intermediate endemicity
  - Have homosexual sex with men
  - Use illegal drugs
  - Work with hepatitis A–infected primates or laboratory specimens
  - Take clotting factor concentrates
- Recommended for people with chronic liver disease
- 2 manufacturers make inactivated hepatitis A vaccines; both brands are given by intramuscular injection.
- A 2-dose schedule is used for the hepatitis A vaccine.
  - Efficacy is >90% after the first dose.
  - Efficacy is ~100% after the second dose.
- Storage
  - Vaccine should arrive unfrozen.
  - Should be stored at temperatures between 2°C and 8°C
  - Shelf life is up to 3 years.

- Contraindications and precautions
  - Hepatitis A vaccine should not be given to individuals who have a history of severe (anaphylactic) allergy to the vaccine or its components, such as alum and phenoxyethanol.
  - Serious adverse events have not been associated with hepatitis A vaccination.
  - The most frequent side effects are local reactions, including soreness at the injection site.

Hepatitis B virus (HBV) vaccine

- Prevents HBV infection and its complications, which include hepatocellular cancer
- Risk factors for HBV infection are lifestyles, occupations, or environments in which contact with blood or other body fluids from infected persons occurs frequently.
- A large proportion of infected individuals were not known to have any risk factor.
- The ACIP recommends hepatitis B vaccination for all unvaccinated children ages 0 to 18 years and makes hepatitis B vaccine available to this group through the Vaccines for Children program.
- Storage
  - Vaccine should arrive with a refrigerant but unfrozen.
  - Vaccine should be refrigerated on arrival and stored at 2°C–8°C.
  - Vaccine should not be frozen.
  - Shelf life is up to 3 years.
- Administration
  - A vaccination series started with one manufacturer's product can be completed with the other manufacturer's product.
  - The vaccine is 80–100% effective at preventing infection.
  - A 3-dose schedule is recommended for active immunization.
    - For routine infant immunization, the initial dose should be given to the newborn before hospital discharge.
    - The minimal intervals between doses are:
      - Between the 1st and 2nd doses—4 weeks
      - Between the 2nd and 3rd doses—8 weeks
      - Between the 1st and 3rd doses—16 weeks
    - The 3rd dose should be administered no earlier than 24 weeks of age.
  - For infants, children, and adolescents through 19 years of age, the dose is 0.5 mL of either the pediatric formulation of Recombivax HB or Engerix B.
  - The seroconversion rate is >95% for infants, children, and adolescents receiving all 3 doses.
- Contraindications and precautions
  - Administration of hepatitis B vaccine is contraindicated for individuals who had a serious (anaphylacti) allergic reaction to a prior dose of hepatitis B vaccine or a vaccine component.

- Serious systemic adverse events and allergic reactions are rare.
  - The most common adverse event after receiving the hepatitis B vaccine is pain at the injection site.
  - Mild systemic symptoms, including fatigue, headache, and irritability, occur in <20% of children.
  - Low-grade fever occurs in up to 6% of children.
- High-risk groups for hepatitis B
  - Native Alaskans, Asian Americans, and Pacific Islanders
  - Children of immigrants or refugee families from countries having high rates of HBV infection
    - Special efforts should be made to vaccinate non–US born and immigrant children.
    - These children also should be screened for HBsAg.
  - Babies born to HBsAg–positive mothers
    - All women should be screened for HBsAg during pregnancy.
    - Women at high risk of HBV infection (eg, intravenous drug users) should be screened again at delivery.
    - The results of hepatitis B testing should be available at the time of delivery so that perinatal transmission can be prevented by administration of both hepatitis B vaccine and HBIg.
    - The regimen is approximately 95% effective in preventing infection.
    - All infants born to women who are HBsAg positive should receive hepatitis B vaccine and HBIg (at a different injection site) within 12 hours of birth, regardless of gestational age or birth weight.
    - For infants weighing <2000 g, this birth dose should not be counted as part of the series; that is, 3 additional doses of hepatitis B vaccine should be given, the first of which should be at 1 month of age.
    - Combination vaccines containing a hepatitis B component, COMVAX and Pediarix, cannot be given to infants before 6 weeks of age.
  - Although these combination vaccines are not licensed for use in infants born to HBsAg-positive mother, ACIP has recommended off-label use of COMVAX or Pediarix after 6 weeks of age to complete the hepatitis B vaccination series for these infants after a birth dose of a single-antigen hepatitis B vaccine.
  - After the hepatitis B immunization series is complete (preferably at 6 months of age), all infants of HBsAg-positive mothers should be tested for the presence of anti-HBs and HBsAg at 9–15 months of age.
  - Infants born to women who were not tested for HBsAg should receive an initial dose of hepatitis B vaccine within 12 hours of birth.
    - The mother should be tested immediately, and if she is positive, then the infant should receive HBIg within 7 days.

- Low-birth-weight infants
  - Hepatitis B vaccination should be postponed if:
    - The mother is HBsAg negative, and
    - The infant weighs <2000 g
  - If the mother's surface antigen status is positive or unknown, these infants should receive immediate vaccination and HBIg, as previously described.

Hib vaccine

- The Hib vaccines in use today are conjugated vaccines.
  - The polysaccharide component of the capsule (polyribosyl-ribitol phosphate [PRP]) is bonded chemically to a protein carrier to enhance immunogenicity (especially in infants) and response to booster doses.
- Available vaccines vary by the carrier protein to which PRP is bonded.
  - Carriers include:
    - A mutant diphtheria toxin (HbOC)
    - Tetanus toxoid (PRP-T)
    - A *Neisseria meningitidis* outer membrane protein complex (PRP-OMP)
- Efficacy is ~97% after 3 doses.
- Storage
  - Hib vaccines should arrive in insulated containers to prevent freezing.
  - They should arrive unfrozen and should be refrigerated immediately and stored between 2°C and 8°C.
  - Freezing reduces or destroys potency.
  - Shelf life is up to 2 years.
- Administration
  - Differences among the vaccines result in slightly different administration schedules.
    - PRP-T (Act-Hib) and HbOC (Hib titer)
      - 4-dose series
      - Given at 2, 4, 6, and 12–15 months of age
    - PRP-OMP (COMVAX, PedvaxHIB)
      - 3-dose series
      - Given at 2, 4, and 12–15 months of age
    - If a child receives different brands of Hib vaccine at 2 and 4 months of age, the Hib vaccine dose should be given at 6 months—even if 1 of the earlier doses was PRP-OMP—and this primary series should be followed by a booster at 12–15 months of age.
  - Hib vaccine is marketed in several combination vaccines, including separate combinations with DTaP and hepatitis B vaccines.
  - The package insert should be consulted for product-specific dosing schedules.
    - The DTaP-Hib combination (TriHibit) is licensed only for the 4th dose of the DTaP-Hib series.
  - Completing the series with a different Hib product from the product used to start the Hib vaccination series is acceptable.
    - Necessitates a 3-dose primary series, after which a booster is given at 12–15 months of age
  - The number of doses needed to complete the Hib series is different for children who have a late start on Hib vaccination or who have a lapsed series.
  - The table Detailed Vaccination Schedule for *Haemophilus Influenzae* Type b Conjugate Vaccines gives a detailed Hib vaccination schedule.
- Adverse events after Hib vaccination are mild and infrequent.
  - 5–30% of children have a local reaction consisting of swelling, redness, or pain.

Detailed Vaccination Schedule for *Haemophilus Influenzae* Type b Conjugate Vaccines[a]

Vaccine	Age at 1st Dose (months)	Primary Series	Booster
PRP-T (ActHIB)	2–6	3 doses, 2 months apart	12–15 months[b]
	7–11	2 doses, 2 months apart	12–15 months[b]
	12–14	1 dose	2 months later
	15–59	1 dose	None
PRP-OMP (PedvaxHIB)	2–6	2 doses, 2 months apart	12–15 months[b]
	7–11	2 doses, 2 months apart	12–15 months[b]
	12–14	1 dose	2 months later
	15–59	1 dose	None

[a] From: Centers for Disease Control and Prevention. Detailed Vaccination Schedule for *Haemophilus influenzae* type b Conjugate Vaccines. Available at www.cdc.gov/vaccines/pubs/pinkbook/downloads/hib.pdf.
[b] At least 2 months after previous dose.

- Systemic adverse events, such as fever, are uncommon.
- Contraindications and precautions
  - History of severe (anaphylactic) allergic reaction after a prior dose of Hib vaccine or a vaccine component
  - Vaccination should be deferred in the event of a moderate to severe acute illness until the patient's health improves.

Influenza virus vaccine

- In 2008 the AAP approved the recommendations to expand the ages for annual influenza vaccination of children to include all youths from 6 months through 18 years of age.
- Annual influenza vaccination is recommended for:
  - Older children with any of the following conditions:
    - Asthma and other chronic pulmonary or cardiovascular system diseases (does not include hypertension)
    - Any condition that can compromise respiratory function or the handling of respiratory secretions or that can increase the risk for aspiration
    - Immunosuppressive conditions, HIV infection, sickle cell disease, and other hemoglobinopathies
    - Chronic metabolic diseases, including diabetes mellitus, renal dysfunction, and long-term aspirin use
  - Persons who live with or care for an individual for whom the vaccine is recommended or an infant who is too young to be vaccinated (ie, <6 months of age)
  - Women who will be pregnant during influenza season
  - Residents of nursing homes and other chronic care facilities
- Currently, influenza immunization can be achieved using an injectable trivalent inactivated vaccine (TIV) or an LAIV.
  - Both vaccines consist of 3 highly purified, egg-grown influenza virus subtypes.
  - The composition is based on the viral strains expected during the winter influenza virus season.
    - TIV consists of either purified surface antigens or viral particles prepared by disrupting the membrane.
    - TIV is licensed for use in persons ≥6 months of age.
    - LAIV is licensed only for use in healthy persons (ie, those without a chronic illness) who are 2–49 years of age and are not pregnant.
- Administration
  - TIV is administered intramuscularly and LAIV is administered intranasally are given in an age-dependent schedule as follows.
    - 6–35 months of age: require 2 doses the first time they receive influenza vaccine, with single annual doses thereafter (TIV dose is 0.25 mL at this stage)
    - 3–8 years of age: require 2 doses the first time they receive influenza vaccine, with single annual doses thereafter (TIV dose is 0.50 mL at this stage)
    - ≥9 years of age: 1 dose annually (TIV dose is 0.50 mL at this stage)
  - For the 2-dose regimen, the minimum interval recommendation between doses of either TIV or LAIV is 4 weeks.
  - In 2008 in addition to the LAIV made by a sole manufacturer, injectable vaccines from 5 manufacturers have been licensed in the US as shown below along with the age category for which the product is licensed.
    - sanofi pasteur (Fluzone): ≥6 months of age
    - Novartis vaccine (Fluvirin): ≥4 years of age
    - GlaxoSmithKline (Fluarix): ≥18 years of age
    - CSL Biotherapies (Afluria): ≥18 years of age
    - ID Biomedical Corporation of Quebec (FluLaval): ≥18 years of age
- Storage
  - All influenza vaccine (TIV and LAIV)
    - Should be stored between 35°F–46°F (2°C and 8°C)
  - FluMist
    - Now refrigerator stable
    - Should be shipped frozen
    - Upon receipt, should be stored in refrigerator between 35°F–46°F (2°C–8°C)
    - Should not be refrozen
  - Additional details on influenza vaccine storage, shipping, and handling can be found on the Web site of the Minnesota Department of Health.
- Adverse events
  - TIV
    - Rarely causes febrile or other systemic reactions
    - Local reactions, including soreness, redness, and induration at the site of the injection, occur in <30% of vaccinees.
    - Immediate hypersensitivity reactions, such as hives, angioedema, allergic asthma, or anaphylaxis, occur rarely after influenza vaccination.
  - LAIV
    - May be associated with coryza or nasal congestion, headache, fever, vomiting, abdominal pain, and myalgias
    - These symptoms are associated more often with the first dose and are self-limited.
- Contraindications and precautions
  - Administration of influenza vaccine is contraindicated for individuals who have had a serious (anaphylactic) allergic reaction to a prior dose of influenza vaccine or a vaccine component (eg, eggs).
  - For details about specific influenza vaccines, consult their package inserts at the US Food and Drug Administration's (FDA) Center for Biologics Evaluation and Research Web site.

MMR vaccine

- A combination of 3 live attenuated vaccines that together protect against measles, mumps, and rubella

- The purpose of the measles and mumps vaccines is to protect against these specific diseases.
- The purpose of the rubella vaccine is to prevent congenital rubella syndrome by preventing the occurrence of rubella, (which itself is a mild disease) in the general population, thereby preventing its spread to susceptible pregnant women.
- MMR is also licensed in combination with varicella vaccine as MMRV (ProQuad, Merck Vaccine Division).
- In the US, only 1 strain of each vaccine virus in MMR is available.
  - Each one is highly immunogenic, leading to seroconversion in ≥90–95% of recipients vaccinated at ≥15 months of age.
- Storage
  - MMR vaccine
    - Should arrive at the office in an insulated container at a temperature <10°C
    - Should be refrigerated on arrival and stored between 2°C and 8°C (never frozen)
    - The shelf life is up to 2 years; the expiration date is marked on the vials.
    - On reconstitution, the vaccine should be stored in a dark place between 2°C and 8°C and must be used within 8 hours.
  - MMRV
    - Must be shipped and stored at ≤4°F (−20°C) at all times
    - Must not be stored at refrigerator temperature at any time
    - Must be administered within 30 minutes of reconstitution
- Administration
  - The AAP and ACIP recommend administration of 2 doses of MMR vaccine for children; these doses are 0.5 mL delivered subcutaneously.
    - The 1st dose should be given at 12–15 months of age.
    - The 2nd dose should be given before elementary school entry (4–6 years of age).
    - The purpose of the 2nd dose is to produce immunity in the small proportion of children who fail to respond to the first.
  - MMRV is approved only for children 12 months through 12 years of age and may be administered whenever MMR or varicella vaccines, or both, are indicated.
- Adverse reactions
  - Because MMR is composed of live attenuated vaccines, if side effects other than those related to allergy occur, they do so 5–12 days after administration.
  - Adverse reactions include:
    - Rash: 5–10% (measles, rubella)
    - Fever: 5–15% (measles)
    - Thrombocytopenia: 1 per 30,000 (measles)
    - Parotitis: rare (mumps)

- Transient arthritis: <1% (rubella)
- Arthralgia: adults, but not children
  - An association between autism and MMR has been postulated but is not supported by scientific evidence.
- Contraindications and precautions
  - Contraindications to MMR vaccination include:
    - History of a severe (anaphylactic) allergic reaction to a prior dose or a vaccine component (eg, neomycin, gelatin)
    - Significant immunosuppression from any cause, including cancer or its treatment, immunodeficiency diseases, or immunosuppressive therapy
    - Asymptomatic HIV infection is not a contraindication to receipt of MMR.
    - Pregnancy
  - Precautions regarding MMR vaccination include:
    - Moderate or severe acute illness (defer vaccination until illness improves)
    - Recent receipt of a blood transfusion, blood products, or immune (γ) globulin
    - A history of thrombocytopenia or thrombocytopenia purpura
  - MMRV
    - Contraindications and precautions include all of those for both MMR and varicella vaccines.

Pneumococcal vaccine—conjugated

- The pneumococcal conjugate vaccine (PCV) is analogous to the Hib conjugate vaccine, in which a protein is joined to the polysaccharide.
- The currently licensed formulation contains 7 serotypes (thus the acronym PCV7) that accounted for most of the invasive pneumococcal diseases in children in the prevaccine era.
- Prelicensure studies of the conjugate vaccine indicated:
  - High efficacy against invasive disease
  - 10% reductions in acute otitis media
  - Reductions in nasopharyngeal carriage of the bacteria
- Postlicensure studies have confirmed marked reductions in invasive pneumococcal disease, as well as possible indirect protection of other populations, such as older adults through herd immunity.
  - For these reasons, the AAP and ACIP recommend that all children should be routinely vaccinated with PCV7 beginning at 2 months of age.
- Special efforts should be made to ensure on-time vaccination of children with medical conditions that put them at increased risk of invasive pneumococcal disease, such as:
  - Sickle cell disease
  - Asplenia
  - HIV infection or other immunocompromising conditions

- Chronic disease (eg, cardiopulmonary disease except asthma, chronic liver disease, or diabetes mellitus)
- Black, American Indian, and Native Alaskan children also are considered to be at high risk.
- Administration
  - PCV7 is administered intramuscularly as a 0.5-mL dose.
  - Administration should begin at 2 months but not earlier than 6 weeks of age.
  - The recommended interval between the subsequent 2 doses is 2 months; the minimal interval is 4 weeks.
  - The booster dose should be given at 12–15 months of age, at least 2 months after the 3rd dose.
  - Recommended schedules vary for children who had a delayed 1st dose or a lapse in vaccination. See tables Recommended Schedule for Use of 7-Valent Pneumococcal Conjugate Vaccine (PCV7) and Recommendations for Use of 7-Valent Pneumococcal Conjugate Vaccine (PCV7).
- Adverse reactions
  - Local reactions (1 in 4) and low-grade fever (1 in 3 with temperature >100.4°F) are common following PCV7.
  - Fever >102.2°F is not common (1 in 50).
  - To date, no serious reactions have been associated with the vaccine.
- Contraindications and precautions
  - A severe (anaphylactic) allergic reaction following a prior dose of PCV7 or its components
  - Vaccination should be deferred for children with a moderate to severe acute illness until the illness improves.

Pneumococcal vaccine—polysaccharide (PPV23)

- The pure polysaccharide pneumococcal vaccine (PPV23) consists of purified capsular polysaccharide antigen from 23 types of pneumococcal bacteria.
- It is given by intramuscular or subcutaneous injection.
- Unlike PCV:
  - Does not reduce nasopharyngeal pneumococcal carriage
  - Does not protect children <2 years of age
- Use of PPV23 is recommended for all persons ≥65 years of age, as well as children ≥2 years of age who have conditions that place them at increased risk of systemic pneumococcal infection.

Recommended Schedule for Use of 7-Valent Pneumococcal Conjugate Vaccine (PCV7)[a]

Age at 1st Dose (months)	Number of Doses in Primary Series	Additional Dose
2–6	3 doses, 2 months apart[b]	1 dose at 12–15 months, at least 8 weeks after the primary series has been completed
7–11	2 doses, 2 months apart[b]	1 dose at 12–15 months, at least 8 weeks after the primary series has been completed
12–23	2 doses, 2 months apart[c]	None
24–59 without high-risk condition	1 dose	None
24–59 with high-risk condition[d]	2 doses, 2 months apart	None
>59	0	None

[a] Among previously unvaccinated infants and children by age at time of first vaccination.
[b] For children vaccinated at age <1 year, the minimum interval between doses is 4 weeks.
[c] The minimum interval between doses is 8 weeks.
[d] High-risk conditions include sickle cell disease, asplenia, HIV infection, chronic illness, cochlear implant, and immunocompromising conditions.

Recommendations for Use of 7-Valent Pneumococcal Conjugate Vaccine (PCV7)[a]

Age at Visit (months)	Previous PCV7 Vaccination History	Recommended Regimen
7–11	1 dose	1 dose at 7–11 mo; another ≥2 mo later at 12–15 mo
	2 doses	Same as above
12–23	1 dose before age 12 mo	2 doses ≥2 mo apart
	2 doses before age 12 mo	1 dose ≥2 mo after the most recent dose
24–59	Any incomplete schedule	1 dose[b]

[a] Among children with a lapse in vaccine administration.
[b] Children with high-risk conditions (eg, sickle cell disease, asplenia, HIV infection, chronic illness, cochlear implant, immunocompromising conditions) should receive 2 doses ≥2 mo apart.

- At least 2 months should separate the last dose of PCV7 and 1st dose of PPV23.
- For children undergoing splenectomy or chemotherapy initiation, vaccination should occur >2 weeks before splenectomy or the start of chemotherapy, if possible.
- Details on the use of PPV23 after vaccination with PCV7 are found on the Centers for Disease Control and Prevention (CDC) Web site.
- Storage
  - Should arrive at the office unfrozen
  - Should be refrigerated immediately on arrival
  - Should be stored between 2°C and 8°C
  - Shelf life is up to 2 years.
- Adverse reactions
  - Mild local reactions in ~50% of recipients
  - Fever or severe local reactions in <1%
- Contraindications and precautions
  - Severe (anaphylactic) allergic reaction following a prior dose of the vaccine or its components
  - Vaccination should be deferred for children with a moderate to severe acute illness until the illness improves.

Polio vaccine

- 2 polio vaccines have been developed: enhanced-potency IPV and OPV.
- Routine polio vaccination in the US is currently accomplished with IPV, which is administered subcutaneously (or intramuscularly) with a dose of 0.5 mL and consists of formaldehyde-killed polio virus.
- OPV is a live attenuated vaccine that is administered orally.
  - Although still used routinely in many countries (eg, Mexico), use of OPV was discontinued in the US in 2000.
- Storage
  - IPV should arrive at the office unfrozen and should be refrigerated between 2°C and 8°C.
  - The shelf life is up to 18 months.
- Administration
  - In many states, 4 polio vaccinations are required before school entry—3 doses in the primary series and 1 supplementary dose.
  - If an all-IPV schedule is used and the 3rd dose is administered after the child's 4th birthday, then no supplemental dose is indicated.
- Adverse reactions
  - No serious adverse effects have been reported following IPV.

Rotavirus vaccine

- Rotavirus is the most common cause of severe gastroenteritis in infants and young children in the US.
- The CDC estimates that rotavirus infection leads to 55,000 hospitalizations each year for acute gastroenteritis.

- In February 2006 an attenuated pentavalent bovine-human rotavirus vaccine (PRV) was licensed for use in the US.
- PRV is expected to cover >80% of the strains that currently are responsible for rotavirus acute gastroenteritis worldwide.
- In large prelicensure studies, PRV was efficacious and well tolerated.
  - The efficacy of the vaccine against rotavirus gastroenteritis caused by G1 through G4 serotypes was 74% against any severity and 98% against severe disease.
  - Use of this vaccine was associated with a 94.5% reduction in G1 through G4 rotavirus–related hospitalizations and emergency department visits in the 1st full rotavirus season after the 3rd PRV dose.
- Schedule
  - The 1st dose should be given between 6 and 12 weeks of age.
  - An interval of 4–10 weeks should pass between doses in the series.
  - All 3 doses should be given by 32 weeks of age.
  - Age should be calculated based on chronological age.
  - Premature infants can be immunized if they are clinically stable and are being or have been discharged from the hospital nursery.
  - If a child spits out or vomits after vaccination, then the dose should not be repeated; the series should simply continue according to the recommended intervals.
- Storage
  - The recommended dose of PRV is 2 mL orally.
  - This dose comes as a liquid in latex-free single-dose tubes.
  - PRV should be transported and stored at 2°C–8°C (36°F–46°F) and protected from light.
- Contraindications and precautions
  - A severe (anaphylactic) allergic reaction after a prior dose of the vaccine or its components
  - Moderate-to-severe acute illness: vaccination should be deferred until the illness improves.
  - Other precautions include:
    - Altered immunocompetence
    - Preexisting chronic gastrointestinal disease
    - History of intussusception
- Adverse reactions
  - Within a week of receiving PRV, children are slightly (1–3%) more likely to have mild, temporary diarrhea or vomiting than unvaccinated children.
  - Unlike a previously licensed rotavirus vaccine, no evidence has been found that PRV causes intussusception or other serious adverse events.
- Other live oral rotavirus vaccines are in development.

Varicella vaccine

- The AAP and ACIP first recommended routine varicella vaccination in 1996.
- Most states now have varicella vaccination requirements for child care and school entry.
- The Oka/Merck strain, a live attenuated vaccine virus developed in the early 1970s in Japan, is the sole vaccine virus strain licensed in the US today.
  - The efficacy of the vaccine is:
    - ~70% for preventing any varicella disease
    - >95% for preventing severe varicella disease
- In 2007 ACIP expanded their recommendations to include
  - A routine 2-dose varicella vaccination program for children (at age 12–15 months and again at age 4–6 years)
  - A second dose for all persons who previously had received only 1 dose
  - Routine vaccination of all healthy persons age >13 years without evidence of immunity
  - Prenatal assessment and postpartum vaccination
  - Expansion of the use of the varicella vaccine for specific groups of HIV-infected children
- Varicella vaccine is also licensed in combination with MMR vaccine as MMRV for use in children 12 months to 12 years of age (see MMR Vaccine section).
- Administration
  - The recommended dose is 0.5 mL injected subcutaneously.
  - For children 12 months to 12 years of age, the recommended minimum interval between the two doses is 3 months.
    - Any dose given >28 days after the first dose is considered valid.
  - For persons ≥13 years of age, the recommended minimum interval is 4 weeks.
  - Varicella vaccine may be given simultaneously with MMR, but, if not given on the same day, at least 28 days should elapse between the administration of the 2 doses.
  - Whether immunity is lifelong is unknown, and the answer to this question is complicated by persistent exposure to circulating wild type varicella virus, which boosts immunity in vaccinated children.
- Storage
  - Varicella vaccine has stringent cold chain and storage requirements.
  - The vaccine should arrive at the office frozen, having been shipped in dry ice, which should still be present in the shipping container.
  - It must be stored in a freezer with a separate door at 5°F or colder.
  - The shelf life of vaccine that is properly handled is 18 months.

- If stored at refrigerator temperatures, then varicella vaccine must be used within 72 hours, and it cannot be refrozen.
  - MMRV must be stored frozen at all times and cannot tolerate refrigerator temperatures.
- After reconstitution, varicella vaccine must be administered within 30 minutes.
- Contraindications and precautions
  - Contraindications include:
    - History of a severe (anaphylactic) allergic reaction to a prior dose or a vaccine component (eg, neomycin, gelatin)
    - Substantial suppression of cellular immunity from any cause, including cancer or its treatment, immunodeficiency diseases, or immunosuppressive therapy (although persons with impaired humoral immunity may be vaccinated).
    - Pregnancy
  - Asymptomatic HIV infection and pure humoral immunodeficiencies (eg, immunoglobulin A deficiency, hypogammaglobulinemia) are not contraindications to receipt of varicella vaccine.
  - Precautions include:
    - Moderate or severe acute illness (vaccination is deferred until illness improves)
    - Receipt of a blood transfusion, blood products, or immune (γ) globulin
    - The manufacturer recommends discontinuing salicylates for 6 weeks after receiving varicella vaccine because of the association between aspirin use and Reye syndrome after acquiring chickenpox.
  - Contraindications and precautions to MMRV include all of those for both MMR and varicella vaccines.
- Adverse reactions
  - Local symptoms, such as pain, soreness, redness, and swelling, which occur in 19% of young children and 24–33% of adolescents
  - A varicella-like rash at the injection site, which occurs within 2 weeks in 3% of first-dose recipients
  - A varicella-like rash at noninjection sites, which occurs within 3 weeks in 4–6% of children
  - The incidence of zoster is less after varicella vaccination than after natural infection, but zoster may be caused by varicella vaccine virus.

Routine adolescent immunization

- A major effort is under way to protect adolescents from vaccine-preventable diseases.
- Routine well-child visits should be established for adolescents to provide vaccines and other preventive care measures.
- 3 main categories of vaccines for adolescents should be considered.
  - Routinely recommended vaccines (discussed below)

- Vaccines needed because of special high-risk conditions (eg, influenza, pneumococcal polysaccharide)
- Vaccines that were missed previously
  - Persons who have had no previous varicella vaccination (or history of disease), <2 doses of MMR, or <3 doses of hepatitis B vaccine

Meningococcal conjugate vaccine

- *N meningitidis* is a much-dreaded cause of meningitis and overwhelming sepsis.
- Freshmen college students living in dormitories are at greater risk than their similarly aged peers.
- In January 2005 a quadrivalent meningococcal conjugate vaccine (MCV4) was licensed in the US for persons aged 11–55 years.
- In 2007 ACIP expanded the recommendations to include routine vaccination of all persons aged 11–18 years with 1 dose of MCV4 at the earliest opportunity.
  - College freshmen living in dormitories
- ACIP also reiterated the recommendation to ensure vaccination of groups with an elevated risk of meningococcal disease.
  - College freshmen living in a dormitory
  - Military recruits
  - Persons with anatomic or functional asplenia
  - Persons with terminal complement component deficiencies
  - Persons who travel to or reside in countries in which *N meningitidis* is hyperendemic or epidemic
  - Microbiologists who are routinely exposed to isolates of *N meningitidis*
- Persons 2–55 years of age who are at increased risk, MCV4 (rather than MPSV4) is the preferred formulation.
- Unlike MPSV4, MCV4 is conjugated (ie, the polysaccharide is linked to a protein); thus, it offers improved duration of immunity.
- Whereas the older polysaccharide vaccine guarded against disease for 3–5 years, the new vaccine may offer protection for a decade.
  - Conjugated vaccines are known to limit disease spread among unvaccinated persons by reducing asymptomatic bacterial carriage among those who are vaccinated.
- MCV4 is serogroup specific against groups A, C, Y, and W-135, similar to the polysaccharide vaccine.
- No vaccine is available against serogroup B disease, which causes >50% of meningococcal disease in young children and 30% of meningococcal disease in adolescents and young adults.
- MCV4 has been shown to have high immunogenicity, with significant titers in 98% of recipients after 1 dose.
- Administration
  - The meningococcal conjugate vaccine is licensed for ages 2–55 years.
  - It is administered intramuscularly at a dose of 0.5 mL.
  - The vaccine can be given concomitantly with other vaccines, including Td or Tdap.
- Storage
  - Vaccine should be stored at temperatures of 2°C–8°C (35°F–46°F) and should not be frozen.
  - It is packaged in single-dose vials.
  - Product that has been frozen should not be used.
- Adverse reactions
  - Common adverse effects from the vaccine include local pain (59%), headache (35%), and fatigue (30%).
  - Guillain-Barré syndrome (GBS)
    - Has been associated with receipt of MCV4
      - Specifically, at a rate of 0.20 per 100,000 person-months, the ratio of the Vaccine Adverse Event Reporting System (VAERS) reporting rate of GBS after MCV4 vaccination to the expected incidence rate was 1.77 (CI=0.96–3.07).
    - Because persons with a history of GBS might be at increased risk for postvaccination GBS, ACIP recommends that persons who have a personal or parental history of GBS should discuss the decision to receive MCV4 with their health care provider.

Tdap vaccine

- Vaccinating adolescents for pertussis is intended to reduce both pertussis morbidity among adolescents and the reservoir of disease.
  - The latter effect presumably will decrease infant mortality, especially among children who are too young to have received the childhood DTaP series.
- 2 Tdap vaccines for adolescents are FDA approved.
  - Adacel (for ages 11–64)
  - Boostrix (for ages 10–18)
  - Both vaccines are indicated only as boosters.
  - Both contain lower amounts of diphtheria toxoid and pertussis antigen than the childhood vaccine (DTaP).
  - Neither is interchangeable with the infant formulation.
  - Both vaccines were shown to produce significant pertussis antibody booster responses in 95–99% of patients and induced similar tetanus-diphtheria antibody responses to Td vaccine.
- Administration
  - The ACIP and AAP recommend that adolescents ages 11–12 years old be given Tdap in place of the Td booster previously given.
  - The committee also recommended that Tdap be given to adolescents ages 13–18 who missed the early adolescent dose of Td.

- Adolescents ages 11–18 who have already been vaccinated with Td are encouraged to receive a dose of Tdap to further protect against pertussis.
- A dose of Tdap is also recommended for adults <65 years of age.
- Although the manufacturers' prescribing information recommends a 5-year interval after a Td vaccination before administering Tdap, ACIP does not recommend any absolute minimum interval between Td and Tdap.
- ACIP suggests administering Tdap regardless of interval since last Td if pertussis immunity is imparative (eg, for health care professionals or for those who have an infant in the household).
- Tdap may be given concomitantly with any other vaccine and is recommended for would management in place of Td.
- If the individual has no history of receipt of the primary DTaP series, then he or she should receive 3 doses of vaccine; the 1st should be with Tdap, and the next 2 should be Td at 4 weeks and 6 months after Tdap.

■ Storage
- The dose for both brands of Tdap is 0.5 mL injected intramuscularly.
  - Boostrix is available in 0.5-mL single-dose vials and syringes.
  - Adacel is available in 0.5-mL single-dose vials.
- Both products should be refrigerated (2°C–8°C [35°F–46°F]) but not frozen.

■ Adverse reactions
- Side effects of Tdap include:
  - Mild pain at the injection site (75–88%)
  - Redness and swelling (11–22%)
  - Low-grade fever
  - Headache
  - Fatigue
- All side effects are similar to those from Td vaccination.

■ Contraindications and precautions
- Contraindications include:
  - A severe (anaphylactic) allergic reaction after a prior dose of the vaccine or its components
  - A history of encephalopathy within 7 days of administration of a pertussis-containing vaccine
- Vaccination should be deferred for persons with a moderate to severe acute illness until the illness improves.

HPV vaccine

■ HPV is the most common sexually transmitted infection in the US, with an estimated 6 million infections each year, 74% of which occur in adolescents age 15–24 years.

■ Although 32–46% of adolescents and young women are infected with HPV, a small percentage go on to develop cervical dysplasia and eventually cervical cancer.

■ Specific subtypes of HPV are high-risk (types 16, 18, 31, and 45 are associated with genital cancers and their precursors) or are low-risk (types 6 and 11 are associated with low grade cervical abnormalities, genital warts and, in infants, laryngeal papillomas).

■ HPV subtypes 16 and 18 are known to be present in ≥70% of cervical cancers, and types 6 and 11 are related to 90% of anogenital warts.

■ The vaccine has been shown to be cost effective when combined with continued Papanicolaou testing.

■ Papanicolaou testing would continue to be recommended because not all HPV types could be included in 1 vaccine.

Other sexually transmitted infections

■ May become available within the next decade

■ Herpes simplex virus (HSV)
- A vaccine against HSV was found to have an efficacy of 74% in HSV-seronegative women, but was not effective for men or HSV-1–seropositive women.
- The potential effect of such a vaccine depends, in large part, on its ability to blunt viral shedding.

■ Chlamydia
- Several vaccines against *Chlamydia trachomatis* are in development, ranging from DNA vaccines to live attenuated vaccines.
- Animal studies are promising, but vaccines for adolescents are still several years away.

Increased Intracranial Pressure

DEFINITION

- Increased intracranial pressure (ICP) is a potentially life-threatening neurologic or neurosurgical emergency.
- Rapidly identifying and managing the cause can prevent serious morbidity and possible death.
- Increased ICP has many causes, and symptoms can be acute, subacute, or chronic.

ETIOLOGY

Causes of increased ICP in children

- Head trauma
  - Cerebral edema
  - Intracerebral hemorrhage
  - Extracerebral hemorrhage (subdural, epidural)
- Vascular causes
  - Arterial or venous infarctions
  - Intracerebral hemorrhage
  - Dural sinus thrombosis
  - Subarachnoid hemorrhage
  - Vascular anomalies (vein of Galen malformation, arteriovenous malformations)
- Neoplastic causes
  - Primary brain tumors
  - Metastatic (intracerebral, meningeal infiltration)
- Hydrocephalus (congenital or acquired, communicating or noncommunicating)
- Pseudotumor cerebri (benign intracranial hypertension)
- Central nervous system infections
  - Meningitis (bacterial, fungal, mycobacterial)
  - Encephalitis (focal or diffuse)
  - Abscess
- Metabolic causes
  - Inborn errors of metabolism (hyperammonemia)
  - Hepatic encephalopathy
  - Diabetic ketoacidosis
  - Renal failure
  - Reye syndrome
  - Hypoxic-ischemic encephalopathy
  - Fluid-electrolyte abnormalities (hyponatremia, hypernatremia)
- Structural causes
  - Craniosynostosis
  - Status epilepticus

Mechanism

- Depending on the cause, intracranial hypertension can be:
  - Chronic (as with pseudotumor cerebri)
  - Acute (as with head trauma resulting in cerebral edema or intracerebral hemorrhage)
- Based on experimental data, 2 primary mechanisms are thought to be involved.
  - Vasogenic extracellular brain edema
  - Delayed reabsorption through the arachnoid villa
- Idiopathic intracranial hypertension may be compounded by secondary exacerbation of intracranial venous sinus compression that results in further reduction of flow across the arachnoid villi.
  - Predominantly affects young obese women of childbearing age

RISK FACTORS

- In the young, risk factors include:
  - Medications
    - Vitamin A in infants
    - Isotretinoin (Accutane)
    - Corticosteroids
    - All-trans-retinoic acid for treatment of promyelocytic leukemia
    - Levothyroxine
    - Tetracycline
    - Trimethoprim-sulfamethoxazole
    - Cimetidine
    - Nalidixic acid
    - Nitrofurantoin
    - Recombinant growth hormone
  - Endocrinopathies
    - Recent weight gain
    - Menstrual irregularity
    - Adrenal insufficiency
    - Cushing disease
    - Hypoparathyroidism
    - Hypothyroidism
    - Excessive thyroxine replacement
  - Chronic renal failure
  - Systemic lupus erythematosus

SIGNS AND SYMPTOMS

Infants

- Acute increased ICP
  - Irritability
  - Poor feeding or emesis
  - Split sutures (especially lambdoid)
  - Bulging fontanelle
  - Altered mental status

- Seizures
- Parinaud sign (upgaze paresis)

■ Chronic increased ICP

- Irritability
- Poor feeding or emesis
- Increased head circumference
- Bulging fontanelle
- Split sutures (especially lambdoid)
- Apparent developmental arrest or regression
- Parinaud sign (upgaze paresis)

Children

■ Acute increased ICP

- Severe, acute headache
- Seizures
- Emesis
- Rapidly deteriorating mental status
- Decerebrate or decorticate posture
- Focal neurologic deficits
- Papilledema
- Pupillary abnormalities
- Autonomic dysfunction (Cushing triad)

■ Chronic increased ICP

- Chronic, progressive headache
- Seizures
- Early morning emesis
- Change in school performance
- Altered mental status
- Cranial neuropathy (eg, sixth cranial nerve palsy)
- Focal neurologic deficits
- Papilledema
- Visual changes

Differentiating between acute and chronic ICP

■ Many of the signs and symptoms of acute and chronic ICP are the same, demonstrating their somewhat nonspecific nature.

■ The temporal pace of development differs between the 2 forms.

■ Acute signs of rapidly increasing ICP result from displaced neuronal tissue through several dural openings, with subsequent compression and ischemic changes to cerebral structures.

- With uncal herniation, in association with supratentorial masses, the uncus is displaced through the tentorial opening, leading to compression of the ipsilateral third nerve and displacement of the peduncles and brainstem laterally.
  - Clinically, the patient is comatose.
  - Ipsilateral pupillary dilation (third nerve palsy)

- Ipsilateral hemiparesis, suggesting a falsely localizing lesion in the contralateral hemisphere

- The pupil reliably localizes the side of the lesion.

- Downward herniation of the cerebellar tonsils through the foramen magnum leads to compression and vascular compromise of the lower brainstem structures (medulla).
  - Patients are comatose.
  - Decorticate or decerebrate rigidity
  - Autonomic (respiratory and circulatory) changes

- Cushing triad (rarely seen clinically)
  - Widened pulse pressure
  - Bradycardia
  - Deep, slow respiration

DIAGNOSTIC APPROACH

■ The key to managing increased ICP is rapidly recognizing intracranial hypertension.

■ History and physical and neurologic examinations are the most important aspects of the initial evaluation.

■ It is critical to obtain information on the pace of illness, to discern the need for urgent versus emergent management.

■ If process is rapidly evolving (eg, impending herniation), stabilizing the patient is essential before proceeding to definitive diagnosis and therapy.

IMAGING

■ Computed tomography (CT) is performed more often than magnetic resonance imaging (MRI).

- MRI provides better anatomic differentiation than CT, but it is frequently unavailable in the emergency setting.

■ If a mass lesion is suspected, neuroimaging (regardless of modality) should include contrast enhancement.

■ Both modalities are effective in evaluating the cause of intracranial hypertension.

■ If the patient is suspected of having a subarachnoid hemorrhage, CT followed by lumbar puncture (LP) remains the mainstay of initial diagnosis.

■ Ultrasonography is a reasonable alternative to CT or MRI in infants suspected of having aqueductal stenosis.

■ Other neuroimaging studies, such as angiography, rarely play a role in the initial diagnostic management of intracranial hypertension.

■ Imaging studies are recommended to screen for mass lesions or hydrocephalus, although most patients have normal scans.

- CT of the head may show small, slit ventricles.

- MRI of the brain with gadolinium enhancement is preferred for its sensitivity in screening other conditions.

- Magnetic resonance venography:
  - Is recommended for suspected dural venous sinus thrombosis

– May show extraluminal narrowing of the transverse sinus that may be a typical feature of pseudotumor cerebri

DIAGNOSTIC PROCEDURES

- LP provides an opportunity to evaluate ICP.
  - LP is performed by inserting a spinal needle into the thecal sac and attaching a manometer.
  - Cerebrospinal fluid (CSF) column height is measured while the patient is in the lateral decubitus position with legs extended.
    - Between 12 and 18 cm is normal.
- If a mass lesion is suspected, withdrawing lumbar CSF may create a pressure gradient intracranially and precipitate herniation syndrome; thus, neuroimaging is generally recommended before LP.
- In children suspected of having meningitis, neuroimaging before LP may unnecessarily delay antibiotic treatment.
  - If meningitis is a serious consideration and a CT scan is still desired, antibiotic therapy should not be delayed.
- Spinal fluid analysis should always include glucose and protein measurement and a total and differential cell count.
- Depending on the clinical situation, other studies can be obtained, including microbial cultures, special stains, and cytology.

TREATMENT APPROACH

- Rapid recognition and stabilization of the patient suspected of having acutely increased ICP is essential in preventing greater morbidity and mortality.
- Goals of early management
  - Decrease ICP without compromising cerebral perfusion
  - Identify the cause so that definitive therapy can be provided
- Neurologically stable patients with evidence of chronically increased ICP
  - Management is directed toward definitive therapy.
    - Evacuation of the chronic subdural hematoma
    - Appropriate tumor management (corticosteroids, surgery or radiation plus chemotherapy or both)
    - Treatment with acetazolamide, loop diuretics, steroids, or lumbar drain in patients with more benign causes of intracranial hypertension

SPECIFIC TREATMENTS

Emergency management

- Assess the airway, breathing, and circulation (the ABCs).
- Obtain a urine dextrostick and, in the case of trauma, expose the patient completely to identify injuries.

- When acute increased ICP is suspected:
  - Stabilize the airway.
    - In most instances, this requires rapid, controlled intubation, taking care to minimize Valsalva maneuvers, which increase ICP further (albeit transiently).
  - Obtain intravenous (IV) access.
    - Use only isotonic solutions, minimizing fluids initially unless circulatory compromise is evident.
  - Measure the vital signs, and assess the neurologic state rapidly and frequently.
  - Position the head at 30 degrees, and maintain midline position if an injury to the cervical spine exists or is suspected.
  - Maintain adequate intravascular volume and blood pressure.
  - Maintain adequate oxygenation.
- Further interventions should be attempted on the basis of the clinical situation.
- The pediatric section of the Society of Critical Care Medicine and the World Federation of Pediatric Intensive and Critical Care issued evidence-based guidelines for acute medical management of severe traumatic brain injury in infants, children and adolescents.
  - These guidelines were adapted from previously published guidelines for adult traumatic brain injury treatment.
  - Interventions to treat intracranial hypertension described here are based on these guidelines.

Monitoring ICP and removing cerebrospinal fluid

- Monitor ICP, especially in traumatic brain injury.
  - Maintaining normal ICP allows maintenance of cerebral perfusion pressure (CPP), oxygenation, and metabolic substrate delivery and prevents cerebral herniation.
  - ICP-targeted protocols and therapies have clearly improved outcomes.
  - Guidelines recommend treatment goals to keep ICP <20 mm Hg and maintain CPP > 40 mm Hg.
- Numerous invasive devices are available to assess ICP.
  - Intraventricular catheters allow CSF drainage, reducing ICP.
    - The disadvantage is higher risk of infection, seizures, and hemorrhage compared with other available devices.
  - Fiberoptic catheter tip pressure transducers or strain gauge devices (Camino catheter or Codman catheter) placed within the brain parenchyma provides effective, continuous monitoring of ICP with minimal morbidity.
  - Intraparenchymal catheters that measure brain tissue oxygenation (PbO$_2$) and oxygen delivery (DO$_2$) (Licox catheter) and microdialysis catheters that allow measurement of substrates, such as pyruvate and lactate, enable monitoring for brain ischemia and can be used in conjunction with ICP monitoring.
  - Jugular bulb indwelling catheters enable measurement

of cerebral venous oxygenation.

- Transcutaneous and transcranial near infrared spectroscopy are used to assess ICP and cerebral perfusion indirectly and noninvasively.

■ In severe traumatic brain injury, standard ICP and CPP monitoring often do not reflect true DO_2.

- Combination of ICP and PbO_2 monitoring (Licox) using PbO_2-directed critical care are associated with improved outcomes.
- High ICP correlates with decreased cerebral DO_2.
- Monitoring ICP and PbO_2 allows early recognition of low oxygen delivery states, enabling appropriate therapeutic interventions.

Hyperventilation

■ Cerebral blood flow is exquisitely sensitive to carbon dioxide levels.

■ Low carbon dioxide levels lead to cerebral vasoconstriction; elevated levels lead to dilation.

■ Early hyperventilation (HV) of the patient with increased ICP decreases cerebral blood volume and ICP.

- The most rapid, effective way to decrease ICP acutely
- This effect is transient; therefore, other methods must be used to maintain normal or near-normal ICP.

■ In general, carbon dioxide should be decreased to the low thirties (mm Hg).

- Further decreases can lead to a significant decrease in cerebral blood flow, producing ischemia and increasing ICP.

■ Failure to respond to HV is often a poor prognostic sign.

■ Evidence suggests that the alkalizing effect of HV—and therefore decreased ICP—can be minimized with IV buffers, such as tris hydroxymethyl aminomethane.

■ HV was recently called into question as possibly causing more harm than good.

- HV induces a more pronounced change in cerebral blood flow than in cerebral blood volume.
- This can lead to a reduction in oxygen pressure despite the beneficial effect on CPP and ICP.
- One study found that aggressive HV had worse outcomes for patients with early, severe head trauma than for those who were normocapnic.
- Although HV is the most rapid method to decrease ICP acutely, aggressive HV is not beneficial for long-term treatment.

■ For intracranial hypertension refractory to other maneuvers, recent guidelines suggest considering:

- Aggressive HV (carbon dioxide pressure <30 mm Hg) for short periods
- Mild HV (carbon dioxide pressure 30–35 mm Hg)

■ For longer periods, HV should be used judiciously with cerebral oxygenation monitoring if possible.

Osmotic agents and diuretics

■ Intravenous osmotic agents (mannitol and glycerol) do not permeate the blood-brain barrier.

■ Mannitol and glycerol are probably equally effective and may be complementary because of their different properties.

■ They draw fluid from the intracellular brain compartment to the vascular space, reducing ICP and allowing increased cerebral perfusion.

■ Traditionally, mannitol is favored over glycerol.

- One study found that although mannitol decreased ICP, it did not improve cerebral oxygen pressure.
- Mannitol is given rapidly in an initial IV bolus of 0.5–1 g/kg.
- After administration, additional boluses 0.25–0.5 g/kg should be given every 2–5 hours, depending on the patient's status.
- Response to IV mannitol is rapid and usually occurs within 10–20 minutes.
- Serum osmolarity should be maintained in the 295- to 320-mOsm/L range.
- Mannitol is excreted renally; thus, it cannot be given in renal failure because it can provoke potentially life-threatening pulmonary edema.

■ Glycerol acts in a similar fashion but is used less often.

- Glycerol has the advantage of being a physiologic agent with caloric value, which is beneficial for nutritional support.
- Because glycerol has less diuretic effect and is not dependent solely on renal function, it can be given to patients with renal insufficiency.
- The main side effect is intravascular hemolysis, which can be prevented by giving a low concentration (<20%) at a slow infusion rate (>1 hour).
- Glycerol is most effective via enteroduodenal administration.
- Direct oral intake or gastric tube administration is less effective.
- Glycerol is usually given as a continuous drip.

■ Loop diuretics, such asfurosemide

- Reduce ICP by provoking a diuresis of water and electrolytes, establishing a gradient between the intravascular compartment and the brain
- Diuretics must be used cautiously in patients with traumatic brain injury and subarachnoid hemorrhage.
  - Volume depletion can worsen outcome.
  - Diuretics are frequently used in combination with osmotic diuretics but are infrequently used alone.
  - Care must be taken when using any of the aforementioned agents to maintain intravascular volume and adequate blood pressure.
  - Electrolytes must be monitored carefully.

Hypertonic saline

■ A more recent treatment for increased ICP is IV administration of 3–23.4% hypertonic saline.

■ IV boluses can reduce ICP and augment CPP for several hours.

- Creates an osmotic gradient and draws water from the intracellular and extracellular spaces into the intravascular compartment

■ Hypertonic saline can be given quickly and requires lower fluid volumes than osmotic agents.

■ No immediate concern exists for volume depletion, as can occur with mannitol.

■ Potential side effects

- Hyperosmolar central pontine myelosis
- Congestive heart failure
- Subdural hematomas
- Coagulopathy (rarely)

■ The trauma guidelines recommend:

- Continuous infusion of 3% saline between 0.1 and 1.0 mL/kg/hour
- Administration on a sliding scale, with the minimal dose needed to maintain ICP under 20 mm Hg

■ Serum osmolarity should be maintained below 360 mOsm/L when using hypertonic saline as the only hyperosmolar therapy, to control brain edema.

Neuromuscular blockade

■ Pancuronium and vecuronium can effectively decrease ICP by preventing maneuvers that increase intrathoracic pressure, such as coughing, straining, or bucking the ventilator.

■ These agents do not provide analgesia or sedation; they should be used in conjunction with analgesic agents and short-acting sedatives.

Temperature control

■ Hyperthermia leads to greater cerebral metabolism; measures should be taken to prevent body temperature elevation.

■ Includes judicious use of:

- Antipyretics
- Cooling blankets
- Antibiotics if infection is suspected

■ Hypothermia decreases cerebral metabolism and may be advantageous in managing increased ICP.

- Shivering should be prevented and efforts made to maintain full cardiorespiratory function.

■ Body temperature should be maintained between 96.8°F and 98.6°F (36°C and 37°C).

Seizure control

■ Seizure activity (clinical or subclinical) places excessive metabolic demand on already compromised brain tissue.

■ Treatment with antiepileptic drugs is necessary for any patient having or suspected of having seizures, especially if neuromuscular blocking agents are to be used.

- To treat acute seizures
  - Diazepam (0.1 mg/kg/dose IV)
  - Lorazepam (0.05–0.1 mg/kg/dose IV)
- For more prolonged therapy

■ If possible, the cause of seizure activity (eg, fever, drug toxicity, hypoglycemia, electrolyte abnormalities) should be identified and treated.

Corticosteroids

■ Corticosteroids remain controversial in managing acutely elevated ICP associated with:

- Head trauma
- Intracerebral hemorrhage
- Ischemic stroke

■ Several controlled studies involving glucocorticoids in head injury did not find any change in outcome or benefit for controlling increased ICP.

- Thus steroids are rarely used to treat increased ICP in patients with head injury.

■ Steroids do have clear utility in managing edema associated with:

- Brain tumors
- Refractory pseudotumor cerebri

■ Mechanism of action is unknown, but hypotheses include stabilizing the blood-brain barrier, enhancing brain energy supplies, decreasing tumor growth, reducing CSF production, and stabilizing cellular membranes.

■ Dexamethasone is generally used.

Glycemic control

■ Hyperglycemia after head injury is associated with a poorer outcome than that for patients who are normoglycemic.

■ Many centers now remove glucose from IV fluids and aggressively treat hyperglycemia.

High-dose barbiturates

■ Treating refractory increased ICP with high doses of barbiturates can sometimes be effective.

■ These agents decrease cerebral blood flow and metabolism.

■ Pentobarbital is given for prolonged therapy.

- IV loading dose of 3–10 mg/kg is given, followed by a maintenance infusion of 1–2 mg/kg/hour.
- Dose should be titrated according to the electroencephalogram, with a goal of obtaining a burst-suppression pattern.
- Therapy should be maintained for ≥24 hours and then tapered.
- Side effects are frequent and include myocardial suppression and hypotension, often requiring pressors.

Images

FIGURE 1. Closed comedones (whiteheads) appear as dome-shaped, flesh-colored papules that often are overlooked.

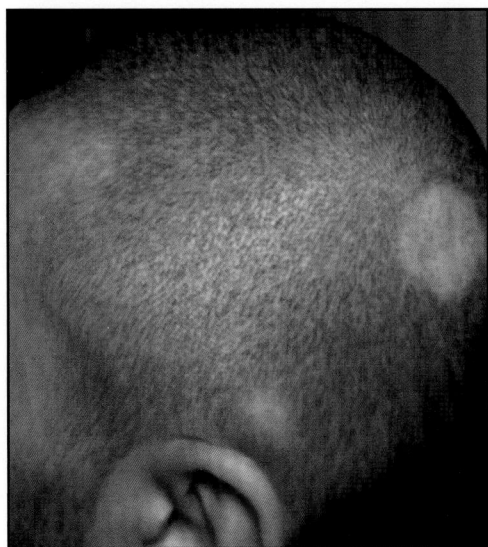

FIGURE 2. Flat warts.

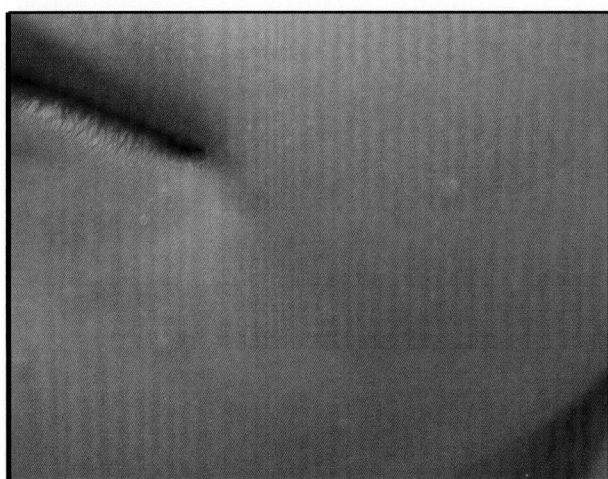

FIGURE 3. Rosacea. (Acne)

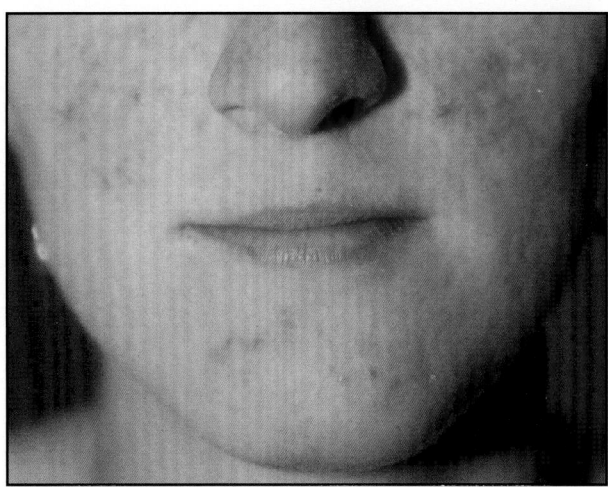

FIGURE 4. This 30-year-old man developed slow expanding hair loss on the scalp 1 month earlier. Although a potassium hydroxide preparation was supposedly positive, he did not improve on topical ciclopiron shampoo and oral itraconazole. At a subsequent visit a month later several new patches were also noted and the diagnosis was switched to alopecia areata. (Reprinted with permission from DermAtlas.org. Courtesy of Manoj Ram, MD.)

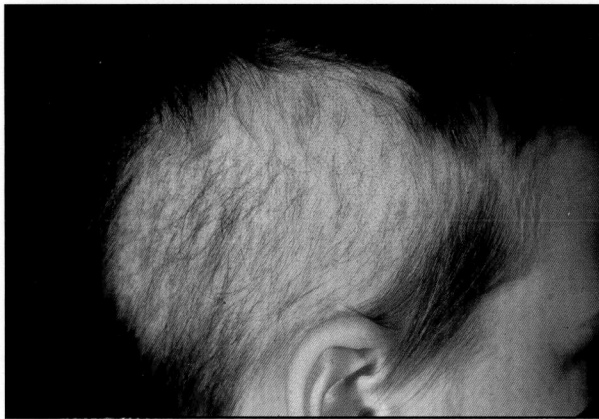

FIGURE 5. Trichotillomania in a 7-year-old boy. (Reprinted with permission. Copyright 2010, Interactive Medical Media, LLC)

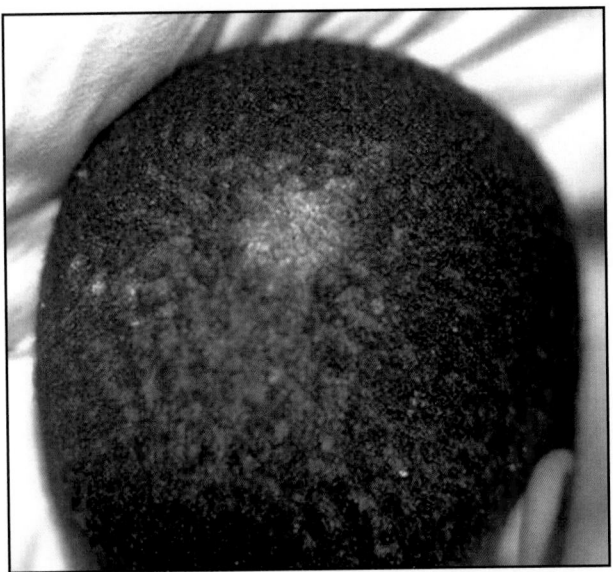

FIGURE 6. A young boy admitted for asthma therapy was incidentally noted to have a scalp lesion. The scaling and focal alopecia suggested the diagnosis of tinea capitis. The child was successfully treated with griseofulvin.

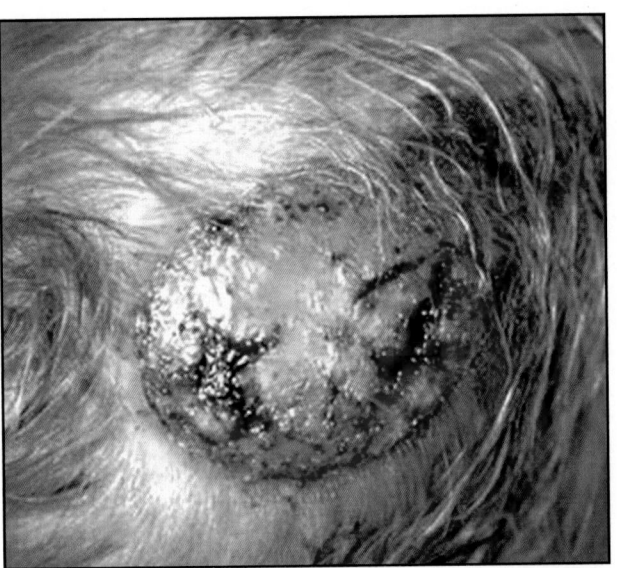

FIGURE 7. A 2½-year-old boy with a kerion secondary to chronic, progressive tinea capitis. (Courtesy of Martin Myers, MD.)

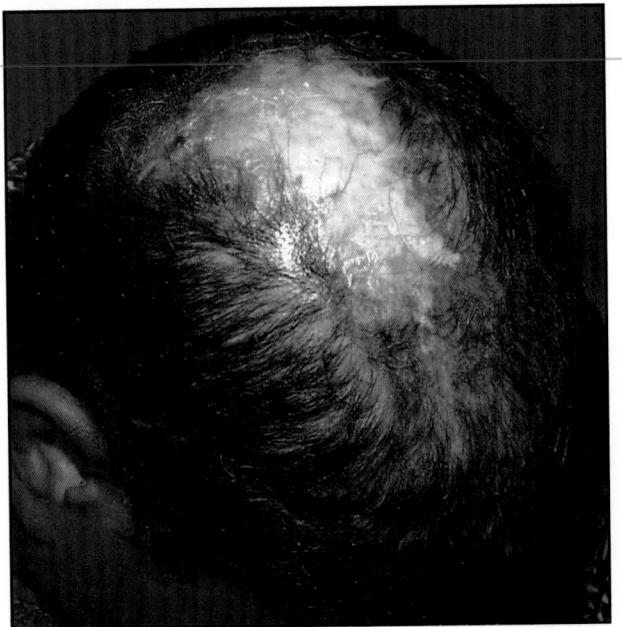

FIGURE 8. This 48-year-old woman had discoid lesions for over 10 years with lesions restricted to sun exposed sites. She had large areas of scarring alopecia. (Reprinted with permission from DermAtlas.org. Courtesy of Kosman Sadek Zikry, MD.)

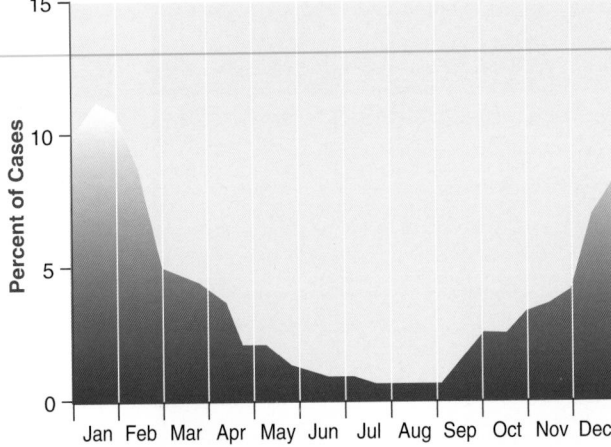

FIGURE 9. Seasonal occurrence of bronchiolitis cases obtained over a 20-year period from a community surveillance program in Monroe County, New York.

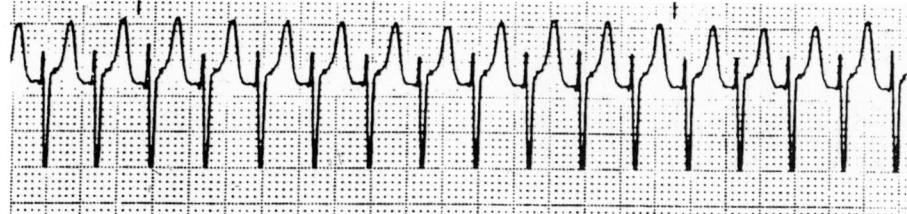

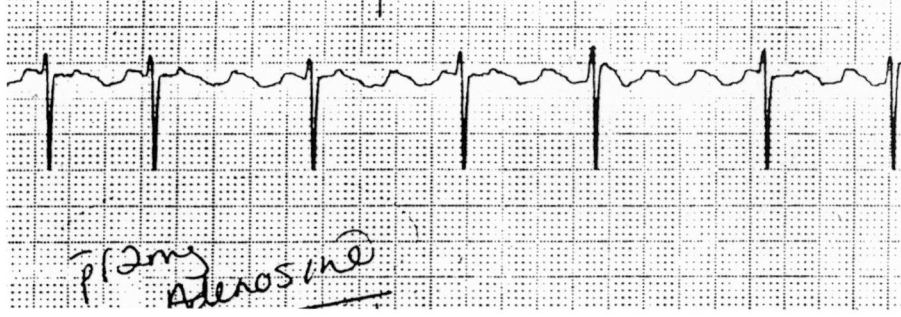

FIGURE 10. Atypical atrial flutter or intraatrial reentry tachycardia before and immediately after adenosine treatment in a 12-year-old boy after a Mustard repair of transposition of the great arteries in infancy. Adenosine produces high-grade AV block revealing but not converting the underlying atypical atrial flutter.

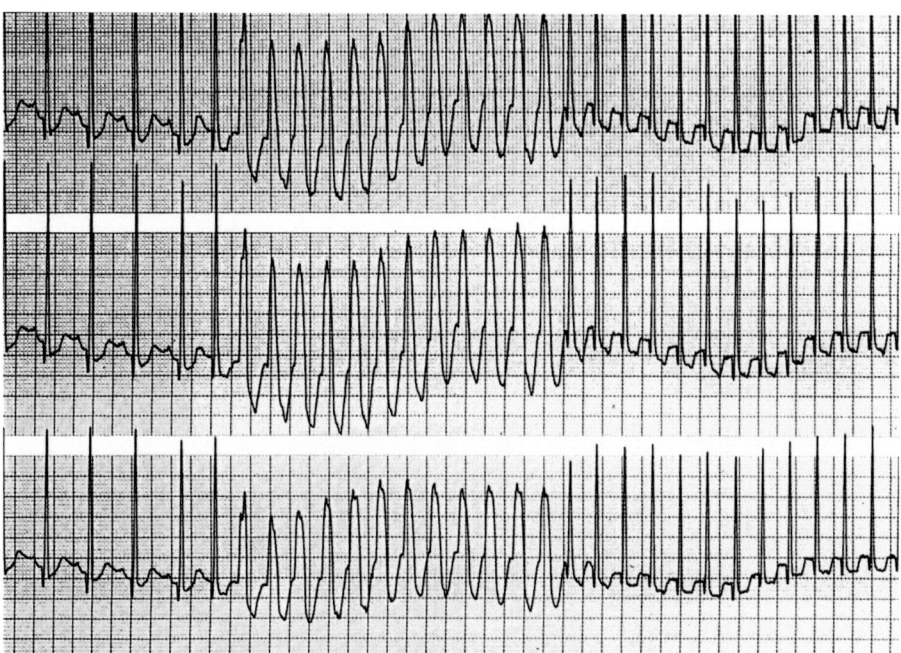

FIGURE 11. Transient aberrant conduction at the onset of SVT during an exercise test in a 14-year-old adolescent. The QRS duration then returns to normal.

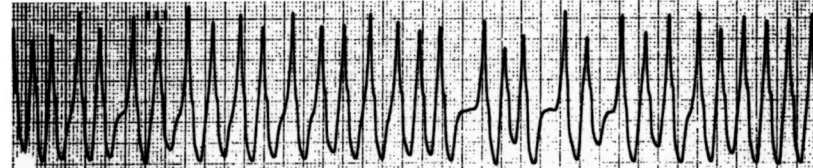

FIGURE 12. Antegrade conduction over an accessory pathway during atrial fibrillation in a 15-year-old boy with syncope. The short RR intervals represent rapid conduction over the accessory connection and a risk for ventricular fibrillation.

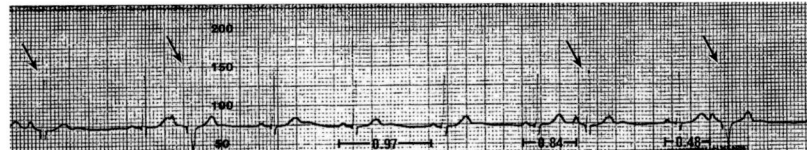

FIGURE 13. Atrial premature contractions (arrows) with normal and aberrated conduction.

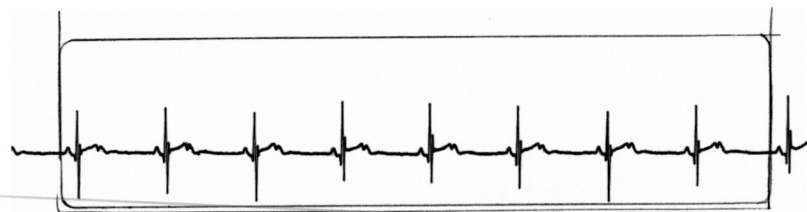

FIGURE 14. Every other beat is a blocked atrial premature contraction (blocked atrial bigeminy) represented by a consistent sharp deflection in the T waves.

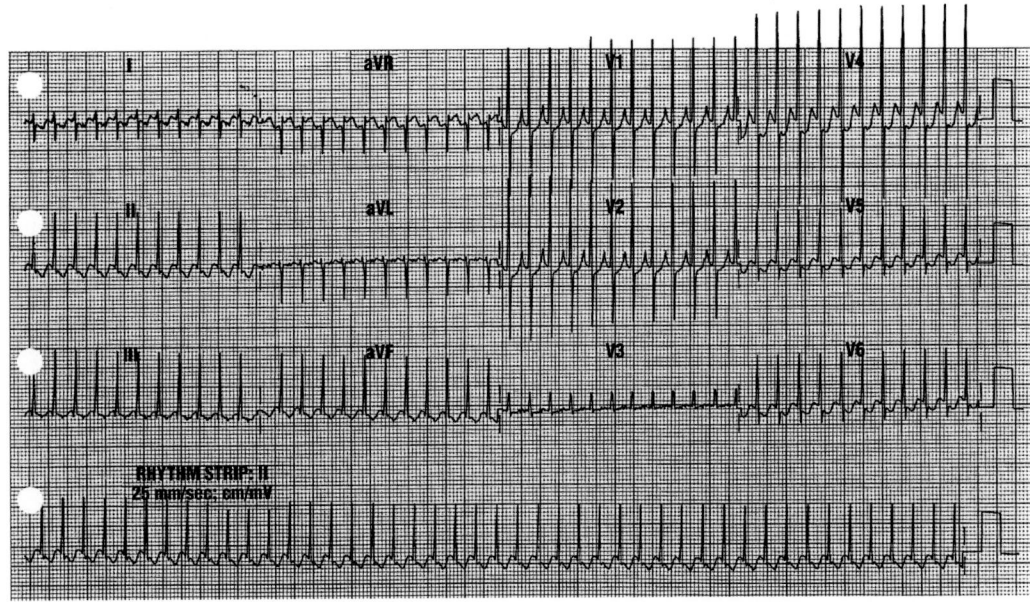

FIGURE 15. Twelve-lead ECG of SVT in a 2-week-old infant. Consistent sharp deflections in the T waves are present in lead III, indicating retrograde atrial activation via an accessory pathway. A repeat ECG after conversion to sinus rhythm did not reveal any preexcitation; therefore a concealed accessory pathway is present.

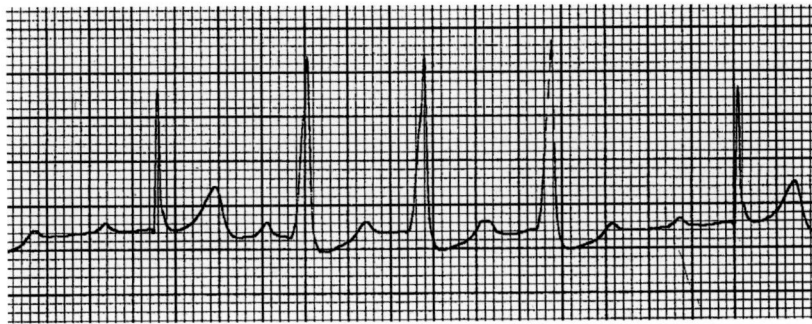

FIGURE 16. Accelerated ventricular rhythm with a ventricular rate of 110 bpm in a healthy 7-year-old girl. First-degree block is present in the sinus beats.

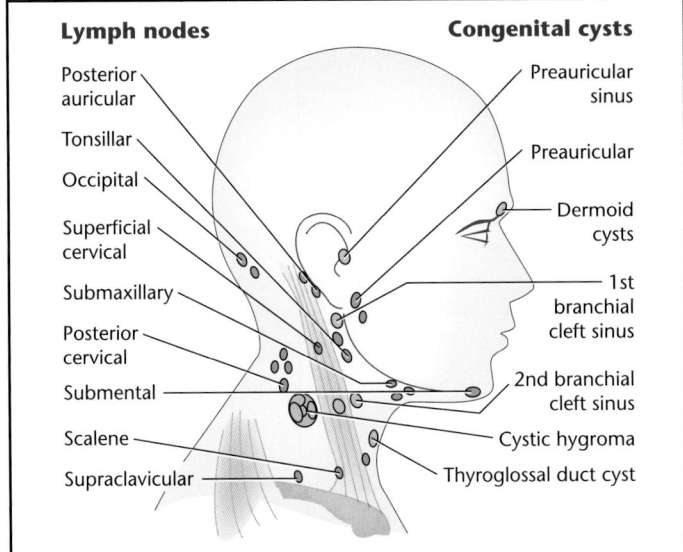

FIGURE 17. Common locations for cystic (orange circles) and lymph nodes (blue circles) of the face and neck.

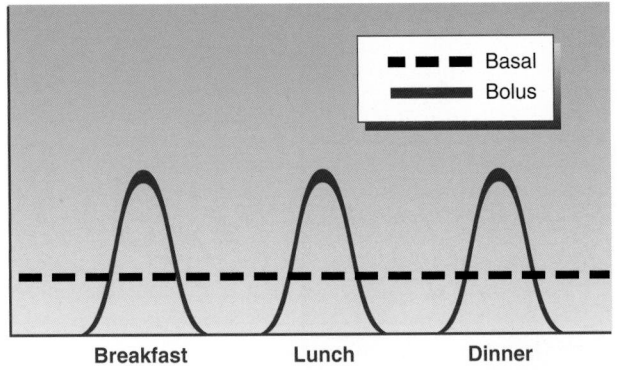

FIGURE 18. Bolus insulin is used to maintain blood glucose in the goal range after a meal. Basal insulin is used to maintain blood glucose in the goal range between meals and overnight.

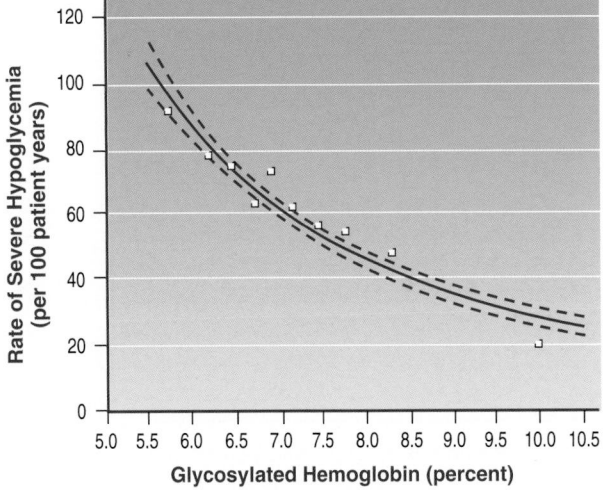

FIGURE 19. Increased risk of severe hypoglycemia with lower HbA1c. (Reproduced from the Diabetes Control and Complications Trial Research Group. The effect of intensive treatment of diabetes on the development and progression of long-term complications in insulin-dependent disbetes mellitus. *N Engl J Med*. 1993:329(14):977–986 Copyright © Massachusetts Medical Society. All rights reserved.)

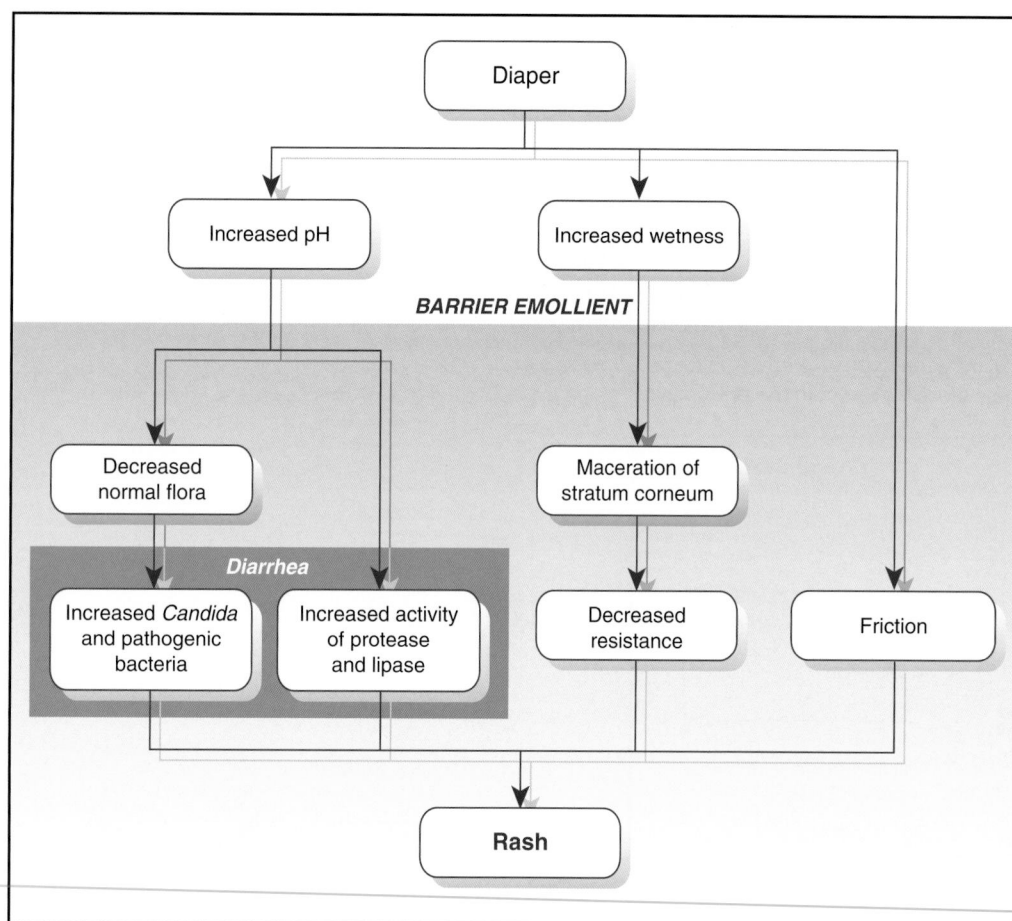

FIGURE 20. Pathogenesis of irritant diaper dermatitis, showing effects of diarrhea and barrier emollient.

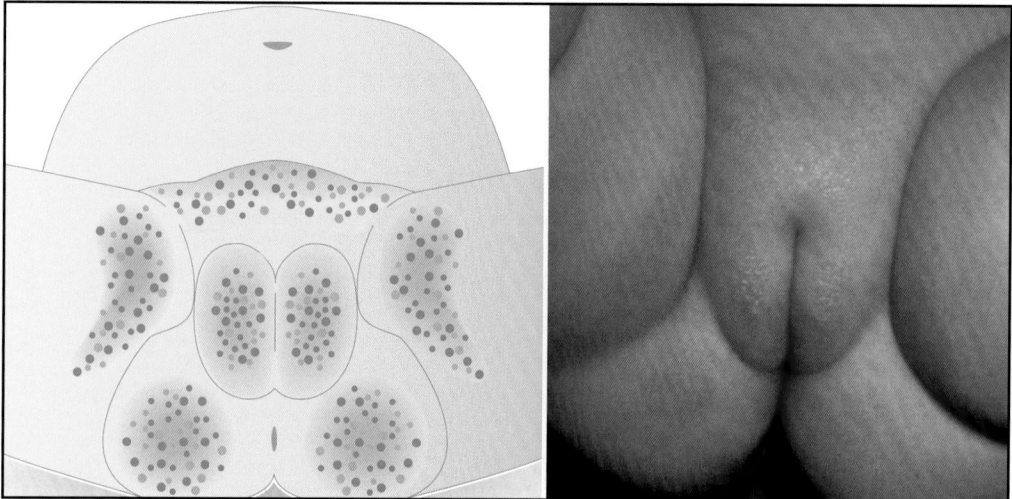

FIGURE 21. Erythematous desquamative pattern of diaper dermatitis.

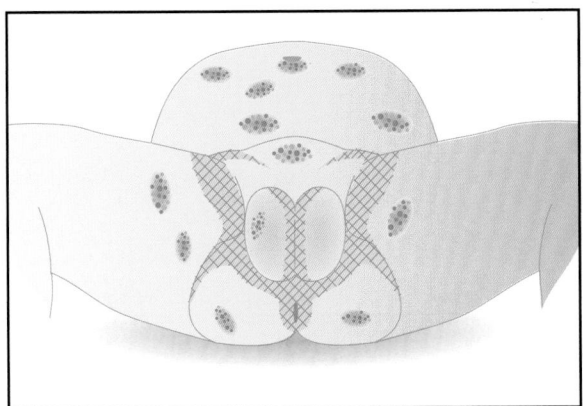

FIGURE 22. Intertriginous pattern of diaper dermatitis.

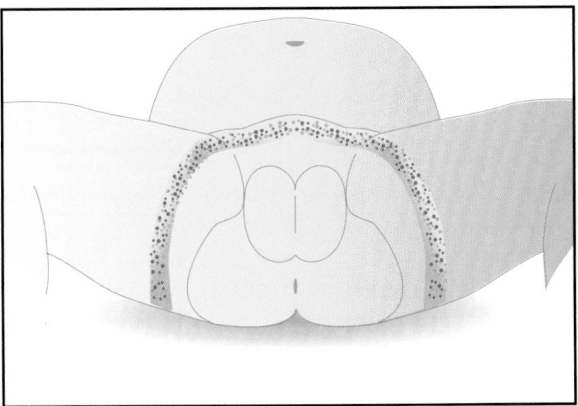

FIGURE 24. Constrictive pattern of diaper dermatitis.

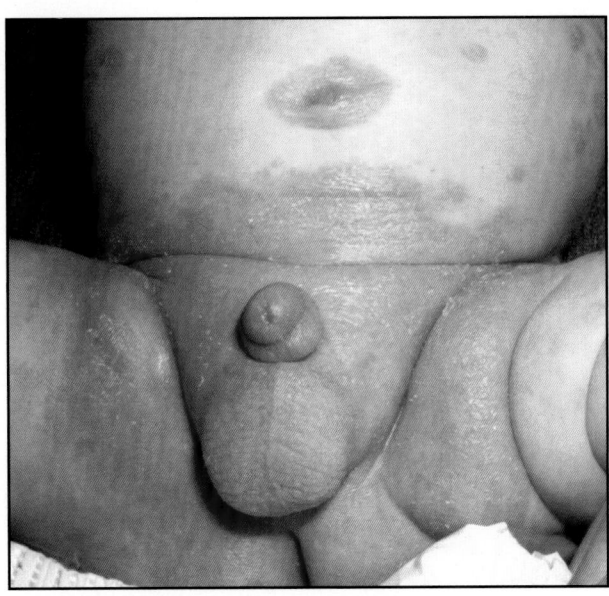

FIGURE 23. Seborrheic dermatitis is characterized by erythematous pattern of diaper dermatitis.

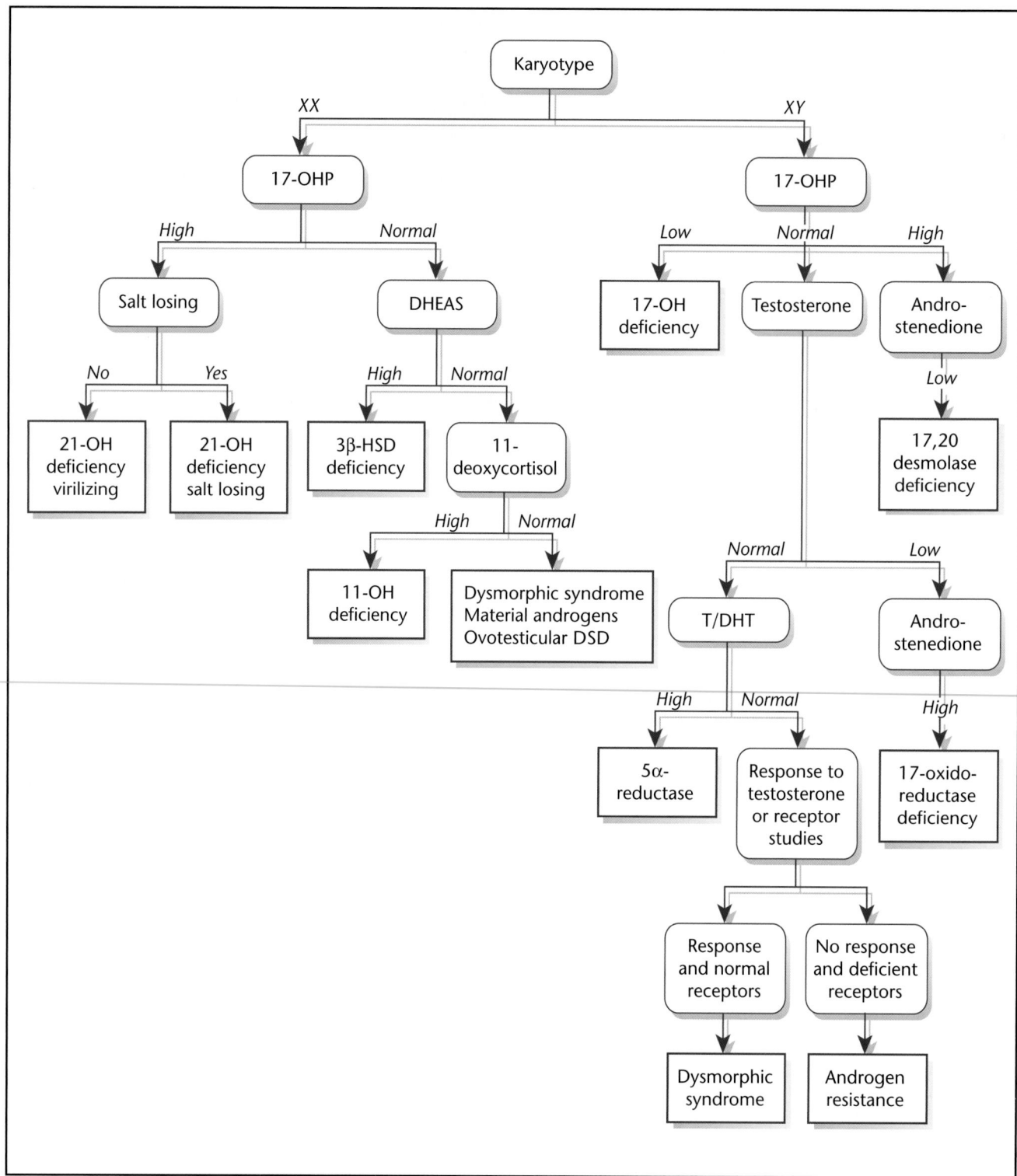

FIGURE 25. Diagnostic algorithm for a child with ambiguous genitalia without palpable gonads is presented for information only. This complex clinical situation requires the assistance of a pediatric endocrinologist for ultimate diagnosis. (Reprinted with permission from Styne D. *Pediatric Endocrinology*. Philadelphia, PA: Lippincott Williams & Wilkins; 2004.)

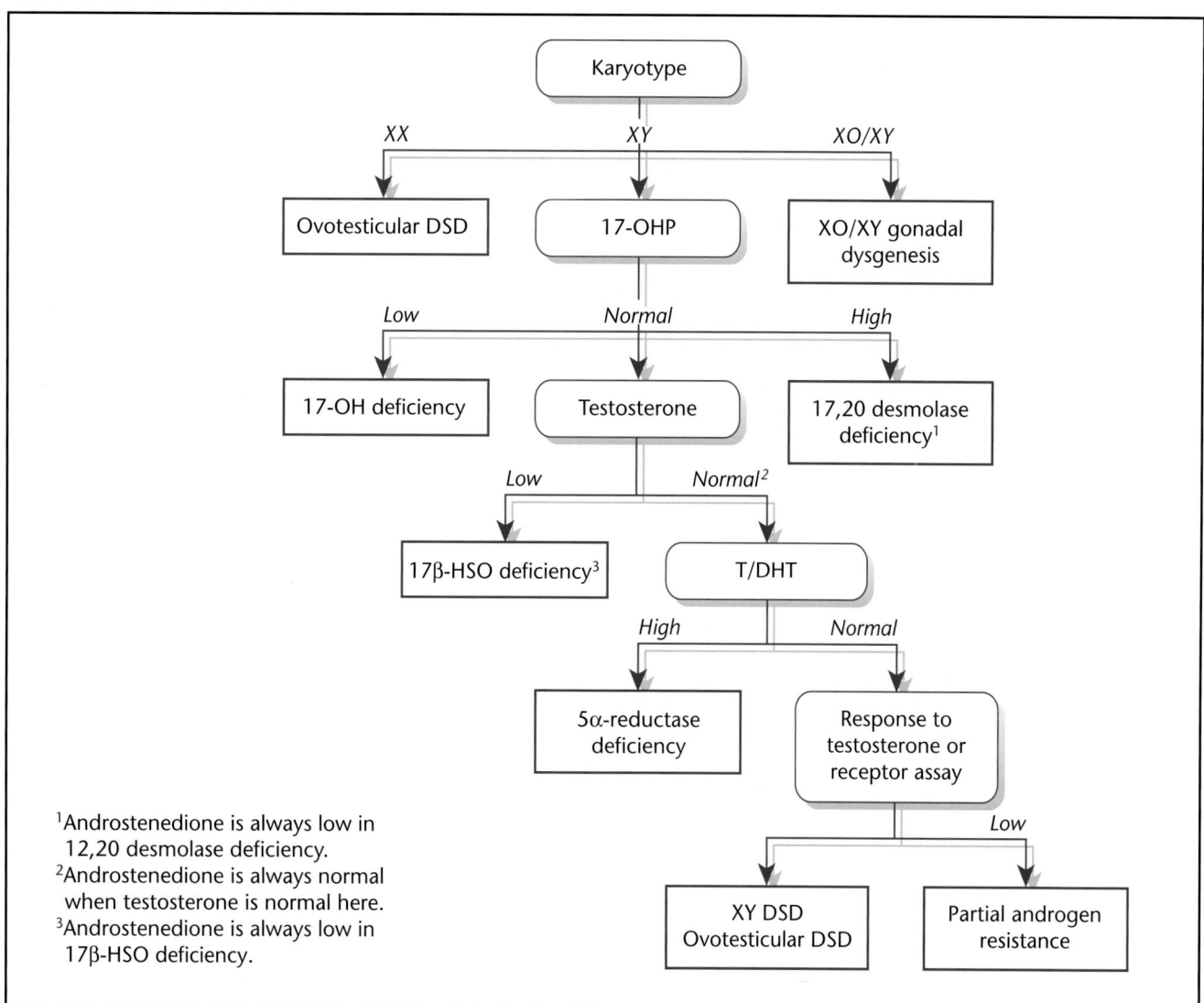

FIGURE 26. Diagnostic algorithm for a child with ambiguous genitalia with palpable gonads is presented for information only. This complex clinical situation requires the assistance of a pediatric endocrinologist for ultimate diagnosis. (Reprinted with permission from Styne D. *Pediatric Endocrinology*. Philadelphia, PA: Lippincott Williams & Wilkins; 2004.)

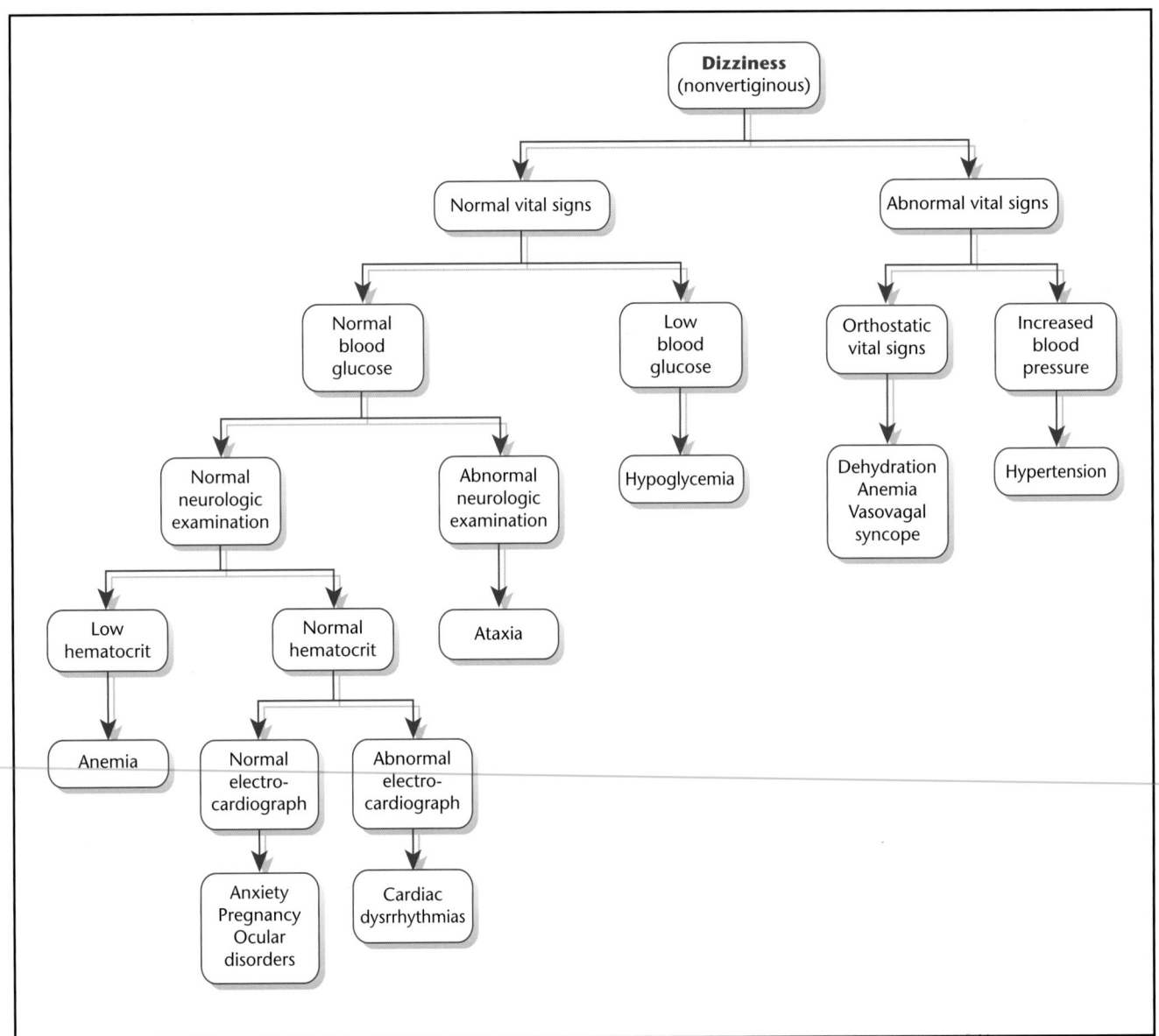

FIGURE 27. Algorithm for the differential diagnosis of dizziness.

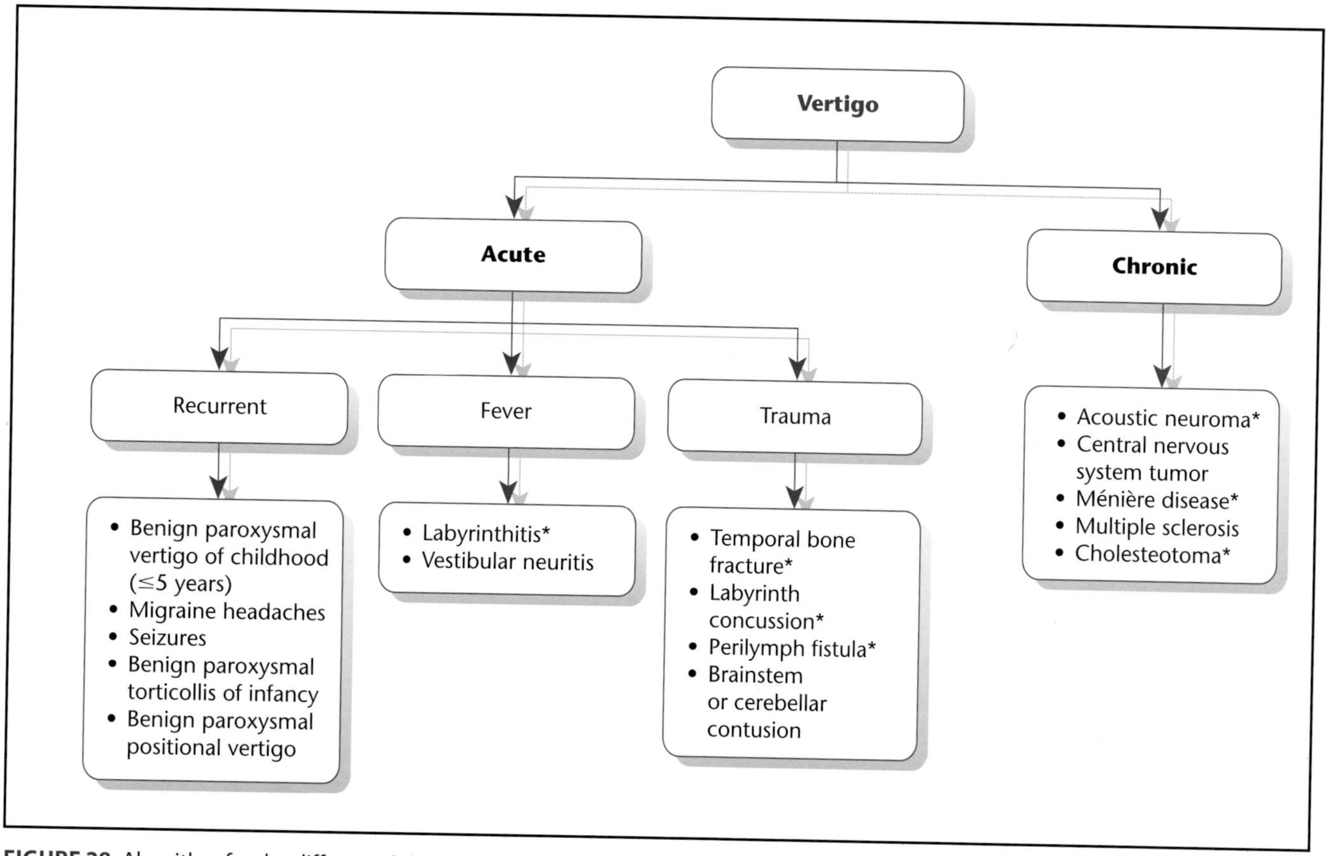

```
                              ┌─────────────┐
                              │   Vertigo   │
                              └─────────────┘
                    ┌─────────────┴─────────────────┐
            ┌─────────────┐                   ┌─────────────┐
            │    Acute    │                   │   Chronic   │
            └─────────────┘                   └─────────────┘
     ┌───────────┼───────────┐                       │
┌──────────┐ ┌──────────┐ ┌──────────┐
│ Recurrent│ │  Fever   │ │  Trauma  │
└──────────┘ └──────────┘ └──────────┘
```

Recurrent
- Benign paroxysmal vertigo of childhood (≤5 years)
- Migraine headaches
- Seizures
- Benign paroxysmal torticollis of infancy
- Benign paroxysmal positional vertigo

Fever
- Labyrinthitis*
- Vestibular neuritis

Trauma
- Temporal bone fracture*
- Labyrinth concussion*
- Perilymph fistula*
- Brainstem or cerebellar contusion

Chronic
- Acoustic neuroma*
- Central nervous system tumor
- Ménière disease*
- Multiple sclerosis
- Cholesteotoma*

FIGURE 28. Algorithm for the differential diagnosis of vertigo. Asterisk denotes an associated hearing loss.

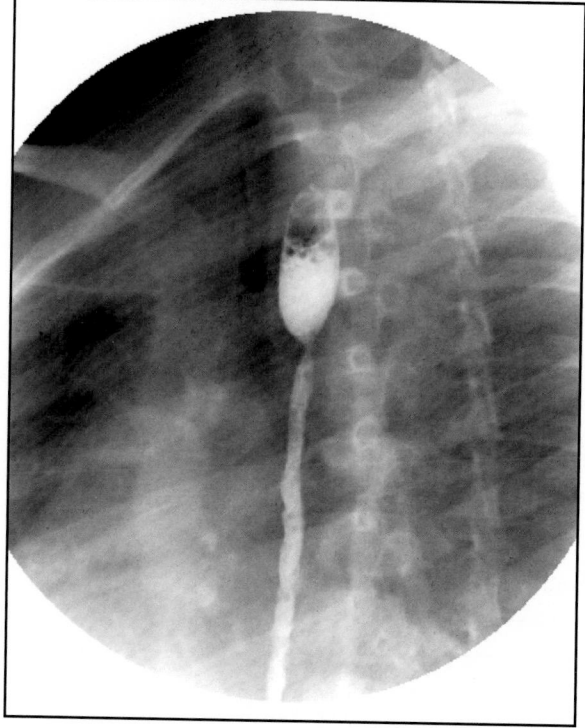

FIGURE 29. Esophagram demonstrating long-segment esophageal stricture after lye ingestion in a 2-year-old girl.

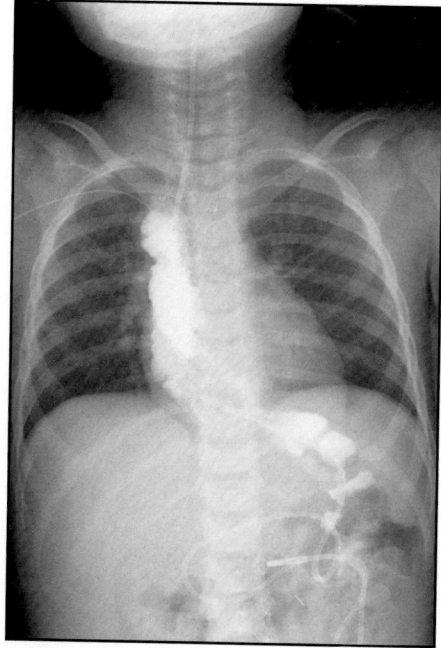

FIGURE 30. Colonic interposition in same child 6 months after injury.

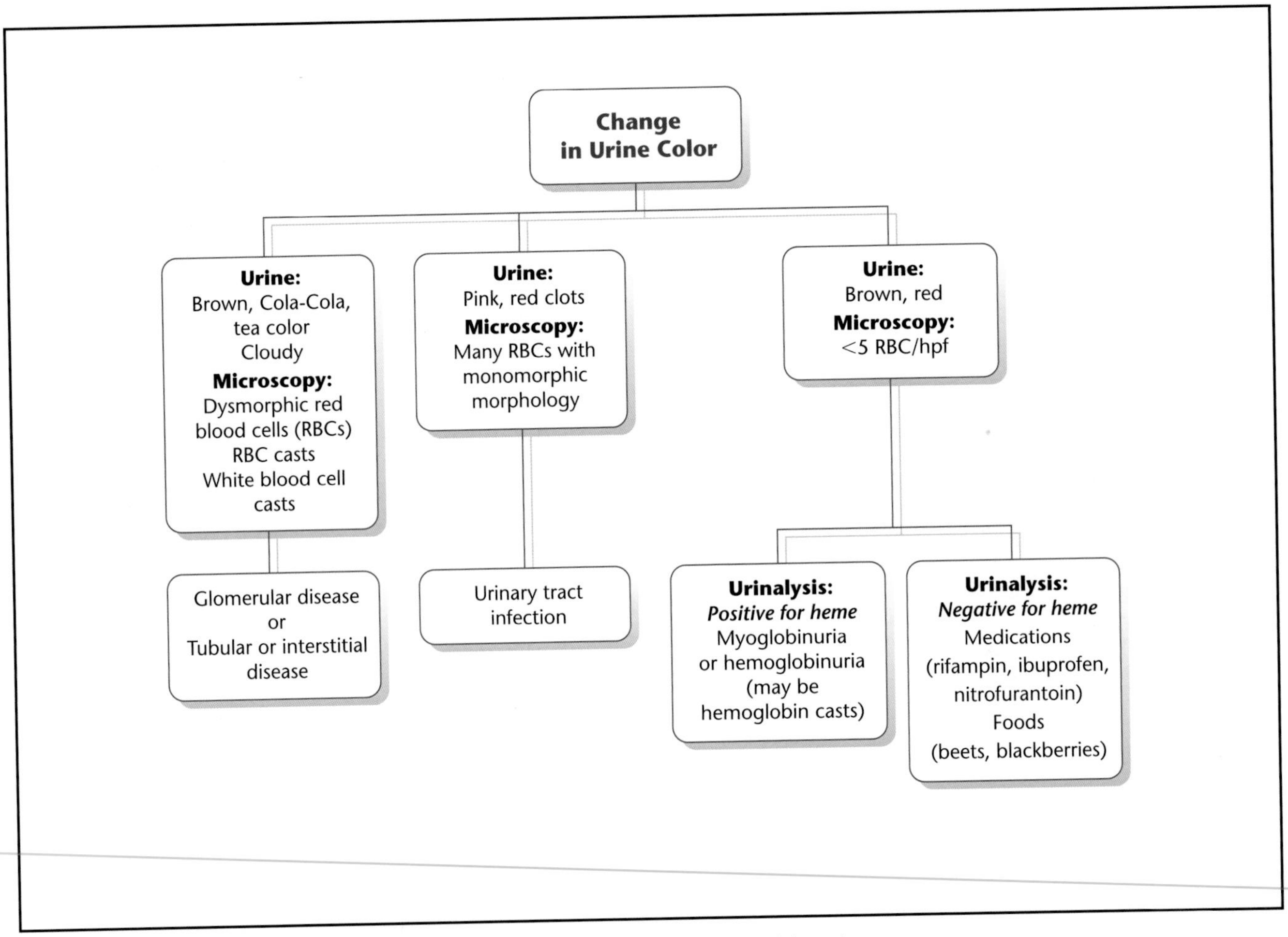

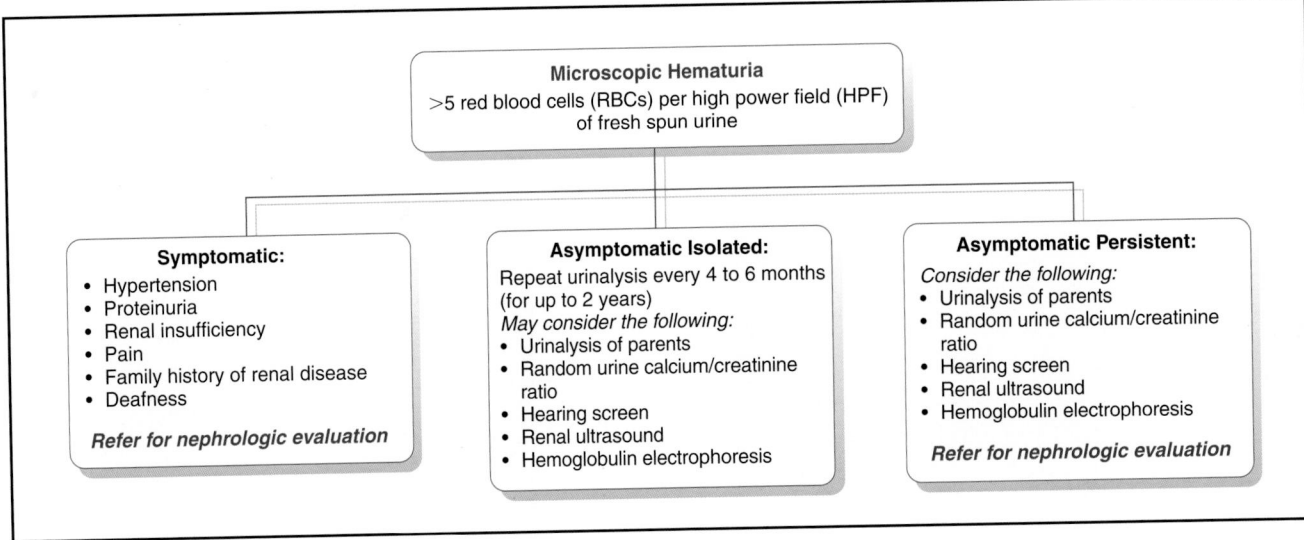

Change in Urine Color

Urine:
Brown, Cola-Cola, tea color
Cloudy
Microscopy:
Dysmorphic red blood cells (RBCs)
RBC casts
White blood cell casts

Urine:
Pink, red clots
Microscopy:
Many RBCs with monomorphic morphology

Urine:
Brown, red
Microscopy:
<5 RBC/hpf

Glomerular disease
or
Tubular or interstitial disease

Urinary tract infection

Urinalysis:
Positive for heme
Myoglobinuria or hemoglobinuria
(may be hemoglobin casts)

Urinalysis:
Negative for heme
Medications (rifampin, ibuprofen, nitrofurantoin)
Foods (beets, blackberries)

FIGURE 31. Evaluation for macroscopic hematuria begins with the examination of the urine.

Microscopic Hematuria
>5 red blood cells (RBCs) per high power field (HPF) of fresh spun urine

Symptomatic:
- Hypertension
- Proteinuria
- Renal insufficiency
- Pain
- Family history of renal disease
- Deafness

Refer for nephrologic evaluation

Asymptomatic Isolated:
Repeat urinalysis every 4 to 6 months (for up to 2 years)
May consider the following:
- Urinalysis of parents
- Random urine calcium/creatinine ratio
- Hearing screen
- Renal ultrasound
- Hemoglobulin electrophoresis

Asymptomatic Persistent:
Consider the following:
- Urinalysis of parents
- Random urine calcium/creatinine ratio
- Hearing screen
- Renal ultrasound
- Hemoglobulin electrophoresis

Refer for nephrologic evaluation

FIGURE 32. Evaluation of microscopic hematuria.

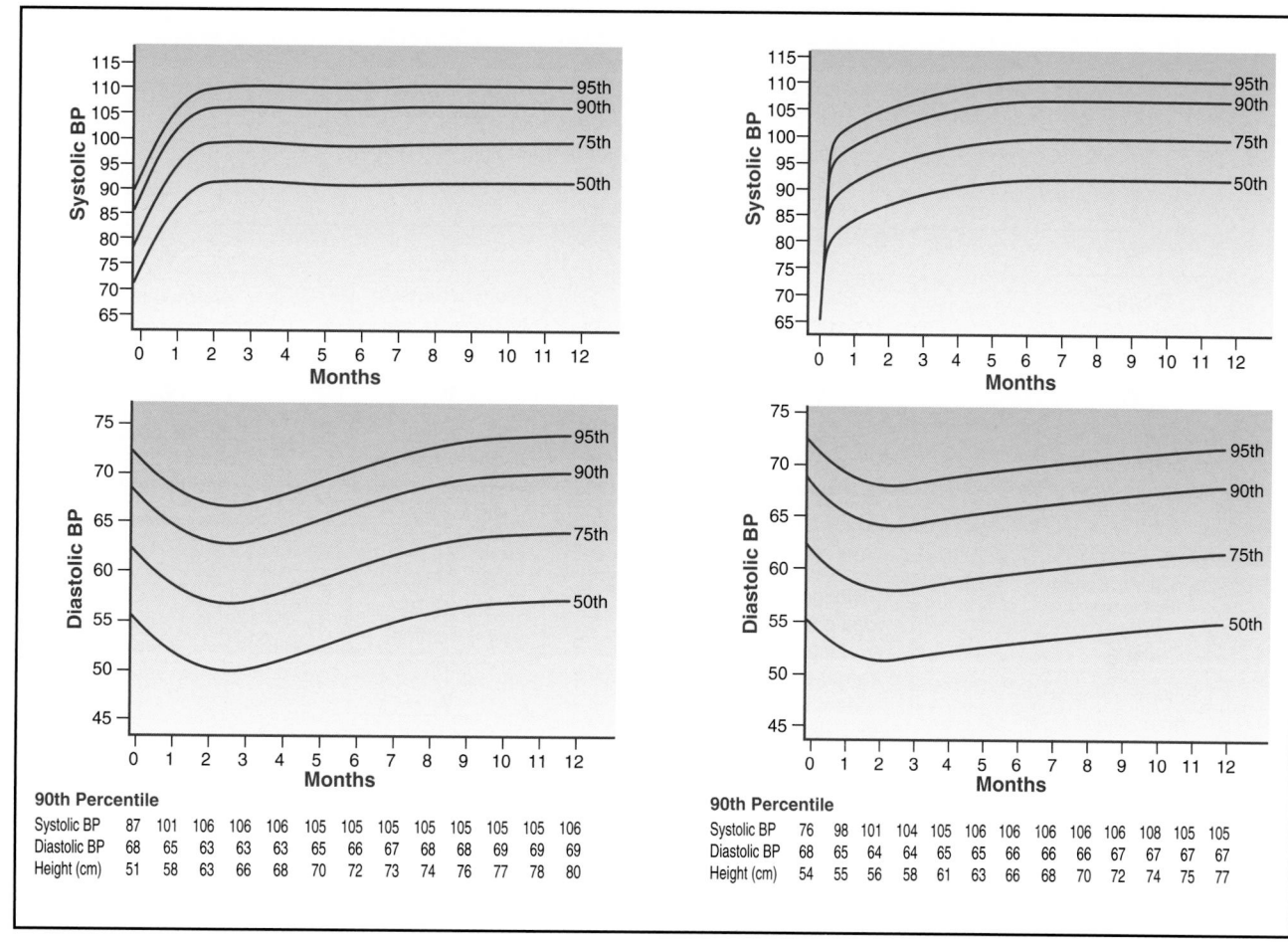

FIGURE 33. Age-, sex-, height-, and weight-specific percentiles of systolic and diastolic blood pressure in boys (left) and girls (right) from birth to 12 months of age. (National Heart, Lung, and Blood Institute. Report of the Second Task Force on Blood Pressure in Children–1987. *Pediatrics.* 1987;79:1–25.)

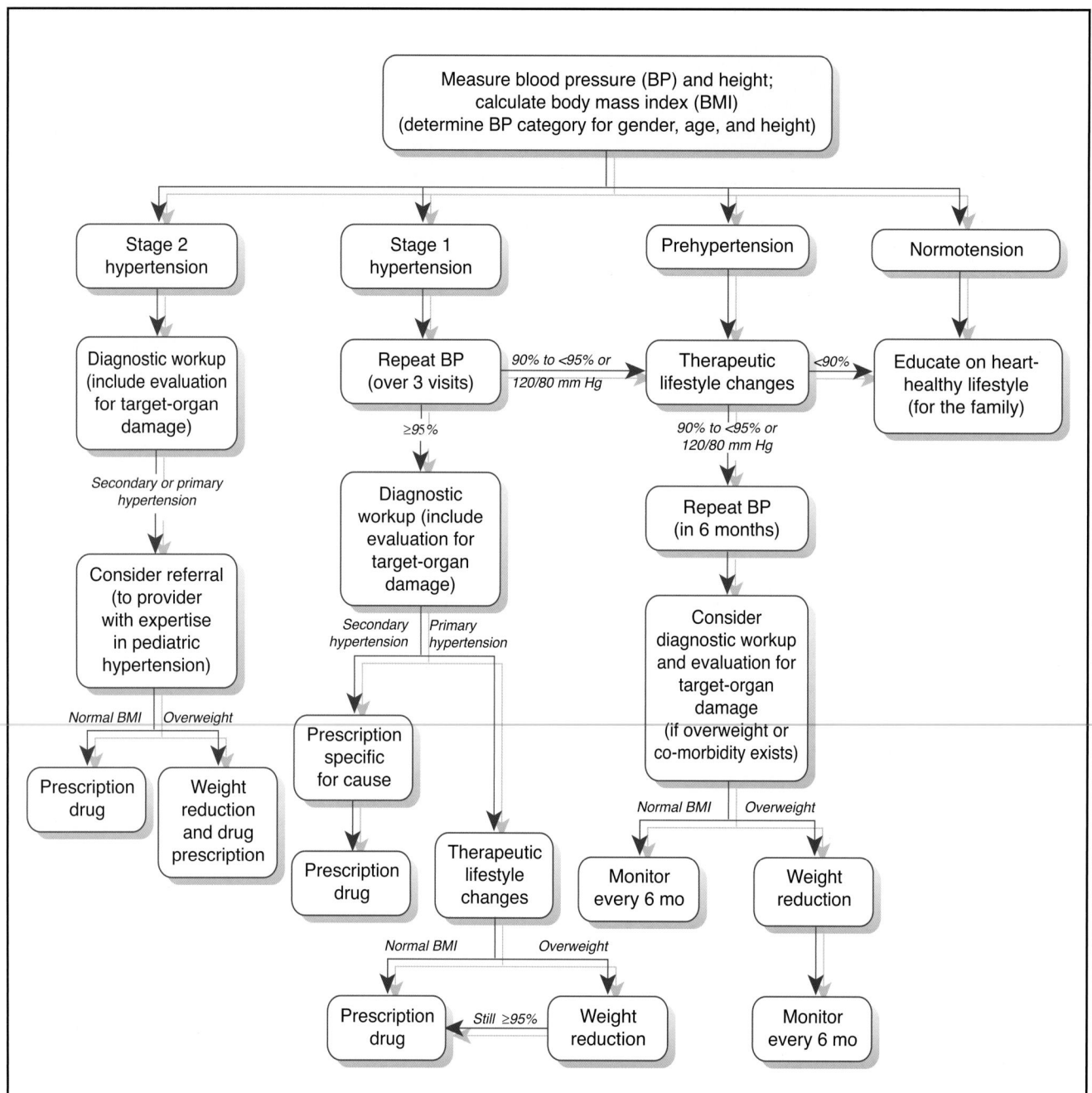

FIGURE 34. Algorithm for diagnosing high blood pressure in children. (Modified from National High Blood Pressure Education Program Working Group on High Blood Pressure in Children and Adolescents. The fourth report on the diagnosis, evaluation, and treatment of high blood pressure in children and adolescents. *Pediatrics*. 2004;114[2]:555–572.)

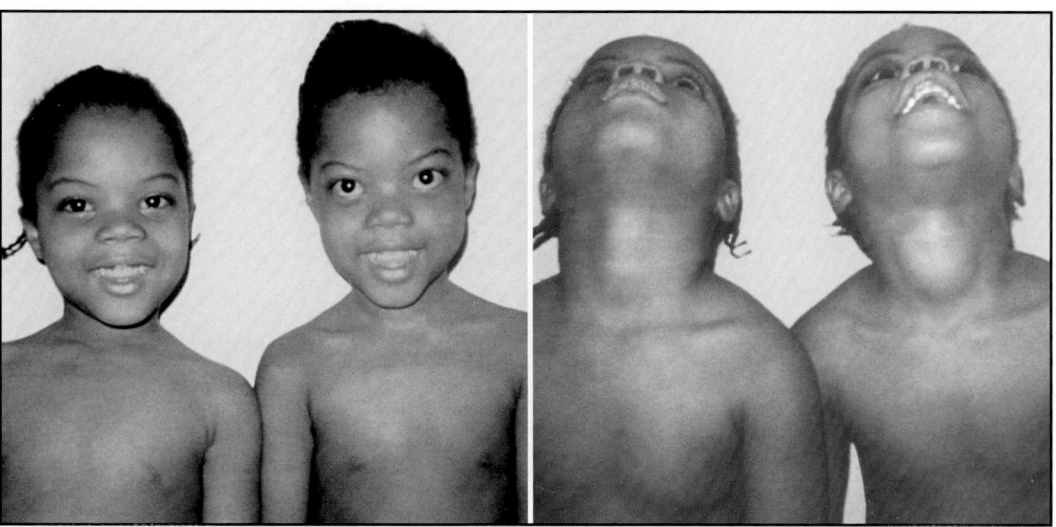

FIGURE 35. The patient on the right exhibits a widened palpebral fissure and goiter; her twin, on the left, was unaffected at the time of this photograph, although later she also developed Graves disease.

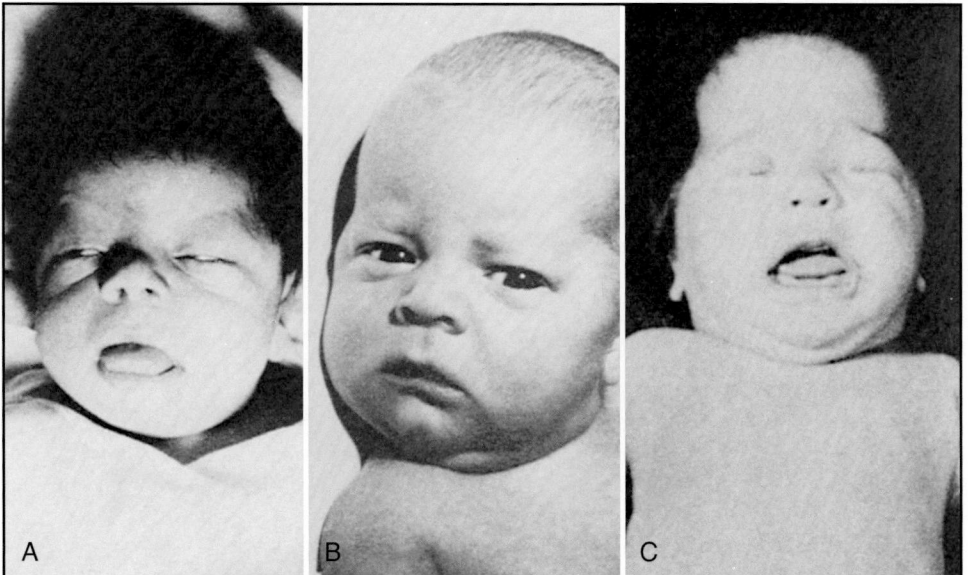

FIGURE 36. A. Normal infant referred at 8 months of age who had clinical signs but no clinical symptoms of congenital hypothyroidism. **B.** Infant with documented primary hypothyroidism at 4 weeks of age. Her clinical features at this age were minimal and included only mild periorbital edema, an enlarged posterior fontanelle, decreased stooling, and abdominal distention. **C.** Infant at age 6 months who has athyreosis and severe congenital hypothyroidism. (From Foley TP Jr. Sporadic congenital hypothyroidism. In: Dussault JH, Walker P, eds. *Congenital Hypothyroidism*. New York, NY: Marcel Dekker; 1983.)

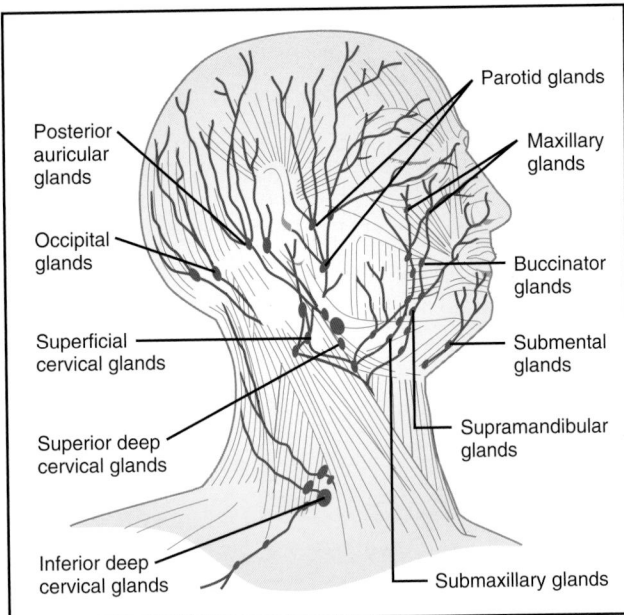

FIGURE 37. Lymph nodes and lymphatics of the head and neck. The nodes in the region below the mandible are designated submaxillary. (Reproduced from *Anatomy of the Human Body* by Henry Gray, 20th edition, with permission from Bartleby.com, Inc.)

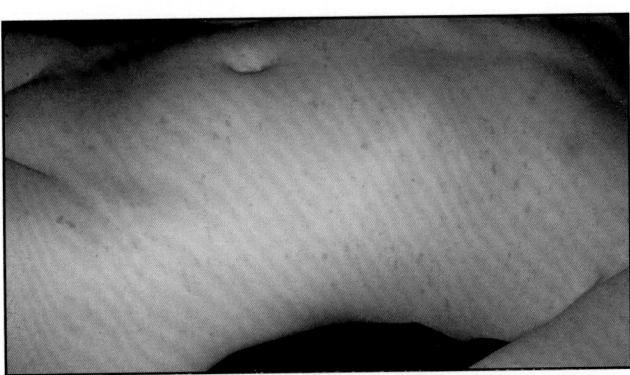

FIGURE 38. A 4-year-old white girl with acute meningococcemia without meningitis with a near uniform distribution of petechiae over the trunk and extremities.

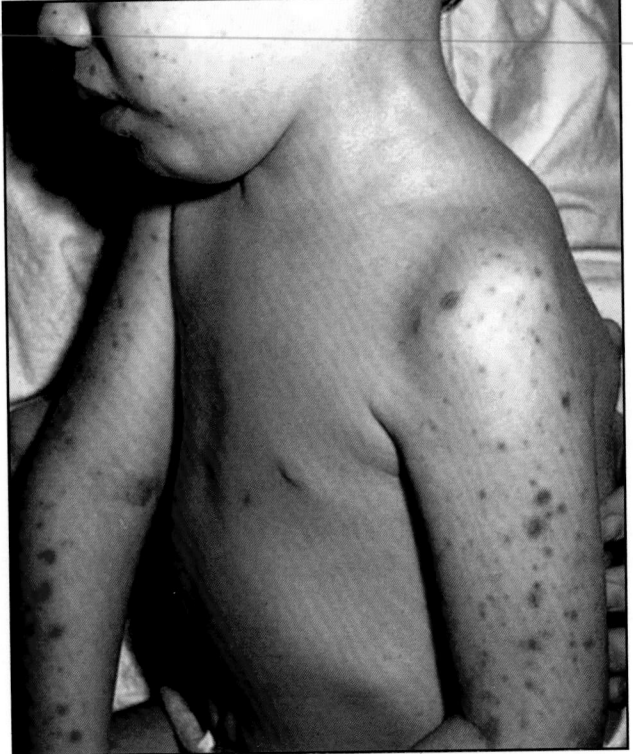

FIGURE 39. Meningococcemia showing striking involvement of the extremities with relative sparing of the skin of the child's body surface.

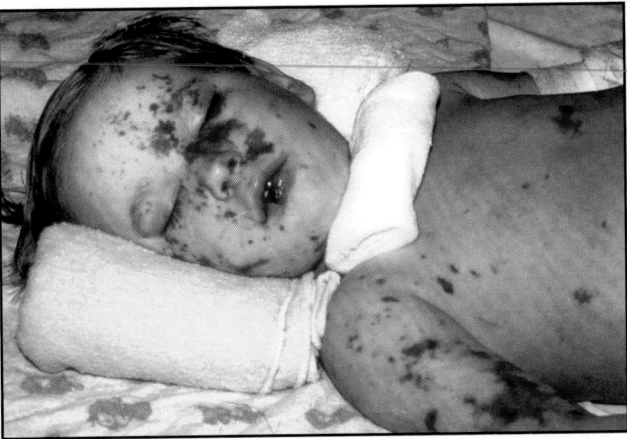

FIGURE 40. Ecchymotic or purpuric rash is the most significant manifestation of meningococcal disease, showing a centrifugal distribution present in the child with fulminant meningococcemia.

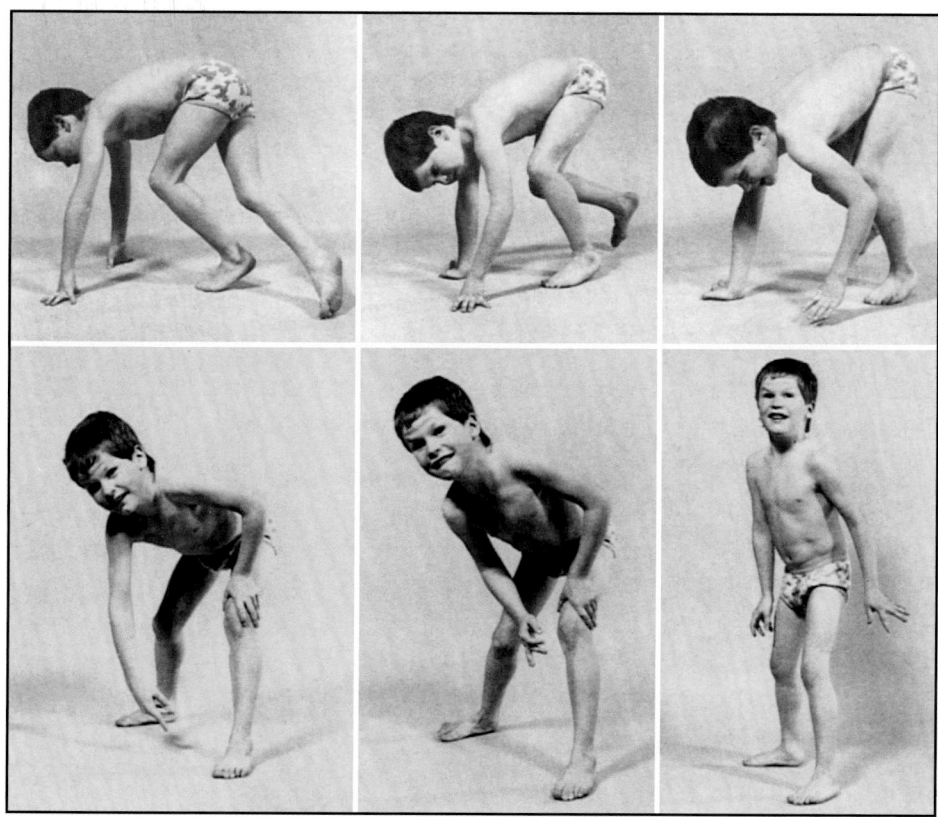

FIGURE 41. Boy who has Duchenne muscular dystrophy demonstrating the sequence of maneuvers that constitutes Gowers sign. The child pushes off the floor with all 4 extremities, then prepares to push up by moving the hands along the floor closer to the feet, and finally places the hands on the thighs and pushes up to the erect position. The maneuver is necessary because of the marked weakness of the hip extension. (Swaiman KF. *Pediatric Neurology: Principles and Practice*. 2nd ed. St Louis, MO: CV Mosby; 1994. Copyright © 1994, with permission.)

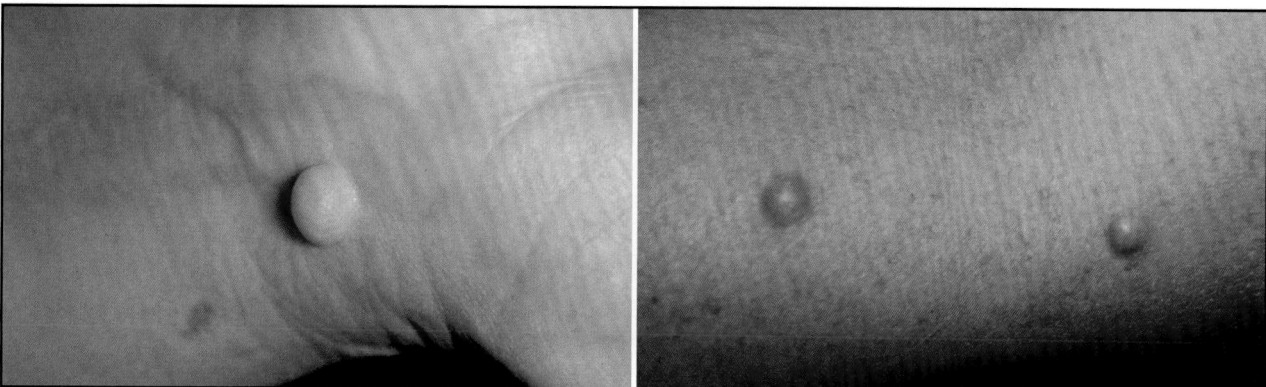

FIGURE 42. Cutaneous neurofibromas in neurofibromatosis type 1.

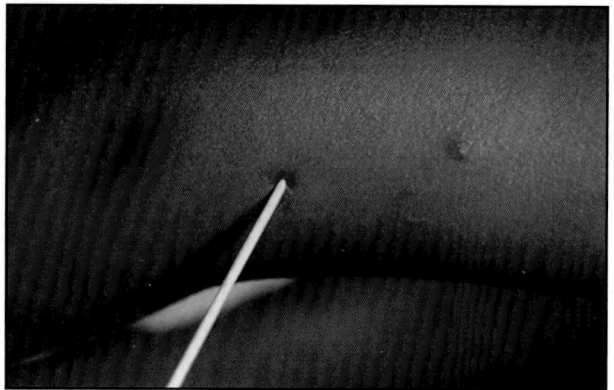

FIGURE 43. Neurofibroma dimpling through underlying dermis.

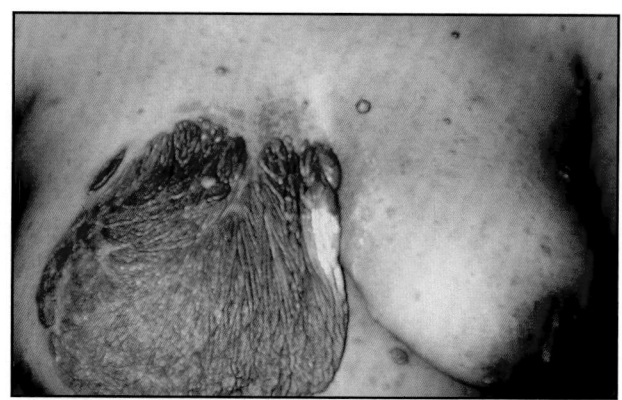

FIGURE 44. Plexiform neurofibroma on a breast.

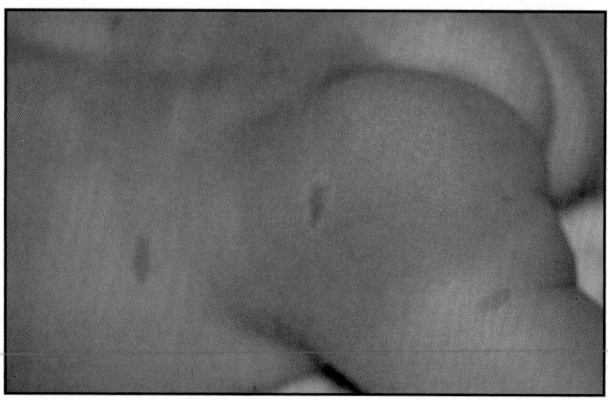

FIGURE 45. Multiple café-au-lait macules on an infant, with coincidental gray Mongolian spot.

FIGURE 46. Multiple schwannomas in neurofibromatosis type 2.

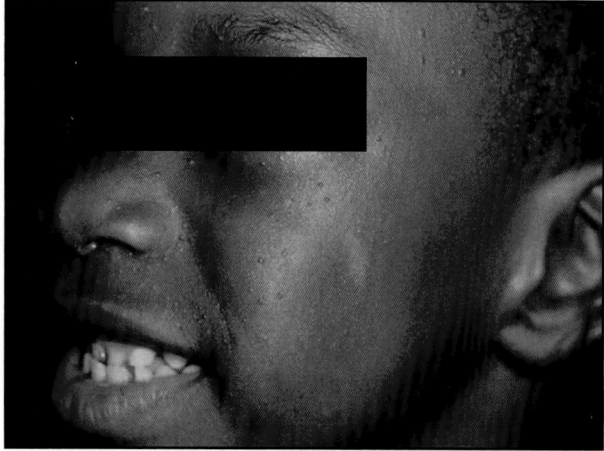

FIGURE 47. Facial angiofibromas and hypomelanotic macules in tuberous sclerosis complex.

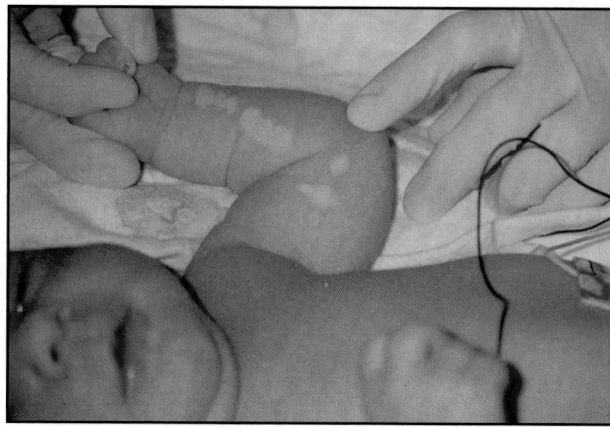

FIGURE 48. Shagreen patch on the arm of an infant with tuberous sclerosis complex.

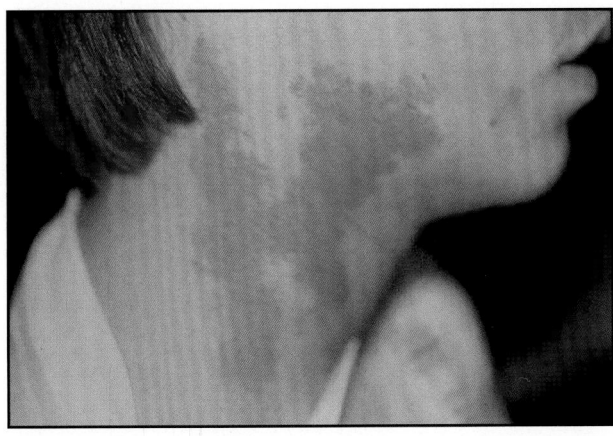

FIGURE 49. Port wine stain on the neck (not associated with Sturge-Weber syndrome).

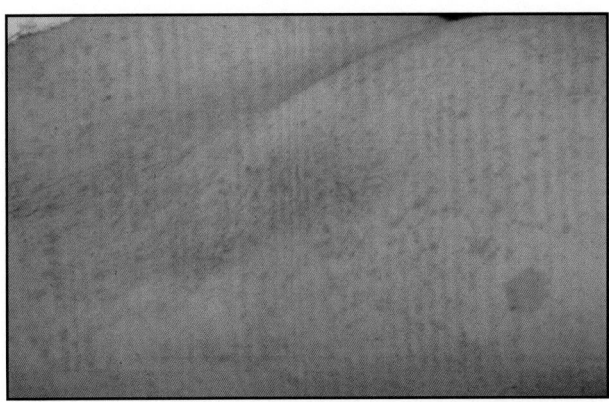

FIGURE 50. Axillary freckling in neurofibromatosis type 1.

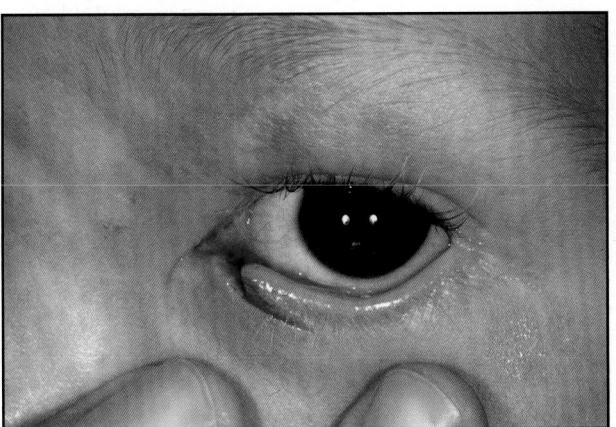

FIGURE 51. Full-thickness injury involving the lid margin and lower canaliculus. The laceration is medial to the lacrimal punctum.

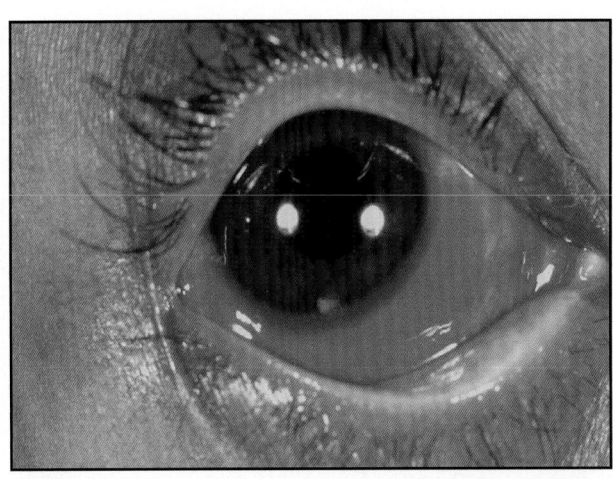

FIGURE 52. Subconjunctival hemorrhage after blunt injury.

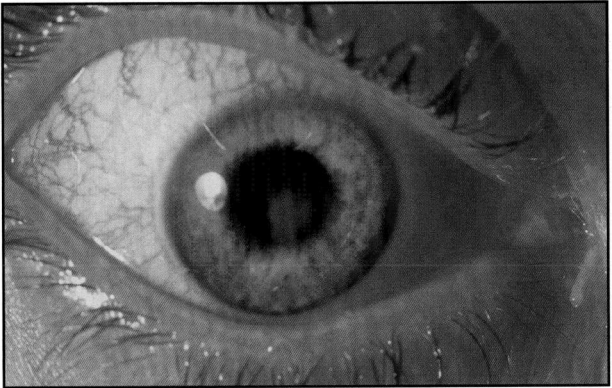

FIGURE 53. Central corneal abrasion is highlighted with fluorescein dye.

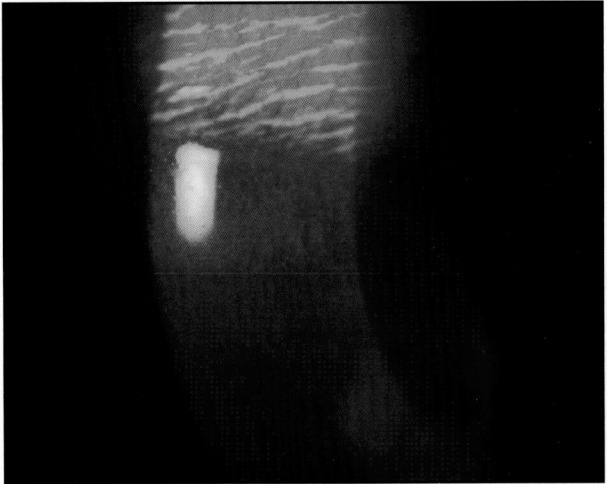

FIGURE 54. Fine, linear abrasions of the superior cornea are luminated with fluorescein dye and the use of a cobalt blue filter.

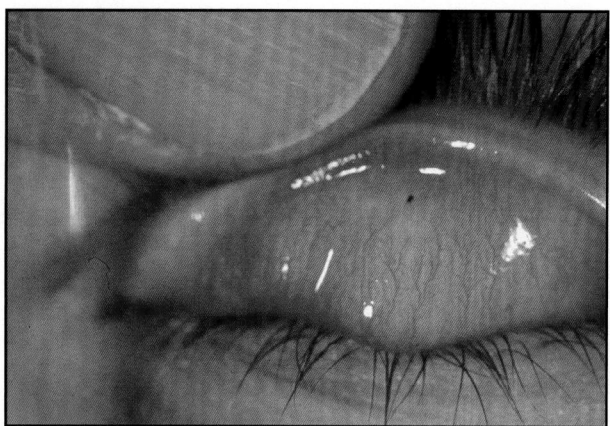

FIGURE 55. Eversion of the upper lid reveals a small particle resting in the superior tarsal conjunctiva.

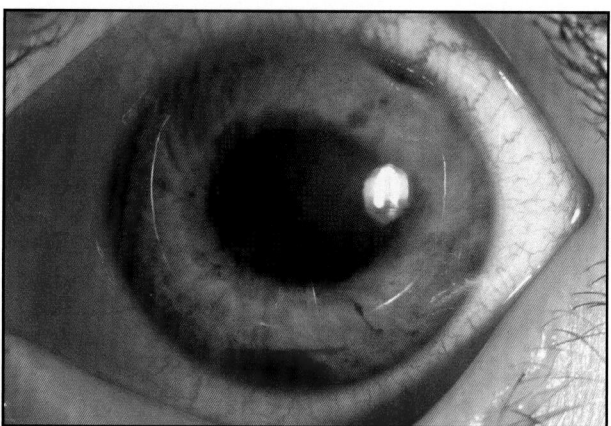

FIGURE 56. Small hyphema is associated with an iris root tear at the 2 o'clock position.

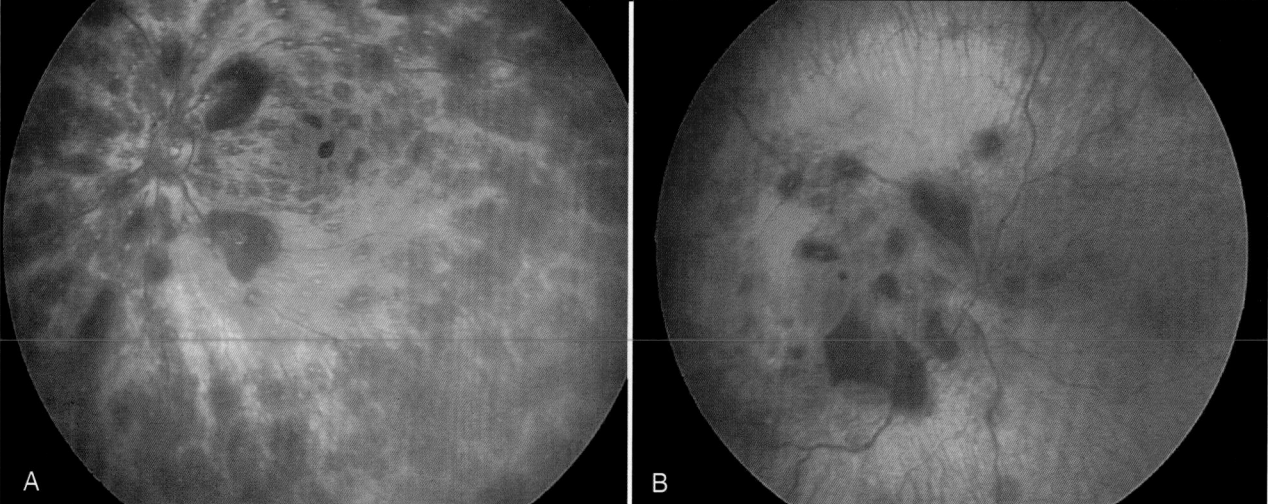

FIGURE 57. A. Severe retinal hemorrhages as the result of a shaking injury. **B.** Moderate retinal hemorrhages as a result of a shaking injury. Preretinal hemorrhages, which obscure the retinal vessels, and intraretinal hemorrhages, which are beneath the retinal vessels, are both visualized.

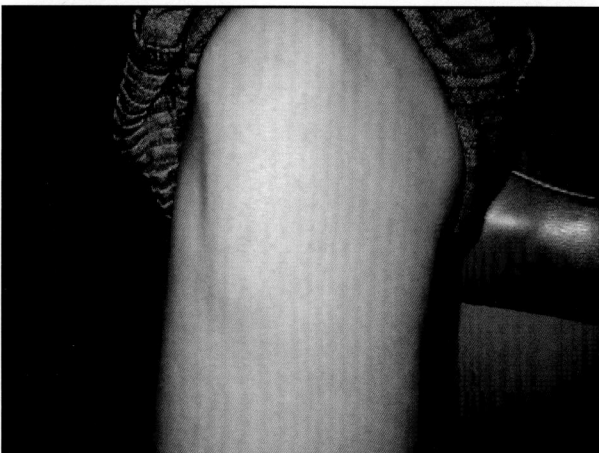

FIGURE 58. Osgood-Schlatter disease.

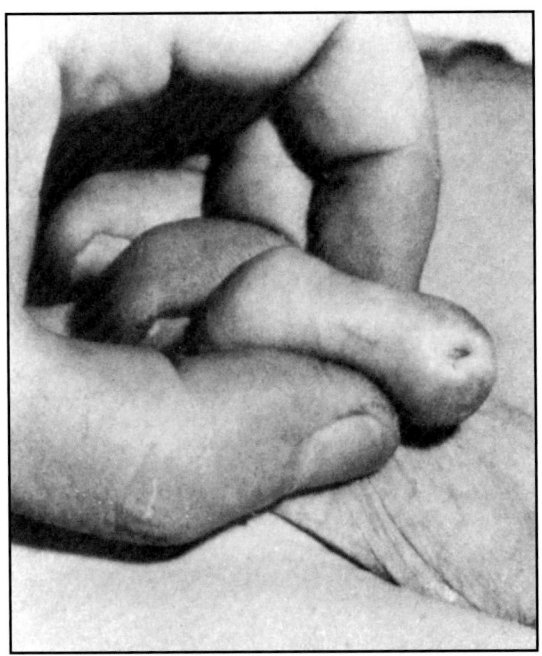

FIGURE 59. Physiologic phimosis. (From Rickwood AMK. Medical indications for circumcision. *BJU Int.* 1999;83[suppl 1]:45–51. Used with permission.)

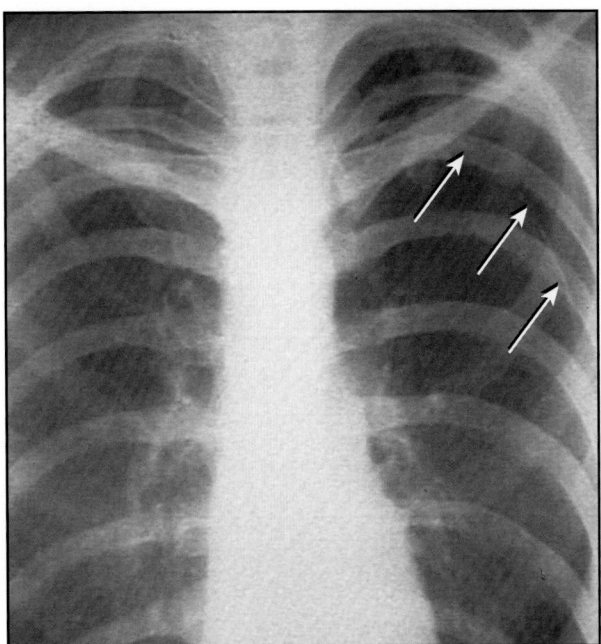

FIGURE 60. Pneumothorax: a white visceral pleural line, separated from the parietal pleura by radiolucent air. (Courtesy of Richard Wiggins, MD.)

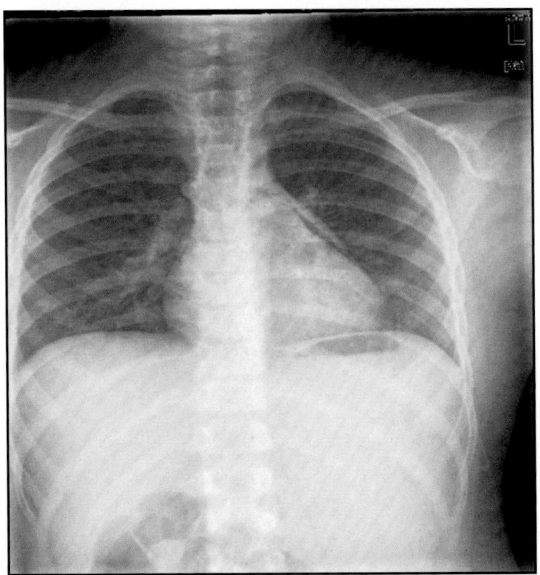

FIGURE 61. Pneumomediastinum. Free air in the mediastinum outlines the left heart border sharply. (Courtesy of Kiran Nandalike, MD.)

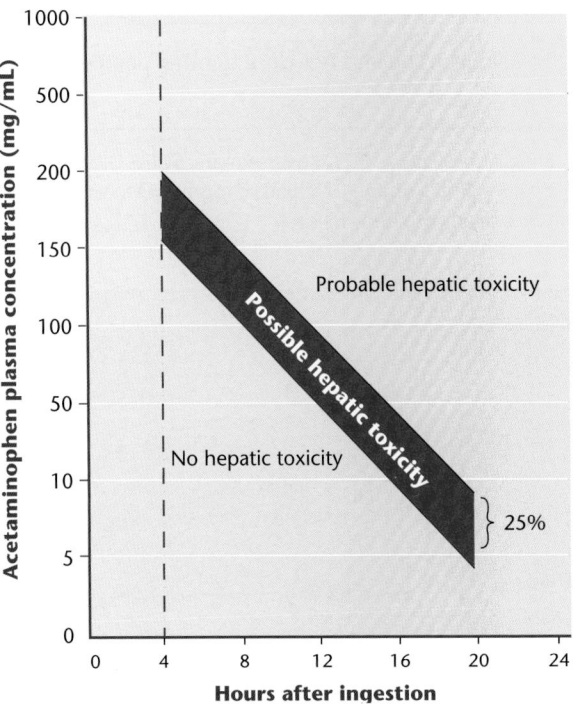

FIGURE 62. Rumack-Matthew nomogram for deciding whether to use N-acetylcysteine (NAC) as an antidote in treating acetaminophen overdose.

	None	Little	Some	Much	Most
1. I get upset, afraid, or sad when something makes me think about what happened.	☐ 0	☐ 1	☐ 2	☐ 3	☐ 4
2. I have upsetting thoughts or pictures of what happened come into my mind when I do not want them to.	☐ 0	☐ 1	☐ 2	☐ 3	☐ 4
3. I feel grouchy, or I am easily angered.	☐ 0	☐ 1	☐ 2	☐ 3	☐ 4
4. I have trouble going to sleep, or I wake up often during the night.	☐ 0	☐ 1	☐ 2	☐ 3	☐ 4
5. I try not to talk about, think about, or have feelings about what happened.	☐ 0	☐ 1	☐ 2	☐ 3	☐ 4
6. I have trouble concentrating or paying attention.	☐ 0	☐ 1	☐ 2	☐ 3	☐ 4
7. I try to stay away from people, places, or things that make me remember what happened.	☐ 0	☐ 1	☐ 2	☐ 3	☐ 4
8. I have bad dreams, including dreams about what happened.	☐ 0	☐ 1	☐ 2	☐ 3	☐ 4
9. I feel alone inside and not close to other people.	☐ 0	☐ 1	☐ 2	☐ 3	☐ 4

FIGURE 63. Abbreviated UCLA Posttraumatic Stress Disorder Reaction Index for DSM-IV. (Copyright Robert S. Pynoos, MD, and Alan Steinberg, PhD, Trauma Psychiatry Program, Department of Psychiatry and Biobehavioral Sciences, University of California, Los Angeles. Used with permission.)

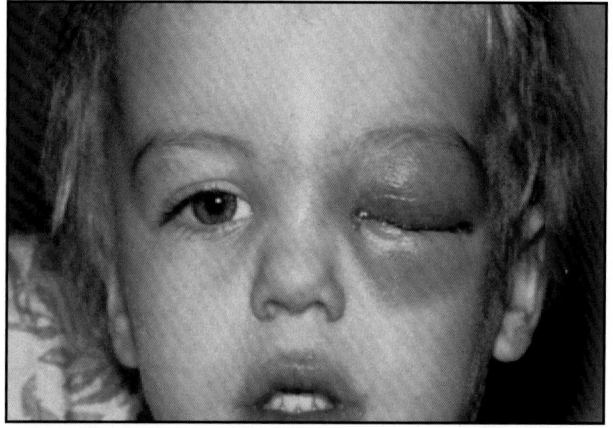

FIGURE 64. A 3-year-old boy with rapid onset of left eyelid swelling and erythema after he incurred a small laceration at the lateral margin of the left eye. He had an upper respiratory tract infection for 10 days. Group A *streptococcus* was recovered from the wound.

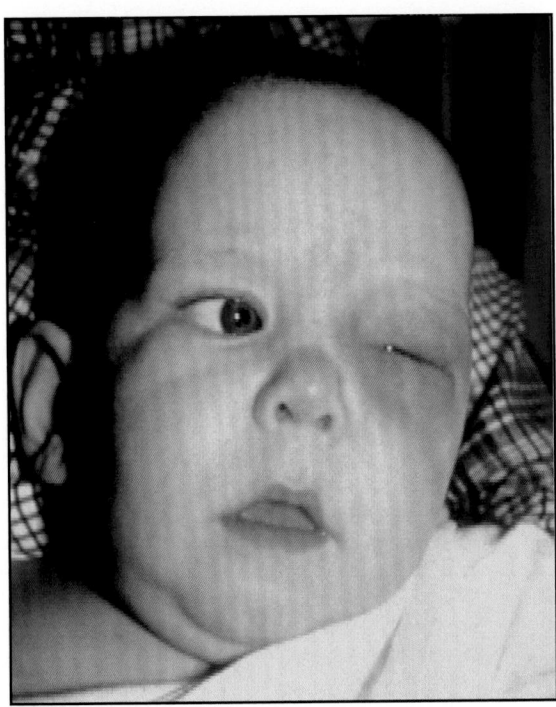

FIGURE 65. A 10-month-old with bacteremic periorbital cellulitis due to *Haemophilus influenzae* type b.

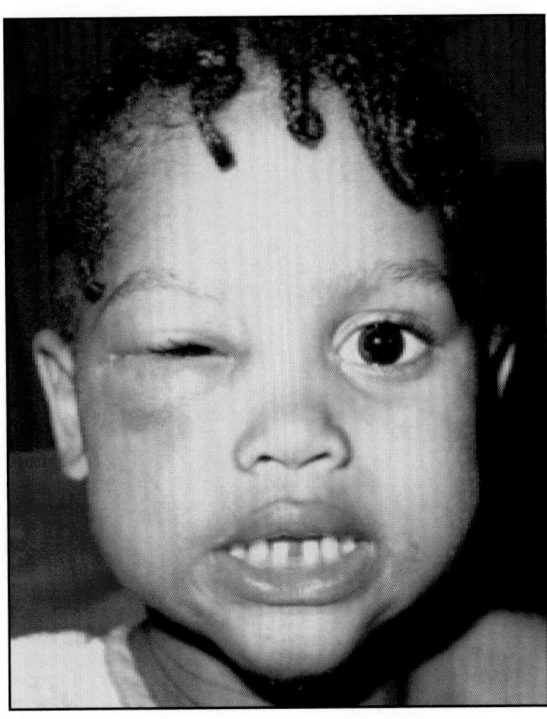

FIGURE 66. A 3-year-old child with inflammatory edema caused by ethmoiditis.

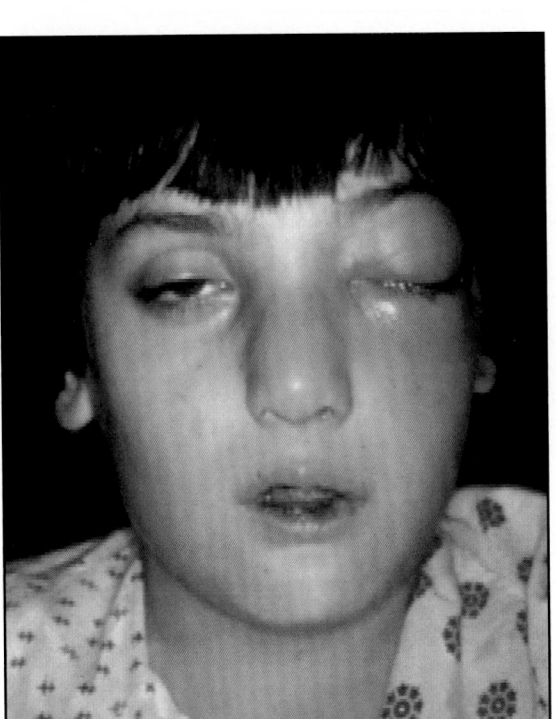

FIGURE 67. A 12-year-old boy with orbital cellulitis. He had a 5-day history of eye pain and progressive swelling of the eyelids, which were markedly erythematous. When his eyelids were retracted, anterior and lateral displacement of the globe and impairment of upward gaze were noted.

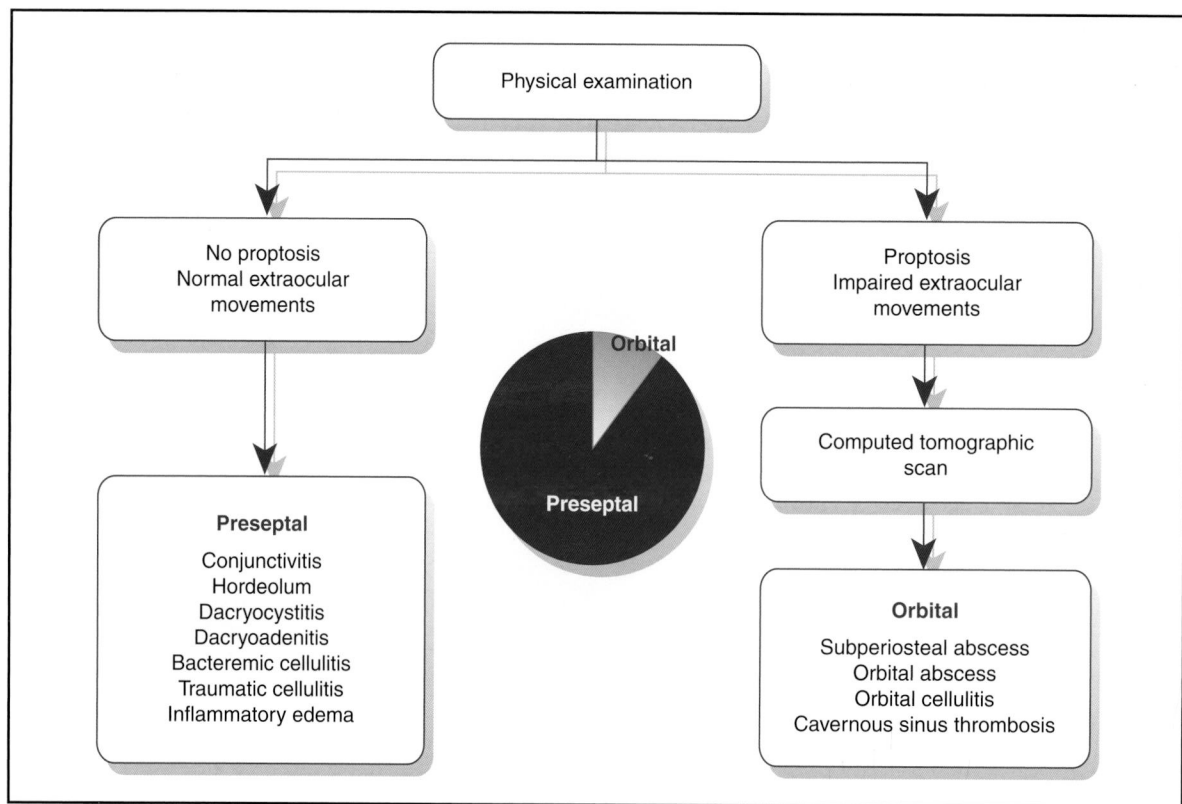

FIGURE 68. Algorithm for the differential diagnosis of the swollen eye.

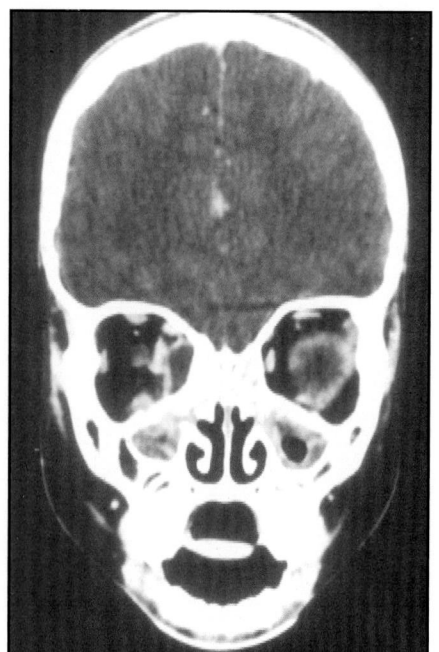

FIGURE 69. Axial computed tomography scan showed a subperiosteal abscess extending from the left ethmoid sinus.

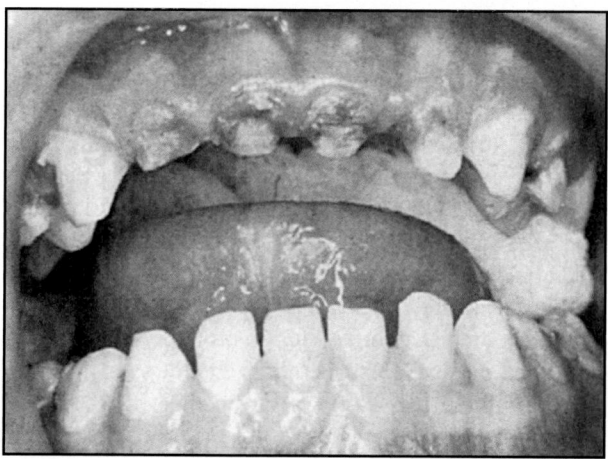

FIGURE 70. Nursing bottle dental caries in a child aged 2½ years.

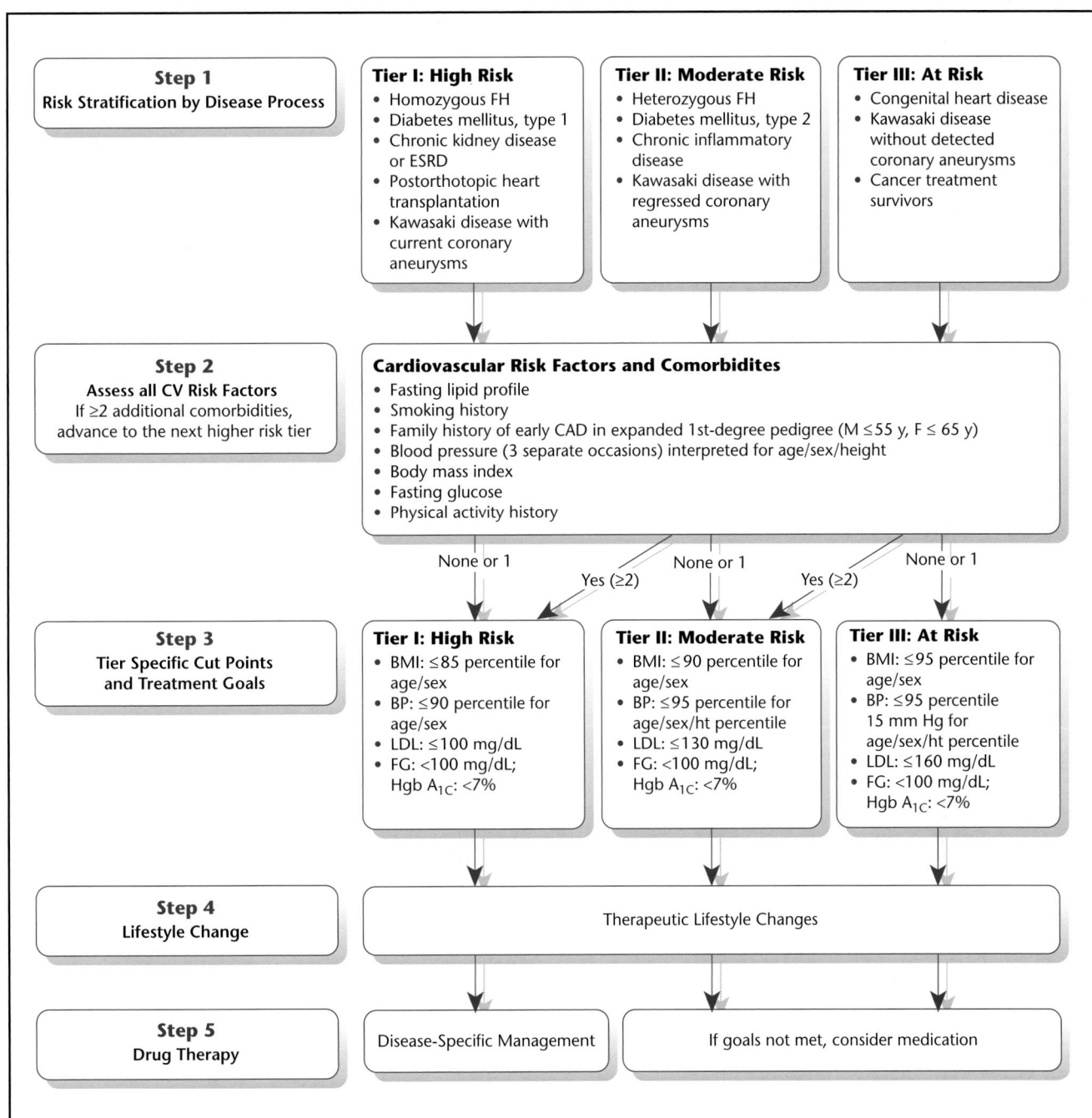

FIGURE 71. High-risk pediatric populations: risk stratification and treatment algorithm. Directions: **Step 1:** Risk stratification by disease process. **Step 2:** Assess all cardiovascular risk factors. If two or more comorbidities exist, then assign patient to the next higher risk tier for subsequent management. **Step 3:** Tier-specific intervention cut points or treatment goals defined. **Step 4:** Initial therapy: for tier I, initial management is therapeutic lifestyle change plus disease-specific management. For tiers II and III, initial management is therapeutic lifestyle change. **Step 5:** for tiers II and III, if goals are not met after initial management, consider medication.

BP, blood pressure; CAD, coronary artery disease; CV, cardiovascular; ESRD, end-stage renal disease; FG, fasting glucose; FH, familial hypercholesterolemia; HgbA1C, hemoglobin A1C; ht, height; LDL, low-density lipoprotein. (Modified from Kavey R-EW, Allada V, Daniels SR, et al. Cardiovascular risk reduction in high-risk pediatric patients: a scientific statement from the American Heart Association Expert Panel on Population and Prevention Science; the Councils on Cardiovascular Disease in the Young, Epidemiology and Prevention, Nutrition, Physical Activity and Metabolism, High Blood Pressure Research, Cardiovascular Nursing, and the Kidney in Heart Disease; and the Interdisciplinary Working Group on Quality of Care and Outcomes Research: endorsed by the American Academy of Pediatrics. *Circulation.* 2006;114[24]:2710–2738.)

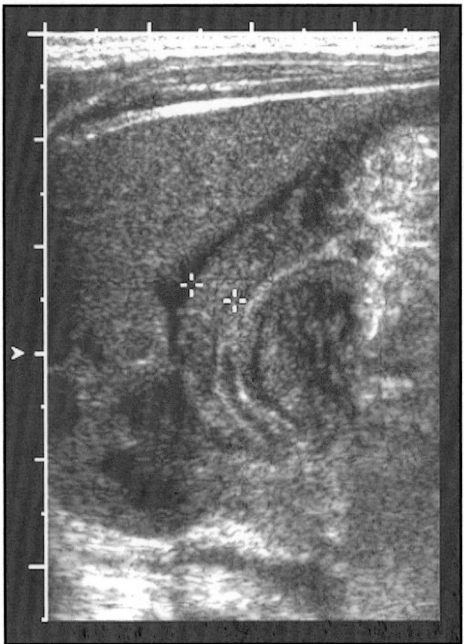

FIGURE 72. Ultrasound of the abdomen shows abnormal thickening (4.5 mm) of pyloric wall, which is consistent with pyloric stenosis.

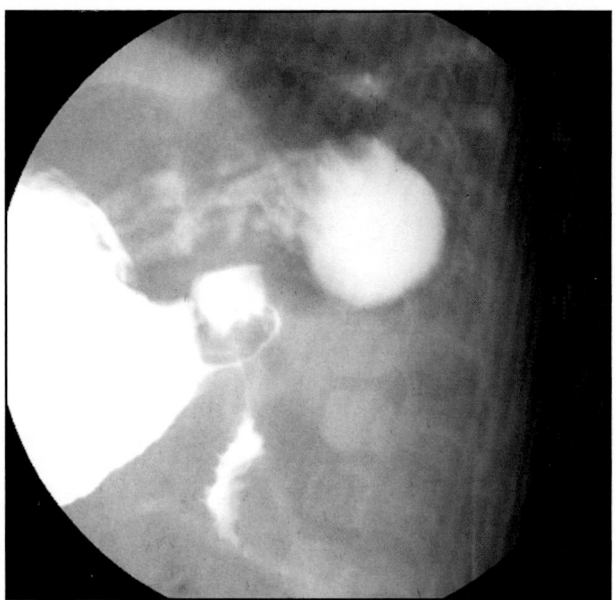

FIGURE 73. Upper gastrointestinal study shows that the pyloric channel is narrowed and elongated with a double-track appearance. This finding is consistent with pyloric stenosis.

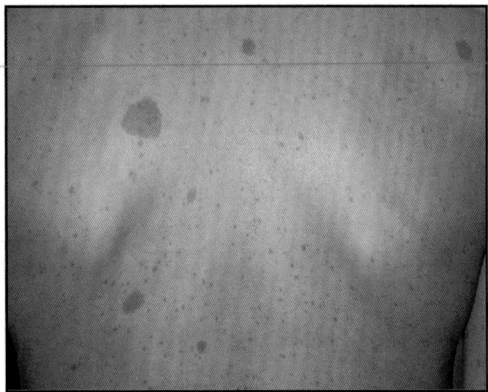

FIGURE 74. Café-au-lait macules in a patient who has neurofibromatosis type 1.

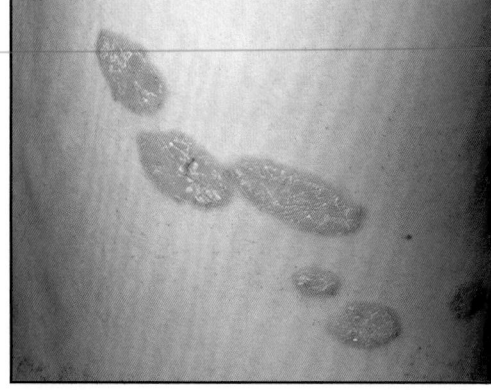

FIGURE 75. Scaling plaques, plateau-like lesions, are observed in psoriasis.

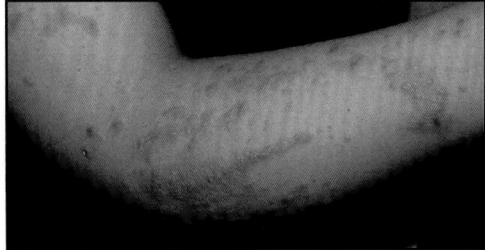

FIGURE 76. A linear arrangement of papules or vesicles often occurs in contact dermatitis caused by poison ivy.

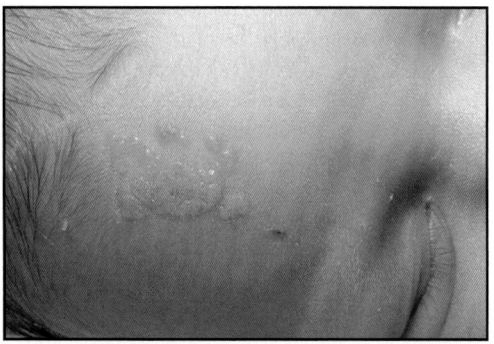

FIGURE 77. Grouped vesicles are characteristic of herpes simplex virus infection on the skin.

FIGURE 78. Lesions of herpes zoster appear in a dermatomal distribution.

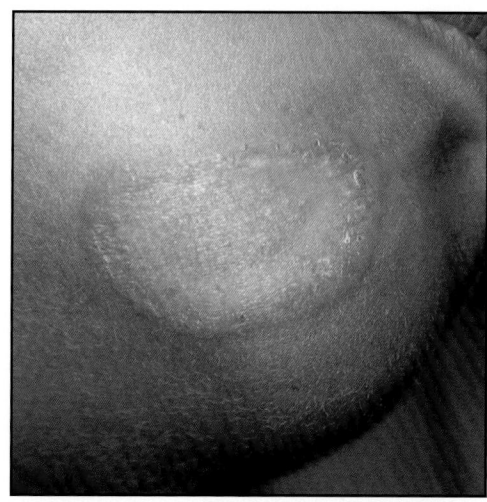

FIGURE 79. An annulus (ie, ring-shaped lesion) is typical of tinea corporis.

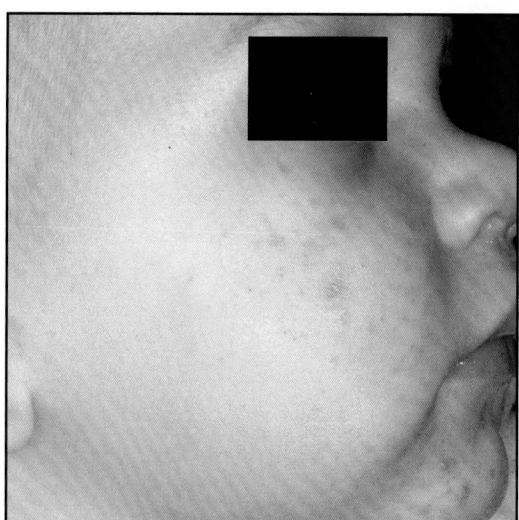

FIGURE 80. Neonatal acne is composed of erythematous papules and papulopustules.

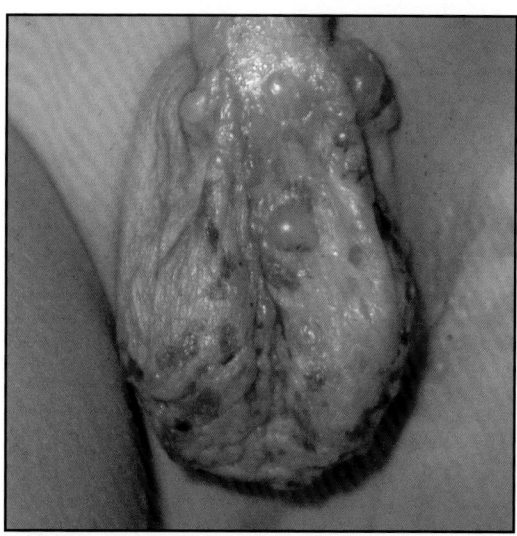

FIGURE 81. Bullae, filled with clear fluid, are observed in chronic bullous disease of childhood.

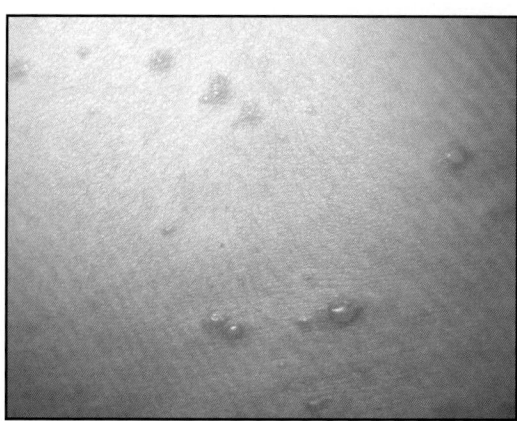

FIGURE 82. Vesicles, as seen here in varicella, are filled with clear or serous fluid.

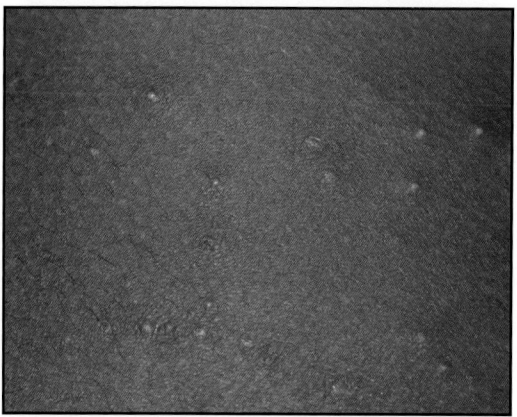

FIGURE 83. Pustules are filled with purulent material. This patient has folliculitis.

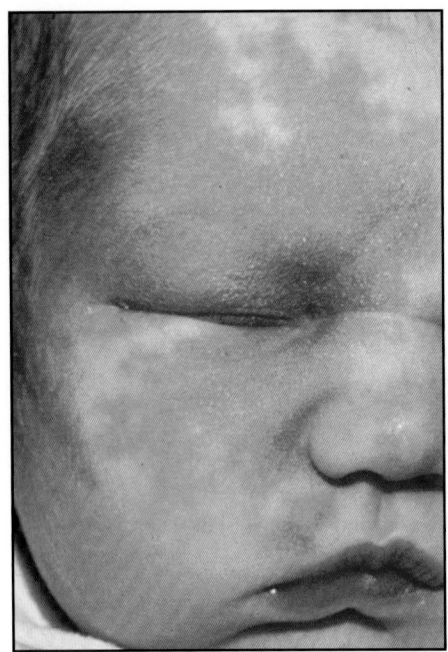

FIGURE 84. A port wine stain is an example of an erythematous patch.

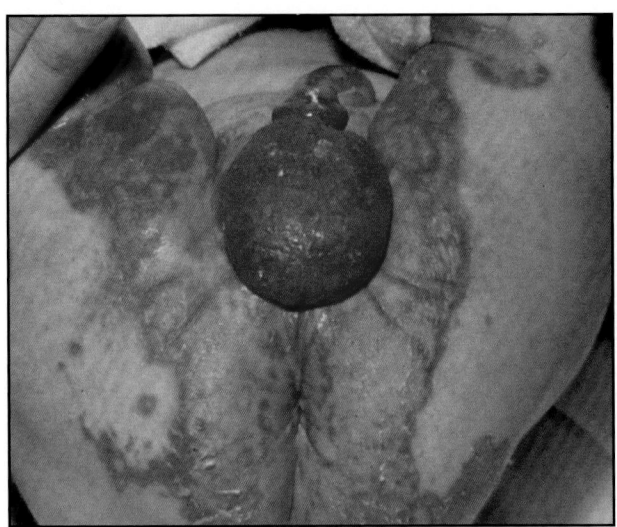

FIGURE 85. Erosions, as seen in this infant who has acrodermatitis enteropathica, represent a superficial loss of epidermis.

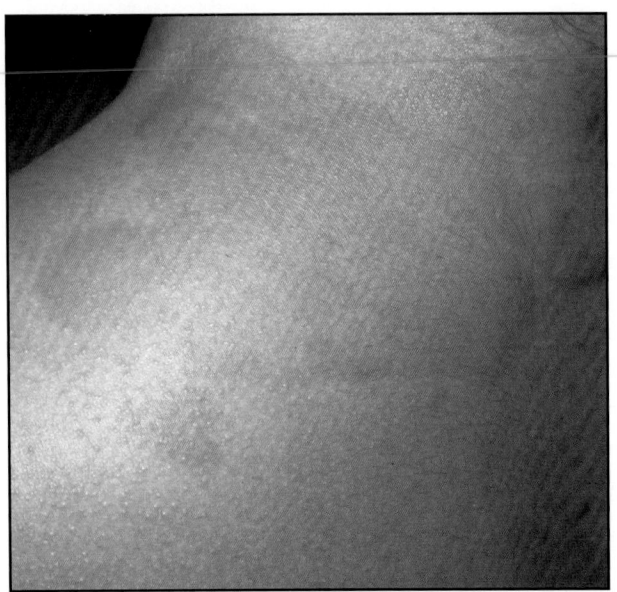

FIGURE 86. Pink wheals in a patient who has urticaria.

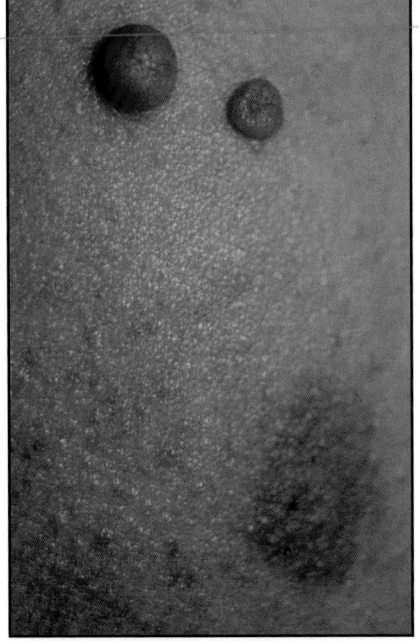

FIGURE 87. Nodules representing neurofibromas in a patient who has neurofibromatosis type 1.

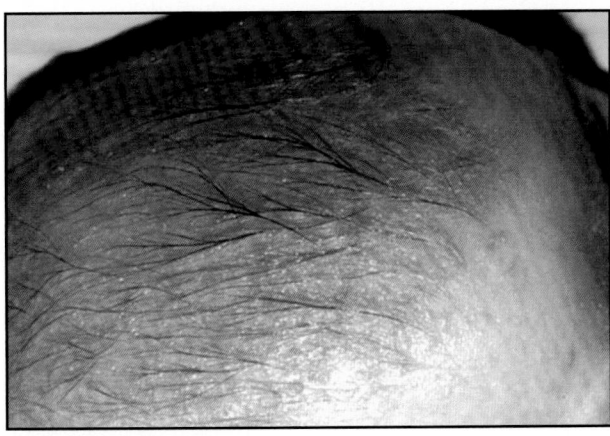

FIGURE 88. Cradle cap.

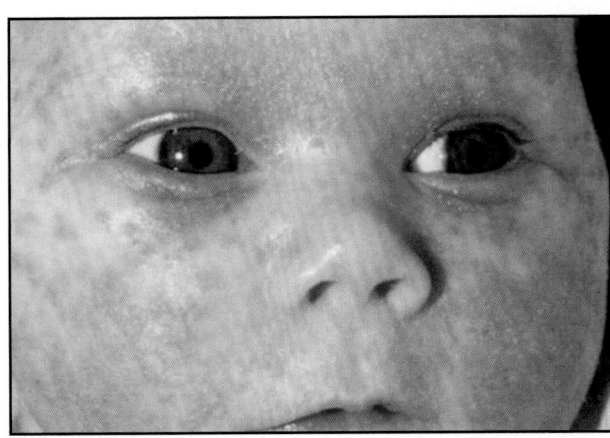

FIGURE 89. Seborrheic dermatitis in the retroauricular creases, eyebrows, and nasolabial folds.

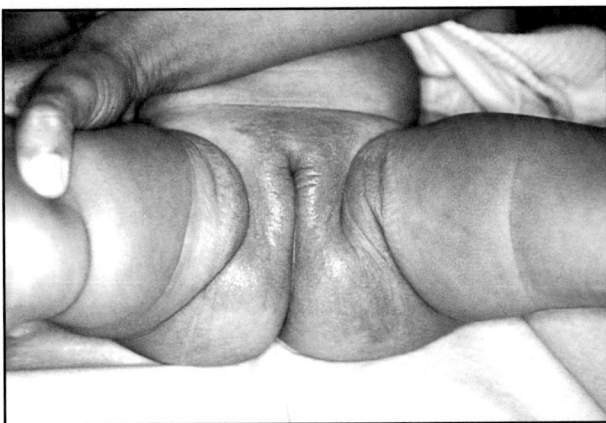

FIGURE 90. Irritant diaper dermatitis.

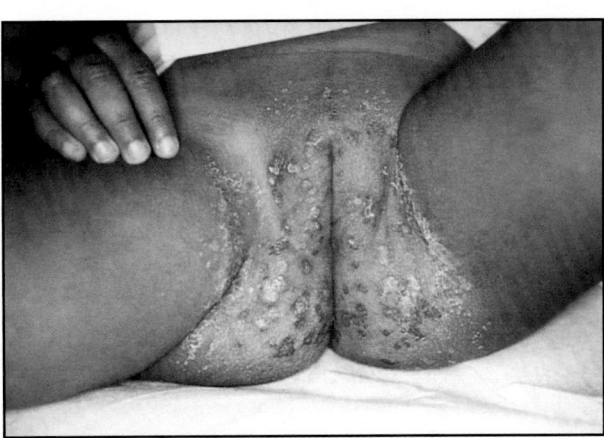

FIGURE 91. Candidal diaper dermatitis.

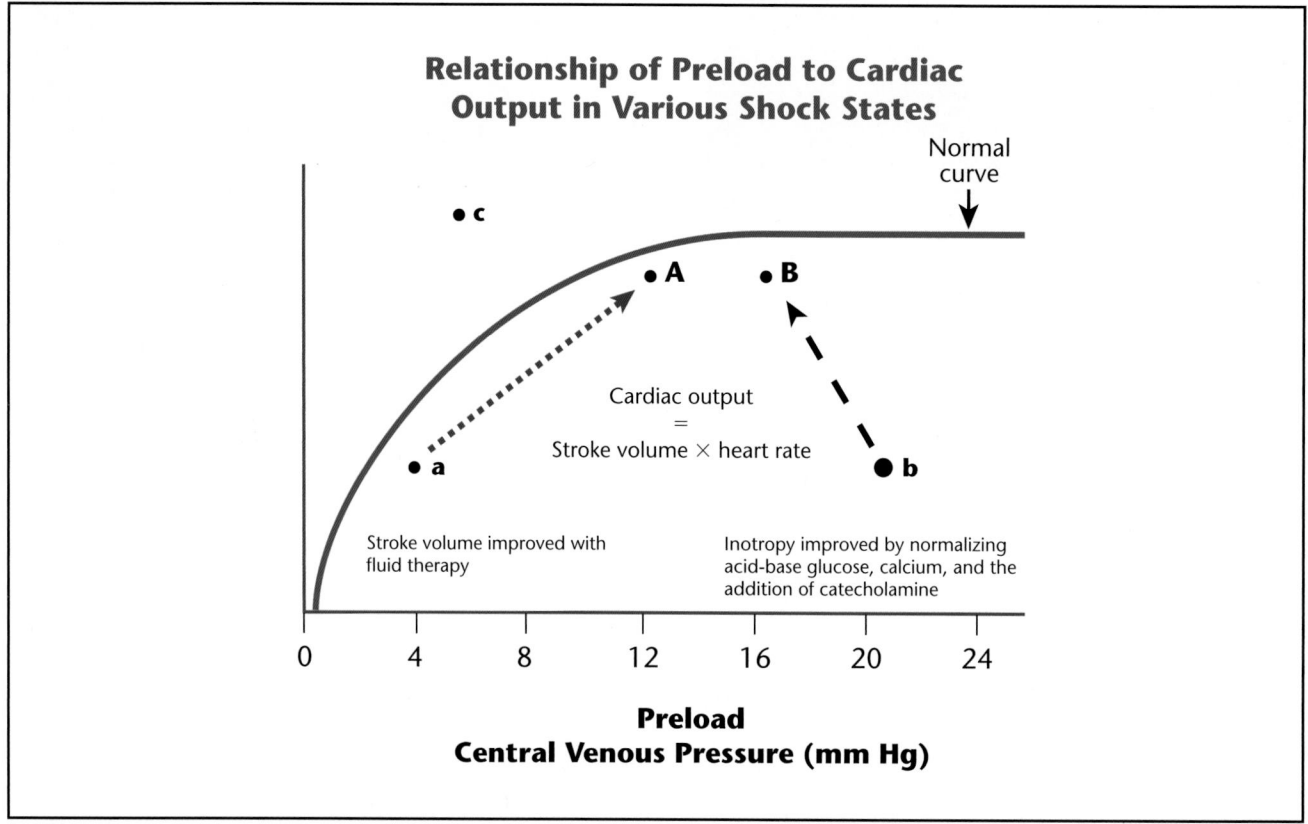

Relationship of Preload to Cardiac Output in Various Shock States

Normal curve

● c

● A   ● B

Cardiac output
=
Stroke volume × heart rate

● a   ● b

Stroke volume improved with fluid therapy

Inotropy improved by normalizing acid-base glucose, calcium, and the addition of catecholamine

0   4   8   12   16   20   24

Preload
Central Venous Pressure (mm Hg)

FIGURE 92. This figure demonstrates the interaction of adequate volume status (preload or central venous pressure) and contractility (cardiac output). **Point a** represents the situation in hypovolemic shock. Fluid administration increases preload and cardiac output increases. **Point b** is a patient with a high preload who would most likely have congestive signs on examination: rales, hepatomegaly, and a low cardiac output state. This condition might be caused by primary cardiogenic shock or with myocardial dysfunction in late stages of septic shock. Evidence of poor perfusion would be obvious on examination: cold clammy skin, prolonged capillary refill rate, and thready, rapid pulses. The restoration of acid-base, glucose, calcium, and magnesium homeostasis and the addition of inotropic agents can improve cardiac patients and return function toward normal. Notably, infants' resting cardiac output is near the maximum, and infants rely on increasing heart rate, whereas adults increase cardiac output by mechanisms intended to increase stroke volume. **Point c** is a patient who is vasodilated, with hyperdynamic cardiac output and relatively low cardiac preload. This scenario would occur in distributive forms of shock: anaphylaxis and septic shock. This state would be reflected in the physical examination by presence of flash capillary refill, bounding cardiac pulses, and a hyperdynamic precordium with tachycardia.

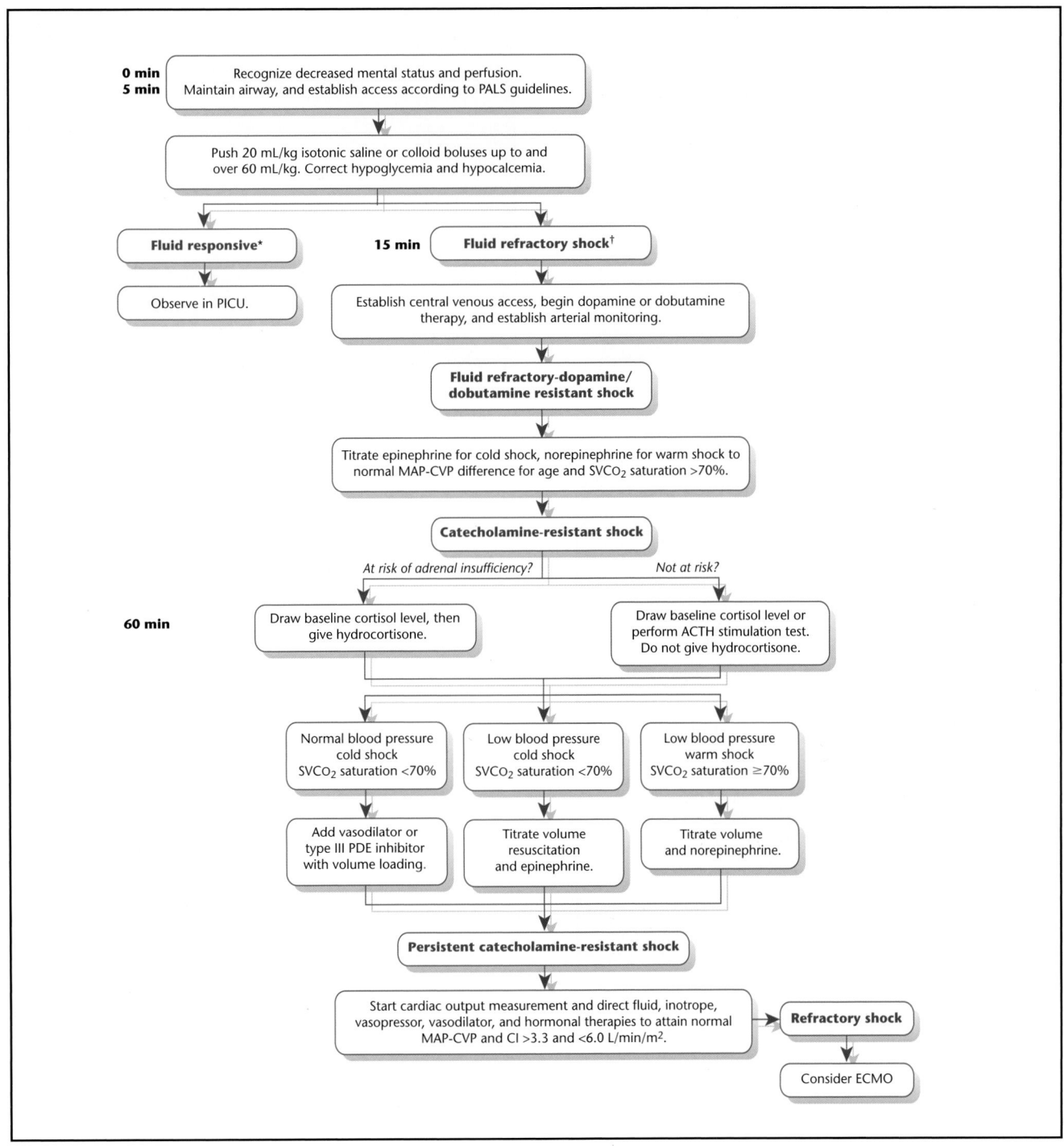

FIGURE 93. American College of Critical Care Medicine Pediatric Advanced Life Support (ACCM-PALS) guidelines for children in septic shock. The 1st hour of care can be crucial to outcome and is easily accomplished in the primary care setting. Recommendations are presented for stepwise management of hemodynamic support in infants and children with goals of normal perfusion and perfusion pressure (MAP-CVP). Proceed to next step if shock persists.

*Normalization of blood pressure and tissue perfusion.

†Hypotension, abnormal capillary refill or extremity coolness.

ACTH, adrenocorticotropic hormone; CI, cardiac index; ECMO, extracorporeal membrane oxygenation; MAP-CVP, mean arterial pressure minus central venous pressure; PALS, pediatric advanced life support; PDE, phosphodiesterase; PICU, pediatric intensive care unit; SVCO$_2$, superior vena cava oxygen.

(Source: Carcillo Ja, Fields AI [task force committee members]. Clinical practice parameters for hemodynamic support of pediatric and neonatal patients in septic shock. *Crit Care Med.* 2002;30:1365–1378.)

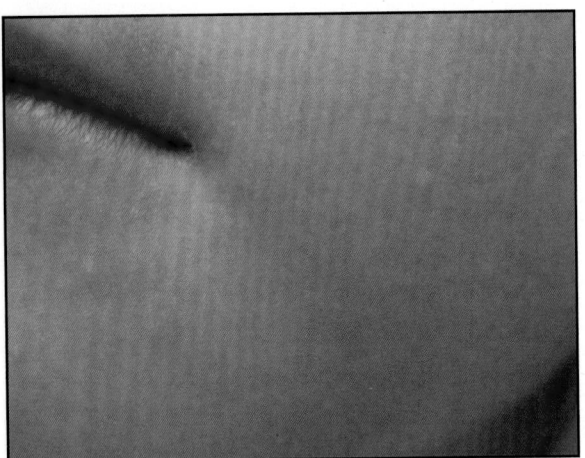

FIGURE 94. Flat warts. Flat warts may be confused with comedones.

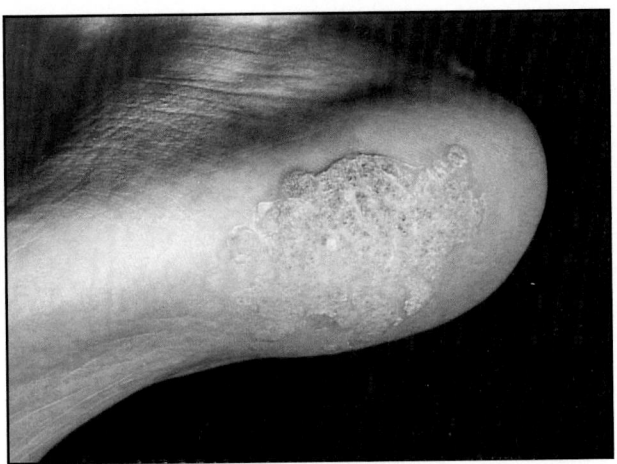

FIGURE 95. A mosaic plantar wart with a roughened surface punctuated with black specks.

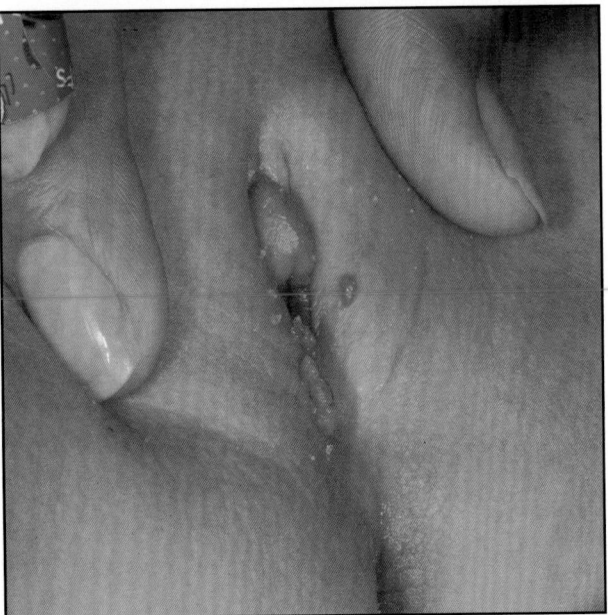

FIGURE 96. Condylomata acuminate appear as skin-colored papules and plaques.

- It is not yet known which patients with refractory increased ICP benefit from this therapy.
- Pentobarbital should be used only when all other medical and surgical therapies failed.

Surgical decompression

- Removing large intracranial masses causing acutely increased ICP can be life saving.
- Surgery may play a role:
  - In decreasing ICP in select patients with large intracerebral hemorrhages by removal of clot
  - In trauma patients with massive edema and contusion
  - In patients who have a large cerebral infarction through craniectomy or decompression of the edematous mass
    - In the latter 2 instances, surgery is performed after all other measures have failed and increased ICP becomes refractory.
  - Surgery should be considered before the ICP critically impairs the CPP.
- Trauma guidelines recommend considering decompressive craniectomy to treat:
  - Severe traumatic brain injury
  - Medically refractory intracranial hypertension, particularly when a potentially recoverable brain injury occurs
- Craniotomy has shown to be effective in reducing ICP and can be associated with favorable outcomes in surviving patients.
  - Mortality in children with severe traumatic brain injury remains high.

Pseudotumor cerebri

- Management is based on symptoms (intractable headache) or when signs of papilledema or visual loss are detected.
- Patients in whom medical therapy fails or those experiencing progressive visual loss may be considered for surgical treatment that includes:
  - CSF shunting procedures (ventriculoperitoneal, ventriculoatrial shunts, or lumboperitoneal shunt) *or*
  - Optic nerve sheath fenestration
- LP is recommended to document opening CSF pressure and may be used therapeutically to decrease ICP by draining CSF.
- Medical management includes carbonic anhydrase inhibitors (acetazolamide) to decrease CSF production.
- Digoxin has been suggested as a similar alternative with the same effect but lesser side effects.
- Patients with severe symptoms or visual loss and those in whom standard medical therapy is failing may benefit from a short course of high-dose corticosteroids (prednisone).

Future trends

- In the future, cerebral protectants may be part of the cocktail in the initial emergent management of acutely increased ICP.
  - Free radical scavengers
  - Excitotoxic amino acid antagonists
  - Lazeroids
  - N-methyl-D-aspartate-receptor antagonists

WHEN TO ADMIT

- Bulging fontanelle
- Altered mental status
- Prolonged seizures
- New focal neurologic deficits
- Moderate to severe papilledema
- Cushing triad (widened pulse pressure; bradycardia; and deep, slow respirations)

WHEN TO REFER

- Macrocephaly or accelerating head growth (crossing percentiles)
- Chronic unremitting headache or new onset of severe headache
- Mild papilledema
- Visual abnormalities (field cuts, diplopia)
- Developmental arrest or regression

COMPLICATIONS

- Herniation of uncus or cerebellar tonsils

PROGNOSIS

- Increased ICP is a major complication that affects morbidity and ultimate outcome in:
  - ≥50% of children with severe head injuries
  - Children who are comatose from other cerebral insults (hypoxia, infections, metabolic disorders)
- Which variables—ICP, CPP, or initial Glasgow Coma Scale score (see table)—are helpful in predicting prognosis remains uncertain.
- Regardless, significant morbidity remains for children with increased ICP.
- Early identification and treatment before a catastrophic increase in ICP will improve outcome in select children with mass lesions or treatable metabolic disorders.

Glasgow Coma Scale [a,b]

Eye-Opening Response		
Score	**>1 Year**	**<1 Year**
4	Spontaneous	Spontaneous
3	To verbal command	To shout
2	To pain	To pain
1	None	None

Motor Response		
Score	**>1 Year**	**<1 Year**
6	Obeys commands	Displays spontaneous response
5	Localizes pain	Localizes pain
4	Withdraws from pain	Withdraws from pain
3	Displays abnormal flexion to pain (decorticate rigidity)	Displays abnormal flexion to pain (decorticate rigidity)
2	Displays abnormal extension to pain (decerebrate rigidity)	Displays abnormal extension to pain (decerebrate rigidity)
1	None	None

Verbal Response			
Score	**>5 Years**	**2–5 Years**	**0–23 Months**
5	Is oriented and converses	Uses appropriate words and phrases	Babbles, coos appropriately
4	Conversation is confused	Uses inappropriate words	Cries, but is consolable
3	Words are inappropriate	Cries or screams persistently to pain	Cries or screams persistently to pain
2	Sounds are incomprehensible	Grunts or moans to pain	Grunts or moans to pain
1	None	None	None

[a] Modified from: Teasdale G, Jennett B. Assessment of coma and impaired consciousness: a practical scale. *Lancet*. 1974;304(7872):81–84. Copyright © Elsevier 1974.

[b] Glasgow Coma Scale score equals sum of best eye opening, motor, and verbal responses. Range is 3–15. Usual definitions of severity of head injury: severe, ≤9; moderate, 9–12; mild, 13–15.

Injury Prevention

BACKGROUND

- Injury is the most significant health problem of childhood and adolescence.
- Injuries cause a majority of deaths of children and adolescents aged 1 to 19 years.
- The major causes of nonfatal injury encompass those that produce fatal injury; these include
  - Motor vehicles
  - Firearms
  - Drowning
  - Suffocation
  - Fires
- Injury results in:
  - Acute morbidity
  - Short- and long-term disability
  - High medical care costs
- Although leading causes of injury death vary by age group, events involving the following are important in every age group:
  - Falls
  - Burns
  - Poisonings
  - Fights
  - Sports
- Injuries are often classified as unintentional or intentional.
  - Strategies that prevent unintentional injury may also prevent some intentional injuries:
    - Locking up firearms
    - Turning down the water heater temperature
  - Some forms of intentional injury are so important as causes of pediatric morbidity and mortality that they demand focused attention:
    - Child abuse
    - Child and adolescent suicide
    - Homicide
  - Causes of intentional injury are extremely complex.
- The number of unintentional childhood injury deaths has been decreasing, partially as a result of the hard work of pediatricians and public health professionals.
- For almost all types of injury, boys are at greater risk than girls.
  - Not yet fully explained but may stem from several factors, including:
    - Innate behavioral differences
    - Societal expectations
    - Exposure
- Children living in poverty are more likely to suffer serious and fatal injury of many types than advantaged children.

GOALS

- Injury control includes:
  - Preventing events that might cause injury
  - Diminishing the likelihood or severity of injury, even though events with injury-causing potential occur
  - Minimizing the after effects of the injury through:
    - State-of-the-art emergency response
    - Medical care
    - Rehabilitation
- Role of the pediatrician:
  - To persuade individuals to decrease risk of injury through education and behavior change strategies
  - To become involved with injury-control advocates through the following activities:
    - Media campaigns
    - Legislation
    - Regulation
    - Litigation
    - Environmental design
    - Cultural change
  - To become involved in research to:
    - Identify risk and protective factors for injury
    - Evaluate preventive interventions
  - For most causes of injury, multiple strategies will need to be applied.

GENERAL APPROACH

- Prevention strategies
  - Active strategies
    - Require involvement of the child or the child's parent every time protection is needed.
      - Example: Seat belts in automobiles
    - Require compliance, but may not be fully used
    - Often least likely to be adopted by the persons at greatest risk
  - Passive (or automatic) strategies
    - Protect the individual whether the person needing protection is mindful of the need and takes appropriate action or not.
      - Example: Automobile airbags
    - Usually favored over active strategies
- Events leading to injury are usually predictable and preventable.
  - Should not be considered as *accidents*, implying a sense of randomness and lack of preventability
  - In some instances, prevention is achieved through:
    - Eliminating injury-producing events
      - Example: building divided highways to reduce motor vehicle crashes

- Eliminating injury even though the event takes place
  - Example: protecting passengers by restraining them in car safety seats
- When energy affects the body acutely at a damaging level, injury results.
  - For most pediatric injuries, the energy is mechanical.
  - Other agents of injury include:
    - Thermal energy
    - Chemical energy
    - Radiation
    - Electrical energy
- Injury prevention
  - Keep energy away from the child.
    - Example: building a bicycle path as an alternative to riding on streets
  - Diffuse energy transfer to tissue over time and/or space so that it does not reach damaging levels.
    - Example: use of bicycle helmet
      - Helmet absorbs and dissipates the forces of the impact.
      - Brain is exposed to a lower level of energy over a longer period.
- Injury-control strategies
  - May be categorized in several ways.
  - Haddon's matrix (see table Haddon's Matrix and Examples of Variables and Injury Prevention Interventions) places strategies in a framework according to:
    - Phase
      - Pre-event
      - Event
      - Post-event

- Factor
  - Human
  - Vector or vehicle
  - Physical environment
  - Socioeconomic environment
- Comprehensive injury-prevention efforts incorporate interventions from multiple matrix cells.

SPECIFIC INTERVENTIONS

Education, engineering, and enforcement

- Education: the most familiar approach to prevention
  - Examples include:
    - Counseling during health supervision visits
    - Public education campaigns
- Engineering: modifying a hazard or the environment to
  - Prevent injuries
    - Reduce the severity of injuries
  - Enactment and enforcement of legislation and regulation can
    - Motivate people to adopt safety-promoting behaviors
    - Require environmental modifications to reduce hazards
    - Facilitate changes in social norms
- Injury prevention is usually most effective when all 3 approaches are incorporated.
  - Example: bicycle helmet use can be promoted through
    - Education in schools
    - Design of more comfortable or attractive helmets
    - Local laws or ordinances requiring helmet use

Haddon's Matrix and Examples of Variables and Injury Prevention Interventions[a]

Phase	Epidemiologic Dimension			
	Human	**Vector or Vehicle**	**Physical Environment**	**Socioeconomic Environment**
Pre-event	Judgment Coordination	Safe storage of firearms Infant walker ban	Bicycle paths Swimming pool barriers	Speed limits Graduated driver licensing
Event	Car safety seat use Use of protective equipment	Airbags Energy-absorbing surfacing on playgrounds	Smoke alarms Highway guard rails	Helmet laws Enforcement of seat belt laws
Post-event	Age Physical condition	Activated charcoal Fuel system integrity	Time to emergency treatment Availability of rehabilitation programs	Training of emergency medical system personnel Cardiopulmonary resuscitation training

[a]Adapted from: American Academy of Pediatrics, Committee on Injury and Poison Prevention. *Injury Prevention and Control for Children and Youth.* 3rd ed. Elk Grove Village, IL: American Academy of Pediatrics; 1997; and Pedialink continuing medical education course, Moving Kids Safely: Introduction to Car Safety Seats.

Injury prevention counseling

- Scientific evidence of positive outcomes in clinical practice.
- Evidence for effectiveness of injury-prevention counseling is stronger in some areas than others, prompting continual calls for:
  - Additional research
  - Improvements in counseling
  - Investment in more passive injury-control strategies
- Counseling is a cornerstone of pediatric practice, but can be daunting.
  - Requires time and expertise
  - Sources of possible injury are very diverse.
  - A pediatrician cannot counsel on all possible risks.
- Injury-prevention can be prioritized based on:
  - Severity of the injury
  - Frequency with which the injury occurs
  - Availability of effective preventive strategies
- Pediatricians will want to:
  - Be sensitive to individual circumstances of patients and families.
  - Customize anticipatory guidance.
    - Recognizing different needs of farm versus city families, various ethnicities
    - Discussing drowning risk if a family has a boat or backyard swimming pool
    - Counseling a family that has 2 automobiles about car safety seats
- The AAP recommends that parents be given advice by the pediatrician about various injury issues, depending on the age of the child
  - Infants
    - Traffic safety: Appropriate use of car safety seats rear-facing in the back seat
    - Burn prevention: Smoke alarms, hot water temperature no higher than 120°F
    - Fall prevention: Window and stairway guards and gates, avoiding walker use
    - Choking and strangulation prevention: Keeping small objects and balloons or plastic bags away from infants, blind and drapery cord safety
    - Drowning prevention: Supervising baths, emptying buckets
    - Safe sleep environment: Back to sleep in a crib that meets current safety standards
    - CPR training: Parent knowledge of infant or child CPR and local emergency medical services (911)
  - Preschoolers
    - Traffic safety: Appropriate use of car safety seats, not leaving children unsupervised in or around cars
    - Burn prevention: Smoke alarm batteries; keeping children away from hot objects
    - Fall prevention: Window and stairway guards and gates; preventing furniture tip-overs
    - Poison prevention: Storage of poisons; poison control phone number (1-800-222-1222)
    - Drowning prevention: Pool fencing; *touch supervision*
    - Firearm safety: Preferably keeping firearms out of the home or at least keeping firearms unloaded and locked separately from locked ammunition
  - School-aged children
    - Traffic safety: Booster seat and seat belt use, avoiding riding on ATVs and in the beds of pickup trucks; safe pedestrian practices; helmets for biking
    - Water safety: Swimming lessons, but no swimming alone; personal flotation devices for boating
    - Sports safety: Safety equipment, physical conditioning, and protective equipment for rollerblading and skateboarding
    - Firearm safety: Preferably keeping firearms out of the home or at least keeping firearms unloaded and locked separately from locked ammunition; asking about firearms in other homes the child visits
  - Adolescents
    - Traffic safety: Seat belt use, role of alcohol in motor vehicle crashes, and minimizing distracted driving; graduated driver licensing; rules for teenage drivers; helmets for biking, motorcycling, and riding an ATV
    - Water safety: Role of alcohol and other drugs in water-related injuries; personal flotation devices for boating
    - Sports safety: Safety equipment; physical conditioning
    - Firearm safety: Preferably keeping any firearms out of the home or at least unloaded and locked separately from locked ammunition
- Counseling about any injury-prevention topic requires both knowledge and counseling skill.
- Counseling technique is not specific to injury prevention.
- Approach can be adapted from existing methods for prompting and supporting healthy behavior change (eg, motivational interviewing).
- Traffic safety is a lifetime issue
  - Car safety seats (see table Appropriate Car Safety Seat Selection Based on Child's Age, Height, and Weight)
    - Motor vehicle crashes are the leading cause of death of children and adolescents.
    - Topic warrants frequent discussion during well-child care.
    - Pediatricians should know how to counsel parents on appropriate car safety seat selection based on developmental milestones.
    - Know where to refer parents for more information.
    - Be familiar with state laws.

Appropriate Car Safety Seat Selection Based on Child's Age, Height, and Weight

If the child is...	Use the following type of car safety seat...	And remember the following...
Younger than 1 year OR under 20 lb	Rear-facing car safety seat (infant-only or convertible)	NEVER place a rear-facing car safety seat in the front seat with an airbag.
Older than 1 year AND over 20 lb	Recommended: rear-facing convertible seat to seat's height or weight (usually 30 or 35 lb) limit Then: forward-facing car safety seat (convertible, combination, or forward-facing only) to seat's height or weight limit	When switching a convertible seat from rear-facing to forward-facing, adjustments are usually needed to the harness, the angle of the seat, and the seat belt.
Too tall or heavy for a forward-facing seat with a harness (often around 4 years of age or 40 lb)	Booster seat	Booster seats must be used with lap and shoulder belts.
Big enough to fit in the adult seat belt (usually around 4' 9" and between 8 and 12 years of age)	None. Use the vehicle's seat belt if it fits properly (shoulder belt across chest and shoulder, lap belt low and snug on thighs, child's back against vehicle seat back and knees bent at edge of vehicle seat).	Children should sit in the back seat until they turn 13 years of age.

a Adapted from: American Academy of Pediatrics, Committee on Injury and Poison Prevention. Selecting and using the most appropriate car safety seats for growing children: guidelines for counseling parents. *Pediatrics.* 2002;109(3):550-553.

- Recognize when state laws often do not reflect best practice in car safety seat use.
- Encourage parents to:
  - Read instruction manuals for their car safety seats and vehicles.
  - Learn how to install and use car safety seats.
- Refer parents to local *child passenger safety technicians.*
- A staff member can complete the 3- to 4- day training course to become a certified technician.
- Teen drivers
  - Motor vehicle–related death rates increase dramatically in adolescence.
  - Novice teen drivers and their passengers are at particularly high risk.
  - Pediatricians can play a key role in helping parents and teens:
    - Negotiate their changing relationship
    - Balance the need to ensure the teen's safety with the teen's growing independence and increasing mobility.
  - Pediatricians should be familiar with their states' laws.
  - A state's graduated driver licensing (GDL) system may provide a good starting point for counseling.
    - Under GDL, teen drivers graduate from a learner's permit to an intermediate/provisional license to a regular driver's license after a required amount of time and demonstration of proficiency.
    - Each stage has its own restrictions.
  - Both parents and teens should be counseled on:
    - Seat belt use

- Dangers of impaired driving
  - Teens and parents should also be encouraged to have a safe ride agreement
    - Teen promises to call the parent rather than driving while impaired or with another impaired driver.
    - Parent agrees to provide a ride home in a nonjudgmental way.
  - Pediatricians can consider having a family develop a parent-teen driving contract that:
    - Specifies restrictions on teen drivers
    - Determines when restrictions will be relaxed
    - Outlines the consequences for violating the restrictions

■ Firearms
  - Second leading cause of death of children and adolescents
  - Pediatricians are often reluctant to counsel on this topic because of concerns about parent reactions.
  - Parents may view such counseling as intrusive or outside the purview of pediatrics.
  - Strategies are available that can make counseling on firearms more palatable to both parents and pediatricians.
    - Families with infants and toddlers
      - Discuss firearms in the context of childproofing and children's natural curiosity.
    - Parents of depressed adolescents
      - Discuss association between presence of firearms in the home and higher risk of teen suicide.
    - Introduce the concept of asking about the presence of guns in other homes where their children spend time.

Insect Bites and Infestations

DEFINITION

- Insect bites and stings
  - Insects and arachnids (mites, ticks, and spiders) are often vectors of serious or fatal disease.
    - Viral encephalitis
    - Malaria
- Infestation
  - Pediculosis (lice)
    - Capitis (scalp)
    - Palpebrum (eyelashes)
    - Corporis (limbs and trunk)
    - Pubis (pubic area)
  - Scabies
    - Highly pruritic dermatosis caused by mites

EPIDEMIOLOGY

- Insect bites
  - Worldwide, malaria is still one of the most common causes of serious childhood morbidity and death.
  - Ticks
    - Most common insect vectors of disease in the US (Lyme disease and other infections)
- Infestation
  - Bedbug infestations
    - Incidence has increased.
    - Epidemic in urban US
  - Pediculosis capitis
    - Outbreaks occur mainly among school-age children.

ETIOLOGY

- Pediculosis
  - Lice are obligate human ectoparasites that create pruritic dermatoses after their bites puncture the skin and inject saliva.
    - The saliva incites inflammation and sometimes hypersensitivity.
    - Lice can transmit diseases, including typhus.
    - Head lice are spread primarily by close personal contact and occasionally by fomites.
    - Body lice are primarily spread by clothing.
- Scabies
  - Infestation with the mite *Sarcoptes scabiei hominis,* causes scabies.
    - The burrowing of the female mite into the stratum corneum initiates infestation.
    - Eggs are laid within the stratum corneum.
    - Over the next 2–6 weeks, itching and papules develop gradually as the eggs hatch and the host develops delayed hypersensitivity.

- Generally spread by close personal contact
  - Usually through persistent or repeated skin-to-skin contact, such as individuals sleeping in the same bed or holding a child closely

RISK FACTORS

- Infestation
  - Sleeping in the same bed or otherwise maintaining close contact
  - Pediculosis pubis is often sexually transmitted.

SIGNS AND SYMPTOMS

Insect bites

- Discrete, erythematous or flesh-colored papules, nodules, or wheals
  - Some bites have central puncta or vesicles; others are capped by pustules or by hemorrhagic or serous crusts.
  - Usually pruritic
  - Excoriations created by scratching are common.
- Often clustered
  - Linear or arcuate pattern, especially when caused by a crawling insect
  - Most commonly found on surfaces not covered by clothing
- Sensitized child (prior exposure)
  - Larger nodules or blisters are a robust reaction to insect- or arachnid-associated toxins.
- Unsensitized child
  - Discomfort varies from mild itch to pain caused by toxin injection.

Pediculosis

- Pediculosis capitis
  - Grayish, crawling, 6-legged louse may be seen in areas of thick terminal hair growth close to the scalp.
    - Louse eggs (nits) may be seen as minute, white-gray fixed attachments to hair shafts.
    - Nits or the insects themselves may be visible on the eyelashes or pubic hair.
  - Pruritus
    - Sometimes accompanied by erythematous papules (bites), 1–2 mm in diameter
    - Noted around the nape of the neck and the hairline, especially posteriorly
  - Other possible signs
    - Cervical adenopathy
    - Urticaria-like changes
    - Involvement of other body areas
  - Family members
    - Should be examined for head lice, especially if combs, towels, and other personal items are shared

- Pediculosis pubis
  - Often sexually transmitted
  - Affected individuals may have othersexually transmitted infections.
- Pediculosis corporis
  - Should be suspected when widespread pruritus is present
  - In most instances, the body louse and nits are not found on the body but in the seams of clothing or bedding.
  - Bites consist of erythematous macules and papules, which are often obscured by the results of scratching.
    - Excoriation
    - Impetiginization
    - Eczematization
    - Overt infection
    - Pigmentation

Scabies

- Highly pruritic dermatosis
  - In the setting of worsening or persistent widespread pruritus, a diagnosis of scabies must be considered, especially if close contacts are also itching.
  - The distribution of skin changes is often the best clue to the diagnosis along with itching that is more widespread than the objective skin findings.
- Varied and protean manifestations
  - Ranges from rare scattered erythematous papules to widespread eczematous dermatitis and excoriations
  - Multiple areas of mite-laden, crusting, possibly infectious complications of any presentation (Norwegian scabies)
  - As eggs hatch, repeated infestation of host leads to more rapid development of itching and other manifestations, often within 24–96 hours.
- Common sites of infestation
  - Digital web spaces
  - Extensor surface of the elbows and knees
  - Flexor aspect of the wrists
  - Axilla
  - Upper trunk
  - Groin
- Infants
  - Involvement of palms and soles, especially with vesicles
  - Skin changes on the face and head
- Burrows created by female mites
  - Help establish diagnosis in some patients
  - Often disguised by excoriations, eczematous reactions, or superimposed infection

- Family members, sexual partners, and other close contacts of index cases should be examined when possible.
  - The patient's history may reveal that several people in a household are itching.
  - Fomites rarely transmit scabies, especially in temperate climates.
  - Although humans may acquire subspecies of scabies mites that infest other mammals, such infestation is self-limiting, as other mite subspecies do not reproduce in human skin.

DIAGNOSTIC APPROACH

- Insect bites
  - Discrete, erythematous, or flesh-colored papules, nodules, or wheals, usually pruritic, suggest the diagnosis of insect or arachnid bites.
- Infestation
  - In pediculosis, the louse and/or nits will be found.
  - Worsening or persistent widespread pruritus suggests scabies.
    - Especially if close contacts are also itching
    - Distribution of skin changes (eg, digital web spaces) is also a clue.

LABORATORY FINDINGS

- Light microscopy
  - Diagnosis of scabies in infants
    - A drop of mineral oil is placed on the skin.
    - Scrapings of burrows or papules from palms or soles are removed by scalpel.
    - Confirmatory ova, mites, or feces are revealed under low magnification.

TREATMENT APPROACH

- Insect bites
  - Topical corticosteroid creams
  - Oral antihistamines
- Pediculosis
  - Head lice
    - Physical removal is as effective as drug treatment.
    - Chemical treatments should be avoided in infants.
  - Body lice
    - 5% permethrin cream
  - All methods depend on following instructions carefully.
  - All methods will need to be repeated.
  - Clothing, bedding, towels, etc must be washed in hot water.
- Scabies
  - Should be treated regardless of symptoms
    - 5% permethrin to the entire body, except the face

SPECIFIC TREATMENTS

Insect bites

- Topical corticosteroid creams plus oral antihistamines
  - Primary treatment
  - Reduces inflammation and pruritus
- Topical antipruritics (calamine) and cold soaks/ice
  - Soothing
- Topical antihistamines should be avoided.
  - Ineffective
  - May cause allergic contact dermatitis
- Oral systemic corticosteroids (rare cases)
  - Sometimes indicated for:
    - Extensive bites
    - Hypersensitivity manifesting as papular urticaria or in other ways that involve >20% of the body
  - ≤1-week course of approximately 0.5 mg/kg of prednisone or equivalent
    - Longer-term or chronic treatment is not indicated for this circumstance alone.
  - Topical therapy should be started at the same time.
    - Prevents rebound phenomenon
  - All contraindications must be excluded.
    - The risk of adverse events, although small with brief treatment courses, must be considered.

Pediculosis

- Head lice, pubic lice
  - Physical removal of lice and eggs
    - Careful, repeated removal of head lice has shown superior results to drugs, even malathion.
    - Kits are available.
  - Chemical treatment
    - Resistance to chemical agents is increasing.
    - Chemical treatments are used only with great caution by pregnant or nursing women and should be avoided by persons with allergies to any component of the treatment.
    - Infants should not be treated unless essential and only with very close supervision.
  - Pyrethrins
    - Several nonprescription preparations are available.
    - Nix cream rinse contains 1% permethrin.
    - A fine-toothed comb can be used to remove nits from hair shafts after chemical treatment.
    - Retreatment is usually necessary about 1 week after the first application to kill lice that have hatched from viable nits that were not killed initially.

- Malathion 0.5% solution
  - Must be left on for 8–12 hours
  - Flammable
- Dimethicone 4%
  - Recently found to be effective
- Other insecticides
  - Lindane (gamma-benzene hexachloride [GBH]) is more toxic and probably less effective with much resistance and should only be used when all other treatment options have failed.
    - California has banned lindane for human use because of its neurotoxicity.
  - Oral ivermectin
    - 2 doses given 7 days apart are effective for treatment of several kinds of lice infestation.
    - This application is an off-label use.
- Body lice
  - Total-body application of 5% permethrin cream (Elimite) for 8–14 hours
    - May be necessary to apply to the hair
  - A limited number of treatments spaced approximately 7 days apart may be required for eradication, using various pediculicides, such as:
    - Permethrin
    - GBH
    - Pyrethrins
    - Vinegar rinse to remove stubborn nits
  - Pruritus
    - May continue for ≥2 weeks after treatment
    - Patients should be advised that itching might continue, so that they do not overtreat themselves through repeated applications.
    - Oral antipruritics, soothing bland lotions, and topical corticosteroids can help.
- Pediculosis palpebrarum
  - Apply plain petrolatum to the eyelashes 3–5 times daily.
    - Treatment is required for approximately 8–10 days.
  - A moustache comb can be used daily to remove lice and nits from the eyelashes.
    - Other infested body areas should be treated simultaneously.
  - If this method fails, physostigmine 0.25% may be similarly applied to eyelashes.
    - Usually curative in 3 or 4 days, but may interfere with vision.

- All potentially infested items should be treated with wet or dry heat (or both)
  - Minimum of 65°C (149°F) for minimum of 15 min (preferably at least 30 min)
    - Clothing
    - Bedding
    - Combs
    - Towels
  - Clothing, stuffed animals, comforters, and other items that cannot be washed or dry cleaned:
    - Store in a sealed plastic bag for 2 weeks.

Scabies

- Should always be treated, regardless of symptoms
  - Patients may be asymptomatic carriers.
  - Chemical treatments are used only with great caution in:
    - Pregnant or nursing women
    - Infants
    - Persons with allergies to any component of the treatment (should be avoided)
- Permethrin 5%
  - Thorough application to the entire body, except the face
  - Treatment of choice because of high efficacy and relatively low toxicity
- Alternate treatments
  - Lindaneor a similar GBH preparation
    - Probably less effective than permethrin
    - Lindane is associated with irritant dermatitis.
    - GBH is associated with adverse reactions and toxicity.
    - Should be dispensed in limited quantities and used only when other treatment options have failed.
    - Parents should be informed about possible neurotoxicity and other complications from organophosphate exposure.
    - Repeated treatments, especially when based only on symptoms, should be actively discouraged.
  - Crotamiton 10% (Eurax)
    - Probably less efficacious
    - Must be applied at least twice
  - Benzyl benzoate
    - Widely used as an inexpensive emulsion, sometimes recommended by the World Health Organization
    - Not available in the US.
- If topical treatment fails or is not feasible
  - Oral ivermectin
    - Highly effective used at appropriate dosing for weight
    - Off-label indication, but widely used for scabies

- Published clinical data in young children are limited
- 2 doses, separated by approximately 1–2 weeks, may be necessary.

- All potentially infested items should be washed immediately after treatment of all individuals in the same household.
  - Minimum of 65°C (149°F) for minimum of 15 min (preferably at least 30 min)
    - Clothing
    - Bedding
    - Combs
    - Towels
- Pruritus and rash
  - Often persist for ≥2–4 weeks after successful eradication of an infestation
    - Treatment should be repeated only when continued infestation with live mites is clearly demonstrated.
  - Pruritus can be treated with oral antihistamines or mild topical agents, such as emollients, pramoxine, or very minimal concentrations of menthol.
  - Nodular scabies, postscabetic nodules
    - Hypersensitivity reaction
    - Red to purple discrete nodules up to 2 cm in diameter on surfaces usually covered by clothing
    - Usually on the genitals or around the axillae
    - Usually respond to topical or intralesional injections of corticosteroids

WHEN TO ADMIT

- The patient has severe systemic allergic reactions to insect bites.
- The patient needs intravenous antibiotics to treat secondary bacterial infection or cellulitis.
- The patient develops noninfectious complications, such as:
  - Acute postinfectious glomerulonephritis
  - Hypertension
- Patient is suspected of having contracted:
  - Viral meningitis
  - Other severe or systemic illness through insect bites

WHEN TO REFER

- Refer to an allergist if:
  - The patient develops a severe allergic reaction to insect bites, especially repeatedly.
  - Hymenoptera allergy is suspected.

COMPLICATIONS

Insect bites

- Infection
  - Impetigo
  - Cellulitis
- Eczematous changes
  - Inflamed plaques
    - From scratching
    - From topical remedies that cause irritant or allergic contact dermatitis, eg, neomycin
- Localized hypersensitivity reactions
  - Papular urticaria
    - Recurrent crops of urticarial (hive-like) papules, nodules, or wheals on exposed surfaces; may be either new or reactivated old bites
    - Occurs in some sensitized individuals
    - Can last weeks or months
    - The patient experiences profound itch, especially if repeatedly scratched or otherwise traumatized.
    - Scratching can leave scarring or postinflammatory pigment change, most often hyperpigmentation.
- Systemic reactions
  - Viral encephalitis or tick-borne disease
    - More thorough follow-up
    - Consideration of hospital observation
  - Bacterial infection
    - Can lead to cellulitis or a multitude of toxin-induced or immune-mediated complications, such as nephritis

Infestation

- Bacterial infection
  - Toxin-producing strains
- Cellulitis
- Systemic treatment may be necessary.
  - Especially in immunosuppressed children

PREVENTION

- Insect bites
  - Cover as much of the body as possible with clothing.
  - Judicious use of repellents
    - *N,N*-diethyl-metatoluamide (DEET) at exposed areas (avoiding children's hands, eyes, and mouth areas)
    - DEET can cause central nervous system and systemic symptoms in children.
    - Usually safe to use intermittently and in moderation at concentrations ≤30% in children >2 months.
    - Alternate repellents may be less effective or toxic.
  - Mosquitoes
    - Avoid potential attractants, such as bright clothing.
    - Use of bed nets impregnated with repellents can be extremely effective in preventing bites.
- Infestation
  - Pediculosis
    - No-nit policies aimed at excluding children from school are ineffective.
      - Such policies penalize children excessively by causing missed school days.

Intellectual Disability

DEFINITION

- *Intellectual disability* is the preferred synonym for mental retardation.
  - The recent change from the term *mental retardation* to *intellectual disability* does not match the current legal definition for entitlement to services for individuals with intellectual disability.
  - However, for individuals who meet diagnostic criteria, the label of mental retardation remains essential to obtaining educational and social services.
    - Therefore, primary care physicians should continue to use this term to assist clients in obtaining appropriate supports.
- American Association on Intellectual and Developmental Disabilities (AAIDD) guidelines for the accurate use of the term *intellectual disability*
  - The level of functioning of an individual should be considered within their particular social and cultural context.
  - Any assessment of cognitive and adaptive ability should take into account communication, as well as sensory, motor, and behavioral functioning.
  - An individual's strengths must be emphasized in assessments and included in support plans.
  - The purpose of assessing limitations is to guide the development of appropriate supports for the individual in question.
  - The provision of individualized supports is expected to improve functioning significantly.
- The AAIDD defines intellectual disability as impairments in cognitive functioning and adaptive behavior that develop before age 18 years.
  - *Cognitive impairment* is defined as performance in the abnormally low range on standard assessments of intelligence.
    - Cognitive impairment implies significantly low scores in all domains of intelligence testing.
    - Widely discrepant scores in various domains would be best defined as learning disability, not intellectual disability.
  - Adaptive impairment is defined by functioning in the abnormally low range on formal measures of adaptive functioning, eg, Vineland Adaptive Behavior Scales.
    - Includes such domains as communication, self-care, home living, social or interpersonal skills, ability to use community resources, self-direction, functional academic skills, work, leisure, health, and safety
- Implicit is the understanding that, although cognitive and adaptive impairments are not reversible, intellectual disability can be ameliorated by environmental modifications and supports.
- *Developmental delay* reflects functioning at <75% of expectations for chronologic age in a particular developmental domain.
  - Some children experience this development in a single domain, whereas others have delays in multiple or all domains.
  - Conceptually, this term suggests the child will at some time make up the delay.
    - Catch-up frequently occurs in the case of delays in isolated domains.
    - The child who is delayed in all domains, frequently described as having *global developmental delay,* is less likely to catch up.
  - In general, psychologists are hesitant to describe children as having intellectual disability until they are approximately at the age of school entry.
    - This hesitation allows parents to focus on interventions that maximize the child's potential while de-emphasizing what the child cannot accomplish.

ETIOLOGY

- In most cases of mild intellectual disability, the cause is multifactorial.
  - No single cause is identified or identifiable.
- In moderate to severe intellectual disability, a single cause may be identified by systematic investigation.

SIGNS AND SYMPTOMS

Intellectual disability, by level of function

- Mild
  - IQ: 55–70
  - 5th-grade academics by 18 years of age
  - Support level: intermittent
  - Adults generally function well independently, are able to work in competitive employment, and manage domestic affairs adequately.
  - Individuals may have difficulty with stress.
  - Individuals with mild intellectual disability usually benefit from the intermittent support of a care coordinator.
- Moderate
  - IQ: 40–55
  - 2nd-grade academics by 18 years of age
  - Support level: limited
  - Most adults are able to work in the community but often require ongoing job coaching, particularly to cope with changes in routine.
  - Adults are typically able to manage many aspects of their domestic life, such as hygiene and taking public transportation, but require some assistance with daily living.
- Severe
  - IQ: 25–40
  - Preschool academics by 18 years of age
  - Support level: extensive

- Individuals with severe intellectual disability typically cannot work in the community.
- Individuals often require significant daily assistance with many aspects of their domestic life.
- Profound
  - IQ: <25
  - Support level: pervasive
  - Individuals with profound intellectual disability cannot work in the community.
  - Individuals require significant daily assistance with many aspects of their domestic life.

Physical examination

- Can provide important clues to the cause of intellectual disability
- In the workup of global developmental delay or intellectual disability, referral for assessment of hearing and vision may be important.
- In addition to determining potential causes of intellectual disability, physical examination:
  - Establishes a connection with the child
  - Aids in assessment of interpersonal interactions

Behavioral symptoms

- Avoidance of diagnostic "overshadowing" or attributing all symptoms to intellectual disability is important.
  - Autism is a common comorbid feature of intellectual disability.
    - Several behavioral symptoms, such as irritability, aggression, and self-injury, are seen in both intellectual disability and autism.
    - Autism occurs at a higher rate in individuals with intellectual disability; a diagnosis of autism prompts differences in management.
    - For this reason, authorities strongly recommend that autism be considered, particularly in the face of characteristic symptoms.
  - Irritability and aggression have long been seen as intrinsic features of intellectual disability, often precluding more meticulous investigation.
    - Frequently, they are symptoms of psychiatric illness, such as depression or anxiety.
  - Self-injury may be a sign of physical illness.
    - For example, hitting the chest may be an indication of undiagnosed gastroesophageal reflux.
  - Apparent hypersexuality may be a manifestation of an uncomfortable erection in the context of inadequate sexuality education.

Nonspecific dysmorphic features associated with anomalous brain development

- Microcephaly
  - Reduced brain growth
- Cranial asymmetry
  - Premature suture fusion vs deforming external forces vs abnormal underlying brain growth
- Hair: absent or multiple (>2) parietal whorls
  - Abnormal brain development between 10 and 16 weeks' gestation
- Cowlick, or anterior upsweep of scalp hair
  - Posterior displacement of junction of parietal and frontal hair streams, resulting from reduced frontal brain development
- Short palpebral fissures
  - Deficient frontal brain growth
- Up-slanted palpebral fissures
  - Relatively deficient frontal brain growth compared with midface
- Low-set ears (top of helix below outer canthi)
  - Reflects delayed morphogenesis, as ears are low set in the early fetus
- Posterior rotation of ears (axis tilted backward >15 degrees)
  - Reflects delayed morphogenesis, as ears are posteriorly rotated in the early fetus
- High-arched mouth
  - Persistent lateral palatal ridges, indicative of oral hypotonia or other oral-motor dysfunction

DIFFERENTIAL DIAGNOSIS

Syndromes associated with intellectual disability

- Down syndrome
  - Brachycephaly
  - Microcephaly
  - Epicanthal folds
  - Brushfield spots
  - Upslanting palpebral fissures
  - Small ears
  - Small nose with low nasal bridge
  - Brachydactyly and clinodactyly
  - Single transverse palmar crease
  - Wide gap and plantar crease between first and second toes
  - Hypotonia
  - Short stature
- Fragile X syndrome
  - High forehead
  - Long jaw or face

- Large protuberant ears
- Velvety palmar skin with dorsal redundancy
- Hyperextensible joints
- Peripubertal macroorchidism
- Early onset overgrowth
- Initial shyness
- Repetitive behaviors and stereotypies
- Fetal alcohol syndrome
  - Microcephaly
  - Short palpebral fissures
  - Maxillary hypoplasia
  - Flat philtrum
  - Thin upper lip
  - Small distal phalanges and small fifth fingernail
  - Joint anomalies of position and function
  - Short stature
- Williams syndrome
  - Stellate iris
  - Short palpebral fissures
  - Medial eyebrow flare
  - Periorbital fullness
  - Flat nasal bridge
  - Anteverted nares
  - Long philtrum
  - Prominent lips
  - Hoarse voice
  - Heart murmur
  - Hyperactive deep-tendon reflexes
  - Friendly personality
  - Hyperactivity
  - Short stature
- Velocardiofacial syndrome
  - Narrow palpebral fissures
  - Cleft palate
  - Velopharyngeal insufficiency
  - Prominent nose with narrow base
  - Abundant scalp hair
  - Long face
  - Retruded mandible
  - Heart murmur
  - Slender, hypotonic limbs with hyperextensible hands and fingers
- Rett syndrome
  - Acquired delay in head growth
  - Acquired diminished eye contact and loss of speech
  - Repetitive purposeless midline hand movements, such as wringing or washing
  - Apraxia
  - Hypotonia, principally in girls

Neurocutaneous findings associated with intellectual disability

- Tuberous sclerosis complex
  - Hypomelanotic macules
    - Oval or ash-leaf shaped, few mm to cm, mostly on trunk or extremities; may occur in infancy
  - Shagreen patches
    - Firm yellow to red clusters of nodules, few mm to cm, on dorsum of body; particularly lumbosacral area; typically occurring at puberty (less commonly before)
  - Facial angiofibroma
    - Pink or red shiny nodules, on face, especially on nasolabial folds, usually appearing between 2 and 5 years of age
  - Forehead fibrous plaque
    - Yellowish-brown or flesh-colored, raised soft or hard plaque, few mm to cm, on forehead or scalp; can occur at any age
  - Periungual fibroma
    - Reddish or flesh colored, arising from nail bed or cuticle, found on toes more often than fingers, usually occurring at puberty or later
- Neurofibromatosis
  - Café-au-lait macules
    - Usually hyperpigmented, but also includes hypopigmented macules ≥5 mm
    - Axillary freckling
      - Small brown macules in axillae and perineum
    - Cutaneous neurofibroma
      - Small, raised, soft, pigmented nodules
- Sturge-Weber syndrome
  - Cranial port-wine stain
    - Light pink to deep purple birthmark, typically involving ≥1 upper eyelid and the forehead

DIAGNOSTIC APPROACH

General

- Diagnosis of intellectual disability requires documentation of impairment of cognition and of adaptive functioning.
- Communicating with families and patients about diagnosis is challenging.
  - Thoughtful communication is essential in helping families acknowledge a diagnosis that is difficult to accept.
  - Acceptance is essential in accessing important services.

- Careful and specific use of diagnostic labels and the consistent use of person-first language shows respect and compassion.
  - To state impairment first, as in *the intellectually disabled child,* implies that disability is the most salient characteristic of the child.
  - Saying the *child with a disability* is preferable.
- The American Academy of Neurology (AAN) has established criteria (below) for diagnosis of intellectual disability; these may be used for the diagnostic workup of intellectual disability and global developmental delay.
- A useful framework (below) for organizing the collection of these data, and for organizing the care plan, is provided by the International Classification of Functioning (ICF).
  - Emphasis on function over diagnostic labels and consideration of environmental factors
  - Congruent with guidelines put forth by the AAIDD
  - For the primary care physician, the ICF can serve as a review of functional status.
- International classification of functioning to organize evaluation and care plan

Guidelines from the AAN

- Cognitive impairment (IQ ≤90)
  - IQ is defined by a mean of 100, with standard deviation of 15.
  - Cognitive impairment is defined as an IQ ≥2 standard deviations below the mean.
- Adaptive impairment
  - Adaptive skills include such domains as communication, self-care, home living, social or interpersonal skills, use of community resources, self-direction, functional academic skills, work, leisure, health, and safety.
  - Adaptive impairment is identified by functioning in the range of impairment in these areas.
    - ≥2 standard deviations below the mean, as measured by formal testing on measures of adaptive functioning, such as the Vineland Adaptive Behavior Scales
- Onset of cognitive and adaptive impairment during the developmental period (<18 years of age)
  - Onset of cognitive and adaptive impairment after the developmental period would be referred to by etiology, for example, as traumatic brain injury.

ICF guidelines to evaluation

- Learning and applying knowledge
  - Elements to include in evaluation: Learning, thinking, problem solving, and decision making
- General tasks and demands
  - Elements to include in evaluation: Carrying out tasks, organizing routines, handling stress

- Communication
  - Elements to include in evaluation: Use of language, signs, and symbols; receiving and producing messages; carrying on conversation; use of communication devices and techniques
- Mobility
  - Elements to include in evaluation: Moving body position or location; transferring from one place to another; carrying, moving, and manipulating objects; walking, running, climbing; using transportation
- Self-care
  - Elements to include in evaluation: Washing, dressing, grooming, eating, drinking, hygiene, health practices
- Domestic life
  - Elements to include in evaluation: Acquiring food, clothing, place to live; household chores; assisting others
- Interpersonal interactions and relationships
  - Elements to include in evaluation: Basic and complex interactions with people, including strangers, friends, relatives, immediate family members, and intimate relations in a socially appropriate manner
- Major life areas
  - Elements to include in evaluation: Carrying out tasks related to education, work, and economic transactions
- Community, social, and civic life
  - Elements to include in evaluation: Recreation and leisure, religion or spirituality, political life or citizenship

LABORATORY FINDINGS

- Karyotype
  - Recommended in all children with moderate to severe global developmental delay or intellectual disability
- Metabolic workup
  - Not generally recommended if newborn screen is documented
  - Recommended with specific family history, consanguinity, regression, or episodic decompensation
- Fragile X syndrome (DNA methylation testing)
  - Recommended in boys with moderate to severe global developmental delay or intellectual disability
  - Particularly recommended when characteristic features are present
- Rett syndrome (*MECP2* gene testing)
  - Recommended in girls with moderate to severe global developmental delay or intellectual disability
  - Particularly recommended when characteristic features are present

- Subtelomeric fluorescence in situ hybridization
  - Before the development of complete genomic hybridization technology, this was the best test for the detection of small subtelomeric rearrangements.
  - This test has been replaced by microarray comparative genomic hybridization.
- Microarray comparative genomic hybridization
  - Consider in moderate to severe global developmental delay or intellectual disability.
  - This test has higher yield when ≥1 of the following features are present.
    - Family history of unexplained moderate to severe intellectual disability
    - Prenatal onset growth retardation
    - Postnatal growth abnormalities, including micro- or macrocephaly or short or tall stature
    - ≥2 dysmorphic facial features or nonfacial congenital anomalies
- Thyroid function testing
  - Recommended if no newborn screen documented or with characteristic symptoms, such as:
    - Late tooth eruption or fontanelle closure
    - Weight for age above height for age
    - Constipation
    - Delayed relaxation phase of deep-tendon reflexes
- Lead testing
  - Levels are found to be elevated at higher rate in children with intellectual disability than in children without.
  - Pica is a behavioral characteristic associated with intellectual disability.

IMAGING

- Brain magnetic resonance imaging
  - Recommended for global developmental delay, although clinical picture should be taken into account
  - Lower yield in mild global developmental delay, which tends to be familial
  - Higher yield with focal or abnormal neurological examination, in the presence of cranial anomalies or neurocutaneous features

DIAGNOSTIC PROCEDURES

- Ophthalmologic assessment
  - Recommended in all children with moderate to severe global developmental delay or intellectual disability

- Audiologic assessment
  - Recommended in all children with moderate to severe global developmental delay or intellectual disability
- Electroencephalography
  - Recommended only if a clinical indication of seizures is present

WHEN TO REFER

- Infants and toddlers failing to meet developmental milestones using standard reference instruments, such as:
  - Ages and Stages Questionnaire
  - Child Development Inventory
  - Parents' Evaluation of Development Status
  - Bright Futures guidelines
- A pediatrician need not conduct formal developmental screening to refer for evaluation through early intervention programs.
- Referrals can be based on objective criteria or clinical judgment.
- Parents who express concerns about their child's development should have their concerns validated by a referral to early intervention services.
- If the primary care physician even suspects developmental delay, erring on the side of caution would be advisable.
- Children with a new diagnosis of global developmental delay or of intellectual disability:
  - Should have a medical evaluation to determine the causes of the delays
  - The primary care physician may wish to refer to subspecialists in genetics, developmental and behavioral pediatrics, or neurodevelopmental disabilities.
- Children of sufficient age who are suspected of having intellectual disability and who have not had a formal psychological assessment should be referred for evaluation of cognitive abilities, academic achievement, and adaptive skills.
  - Families may obtain such testing free of charge through their local school district by making a formal request for a multidisciplinary evaluation.
  - Primary care physicians can support families in this endeavor by providing references to the process of requesting an evaluation through the school district.
  - Families may obtain an independent psychological evaluation from a private psychologist.

Iron-Deficiency Anemia

DEFINITION

- Iron-deficiency anemia (IDA) is the most common nutritional deficiency worldwide.
- Children with iron deficiency in infancy continue to have poor cognition and school achievement and increased behavior problems into middle childhood.
- Iron deficiency is associated with deficits in work productivity.
- Severe anemia is associated with maternal and child mortality.
- Prevention of iron deficiency is therefore an important public health issue.
- Iron deficiency occurs when total body iron content is diminished.
- When absorption exceeds losses, iron surplus is stored in the reticuloendothelial system.
  - Liver
  - Spleen
  - Bone marrow
- Iron is removed from the reticuloendothelial storage pool to compensate for negative iron balance.
- Development of iron deficiency proceeds through a series of overlapping stages:
- Stage 1
  - The first stage of iron deficiency is storage iron depletion.
  - Anisocytosis and an increased percentage of microcytic cells are the first hematologic abnormalities.
  - During this stage, no deficit of iron supplied to the erythroid marrow for red blood cell (RBC) production occurs.
- Stage 2
  - If the negative iron balance continues, iron-deficient erythropoiesis (IDE) will occur.
  - Mean corpuscular volume (MCV) and mean corpuscular hemoglobin (MCH) decrease.
  - During this stage, erythroid iron supply is diminished, but hemoglobin concentration remains in the normal range.
- Stage 3
  - If the negative iron balance persists, IDA finally develops.
  - The third stage is characterized by a decrease in the hemoglobin concentration and reduction in RBC size and hemoglobin content.
  - Hematologic abnormalities in iron deficiency progress as impairment of hematopoiesis progresses.
  - Characterized by:
    - Low MCH
    - Hemoglobin concentration <9 g/dL
    - Transferrin saturation <16%

EPIDEMIOLOGY

- In the US
  - Common, despite the generally good standard of nutrition and the widespread use of iron-fortified foods
  - Most common among women and young children
- Age
  - IDA is most prevalent among:
    - Toddlers age 1–2 years (7%)
    - Adolescent girls
    - Adult women age 12–49 years (9–16%)
- Race/ethnicity
  - Prevalence is 2 times higher among African-American and Latino-American women (19–22%) than among white women (10%).
  - Prevalence remains higher than the goal of national health objectives for 2010 to reduce iron deficiency in vulnerable populations by 3–4 percentage points.

ETIOLOGY

- The 4 most important factors in the development of iron deficiency in children are:
  - Iron endowment at birth
  - Iron needs during rapid body growth
  - Exogenous iron absorption
  - Blood loss

Causes of iron deficiency

- Inadequate iron absorption
  - Diet low in bioavailable iron
    - Formula not fortified with iron
    - Cow's milk before the age of 6 months
    - Strict vegetarian diet
    - Poor dietary habits in adolescents
  - Impaired absorption
    - Intestinal malabsorption
    - Gastric surgery
    - Hypochlorhydria
- Increased iron requirements
- Blood loss
  - Menstruation
  - Gastrointestinal tract
    - Milk enteropathy
    - Food sensitivity
    - Inflammatory bowel disease
    - Meckel diverticulum
    - Peptic ulcer disease

- Reflux esophagitis
- Hookworms
- Cancer
- Genitourinary tract
- Respiratory tract
  - Idiopathic pulmonary
  - Hemosiderosis
  - Cystic fibrosis
  - Pulmonary tuberculosis
- Cardiac
  - Hemosiderinuria due to cardiac hemolysis
- Blood donation
- Pregnancy
- Growth
  - Prematurity
  - Infancy
  - Adolescence

During gestation

- Fetal iron stores in newborns are related to maternal iron status, and the maternal-fetal unit is dependent on exogenous iron.
- The ratio of iron content to weight in the human fetus remains constant throughout gestation.
- The healthy full-term newborn has sufficient iron stores to last for 6 months, if sufficient small amounts of iron are ingested from the diet.
- The infant's iron endowment can be compromised by blood loss during pregnancy or the perinatal period.
- Common causes of blood loss include:
  - Third-trimester bleeding
    - Abruptio placentae
    - Placenta previa
    - Fetomaternal hemorrhage
    - Twin-to-twin transfusions

During growth

- Iron is needed not only for many metabolic functions and tissue replacement, but also for growth.
- Growth rates vary with age and are maximal during infancy and adolescence, the same periods associated with the highest frequency of iron deficiency.
- Blood loss causes iron deficiency in children less frequently than in adults.
- In infancy and childhood, iron deficiency caused by blood loss is most commonly associated with the ingestion of unprocessed cow's milk and with parasitic infections.
  - Hypersensitivity to whole cow's milk causes an exudative enteropathy and frequently leads to gastrointestinal blood loss.

- Less common causes of blood loss in children include:
  - Meckel diverticulum
  - Intestinal duplication
  - Peptic ulcer disease
  - Hereditary hemorrhagic telangiectasia
  - Long-term use of medications that prolong the bleeding time (eg, aspirin)

RISK FACTORS

- Gestational conditions that result in lower newborn iron stores include:
  - Severe maternal iron deficiency
  - Maternal hypertension with intrauterine growth retardation
  - Maternal diabetes mellitus
- Stable, very low–birth-weight premature infants are also at risk for early postnatal iron deficiency because they:
  - Accrete less iron during gestation
  - Grow more rapidly after birth
  - Typically are undertreated with enteral iron

SIGNS AND SYMPTOMS

History

- The onset and progression of iron deficiency are usually gradual.
- Most children will not have major symptoms.
- Iron deficiency in infants and children is associated with:
  - Generalized weakness
  - Irritability
  - Easy fatigability
  - Headaches
  - Poor feeding
  - Anorexia
  - Pica
  - Poor weight gain

Physical examination

- The physical examination is usually unremarkable except for marked pallor of the mucous membranes and skin.
- Other physical findings associated with IDA but rarely observed include:
  - Mild hepatosplenomegaly
  - Lymphadenopathy
  - Glossitis
  - Stomatitis
  - Blue sclerae
  - Koilonychia (spoon-shaped nails)

DIFFERENTIAL DIAGNOSIS

- Iron deficiency must be distinguished from other hypochromic microcytic anemias.
- Serum transferrin receptor levels help discriminate iron deficiency from the anemias of chronic disease.

Thalassemia trait

- IDA and thalassemia trait are the most common causes of mild microcytic anemia with hemoglobin level ≥9 g/dL.
- The RBC count is often increased above normal despite the presence of a mild anemia and microcytosis in thalassemia trait, whereas it is reduced in IDA.
- The RBC distribution width (RDW) is increased in iron deficiency.
- The Mentzer index, defined as the MCV divided by the RBC count in millions, can help distinguish the anemia of iron deficiency from that of ß-thalassemia trait.
  - In IDA, the Mentzer index is often >13.5.
  - In ß-thalassemia trait, it is <11.5, with 82% specificity.
  - The RDW index (RDWI) is calculated using the formula RDWI = (MCV ÷ RBC × RDW)
    - An RDWI ≥220 is indicative of IDA.
    - An RDWI <220 is indicative of thalassemia trait, with a specificity of 92%.
- The RBC count and RDWI are the most reliable discrimination indices in differentiation between ß-thalassemia trait and IDA.
- If α- and ß-thalassemia trait or hemoglobin E disease is suspected, the diagnosis can be established by:
  - Review of the newborn screen
  - Performing hemoglobin electrophoresis (only in case of ß-thalassemia and not α-thalassemia)
    - Because thalassemia trait is frequently not associated with a hemoglobin level <9 g/dL, it is not included in the differential diagnosis in severe anemia.
    - The diagnosis of α-thalassemia trait can be assumed when a patient with a familial hypochromic microcytic anemia has normal results of iron studies (including ferritin), normal levels of hemoglobin (Hb) A_2 and Hb F, and normal hemoglobin electrophoresis.
    - It is a diagnosis of exclusion, except in the newborn period, when infants with a-thalassemia trait have 3–10% Hb Barts (γ_4), which may be detected in the newborn screen.

Hb H disease

- Hb H disease, another form of α-thalassemia, results from deletion of 3 of the 4 α-globin genes.
- It is characterized by hypochromia and microcytosis.
- A mild hemolytic component is present from instability of the ß-chain tetramers (Hb H) resulting from a deficiency of α-globin chains.
- Beyond infancy, Hb H is readily identified by hemoglobin electrophoresis.
- During the newborn period, the moderately severe α-globin deficiency allows accumulation of more γ chains, and the concentration of Hb Barts is >20%.

Anemia of chronic disease or inflammation

- Inflammation impairs the supply of iron to the plasma and ultimately results in a form of anemia called *anemia of chronic disease* or *anemia of inflammation*.
  - It is usually normocytic, although it may occasionally be slightly microcytic.
  - Because inflammation alters screening tests for iron status in the same manner as true iron deficiency, the distinction between anemia of chronic disease and IDA requires tissue-related iron measurements.
  - Usefulness of the serum ferritin in the diagnosis of IDA is compromised by the effect of inflammation on the value.
  - Consequently, a serum ferritin concentration >30 mg/L in an anemic patient does not exclude IDA in the presence of chronic inflammation.
- C-reactive protein level is generally considered to be the best laboratory marker of inflammation.
  - If it is <30 mg/L, the inflammation is generally considered unlikely to be sufficient to increase the serum ferritin level.
  - Suggested ferritin levels of <40 mg/L and <70 mg/L are used to diagnose IDA in anemic patients without and with inflammation, respectively.
  - The serum transferrin receptor (sTfR) measurement for identifying IDA is one in which the concentration is not affected by inflammation.
  - Use of the sTfR/ferritin ratio further improves the specificity of the diagnosis of IDA and may eliminate the need for bone marrow examination for assessment of iron stores.

Lead poisoning and anemia

- Lead poisoning and IDA are both associated with high levels of RBC zinc protoporphyrins (ZnPP).
- Iron deficiency and lead poisoning frequently coexist.
- Although the nature of their relationship is not completely elucidated, characterization of a common iron-lead transporter and epidemiologic studies among children strongly suggest that iron deficiency may increase susceptibility to lead poisoning.
- In cases of lead poisoning associated with iron deficiency, the RBCs are morphologically similar, but coarse basophilic stippling of the RBCs is frequently prominent.
- Increases in blood lead, ZnPP/heme (ZnPP/H) ratio, and urinary coproporphyrin levels are seen.

Laboratory Abnormalities in the Three Stages of Iron Deficiency[a]

	Normal Iron States	Stage 1 Storage Iron Depletion	Stage 2 Transport Iron Depletion	Stage 3 Functional Iron Depletion (Iron Deficiency Anemia
Hemoglobin	N	N	↑	↓
Serum iron	N	N	↓	↓
TIBC	N	N	↑	↑
Ferritin	N	↓	↓	↓

Abbreviation: N, normal.

[a] Adapted from: Rodak BF, Fritsma GA, Doig K. *Hematology Clinical Principles and Applications.* 3rd ed. Philadelphia, PA: WB Saunders; 2007. Copyright © Elsevier 2007.

[b] ↑, increased; ↓, decreased.

DIAGNOSTIC APPROACH

- Diagnosis of iron deficiency is made by the combination of:
  - RBC indices
  - Serum transferrin saturation
  - Ferritin
- Transferrin saturation and ferritin may be altered by:
  - Infection
  - Inflammation
  - Cancer
  - Starvation
- Although absence of iron stores in the bone marrow remains the gold standard for a diagnosis of iron deficiency, this test is rarely used because of patient discomfort and the difficulty of standardizing bone marrow iron stain.
- Once IDA is diagnosed, efforts should be undertaken to establish its cause.
- A therapeutic iron trial has been proposed as a convenient method to diagnose iron deficiency in patients with anemia.
  - This approach is reasonable in otherwise healthy individuals.
  - Making a definitive laboratory diagnosis at the outset is preferable for those at high risk of deficiency, such as:
    - Infants
    - Teenage girls
    - Pregnant women

LABORATORY FINDINGS

- Specific laboratory findings are associated with each of the 3 stages of iron deficiency.
- Laboratory test findings characteristic of each stage are summarized in table Laboratory Abnormalities in the Three Stages of Iron Deficiency.
- Tests demonstrate either a reduced supply of plasma iron or poor hemoglobinization of circulating RBCs.

- Definitive tests identify IDA by measuring iron-related proteins derived from either iron storage compartment in macrophages or iron utilization compartment in RBC precursors.

Screening measurements

Hemoglobin concentration

- The most commonly used screening test for iron deficiency
- Someone with normal body iron stores must lose a large portion of body iron before hemoglobin falls below laboratory definitions of anemia.
- Low hemoglobin does not distinguish among the causes of anemia other than iron deficiency, so additional testing is required.

Serum iron and transferrin saturation

- Serum iron levels normally fluctuate daily, with maximal levels occurring in the morning and minimal levels in the evening.
- Total iron-binding capacity (TIBC) varies less than serum iron but is harder to measure accurately.
- Normal TIBC is 250–400 mg/dL, but as serum iron levels decrease, TIBC increases to ≥450 mg/dL.
- Iron and TIBC measurements are useful in distinguishing IDA from anemia of chronic disease.
- Serum iron levels decrease with both, but TIBC levels also decrease in chronic disease states (table Laboratory Findings Associated With the Differential Diagnosis of Microcytic Anemias).
- Degree of iron saturation of plasma transferrin is calculated as follows: transferrin saturation = (serum iron concentration ÷ TIBC) × 100.
- Serum iron and TIBC levels help confirm the diagnosis of iron deficiency, with a low serum iron and a high transferrin level, resulting in a transferrin saturation <10–15%.
- Transferrin levels are increased in iron-deficiency states because of increased hepatic synthesis of the protein and greater liberation of apotransferrin (the transport protein without iron) from hemoglobin-synthesizing sites.

Laboratory Findings Associated With the Differential Diagnosis of Microcytic Anemias[a]

Finding	Iron Deficiency	Lead Poisoning	ß-Thalassemia Trait	Chronic Disease
Ferritin	↓	Normal	Normal	↑
Serum iron	↓	Normal	Normal	↓
Total iron-binding capacity	↑	Normal	Normal	↓
Erythrocyte zinc protoporphyrin	↑	↑↑	Normal	↑
Red blood cell distribution width	↑	Normal	Normal	Normal
Serum transferrin receptor	↑	Normal	↑	Normal

[a]↑, increased; ↑↑, very increased; ↓, decreased. Iron deficiency and lead poisoning frequently co-exist.

Red Blood Cell Indices During Infancy and Childhood[a]

Age		Hemoglobin (g/dL)		Hematocrit (%)		Reticulocytes (%)	MCV (fL)
		Mean	Range	Mean	Range	Mean	Lowest
Child	Cord blood	16.8	13.7–20.1	55	45–65	5.0	110
	2 wk	16.5	13.0–20.0	50	42–66	1.0	107
	3 mo	12.0	9.5–14.5	36	31–41	1.0	80
	6 mo–6 yr	12.0	10.5–14.0	37	33–42	1.0	70–74
	7–12 yr	13.0	11.0–16.0	38	34–40	1.0	76–80
Adult	Female	14	12.0–16.0	42	37–47	1.6	80
	Male	16	14.0–18.0	47	42–52	1.6	80

Abbreviations: MCV, mean corpuscular volume; WBC, white blood cells.
[a] Modified from: Behrman RE. *Nelson Textbook of Pediatrics*. 17th ed. Philadelphia, PA: WB Saunders; 2004. Copyright © Elsevier 2004.

- This relatively inexpensive measurement is widely available.
- Marked diurnal variation in plasma iron values and numerous clinical disorders that affect transferrin saturation limit its use in the clinical setting.
- Transferrin saturation
  - Normal or high transferrin saturation is useful for excluding IDA.
  - Low transferrin saturation is useful for identifying IDA.

RBC indices

- Development of electronic counters has made use of RBC indices widely available for initial screening of infants and children.
- These tests are highly reproducible and less subject to sampling error compared with hemoglobin determinations because tissue fluid dilution does not affect RBC size.
- RBCs become smaller than normal (decreased MCV), and their hemoglobin content decreases (decreased MCH).
- RDW approximates the standard deviation of the RBC size variation.

- Normal RDWs occur in the range of 12–17%.
- In IDA, a marked dispersion exists in cell volumes (sizes), such that the RDW increases.
- RBC indices in infancy and childhood are described in table Red Blood Cell Indices During Infancy and Childhood.

ZnPP

- A simple and reliable measurement of IDE is the RBC ZnPP, a product of abnormal heme synthesis.
- Normally, a trace of zinc rather than iron is incorporated into protoporphyrin during the final step of heme biosynthesis.
- In states of IDE, ZnPP formation is enhanced.
- An increase in the ZnPP/H ratio >80 mcmol/mol is a sensitive, specific, and cost-effective test for identifying preanemic iron deficiency.
- A major advantage is the ability to measure the ZnPP/H ratio directly on a drop of blood using a portable instrument called a *hematofluorimeter*.
- Initially, ZnPP was erroneously characterized as metal-free protoporphyrin or free RBC protoporphyrin or RBC protoporphyrin.

- Now, most presumed metal-free protoporphyrin in RBCs is known to be largely an artifact of older analytical procedures (still used in some laboratories).
- Because approximately 95% of the nonheme protoporphyrin in RBCs is ZnPP, this procedure should not create a diagnostic problem.
- The ZnPP/H ratio is an indicator of iron available to developing RBCs in bone marrow regardless of the cause, such as iron deficiency, inflammation, or functional iron deficiency such as in chronic renal failure.
- Another significant limitation of ZnPP are with lead toxicity and the normal range with environmental lead exposure, infections, inflammatory diseases, and protoporphyria.
- However, the ZnPP/H ratio is not increased in thalassemia trait, which makes ZnPP/H ratio determinations helpful in distinguishing iron deficiency from α- or ß-thalassemia trait, in addition to its use screening for IDA (table Laboratory Findings Associated With the Differential Diagnosis of Microcytic Anemias).

Reticulocyte hemoglobin

- The mean reticulocyte hemoglobin content is analogous to the RBC mean corpuscular hemoglobin, but with the advantage of monitoring hemoglobinization of the most recently produced RBCs.
- A reticulocyte hemoglobin concentration <26 pg is an early indicator of iron-restricted hematopoiesis and IDA in children.
- The diagnostic power of reticulocyte hemoglobin is limited in patients with high MCV or with RBC disorders, such as thalassemia.

Peripheral blood smear

- Examination of the blood smear in IDA reveals:
  - Hypochromic microcytes
  - Poikilocytes
  - Elliptocytes
  - Target cells
- Presence of basophilic stippling suggests associated lead poisoning.
- RBC changes seen on the blood smear are not specific for iron deficiency.
- Leukocyte count and morphology in IDA are usually normal.
- Both thrombocytosis and thrombocytopenia occur with iron deficiency.
  - Thrombocytopenia is more common in severe iron deficiency and resolves once iron therapy is begun.

Definitive tests

- Absence of stainable iron in bone marrow is a definitive test for IDA but is not routinely applicable for obvious reasons.

- The 2 key definitive measurements for diagnosing iron deficiency are serum ferritin, which measures the size of iron stores, and serum transferrin receptor, which measures the extent of tissue iron deficiency.
  - Serum ferritin
    - Definitive serum ferritin levels vary with age during infancy and childhood.
    - In healthy individuals, serum ferritin levels reflect body iron stores.
    - Levels <30 ng/L indicate iron deficiency.
    - Ferritin is an acute-phase reactant.
    - Serum ferritin levels are increased during infections, inflammatory processes, liver disease.
    - Although low serum ferritin is diagnostic of iron deficiency, high ferritin associated with inflammation or liver disease does not rule out concomitant iron deficiency.
  - sTfR
    - Proteolytic cleavage of transferrin receptors can be measured in serum as sTfR.
    - sTfR directly correlates with total mass of erythroid precursor.
    - sTfR is high in iron deficiency and in conditions resulting in increased production of RBCs, including thalassemia and sickle cell disease.
    - Because sTfR is not affected by inflammation, it is useful in distinguishing iron deficiency from chronic inflammatory states that do not have high sTfR (table Laboratory Findings Associated With the Differential Diagnosis of Microcytic Anemias).
    - Infants have higher baseline sTfR levels than children and adults, indicating the need to establish age-specific reference values.
    - The ratio of sTfR to serum ferritin has been shown to have excellent performance in estimating body iron stores but is limited by lack of standardization.

Bone marrow iron

- The staining of a normal bone marrow aspirate sample with Prussian blue dye reveals the presence of iron in RBC precursors (normoblasts) and serves as a reliable index of body iron stores.
- In iron deficiency, the number of iron granules in normoblasts is decreased, and stainable iron in the marrow aspirate is almost completely absent.

TREATMENT APPROACH

- The treatment of choice for iron deficiency is oral administration of iron.

SPECIFIC TREATMENTS

Oral administration of iron

- Although various iron salts are available, ferrous sulfate is inexpensive and well tolerated, although adverse effects may occur, such as:
  - Nausea
  - Dyspepsia
  - Constipation
  - Diarrhea
- Adverse effects can be managed by administering the iron with or immediately after meals.
- If symptoms persist, reductions in the amount of iron in each dose or reduction in frequency to a single daily dose may help control side effects.
- If intolerance is persistent, then switching to ferrous gluconate may be helpful.
- Iron polysaccharide complex has the advantage of availability as tablets or elixir and is well tolerated.
- Approximately twice as much iron is absorbed on an empty stomach as at mealtime.
- Consumption of milk should be limited, allowing increased intake of iron-rich foods and reduction of blood loss from intolerance to cow's milk proteins.
- Soy-based formulas can lead to blood loss, so children with milk enteropathy should be switched to a primary diet of iron-containing solids.
- In the absence of ongoing blood losses, response to iron therapy is rapid and predictable.
- Response of decreased irritability and increased appetite has been noted within 12–24 hours (table Responses to Iron Therapy in Iron-Deficiency Anemia).
- Reticulocyte response peaks 5–7 days after the institution of iron therapy.
- In an otherwise healthy individual, recovery from anemia is approximately two-thirds complete within 1 month.
- Hemoglobin should be measured again at 1 month to check therapeutic progress and to emphasize compliance.
- If after 4 weeks anemia does not respond to iron treatment despite compliance and absence of acute illness, then anemia can be further evaluated by using other laboratory tests, including MCV, RDW, and serum ferritin concentration.
- Serum ferritin concentration ≤15 mcg/L confirms iron deficiency, and a concentration >15 mcg/L suggests that iron deficiency is not the cause of the anemia.
- Once diagnosis is confirmed, either by a response to a therapeutic trial or by further tests, oral therapy with elemental iron at 3–6 mg/kg per day should be continued for 2–3 months after normal hemoglobin levels have been restored.

Responses to Iron Therapy in Iron-Deficiency Anemia[a]

Time After Iron Administration	Response
12–24 hr	Replacement of intracellular iron enzymes; subjective improvement; decreased irritability; increased appetite
36–48 hr	Initial bone marrow response; erythroid hyperplasia
48–72 hr	Reticulocytosis, peaking at 5–7 days
4–30 day	Increase in hemoglobin level
1–3 mo	Repletion of stores

[a] From: Behrman RE. *Nelson Textbook of Pediatrics.* 17th ed. Philadelphia, PA: WB Saunders; 2004. Copyright © Elsevier 2004.

- This regimen allows the repletion of body iron stores.
- Anemia, microcytosis, and increased free RBC protoporphyrin levels are corrected completely with 3–5 months of treatment.

Intramuscular or intravenous iron

- Use of intramuscular or intravenous iron is rarely warranted.
- Parenteral iron administration may be indicated.
  - If ongoing blood loss exceeds the body's ability to replenish iron stores through oral absorption
  - In the presence of iron malabsorption
  - When the patient cannot tolerate or will not take oral iron preparations
- Intramuscular injections are painful, and skin discoloration is common.
- Anaphylactic reactions have occurred with both intramuscular and intravenous injection, and deaths have been reported.
- Parenteral treatment should therefore be used only when oral therapy is not possible, eg, in patients with inflammatory bowel disease.
- 3 drugs are licensed in the US.
  - Iron dextran has been used for several years but is associated with significant risks.
  - Iron sucrose and iron gluconate may have a better safety profile than iron dextran.

Blood transfusion

- Blood transfusion is indicated only when severe anemia leads to congestive heart failure and cardiovascular compromise.
- If a blood transfusion is clinically warranted, then packed RBCs should be given slowly or a partial exchange transfusion performed.
- Vital signs should be monitored carefully.

Failure to respond to therapy

■ When a patient fails to respond to oral iron treatment, the following factors should be considered:

- Noncompliance with oral therapy
- Inadequate iron dose
- Persistent or unrecognized blood loss
- Malabsorption of iron (eg, primary gastrointestinal disease)
- Other diagnoses (eg, α- or ß-thalassemia trait and Hb E disease)
- Poor iron utilization (eg, chronic inflammatory disease, sideroblastic anemia, lead poisoning, congenital atransferrinemia)

WHEN TO ADMIT

■ The patient exhibits signs of cardiac failure.

■ The patient requires intravenous iron.

■ The patient has moderate to severe blood loss.

WHEN TO REFER

■ The cause of anemia is unknown.

■ Gastrointestinal blood loss is suspected.

■ Anemia is not explained by nutritional imbalance.

■ Anemia is refractory to treatment.

■ The patient requires intravenous iron.

■ The diagnosis of iron deficiency is questionable.

FOLLOW-UP

■ After an iron therapy is initiated, the patient should be re-evaluated at 1 month to see whether there is response.

- If, despite compliance, there is no response to treatment, an alternate diagnosis should be considered.

COMPLICATIONS

■ Iron is an important ingredient of hemoglobin and is involved in numerous cellular processes.

■ Children with iron deficiency in infancy have:

- Poor cognition
- Poor school achievement
- Increased behavior problems into middle childhood

■ Iron deficiency is also associated with deficits in work productivity.

■ Severe anemia is associated with maternal and child mortality.

PROGNOSIS

■ Prognosis for nutritional iron deficiency is good.

PREVENTION

■ Prevention of iron deficiency is an important public health issue.

■ Iron balance is maintained by regulation of iron absorption.

- The amount absorbed depends both on amount and bioavailability of dietary iron and on regulation of iron absorption by the intestinal mucosa.
- Most dietary iron occurs in the nonheme form and is much less bioavailable than that in heme proteins.
- The iron in hemoglobin and myoglobin is particularly bioavailable; up to 30% is directly absorbed by the gastrointestinal tract.
- Human milk and cow's milk contain small amounts of iron (0.5–1 mg/1000 mL).
  - However, 50% of the iron in human milk is absorbed, compared with only 10% in cow's milk.
  - Full-term infants who are exclusively breastfed for the first 6–9 months do not become iron deficient.
- Nonheme iron absorption is inhibited by:
  - Bran in cereals
  - Polyphenols in many vegetables
  - Tannins in tea
- Addition of solids to an infant's diet can greatly impair iron absorption and puts the infant at risk for developing iron deficiency.
  - The introduced solids should contain abundant amounts of iron (eg, iron-fortified cereals).

■ Increased iron intake among infants has resulted in a decline in childhood IDA in the US.

■ Consequently, use of screening tests has become a less efficient means of detecting iron deficiency in some populations, whereas for women of childbearing age, iron deficiency has remained prevalent.

■ The Centers for Disease Control and Prevention (CDC) has developed recommendations for primary prevention of iron deficiency through appropriate dietary intake and secondary prevention through detecting and treating IDA.

CDC recommendations

Primary prevention of iron deficiency in infants, children, and adolescents

■ Breastfeeding and iron-fortified formula

- Encourage exclusive breastfeeding of infants (without supplementary liquid, formula, or food) for 4–6 months after birth.
- When exclusive breastfeeding is stopped, encourage use of an additional source of iron (approximately 1 mg/kg daily), preferably from supplementary foods.
- For infants <12 months who are not breastfed or who are partially breastfed, recommend only iron-fortified infant formula as a substitute for human milk.

- For breastfed infants who receive insufficient iron from supplementary foods by age 6 months (ie, <1 mg/kg daily), suggest 1 mg/kg daily of iron drops.

- For breastfed infants who were preterm or who had low birth weight, recommend 2–4 mg/kg daily of iron drops (to a maximum of 15 mg/day) starting at 1 month after birth and continuing until 12 months after birth.

- Encourage use of only human milk or iron-fortified infant formula for any milk-based part of the diet (eg, in infant cereal) and discourage use of low-iron milks (eg, cow's milk, goat's milk, soy milk) until age 12 months.

- Suggest that children age 1–5 years consume no more than 24 oz of cow's milk, goat's milk, or soy milk each day.

■ Solid foods

- At age 4–6 months or when the extrusion reflex disappears, recommend that infants be introduced to plain, iron-fortified infant cereal.

- ≥2 servings per day of iron-fortified infant cereal can meet an infant's requirement for iron at this age.

- By approximately age 6 months, encourage 1 feeding per day of foods rich in vitamin C (eg, fruits, vegetables, juice) to improve iron absorption, preferably with meals.

- Suggest introducing plain, pureed meats after age 6 months or when the infant is developmentally ready to consume such food.

■ Adolescent girls and nonpregnant women

- Encourage adolescent girls and women to eat iron-rich foods and foods that enhance iron absorption and to optimize their dietary iron intake.

Screening for iron deficiency in infants, children, and adolescents

■ Anemia screening before age 6 months for preterm infants and low–birth-weight infants who are not fed iron-fortified infant formula

■ Annual assessment of children age 2–5 years for risk factors for IDA (eg, a low-iron diet, limited access to food because of poverty or neglect, special health care needs)

■ Assessment at age 9–12 months and 6 months later (at age 15–18 months) for infants and young children for risk factors for anemia

- Preterm or low birth weight infants

- Infants fed a diet of non–iron-fortified infant formula for ≥2 months

- Infants introduced to cow's milk before age 12 months

- Breastfed infants who do not consume a diet adequate in iron after age 6 months (ie, who receive insufficient iron from supplementary foods)

- Children who consume ≥24 oz daily of cow's milk

- Children with special health care needs (eg, children who use medications that interfere with iron absorption and children who have chronic infection, inflammatory disorders, restricted diets, or extensive blood loss from a wound, an accident, or surgery)

■ In populations of infants and preschool children at high risk for IDA (eg, children from low-income families, children eligible for the Special Supplemental Nutrition Program for Women, Infants, and Children, migrant children, or recently arrived refugee children), screen all children for anemia between ages 9 and 12 months, 6 months later, and annually from age 2–5 years.

■ Starting in adolescence, screen all nonpregnant women for anemia every 5–10 years throughout their childbearing years during routine health examinations.

■ Annually screen for anemia women with risk factors for iron deficiency (eg, extensive menstrual or other blood loss, low iron intake, a previous diagnosis of IDA).

Irritability

DEFINITION

- Irritability is excessive response to a stimulus.
- Not a quantifiable symptom
  - Includes episodes of crying or fussiness despite attempts to comfort

MECHANISM

- May result from:
  - Lack of vital nutrients (eg, oxygen, glucose)
  - Presence of noxious stimuli (eg, pain, toxins)
  - An emotional state (eg, anger, frustration)
- Causes and manifestations may be different in infants, children, and adolescents.

HISTORY

- Acute irritability may be associated with life-threatening illnesses requiring urgent intervention and stabilization before a search for the cause can begin.
- A parent who seeks care for an infant who is fussier than usual may arrive with a child who is in shock, in respiratory distress, or having a seizure.
- If the child's condition is not immediately life-threatening, then a complete history and thorough physical examination are the first steps in the evaluation of irritability, and, in many cases, will reveal the cause of the symptom.

PHYSICAL EXAM

- A thorough head-to-toe examination, including special attention to the eyes, ears, digits, and genitalia, is essential to establish a diagnosis.
- Irritability and nonspecific crying episodes may be related to:
  - Foreign body in the ear or nose
  - Corneal abrasion
  - Hair wrapped around a digit or penis
  - Diaper rash
  - Nonspecific vaginitis
  - Balanitis
  - Insect and spider bites or stings
  - Vaccination pain
- A systematic search for injuries should be performed on any child with a history of trauma.
  - Inflicted injuries are more difficult to diagnose.
  - Signs may be subtle, and the history often is misleading.
  - Causes may be easily apparent, such as fractures or dislocations.

DIFFERENTIAL DIAGNOSIS

Acute irritability in the ill-appearing child

Central nervous system

- Children <2 years are at high risk for significant brain injury after accidental head trauma.
  - Overall rates of brain injury are:
    - Approximately 12% in the 0- to 2-month age group
    - 6% in the 3- to 11-month age group
    - 2% in infants >12 months of age
  - A history of a fall is often found.
  - A high index of suspicion should be maintained in infants <3 months.
- Concussion may be sustained from sports-related injuries.
  - The term *postconcussive syndrome* refers to a constellation of acute symptoms, which can be:
    - Somatic (headache, dizziness, blurriness)
    - Emotional (irritability, anxiety)
    - Cognitive (concentration and memory difficulties)
  - The term *second impact syndrome* has been proposed for an athlete who:
    - Has sustained a concussion and then sustains a second head injury before symptoms associated with the first have fully cleared
    - These athletes are at risk for a catastrophic outcome, such as permanent disability or death.
- Brain tumor
  - Increased intracranial pressure (ICP) from a brain tumor may produce acute irritability and altered behavior without the usual preceding symptoms, such as headache or loss of coordination.
  - Diagnosis may be delayed in young children because their symptoms are subtle (eg, headache, irritability, or drowsiness) or similar to those of more common illnesses, such as gastrointestinal disorders (eg, vomiting).
- Hydrocephalus
  - Causes increased ICP
  - Often occurs in infancy with irritability, vomiting, a tense or bulging fontanel, and an increasing head circumference that crosses percentile lines
  - Older children usually complain of headaches.
  - Obstruction, infection, or malfunction of the ventriculo-peritoneal shunt may lead to over- or underdrainage, initially causing irritability, headache, vomiting, or lethargy.
- Undiagnosed migraine headache may be the reason for irritability in the preverbal child.
  - Migraine headaches occur in 8–12% of children <3 years.
- Seizures
  - Children with seizures, especially unwitnessed, may appear irritable during an aura or the postictal phase.

- Neonatal seizures
  - More common in preterm infants than term infants
  - May have only subtle symptoms
    - Ocular or pedaling movements
    - Lip smacking
    - Apnea
- Nonconvulsive status epilepticus, which includes absence and partial complex seizures, is a relatively rare cause of abnormal behavior.
  - Produces continuous or intermittent seizure activity in the absence of any motor component and without a return to baseline for >30 minutes
  - Irritability and a change in behavior or mental status may be associated findings.
- Infant botulism
  - Initial findings may include:
    - Difficulty in feeding
    - Irritability
    - Lethargy
    - Weak cry
    - Constipation
  - Findings in advanced disease may include:
    - Drooling
    - Dysphagia
    - Loss of head control
    - Respiratory distress and flaccid paralysis from progressive bulbar involvement

Infections

- Bacterial infection should be suspected in a child with fever- and irritability.
  - In infants and children, the most common bacteria are *Streptococcus pneumoniae*, *Neisseria meningitidis*, and *Haemophilus influenzae* type B.
- Meningitis
  - Infants with meningitis may have irritability, lethargy, and poor feeding.
  - If the fontanelle is still open, it may be bulging.
  - Group B streptococci and gram-negative bacilli are the most common causes in neonates.
- Irritability and decreased movement of a limb should raise concern for osteomyelitis.
  - Swelling and erythema of the soft tissue overlying the bone may exist, often with a history of preceding trauma.
- Joint pain, fever, irritability, and a limp should raise concern for septic arthritis.
  - Examination reveals erythema, swelling, or warmth over the affected joint, with restricted movement.

- With septic arthritis of the hip, swelling and redness may not be visible, and the pain may be referred to the knee.
- An orthopedist should be consulted for possible surgical drainage.
- Children with Kawasaki disease, a vasculitis triggered by an unknown infectious agent, are often more irritable than patients with other febrile illnesses.
- Occult sepsis, urinary tract infections, and pneumonia also can produce irritability, along with fever and other signs that cause a patient to appear toxic.

Trauma

- Shaken baby syndrome
  - Occurs most commonly in children <2 years
  - The rotational forces sustained during shaking cause movement of the brain within the subdural space and tearing of the bridging veins.
  - Clinical signs may be poor feeding, vomiting, lethargy, or irritability.
- Blunt trauma
  - In infants and young children, pressure from the lap belt of a restraint system in a motor vehicle crash or other blunt abdominal trauma can lead to intraabdominal bleeding, initially displayed as irritability from tissue hypoperfusion and pain.
- Occult fracture

Acute abdomen

- Intussusception is most common between the ages of 3 months and 5 years, with a peak incidence at 6–11 months.
  - The child appears colicky, cries, and may draw the knees upward toward the chest; this may last a few minutes and then subside.
  - The child often looks better between episodes, and irritability gradually increases and vomiting becomes more frequent and sometimes bilious.
  - The classic triad is intermittent colicky abdominal pain, vomiting, and bloody mucous stools.
    - This triad is present in only 20–40% of cases.
    - ≥2 of these findings are present in approximately 60% of patients (see Acute Surgical Abdomen).
- Malrotation with midgut volvulus peaks during the first month of life but can occur anytime in childhood.
  - The neonate will be irritable initially.
  - As bowel becomes obstructed and necrotic, bilious vomiting and shock may result from perforation.
- Appendicitis is the cause of abdominal pain in 2–3% of children seen in ambulatory clinics or emergency departments.
  - Abdominal pain in a young child may first manifest as irritability, before the appearance of nausea, vomiting, fever, and right lower quadrant tenderness.

- Perforation rates for appendicitis are higher in children (30–60%) than in adults.
- Because the omentum is less developed in children, perforations are less likely to be walled off or localized.

■ Hypertrophic pyloric stenosis may become symptomatic as early as the first week of life and as late as the fifth month.

- Symptoms begin with nonbilious vomiting after feeding.
- As the disease progresses, vomiting becomes projectile.
- The baby may appear normal initially, but hunger makes the infant irritable, and signs of dehydration eventually become apparent.

■ Necrotizing enterocolitis typically is seen in premature infants in their first few weeks of life.

- It may be seen rarely in full-term infants, within the first 2 weeks after birth, particularly with a stressor, such as infection or anoxic event.
- Infants are ill-appearing, irritable, and lethargic, with distended abdomen and bloody stools.

■ Inguinal hernia

- 60% of incarcerated inguinal hernias occur during the first year of life, with symptoms of irritability, vomiting, and pain in the groin and abdomen.
- Testicular examination is imperative in all boys with irritability or abdominal pain.
  - On examination, a nonfluctuant tender mass is present in the inguinal region and may extend down into the scrotum.
- With the onset of ischemia of the involved bowel, pain becomes more intense and localized to the scrotum, and the infant may have bilious vomiting with the presence of bloody stools.

■ Irritability with scrotal pain also may result from epididymitis, torsion of the testis, or torsion of the appendix testis.

Cardiac system

■ Acute myocarditis

- 3 phases have been identified in the pathogenesis.
  - Viral replication
  - Autoimmune injury to myocytes
  - Dilated cardiomyopathy

■ Anomalous left coronary artery originating from the pulmonary artery

- Occurs in early infancy with irritability during or soon after feedings
- Associated signs may include poor weight gain, diaphoresis, a murmur, and respiratory distress.

■ Supraventricular tachycardia

- May cause irritability and poor feeding

Hypoxic or ischemic events

■ Carbon monoxide (CO) poisoning and methemoglobinemia cause irritability in response to hypoxia.

- A history of smoke inhalation and exposure to an indoor gas stove or to automobile exhaust fumes is indicative.
- Early findings with CO poisoning are influenza-like: headache, irritability, and dizziness.
- Prolonged exposure may result in altered mental status.

■ Methemoglobinemia

- Characteristic blue-gray cyanosis that is not improved with oxygen, despite normal arterial oxygen tension, and chocolate brown appearance of arterial blood are the hallmarks of methemoglobinemia.
- In infancy it may be hereditary; the hereditary form usually is mild.
- May be acquired, related to:
  - Hypoxic events
  - Medication use (sulfonamides, topical anesthetics, metoclopropamide)
  - Ingestion of products containing nitrites and nitrates (contaminated well water or foods with naturally occurring nitrates, such as spinach, green beans, carrots, and squash)
  - Diarrhea, probably caused by the nitrite-forming bacteria in the gut

■ Sickle cell anemia

- Ischemia may cause a painful vasoocclusive crisis.
- Initial presentation in infants and younger children usually is irritability and dactylitis, and painful swelling of the hands and feet as a result of vascular stasis and ischemia.

Metabolic system

■ Hypoglycemia, hypo- or hypernatremia, hypo- or hypercalcemia, hypomagnesemia, and inborn errors of metabolism can all cause irritability.

■ Hypoglycemia is defined as a glucose level ≤40 mg/dL.

- Can be a primary process
- Can be caused by sepsis, ingestion, or cardiac or respiratory failure

■ Hyponatremia can result from gastrointestinal losses or water intoxication.

■ Hypernatremia is seen with diarrhea in which the water losses exceed salt loss, when replacement fluid has too high a sodium content, or with improper preparation of infant formula.

■ Hypocalcemia

- In the newborn period, may cause irritability, poor feeding, and lethargy
- Later in infancy and during childhood, it is seen with rickets.

■ Hypercalcemia is a rare electrolyte disturbance resulting from hyperparathyroidism, vitamin D intoxication, or idiopathic causes.

■ Hypomagnesemia is found with hypocalcemia.

■ Inborn errors of metabolism that cause irritability are those in which a toxic intermediate accumulates.

● Organic and aminoacidemias and urea cycle disorders result in metabolic acidosis or hyperammonemia.

– Symptomatic in the first few weeks of life, with vomiting, poor feeding, irritability, and lethargy

● When a milder degree of enzyme dysfunction is present, clinical disease may be triggered by a bacterial or viral illness.

Toxins and drugs

■ Life-threatening intoxications may result from:

● Heavy metals, such as lead and mercury

● Drugs of abuse, such as cocaine and alcohol

● Envenomations by scorpions and snakes

● Overdoses of or idiosyncratic reactions to medications

● Contact with agricultural, industrial, or household chemicals

■ Thorough questioning about recent use of lawn chemicals, pesticides, and cleaning products may be the only clues to these factors as a cause of irritability, because many are not detected by standard toxicologic screening.

■ Prescribed or over-the-counter medications may cause irritability, even when used as directed and certainly when overused.

● ß-Agonists

● Antiepileptics

● Decongestants

● Antihistamines

● Antitussives

● Various cold medicines

■ Certain drugs of abuse are known to cause irritability.

● Cocaine

● Alcohol

● Phencyclidine hydrochloride

● Inhalants

■ Exposure in infants and children may occur:

● By passive means

– Transplacentally

– By ingestion of human milk

– By inhalation

● By accidental ingestion

■ A positive history may be difficult to elicit, and toxicologic screen may not always be helpful; thus, a strong index of suspicion is needed.

■ Substance use or withdrawal should be considered in the differential diagnosis when any adolescent has chronic persistent irritability.

■ In rare instances, intentional poisoning may be the cause of a child's distress.

■ Irritability and intermittent fever sometimes indicate leukemia with bone pain.

● Cancer of all sorts may have a component of irritability among their symptoms and must be considered carefully when no other diagnosis is forthcoming.

Acute irritability in the well-appearing child

■ Irritability in infants has been attributed to a variety of causes of pain or discomfort that may become obvious during the evaluation.

■ Dental caries and teething may cause an infant to be fussy or irritable (see Prevention of Dental Caries).

● Teething may be accompanied by loose stools but not fever.

■ Acute otitis media is a common cause of irritability, with or without fever, in children <2 years and in those attending child care.

■ Gastroesophageal reflux

● Particularly common in the first year of life

● May be asymptomatic

● May be indicated by postprandial irritability, recurrent vomiting, and inadequate weight gain

■ Other sources of irritability and nonspecific crying episodes may be related to:

● A foreign body in the ear or nose

– If present for a prolonged period, results in foul-smelling discharge

– Disk batteries need to be removed emergently because they may leak and can cause tissue destruction.

– An insect in the ear canal can make a child very irritable and may be removed after first killing the insect with mineral oil or lidocaine.

● Corneal abrasion

– Foreign bodies under the eyelid, inward-turned eyelashes, or eye scratching may cause corneal abrasion.

■ Irritability, increased tearing, conjunctival injection, and photophobia

■ The foreign body may be removed by a moistened cotton-tipped applicator or by irrigation.

● A hair tourniquet around the digit or genitals can cause pain and irritability.

– Thorough examination of creases is essential; prolonged constricting bands may compromise distal circulation.

● In some instances, the source of a child's irritability will be found only on thorough examination of the genitalia, which may reveal evidence of vaginitis, balanitis, or anal fissure.

● Diaper dermatitis, common after a diarrheal illness, with *Candida* infection or as an allergic reaction to the diaper material

● Insect and spider bites or stings

- Infants may be irritable after vaccination, with local erythema, swelling, and tenderness at the injection site.
  - Persistent, inconsolable crying lasting ≥3 hours within 48 hours of receiving whole-cell pertussis DTP vaccine has been reported but not with the newer acellular pertussis DTaP vaccine.

Chronic irritability

- Chronic irritability may be recurrent or persistent.
  - Psychosocial causes are most common.
  - Toxic, neurologic, metabolic, and miscellaneous causes
  - Abuse and neglect
- Irritability as a chronic feature of a child's behavior may indicate significant problems with familial relationships and the ability to master the environment.
  - Infants may be irritable because of maternal-infant temperament mismatches, maternal depression, or stress within the family.
- An older child or adolescent who has a psychiatric problem, such as depression, psychosis, autism, posttraumatic stress disorder, or substance abuse, may be described as "irritable."

Chronic recurrent irritability

- Colic
  - Usually occurs in infants <3 months
  - Characterized by paroxysms of screaming, which may persist for several hours
  - Criteria for the diagnosis
    - Crying for ≥3 hours per day
    - For ≥3 days per week
    - Over >3 weeks
  - Typically peaks at 6 weeks and abates by 3–4 months
- Constipation
  - Associated with inadequate fluid intake, low-fiber diet, dietary changes, and toilet training
  - Large, hard stools can result in anal fissures, which make the situation worse as the child becomes even more reluctant to use the bathroom because of the pain.
- Food allergy
  - Affects approximately 6–8% of infants and young children and approximately 3.5–4% of adults
  - The most common food allergens include cow's milk, eggs, peanuts, wheat, and shellfish.
  - Milk protein allergy usually is seen in the first few months of life.
    - Children are irritable and have blood-streaked stools, although they are otherwise healthy.
    - Treatment involves switching to hypoallergenic formulas derived from cow's milk, then gradually advancing to an unrestricted diet by 9–12 months of age.

- Sleep disturbance
  - Night terrors
    - Typically occur between 2 and 4 years of age during non–rapid eye movement sleep
    - Usually begin with sudden and prolonged periods of inconsolable crying and end spontaneously, with the child rapidly returning to sleep
  - Nightmares
    - A nightmare occurs during rapid eye movement sleep, characterized by a frightening dream, which fully awakens the child; return to sleep is delayed.
    - Vivid recollection of dream appropriate to the child's developmental and maturational stage
- Neurologic disorders
  - Brain tumors
  - Migraine headaches
  - Seizures
  - Postconcussion syndrome
    - Particularly distressing to families because head injury may have occurred months or years before and may have seemed minor, yet irritability and behavior changes may be persistent

Chronic persistent irritability

Psychosocial disorders

- Attention-deficit/hyperactivity disorder is the most commonly diagnosed biological-behavioral disorder of childhood, occurring in approximately 6–9% of school-age children.
  - Children may have coexisting externalizing disorders (conduct disorder and oppositional defiant disorder) and internalizing disorders (depression and anxiety disorders).
  - A common presentation in infants and young children may be irritability from frustration as a result of family and peer relationships, propensity to accidental injury, and difficulty with academic work.
- Autistic disorder usually occurs in children <3 years.
  - Early symptoms include irritability, deficits in verbal and social interaction, repetitive behaviors, failure to participate within groups, and hours spent in solitary play.
- Children with cognitive impairments
  - Children with severe cognitive impairments cannot verbalize what they are experiencing.
    - Although caregivers are usually adept at reading a child's body language and behaviors to know when the child is in pain, they often cannot identify the specific cause.
    - These children are likely to experience pain from the same sources as unimpaired children (eg, teething, sore throat, headache, minor trauma) but are at risk for additional sources of pain and discomfort.
    - Constipation, muscle spasms, and irritation from feeding tubes are frequent causes of irritability.

- In children with spastic quadriplegia, pathologic fractures are a common finding, related to limb rigidity, joint contractures, bone demineralization, and anticonvulsants.
- Children with cognitive impairments often receive multiple drugs for seizures, respiratory conditions, and constipation, with a high incidence of behavioral side effects (irritability, aggression, and hyperactivity).
- A wide variety of chronic disorders have irritability as a prominent or sole component.
- Hormonal effects associated with adolescence in both boys and girls can cause moodiness and irritability.

LABORATORY EVALUATION

- Infection
  - Cultures
  - Complete blood count
  - Erythrocyte sedimentation rate
  - C-reactive protein
- Metabolic system
  - Glucose
  - Electrolytes
  - Anion gap calculation
  - Ammonia
- Toxins and drugs
  - Blood and urine screening
- Acute myocarditis
  - Serum troponin level
- Carbon monoxide poisoning
  - Arterial measurement of carboxyhemoglobin

IMAGING

- Unexplained irritability or lethargy, or a scalp hematoma in an irritable child, protracted vomiting, or neurologic deficits, all warrant computed tomography of the head.
- Plain films, ultrasonography, magnetic resonance imaging, and bone scanning can be helpful in the evaluation of:
  - Suspected bone abnormalities
    - Fractures
    - Osteomyelitis
    - Infarction in sickle cell disease
  - Joint processes
    - Septic arthritis, particularly of the hip
    - Trauma

- Plain films of the abdomen can be helpful in diagnosing:
  - Necrotizing enterocolitis (pneumatosis intestinalis)
  - Malrotation with midgut volvulus
- Ultrasonography and computed tomography can be helpful with intraabdominal processes:
  - Appendicitis
  - Intussusception
  - Pyloric stenosis
  - Blunt abdominal trauma
- Acute myocarditis
  - Echocardiogram will show reduced ventricular function.
- Anomalous left coronary artery originating from pulmonary artery
  - Cardiomegaly on radiograph is almost universal.

DIAGNOSTIC PROCEDURES

- Corneal abrasion
  - Diagnosis is made by Wood lamp examination after instillation of fluorescein into the eye.
- Acute myocarditis should be considered in an irritable child with tachycardia, especially if accompanied by poor perfusion.
  - Electrocardiography may reveal sinus tachycardia with low-voltage QRS complexes, arrhythmias, and ST changes.
- Anomalous left coronary artery originating from pulmonary artery
  - Myocardial ischemia on electrocardiographic examination is almost universal.
- Nonconvulsive status epilepticus
  - Electroencephalography can be diagnostic.

TREATMENT APPROACH

- Treatment is based on the cause of irritability.

WHEN TO ADMIT

- Infants <1 month of who are irritable, for evaluation and observation
- Children in whom child abuse and neglect are suspected
- Children with a life-threatening condition, such as meningitis or brain tumor, that causes irritability

Jaundice

DEFINITION

- *Jaundice* is a yellowish discoloration of skin, sclerae, and mucous membranes that results from an increase in the serum concentration of bilirubin.
- Jaundice becomes evident at serum bilirubin concentrations:
  - >3 mg/dL in older children
  - >5 mg/dL in newborns
- *Hyperbilirubinemia* is defined as total serum bilirubin concentration >1.5 mg/dL.
  - Typically characterized by the fraction of bilirubin that is increased, unconjugated (indirect), or conjugated (direct)
  - Normal conjugated fraction accounts for <5% of total serum bilirubin.
  - *Conjugated hyperbilirubinemia* refers to direct bilirubin concentration >2 mg/dL or >20% of the total bilirubin concentration.
  - Conjugated hyperbilirubinemia should always be considered important because it suggests liver or biliary tract dysfunction.
- *Neonatal hepatitis* refers to infants <3 months who have cholestatic jaundice with nonspecific histologic features of hepatic inflammation and no defined cause.
  - The number of patients categorized as having neonatal hepatitis has been decreasing with:
    - Better understanding of the causes of neonatal cholestasis
    - Availability of many new advanced diagnostic techniques

EPIDEMIOLOGY

- Prevalence
  - All newborn infants have a total bilirubin level greater than an adult's normal limit of 1.5 mg/dL.
  - >50% of newborn babies will develop clinical jaundice in the first week of life.
    - Most have unconjugated hyperbilirubinemia.
  - Hemolysis
    - ABO incompatibility occurs in approximately 15% of all pregnancies.
    - Results in hemolytic disease in ~3% of newborns, with <0.1% of infants needing exchange transfusion
    - In the US, Rh negative genotype seen in:
      - 15% of white persons
      - 5% of black persons
      - <1% of Asian persons
    - Rh incompatibility occurs in ~1.06 per 1000 live births.
    - Prophylactic use of RhoGAM (anti-D γ-globulin) in Rh-negative mothers has decreased incidence of hemolytic disease to <0.11% of Rh-negative pregnancies.

- Polycythemia
  - 1–5% of newborns
  - Unconjugated hyperbilirubinemia develops in 2–22% of affected babies.
- Parenteral nutrition
  - 30–50% of infants and 80% of preterm babies who receive total parenteral nutrition (TPN) for >2 weeks develop cholestatic jaundice.
- α1-Antitrypsin deficiency
  - Found in 1 in 1600–2000 live births
- Galactosemia
  - Occurs in 1 per 60,000
- Gilbert syndrome
  - Affects 7% of the general population

MECHANISM

- Bilirubin is the end product of heme degradation.
- Heme is produced from the breakdown of hemoglobin (70–80%) and other hemoproteins (20–30%).
- The conversion from heme to bilirubin follows a 2-step process that occurs mainly in the reticuloendothelial cells of the spleen, liver, and bone marrow.
  - Heme is converted to biliverdin by the microsomal enzyme heme oxygenase
  - Biliverdin is converted to bilirubin by the cytosolic enzyme biliverdin reductase.
  - This unconjugated bilirubin is a hydrophobic compound that is:
    - Tightly bound to serum albumin
    - Transported to the liver for conjugation and clearance
- Metabolism of bilirubin in the liver follows 4 distinct steps.
  - Bilirubin is taken up across the sinusoidal (basolateral) membrane of the hepatocyte by a membrane receptor carrier.
  - Bilirubin then binds to ligandin, an intracellular binding protein and is conjugated with glucuronic acid in the endoplasmic reticulum by the enzyme bilirubin uridine diphosphate-glucuronosyl transferase (BUGT) to form bilirubin mono- and diglucuronides.
    - The isoform *UGT1A1* is responsible for bilirubin conjugation.
    - Different mutations in the gene for this enzyme have been found in such diseases as Gilbert syndrome and Crigler-Najjar syndrome.
  - Water-soluble bilirubin glucuronides are excreted into bile through the apical canalicular membrane.
    - This process is mediated by an adenosine triphosphate-dependent export pump.

- Genetic mutations in the gene for this pump are found in cystic fibrosis and in Dubin-Johnson and Rotor syndromes.
- Almost all bilirubin in adult human bile is of the conjugated form.
  - 15% as bilirubin monoglucuronides
  - 85% as diglucuronides
- Neonates have a higher concentration of bilirubin monoglucuronides in their bile because of lower BUGT enzyme activity.
  - Monoglucuronides are easily deconjugated and reabsorbed in the intestine.

- Excreted bilirubin is further metabolized by intestinal bacteria to form urobilinoids, which are then eliminated in the feces.
  - This prevents intestinal reabsorption of bilirubin.
  - Bilirubin glucuronides can also be deconjugated by bacterial or tissue ß-glucuronidase in the intestine and then reabsorbed in the terminal ileum, a process known as *enterohepatic circulation.*
  - Newborns are more likely to absorb bilirubin from the intestine because they lack bacterial flora to form nonabsorbable urobilinoids.
  - Conditions that delay passage of meconium, which contains large amounts of bilirubin and ß-glucuronidase, can result in neonatal hyperbilirubinemia.
  - Breast milk contains high levels of ß-glucuronidase, which may be a contributing factor in the development of breast milk jaundice.
- Direct bilirubin consists of 2 components.
  - Conjugated bilirubin
  - δ-bilirubin
    - Conjugated bilirubin-albumin compound formed when bilirubin glucuronides reflux into systemic circulation and covalently bind to albumin
  - The terms *direct* and *conjugated* bilirubin are used interchangeably.
- α-, ß-, and γ-bilirubin correspond to unconjugated, mono-conjugated, and diconjugated forms.
  - δ-Bilirubin is clinically important because it is not excreted in bile or urine until albumin is degraded.
  - This accounts for prolonged direct hyperbilirubinemia occasionally observed after restoration of normal bile flow.

HISTORY

- A detailed history is essential when evaluating a patient with jaundice.
- Special attention should be paid to the presence of:
  - Fever
  - Viral prodrome
  - Abdominal pain or distention
  - Acholic stools
  - Dark urine
  - Pruritus
- In patients with neonatal jaundice, focus on:
  - Prenatal history
  - Quality of prenatal care
  - Maternal blood test results
  - Birth history
- In older children, focus on:
  - Patient's age at onset of jaundice
  - Associated signs and symptoms before and during the period of jaundice
  - Exposure to hepatotoxic agents
- Detailed family history should include:
  - Information about the presence of persistent jaundice
  - Chronic liver diseases
  - Hemolysis
  - Metabolic diseases
- Goals of initial evaluation are to distinguish:
  - Acute from chronic liver diseases
  - Intrahepatic processes from extrahepatic biliary tract obstruction
  - Primary liver diseases from systemic diseases

PHYSICAL EXAM

- Patients with jaundice from unconjugated hyperbilirubinemia have bright yellow–colored skin.
- Patients with jaundice from conjugated hyperbilirubinemia have dark yellow-greenish–colored skin.
- Patients should undergo a complete physical examination, with special focus on:
  - General appearance
  - Growth and development
  - Signs of cardiovascular dysfunction
  - Neurologic signs
  - Organomegaly
- The size and character of the liver should be determined.
  - The newborn or infant liver is a large organ relative to body size.
    - In newborns, mean liver span is 5.9 cm along the mid-clavicular line, calculated by measuring the distance between the percussed upper and palpated lower liver edge.
    - Normal infant liver may be palpable and is typically <2 cm below the right costal margin.

- Consistency and character of the liver edge may help determine nature of underlying liver disease.
    - Enlarged liver resulting from an acute intrahepatic process is usually tender but soft.
    - Cirrhotic liver may have a hard and irregular edge, but its edge is not always palpable.
- Thorough abdominal examination to identify:
    - Enlarged spleen
        - In newborns and infants, the tip of the spleen can normally be palpated below the left costal margin.
        - Splenomegaly in a patient with underlying liver disease implies portal hypertension, especially in the presence of ascites and a prominent abdominal cutaneous venous pattern.
    - Other abdominal masses
    - Areas of tenderness
    - Ascites
    - Abdominal cutaneous venous pattern
    - Other physical findings may indicate a particular cause, such as:
        - Xanthomas in primary biliary cirrhosis
        - Kayser-Fleischer rings in Wilson disease
        - Characteristic facial features and posterior embryotoxon in Alagille syndrome

DIFFERENTIAL DIAGNOSIS

General

- Differential diagnosis of jaundice is categorized as either unconjugated or conjugated hyperbilirubinemia in 2 age groups:
    - Newborn and young infants
    - Older infants and children
- Unconjugated hyperbilirubinemia is common in neonates but relatively rare thereafter.
    - Typically transient and benign, but marked increases of bilirubin can be toxic to the central nervous system.
- Conjugated hyperbilirubinemia is always pathological.
    - When present in young infants, it is often related to:
        - Primary hepatobiliary disorders
        - Systemic or metabolic diseases
        - Genetic defects in bilirubin or bile acid metabolism or transport.
    - More prevalent in older children
        - Viral hepatitis
        - Drug- or toxin-induced liver damage

Jaundice in newborns and young infants

Unconjugated hyperbilirubinemia

- Nonphysiological jaundice should always be considered in neonatal jaundice.

- A pathological cause suggested by:
    - Early onset
    - Rapid progression
    - Persistence beyond 2 weeks of life
    - Association with other signs or symptoms
- In most instances, pathological unconjugated hyperbilirubinemia results from either excessive production of bilirubin or abnormal hepatic clearance of bilirubin.

Increased production of bilirubin

- Hemolysis (ABO or Rh incompatibility, erythrocyte defects, erythrocyte enzyme defects, disseminated intravascular coagulopathy)
- Weakly positive direct Coombs test, high reticulocyte count, spherocytes on blood smear, and high levels of unconjugated bilirubin.
    - The most common cause of excessive bilirubin production in neonates
    - Usually observed within the first 24 hours of life
    - Often seen in association with maternal-fetal blood type incompatibility (ABO or Rh incompatibility)
        - Positive direct Coombs test, high reticulocyte count, spherocytes on blood smear, and high levels of unconjugated bilirubin
        - ABO incompatibility is usually seen in newborn infants with blood type A or B born to blood type O mothers.
        - Hemolytic disease in Rh incompatibility usually develops when an Rh-negative mother has become sensitized after exposure to Rh-positive fetal blood during a previous pregnancy.
        - Rh incompatibility is less common and usually more severe than ABO incompatibility.
        - Affected infants usually experience onset of jaundice in the first hours of life, and have anemia and hepatosplenomegaly.
        - In severe cases, the infant may be born with fetal hydrops from intrauterine hemolysis.
- Hemoglobinopathies
    - Polycythemia
        - Can cause an increase in bilirubin production as a result of absolute increase in erythrocyte mass
    - α-thalassemia
        - Suspect in newborns with jaundice and moderate hypochromic, microcytic, hemolytic anemia
    - Erythrocyte enzyme defects
        - Erythrocyte enzyme defects, such as glucose-6-phosphate dehydrogenase (G6PD) or pyruvate kinase deficiency, may cause hemolysis at any age.

- G6PD deficiency is often benign in the newborn period; however, clinically important hemolysis and jaundice may develop in the presence of oxidant stressors, such as infections.
- Cephalohematoma resorption
  - Increased bilirubin production caused by rapid breakdown of erythrocytes in the extravascular space

Decreased hepatocellular uptake or conjugation

- Prematurity
- Congenital hypothyroidism
  - Presumably caused by delayed maturation of BUGT
- Physiological jaundice of the newborn
- Breast milk jaundice
  - Usually occurs in a thriving breastfed newborn during the second and third weeks of life
  - Thought to be related in part to inhibition of BUGT activity by compounds found in breast milk
- Drugs
  - Aspirin, cephalosporins, and sulfonamides can impair bilirubin transport by altering bilirubin-albumin binding
  - Rifampincan inhibit hepatocellular uptake of bilirubin.
- Gilbert and Crigler-Najjar syndromes
  - Gilbert syndrome is a common inherited condition characterized by mild unconjugated hyperbilirubinemia.
    - An insertional mutation of the *UGT1A1* gene results in a reduced level of expression of the gene.
    - Gilbert syndrome is usually diagnosed during or after adolescence.
  - Crigler-Najjar syndrome is a rare familial form of unconjugated hyperbilirubinemia caused by mutations in the gene encoding BUGT1.
    - Leads to either absent (type 1) or decreased (type 2) BUGT activity.
    - Type 1 is an autosomal-recessive disease and exhibits in the first hours of life with severe nonhemolytic jaundice.
    - Type 2 is an autosomal-dominant disease with less severe jaundice and may improve with phenobarbital to promote bile flow.

Conjugated hyperbilirubinemia

- Also known as *cholestatic jaundice*, regardless of cause
- Usually associated with liver dysfunction, and always pathological
- It can result from:
  - Impaired bile formation by the hepatocyte
  - Obstruction to the flow of bile through the intrahepatic or extrahepatic biliary tree from
    - Primary hepatobiliary disorders
    - Genetic or metabolic diseases

- Systemic infections
- Drug toxicity

Liver diseases

- Acute liver damage (ischemia, hypoxia, acidosis)
  - Conditions that alter systemic circulation, such as cardiopulmonary arrest, shock, and severe metabolic acidosis, may lead to an acute ischemic insult to the liver and necrosis of hepatocytes.
  - Affected patients have a marked and rapid increase in serum aminotransferase levels and direct hyperbilirubinemia within 24–48 hours after the insult.
  - In most, liver function will normalize once the initial insult is corrected.
  - A small number of patients may develop acute liver failure.
- Infection
  - Sepsis
    - The most frequently associated bacterial organisms are *Escherichia coli*, *Streptococcus* group B, and *Listeria monocytogenes*
  - TORCH (toxoplasmosis, other agents, rubella, cytomegalovirus, herpes simplex)
    - Low birth weight, hepatosplenomegaly, cutaneous manifestations, and ophthalmologic and central nervous system involvement
    - Diagnosis is often made by virus culture, serologic titers, imaging studies, and ophthalmologic examination.
    - Anemia, thrombocytopenia, increased aminotransferase levels, and cholestasis
    - Other infections, such as HIV and hepatitis B and C, have decreased with improved prenatal screening.
  - Urinary tract infections
- Viral or other hepatitis
- TPN–related liver disease
  - Factors thought to contribute include lack of enteral feeds, immaturity of the hepatobiliary system, infused nutrient composition, and sepsis.
  - In most infants, liver function abnormalities usually resolve within 4–6 months after discontinuation of TPN.
  - In severe cases, progression to end-stage liver disease may occur.
- Metabolic liver disease (galactosemia, neonatal hemochromatosis, α_1-antitrypsin deficiency, tyrosinemia, mitochondrial defects)
  - Neonatal hemochromatosis
    - Typical laboratory findings include increased ferritin and transferrin saturation and relatively low transferrin levels.
    - Liver aminotransferase levels can be slightly increased or even normal.

J

- Tyrosinemia type 1
  - Markedly increased α-fetoprotein level
  - Presence of succinylacetone in urine or blood is pathognomonic.
- Hormones and drugs

Obstruction of biliary system

- Congenital anomalies (biliary atresia, choledochal cyst)
  - *Extrahepatic biliary atresia* (EHBA) is an idiopathic, destructive, inflammatory process of both the intra- and extrahepatic bile ducts.
    - One of the few causes of neonatal cholestasis that can be treated with surgery
    - Infants typically exhibit symptoms of cholestatic jaundice and acholic stools when they are approximately 2–4 weeks of age.
    - In early stages, the stool may still have some bile pigment.
    - When EHBA is suspected, exploratory laparotomy with intraoperative cholangiography should be performed to confirm the diagnosis.
      - Patients then undergo hepatoportoenterostomy, or the Kasai procedure.
      - The highest success rate of reestablishing bile flow after surgery is seen when the procedure is performed before the child is 8 weeks of age.
  - Choledochal cysts are rare congenital anomalies characterized by varying degrees of cystic dilation of the intra- or extrahepatic biliary tree.
    - May be detected at any age; 18% of cases are diagnosed during the first year of life.
    - Classic presentation of jaundice, abdominal pain, and right epigastric mass is often not observed in infants and young children.
  - *Alagille syndrome*, also known as *arteriohepatic dysplasia*, is inherited as an autosomal-dominant condition with variable penetrance.
    - Characterized by paucity of intrahepatic bile ducts, peripheral pulmonary stenosis, butterfly vertebrae, posterior embryotoxon, and peculiar faces.
    - Jaundice and pruritus are often the main clinical features during infancy.

Defects of bilirubin metabolism or transport

- Progressive familial intrahepatic cholestasis
  - Identified as a distinct group of conditions involving intrahepatic cholestasis from bile acid transport defects leading to impairment of bile excretion.
    - Affected patients often develop jaundice in the 1st few months of life.
    - They may also have severe pruritus, growth failure, fat-soluble vitamin deficiency, abnormal coagulation profile, and increased serum bile acids.

  - Disease usually progresses to cirrhosis and liver failure early in life.
- Dubin-Johnson syndrome, Rotor syndrome
- *Galactosemia* is an inborn error of galactose metabolism inherited as an autosomal-recessive trait.
  - Can affect many organs, including the liver, kidneys, brain, eyes, intestines, and gonads
  - Hepatocellular damage is caused by accumulation of toxic metabolites of galactose-1-phosphate and galactitol in the liver.
  - Clinical presentation varies from mild liver disease to fulminant liver failure in the neonatal period.
  - Jaundice and hepatomegaly can develop in association with vomiting, diarrhea, poor feeding, or *E coli* sepsis.
- Other inborn errors of carbohydrate metabolism, such as hereditary fructose intolerance and certain types of glycogen storage diseases, can also have jaundice as part of their clinical picture.
  - Onset of symptoms rarely occurs during early infancy.
- *Neonatal hemochromatosis* is a rare idiopathic syndrome characterized by liver disease of prenatal onset and excess iron deposition in extrahepatic sites.
  - Infants are usually born early and have experienced intrauterine growth retardation.
  - In most, signs and symptoms of acute liver failure are present at birth or develop soon thereafter.
  - Clinical presentation includes hypoglycemia, hypoalbuminemia, profound coagulopathy, and cholestatic jaundice.
  - The diagnosis should be considered in every case of neonatal liver failure.
- *α₁-Antitrypsin deficiency* is a genetic disorder, with the homozygous PiZZ genotype.
  - Only 10% of patients with α_1-antitrypsin deficiency develop signs and symptoms of liver disease.
  - The most common genetic cause of neonatal liver disease
  - Typically shows in the first few months of life with jaundice, although onset of liver disease can occur later in life
  - Injury to the liver is thought to be the result of the hepatotoxic effect of retained mutant α_1ATZZ molecule in the endoplasmic reticulum of the hepatocyte.
- *Tyrosinemia type 1*, also known as *hepatorenal tyrosinemia*, is a rare disorder that can affect the liver, kidneys, and peripheral nerves.
  - Deficiency of fumarylacetoacetate hydrolase, an enzyme involved in tyrosine degradation, results in tissue accumulation of tyrosine and other intermediate metabolites.
  - Clinical findings range from severe liver disease or acute liver failure in early infancy to chronic liver disease in older children.

- Tyrosinemia should be suspected in patients who exhibit signs and symptoms of liver disease, especially when associated with acute neurologic symptoms, such as excruciating pain, weakness, and paralysis.
- Early diagnosis is important because specific medical therapy will improve quality of life and delay disease progression.

- Primary mitochondrial hepatopathies are caused by a variety of defects, including mitochondrial DNA depletion, respiratory chain defects, fatty acid oxidation defects, and mitochondrial membrane enzyme defects.

  - Patients commonly have neuromuscular problems and may have marked lactic acidosis.
  - Symptoms usually develop within the first few months of life.

Jaundice in older infants and children

- In this age group, jaundice is an unusual sign and may suggest a serious clinical condition.

Unconjugated hyperbilirubinemia

- In general, unconjugated hyperbilirubinemia is rarely seen in older infants and children.
- Hemolysis: erythrocyte defects, erythrocyte enzyme defect (G6PD), disseminated intravascular coagulopathy
- Gilbert syndrome

  - A benign disorder inherited as an autosomal-dominant trait, although an autosomal-recessive pattern has also been described.
  - Jaundice does not typically develop until after puberty
  - Jaundice is usually intermittent and more evident with fasting.
  - Patients usually have mild indirect hyperbilirubinemia with otherwise normal liver function tests and no evidence of ongoing hemolysis.

Conjugated hyperbilirubinemia

Liver disease

- Viral hepatitis (hepatitis A, B, C, E)

  - Acute viral hepatitis is the most common cause of jaundice in older children.
  - Hepatitis A
    - In older children and adolescents, jaundice is a common manifestation
    - Children <5 years tend to be anicteric.
    - Rarely causes fulminant liver failure
  - Hepatitis E has a clinical course similar to that of hepatitis A.
    - Should be suspected in children with a history of recent travel to India or South Asia
  - Hepatitis B or C infection is usually anicteric and chronic in children.

- Other viruses (eg, Epstein-Barr virus, cytomegalovirus, adenovirus, enterovirus) can also cause acute hepatitis.

  - Jaundice is a common presenting feature.

- Toxins and drugs (ethanol, acetaminophen, isoniazid, phenytoin)

  - Initially suspected on the basis of circumstantial evidence
  - Classified into 3 types, according to the different clinical features
    - Hepatitic
      - Acetaminophen overdose can cause acute hepatitis with zonal hepatocyte necrosis; jaundice develops when hepatocellular damage is sufficiently severe.
    - Cholestatic
      - Cholestasis is more prominent when damage to bile duct epithelial cells results in an impaired bile flow.
      - Can be caused by many different drugs, including estrogen or oral contraceptive pills, erythromycin, cyclosporine, and haloperidol.
    - Mixed hepatitic-cholestatic
  - Most cases of drug-induced liver damage spontaneously resolve once the drug responsible for the injury is withdrawn.

- Autoimmune hepatitis (AIH)

  - Cause unknown
  - Usually progresses to cirrhosis if not promptly diagnosed and treated
  - Should always be considered in a child with jaundice associated with increased liver aminotransferase levels
  - Jaundice is present in more than one half of patients with AIH.
  - Hyperglobulinemia and autoantibodies, such as anti-nuclear antibody, anti–smooth muscle antibody, and anti–liver kidney microsomal antibody, may be found.
  - When present, anti–liver kidney microsomal antibody categorizes the disease as AIH type 2.
  - AIH type 1 usually has an insidious course.
    - Patients are likely to come to attention at an older age, some already with cirrhosis.
  - AIH type 2 may have a more fulminant course, even first exhibiting as acute liver failure.

- Metabolic liver disease (α_1-antitrypsin deficiency, tyrosinemia, Wilson disease, mitochondrial defects)

  - *Wilson disease* is an autosomal-recessive disorder of human copper metabolism, usually found in children >5 years.
  - Mutations in the *ATP7B* gene lead to impaired biliary excretion of copper, resulting in progressive accumulation of copper in the liver and subsequently in other organs and tissues.

J

- Hemolytic anemia, Kayser-Fleischer rings in the eyes, and neuropsychiatric symptoms are manifestations of the disease.
- Copper deposition in liver can result in acute or chronic hepatitis, cirrhosis, or fulminant liver failure.
- Markedly increased bilirubin is typically found in patients with Wilson disease who have fulminant liver failure.
- Nonalcoholic fatty liver disease
- Acute liver damage: ischemia, hypoxia, acidosis
- TPN related
- Pregnancy related (acute fatty liver of pregnancy, preeclampsia)
- Cancer
  - Infiltrative cancers may occur rarely and can cause jaundice at any age.

Obstruction of the biliary system

- Choledochal cyst
- Cholelithiasis or choledocholithiasis
  - Most common cause of biliary obstruction in children
  - Often found in patients with an underlying hemolytic disease
  - Isolated gallstone disease can occur:
    - In infants, jaundice is the most common presentation.
    - Older children usually experience vomiting and right upper quadrant pain, with or without jaundice.
- Cholecystitis
- Diseases of the bile ducts (primary sclerosing cholangitis, AIDS cholangiopathy)
  - Primary sclerosing cholangitis is characterized by stenosis, dilatation, and fibrosis involving the intrahepatic or extrahepatic biliary tree or both.
    - Most common form of chronic liver disease in children with inflammatory bowel disease.
    - Clinical presentation is highly variable, with cholestatic jaundice developing in <50% of affected patients.

Bilirubin metabolism or transport defects

- Progressive familial intrahepatic cholestasis
- Dubin-Johnson syndrome
  - Recessively inherited disorder caused by mutations in gene encoding for the canalicular transporter for conjugated bilirubin that results in an impaired secretion of conjugated bilirubin
  - Chronic jaundice is the main clinical manifestation.
  - Serum bile acids are normal.
  - Can be precipitated by pregnancy or the use of oral contraceptives

- Rotor syndrome
  - Clinically similar to Dubin-Johnson syndrome, but involving impairment of liver storage capacity rather than a defect in bilirubin secretion
  - Inherited as an autosomal-recessive disorder
- In both Dubin-Johnson syndrome and Rotor syndrome, conjugated hyperbilirubinemia is noted without abnormalities in other liver function tests.

LABORATORY EVALUATION

- Serum bilirubin is conventionally measured by spectrophotometry based on the Van den Bergh (diazo) reaction.
  - Conjugated (direct) bilirubin reacts rapidly with diazo reagents.
  - Unconjugated (indirect) bilirubin reacts slowly.
  - Indirect bilirubin is calculated as the difference between total bilirubin and direct bilirubin fraction.
  - Direct bilirubin consists of conjugated bilirubin and δ-bilirubin.
    - High-pressure liquid chromatography can measure δ-bilirubin, as well as α-, ß-, and γ-bilirubin.
- Initial laboratory studies in the evaluation of jaundice include:
  - Complete blood count
    - Useful in detecting hemolysis, indicated by the presence of anemia with fragmented erythrocytes (schistocytes) and increased reticulocytes on the smear
    - Thrombocytopenia is typically seen in patients with portal hypertension and hypersplenism.
  - Liver function tests
    - Isolated hyperbilirubinemia with otherwise normal liver function suggests hemolytic disease or bilirubin metabolism defects.
  - Coagulation profile
- Aspartate aminotransferase (AST) and alanine aminotransferase (ALT) levels are the most frequently used markers of hepatocellular injury.
  - ALT is a more specific indicator of hepatocyte injury because AST may be increased with hemolysis and myocardial or skeletal muscle injury.
  - In general, marked increase in AST and ALT occurs in severe viral hepatitis, acute toxin- or drug-induced hepatic necrosis, or ischemia.
  - Mild increase of AST and ALT is seen in nonalcoholic fatty liver disease, chronic viral hepatitis, and drug toxicity.
  - Declining AST and ALT levels indicate hepatocyte recovery.
    - In the course of fulminant liver failure, if seen in association with a worsening liver synthetic function, decreasing AST and ALT levels may be an ominous sign of massive hepatic necrosis, with few viable hepatocytes remaining to further release these enzymes.

- AST and ALT are less useful in patients with chronic end-stage liver disease because they can be normal or only slightly increased in the presence of marked fibrosis of the liver.
- Alkaline phosphatase and γ-glutamyltransferase (GGT) are 2 useful markers for intra- and extrahepatic cholestasis.
  - In most hepatobiliary diseases, both GGT and alkaline phosphatase are increased.
  - In progressive familial intrahepatic cholestasis (types 1 and 2), a normal or low GGT is observed in the presence of a high alkaline phosphatase.
  - Isolated increase of alkaline phosphatase may be seen in patients with nonhepatobiliary diseases, such as bone disorders.
  - Normal GGT values in newborn infants may be 5–8 times greater than those in adults.
- Prothrombin time (PT) and albumin are used to evaluate hepatic synthetic function.
  - Abnormal PT results from impaired hepatic synthesis of coagulation factors I, II, V, VII, and X or deficiency of vitamin K (or both).
  - Parenteral administration of vitamin K generally normalizes a prolonged PT in patients with vitamin K deficiency associated with cholestatic jaundice but not in patients with hepatocellular disease.
  - In acute liver disease, markedly increased PT suggests the possibility of fulminant liver failure.
  - Hypoalbuminemia may be seen in patients with acute and chronic liver diseases.
  - In the early stages of acute liver disease, serum albumin may not be a reliable indicator of hepatic synthetic function because it has a long half-life(~21 days).
- Based on clinical information and results of initial tests, further evaluation, including imaging studies, may be warranted.
- Additional studies may include:
  - Blood and urine cultures
  - Viral serologic studies
  - Toxin and drug screen
  - Autoimmune markers
  - α₁-antitrypsin phenotype
  - Ceruloplasmin
  - Urine succinyl acetone
  - Serum bile acids
- In jaundiced newborns or young infants with abnormal liver function tests, TORCH titers should also be obtained.

IMAGING

- Ultrasonography is the most useful initial imaging modality in the assessment of the intra- and extrahepatic biliary system in patients with jaundice.

- Suggests such causes of jaundice as:
  - Biliary atresia
  - Choledochal cyst
  - Hepatic cystic lesions
  - Cholelithiasis
  - In EHBA:
    - Can exclude other causes of cholestasis, such as choledochal cysts, gallstones, or biliary sludge.
    - Absence of gallbladder or appearance of the triangular cord sign at the hilar region is suggestive of EHBA.
    - Presence of a gallbladder on sonography does not exclude EHBA.
- Computed tomography may be preferred for
  - General anatomic information of the hepatobiliary system
  - Assessing possible noncystic hepatic lesion
- Nuclear scintigraphy, useful in
  - Differentiating biliary atresia from other causes of neonatal cholestasis
  - Diagnosis of acute cholecystitis and chronic acalculous cholecystitis in older children
    - By calculation of gallbladder ejection fraction
- Magnetic resonance imaging (MRI) cholangiopancreatography
  - Noninvasive study that identifies abnormalities of the intra- and extrahepatic biliary system.
- Endoscopic retrograde cholangiopancreatography provides information similar to that of MRI.
  - Invasive and should be reserved for patients who need a possible therapeutic intervention
    - Biliary stent placement
    - Sphincterotomy

DIAGNOSTIC PROCEDURES

- Liver biopsy provides information on the histology and architecture of the liver.
  - Percutaneous liver biopsy is most commonly used in patients with persistently abnormal liver function tests, especially when conventional laboratory and imaging studies do not lead to a firm diagnosis.
  - Use of liver biopsy to diagnose acute hepatitis or acute cholestatic jaundice is limited because the histologic changes may be nonspecific.
  - In fulminant liver failure, percutaneous liver biopsy is contraindicated because of high risk of bleeding; when needed, transjugular liver biopsy under radiographic guidance should be performed.
- EHBA
  - Percutaneous liver biopsy is an essential procedure in suspected EHBA.

- Main histopathological features observed are bile duct proliferation and fibrosis.
■ Neonatal hemochromatosis
  - The diagnosis is made by punch biopsy of the lower-lip mucosa; the sample is analyzed for iron deposition in salivary glands.
■ Dubin-Johnson syndrome
  - Characteristic brown to black discoloration of the liver, the result of pigment deposition in the lysosomes
■ Dubin-Johnson syndrome, Rotor syndrome
  - Liver histologic findings are otherwise normal in both syndromes.

TREATMENT APPROACH

■ Treatment of newborns with unconjugated hyperbilirubinemia is based on revised guideline published by the AAP.
  - Provides a framework in detecting neonatal hyperbilirubinemia and preventing kernicterus in term and near-term newborn infants
  - Emphasizes the importance of:
    - Systematic assessment of the risk of severe hyperbilirubinemia
    - Close follow-up
    - Prompt intervention when necessary

SPECIFIC TREATMENT

Direct hyperbilirubinemia

■ Management should focus on correcting the underlying cause, optimizing nutrition, and controlling pruritus.
■ Malabsorption of fat and fat-soluble vitamins is commonly seen in patients with cholestasis because they have impaired bile acid secretion.
■ A diet high in medium-chain triglycerides should be used to promote growth in children with chronic cholestasis.
  - Medium-chain triglycerides are relatively water soluble and directly absorbed into the portal system, unlike long-chain triglycerides, which require bile acid micelles for solubilization.
■ Supplementation of fat-soluble vitamins A, D, E, and K is essential.
  - Serum vitamin levels should be routinely monitored because patients may still have biochemical evidence of fat-soluble vitamin deficiency despite supplementation.

Cholestasis-associated pruritus

■ Several different therapeutic agents have been used with very little success.
■ Choleretic agents, such as ursodeoxycholic acid and phenobarbital, increase bile flow, decreasing serum level of bile acid.
  - These agents have shown some beneficial effect in relieving pruritus.

■ Other agents have been shown to reduce pruritus in some patients.
  - Cholestyramine, a bile acid–binding resin
  - Rifampin, an antibiotic used to treat tuberculosis

Liver transplantation in children

■ Accepted therapy for many life-threatening liver diseases
■ Whole-liver, split-liver, and living donor transplantations have been successfully used to treat both infants and older children.
■ Current survival rates for children after liver transplantation are:
  - 90% at 1 year
  - 85% at 3 years
■ Early referral and transfer to a liver transplant center are important to good outcome.
■ EHBA with a failed Kasai procedure is the most common reason children undergo liver transplantation.
■ Other indications include:
  - α_1-antitrypsin deficiency
  - Fulminant liver failure
  - Chronic hepatitis
  - Metabolic liver disease
  - Cirrhosis of unknown origin

WHEN TO REFER

■ Unexplained jaundice
■ Direct hyperbilirubinemia at any age
■ Jaundice with persistent or unexplained abnormal liver function tests
■ Jaundice with hepatomegaly or splenomegaly

WHEN TO ADMIT

■ Jaundice in an ill patient
■ Poor feeding tolerance and intravenous hydration
■ Need for intravenous antibiotics
■ Inpatient management of underlying conditions
■ Impending acute liver failure

COMPLICATIONS

■ If the underlying liver condition which results in hyperbilirubinemia is not diagnosed early and treated properly, it may lead to hepatic failure

PROGNOSIS

■ Prognosis depends on the underlying cause of direct or indirect hyperbilirubinemia.

PREVENTION

■ Hepatitis A and hepatitis B can be prevented by vaccinating all children.

Joint Pain

DEFINITION

- *Arthralgia* is joint pain, the subjective experience of pain |referable to a bony articulation.
  - In a young child, it might be inferred from the patient's refusal to move a particular extremity or joint.
- *Arthritis* is an inflamed joint.
  - Redness
  - Warmth
  - Swelling
  - Tenderness
  - Pain with motion
  - Can be accompanied by loss of motion
- All that is arthralgia is not arthritis.

EPIDEMIOLOGY

- Juvenile idiopathic arthritis (JIA)
  - Prevalence
    - 0.1–1 child per 1000 children worldwide
  - Age
    - Systemic-onset disease is typically seen in children 1.5–2 years of age.
    - Onset of JIA can occur through late adolescence.
- Reactive arthritis (previously called *Reiter syndrome*)
  - Sex
    - More common in boys than in girls

MECHANISM

- Onset of joint pain can be sudden or indolent (over days or weeks).
  - When sudden, an associated history of a fall or direct blow to the joint suggests a traumatic cause.
- Presence of fever indicates:
  - Infectious process (eg, septic arthritis)
  - Systemic inflammatory disease (eg, systemic-onset JIA)
- Fractures and dislocations are common causes of joint pain.

HISTORY

- A complete history is indispensable in initial assessment of joint pain.
- A common symptom is loss of motion in a joint, with or without obvious swelling.
  - Further clues are time of day the stiffness occurs and its duration.
  - In JIA, patients typically experience joint stiffness when waking up in the morning (lasting 30 minutes to several hours).
  - Hypermobility syndrome or other mechanical, noninflammatory condition causes pain and stiffness at the end of a vigorous day.

PHYSICAL EXAM

- The physical examination can substantiate or alleviate suspicions raised during history taking.
- Distinguishing between arthralgia and arthritis is essential.
- In systemic-onset JIA, in addition to fever, other distinguishing signs are:
  - Rash
  - Mucous membrane involvement
  - Lymph node inflammation or enlargement
- See Differential Diagnosis for condition-specific physical examination findings.

DIFFERENTIAL DIAGNOSIS

- Differential diagnosis should begin by determining whether disease is rheumatic or nonrheumatic.
- Most rheumatic diseases cause joint pain and tend to be chronic (often with waxing and waning courses).
- Many of the nonrheumatic diseases are acute in onset and short in duration, given appropriate therapy.

JIA

- JIA is also called *Still disease*, previously called *juvenile rheumatoid arthritis*.
- Clinical presentation
  - Can be limited to ≤4 joints, or include a greater number
  - Usually large joints (oligoarticular disease)
  - Both large and small joints might be involved (polyarticular disease)
  - The systemic and at times initially fulminant form is called *systemic-onset disease.*
    - Marked by high, spiking fevers
    - Typical salmon-pink, maculopapular, evanescent rash
    - Lymph node, spleen, and liver enlargement
    - Subcutaneous nodules
    - Anemia
    - General malaise
  - Systemic findings can precede onset of joint involvement.
    - Arthritis must be present for ≥6 consecutive weeks to establish diagnosis of any of the subgroups of JIA.
  - Among patients with any subtype of JIA:
    - The clinician may glean only a history of ill-defined arthralgias and stiffness
    - Physical examination may reveal:
      - Contractures of the elbows, knees, and wrists
      - Limitation of cervical motion
      - Iridocyclitis and keratopathy

Acute rheumatic fever

- Usually involves large joints (eg, knees)
- Typically migratory
- Joints tender to palpation
- Signs of marked inflammation are commonly present, but arthralgia alone may be seen.

Ankylosing spondylitis (spondyloarthropathy)

- Can involve large joints of the lower extremities
- Typified in late adolescence by involvement of the sacroiliac joint
  - Seen on radiographs or magnetic resonance imaging
  - Pain elicited on palpation or compression over the joint
  - HLA-B27 transplantation antigen seen in 90% of patients

Reactive arthritis

- Previously called *Reiter syndrome*
- Triad of urethritis, conjunctivitis, and arthritis
- Often triggered by an episode of enteritis
- Diagnosis depends on excluding direct infectious causes of the inflammation.
- Arthritis predominantly occurs in large joints.

Psoriasis

- Characteristic involvement of the skin, or a history of psoriatic skin disease in the family
- Affected patients do not show rheumatoid factor.

Rheumatic diseases

- Systemic lupus erythematosus
  - Can cause chronic joint pain in adolescent girls
    - Joints may be stiff and painful.
    - Joints may show frank signs of inflammation.
- Dermatomyositis
  - Can cause inflamed joints in addition to muscle and skin involvement
- Scleroderma
- Mixed connective-tissue disease
- Kawasaki disease

Infectious diseases

- Acute bacterial infection (septic arthritis)
  - A medical emergency
  - The usual manifestation is rapid onset of pain in a joint, typically accompanied by fever.
  - The joint is red, warm, swollen, and exquisitely tender to palpation or with movement.
- Systemic bacterial infections
  - Notably caused by *Neisseria gonorrhoeae* and *Neisseria meningitidis*

- Can produce arthritis, although organisms not usually isolated from the joint
- Other bacterial infections that can involve the joints
  - Brucellosis
  - Leptospirosis
  - Tularemia
  - Rocky Mountain spotted fever
  - Rat-bite fever
  - Mycobacteria and fungal agents, particularly in immuno-compromised individuals
  - *Borrelia burgdorferi* (Lyme disease)
    - Recurrent attacks of inflammation of the large joints (85–90% of cases involve the knee)
    - Each recurrence usually lasts 1 or 2 weeks.
    - Symptoms may persist for several months; chronic arthritis of the knee has been reported.
- Osteomyelitis: acute bone infection
  - If a long bone next to a joint (eg, the distal femur and knee) is infected
    - The patient may describe pain in the joint.
    - Sterile effusion may be present.
  - Although unusual, infection can directly invade the joint space from the bone, particularly in young children.
- Diskitis
  - Disorder characterized by back pain and tenderness over the spinous process contiguous to the involved disk space
    - Causes joint pain, sometimes with low-grade fever, but often with none
    - Often, no culture-proven cause can be found.
    - Presentation can involve sensory and motor complications.
    - Epidural abscess must be considered in the differential diagnosis.
- Congenital syphilis
  - In infants, painful bony lesions and refusal to move the involved limb (Parrot pseudoparalysis), along with other associated stigmata
  - Adolescents born with this disease can develop bilateral knee effusions (Clutton joints).
- Nonbacterial organisms that cause joint disease
  - Viruses
    - Rubella
    - Mumps
    - Chickenpox
    - Adenovirus
    - Epstein-Barr virus
      - Signs of viral syndrome (rash, fever, mucous membrane involvement) usually precede joint involvement.

– Infectious hepatitis can cause arthritis before overt hepatic involvement.

- Rubella immunization causes arthralgia and arthritis in up to 3% of recipients; sequelae are rare.

Noninfectious causes

- Inflammatory bowel disease
  - Large-joint involvement
    – Pain alone or pain with inflammation
  - Joint symptoms may precede the appearance of bowel disease.
  - Activity of the bowel disease may or may not correlate with joint flare-ups.
- Sarcoidosis
- Polyarteritis nodosa
- Marfan syndrome
- Vasculitic disorders
  - Henoch-Schönlein purpura
    – Fever
    – Abdominal pain (with or without melena)
    – Purpuric lesions of the buttocks and lower extremities
    – Warm, swollen, painful, tender joints (usually knees and ankles)
- Hematologic disorders
  - Hemophilia
  - Sickle cell disease
    – Hand-foot syndrome: type of vasoocclusive crisis that is a common initial presentation in children 1–4 years of age
- Hyperuricemia and subsequent joint disease may be seen with:
  - Leukemia (with chemotherapy producing sudden lysis of cells)
  - Hemolytic anemia
  - Glycogen storage disease
  - Lesch-Nyhan syndrome
- Polyarthritis after traumatic pancreatitis
- Infantile cortical hyperostosis (Caffey disease)
  - In infants <6 months of age
  - Fever
  - Irritability
  - Increased erythrocyte sedimentation rate
  - Tender swellings of facial, trunk, and limb bones
- Toxic (transient) synovitis of the hip

Systemic autoinflammatory diseases

- A common feature is periodic fever without infectious cause.
  - Familial Mediterranean fever
  - The cryopyrinopathies

- TRAPS (tumor necrosis factor receptor–associated periodic syndrome)
- Hyper–immunoglobulin D syndrome

Hypermobility syndrome

- Increased joint laxity with vigorous activity, especially when requiring extremes of joint flexion and extension patient can experience significant arthralgia
- Diagnosis is made by physical examination and observation ≥3 of these 5 signs.
  - Hyperflexion of the wrist, bringing the thumb in contact with the volar surface of the forearm
  - Hyperextension of the fingers to parallel with the forearm
  - Hyperextension of the elbow to at least –10 degrees
  - Hyperextension of the knee to at least –10 degrees
  - Hyperflexion of the spine such that with forward flexion, the palms can be placed flat on the ground with the feet together and without flexing the knees
- Arthralgia may be present in only 1 or 2 of these sites, with hypermobility only in the joints that are painful.
- All laboratory and radiologic studies are normal.

Chondromalacia patellae (patellofemoral pain syndrome)

- Knee pain, experienced as the patella moves in the patellofemoral groove, is usually related to activity.
- Results from irregularity of the cartilage on the underside of the patella

Growing pains

- Discomfort in the lower limbs and joints
- Often worse at night
- Adolescent girls with fibromyalgia syndrome can experience diffuse arthralgia, but pain is more typically muscular or periarticular.

Physical abuse

- Consider whenever signs of trauma are evident.
- Accidents representing neglect on the part of parents or guardians need to be pursued.
- Any suspicious history or circumstance demands complete investigation.

LABORATORY EVALUATION

- Erythrocyte sedimentation rate
- C-reactive protein
- Complete blood count
- Antinuclear antibody test
  - Among children with JIA, those with oligoarticular disease are most likely to have a positive result.
- Rheumatoid factor titer
  - Present in only a small subset of children with polyarticular JIA

- Serum immunoglobulin levels
- Blood cultures may yield growth of the organism, occasionally in the absence of a positive joint fluid culture.

IMAGING

- Radiographs of joints are not routinely helpful with diagnosis.
- They can be useful in evaluating surrounding soft tissue and bones.

DIAGNOSTIC PROCEDURES

- Arthrocentesis for septic arthritis and analysis of the fluid for:
  - Appearance (opaque)
  - Viscosity (usually low)
  - Mucin clot (friable)
  - Cell count (>100,000 leukocytes/mm with ≥80% polymorphonuclear cells)
  - Glucose (usually low, much less than in serum)
  - Protein (high)
  - A portion of the fluid should be Gram stained to assess for bacterial organisms.
  - Cultures can direct definitive antimicrobial therapy.
    - *Staphylococcus aureus* and *Streptococcus* organisms are likely to be the causative organisms.

TREATMENT APPROACH

- Management focuses on:
  - Subduing inflammation
  - Preserving normal range of joint motion and strength
- Septic arthritis demands immediate arthrocentesis for diagnosis and therapy.
- Systemic bacterial infection
  - After joint aspiration and establishment of strong suspicion of purulent arthritis, the child should be hospitalized and appropriate intravenous antibiotic therapy initiated.
  - Prompt, aggressive therapy usually brings about recovery without adverse side effects, although some foci, such as the hip joint, can remain persistent problems.
- Surgery is used mostly in joint reconstruction or prosthetic replacement.

SPECIFIC TREATMENT

- Nonsteroidal antiinflammatory drugs (NSAIDs) are used as initial therapy.
- For children with JIA, methotrexate plays a central role in therapy beyond NSAIDs.
- Other long-acting agents
  - Anti–tumor necrosis factor-α agents
  - Anti-interleukin-1 drugs in systemic-onset JIA
- Systemic corticosteroids are used less frequently and at lower doses than in the past.

- For patients with a single persistently active joint, intra-articular corticosteroids (eg, triamcinolone hexacetonide) can be effective.
- Growing pains
  - A bedtime dose of an NSAID can help alleviate this pain until it resolves by itself.
- Hypermobility syndrome
  - Treated with NSAIDs and reassurance
  - For some patients, exercises to increase muscle strength and tone can be beneficial.
- Chondromalacia patellae
  - Exercises that strengthen the quadriceps femoris and adductor muscles can produce marked improvement.
  - NSAIDs or analgesics (or both taken together) may also be administered.

WHEN TO REFER

- Orthopedics
  - Fracture
  - Ligamentous or cartilage injury to joint
  - Continuous pain in a joint with deformity
- Rheumatology
  - Suspicion of JIA or other rheumatologic disorder
- Infectious diseases
  - Septic arthritis
  - Lyme disease; other spirochetal infection
  - Osteomyelitis
- Hematology
  - Sickle cell disease
  - Hemophilia
- Gastroenterology
  - Joint symptoms associated with inflammatory bowel disease
- Occupational or physical therapy
  - Joint disease complicated by contractures, weakness, poor function
  - Hypermobility syndrome
- Mental health
  - Suspicion of somatization or conversion disorder

WHEN TO ADMIT

- Fracture requiring open fixation or traction
- Systemic-onset JIA with macrophage activation syndrome
- Septic arthritis
- Osteomyelitis
- Severe sickle cell pain crisis
- Inadequate response to outpatient occupational or physical therapy and to rehabilitation

FOLLOW-UP

- For ongoing joint problems, issues related to chronic pediatric disease must be addressed.
  - The child may be unable to keep up with peers in physical activity.
  - The child may need to make many health care visits or be hospitalized, which may result in school absences.
  - Environmental stress in addition to stress caused by the disease can exacerbate various chronic conditions, such as may occur in children with JIA.
  - Children should be provided with the services of a specialized social worker, counselor, or psychologist.
  - Family resources (both emotional and financial) need to be assessed and support provided when needed.
  - Discussion groups or support groups composed of these children and their families can be helpful.
  - Major problems of body image and feelings of lack of independence must be dealt with appropriately.

COMPLICATIONS

- Long-term psychosocial sequelae also may develop from chronic joint problems.

PROGNOSIS

- Reactive arthritis
  - Usually, recovery is seen within a few months.
  - There may be a more chronic and relapsing course that can progress to ankylosing spondylitis.

J

Juvenile Idiopathic Arthritis

DEFINITION

- Juvenile idiopathic arthritis (JIA) is an uncommon collection of clinical syndromes that have the common feature of chronic childhood arthritis.
  - Previously referred to as *juvenile rheumatoid arthritis* or *juvenile chronic arthritis*
  - Term refers to any child <16 years who has:
    - Persistent arthritis of ≥1 joints
    - Condition lasting for >6 weeks
    - All other diseases have been excluded
  - JIA is classified further into 7 subtypes.
    - Most patients fit into systemic-onset, oligoarthritis, or polyarthritis based on the clinical course over the first 6 months of illness.
- Arthritis is defined as being present when:
  - Intraarticular swelling or effusion is present *or*
  - ≥2 of the following occur:
    - Joint pain or tenderness with motion
    - Limitation of joint motion
    - Increased warmth overlying the joint
- *Arthralgia* is joint pain, which is a relatively frequent symptom in children.
- Rheumatologic disorders with arthritis
  - Juvenile ankylosing spondylitis and other spondylo-arthropathies can present as a subtype of JIA at onset, especially in an older child who is human leukocyte antigen (HLA) B27 positive.
  - Acute rheumatic fever has seen a resurgence in the past 2 decades.
    - Patients can experience both arthralgia and arthritis, classically characterized as migratory.
  - Systemic lupus erythematosus has arthritis as 1 of its major manifestations.
    - Can be differentiated from JIA by other systemic features and specific laboratory test abnormalities
    - Sex distribution is equal in younger children, but a female preponderance is found after puberty.
  - Dermatomyositis is characterized by inflammatory muscle involvement rather than by arthritis.
    - Joint inflammation and contractures may be present.
  - Scleroderma is occasionally associated with arthritis.
    - Classic dermatologic and other manifestations distinguish it from JIA.

EPIDEMIOLOGY

- Prevalence
  - The most common of the pediatric rheumatic diseases
  - The true incidence and prevalence are unknown.
  - Best estimate of prevalence is ~0.5–1 case per 1000 children; ~40,000–100,000 children in the US have JIA at any given time.
  - Systemic-onset JIA affects ~15% of children who have JIA.
  - Polyarticular JIA affects 30–35% of children with JIA.
    - Subgroups include immunoglobulin (Ig) M rheumatoid factor (RF)–positive (~10% of the total) and IgM-RF–negative (~25%)
    - Positive RF in a child <7 years is rare.
  - Oligoarticular JIA affects 50–60% of children with JIA.
    - 5–10% of all patients who have JIA have persistent oligoarthritis.
    - 20–25% of all children with oligoarthritis have extended oligoarthritis.
- Age
  - Peak age at onset is between 2 and 4 years of age for all subtypes taken collectively, with a smaller peak later in childhood.
  - Systemic-onset JIA usually begins at an early age, although it has even been recognized in adults (adult-onset Still disease).
- Sex
  - General female predominance, but not in all subtypes
  - Systemic-onsest JIA is slightly more common among boys than girls.

ETIOLOGY

- The exact cause of JIA is unknown.
- Concept of genetic predisposition for the development of inflammatory arthritis that may be triggered by any of several events, such as trauma, infection or emotional stress
  - HLA-DR5 and -DR8 in younger girls with oligoarticular JIA
  - HLA-DR4 in RF-positive polyarticular JIA
  - HLA-B27 in older boys with enthesitis-related JIA
- Research is under way on:
  - Immunologic abnormalities involving autoantibodies
  - Cytokines
  - Immunoregulation
  - Function of and communication between T and B lympho-cytes and antigen-presenting cells
  - Precise nature of these interactions and their role in development of JIA remain unknown, but the success of specific cytokine-directed therapy (eg, etanercept, anakinra) supports involvement of proinflammatory mediators.

SIGNS AND SYMPTOMS

General

■ The presence of arthritis or inflammation within the joint is an absolute criterion for diagnosing JIA.

■ Younger children rarely complain of joint pain but may:

● Become irritable

● Stop walking or using an extremity

● Regress in their behavior

■ Other symptoms include:

● Decreased appetite

● Malaise

● Inactivity

● Morning stiffness

● Nighttime joint pains

● Failure to thrive

■ Features that may be present in children who have chronic arthritis (varying with the subtype) include:

● Fever

● Rash

● Lymphadenopathy

● Hepatosplenomegaly

● Polyserositis

● Subcutaneous (rheumatoid) nodules

● Vasculitis

● Growth retardation

■ Pattern and number of involved joints are important in classifying the disease.

Systemic-onset JIA (Still disease)

■ The hallmark of systemic-onset JIA is its extraarticular manifestations.

■ The eventual presence of arthritis is still necessary to confirm diagnosis.

■ The systemic features may persist for months and occur or recur independently of the arthritis.

● Daily intermittent fevers

– Rectal temperature reaches as high as 40°C–41°C (104°F–106°F).

– Most often in the afternoon

– Returning to normal or subnormal levels (known as aquotidian fever pattern)

– Children frequently complain of myalgias or arthralgias when they are febrile, but they may have few symptoms when the fevers resolve.

● Evanescent, salmon-colored rash often accompanies fevers.

– Lesions are small macules or papules.

– Frequently with central clearing

– Often appear in areas of increased heat (eg, axilla)

● Mild abrasion of unaffected skin can precipitate appearance of the rash (Koebner phenomenon).

● Polyserositis in the form of pericarditis or pleuritis

– These serosal effusions are rarely symptomatic or clinically significant.

● Enlargement of the lymph nodes, liver, and spleen may suggest the presence of cancer.

● Arthritis may occur at any time after the onset of disease.

– In some, it appears only days to weeks after the systemic signs occur.

– Tends to be polyarticular, involving both large and small joints

– Can be persistent, destructive, and severe

■ Clinical course is extremely variable.

● A single systemic episode may last weeks to months, with few joint problems.

● Multiple systemic episodes may precede development of arthritis.

● Can be oligoarticular but is more commonly polyarticular

■ Macrophage activation syndrome

● An unusual but potentially fatal complication of systemic-onset JIA

● Rapidly progessive and difficult to distinguish from a flare of JIA

● Characterized by:

– Intravascular consumption coagulopathy

– Dramatically elevated ferritin (>10,000 ng/mL)

– Paradoxically decreased erythrocyte sedimentation rate (ESR)

– Decreased fibrinogen

– Increased triglyceride levels

– Pancytopenia

– Hepatic failure

● Diagnosis confirmed by bone marrow biopsy

● Rapid intervention is necessary

Polyarticular JIA

■ Systemic features in polyarticular JIA are usually mild and include:

● Low-grade fever

● Easy fatigability

● Slowing of growth

– Growth problems may be local (eg, micrognathia) or generalized

– Can occur regardless of whether the child receives corticosteroid treatment

J

- Discrepancies between height and weight can help with diagnosis.
  - For example, children who have polyarticular arthritis may be of low weight for height, whereas children who have systemic-onset JIA tend to be average in weight for height.
- Chronic uveitis

■ Arthritis symptoms
  - Most often chronic, symmetrical, and involving ≥5 joints
  - Any joint can be affected.
  - Nearly all children have wrist involvement; small joint involvement of hands and feet is common.

RF-positive polyarticular JIA

■ Patients with IgM RF-positive polyarticular JIA are:
  - Most often >8–10 years
  - More likely to be girls than boys
  - Similar clinically to patients with adult rheumatoid arthritis

■ Arthritis symptoms are:
  - Severe
  - Rapidly progressive
  - Erosive
  - Crippling
  - Subcutaneous rheumatoid nodules
  - Rheumatoid vasculitis

RF-negative polyarticular JIA

■ Children with IgM RF-negative polyarticular JIA are usually younger.

■ Because their arthritis starts earlier, it can lead to deformities and problems as a result of:
  - Tendency to develop flexion contractures
  - Subluxations at the involved joints

■ Compared with adults, hand involvement affects interphalangeal joints more often than metacarpophalangeal joints.

■ Ulnar deviation of the fingers is much less common in children.

■ Ulnar deviation and subluxation at the wrist may occur.

■ More frequently seen in children
  - Flexion contractures
  - Boutonniere (buttonhole) deformities
  - Radial deviation of the fingers

■ Arthritis of the apophyseal joints of the cervical spine is common.
  - Can lead to rapid and significant limitation of extension and rotation

■ These children are at the highest risk for local and generalized growth problems.

Oligoarticular JIA

■ Involves ≤4 joints, most often the large (eg, knee, ankle, elbow)

■ Typically asymmetrical in distribution

■ Important in distinguishing this form of JIA
  - Pattern and course of joint involvement
  - Number of joints involved

■ Systemic features are infrequent and mild.

■ Oligoarticular JIA can be subdivided further into persistent and extended oligoarticular subtypes.

■ Persistent oligoarthritis
  - Occurs classically in girls <6 years of age
  - Involves the large joints
  - Higher risk for chronic uveitis, particularly when positive for antinuclear antibodies (ANA)
  - Systemic signs and symptoms, except for uveitis, are few.
  - These children generally function well and only rarely complain of significant pain.
  - Little erosive joint damage occurs, even though patients may have ongoing arthritis for many years.
  - At risk for long-term problems, including:
    - Leg-length discrepancies (especially with asymmetrical knee joint involvement)
      ■ Growth centers around the arthritic knee can become more active because of the inflammatory-associated hyperemia, resulting in increased growth of that leg.
    - Muscle atrophy
      ■ As a result of changes in the child's biomechanics, decreased quadriceps mass on the affected side is frequently found.

■ Extended oligoarthritis
  - ≤4 joints involved within first 6 months of disease
  - At a variable time after the initial 6 months, children develop arthritis in more joints.
  - Genetic makeup
    - Higher frequency of HLA-DR1 than in persistent oligoarthritis
  - Higher occurrence of erosive disease than in persistent oligoarthritis
  - Additionally involved joints are often:
    - Wrists
    - Fingers
    - Other smaller joints
  - Chronic uveitis still occurs, although less frequently.

Enthesitis-related arthritis

■ A newer classification that includes children who previously were classified as late-onset oligoarthritis

- Complaints and findings of enthesitis (inflammation of the attachment of a tendon, ligament, fascia, or capsule to bone) are a hallmark of this group and may predate joint problems.
- Subgroup includes children with:
  - Arthritis and enthesitis *and*
  - ≥2 of the following:
    - Sacroiliac joint pain or inflammatory spinal pain (or both)
    - Presence of HLA-B27
    - History of relatives with HLA-B27–associated disease
    - Anterior uveitis usually associated with pain, redness, or photophobia
    - Onset of arthritis in a boy >8 years
- More frequently occurs in the lower extremities, involving the knees and ankles; occasionally in toes (resulting in so-called sausage toe, or dactylitis)
- Patients may progress to:
  - Ankylosing spondylitis
  - Reactive arthritides
  - Arthritis associated with inflammatory bowel disease

Psoriatic arthritis

- An additional classification subtype of JIA
- Similar to enthesitis-related arthritis in that large joint inflammation, enthesitis, and dactylitis are often found
- Psoriasis must be present in the patient or in family members.
  - Thus a child can have psoriatic arthritis in the absence of skin disease.
  - Psoriatic rash can appear at some time after the onset of joint disease.
- Pitting of the fingernails or toenails can identify psoriatic arthritis in the child with characteristic musculoskeletal findings, but no skin eruption.

Undifferentiated arthritis

- Children who do not meet the criteria for ≥1 subtype

DIFFERENTIAL DIAGNOSIS

- Diseases to be considered in the differential diagnosis of JIA
  - Rheumatic diseases of childhood
    - Autoinflammatory diseases
    - Acute rheumatic fever
    - Systemic lupus erythematosus
    - Juvenile ankylosing spondylitis
    - Polymyositis and dermatomyositis
    - Vasculitis
    - Scleroderma
    - Mixed connective-tissue disease/overlap
    - Kawasaki disease
    - Behçet syndrome
    - Postinfectious reactive arthritis
    - Reactive arthritis
    - Reflex sympathetic dystrophy (complex regional pain syndrome type II)
    - Fibromyalgia syndrome
  - Infectious diseases
    - Bacterial arthritis
      - Must be considered if the child has a single inflamed joint
      - *Haemophilus influenzae* type b has decreased markedly in incidence in children <2 years of age with universal immunization.
      - *Neisseria gonorrhoeae*, particularly in adolescence
      - Staphylococci may be found at any age.
      - Lyme disease (*Borrelia burgdorferi* infection) in endemic areas.
    - Viral or postviral arthritis
      - Parvovirus
      - Rubella
      - Hepatitis B
    - Fungal arthritis
    - Osteomyelitis
    - Postinfectious reactive arthritis
      - From a gastrointestinal bacterial infection (eg, *Shigella, Salmonella, Campylobacter,* or *Yersinia* organisms)
  - Neoplastic diseases
    - Leukemia
    - Lymphoma
    - Neuroblastoma
    - Primary bone tumors
  - Noninflammatory disorders
    - Trauma
    - Avascular necrosis syndromes
    - Osteochondroses
    - Slipped capital femoral epiphysis
    - Diskitis
    - Patellofemoral dysfunction (chondromalacia patellae)
    - Toxic synovitis of the hip
    - Overuse syndromes
  - Hematologic disorders
    - Sickle cell disease
    - Hemophilia
  - Miscellaneous
    - Inflammatory bowel disease
    - Chronic recurrent multifocal osteomyelitis

J

- Sarcoidosis
- Collagen (connective tissue) disorders
  (eg, Ehlers-Danlos syndrome, Marfan syndrome)
- Growing pains
- Psychogenic arthralgias (conversion reactions)
- Hypermobility syndrome
- Villonodular synovitis
- Foreign-body arthritis

DIAGNOSTIC APPROACH

- Because the diagnosis of JIA is based on clinical findings, history and physical examination are paramount.
- The hallmark of JIA is its chronic nature, and the best initial strategy is often careful, watchful waiting.
- The primary care physician can avoid mislabeling other transient entities as JIA by:
  - Meeting the criterion of sustained arthritis (>6 weeks)
  - Excluding other possible diseases

LABORATORY FINDINGS

- No unique or specific diagnostic laboratory tests yet exist.
- Systemic-onset JIA
  - High leukocyte count, with predominance of band forms and polymorphonuclear leukocytes
  - Most patients are anemic.
  - Thrombocytosis
  - Significant increases of acute phase reactants (eg, ESR and C-reactive protein level)
  - RF and ANA tests are rarely positive.
  - Serum immunoglobulin and complement levels are usually normal.
    - May be elevated, reflecting the degree of inflammation
    - Sometimes indicate a vasculopathy and an intravascular consumption coagulopathy
      - With intravascular consumption coagulopathy, need to rule out macrophage activation syndrome
- RF-positive polyarticular JIA
  - Cyclic citrullinated protein can be used to assess disease severity and potential for joint destruction.
  - An elevated serum level would serve as reason to institute early and aggressive therapy.
- Persistent oligoarthritis
  - Few laboratory abnormalities will be found except for positive ANA.
    - When positive, the ANA titer is typically low.
  - Mild increases in leukocyte count and ESR or low-grade anemia may be observed, but these tests are most often normal.

- HLA-DR5 gene markers appear to confer increased susceptibility for persistent oligoarthritis; HLA-DR1 and -DR4 are underrepresented in this group.
- Enthesitis-related arthritis
  - Abnormal laboratory tests are found infrequently.
  - Mild to moderate increase in the ESR is common.

DIAGNOSTIC PROCEDURES

- If any question exists as to an intraarticular septic process, arthrocentesis must be performed to establish the diagnosis.

TREATMENT APPROACH

- JIA is a chronic illness, and no current mode of therapy is curative.
- The patient's management should be individualized for:
  - Disease subtype
  - Extent of activity
  - Clinical course to date
  - Family situation
- Pharmacologic therapy is only 1 aspect of treatment for children with JIA.
- Drug therapy is not yet curative but can suppress the inflammatory activity in many children.
- 5 major categories of drug therapy are available.
  - Nonsteroidal antiinflammatory drugs (NSAIDs)
  - Disease-modifying antirheumatic drugs (DMARDs)
  - Corticosteroids
  - Immunosuppressive drugs
  - Agents with immune- and cytokine-modulating effects (biological agents)
- A multidisciplinary team approach is the most effective approach.
- The goal of therapy is to attain the highest possible level of physical and psychological function for the child.
- In addition to an attentive and understanding primary care physician, the patient and family need:
  - Family counselor, social worker, and psychologist or similar mental health professional to help them adjust to this chronic illness
    - Feelings of denial, guilt, and frustration at the time of the diagnosis and throughout the course of the disease are common.
    - Siblings frequently find difficulty to cope with the special and extensive treatment the affected child may receive.
- Periodic depression and anger are frequent, especially in the early stages, and again as the patient enters adolescence.
- Poor maternal function, maternal depression, and social isolation are risk factors for poor psychosocial outcomes; a sense of control and mastery are important positive factors.

■ Most children with JIA can do well in school; thus, all efforts should be made to keep them enrolled.

- Some school adjustments may be necessary, such as different transportation or physical education (or both) and allowing extra time between classes.

- 2 sets of books, 1 for school and 1 for home, reduces the work of carrying books.

- The primary care physician or pediatric rheumatology team may have to advocate within the school to ensure services.

■ Preparation for eventual independent living and vocations must begin in childhood to reduce potential barriers.

- Anticipatory guidance about transitional issues should start in childhood and early adolescence.

■ The child with mild disease and a hidden disability may have problems coping, adapting, and trying to accomplish unrealistic goals of a society that does not recognize the disability.

■ Any chronic illness imposes many additional stresses on the entire family.

SPECIFIC TREATMENTS

NSAIDs

■ NSAIDs currently approved by the US Food and Drug Administration (FDA) for use in children

- Individual responses to NSAIDs vary widely, and if a child does not improve within 4–6 weeks, then trying a different NSAID is reasonable.

- Salicylates
  - No longer the initial NSAIDs of choice because of concerns regarding Reye syndrome
  - Other agents have emerged that are essentially equivalent in efficacy and toxicity.

- Indomethacin
- Tolmetin sodium
- Naproxen
- Ibuprofen
- Celecoxib
- Meloxicam

■ NSAIDs not approved by the FDA for use in children
- Diclofenac sodium
- Fenoprofen
- Flurbiprofen
- Ketoprofen
- Phenylbutazone
- Pirprofen
- Piroxicam
- Meclofenamate sodium
- Sulindac

■ NSAIDs available in liquid form for younger children who have trouble swallowing pills
- Naproxen
- Ibuprofen
- Indomethacin
- Meloxicam

■ Cyclooxygenase II (COX-2)–selective inhibitors interfere only with COX-2 and decrease the prostaglandin production that mediates inflammation, in a gastroprotective manner.

- Reduces the risk of gastric erosion or ulcer formation, or both

- As a result of cardiovascular safety questions, many were removed from the market.

- Celecoxib remains available in the US.

- Meloxicam is predominantly COX-2 selective and is available in a generic preparation.

DMARDs and cytotoxic/immunosuppressive drugs

■ If a child does not quickly respond to NSAID therapy alone or is in a high-risk category, more aggressive interventions are necessary.

■ Moving quickly to DMARDs and/or biologic agents, as well as performing intraarticular corticosteroid injections, appears to achieve the goal of no inflammation with great effectiveness.

■ Methotrexate

- Essentially replaced intramuscular and oral gold, D-penicillamine, and hydroxychloroquine as primary second-line agent of JIA treatment

- Competitive inhibitor of dihydrofolate reductase, which exerts both antiinflammatory and immunosuppressive effects on arthritis

- Efficacy and dose response have been well established.

- Hepatic, bone marrow, gastrointestinal, pulmonary, and teratogenic adverse effects may result.

  - To detect liver or hematopoetic adverse effects, laboratory monitoring every 4–8 weeks is suggested.

  - Administration of folic (or folinic) acid may decrease some of methotrexate's adverse effects, such as nausea and oral ulcers.

■ Leflunomide

- Immunosuppressive agent that inhibits pyridine synthesis and suppresses tumor necrosis factor-α (TNF-α)–induced cellular responses

- Shown to have beneficial effects similar to methotrexate

- Teratogenic effects are possible

- Requires ongoing monitoring

- Not FDA-approved for use in treating JIA

- Sulfasalazine
  - Has seen a resurgence, but should not be used in anyone:
    - Sensitive to sulfa drugs or salicylates
    - Whose renal or hepatic function is impaired
    - Who has such conditions as glucose-6-phosphate dehydrogenase deficiency
  - Adverse effects caused by sulfasalazine
    - Rashes
    - Nausea
    - Vomiting
    - Dyspepsia
    - In boys, a reversible decrease in sperm count
    - Bone marrow depression rarely occurs.
- Other immunosuppressive agents occasionally administered in specific patients, but not currently the standard
  - Intravenous immunoglobulin
  - Azathioprine
  - Chlorambucil
  - Cyclophosphamide
  - Cyclosporine
  - Thalidomide

Biologic agents

- Considered standard to add a TNF-α blocker to the regimen of any child with JIA:
  - Who has not responded to previously administered DMARD therapy
  - When tapering the dose of corticosteroids is not possible without precipitating a flare of the disease
- Testing for tuberculosis is recommended before starting because these agents can interfere with immune response.
- Adverse effects
  - Injection site pain or reactions
  - Increased risk of infection
  - Possible increased risk of other autoimmune conditions or neoplasms
- Long-term effects are not yet known.
- Etanercept, adalimumab, and infliximab
  - Blocks activity of TNF-α (a major proinflammatory cytokine)
  - Etanercept and adalimumab are approved for use in children with JIA.
  - Demonstrated dramatic improvements in condition of children and adults with arthritis
  - A child who has not responded or has had an adverse effect to 1 agent may still respond to another because each is slightly different.

- Interleukins 1 and 6 (IL-1 and IL-6) are cytokines that play a significant role in JIA treatment.
  - Systemic-onset JIA is more of an IL-1- or IL-6- (or both) driven condition.
    - Often responds better to blocking these cytokines than TNF-α
- Anakinra
  - IL-1–receptor antagonist
  - Proven effective in children who have not responded adequately to TNF-α inhibitors
  - Should not be administered in combination with a TNF-α inhibitor or any other biologic agent
- Abatacept
  - Recently approved for treating children with JIA
  - Selectively modulates the CD80/CD86:CD28 costimulatory signal required for full T-cell activation
  - Demonstrated efficacy in both children and adults with arthritis who have not responded adequately to TNF-α inhibitors
- Rituximab
  - Monoclonal antibody directed against the CD20 marker on B-lymphocytes
  - Currently approved for adults not responding to TNF-α blockade
  - Not yet determined for use in children

Corticosteroids

- Monoclonal antibodies have rendered systemic corticosteroid use in JIA much less necessary.
- Corticosteroids remain important and effective medications, and use should follow these maxims.
  - They should be administered only when other agents have failed or when the child is seriously ill or has progressive severe chronic anterior uveitis unresponsive to local or other systemic therapy.
  - As small a dose as possible should be administered.
  - Their use should be tapered and discontinued as soon as possible.
- Corticosteroids are effective antiinflammatory agents but do not alter the course of the disease.
- Can be extremely difficult to discontinue in children with JIA
- Long-term use is associated with many serious adverse effects, including:
  - Immunosuppression
  - Osteoporosis
  - Growth retardation
- Small daily doses of prednisone may be effective in treating pain and stiffness.
- Higher doses may be needed to manage systemic features, such aspericarditis.

- High-dose intravenous pulse corticosteroid therapy can be useful in dire situations but is not more effective as chronic therapy.
- Intraarticular corticosteroids now play a larger role, especially oligoarticular JIA.
  - Can be effective in controlling acute problems associated with 1 or several active joints
  - Usually used in combination with systemic, ongoing therapy
- Children with a painful or swollen joint frequently respond to arthrocentesis and instillation of a long-acting corticosteroid preparation (eg, triamcinolone hexacetonide).
  - This procedure should not be performed >3 or 4 times per year.
  - The physician should be absolutely certain that concomitant infectious arthritis is not the cause of the acute joint problem.
  - Early use of intraarticular corticosteroids may even have the potential to modify the course of JIA.

Physical and occupational therapy

- Crucial adjuncts to:
  - Maintain strength and range of motion
  - Prevent contractures
  - Allow the best possible quality of life
- All patients should be given a home program of therapy that is reviewed and updated regularly.
- Heat therapy often helps minimize morning stiffness.
  - Warm baths or using a sleeping bag at night
- Swimming is an excellent exercise; affected children should be encouraged to swim and to participate in as many other activities as possible.
- Normal play is a form of physical and occupational therapy.
- The orthopedist's contribution ranges from the application of splints to operative tendon releases and capsulotomies.
  - Some children may require joint resurfacing or joint replacement surgery.
  - The orthopedist's perspective is an important part of disease management.

WHEN TO ADMIT

- Children with systemic-onset JIA who develop severe chest pain with shortness of breath (suggesting pericarditis with hemodynamic compromise) or a change in voice quality and difficulty breathing (suggesting cricoarytenoid arthritis)
- Children with chronic arthritis who are receiving corticosteroid therapy and develop signs of severe infection
- Children with chronic arthritis who are receiving NSAIDs and have acute anemia and melanotic stools

- Children with longstanding polyarticular arthritis complicated by multiple joint contractures and weakness and who require a period of inpatient rehabilitation (eg, physical and occupational therapy)

WHEN TO REFER

- Children with persistent oligoarticular or polyarticular joint inflammation
- Children with spiking fevers and rash but no obvious infectious cause
- Children with persistent joint pain, limp, or asymmetrical use of an extremity for which no explanation has been found

FOLLOW-UP

- Risk of uveitis decreases with time and varies by JIA subtype and age at diagnosis.
  - Prescribed intervals between examinations vary, eventually lengthening after several years if no uveitis is present (see table Frequency of Ophthalmologic Examination in Patients With Juvenile Rheumatoid Arthritis).
  - Persistent oligoarticular JIA
    - Regular ophthalmologic evaluation for uveitis, including slit-lamp examinations, should be:
      - Instituted early
      - Performed every 4–6 months
      - Continued indefinitely
  - Children with extended oligoarthritis should be monitored closely, although uveitis is more common in children with the persistent type.

Complications

- Joint related
  - Pain
  - Loss of mobility
  - Impaired growth
  - Leg length discrepancy
  - Muscle atrophy
  - Destructive arthropathy
- Uveitis
- Psychosocial effects
- Treatment side effects

PROGNOSIS

- JIA is rarely fatal, and in general the long-term prognosis is good.
- Approximately 60–75% of children will undergo remission at some point; many children will experience permanent remission.
- Most children with JIA will complete school, be gainfully employed, and raise families.

J

Frequency of Ophthalmologic Examination in Patients With Juvenile Rheumatoid Arthritis[a,b]

Type	ANA	Age at Onset (yr)	Duration of Disease (yr)	Risk Category	Eye Examination Frequency (mo)
Oligoarthritis or polyarthritis	+	≤6	≤4	High	3
	+	≤6	>4	Moderate	6
	+	≤6	>7	Low	12
	+	>6	≤4	Moderate	6
	+	>6	>4	Low	12
	−	≤6	≤4	Moderate	6
	−	≤6	>4	Low	12
	−	>6	NA	Low	12
Systemic disease (fever, rash)	NA	NA	NA	Low	12

Abbreviations: ANA, antinuclear antibodies; NA, not applicable.

[a] From: Cassidy J, Kivlin J, Lindsley C, et al, American Academy of Pediatrics, Section on Rheumatology and Section on Ophthalmology. Ophthalmologic examinations in children with juvenile rheumatoid arthritis. *Pediatrics.* 2006;117(5):1843–1845.

[b] Recommendations for follow-up continue through childhood and adolescence.

- Patterns of disease activity
  - Persistent active arthritis and destructive arthropathy
  - Active disease, then remission
  - Polycyclic diseases characterized by acute flares of activity followed by temporary remissions
  - Low-grade continued disease activity with little if any joint destruction
- Oligoarticular JIA
  - Children with oligoarticular arthritis and no chronic anterior uveitis have the best prognosis.
  - 40–50% of children undergo complete remission.
  - Persistent oligoarthritis
    - The course can be extremely variable.
    - Some children have a single episode; others may have recurrent exacerbations and remissions.
    - This group has the fewest musculoskeletal complications and more long-term remissions.
  - Extended oligoarthritis
    - Fewer children in this subgroup enter a prolonged remission than do those with persistent oligoarthritis, and they fare better than children with polyarthritis-onset disease.

- Systemic-onset JIA
  - 25–30% undergo complete remission.
  - Younger children with systemic-onset and polyarticular arthritis have a poorer articular prognosis.
  - Poor prognostic signs include:
    - Continued presence of systemic features
    - Platelet count >600,000 cells/mm 6 months after onset
  - At least one-third of these children will develop severe arthritis.
- Polyarticular JIA
  - 25–30% undergo complete remission.
  - RF-negative polyarticular JIA
    - Overall better prognosis than children with RF-positive polyarticular JIA
    - Typically respond better to therapy and have a lower frequency of severe, early, crippling arthritis, but may develop significant problems

Kawasaki Disease

DEFINITION

- An acute, multisystem vasculitis of infancy and early childhood
- Characterized by:
  - High fever
  - Rash
  - Conjunctivitis
  - Inflammation of the mucous membranes
  - Erythematous induration of the hands and feet
  - Cervical adenopathy
- Formerly known as *mucocutaneous lymph node syndrome*

EPIDEMIOLOGY

- Prevalence
  - For children ≤8 years in the continental US
    - 32.5 cases per 100,000 in those of Asian or part Asian descent
    - 16.9 per 100,000 in blacks
    - 11.1 per 100,000 in Hispanics
    - 9.1 per 100,000 in whites
  - Recurrent cases
    - 0.3–5% in Japan
    - 1–2% in the US
- Age
  - Most common during the 2nd year of life
  - More than 80% of all cases occur in children <5 years.
  - Uncommon beyond 9 years of age
- Sex
  - Boys are affected more commonly than girls, with a male-to-female ratio of nearly 1.5:1.
- Geographic distribution
  - Most prevalent in Japan and in children of Japanese ancestry, but distribution is worldwide
- Seasonality
  - More common in winter and spring
  - Numerous temporal clusters have been reported in the US and Japan, suggesting an infectious cause.

ETIOLOGY

- No specific cause has been established, although clinical features suggest an infectious process.
  - The most recent theory is that toxin-producing staphylococcal or streptococcal bacteria are the primary cause.
  - These agents are attractive candidates because of the similarity of Kawasaki disease to illnesses such as staphylococcal toxic shock syndrome and streptococcal toxic shock syndrome.

RISK FACTORS

- Intravenous immunoglobulin (IVIG) therapy for first episode may increase risk of recurrence within the following 12 months.
- Sibling with the disease
  - Incidence is higher in twins than in nontwin siblings.
    - Not significantly different between monozygotic twins and dizygotic twins
  - The interval between sibling cases is <10 days in 54% of cases; onset sometimes occurs on the same day.
    - Suggests a common exposure to an infectious agent in a genetically predisposed population

SIGNS AND SYMPTOMS

Typical Kawasaki disease

Criteria

- Fever of unknown cause lasting ≤5 days *and*
- At least 4 of the 5 following principal features:
  - Changes in extremities
    - Acute: erythema of palms, soles; edema of hands, feet
    - Subacute: periungual peeling of fingers, toes in weeks 2 and 3
  - Polymorphous exanthem
  - Bilateral bulbar conjunctival injection without exudate
  - Changes in lips and oral cavity: erythema, lips cracking, strawberry tongue, diffuse injection of oral and pharyngeal mucosae
  - Cervical lymphadenopathy (diameter >1.5 cm), usually unilateral
- Other illnesses with similar features must be excluded.
- Cervical lymphadenopathy is the least common of the principal features.
- Coronary artery abnormalities detected by 2D echocardiography or coronary angiography in a patient with fever for ≥5 days, even with <4 criteria, fulfill the diagnosis.
- Patients with ≥4 criteria can be diagnosed on day 4 of illness.
- Other findings
  - Cardiovascular
    - Congestive heart failure
    - Myocarditis
    - Pericarditis
    - Valvular regurgitation
    - Coronary heart abnormalities
    - Aneurysms of medium-size noncoronary arteries
    - Raynaud phenomenon
    - Peripheral gangrene

- Musculoskeletal
  - Arthritis
  - Arthralgia
- Gastrointestinal
  - Diarrhea
  - Vomiting
  - Abdominal pain
  - Hepatic dysfunction
  - Hydrops of gallbladder
- Central nervous system
  - Extreme irritability
  - Aseptic meningitis
  - Sensorineural hearing loss
- Genitourinary
  - Urethritis/meatitis
- Other
  - Erythema
  - Induration at Bacille Calmette-Guérin inoculation site
  - Anterior uveitis (mild)
  - Desquamating rash in groin

Phases

- The course of the disease can best be described as triphasic.
- Symptoms are not all apparent simultaneously, but the timing of their appearance is remarkably constant.
- Acute phase
  - Fever
  - Oropharyngeal erythema
  - Swelling of the hands and feet
  - Polymorphous erythematous rash
  - Cervical lymphadenopathy
- Subacute phase
  - Begins after 10–12 days of the illness, when fever, rash, and lymphadenopathy fade
  - Characterized by:
    - Lip cracking and fissuring
    - Unusual desquamation of the skin, beginning at the subungual and periungual regions of the fingers and toes
      - Occurs in nearly all cases 2–3 weeks after the onset and after early signs involving the extremities have disappeared
      - May progress to complete peeling of palms and soles, but exfoliation generally does not extend to remainder of body surface
    - Onset of arthralgias or arthritis (or both), thrombocytosis, and cardiac disease
- Convalescent stage
  - Usually begins ~25 days after onset

- Characterized by:
  - Absence of clinical signs of disease
  - Persistence of residual inflammation, marked by elevated erythrocyte sedimentation rate (ESR)

Symptoms

- Fever is the most prominent symptom of the acute phase of the disease.
  - High-spiking remittent pattern in the range of 38.4°C (101.1°F) to >40°C (104°F)
  - Persists despite use of empirical antibiotics, corticosteroids, and standard doses of antipyretics.
  - Is present on average for ~12 days, although prolonged courses of up to 5 weeks have been reported; defervescence occurs over 1–3 days.
- Conjunctival hyperemia
  - Discrete engorgement of the bulbar conjunctivae blood vessels (without associated discharge, exudate, keratitis, chemosis, or pseudomembrane formation) and an anterior uveitis develop shortly after the onset of fever.
  - The cornea, lens, and retina are not involved.
- Early oropharyngeal signs include dryness and reddening of lips and of buccal and pharyngeal mucosa.
  - Absence of aphthous ulceration or hemorrhagic bullae is noticeable.
  - A "strawberry tongue" often is present.
  - Later, as intensity of the erythema subsides, lips usually become cracked and fissured.
- The most characteristic and unique feature of Kawasaki disease relates to changes that occur in the hands and feet.
  - Early on, they become diffusely indurated and swollen; overlying skin develops a woody firmness suggestive of acute scleroderma.
  - The palms and soles usually become erythematous or purplish.
  - Fusiform swelling of the fingers also occurs, which limits the child's ability to grasp objects.
  - Feet are painful to the touch, and many children will refuse to stand or walk.
  - During convalescent phase, deep transverse grooves (Beau lines) may appear across the fingernails and toenails, presumably as a result of arrested growth during the illness.
- A polymorphous, erythematous rash appears 1–5 days after the onset of fever.
  - Usually begins on the extremities and spreads centripetally
  - The 3 most common patterns of rash are
    - Maculopapular (morbilliform)
    - Erythema multiforme-like with iris lesions
    - Scarlatiniform
  - The rash may be coalescent, producing large, irregular, raised plaques, and may be pruritic.

K

- Vesicles, pustules, and bullae are not seen.
- The rash is not petechial or purpuric.
- Rash usually fades within 1 week but occasionally persists longer or recurs.
  - Lymphadenopathy
    - Typically involves a single cervical node measuring >1.5 cm in diameter.
      - The node usually is not tender or warm and does not become fluctuant.
      - The lymph node diminishes in size with defervescence of the disease.
    - Generalized lymphadenopathy does not occur.
    - The least often seen of the major criteria
      - Occurs in only ~60% of patients in most US series.
  - Other features of Kawasaki disease may be noted.
    - Sterile pyuria occurs more often than lymphadenopathy in most US cases.
      - 10–100 white blood cells (WBCs) per high-power field may be observed on a clean-catch voided urine specimen.
      - No WBCs will be seen on a bladder aspiration specimen, because the sterile pyuria is caused by urethral inflammation or ulceration.
  - Occasionally, trace proteinuria or hematuria
  - Irritability, mild meningismus, and lethargy are seen in nearly all patients with Kawasaki disease, and nearly all probably have aseptic meningitis.
  - Cerebrospinal fluid (CSF) typically shows 25–100 WBCs/mm³ with normal amounts of glucose and protein.
  - Diarrhea is seen in approximately 50% of patients.
    - Passing 5–15 stools per day for 2–7 days during the acute or subacute phase is common.
    - Stools do not contain polymorphonuclear cells and do not test positive for occult blood.
  - Either arthralgias, arthritis, or both occur in 30–40%.
    - Large joints, particularly the knees and ankles, are involved most often.
    - Usually, no more than 2 or 3 joints will be affected.
    - Joint symptoms occur 8–12 days after the onset of disease.
    - Joint fluid, if analyzed, reveals findings similar to those of rheumatoid arthritis.
  - Pneumonia, tympanitis, photophobia, and mild liver dysfunction are observed somewhat less commonly.
  - Acute hydrops of the gallbladder, jaundice, convulsions, encephalopathy, Bell palsy, hearing loss, pancreatitis, orchitis, and pleural effusions are seen rarely but also are associated complications of Kawasaki disease.
  - Cardiovascular system findings
    - Disease mortality results from coronary artery aneurysm rupture or occlusion.

- During the acute phase, tachycardia and gallop rhythms may appear.
- However, the most serious manifestations of cardiac involvement occur during the subacute phase.
- Manifestations may include:
  - Serious arrhythmias
  - Congestive heart failure
  - Pericardial effusion
  - Mitral insufficiency
  - Myocardial ischemia or infarction
  - Infants <6 months of age with Kawasaki disease
    - High risk for coronary abnormalities
      - This group is at highest risk (≥50%) for coronary artery lesions if untreated.
      - Echocardiography should be considered in any infant aged <6 months with fever of >7 days, laboratory evidence of systemic inflammation, and no other explanation for the febrile illness.

Atypical Kawasaki disease

- Severe or even fatal coronary abnormalities can develop after illnesses that resemble but do not fulfill the classic diagnostic features of Kawasaki disease.
- Should be considered in:
  - Infants and children with unexplained fever for >5 days and 2 or 3 of the principal diagnostic criteria
    - Young infants may have fever only.
  - Children (<1 year and teens) with fever for >7 days, rash with or without nonexudative conjunctivitis
- Laboratory results are similar to those of classic cases.
- Patients may display
  - Prolonged high fever
  - Nonspecific rash
  - Arthralgia or arthritis
  - Fissuring of the lips
  - Nonexudative conjunctivitis
  - Extreme irritability
- Atypical Kawasaki disease occasionally can produce prolonged fever for ≥5 days in the absence of other clinical criteria for the illness.
- In other patients, unilateral cervical adenopathy refractory to antibiotic therapy indicates that atypical Kawasaki disease may be present.
- In infants <6 months of age, atypical Kawasaki disease is likely to produce the same subtle manifestations seen in typical Kawasaki disease.
  - Usually lack full diagnostic criteria
  - Manifestations often subtle: fever, rash, and cerebral spinal fluid pleocytosis may be misdiagnosed as viral meningitis

K

- High risk for coronary abnormalities
  - This group is at highest risk (≥50%) for coronary artery lesions if untreated.
  - Echocardiography should be considered in any infant aged <6 months with fever for >7 days, laboratory evidence of systemic inflammation, and no other explanation for the febrile illness.

DIFFERENTIAL DIAGNOSIS

- The clinical picture of Kawasaki disease, after all major features have exhibited, is not difficult to differentiate from other mucocutaneous syndromes.

- In the first days of the illness, a whole spectrum of acute febrile diseases might be considered.
- By 3–5 days after onset, certain clinical features may be singled out as compatible with other diagnoses—eg, strawberry tongue, which is suggestive of streptococcal infection.

- 2 conditions most commonly mimic Kawasaki disease: streptococcal and staphylococcal scarlet fever.
  - However, if all the signs and symptoms are considered carefully, then the diagnosis is readily apparent.
- The clinical features of Kawasaki disease and other mucocutaneous disorders are compared in the table below.

Clinical Features of Kawasaki Disease and Other Mucocutaneous Diseases

	Kawasaki Disease	Stevens-Johnson Syndrome	Streptococcal Scarlet Fever	Staphylococcal Scarlet Fever	Staphylococcal Toxic Shock Syndrome	Leptospirosis
Age (yr)	Usually <5	Usually 3–30	Usually 5–10	Usually 2–8	Usually adolescent	Usually >2
Fever	Prolonged	Prolonged	Variable	Variable	Usually <10 days	Variable
Eyes	Hyperemia of ocular conjunctivae; uveitis	Catarrhal conjunctivitis; chemosis; iritis; uveitis; panophthalmitis	No change	Hyperemia of ocular conjunctivae	Hyperemia of ocular conjunctivae	Hyperemia of ocular conjunctivae; uveitis
Lips	Red, dry, fissured	Erosions; crusted, fissured, bleeding	No change	No change	Red	No change
Oral cavity	Diffuse erythema; strawberry tongue	Erythema; bullae, ulcers, pseudomembrane formation	Pharyngitis; palatal petechiae; strawberry tongue	Pharyngitis	Erythema; pharyngitis	Pharyngitis
Peripheral extremities	Erythema of palms and soles; indurative edema; periungual, palmar, and plantar desquamation	No change	Periungual desquamation	No change	Swelling of hands and feet; dry gangrene	Gangrene of hands and feet (rare)
Exanthem	Erythematous, polymorphous	Erythematous, polymorphous; iris lesions, vesicles, bullae, crusts	Finely papular erythroderma; Pastia lines; circumoral pallor	Finely papular erythroderma; Pastia lines	Erythroderma	Erythematous, maculopapular, petechial, or purpuric
Cervical lymph nodes	Nonpurulent swelling; unilateral (frequent)	Nonpurulent swelling (occasional)	Nonpurulent or purulent swelling (frequent)	Nonpurulent or purulent swelling (occasional)	No change	Nonpurulent swelling (infrequent)
Other	Meatitis; diarrhea; arthralgia and arthritis; aseptic meningitis; rhinorrhea (uncommon): ECG changes	Malaise; cough, rhinorrhea, pneumonitis; vomiting; arthralgia; recurrent episodes	Malaise; vomiting; headache		Headache; confusion; hypotension; icteric hepatitis; diarrhea; coagulopathy; renal injury	Headache myalgia; abdominal pain; icteric hepatitis; meningitis

Abbreviation: ECG, electrocardiogram.

■ Other conditions that share some aspects of Kawasaki disease include:

- Ratbite fever
- Rubella
- Rubeola
- Infectious mononucleosis
- Toxoplasmosis
- Juvenile rheumatoid arthritis
- Systemic lupus erythematosus
- Behçet syndrome
- Acrodynia (mercury poisoning)
- Febrile drug reactions, especially those caused by anticonvulsants

■ The similarities between fatal Kawasaki disease and fatal infantile polyarteritis nodosa are striking.

- Pathologically, the 2 diseases cannot be distinguished.
- The exact relationship between them, however, is undetermined.
- The clear differentiating feature is that Kawasaki disease rarely is fatal (<1% mortality), whereas infantile polyarteritis nodosa is a pathological diagnosis made at autopsy.

LABORATORY FINDINGS

■ No pathognomonic laboratory findings

■ Certain laboratory abnormalities that are seen commonly can help establish the diagnosis.

- In the acute phase, most patients exhibit an elevated WBC count with an associated left shift.
  - WBC counts of 15,000–20,000/mm^3 are common and may remain elevated for 1–3 weeks.
- Other laboratory abnormalities commonly seen in the acute phase include:
  - Elevated ESR (mean >55 mm/hr)
  - Increased C-reactive protein (CRP) and ß$_2$-globulin
  - Mild normochromic, normocytic anemia
  - Slight elevations of the liver enzymes
  - Slight decrease in erythrocyte and hemoglobin levels
- Many patients demonstrate sterile pyuria and CSF pleocytosis.
- In weeks 2–3 of illness, patients characteristically develop significant thrombocytosis, with platelet counts averaging >700,000/mm^3.

■ Importantly, results of several laboratory studies are negative.

- Routine cultures of blood, CSF, urine, throat, and lymph node aspirates reveal no growth or normal flora.
- Serologic studies for bacterial and viral agents are negative, including the antistreptolysin titer.
- Antinuclear antibodies, rheumatoid factor, and other autoantibodies are absent.

IMAGING

■ Echocardiography

- Should be considered in any infant <6 months with
  - Fever for >7 days
  - Laboratory evidence of systemic inflammation
  - No other explanation for the febrile illness
- Baseline echocardiogram should be performed as soon as the diagnosis of Kawasaki disease is suspected.
  - To evaluate cardiac function and the anatomy of the coronary arteries
    - Coronary artery abnormalities usually are apparent by the 3rd or 4th week of the illness.
    - Coronary artery disease rarely, if ever, develops after 6–8 weeks, although late-onset valvular disease has been reported.
  - To assess for the presence or absence of pericardial effusion
  - May reveal:
    - Decreased left ventricular contractility
    - Mild valvular regurgitation (mitral regurgitation)
    - Pericardial effusion
- Cases of atypical Kawasaki disease followed by typical coronary artery involvement have led to the suggestion that an echocardiography examination be performed in children with prolonged unexplained febrile illnesses associated with subsequent peripheral desquamation.
  - Although aneurysms rarely form before day 10 of the illness, perivascular brightness, ectasia, and lack of tapering of the coronary arteries can be seen in the acute stage of disease.

DIAGNOSTIC PROCEDURES

■ Electrocardiography

- In the acute phase, may reveal
  - Sinus tachycardia
  - Nonspecific ST segment and T wave changes
  - Evidence of mild left ventricular hypertrophy
- In the subacute phase
  - Myocardial infarction patterns may be observed infrequently.

TREATMENT APPROACH

■ Treatment should begin as soon as the diagnosis is established and as early as possible in the course of the illness.

■ IVIG with aspirin

- The best available therapy for preventing coronary artery abnormalities
- Should be administered to all patients diagnosed within the first 10 days of the illness

K

SPECIFIC TREATMENTS

Aspirin

■ Aspirin, given in high doses (80–120 mg/kg/day), reduces the length and severity of Kawasaki disease during the acute phase.

• Aspirin used early in the course of the disease may reduce coronary artery involvement.

• Salicylate levels should be checked to avoid toxicity.

• Defervescence is accompanied by improvement in gastrointestinal absorption of aspirin.

– Dosages should be reduced to 30–50 mg/kg/day after fever subsides and continued until the ESR has returned to normal.

– Thereafter, aspirin should be prescribed because of its antithrombotic effects at 3–5 mg/kg/day until the platelet count has returned to normal.

• If coronary aneurysms are recognized, then salicylates (3–5 mg/kg/day) should be continued until careful follow-up electrocardiograms demonstrate aneurysm resolution.

IVIG

■ High-dose IVIG may prevent coronary artery lesions in Kawasaki disease.

• 400 mg/kg/day for 4 consecutive days initially was shown to be effective, but a single dose of 2 g/kg infused over 10–12 hr has replaced the 4-day regimen.

• No apparent difference exists in efficacy among particular IVIG products currently commercially available.

• Patients should be monitored carefully during IVIG infusions for signs of anaphylaxis and immune hemolysis.

• 80–90% of children treated with IVIG respond favorably with decreased fever and reduction in mucocutaneous findings.

– Remainder have persistent or recurrent fever, with or without mucocutaneous signs.

• If ongoing fever cannot be attributed to another cause, then the assumption should be made that Kawasaki disease is persisting or has relapsed.

– Because fever may be viewed as a sign of continued vasculitis, retreatment with IVIG is advocated.

– Most patients treated again after failure of a single dose of IVIG therapy will respond to retreatment.

– Patients who remain symptomatic beyond the 10th day still may benefit from IVIG.

– Decision to administer IVIG later than the 10th day of the illness must be individualized.

Other therapeutic options

■ Corticosteroids

• Previously believed dangerous as therapy for Kawasaki disease based on an early study in Japan in which 65% of patients treated with oral prednisolone developed coronary artery aneurysms.

• Subsequent studies have not confirmed a detrimental effect of corticosteroids, and some patients have benefited.

• If IVIG therapy fails (particularly after 2 treatments), then patients are at high risk for developing severe coronary artery complications, including death.

– Such patients may benefit from 1–3 pulse-doses of methyl prednisolone at 30 mg/kg per dose.

– This therapy should be reserved for patients who are clearly refractory to more established treatments (ie, failure of 2 doses of IVIG).

■ Plasmapheresis and exchange transfusion have been reported to be of benefit in patients with Kawasaki disease, but these treatments are cumbersome and more involved.

■ Antibiotics are not useful.

WHEN TO ADMIT

■ All patients with Kawasaki disease should be admitted for treatment.

WHEN TO REFER

■ Patients suspected of having atypical or incomplete Kawasaki disease

■ Patients with Kawasaki disease who have not responded to 2 doses of IVIG

■ Patients who have developed complications such as coronary dilatation and aneurysm.

FOLLOW-UP

■ For long-term management of patients with Kawasaki disease, a risk stratification scheme may be of benefit

■ Level I risk: no coronary artery abnormalities at any stage of the illness

• The primary care physician may fully assume care after the 1-year anniversary of Kawasaki disease onset.

• Physical activities should not be restricted.

■ Level II risk: transient coronary artery ectasia followed by regression

• A pediatric cardiologist should be consulted every 1–2 years.

• At least 1 stress test evaluating myocardial functioning should be performed at ~10 years of age.

■ Level III risk: small to medium solitary coronary artery aneurysm

• Daily low-dose aspirin therapy

• Annual cardiac follow-up with echocardiography and electrocardiography

• Periodic stress tests recommended

■ Level IV risk: ≥1 giant aneurysms or multiple aneurysms without obstruction

• Low-dose aspirin therapy should be maintained.

• Low-dose warfarin should be considered.

- Coronary angiography may be considered 6–12 months after the acute disease has resolved, to delineate coronary artery anatomy.
- Physical activities should be modified to minimize the risk of hemorrhage.
- Strenuous or competitive sports should be avoided.
- Level V risk: coronary artery obstruction (thrombosis or stenosis)
  - Daily low-dose aspirin
  - Warfarin should be considered.
  - Patients should be evaluated for indications for bypass graft surgery.
  - Mild to moderate recreational physical activities are permitted.

COMPLICATIONS

- Coronary artery aneurysm
  - The major complication of Kawasaki disease
  - Risk increased if:
    - Fever lasts for >14 days
    - Fever pattern is biphasic
    - Skin rash has biphasic pattern
    - Maximum WBC count is 30,000/mm^3
    - Maximum ESR is 101 mm/hr
    - ESR or CRP does not normalize until day 30 of the illness
    - Biphasic elevation of ESR or CRP
    - Increased Q/R ratio in leads II, III
    - aVF >0.3
  - More common in
    - Boys
    - Children <1 year of age
    - Children who have a triphasic fever pattern or fever for >2 weeks when a gallop rhythm or other arrhythmia is noted or when the ESR exceeds 50 mm/hr
  - If IVIG is not administered, aneurysms occur in 15–25% of cases.
  - Usually apparent by echocardiogram during the subacute phase of the illness.
  - Most patients who have aneurysms are asymptomatic.
    - In some cases, formation of an aneurysm, particularly a giant aneurysm (>8 mm in diameter), is followed by thrombosis or rupture, resulting in a fatal myocardial infarction.
  - Some authorities treat patients with giant aneurysms with a regimen of low-dose warfarin in combination with low-dose aspirin.

- In children <7 years, a radionuclide scan may help identify areas of mild cardioischemia.
  - When echocardiography, angiography, or radionuclide scanning detects thrombi occluding a significant portion of main branches of coronary arteries, thrombolytic therapy should be instituted.
- Myocardial infarction
  - Risk increased by
    - Male gender
    - Age at onset <1 year
    - Hemoglobin <10 g/dL
    - Red blood cell count <3.5 million
    - Maximum WBC count >26,000/mm^3
    - Maximum ESR >50 mm/hr
    - Cardiomegaly
    - Arrhythmia
    - Recurrence of disease
  - Bypass surgery should be undertaken.
- Hydrops of the gallbladder
  - A rare complication of Kawasaki disease
  - Occurs in ~3% of cases
  - Seen most commonly in children who are jaundiced
  - Becomes evident during the acute phase of the illness
  - Is diagnosed best by ultrasound on recognition of a right upper quadrant abdominal mass
  - Pathogenesis is unknown.
  - Resolves spontaneously in convalescence

PROGNOSIS

- Mortality rate is 0.3%.
- Death occurs almost exclusively in children who have giant aneurysms, largely as a result of coronary artery thrombosis, massive myocardial infarction, and cardiogenic shock.
- Eighty percent of children whose aneurysms are small to moderate in size have complete resolution without apparent sequelae within 5 years.
- The remaining children may experience persisting aneurysms, coronary artery stenosis or obstruction, or aortic regurgitation.
  - Emerging evidence suggests that a portion of this last group of children may be at risk for subsequent development of significant cardiovascular disease such as coronary arteriosclerosis or persistent aneurysms, placing some at risk for sudden death from aneurysm rupture or thrombosis, cardiac arrhythmias, angina, or hypertension.
- Almost always self-limited and without complications, which should be emphasized to the parents
  - Even if coronary artery aneurysms do develop, they resolve spontaneously in >50% of patients in 2 years and 80% in 5 years.

K

Labial Adhesions

DEFINITION

- Labial adhesions are membranous structures that develop as a result of fusion of the adjacent mucosal surfaces of the labia minora.
- Also known as *labial agglutination* or *synechia vulvae*

EPIDEMIOLOGY

- Prevalence
  - Among preadolescent girls in a general pediatric setting, ranges from ~2% identified by inspection alone to 39% identified with inspection plus magnified photographic vulvar images
  - Found in 15.6% of girls referred to a gynecology clinic for various hymenal findings documented during well-child evaluations
- Age
  - Healthy, postpubescent young women do not develop labial adhesions.
  - Most common in prepubertal girls <5 years of age
  - Decreased in older preadolescent girls, most likely because of:
    - An increase in endogenous estrogen levels during the prepubertal period
    - Improved hygiene
  - Rare in neonates
    - Maternal estrogen is presumed to have a protective influence.

ETIOLOGY

- The exact cause of labial adhesions is not known.
  - They may be the result of fusion of the adjacent mucosal surfaces of the labia minora; the cause of this fusion is unknown.
  - Usually considered a nonspecific finding
  - Probably due to chronic irritation and inflammation of the hypoestrogenic vulva
- Triggers for chronic inflammation include:
  - Physical or chemical trauma
  - Infection (*Candida albicans*, *Enterobius vermicularis*, various bacteria)
  - Poor hygiene
  - Sexual abuse
- During healing of the irritated area, the medial edges of the labia minora adhere to each other, forming an adhesion.

RISK FACTORS

- Poor hygiene
- Physical or chemical trauma
- Infection (*Candida albicans*, *Enterobius vermicularis*, various bacteria)

- Sexual abuse
- Trauma
- Herpesvirus infection
- Episiotomy
- Chemotherapy
- Graft-versus-host disease

SIGNS AND SYMPTOMS

- Labial adhesions often are asymptomatic.
  - Discovered at routine well-child visits
  - Brought to the attention of the pediatrician by the child's caregiver
- If the adhesions partially dehisce, the child may experience
  - Spotting of a minute amount of blood
  - Irritation
- Uncommon symptoms:
  - Pain with urination
  - Vaginal pain
  - Pain with ambulation
  - Urinary retention
  - Altered urinary stream
  - Other symptoms suggestive of urinary tract infection
  - History of recurrent urinary tract infection
- The membranous structure can vary from thin and transparent to thick and fibrous.
- Any degree of labial involvement can occur, including covering of the urethral meatus.

DIFFERENTIAL DIAGNOSIS

- Conditions that may be confused with labial adhesions include:
  - Ambiguous genitalia
  - Vaginal agenesis
  - Imperforate hymen
  - Septated hymen
- Physical examination easily differentiates these entities.
  - A line of demarcation between the clitoral hood and labia minora is:
    - Present with labial adhesions
    - Not present with ambiguous genitalia secondary to androgen excess
  - In vaginal agenesis and hymenal variants, the labia are normal and unfused.
    - The characteristic findings of these entities are located in the vaginal introitus.

DIAGNOSTIC APPROACH

- The condition is diagnosed by visual inspection of the vulva.
  - Includes hymenal examination in the supine frog-leg or prone knee-chest position
- The labia majora should be gently stretched apart.
  - A membrane of variable length and thickness is seen in the midline.
  - A small opening near the clitoris allows the outflow of urine.
- A line of adhesion between the 2 nonrugated labia minora or raphae also may be seen.

LABORATORY FINDINGS

- Urinalysis and urine culture if the child has accompanying symptoms, such as
  - Pain on urination or ambulation
  - Altered urinary stream
  - Urinary retention
  - History of urinary tract infections

TREATMENT APPROACH

- If the child has no accompanying symptoms, labial adhesions should not be treated.
- Any documented urinary tract or vulvar infection should be treated accordingly.

SPECIFIC TREATMENTS

Uncomplicated

- If the child has no accompanying symptoms, labial adhesions should not be treated.
- Parents should be given an opportunity to visualize the adhesion so they are not surprised and concerned about the unusual appearance of the vulva.
- Reassurance of the benign, self-limiting nature of this condition and education about potential symptoms should be provided.

Complicated

- The first-line treatment of the complicated labial adhesion is topical estrogen.
  - Goal: to use the least amount of medication that will achieve separation of the adhesion
  - 0.625 mg conjugated estrogen cream (Premarin Vaginal Cream, Wyeth Ayerst)
    - Applied to the adhesion and labial edges with a fingertip or cotton swab
    - Gentle traction should be placed on the opposing labia during the application.
    - Specific optimal dosing and length of treatment are unknown; twice-daily application for 2 weeks is a reasonable starting point.

- Treatment produces thinning of the line of fusion.
  - Facilitates manual labial separation in the office
  - Highly effective for most thin, transparent adhesions
  - Less effective in dense and fibrous or long-standing adhesions
  - Even dense adhesions should be treated initially with topical estrogens
  - Possible adverse effects of topical estrogen
    - Breast budding and tenderness
    - Vulvar hyperpigmentation
    - Local irritation
    - All these effects are reversible on discontinuation of the medication.
  - After labia are separated
    - Topical lubricant (eg, white petroleum jelly) applied daily for several months
    - To ensure complete healing and persistent separation
  - Treatment with estrogen cream is considered unsuccessful if:
    - Labial separation has not occurred within 8 weeks.
    - The child suffers untoward effects from the estrogen and cannot continue using it.
  - Topical anesthetic is applied to the affected area.
  - Firm traction on the opposing edges of the labia minora is applied to separate the fused edges.
  - Edges should be smoothly peeled away from each other.
  - After separation, a lubricant should be applied to the affected area daily for several months to prevent readherence.
  - Warm soaks or sitz baths in the days after separation may provide relief if vulva is irritated.
- Manual separation if estrogen therapy is unsuccessful
  - Topical anesthetic is applied to the affected area.
  - Firm traction on the opposing edges of the labia minora is applied to separate the fused edges.
  - Edges should be smoothly peeled away from each other.
  - After separation, a lubricant should be applied to the affected area daily for several months to prevent readherence.
  - Warm soaks or sitz baths in the days following separation may provide relief if the vulva is irritated.
- Surgical treatment is rarely required.
  - Surgical lysis by a pediatric urologist or gynecologist while under general anesthesia
  - For thick labial adhesions that cannot be separated by the previously described treatments or adhesions associated with complications

- The decision to treat labial adhesions with surgery is made by weighing:
  - Significance and severity of symptoms after less aggressive treatments
  - Risks of general anesthesia
- Postoperative care includes:
  - Sitz baths in the immediate postoperative period
  - Application of topical lubricant for several months

WHEN TO REFER

- A symptomatic child with persistent or recurrent labial adhesions should be referred to a pediatric urologist or gynecologist for surgical lysis if she has:
  - A history of urinary tract infections
  - Urinary retention
  - Altered urinary stream
  - Dysuria
  - Pain with ambulation
  - Failed topical estrogen therapy

PROGNOSIS

- The condition is self-limiting.
- Spontaneous resolution in affected individuals has been reported to occur in
  - 50% of cases within 6 months
  - 90% of cases within 12 months
  - 100% of cases within 18 months

PREVENTION

- Explain the value of proper hygiene of the vulva.
- Educate the parents about practices to help their child avoid recurrent labial adhesions
  - Wiping front to back after urination or defecation
  - Wearing cotton underwear
  - Avoiding application of detergents in the genital area
  - Avoiding wet, tight clothing against the vulva for prolonged periods

L

Language and Speech Assessment

BACKGROUND

- Each child who enters school is assumed to have a well-developed system of spoken language skills.
  - This system is the foundation for social interaction and higher levels of communication.
- Children with early language problems are at an increased risk for later reading problems.
  - In a 5-year follow-up study of 3-year-old children, as many as 50% of those with preschool articulation or phonologic disorders were receiving some type of special education by the third grade.
- Children identified in second or third grade as needing special assistance in reading, spelling, writing, and math previously exhibited:
  - Slow development of spoken words
  - Unintelligible speech at age 3 years
  - Word-finding difficulties

GOALS

- Fundamental question to ask:
  - "Is the child I am examining, who appears to be slow in speech or language development, simply at the low end of the normal continuum (and presumably will catch up without professional assistance), or is this a child who is at risk for later learning difficulties?"
    - The age at which typical children achieve spoken language milestones varies.
  - Interventionists see these children only after problems are suspected and referrals are made.
    - Speech-language pathologists
    - Occupational therapists
  - Nurses and primary care physicians are often the only trained professionals who monitor young children on a regular basis before school entry at a variety of sick and well visits.
  - Access to young children carries with it a responsibility to make early and appropriate referrals to specialists trained to perform comprehensive evaluations.

GENERAL APPROACH

- A child's communication competency may be assessed using a validated screening instrument.
  - The emergence of certain critical speech and language abilities follows a relatively stable timetable.
  - The purpose of screening is not to diagnose but to identify children in need of further testing.
- Children who are identified as having a concern should be referred for evaluation by a developmental specialist or a speech-language pathologist.
  - Benefits of referral
    - Assurance of early intervention

- Regular and appropriate reassessment of children whose developmental status remains uncertain
- Objective baseline data for measurement of progress over time
  - Delayed onset of language may be the first indication of more global developmental delays.
- Children develop communication skills long before the onset of first words.
  - Wave good-bye months before saying "bye-bye"
  - Raise their hands to be held before saying "up"
  - Shake their head before saying "no"
- Within the first year of life, the normally developing infant progresses from a reflexive newborn to a purposeful communicator.
  - Preverbal red flags may indicate potential developmental problems.
    - Failure to smile or show joyful expressions by 6 months
    - No reciprocal turn taking with sounds and facial expressions by 9 months
    - No pointing or reaching to communicate by 12 months
- Preschool speech and language development
  - By age 3 years, most children have a spoken vocabulary of >500 words.
    - Routinely speak in 3- and 4-word sentences
    - Some basic rules of grammar are finely tuned.
      - Plural, possessive, and past tense forms of words are emerging.
      - Use of pronouns, such as *I, me, you,* and *mine,* is common.
    - 3-year-olds demonstrate an appropriate understanding of *why?* questions.
      - Appreciation of cause and effect
    - The speech of a 3-year-old is highly intelligible.
      - Parents and most strangers have little difficulty understanding the child.
      - Frequent mispronunciations do not impair understanding.
      - 3-year-olds have the capacity to carry on a reasonable conversation with an adult.
  - The language of 4-year-olds approaches adult competency in grammatical skill.
    - Unlike 2- and 3-year-olds, 4-year-olds speak in complete sentences.
      - They rarely omit words from the 4- and 5-word sentences that are typically produced.

– 4-year-olds do not have as many different ways to say the same things as do older children.

■ They usually have at least one way to express all thoughts and desires.

– The vocabulary of a 4-year-old is extensive.

■ By this age, most children can:

o Recognize and name several colors

o Count to 10 by rote

o Understand the prepositions *in, on, under, beside, in front,* and *in back* (understanding of *behind* at 5 years)

o Answer complex questions, such as *How much? How long?* and *What if...?*

– 3- and 4-year-olds are beginning to formulate questions using mature constructions.

■ For example, *Is it broken?*

• By age 5 years, children have developed most of the language-based concepts that are important for schooling.

– Sort and classify objects by category

– Name all the basic colors

– Understand the concept of time (and answer *when* questions)

– Understand the concept of numbers up to 10 integers

– The acquisition of individual speech sounds should be fully developed by age 5 years, with the exception of *th*.

– Occasional mispronunciations are usually restricted to:

■ Sound blends (*truck, sprinkle*)

■ Difficult-to-pronounce, multisyllabic words

SPECIFIC INTERVENTIONS

Late talkers

■ The term *late talker* or *slow expressive language development* refers to children who:

• Have <50 spoken words and no word combinations by 24 months of age with otherwise normal:

– Receptive language

– Cognitive and social-emotional development

– Adaptive behavior

■ Research appears inconclusive regarding the long-tem outcomes.

• Some of the literature suggests that 40–50% continue to exhibit expressive language delays throughout the pre-school years.

• 25% will exhibit problems well into elementary school.

■ Positive predictors of children who will outgrow their delayed speech are:

• Age-appropriate development in receptive language, cognitive, and self-help skills

• Lack of oral-motor concerns

• Lack of social or interactive concerns

• Appropriate play skills

• Lack of family history of speech-language disorders or learning disabilities

■ The emergence of 2-word phrases is a significant milestone in language learning.

• Rudimentary rules of grammar are first evidenced.

• Normally developing children begin producing 2-word combinations as early as 18 months.

– Failure to achieve this milestone by 24 months indicates a risk for later language-based difficulties.

– Child should be referred for further testing.

• To many parents, the child's production of *hot dog, choo-choo,* and *merry-go-round* represent word combinations.

– Instead, they are simply learned labels of objects and thus considered single words.

• Ask, "Can you give me an example of some of your child's word combinations?"

– Helps parents give a clearer picture of the child's language abilities.

– Common early 2-word combinations include:

■ *No juice*

■ *What that*

■ *My cup*

■ *Look, kitty*

Mispronunciation

■ Children commonly mispronounce certain sounds or have problems producing particular words with difficult sound combinations.

■ The mastery of speech sounds is a gradual process that takes place over 6–7 years.

■ As children master various sounds and sound combinations, their speech becomes more adult-like.

■ Normally developing children are easily understood by their caregivers.

• Regardless of the frequent errors in pronunciation

• Complaints by parents that they cannot understand their child's speech suggests a pattern of mispronunciation so unusual and unpredictable that it is not characteristic of normal mispronunciations.

■ The reaction of the child regarding speech intelligibility is equally important.

• Many children with unintelligible speech become frustrated by their inability to communicate effectively.

– They cease talking and resort to gestures and pantomime to fulfill their communicative needs.

- Children with childhood apraxia of speech (CAS) often exhibit frustration.
  - CAS is the inability to program voluntary movements of the articulators in absence of paralysis, paresis, incoordination.
  - Such children often:
    - Have mastered only 1 or 2 speech sounds
    - Exhibit groping while attempting to search for the correct tongue placement
    - Have great difficulty imitating simple words
  - CAS is often misdiagnosed as expressive language disorder because of the child's frequent nonverbal nature.

Screening for hearing loss

- Hearing screening is an integral part of any developmental evaluation.
- Normal speech and language development requires an intact auditory system.
- The Joint Committee on Infant Hearing has endorsed early detection of hearing loss and early intervention.
- A national program of universal newborn hearing screening has been implemented.
  - This program provides the opportunity for infants with significant hearing impairment to have early identification and intervention.
  - Children who fail neonatal hearing screening are given additional in-depth assessment.
    - Intervention can begin in the first 3–4 months.
- Among toddlers and preschoolers, parental concern was identified as a significant factor in the identification of 70% of children with hearing impairment.
  - Toddlers <3 years of age may be difficult to screen.
    - Should be tested using physiologic methods, such as:
      - Brainstem audiometry
      - Tympanometry
    - Screening stimuli that do not have calibrated levels or frequency information or that rely on behavioral observation are not recommended.
      - For example, rattles, music toys, other noisemakers
  - For children 3–5 years of age, play audiometry and tympanometry may be helpful.
    - In play audiometry, children are trained to provide an operant response to a sound that establishes an estimate of hearing acuity.
- The American Speech-Language-Hearing Association recommends hearing screening:
  - At birth
  - On initial entry into school
  - Annually through the third grade

- Repeat testing in the 7th and 11th grades
- These school screening tests should be completed at 20 dB for 1000, 2000, and 4000 Hz under earphones.
- Any child with a speech and language delay should have hearing screening using:
  - Age-appropriate method
  - Tympanometry
  - Otologic evaluation
- Sensorineural hearing losses in children should be identified as early as possible.
  - Reduces the effect of hearing loss on speech and language development
- Hearing-impaired children who receive appropriate amplification and intervention before 6 months of age have significantly better language scores than those receiving intervention after 6 months.
- For the mild or moderately hearing-impaired infant:
  - Traditional hearing amplification and aural habilitation is provided by audiologists and speech-language pathologists.
- Options for severely impaired infants and children may include:
  - Referral for consideration of cochlear implant surgery
  - Specialized postoperative aural habilitation
  - Families who strongly identify with deaf culture may rightfully not choose this option for their infants and young children.

Acquired communication disorders

- Acquired communication disorders can be secondary to:
  - Stroke
  - Seizure disorder
  - Meningitis
  - Other diseases
  - Brain trauma (cause of the majority of childhood-acquired speech and language disorders)
- A brain injury often interferes with acquisition of new knowledge and skills.
  - Older children have the advantage of greater knowledge acquired before the brain injury.
  - Younger children must gain more new knowledge and skills with a brain developing with injured areas.
- Traumatic brain injury (TBI) can result in a focal or, more often, a diffuse brain injury with sequelae that include:
  - Speech disorders
    - Apraxic speech, characterized by difficulty initiating and programming speech
    - Dysarthric speech resulting from paralysis or paresis of oral or pharyngeal musculature; may contribute to a secondary swallowing or dysphagic disorder

L

- Communication disorders
- Swallowing problems
- Language disorders
  - Disorganized, tangential, wandering discourse
  - Imprecise language
  - Word-retrieval difficulties
  - Disinhibited, socially inappropriate language, with ineffective use of contextual cues
  - Restricted output and lack of initiation
  - Difficulty comprehending extended language in spoken or written form and detecting main ideas
  - Difficulty understanding abstract language, including indirect or implied meaning
  - Inefficient verbal learning caused by reduced memory ability
- These problems are different from the grammatical difficulties typical of children who have developmental problems.
- They are frequently misunderstood and not seen as being symptomatic of a language disorder.
- Standardized testing may not be sensitive to the social communication and language effects of TBI.
- Clinical evaluation of speech and language function is essential to determine the need for rehabilitative or specialized educational intervention.
- Children with TBI should be referred for a speech-language-cognitive assessment if any memory, learning, comprehension, or attention problems are reported.
  - Consequences of speech, language, and related cognitive function are often difficult to identify through screening procedures.
- Therapeutic intervention goals may be rehabilitative or compensatory.
  - Necessary for cognitive processing and language functioning
    - Rehabilitation of attention
    - Awareness

- Perception
- Memory
- Learning
- Organization
- Social cognition
- Problem solving
- General executive system functioning
- Compensatory techniques may include:
  - Memory devices
  - Organizational patterning
  - Referent cues
- Stimulating speech programming and muscular strengthening may improve oral communication.
  - Compensatory techniques may be required in the form of augmentative communicative devices.
    - Communication boards
    - Computerized speech

WHEN TO REFER

- No smile or joyful expression by 6 months
- No reciprocal turn-taking, with sounds and facial expressions, by 9 months
- No babbling, pointing, or gestures by 12 months
- No spoken words by 15 months
- No 2-word combinations by 24 months
- Inability of parents to understand their child's speech at 30 months
- Continued poor intelligibility at 36 months of age
- Difficulty answering *why* questions by 48 months of age
- Poor ability to associate letters with their sounds by the end of kindergarten
- Parents voice concern about their child's hearing, speech, or language
- Any regression in speech, language, or social skills at any age

Leukemias

DEFINITION

- Leukemias are a heterogeneous group of disorders classified by immunophenotype and subclassified primarily on the basis of prognostic features.
- *Acute leukemias* are defined as a clonal expansion of hematopoietic progenitor cells (blasts), such that the number of these cells exceeds:
  - 25% of the total nucleated-cell population in the marrow for acute lymphocytic leukemia (ALL)
  - 20% for acute myelogenous leukemia (AML)
- *Chronic leukemia* is a hyperproliferation of mature hematopoietic elements.
  - Classified as either chronic myelogenous leukemia (CML) or chronic lymphocytic leukemia (CLL)
- *Juvenile myelomonocytic leukemia* (JMML) is a clonal disorder of early childhood.
- *Myelodysplastic syndromes* (MDS) are clonal disorders of ineffective or abnormal hematopoiesis that frequently precede AML or aplastic anemia.
- Chloromas, or granulocytic sarcomas, are solid collections (tumors) of malignant cells in patients with AML.

EPIDEMIOLOGY

- Prevalence
  - Leukemia is the most common cancer of childhood.
    - Leukemias account for one-quarter of all childhood cancers.
  - Frequency of leukemias in children
    - ALL: 80%
    - Of those with ALL:
      - Early pre-B cell: 60–65%
      - Pre-B cell: 15%
      - Mature B cell: <5%
      - Pre-T cell: 10–15%
    - AML: 16%
    - CML: 3%
    - CLL: <1%
  - Extramedullary leukemia
    - As many as 20% of patients will have evidence of disease in the central nervous system (CNS).
  - Mixed-lineage leukemia (MLL)
    - Translocations involving the *MLL* gene at 11q23 and >30 potential partner chromosomes can be found in 6% of childhood ALL cases.
  - The t(4;11)(q21;q23) mutation resulting in the *MLL-AF4* fusion product is commonly seen in infant ALL.
- Incidence
  - 40 cases per 1,000,000 children in the US annually
  - In the US, leukemia will be diagnosed in >3000 children <20 years of age each year.

- Age
  - Peak incidence is ~4 years of age.
    - Due almost entirely to ALL
  - AML is equally distributed among patients 0–10 years of age.
    - Slight increase in incidence in adolescence
  - T-cell ALL is also more common during adolescence.
    - Diagnosed in nearly 40% of children 10–18 years of age with ALL
  - JMML occurs at a median age of 1.8 years.
- Race/ethnicity
  - ALL is more common among white persons than black persons in the US.
  - AML has an equal distribution among all ethnic groups.
  - Early reports of worse outcomes for black persons with leukemia have been refuted in recent publications.
- Sex
  - Incidence of leukemia is slightly higher among boys than girls.
  - The ratio of boys with leukemia to girls with leukemia is greatest during adolescence.
    - Particularly in patients with T-cell ALL

ETIOLOGY

- The cause of most leukemias is multifactorial, including genetic, immune, infectious, and environmental factors.
  - DNA damage and inadequate DNA repair is the initial insult.
- Genetic factors
  - Predisposition to childhood leukemia may be inherited, as indicated by:
    - An association of leukemia with various constitutional chromosomal abnormalities
    - Reports of familial leukemias
    - Several reported karyotypic abnormalities in leukemia cells
  - Patients with Down syndrome (trisomy 21) have a 15-fold increased risk of leukemia compared with patients without trisomy 21.
  - Patients with autosomal-recessive chromosomal fragility disorders, such as Bloom syndrome, ataxia telangiectasia, and Fanconi anemia, have a well-documented high incidence of leukemia.
  - Concordance of both AML and ALL in monozygotic twins is estimated to be as high as 25%.
- Environmental factors
  - Risk of leukemia after exposure to ionizing radiation is well established.
  - Environmental influences in leukemogenesis are likely to be complex and multifactorial.

- Investigators have examined the role of:
  - Toxins
  - Electromagnetic fields
  - Pesticides
  - Nitrites
  - Population mixing
  - Seasonal and climatic variations
  - Birth weights
  - Socioeconomic status
  - Breastfeeding
  - Maternal history of fetal loss in leukemogenesis
  - Little conclusive evidence exists.
- Equally unclear is the role of in utero and childhood infections in the pathogenesis of childhood leukemia.
- Most studies evaluating childhood vaccination and leukemia demonstrated a protective effect.
- MDS may occur spontaneously or after exposure to:
  - Radiation
  - Epipodophyllotoxin
  - Alkylators

RISK FACTORS

- Factors associated with a higher risk of leukemia
  - Genetic predisposition
    - Siblings of patient with a childhood leukemia
    - Down syndrome
    - Fanconi anemia
    - Bloom syndrome
    - Ataxia telangiectasia
    - Paroxysmal nocturnal hemoglobinuria
    - Congenital hypogammaglobulinemia
    - Wiskott-Aldrich syndrome
    - Neurofibromatosis
    - Klinefelter syndrome
    - Shwachman-Diamond syndrome
  - Environmental exposures
    - Ionizing radiation (therapeutic or environmental exposure)
    - Epipodophyllotoxin or alkylator-based chemotherapy
- Extramedullary leukemia
  - Greatest risk for CNS disease is in patients with:
    - T-cell ALL
    - Age <2 years
    - Monoblastic forms of AML

SIGNS AND SYMPTOMS

ALL and AML

- Signs and symptoms are similar to common symptoms in children with benign illnesses.
- Presenting clinical features
  - Fever
    - ALL: 61%
    - AML: 34%
  - Pallor
    - ALL: 55%
    - AML: 25%
  - Petechiae, purpura, bleeding
    - ALL: 8%
    - AML: 33%
  - Anorexia or weight loss
    - ALL: 33%
    - AML: 22%
  - Fatigue, malaise
    - ALL: 30%
    - AML: 19%
  - Bone or joint pain
    - ALL: 38%
    - AML: 18%
  - Lymphadenopathy
    - ALL: 50%
    - AML: 14%
  - Hepatosplenomegaly
    - ALL: 68%
    - AML: 55%
  - Swollen gingivae
    - AML: 8%
  - Cough, dysphagia
    - AML: 41%
  - Recurrent infection
    - AML: 3%
  - Neurologic symptoms
    - ALL: 3%
    - AML: 10%
- Extramedullary leukemia
  - CNS disease
    - Few children have symptoms of disease at diagnosis, including vomiting, headache, and lethargy.
    - Papilledema and cranial nerve palsies can be present.
      - Cranial nerve palsies typically reflect meningeal infiltration of leukemic cells rather than increased intracranial pressure.

- Painless enlargement of 1 or both testicles has been reported in <5% of boys with leukemia and is more common in ALL (particularly T-cell ALL) than AML.
- Chloromas
  - Can occur anywhere, including:
    - Skin
    - CNS
    - Bones
  - Rarely, chloromas can occur independent of or before evidence of bone marrow disease.

CML

- Typically produces leukocytosis marked by myeloid progenitor cells at all levels of differentiation, and thrombocytosis
- Hepatosplenomegaly is present in a majority of patients.
- Fatigue, weight loss, bone pain, and low-grade fevers may be present for weeks to months.
- In most patients, CML is diagnosed in the chronic phase (cytogenetic evidence of disease with <5% blasts in the marrow) or the accelerated phase (cytogenetic evidence of disease with 5–30% blasts in the bone marrow).
- Blast crisis indicates more advanced disease and is indistinguishable from AML, with the exception of the presence of the Ph chromosome.

JMML

- Hallmarks of the disease at diagnosis include:
  - Marked hepatosplenomegaly
  - Peripheral blood monocyte count $>1 \times 10^9$/L
  - Myeloid precursors in the peripheral blood
  - Chronic infections
  - Lymphadenopathy
  - Rash (eczema, xanthomas, café-au-lait spots)
  - Failure to thrive

DIFFERENTIAL DIAGNOSIS

- Differential diagnosis of individual or concurrent cytopenias/cytosis includes several common infectious and noninfectious diseases of childhood.
- Nonmalignant diseases
  - Juvenile idiopathic arthritis
  - Systemic lupus erythematosus
  - Infectious mononucleosis
  - Immune thrombocytopenia purpura
  - Aplastic anemia
  - Pertussis, parapertussis
  - Benign lymphocytosis
  - Leukemoid reaction
  - Sepsis
  - Osteomyelitis
- Malignant diseases
  - Metastatic bone marrow disease in retinoblastoma
  - Neuroblastoma
  - Ewing sarcoma
  - Rhabdomyosarcoma
  - Lymphoma
- Many more common illnesses than leukemia produce:
  - Fever
  - Rash
  - Lymphadenopathy
  - Hepatosplenomegaly
  - Mild cytopenias
  - Lymphocytosis
- Appearance of atypical and variant lymphocytes on the peripheral blood smears of children with such infections as Epstein-Barr virus, pertussis, and parapertussis often bring leukemia into the differential diagnosis.
- Such diseases as systemic lupus erythematosus and juvenile idiopathic arthritis may be associated with bone or joint pain and cytopenias that are indistinguishable from acute leukemia.
- For many diseases, eliminating leukemia from the differential diagnosis becomes of paramount importance.
  - In specific diseases that require use of corticosteroids:
    - Systemic lupus erythematosus
    - Juvenile idiopathic arthritis
    - Immune thrombocytopenia purpura
    - Hemolytic anemia
    - Infectious processes precipitating an acute asthma exacerbation
  - In these instances, if leukemia is possible or probable, referral to a hematologist may be necessary.
  - Inadvertent administration of corticosteroids may impair or delay the diagnosis of leukemia and may necessitate more intensive high-risk chemotherapy for patients with otherwise standard-risk disease.
- Mature B-cell leukemias are indistinguishable from Burkitt lymphoma with bone marrow involvement.

LABORATORY FINDINGS

General

- Leukocyte count may be normal, increased, or decreased in a patient with newly diagnosed leukemia.
  - Leukocyte count (per mcL)
    - <10,000 (53% ALL, 39% AML)
    - 10,000–49,000 (30% ALL, 29% AML)
    - >50,000 (17% ALL, 32% AML)
- Anemia and thrombocytopenia are common but not always present.

- Hemoglobin (g/dL)
  - <7 (43% ALL, 41% AML)
  - 7–11 (45% ALL, 48% AML)
  - >11 (12% ALL, 11% AML)
- Platelet count (per mcL)
  - <20,000 (28% ALL, 15% AML)
  - 20,000–99,000 (47% ALL, 67% AML)
  - >100,000 (25% ALL, 18% AML)
  - Coagulopathy (17% AML)
- Blasts may or may not be present on the peripheral blood smear.
- Continued close follow-up or referral to a hematologist should be guided by clinical evidence and laboratory findings.

Tumor lysis syndrome

- Other abnormal laboratory findings include measures of tumor burden and cell turnover.
  - Increased potassium
  - Increased phosphorus
  - Decreased calcium
  - Increased uric acid
  - Increased lactate dehydrogenase
- Usually most severe after administration of chemotherapy, signs of tumor lysis syndrome may be present at diagnosis because of rapid proliferation and destruction of leukemic cells.
- Patients at risk for significant electrolyte abnormalities and renal failure are those with evidence of high tumor burden, especially if an extramedullary tumor mass is present.
  - High leukocyte count
  - Massive organomegaly
  - Mature B-cell leukemia (Burkitt type)
- With appropriate preemptive management, clinically significant tumor lysis syndrome is rare in childhood leukemias.

IMAGING

- Mediastinal masses are present in 5–10% of children with leukemia, especially older boys, who are more likely to have T-cell leukemia.
- Chest radiography is necessary in all patients with suspected acute leukemia.
  - Should be performed before administration of anesthesia for any procedures
  - Radiographs of long bones frequently demonstrate evidence of leukemic infiltration of the periosteum and bone.
  - Patients with particularly high leukemic cell burdens may appear osteopenic.
  - Others may demonstrate signs of:
    - Subperiosteal new bone formation
    - Radiolucent bands in the metaphysis (leukemic lines)
    - Discrete osteolytic lesions
    - Growth arrest lines

DIAGNOSTIC PROCEDURES

- Cases in which the index of probability is sufficient require a more definitive bone marrow aspiration and biopsy.
- If the leukemic cell burden is sufficient to elicit clinical symptoms, findings on a bone marrow evaluation will not be subtle.
  - Identifying patients with signs and symptoms severe enough to warrant bone marrow evaluation (frequently requiring anesthesia in younger children) can be challenging.

CLASSIFICATION

Immunophenotypic classification

- Classification of leukemia by immunohistochemical or immunoflow cytometric detection of lineage-specific antigens allows precise and biologically relevant description of the leukemia cells.
- Surface and cytoplasmic antigens differentially expressed on cells of myeloid or lymphoid origin can be used to reliably distinguish AML from ALL and to subclassify within each lineage.
- Classification and immunophenotype of ALL (TdT = terminal deoxynucleotidyl transferase)
  - Early pre-B cell, CD10–
    - Common features of immunophenotype: CD10–, CD19+, CD20+, TdT+
    - Prevalence: 5.2%
    - Common in infants <1 year of age, associated with t(4;11)
  - Early pre-B cell, CD10+
    - Common features of immunophenotype: CD10+, CD19+, CD20+, TdT+
    - Prevalence: 63.1%
    - Peak incidence in early childhood
  - Pre-B cell
    - Common features of immunophenotype: CD10+/–, CD19+, CD20+, TdT+, cytoplasmic immunoglobulin+
    - Prevalence: 15.5%
    - Clinically similar to early pre-B-cell ALL
  - Mature B cell
    - Common features of immunophenotype: CD19+, CD20+, TdT+, surface immunoglobulin+
    - Prevalence: 3.9%
    - Burkitt-type leukemia, treated differently than pre-B-cell ALL
  - Pre-T cell
    - Common features of immunophenotype: CD2+, CD3+, CD7+, TdT+
    - Prevalence: 12.3%

L

- More common in adolescents and in boys
- Associated with high leukocyte count and bulky extramedullary disease, particularly a mediastinal mass

Classification of AML

- French-American-British classification
  - M1: AML without maturation (24%)
  - M2: AML with maturation (23%)
  - M3: Promyelocytic leukemia (5%)
  - M4: Myelomonocytic (27%)
  - M5: Monocytic (10%)
  - M6: Erythroleukemia (2%)
  - M7: Megakaryocytic (7%)
- World Health Organization Classification
  - AML with recurrent genetic abnormalities
    - t(8;21)(q22;q23), (AML/ETO)
    - AML with abnormal marrow eosinophils and inv 16(p13q22), or t(16;16)(p13;q22), CBFß/MYH11
    - APML with t(15;17)(q22;q12), (PML/RARa) and variants
    - AML with 11q23 abnormalities
  - AML with multilineage dysplasia
    - After MDS or myeloproliferative diseases
    - No antecedent MDS or myeloproliferative disease, but dysplasia in 50% of cells
  - Therapy-related AML and MDS
    - Alkylating agent, radiation related
    - Topoisomerase II–inhibitor related
  - AML not otherwise categorized
    - Apply FAB categories
- The European Group for the Immunologic Classification of Leukemias developed a scoring system of lineage specificity for different markers to distinguish AML from ALL
  - The following abbreviations are used in this section: cy, cytoplasmic; mem, membrane; MPO, myeloperoxidase; TCR, T-cell receptor; TdT, terminal deoxynucleotidyl transferase.
  - Biphenotypic or mixed-lineage leukemia is defined as a score = 2 in 2 separate lineages.
  - Points: 2
    - B-cell ALL: cyCD79
    - T-cell ALL: cyCD3 or memCD3
    - AML: MPO
  - Points: 2
    - B-cell ALL: cyCD22
    - T-cell ALL: cyCD3 or memCD3
  - Points: 2
    - B-cell ALL: cyIgM
    - T-cell ALL: Anti-TCR

- Points: 1
  - B-cell ALL: CD19
  - T-cell ALL: CD2
  - AML: CD117
- Points: 1
  - B-cell ALL: CD20
  - T-cell ALL: CD5
  - AML: CD13
- Points: 1
  - B-cell ALL: CD10
  - T-cell ALL: CD8
  - AML: CD33
- Points: 1
  - T-cell ALL: CD10
  - AML: CD65
- Points: 0.5
  - B-cell ALL: TdT
  - T-cell ALL: TdT
  - AML: CD14
- Points: 0.5
  - B-cell ALL: CD24
  - T-cell ALL: CD7
  - AML: CD15

Cytogenetic and molecular markers for AML and ALL

- Common cytogenetic abnormalities of childhood leukemias
  - ALL
    - Karotype: t(12;21)(p13;q22)
      - Fusion gene: TEL/AML1
      - Frequency in childhood leukemia: 25–30% of ALL
    - Karotype: 11q23 abnormalities
      - Fusion gene: Multiple MLL fusion genes are reported.
      - Frequency in childhood leukemia: 6% of ALL
    - Karotype: t(1;19)(q23;q13)
      - Fusion gene: E2A/PBX
      - Frequency in childhood leukemia: 5% of ALL
    - Karotype: t(12;21)(p13;q22)
      - Fusion gene: TEL/AML1
      - Frequency in childhood leukemia: 25% of ALL
    - Karotype: t(9;22)(q34;q11)
      - Fusion gene: BCR/ABL
      - Frequency in childhood leukemia: 3–5% of ALL
    - Karotype: Hyperdiploidy
      - Fusion gene: --
      - Frequency in childhood leukemia: 30% of ALL

L

- AML
  - Karotype: t(8;21)(q22;q22)
    - Fusion gene: *AML1/ETO*
    - Frequency in childhood leukemia: 10–15% of AML
  - Karotype: inv16(p13;q22)
    - Fusion gene: *CBFB-MYH11*
    - Frequency in childhood leukemia: 6-12% of AML
  - Karotype: t(15;17)(q22;q21)
    - Fusion gene: *APML/RARα*
    - Frequency in childhood leukemia: 8–10% of AML
  - *HOX11* over expression is a common abnormality in T-cell ALL and is identified in 5–10% of patients.
- Cytogenetic and molecular markers in ALL include:
  - Ploidy
  - Mixed-lineage leukemia (*MLL*)
  - E2A/PBX
  - BCR-ABL
  - *TEL/AML1*
- Cytogenetic and molecular markets in AML include:
  - PML/RARα
  - Core-binding factor

JMML

- Bone marrow aspiration will reveal:
  - Hypercellularity with a predominance of all stages of granulocyte maturation
  - Blast count <20%, similar to the findings in CML, with 1 key exception:
    - Patients with JMML do not harbor the Ph chromosome.
- With the exception of proving that no Ph chromosome is present, bone marrow aspiration is not diagnostic in JMML, as it is in the acute leukemias.

Myelodysplasia

- Diagnosis is based on identification of:
  - Dysplastic features in the bone marrow
  - Characteristic cytogenetic abnormalities
- Further classification is based on the number of blasts present in the marrow.
  - Used primarily to predict progression to AML

TREATMENT APPROACH

Pharmacogenetics

- Genetic polymorphisms in specific genes that are responsible for regulating drug metabolism, transport, and target expression can have a profound effect on both therapeutic and toxic responses to leukemia therapies.

- Understanding the incidence and implication of polymorphisms affecting drug metabolism and distribution will ultimately help control for individual variability in leukemia treatment protocols, with the goal of further reducing toxicity while maximizing efficacy.

Thiopurine metabolism

- 1 in 300 individuals will have 2 alleles with thiopurine *S*-methyltransferase (TPMT) polymorphisms, resulting in very low TPMT enzyme activity.
- 10% of individuals will have intermediate enzyme activity, resulting from 1 abnormal allele.
- Nearly 90% of the population is wild type and defined as having normal enzyme activity.
- All patients with low activity, 35% of patients with intermediate activity, and 7% of patients with wild-type activity require 6-mercaptopurine (6-MP) dose reductions.
- Higher doses of 6-MP are associated with improved outcomes, and defective TPMT metabolism is associated with a higher incidence of topoisomerase II inhibitor–induced secondary AML and a higher risk of brain tumors in patients who receive concomitant radiation therapy.
- Commercially available genotype and phenotype analysis of the TPMT enzyme helps guide current thiopurine therapy.
- Direct clinical applications of these relatively recent pharmacogenetic discoveries are clear.

Antifolate metabolism

- Antifolates remain essential in the treatment of ALL.
- Polymorphisms in methotrexate (MTX) transport, metabolism, and target expression may all effect leukemia cell sensitivity to MTX and illustrate how multiple polymorphisms may alter efficacy and toxicity of a single drug.
- Reduced folate carrier (RFC) is an active transport system for MTX.
- Decrease in RFC expression will lead to decreased MTX accumulated intracellularly.
- Though not yet correlated to RFC function, specific RFC polymorphisms are associated with a worse outcome with standard therapy for ALL.
- MTX is a tight-binding inhibitor of dihydrofolate reductase.
  - The concentration of MTX required to achieve inhibition of enzyme activity increases in direct proportion to the amount of the enzyme in target cells.
- Amplification of the dihydrofolate reductase gene is seen in 30% of patients with relapsed ALL but only 10% of patients with newly diagnosed ALL.
- Polymorphisms of other enzymes involved in MTX metabolism that are implicated in pediatric ALL include:
  - Methylenetetrahydrofolate reductase (an enzyme responsible for the reduction of 5,10-methylenetrahydrofolate to 5-methlytetrahydrofolate)
  - Thymidylate synthase (a target of MTX)

- In addition to the enzymes specifically involved in metabolism of MTX and thiopurines, several detoxifying enzyme systems have profound effects of a broader range of chemotherapeutic agents.
  - Cytochrome P450 enzymes are involved in the activation or inactivation of a variety of anticancer agents.
  - Polymorphisms in the cytochrome system have been implicated both in treatment efficacy and in toxicities, including vincristine neuropathies and treatment-related leukemias.
  - Implications of polymorphisms in glutathione S-transferase enzymes, glucocorticoid receptors, vitamin D receptor, and others are more controversial and not clearly defined.

SPECIFIC TREATMENTS

ALL

- Risk-stratified therapy
  - Today, risk-adapted therapies based on clinical features (age, leukocyte count, and response to induction therapies) and biological features (ploidy and mutations of known prognostic significance) are used to maximize response and cure rates while minimizing long-term side effects.
  - Importance of T cell–directed therapy is underscored by:
    - Greater sensitivity of T-lineage cancers to asparaginase
    - A new antimetabolite, ara-G (nelarabine)
    - Relative resistance of these cells to low doses of MTX
- Principles of treatment
  - Leukemia cell infiltration in marrow space and other organ systems in patients with newly diagnosed ALL may result in pancytopenia and many systemic symptoms.
  - Resolution of symptomatic disease and recovery of normal bone marrow function can only be achieved with the administration of potentially myelosuppressive and immunosuppressive chemotherapy.
  - Therapy is frequently divided into 4 phases.
    - Remission induction
    - Delayed intensification
    - Extramedullary disease treatment or prophylaxis
    - Maintenance

Remission induction

- 3 drugs are used in standard-risk patients.
  - Vincristine
  - Asparaginase
  - Corticosteroid
- In high-risk patients, the same 3 drugs are used, with the addition of:
  - Daunorubicin
- The goal is to induce complete remission.

- With current chemotherapeutic regimens, remission induction is possible in >95% of children with ALL.
- Many protocols follow an induction phase with a consolidation phase heavy in antimetabolites to secure or consolidate remission.

Delayed intensification

- A second phase of intensified chemotherapy similar to the induction and consolidations phases
- The addition of a delayed-intensification phase has led to significant improvement in survival in all patients with childhood ALL.
- Survival among patients with high-risk leukemia may be further improved by augmenting the regimen with a second delayed intensification phase.

Extramedullary disease treatment or prophylaxis

- Trials have demonstrated that CNS radiation may be reduced (to 1200–1800 cGy) or eliminated in patients with low-risk B-cell ALL with a rapid early response to induction therapy.
- Elimination of cranial radiation in patients with T-cell ALL has not proven feasible.
- Reduction in cranial radiation is designed to reduce long-term endocrine and cognitive effects and reduce the risk of secondary cancer.
- Intensified intrathecal therapy and high-dose MTX are associated with late cognitive side effects even when administered without radiation therapy.
- Optimal CNS treatment and prophylactic regimens in childhood ALL are not yet clearly defined, but current widely used strategies are associated with significantly fewer side effects than previous efforts.

Maintenance

- Unlike treatment paradigms for most cancers, successful therapy for childhood ALL includes a protracted maintenance period.
- Components of maintenance therapy vary between cooperative group studies.
- Attempts to reduce therapy to <24 months have never been successful.
- In the current Children's Oncology Group studies, boys with standard-risk ALL receive 3 years of postremission therapy.
- Boys with high-risk disease (therapy is intensified up front) and all girls with ALL receive 2 years of postremission therapy.
- Maintenance consists of:
  - Daily oral mercaptopurine
  - Weekly oral MTX
  - Monthly intravenous vincristine
  - Monthly 5-day oral corticosteroid pulses
  - Intrathecal therapy once every 3 months

- Therapy is adjusted to maximize the dose within a range that maximizes the antileukemic effect and minimizes toxicity, including myelosuppression and immunosuppression.
- Many children on maintenance chemotherapy may return to school and normal daily activities.

Infant acute lymphoblastic leukemia

- Incremental improvement in survival with intensified chemotherapy approaches has prompted several investigators to consider bone marrow transplantation in first remission for infants.
- Transplantation poses several problems, including:
  - Matched siblings are not usually available.
  - Total-body radiation is associated with significant long-term side effects in young infants.
- Continuous intensified multiagent chemotherapy may improve event-free survival for many infants, reserving the use of bone marrow transplantation only in the setting of relapse or abnormalities involving 11q23 in younger infants.

BCR-ABL

- Matched-sibling bone marrow transplantation is now recommended for children in first remission.
  - The role of specific tyrosine kinase inhibitors, such as imatinib mesylate, are currently being evaluated.

TEL/AML1

- Patients with the *TEL/AML1* translocation do very well with conventional therapy.
  - May be preferentially sensitive to protocols containing augmented therapy with asparaginase
- Patients with *TEL/AML1*–positive leukemias tend to have relapse late.
  - Salvage after relapse remains excellent.

AML

- >90% of patients achieve complete remission with cytarabine and daunorubicin in combination with either etoposide or thioguanine.
- Attempts to improve remission induction rates and long-term survival by substituting idarubicin or mitoxantrone for daunorubicin or by increasing the dose of cytarabine have largely proven to be of similar efficacy and occasionally greater toxicity.
- Alternative approaches under investigation include the introduction of monoclonal antibodies directed against CD33, a surface antigen expressed on most myeloid neoplasms.
- Intensive postremission therapies have been developed using multiagent regimens cycled every 4–6 weeks.
- No randomized head-to-head comparisons of regimens have been made.
  - None has succeeded in improving long-term, event-free survival beyond 60%.

- Allogeneic stem cell transplantation has been extensively evaluated.
  - Most studies nonrandomly assign patients with matched-sibling donors to undergo transplantation and those without sibling donors to continue with conventional chemotherapy.
  - Relapse-free survival is generally better in patients who undergo transplantation, but overall survival is comparable because of transplant-related mortality.
  - Stem cell transplantation (SCT) is currently not recommended in first remission among patients with t(8;21), t(9;11), t(15;17) and *inv* 16, all favorable cytogenetic features.

Relapsed leukemias
ALL

- Despite development of successful therapies in childhood leukemias, 20–25% of children with ALL and 50% of children with AML have relapse after chemotherapy treatment.
- In most children with relapsed leukemia, long-term, event-free survival is <50%, even with SCT.
- 2 reliable predictors of survival after relapse are:
  - Duration of the first remission (improved survival after a longer first remission)
  - Phenotype (relapse B-lineage leukemias are more curable than T-lineage leukemias)
- According to the Berlin-Frankfurt-Munste (BFM) group, patients with late relapse tend to do better with both chemotherapy and SCT.
  - Very early relapse occurs after a first remission of <18 months.
  - Early relapse occurs after a first remission of >18 months but <6 months after completion of therapy.
  - Late relapse occurs after a first remission of >18 months and >6 months after completion of therapy.
- In the Children's Cancer Study Group:
  - Bone marrow relapse occurred in 539 patients (12%).
  - CNS relapse in 194 patients (4%)
  - Testicular relapse in 56 patients (1.5%)
  - Overall 3-year survival after marrow relapse was 28% for CNS relapse and 60% for testicular relapse.
- Remission reinduction after relapse is relatively good, but overall survival remains poor owing to a lack of effective therapies.
- Most studies comparing SCT to chemotherapy approaches demonstrate an advantage to SCT.
  - These studies typically include significant selection bias (based on donor availability and response to remission reinduction).

AML

- As in ALL, hematologic relapse is the most common adverse event in patients with AML.
- Approximately 30–40% of patients who achieve remission will have relapse.
  - 25% will have residual disease after intensive induction therapy.
- Many patients with AML undergo SCT in first remission.
  - As many as 40–50% still have relapse.
  - Their relapse therapy may be severely limited or complicated by posttransplant toxicities.
- Remission reinduction rates for all patients with AML in first relapse ranges from 50–80% using multiagent chemotherapy.
- Overall survival after relapse is 30–40%.
- In ALL, a subset of patients may be found who had late relapse that may still be salvaged with conventional chemotherapy.
- The only curative alternative for patients with relapsed AML is SCT.

Acute promyelocytic leukemia

- When treated with standard AML therapy, patients fared poorly.
- Recent regimens intensifying anthracycline dose in induction and incorporating retinoic acid, mercaptopurine, and MTX into maintenance therapy have led to 5-year survival rates >80%.

CML

- Until recently, standard therapy for CML in children and adults included:
  - Hydroxyurea
  - Interferon
  - Low-dose cytarabine
- More recently, imatinib mesylate was developed as a specific inhibitor of *BCR-ABL* tyrosine kinase.

Imatinib mesylate

- Imatinib mesylate has been established as the standard of care for CML.
- ~60% of patients with disease that is refractory to interferon achieved major cytogenetic response with imatinib, with infrequent hematologic toxicities.
- Imatinib is most effective in patients with chronic-phase CML (76% major cytogenetic response rate reported) compared with the accelerated phase or blast crisis.
- Limited data are available on imatinib mesylate in children; however, preliminary data are promising.
- In the current era of imatinib mesylate therapy, once-unattainable cytogenetic and molecular remissions are not only possible but also expected.

- Durable remissions on imatinib mesylate therapy are likely to extend beyond the first year after diagnosis, making delay of transplantation possible, especially in patients without an appropriate donor and in very young children.

SCT

- The only proven curative strategy for children with CML is allogeneic SCT.

JMML

- The European Working Group of MDS in Childhood reported 5-year event-free survival in approximately 50% of children with JMML who received a transplant from matched-related and matched-unrelated donors.
- The role of conventional chemotherapy before transplantation or in patients without an appropriate donor is not clearly defined.
- Most European trials typically use mercaptopurine or no drug therapy.
- Current Children's Oncology Group trials in the US administer:
  - Cytarabine
  - Fludarabine
  - Retinoic acid
- Granulocyte-macrophage colony-stimulating factor agonists and farnesyltransferase inhibitors are currently under evaluation.

MDS

- AML that occurs after MDS is typically more difficult to treat than de novo AML.
- The only available therapy for AML includes supportive care and SCT.

WHEN TO REFER

- The role of the pediatrician does not end with the initial referral to an oncologist.
- Much of the treatment for ALL is given on an outpatient basis.
  - Patients should be seen periodically by their pediatrician throughout treatment.
- As the number of long-term survivors among patients with leukemias increases, so will the role of the general pediatrician.
  - Understanding biology, treatment, prognosis, and short- and long-term side effects of childhood leukemias is necessary for primary care physicians.
- Referral for an endocrine evaluation should be considered for all survivors of childhood leukemia with short stature.

COMPLICATIONS

- Long-term side effects of treatment need to be anticipated, monitored, and treated effectively.

Cognitive function

- Changes in cognitive function after cranial radiation are among the most well-studied side effects.
- Radiation-induced white-matter changes may result in:
  - Deficits in speed of information processing
  - Potentially progressive decrements in IQ testing
  - Poor school performance
- Age at the time of treatment and total dose of radiation administered are the most reliable predictors of late cognitive effects.
- Patients receiving cranial radiation at <5 years, and especially <3 years, are more susceptible to resultant cognitive deficiencies.
- Other significant observations include a dose-dependent effect between cognitive deficiencies after 1800, 2400, and 3600 cGy cranial radiation.
- Many recent treatment regimens attempt to:
  - Eliminate cranial radiation for patients at the lowest risk for CNS recurrence
  - Reduce the dose of radiation to 1200 or 1800 cGy for patients at highest risk for CNS recurrence
- Intensifying intrathecal therapy has proven to be effective prophylaxis against CNS recurrence while maintaining baseline long-term cognitive function.

Cardiac effects

- Anthracyclines will probably remain a crucial component of effective therapy for ALL and AML.
- Incidence and severity of cardiac toxicity relate to:
  - Cumulative dose of anthracycline
  - Concomitant use of mediastinal radiation
  - Use of cyclophosphamide or ifosfamide
  - Younger age at diagnosis
- Most current treatment regimens in childhood cancer are capped at a total cumulative anthracycline dose of 350–400 mg/m^2 to reduce late cardiac toxicities.
  - Most ALL treatment regimens do not approach this level.
- The following are associated (in addition to cumulative dose) with a higher risk of late cardiac toxicities.
  - Bolus infusion of anthracycline (as compared with continuous infusion)
  - Female sex
  - Young age at diagnosis
- Cardiac toxicities may affect function or rhythm, or both, and may be asymptomatic until years after completion of therapy, usually exhibiting at times requiring rapid increases in cardiac output (eg, puberty, pregnancy, weight training).
- Patients receiving high cumulative doses of anthracycline should maintain diligent follow-up, especially if echocardiographic abnormalities are detected before completion of therapy.

- Patients with no detectable abnormalities should undergo electrocardiography and echocardiography at least every 2–3 years.

Endocrine effects

- Craniospinal radiation may reduce adult standing height as a result of deficient growth of the vertebral bodies after spinal radiation and growth hormone deficiency after cranial radiation.
- For many patients, growth hormone supplementation may be necessary and effective.
- Osteoporosis after corticosteroid administration is a significant problem that may affect growth.
- Infertility is a significant concern after chemotherapy (especially with alkylator-based regimens) and radiation (especially boys who required testicular radiation).
  - Abnormal gonadal development and function may result from direct damage to the gonads after radiation or to the hypothalamic-pituitary axis after cranial radiation.
  - With higher cumulative doses of alkylators, boys (especially those in puberty at the time of treatment) are more likely than girls to be infertile.

Second malignant neoplasms

- Risk and development of a second cancer is a devastating side effect of both chemotherapy and radiation therapy for childhood ALL.
  - Risk is significantly less than that reported for other childhood cancers.
- Cumulative incidence of any second neoplasm in survivors of childhood leukemia is reportedly 1.18% at 10 years (95% confidence interval, 0.8–1.5%).
  - 7.2-fold increased risk above the general population
- Cranial radiation, relapse, and female gender have all been associated with an increased risk for developing a second cancer.
- Secondary CNS cancers are most common.
  - Secondary leukemias and myelodysplasia, soft-tissue sarcomas, brain tumors, and solid tumors are all reported.
- Deficiencies in TPMT may predispose patients to secondary brain tumors.
  - In protocols incorporating high doses of antimetabolites, the 8-year cumulative incidence of secondary brain tumors among TPMT-deficient children was 43%.
  - Patients with normal TPMT activity had an 8-year cumulative incidence of secondary brain tumors of 8.3%.
  - This exceptionally high incidence of secondary brain tumors in both groups probably reflects the concomitant use of cranial radiation and high-dose antimetabolites.
  - Identification of the possible late side effects of leukemia therapy has been key in the development of risk-stratified therapy.

- Reducing cumulative doses of agents with significant short- and long-term side effects while maintaining excellent cure rates in children with ALL has been an important accomplishment.

PROGNOSIS

- ALL

  - Leukemia cells that express aberrant myeloid markers but do not meet strict criteria for biphenotypic leukemia historically yield an inferior outcome.

  - T-cell phenotype is associated with an inferior outcome, although older age, male sex, and extramedullary disease frequently associated with T-cell ALL may partly account for the greater risk for relapse.

  - Identification of leukemia cells in the CNS at diagnosis continues to be an adverse prognostic feature of childhood ALL despite attempts to intensify intrathecal therapy and CNS irradiation.

  - Independent of the increased incidence of T-cell ALL among boys, girls appear to do better with less therapy.

    - In recent studies that intensify therapy for boys, the differences in survival among boys and girls are still apparent, although significantly reduced.

    - The reason for these sex differences is not known.

  - See table Common Prognostic Features of the Acute Leukemias.

- Response to induction therapy is predictive of outcome and used to stratify patients for more intensified therapy when necessary.

  - After 7 days of therapy, patients with <5% blasts in their marrow have event-free survival of 80%, whereas those with >25% blasts in the marrow have event-free survival of 68%.

  - Among patients with a slow early response to induction therapy, those who receive intensified therapy will have an improved outcome compared with those who remain on standard therapy.

- Addition of a delayed-intensification phase by the BFM group has led to significant improvement in survival in all patients with childhood ALL.

Common Prognostic Features of the Acute Leukemias[a]

		Clinical Features	**Cytogenetics**
B-cell-precursor ALL	*Favorable*	Age between 1 and 9.99 years	t(11;22)(p13;q22), *TEL/AML1* fusion
			Hyperdiploidy (>50 chromosomes)
			Trisomies 4, 10, and 17
	Unfavorable	Age >10 years	Philadelphia chromosome
		Initial leukocyte count >50,000 cells/mcL	*MLL* rearrangements in infants
		Poor response to induction therapy	
		Extramedullary disease	
T-cell precursor ALL	*Favorable*	Good response to steroids[b]	*HOX11* overexpresssion
			t(11;19) *MLL-ENL* fusion
	Unfavorable	Poor early response to treatment	—
		Low-intensity chemotherapy regimens	
T-cell precursor AML	*Favorable*	Acute promyelocytic leukemia	t(8:21) *AML1-ETO* fusion
		AML in Down syndrome	inv(16) or t(16;16)(p13;q22)
			t(15;17)(q22;q21), *APML/RARα* fusion
	Unfavorable	Leukocyte count >100,000 cells/mcL	Monosomy 7 (7q–)
		Secondary AML or AML after MDS	

Abbreviations: ALL, acute lymphocytic leukemia; AML, acute myelogenous leukemia; MDS, myelodysplasia.

[a] Adapted from: Pui CH, Schrappe M, Ribeiro RC, et al. Childhood and adolescent lymphoid and myeloid leukemia. *Hematology Am Soc Hematol Educ Program*. 2004:118–145.

[b] With kind permission from Springer Science + Business Media. *Annals of Hematology*. Evolution of BFM trials for childhood ALL, 83,2004;S121–S123, Schrappe M.

- Subsequent trials in the US and Europe have confirmed the importance of postinduction intensification in the long-term survival of patients with ALL.
- Survival among patients with high-risk leukemia may be further improved by augmenting the regimen with a second delayed intensification.

■ Infant ALL
  - Infants have a higher incidence of relapse, death from toxicity, and long-term side effects compared with older children.
  - Studies with intensified therapy in infants demonstrated event-free survival:
    - <10% in those <6 months of age
    - 40% in those >6 months of age.

■ Early-cell ALL has poor outcome.

■ Pre-B-cell ALL
  - Recent intensification of therapy has improved survival.

■ Historically, T-cell ALL is associated with a less favorable prognosis.
  - Poor prognosis has largely been eradicated because of intensification of therapy for patients with T-cell ALL.

■ Ploidy
  - Event-free survival in patients with hyperdiploid leukemia cells exceeds 75–90%, making it a reliable marker of a good prognosis.
  - Patients with simultaneous trisomies of chromosomes 4, 10, and 17 have a 7-year event-free survival >90%.
  - Patients with <46 chromosomes (hypodiploidy) have a worse prognosis.
  - Event-free survival for patients with 33 to 44 chromosomes is 40%.
  - For patients with <28 chromosomes, event-free survival is 25%.

■ MLL
  - The t(4;11)(q21;q23) mutation resulting in the *MLL-AF4* fusion product is associated with an event-free survival of only 20–25%.
  - In children >1 year of age, the negative impact of *MLL* gene rearrangements on survival is less.
  - The t(11;19)(q23;q13.3) translocation fusing *MLL* with the *ENL* locus on chromosome 19 is associated with a favorable prognosis in T-cell ALL.

■ *BCR-ABL*
  - Ph+ childhood ALL remains one of the most difficult subsets to cure.
    - Long-term, event-free survival of <50%.

AML

■ Event-free survival rate in childhood AML has reached a plateau at 60% despite aggressive intensification of therapy.

■ Individualized treatment regimens have worked to improve survival rates significantly in children with acute promyelocytic leukemia but have done little for other subsets of AML.

■ >90% of patients will obtain complete remission with cytarabine and daunorubicin in combination with either etoposide or thioguanine.

■ Allogeneic STC
  - Relapse-free survival is generally better in patients who undergo transplantation, but overall survival is similar because of transplant-related mortality.
  - Among patients with t(8;21), t(9;11), t(15;17), and *inv* 16, all favorable cytogenetic features, STC is currently not recommended in first remission (reviewed in 52 studies).

CML

■ Survival after SCT for CML is reported to be 70–80% with a matched-sibling donor and 40–60% when unrelated donors are used.

JMML

■ The natural history of JMML, if untreated, is death within a median of 1 year.

■ At age >2 years, thrombocytopenia and high hemoglobin F at diagnosis are predictors of more aggressive disease.

MDS

■ Life-threatening complications may occur in a minority of patients.
  - Most experience spontaneous remission within a few months.

■ ~25% will develop leukemia within 1–3 years.

Limp

DEFINITION

- Abnormal gait pattern
  - Common presenting symptom in pediatric primary care offices and emergency departments
  - Most commonly associated with trauma, but has many possible benign or life-threatening causes
- Types of limp
  - Antalgic gait: shortened stance time on affected side caused by pain on weight bearing, with shortened swing phase on the contralateral side
  - Trendelenburg gait
    - Hip girdle drops on the affected side, and the trunk moves over the affected side to maintain balance.
    - If the problem is bilateral, the trunk swings from side to side.
  - Circumduction (vaulting): straight-legged walking
  - *Steppage equinus* gait: foot drop caused by peroneal nerve injury or weakness of the tibialis anterior muscle
  - Toe-walking
  - Waddling: wide-based stance

EPIDEMIOLOGY

- See Differential Diagnosis for causes of limp by age group.
- Legg-Calvé-Perthes disease (avascular necrosis of the femoral head)
  - 5 times more likely in boys than in girls
- Slipped capital femoral epiphysis (SCFE)
  - Most common among adolescents, often during or just before the pubertal growth spurt (age 10–15 years)
  - Boys are affected more often than girls (3:2).
    - Obesity and tall stature are risk factors.

MECHANISM

- Antalgic gait
  - Caused by pain on weight bearing, possibly as a result of:
    - Mechanical difficulties
    - Inflammatory processes
    - Infectious processes
    - Specific hip disorders
    - Cancer
    - Hematologic disorders
- Trendelenburg gait
  - Caused by hip abductor weakness or hip joint instability
    - Inflammatory processes
    - Infectious processes
    - Specific hip disorders

- Circumduction (vaulting)
  - Caused by joint pain/stiffness or muscle weakness
    - Inflammation
    - Infection
    - Pain
  - Leg-length discrepancy (true or functional)
- Steppage (equinus) gait: due to peroneal nerve injury or weakness of the tibialis anterior muscle (eg, Guillain-Barré syndrome)
- Toe-walking: result of real or functional leg-length discrepancy
  - Contractures
  - Muscle spasms
- Waddling: results from bilateral hip disease or neuro-muscular disease
- Stooped and shuffle gaits (symmetric or asymmetric)
  - Caused by peritoneal inflammation
    - Pelvic inflammatory disease
    - Appendicitis
    - Salpingitis
    - Psoas abscess

HISTORY

- Important historical points
  - Duration of limp
  - Antecedent trauma and activity
  - Associated or preceding symptoms
    - Fever
    - Viral illness
    - Rash
      - Recurrent fevers, rash, and joint pain suggest an inflammatory process, eg, juvenile idiopathic arthritis).
    - Weight loss
  - Changes in exercise patterns
  - Possible trauma
    - If the nature or degree of child's injury does not fit the history given, nonaccidental injury should be considered and further evaluated.
- Recent vaccinations
  - Adolescent girls who receive rubella vaccination may develop transient but painful reactive arthritis 1–2 weeks after vaccination.
- History of influenza-like illness and erythematous rash with central clearing
  - Evaluate for Lyme disease.

■ Physical activities
- Athletes, especially runners
  - Stress fractures
  - Patellofemoral arthralgia syndrome
- Overuse syndromes due to repetitive microtrauma to:
  - Tibia (Osgood-Schlatter disease)
  - Calcaneus (Sever disease)
  - Patella (patellofemoral arthralgia syndrome)
- Sudden increase in the amount or duration of exercise is frequently associated with injury.

■ Consider underlying hematologic disorders.
- Hemarthrosis from hemophilia in a boy with a swollen, painful knee and family history of bleeding problems
- Vasoocclusive pain crisis in a black patient with a history suggesting sickle cell disease

PHYSICAL EXAM

■ Physical examination should be tailored on the basis of patient history.
- If there is any indication of systemic illness, a complete examination should be conducted.
- If there are no systemic signs, most of the examination can be directed toward the back and lower extremities.
- Thigh or knee pain:
  - May be referred from a hip process
  - Requires thorough evaluation of the hip joint

■ Determining the gait abnormality is crucial.
- Observe the patient's gait with good visibility of feet, leg, and pelvis.
- In younger children, useful information may be gained by observing the child before entering the examination room or when the child is engaged in other activities.

■ Leg examination
- To localize the cause, look for:
  - Erythema
  - Warmth
  - Bruising
  - Swelling
  - Muscle atrophy
  - Asymmetry
- Erythema, warmth, and swelling suggest an infectious or inflammatory process of subcutaneous tissue, muscle, bone, or joint.
- Palpation along the limb from lower spine to the toes may localize pain.
  - Pinpoint tenderness is found most often with fractures or osteomyelitis.

■ If hip or upper thigh appear involved, then examine:
  - Lower spine
  - Paraspinal areas
  - Abdomen
  - Inguinal areas

■ Joint examination
- Each joint should be examined systematically for:
  - Infection or inflammation, suggested by erythema, warmth, and swelling
  - Pain
  - Range of motion (both active and passive)
    - Limited range of motion at the joint suggests an intraarticular process.
- Infected or inflamed hip joints
  - Tend to be held in the position of most comfort (affected leg flexed, abducted, and externally rotated to decrease pressure in the hip joint), even to the extent of pseudoparalysis
  - Are painful with direct compression into the joint
  - Hip joints in particular should be assessed for both external and internal rotation.
- Knee joint
  - Evaluate for the presence of an effusion.
  - Evaluate for patellar pain with pressure.
  - Assess stability for ligamentous injury.
  - Pain with active, but not passive, range of motion suggests a muscle or tendon injury.

■ Musculoskeletal examination
- Leg-length discrepancy (true or functional)
  - Measure both legs from the anterior superior spine of the ilium to distal end of the ipsilateral medial malleolus.
  - Developmental dysplasia of the hip (DDH) results in functional leg-length discrepancy.
    - Significantly better prognosis if diagnosed in infancy
    - In infants, asymmetric skin folds suggest a leg-length discrepancy and are a characteristic finding of unilateral DDH.
  - The Galeazzi test should be performed to evaluate for DDH or other leg-length discrepancy.
    - The patient lies supine, with ankles to buttocks, hips and knees flexed.
    - Test is positive if the knees are at different heights.

■ General examination
- General appearance
- Temperature
- Presence of a rash that may suggest a systemic cause
- Bruising or scars that suggest nonaccidental injury

DIFFERENTIAL DIAGNOSIS

- Approaching a diagnosis by the type of gait abnormality allows a well-organized approach to evaluation and management.

Differential diagnosis, by disease type and gait pattern

- **A** (antalgic), **T** (Trendelenburg), **C** (circumduction), **S** (stepping), **E** (equinus)
- **M**echanical
  - Soft-tissue injury, including bruising, strains, and foreign body (A)
  - Skeletal fracture, including stress or overuse fracture (A)
  - Toddler's fracture (A)
  - Apophysitis of tibial tuberosity (Osgood-Schlatter disease) or calcaneum (Sever disease) (A)
  - Chondromalacia patellae (A)
  - Spondylolisthesis and spondylolysis (A)
- Inflammatory
  - Reactive arthritis, including transient synovitis of the hip (A, T, possibly C)
  - Juvenile idiopathic arthritis (A, T, possibly C)
  - Myositis (A, T)
  - Other connective tissue disease (eg, systemic vasculitis, systemic lupus erythematosus) (A, T)
  - Chronic recurrent multifocal osteomyelitis (A, T)
- Infection
  - Skeletal, including osteomyelitis and septic arthritis (A, T, possibly C)
  - Diskitis (A)
  - Soft-tissue infection (A, T, possibly C)
  - Abdominal sepsis, including psoas abscess, appendicitis, peritonitis (A, T)
  - Inguinal lymphadenitis (A)
- Specific hip disorders
  - Legg-Calvé-Perthes disease (A, T)
  - SCFE (A, T)
    - May have dull aching in the hip or leg and pain occurring only with exercise
    - Diagnosis of SCFE is delayed in as many as 30% of cases, leading to increased difficulties with treatment.
  - Idiopathic chondrolysis (A, T)
- Congenital
  - DDH (T)
  - Congenital talipes equinovarus (E)
  - Congenital short femur (C)
  - Skeletal dysplasias (A, T, C)

- Malignant disease
  - Leukemia (A)
  - Bone neoplasia (eg, osteoid osteoma, osteoblastoma osteosarcoma, Langerhans cell histiocytosis) (A)
  - Spinal cord tumor (A)
- Metabolic
  - Rickets (A)
- Other
  - Neurologic and neuromuscular disease (T, C)
  - Hematologic disease (eg, hemophilia, sickle cell disease) (A)
  - Tarsal coalitions (A)
  - Chronic pain syndromes (A, C, T, S, E)
  - Idiopathic or conversion disorder (usually bizarre gait) (A, C, T, S, E)
- Further narrowing of the differential diagnosis depends on:
  - Time course
  - Associated signs and symptoms
  - Age (see below)
  - Physical examination

Causes of limp, by age

- Toddler (1–3 years)
  - Antalgic gait
    - Infection
      - Septic arthritis: hip, knee
      - Osteomyelitis
      - Diskitis
    - Trauma
    - Accidental
    - Nonaccidental
    - Toddler's fracture
    - Neoplasia
  - Trendelenburg gait
    - Hip dislocation
    - Neuromuscular disease
    - Cerebral palsy
    - Poliomyelitis
- Childhood (4–10 years)
  - Antalgic gait
    - Infection
      - Septic arthritis: hip, knee
      - Osteomyelitis
      - Diskitis
    - Reactive arthritis, including transient synovitis of the hip
    - Legg-Calvé-Perthes disease
    - Tarsal coalition

- Rheumatologic disorder
- Juvenile idiopathic arthritis
- Acute rheumatic fever (ARF)
- Trauma
- Neoplasia
- Trendelenburg gait
  - Hip dislocation
  - Neuromuscular disease
  - Cerebral palsy
  - Poliomyelitis
- Adolescence (>11 years)
  - Antalgic gait
    - SCFE
    - Rheumatologic disorder
    - Juvenile idiopathic arthritis
    - Trauma: fracture, overuse
    - Tarsal coalition
    - Neoplasia
  - Trendelenburg gait
    - Neuromuscular disease

LABORATORY EVALUATION

- If history and physical examination suggest an infectious, inflammatory, or neoplastic cause
  - Complete blood cell count with differential
  - Erythrocyte sedimentation rate (ESR)
    - ESR <20 mm/hour: unlikely to be associated with serious infectious, inflammatory, or neoplastic causes
  - C-reactive protein (CRP) level
  - In febrile or ill-appearing patients: blood culture
    - Positive in up to 50% of cases of septic arthritis and osteomyelitis
- Tests to distinguish between hip septic arthritis (requires urgent joint drainage and parenteral antibiotic treatment) and transient synovitis (treated symptomatically)
  - Difficult because there can be significant overlap of history, physical examination findings, laboratory results, and radiologic findings
    - Leukocyte count, ESR, and CRP level all tend to be increased in septic arthritis.
  - CRP may be clinically useful as a negative predictor.
    - If the CRP level is <1.0 mg/dL, the patient probably does not have septic arthritis.
  - Septic arthritis
    - Temperature >37°C
    - ESR >20 mm/hour
    - CRP level >1.0 mg/dL

- Leukocyte count >11,000 cells/mm^3
- Radiographic finding of >2-mm difference between affected and unaffected hips
- If 4 or 5 of these factors are present, likelihood of septic arthritis is very high (85–99%).
- If joint sepsis is suspected:
  - Aspirate joint fluid (should be done by an orthopedic surgeon).
  - Obtain Gram stain, culture, and cell counts to guide diagnosis and treatment.
  - If gonococcal arthritis is a consideration, vaginal, anal, and throat specimens should be sent for culture.
- Additional tests for specific diagnoses
  - Lyme titers if history of:
    - Preceding erythema migrans rash
    - Fever and malaise
    - Arthritis
    - Travel or residence in a Lyme disease–endemic area
  - Rheumatologic workup, with history of:
    - Recurrent fevers, rash, and joint pain
    - Antinuclear antibody titer
    - Possibility of ARF should be evaluated with antistreptolysin O titer if:
      - Recent pharyngitis (previous 2–4 weeks)
      - Migrating arthritis
      - Rash
      - Possible chest discomfort (caused by carditis)
      - ARF is most common in children 4–9 years of age.

IMAGING

- Radiography (plain film)
  - Useful to diagnose:
    - Fractures
    - Hip disease
    - Spinal abnormalities
    - Foot disease (eg, tarsal coalition)
  - ≥2 views of affected area are essential.
  - Suspected hip disease
    - Anteroposterior and frog-leg lateral (Lauenstein) views of the pelvis
  - Hips
    - Radiographic evidence of >2-mm difference between affected and unaffected hip is associated with septic arthritis if temperature is >37°C and laboratory values are suggestive.

- SCFE
  - Characteristic appearance of ice cream falling off the cone at the affected femoral head
  - Seen best on Lauenstein (frog-leg) films, in which the displaced femoral head is more apparent
- DDH
  - Femoral head out of position and abnormal development on both sides of the joint (acetabulum and femoral head)
- Cancer (Ewing sarcoma, osteosarcoma)
- Multiple lesions of Langerhans cell histiocytosis
  - Additional imaging is needed for further assessment.
- Legg-Calvé-Perthes disease
  - Approximately 5 months after initial ischemia, anteroposterior radiographs of the pelvis show dense femoral epiphysis and apparent widening of the medial joint space.
- Osteomyelitis
  - Findings are not usually apparent until ≥10 days after onset of symptoms.

■ Ultrasonography of hip
- To assess for joint effusion
- If there is significant effusion, aspiration is required to differentiate among inflammation, infection, and hemorrhage.

■ Bone scintigraphy
- Uptake of technetium-99m is increased at sites of increased blood supply or bone turnover.
- Useful to diagnose
  - Osteomyelitis
  - Recurrent multifocal osteomyelitis
  - Diskitis
  - Stress fracture
  - Osteoid osteoma
  - Legg-Calvé-Perthes disease
  - Neoplasms

■ Computed tomography in evaluation of bones
- Tarsal coalition
- Spondylolisthesis or spondylolysis
- Osteoid osteoma

■ Magnetic resonance imaging is useful to evaluate:
- Intraspinal lesions (diskitis, soft-tissue neoplasms, bone marrow disease)
- Legg-Calvé-Perthes disease (if early)

DIAGNOSTIC PROCEDURES

■ Joint aspiration may be required in case of septic arthritis.
- Aspiration of the osteomyelitis site may be performed to identify organism and to determine the sensitivity of those organisms.

SPECIFIC TREATMENT

Mechanical or musculoskeletal problems

■ Unless evaluation suggests fracture or ligament damage, treat with:
- Rest
- Ice (in initial 48–72 hours after trauma)
- Compression
- Elevation
- Mild analgesics

■ If severe or persistent symptoms, orthopedic involvement may be indicated.

■ Fracture, ligament, and tendon injury require appropriate orthopedic referral and treatment.

Infection

■ High morbidity

■ Septic arthritis
- Surgical emergency
- Necessitates emergent orthopedic involvement for diagnosis and therapeutic aspiration

■ Septic arthritis and osteomyelitis
- Broad-spectrum parenteral antibiotics, including coverage for methicillin-resistant *Staphylococcus* if present in the community
- Treat until significant clinical improvement takes place.
  - Decreased ESR level
  - Decreased leukocyte count
  - Negative blood culture
  - Afebrile
  - CRP level should be monitored regularly because it decreases rapidly with effective antimicrobial treatment.
- When the patient has clinically improved and in consultation with a pediatric infectious disease specialist, oral antibiotics can be considered 3–4 weeks if:
  - The organism is susceptible.
  - Outpatient compliance is excellent.
  - The patient is monitored closely.

Specific hip disorders

■ Legg-Calvé-Perthes disease
- Intermittent synovitis with discomfort may occur, requiring limitation of normal activity, bracing, or casting.

■ SCFE
- Treatment consists of pinning the femoral epiphysis for stabilization.

Inflammation

■ Treatment of transient synovitis of the hip is symptomatic, usually requiring some limitation of activity.
- Transient synovitis is self-limited, and full recovery is anticipated, usually within weeks.

L

■ Arthritis (juvenile idiopathic arthritis, ARF, Lyme arthritis, and systemic lupus erythematosus)

- Consultation with a rheumatologist may be beneficial.
- Depending on laboratory test results, treatment consists of:
  - Antiinflammatory agents for autoimmune processes
  - Antibiotics for disseminated Lyme disease

Developmental or acquired conditions

■ Referral to an orthopedist is needed for treatment.

WHEN TO REFER

■ Refer if clinical, radiographic, or laboratory concern for:

- Fracture
- Septic arthritis
- Osteomyelitis
- DDH
- SCFE
- Neoplastic disease
- Appendicitis or psoas abscess
- Persistent limp of unclear cause

WHEN TO ADMIT

■ Patients with septic arthritis and osteomyelitis need to be hospitalized for intravenous antibiotic administration, at least in the beginning of therapy.

FOLLOW-UP

■ Patients with transient synovitis need to be followed closely because the signs and symptoms of transient synovitis and septic arthritis overlap.

- Misdiagnosis may delay therapy for septic arthritis.

PROGNOSIS

■ DDH

- Prognosis is best in children diagnosed in early infancy and with mild dysplasia.
- If not diagnosed early, DDH may result in a limp in an infant or toddler learning to walk.

■ Legg-Calvé-Perthes disease

- Self-limited, with resolution in 18–24 months
- Intermittent synovitis with discomfort may occur, requiring limitation of normal activity, bracing, or casting.

L

Loss of Appetite

DEFINITION

- Loss of appetite (anorexia) is a common symptom in children.
- A transient loss of appetite is often associated with acute illness.
- Prolonged loss of appetite, when associated with poor weight gain or weight loss, may signify a serious or chronic illness.
- In infants, it is difficult to differentiate between loss of appetite and poor feeding.
- This is distinct from, but closely related to, failure to thrive.

MECHANISM

- Mechanisms regulating hunger and satiety are not completely understood.
- Appetite is regulated by the hypothalamus.
  - *Satiety center* in the ventromedial hypothalamus
  - *Feeding center* in the lateral hypothalamus
- Central control of appetite is influenced by:
  - Anticipation of a pleasurable meal
  - Visual and taste sensations
  - Ambient temperature
  - Changes in blood levels of glucose or other nutrients
  - Limbic signals from higher central nervous system (CNS) regions
- Initiators of satiety include:
  - Vagal input from gastric distention
  - Cholecystokinin from the intestine and CNS
  - Other humoral factors, including insulin, glucagon, endorphins
- Changes in appetite may be mediated by the interaction of hormones, with changes in leptin/ghrelin levels influencing the release of CNS neuropeptides, including neuropeptide Y, melanocyte-stimulating hormone, and the orexins.
  - Leptin
    - Produced in adipose cells
    - Appears to suppress appetite
  - Ghrelin
    - Produced by endocrine cells in the stomach and gastrointestinal (GI) tract
    - Appears to stimulate appetite
- Cytokines are key mediators of appetite suppression in both acute and chronic illnesses.
  - Interleukin-1ß and tumor necrosis factor-α have been shown to induce anorexia by acting directly on the hypothalamus.
  - Effects on the peripheral nervous system and on hormone levels also occur.
- The set point for body fat content may be individualized.

HISTORY

- Review diet and consumption history of the child and family.
- Adequate evaluation of nutritional intake requires caloric assessment.
- Assess parental expectations.
- Take a careful birth, family, medical, and medication history.
- For infants:
  - Assess for sick contacts and exposure to illness.
  - Discuss GI symptoms, such as emesis; constipation; diarrhea; and amount, frequency, and character of stools.
  - Evaluate for other indications of feeding intolerance, including rashes.
  - Compare caloric intake with estimated caloric needs.
  - Assess feeding effort and coordination.
  - If formula-feeding:
    - Discuss the proportions in which formula is constituted.
    - Estimate total caloric intake from volume of formula and caloric density of formula (standard is 20 kcal/oz).
  - If breastfeeding, assess:
    - Perceived adequacy of maternal milk production
    - Ability of infant to breastfeed
- For children and adolescents:
  - Assess intake and output.
  - Discuss whether eating leads to symptoms, such as pain, emesis, diarrhea, and fatigue.
  - Discuss quantity and type of stools.
  - Assess body image, social context, and stressors
  - Consider substance abuse
  - Consider HEADSSS assessment (home, education, activities, drugs, sexuality, suicide/depression, safety)

PHYSICAL EXAM

- Vital signs
  - Assess temperature.
  - Consider heart rate, blood pressure, and orthostatic vital signs.
  - Weigh the individual and plot on a growth chart.
    - Consider serial weights for computation of growth velocities.
  - With breastfed infants, consider weighing infant before and after feedings.
  - In children ≥2 years of age, compute body mass index, body mass index percentile, and weight for length/height
- Physical examination
  - Assess mental status.
  - Assess volume status and for anemia (eg, pale conjunctiva).
  - Examine oral mucosa for thrush, ulcerations.
  - Examine nose and palate.

- Assess cardiorespiratory status.
- Assess the abdomen for organomegaly.
- Look for signs of malnutrition or vitamin deficiencies (eg, lanugo).
- Look for clinical findings related to genetic disorders (eg, Down syndrome, Turner syndrome).
- Oral aphthous ulcers may be related to Crohn disease.
- Discoloration of teeth may be related to purging behaviors.
- Assess for toxidromes in adolescents.

DIFFERENTIAL DIAGNOSIS

Newborn period

- Poor oral intake by an infant developmentally capable of feeding has a broad differential diagnosis that includes:
  - Infection
    - Sepsis
    - Meningitis
    - Urinary tract infection
    - Perinatal infection
    - Oral thrush, herpangina
  - CNS abnormality or disease
  - Cardiac disease (eg, congestive heart failure, cyanotic heart disease)
  - Structural or functional craniofacial or GI abnormality (eg, choanal atresia, cleft palate, velopharyngeal insufficiency)
  - Renal failure
  - Metabolic or genetic issues (eg, inborn error of metabolism, Down syndrome, Präder-Willi syndrome)
  - Endocrine disorders (eg, congenital hypothyroidism)
  - Drug intoxication (including maternal substance abuse, perinatal administration of opioids or magnesium)

Organic disease in children and adolescents

- Infections, acute or chronic
- Neurologic causes
  - Cerebral palsy
  - Congenital degenerative disease (eg, neurodegenerative disorders, spinomuscular atrophy, muscular dystrophy)
  - Hypothalamic lesion
  - Increased intracranial pressure, including brain tumor
  - Static encephalopathy
- Cardiac causes
  - Congestive heart failure
  - Cyanotic heart disease
- GI causes
  - Significant GI disease commonly leads to poor appetite.
    - However, anorexia may result from disease that is distant from the bowel.
  - Oral or esophageal lesions (eg, thrush, herpes simplex)
  - Gastroesophageal reflux
  - Eosinophilic esophagitis
  - Dietary protein intolerance
  - Bowel obstruction, especially with gastric or intestinal distention
  - Short-bowel syndrome
  - Inflammatory bowel disease
  - Celiac disease
  - Constipation
  - Esophageal motility disorder (eg, cricopharyngeal dysfunction, achalasia, connective tissue disorder)
- Metabolic causes
  - Renal failure, renal tubular acidosis, or both
  - Liver failure
  - Inborn errors of metabolism
  - Lead poisoning
- Endocrine
- Nutritional causes
  - Marasmus
  - Iron deficiency
  - Zinc deficiency
- Drugs
  - Morphine
  - Digitalis
  - Antimetabolites
  - Methylphenidate
  - Amphetamines
- Prolonged restriction of oral feedings, beginning in the neonatal period
- Tumor
- Chronic febrile conditions (eg, rheumatoid arthritis, rheumatic fever)

Psychological factors

- Emotional deprivation
  - Common cause of failure to thrive
  - Thorough social history is essential to the evaluation.
  - Early observation of parent-infant interaction in the hospital, including feeding techniques, may be helpful.
- The infant may not be interested when feedings are introduced by mouth.
  - Mother and infant may require training.
    - Typically provided by occupational therapist, physical therapist, or speech pathologist
  - The infant may require gradual advancement of an oral diet.

- Anxiety, fear, depression, or mania (limbic influence on the hypothalamus) may affect feeding.
- If meals produce discomfort (abdominal pain, nausea, diarrhea, bloating, urgency, dumping syndrome), poor feeding may be a result of avoidance.
- Anorexia nervosa
- Excessive weight loss and food aversion in athletes, simulating anorexia nervosa

LABORATORY EVALUATION

- Evaluation is guided by clinical suspicion.
- In infants, ensure that newborn screening has been performed.
- Because the differential diagnosis is broad, the workup is nonspecific.
- Studies may include:
  - Blood chemistries
  - Complete blood count
  - Blood, cerebrospinal fluid, and urine for:
    - Viral studies
    - Bacterial studies
  - Stool studies for:
    - Reducing substances
    - Collections for fat quantification
    - Guaiac
  - Serum studies
    - Ammonia
    - Liver function tests (including albumin)
    - Vitamin and mineral levels
  - Serum and urine amino/organic acid testing
  - Therapeutic drug monitoring
  - Toxin screens
  - Chromosome count
  - Specific genetic testing

IMAGING

- Imaging is guided by clinical suspicion.

DIAGNOSTIC PROCEDURES

- Diagnostic procedures may be performed as guided by clinical suspicion.
  - Upper endoscopy with biopsy
  - Colonoscopy
  - Sweat chloride testing
  - Esophageal motility testing
  - pH probes

TREATMENT APPROACH

- Serial evaluations of weight and intake are the cornerstones of assessing appetite.
- Assess parental expectations to ensure that they are realistic, especially in the setting of a normal growth pattern.
- If growth is poor, a systematic evaluation in the case of failure to thrive can be extensive.
- Includes:
  - Assessment of bone age (imaging or teeth)
  - Parental growth patterns
  - Mid-parental height
  - Nutrition
  - Environmental influences

SPECIFIC TREATMENT

- Treatment that improves symptoms may result in rapid improvement in appetite.
- In infants, lactation consultation as indicated and available
- Enlist the help of a nutritionist to plan diets and supplementation.
  - Foods more acceptable to the child
  - High-calorie milkshakes or snacks
  - Commercial high-calorie supplements
- Medications can be used to stimulate appetite.
- Occasionally, children will require feeding supplementation.
  - Consider placement of nasogastric, gastric, and jejunal feeding tubes.

Appetite stimulants

- Cyproheptadine
  - Does not seem to affect appetite in all children treated
  - When successful, response is dramatic.
- Megestrol acetate
  - Progesterone derivative
  - Has been administered for cancer-related anorexia, primarily in adults
  - Potential side effects include adrenal insufficiency.
  - Weight gained may be largely from increased fat mass.

Feeding supplementation

- Initial nasogastric or nasoduodenal nutrient infusion
  - May be necessary to promote growth in some disorders (ie, congenital heart disease)
  - Place gastrostomy tube if prolonged supplementation is required.
- Parenteral nutrition
  - May be indicated in specific situations
  - Expertise with this modality and close supervision are required.

- Caretakers need special training if parenteral nutrition is to be provided at home.
- Refeeding after severe malnutrition requires careful consideration of potential cardiac and metabolic complications and may require inpatient monitoring.

WHEN TO REFER

- Loss of appetite without an obvious explanation, especially in association with weight loss or failure to thrive
- Anorexia nervosa

WHEN TO ADMIT

- Weight lossor lack of weight gain unresponsive to outpatient management

- To initiate enteral or parenteral feeding because of inadequate oral intake
- Significant metabolic derangements caused by prolonged malnutrition

FOLLOW-UP

- Patients with failure to thrive need close monitoring of their calorie intake and weight gain.

Lyme Disease

DEFINITION

- Lyme disease is a tickborne infectious disease.

EPIDEMIOLOGY

- Lyme disease was first recognized in 1975 after an investigation of a cluster of arthritis cases among children in Lyme, Connecticut.
- Prevalence
  - The most common tickborne infectious disease in the US
  - 23,305 cases were reported to the Centers for Disease Control and Prevention in 2005.
- Geographic distribution
  - Lyme disease has been reported in almost every state.
    - 95% of all cases are concentrated in 11 states from 3 geographic regions.
      - The Northeast from Maine to Maryland
      - The Midwest in Wisconsin and Minnesota
      - The West in Northern California and Oregon
    - The occurrence of disease corresponds with the distribution of the tick vectors *Ixodes scapularis* in the East and Midwest and *Ixodes pacificus* in the West.

ETIOLOGY

- In 1975 the black-legged deer tick *I scapularis* was implicated as the vector of this disease.
- In 1982 a spirochete, *Borrelia burgdorferi,* was detected in the midgut of the tick and identified as the etiologic agent.
- *B burgdorferi* live in mice, squirrels, and other small animals and are transmitted among these animals and to humans by the bite of the tick.
  - The tick lives for 2 years and has 3 stages: larvae, nymph, and adult.
  - A blood meal is required at each stage of development.
  - When the tick feeds on an infected animal, the spirochete is acquired; when the tick feeds again, the spirochete can be transmitted to a new host.
  - Although deer are important for maintaining the tick population, deer do not become infected by the spirochete.
- No causal relationship between maternal Lyme disease and congenital disease has been documented.
- No evidence exists to support transmission of *B burgdorferi* via human milk.

RISK FACTORS

- Most cases of human Lyme disease are acquired in June, July, or August, when the nymphal stage is most active and human outdoor activity is greatest.

SIGNS AND SYMPTOMS

- The clinical manifestations of Lyme disease vary with the time that elapses after inoculation by the tick.

- The infection has thus been divided into:
  - Early localized phase
  - Early disseminated phase
  - Late-stage disease

Early localized phase

- Erythema migrans (EM) is the most common manifestation of early Lyme disease.
- Approximately 70–80% of patients exhibit or have a history of a skin lesion at the site of the tick bite.
- Macule gradually expands over several days to a large erythematous lesion that may increase in size to ≥5 cm, sometimes with central clearing.
- Early lesions may not have central clearing or the characteristic target-like appearance.
- Rash may be warm but is not painful.
- Influenza-like symptoms may accompany the skin lesion, including:
  - Malaise
  - Fatigue
  - Headache
  - Arthralgia
  - Myalgia
  - Fever
  - Regional lymphadenopathy
- Cough, rhinorrhea, vomiting, or diarrhea are not typical.
- Rash typically appears within 7–14 days (range, 3–30 days) of the tick bite and, if untreated, resolves within 3–4 weeks.

Early disseminated phase

- In the absence of antimicrobial therapy, spread of the spirochete may occur, producing the disseminated phase of early Lyme disease.
- Within days or weeks, in an untreated person, early disseminated disease may produce:
  - Multiple secondary EM lesions
  - Bell palsy
  - Lymphocytic meningitis
  - Conjunctivitis
- Common systemic symptoms include:
  - Arthralgia
  - Myalgia
  - Headache
  - Fatigue
- Serum antibody to *B burgdorferi* is usually not present during this phase, as antibody is not detectable until 3–4 weeks have passed.
- The spirochete is cultured from the skin more easily during early infection than at any other time in the illness.

- Approximately 60% of untreated patients will develop mono-articular or oligoarticular arthritis, which generally involves the knees.
- Approximately 5–10% of untreated patients will develop neurologic manifestations.
  - Nervous system involvement may include:
    – Cranial neuropathy (especially unilateral or bilateral facial palsy)
    – Radiculopathy
  - Central nervous system involvement may include lymphocytic meningitis.
  - Encephalopathy associated with late-stage Lyme disease consisting of mild abnormalities of memory and cognitive function is poorly understood and is a rare occurrence.
- <5% of untreated patients will develop cardiac disease.
  - Cardiac involvement is characterized most commonly by varying degrees of atrioventricular block but may include myopericarditis.
  - Hospitalization is appropriate for patients with syncope, dyspnea, or chest pain.
  - Complete heart block is usually brief, and only temporary cardiac pacing is needed.
- In untreated persons, symptoms involving the joints, central nervous system, or heart reflecting spread of the spirochete to other parts of the body may occur months after the tick bite.

Late-stage disease

- Late-stage disease most commonly produces recurrent pauciarticular arthritis that involves the knees.
- Peripheral or central nervous system involvement is rare.
- Late-stage disease is uncommon in children who receive antimicrobial therapy early in the disease.

DIFFERENTIAL DIAGNOSIS

- The same tick that transmits *B burgdorferi* also can transmit *Anaplasma phagocytophilum* (the agent of ehrlichiosis) and *Babesia microta* (the agent of babesiosis), either as a mixed infection or as a single infection.
  - Ehrlichiosis or anaplasmosis should be suspected in the appropriate epidemiologic setting in a patient with:
    – Fever
    – Chills
    – Headache
    – Thrombocytopenia
    – Leukopenia
    – Increased liver enzyme levels
  - Babesiosis in symptomatic patients may produce:
    – Fever
    – Malaise
    – Chills
    – Sweating episodes

- Additional differential diagnosis
  - Pauciarticular juvenile arthritis
  - Septic arthritis
  - Acute rheumatic fever
  - Fibromyalgia syndrome
- Other considerations
  - Aseptic meningitis caused by enterovirus infection
  - Bell palsy
  - A peripheral neuropathy not caused by *B burgdorferi*
  - Multiple sclerosis

DIAGNOSTIC APPROACH

- Some patients with Lyme disease may offer no history of a tick bite and EM.
- During summer months in an endemic area, Lyme disease should be considered in a patient who has lymphocytic meningitis or arthritis involving the knee.
- EM can be diagnosed in a person who lives in or has traveled to an endemic area and generally is a sufficient basis for a clinical diagnosis without laboratory confirmation.

LABORATORY FINDINGS

- Serologic testing in a person with typical EM is generally discouraged because of the lack of sensitivity at this early stage of disease.
  - As many as 60% of cases will have a false-negative test result at this stage.
  - However, not all patients with Lyme disease will develop EM, and many may not recall a tick bite.
- Serologic testing may be useful in the few patients in whom a diagnosis is uncertain, particularly when symptoms have been present for more than several weeks.
- A 2-tier approach to serologic testing for Lyme disease should be used with both acute- and convalescent-phase serum specimens.
  - Initial testing is conducted using an enzyme immunoassay.
  - If positive or equivocal results are obtained, then a standardized Western immunoblot for both Lyme-specific immunoglobulin M (IgM) and IgG should be performed, using the same serum specimen for tier 1 and tier 2 testing.
  - An IgM immunoblot is considered positive if 2 of 3 bands are present.
  - An IgG immunoblot is defined as positive if 5 of 10 bands are detected.
  - In endemic areas, a positive immunoblot result is not always due to an active *B burgdorferi* infection and may reflect previous infection.
  - 2-tier testing should be used because of the high sensitivity but low specificity of the commercial enzyme immunoassays used in the first step.

- Testing by immunoblot should not be performed without first performing an enzyme immunoassay.
- Laboratory testing should not be performed for people who do not have symptoms of Lyme disease.
- Testing of individual ticks is not useful for deciding whether antibiotic therapy should be initiated after a tick bite.
- Other laboratory tests that should not be used include:
  - Urine antigen assays
  - Immunofluorescence staining for cell wall–deficient forms of *B burgdorferi*
  - Lymphocyte transformation assays

CLASSIFICATION

- The infection can be classified as:
  - Early localized phase
  - Early disseminated phase
  - Late-stage disease

SPECIFIC TREATMENTS

Pharmacotherapy

- Patients with early localized or early disseminated disease who do not have neurologic or cardiac involvement should be treated for 14–21 days with doxycycline (for children ≥8 years of age)
  - Pregnant or lactating women should not be treated with doxycycline.
  - An advantage of doxycycline is efficacy against the agent of human granulocytic ehrlichiosis, which may be a coinfecting microbe.
- Amoxicillin should be used for children <8 years of age and in pregnant women.
- Cefuroxime axetil is a third drug of choice for patients not able to take the above drugs.
- Clinical trials of patients with EM show resolution of symptoms in >90% of patients treated with doxycycline, amoxicillin, or cefuroxime axetil.
- Macrolide antibiotics are less effective than other antimicrobial agents and should be reserved for patients who cannot take preferred agents.
- Intravenous ceftriaxone is not superior to oral agents, except in patients with neurologic or cardiac involvement.
- Oral antimicrobial agents are effective for treating multiple EM and uncomplicated Lyme arthritis.
- Oral agents can be used to treat most people with facial nerve palsy.
- Central nervous system involvement, such as meningitis, should be treated with parenteral antibiotic therapy.
- Although first-degree atrioventricular block usually responds to oral therapy, higher-grade blocks are usually treated with parenteral ceftriaxone or penicillin.

- Persistent or recurrent arthritis should be treated with either parenteral ceftriaxone or penicillin.
- Specific dosages and durations are given in table Treatment Regimens for Lyme Disease.

Vaccine

- In 1998 the US Food and Drug Administration (FDA) approved a vaccine against Lyme disease (LYMErix) for individuals 15–70 years of age.
- In 2002 the vaccine was withdrawn and is no longer available.

Prophylaxis after a tick bite

- Clinical practice guidelines for prevention of Lyme disease after a tick bite suggest that the following conditions be satisfied.
  - The biting tick is identified as *I scapularis,* with an estimated attachment time >36 hours based on the size of the engorged tick.
  - Prophylaxis can be started within 72 hours of tick removal.
  - Local rates of tick infection by *B burgdorferi* exceed 20%.
  - The use of doxycycline is not contraindicated.
    - Doxycycline is the only antibiotic shown to be effective for postexposure prophylaxis.
  - No data are available to support amoxicillin use in this setting.

WHEN TO ADMIT

- Cardiac involvement
- Meningitis or encephalopathy

WHEN TO REFER

- Cardiac involvement (heart block, pericarditis, myocarditis)
  - Neurologic involvement (except isolated facial palsy in patient with definite Lyme disease)
  - Nonspecific clinical history but positive or equivocal laboratory testing
  - Persistent arthritis

COMPLICATIONS

- Chronic pauciarticular arthritis
- Heart block
- Meningitis
- Cranial neuropathy
- Radiculopathy

PREVENTION

- Ticks are most likely to be located in wooded and bushy areas with high grass.
- When walking in a tick-infested area, people should walk in the center of the path to avoid contact with grass and brush.

L

Recommended Treatment of Lyme Disease in Children[a]

Disease Category		Drug(s) and Dose[b]
Early localized disease[b]	8 y of age or older	Doxycycline, 100 mg, orally, twice a day for 14–21 days[c]
	Younger than 8 y of age or unable to tolerate doxycycline	Amoxicillin, 50 mg/kg per day, orally, divided into 3 doses (maximum 1.5 g/day) for 14–21 days
		OR
		Cefuroxime, 30 mg/kg per day in 2 divided doses (maximum 1000 mg/day) or 1.0 g/day for 14–21 days
Early disseminated and late disease	Multiple erythema migrans	Same oral regimen as for early localized disease, but for 21 days
	Isolated facial palsy	Same oral regimen as for early localized disease, but for 21–28 days[d,e]
	Arthritis	Same oral regimen as for early localized disease, but for 28 days
	Persistent or recurrent arthritis[f]	Ceftriaxone sodium, 75–100 mg/kg, IV or IM, once a day (maximum 2 g/day) for 14–28 days
		OR
		Penicillin, 300 000 U/kg per day, IV, given in divided doses every 4 h (maximum 20 million U/day) for 14–28 days
		OR
		Same oral regimen as for early disease
	Carditis	Ceftriaxone or penicillin: see persistent or recurrent arthritis
	Meningitis or encephalitis	Ceftriaxone[g] or penicillin: see persistent or recurrent arthritis, but for 14–28 days

Abbreviations: IV, intravenously; IM, intramuscularly.

[a]Modified from: American Academy of Pediatrics. Lyme disease. In: Pickering LK, Baker CJ, Kimberlin DW, Long SS, eds. *Red Book: 2009 Report of the Committee on Infectious Diseases.* 28th ed. Elk Grove Village, IL: American Academy of Pediatrics; 2009:434.

[b]For patients who are allergic to penicillin, cefuroxime and erythromycin are alternative drugs.

[c]Tetracyclines are contraindicated in pregnancy.

[d]Corticosteroids should not be given.

[e]Treatment has no effect on the resolution of facial nerve palsy; its purpose is to prevent late disease.

[f] Arthritis is not considered persistent or recurrent unless objective evidence of synovitis exists at least 2 months after treatment is initiated. Some experts administer a second course of an oral agent before using an IV-administered antimicrobial agent.

[g]Ceftriaxone should be administered IV for treatment of meningitis or encephalitis.

- Insect repellent containing *N,N*-diethyl-metatoluamide (DEET) should be applied to skin and clothing.
  - DEET-containing compounds can be used for children >2 months, should not be applied to the face or hands, and should be removed from skin with soap and water once the risk of exposure is over.
- Permethrin kills ticks on contact and can be applied to clothing but should not be applied directly to skin because it is inactivated by skin lipids.
- Long pants and sleeves will help keep ticks off skin.
- Light-colored clothing makes the task of spotting ticks easier.

- Daily tick checks should be performed.
- If a tick is attached for <24 hours, the risk of acquiring Lyme disease is extremely small.
- Attached ticks should be removed as soon as possible using fine-tip forceps.
- Vaccine
  - In 1998 the FDA approved a vaccine against Lyme disease (LYMErix) for individuals 15–70 years of age
  - In 2002 the vaccine was withdrawn and is no longer available.

Lymphadenopathy

DEFINITION

- Lymphadenopathy is defined as any lymph node enlargement.
- All lymph nodes that are palpable are technically considered to be enlarged but may not be clinically significant.
- Enlargement of =1 lymph nodes is a common finding in childhood.
  - Nodes in the cervical chain, occipital, and inguinal areas drain regions that are commonly infected in childhood.
  - These nodes often are mildly enlarged (<1 cm in diameter) in children who are otherwise healthy.

EPIDEMIOLOGY

- Prevalence
  - For prevalence by age, see table Prevalence of Lymphadenopathy by Age.
- Age
  - Small occipital and postauricular nodes are common in infants but not in older children.
  - Cervical and inguinal nodes are common after age 2 years.

MECHANISM

- The lymphatic system includes:
  - Lymph nodes
  - Spleen
  - Thymus
  - Tonsils
  - Waldeyer ring
  - Appendix
  - Peyer patches in the intestine

- Potentially palpable lymph node groups and their drainage areas:
  - Occipital: posterior scalp, neck
  - Anterior auricular, parotid: lateral pinna, frontotemporal, eyelids
  - Posterior auricular: mastoid area and pinna
  - Superior (anterior) cervical: posterior scalp and neck, tongue, pharynx, larynx
  - Inferior (posterior) cervical: posterior scalp, neck, pectorals, and arm
  - Submental: apex of tongue and lower lip
  - Submaxillary: tongue, buccal cavity, lips, and cheek
  - Supraclavicular:
    - *Right:* inferior neck and mediastinum
    - *Left:* inferior neck, mediastinum, and upper abdomen
  - Mediastinal, hilar
    - *Anterior:* thymus, pericardium
    - *Posterior:* esophagus, pericardium, liver surface
    - *Hilar:* lungs
  - Axillary: greater part of arm and shoulder; superficial, anterior, and lateral thoracic and upper abdominal wall
  - Epitrochlear: hand, forearm, and elbow
  - Abdominal: abdominal organs to various mesenteric nodes and to retroperitoneal nodes
  - Inguinal, femoral: leg and genitalia
- Location of the lymphatics of the head and neck and lymph node drainage are shown in Figure 37 on page F16.

Prevalence of Lymphadenopathy by Age[a]

Age	Number of Patients	Palpable Nodes								No Palpable Nodes	
		Occipital		Postauricular		Submandibular		Cervical			
		Number	(%)	Number	(%)	Number	(%)	Number	(%)	Number	(%)
0–6 mo	52	17	(32)	7	(13)	1	(2)	1	(2)	32	(62)
7–12 mo	31	8	(26)	4	(13)	1	(3)	8	(26)	16	(52)
13–23 mo	39	4	(10)	3	(7)	7	(18)	11	(28)	20	(52)
2 years	35	3	(8)	2	(6)	7	(20)	16	(45)	11	(32)
3 years	27	2	(7)	0	(0)	7	(26)	9	(33)	11	(41)
4 years	20	0	(0)	0	(0)	5	(25)	11	(55)	7	(35)
5 years	19	0	(0)	1	(5)	4	(21)	12	(63)	5	(26)
Total	**223**	**34**	**(15)**	**17**	**(8)**	**32**	**(14)**	**68**	**(30)**	**102**	**(45)**

a From: Herzog LW. Prevalence of lymphadenopathy of the head and neck in infants and children. *Clin Pediatr (Phila)*. 1983;22:485–487.

HISTORY

- Inquire about:
  - Exposures
  - Medications
  - Weight loss
  - Fever
  - Night sweats
  - Bone pain
  - Localized infection
    - Dental abscess
    - Mastoiditis
    - Scalp infection
    - Insect bite
    - Cat scratch
    - Pharyngitis
  - Systemic diseases
    - Infectious mononucleosis
    - Juvenile idiopathic arthritis
    - HIV

PHYSICAL EXAM

- The physical examination should include all palpable nodes.
- Determine whether any lymph node or lymph node aggregate or chain is abnormal and requires further assessment.
- Abnormal lymph node: enlarged, tender, warm to touch, fluctuant, fixed to skin or underlying structures
  - Any abnormal node
    - Determine whether the node is benign, primarily inflammatory, or malignant.
  - Fluctuance and signs of inflammation surrounding a group of enlarged lymph nodes:
    - Strongly suggest an infectious cause, primarily bacterial
    - Are helpful in reaching a diagnosis, particularly if an infectious source is found distal to the node area
  - No inflammation, firm consistency, and nodes that are not mobile indicates possible cancer.
    - Lymphoma
    - Sarcoma
    - Neuroblastoma
  - Hard, fixed nodes
    - Seen more often in adults with metastatic carcinoma
  - Nodes that are more matted than hard indicative of:
    - Hodgkin disease
    - Lymphoma
  - Nodes associated with neuroblastoma, rhabdomyosarcoma, and other childhood cancers may mimic the findings in adults.

DIFFERENTIAL DIAGNOSIS

- See table Entities Associated With Lymphadenopathy for diseases associated with lymphadenopathy.
- Anatomic location of mediastinal masses and associated conditions
  - Anterior mediastinum
    - Lymphoma
    - Thymoma
    - Malignant germ cell tumor
    - Benign teratoma
    - Substernal goiter
    - Thymic hyperplasia
    - Thymic cyst
    - Mesenchymal tumors
  - Middle mediastinum
    - Lymphoma
    - Tuberculosis
    - Sarcoidosis
    - Histoplasmosis
    - Castleman disease
    - Bronchogenic cyst
    - Sarcoma
  - Posterior mediastinum
    - Neuroblastoma
    - Ganglioneuroma
    - Neurofibroma
    - Primitive neuroectodermal tumor
    - Sarcoma
    - Germ cell tumor
    - Schwannoma
    - Duplication cyst
- In hilar or mediastinal adenopathy
  - Assess promptly for neoplastic or granulomatous causes.

LABORATORY EVALUATION

- Complete blood count
  - Reactive lymphocytes
    - Infectious mononucleosis
  - Granulocytosis with a shift to the left
    - Systemic bacterial infection
  - Bicytopenia (eg, anemia, granulocytopenia, and/or thrombocytopenia)
    - Hematologic cancer, such as leukemia or lymphoma
    - Metastatic disease involving the bone marrow, such as neuroblastoma

Entities Associated With Lymphadenopathy

Infections		Generalized	Cervical	Other Regional
Viral	Respiratory viruses (adenoviruses, picornaviruses, respiratory syncytial virus, parainfluenza, influenza, coronaviruses)		1–3+	
	Epstein-Barr virus	2–3+	3+	+
	Cytomegalovirus	2+	2+	
	Primary human herpesvirus type 6		+	2–3+ (postoccipital)
	Parvovirus B19	1–2+		2+
	Human immunodeficiency virus	2–3+	+	+
	Rubella	2+	3+	+
	Rubeola	1–2+	3+	
	Varicella-zoster	1–2+	+	+
	Herpes simplex virus		3+	1–2+ (genital infection)
	Human herpesvirus type 8	2–3+	2–3+	+
	Hepatitis A	+	2+	
Bacterial	*Staphylococcus aureus*		3+	2–3+
	Streptococcal pyogenes	+	3+	2–3+
	Bartonella henselae (cat-scratch disease)	+		2–3+
	Bartonella bacilliformis (Oroya fever, verruga peruana)	3+	3+	3+
	Yersinia enterocolitica	+		3+
	Salmonella typhi	2–3+		2+
	Tularemia	+	3+	2+
	Brucellosis	2–3+	+	+
	Anaerobic infections			
	Dental, gingival infections		2–3+	2–3+
	Postanginal sepsis		2–3+	
	Mycobacteria			
	Mycobacterium tuberculosis	+	2–3+	2–3+
	Atypical mycobacteria		2–3+	2–3+
	Spirochetal			
	Syphilis	2–3+	+	+
	Lyme disease			+
	Leptospirosis	3+	+	+
Rickettsia/chlamydia	Lymphogranuloma venereum			3+
	Ehrlichiosis	2–3+		
	Rickettsia tsutsugamushi	3+	2–3+	3+

continued

Entities Associated With Lymphadenopathy, *continued*

Infections		Generalized	Cervical	Other Regional
Protozoan	Toxoplasmosis	+	3+	+
	Malaria	+		
Parasitic **(Toxocara canis, Toxocara cati, Baylisascaris pyocyonis, Trichinella spiralis, filiaris)**	Myiasis	1–2+	+	1–2+
			+	1–2+
Fungal	Histoplasmosis	1–3+	+	1–2+
	Coccidiomycosis	1–3+	+	1–2+
	Tinea capitis			2–3+
Immunizations	Viral	+		+
	Typhoid	+		+
	Bacille Calmette-Guérin			1–3+
Neoplastic	Leukemia	1–2+		
	Lymphoma	1–3+	2–3+	2–3+
	Hodgkin's disease		2–3+	2–3+
	Metastatic, solid tumors (neuroblastoma, Wilms tumor, Ewing sarcoma, rhabdomyosarcoma)	1–2+		1–2+
Histiocytoses	Langerhans cell histiocytosis		1–3+	
	Malignant histiocytosis		1–2+	1–2+
	Sinus histiocytosis (Rosai-Dorfman disease)		3+	
	Hemophagocytic syndromes	1–2+	2+	
Immunologic	Deficiency syndromes	1–2+	1–2+	2–3+
	Autoimmune lymphoproliferative syndrome	2–3+		
	Serum sickness	2+	+	+
	Ommen syndrome	1–2+	+	+
	Juvenile rheumatoid arthritis	1–2+	+	+
	Atopic disease, eczema	2–3+	2+	2–3+
	Castleman disease	1–3+	3+	2–3+
Medications **(phenytoin and others)**		1–2+		
Storage diseases **(Gaucher, Niemann-Pick disease)**		2–3+		1–3+
Granulocyte defects	Chronic granulomatous disease	+	1–2+	2–3+
	Leukocyte adhesion deficiencies		1–3+	1–3+
	Chédiak-Higashi anomaly		1–3+	1–3+
Other	Kawasaki disease		2–3+	
	Hemoglobinopathic conditions	+	1–2+	
	Hemophilia with HIV	2–3+	+	+
	Sarcoidosis	2–3+	+	1–2+
	Gianotti-Crosti syndrome	3+	+	+

Entities Associated With Lymphadenopathy, *continued*

Infections		Generalized	Cervical	Other Regional
Other, continued	Necrotizing lymphadenitis (Kikuchi lymphadenitis, Fujimoto necrotizing lymphadenitis)	+	2–3+	2–3+
	Insect bites		+	+
	Kimura		2–3+	1–2+
	Addison disease	1–2+		
	Hyperthyroidism	1–3+		

- Nucleated erythrocytes and immature granulocytes (leuko-erythroblastic blood picture) on the blood film
  - Bone marrow irritation, with premature release of blood cell precursors
  - Metastatic diseases
    - Neuroblastoma
    - Rhabdomyosarcoma
  - Immunologic vasculitis
  - Granulomas (mycobacteria) in the marrow
- Isolated leukopenia and neutropenia
  - Viral infections
  - Severe bacterial infections (particularly in infants)
- Serologic assessment
- Antigen detection
- Polymerase chain reaction
- C-reactive protein
- Erythrocyte sedimentation rate
- Anaerobic and aerobic culture of material obtained from biopsy or aspiration
  - Including special stains, eg, Worthin-Stern-Silver stain for cat-scratch disease

IMAGING

- Chest radiograph
  - The sensitivity and specificity of methods to define chest (mediastinal or hilar) lymphadenopathy are variable.
  - In 1 study of patients thought to have tuberculosis, the chest radiograph was 67% sensitive and 59% specific compared with spiral chest computed tomography (CT) with contrast.
- A variety of imaging modalities may be used, including ultrasonography, CT, magnetic resonance imaging (MRI), nucleotide or positron emission tomographic scanning, and scintigraphy.
- Specific regions studied include:
  - Abdomen
    - Retroperitoneal, periportal, and celiac nodes
    - Nodes of the splenic hilum
  - Spleen
    - Ultrasonography or CT
  - Abdominal and pelvic lymph nodes
    - Ultrasonography, CT, MRI

DIAGNOSTIC PROCEDURES

- Intradermal skin tests
  - When mycobacterial infection is suspected
- Biopsy
  - Should be performed at a medical center that specializes in the care of children
  - For significant adenopathy
    - If no evidence of infection or other cause exists
    - If mediastinal or hilar nodes are enlarged
  - Biopsy sample should encompass the central mass of the enlarged nodes to avoid misdiagnosis of reactive inflammation in adjacent nodes.
  - For suspicion of tuberculosis
  - Needle aspiration should be avoided to prevent spread of the infection and creating a track; excisional biopsy is required.
  - Prompt biopsy is recommended in significantly enlarged, unexplained lymph nodes.
    - Even in the absence of mediastinal or hilar adenopathy
    - Allows institution of appropriate therapy
- Fine-needle aspiration biopsy
  - Reserved for surgically inaccessible nodes; not recommended for biopsy of superficial, accessible nodes
  - May be useful for intrathoracic nodes to avoid thoracotomy
  - Acute cervical adenitis
    - Acutely inflamed, sometimes fluctuant, node demonstrates the infecting organism in two-thirds or more of cases.
  - Negative findings are not definitive.
- The pathology of Hodgkin disease, lymphoma, and other similar round-cell tumors may be difficult to establish.
  - Requires the assessment of a pediatric pathologist who has experience in these diseases

L

- Precise diagnosis may require:
  - Immunophenotyping
  - Cytogenetic analysis
  - Molecular studies of gene rearrangement
  - Electron microscopy

TREATMENT APPROACH

- If a bacterial source for localized adenopathy (eg, pharyngitis, cervical nodes) is suggested, a limited course of 7–10 days of antibiotic therapy may be tried.
- Further evaluation should be carried out promptly, if the nodes have not regressed significantly after the trial.
- Treatment of neoplastic causes is, in most instances, oriented toward cure.

SPECIFIC TREATMENT

Infectious disease

- Therapy for lymphadenitis depends on the cause or most likely cause.
- Infection with group A ß-hemolytic streptococci or *Staphylococcus aureus*
  - In children beyond the neonatal period who have acute localized adenitis, particularly cervical adenitis
    - Antibiotics directed at group A streptococci and penicillinase-producing strains of *S aureus*
  - Community-acquired methicillin-resistant *S aureus*
    - Treatment should include an antibiotic to cover methicillin-resistant *S aureus*.
  - For most patients, oral therapy is adequate.
    - Typical length of treatment is 10–14 days.
    - Treatment should be continued for ≥5 days after signs of acute inflammation have subsided.
  - For patients who have suppurative adenitis from these organisms, drainage is not only diagnostic (by culturing the exudate) but also therapeutic.
  - Parenteral antibiotic therapy is required in patients who do not respond to oral therapy.
    - Even with a drug to which the organism is sensitive
- Anaerobic infection
  - Therapy depends on location of the adenitis and type of organism.
  - Most anaerobic infections of the cervical and submental areas are associated with mouth flora; most are sensitive to penicillin.
  - Alternative therapy
    - Clindamycin
    - Amoxicillin-clavulanate
    - Metronidazole
    - Some cephalosporins

- *Mycobacterium tuberculosis* and atypical mycobacteria may be difficult to differentiate.
  - Many strains of atypical mycobacteria are resistant to the usual antitubercular chemotherapy.
  - If tubercular infection is suspected, excisional biopsy may be required.
  - Appropriate therapy for *M tuberculosis* should be initiated while awaiting identification and sensitivities of the organism.
    - Adenitis that is thought to be tubercular should not be incised or drained.
- Cat-scratch disease (*Bartonella* species, especially *B henselae*) is usually self-limited.
  - Some antibiotics, alone or combined, may be of clinical benefit
    - Azithromycin
    - Erythromycin
    - Rifampin
    - Trimethoprim-sulfamethoxazole
    - Doxycycline
    - Parenteral aminoglycosides
  - For markedly enlarged, tender, and fluctuant nodes:
    - Aspiration may help relieve symptoms.
    - Incision and drainage should be avoided.
- For severe primary herpes simplex virus infection with localized adenitis (unusual)
  - Treatment with oral acyclovir to shorten the clinical course

Neoplastic disease

- Effectiveness of therapy is markedly improved for:
  - Lymphocytic and myelocytic leukemia
  - Lymphomas
  - Wilms and other tumors
- For specific treatment of childhood cancer, see Cancers in Childhood.

WHEN TO REFER

- History and physical examination do not suggest an infectious cause.
- Potentially infectious nodes have not responded to a course of antibiotics.
- Mediastinal or hilar adenopathy is present.
- When biopsy is considered
  - Biopsies should be performed only at a center specializing in the care of children.

WHEN TO ADMIT

- When biopsy requires hospitalization (mediastinal or hilar biopsy)
- When biopsy results require inpatient treatment or further evaluation
- When an infection requires intravenous therapy

Macrocephaly

DEFINITION

- Macrocephaly is defined as a head circumference >2 standard deviations above the mean (approximately the 97th percentile) based on age and sex.

MECHANISM

- Head size
  - Can be influenced by different components that make up the cranial cavity
  - Most common causes are:
    - Hydrocephalus
    - Enlarged brain (megalencephaly)
    - Thickened skull
    - Space-occupying lesions
  - Conditions are not mutually exclusive; children may have >1 underlying factor.
- Hydrocephalus
  - Causes include:
    - Intracranial hemorrhage
    - Meningomyelocele
    - Dandy Walker malformation
    - Aqueductal stenosis
    - Malignancy
    - Space-occupying lesions
    - Benign accumulation of extracranial fluid
  - Conventionally, classified as either communicating or noncommunicating.
    - Communicating hydrocephalus, results from:
      - Impaired absorption of cerebrospinal fluid by the arachnoid villi because of meningeal irritation caused by:
        - Meningitis
        - Trauma
        - Malignant infiltration
      - Overproduction of cerebrospinal fluid from a choroid plexus papilloma (less common)
    - Noncommunicating or obstructive hydrocephalus
      - Marked by enlargement of the ventricular system proximal to the site of an obstruction
      - Obstruction may be an anatomic defect (such as aqueductal stenosis) or the result of a tumor, infection, or infiltrate.
      - Congenital aqueductal stenosis may occur sporadically or be transmitted by X-linked inheritance.
      - Hydrocephalus with Chiari type II defect is present in 80% of children with myelomenigocoele.

- In Dandy Walker malformation, a cystic dilatation of the fourth ventricle with hypoplasia of the cerebellar vermis and a variety of other cranial malformations, macrocephaly is the first clinical manifestation.
    - In many cases, classification of hydrocephalus as either communicating or noncommunicating may not be clear-cut.
      - Hemorrhage and intrauterine infections, for example, may lead to both communicating and noncommunicating hydrocephalus.
    - Intraventricular hemorrhage occurs in approximately 15% of premature infants with birth weight <1500 g.
- Megalencephaly
  - Megalencephaly—metabolic
    - In metabolic megalencephaly, enlargement of the brain is caused by an inborn error of metabolism that leads to the abnormal deposition of some substrate in the brain.
      - Most such inborn errors are autosomal-recessive disorders.
      - Produce significant developmental delays, psychomotor regression, and an enlarging head that may cross percentiles over time
    - Examples of metabolic conditions causing macrocephaly:
      - Mucopolysaccharidoses
        - Hurler syndrome is the most severe form of mucopolysaccharidoses
          - Results from a deficiency of a-L-iduronidase
      - Canavan disease
        - A leukodystrophy that predominantly affects Ashkenazi Jews
        - Caused by a deficiency of aspartoacylase
      - Alexander disease
        - A rare, mostly sporadic condition
        - Characterized by abundant accumulation of glial fibrillary acidic protein in Rosenthal fibers
      - Glutaric aciduria
  - Megalencephaly—anatomic
    - Overgrowth syndromes
    - Neurocutaneous syndromes
    - Achondroplasia
    - Autism
    - Fragile X syndrome
  - Megalencephaly—idiopathic (benign)
- Skull thickening and skull abnormalities
  - Thalassemia
  - Cleidocranial dysostosis and other skeletal disorders

- Space-occupying lesions
  - Vascular malformations
  - Intracranial tumors
  - Subdural effusion
  - Subdural hematoma

HISTORY

- Review previously measured head circumferences.
  - Determine whether a child has had any change in pattern or percentiles of head circumferences over time.
- A large head circumference at birth:
  - Presupposes a cause of prenatal origin
  - Necessitates a detailed prenatal history
  - Conditions that may cause congenital macrocephaly
    - X-linked aqueductal stenosis
    - Overgrowth syndromes
- An abnormally enlarging head postnatally in a child with neurodevelopmental problems is a clue to an acquired condition, such as:
  - Acquired hydrocephalus
  - A possible metabolic disorder
- History should explore:
  - Delays in developmental milestones
  - Regression in motor, language, and social skills
  - Seizures
  - Signs of increased intracranial pressure
    - Lethargy
    - Vomiting
    - Behavioral changes
- A family history of any genetic, neurologic, and developmental condition may be a red flag for similar disorders.
- A history of otherwise normal parents and siblings with large heads can be reassuring.

PHYSICAL EXAM

- Physical examination of the child with macrocephaly should focus on:
  - Accurate measurement of the head circumference and assessment of the pattern of head growth
  - Inspection and palpation of the skull
  - Comparison of the head circumference with other growth parameters
  - Presence or absence of dysmorphic features
  - Presence or absence of congenital abnormalities involving other organ systems
  - Thorough neurologic and developmental assessment, including a check for signs of increased intracranial pressure

- Monitoring of head size must be performed periodically during health care maintenance visits.
  - In the presence of a rapid enlargement in head circumference, more frequent monitoring is necessary.
  - Measurements should be plotted on the appropriate head circumference charts.
  - A disproportionately enlarged head relative to height and weight may indicate a primary neurologic disorder.
  - Measuring the size of the fontanelles and palpating sutures are important.
    - Significant hydrocephalus in infants may produce a bulging anterior fontanelle and separation of cranial sutures, which are uncommon in anatomic megalencephaly.
  - A vein of Galen arteriovenous malformation may produce a cranial bruit on auscultation.
  - Because macrocephaly is a feature of many genetic syndromes, dysmorphic features and other organ involvement should be noted.
  - Examination of the skin may reveal:
    - Café-au-lait spots
    - Axillary freckling
    - Ash-leaf spots
    - A whorled pattern of pigmentation that may indicate a neurocutaneous disorder
  - Careful neurologic examination is critical and may reveal:
    - Abnormalities in muscle tone and posture
    - Asymmetries
    - Persistence of primitive reflexes
    - Hyperreflexia
  - Developmental assessment may reveal:
    - Cognitive impairment
    - Autistic features
    - Learning disabilities
    - Behavioral difficulties

DIFFERENTIAL DIAGNOSIS

Hydrocephalus

- Enlargement of the ventricular system
- May be congenital or acquired
- Clinical presentation is influenced by:
  - Age of onset
  - Underlying condition causing the hydrocephalus
- Infants
  - Enlarging head circumference is the most obvious finding because cranial sutures have not fused.

- In older children whose sutures have fused:
  - Significant head enlargement does not occur.
  - Other signs and symptoms of increased intracranial pressure may occur.
    - Headaches
    - Vomiting
    - Papilledema
  - Hydrocephalus with intraventricular hemorrhage
- Intraventricular hemorrhage occurs in approximately 15% of premature infants with birth weight <1500 g.
- Although subtle changes in head circumference may be present, macrocephaly is not always evident in infants with intraventricular hemorrhage.
- Grade III and IV hemorrhages are associated with poorer neurodevelopmental outcomes than grade I and II hemorrhages.
  - An estimated 35% and 90% of affected children, respectively, show neurologic sequelae.
- Hydrocephalus with Chiari type II defect
  - Present in 80% of children with myelomenigocoele
- Dandy Walker malformation
  - Cystic dilatation of the fourth ventricle with:
    - Macrocephaly—commonly the first manifestation
    - Hypoplasia of the cerebellar vermis
    - Various other cranial malformations
  - Head size may be normal at birth, but acceleration in head growth is noted in the majority of children by 1 year.
    - Sometimes shows prominence of the posterior part of the skull
- Congenital aqueductal stenosis
  - May occur sporadically or be transmitted by X-linked inheritance
  - Severe hydrocephalus may:
    - Complicate labor and delivery with cephalopelvic disproportion
    - Lead to signs and symptoms of increased intracranial pressure after birth
- Benign accumulation of extracranial fluid
  - May be seen in many children with macrocephaly who have an unremarkable neurologic examination
  - The exact nature of fluid collection is not clearly established and is variously called:
    - Benign macrocephaly
    - External hydrocephalus
    - Benign extracerebral fluid collections
    - Benign subdural collections
    - Benign enlargement of the subarachnoid space
  - Fluid collection is most evident in the prefrontal area.

- In some cases, there is mild nonprogressive dilation of the ventricular system.
- Brain size is normal.
- Normal or large head circumferences at birth
- In succeeding months, head circumference grows to >98th percentile and then generally parallels the normal growth curves.
- Large head size is an isolated feature; the affected child has an otherwise normal neurologic examination and age-appropriate development.
  - Transient early developmental delays may be seen, especially in the first year of life.
- Condition appears to be self-limited, with normalization of CT findings usually by 2.5 years of age.
- Relationship to benign megalencephaly has not been established and is not fully understood.

Megalencephaly

- Benign or idiopathic megalencephaly
  - Large head
  - No significant collection of extraventricular or intraventricular fluid
  - Normal neurologic examination and developmental history
  - No signs of increased intracranial pressure
  - Family history of large head sizes in normal adult megalencephaly
  - Although these individuals have been thought to develop normally, recent evidence suggests they may exhibit mild neurodevelopmental dysfunction, such as incoordination and visual-motor weaknesses.
- Anatomic megalencephaly
  - Usually associated with neurodevelopmental impairment
  - The brain is abnormally large because of an increase in the size and number of its cells.
- Overgrowth syndromes
  - Generalized increase in body size with macrocephaly; usually present at birth
- Sotos syndrome
  - Facial dysmorphism
  - Neurodevelopmental deficits, such as poor coordination and behavioral problems
  - Macrocephaly may reflect a combination of:
    - Megalencephaly
    - Ventricular enlargement
    - Midline anomalies
- Neurocutaneous syndromes, such as
  - Neurofibromatosis
  - Tuberous sclerosis

M

- Hypomelanosis of Ito
- Associated with megalencephaly in addition to characteristic skin findings, intracranial conditions, and neurodevelopmental problems.
- Achondroplasia
  - Megalencephaly
  - Short stature
  - Shortened proximal arms and legs (rhizomelia)
  - Dysmorphic facial features
  - Normal intelligence
  - Risk for:
    - Hydrocephalus
    - Obstructive sleep apnea
    - Central apnea
    - Spine and joint problems
- Hurler syndrome
  - Enlarging head that quickly crosses percentiles during infancy
  - Coarse facial features
  - Frontal bossing
  - Corneal clouding
- Infantile form of Canavan disease
  - Irritability
  - Poor visual fixation
  - Head lag
  - Motor delay
- Alexander disease
  - Macroencephaly
  - Spasticity
  - Seizures
  - Developmental regression
- Autism
  - Compared with the general population, a disproportionately large number of autistic children have enlarged head circumferences.
  - The pattern of brain growth in some autistic children appears to be abnormal, with:
    - Acceleration of head growth in early childhood
    - Hyperplasia in cerebral gray matter and cerebral and cerebellar white matter
    - Slight decrease in brain volume during adolescence
  - The relationship between acceleration in head growth and concomitant developmental (social and language) regression (in approximately a third of autistic patients) remains unclear.

- Fragile X syndrome
  - Macrocephaly
  - Longish face with prominent ears
  - Joint hyperextensibility
  - Enlarged testes
  - Family history on the mother's side of:
    - Intellectual disability
    - Developmental and behavioral problems
    - Autistic behaviors

Thickening of the skull

- Hemolyticanemia (such as ß-thalassemia)
  - May exhibit frontal bossing attributable to extracranial hematopoieses of skull bones
- Cleidocranial dysostosis
  - Autosomal disorder of abnormal bone formation characterized by:
    - Delayed closure of fontanelles
    - Widening of the head circumference
    - Other skeletal abnormalities

Space-occupying lesions

- Arteriovenous malformation
- Brain tumors
- Subdural effusion as a complication of bacterial meningitis in infants may produce:
  - Enlarging head circumference
  - Bulging anterior fontanelle
  - Signs of increased intracranial pressure

LABORATORY EVALUATION

- Metabolic testing
  - Available to identify many of the storage diseases
  - Recommended in a child exhibiting developmental regression
- Genetic and chromosomal testing
  - For suspected cases of genetic disorders

IMAGING

- Neuroimaging
  - Procedure of choice in evaluating for macrocephaly
- Magnetic resonance imaging
  - Most informative
  - Good for identifying:
    - Gray and white matter disease (eg, leukodystrophy)
    - Migration defects
    - Hydrocephalus
    - Posterior fossa lesions

- Computed tomography
  - Can identify:
    - Hydrocephalus
    - Intracranial calcifications
    - Hemorrhages
- Head ultrasonography
  - For infants with open fontanelles, useful in identifying:
    - Intraventricular hemorrhage
    - Hydrocephalus
    - Intracranial tumors
- Skeletal survey
  - May reveal:
    - Bone age abnormalities in the overgrowth syndromes
    - Abnormalities that may be present in the mucopolysaccharidoses
    - Bone dysplasias

TREATMENT APPROACH

- Management of macrocephaly depends on its cause.

SPECIFIC TREATMENT

Shunting

- Treatment of choice for significant and progressive hydrocephalus
- Complications are not rare and continue to be challenging in the care of these children owing to:
  - Infection
  - Obstruction
  - Malfunction
- Risks are even greater in premature infants, asymptomatic, or mildly symptomatic patients.
- Dandy Walker cysts
  - Dual shunting has been recommended to drain both the hydrocephalus and the posterior fossa cyst.

Lumbar puncture

- Serial lumbar punctures may be used as initial therapy.

Medical management

- Carbonic anhydrase inhibitors
- Other diuretics

Other

- Children suspected to have inborn errors of metabolism:
  - Should be referred for genetic evaluation, treatment, and counseling
  - Treatment for these conditions is mainly supportive and symptomatic.
  - Bone marrow transplantation and enzyme replacement therapy are promising interventions for certain disorders.
- Anatomic megalencephaly
  - The association with developmental and cognitive problems warrants early intervention and special education services.
- Benign accumulation of extracranial fluid and idiopathic megalencephaly
  - Serial measurement of the head circumference
  - Ongoing clinical assessments

WHEN TO REFER

- Head circumference >2 standard deviations above the mean
- Head circumference that is crossing percentiles or growing rapidly
- Dysmorphic features
- Abnormal neurologic examination
- Regression in developmental skills or significant developmental delay

WHEN TO ADMIT

- Signs of increased intracranial pressure or mental status change
- Shunt infection or malfunction

M

Malocclusion

DEFINITION

- In normal occlusion, maxillary and mandibular molars appropriately interdigitate, allowing anterior teeth to sit in correct alignment with the maxillary incisors slightly overlapping those in the mandible and resulting in a closed bite.
- Class I malocclusion
  - Maxillary and mandibular molars normally interdigitate.
  - Crowding or misalignment exists in other oral positions.
- Class II malocclusion
  - Maxillary molars are anterior to mandibular molars, allowing anterior teeth to appear to jut out over the lower ridge.
- Class III malocclusion
  - Mandibular molars are anterior to maxillary molars, giving the appearance of a protruding jaw.
- Abnormal dental occlusion may predispose individuals to health risks.
  - Dental caries
  - Periodontal disease
  - Increased susceptibility to trauma or root resorption
  - Disturbances of physiologic functioning linked to malocclusion
    - Muscular dysfunction
    - Speech defects
    - Masticatory disturbances

EPIDEMIOLOGY

- The incidence of malocclusion in school-age children and adolescents may be ≥90%.
  - The National Health and Nutrition Survey (NHANES I; 1963–1965) examined 7400 children 6–11 years of age.
    - 14.2% had severe or very severe malocclusion.
  - NHANES III survey (1988–1991)
    - 15% of adults had malocclusion severe enough to affect social acceptability and function.
- Slightly <60% of individuals across all racial groups might benefit from orthodontic treatment.
  - Prevalence of therapy by race or ethnicity
    - 30% of white youth
    - 11% of Mexican Americans
    - 8% of black persons
  - Higher-income youths are more likely to receive orthodontic care.

MECHANISM

- Involves both genetic and environmental factors
- The cause of malocclusion is clearly identifiable in only approximately 5% of cases.

- Nasal obstruction has been linked to the development of a high-arched palate and posterior crossbite, especially when caused by enlarged tonsils or adenoids.
- Pacifiers, thumb sucking, and finger sucking play a role.
  - Children develop nonnutritive sucking habits during infancy.
  - By 4 or 5 years of age, most have stopped the practice, but as many as 5.9% continue into school age.
  - If sucking continues into the periods of mixed and permanent dentition, the potential for developing malocclusion is increased.
  - Anterior open bite, excessive overjet, posterior crossbite, and other malocclusions have been reported in association with sucking habits.
  - Children who have such habits may show no abnormalities.
  - Thumb sucking may be preferable to finger sucking because fewer physical stresses are exerted on the teeth.
    - Results of several studies of nonnutritive sucking from many countries are mixed regarding whether digit sucking is more or less deleterious than use of a pacifier.
  - Nearly all studies showed increased incidence of malocclusion among children who have prolonged sucking habits compared with those who do not.
  - Abnormal bite may revert to normal after the habit is stopped.
  - Functional exercisers, such as the Nuk nipple or pacifier, have no apparent advantage.

PHYSICAL EXAM

- Orthodontic treatment may be hindered by the fact that evaluation lacks a universally acceptable and quantitative classification system.
- Initial assessment
  - Observe both the maxillary and the mandibular arches with the child's mouth open.
  - Determine whether the teeth are crowded or have excess space between them.
    - Crowding increases over time.
    - Excess space may improve or worsen.
    - Excess space, especially between upper lateral incisors and canines, and between lower canines and first deciduous molars, is the norm in young children with primary dentition and allows room for eruption of permanent teeth.
- Posterior teeth are assessed with teeth set in the biting position.
  - The tongue should not be visible between the upper and lower teeth.
    - The presence of such a space or the contrasting problem of a deep bite (lower incisors biting on palatal gingiva) nearly always requires treatment.

- Maxillary teeth should overlap their mandibular partners slightly in the lateral plane and should be placed slightly anteriorly (~ one-half a tooth width).
- Posterior crossbites where posterior maxillary teeth are either medial or lateral to corresponding mandibular teeth rarely self-correct.

■ Problems with anterior dentition
- Readily apparent when the patient smiles

■ Occasionally, ≥1 permanent teeth may erupt before the corresponding primary teeth have been shed.
- Often the incisors
- Gives a double row of teeth
- Causes much parental concern
- Normal tongue movements usually ensure correct final placement of the permanent teeth.

TREATMENT APPROACH

■ Few data link maloccluded primary dentition with maloccluded permanent teeth.
- Anterior crossbite may interfere with ultimate maxillary growth and tooth position.
  - Upper lateral incisors erupt behind the lower ones *or*
  - Upper posterior teeth erupt medial to the lower ones.
- Absence of normal spacing in primary dentition almost always leads to severe crowding of the permanent teeth.
  - Children who have such conditions should be referred to an orthodontist early.

■ Considerable controversy exists over whether treatment of other abnormalities, such as overbite or class III malocclusions, should:
- Begin early during the period of mixed dentition
- Be delayed until adolescence

■ In general, 2 stages of treatment are required, so an early start may increase the total time the child wears braces without necessarily resulting in a superior outcome.

■ Data supporting treatment outcomes are scanty and/or conflicting.

■ Posterior crossbite should be treated during primary or early mixed stages of dentition.
- Timely treatment establishes optimal function to normalize dental, skeletal, and neuromuscular growth.

■ Anterior dentition problems
- Open bite, with space visible between upper and lower arches, and underbite are difficult to treat.
- Overbite (buck teeth) or anterior crossbite can be corrected easily.

■ Eruption of permanent teeth before primary teeth have been shed
- Extraction is rarely necessary.
- Primary teeth are almost always shed by age 8 years.

■ Temporomandibular joint (TMJ) dysfunction
- Increasingly cited as a possible cause of headache and other symptoms in school-age children and adolescents
- Some studies show a high incidence of signs referable to the TMJ, but usually without symptoms of TMJ dysfunction.
- Joint sounds with movement or condyle position do not correlate well with symptomatic TMJ dysfunction that requires treatment.
- There is no convincing evidence that malocclusion or orthodontic therapy is related to development of TMJ symptoms.

■ Most patients seek orthodontic treatment because of malocclusion's effect on their appearance.

WHEN TO REFER

■ The decision to refer is difficult because objective referral guidelines are few.
- Treatment nearly always results in improved appearance.
- Posterior crossbites rarely self-correct, and treatment during the stage of primary or mixed dentition may be optimal to promote normal development of the teeth, bones, and muscular structures.
- Absence of normal dental spacing in the primary dentition requires early referral, especially if any primary tooth is lost or fails to erupt.

■ Assess the patient's and family's expectations, as well as willingness to comply with the discomfort and cost of treatment, before arranging for referral.

M

Meningitis

DEFINITION

- Meningitis, or inflammation of the meninges, is most often caused by an infectious agent and less commonly by a chemical (medication) or cancer.
- Bacterial meningitis, also known as *pyogenic meningitis,* is often quickly fatal, making early diagnosis and treatment essential.
- *Aseptic meningitis* refers to inflammation of the meninges without the presence of visible microorganisms on routine Gram staining.
  - Not synonymous with *viral meningitis,* although the 2 terms are often used interchangeably
- Neonatal meningitis is considered separately because:
  - Agents that cause it are unique.
  - It is more often fatal than meningitis in the older child.

EPIDEMIOLOGY

- Incidence
  - Neonatal meningitis occurs in 0.2–1 per 1000 live births.
  - Between 1987 and 1997, the incidence of *Haemophilus influenzae* type b (Hib) meningitis decreased from 40 cases per 100,000 children <5 years of age to 1 case per 100,000.
  - Current annual estimates are as low as 0.1 cases per 100,000.
  - Aseptic meningitis (predominantly caused by enteroviruses) ranges from 1.5–4 cases per 100,000 population.
- Age
  - In the US
    - As many as 300–400 cases per 100,000 live births
    - 141 per 100,000 during the second month of life
    - <50 per 100,000 in the second year of life
  - Until recent years, a second peak occurred at 6–8 months, nearly 180 per 100,000 infants.
    - Due to Hib
    - Has declined dramatically since Hib conjugate vaccines were approved for use
  - The decline in Hib meningitis has converted bacterial meningitis to a disease of adults.
    - Median age at diagnosis of 25 years in 1995 compared with 15 months in 1985
  - Few reported cases of aseptic meningitis occur in persons >30 years of age.

ETIOLOGY

- Aseptic meningitis
  - Nonpolio enteroviruses cause 85% of cases in the US.
  - Fungi, parasites, reactions to medications, and atypical bacteria not well seen on Gram staining represent other causes.

Post-neonatal meningitis (after age 1 month)

- Bacterial meningitis
  - Most cases are caused by:
    - *Neisseria meningitidis*
    - *Streptococcus pneumoniae*
    - Hib
      - In regions where pneumococcal and Hib conjugate vaccines are widely used, *S pneumoniae* and Hib are the cause increasingly less often.
      - All 3 pathogens can be isolated from the throat or nasopharynx of healthy individuals.
      - Most studies of microorganism carrier states suggest that children at highest risk for disease are also the most likely to be colonized; however, does not always cause meningitis.
  - The successful meningeal pathogen must follow several sequential steps.
    - Nasopharyngeal mucosal colonization is facilitated by various microbial-binding adhesins and secreted enzymes.
    - Invasion across the epithelium, followed by survival of bacteria in the bloodstream, evading the action of alternative complement pathway
    - Finally, bacteria must invade the cerebrospinal fluid (CSF) by crossing the blood-brain barrier.
  - Meningitis may occasionally occur after head trauma.
    - Particularly fractures of the paranasal sinuses or middle ear
    - The pathogens most often associated are *S pneumoniae* and *H influenzae.*
    - Posttraumatic meningitis can recur if CSF leakage persists.
  - Meningitis can occur by direct spread from a congenital dermal sinus that communicates with the central nervous system (CNS).
  - Meningitis can develop after neurosurgery and is not uncommon after procedures performed to shunt ventricular fluid.
    - Coagulase-negative staphylococci are most often associated with shunt infections.
  - Cochlear implantation is a risk factor.

Neonatal meningitis

- Causes have changed since 1970, and clinicians should be alert to the possibility of future shifts.
  - Group B ß-hemolytic streptococci (*Streptococcus agalactiae*) and *Escherichia coli* account for 50–66% of cases of neonatal meningitis.
  - *Listeria monocytogenes* for approximately 1–5%.

- Neonatal sepsis and meningitis caused by non–group D α-hemolytic streptococci and coagulase-negative staphylococci have been reported.

■ Antimicrobial prophylaxis of pregnant women is now performed in the US who are found to be carrying group B ß-hemolytic streptococci at term or those with fever, premature labor, prolonged rupture of membranes.

SIGNS AND SYMPTOMS

Bacterial meningitis

■ Fever is usually present in bacterial meningitis.

■ Absence of fever in a child with signs of meningeal irritation does not preclude the diagnosis.

■ Inflammation of the meninges can be characterized by:
- Irritability
- Anorexia
- Headache
- Nausea
- Vomiting
- Confusion
- Back pain
- Nuchal rigidity
- Photophobia

■ The Kernig and Brudzinski signs can be assessed during physical examination to demonstrate meningeal inflammation.
- Kernig sign
  - Extend the leg at the knee of the supine patient while the hip is flexed at 90 degrees.
  - When positive, the maneuver causes extensor spasm of knee and pain in hamstrings when the lower leg is extended to approximately 135 degrees.
- Brudzinski sign
  - Flex the neck of the patient in the supine position.
  - When positive, the patient will involuntarily flex hips and knee.
  - Stiffness of neck is a sensitive (80–98%) indicator of true bacterial meningitis in children, adolescents, and adults.

■ In a young infant, signs of meningeal inflammation can be minimal or absent.
- In patients <12 months of age, absence of nuchal rigidity must not be used to exclude meningitis.
- Distinguishing nuchal rigidity from voluntary movement and guarding can be difficult in a sick infant with irritability.
  - In this case, additional signs may be helpful: lethargy, poor feeding, restlessness.

- Lay the infant near the edge of the examining table, with the head supported by the examiner's hand but gently extended off edge of table.
  - The natural tendency for an infant in this position will be to try to lift the head.
  - The examiner can feel whether nuchal rigidity is preventing flexion of the neck rather than voluntary guarding or noncooperation.

■ Signs of increased intracranial pressure may be seen.
- Headache
- Bulging fontanelle

■ Papilledema is uncommon.
- When present, other causes should be sought.
- Bacterial meningitis progresses so quickly that the time needed for papilledema to develop may not be sufficient.

■ Cranial nerve involvement occurs with bacterial meningitis; although often transient, it can be permanent.

■ The auditory nerve is often affected.
- Deafness
- Disturbances of vestibular function

■ Blindness is rare but has been reported.

■ Children may have paralysis of extraocular or facial nerves.

■ The degree of CNS derangement observed with bacterial meningitis ranges from irritability to coma.
- Approximately 15% of children with bacterial meningitis are comatose or semicomatose at the time of hospitalization.
  - Occurs more often with *S pneumoniae* or *N meningitidis* than with Hib
- Seizures occur before or within 1–2 days after admission in approximately 30% of patients.
- Focal neurologic signs correlate with persistent abnormal neurologic and developmental examinations 1 year after discharge in approximately 16% of patients.

■ Subdural effusions occur in approximately 50% of children with bacterial meningitis.
- Seldom clinically significant
- Effusions need not be sought through subdural taps or computed tomography (CT) unless focal neurologic signs or signs of increased intracranial pressure develop.
- Infection of subdural effusions is extremely rare.

■ Arthralgia and myalgia often occur, particularly in those with meningococcemia.

■ Vasculitis can be seen in children with any type of bacterial meningitis.
- Petechiae and purpura are more commonly associated with meningococcal disease.
- Children who have such rashes should be considered in imminent danger of developing septic shock.

M

- Clinical signs associated with neonatal meningitis are nonspecific.
  - Neonates with meningitis often have apneic episodes or feed poorly, and they can exhibit:
    - Hyperthermia or hypothermia
    - Irritability or lethargy
    - Respiratory distress or diarrhea (or both)
    - Nuchal rigidity (rarely)
    - Bulging fontanelle
- The neonate has a limited repertoire of clinical responses to disease or insult.
  - Most sick neonates therefore receive a diagnostic evaluation for sepsis, including lumbar puncture, and antimicrobial agents are initiated pending culture results.
- Cytology and chemistry of the CSF in neonates have a much broader normal range than children in other age groups, especially during first week of life.
  - Any single test result may not appear abnormal.
  - Infants who have bacterial meningitis rarely have completely normal CSF at examination.
  - During the first 24 hours of life, isolated meningitis without sepsis occurs rarely enough that lumbar puncture has sometimes been omitted for infants appearing septic on day of birth.
    - May lead to missed cases of both early-onset and late-onset meningitis
    - As many as 25% of neonates with meningitis have been found to have sterile blood cultures despite positive CSF cultures.
    - The proportion of such cases might increase as antibiotic prophylaxis is given to mothers and babies in the peripartum period.
    - In general, if possible, any infant thought to have sepsis or meningitis should undergo lumbar puncture.

Aseptic meningitis

- Infants and children who have aseptic meningitis caused by enteroviruses may exhibit the following.
  - Acute fever
    - Temperature is usually 38.0°C–40.5°C (100.4°F–105°F) for 4–5 days.
  - Irritability
  - Lethargy
  - Upper respiratory tract symptoms
  - Headache
  - Photophobia
  - Nausea
  - Vomiting
  - Rashes

- In general, a child with viral meningitis does not appear as critically ill as a child with bacterial meningitis.
  - Less likely to have meningeal signs
- Aseptic meningitis is likely when CSF pleocytosis ranges from 10–500 cells/mcL that are predominantly lymphocytes.
  - CSF protein level is mildly high, at 50–150 mg/dL.
  - CSF glucose concentration is normal.

Viral meningitis

- Early in the course of viral meningitis, polymorphonuclear neutrophils can predominate in the CSF.
  - Transition from a predominance of polymorphonuclear neutrophils to lymphocytes usually occurs rapidly.
  - Repeat lumbar puncture after 8–12 hours may show transition.
- Tuberculous and fungal meningitis generally have gradual onsets of illness over days to weeks.
- Hypoglycorrhachia (low CSF glucose level) rarely occurs with viral meningitis caused by:
  - Enteroviruses, mumps
  - Herpes simplex
  - Eastern equine encephalitis viruses
  - Hypoglycorrhachia caused by these viruses tends to result in CSF glucose concentrations that equal approximately 30% of simultaneous blood glucose concentration.
    - Bacterial meningitis usually results in CSF glucose concentrations of <30% of blood glucose.
    - CSF glucose concentration can also be low with tuberculous and fungal meningitis.
- Many physicians are reluctant to obtain specimens for viral culture because they believe that isolating viruses takes too long to affect management.
  - Diagnosis of enteroviral meningitis frequently results in discontinuation of antimicrobial therapy and early discharge from the hospital.
  - Therefore, when viral meningitis is a possibility, CSF should be cultured for viruses, as should nasopharyngeal or throat and rectal swab specimens.
  - Isolation of a virus from a site other than CSF can be misleading.
    - Taken in the context of other clinical and laboratory findings, a presumptive diagnosis often can be made when virus is isolated from ≥1 sites.
- Polymerase chain reaction (PCR) holds much promise as a rapid and sensitive method of diagnosing meningitis caused by:
  - Enteroviruses
  - Herpesviruses
  - Possibly other viruses

- PCR amplification of enteroviral RNA from CSF and serum appears to have good sensitivity, specificity, and predictive value.
  - Where PCR for enterovirus is available, it may substitute for viral culture in many cases.

DIFFERENTIAL DIAGNOSIS

- Signs and symptoms suggesting meningeal inflammation or increased intracranial pressure can be seen with other CNS infections.
  - The most common cause of meningeal inflammation is enteroviral aseptic meningitis.
- Aseptic meningitis can also be caused by:
  - Lyme disease spirochetes *(Borrelia burgdorferi)*
  - *Mycobacterium tuberculosis*
  - Fungi
  - Parasites
  - Inflammatory conditions
- Meningitis or meningoencephalitis may also be present in patients with:
  - Rocky Mountain spotted fever
  - Kawasaki disease
  - Cat-scratch disease
  - Toxic shock syndrome
- Meningitis often is associated with or occurs after:
  - Mumps
  - Rubeola
  - Rubella
  - Varicella
  - Infectious mononucleosis
  - Roseola
  - Erythema infectiosum
- The following conditions can mimic bacterial meningitis.
  - Brain abscess
  - Epidural abscess
  - Primary amebic meningoencephalitis
  - Embolic diseases (eg, endocarditis, thrombophlebitis)
  - Venous sinus thrombosis
  - Space-occupying lesions
  - Reactions to medications
    - Intravenous immunoglobulin
    - Intravenous monoclonal antilymphocyte antibody
    - Oral trimethoprim-sulfamethoxazole
    - Some oral nonsteroidal antiinflammatory drugs
  - Ingestion of toxins (eg, lead)
  - Spider bites

- Pemphigus
- Behçet syndrome
- Eosinophilic meningitis is rarely seen; the differential diagnosis includes reactions to:
  - Ventriculoperitoneal shunts
  - Unusual presentations of bacterial or *Toxoplasma* infection
  - Parasitic roundworms
- Conditions that can simulate a clinical picture of meningitis but that usually have normal CSF findings include:
  - Pharyngitis
  - Retropharyngeal abscess
  - Cervical adenitis
  - Cervical spine arthritis or osteomyelitis
  - Pyelonephritis
  - Pneumonia
  - Torticollis
  - Tetanus
  - Oculogyric crisis
- Selected causes of asceptic meningitis
  - Viruses
    - Common
      - Enteroviruses
      - Arboviruses
      - Herpes simplex type 2
      - Human herpesvirus 6
    - Uncommon
      - HIV-1
      - Epstein-Barr virus
      - Lymphocytic choriomeningitis virus
      - Mumps
    - Rare
      - Adenovirus
      - Varicella-zoster virus
      - Cytomegalovirus
      - Measles
      - Rubella
      - Parvovirus B19
      - Influenza A and B
  - Bacteria
    - Common
      - Pyogenic (partially treated)
      - *M tuberculosis*
      - *B burgdorferi*
      - *Mycoplasma pneumoniae*
      - *Leptospira* species

- Uncommon
  - *Treponema pallidum*
  - *Borrelia* species
  - *Bartonella henselae*
  - *Rickettsia rickettsii*
  - *Ehrlichia canis*
- Rare
  - *Chylaydophila psittaci*
  - *Chlamydophila pneumoniae*
  - *Rickettsia prowazekii*
  - *Coxiella burnetii*
  - *Brucella abortus*
  - *Streptobacillus moniliformis*
- Fungi
  - Common
    - *Candida* species
    - *Cryptococcus neoformans*
    - *Histoplasma capsulatum*
    - *Coccidiodes immitis*
  - Uncommon
    - *Blastomyces dematitidis*
  - Rare
    - Various molds
- Parasites
  - Uncommon
    - *Toxoplasma gondii*
    - Neurocysticercosis
  - Rare
    - *Angiostrongylus cantonensis*
    - *Baylisascaris procyonis*
    - *Strongyloides stercoralis*
    - Free-living amoebae
- Miscellaneous
  - Common
    - Parameningeal infections
    - Kawasaki disease
    - Foreign bodies (CSF shunts)
    - CNS leukemia, tumors
    - Acute disseminated encephalomyelitis
  - Uncommon
    - Medications (trimethoprim-sulfamethoxazole, intravenous immunoglobulin, ibuprofen)
    - Systemic lupus erythematosus

- Rare
  - Sarcoidosis
  - Behçet syndrome
  - Heavy metal poisoining
- "Common," "uncommon," and "rare" refer to relative frequencies within each broad category of etiologic agents (eg, viruses, bacteria).
- Overall, enteroviruses cause ≥85% of aseptic meningitis cases diagnosed in children in the US.
- Arboviruses cause approximately 5%; all other causes combined account for the remaining ≤10% of cases.

■ Syndrome of aseptic meningitis consists of a clinical picture of meningitis with CSF pleocytosis and absence of bacteria on Gram stain or culture.
- Aseptic meningitis is usually caused by a virus; treatable causes should be considered in the differential diagnosis.
- Nonpolio enteroviruses cause 85% of cases of aseptic meningitis in the US.
- Mumps and polio should be considered in other areas of the world where they are still endemic.
- Longer duration of symptoms has been associated with Lyme disease meningitis, especially if accompanied by erythema migrans or cranial neuropathies.

■ West Nile virus infection may cause:
- Aseptic meningitis
- Meningoencephalitis
- Acute flaccid paralysis

DIAGNOSTIC APPROACH

■ The clinical situation should influence the amount of data required before a therapeutic decision is made.

■ Interpretation of CSF findings in context of clinical manifestations usually differentiates bacterial meningitis from other diseases.
- If CSF from an ill, febrile child is turbid or purulent, then antimicrobial therapy should be initiated as treatment for bacterial meningitis before further laboratory results are available.

■ In partially treated meningitis, antibiotics have been provided before lumbar puncture is performed.
- Renders Gram staining and bacterial culture less useful (because of the possibility of temporary bacterial sterilization)

■ Distinguishing partially treated bacterial meningitis with false-negative CSF cultures from aseptic meningitis can be difficult.
- Accompanying CSF laboratory studies may be of assistance.
  - Leukocyte count and differential
  - CSF protein and glucose concentrations

M

- Reasons for delaying lumbar puncture
  - Clinically important cardiorespiratory compromise, most often observed in the neonate
  - Signs of significantly increased intracranial pressure
    - Retinal changes
    - Altered pupillary responses
    - Increased blood pressure with associated bradycardia and hyperpnea (Cushing triad)
    - Focal neurologic signs during the physical examination
  - Infection in the skin, soft tissues, or epidural area at the site of lumbar puncture
  - Suspicion or history of bleeding disorders
    - Hemophilia
    - Severe thrombocytopenia
- In the circumstances above, blood cultures should be obtained.
  - Antibiotics are provided empirically without performing a lumbar puncture.
  - In cases of suspected increased intracranial pressure:
    - Arrangements should be made for cranial CT with and without contrast enhancement during or immediately after antibiotic administration.
    - If imaging suggests that it would be safe to proceed, then lumbar puncture may follow.
    - Performing CT routinely before lumbar puncture is not necessary in patients with suspected meningitis.

LABORATORY FINDINGS

General tests

- The initial laboratory examination should include:
  - CSF examination and culture
  - Blood culture
  - Measurement of serum electrolyte and glucose concentrations
  - Complete blood count and platelet count
  - Measurement of urine specific gravity
- If the patient has petechiae or purpura or is in shock, then the laboratory tests should include:
  - Partial thromboplastin time
  - Prothrombin time
  - Measurement of fibrinogen- or fibrin-breakdown products

CSF

- Most experts suggest that the following tests should be performed on CSF from all samples drawn by lumbar puncture.
  - Gram stain
  - Bacterial culture
  - Cell count
  - Differential cell count
  - CSF concentrations of total protein and glucose
- If the nucleated blood cell count of CSF is not >6 cells/mcL, the only other tests likely to be useful in diagnosing bacterial meningitis are Gram stain and culture.
- If only a small amount of CSF is obtained, the most important tests to perform are Gram stain and bacterial culture.
- If possible, blood glucose should be measured just before lumbar puncture is performed to determine the ratio of CSF to blood glucose.
  - Measuring the blood glucose level before lumbar puncture is best because stress of the procedure can temporarily increase it.
- CSF should be cultured on chocolate and blood agar plates and in broth.
  - Generally, bacterial cultures will be positive within a few days if pathogens are present.
- The causative agent may be identified by latex agglutination reactions or counterimmunoelectrophoresis to detect soluble capsular antigens in CSF, and in serum or concentrated urine if needed.
  - These tests are rapid but should not be viewed as essential; the negative predictive value does not approach 100%, and they are not that useful in directing patient care.
  - Rapid diagnostic tests are likely to be truly valuable only in patients who have received significant amount of anti-biotics ≥24 hours before lumbar puncture.
- Distinguishing CSF abnormalities caused by infection from those associated with traumatic lumbar puncture:
  - Common clinical practice is to use the ratio of erythrocytes to leukocytes to correct the observed CSF leukocyte count, either by subtraction or by examination of the ratio of observed to expected cells.
  - Despite this apparently sound theoretical basis, in practice, calculations are generally not helpful when deciding whether to proceed with antibiotic therapy.
  - Bacterial or viral cultures will yield a more definitive answer relatively quickly.

Representative CSF findings in neonates without meningitis

- Age: 0–7 days
  - Full-term neonates (mean range)
    - Leukocytes/mcL: 8 (1–30)
    - Polymorphonuclear neutrophils: 5% of leukocytes
    - Protein: 81 mg/dL
    - Glucose: 46 mg/dL
    - CSF/blood glucose: 0.73%
  - Preterm neonates (mean range)
    - Leukocytes/mcL: 4 (1–10)
    - Polymorphonuclear neutrophils: 7% of leukocytes
    - Protein: 150 (85–222) mg/dL

M

– Glucose: 72 (4–96) mg/dL

– CSF/blood glucose: not reported

■ Age: 8–28 days

• Full-term neonates (mean range)

– Leukocytes/mcL: 6 (0–18)

– Polymorphonuclear neutrophils: 3% of leukocytes

– Protein: 64 mg/dL

– Glucose: 51 mg/dL

– CSF/blood glucose: 0.62%

• Preterm neonates (mean range)

– Leukocytes/mcL: 7 (0–44)

– Polymorphonuclear neutrophils: 9% of leukocytes

– Protein: 148 (54–370) mg/dL

– Glucose: 64 (33–217) mg/dL

– CSF/blood glucose: not reported

Blood cultures

■ Blood cultures should be obtained for all children suspected of having bacterial meningitis.

• Positive in 80–90% children who have not previously received antimicrobial agents and have meningitis caused by Hib, *S pneumoniae*, or *N meningitidis*

Partially treated meningitis

■ Leukocyte counts in CSF, percentage of polymorphonuclear cells, and glucose and protein concentrations in patients with partially treated bacterial meningitis do not greatly differ from those in patients who were not previously treated.

■ Even children who have received intravenous antibiotics for 44–68 hours have CSF findings still characteristic of bacterial meningitis.

■ Cultures of CSF from pretreated children with bacterial meningitis frequently grow Hib.

• Pneumococci and meningococci grow less often after pretreatment.

• Some patients who have partially treated bacterial meningitis will have CSF findings indistinguishable from classic findings of aseptic meningitis.

IMAGING

■ Herniation of the brain associated with meningitis has been observed before lumbar puncture and in the presence of normal cranial CT.

■ Nevertheless, lumbar puncture should be performed cautiously if significantly increased intracranial pressure is suspected.

■ Obtaining CT before lumbar puncture in selected patients is reasonable, especially in children or adults with a history of:

• Immunosuppression

• Hydrocephalus

• Ventricular shunts

• Head trauma

• Those who have focal neurologic signs

• Those with signs of greatly increased intracranial pressure

■ Radiographs may help in identifying suspected bone or joint infection in selected patients.

■ Radionuclide and CT studies play a role in complicated cases of meningitis.

• May be helpful for decisions on management later during the course of therapy

• Useful for evaluating selected cases of prolonged (primary) or recurrent (secondary) fever

■ CT should not be routinely done as a result of prolonged or secondary fever; results are unlikely to affect clinical management.

DIAGNOSTIC PROCEDURES

■ When meningitis is suspected in a patient without papilledema, lumbar puncture should be performed.

• Opening pressure should be measured and the CSF examined immediately.

■ In general, lumbar puncture should be performed whenever the diagnosis of meningitis is known or suspected.

• Children <12 months, and perhaps those <18 months, with a first febrile seizure should undergo lumbar puncture to exclude meningitis or atypical febrile seizure.

■ Herniation of the brain on removal of a small amount of CSF is rare in meningitis, especially in infants with open fontanelles.

■ If lumbar puncture was not initially performed or was contraindicated, the procedure may be reconsidered after:

• The patient has been stabilized.

• Contraindications have been resolved.

■ Lumbar puncture may be performed even 12–24 hours after initiation of antimicrobial therapy.

• Interpretation of CSF leukocyte counts and protein and glucose concentrations may be helpful in discerning the likelihood of true bacterial meningitis.

TREATMENT APPROACH

■ The severity of illness at the time the patient seeks care can predict morbidity and should dictate immediate management.

■ Therapies that are crucial for all patients with bacterial meningitis

• Fluid management

• Possible antiinflammatory adjunctive treatments

• Antimicrobial therapy

■ Acute bacterial meningitis is always a medical emergency.

■ All infants and children with an altered state of consciousness should be observed closely and need for intensive care anticipated.

- As soon as bacterial meningitis is diagnosed, intravenous administration of appropriate antimicrobial agents and possibly antiinflammatory agents should begin.
- Management of the child who is awake and has stable cardiorespiratory vital signs consists primarily of:
  - Administering antimicrobial agents and fluids and careful monitoring for:
    - Changes in level of consciousness
    - Development of seizures
    - Changes in vital signs
    - Development of the syndrome of inappropriate secretion of antidiuretic hormone (SIADH)
- Other therapies should be considered in more critically ill children.
- Seizures should be treated with appropriate anticonvulsants.
  - An open airway that provides good oxygenation should be ensured.
- Patients who are in a profound coma or whose level of consciousness deteriorates while receiving therapy should be evaluated for complications.
  - Cerebral abscess
  - Obstructive hydrocephalus
  - Increased intracranial pressure
  - CT of the brain with and without contrast is helpful in determining the diagnosis in such cases.
- If increased intracranial pressure is a major clinical concern and treatment has been initiated or is anticipated, a neurosurgeon should be consulted and an intracranial pressure monitoring device placed.
  - All children with bacterial meningitis have some increase in intracranial pressure.
  - Monitoring devices are not required for most patients.
  - If an intraventricular catheter can be placed, then increased intracranial pressure can often be treated by removing CSF.
    - Placement of a pressure transducer affords continuous intracranial monitoring, so that mannitol and hyperventilation can be used as necessary to decrease pressure and maintain cerebral perfusion.
    - Decreased inflammation and increased cerebral perfusion probably account for the benefits reported by some investigators with dexamethasone therapy.

SPECIFIC TREATMENTS

Fluid therapy

- Traditionally, fluids were restricted to two-thirds of total daily maintenance amount in patients who had bacterial meningitis.
  - To minimize brain edema and prevent SIADH, which has been reported to occur in 29–88% of cases of bacterial meningitis.

- Some studies have found that plasma antidiuretic hormone concentrations return to normal in patients with bacterial meningitis who receive replacement plus maintenance fluids for 24 hours.
  - Concentrations remain high in patients restricted to two-thirds of maintenance requirements.
- Dehydration probably produces appropriate increase of antidiuretic hormone, but SIADH may still occur in nondehydrated or fluid-replete children.
  - SIADH occurs in bacterial meningitis; however, no firm evidence has been found that fluid restriction prevents it.
- Maintenance fluids are believed necessary to perfuse, oxygenate, and deliver host defenses to the CNS.
- Obvious fluid deficits should be rapidly corrected.
- Serum sodium concentrations should be closely monitored several times during the first 24 hours of therapy, along with measurements of urine specific gravity.
  - If the serum sodium concentration decreases to <125 mEq/L, the test should be repeated as soon as possible.
  - If the serum sodium concentration is still <125 mEq/L, fluids should be restricted to keep the vein open until serum electrolyte concentrations have been corrected.
  - Otherwise, for bacterial meningitis, providing routine maintenance fluids at approximately 80% of maintenance rate after fluid repletion and advancing to full maintenance rates as serum sodium increases to >135 mEq/L seems to be appropriate.
- The period of fluid restriction may only needs to be ≤1 day.

Anti-inflammatory therapy

- Use of glucocorticoids as adjunctive therapy in patients who have bacterial meningitis continues to be controversial.
  - Dexamethasone most likely improves hearing and neurologic outcomes of children with bacterial meningitis caused by Hib.
  - The usefulness of dexamethasone therapy in children with bacterial meningitis in children and adults caused by S pneumoniae or N meningitidis is less certain.
- Glucocorticoid therapy may also cause:
  - Gastrointestinal bleeding
  - Decreased penetration of antimicrobial agents into the CSF
  - Obfuscation of the clinical assessment of children's response to therapy
- Dexamethasone may be beneficial when administered before or within 1 hour of the first dose of antimicrobial agents to children ≥6 weeks of age with Hib meningitis.
- Dexamethasone should be considered for children who have pneumococcal meningitis, although uncertainty exists regarding benefits and risks.

M

Antimicrobial therapy

- Empirical guides to therapy are primarily based on age because knowing which causative agent is present at the time of diagnosis of bacterial meningitis is difficult.
  - Adjustment to therapy can be made as conjugate vaccination history and results of CSF Gram stain and culture are confirmed.

Empirical therapy for bacterial meningitis pending culture and susceptibility data

- Age: 0–1 mo
  - Likely pathogens
    - *Streptococcus agalactiae*
    - *E coli*
    - *Listeria monocytogenes*
  - Antimicrobial agent
    - Ampicillin + cefotaxime *or* ampicillin + aminoglycoside
- Age: 1–3 mo
  - Likely pathogens
    - *S agalactiae*
    - *L monocytogenes*
    - *S pneumoniae*
    - *N meningitidis*
    - Hib
  - Antimicrobial agent
    - Ampicillin + (cefotaxime *or* ceftriaxone) *plus* vancomycin
- Age: 3 mo–21 yr
  - Likely pathogens
    - *S pneumoniae*
    - *N meningitidis*
    - Hib (if not vaccinated)
  - Antimicrobial agent
    - (Ceftriaxone *or* cefotaxime) *plus* vancomycin

Specific therapy

- Pathogen: *S agalactiae*
  - Therapy: Ampicillin or penicillin G for 14–21 days; first 3 days, add gentamicin
- Pathogen: *L monocytogenes*
  - Therapy: Ampicillin for 14–21 days; first 3 days, add gentamicin
- Pathogen: *S pneumoniae*
  - Therapy
    - Penicillin MIC <0.1 mcg/mL and ceftriaxone or cefotaxime MIC ≤.5 mcg/mL: penicillin G or ampicillin for 10–14 days
    - Penicillin MIC ≥0.1 mcg/mL and ceftriaxone or cefotaxime MIC ≤0.5 mcg/mL: ceftriaxone or cefotaxime for 10–14 days

- Penicillin MIC ≥0.1 mcg/mL and ceftriaxone or cefotaxime MIC 1.0 mcg/mL: (ceftriaxone or cefotaxime) + vancomycin for 10–14 days
- Penicillin MIC ≥0.1 mcg/mL and ceftriaxone or cefotaxime MIC ≥2.0 mcg /mL: (ceftriaxone or cefotaxime) + vancomycin ± rifampin for 10–14 days

- Pathogen: *N meningitidis*
  - Therapy
    - Penicillin G for 7 days
    - Alternatives: ampicillin, ceftriaxone, cefotaxime
- Pathogen: Hib
  - Therapy
    - Ceftriaxone or cefotaxime for 10 days
    - Alternative: ampicillin if isolate is susceptible

Antimicrobial dosage, in mg/kg/day

- Ampicillin
  - 0–7 days: 150–200 divided every 8 hr
  - 8–28 days: 200–300 divided every 6 hr
  - Infants and children: 200–300 divided every 6 hr
- Cefotaxime
  - 0–7 days: 100 divided every 12 hr
  - 8–28 days: 200 divided every 8 hr
  - Infants and children: 200–300 divided every 6 hr
- Ceftriaxone
  - 0–7 days: Not recommended
  - 8–28 days: 80–100 divided every 12–24 hr
  - Infants and children: 80–100 divided every 12–24 hr
- Gentamicin
  - 0–7 days: 5 divided every 12 hr
  - 8–28 days: 7.5 divided every 8 hr
  - Infants and children: 7.5 divided every 8 hr
- Penicillin G
  - 0–7 days: 100,000–150,000 Units divided every 12 hr
  - 8–28 days: 150,000–200,000 U divided every 6 hr
  - Infants and children: 300,000–400,000 U divided every 4–6 hr
- Rifampin
  - 0–7 days: 10 divided every 12 hr
  - 8–28 days: 20 divided every 12 hr
  - Infants and children: 20 divided every 12 hr
- Vancomycin
  - 0–7 days: 20 divided every 12 hr
  - 8–28 days: 30 divided every 8 hr
  - Infants and children: 40–60 divided every 6 hr

Antimicrobial selection

- Dexamethasone can decrease CSF penetrance (and thus the activity) of vancomycin, and some experts therefore advise that:
  - Dexamethasone should be omitted altogether *or*
  - Rifampin *plus* vancomycin *plus* a third-generation cephalosporin should be used with dexamethasone.
- Up to 40% of pneumococcal isolates may be resistant to penicillin at some level.
  - Many also are resistant to third-generation cephalosporins.
  - Therefore, infants and children suspected of having bacterial meningitis caused by pneumococci should receive vancomycin in addition to either ceftriaxone or cefotaxime.
- As soon as the antimicrobial susceptibility of an isolate is known, vancomycin should be discontinued if the isolate is susceptible to penicillin or if it is nonsusceptible to penicillin but still susceptible to third-generation cephalosporins.
  - Vancomycin is continued with ceftriaxone or cefotaxime for isolates found to be nonsusceptible to both penicillin and the third-generation cephalosporins.
    - Rifampin is added to the combination in some circumstances.
    - Consultation with an infectious diseases subspecialist is suggested.
- In areas with low prevalence of penicillin-nonsusceptible pneumococci, providing a third-generation cephalosporin alone (without vancomycin) for empiric therapy is reasonable.
  - Especially when examination of the CSF Gram stain shows absence of gram-positive cocci
  - Suspected or proven Hib disease may be treated reliably with either ceftriaxone or cefotaxime.
  - Ampicillin may be used only if the isolate is known to be susceptible.
  - Disease caused by *N meningitidis* is treated with:
    - Penicillin G at high doses *or*
    - Ampicillin *or*
    - A third-generation cephalosporin
- Meningitis caused by *N meningitidis* is usually treated for 7 days.
  - That caused by Hib is treated for 10 days.
  - That caused by *S pneumoniae* is treated for 10–14 days.
    - A 7-day course of antimicrobial therapy for uncomplicated Hib and *S pneumoniae* meningitis may also be effective.
  - Chloramphenicol is now rarely used in the industrialized world.
  - If an alternative agent beyond ampicillin or third-generation cephalosporins is required, then meropenem may be administered.
    - Consultation with an infectious diseases specialist is suggested.

Assessment of therapeutic success

- Most failures are caused by:
  - Inadequate therapy with the correct antimicrobial agent
  - Resistant organisms
  - Long delay in diagnosis
- Repeat lumbar puncture performed after therapy is completed does not reflect the adequacy of therapy or predict likelihood of recurrence.
  - Usually not indicated
  - Delay in sterilizing the CSF beyond 24–36 hours has been associated with adverse outcomes; therefore, another lumbar puncture may be performed at that time.
  - Repeat lumbar puncture at 24–48 hours is indicated if drug-resistant *S pneumoniae* is present, especially if dexamethasone is administered.

Neonatal meningitis

- Principles of antimicrobial therapy are the same as for infants and children.
  - Because organisms are different, antimicrobial selection must be adjusted.
- The ideal antimicrobial agent would be effective against:
  - *E coli* and other enteric organisms
  - Group B ß-hemolytic streptococci and other gram-positive organisms
- Cefotaxime and ceftriaxone are extremely active against organisms that usually cause neonatal meningitis, with the exception of *L monocytogenes*.
  - Ceftriaxone has a much longer serum half-life than cefotaxime.
  - Ceftriaxone is highly protein bound and can displace unconjugated bilirubin from albumin, and thus is generally not used in:
    - Premature infants at risk for kernicterus
    - Term infants with hyperbilirubinemia
  - No formal comparison has been made of these newer agents with the historical regimen of ampicillin plus an aminoglycoside, such as gentamicin.
- Cefotaxime plus ampicillin (to empirically treat *Listeria*) should be used to treat suspected neonatal meningitis.
  - Some authorities would add gentamicin as a third agent if gram-negative enteric meningitis were thought likely.
- Some enteric pathogens, such as *Pseudomonas aeruginosa* and Enterobacteriaceae, readily become resistant to third-generation cephalosporins.
  - These antibiotics should not be used empirically for all cases of suspected sepsis in neonates.
  - Choice of empiric ampicillin with gentamicin remains appropriate when the CSF appears normal.
- Intraventricular antimicrobial therapy
  - Its role remains uncertain, and it may even be harmful.

M

- Other therapeutic considerations are the same for neonates as for infants and children with bacterial meningitis.
  - No data support use of dexamethasone in infants <6 weeks of age.
- Head circumference should be measured serially to detect early signs of hydrocephalus.
- Conflicting data have been reported regarding whether intravenous immunoglobulin is helpful.
  - At present, it does not have a defined role.

Aseptic meningitis

- Mainly supportive
- Meningoencephalitis caused by herpes simplex or varicella-zoster viruses should be treated with acyclovir.
- Aseptic meningitis caused by 1 of the other less common organisms may require specific therapy.
- Pleconaril, an antienteroviral agent, has been evaluated in both adults and children with enteroviral meningitis.
- This or other similar drugs may be useful in the future, but clinical development of pleconaril has been halted at present.

WHEN TO ADMIT

- All patients with suspected or proven meningitis should be hospitalized for evaluation and management.
- Patients with bacterial meningitis should be transferred to a facility experienced in management of critically ill children, with availability of consultation by pediatric critical care, infectious diseases, neurologic, and neurosurgical subspecialists, which is especially important for newborns with neonatal meningitis.
  - Treatment must begin at the referral hospital, however.
- Infants and toddlers with viral meningitis may continue to be hospitalized at primary care level hospital; transfer to a referral facility may be required for complicated cases (eg, uncertainty in diagnosis, slow resolution, presence of immune compromise).
- Older children and adolescents with viral meningitis do not always require hospitalization if the CSF evaluation strongly suggests that bacterial disease is not present, if adequate hydration and pain control can be undertaken at home, and if follow-up with the physician can be ensured.

WHEN TO REFER

- All patients with bacterial meningitis should be treated in consultation with pediatric infectious disease subspecialists, and pediatric neurologic, critical care, and neurosurgical subspecialists should be available if required.
- Patients with viral meningitis may be managed by the primary care physician, unless unusual features or complications are present (eg, immune compromise, unexpected severity, slow resolution of illness, possibility of nonviral aseptic meningitis).

- Patients with neonatal meningitis should be referred to pediatric infectious diseases, newborn medicine, and neurologic subspecialists.

COMPLICATIONS

- Early in the course of bacterial meningitis, the following may occur:
  - Increased intracranial pressure
  - Septic shock
  - Disseminated intravascular coagulation
  - Cardiorespiratory arrest
- Subdural effusions occasionally cause seizures or focal neurologic deficits.
  - In such cases, fluid should be removed by subdural taps.
  - Such effusions are rarely infected directly.
    - Subdural empyemas are occasionally reported.
- SIADH can also complicate bacterial meningitis.
  - Thus the patient should be monitored carefully for this complication.
  - If it occurs, fluid should be sharply restricted.
- Brain abscess is extremely rare after bacterial meningitis, except in neonates with meningitis caused by *Citrobacter* or certain *Enterobacter* species.
- Complications of neonatal meningitis are similar to those seen among older infants but are perhaps more common.
  - Hydrocephalus
  - Deafness
  - Blindness

PROGNOSIS

- Encephalitis mortality
  - Despite the appropriate use of bactericidal antibiotics, the mortality rate for bacterial meningitis remains 5–10%.
  - Case-fatality rate for neonates generally ranges from 20–25%.
  - In general, mortality is lower for full-term infants than for low–birth-weight infants (<2500 g).
    - The case-fatality rate may approach 50% in low–birth-weight infants with gram-negative enteric meningitis.
  - The case-fatality rate falls to approximately 5% for neonates who survive the first 24 hours.
  - Mortality of bacterial meningitis varies by pathogen.
    - 21% for *S pneumoniae*
    - 3% for *N meningitidis*
    - 6% for Hib
- Approximately 15–25% of survivors will have long-term morbidity, including:
  - Developmental delay
  - Seizure disorder

- Spasticity
- Hearing loss

■ Approximately 65% of survivors of coliform meningitis are normal 3–7 years after illness.
  - Approximately 15–30% have mild to moderate neurologic sequelae.
  - 5–10% have major sequelae.
■ Approximately 50% of group B ß-hemolytic streptococcal meningitis survivors are normal.
  - 20% have mild to moderate sequelae.
  - 15–30% have major sequelae, such as:
    - Hydrocephalus
    - Seizures
    - Profound intellectual disability
■ As many as 80% of neonates who have gram-negative enteric meningitis caused by either *Citrobacter* or certain *Enterobacter* species will develop single or multiple brain abscesses.
  - Unusual in meningitis caused by any other organism
  - Routine follow-up with cranial CT is indicated for neonates with meningitis or sepsis caused by *Citrobacter* species or *Enterobacter sakazakii.*
  - All infants recovering from meningitis should have careful audiologic testing and close evaluation for attainment of developmental milestones.
■ Outcome of aseptic meningitis relates to both the causative agent and the child's age.
  - Patients with enteroviral meningitis usually recover completely.
  - However, some studies have reported low intelligence and delayed speech development after enteroviral meningitis in very young infants.
  - In light of these findings, the prognosis for an infant <3 months of age is somewhat guarded.
  - The child's development should be monitored carefully.
  - In general, when encephalitis accompanies aseptic meningitis, the clinical course is more severe and the chance of sequelae increases.
■ Predicting long-term sequelae for an individual child is difficult at the time of hospital discharge.
  - Some children who are apparently normal are later found to have hearing or learning deficits or develop a seizure disorder.
  - Conversely, some children expected to have a dismal prognosis based on abnormal neurologic examinations make remarkable gains.
  - The practitioner should be guardedly optimistic with family while remaining sensitive to possible sequelae.

■ Hearing should be tested formally before discharge from the hospital.
  - Most sensorineural hearing loss can be detected at this time.
  - The rate of persistent bilateral or unilateral sensorineural hearing loss is:
    - 31% after pneumococcal meningitis
    - 10.5% after meningococcal meningitis
    - 6% after Hib meningitis
  - In young infants, auditory brainstem response or otoacoustic emissions testing is necessary for screening.
  - In older toddlers and children, conditioned response, play, or conventional audiometry may be performed.
  - Current thinking asserts that much of the hearing loss in meningitis occurs soon after infection.
    - This may explain why not all studies have shown reduction of hearing loss by dexamethasone therapy.
■ Timing of other neurologic sequelae is less certain.

PREVENTION

■ Some contacts of patients who have *N meningitidis* or Hib meningitis are at increased risk for the disease and should therefore receive prophylaxis.
■ Whether all contacts of patients who have Hib meningitis should receive prophylaxis remains controversial.
■ The AAP recommends that rifampin be provided to all household contacts, including adults, in households that have ≥1 contact <4 years of age whose immunization status against Hib is incomplete
  - Definition of complete immunization depends on the age of the individual involved.
  - A household contact is:
    - Anyone who resides with the index patient or
    - A nonresident who has spent ≥4 hours a day with index patient for 5 of the 7 days before the patient was hospitalized
■ Prophylaxis for all household contacts, regardless of age, is provided in households with a child <12 months of age.
  - Prophylaxis for nonhousehold contacts of Hib disease does not appear to be necessary.
  - The index patient should receive rifampin either during or at completion of treatment for Hib or meningococcal meningitis, unless ceftriaxone was used for treatment.
    - Many authorities still recommend that the index patient should receive rifampin either during or at completion of treatment for Hib or meningococcal meningitis.
■ The 1990s marked the beginning of conjugate vaccine era.
  - With widespread use, these vaccines have dramatically decreased the incidence of invasive Hib disease.

M

- Similarly, use of pneumococcal and meningococcal polysaccharide-protein conjugate vaccine promises a marked decrease in invasive pneumococcal and meningococcal infection.
■ 1 of 3 Hib conjugate vaccines or 1 of 3 Hib conjugate–containing combination vaccine products is routinely provided to US infants beginning at 2 months of age.
■ Pneumococcal conjugate vaccine is recommended for routine universal administration to infants and children <2 years of age.
  - Pneumococcal conjugate vaccine is also suggested for high-risk children 2–5 years of age, including children with:
    - Sickle cell disease
    - Functional or anatomic asplenia
    - Immunosuppression
    - Cancer
    - Chronic renal disease
    - Chronic cardiopulmonary disease
    - CSF leaks
    - Diabetes

■ At present, tetravalent meningococcal polysaccharide conjugate vaccine is routinely used only for children and adults at high risk of disease, including:
  - Young adolescents 11–12 years of age
  - Teens on entry to high school (15 years)
  - College freshmen (especially those living in dormitories)
  - Certain travelers
  - Those with sickle cell disease, functional or anatomic asplenia, immunosuppression, CSF leaks
■ Meningococcal conjugate vaccine is:
  - Used as an adjunct to chemoprophylaxis in outbreak control
  - Undergoing clinical trials for safety and immunogenicity in US children as young as 2 years

M

Meningococcemia

DEFINITION

- Meningococcemia is a consequence of infection with *Neisseria meningitidis* and a classic example of fulminant bacterial sepsis.

EPIDEMIOLOGY

- Incidence
  - Approximately 2600 cases of meningitis and sepsis are reported annually in the US.
    - Meningococcal infection the leading cause.
- Prevalence
  - The Centers for Disease Control and Prevention reported 1.1 cases of meningococcal disease per 100,000 people between 1992 and 1996.
  - Invasive meningococcal disease is relatively uncommon.
  - ~5–30% of adolescents and adults in nonepidemic conditions are colonized.
- Age
  - Highest incidence of disease consistently found in infants
    - Peak attack rate for infants is 15.9 cases per 100,000 population.
    - 20–25% of all cases of meningococcal disease occur in children <2 years.
  - Second smaller peak of disease is found in adolescents and young adults.
- Geographic distribution
  - *N meningitidis* causes both epidemic and endemic disease worldwide.
- Seasonal occurrence
  - Varies with the seasons
  - Winter and spring peak time of disease in the US
- Special populations
  - Subgroups, such as military recruits, can have rates of invasive meningococcal disease as high as 80%.
  - High carriage rates in household contacts of infected patients
- Serogroups of meningococcus
  - Historically, the majority of cases of invasive meningococcal disease in the US have been caused by serogroup B meningococcus.
  - In the mid-1990s
    - Organisms of serogroup B and C were each identified in approximately 35% of cases.
    - Serogroup B
      - 40% of disease occurred in children <2 years.
    - Serogroup C
      - 57% of disease occurred in persons between 2 and 30 years of age.
    - Serogroup Y
      - Accounted for 26% of isolates
      - Associated with older age groups and the clinical syndrome of pneumonia

ETIOLOGY

- *N meningitidis*
  - An aerobic gram-negative coccus found only in the human nasopharynx
  - Spread from person to person via respiratory droplets or direct contact with secretions
  - Thirteen serogroups have been identified on the basis of the antigenic structure of the capsular polysaccharide.
    - Five are responsible for the majority of human disease: serogroups A, B, C, Y, and W-135.
  - Additional methods of typing outer membrane proteins and lipooligosaccharides have lead to classifications of serosubtypes, serotypes, and immunotypes that are useful in epidemiologic investigations.

SIGNS AND SYMPTOMS

- Early symptoms (first 12 hours) (see table Cumulative Proportion of Children Developing Clinical Features During the Course of Meningococcal Disease)
  - Leg pain
  - Thirst
  - Diarrhea
  - Abnormal skin color (pallor)
  - Breathing difficulty
  - Cold hands and feet
- Classic symptoms
  - Hemorrhagic rash
  - Neck pain or stiffness
  - Photophobia
  - Bulging fontanelle
  - Irritability or lethargy (~50%)
  - Vomiting (~35%)
  - Shock (~42%)
- Late symptoms
  - Confusion or delirium
  - Seizure
  - Unconsciousness
- Less frequent symptoms
  - Delirium
  - Headache
  - Coryza
  - Diarrhea
  - Myalgia
  - Hypothermia

Cumulative Proportion of Children Developing Clinical Features During the Course of Meningococcal Disease[a]

		Fatal Cases (*n*=103)	Nonfatal Cases (*n*=345)	Overall (95% Confidence Interval)	Median Hour of Onset
Early Symptoms	Leg pain	22.3%	38%	36.7% (28–47)	7
	Thirst	41.7%	40.6%	40.7% (31–50)	8
	Diarrhea	54.4%	44.6%	45.2% (36–56)	9
	Abnormal skin color	73.8%	53.9%	55.1% (45–65)	10
	Breathing difficulty	75.7%	58.0%	59.1% (50–69)	11
	Cold hands and feet	81.6%	75.7%	76.1% (67–85)	12
Classic Symptoms	Hemorrhagic rash	94.2%	88.4%	88.8% (82–95)	13
	Neck pain or stiffness	94.2%	91.6%	91.8% (86–97)	13
	Photophobia	94.2%	92.5%	92.6% (87–97)	15
	Bulging fontanelle	94.2%	93.0%	93.1% (88–98)	15
Late Symptoms	Confusion or delirium	94.2%	95.1%	95.0% (90–99)	16
	Seizure	96.1%	95.4%	95.4% (91–99)	17
	Unconsciousness	97.1%	95.9%	96.0% (92–99)	22

[a] From: Thompson MJ, Ninis N, Mayon-White R, et al. Clinical recognition of meningococcal disease in children and adolescents. *Lancet.* 2006;367(9508):397–403. Copyright © Elsevier 2006.

■ Rash
  • Type and duration provide important information about the course and prognosis of the disease.
  • Tender, pink maculopapular rash
    – Seen early in the infection
    – Similar to that seen in rubella, secondary syphilis, or disseminated gonorrhea
    – Can appear on any part of the skin
    – Often fades rapidly with treatment
    – Patients who have this type of manifestation are less likely to have a fulminant course.
  • Generalized petechial rash (see Figure 38 on page F16)
    – Usually associated with meningococcal disease (see Figure 39 on page F16)
    – Initially, lesions are discrete and 1–2 mm in diameter.
    – Most prominent on the distal extremities, including the palms and soles
    – Found in clusters where clothing puts pressure on the skin
    – Scrapings of lesions reveal the organism approximately 70% of the time.
  • Ecchymotic or purpuric rash
    – Meningococcemia is the most common cause of purpura.
    – Most ominous manifestation of meningococcal disease
    – A centrifugal distribution is usually present in cases of fulminant meningococcemia (see Figure 40 on page F16).

    – Patients with purpura fulminans have a 20–50% mortality rate.
    – The case-fatality rate also is significantly higher in a febrile child with purpura or petechiae that have been present for <12 hours.

DIFFERENTIAL DIAGNOSIS
■ Other infectious and noninfectious diseases that manifest in petechiae or purpura include:
  • Viruses
    – Varicella-zoster virus
    – Cytomegalovirus (congenital infection)
    – Variola virus
    – Coxsackievirus
  • Echoviruses
    – Colorado tick fever virus
    – Rubella virus
    – Measles virus
    – Alpha viruses (eg, Ross River fever)
    – Lassa virus
    – Marburg viruses
  • Nonviral agents
  • *Rickettsia typhi* (murine typhus)
  • *Rickettsia prowazekii* (epidemic typhus)
  • *Rickettsia rickettsii* (Rocky Mountain spotted fever)
  • *Ehrlichia canis*

- *Mycoplasma pneumoniae*
- *Streptococcus pyogenes* (scarlet fever)
- *Streptococcus pneumonia*
- Enterococcal and viridans group streptococci (endocarditis)
- *Neisseria gonorrhoeae*
- *Neisseria meningitides*
- *Moraxella catarrhalis*
- *Haemophilus influenzae*
- *Streptobacillus moniliformis* (rat-bite fever)
- *Pseudomonas aeruginosa* (erythema gangrenosa)
- *Yersinia pestis* (plague)
- *Bartonella henselae* (cat-scratch disease)
- *Treponema pallidum* (congenital syphilis)
- *Borrelia* species (relapsing fever)
- *Trichinella spiralis* (trichinosis)
- *Toxoplasma gondii* (congenital toxoplasmosis)
- Miscellaneous
  - Henoch-Schönlein purpura
  - Immune thrombocytopenic purpura
  - Kawasaki disease
  - Serum sickness
  - Poisons
  - Erythema multiforme
  - Erythema nodosum
  - Systemic lupus erythematosus
- In a clinical study of >200 children in an emergency department with a nonblanching rash:
  - 11% were found to have meningococcal disease
  - Children with meningococcemia were more likely to:
    - Be judged ill by the investigators
    - Have fever >38.5°C
    - Have a purpuric rash
    - Have a capillary refill time of >2 seconds
- In a similar study:
  - 15% of children with fever and hemorrhagic rash had documented invasive meningococcal disease.
  - 45% did not have a specific diagnosis identified.
    - Presumably most of these had self-limited viral illnesses.
  - The following were highly associated with a diagnosis of invasive meningococcal disease:
    - Poor general condition
    - Presence of nuchal rigidity
    - >2-mm maximal diameter of skin hemorrhages
    - Generalized distribution of the rash
- These 2 studies confirmed absence of meningococcal disease in children with petechial rashes confined to the area of superior vena cava distribution (above the nipple line).

DIAGNOSTIC APPROACH

- Symptoms of meningococcal disease are nonspecific.
- Clinicians must maintain a high index of suspicion.
- Median time between onset of symptoms and hospitalization for pediatric patients is 13–22 hours.
- Early recognition of meningococcemia is challenging, but it is an important determinant of survival.
- The majority of children with invasive meningococcal disease have an illness with symptoms and signs lasting only a few hours to a day.
  - In general, the children have no significant medical history.
  - Approximately 25% may report a recent respiratory illness.
- Physical examination of a child or adolescent with suggested meningococcemia:
  - Should be performed expeditiously and with close attention to vital signs and skin findings.
  - The following need to be evaluated to determine the presence of shock:
    - Adequacy of respiration
    - Central and peripheral circulation
    - Mental status
- Frequent reassessments are warranted.

LABORATORY FINDINGS

- Initial laboratory tests should include:
  - Blood culture
  - Complete blood count and differential
  - Partial thromboplastin time
  - Prothrombin time
  - Measurement of fibrin breakdown products
  - Serum chemistries

DIAGNOSTIC PROCEDURES

- Lumbar puncture should be performed in a stable patient to:
  - Examine the cerebral spinal fluid for organisms
  - Obtain cultures
  - Assess the prognosis
- In an unstable patient, lumbar puncture should be deferred.

TREATMENT APPROACH

- Patients with signs and symptoms of invasive meningococcal disease should have aggressive monitoring and treatment as soon as the diagnosis is reasonably thought to be present.
- Do not withhold antibiotic therapy while waiting to obtain cerebrospinal fluid.
- Treatment regimen for children with meningococcemia includes:
  - Antibiotics

M

- Invasive monitoring of:
  - Hemodynamic function
  - Neurologic function
  - Respiratory function
- If the patient must be transported to a pediatric intensive care unit:
  - Blood should be drawn.
  - Antibiotics should be given.
  - Intravenous access should be secured.
  - The patient should be attended during transport by a physician prepared to treat shock.
    - The disease may worsen when endotoxin is liberated after antibiotic therapy.

SPECIFIC TREATMENTS

Antibiotics

- Recommended regimen
  - Aqueous penicillin G 250,000 U/kg of body weight/day in 4–6 divided doses.
    - A small number of meningococcal isolates with intermediate susceptibility to penicillin have been identified in the US.
    - No resistance to penicillin has been reported.
  - Alternative antibiotics if penicillin allergy is present
    - Ceftriaxone
    - Cefotaxime
    - Chloramphenicol
  - Continue antibiotic therapy for 5 afebrile days or 7 days total.
  - Rifampin (10 mg/kg per dose given twice a day for 2 days)
    - Prescribed at the end of the course of penicillin
    - Eliminates carriage of the organism from the nasopharynx
    - Not necessary if the patient has been treated with a third-generation cephalosporin (also effective in eliminating carriage)

Supportive therapy and critical care

- Aggressive supportive therapy in a pediatric intensive care setting
- Invasive monitoring of hemodynamic, neurologic, and respiratory function
- Mechanical ventilation to treat respiratory failure
- Maintenance of optimal plasma expansion with intravenous fluids
  - First step in stabilizing the circulatory system
  - Large amounts of fluid may be needed because of capillary leak associated with endotoxic shock.
  - Multiple transfusions with platelets and fresh-frozen plasma may be necessary to correct coagulopathy.

- Several studies have demonstrated that myocardial dysfunction precedes shock in adult and pediatric patients with meningococcal sepsis.
  - Believed to be caused by endotoxemia
  - Use of inotropic agents is recommended to:
    - Reverse myocardial depression
    - Improve tissue perfusion
  - Supportive measures for severe purpura
    - Treatments aimed at relieving the ischemic complications associated with vasculitis
  - Prevention of gangrenous necrosis
    - Mechanism of action is thought to be vasodilatation of partially occluded vessels via sympathetic blockade.
    - Continuous epidural anesthesia may help in improving perfusion of the lower extremities.
    - If there is no evidence of coagulopathy, an anesthesiologist can perform this type of regional block with an indwelling catheter in the caudal space.

Experimental therapies

- Systemic thrombolytic therapy with recombinant tissue plasminogen activator
  - Used in a limited number of patients in an attempt to dissolve microthrombi and restore organ and tissue perfusion
  - Risks of bleeding complications caused by this intervention have not been fully evaluated.
  - Not recommended for use outside of a research setting
- Topical administration of nitroglycerin
  - Reported to be useful in restoring blood flow to limited areas of skin and superficial tissues
  - No notable adverse effects
  - Has not been systematically studied
- Plasmapheresis
- Whole-blood exchange
- Extracorporeal membrane oxygenation
- Continuous venovenous hemodiafiltration
  - Designed to interrupt the disease process pathophysiology via interference with both endotoxin and the secondary mediators of inflammation induced by endotoxin
  - Studies have shown a correlation between plasma levels of endotoxin or tumor necrosis factor and multiorgan failure or disease severity.
- Recombinant human bactericidal–permeability-increasing protein (rBPI$_{21}$)
  - N-terminal fragment of a human protein naturally found in the azurophilic granules of polymorphonuclear leukocytes.
  - In a preliminary trial of rBPI$_{21}$ in children who had severe meningococcemia, mortality was reduced compared with historical controls.

- A large, randomized, placebo-controlled trial of this product in children with invasive meningococcal disease demonstrated:
  - Lower incidence of multiple and severe amputations
  - Improved functional outcome
  - Less need for blood product support
  - No substantial benefit in mortality
- On the basis of this study, the product remains in clinical development.
- Not available for general use
- Reports have associated purpura fulminans induced by sepsis with:
  - Acquired deficiencies of the natural anticoagulation factor proteins C and S and deficiency in the activation pathway for protein C
  - Drotrecogin alfa (activated) is an activated protein C compound licensed for use in adults with severe sepsis and organ dysfunction.
  - Although efficacy has been demonstrated in adult populations, a recent pediatric trial of this compound was halted because of:
    - Concerns over lack of benefit
    - Increased number of intracranial hemorrhages in patients receiving the product
- High-dose steroids
  - Use in children with meningococcal disease remains controversial.

WHEN TO ADMIT

- A febrile child who has purpura or petechiae present for <12 hours should be managed as a medical emergency.

COMPLICATIONS

- 15–40% of patients develop a complication of infection that may be categorized broadly as suppurative, neurologic, ischemic, or allergic.
- Suppurative complications
  - Subdural effusions
  - Subdural empyema
  - Acute suppurative arthritis
  - Occur in approximately 9% of children
- Neurologic sequelae
  - Deafness is the most common (2–6%).
- Ischemic complications
  - Gangrenous necrosis of the skin or extremities
  - Require skin grafting or amputation
  - Percentage of survivors varies from 3–20%.
- Arthritis and pericarditis
  - Most common sequelae
  - Reported in 4–10% of pediatric cases

- Thought to be caused by an allergic phenomenon with immune complex deposition rather than a direct invasion of the heart or joints by the organism
- Allergic arthritis and pericarditis
  - Late in onset
  - More common in adults than in children
  - Symptoms are usually self-limited.
  - Specific therapy is generally not required.
    - Drainage of pericardial or joint fluid occasionally is necessary.
- Complement deficiency
  - Not a true complication
  - Reported in approximately 15% of adolescents and children who have meningococcal disease
  - Creates high risk for recurrent episodes of invasive infection
  - Screening with a total hemolytic complement assay should be considered in any pediatric patient with meningococcemia.
- Several studies have shown an association between meningococcal disease and influenza and other viral respiratory infections.
  - The exact nature of the interaction is not clear.
- 50% of cases of invasive meningococcal disease are associated with meningitis.
- Approximately 35% of cases of invasive meningococcal disease are classified as sepsis without central nervous system involvement.

PROGNOSIS

- The majority of children who survive meningococcal disease recover completely.
- Overall mortality in meningococcal disease is 5–15%.
- Children with the severe form of the disease can progress from a state of good health to death in hours, regardless of whether meningitis is present.
- Occult or chronic meningococcemia is occasionally detected.
- Subgroups of patients (eg, those with fulminant meningococcemia) can have fatality rates as high as 50–80% despite aggressive intensive care therapy.
- Investigators have attempted to predict the outcome for individual patients who have meningococcal disease on the basis of laboratory and clinical data.
  - These scoring systems are used to:
    - Determine which patients might benefit from more aggressive or experimental therapies
    - Help evaluate the usefulness of newer treatments
- In 1966 Stiehm and Damrosch developed a prognostic score.
  - Patients who had ≥3 of the following signs or symptoms had fatality rates of ≥85%, and scores were then validated.
    - Presence of petechiae for <12 hours before admission
    - Shock

M

– Absence of meningitis
– Normal or low leukocyte counts
– Normal or low erythrocyte sedimentation rates
■ Glasgow Meningococcal Septicemia Prognostic Score
  ● Designed for rapid bedside assessment without the need for multiple laboratory tests
  ● Maximum score 15
    – Blood pressure <75 mm Hg systolic, age <4 years and <85 mm Hg systolic, age >4 years: 3 points
    – Skin to rectal temperature difference >3°C: 3 points
    – Modified Glasgow Coma Scale score <8 or deterioration of at least 3 points in 1 hour: 3 points
    – Clinical deterioration in hour before scoring: 2 points
    – Absence of meningitis: 2 points
    – Extending purpuric rash or widespread ecchymoses: 1 point
    – Base deficit (capillary or arterial) >8.0: 1 point
  ● The scale was tested retrospectively in 123 children with meningococcemia.
    – A score ≥10 had a positive predictive value of 87.5% and a negative predictive value of 100%.
  ● Scoring systems are used to determine
    – Which patients might benefit from more aggressive or experimental therapies
    – Usefulness of newer treatments

PREVENTION

■ Natural immunity can be developed by colonization with:
  ● Pathogenic and nonpathogenic *Neisseria*
  ● Other gram-negative organisms that have similar capsular polysaccharides
■ Antimicrobial chemoprophylaxis is an integral component in the control of invasive meningococcal disease.
■ Studies have demonstrated that household, child care, and preschool contacts of patients who have invasive disease have a rate of infection approximately 100–800 times that of the general population.
  ● 50% of secondary cases occur within 5 days of the index case.
  ● 70% occur within 1 week.
■ Rifampin
  ● Highly effective in eliminating carriage of the meningococcus from the nasopharynx
  ● AAP recommends that all household, child care, or preschool contacts or anyone directly exposed to a patient's secretions be given rifampin within 24 hours of recognizing the primary case.
  ● For children ≥1 month of age: 10 mg/kg per dose (maximal adult dose is 600 mg) every 12 hours for 2 days

  ● For infants <1 month of age: 5 mg/kg per dose every 12 hours for 2 days
  ● Not recommended for use in pregnant women
■ Alternative chemoprophylactic agents
  ● Ceftriaxone
    – For children <15 years of age: 125 mg IM in a single dose
      ■ Dilute with 1% lidocaine to decrease pain at the injection site.
    – For adolescents ≥15 years of age: 250 mg IM in a single dose
    – Not recommended for widespread chemoprophylactic use
    – A single 250-mg IM dose is safe for pregnant women.
  ● Ciprofloxacin
    – Can be used in older adolescents and young adults
    – Has the advantage of being administered as a single oral 500-mg dose
    – For patients ≥18 years of age: 500 mg orally in a single dose
    – Not recommended for anyone <18 years
    – Not recommended for widespread chemoprophylactic use
    – Not approved for children or pregnant women
■ Vaccination
  ● Licensed for use in January 2005 for individuals 11–55 years of age
  ● The Centers for Disease Control and Prevention's Advisory Committee on Immunization Practices recommend adding meningococcal conjugate vaccine to the routine immunization schedule for all children at age 11–12 years.
  ● Vaccine contains purified capsular polysaccharide of serogroups A, C, Y, and W-135 conjugated to diphtheria toxoid.
    – The conjugated protein elicits a T cell–dependent antibody response and induces immunologic memory.
  ● In a trial comparing meningococcal polysaccharide vaccine with the new conjugate meningococcal vaccine among >800 children age 11–18 years who received conjugate vaccine:
    – 82–97% of children achieved ≥4-fold increases in serum bactericidal antibody titers.
    – 98.6–99.8% achieved protective levels to all 4 serogroups.
    – Adverse reactions were mild and infrequent, usually limited to local reactions and fever.
■ Group B meningococcal disease
  ● No vaccine available
  ● Group B capsule not strongly immunogenic in humans
  ● Has been found to share cross-reacting antigens with human neural tissue
  ● Attempts to create vaccine by using outer membrane proteins are ongoing.
  ● Studies aimed at evaluating the immunogenicity and safety of the new meningococcal conjugate vaccine in younger age groups are under way.

Meningoencephalitis

FOUNDATION

- Infection of the meninges and underlying brain parenchyma can be classified as septic or aseptic.
  - Septic
    - Traditionally termed *bacterial meningitis*
    - Characterized by high fever, coma, and purulent cerebrospinal fluid (CSF)
  - Aseptic
    - Aseptic meningitis
    - Encephalitis
    - Most often caused by viruses, but occasionally caused by parasites, spirochetes, rickettsia, and prions

EPIDEMIOLOGY

- Incidence of meningoencephalitis is unknown.
  - Centers for Disease Control and Prevention tallied 2840 cases of arboviral encephalitis (367 children) in 2004.
  - Approximately 75,000 cases of aseptic meningitis occur annually.
  - Difficulty in identifying the specific agent in each suspected case makes precision impossible.
- Polio
  - In the US, occurs primarily in:
    - Immigrant children
    - Immunodeficient children
    - In small communities of unimmunized children
  - Continues to cause epidemics in developing countries where clean water and sewage treatment facilities are lacking
- Herpes simplex virus (HSV)
  - HSV encephalitis has a bimodal age distribution.
    - One-third of cases occur in childhood.
- Arbovirus meningoencephalitis
  - Typically occurs in epidemics during the summer and early fall
- Rabies
  - 50,000 deaths estimated worldwide
    - Frequently in children who are bitten by rabid dogs
  - In the US, pediatric rabies infections are attributed most often to rabid bats, raccoons, and cats.
- West Nile virus (WNV)
  - 2866 West Nile neuroinvasive cases were reported in 2003.
    - 8% were fatal.
  - Cases of WNV encephalitis have been reported in children.
- Measles virus
  - Causes meningoencephalitis in approximately 1 in 1000 cases

- In 2003, 56 confirmed measles cases were reported in the US.
- Varicella-zoster virus (VZV)
  - In US, more deaths occur as complication of varicella infection than from all other disorders for which immunizations exist.
- Congenital rubella syndrome
  - Cases have declined from 57,686 in 1969 to 271 in 1999.
  - Rubella in US now primarily affects infants born to foreign-born women.
- Rocky Mountain spotted fever (RMSF)
  - In one study, 81% of 16 patients with RMSF were children.
  - In summer of 2003, 3 fatal cases of RMSF were reported in children.
- Congenital toxoplasmosis
  - An estimated 400–4000 cases occur each year.
- Congenital syphilis
  - In 2003, 413 cases related to absent or late prenatal care were reported.
  - Rate has sharply declined in recent years.
  - Congenital syphilis is more common in the southern US.
    - Possibly because of more women with inadequate prenatal care.
- New-variant Creutzfeldt-Jakob disease (CJD)
  - Related to bovine spongiform encephalopathy (BSE), which is endemic in the United Kingdom

ETIOLOGY

- Enteroviruses
  - Common cause of aseptic meningitis in infants
  - May also cause encephalitis
  - Nonpolio enteroviruses include:
    - Coxsackieviruses A and B
    - Echoviruses
  - Progression to meningoencephalitis is uncommon with most enteroviral infections.
  - When it does occur, it is usually mild, self-limited disease.
  - May infect a fetus transplacentally
- HSV
  - Neonatal infection results from passage through an infected birth canal.
  - In neonate, HSV may produce:
    - Cutaneous disease
    - Meningoencephalitis
    - Disseminated disease
- Arboviruses
  - Arboviral infections caused by *Bunyavirus* species and togavirus are transmitted to humans by arthropods.

- Other viral diseases transmitted by vectors
  - Colorado tick fever is a reovirus transmitted by rodent arthropods.
  - Lymphocytic choriomeningitis (arenavirus) is transmitted directly to humans by infected laboratory or domestic rodents.
  - WNV
  - Principally transmitted by *Culex* mosquitoes
  - Occurs mostly in older adults; cases of intrauterine transmission and possible transmission through breastfeeding have occurred
- Rabies
  - Transmitted by bite, scratch, or droplet from infected wild animal (eg, raccoon, bat) or unimmunized domestic animal
  - Rabies has been documented after transplantation.
- Common childhood viral infections can occasionally cause meningoencephalitis.
  - Rubella
  - Adenovirus
  - Influenza
  - Cytomegalovirus (CMV)
  - Epstein-Barr virus (infectious mononucleosis)
  - Measles
- VZV
  - May cause mild encephalitis or a focal cerebellitis with prominent ataxia
- AIDS
  - Noteworthy for meningoencephalitides caused both by HIV and by unusual organisms, such as:
    - *Toxoplasma gondii*
    - *Candida albicans*
    - Epstein-Barr virus
- Fungi, spirochetes, and parasites
  - Nonviral causes of meningoencephalitis include infectious and noninfectious conditions associated with CSF pleocytosis.
    - Amebic meningoencephalitis may result from swimming in freshwater rivers or lakes infected with *Naegleria*.
  - RMSF
    - Transmitted by *Dermacentor* ticks
  - Toxoplasmosis
    - Causes cerebral calcifications, microcephaly, and seizures
      - Resulting from transplacental infection by the protozoa *T gondii* to the fetus
    - Transmitted to humans through ingestion of inadequately cooked meat or ingestion of oocysts from cat feces

- Prions
  - Transmissible spongiform encephalopathies include:
    - Kuru
      - Children of the Fore tribe of New Guinea
    - BSE
      - Cattle
    - CJD
      - Humans
      - CJD has been transmitted to children through administration of cadaveric growth hormone.

RISK FACTORS

- The developing nervous system may be more susceptible to viral infection.
  - Pediatric patients are thus more likely to sustain serious sequelae.
- WNV
  - Risk for WNV encephalitis increases with age and immunosuppression.
  - Possible transmission through breastfeeding has occurred.
    - However, mothers should continue breastfeeding even in areas with WNV transmission.
  - Most women infected with WNV during pregnancy have delivered apparently healthy infants, although exceptions have been reported.
- Susceptibility to new-variant CJD may be highest in teenagers.

SIGNS AND SYMPTOMS

General features

- Most viruses spread via the bloodstream to the choroid plexus and from there to brain parenchyma.
  - Rabies and HSV travel in a retrograde manner via peripheral nerves.
- The course of meningoencephalitis depends on virulence of the organism.
  - Typically, children with aseptic meningitis have:
    - Intense headache
    - Meningismus
    - Photophobia, but a clear sensorium
  - In contrast, amoebae, fungi, and the viruses causing Eastern equine encephalitis, HSV, or rabies may cause:
    - Cerebral or brain stem dysfunction
    - Seizures
    - Increased intracranial pressure
    - Death

M

- Presenting signs and symptoms produced by viruses are often protean and include:
  - Fever
  - Chills
  - Myalgia
  - Headache
- Differences in seasonal occurrence, clinical course, and outcome allow differentiation of some disorders.
- Encephalitis may produce focal neurologic findings.
  - If the spinal cord is involved, the patient may have:
    - Symmetrical limb paralysis
    - Transverse sensory symptoms
    - Bowel and bladder dysfunction
- Viral infection of the central nervous system may be occult.
  - CSF pleocytosis may or may not be present in meningoencephalitis.

Specific viruses

- HSV commonly produces a necrotizing encephalitis.
  - Mothers of infected infants often have no symptoms of herpes infection during or before gestation.
    - Makes diagnosis of neonatal infection more difficult
  - Herpes simplex encephalitis is classically heralded by temporal lobe seizures and olfactory hallucinations.
- VZV and Epstein-Barr virus
  - May infect cerebellum, producing an acute ataxia
- Congenital syphilis
  - Rash develops on palms and soles in many instances.
- Arboviruses
  - California virus encephalitis
    - Suspect in a child living in a known endemic region with signs of fever and cerebrocortical dysfunction.
    - The course is usually mild, with a fatality rate <5%.
  - Western equine encephalitis
    - Primarily in infants
    - More severe syndrome than California virus
  - Eastern equine encephalitis has a predilection for infants and young children.
  - St Louis encephalitis occurs most often in epidemic form.
    - Produces illness in adults more often than in children
  - The virus that causes Colorado tick fever produces dengue-like illness.
- Rabies
  - Long incubation period

- Measles viruses
  - Meningoencephalitis within 4–7 days after onset of rash
    - The severity of neurologic illness (including irritability, drowsiness, and ataxia) does not seem to be related to the intensity of systemic illness.
- Rubella
  - Mild febrile exanthem of childhood with prominent arthralgia
  - As many as one-half of individuals are asymptomatic.
  - Infection during first trimester of pregnancy may result in congenital rubella syndrome.
  - A child affected with rubella in utero may be infectious for ≥12 months.
- Mumps meningoencephalitis
  - May occur without parotitis, before the appearance of parotitis, or after it has resolved

DIFFERENTIAL DIAGNOSIS

- Laboratory tests require time to establish diagnosis of meningoencephalitis.
  - The clinician must consider the differential diagnosis carefully.
- Metabolic encephalopathy resulting from Reye syndrome or from lead, alcohol, or other toxins
  - Can be ruled out by appropriate laboratory investigations
- Brain abscess
  - The clinical course is usually slower.
  - Focal findings may be prominent.
  - History of sinus infection, bronchiectasis, or congenital heart disease may be elicited.
- Myelitic form of viral nervous system infection may be mimicked by mass lesion or Guillain-Barré syndrome.
- Congenital lymphocytic choriomeningitis mimics congenital toxoplasmosis or CMV infection with chorioretinopathy, hydrocephaly, or microcephaly.

DIAGNOSTIC APPROACH

- Every attempt should be made to identify the offending organism to:
  - Help determine prognosis
  - Document potential epidemic outbreaks

LABORATORY FINDINGS

- Typical CSF alterations among patients with meningo-encephalitis consist of:
  - Mild pleocytosis
  - Slight increase in protein level
  - No alteration in glucose concentration

M

- Erythrocytes in the CSF may indicate hemorrhagic brain necrosis.
  - Commonly seen with HSV infections and Eastern equine encephalitis
- Predominance of mononuclear cells in CSF is the exception in acute bacterial meningoencephalitis.
  - May be present with:
    - Syphilis
    - Lyme disease
    - Listeriosis
    - Tuberculosis
- Polymerase chain reaction
  - Powerful tool in identifying enterovirus, mumps virus, CMV, VZV, and other viruses
  - Polymerase chain reaction of CSF in patients with herpes simplex encephalitis is 98% specific and 94% sensitive.
  - Rapid-screening test for Epstein-Barr virus (Monospot) is available at most hospitals.
- Typical CSF findings in meningoencephalitis and bacterial meningitis
  - Viral meningoencephalitis
    - Leukocytes
      - Initial predominance of polymorphonuclear neutrophils, followed by shift to mononuclear cells
      - Range, 0–2000 cells/mm^3
    - Glucose
      - >50% of serum concentration
    - Protein
      - Mild to moderate increase
      - Range, usually <200 mg/dL
    - Gram stain
      - Negative
  - Bacterial meningitis
    - Leukocytes
      - Predominantly neutrophils
      - Range, 0–200,000 cells/mm^3
    - Protein
      - Marked increase
      - Range, usually >150 mg/dL
    - Gram stain
      - Usually reveals bacteria

IMAGING

- Magnetic resonance imaging
  - Viral encephalitis shows:
    - Diffuse scattered or confluent areas of T2-weighted hyperintensities that are isointense or hypointense on T1-weighted imaging

- In more severe cases, increased intracranial pressure (ventricular compression) or cerebral cortical enhancement
- Temporal lobe enhancement or necrosis may be evidence of HSV infection.

DIAGNOSTIC PROCEDURES

- Electroencephalography
  - Periodic pattern in infant with partial motor seizures and signs of meningoencephalitis is diagnostic of HSV encephalitis.
- Biopsy
  - Newborns with cutaneous vesicles thought to have herpes simplex meningoencephalitis need not undergo brain biopsy to establish the diagnosis.
  - Attempts should be made to isolate the virus from throat, eye, or cutaneous lesions or from blood, urine, stool, and CSF.

TREATMENT APPROACH

- Treatment of patient with meningoencephalitis is supportive and includes:
  - Reducing high intracranial pressure
  - Providing respiratory support
  - Treating seizures
  - Maintaining fluid and electrolyte balance
    - Two-thirds of infants with aseptic meningitis develop inappropriate secretion of antidiuretic hormone.
- Corticosteroids have not proved useful in treating meningoencephalitis and may blunt host defenses.

SPECIFIC TREATMENTS

HSV infection

- Specific treatment of acute viral infections of the nervous system is indicated in herpes simplex infections of the central nervous system.
  - Although it is nephrotoxic, acyclovir is the drug of choice.
    - Generally well tolerated by neonates and children with renal dysfunction

CMV infection

- Ganciclovir has been approved for use in CMV infections.
- α-Interferon has been used as prophylaxis against CMV in immunocompromised children, but not as adjunct therapy in meningoencephalitis.

HIV infection

- 17 HIV drugs are currently available, including:
  - Nucleoside and nonnucleoside reverse transcriptase inhibitors
  - Protease inhibitors
  - Fusion inhibitors

M

- Intravenous immunoglobulin may be of benefit.
  - Known to contain viral antibodies for specific viral infections
  - Nonspecific immunoglobulin preparations have been used as replacement therapy or as adjuncts to treatment of meningoencephalitis in immunodeficient patients.
  - Immunoglobulin therapy for overwhelming viral sepsis remains controversial.

VZV infection

- α-Interferon has been used as prophylaxis against VZV in immunocompromised children.
  - Not as adjunct therapy in meningoencephalitis

WHEN TO ADMIT

- Patients with meningoencephalitis who have increased intracranial pressure, intractable seizures, and altered mental status must be admitted

WHEN TO REFER

- Patients with meningoencephalitis who have increased intracranial pressure, intractable seizures, and altered mental status must be managed with the help of infectious diseases and critical care medicine specialists.

ONGOING CARE

- Every child who has a documented or suspected viral nervous system infection must be carefully monitored.
  - Auditory aftereffects
  - Visual aftereffects
  - Cognitive aftereffects
  - These children are at risk for cerebral cortical dysfunction.

COMPLICATIONS

- The more benign meningoencephalitides of infancy (ie, those caused by enteroviral infection)
  - May result in substantial reductions in head circumference, intelligence, and learning ability
- California encephalitis
  - Causes emotional or learning disorders in 15% of affected children
- Epstein-Barr virus
  - Focal epilepsy may be a sequelae of a mild encephalitis caused by Epstein-Barr virus.
- Measles
  - An unusual syndrome of dementia and myoclonic seizures can develop in school-aged children many years after measles infection or immunization.
    - Results from persistent measles infection known as *subacute sclerosing panencephalitis*
  - Syndrome of subacute measles encephalitis has also been reported in immunosuppressed individuals.

PROGNOSIS

- Eastern equine encephalitis
  - Usually fatal
  - Patients who survive are severely impaired.
- Western equine encephalitis
  - Associated with complete recovery in adults
  - Causes death in 20% of children
  - Has a high prevalence of neurologic sequelae among survivors
- HSV necrotizing encephalitis
  - 50–70% of untreated cases are fatal.
  - Two-thirds of patients who survive have neurologic sequelae.
- Measles meningoencephalitis
  - Mortality approximates 10%.
  - As many as one-half of survivors may have neurologic sequelae.
- Rabies
  - Has highest case fatality of any infection
  - Invariably produces meningoencephalitis
  - All but 1 of the reported cases of rabies encephalitis have been fatal.
- Mumps meningoencephalitis
  - Mild illness that generally has a good prognosis
- RMSF
  - Case-fatality rate may be as high as 30%.

PREVENTION

- Prevention is the most cost-effective method of reducing morbidity and mortality caused by viral meningoencephalitis.
- Immunization
  - Has reduced, but not eliminated, poliomyelitis
  - Has made rubella, mumps, and measles meningoencephalitis uncommon
  - Repeat measles immunizations of older children should reduce the incidence of measles encephalitis and subacute sclerosing panencephalitis further.
- Use of varicella vaccine may reduce incidence of VZV infections.
- Prohibition of beef products in cattle feed has reduced incidence of both new-variant CJD and BSE.
- Mosquito and other insect controls

M

Microcephaly

DEFINITION

- *Microcephaly* refers to having a head size ≥2 standard deviations below the mean (below the third percentile).
  - Norms based on age and sex
  - May be neurologically normal, especially if very close to the third percentile curve
  - Head size >3 standard deviations below the mean (~0.2 percentile) is probably associated with neurologic impairment.
- *Micrencephaly* refers to having a small brain.
  - Leads to a small head size
- Compare with *craniosynostosis*—premature closure of sutures (with normal brain growth).

EPIDEMIOLOGY

- Prevalence
  - By definition, approximately 2.5% of all children are microcephalic.

MECHANISM

- Microcephaly is a clinical finding, and the mechanism for development of microcephaly depends on its cause.
- Possible causes include:
  - Small brain/abnormal brain development
  - Genetic syndromes
  - Intrauterine environment
  - Infections (meningitis)
  - Severe malnutrition
  - Traumatic brain injury, including shaken baby syndrome
  - Craniosynostosis

HISTORY

- Medical history, including
  - Previous infections, such as meningitis
  - Results of neuroimaging studies
- Review of systems, including:
  - Feeding difficulties
  - Seizures
- Family history
  - Construct a pedigree, noting genetic syndromes, miscarriages, and microcephaly.
- Prenatal history
  - Explore potential toxin exposure (alcohol, drugs).
  - Review maternal health during pregnancy.
  - Review records and assess the likelihood of intrauterine infections.
  - Review records and assess the likelihood of placental insufficiency.

- Discuss psychosocial factors, including history of prenatal care and maternal education.
- Developmental history
  - Include a chronology of developmental milestones.
  - Assess the child's current function and behavior.
  - Note any developmental regression.

PHYSICAL EXAM

Vital signs and anthropomorphics

- Measure stature, weight, and head circumference.
  - Perform these at each well-child visit.
  - Measure head circumference with a flexible, nonstretchable tape.
    - Measure above the supraorbital ridges and across the occipital prominence.
    - This occipitofrontal circumference correlates with brain volume.
    - Consider repeating suspicious measurements yourself.
  - Plot measurements on standardized charts.
    - Centers for Disease Control and Prevention growth charts from 2000 include curves for the 3rd and 97th percentiles.
    - Adjust head circumference for prematurity until approximately 2 years of age.
      - In infants with birth weight <1000 g, use corrected age until 3 years of age (or until growth has caught up to normal).
    - Use charts specific to special populations when indicated (eg, Down syndrome, Williams syndrome, achondroplasia, very–low-birth-weight infants)
    - For children >36 months, may use head circumference curves developed by Nellhaus
  - Measuring over time allows early identification of when percentiles are crossed, even if measurements are still within normal ranges.
  - Disproportionately small head circumference, with respect to stature and weight, may indicate a central nervous system condition.
- Measure head circumferences of other family members as possible.
- Evaluate heart rate, respiratory rate, and blood pressure for Cushing triad (bradycardia, irregular respirations, hypertension).

Physical examination

- Inspect and palpate skull, looking for asymmetry and bony ridges.
  - Bony ridges may suggest craniosynostosis.
- Examine for features of genetic conditions.
  - Characteristic facies (eg, Seckel syndrome, Down syndrome, de Lange syndrome)

- Evidence of involvement of other organ systems, such as:
  - Ocular abnormalities (eg, colobomas, cataracts)
  - Congenital heart disease
  - Genitourinary abnormalities (eg, cryptorchidism)
- Examine for neurologic abnormalities indicative of potential central nervous system malformation
  - Pupils, extraocular muscles, visual fields, smell, and cranial nerve functions
  - Funduscopic examination for papilledema
  - Assess for asymmetries, abnormalities in muscle tone, posture, strength, and reflexes.

DIFFERENTIAL DIAGNOSIS

- Asymptomatic familial microcephaly
  - Small head size in context of normal development, normal neurologic examination, and family history
- Genetic causes (primary microcephaly)
  - Small brain/abnormal brain development
    - Microcephaly vera ("true microcephaly")
      - Brain size usually 3 standard deviations below the mean
      - Brain architecture grossly normal
      - Patients almost always have mental retardation but have otherwise unremarkable neurologic examination.
      - May see sloping forehead and prominent ears
    - Microcephaly with severe neurologic impairment (seizures, spasticity, and/or global developmental delays)
      - More common than microcephaly vera
      - Neuroimaging may identify abnormal brain architecture
  - Genetic syndromes
    - Miller-Dieker lissencephaly (17p; deletion/mutation of *LIS1* gene)
      - Small smooth brain/lissencephaly, facial dysmorphism, severe mental retardation
    - Seckel syndrome (multiple possible loci: 3q, 18, 14q; autosomal recessive)
      - Low birth weight, intrauterine growth restriction
      - Growth delays after birth resulting in short stature
      - Bird-headed appearance ("beak-like" protrusion of nose, abnormally large eyes, narrow face, malformed ears, small jaw)
      - Varying degrees of intellectual disability
    - Rubinstein-Taybi syndrome (22q, 16p; autosomal dominant; mutation in CREB binding protein)
      - Characteristic facial features, moderate to severe mental retardation, broad thumbs and toes

- Other findings may include coloboma, cataract, congenital heart disease, renal abnormalities, and cryptorchidism.
    - Trisomy 21
      - Distinct facial features, congenital heart anomalies, and growth retardation
    - Trisomy 13
    - de Lange syndrome (multiple possible loci: 5p, Xp, 10q; mutation in cohesin complex)
      - Growth retardation; hirsutism; and unusual facial features, such as synophrys and low anterior hairline
      - Microcephaly is almost always present at birth.
    - Rett syndrome (X chromosome; mutation in gene encoding MECP2)
      - Condition of decelerating head growth, almost exclusively in females; majority of cases appear to be sporadic
      - Developmental regression, autistic features, and unusual hand mannerisms (hand-wringing and hand-washing movements)
- Environmental causes (secondary microcephaly)
  - Intrauterine environment/perinatal time frame
    - Teratogens
    - Fetal alcohol syndrome
      - Intrauterine growth restriction
      - Small palpebral fissures, smooth philtrum and thin upper lip
      - Heart and eye defects
      - Behavioral and cognitive deficits
    - Maternal metabolic disease
      - Untreated maternal phenylketonuria and hyperphenylalaninemia may produce findings similar to those of fetal alcohol syndrome: facial dysmorphism, intellectual disability, and heart defects.
    - Intrauterine infections (eg, TORCH [toxoplasmosis, other agents, rubella, cytomegalovirus, and herpes simplex])
    - Maternal health problems
    - Intrauterine irradiation
    - Hypoxic-ischemic encephalopathy
      - Severe perinatal asphyxia is an important cause of acquired microcephaly
      - Normal head circumference at birth, but head growth decelerates
      - May be detected as early as 6 weeks of age; these infants develop significant neuromotor and cognitive deficits.
  - Infections
    - Meningitis
  - Severe malnutrition
  - Traumatic brain injury, including shaken baby syndrome

M

- Craniosynostosis (multiple sutures; problem of skull, not brain)
  - Head circumference may be small at birth, or head growth may abruptly cease during infancy.
  - Asymmetric skull with bony ridging in the areas of fused sutures
  - Increased intracranial pressure may be present.

LABORATORY EVALUATION

- Laboratory evaluation is guided by clinical suspicion.
- In children with possible intrauterine infection
  - Test for perinatal infections
    - Toxoplasmosis
    - Rubella
    - Cytomegalovirus
    - Syphilis
    - HIV
    - Herpes
  - Ophthalmologic and audiologic evaluations
- If a genetic syndrome is suspected, perform a focused evaluation, consulting experts in genetics as needed.
  - Karyotype
  - Genetic testing is available for:
    - Miller-Dieker syndrome
    - Rett syndrome

IMAGING

- Neuroimaging may help to identify abnormal brain architecture, such as:
  - Holoprosencephaly
  - Lissencephaly
  - Schizencephaly
  - Pachygyri
  - Polymicrogyri
  - Heterotopias
  - Midline defects (agenesis of corpus callosum)
- Imaging modalities include:
  - Magnetic resonance imaging (MRI)
    - Use when the following are suspected.
      - Gray and white matter disease
      - Migration defects, such as lissencephaly, pachygyria, and polymicrogyria
      - MRI is limited in its ability to study bone and calcifications.
  - Computed tomography
    - Use when the following are suspected.
      - Intracranial calcifications due to intrauterine infections
      - Skull abnormalities, as seen with premature fusion of cranial sutures
      - Ventricular system abnormalities

- Radiography of the skull
  - Can demonstrate intracranial calcifications
  - Can show characteristic bone findings in craniosynostosis
  - Cannot detect abnormalities in brain structure
- Ultrasonography
  - Useful in infants because of open fontanelles

TREATMENT APPROACH

- Treatment is largely supportive, with targeted therapies to address functional disabilities.
- Refer to early intervention and special education services as needed.

SPECIFIC TREATMENT

- Children with microcephaly may have multiple medical issues; treatments depend on the individual.
- There is a reported risk of cardiac arrhythmia with use of succinylcholine in children with Rubinstein-Taybi syndrome.

WHEN TO REFER

- Head circumference >2 standard deviations below the mean (especially >3 standard deviations)
- Deceleration of head growth
- Dysmorphic features
- Abnormal neurologic examination and development
- Regression in motor, language, and social skills
- Seizures
- Suspected craniosynostosis

WHEN TO ADMIT

- Signs of increased intracranial pressure
- Mental status changes

FOLLOW-UP

- Children with microcephaly may require close follow-up for developmental issues.

PREVENTION

- Prevention
  - Appropriate prenatal care
  - Maternal education and nutrition
  - Avoidance of teratogenic substances
  - Screening for intrauterine infections
  - Management of maternal health conditions
- Genetic counseling may be offered to parents if genetic disorders are identified.

Mononucleosis and Epstein-Barr Infections

DEFINITION

- Epstein-Barr virus (EBV) is a member of the herpesvirus group.
- EBV infections can produce infectious mononucleosis.

EPIDEMIOLOGY

- Prevalence
  - Infection with EBV is extremely common.
- Age/socioeconomics
  - EBV antibodies are developed in:
    - 70–90% of children from low socioeconomic groups by 5 years of age
    - 40–50% of children from high socioeconomic groups
  - Primary infections that do not occur until adolescence and young adulthood are much more likely to produce infectious mononucleosis.
  - Annual incidence (~1 in 2,500 students) of infectious mononucleosis is highest among white high school and college students.
- Geographic distribution
  - In Africa, a strong association exists between infection with EBV and development of Burkitt lymphoma and nasopharyngeal carcinoma.
    - This association is less clear in Western countries, where infection with EBV occurs at a later age.
  - In the US, interest in EBV infection centers on the typical clinical syndrome: infectious mononucleosis.
    - Studied for emerging relationship with an increasing number of tumors, noted for the most part in immunocompromised patients
- Transmission
  - In a study of families that have a childhood index case of infectious mononucleosis, seroconversion occurred in 34.6% of susceptible siblings over several months.
  - The rate of transmission of the EBV infection was relatively low and slow.
    - Development of infectious mononucleosis was high (55.6%) in sibling contacts who showed seroconversion.
  - Secondary infection in typical college settings is even lower.

ETIOLOGY

- Infection follows entry of the EBV into the oropharynx.
  - Recovery from this site can be documented up to 16 months after illness.
- EBV establishes latency in the epithelial cells of the oropharynx.
  - Virus is periodically shed from this site throughout an individual's lifetime.

RISK FACTORS

- Transmission from one individual to another appears to occur most often through mixing of saliva.
  - Described as the *kissing disease*
- In the absence of such contact, transfer of infection is unlikely.

SIGNS AND SYMPTOMS

- In childhood, EBV infection is usually inapparent clinically or characterized by a nonspecific, uncomplicated episode of upper respiratory tract infection or pharyngitis.
- The incubation period is 2–6 weeks (usually 20–30 days).
- Classic signs of infectious mononucleosis
  - Fever
  - Sore throat
  - Lymphadenopathy
- This constellation of symptoms and signs may be preceded by vague symptoms of:
  - Fatigue
  - Malaise
  - Anorexia
- Infectious mononucleosis is the result of a systemic viral infection.
  - Virtually every organ system may be involved.
- Clinical manifestations compatible with infectious mononucleosis include:
  - Fever
    - Usually not higher than 103°F (39.5°C)
  - Lymphadenopathy
    - Most striking feature of the illness
    - Can be limited to the cervical nodes
    - Can involve virtually all lymph node groups
    - Posterocervical adenopathy is noted most frequently.
    - The lymph nodes are not tender and do not demonstrate other signs of inflammation.
  - Sore throat/tonsillopharyngitis
    - Can be excruciating
    - Frequently accompanied by tonsillar exudate and a palatal enanthem or a grayish necrosis of the tonsillar surfaces in adolescents
  - Splenomegaly
    - Some patients do not have any palpable splenic enlargement.
  - Hepatomegaly
    - Liver enzyme levels are elevated in virtually all patients.
    - Frequency of jaundice is low.
  - Rhinitis, cough

- Rash
  - In approximately 20% of children
  - Erythematous
  - Petechial
  - Erythema multiforme–like
  - Urticarial
  - Scarlatiniform
  - In 70–90% of young adult patients treated with ampicillin and can appear after the medication has been discontinued
- Abdominal pain
- Eyelid edema
  - In approximately 25%
- Severity of illness is extremely variable.
  - Some individuals may have relatively few manifestations of infection.
  - Others will demonstrate virtually all symptoms.
- Clinical manifestations last approximately 2–3 weeks.
  - Peak involvement during the second week

DIFFERENTIAL DIAGNOSIS

- Massive enlargement of the spleen should suggest an alternative diagnosis.
- EBV-negative infectious mononucleosis
  - Symptoms similar to those of EBV infection can be produced by:
    - Rubella
    - Hepatitis
    - Toxoplasmosis
    - Cytomegalovirus
    - Human herpesvirus-6
    - Adenovirus infections
    - Systemic lupus erythematosus
    - Drug reactions
  - Negative EBV titers and heterophil antibody responses strongly suggest one of these other agents or conditions as the cause.
  - In hepatitis:
    - Heterophil test can give a false-positive result.
    - Liver enzyme levels generally are much more elevated than those seen with infectious mononucleosis.
    - Results of serologic tests for hepatitis will be positive.
  - Rubella titers in rubella infection will be positive.
  - Cytomegalovirus can be cultured from urine as the cause of illness.

- Illnesses that mimic infectious mononucleosis but lack serologic confirmation of EBV should be classified as heterophil-negative infectious mononucleosis rather than atypical mononucleosis.
  - Cause of most of these cases is unknown.

DIAGNOSTIC APPROACH

- Diagnosed by the presence of a triad of findings
  - Clinical
  - Hematologic
  - Serologic
- Minimal hematologic features should include:
  - Lymphocytosis ≥50% of all leukocytes
  - Atypical lymphocyte count ≥10% of all leukocytes

LABORATORY FINDINGS

- General laboratory findings usually include a decrease in the number of granulocytes and platelets.
- Paul-Bunnell antibody, a heterophilic immunoglobulin (Ig)M antibody produced by humans during infection, is the cornerstone of laboratory diagnosis.
  - Will be present in ≤50% of children <4 years
  - Among school-age children and young adults, detectable 80–90% of the time during the second week of clinical illness
  - Heterophil response will be brief and minimal or will occur late in the illness.
    - Shows negative results early in the course of the illness
  - Commercial diagnostic kits rely on differential adsorption to detect the heterophil antibody.
    - Readily available and easy to use in a physician's office
    - 96–99% sensitive
    - Give a result in 2 minutes
    - False-positive results have been reported in cases of:
      - Rubella
      - Hepatitis
      - Serum sickness
      - Drug reactions
      - Systemic lupus erythematosus
      - Improper use of the kit
      - Inaccurate interpretation of the agglutination reaction
    - Magnitude of the heterophil antibody titer does not correlate with clinical severity.
    - Repeat testing, once a positive test result is obtained, provides no additional information beyond that gained from clinical assessment.
- If heterophil test results are negative and infection is strongly suspected, confirmation of EBV infection should be sought by other serologic tests.

Interpretation of Epstein-Barr Virus Serology[a,b]

	Heterophil Antibody	Epstein-Barr Virus Antibodies			
		VCA-IgM	VCA-IgG	EA	EBNA
No infection	–	–	–	–	–
Acute infection	+/–	+	+ (>1:320)	+/–	–
Past infection	–	–	+ (1:80–1:160)	+/–	+

Abbreviations: EA, early antigen; EBNA, IgG antibody to Epstein-Barr nuclear antigen; VAC-IgG, IgG antibody to viral capsid antigen; VCA-IgM, IgM antibody to viral capsid antigen.
[a] From: Sumaya CV, Ench Y. Epstein-Barr virus infectious mononucleosis in children. I. Clinical and general laboratory findings. *Pediatrics.* 1985;75(6):1003–1010.
[b] Other patterns may occur in an individual patient; the above profile is for a typical individual.

- Patients who have negative heterophil test results will have antibodies against specific components of the virus if EBV is the cause of illness.
- A variety of antibodies directed against various portions of EBV can be detected.
- 4 different antibodies define the EBV serologic profile.
  - IgG antibody to the viral capsid antigen (VCA-IgG)
  - IgM antibody to viral capsid antigen (VCA-IgM)
  - IgG antibody to early antigen (EA)
  - IgG antibody to Epstein-Barr nuclear antigen (EBNA)
    - Includes 2 patterns: diffuse and restricted
    - These antibodies usually appear in an individual who acquires a primary EBV infection.
  - The pattern of antibody responses can help determine the date of EBV infection onset.
  - In most cases, an individual develops a VCA-IgM antibody (or VCA-IgG antibody) response in the acute period after an EBV infection.
  - IgG antibodies to the VCA persist for life.
  - VCA-IgM tends to disappear in 2–3 months.
  - Height of the VCA-IgG response decreases as the acute infection resolves.
    - Serial measurements of antibody titers are not clinically beneficial.
  - EA response peaks at 3–4 weeks into the illness.
    - Initially thought to persist only for several months
    - Was considered a good marker for an acute or recent infection
    - Recent evidence suggests that the EA response may persist for years in some children and may not develop at all in others.
  - EBNA antibody response usually appears several weeks to months after a primary infection.
    - Thought to be a marker for a past or convalescent infection

  - Must be interpreted in light of the clinical situation
    - A large number of children develop this response in the acute phase of their infection.
    - 10–20% of individuals never develop detectable levels of antibody to EBNA.
- Children who acquire EBV infections typically develop antibodies in the same sequential pattern.
  - Not all patients follow the same pattern.
- Clinical judgment remains important in the interpretation of such findings.
- Interlaboratory variability in results of EBV antibody testing has been observed.
  - Reliability of tests is suspect in some cases.
  - If both heterophil test and specific serologic findings are negative, a non-EBV infectious mononucleosis–like illness should be suspected.
- The table above provides an interpretation of EBV serology.

TREATMENT APPROACH

- Most patients who have infectious mononucleosis recover uneventfully.
- Physicians need do little except:
  - Establish the diagnosis.
  - Explain the nature of the illness.
  - Reassure parents.
- No specific therapy is indicated.
- Patients should rest to the extent that they believe necessary.
- As long as the patient can consume adequate amounts of fluids and calories, hospitalization is unnecessary.
- To minimize the danger of splenic rupture, ambulatory patients should avoid strenuous physical exercise or contact sports for 1 month or until the spleen is no longer palpable.
- Patients who have a late-onset heterophil antibody response appear to have a prolonged convalescence.
- Accounts are rare but increasing of infectious mononucleosis episodes that are severe or fatal or result in significant long-lasting problems.

M

- Most of these patients had some form of immunological abnormality.
  - X-linked lymphoproliferative syndrome
  - Renal or bone marrow transplant
  - Chédiak-Higashi syndrome
- Definitive management of these patients remains unclear.

SPECIFIC TREATMENTS

Corticosteroids

- Corticosteroids are of unproved value in treating this illness.
  - Should not be used routinely merely to make the patient feel better
- Controlled studies documenting efficacy are lacking.
- Most clinicians believe that their use is justified in treating:
  - Severe hemolytic anemia
  - Significant airway obstruction secondary to tonsillar hypertrophy
  - Thrombocytopenia
- Some authorities suggest using corticosteroids if neurologic involvement is significant.
  - Proof of efficacy is not available.
- High-dose, short-term courses of steroids have been used with dramatic improvement typically noted over 24–72 hours.
  - Dexamethasone: 0.25 mg/kg every 6 hours
  - Methylprednisolone: 1 mg/kg every 6 hours
  - Oral prednisone: 40 mg/day

Antiviral agents

- Acyclovir has good activity against EBV in vitro.
  - Has not been shown to be beneficial in several clinical trials
  - At this time, routine use is not recommended.
- Several antivirals (acyclovir, ganciclovir, vidarabine) and immunomodulating agents (interferon-γ, interferon-α, interleukin-2) have been used in severe EBV infections.
  - Varying degrees of success
- Pharyngitis of infectious mononucleosis can be indistinguishable from that of streptococcal pharyngitis, and culture specimens of the pharynx should be obtained.
- Patients who have positive culture findings should be treated accordingly.
- Clinician should avoid using ampicillin or amoxicillin when EBV infection is suspected.
  - Rash develops in most young adults with EBV infection who receive this drug.
- Ampicillin effect has not been well demonstrated in young children with infectious mononucleosis.

Experimental approaches

- Approaches under investigation for the treatment of EBV-associated lymphoproliferative disease include:
  - Bone marrow transplantation
  - Treatment with monoclonal antibodies
  - Infusions of donor peripheral leukocytes

WHEN TO ADMIT

- Hospitalization may be necessary in the presence of:
  - Airway compromise
  - Splenic rupture
  - Neurologic complications
  - Severe hemolytic anemia
  - Thrombocytopenia

WHEN TO REFER

- Consultation with appropriate subspecialists for the complications listed below would be warranted.
  - Airway compromise
  - Splenic rupture
  - Neurologic complications
  - Severe hemolytic anemia
  - Thrombocytopenia

FOLLOW-UP

- Many patients with chronic fatigue syndrome date the onset of their illness to an episode of infectious mononucleosis.
- Virologic and clinical studies have confirmed that active EBV infection is not responsible for the illness.
- At present, no single infectious or other cause has been identified for chronic fatigue syndrome.

COMPLICATIONS

- Death occurs in approximately 1 in 3000 cases.
  - True complication and death rates during this illness are uncertain.
  - Many reports do not include strict diagnostic criteria for infectious mononucleosis.
- Relative frequencies (approximate) of more common complications associated with this illness from one study
  - Pneumonia—5%
  - Severe airway obstruction—3.5%
  - Seizures—4%
  - Meningitis, encephalitis—2%
  - Peripheral facial nerve paralysis—1%
  - Guillain-Barré syndrome—1%
  - Thrombocytopenia with hemorrhages—3.5%

M

- Hemolytic anemia—1%
- Bacteremia—1%
- Recurrent tonsillopharyngitis—3%
- Jaundice—2%
- Glomerulonephritis —1%
- Orchitis—1%

■ Abdominal pain is an infrequent symptom of this illness.

- Its appearance, particularly if severe and in the left upper quadrant, should alert the clinician to the possibility of impending or actual splenic rupture.

■ Fatal cases of Reye syndrome associated with serologic evidence of EBV infection have been reported.

■ EBV infection and cancer

- Some have speculated that EBV infection might be oncogenic in the US.
- Some cases of leukemia occurring shortly after the onset of infectious mononucleosis have been reported.
  - No other evidence exists to support this speculation.
- The association between EBV and classic Burkitt lymphoma is not as strong in the US as in Africa.

- The EBV genome can be detected in approximately 50% of Reed-Sternberg cells found in patients with the mixed cellularity form of Hodgkin lymphoma.
  - Whether EBV is a causal agent, or even a cofactor, is unknown.
- EBV has also been associated with several lymphoreticular cancers in patients with AIDS.
  - Malignant B-cell lymphoma
  - Colonic lymphoid hyperplasia
- EBV has been associated with:
  - Oral hairy leukoplakia
  - Lymphoid interstitial pneumonitis in individuals with AIDS
- The precise relationship between EBV and cancer remains unknown and is the subject of intense investigation.

PREVENTION

■ Secondary infection in typical college settings is low.

- Strict isolation of the patient is unnecessary.
- Separation of drinking and eating utensils should suffice.

M

Mood Disorders

DEFINITION

- Mood disorders include major depressive disorder, dysthymic disorder, adjustment disorder, bipolar affective disorder, and cyclothymic disorder.
- Major depressive disorder requires ≥2 weeks of depressed mood more than one-half of the time and 4 additional depressive symptoms.
- Dysthymic disorder may have periods of depression interspersed with normal mood.
- Adjustment disorder is a mild, self-limited disturbance of mood that follows a serious life stressor.
- Manic symptoms with dysthymia is diagnosed as bipolar affective disorder.
- Manic symptoms with major depression is diagnosed as cyclothymic disorder.

EPIDEMIOLOGY

- Age
  - Relatively rare in prepubertal children; point prevalences range from 1.8–2.9%
  - Incidence is 3–4 times more common in adolescence.
    - Approximately 3–8% experience depression.
    - Bipolar disorder is diagnosed in 1–2%.
    - Bipolar spectrum is diagnosed in 5–7%.
    - Rate of bipolar disorder is twice as high in adolescents as in prepubertal children.
- Sex
  - Sex ratio for affectively ill prepubertal children approaches unity.
  - Depression among adolescents is 2–3 times more common among girls than boys.
  - Earlier onset of puberty may be associated with an increased risk of depression, especially in girls.

ETIOLOGY

- Childhood depression is associated with:
  - Serotonergic and noradrenergic neurotransmission abnormalities, as demonstrated by altered response to neuroendocrine challenges
  - Structural and functional alterations in the prefrontal cortex and the limbic system
- Genetics
  - Adoption, twin, and linkage studies support a genetic component.
  - Genetic epidemiologic studies suggest that depression results from an interaction between genetic vulnerability and accumulated stressful life events.

RISK FACTORS

- Depression
  - Family history
    - ≥1 parent with a history of depression
    - Earlier age of onset of depression in parent(s)
    - Family history of bipolarity or recurrent unipolar disorder
    - Previous psychiatric disorder and family history of depression predispose to the development of depression following bereavement.
  - Age
    - In girls, early onset of puberty may be a risk factor.
  - Severe stressors, such as physical or sexual abuse
  - Exposure to family and community violence
  - Anxiety disorders
  - Medications
    - Antihypertensive agents
    - Steroids
    - Phenobarbital
  - Chronic illnesses
    - Epilepsy
    - Inflammatory bowel disease
    - Juvenile-onset diabetes

SIGNS AND SYMPTOMS

Criteria for diagnosis of a major depressive episode

- ≥5 of the following symptoms during the same 2-week period, representing a change from previous functioning (must have 1 of first 2):
  - Depressed mood most of the day, nearly every day, indicated by either:
    - Subjective report (eg, feels sad or empty)
    - Observation by others (eg, appears tearful or irritable)
  - Markedly diminished interest or pleasure in most or all activities most of the day, nearly every day, by:
    - Subjective account
    - Observation made by others
  - Significant weight loss without dieting, or weight gain (change in body weight >5% in 1 month), or decrease or increase in appetite nearly every day
    - Consider failure to make expected weight gains as weight loss.
  - Insomnia or hypersomnia nearly every day
  - Psychomotor agitation or retardation nearly every day:
    - Observable by others, not merely subjective feelings of restlessness or being slowed down
  - Fatigue or loss of energy nearly every day

- Feelings of worthlessness or excessive or inappropriate guilt
  - May be delusional nearly every day
  - May not merely be self-reproach or guilt about being sick
- Diminished ability to think or concentrate, or indecisiveness nearly every day, either by:
  - Subjective account
  - Observations of others
- Recurrent thoughts of death (not just fear of dying), recurrent suicidal ideation without a specific plan, suicide attempt, or specific plan for committing suicide
■ Symptoms do not meet criteria for a mixed episode.
■ Symptoms cause clinically significant distress or impairment in social, occupational, or other important areas.
■ Symptoms are not due to physiologic effects of:
  - A substance (eg, a drug of abuse, a medication)
  - General medical condition (eg, hypothyroidism)
■ Symptoms are not better accounted for by bereavement (ie, after the loss of a loved one).
■ Symptoms persist for >2 months or are characterized by marked functional impairment, morbid preoccupation with worthlessness, suicidal ideation, psychotic symptoms, or psychomotor retardation.

Criteria for diagnosis of dysthymic disorder

■ Depressed mood most of the day, for more days than not
  - In children and adolescents, mood can be irritable or depressed.
  - Duration must be ≥1 year.
■ Presence, while depressed, of ≥2 of the following:
  - Poor appetite or overeating
  - Insomnia or hypersomnia
  - Low energy or fatigue
  - Low self-esteem
  - Poor concentration or difficulty making decisions
  - Feelings of hopelessness
■ During the 1-year period of the disturbance, the person has never been free of the above symptoms for ≥2 months at a time.
■ No major depressive episode during 1 year of the disturbance
  - Disturbance is not better accounted for by chronic major depressive disorder or by major depressive disorder in partial remission.
  - After the initial year of dysthymic disorder, episodes of major depressive disorder may be superimposed.
    - Both diagnoses may be given when the criteria for a major depressive episode are met.
■ Patient has never had a manic, mixed, or hypomanic episode, and criteria for cyclothymic disorder have never been met.
■ The disturbance does not occur exclusively during the course of a chronic psychotic disorder (eg, schizophrenia or delusional disorder).

■ Symptoms are not due to the physiologic effects of:
  - A substance (eg, a drug of abuse, a medication)
  - A general medical condition (eg, hypothyroidism)
■ Symptoms cause clinically significant distress or impairment in social, occupational, or other important areas of functioning.

Criteria for diagnosis of adjustment disorder with depressed mood

■ Development of emotional or behavioral symptoms in response to an identifiable stressor(s) within 3 months of the onset of the stressor(s)
■ Clinically significant symptoms or behaviors, evidenced by either:
  - Marked distress in excess of what would be expected from exposure to the stressor
  - Significant impairment in social or occupational (academic) functioning
■ The disturbance does not meet the criteria for another specific axis I disorder and is not merely an exacerbation of a preexisting axis I or axis II disorder.
■ Symptoms do not represent bereavement.
■ Once the stressor (or its consequences) has terminated, the symptoms do not persist for more than an additional 6 months.

Criteria for diagnosis of bipolar disorder

■ Past or current history of a manic episode, characterized by:
  - Distinct period of abnormally and persistently elevated, expansive, or irritable mood, lasting ≥1 week (or any duration where hospitalization is necessary)
    - During the period of mood disturbance, ≥3 of the following have persisted (4 if the mood is only irritable) and have been present to a significant degree.
      ■ Inflated self-esteem or grandiosity
      ■ Decreased need for sleep (eg, feels rested after only 3 hours of sleep)
      ■ More talkative than usual, or pressure to keep talking
      ■ Flight of ideas or subjective experience that thoughts are racing
      ■ Distractibility (ie, attention too easily drawn to unimportant or irrelevant external stimuli)
      ■ Increase in goal-directed activity (either socially, at work or school, or sexually) or psychomotor agitation
      ■ Excessive involvement in pleasurable activities that have a high potential for painful consequences (unrestrained buying sprees, sexual indiscretions)
■ Symptoms do not meet criteria for a mixed episode.
■ Mood disturbance includes either:
  - Marked impairment in academic functioning or in usual social activities or relationships with others

M

- Necessity for hospitalization to prevent harm to self or others
- Psychotic features

■ Symptoms are not due to the direct physiologic effects of:
- A substance (eg, a drug of abuse, a medication)
- Other treatment
- General medical condition (eg, hyperthyroidism)

Criteria for diagnosis of cyclothymic disorder

■ For ≥1 year, numerous periods with hypomanic symptoms and numerous periods with depressive symptoms that do not meet criteria for a major depressive episode

■ During the 1-year period, the patient has not been free of the above symptoms for ≥2 months at a time.

■ No major depressive episode, manic episode, or mixed episode has been present during 1 year of the disturbance. The symptoms are not better accounted for by schizoaffective disorder and are not superimposed on:
- Schizophrenia
- Schizophreniform disorder
- Delusional disorder
- Psychotic disorder not otherwise specified

■ Symptoms are not due to the direct physiologic effects of:
- A substance (eg, a drug of abuse, a medication)
- A general medical condition (eg, hyperthyroidism)

■ Symptoms cause clinically significant distress or impairment in social, occupational, or other important areas of functioning.

DIFFERENTIAL DIAGNOSIS

■ Within depressive disorders, the main differential diagnosis is among the triad of dysthymia, depression, and adjustment disorder with depressed mood.
- Dysthymia
  - More chronic and intermittent depression than major depression
  - The 2 disorders can coexist (so-called double depression).
- Adjustment disorder with depressed mood
  - Less severe mood disturbance
  - Fewer symptoms
  - Self-limited compared with dysthymia or major depression
- If a life stressor precedes a syndrome of depression, the presence of the stressor does *not* invalidate the diagnosis of major depressive disorder.

■ Symptoms of bereavement may be hard to distinguish from depressive symptoms.
- Depression is diagnosed if bereavement is associated with:
  - Functional impairment
  - Suicidal ideation

- Psychotic features
- Feelings of worthlessness
- Prolonged course

■ Other psychiatric disorders that may have associated mood disturbances
- Learning disabilities or attention-deficit/hyperactivity disorder (ADHD)
  - Patients may have poor self-esteem and feel demoralized.
  - Depression should not be diagnosed in these patients unless they meet the criteria for the syndrome.
  - Poor concentration is characteristic of both ADHD and depression.
    ■ ADHD usually has an earlier onset and is not associated with anhedonia or social withdrawal.
- Anxiety disorder
  - Children are often dysphoric when separated from their parents.
  - In the absence of premorbid depression, reunion with the parent relieves the dysphoria.
- Patients who are anorectic, particularly if malnourished, may show a markedly depressed affect.
  - Depression should not be diagnosed until nutritional status has been normalized.
- Abusers of drugs and alcohol often show disturbances of mood.
  - Mood disorder may antedate and even predispose the individual to substance abuse.
  - Mood disorder is often secondary to substance abuse and subsides within a month of detoxification.
- Distinguishing depression from chronic medical illness can be difficult.
  - Depression may be higher in certain illnesses.
    ■ Chronic illness may affect sleep, appetite, and energy similarly to depression.
  - Feelings of guilt, worthlessness, hopelessness, and suicidal thoughts are unlikely to be attributable to the illness itself.
    ■ If present, strongly suggest a depressive disorder
- Mania
  - Abuse of stimulants (eg, cocaine, amphetamine) can mimic symptoms of mania.
  - The irritability of mania also can be seen in depression.
    ■ Distinguishing depression from mania rests on whether the preponderance of associated symptoms is more consistent with mania or with depression.
  - Euphoria, increased energy, and increased sexuality are much more common in patients with bipolar disorder than in those with unipolar (ie, only experiencing depression) disorder.

– Irritability, anger, and poor judgment also may be prominent features of conduct disorder.

  ■ Lack of changes in energy, sleep, sexuality, and thought patterns generally exclude mania as a diagnosis.

– Features of ADHD may suggest mania, but patients with mania are more likely to:

  ■ Have mood swings and alterations in sleep and appetite

  ■ Show hypersexuality and inappropriate joking and punning

– Severe clinical deterioration of a patient with an attention-deficit disorder after a trial of stimulants suggests bipolar disorder.

  ■ Particularly with some of the manic clinical features mentioned earlier or with a positive family history of mania

• Sexually abused children

– May show sexually provocative behavior and depressed mood

– However, euphoria or increased energy in the absence of bipolar disorder is rarely seen.

DIAGNOSTIC APPROACH

■ Both child and parent usually contribute important information used in diagnosing depression.

• The child is likely to be the most accurate reporter of symptoms referring to an internal state, such as:

– Depressed mood

– Anhedonia

– Guilt

– Worthlessness

– Suicidal thoughts

• The parent may be able to note externally validated symptoms, such as:

– Irritability

– Decline in school performance

– Listlessness

– Withdrawal from social and other pleasurable activities

– Weight loss

■ Mood disorder is classified on the basis of 3 factors:

• Severity

• Course

• Presence or absence of mania

■ Suspicion for depression should be high when the patient exhibits substantial alteration of mood with evidence of a decline in function.

■ Important in identifying mood disorder is to recognize that the depressed mood may be described as grouchy, mad, or bored rather than sad.

■ A brief self-report, the *Mood and Feelings Questionnaire*, can be useful in identifying which children have depression and need more specialized treatment.

TREATMENT APPROACH

■ Mood disorders are best managed by collaboration among a pediatrician, mental health specialist, and child psychiatrist.

■ Generally, psychiatric intervention has 3 components.

• Psychoeducation

• Psychotherapy

• Pharmacotherapy

■ Most patients with mood disorder can be managed as outpatients.

■ Family psychoeducation approaches depression as a chronic illness, aiming to instruct the family about the nature and course of the illness.

• This is likely to improve adherence with treatment.

• May reduce the rate of relapse

• Psychoeducation reduces the tensions of living with a person with mood disorder by altering familial expectations.

– Parents' accepting the illness and making appropriate expectations of the patient and of themselves

• Psychoeducation should enable the child and family to:

– Identify early signs of recurrence

– Seek treatment before recurrent disorder becomes severe and chronic

• Identification and treatment of parental depression are critical.

– Evidence suggests that parental depression may prolong the child's depressive episodes and interfere with recovery.

■ Depressed patients with a family history for bipolar disorder should be treated initially with psychotherapy.

• If they require an antidepressant, they should be monitored closely for emergent manic symptoms.

• Other side effects include:

– Drowsiness

– Extrapyramidal symptoms

– Galactorrhea

– More rarely, tardive dyskinesia

■ Treatment for bipolar disorder includes:

• Mood stabilizers for prophylaxis and acute treatment of manic or depressive episodes

• Encouragement of continued treatment after normalization of mood

– Psychoeducation for the patient and family is key.

M

SPECIFIC TREATMENTS

Cognitive-behavioral therapy (CBT) for depression

■ Brief CBT (3 months) is more efficacious than credible alternative treatments (family, supportive, or relaxation therapies) for adolescent depression.

■ Group CBT is helpful both for treating depression and for preventing depression in at-risk youth.

■ Combination of CBT and medication
  ● Results in highest remission rate and a trend toward lower rates of suicidal adverse events
  ● In more severe depression, may be no better than fluoxetine alone

■ Interpersonal psychotherapy is efficacious in treating adolescent depression.
  ● Has not been compared with antidepressant medication

Pharmacologic treatment for depression

Selective serotonin reuptake inhibitors (SSRIs)

■ Somewhat effective
  ● The strongest data support the use of fluoxetine.
    – The only SSRI with US Food and Drug Administration (FDA) approval for treatment of pediatric depression

■ Standard approach
  ● The equivalent of 10 mg of fluoxetine for 1 week, then increase to 20 mg for 3 more weeks
    – If the patient does not show an adequate clinical response to increase, the dose is increased to 40 mg.

■ Adolescents who do not respond to the first SSRI
  ● The standard is to try another SSRI at an adequate dose for 6–8 weeks.
  ● Establishing adherence and ruling out possible medical problems, such as hypothyroidism that might contribute to lack of response, are important.
  ● If patient shows partial response, consider augmentation with lithium, which is effective in adults.
  ● If there is complete lack of response, switch to another type of agent, such as bupropion.
  ● Addition of psychotherapy may enhance treatment response.

■ The FDA has determined that SSRIs are associated with an increased risk of suicidality (ie, suicidal ideation and behaviors) compared with placebo.
  ● Recommends close monitoring for clinical response and adverse events during the early phase of treatment
    – Weekly for the first month
    – Every other week for the next 2 months
    – Monthly thereafter

● This adverse effect emerges early in treatment.
    – Most often characterized by new-onset or worsening suicidal ideation; a suicidal threat; or much more rarely, a suicide attempt
  ● In the FDA's review of clinical trials involving ≥4300 pediatric patients, no suicides occurred.
    – The rate of emergent or worsening suicidality was, on average, 4% in the antidepressant group and 2% in the placebo group.
  ● Although many more patients will benefit from SSRIs than will experience suicidality, SSRIs should be prescribed only:
    – When patients and families understand the risks and benefits, *and*
    – The physician can monitor progress and side effects on a regular basis.

■ 2–5% of patients treated with SSRIs develop manic symptoms.
  ● Expansive mood
  ● Racing thoughts
  ● Increased energy
  ● Decreased need for sleep
  ● Increased risk taking
  ● Risk is higher in younger patients and in persons with a positive family history for bipolar disorder.

Tricyclic antidepressants

■ An older type of antidepressant

■ Should not be prescribed as a first-line treatment because:
  ● Not efficacious for treating pediatric depression
  ● Are potentially lethal in overdose

Pharmacologic treatment for bipolar disorder

■ If the patient is exhibiting acute mania, administer either:
  ● Lithium *or*
  ● Anticonvulsant mood stabilizers (divalproex or carbamazepine) *or*
  ● Atypical neuroleptics (risperidone and quetiapine)

■ If the patient is exhibiting psychotic mania
  ● Lithium, divalproex, or carbamazepine combined with an atypical neuroleptic agent is recommended.
  ● If the patient has partial response to monotherapy, adding a second agent from the above group is recommended.

■ Treatment of depression in a patient with bipolar disorder requires relieving depression and prophylaxis against mania.
  ● Mood stabilizers and atypical neuroleptics have some antidepressant properties.
  ● Depressed patients with bipolar disorder often require the addition of an antidepressant.
    – This should always be prescribed *after* adequate coverage with a mood-stabilizing agent.

M

- Family interventions to improve communication, problem solving, and coping with having a bipolar family member may improve outcome.
- Mood-stabilizing agents have significant medical complications requiring close management.
  - Lithium
    - Causes weight gain; acne; hypothyroidism; and, rarely, renal damage
    - Therapeutic levels are between 0.6 and 1.0 mEq/L.
      - Should be monitored to assess compliance and prevent toxicity
    - Monitor every 4–6 months for hypothyroidism.
    - Monitor renal function annually with a blood urea nitrogen test, creatinine test, urinalysis, and creatinine clearance test.
  - Divalproex
    - Causes weight gain, can affect hepatic and hemopoietic function, and has been associated with polycystic ovarian disease
    - Requires periodic assessment of liver function and blood and platelet counts
  - Carbamazepine
    - Less frequently used because of its greater sedative effects and risk of hemopoietic side effects
  - Atypical neuroleptics typically cause weight gain.
    - Before prescribing, weight, body mass index, fasting blood glucose level, and lipid levels should be documented.
    - Weight and body mass index should be monitored closely.
- Lamotrigine
  - Anticonvulsant that has been demonstrated to be helpful for treating and preventing adult bipolar depression
    - Has not yet been carefully studied in children
  - Has a very benign side effect profile except, for the rare but very serious complication of Stevens-Johnson syndrome
    - For this reason, practitioners titrate this medication very slowly and monitor carefully for rashes.

WHEN TO ADMIT

- Inpatient admission is suggested if patient is:
  - Psychotic *or*
  - Acutely suicidal *or*
  - Acutely manic or in a mixed state *or*
  - Abusing substances *or*
  - Unresponsive to outpatient intervention

WHEN TO REFER

- Consider referring patients who have either:
  - Chronic, complex, or severe disorder, exhibited by:
    - Comorbidity
    - Suicidality
    - Psychosis
    - Bipolar-type depression

FOLLOW-UP

- After termination of CBT or pharmacotherapy, risk of relapse is high.
- Patient should continue treatment at a lower frequency of contact for 6 months after recovery is achieved.
  - For CBT, this consists of monthly visits or booster sessions.
  - For pharmacotherapy, continue treatment at same dose for at least 6 months after recovery.
  - Critical in treating early-onset depression because getting depressed patients well is not enough; keeping them well is crucial.

PROGNOSIS

- Untreated major depressive disorder lasts an average of 7.2 months.
- Untreated dysthymic disorder lasts an average of 45.9 months.
- Patients with both major depressive disorder and nonaffective morbidity (eg, additional diagnoses of conduct disorder, attention-deficit disorder) may have a prolonged course, as do depressed youth whose parents also are depressed.
- Recurrence of depression
  - 40% of depressed children experience recurrence within 2 years.
  - Nearly 75% have recurrence within 5 years.
  - Earlier age of onset and co-occurrence of a preexisting dysthymic disorder increase risk for major recurrences.
- Compared with nondepressed peers, depressed adolescents show greater risk of:
  - Academic, occupational, and interpersonal impairment
  - Tobacco and substance abuse
  - Obesity
- Residual social impairment may be related to unresolved depression.
  - However, many adverse outcomes are due to risk factors seen for depression and other conditions (eg, abuse, family discord, parental substance abuse).
- Depression confers increased risk for completed and attempted suicide, in both male and female adolescents.
- Girls are more likely to attempt suicide, but boys are more likely to complete suicide.

M

Muscular Dystrophy

DEFINITION

- Muscular dystrophies are a group of slowly progressive inherited diseases with specific patterns of muscle wasting and weakness.

EPIDEMIOLOGY

- Duchenne dystrophy
  - Most common pediatric muscular dystrophy
  - Prevalence: 1:3500 male births
- Becker dystrophy
  - Prevalence: 1:35,000 male births
- Myotonic dystrophy
  - Prevalence: 1:8000 all births
- Facioscapulohumeral dystrophy
  - Prevalence: 1:20,000 of all births
- Fukuyama-type congenital muscular dystrophy
  - Prevalence: 1:18,000 of all births
- Congenital muscular dystrophy
  - Prevalence unknown
- Emery-Dreifuss muscular dystrophy
  - Prevalence: 1:100,000 of all births

ETIOLOGY

- Duchenne dystrophy
  - Due to absence of dystrophin
    - A large cytoskeletal protein that attaches to the inner surface of the muscle fiber membrane as part of a complex of glycoproteins
    - Also part of the inner membrane structure of smooth and cardiac muscle and of certain cells in the central nervous system and in specialized connective tissues, such as the myotendinous junctions
  - X-linked recessive; $XP21$ region encodes for the protein dystrophin
    - Large deletions occur in approximately two-thirds of cases.
    - Additionally, smaller point mutations occur in ~30% of patients.
    - No consistent relationship exists between the size of the gene mutation and clinical severity.
- Becker dystrophy
  - Marked deficiency of dystrophin
  - X-linked recessive; $XP21$ region encodes for the protein dystrophin
    - Large deletions occur in more than two-thirds of cases.
    - Additionally, smaller point mutations occur in ~15% of patients.

- Myotonic dystrophy
  - Autosomal-dominant; chromosome 19
  - Abnormal expansion of CTG trinucleotide repeat in the 3'nontranslated region of a gene coding for a serine/threonine kinase
- Facioscapulohumeral dystrophy
  - Autosomal dominant; most cases localize to chromosome 4
  - Deletion of a variable quantity of 3.3-kb tandem repeats at $4q35$
- Fukuyama-type congenital muscular dystrophy
  - Autosomal recessive; chromosome 9, $q31-33$ region for most cases
  - 3-kb insertion of 3'noncoding region of gene encoding fukutin; mutation-caused instability of messenger RNA for fukutin
- Congenital muscular dystrophy
  - Autosomal recessive; chromosome $6q22-23$ region, laminin α2 gene
  - Complete (or partial) loss of merosin (laminin α2) in both muscle and skin
- Emery-Dreifuss muscular dystrophy
  - X-linked recessive form $Xq28$ and autosomal-dominant form $1q21.3$
  - The X-linked form involves gene for emerin and dominant form gene for lamins A and C.

SIGNS AND SYMPTOMS

Duchenne dystrophy

- Slowly progressive muscle-wasting disease marked by symptoms that develop before 5 years of age
  - Presents typically at 2–4 years of age
- Early symptoms
  - Cannot run or keep up with peers
  - Can take only 1 step at a time
  - Weakness of forward head flexion that persists beyond infancy
    - Accompanied by slowed motor development
  - Muscles affected early in course of disease are:
    - Proximal hip and shoulder girdle
    - Anterior neck
    - Abdominal
- Progressive gluteal and shoulder girdle muscular weakness
  - Widened stance
  - Lumbar lordosis
  - Forward thrusting of abdomen
  - Winging of scapulae

- Patients:
  - Never run normally
  - Put their hands on their knees to rise from the floor (see Figure 41 on page F17) and to assist in climbing steps
  - Have difficulty keeping up with peers
    - More apparent as children enter nursery school and kindergarten
    - May appear clumsy, or fall more easily
    - Complain of tiredness and calf cramps
- Mild cognitive deficits are common.
  - The patient may appear to be intellectually disabled; thus, the diagnosis of Duchenne dystrophy may be overlooked.
- Hip and knee extensor weakness develops gradually in middle childhood.
  - Patients often toe-walk to use the power of the gastrocnemius to help stabilize knee extension.
  - Reliance on calf muscles during ambulation contributes to typical hypertrophy of calf muscles.

Becker dystrophy

- Presentation is similar, but onset is later and symptoms are milder.
- Fatigue or marked thigh weakness
- Trouble climbing steps
- Occasional calf or thigh cramps

Myotonic dystrophy

- Congenital form
  - Floppy infant
  - Poor suck
  - Weak respiratory effort
  - Talipes
- Childhood form
  - Bifacial weakness
  - Slurred speech
  - Impaired hearing
  - Intellectual disability

Facioscapulohumeral dystrophy

- Congenital form (rare)
  - Bifacial weakness
  - Ophthalmoparesis (sometimes)
  - Occasionally floppy
  - Deafness
- Childhood form (more common)
  - Mild facial weakness
  - Weakness of scapular fixator muscles

Fukuyama-type congenital muscular dystrophy

- Develops in infancy
- Floppy infant

Congenital muscular dystrophy

- Develops in infancy
- Floppy, contractures

Emery-Dreifuss muscular dystrophy

- Onset in middle to late childhood
- Mild elbow contractures
- Mild weakness of triceps, biceps, and scapular fixator muscles
- Occasionally presents as isolated cardiomyopathy
- Can produce severe cardiac complications that require urgent treatment
  - Cardiac symptoms may prompt medical evaluation before muscle weakness or contractures occur.

DIFFERENTIAL DIAGNOSIS

- Awareness that there are a variety of uncommon muscular dystrophies helps parents and patients understand that different tests may be necessary to establish the specific diagnosis, prognosis, and plan of treatment.

Muscular dystrophies

- Duchenne dystrophy
- Becker dystrophy
- Myotonic dystrophy
- Facioscapulohumeral dystrophy
  - Rare in infancy, occasional in childhood, usually seen in adults
  - Early-onset cases of facioscapulohumeral dystrophy may resemble Duchenne dystrophy.
    - Facioscapulohumeral dystrophy causes only a mild to moderate increase in creatine kinase (CK) or creatine phosphokinase.
- Fukuyama-type congenital muscular dystrophy
- Congenital muscular dystrophy
- Emery-Dreifuss muscular dystrophy
  - Clinically and genetically distinct from, but occasionally confused with, Becker dystrophy
  - Presents with the triad of:
    - Joint contractures that begin in early childhood
    - Slowly progressive muscle weakness
    - Cardiac involvement
- Limb-girdle muscular dystrophy (see tables Autosomal-Dominant Forms of Limb Girdle Muscular Dystrophy [LGMD 1A-D] and Autosomal-Dominant Forms of Limb Girdle Muscular Dystrophy [LGMD 2G-I])

M

Autosomal-Dominant Forms of Limb Girdle Muscular Dystrophy (LGMD 1A-D)[a]

Characteristic	LGMD 1A	LGMD 1B	LGMD 1C	LGMD 1D
Age at onset	18–35 yr	4–38 yr (half of the cases in childhood)	~5 yr	<25 yr
Gene location (chromosome)	*5q31*	*1q21.2*	*3p25*[b]	*6q23*
Protein	Myotilin	Lamin A/C	Caveolin 3	Unknown
Serum creatine kinase	Normal or 2–5× normal	Normal or 2–5× normal	Often >10× normal	22–5× normal
Muscle biopsy	Fiber size variation; moth-eaten fibers; increased internal nuclei; occasional necrotic and regenerating fibers	Fiber size variation; increased internal nuclei; mild endomysial fibrosis; occasional necrotic and regenerating fibers	Similar findings to 1A and 1B; absence or deficiency of caveolin 3 on immunocytochemistry	Similar findings to 1A and 1B
Clinical features	Proximal weakness: occasional dysarthria; slow progression; Achilles tendon contractures; may show anticipation	Cardiac disturbances prominent; proximal weakness; slow progression; may be allelic to autosomal dominant locus for Emery-Dreifuss dystrophy	Proximal weakness; calf hypertrophy; muscle pain on exertion; variable progression; muscle cramps	Cardiac conduction disturbances prominent; proximal weakness; problems worse in boys

[a] Each of these has been described in a single family. Linkage analysis has excluded other known LGMD loci, but new causative genes have not yet been identified.
[b] Mutations alter the scaffolding domain of the protein.

Autosomal-Recessive Forms of Limb Girdle Muscular Dystrophy (LGMD 2G-I)

Characteristic	LGMD 2G	LGMD 2H	LGMD 2I
Age at onset	9–15 yr	1–27 yr	Early childhood to 27 yr (61% <5 yr)
Genetics	Chromosome 17q12; mutation found in the gene encoding the sarcomeric protein telethonin	D487N homozygous mutation in the *TRIM 32* gene, *9q31-0.34-1* coding for a E3 ubiquitin ligase responsible for posttranslational regulation of protein levels	Chromosome 19q13.3 fukutin-related protein gene
Serum creatine kinase	Usually <5× normal; may be >10× normal early in the disease	From near normal to 20× normal	Markedly increased, 5–70× normal
Muscle biopsy	Rimmed vacuoles in some patients	Mild dystrophic changes (fiber size variation, degeneration/regeneration); fiber splitting, internal nuclei; endomysial fibrosis	Dystrophic changes; type I fiber predominance; reduced staining for merosin (α2 chain of lamin)
Clinical features	Anterior tibialis weakness early in the course in some patients	Proximal lower limb weakness; weakness of facial muscles with flat smile; slow progression (patients remain ambulatory through midadulthood)	Severe limb girdle weakness; cardiac failure (30–50%) and respiratory failure (30%)

M

- Occurs during childhood or in the teens, and on superficial evaluation, resembles Duchenne dystrophy
- Most forms progress more slowly than Duchenne dystrophy, and prognosis differs.

Other diseases with similar presentation to muscular dystrophies

- Variants of spinal muscular atrophy
  - Spinal muscular atrophy produces no increase or only mild increase in creatine phosphokinase.
  - Hypertrophy of calf muscles
- Cerebral palsy
  - Pattern of walking and presence of mild cognitive deficits can lead to an incorrect diagnosis of cerebral palsy.
  - Misdiagnosis delays effective treatment
- Myasthenia gravis
  - More rapid development of weakness
  - Ptosis, ophthalmoparesis, and facial weakness
- Inflammatory myopathy
  - More rapid development of generalized weakness
  - Skin rash
- Chronic demyelinating polyneuropathy
  - Absence of ankle reflexes
  - More generalized weakness
  - More rapid course
  - No marked increase of CK
  - Abnormally slowed nerve conductions
- Hypothyroidism
  - Symptoms usually more generalized
  - May be identified by blood tests
  - Does not cause high CK levels that occur in Duchenne dystrophy
- Carnitine deficiency
  - Symptoms usually more generalized
  - May be identified by blood tests
  - Does not cause high CK levels that occur in Duchenne dystrophy

The floppy infant

- Floppy infants can have markedly increased serum CK levels.
  - Newborns or infants with Duchenne dystrophy also have a marked increase in CK, but they are not floppy.
- The floppy infant without an infectious, toxic, or metabolic disorder that causes muscle destruction to account for marked increase of serum CK level:
  - Usually has one of the severe childhood autosomal-recessive forms of congenital muscular dystrophy:
    - Fukuyama-type muscular dystrophy
    - Congenital muscular dystrophy

- Certain congenital myopathies may be marked by floppiness.
  - These infants do not have significantly increased CK levels.

DIAGNOSTIC APPROACH

- Complete history
  - Almost always distinguishes muscular dystrophy from other conditions that cause proximal weakness without sensory findings in childhood
- In suspected cases, serum CK should be measured first.
  - A marked increase is suggestive of a muscular dystrophy.
    - Detailed discussion of natural history of Duchenne dystrophy or procedures for screening at-risk family members for carrier status is premature and best initiated after neurologic consultation and specific diagnostic data are available.
- The clinician should refer the patient for further evaluation to a neurologist skilled in the care of patients with neuromuscular disease.

LABORATORY FINDINGS

- A continuously updated list of laboratories and tests available for genetic diagnosis of the muscular dystrophies can be found at GeneTests.

Duchenne dystrophy

- Serum creatine phosphokinase level 10× above normal
- If suspicion is high, perform DNA screening first.
  - If negative, perform muscle biopsy.
- Leukocyte DNA testing
  - DNA is screened for deletions, which are found in 60–70% of patients.
  - If a deletion is found, deletion tests are performed in at-risk family members.
  - If no deletion is found, DNA sequencing for point mutation should be performed.

Becker dystrophy

- Serum creatine phosphokinase level 5–10× above normal
- Leukocyte DNA testing
  - DNA is screened for deletions, which are found in 60–70% of patients
  - If a deletion is found, deletion tests are performed in at-risk family members.
  - If no deletion is found, DNA sequencing for point mutation should be performed.

Myotonic dystrophy

- Serum creatine phosphokinase level ranges from normal to 2–5× above normal.

M

- Leukocyte DNA testing
  - Southern blot analysis is performed to identify abnormally large expansion of CTG repeats in the gene; most childhood cases show abnormal CTG repeat enlargements (eg, 500–4000 repeats), whereas normal alleles have 5–30 repeats.
  - If normal, polymerase chain reaction is performed to search for smaller expansion of the repeat.

Facioscapulohumeral dystrophy

- Serum creatine phosphokinase level 2–5× above normal
- DNA analysis is available to identify the 3.3-kb deletions.
  - Should perform before obtaining muscle biopsy if clinical suspicion is high

Fukuyama-type congenital muscular dystrophy

- Serum creatine phosphokinase level >10× above normal

Congenital muscular dystrophy

- Serum creatine phosphokinase level >10× above normal
- Genetic testing available at select laboratories for some forms of congenital muscular dystrophy

Emery-Dreifuss muscular dystrophy

- Serum creatine phosphokinase level 5–10× above normal
- Genetic testing is available at selected laboratories.

DIAGNOSTIC PROCEDURES

Duchenne dystrophy

- Muscle biopsy
  - Active myopathy
  - Absence of dystrophin
  - Severe reduction in dystrophin-associated proteins
  - Helps distinguish among many of the autosomal-dominant and autosomal-recessive forms of limb-girdle muscular dystrophy that are clinically similar to Duchenne dystrophy
- Electrodiagnostic testing
  - Normal nerve conductions

Becker dystrophy

- Muscle biopsy
  - Moderately active myopathy
  - Absence or deficiency of dystrophin
  - Reduction in dystrophin-associated proteins
- Electrodiagnostic testing
  - Normal nerve conductions; mildly myopathic electromyogram (EMG)

Myotonic dystrophy

- Muscle biopsy
  - Increased central nuclei atrophy of type I fibers
  - Ringbinden
  - Subsarcolemma masses

- Electrodiagnostic testing
  - Normal nerve conductions
  - Myotonic discharges are present in children and adults but are often absent in infants (EMG should be performed on the mother).

Facioscapulohumeral dystrophy

- Muscle biopsy
  - Nonspecific myopathy
  - Up to 30% have mononuclear inflammation.
- Electrodiagnostic testing
  - Normal nerve conductions; EMG occasionally myopathic, often within normal limits

Fukuyama-type congenital muscular dystrophy

- Muscle biopsy
  - Mixture of necrotic and regenerating fibers, fibrosis, and an increased number of small fibers
- Electrodiagnostic testing
  - Normal nerve conductions; myopathic EMG

Congenital muscular dystrophy

- Muscle biopsy
  - Dystrophic changes with adipose and connective tissue replacement
  - Often prominent inflammatory infiltrates
- Electrodiagnostic testing
  - Normal nerve conductions; myopathic EMG

Emery-Dreifuss muscular dystrophy

- Muscle biopsy
  - Mild to moderate active myopathy
  - Occasional atrophic type 1 fibers
- Electrodiagnostic testing
  - Normal nerve conductions; EMG often normal in early stages

TREATMENT APPROACH

Duchenne dystrophy

- Goals
  - Maintain ambulation for as long as possible.
  - Optimize development of the patient's cognitive abilities.
  - Anticipate complications.
- Develop an individualized care plan for each stage of disease.
  - The patient and family need to work closely with physicians, schoolteachers, physical educators, and physical and occupational therapists to develop a plan.

- Muscular Dystrophy Association clinics offer multiple services to patients.
  - Orthopedic care, physical therapy, occupational therapy, and neurologic care are coordinated by a neuromuscular specialist.
    - Typically, services are provided in a clinic financed partly by the Muscular Dystrophy Association.
  - Role of primary care physician remains critical.
    - The pediatrician usually provides routine care of upper respiratory infections, as well as treatment for other common medical problems.

SPECIFIC TREATMENTS

Duchenne dystrophy

- Prednisone is the only effective therapy.
  - Administered daily to maintain or stabilize muscle strength and function
    - Muscle strength begins to increase after only 10 days of treatment; maximal response after 3 months of therapy.
    - Muscle mass increases 10% after 3 months of treatment.
    - Rate of muscle breakdown declines in association with maintenance of normal rate of muscle protein synthesis.
  - Treatment is preferably monitored by or coordinated with a specialized neuromuscular center.
  - Appears to maintain respiratory muscle power even in late stages of disease
  - Has reduced number of patients who develop respiratory failure
  - Has decreased need for: tendon release surgery, long-leg bracing, spinal stabilization surgery for scoliosis
  - The mechanism responsible for beneficial effect is unknown.
  - Side effects
    - Most common
      - Excessive weight gain
      - Mood disturbances (more aggressive, more tearful)
      - Cushingoid facial appearance
    - Serious side effects are uncommon, but may include:
      - Compression fractures of the spine
      - High blood pressure
      - Gastrointestinal bleeding
      - Severe infections
      - Diabetes
    - Some patients develop small, dot-shaped cataracts.
    - Some patients experience decreased linear growth
      - Probably helps maintain ambulation

- Azathioprine immunosuppressive therapy
  - Has been used, but confers no beneficial effect
- Lightweight long-leg bracing
  - Often helpful by 10–12 years of age
  - Prolongs weight-bearing and ambulation, both of which delay the development of joint contractures and scoliosis
- Gene therapy
  - Discovery of the gene in Duchenne dystrophy has raised hopes that direct gene therapy, by either local injection or viral vector, will prove feasible.
- Other advances in research include:
  - Stem cell therapy
  - Treatments to "read through" certain types of mutations

WHEN TO ADMIT

- Before surgery
  - For medical, cardiology, and pulmonary consultations
- After surgery
  - For 24 hours (or longer, depending on type of surgery) to monitor cardiac and pulmonary function
- For evaluation and management of pneumonia or respiratory insufficiency, especially in:
  - Nonambulatory patients with Duchenne dystrophy
  - Patients with advanced cardiomyopathy with cardiac failure

WHEN TO REFER

- Neuromuscular clinic or specialist
  - When diagnosis of Duchenne dystrophy is strongly suspected (eg, symptoms and high CK levels)
  - To facilitate workup
  - Once diagnosis is confirmed
    - A neuromuscular specialist should take responsibility for initial description of course of Duchenne dystrophy and treatment options.
- Genetic counselor
  - After the diagnosis of Duchenne dystrophy is established
  - Offered to family members of patients, especially at-risk carrier women
- Cardiologist
  - After the patient with Duchenne dystrophy becomes wheelchair bound
  - To obtain a baseline cardiologic evaluation
  - In late stages of disease for monitoring of cardiac function and management of cardiomyopathy
  - Before surgery

M

- Pulmonologist
  - Pulmonary consultation before and after general anesthesia is integral part of any elective surgery.
    - Includes training patient and home care providers in use of assisted coughing techniques and nasal bilevel positive airway pressure to:
      - Hasten recovery after general anesthesia
      - Decrease likelihood of postoperative pneumonia
  - After the patient with Duchenne dystrophy becomes wheelchair bound
  - To obtain a baseline pulmonary evaluation
  - In late nonambulatory stage of disease
    - To monitor and manage respiratory failure
- Orthopedic surgeon
  - Can help guide timing of use of long-leg bracing
  - Can discuss possible need for surgery to lengthen Achilles tendons
  - Can monitor severity of contractures, as well as degree of spinal curvature
    - Orthopedic consultation is especially important in early nonambulatory stage of Duchenne dystrophy, when contractures and spinal curvature become prominent.
  - After the patient with Duchenne dystrophy becomes wheelchair bound
  - To obtain a baseline orthopedic consultation
  - For consideration of scoliosis surgery
  - For release of heel cord contractures
- Physical and/or occupational therapist
  - Patients usually receive this care in their schools.
  - During ambulatory stage of Duchenne dystrophy, to develop a heel cord stretching program and an individualized exercise program
  - In the late ambulatory stage of Duchenne dystrophy, when the patient may appear to be close to becoming wheelchair limited
  - To be fitted with adaptive equipment and long-leg braces
  - To evaluate and manage contractures
- Dietitian
  - During ambulatory stage of Duchenne dystrophy
    - Particularly in patients receiving corticosteroid treatment
  - To help manage weight gain
  - To establish healthy eating patterns
- Neuropsychologist
  - During ambulatory and nonambulatory stages of Duchenne dystrophy
    - Patients are at risk for emotional, cognitive, and behavioral problems.

- For patients:
  - With borderline intellectual abilities
  - With cognitive or behavioral abnormalities
- For patients and family members who need end-of-life counseling

FOLLOW-UP

- Monitoring for side effects of prednisone
  - Patients are seen every 3 months for:
    - Weight check
    - Blood pressure check
    - Pulse check
    - Forced vital capacity check
    - Urinalysis
    - Assessment of neuromuscular functioning
  - Each visit includes measures to help guide the physician in adjusting the dose of prednisone.
    - Timed function tests
      - Time needed to travel 30 feet, to arise from supine to standing position, and to climb 4 standard steps
    - Muscle strength evaluation
      - Shoulder abductors
      - Elbow flexors and extensors
      - Knee extensors
      - Hip flexors and extensors
  - Blood count and serum electrolyte levels are measured at 6-month intervals.

COMPLICATIONS

- See table Complications and Treatment of Muscular Dystrophies.

Duchenne dystrophy

- In middle and late nonambulatory stages, minor medical problems can provoke major complications.
  - Contractures and scoliosis
    - Develop when the patient becomes wheelchair bound
    - Do not appear at a specific age
    - Depend on patient's functional status
    - Usually begin to develop at ankles and elbows (flexion)
  - Respiratory problems
    - Mild cold may lead to atelectatic pneumonitis and acute respiratory insufficiency.
    - Chronic constipation can produce respiratory compromise in later stages due to abdominal distention and upward pressure on diaphragm.
    - An effective regimen to maintain regular bowel movements becomes important in routine care.

Complications and Treatment of Muscular Dystrophies in Childhood

Characteristic	Duchenne Dystrophy	Becker Dystrophy	Myotonic Dystrophy	Facioscapulohumeral Dystrophy	Fukuyama-Type Congenital Muscular Dystrophy	Congenital Muscular Dystrophy: Primary Deficiency of Merosin	Emery-Dreifuss Muscular Dystrophy
Muscle weakness	Treatment with prednisone slows or stabilizes muscle strength; lightweight long-leg bracing maintains ambulation in later stages.	No controlled studies of prednisone treatment; bracing is helpful in late stages.	No specific therapy; braces for foot drop; children can usually participate in gym in school.	No specific treatment; patients should avoid lifting with arms fully extended and abducted; braces are sometimes needed.	No specific treatment; bracing and physical therapy are useful in some patients.	Same as Fukuyama-type congenital muscular dystrophy	No specific treatment; skeletal muscle weakness often is relatively mild compared with cardiac problems and does not limit function.
Respiratory problems	Forced vital capacity is monitored (in later stages, atelectasis pneumonitis is common); colds are treated aggressively; if signs of respiratory failure develop, nasal or oral ventilation should be considered.	Uncommon until late stages; management then as with Duchenne dystrophy	For congenital cases, ventilation is often needed; the prognosis for survival is poor if the patient is ventilator dependent at >4 weeks of age; otherwise management is as for Duchenne dystrophy.	Uncommon	As with Duchenne dystrophy; patients often die of respiratory failure late in childhood or in early teens.	Same as Fukuyama-type congenital muscular dystrophy	Mild other than symptoms related to cardiac dysfunction
Cardiac problems	Occasionally, cardiomyopathy leads to congestive heart failure; afterload-reducing therapy often helps; patient should be monitored for intracardiac clots.	Occasionally, severe cardiomyopathy develops; treatment is the same as for Duchenne dystrophy.	Occasionally, tachyarrhythmias or heart block develops in childhood forms, and pacemaker treatment is indicated.	Uncommon	Uncommon	Uncommon	Frequent cardiac conduction defects; atrial paralysis, cardiac arrest, and sudden death are common; pacemaker treatment and preventive therapy for cardiac emboli are often necessary.
Orthopedic problems	Achilles tendon contractures respond to stretching in early stages; later tendon release surgery is often necessary; contractures at the hips, knees, elbows, and wrists usually develop after the patient becomes wheelchair bound; scoliosis often develops when patients stop ambulating; spinal stabilization surgery helps maintain use of the arms.	Uncommon; contractures are much less common than in Duchenne dystrophy.	Talipes deformity requires treatment with stretching and orthotic support; occasionally, surgery is necessary.	Occasionally, knee effusion and low back pain develop as a result of weakness; conservative care measures are effective; in late stages, surgery to stabilize the scapula may be performed, but surgery is uncommon.	Contractures develop in 70% of patients by 3 months of age at the ankles, knees, and hips.	Contractures, especially feet and hips	Contractures, especially in the elbows and ankles, occur early and respond somewhat to physical therapy; surgical release of Achilles tendon may be necessary; some patients develop a rigid spine syndrome, for which no effective therapy is available.

M

M

Complications and Treatment of Muscular Dystrophies in Childhood

Characteristic	Duchenne Dystrophy	Becker Dystrophy	Myotonic Dystrophy	Facioscapulohumeral Dystrophy	Fukuyama-Type Congenital Muscular Dystrophy	Congenital Muscular Dystrophy: Primary Deficiency of Merosin	Emery-Dreifuss Muscular Dystrophy
Nervous system problems	Increased incidence of cognitive and behavioral problems; some patients improve with small doses of methylphenidate.	Uncommon	Intellectual disability is common, especially in congenital cases, and special classroom care is needed; hearing deficits are common and may require hearing aids; facial weakness, dysarthria, and hearing problems exaggerate the impression of intellectual disability.	Uncommon; in rare cases, the infant-onset form of the disease occurs in association with hearing loss, retinal disease, or both.	Generalized or focal seizures occur in most patients; anticonvulsant therapy is necessary; intellectual disability is common; most patients have microcephaly, polymicrogyria, pachygyria, and heterotopias.	Intellectual disability is common; magnetic resonance imaging of head shows increased signal from white matter on T2-weighted images; occipital agyria	Caused only by stroke from heart block or cardiac emboli
Gastrointestinal problems	Constipation is common, especially late in the disease; careful dietary monitoring, stool softeners, and good water intake (urine specific gravity 1.007–1.010) are usually effective; occasionally acute gastric dilation occurs; it resolves over 2–3 days with nasogastric tube decompression of the stomach and intravenous hydration.	Uncommon	Spastic colon–type symptoms with abdominal pain are common; occasionally, these symptoms improve with antimyotonia therapy with mexiletine; eating small portions at each meal diminishes tendency to aspirate.	Uncommon	Uncommon	Uncommon	Uncommon

- Respiratory insufficiency often develops in late stages.
  - Forced vital capacity declines, usually into the range of 600–1000 mL.
- Management options include nasal ventilation rather than positive pressure ventilation via tracheostomy.
- Assistive cough devices (insufflator-exsufflator) may be helpful in speeding recovery from episodes of bronchitis and pneumonia.
- Ventilatory care usually is coordinated among pediatrician, neuromuscular specialist, pediatric pulmonologist, and patient and family.
- Cardiac problems
  - In late stages, patients occasionally develop cardiomyopathy.
    - Chest radiography reveals a dilated heart.
    - Cardiac ejection fraction decreases to 10–20% of normal.
  - Heart failure often exacerbated by coexisting respiratory insufficiency
  - Ventricular or atrial clots (or both) may be present.
  - Long-term anticoagulant therapy is necessary.
- Gastrointestinal system: acute gastric dilation
  - Infrequent complication occurring in late stages of disease
  - Typically occurs in association with idiopathic metabolic acidosis
  - Responds rapidly to nasogastric tube decompression of stomach and intravenous hydration

- Caution must be used with intravenous repletion of potassium.
  - In late stages of disease, the patient's muscle mass is considerably diminished and is not available to buffer an acute rise in extracellular potassium.
- Cause of gastric dilation is unknown.
  - Probably results, along with chronic intestinal hypomotility (constipation), from deficiency of dystrophin in smooth muscle of gastrointestinal tract.
- Treatment
  - Good hydration
  - Balanced dietary intake
  - Regular bowel habits

PROGNOSIS

Duchenne dystrophy

- Without prednisone treatment, most patients will become wheelchair bound between 10 and 12 years of age.
- With close follow-up, patients have been kept stable or have had only mild progression of muscle weakness for periods exceeding 5 years.

Becker dystrophy

- Patients can ambulate beyond age 15 years.

Fukuyama-type congenital muscular dystrophy

- Slow improvement up to 6–8 years of age, then a decline

M

Nephritis

DEFINITION

- *Nephritis* refers to noninfectious inflammation of the kidney parenchyma, which may involve primarily the glomerulus (glomerulonephritis), the interstitium (interstitial nephritis), or both.
- Acute glomerulonephritis
  - Most commonly, acute poststreptococcal glomerulonephritis (APSGN)
  - Henoch-Schönlein purpura (HSP) is small-vessel vasculitis that most often affects children.
  - Rapidly progressive glomerulonephritis (RPGN) is a variant of acute glomerulonephritis characterized by:
    - Symptoms of acute nephritis
    - Relentless progression to renal failure over days or weeks
- Chronic glomerulonephritis is associated with variety of conditions.
  - Immunoglobulin (Ig)A nephropathy (Berger disease)
  - Benign familial hematuria
  - Alport syndrome
  - Nephritis of systemic lupus erythematosus (SLE)
  - Membranoproliferative glomerulonephritis (MPGN), also called *mesangiocapillary glomerulonephritis,* is a chronic inflammatory disease of the kidney with poor prognosis.
  - Interstitial nephritis
    - Inflammation of the interstitium
    - Much less common than glomerular inflammation

EPIDEMIOLOGY

- Poststreptococcal nephritis
  - May happen at any age, but peak incidence at age 7 years
  - Slight predominance among boys
  - Geography
    - Following streptococcal pharyngotonsillitis, more common in temperate regions
    - Following streptococcal skin infections, more common in tropical and subtropical climates
- Acute glomerulonephritis
  - Of 487 children <15 years of age who underwent renal biopsy, 43% had glomerulonephritis.
    - Only 8.4% of these had a classical nephritic picture with hematuria, hypertension, oliguria, edema, and reduced glomerular filtration rate.
- SLE nephritis
  - Seen mainly in young women during childbearing years
  - 20% of cases involve children.
- IgA nephropathy
  - Males affected more often than females
  - Less frequent in black persons than in white persons

- Primary MPGN
  - Average age of onset, approximately 9 years

ETIOLOGY

- APSGN
  - Consequence of immune response to a nonrenal infection with some strains of group A ß-hemolytic streptococci
    - Types 12 and 49 are the strains most commonly associated with nephritis.
    - Risk of nephritis may differ according to site of infection and the particular M type.
- Nonstreptococcal acute glomerulonephritis
  - Viruses suspected of causing acute glomerulonephritis include:
    - Varicella
    - Echovirus 10
    - Coxsackieviruses
    - Viruses that cause infectious mononucleosis
    - Measles
    - Mumps
- RPGN
  - Most cases are the result of glomerular disease.
  - May be caused by:
    - Acute interstitial nephritis stemming from pyelonephritis
    - Hypersensitivity to certain drugs
- SLE may cause acute glomerulonephritis.
- IgA nephropathy
  - Cause is unknown
  - Abnormal glycosylation of the hinge region of the IgA antibody molecule is a possible mechanism.
- Benign familial hematuria
  - Inherited as an autosomal-dominant trait
- Alport syndrome
  - Inherited as an X-linked–dominant trait in 80–85% of cases
    - Caused by a mutation of the gene encoding the α-5 chain of type-IV collagen
    - The particular type of mutation may influence the severity of the clinical expression of the disease.
  - X-linked Alport syndrome with leiomyomatosis
    - Due to deletions involving the contiguous genes encoding the α-5 and α-6 chains of type-IV collagen
  - Autosomal-recessive Alport syndrome
    - Related to mutations in the genes encoding the α-3 and α-4 chains of type-IV collagen on chromosome 2
  - Autosomal-dominant Alport syndrome
    - Linked to the region of chromosome 2 containing the genes encoding the α-3 and α-4 chains of type-IV collagen

- MPGN
  - Cause usually unknown
  - Some forms are associated with immune complex deposition in the glomeruli.
  - Type-1 MPGN
    - Thought to be mediated by immune complex formation and deposition, with activation of the classical pathway of complement
  - Types 2 and 3
    - Complement consumption is thought to be the result of the presence of circulating autoantibodies (nephritic factors [NFs]) that stabilize C3 convertases activating the alternative (NF_a) and terminal (NF_t) pathways of complement activation, respectively.
- Interstitial nephritis
  - Often caused by an immune reaction to drugs

RISK FACTORS

- Streptococcal pharyngotonsillitis, especially in temperate regions
- Streptococcal skin infections, especially in tropical and subtropical climates
- SLE

SIGNS AND SYMPTOMS

General

- Periorbital or pretibial edema
- Changes in eye grounds
- Uremic odor to the breath
- Pleural or pericardial friction rubs
- Ascites
- Costovertebral angle tenderness
- Joint swelling or tenderness
- Vasculitic rashes
- Hematuria, microscopic or macroscopic
- Proteinuria
  - Proteinuria can range from mild to nephrotic range.
  - The finding of hematuria and proteinuria together strongly suggests underlying glomerular inflammation.
- Erythrocyte casts in the urine

Acute glomerulonephritis

- Abrupt onset of:
  - Hematuria
    - Often grossly visible as tea-colored or cola-colored urine
    - May be microscopic only
    - Erythrocyte casts and dysmorphic erythrocytes, although several urine samples may have to be examined
  - Proteinuria

- Hypertension
- Edema
- APSGN
  - Characteristically occurs:
    - 8–14 days after pharyngeal infection *or*
    - 14–21 days after a skin infection
  - Two-thirds of patients exhibit macroscopic hematuria.
  - Usually oliguria
  - Rarely, anuria
  - Edema that is usually periorbital and, rarely, severe
  - Signs of congestive heart failure
  - Hypertension
    - If severe, may produce headache, drowsiness, vomiting, personality and visual changes, and convulsions
  - Anorexia
  - Pain in the abdomen or flank are common, although palpation of the abdomen usually does not reveal significant findings.
  - Costovertebral angle tenderness

HSP nephritis

- Palpable purpuric lesions
- Arthritis
- Abdominal pain
- Gastrointestinal bleeding
- Not all manifestations need be present at the same time.

IgA nephropathy

- Characteristically, sudden onset of painless gross hematuria concomitant with an infection, usually of the respiratory tract
  - May be associated with flank pain
  - Usually clears within a few days to a week as the infection resolves
  - Frequently recurs with subsequent infections
  - Microscopic hematuria may persist with or without proteinuria between episodes.
  - Urine may clear totally.
- Some patients may have nephrotic syndrome or acute renal failure at presentation.

Benign familial hematuria

- Persistent asymptomatic microscopic hematuria in the absence of:
  - Hearing loss
  - Proteinuria
  - Progressive renal impairment

Alport syndrome

- Persistent microscopic hematuria is found early in all affected male patients.

N

- Most female patients have intermittent microscopic hematuria.
- Macroscopic hematuria is often seen at time of respiratory infection.
  - In up to 70% of male patients
  - In 33% of female patients
- Proteinuria in males; nephrotic range in approximately 30%
- Sensorineural hearing loss
  - Progressive starting with high frequencies
  - Affects male patients more than female patients
- Eye abnormalities in approximately 50% of patients
  - Anterior lenticonus
  - Retinal abnormalities
  - Corneal ulcerations
- Two-thirds of patients with the autosomal-recessive form develop hearing loss.
- Half the carriers of the abnormal gene also have microscopic hematuria.

SLE nephritis

- Initial symptoms may be vague; a high index of suspicion is warranted.
- Initially may have constitutional, cutaneous, or musculo-skeletal symptoms, such as:
  - Fever
  - Malaise
  - Rash
  - Arthritis
- Isolated hematuria
- Hematuria with proteinuria
- Nephrotic syndrome
- Hypertension
- Rapidly progressive renal failure

MPGN

- Hematuria in 60–100%
- Hypertension in 42–67%
- Decreased renal function in 17–50%
- Nephrotic syndrome in 50–67%
  - Some may not have significant hematuria.

DIFFERENTIAL DIAGNOSIS

- Nonstreptococcal glomerulonephritis
  - No effective way to differentiate from other nephritides that progress to renal failure, except observation of clinical course

- Glomerulonephritides with low complement levels
  - APSGN
    - Failure of complement levels to normalize by 8 weeks suggests another form of nephritis, such as MPGN, nephritis of chronic infection, or SLE nephritis.
  - SLE nephritis
  - MPGN
  - Nephritis of chronic infection
  - Cryoglobulinemia
- RPGN with immune complex
  - Postinfectious reaction
    - Streptococcal infection
    - Visceral abscess
    - Other
  - Collagen-vascular disease
    - SLE
    - HSP
    - Mixed cryoglobulinemia
  - Primary renal disease
    - IgA nephropathy
    - MPGN
    - Unknown cases (ie, idiopathic)
- RPGN with no immune deposit
  - Unknown cause
  - Vasculitis
    - Microscopic polyangiitis
    - Wegener granulomatosis
    - Hypersensitivity vasculitides
  - Hemolytic-uremic syndrome
- RPGN with anti–glomerular basement membrane antibody
  - With lung hemorrhage (Goodpasture syndrome)
  - Without lung hemorrhage
  - Complicating membranous nephropathy
- Acute glomerulonephritides characterized by no or mild renal failure
  - More common
    - APSGN
    - HSP with nephritis
      - IgA nephropathy is difficult to differentiate morpho-logically from HSP.
      - Has led to speculation that HSP is a form of IgA nephropathy with systemic findings
    - Postinfectious (nonstreptococcal) glomerulonephritis
    - Interstitial glomerulonephritis
    - Radiation nephritis

- Less common
  - Acute episodes in patients with chronic glomerulonephritis
  - Hemolytic-uremic syndrome (milder cases)
  - MPGN (some)
  - SLE nephritis (some)
- Only a family history of lack of progressive renal impairment, deafness, and eye findings distinguishes benign familial hematuria from early Alport syndrome.
- IgA nephropathy
  - Simultaneous onset of upper respiratory tract infection with gross hematuria helps differentiate this from APSGN, in which delay between infection and hematuria is the rule.
  - Absence of a rash, abdominal pain, and arthritis helps differentiate from HSP nephritis.

DIAGNOSTIC APPROACH

- If nephritis is suspected:
  - Blood pressure should be monitored carefully and frequently and compared with normal values for sex, age, and height percentile.
  - Weight should be measured.
    - Significant weight gain might suggest fluid retention.
  - Poor growth with crossing height percentiles with inappropriate weight gain or loss might suggest a chronic renal disorder.
- Follow up with appropriate laboratory, imaging, and biopsy studies.

LABORATORY FINDINGS

General

- Initial laboratory evaluation should include:
  - Urinalysis with microscopy
  - Serum electrolytes
  - Blood urea nitrogen
  - Creatinine
  - Calcium
  - Phosphorous
  - Albumin
  - Liver enzymes
  - Complete blood count with platelets
  - Complement levels
    - Decreased levels of the third component of complement (C3) and on occasion, fourth component (C4) can help narrow the differential diagnosis by distinguishing the hypocomplementemic nephritides from those with normal complement levels.
  - Antinuclear antibody

- Antistreptolysin O or other antibodies to streptococcal antigens
- For SLE nephritis, Wegener granulomatosis, microscopic polyangiitis, and some cases of membranoproliferative glomerulonephritis or membranous nephropathy:
  - Anti–double-stranded DNA
  - Antineutrophil cytoplasmic antibodies
  - Hepatitis B and C serologic tests
- Urine culture should be obtained if unclear diagnosis versus pyelonephritis

Acute glomerulonephritis

- Leukocytes on microscopy and positive test for leukocyte esterase are often found and suggest inflammation.

APSGN

- Urine usually tea colored and opaque
- Urine specific gravity generally increased
- Proteinuria
  - Usually parallels degree of hematuria
  - Rarely reaches the nephrotic range (>40 mg/m^2 per hour or >3.5 g/day in older children and adults)
- Microscopic urine examination
  - Usually reveals erythrocytes and leukocytes, and granular or cellular casts
  - Identifiable erythrocyte casts and dysmorphic erythrocytes may or may not be present, so serial urine specimens may need to be examined.
- Serum complement levels
  - Reduced C3 in 80% of patients
  - Early in the course, reduced C4 in 50%
- Erythrocyte sedimentation rate usually elevated
- In severe oliguria, azotemia and acidosis may be seen.
- Plasma volume usually expanded, causing decrease in serum protein, hemoglobin, and hematocrit
- Antistreptolysin O titer
  - Elevated in 80% of patients
  - Increases in titer are less common in patients who have skin infection or who receive early treatment with antibiotics.
- Other streptococcal antibodies (antihyaluronidase, antideoxyribonuclease B) are present in 80–90% of patients.

IgA nephropathy

- Findings are often normal except for abnormal urinalysis

Benign familial hematuria

- All laboratory results usually normal except for urinalysis
- Presence of hematuria in otherwise asymptomatic family members suggests the diagnosis.

N

Alport syndrome

- Laboratory findings:
  - Reflect degree of renal impairment
  - May vary from normal early on to advanced renal failure as disease progresses
- Blood urea nitrogen and creatinine levels become elevated with advancing disease.
- Serum electrolytes may become abnormal.
- Hypoalbuminemia may occur in some patients who develop nephrotic syndrome.
- Serum complement level is usually normal.

SLE nephritis

- Antinuclear antibodies positive in most
- Anti–double-stranded DNA positive in many patients with renal involvement
- Serum complement components frequently decreased
- Renal disease may be characterized by:
  - Elevation of serum urea and creatinine levels
  - Decrease in serum albumin levels in the setting of nephrotic-range proteinuria
- Findings on urinalysis vary greatly.
  - Isolated hematuria
  - Hematuria with proteinuria
  - Nephrotic-range proteinuria
- Pyuria reflects the underlying glomerular inflammation.
- Erythrocyte, leukocyte, and renal tubular epithelial cell casts frequently seen
- Coombs-positive anemia
- Leukopenia
- Thrombocytopenia
- Antiphospholipid antibodies; risk factor for thrombotic complications

MPGN

- Serum C3 is depressed in 67–75% of patients.
- Blood urea nitrogen and creatinine values may be elevated.
- Albumin level may be low in severe cases.
- Anemia is common.
- Electrolyte disturbances if renal insufficiency is present
  - Urinalysis most commonly shows both hematuria and proteinuria.
    - Proteinuria may reach the nephrotic range.
    - Hematuria may be macroscopic.
    - Cellular casts are a common finding.

Interstitial nephritis

- Peripheral eosinophilia may or may not be seen.
- If present, urinary eosinophils are demonstrated on Hansel stain.

IMAGING

- APSGN
  - Chest radiography in patients with significant fluid retention and hypertension may reveal:
    - A large heart with prominent pulmonary vasculature
    - Pulmonary edema
    - Rarely, pleural effusions
  - Ultrasonography is nonspecific, usually revealing bilaterally enlarged echogenic kidneys.

DIAGNOSTIC PROCEDURES

- Alport syndrome
  - Renal biopsy may help establish diagnosis if family history is unclear or in patient with a new mutation.
- RPGN
  - Although characteristic clinical and laboratory features may suggest specific causative factors, renal biopsy often is indicated to diagnose and to determine extent of disease.
- Interstitial nephritis
  - Renal biopsy is often necessary to confirm the diagnosis.

SPECIFIC TREATMENTS

APSGN

- Most often resolves spontaneously
  - Must be aggressive in treating symptoms that ocurr in the acute phase of the illness
    - Hypertension
      - Mild hypertension may resolve spontaneously.
      - More severe hypertension should be controlled with quick-acting antihypertensive agents.
    - Oliguria and resulting vascular overload
      - Diuretics
    - Pulmonary edema
    - Encephalopathy
  - Control of severe hypertension often requires either:
    - Intravenous sodium nitroprusside
    - Labetalol
    - Nicardipine
    - Fenoldopam
    - Oral minoxidil
    - Slower-acting, less potent antihypertensive drugs are not good initially but can be substituted once blood pressure has been acutely stabilized.
  - Occasionally, a patient develops acute renal failure severe enough to require dialysis.
  - A 10-day course of antibiotics is usually given to eradicate any remaining group A ß-hemolytic streptococci and prevent transmission of the organism.

- Close contacts should be screened for streptococcal infection and treated if present.

RPGN

- Treatment depends on particular diagnosis, which is often determined by kidney biopsy.
- Plasmapheresis may be helpful in resistant forms of RPGN.
  - Anti-glomerular basement membrane antibody disease
  - Atypical forms of hemolytic-uremic syndrome
  - Thrombotic thrombocytopenic purpura

Other

- Fulminant SLE nephritis, MPGN, IgA nephropathy, HSP nephritis
  - Methylprednisolone pulses frequently are given initially, followed by oral or intravenous alkylating agents.
- IgA nephropathy
  - Suggested regimens for poor prognostic indicators
    - Long-term, alternate-day prednisone, with or without methylprednisolone pulses
    - Mycophenolate mofetil
  - Control of hypertension is essential
- Benign familial hematuria
  - No treatment is indicated.
- Alport syndrome
  - Treatment is supportive, with medical management of hypertension and complications of renal insufficiency.
  - Dialysis or transplantation is instituted when medical management is no longer sufficient.
  - Audiologic screening can identify hearing impairment early for timely implementation of hearing-augmentation services.
- SLE nephritis
  - High-dose corticosteroid therapy is the mainstay of treatment but is associated with considerable morbidity.
    - Pulse methylprednisolone is used to treat rapidly progressive lupus glomerulonephritis.
  - Oral or pulse intravenous cyclophosphamide frequently is recommended for treatment of World Health Organization class III, IV, and sometimes V renal disease.
  - Azathioprine and mycophenolic acid have been used as steroid-sparing agents.
    - Mycophenolic acid may allow decreasing exposure to, or even substitute for, cyclophosphamide, thus preventing significant side effects, particularly on fertility.
  - Cyclosporine
    - Variable results
    - Renal biopsy should be performed before therapy is begun.
    - Patients are managed best by a team trained in dealing with all aspects of this disease.

- MPGN
  - Treatment is controversial.
  - High-dose, long-term, alternate-day prednisone therapy showed renal survival of 82% at 10 years and 56% at 20 years.
  - Some differences in clinical course and response to treatment may be seen according to the type of MPGN.

WHEN TO ADMIT

- Severe hypertension
- Renal failure with significant electrolyte disturbances
- Congestive heart failure from volume overload
- Oliguria or anuria
- Rapidly progressive renal failure

WHEN TO REFER

- Acute glomerulonephritis with significant complications
- Acute glomerulonephritis that is not following a typical course expected of APSGN
- Failure of complement level to normalize within 6–8 weeks in suspected acute glomerulonephritis
- Rapidly progressive course
- Glomerulonephritis with the development of nephrotic syndrome
- Persistent hematuria and proteinuria
- Persistent hypertension
- Elevated creatinine level for age
- Family history of renal failure or deafness
- Any chronic glomerulonephritis

PROGNOSIS

- APSGN
  - Nephrotic-range proteinuria or extensive crescents by biopsy portend a poor prognosis.
  - >95% of children recover.
  - For most children, the critical period is early in the illness, when potentially fatal hypertension or fluid overload presents a danger.
  - Some patients with severe involvement, evidenced by nephrotic-range proteinuria or the presence of extensive glomerular crescents on biopsy, have some residual damage or may progress to end-stage renal failure.
  - Recurrences of APSGN are rare.
- IgA nephropathy
  - 10–30% are anticipated to progress to renal failure over the course of several decades.
  - Progression is related to:
    - Higher amounts of proteinuria
    - Presence of hypertension

N

- Renal insufficiency at presentation
- Severity of histologic changes found on kidney biopsy

■ Alport syndrome

- Renal disease and hearing loss are progressive.
- Families carrying large DNA deletions or stop codons leading to truncated proteins may be at risk for more severe disease than those with mutations leading to an amino acid substitution.
- 3–4% of patients receiving a kidney transplant develop anti-glomerular basement membrane nephritis, leading to loss of the transplanted kidney in 75% of cases.

■ SLE nephritis

- Renal survival in childhood lupus nephritis ranges from 29–71% at 10 years.
- Patients with World Health Organization class IV diffuse proliferative glomerulonephritis have the poorest renal outcome.
- Predictors of poor renal prognosis
  - Sclerosis on biopsy specimens
  - Hypocomplementemia
  - Decreased renal function
  - Nephrotic-range proteinuria
  - Persistent hypertension

■ MPGN

- 50% reach end-stage renal failure within approximately 11 years of diagnosis.
- 90% reach end-stage within 20 years.
- Poor prognostic indicators
  - Nephrotic-range proteinuria
  - Renal insufficiency
  - Hypertension
  - Sclerosis on biopsy examination
- Type 1 MPGN has a better prognosis than the other 2 types.

■ Interstitial nephritis

- The combination of interstitial nephritis with severe glomerulonephritis has a much more guarded prognosis, since combined involvement reflects greater severity of renal disease.
- Interstitial inflammation tends to heal by fibrosis, damaging segments of the remaining kidney.

N

Nephrotic Syndrome

DEFINITION

- Syndrome with clinical findings of:
  - Heavy proteinuria
  - Hypoalbuminemia
  - Edema (often frank anasarca)
  - Hyperlipidemia
- Nephrotic syndrome may result from underlying systemic disease or manifest as a primary idiopathic renal disorder.

EPIDEMIOLOGY

- Incidence
  - Idiopathic nephrotic syndrome in children seen in 2–7 cases per 100,000 children annually
- Sex
  - 2:1 ratio of male to female children
  - Affects male to female adolescents and adults equally
- Children 3 months to 16 years
  - 76% have minimal change nephrotic syndrome (MCNS).
    - Occurrence peaks between 2 and 5 years of age.
  - 7–25% have focal segmental glomerulosclerosis (FSGS).
  - 2–5% have diffuse mesangial hypercellularity or mesangial proliferation.
  - 7% have membranoproliferative glomerulonephritis (MPGN).
  - 1% have membranous nephropathy.
  - Adolescents are more likely than younger children to have a more aggressive cause, such as FSGS, MPGN, or membranous nephropathy.
- Race
  - Black and Hispanic adolescents are more likely than white adolescents to have FSGS and to progress to end-stage renal disease.
  - In a predominantly black and Hispanic population of nephrotic adolescents:
    - 55% had FSGS.
    - 20% had MCNS.
    - 7% had MPGN.

ETIOLOGY

- Filtration barriers are variably altered, depending on the severity and nature of the underlying disease process.
  - Examples of alterations in the filtration barrier include:
    - Loss of negative charge seen in MCNS
    - Altered organization of glomerular basement membrane components in Alport syndrome
    - Mutations of genes encoding proteins associated with glomerular podocytes
- Changes in barriers allow passage of large quantities of plasma proteins into the urine, which may lead to a decrease of proteins in the blood.

- Development of edema has been explained by massive loss of plasma proteins, in particular albumin, in the urine.
  - Development of hypoalbuminemia leads to decreased plasma oncotic pressure and leakage of fluid from the vascular space into the interstitium.
  - Subsequent decrease in circulating blood volume
    - Stimulates the renin-angiotensin-aldosterone system
    - Leads to avid sodium retention
    - Produces a nonosmotic stimulus for vasopressin secretion and free-water reabsorption
  - This scenario does not explain edema formation in all nephrotic patients.
    - In patients who experience remission, diuresis often begins as proteinuria is resolving but before plasma albumin levels normalize.
    - Primary sodium retention has been demonstrated with onset of proteinuria (but before development of hypoproteinemia) in some experiencing relapse.
    - Would lead to expansion of vascular volume and development of edema

RISK FACTORS

- Disease processes associated with FSGS lesions
  - Diabetic nephropathy
  - Sickle cell disease
  - HIV nephropathy
  - Glomerulonephritides
    - IgA nephropathy
    - MPGN
    - Lupus nephritis

DIAGNOSIS

SIGNS AND SYMPTOMS

- Gradual or more acute edema and inappropriate weight gain
  - Periorbital edema when arising in the morning
    - Resolves during the day
    - Often mistaken for allergy
  - Clothing may be tight.
  - Socks may leave indentations in the skin of shins and ankles.
- The abdomen may be distended, and a fluid wave may be discernible on examination.
- Breath sounds may be decreased at lung bases due to accumulation of pleural fluid.
- May see:
  - Gallop on auscultation of the heart
  - Rales over the lung fields
  - Hepatomegaly

- Boys may develop significant scrotal swelling.
- Girls may develop labial swelling.
- Decreased frequency of urination
  - Dark, amber-colored, concentrated-appearing urine
  - Urine appears to foam when voided.
- Hypertension (in 16%)
  - Marked hypertension suggests underlying glomerulonephritis.
- Specific changes due to nephrotic syndrome
  - MCNS, also known as *lipoid nephrosis* or *nil disease,* is the most common pathologic diagnosis in nephrotic children.
    - Hematuria in approximately 13%
    - Hypertension in 10–20%
    - Relapses are common, but long-term prognosis is excellent.
  - Membranous nephropathy
    - Rare in children and adolescents (1% of children with nephrotic syndrome)
    - Spontaneous remissions occur in most, but remission may not occur for several years.
    - 13% of affected children progress to end-stage renal failure.

DIFFERENTIAL DIAGNOSIS

- Causes of primary nephrotic syndrome
  - MCNS
  - FSGS
  - Mesangial hypercellularity
  - MPGN
  - Membranous nephropathy
- Causes of secondary nephrotic syndrome
  - Inherited diseases
    - Congenital nephrotic syndrome (see below)
    - Diffuse mesangial sclerosis
    - Alport syndrome
    - Nail-patella syndrome
    - Lowe syndrome
  - Vasculitides
    - Lupus nephritis
    - Henoch-Schönlein purpura nephritis
    - Wegener granulomatosis
    - Goodpasture syndrome
  - Postinfectious
    - Poststreptococcal
    - HIV
    - Hepatitis B and C
    - Malaria

- Syphilis
- Intrauterine infections
- Other viruses and bacteria
  - Drugs and toxins
    - Nonsteroidal antiinflammatory drugs
    - Gold
  - Diabetes mellitus (rare in children)
- Mutations of certain genes are implicated in the development of hereditary forms of the nephrotic syndrome.
  - Congenital nephrotic syndrome presents in the first 3 months of life.
    - Finnish type is an autosomal-recessive disorder caused by mutations in the *NPHS1* gene encoding nephrin, or the *NPHS2* gene encoding podocin (podocyte membrane protein).
  - Diffuse mesangial sclerosis
    - May be part of Denys-Drash syndrome
    - Onset in first months of life with rapid progression to end-stage kidney failure, male pseudohermaphroditism, and Wilms tumor
    - Associated with mutations of the *WT1* gene
  - Podocin mutations
    - Some are associated with a steroid-resistant, autosomal-recessive form of FSGS in older children with a rapid progression to renal failure.
    - Mutations in the *ACTN4* gene encoding a-actinin result in an autosomal-dominant form of FSGS, with onset during early childhood and slow progression to renal failure.

LABORATORY FINDINGS

- Urinalysis is the first test to be done in a child with edema.
  - Significant proteinuria
- Significant microscopic hematuria or gross hematuria
  - Up to 25% of children with primary nephrotic syndrome will have 3–5 erythrocytes per high-power field.
  - Glycosuria suggests underlying tubular injury and may be seen with FSGS.
- Blood urea nitrogen and creatinine values are generally normal or only slightly increased in primary nephrotic syndrome.
- Serum total protein and albumin levels are low.
- Mild hyponatremia may be present
- Total calcium levels are low; ionized calcium levels are usually normal.
- Serum cholesterol level is usually increased.
- Third component of complement (C3) is generally normal.
  - A low level suggests MPGN, poststreptococcal glomerulonephritis, or lupus nephritis.

- Tests to quantify urinary protein losses
  - 24-hour urine collection
    - Nephrotic-range proteinuria = urinary protein excretion >40 mg/m^2 per hour or 1 g/m^2 per day in children
  - In incontinent children, urine protein-to-creatinine ratio on a random urine sample
    - Ratio (mg/mg) >2:1 on a random urine sample is considered nephrotic.
  - Urinary protein quantification is helpful for monitoring the response to treatment of children with resistant forms of nephrotic syndrome.

IMAGING

- Chest radiography
  - Usually shows small cardiac silhouette and, in severe cases, pleural fluid
  - Cardiomegaly may be seen in patients with increased intravascular volume.

TREATMENT APPROACH

- Clinical response to corticosteroids is informative in determining long-term outcome.
  - 85% respond to a trial of prednisone.
    - 75% respond within 2 weeks of initiating therapy.
    - 94% respond by 4 weeks.
  - Biopsy findings do not predict which children with MCNS will be corticosteroid resistant or which with FSGS will be responsive.
  - Patients who achieve remission on steroids (whether they have MCNS or FSGS) do not progress to renal failure if they remain responsive to corticosteroid therapy.
- Children age 1–6 years (most likely to have MCNS) with new onset of typical, pure nephrotic syndrome should be given a trial of corticosteroids.
  - Depending on the treatment regimen, 36–61% of children will have a relapse within first year of initial episode.
    - Relapse = urine tests ≥2+ for protein on 3 consecutive days
    - Relapses are usually triggered by intercurrent illnesses or allergies.
    - Parents can be taught to use albumin test sticks or sulfosalicylic acid at home to monitor urinary protein excretion.
- Children who have relapse while corticosteroids are being tapered or within 2 weeks of completing a course of corticosteroids are considered corticosteroid dependent and may develop toxicity.
  - Second-tier therapies for difficult cases should be discussed with a pediatric nephrologist.

- Children who fail to respond to initial or subsequent courses of corticosteroids have corticosteroid-resistant nephrotic syndrome and a more guarded prognosis.
  - Consult with a pediatric nephrologist for consideration of a renal biopsy and more aggressive treatment.
- Salt intake should be restricted in edematous children.
- Water intake should be restricted only if:
  - Significant hyponatremia develops.
  - Edema is intractable.
- Diuretics should be used judiciously.
- Treatment of membranous nephropathy is controversial.
  - High rate of spontaneous remission
  - Consider treatment with high-dose corticosteroids (oral or intravenous), alone or combined with cytotoxic agents, if the patient has:
    - Renal insufficiency
    - Persistent heavy proteinuria
    - Hypertension
    - Sclerosis on biopsy
- Treatment for congenital nephrotic syndrome
  - Supportive, but must be aggressive
  - Until kidney transplantation can be done, treatment may include:
    - Intensive nutritional support
    - Nephrectomy
    - Maintenance on dialysis

SPECIFIC TREATMENTS

Corticosteroids

- Prednisone, 2 mg/kg daily or 60 mg/m^2 daily (maximum, 60–80 mg/day) for 4–6 weeks
  - Usually given in divided doses
  - Can also be given as a single morning dose
    - Followed by single dose of 1.3 mg/kg or 40 mg/m^2 for an additional 4–6 weeks given in the morning on alternate days
  - Decreased frequency of relapses in the first year and a lower total steroid dose if:
    - Daily prednisone is given initially for 6 weeks
    - Followed by 6 weeks of alternate-day prednisone
    - Tapered off over an additional 4 weeks
- Treatment of relapse
  - Prednisone, 2 mg/kg daily or 60 mg/m^2 daily until urine is free of protein for 3 consecutive days
  - Dose then changed to 40 mg/m^2 on alternate days for 4 weeks
  - Tapered off over an additional 4 weeks

N

- Complications of corticosteroid therapy
  - Development of cushingoid features
  - Cataract formation
  - Glaucoma
  - Gastritis
  - Peptic ulcer disease
  - Pancreatitis
  - Hypokalemia
  - Hypertension
  - Increased risk of infection
  - Behavioral changes
  - Growth delay if treatment is prolonged

Other pharmacologic agents

- Angiotensin-converting enzyme inhibitors or angiotensin-receptor blockers
  - Can be tried in resistant nephrotic syndrome, even in the presence of normotension
  - High doses of angiotensin-converting enzyme inhibitors may decrease progressive sclerosis.
- Diuretics
  - Furosemide, alone or in combination with a thiazide diuretic, is used to treat clinically significant edema.
  - Intravenous albumin followed by intravenous furosemide when edema is severe:
    - Interferes with ambulation
    - Compromises respiratory status
    - Causes tissue breakdown
  - Renal function and urine output are fairly well maintained.
  - Patients must be monitored closely during infusion for signs of intravascular overload.
    - Rales
    - Cardiac gallop
    - Hepatomegaly
  - Treatment can be used in the severely edematous, corticosteroid-resistant nephrotic patient in whom cyclosporine therapy is being considered for improvement of renal perfusion and prevention of acute renal failure.

Secondary/tertiary/complementary treatment for difficult cases

- Cyclophosphamide, chlorambucil
  - Can induce prolonged remission
- Intravenous nitrogen mustard
  - Can be considered in noncompliant patients
- Cyclosporine or tacrolimus
  - Can be used as a corticosteroid-sparing agent in patients who do not respond to an alkylating agent

- Can cause acute and chronic renal injury
  - Acute renal failure can occur in severely nephrotic patients on cyclosporine who have markedly decreased intravascular volume.
- Methylprednisolone infusions
- Levamisole
  - Has been used to decrease corticosteroid doses in patients who experience frequent relapse
- Mycophenolate mofetil
  - Some success as a corticosteroid-sparing agent
  - Side effects include:
    - Bone marrow suppression
    - Gastrointestinal upset
- Angiotensin-converting enzyme inhibitors
- Angiotensin-receptor blockers
- Nonsteroidal antiinflammatory drugs
  - Used to decrease proteinuria in resistant nephrotic syndrome
  - Can lead to acute renal failure in children with significantly decreased intravascular volume
  - Can cause salt retention and edema
  - Risk of renal failure, especially in patients with decreased intravascular volume
- Complications of cytotoxic agents (eg, cyclophosphamide, chlorambucil, nitrogen mustard)
  - Increased risk of infection
  - Cancer
  - Sterility
    - With higher doses than those typically used for nephrotic syndrome
    - After repeated or prolonged courses
  - Hemorrhagic cystitis (cyclophosphamide)
    - Encourage large fluid intake and frequent voiding.
  - Induction of seizures (chlorambucil)

WHEN TO ADMIT

- Initial episode for teaching of parents, especially if complications are present
- Anasarca interfering with ambulation or compromising ventilation
- Pleural effusions or ascites interfering with ventilation
- Signs of volume overload (congestive heart failure)
- Infection (eg, severe cellulitis, peritonitis)
- Significant hypertension
- Significant electrolyte abnormalities
- Compromised renal function
  - May require dialysis to manage edema, electrolyte disturbances, and uremia

N

WHEN TO REFER

- Complicated nephrotic syndrome
- Outside the expected age range (<1 year or >10 years of age)
- Accompanied by signs of glomerulonephritis (renal insufficiency, hypertension, hematuria, hypocomplementemia)
- Refractory edema
- Frequently relapsing nephrotic syndrome
- Corticosteroid-dependent nephrotic syndrome
- Corticosteroid-resistant nephrotic syndrome

COMPLICATIONS

- Infections
  - Spontaneous bacterial peritonitis
  - Sepsis
  - Cellulitis
  - Pneumonia
    - Children with recurrent nephrotic syndrome should receive multivalent pneumococcal vaccination.
  - *Staphylococcus pneumoniae* and gram-negative bacteria are responsible for most infections in nephrotic syndrome.
  - Predisposing factors for the development of bacterial infections
    - Tissue edema
    - Immunosuppressive therapies
- Thromboembolism
  - Deep-vein thrombosis
  - Pulmonary embolism
  - Renal-vein thrombosis
  - Arterial thrombosis
  - Contributory factors include:
    - Increased plasma levels of procoagulant factors
    - Urinary loss of inhibitors of coagulation
    - Thrombocytosis
  - Predisposition to thrombus formation may be exacerbated by decreased intravascular volume, especially in the face of vigorous forced diuresis.
- Hyperlipidemia
  - In unremitting nephrotic syndrome, increased plasma lipids may contribute to cardiovascular morbidity; treatment of lipid abnormalities should be considered.

PROGNOSIS

- Approximately 25% of children who have relapse follow a frequently relapsing course, ie, either:
  - 2 relapses within 6 months of completing a course of corticosteroids *or*
  - 3 relapses within 1 year
- Prognosis of congenital nephrotic syndrome
  - Depends on the underlying cause
  - Guarded for congenital nephrotic syndrome of the Finnish type, with significant morbidity and mortality from complications
    - Malnutrition
    - Infection
    - Thrombotic events caused by massive protein losses
- Membranous nephropathy, poor prognostic factors
  - Persistent heavy proteinuria (>8 g/day for >6 months)
  - Hypertension
  - Increased creatinine
  - Significant scarring on biopsy

N

Nervousness

DEFINITION

- Feelings, such as anxiety or nervous stomach, that occur as symptoms without any readily discernible underlying pathophysiologic abnormality
- Nonspecific symptoms may be associated with another condition, eg:
  - Anorexia
  - Restlessness at night
  - Sluggishness
  - Overactivity
- A physical problem, with a variety of possible causes, is implied but often not at the root of the complaint.

MECHANISM

- Nervousness may have a physical cause.
  - Caffeine consumption
  - Endocrine disorder
  - Allergy
- Nervousness may result from:
  - Emotional distress
  - Psychological distress

HISTORY

- Complete history and thorough physical examination are needed.
  - The problem is difficult to define; thus adequate time is more important than urgency for:
    - Complete history
    - Thorough physical examination
    - Discussion of the problem in depth
- Ask what accompanies the nervousness.
  - Anorexia
  - Restlessness at night
  - Sluggishness
  - Overactivity
- Inquire about:
  - Caffeine ingestion (colas and coffee)
  - Use of drugs
- Evaluate concomitant findings that may indicate:
  - Attention-deficit disorder with or without hyperactivity
  - Anxiety disorder, such as separation anxiety or school phobia
  - Somatization of depression
  - Autism*
  - Childhood psychoses*
  - Obsessive-compulsive and manic-depressive disorders*
  - Panic attacks*
  - Tourette syndrome*

- More serious psychiatric problems, denoted with an asterisk (*), are rarely defined by families as nervousness alone.

PHYSICAL EXAM

- Even if the patient has no physical disorder, other problems may be evident.
  - Emotional tension
  - Restlessness, agitation
  - Fearful apprehension
  - Acute uneasiness
  - Undue excitability
  - Excessive irritability

DIFFERENTIAL DIAGNOSIS

- Nervousness is often part of the constellation of symptoms from:
  - Endocrine disorders
    - Hyperthyroidism
    - Hypoglycemia
    - Addison disease
  - Disorders associated with pruritus
    - Dermatitis
    - Pinworm infestation
    - Allergy
  - Disorders associated with palpitations
    - Mitral valve prolapse
    - Paroxysmal tachycardia

LABORATORY EVALUATION

- Laboratory investigations need to rule out conditions that cause nervousness.
  - Hyperthyroidism
  - Hypoglycemia
  - Addison disease
  - Pinworm infestation
  - Allergy
  - Mitral valve prolapse
  - Paroxysmal tachycardia

TREATMENT APPROACH

- If a conscientious search for biopsychosocial cause is unsuccessful, nervousness becomes even more difficult to manage.
- If the physician cannot provide the necessary time and effort, refer the patient to ease the morbidity associated with symptoms.

WHEN TO REFER

- Persistent, recurrent symptoms unresponsive to repeated physician reassurance
- Unremitting symptoms that interfere with family, school, and social functioning

Neurocutaneous Syndromes

DEFINITION

- A heterogeneous group of conditions in which abnormalities of skin and nervous system predominate
- Prototypical neurocutaneous conditions
  - Neurofibromatosis
  - Tuberous sclerosis
  - Von Hippel-Lindau disease
- Several other genetic or developmental anomaly syndromes share the phenotypic association of cutaneous and neurologic abnormalities.
  - Sturge-Weber syndrome
  - Ataxia-telangiectasia
  - Incontinentia pigmenti
  - Hypomelanosis of Ito
  - Epidermal nevus syndromes
- Neurofibromatosis (NF) is divided into 7 types.
  - NF-1 and NF-2 are different conditions with only minimal overlap.
    - Both are autosomal-dominant disorders with high penetrance but variable phenotypic expression.
  - NF-1 (von Recklinghausen disease)
  - A complex disorder with neurologic, cutaneous, skeletal, vascular, and endocrinologic abnormalities
    - Neurofibromas are benign tumors that:
      - Appear in late childhood
      - Grow in response to hormonal changes
      - Proliferate with age
      - May compromise local function by mass effect
  - NF-2
    - A tumor syndrome defined by the presence of bilateral vestibular schwannomas
    - Also known as *multiple inherited schwannomas, meningiomas,* and *ependymoma syndrome*
  - NF-3 (mixed) and NF-4 (variant)
    - Autosomal dominant
    - Resemble NF-2
    - More cutaneous NFs
    - Greater risk of optic gliomas, neurilemmoma, meningiomas
  - NF-5 (segmental)
    - Skin lesions are located on a single body segment (eg, leg)
    - Somatic mosaicism
  - NF-6
    - Café-au-lait macules (CALMs)
    - CALM is only disease manifestation
    - Requires 2 generations to diagnose
  - NF-7
    - Late-onset
    - Symptoms manifest in the 20s
    - Not known whether it is heritable
- Tuberous sclerosis complex (TSC), or Bourneville disease
  - Autosomal dominant multisystem disorder
  - Characterized by perturbed cellular growth and differentiation in the brain, heart, kidneys, skin, eyes, and other tissues
- Sturge-Weber syndrome (SWS), or encephalotrigeminal angiomatosis
  - Rare sporadic disorder
  - Characterized by:
    - Upper facial port wine stain (PWS)
    - Ipsilateral ocular abnormalities
    - Ipsilateral leptomeningeal angiomatosis
  - Only 1 or 2 of the triad features may be present.
  - Leptomeningeal involvement is defining element.
- Von Hippel-Lindau disease (VHL) is an autosomal-dominant multiorgan familial cancer syndrome.
  - Subtype 1
    - High risk for hemangioblastoma, renal cell carcinoma, pancreatic cyst or tumor
    - Low risk for pheochromocytoma
  - Subtype 2a
    - High risk for hemangioblastoma, pheochromocytoma
    - Low risk for renal cell carcinoma, pancreatic cyst or tumor
  - Subtype 2b
    - High risk for hemangioblastoma, renal cell carcinoma, pheochromocytoma, pancreatic cyst or tumor
  - Subtype 2c
    - High risk for pheochromocytoma
    - Low risk for hemangioblastoma, renal cell carcinoma, pancreatic cyst or tumor
- Ataxia-telangiectasia (A-T), or Louis-Bar syndrome
  - Autosomal-recessive progressive neurodegenerative disorder

EPIDEMIOLOGY

- NF
  - Prevalence
    - NF-1 occurs in ~1 in 3500.
    - NF-2 occurs in ~1 in 40,000.
    - No race or gender predilection has been found.
    - Approximately one-half of cases of each condition represent new mutations.

- Age
  - NF-2
    - Average age at onset of symptoms is ~20 years.
    - Average age at diagnosis is 28 years.
    - 18% of patients show symptoms before age 15 years.
- TSC
  - Prevalence
    - Approximately 1 in 6000
- SWS
  - Prevalence
    - ~1 in 50,000 live births
  - No gender predilection has been found.
- VHL
  - Prevalence
    - 1 in 40,000 live births
  - Inherited in 80% of patients; 20% represent new mutations.
  - >90% penetrance by age 65 years
- A-T
  - Prevalence
    - 1 in 40,000 in the US
    - 1 in 300,000 in the UK

ETIOLOGY

- NF-1
  - Loss of function mutation in the neurofibromin tumor suppressor gene is thought to be responsible for most clinical features.
- NF-2
  - Precise mechanism of tumor formation is uncertain.
- TSC
  - Results from mutations in 1 of 2 genes:
    - *TSC1* encodes hamartin.
    - *TSC2* encodes tuberin.
  - Mutations of *TSC1* are more common in familial cases.
    - Seem to result in less severe disease
- SWS
  - Thought to result from:
    - Failed regression of the cephalic venous plexus
  - Only a few case reports have suggested familial occurrence.
  - Appears to result from somatic mosaicism
    - Supported by discordance between monozygotic twins
- VHL
  - Almost all patients with VHL have germ-line mutations in the VHL gene (found on chromosome 3) and secondary somatic mutations (Knudson's 2-hit hypothesis)

- Subdivided into 2 major categories based on the type of mutation
  - Type 1 disease: mutations are premature termination mutations or deletions, not associated with significant risk for pheochromocytoma.
  - Type 2 disease: characterized by missense mutations; pheochromocytoma is a predominant tumor in type 2 disease.
- A-T
  - Caused by mutations in the *ATM* (A-T, mutated) gene
  - Loss of *ATM* function leads to:
    - Accumulation of defective DNA
    - Inability to repair or eliminate genetically defective cells
  - Defective DNA repair explains the sensitivity to ionizing radiation.
  - Inability to remove damaged cells has been postulated as a cause of many of the diverse abnormalities in A-T.
  - Cancer has been linked to genomic instability.

SIGNS AND SYMPTOMS

NF-1

- Characteristic lesion is the neurofibroma.
  - Proliferation of Schwann cells and fibroblasts
- Small neurofibromas appear as:
  - Pink to flesh color to brown papules
  - Soft, spongy texture (see Figure 42 on page F17)
  - Gentle downward pressure can cause these lesions to sink through the underlying dermis and create a dimple (see Figure 43 on page F18).
- Size and number vary greatly.
- Slight predilection for trunk involvement, but neurofibromas can occur anywhere on the body.
- Plexiform type (seen in ~50% of patients)
  - Variant of neurofibroma
  - Can be large
  - Can cause considerable disfigurement
  - Highly variable masses
    - Sometimes soft and spongy in texture, other times feels like a bag of rope
  - May have surface hyperpigmentation or remain flesh-colored
  - Overlying skin
    - May be somewhat thickened
    - May exhibit increased hair growth
  - Often produce soft tissue masses
  - Figure 44 on page F18 shows plexiform neurofibroma on a breast.

- Earliest features often are CALMs.
  - Tan, oval macules
  - Smooth margins
  - No surface texture change
  - Remain flat
  - No increased hair growth
  - May vary in size and shape
  - May increase in number and size with age
  - Figure 45 on page F18 shows multiple CALMs on an infant, with coincidental gray Mongolian spot.

NF-2

- Characteristic vestibular schwannomas lead to progressive deterioration of hearing.
- Patients may develop:
  - Intracranial or spinal meningiomas
  - Ependymomas
  - Astrocytomas
  - Neurofibromas
  - Schwannomas of the cranial, spinal, and peripheral nerves
  - Cutaneous schwannomas (with minimal clinical impact)
- Ependymomas and astrocytomas are seen in up to 33% of patients.
- Peripheral schwannomas may arise from any nerve (see Figure 46 on page F18).
  - May produce pain or sensory or motor dysfunction
- Patients may develop peripheral neuropathy not related to tumor growth.
- Seizure disorders are uncommon.
- Cognitive impairment is not a feature.
- Ocular findings include:
  - Juvenile posterior subcapsular lens opacities
  - Retinal hamartomas
  - Cortical wedge opacities

TSC

General

- Classic triad includes:
  - Seizures
  - Intellectual disability
  - Facial angiofibromas
- Seizures and facial lesions occur frequently.
- Mental function often is normal or only slightly impaired.
  - ~50% of patients with TSC have normal intelligence.
  - ~30% have profound intellectual disability
- Hallmark of TSC is the development of hamartomas in the various organ systems involved.

- An international consensus conference in 1998 revised diagnostic criteria, based on new understanding of disease and its underlying pathophysiological features.
  - Major criteria
    - Facial angiofibroma or forehead plaque
    - Ungual or subungual fibroma
    - >3 hypomelanotic macules
    - Connective tissue nevus (Shagreen patch)
    - Cortical tuber
    - Subependymal nodule
    - Subependymal giant-cell astrocytoma
    - Multiple retinal hamartomas
    - Cardiac rhabdomyoma
    - Renal angiomyolipoma
    - Lymphangiomyomatosis
  - Minor criteria
    - Dental enamel pits
    - Hamartomatous rectal polyps
    - Bone cysts (radiographic evidence sufficient)
    - Cerebral white matter migration lines
    - Gingival fibromas
    - Retinal achromic patch
    - Nonrenal hamartomas
    - Multiple renal cysts
    - Confetti skin lesions
- Diagnosis for TSC
  - Definitive: 2 major, or 1 major + 2 minor criteria
  - Probable: 1 major criterion + plus 1 minor criterion
  - Possible: 1 major or ≥2 minor criteria
- TSC has no pathognomonic feature.
- Individual features may occur in isolation.
  - Primary care physician must consider the diagnosis of TSC only if:
    - >1 organ system is involved.
    - Different lesion types occur in a single system.
- Central nervous system manifestations (CNS) are the most common and often most disabling aspect of TSC.
- Neurologic features include:
  - Seizures
  - Cognitive disability
  - Behavioral disturbances

Seizures

- Occur in 80–90% of patients
- All types of seizures except classic absence seizures have been reported.

N

- Infantile spasms
  - Seen in approximately one-third of infants.
    - The presenting feature in 70% of cases
    - Thorough description of the clinical and electroencephalographic findings in infantile spasms is found in Seizure Disorders.
    - Children with infantile spasms are likely to have cognitive disability, corresponding to increased cortical hamartoma (tuber) burden.

Cognitive impairment

- Seizure onset and severity are closely associated with severity of cognitive impairment.
  - Early onset of seizures or infantile spasms is associated with poor cognitive outcome.
- Most patients with TSC and cognitive disability have epilepsy.
  - Many patients with TSC and seizures have normal intellect.
- Presence of ≥7 cortical tubers on magnetic resonance imaging (MRI) confers a 5-fold increase in risk of moderate to profound cognitive impairment.
  - A few patients with multiple tubers and normal intellect have been reported.
- Autism spectrum disorder is more common in TSC.
  - Estimates of prevalence range from 17–68%.
  - Autism spectrum disorder is much more common in children with global cognitive impairment in TSC (>60%), compared with only 6% among TSC children with normal cognitive function.
  - Almost all children with autism spectrum disorder and TSC have epilepsy.
  - Patients with autism and TSC do not exhibit the male preponderance seen in autism without TSC.
  - TSC is found in up to 4% of children with autism spectrum disorder.
  - TSC is the underlying genetic condition in 14% of children with autism and seizures.

Behavioral abnormalities

- Behavioral abnormalities include:
  - Severe temper tantrums
  - Restlessness
  - Impulsivity
  - Attention deficit with hyperactivity
  - Self-injury
  - Anxiety
  - Depression
- Among children with TSC and a history of infantile spasms and autism, 69% exhibit behaviors disruptive to the family by age 5 years.
- Anxiety disorder is seen in up to 59% of adults.
- Depression is seen in 35% of adults.

- Learning disabilities have been noted frequently in TSC.
  - No systematic studies are available to date.

Neuropathology

- Neuropathologic findings responsible for many of the symptoms of TSC include:
  - Tubers
  - Subependymal nodules
  - Subependymal giant cell astrocytomas
- Cortical tubers are nodular areas of gray and white matter dysplasia.
  - Often seen on the apex of a gyrus
  - Tubers are present in >95% of patients with TSC.
  - Tubers have been noted as early as 20 weeks' gestation.
  - Known to persist throughout life
  - No risk of malignant degeneration exists.
  - Tubers function as epileptogenic foci.
- Subependymal nodules are present in up to 80% of patients with TSC.
  - Arise from the lateral and 3rd ventricle walls
  - Often protrude into the lumen
  - Can be present before birth
  - Sometimes may be noted on imaging studies during infancy
- Subependymal giant cell astrocytomas may be symptomatic.
  - Occur in up to 14% of patients with TSC
  - Seem to arise from subependymal nodules
  - Continue to grow during childhood
  - May produce focal neurologic deficits or obstructive hydrocephalus

Cutaneous manifestations

- Skin findings are the most consistent features of TSC.
  - Hypomelanotic macules
    - Found in >90% of patients with TSC
    - Formerly known as *ash leaf spots*
    - May be present at birth (see Figure 47 on page F18)
    - In lighter-skinned individuals, may be visible only with a Wood lamp
    - Usually larger than 1 cm
    - Have a characteristic leaf shape: oval with 1 blunt end and 1 pointed end
    - At least 3 lesions must be visible for diagnostic significance.
  - Hypomelanotic macules
    - Seen most commonly on the trunk, but may occur anywhere
    - Fine, stippled hypopigmentation on the extremities is known as *confetti lesions*.
    - When hypomelanotic macules occur on hair-bearing surfaces, associated poliosis (white hair) may be found.

- Facial angiofibromas
  - Noted in 70–75% of individuals
  - Formerly known as *adenoma sebaceum*
  - Small, discrete, shiny pink to reddish papules develop by ~5 years of age.
  - Increase in number and size into the teenage or early adult years (see Figure 47 on page F18)
  - Initially distributed over the malar areas
  - Often spread to chin and nasolabial folds during puberty
- Forehead plaques
  - Flesh-colored to erythematous fibrotic plaques on the forehead or frontal scalp in ~19% of patients.
  - Appear later than angiofibromas
- Shagreen patches (see Figure 48 on page F18)
  - Connective tissue nevi seen in 20–50% of patients
  - Flesh-colored
  - Slightly raised
  - Irregularly shaped plaques
  - Prominent follicles
  - Cobblestone texture
  - Most often on the lower back
  - Usually noted in later childhood
- Ungual and subungual fibromas
  - Firm flesh-colored to red papules that develop beside or beneath the nails
  - Lesions under the nail may appear as a longitudinal ridge or groove.
  - Toenail involvement is more common.
  - Typically appear during puberty

Cardiac manifestations

- Cardiac rhabdomyomas are present in one-half to two-thirds of infants with TSC.
- Usually remain asymptomatic and decrease in size over time
- Often multiple
- Often diagnosed on prenatal ultrasound

Ocular manifestations

- Retinal hamartomas
  - Seen in 50–87% of patients with TSC
  - Most remain asymptomatic.
  - May be bilateral in up to 50%
  - Three clinical types include
    - Raised mulberry-like calcified nodule
    - Flat translucent gray patch
    - Transitional lesion with mixed features
- Factors that may lead to loss of vision include:
  - Involvement of the macula
  - Enlargement of the hamartoma

- Vitreous hemorrhage
- Retinal detachment
- Other ocular findings may include:
  - Retinal pigment anomalies
  - Strabismus
  - Cataracts
  - Colobomas
  - Iris depigmentation
  - Eyelid angiofibromas

Renal manifestations

- Renal lesions occur in 80% of patients.
- May include angiomyolipoma, cysts, and renal cell carcinoma (RCC)
- Prevalence increases with age.
- Angiomyolipomas develop in 55–75% of patients >10 years.
- Bilateral and multiple tumors are common.
- Small lesions may remain asymptomatic.
- Lesions >4 cm pose risks of:
  - Severe hemorrhage
  - Hypertension
  - Renal insufficiency
- Renal cysts occur in ~17% of children and 47% of adults.
- Solitary epithelial cysts are the most common.
- ~3–5% of patients with TSC will develop polycystic kidney disease as a contiguous gene deletion syndrome.
  - *TSC2* gene is adjacent to the adult polycystic kidney disease gene *PKD1* on chromosome 16.
  - Polycystic kidney disease may lead to renal insufficiency in late adolescence.

Pulmonary manifestations

- Symptomatic lymphangiomyomatosis occurs in 1–2%, almost exclusively in young women.
- Radiographic evidence of lymphangiomyomatosis may be seen in 26–39% of women.
- Main clinical findings include:
  - Spontaneous pneumothorax
  - Dyspnea
  - Cough
  - Hemoptysis

Vascular manifestations

- Arterial dysplasia seen most often in renal angiomyolipomas
- Also has been reported with basilar artery and aortic aneurysms

Dental manifestations

- Gingival fibromas occur in ~50% of adults with TSC.
- Almost all patients with TSC have dental enamel pits in permanent teeth.

N

- Dental pits rarely cause problems.
- Extensive fibromas may result in malocclusion or abnormal tooth eruption.

SWS

General

- Exhibits at birth
- Upper facial capillary malformation (PWS), involving the area of skin innervated by the ophthalmic (V1) division of the trigeminal nerve
  - Area includes:
    - Forehead
    - Brow ridge
    - Upper eyelid
    - Possibly the lower eyelid
  - Lower areas of the face (V2 or V3 distributions) also may be involved.
    - No apparent significant risk of SWS exists in the absence of V1 involvement.
  - Unilateral PWS is the rule.
    - Only 10–30% have bilateral PWS.
    - With unilateral facial PWS, the risk of SWS is ~8%.
    - If bilateral PWS is present, the risk is much higher.
  - One of the more useful clinical clues seems to be eyelid involvement, a significant predictor of disease.
  - PWSs are pink to red blanching macules to patches with variable irregularity of the borders (see Figure 49 on page F19).
    - They are capillary malformations.
    - Remain fixed in location
    - Show no tendency to evolve or involute over time
    - Growth should be commensurate with the child's growth.
    - With age, the PWS may thicken and darken, becoming somewhat cobblestoned by adulthood.

Ocular manifestations

- May include:
  - Glaucoma
  - Vascular anomalies of the globe
    - Conjunctiva
    - Episclera
    - Retina
    - Choroid
  - Buphthalmos
  - Iris heterochromia
  - Retinal detachment
  - Retinal pigment degeneration
  - Cataract
  - Optic disc coloboma

- Glaucoma is the most common ocular problem.
  - Occurs in up to 70% of patients
  - Usually ipsilateral to the PWS
  - May be bilateral, even if the PWS is unilateral
  - Glaucoma may develop from birth to the 5th decade.
  - Median age at onset is 5 years.
  - Develops in infancy to early childhood in 60%
  - Development in infancy, when the globe is more sensitive to increased intraocular pressure, may lead to:
    - Increased corneal diameter
    - Buphthalmos
    - Iris heterochromia
  - Choroidal hemangioma ipsilateral to the PWS is seen in up to 71% of patients.
  - Over time, retinal changes can lead to visual field defects and vision loss.

Neurologic manifestations

- Neurologic features may include:
  - Seizures
  - Focal neurologic deficits
  - Developmental delay
  - Progressive intellectual disability
  - Headaches
- Seizures are the most common neurologic problem.
  - Occur in 75–83% of patients
  - ~75% of seizure disorders develop in the first 2 years of life.
  - Partial motor seizures are the most common type (40%).
  - Generalized tonic-clonic, atonic, and absence seizures may also occur.
  - Infantile spasms may be the presenting seizure type.
  - Seizures tend to worsen with age, becoming more frequent, severe, and complex
  - Seizures may be provoked by febrile episodes.
  - Status epilepticus may occur in up to one half of these children.

Developmental and behavioral problems

- Developmental delays are seen in up to one-half of patients.
  - Early milestones often normal
  - Decline in function noted over time
  - Some of the cognitive decline occurs during periods of encephalopathy after prolonged or severe seizures.
  - Others experience decline in function as a result of recurrent strokelike episodes.
  - Factors that seem to correlate best with developmental delay and its severity are presence of:
    - Bilateral cerebral lesions
    - Degree of cerebral atrophy

- Presence of intractable seizures
- Multiple seizure types
- Early onset of seizures (controversial)
- In the absence of seizures, cognitive development is normal.
- 85% of patients with seizure onset after age 4 years have normal intelligence.

- Psychological manifestations of SWS may include:
  - Attention-deficit/hyperactivity disorder (ADHD)
  - Irritability
  - Social problems
- Inattentive and oppositional behaviors may be noted.
- ~85% of patients who have cognitive disability exhibit emotional or behavioral problems.
  - Aggressive behavior toward others
  - Self-abuse
- Headache, including migraine, is seen in 30–45%.
  - Median age at onset is 8 years.
  - Migraines may be associated with:
    - Visual aura
    - Visual field defects

VHL

General

- Most common tumors
  - Cerebellar
  - Spinal
  - Retinal hemangioblastomas
- Other associated tumors
  - Renal cysts
  - RCC
  - Pheochromocytoma
  - Pancreatic cysts
  - Neuroendocrine tumors
  - Endolymphatic sac tumors of the inner ear
  - Cystadenomas of the epididymis or broad ligament

CNS manifestations

- CNS hemangioblastomas are the most common tumors in VHL (21–72%).
  - Occur most commonly in the cerebellum (63%)
    - Followed by the spinal cord (32%) *and*
    - Brainstem (5%)
  - Mean age at presentation is 33 years.
  - Tumors may develop in childhood through the 4th decade of life.
  - Slow-growing benign tumors produce symptoms largely by mass effect or obstructive hydrocephaly.

- Cerebellar tumors may present with:
  - Headache
  - Nausea
  - Vomiting
  - Vertigo
  - Slurred speech
  - Broad-based gait
- Clinical signs may include:
  - Papilledema
  - Nystagmus
  - Ataxia
  - Dysmetria
- Spinal hemangioblastomas may produce:
  - Back pain
  - Numbness
  - Pain or weakness in arms or legs
  - Posterior column proprioceptive defects
  - Bowel and bladder dysfunction
- CNS hemangioblastomas tend to exhibit alternating periods of growth and stability.
  - Low-level chronic symptoms may worsen acutely during a critical growth phase.

Ocular manifestations

- Retinal hemangioblastomas (capillary hemangiomas) develop in more than one-half of patients with VHL.
  - Most have solitary tumors
  - Approximately one-third have multiple lesions.
  - One-half of patients have bilateral retinal tumors
    - Most develop in the 2nd to 3rd decade of life.
  - Mean age at diagnosis is 25 years.
  - Retinal tumors may develop at any time from infancy to the 9th decade.
  - Patients may experience painless loss of visual acuity or visual field defects.
  - They may remain asymptomatic.
  - Exudation or hemorrhage from the hemangiomas may lead to:
    - Macular edema
    - Retinal detachment
  - Secondary changes in the anterior chamber may lead to:
    - Glaucoma
    - Cataract

Renal manifestations

- Renal cysts are seen in approximately one-half of patients.
- Often multiple and bilateral
- May remain asymptomatic

- Stable lesions may not require intervention.
- RCC develops in 75% of patients by age 60.
- RCC is seen in patients with type 1 or type 2b disease.
  - Usually develops after 20 years of age
  - Often earlier than with sporadic renal carcinoma
  - Lesions often are multiple and bilateral.
  - Tumors may be associated with cysts.
  - May have better 10-year survival than sporadic RCC
  - Symptoms may include:
    - Hematuria
    - Flank pain
    - Flank mass
  - By the time symptoms develop, metastases are present in 30–50% of patients.

Endocrine system

- Pheochromocytoma occurs in 10–24% of persons with type 2 disease.
  - May be the only manifestation of VHL (type 2c)
  - VHL accounts for ~20% of all pheochromocytomas.
  - Mean age at presentation is 27 years.
  - Tumors may be present even before age 10 years.
  - Pheochromocytoma in VHL differs from sporadic tumors by:
    - Occurring at an earlier age
    - Developing multiple, bilateral, and extraadrenal tumors
  - Only 5% of VHL pheochromocytomas are malignant.
  - Clinical features may include:
    - Hypertension (paroxysmal or sustained)
    - Palpitations
    - Sweating
    - Flushing
    - Headache
    - Tachycardia
    - Pallor
    - Nausea
  - Pancreatic cysts or tumors occur in ~90% of patients with VHL.
    - Rarely cause disease
  - Benign adenomas occur in ~12% of patients with VHL.
  - ~5–10% of patients with VHL develop neuroendocrine islet cell tumors.
    - May be multifocal
    - May metastasize in 10–20% of patients
  - Average age at diagnosis of pancreatic lesions is 41 years.
  - Islet cell tumors may be seen as early as 10 years of age.
  - Most pancreatic lesions are asymptomatic.
    - Found during routine imaging surveillance.

- ~10% will develop endolymphatic sac tumors.
  - Cystadenomas arising from the inner ear labyrinth ectoderm may cause:
    - Deafness
    - Tinnitus
    - Vertigo
  - Facial nerve and vocal paralysis may result from progressive tumor growth.
- Cystadenomas may develop in the epididymis in men and the uterine broad ligament in women.
  - Usually asymptomatic

A-T

- Consanguinity is common.
- Characteristic features
  - Progressive decline in cerebellar function
  - Oculocutaneous telangiectasia
  - Immunodeficiency
  - Susceptibility to cancer
  - Sensitivity to ionizing radiation
- Infants are normal.
  - Begin to walk at approximately 12 months of age
  - By age 2–3 years, develop unsteady gait and staggering
- By age 10 years, most require wheelchairs for mobility; they have slow reflexes and tend to fall.
- Ocular apraxia develops in early childhood.
  - Difficulty with voluntary eye movement
  - May be confused with absence seizures in infants
  - Dysarthric speech often is present early in childhood.
    - Can be difficult to assess
- Telangiectasias (tortuous dilated capillaries) develop several years after the onset of neurologic symptoms on:
  - Bulbar conjunctiva
  - Nasal bridge
  - Ears
  - Neck
  - Knuckles
  - Antecubital and popliteal fossae
- Immunodeficiency varies.
  - May be severe in approximately one-third of patients.
  - Many patients have reduced numbers of T lymphocytes with poor mitogen response.
  - Low serum levels are noted despite normal to high numbers of B cells.
    - Immunoglobulin (Ig) E (80% of patients)
    - IgG_2 (80%)
    - IgA (60%)
  - IgM levels vary widely, at times rising enough to create a hyperviscous state

- Some patients exhibit poor immune response to pneumococcal polysaccharides.
- Patients with severe immunodeficiency may develop recurrent sinopulmonary infections.
- Opportunistic organisms are not a problem in patients with A-T.

DIFFERENTIAL DIAGNOSIS

NF-1

- CALMs are often the earliest presenting feature.
  - Up to 25% of normal individuals may have 1–3 CALMs.
  - Up to 40% of people with > 6 CALMs never progress to NF-1.
- Multiple CALMs may be present in the following conditions:
  - NF-1
    - Clinical features
      - Axillary freckling
      - Cutaneous NFs
      - Plexiform NFs
      - Lisch nodules
      - Optic glioma
      - Bony abnormalities
      - Positive FH
      - Present in 95% of patients with NF-1; must have >6 CALMs (>5 mm before puberty; >15 mm after puberty)
  - Watson syndrome
    - Other clinical features
      - Pulmonic stenosis
      - Intellectual disability
      - Axillary freckling
      - Axillary freckling only in NF-1 and Watson syndrome type 1
  - McCune-Albright syndrome
    - Other clinical features
      - Polyostotic fibrous bony dysplasia
      - Precocious puberty
      - Hyperthyroid
      - Cushing syndrome
      - Usually large-segment CALM with irregular border (coast of Maine).
  - Russell-Silver syndrome
    - Other clinical features
      - Short stature
      - Skeletal asymmetry
      - Abnormal pubertal development

- Bloom syndrome
  - Other clinical features
    - Malar facial erythema and telangiectasia
    - Photosensitivity
    - Long, narrow face with prominent nose
    - Short stature
    - Hypogonadism
    - Malignancy risk
    - Facial photosensitivity with multiple CALMs triggers evaluation
- Tuberous sclerosis
  - Other clinical features
    - Hypopigmented macules
    - Facial and periungual angiofibromas
    - Seizures
    - Intellectual disability
    - Renal and cardiac hamartomas
    - Hypopigmented macules more common; mixture very concerning for tuberous sclerosis complex
- Noonan syndrome
  - Other clinical features
    - Hypertelorism
    - Webbed neck
    - Short stature
    - Leg lymphedema
    - Pulmonic stenosis
    - Hypogonadism

TSC

- Does not have a pathognomonic lesion
- Fulfillment of diagnostic criteria is of paramount importance.
- Facial angiofibromas once were considered diagnostic.
  - Now known to occur in multiple endocrine neoplasia syndrome type 1

SWS

- Isolated (ie, nonsyndromic) facial PWS
  - Unilateral forehead PWS has no underlying syndrome in 92% of patients.
  - Bilateral PWS has a much higher likelihood of association with SWS.
- Wyburn-Mason syndrome
  - Rare disorder consisting of retinal and CNS arteriovenous malformations associated with upper facial PWS.
  - Symptoms include:
    - Headaches
    - Seizures
    - Focal neurologic deficits

N

– Retinal hemorrhage

– Subarachnoid hemorrhage

VHL

- CNS hemangioblastomas create symptoms by mass effect.
- Similar to many other tumors, cysts, and obstructive hydrocephalus
- Evaluation of mass effect with neurologic symptoms should reveal characteristic radiologic findings of hemangioblastomas.
- Differential diagnosis of retinal capillary hemangiomas
  - VHL
    – Orange-red circumscribed tumors
    – Pair of prominent vessels
    – Stellate macular exudates
    – Retinal or subretinal exudates
  - Coat disease
    – Diffuse retinal vascular anomaly
    – Retinal or subretinal exudates
  - Wyburn-Mason syndrome
    – Dilation and tortuosity of retinal arteries and veins, but no intervening hemangioma
    – No retinal or subretinal exudates
  - Retinal cavernous hemangioma
    – Cluster of small dilated vessels around central vein
    – Lacks prominent feeder vessels
    – No retinal or subretinal exudates
  - Vasoproliferative tumor of the retina
    – Pink to yellow retinal tumor
    – Lacks dilated feeder vessels
    – Lacks stellate macular exudates
    – Retinal or subretinal exudates (nonstellate)
- Differential diagnosis of renal cysts includes the diagnosis of polycystic kidney disease.
- Pheochromocytoma may occur sporadically or in the setting of
  - VHL
  - Multiple endocrine neoplasia 2a or 2b with associated medullary thyroid carcinoma
  - Neurofibromatosis
  - Succinate dehydrogenase subunit mutations

A-T

- A-T
  - Early ataxia, oculomotor apraxia, progressive neurologic decline
  - Increased α-fetoprotein
  - Cancer risk

- Immune deficiency
- Sensitivity to radiation
- Ataxia-telangiectasia–like disorder (*hMRE11* mutation)
  - Ataxia early
  - No telangiectasia
  - No increase in α-fetoprotein
  - No cancer risk
  - No immune deficiency
  - Sensitivity to radiation
- Nijmegen breakage syndrome
  - Microcephaly, intellectual disability
  - No telangiectasia
  - No increase in α-fetoprotein
  - Cancer risk
  - Immune deficiency
  - Sensitivity to radiation
- Ataxia oculomotor apraxia I
  - Early ataxia, progressive neurologic decline
  - No telangiectasia
  - No increase in α-fetoprotein
  - No cancer risk
  - No immune deficiency
  - No sensitivity to radiation
- Ataxia oculomotor apraxia II
  - Late-onset ataxia
  - No telangiectasia
  - Increased α-fetoprotein
  - No cancer risk
  - No immune deficiency
  - No sensitivity to radiation

DIAGNOSTIC APPROACH

NF-1

- Cannot be diagnosed clinically until ≥2 of the major diagnostic criteria are met:
  - >6 café-au-lait spots
    – >5 mm in prepubertal child
    – >15 mm after puberty
  - Axillary or inguinal freckling
  - ≥2 neurofibromas of any type or = 1 plexiform neurofibroma
  - Optic pathway glioma
  - ≥2 Lisch nodules
  - Characteristic bony lesion: sphenoid wing dysplasia, or thinning of the cortex of long bones—with or without pseudoarthrosis
  - First-degree relative with NF-1

- History
  - Should include age-appropriate questions about:
    - Development
    - Language and learning
    - Socialization
    - Self-esteem
  - Family history is of paramount importance in the initial evaluation of a child with CALMs only.
- Physical examination
  - Should start with a thorough skin survey for CALMs
  - Thorough examination of the entire skin surface should also reveal the presence of plexiform neurofibromas.
    - May be present at birth
    - May develop in the 1st few years of life
- Evaluation for possible NF-1 depends on age.
  - Many features develop over time.
  - CALMs are present at birth and will increase in size and number for the first 5–7 years.
  - Bowing of the long bones (especially tibia) and cutaneous plexiform neurofibromas typically are visible within the 1st year of life.
  - Axillary (see Figure 50 on page F19) and inguinal freckling, optic gliomas, and scoliosis may not be apparent until age 7 years.
  - Cutaneous neurofibromas and iris Lisch nodules usually appear during or after the teenage years.

NF-2

- History should include
  - Vision or hearing changes
  - Tinnitus
  - Vertigo
  - Gait disturbances
  - Decreased facial sensation
  - Facial weakness or twitching
  - Hoarseness
  - Dysphagia
  - Headaches
- Family history of NF-2 is crucial for diagnosis
- Definite NF-2
  - Bilateral vestibular schwannomas *or* 1st degree relative with NF-2 *plus*
    - Unilateral vestibular schwannomas or any 2 of the following:
      - Meningioma
      - Schwannoma
      - Glioma
      - Neurofibroma
      - Juvenile posterior subcapsular cataract

- Probable NF-2
  - Unilateral vestibular schwannoma *plus* multiple meningiomas *or* any 2 of the following:
    - Meningioma
    - Schwannoma
    - Glioma
    - Neurofibroma
    - Juvenile posterior subcapsular cataract
  - *Or* any 2 of the following:
    - Schwannoma
    - Glioma
    - Neurofibroma
    - Juvenile posterior subcapsular cataract
- Physical examination should focus on
  - Vision
  - Hearing
  - Cranial and peripheral nerve function
  - Younger patients often have
    - Headache
    - Tinnitus
    - Cranial nerve symptoms
    - Skin or spinal tumors before the onset of hearing loss
  - Eye examination should assess the presence of lens opacities.
  - Cranial nerve examination should specifically address:
    - Trigeminal nerves
    - Facial nerves
    - Auditory nerves
  - Neurologic examination should assess:
    - Balance
    - Gait
    - Deep tendon reflexes
  - At the skin examination, the physician should note the presence of:
    - Neurofibromas
    - CALMs
    - Cutaneous schwannomas
      - Present in approximately one-half of patients.
      - May be subcutaneous nodules or plaques with thickened texture and occasional hair growth
      - May be surface pink to flesh-colored papules (see Figure 46 on page F18)

TSC

- History
  - In infants, seizures often are the 1st symptom.
  - Any infant with new-onset seizures should have a detailed history, including:

N

- Skin lesions
- Developmental milestones
- Family history
- Initial examination should include:
  - Wood lamp examination of the entire skin surface
  - Funduscopic examination for hamartomas
  - Thorough neurologic examination

SWS

- Infants with facial PWS on the forehead and eyelids should be evaluated for the possibility of SWS.
- Evaluation should include ophthalmologic examination.
  - If eye findings or any other typical clinical features such as seizures are present, then neuroimaging is mandatory.
- Routine MRI may be performed even in the absence of seizures.
- History
  - Earliest manifestation is the PWS present at birth.
  - Relevant history in a child with facial PWS includes:
    - History of seizures
    - History of eye or vision problems
    - Concerns about development
  - Older children should be asked about:
    - Headaches
    - Vision changes
    - Episodes of weakness
    - School progress
- Physical examination
  - Should include a thorough eye examination.
    - Clues to early glaucoma
      - Difference in sizes of cornea or globe
      - Iris heterochromia
    - Presence of PWS on eyelids should be noted.
    - Auscultation of the orbits, fontanelles, and temples should be performed to detect bruits.
    - Funduscopic examination may reveal the characteristic "ketchup stains" of choroidal angiomas.
    - Tortuous vessels or colobomas should be noted.
  - Neurologic examination should search for focal deficits.
  - Developmental evaluation is important.
    - Particularly if the child has a seizure history
  - Observation of an infant should specifically address the presence of a head turn or early handedness.
    - Potential clues to visual field cuts

VHL

- Diagnosis established in a patient who has:
  - 1 characteristic tumor and positive family history
  - Hemangioblastoma *plus* 1 other tumor when the family history is negative

- History
  - Most important historical information is family history
    - 80% of cases are familial
  - Changes in vision
  - Development of neurologic symptoms
    - Clumsiness
    - Broad-based gait
    - Hearing loss
    - Slurring of speech
    - Pain
    - Numbness or weakness in limbs
  - Loss of bowel or bladder control after complete toilet training
  - Hematuria or flank pain
  - Heart palpitations
  - Flushing
  - Sweating spells
  - Episodic nausea and vomiting
- Physical examination should include:
  - Blood pressure evaluation
  - Thorough eye examination
  - Thorough neurologic examination with particular attention to cerebellar and spinal functions
  - Observation of gait
  - Test of balance
  - Observation of deep tendon reflexes
  - Test for sensation

A-T

- Earliest manifestation of A-T is the ataxia.
  - Begins as broad-based gait or staggering
  - Evident by age 2–3 years
- Any other history should focus on:
  - Additional neurologic symptoms
  - Developmental milestones
- Family history should include:
  - Neurologic problems
  - Consanguinity in the family
- Examination should focus on neurologic findings.
  - Include cerebellar function
  - Difficult to assess in young children
  - Voluntary visual tracking of objects will often reveal the early development of oculomotor apraxia.
  - In older children, telangiectasia may be noted on:
    - Bulbar conjunctiva
    - Skin of the neck
    - Face

– Ears

– Extremity flexures

■ Examination also should include:

- Thorough lymph node examination

- Abdominal evaluation for hepatosplenomegaly

LABORATORY FINDINGS

NF-1

■ Routine laboratory testing is unnecessary.

■ In cases of uncertain diagnosis, test for gene mutations.

- Complementary series of analyses is available, including:

  – Premature truncation test

  – Heteroduplex analysis

  – Fluorescent in situ hybridization assay

- This tiered analysis provides a sensitivity of 95%.

NF-2

■ Should always include formal audiologic testing for sensorineural hearing loss

■ Once the diagnosis is established, audiometry should be repeated every 6–12 months.

- Annual screening appropriate for:

  – Children at risk

  – Asymptomatic children with a detected mutation

■ Genetic testing for the mutations is available on a clinical basis.

- Sensitivity is low:

  – 34% in sporadic mutations

  – 54% if familial

- High false-negative rate

TSC

■ Once diagnostic criteria are fulfilled, molecular testing can be performed to determine the specific mutation.

■ 15–20% of patients who fulfill TSC diagnostic criteria have no identifiable mutations.

■ Clinical gene testing is available by using combined techniques such as:

- Denaturing high-performance liquid chromatography

- Heteroduplex analysis

■ Mutation detection rate is only 85%, even with combined methods.

SWS

■ Routine laboratory testing is not useful.

VHL

■ Should begin with molecular testing for the specific mutation

- Phenotypic profile and tumor risk are directly related to the types of mutation.

■ Subsequent laboratory evaluation for patients with type 2 disease should consist of:

- Annual screening for plasma or urine catecholamines and metanephrines

- Begin at age 10 years

A-T

■ Serum α-fetoprotein

- Increased in >95% of patients

- Serum α-fetoprotein increase is only useful after age 2 years

  – Some unaffected children have persistent mild increases beyond the neonatal period.

■ Karyotyping rarely is normal in A-T.

- Often shows translocations between chromosomes 7 and 14

■ Quantitative immunoglobulins may show low levels of:

- IgE

- IgA

- IgG2

■ IgM is normal or high.

■ Quantitative T- and B-cell numbers reveal:

- Low levels of T cells

- Normal to slightly high levels of B cells

■ Radiosensitivity test currently available is the colony survival assay.

- Uses the patients' transformed lymphocytes.

- Requires ~3 months to complete

■ Gene testing is not useful unless the family mutation is known.

- *ATM* is a huge gene with 66 exons and >400 known mutations

  – None with a frequency >3%

■ Measurements of the ATM protein from the transformed lymphocyte cell line also is possible by immunoblotting.

IMAGING

NF-1

■ Routine neuroimaging usually is not undertaken.

■ Evidence of scoliosis or long bone anomaly merits plain-film radiography.

- Scoliosis may require MRI or computed tomography (CT) to:

  – Define the extent

  – Help map surgical intervention

■ Head MRI is indicated for evaluation of:

- Focal neurologic changes

- New-onset seizures

- Severe headaches

N

- Vision changes
- Proptosis
- Short stature
- Rapid change in head circumference
- Plexiform lesions
- Severe cognitive deficits
- Precocious or delayed puberty

■ Cranial MRI is indicated to evaluate for possible optic pathway glioma once symptoms have developed.
  - Routine imaging before symptom onset is not indicated.
  - Once optic gliomas are diagnosed, MRI should be obtained:
    - Every 2 years
    - With any symptom change to age 10 years

■ One unusual finding is the presence of unidentified bright objects on T2-weighted sequences of cranial MRI.
  - These lesions are present in 60–90% of children, but only ~30% of adults.
    - Their significance is uncertain.
  - Controversial evidence suggests that some learning disabilities correlate with presence and specific locations of unidentified bright objects.

■ MRI is useful to assess for radiculopathy.
  - Neurofibromas have a propensity to develop along or within the spine, often impinging on nerve roots.

■ MRI is the mainstay of evaluation of plexiform neurofibromas.

■ Development of pain, or any focal neurologic deficit, warrants an MRI.
  - Particularly important if pain develops in a plexiform neurofibroma, where pain may herald malignant change.

■ Positron emission tomographic (PET) scanning may be of more value in distinguishing benign from malignant lesions.

■ Imaging is useful in evaluation of cerebrovascular disease and renal artery stenosis.

NF-2

■ Routine screening MRI of the brain is required for any patient with:
  - Unilateral vestibular schwannoma
  - Multiple intracranial or spinal tumors
  - 1st-degree relative with NF-2
  - Child with meningioma

■ Any child at risk for NF-2 should have a screening brain MRI annually beginning at age 7 years.

■ Gadolinium-enhanced MRI with thin cuts through the internal auditory canals for assessment of vestibular schwannomas

■ Spinal MRI should be considered if any symptoms or neurologic deficits are noted.

TSC

■ Initial imaging studies include:
  - Brain studies (MRI or CT)
  - Echocardiography
  - Renal ultrasound

■ Cortical tubers are best evaluated by MRI.

■ Subependymal nodules may be seen in infancy on MRI as T1-weighted hyperintense nodules.
  - By age 1 year, the subependymal nodules contain calcium and may be visualized with CT scanning.

■ MRI may be useful to identify subependymal giant cell astrocytomas.
  - Radiologic distinction from subependymal nodules is difficult.

■ Renal lesions in older children and adults may be evaluated by ultrasound, CT, or MRI.

■ Chest CT is indicated for all women with TSC to evaluate for possible pulmonary lymphangiomyomatosis.

SWS

■ Leptomeningeal enhancement, with or without cortical atrophy, is the radiologic hallmark of SWS.
  - Gadolinium-enhanced MRI is the most sensitive imaging modality to evaluate for leptomeningeal angiomatosis.
  - Leptomeningeal involvement is ipsilateral to the PWS.
  - May be seen before calcifications develop
  - Calcification of adjacent gyri may give the classic "tram track" appearance seen on CT and even plain-film radiographs.
  - Involvement of the parietal and occipital lobes often is noted before frontal or temporal findings.
  - PET and single-photon emission CT may reveal areas of altered metabolism and hypoperfusion.

■ Choroidal hemangioma almost always is associated with leptomeningeal lesions.
  - Makes CNS imaging mandatory

■ Choroidal angiomas are best visualized with MRI.

VHL

■ MRI with gadolinium contrast is the modality of choice for most features of VHL.

■ Hemangioblastomas of the cerebellum are usually subpial in location.
  - May appear as a solid enhancing mass with or without surrounding fluid space
  - May appear as a more complex tissue or fluid mass
  - Spinal hemangioblastomas are solid enhancing intramedullary masses, frequently associated with a surrounding fluid filled syrinx that enlarges and displaces the cord.

■ Renal cysts may be found on MRI, ultrasound, or CT.

A-T

- Imaging is limited.
- Cranial MRI will reveal gradual cerebellar atrophy, which is almost always noted by age 10 years
- Imaging with radiation should be considered carefully because of these patients' extreme radiosensitivity.
- Adult female patients and carriers should be screened for breast cancer with regular examinations and ultrasound.
  - Do not use mammograms.

DIAGNOSTIC PROCEDURES

- TSC
  - Should include an electrocardiogram, as well as echocardiogram, because of risk for dysrhythmias
    - Especially in infants or children with evidence of cardiac rhabdomyomas
- SWS
  - Evaluation of seizures should include electroencephalography.
    - Typical findings include:
      - Asymmetry, with background slowing and reduced voltage in the affected hemisphere
      - Asymmetry becomes more prominent with the progressive cerebral atrophy.

TREATMENT APPROACH

NF-1

- Management should focus on the organ system involved, given the wide variability of expression.
- Genetic counseling should be provided for all NF-1 families.
  - Affected individuals have a 50% chance of transmission with each pregnancy.
- Careful attention should also be paid to the long bones of the lower leg.
  - Congenital tibial dysplasia is an early finding in up to 5% of children with NF-1.
  - Any curvature or nodularity of the tibia is worrisome, as is any length discrepancy.
- Head circumference should be monitored at each visit.
  - ~50% of children with NF-1 have macrocephaly.
- Thorough developmental evaluation should be undertaken at each visit and repeated at regular intervals, with preschool attention to:
  - Language
  - Visual motor skills
  - Learning
- Examination of the back for evidence of scoliosis should start by age 2 years.
  - Scoliosis appears at an earlier age in NF-1.

- Severe dystrophic form of kyphoscoliosis can appear between 3–5 years of age.
- Regular blood pressure assessment should begin by age 2 years.
- Ophthalmologic evaluation should be obtained annually to age 10 years.
  - Assess for the presence of optic pathway glioma
  - Grade-1 pilocytic astrocytomas
    - Present in ~15% of children with NF-1 under age 10
    - May produce proptosis, strabismus, papilledema, or vision loss
  - If the optic chiasm is involved, hypothalamic extension can produce an endocrinopathy.
    - Results in precocious or delayed puberty
    - Development of precocious puberty should prompt evaluation for an optic glioma.
  - Other ocular findings may include:
    - Congenital ptosis
    - Orbital asymmetry (result of sphenoid wing dysplasia)
- School-aged children should be assessed for:
  - Limb asymmetry
  - Long bone bowing
  - Scoliosis
  - Cutaneous neurofibromas
- School performance should be addressed, with particular attention to:
  - Learning disabilities
  - ADHD
  - Self-esteem
  - Socialization
- Teens should be assessed for:
  - Limb asymmetry
  - Scoliosis
  - Neurofibromas
  - Hypertension
  - Iris hamartomas (Lisch nodules)
    - Tan to brown papules that usually appear in the teenaged years
    - Found in slit-lamp ophthalmologic evaluation
    - Have minimal impact other than support of diagnosis
  - Complaint of pain
    - Particularly pain associated with focal neurologic deficit or arising from a plexiform tumor
    - Should be thoroughly evaluated by examination and imaging studies.
  - School performance
  - Socialization
  - Self-esteem

N

NF-2

- Most important aspect is early diagnosis so surgery to preserve hearing can be performed.
- Advanced tumors may prevent the preservation of hearing.
  - May lead to complete deafness
  - Creates need for either cochlear or auditory brainstem implants
    - Cochlear implants seem to be better than auditory brainstem implants.
- Once a diagnosis is made, the child should be evaluated by:
  - Ophthalmology
  - Otolaryngology
  - Audiology
  - Imaging

TSC

- 2 basic principles
  - Establishing correct diagnosis
  - Long-term follow-up for later manifestations
- Genetic counseling is mandatory for families and patients.
  - Disorder is autosomal dominant
    - Affected individuals have a 50% risk of affected offspring.
  - Germ-line mutations occur in ~2% of patients.
    - Seemingly unaffected parents with a single affected child have ~2% risk of having another affected child.
- Older children should be screened for:
  - Seizure disorder
  - Developmental delay
  - Autism spectrum disorders

SWS

- Seizure control is the most important aspect of management.

VHL

- Once a diagnosis is established, tumor screening and regular imaging and ophthalmologic examinations are indicated.
  - First-degree relatives should be screened for tumors.
- Annual eye examinations, including dilated funduscopy, should begin by age 6 years.
- Annual cranial and spinal MRI should begin by age 10–11 years.
- Abdominal imaging for kidneys and possible pheochromocytoma should begin by age 15–18 years.
  - May consist of ultrasound, CT, or MRI
  - MRI is best modality for finding all the possible intra-abdominal tumors.
- Hearing loss or tinnitus should be evaluated.
  - By MRI with thin sections through the ear structures
  - By formal audiologic examination

A-T

- Most important aspects of therapy include:
  - Family and patient counseling
  - Support
  - Rehabilitation
  - Assistance with the progressive ataxia

SPECIFIC TREATMENTS

NF-1

- Neurofibromas present unique management issues.
  - Smaller lesions may become painful or may interfere with activities as a result of location.
  - Plexiform lesions can be disfiguring.
  - Numerous or large lesions may exert a profound effect on self-esteem and socialization.
  - Surgical excision may be necessary for problematic tumors.
- Sudden development of pain or focal neurologic deficit in plexiform tumors may represent malignant degeneration.
- Malignant peripheral nerve sheath tumors (formerly called *neurofibrosarcoma*) develop in 5–13% of patients, with devastating effect.
  - Often multicentric
  - Metastasize quickly
  - Usually fatal within a year
- Other malignant tumors are seen with an overall incidence 3% higher than the general population, including:
  - Leukemia, especially juvenile myelomonocytic leukemia
  - Rhabdomyosarcoma
  - Pheochromocytoma (an adult-onset tumor)
  - Carcinoid (an adult-onset tumor)

NF-2

- Screening examinations, audiometry, and imaging should be repeated at least annually starting at age 7 years.
- Children of a parent with NF-2 should have:
  - Annual ophthalmologic examinations starting in infancy
  - Neurologic and audiometric examinations annually from age 7 years
- Most patients should be encouraged to learn sign language as preparation for possible future complete hearing loss

TSC

- Treatment of epilepsy in TSC is the same as in other forms of epilepsy, with 1 exception:
  - Infantile spasms in TSC do not respond as well to adrenocorticotropic hormone as infantile spasms without TSC.
  - Irreversible γ-aminobutyric acid transaminase inhibitor vigabatrin is much more effective.
    - Response rates up to 96% in infants with TSC and infantile spasms

– Vigabatrin is not currently approved by the US Food and Drug Administration because of potential severe ophthalmic toxicity.

– Vigabatrin may be considered despite its toxicity because of potentially devastating cognitive impact of uncontrolled infantile spasms.

SWS

- Seizure control
  - Prophylactic anticonvulsant therapy may be useful for infants with extensive intracranial disease.
  - Carbamazepine and oxcarbazepine are useful first-line anticonvulsants for SWS.
  - Other options include
    – Valproic acid
    – Topiramate
    – Phenobarbital
    – Phenytoin
    – Vigabatrin
  - Refractory seizures in SWS may lead to consideration of seizure surgery.
    – Hemispherectomy has been found to be effective in reducing refractory seizures.
  - Fevers should be treated aggressively to prevent the triggering of seizures.
- Hydration status should be monitored.
  - Especially during gastrointestinal illness
  - Dehydration may create intravascular sludging and further compromise the cerebral circulation.
- Antipyretic agents should be given prophylactically with immunizations.
- Iron-deficiency anemia should be corrected.
- Low-dose aspirin is suggested for prevention of stroke-like episodes.
- Prevent headaches through avoidance of:
  - Fatigue
  - Sleep deprivation
  - Stress
  - Minor head trauma
  - Ibuprofen is useful in management of common headaches.
  - Migraines may require sumatriptan.
- Glaucoma may be managed medically in most patients with:
  - ß-adrenergic blockers
  - Carbonic anhydrase inhibitors
  - Surgical approaches are not usually required.
- PWSs may be treated effectively with pulsed dye laser.

VHL

- Surgical excision generally is considered the best treatment for most symptomatic VHL tumors.

- CNS hemangioblastomas that remain stable and asymptomatic may be followed by serial imaging.
- Proper management for asymptomatic but radiologically progressive lesions is a matter of debate.
- Spinal hemangioblastomas and large or symptomatic intracranial tumors usually are resected.
- Small retinal lesions are often treated with laser photocoagulation.
  - Larger lesions may require
    – Cryotherapy
    – Brachytherapy
    – Vitreoretinal surgery
- Screening for eye lesions is of critical importance.
- Small renal tumors (<3 cm) are often followed by serial imaging.
  - Larger lesions may be addressed by partial nephrectomy.
  - Radical nephrectomy is rarely indicated.
- Symptomatic pheochromocytomas require excision.

A-T

- Speech, physical, and occupational therapy should be obtained early.
  - Speech therapy may help with:
    – Communication
    – Swallowing difficulties
  - Physical and occupational therapy can help with:
    – Mobility
    – Safety
    – Daily living skills
- Careful monitoring is crucial for the recurrent infection and cancer risks.
- Recurrent sinopulmonary infections should be treated aggressively.
  - Aspiration should be anticipated.
- Emotional support is crucial for:
  - Depression
  - Anger
  - Isolation

WHEN TO ADMIT

- NF
  - Sudden neurologic decline
  - Uncontrollable seizures
- TSC
  - Sudden neurologic deterioration
  - Intractable seizures
  - Gross hematuria
  - Heart failure or dysrhythmia

N

- SWS
  - Refractory seizures
- VHL
  - Hypertension crisis with pheochromocytoma
  - Sudden neurologic deterioration
- A-T
  - Severe pulmonary infection, especially if respiratory distress is present
  - Severe aspiration event

WHEN TO REFER

- NF-1
  - Pediatric ophthalmologic evaluation beginning in the first year
  - Neurologic evaluation if seizures are difficult to manage
  - Neurodevelopmental testing if evidence of:
    - Learning disability
    - ADHD
    - Speech delay
  - Surgical referral for symptomatic neurofibromas, renovascular hypertension
- NF-2
  - Hearing loss
  - Gait or balance difficulty
  - Headache
  - Tinnitus
- TSC
  - Ophthalmologic screening
    - In infancy if TSC is suspected
  - Neurologic screening
    - When seizures are hard to manage or progressive
  - Surgery
    - Symptomatic or progressive renal lesions >4 cm
  - Neurodevelopmental testing
    - At diagnosis
- SWS
  - Ophthalmologic evaluation
    - Any infant with forehead and eyelid PWS
  - Neurologic evaluation
    - Difficult seizure management
- VHL
  - Ophthalmologic examination
    - By age 6 years

- Neurologic examination or neurosurgery
  - On detection of CNS tumors
- General surgery
  - On detection of intraabdominal tumors
- A-T
  - Neurologic examination
    - On development of ataxia
  - Speech therapy
    - On development of speech or swallowing difficulty
  - Physical and occupational therapy
    - Before ataxia becomes severe

FOLLOW-UP

TSC

- Neurobehavioral assessment and monitoring
  - Routine formal testing should be performed at age-appropriate levels in:
    - Infancy
    - Preschool
    - Early school age
    - Periodically into adulthood
  - Identify cognitive and behavioral issues as early as possible.
  - Any regressive behavior or new cognitive dysfunction should prompt urgent reevaluation.
- Brain and abdominal imaging should be performed at least every 3 years.
  - More often if lesions exhibit progressive growth or if any acute change in symptoms occurs:
    - Sudden neurologic or cognitive decline
    - Hypertension
    - Hematuria
  - Annual brain MRI is suggested to age 21 years.
  - Annual renal imaging is suggested for monitoring of angiomyolipomas.
  - Serial renal ultrasound is adequate if maximal lesion size is <4 cm.
  - Larger renal lesions should be assessed by Doppler or MRI or magnetic resonance angiography for abnormal vasculature.
  - Chest CT is indicated for all women with TSC to evaluate for possible lymphangiomyomatosis.
  - Women with lung lesions should have annual pulmonary function tests.

N

COMPLICATIONS

NF-1

- Optic pathway gliomas develop in 15–20% of patients at a mean age of 4.2 years.
  - Annual ophthalmologic monitoring from the 1st year of life and continue to age 10 years, checking for:
    - Vision change
    - Afferent pupillary defect
    - Change in funduscopic examination findings
  - Other ocular findings may include:
    - Congenital ptosis
    - Congenital glaucoma
    - Pulsating exophthalmos
  - If optic pathway glioma is present, MRI evaluation should be repeated every 2 years until age 10 in addition to annual ophthalmologic examination.
  - Precocious or delayed puberty may be a later clinical sign of optic glioma extending from the chiasm into the hypothalamus and should prompt reevaluation and MRI.
- Hormonal surges
  - Should be discussed with preteens and teens
  - Factors likely to cause increases in both size and number of neurofibromas
    - Oral contraceptives
    - Puberty
    - Pregnancy
- Neurodevelopment
  - Headaches occur in 20% of patients.
    - Usually migraines that respond well to standard therapy such as amitriptyline or topiramate
  - Seizures occur in 4–10%.
    - Management should be directed toward the specific seizure type.
  - Hearing loss, usually unilateral, occurs in ~10% of patients.
  - Various learning disabilities are observed in 35–65% of children:
    - Math and reading comprehension problems
    - Visual perception deficits
    - Delays in both gross- and fine-motor skills
    - Speech and language delays in ~50%
    - ADHD is common, occurring in ~50%.
  - Various behavioral problems, often in association with a comorbid diagnosis of ADHD
    - Anxiety
    - Depression
    - Social problems
    - Aggression
    - Unusual behaviors
- Vascular disease is more common and may include:
  - Congenital heart defects
  - Hypertension
  - Occlusive arterial disease
  - Aneurysms
  - Arteriovenous fistulae
- Hypertension
  - In young children as a result of renal artery stenosis in 1% of patients
  - In adults as primary hypertension or associated with pheochromocytoma
  - Workup should include:
    - Renal angiography in children
    - Urine catecholamine levels in adults
- Bone abnormalities
  - Range from skeletal dysplasia to nonossifying fibroma to short stature to kyphoscoliosis
  - Long bone dysplasia (especially tibial) may be seen during the first year of life.
    - May present as bowing or, rarely, pseudoarthrosis (nodule at the site of a healing pathological fracture)
    - Pseudoarthrosis occurs in only 3%.
  - Nonossifying fibromas occur in late childhood to the teen years.
    - May lead to pathological fracture, particularly in the femur, tibia, and humerus
  - Scoliosis is seen in 10%.
    - May develop earlier than in the general population
  - Aggressive dystrophic form may develop between 3–7 years of age

TSC

- Heart failure in infancy
- Various dysrhythmias
  - Wolff-Parkinson-White syndrome
- Renal cell carcinoma is a less common but potentially severe complication.
  - Lifetime risk is the same in TSC as in the general population
  - Average age of onset is 28 years in TSC.
  - Average onset is 52 years in general population.
  - Overall morbidity of renal lesions is predominantly related to angiomyolipomas.
- Symptomatic lymphangiomyomatosis
  - Often progressive
  - Leading cause of death among women with TSC

N

SWS

■ Some patients may develop sudden stroke-like episodes of weakness, even in the absence of seizures.
- May be transient
- May leave permanent hemiplegia

■ Hemianopsia may develop in up to one half of patients.

VHL

■ Major causes of death are:
- Renal cell carcinoma
- Complications from CNS hemangioblastomas

A-T

■ Patients with A-T are at higher risk (one third) for developing cancer.
- In children, acute lymphoblastic leukemia predominates.
- Other lymphoid tumors include
  - B-cell non-Hodgkin lymphoma
  - T-cell lymphoma
  - Hodgkin disease
- Older children sometimes develop
  - T-prolymphocytic leukemia
- Adults tend toward nonlymphoid cancers such as
  - Breast
  - Stomach
  - Ovarian
  - Liver
  - Uterus
  - Melanoma
  - Basal cell skin cancer
- Women who are *ATM* mutation carriers have a 5-fold increase in risk of breast cancer compared with the normal population.
- ~15% of patients with A-T die of lymphoid malignancies during childhood.

■ Patients with A-T are susceptible to injury by ionizing radiation and radiomimetic chemotherapeutic drugs.
- Because of the inability to repair defective DNA, this susceptibility complicates therapy for the various malignancies.
- Exposure to these agents poses life-threatening risk to patients with A-T.

PROGNOSIS

NF-1

■ Life expectancy is approximately 10–15 years shorter compared with the general population.

■ Malignancy and vascular disease are the leading causes of death.

TSC

■ Large numbers of tubers are associated with worse overall prognosis.
- Infantile spasms
- Cognitive impairment
- Difficult seizure control

■ Presence and number of subependymal nodules do not seem to correlate with severity of neurologic symptoms.

■ With any type of seizures, better control seems to improve prognosis.
- Seizures become refractory to treatment in up to 50% of children with TSC.

SWS

■ Earlier onset may predict worse outcome.
- Poor seizure prognosis
- More difficult seizure control
- Higher risk of cognitive impairment

■ No definite link exists between age at onset and neurologic outcome.

■ Bilateral leptomeningeal angiomatosis (7–26% of patients) has poor neurologic prognosis.

VHL

■ Visual prognosis is better when ocular lesions are detected before development of symptoms.

A-T

■ Life expectancy varies.

■ Survival into the 6th decade is likely.

■ Leading causes of death are:
- Malignancy
- Infection
- Pulmonary failure
  - From combined recurrent infection and recurrent aspiration

Nonconvulsive Periodic Disorders

DEFINITION

- A variety of paroxysmal nonepileptic disorders occurring in children with a wide range of clinical features that mimic seizures
- Distinguishing these from seizures is important so that the child is not treated inappropriately with anticonvulsants.
  - Syncope (fainting) is an acute and transient loss of consciousness caused by reduced cerebral perfusion.
  - Benign paroxysmal vertigo is a disorder characterized by brief attacks of vertigo.
  - Shuddering attacks or shivering episodes are a benign movement disorder.
  - Benign neonatal sleep myoclonus is sleep-related myoclonus (jerking of limbs) in neonates.
  - Night terrors or sleep terrors are a sleep disorder with some features that mimic partial complex seizures.
  - Narcolepsy is a sleep-wake disorder characterized by excessive and inappropriate periods of sleep during the day.
    - Interrupts activities
    - Does not diminish in response to adequate amounts of sleep at night
    - Naps may last from a few minutes to >1 hour.

EPIDEMIOLOGY

- Breath-holding spells (infantile syncope)
  - 2 types: cyanotic and pallid
  - Prevalence
    - ~5% of children
  - Age
    - Episodes typically begin between 6 and 18 months of age.
    - Spells may begin in the first few weeks of life.
    - Frequency of episodes ranges from once a year to several times daily.
- Syncope
  - Prevalence
    - Relatively common
  - Age
    - Particularly seen among teenagers
- Benign paroxysmal vertigo
  - Age
    - Symptoms usually appear within the first 3 or 4 years of life.
  - Frequency of episodes varies from 1 episode every few months to several weekly.
- Shuddering attacks
  - Prevalence
    - Occurs in many children at one time or another
  - Age
    - Episodes may start as early as a few months of age or not until later in childhood.
  - The number of episodes usually declines gradually.
- Night terrors
  - Prevalence
    - Occur in up to 6% of children
  - Age
    - A peak incidence in late preschool and early school-age children
- Narcolepsy
  - Prevalence
    - Estimated at 0.02–0.05%
  - Age
    - Onset usually occurs in the second decade.
    - Has been reported in children as young as 3 years
  - Sleep studies show that with narcolepsy rapid eye movement (REM) sleep occurs within 15 minutes of sleep onset.
    - In healthy patients, 90 minutes of non-REM sleep precede the first REM period.

MECHANISM

- Syncope
  - Postural hypotension can precipitate an episode.
    - May occur after a sudden change from a sitting or reclining position to a standing position
  - Common provoking stimuli
    - Emotional upset
    - Fright
    - Overheating
  - Cardiac disorders may cause syncope by reducing cardiac output and causing cerebral hypoxia.
    - Arrhythmias
    - Aortic stenosis
    - Severe cyanotic heart disease
  - In rare cases, episodes of syncope have been reported with:
    - Swallowing
    - Coughing
    - Urinating
    - Defecating
  - Clonic movements after the initial episode occur as a result of cerebral ischemia rather than epileptiform discharges from the brain.

- Shuddering attacks
  - The pathophysiologic mechanism is unclear.
  - Attacks have been postulated to be an expression of an essential tremor.
- Breath-holding
  - Cyanotic
    - Evaluation of children who have severe cyanotic breath-holding spells has shown an underlying autonomic system dysregulation.
    - This may contribute to the pathophysiologic features of the episodes.
  - Pallid
    - A vasovagal phenomenon
    - The precipitating event induces a vagally mediated asystole, which then leads to cerebral ischemia.
    - The clonic jerks are caused by cerebral hypoxia and are not caused by epileptiform discharges from the brain.
- Night terrors
  - Caused by a rapid partial arousal from deep, slow-wave sleep
  - Night terror triggers include:
    - Febrile illness
    - Sleep deprivation

HISTORY

- A thorough history is often all that is needed to make the diagnosis.
  - A few patients may require more extensive evaluation.
- Breath-holding spells
  - The most important features of the evaluation are:
    - History of the episode
    - Surrounding events
    - Familial incidence of breath-holding spells is high; parents should be questioned about episodes in other family members.
- Syncope
  - Obtain a description of the event by the patient and an observer.

DIFFERENTIAL DIAGNOSIS

- Breath-holding spells can be divided into 2 types: cyanotic and pallid.
  - Cyanotic
    - More common than the pallid form
    - Usually precipitated by frustration or anger
    - During spells, children cry vigorously and then hold their breath in expiration.

- Apnea is followed by cyanosis, with opisthotonic posturing and loss of consciousness.
- Recovery is usually quick, with return of respiration and consciousness within 1 minute.
  - Pallid
    - Usually provoked by sudden fright or minor injuries
    - The child gasps or cries briefly and then abruptly becomes quiet.
      - The child loses consciousness, has pallor, and becomes limp.
      - The child may develop clonic jerks.
      - The child may fall and hit the occiput.
- Syncope
  - Patients have presyncopal symptoms that may include:
    - Light-headedness
    - Anxiety
    - Sweating
    - Nausea
    - Generalized numbness
    - Visual changes described as constriction or darkening of vision
    - Observers notice marked pallor and clammy skin.
  - Presyncopal symptoms are followed by loss of consciousness and slumping to the floor.
    - Once the patient is recumbent and cerebral perfusion is restored, consciousness returns within a few seconds.
    - If patient is held with the head above the body and cerebral perfusion is not restored, clonic movements may occur.
    - Patients may be tired but are not disoriented or confused after an episode of syncope.
- Benign paroxysmal vertigo
  - Characterized by abrupt onset
    - The child appears fearful and cannot maintain normal posture and gait.
    - The child may seek support and clutch the parent, then abruptly sit down or fall.
    - In severe cases, the child may be limp and incapable of using the extremities.
    - Pallor and diaphoresis are usually apparent.
    - Vomiting and nystagmus sometimes occur.
  - An episode typically lasts <30 seconds.
    - In rare cases, may last a few minutes
    - A brief period of postural instability may follow that usually resolves within a few minutes.
    - Consciousness is not altered during the episode.
    - The child rarely feels sleepy afterwards.

- History and physical examination usually differentiate from:
  - Brain stem lesions
  - Posterior fossa tumors
  - Epilepsy
- Benign neonatal sleep myoclonus
  - Myoclonic jerks begin in the first month of life, sometimes as early as the first day.
  - Myoclonus presents only during quiet sleep and disappears when the infant awakens.
  - Jerks occur every 2–3 seconds for several minutes and have been reported to last up to 12 hours.
  - Jerking movements may begin bilaterally or start in 1 extremity, then progress to involve the other extremities.
  - Neonatal sleep myoclonus is differentiated from seizure disorder by:
    - History of episodes during sleep only
    - Normal electroencephalogram
- Night terrors
  - Affected children often have a family history of either night terrors or another sleep disorder.
  - Episodes usually occur during the first 2 hours after falling asleep.
  - Child sits up in bed abruptly and screams or talks unintelligibly.
  - If the child's eyes are open, they have a glazed look.
  - During the episode, the child appears to be hallucinating and does not respond to parents.
  - Response of the sympathetic nervous system includes tachycardia and diaphoresis.
  - In some cases, the child may sleepwalk.
  - Episode usually lasts 10 minutes; the child then relaxes and abruptly falls back to sleep.
  - On awakening, the child does not remember the episode.
  - Nightmares should be differentiated from night terrors.
    - Nightmares occur during REM sleep.
    - Nightmares are associated with easy arousal and recall of the content, or at least the occurrence of the nightmare.

LABORATORY EVALUATION

- Laboratory evaluation is seldom needed for any of these disorders.
- Narcolepsy
  - A strong association exists between narcolepsy and the human leukocyte class II antigen DQB1*0602.
  - Human leukocyte antigen typing may be helpful but is not diagnostic.
  - Neuropeptides may be absent on cerebrospinal fluid studies.

DIAGNOSTIC PROCEDURES

- Syncope
  - If atypical features are present, electroencephalography or a cardiac evaluation, including Holter monitoring, may be appropriate.
    - Absence of a precipitating factor
    - Confusion after the episode
  - Evaluation with tilt-table testing can be helpful for children who have unexplained syncope.
- Narcolepsy
  - Sleep studies are important in diagnosing narcolepsy.

TREATMENT APPROACH

- In general, the approach with the majority of the nonconvulsive periodic disorders is to:
  - Educate the parents about the disorder
  - Reassure parents that disorder will not lead to intellectual disability or epilepsy
  - Explain that most of the disorders are time-limited and will resolve on their own
- Narcoplepsy is the exception.
  - It is a lifelong disorder that must be accurately diagnosed and subsequently treated.

SPECIFIC TREATMENT

Breath-holding spells

- Treatment is directed mainly at reassuring the family of the benign nature of the episodes.
- Emphasize that the episodes are not seizures and do not lead to intellectual disability or epilepsy.
- Anticonvulsants should not be used.
  - They are not effective in treating either cyanotic or pallid breath-holding spells.
- Cyanotic episodes
  - Often precipitated by temper tantrums, anger, and frustration
  - Advice about behavior management may be helpful.
- Pallid breath-holding spells
  - Anemia has been described as a contributing factor.
  - Treating anemia may reduce the incidence of the episodes.
  - Atropine is effective for pallid breath-holding episodes; however, its use is rarely warranted.

Syncope

- Teach the patient and family about managing an episode.
- When patients have presyncopal symptoms:
  - They should sit or lie down as soon as symptoms begin to prevent progression to loss of consciousness.
  - If the patient loses consciousness, place the child in a recumbent position, with the head lower than the trunk.

N

- Parents should be cautioned against picking up a child who has fainted, as this may prolong the period of unconsciousness.

Benign paroxysmal vertigo

- In most cases, no treatment is necessary.
- Anticonvulsants are not effective.
- Antihistamines have been used in some patients who have frequent episodes.
  - Some have noted an apparent reduction in the number of episodes.
  - Assessing the effect of therapy accurately is difficult because frequency of attacks varies.

Shuddering attacks

- In most cases, no treatment is necessary.
- If episodes are severe and interfere with activities, treatment with propranolol may be helpful.
- Anticonvulsants are ineffective and should not be used.

Benign neonatal sleep myoclonus

- No treatment is necessary.
- Reassure parents that these infants do not subsequently develop epilepsy or cognitive delay.

Night terrors

- The nature of the episodes should be explained to the parents.
- Parents tend to try to wake and reassure the child.
  - Attempts to awaken the child are not helpful and may increase agitation.
- Parents should be told that the child is not aware of their presence.
- If the child is sleep deprived as a result of night terrors, parents should take steps to increase the amount of sleep the child is getting.
- If night terrors persist despite adequate sleep:
  - A sleep study may be needed to evaluate for obstructive sleep apnea, which can trigger night terrors.
- In most cases, no medication is indicated.
  - If episodes are frequent or severe, medications may be helpful.
    - Benzodiazepines
    - Imipramine
    - L-5-Hydroxytryptophan

Narcolepsy

- Central nervous system stimulants help reduce the frequency of naps.
  - Methylphenidate
  - Modafinil

- Tricyclic medications are used to treat cataplexy and the other associated symptoms.
  - Imipramine

WHEN TO REFER

- If a diagnosis cannot be made by history and physical examination
- If a need exists for subspecialty expertise

WHEN TO ADMIT

- Admission may be necessary it the child needs video electro-encephalographic monitoring to evaluate an episode.

COMPLICATIONS

- Narcolepsy
  - In addition to the excessive daytime sleep, patients often have:
    - Cataplexy, a transient partial or complete loss of tone
      - Often triggered by an emotional reaction, eg, laughter or fright
      - The individual does not lose consciousness.
    - Sleep paralysis
      - Occurs as the patient falls asleep or awakens
      - Characterized by the inability to move or speak
    - Hypnagogic hallucinations
      - Occurs while falling asleep
      - Can be auditory or visual
      - May be very frightening to a child

PROGNOSIS

- Breath-holding spells (either cyanotic or pallid) have an excellent prognosis.
  - Most children outgrow such episodes by school age.
- Benign paroxysmal vertigo attacks usually stop spontaneously over a few years.
  - Some children may later develop migraine headaches.
- Benign neonatal sleep myoclonus usually diminishes gradually during the first 6 months of life.
  - Rarely lasts >3 years
- Narcolepsy is a lifelong condition that needs to be monitored and treated.

Obesity and Metabolic Syndrome

DEFINITION

- Definitions of *overweight* and *obesity* are based on body mass index (BMI).
  - BMI = weight in kilograms divided by height in meters squared
    - Approximates a person's body fat
    - Correlates well with medical complications associated with obesity
    - Easily calculated from standard measurements obtained during health care visits
    - In children, body fat changes throughout development, so BMI percentile must be used.
- For children and adolescents in US, terms *at risk for overweight* and *overweight* have been used instead of *overweight* and *obese*.
  - At risk for overweight: BMI between the 85th and the 95th percentiles for age and sex
  - Overweight: BMI at or above the 95th percentile
- In 2007 an expert committee consisting of representatives from 15 national health care associations recommended changing to different terminology.
  - When BMI is between the 85th and 94th percentile, "overweight" should replace "at risk of overweight."
  - When BMI is at or above the 95th percentile, "obesity" should replace "overweight."
- Metabolic syndrome (syndrome X)
  - Cluster of metabolic abnormalities that leads to cardiovascular disease and increased risk of mortality

EPIDEMIOLOGY

- Prevalence of obesity
  - Has dramatically increased worldwide in developed and underdeveloped countries
    - Only the very poorest geographic areas, where food scarcity is widespread (eg, Haiti and sub-Saharan Africa), have yet to be affected.
    - In US in last 2 decades
      - 3-fold increase in obesity in children age 12–19 years
      - Doubling of obesity in children age 6–11
- Age
  - Children and adolescents age 6–19 years: 16% have a BMI >95th percentile.
    - Children age <5 years: >10% have a BMI >95th percentile.
- Ethnicity
  - Between 1986 and 1998, black and Hispanic youth showed increases in obesity prevalence more than double that of non-Hispanic white youth.

- Geographic factors
  - Children living in southern states showed greater increases in obesity prevalence than those in northern and western states.
- Socioeconomic status (SES)
  - Poverty is a risk factor for obesity in non-Hispanic white adolescents.
  - No SES-obesity relationship has been found in Hispanic children.
  - Higher SES is associated with higher rates of overweight and obesity in black persons.
- Sex
  - Risk for obesity varies by ethnicity.
  - Hispanic boys are more likely than Hispanic girls to be overweight.
  - Black girls are more likely than black boys to be overweight.
- Prevalence of metabolic syndrome
  - Increasingly recognized in children and adolescents as prevalence of overweight rises in these age groups
  - Data from the National Health and Nutrition Examination Survey (1988–1994) estimates the prevalence of metabolic syndrome to be as high as 30% in obese adolescents 12–19 years of age.
- Costs
  - The current epidemic of obesity poses a significant threat to health care systems already struggling with escalating costs.
  - The US Surgeon General predicted that costs related to obesity will overtake those of tobacco.
    - Based on alarming increased expenses associated with obesity and related conditions
  - Current costs for obese patients exceed by 36% those of patients who are not obese.
  - Medication expenses are 77% higher for obese compared with non-obese individuals.
  - Obesity is associated with increased numbers of medical diagnoses and medications.
    - Leading to increased medical costs comparable to 20 years of aging
  - These figures do not attempt to capture costs of psychological morbidity.

ETIOLOGY

- Weight gain is caused by a positive energy imbalance.
  - Increased caloric intake, decreased energy expenditure, or a combination of the 2
  - A sustained positive balance of 100 calories per day leads to weight gain of 10 lb/year.

- Overweight and normal-weight children do not differ by metabolic rate.
  - Overweight adolescents have higher total daily energy expenditures and resting energy expenditures than adolescents who are not overweight.
    - Overweight children need to eat more to maintain their higher body weight.
- Leptin
  - Hormone that acts on hypothalamus to regulate hunger and satiety
  - Serum levels correlate with adiposity in children and adults.
  - Whether increased adiposity results in decreased leptin production or whether primary leptin deficiency is followed by weight gain is unclear.
  - Leptin resistance or deficiency results in increased food intake in animal models.
  - The role of hormones and neurotransmitters in human energy regulation remains poorly understood.

RISK FACTORS

- Genetic and family influences
  - The rapid increase in obesity over the past 20 years demonstrates the significance of lifestyle and societal influences.
  - Shared family conditions support the importance of causal environmental factors.
- Family environment and food preferences
  - Children of overweight parents are more likely than children of normal-weight parents to prefer high-fat foods.
  - Children with higher BMI consume less at breakfast and more at dinner than their normal-weight peers.
  - Skipping breakfast is associated with poorer food choices and increased risk for obesity.
  - Families who eat meals together consume less fried food and carbonated beverages and more fruits and vegetables.
- Recent environmental changes may be related to population-level increases in obesity.
  - Urbanization
    - Increased reliance on motorized transport
    - Less outdoor play time
  - Technologic advances
  - Easy access to calorie-dense foods
- Eating behaviors
  - Overeating in response to environments that interfere with normal regulatory mechanisms
    - Extremes of parental behavior (neglect and overinvolvement)
    - Use of food to comfort children
    - Prompting children to finish what is on their plate may impair the ability to self-regulate appetite and satiety.

- Food insecurity
  - Malnutrition during gestation and early infancy is associated with both stunting and obesity.
    - Possible mechanisms
      - Excess deposition of fat in subsequent times of nourishment
      - Preference for high-fat foods, overeating when food is plentiful
    - Individuals may develop increased sensitivity to hunger- and satiety-related hormones and neurotransmitters, resulting in fat deposition in response to early life stress.
- American diet
  - Large portion sizes
  - Greater intake of calorie-dense beverages and juice
  - Increases in consumption of fast-food
  - School lunches (usually contain >30% of calories from fat)
  - Vending machines in schools
- Parental obesity
  - For children <3 years of age, parental weight is a better predictor of adult obesity than the child's actual weight.
    - This effect lessens with age; toward adolescence, the child's weight becomes an equal predictor at school age and a more important predictor.
    - Overweight and normal-weight children with 1 obese parent are at twice the risk of adult obesity.
- Smaller family size
- Single-parent families
- Parental neglect
- Overparenting
- High prepregnancy maternal BMI
- Higher birth weight
- Servings of sugar-sweetened beverages
- Television time >3 hours per day is associated with a higher average BMI.

SIGNS AND SYMPTOMS

- Clinical manifestations of metabolic syndrome
  - Obesity
    - Excess body fat
    - Increased visceral fat
    - Central fat distribution
  - Insulin resistance
  - Dyslipidemia/hypertriglyceridemia
  - Hypertension
  - Glucose intolerance or non–insulin-dependent diabetes mellitus

DIFFERENTIAL DIAGNOSIS

- Primary medical causes of obesity are rare.
- Endocrine and genetic causes of obesity often cause short stature or cognitive impairment.
  - Hypothyroidism
    - Associated with short stature
    - Weight gain, fatigue, constipation, cold intolerance, myxedema
    - Testing: thyroid-stimulating hormone, free thyroxine
  - Cushing syndrome
    - Short stature
    - Central obesity, hirsutism, moon face, plethora, hypertension
    - Testing: dexamethasone suppression test
  - Pseudohypoparathyroidism
    - Short stature
    - Short metacarpals, subcutaneous calcifications, dysmorphic facies, intellectual disability, hypocalcemia, hyperphosphatemia
    - Testing: urinary cyclic adenosine monophosphate after synthetic parathyroid hormone infusion
  - Growth hormone deficiency
    - Short stature
    - Fatigue
    - Testing: evoked growth response, insulinlike growth factor-1 (IGF-1)
  - Down syndrome
    - Short stature
    - Dysmorphic facies, intellectual disability
    - Testing: karyotyping
  - Turner syndrome
    - Short stature, web neck
    - Testing: karyotyping
  - Präder-Willi syndrome
    - Cognitive impairment
    - Hypogonadism, small hands and feet
    - Testing: FISH *15q11* microdeletion (70% of cases)
  - Bardet-Biedl syndrome
    - Cognitive impairment
    - Retinitis pigmentosa, renal abnormalities, polydactyly, hypogonadism
    - Testing: *BBS1* gene
  - Biemond syndrome
    - Cognitive impairment
    - Iris coloboma, hypogonadism, polydactyly
    - Testing: clinical
  - Alstrom syndrome
    - Cognitive impairment
    - Retinitis pigmentosa, diabetes mellitus, and hearing loss
    - Testing: *ALMS1* gene

DIAGNOSTIC APPROACH

- The Centers for Disease Control and Prevention provides age- and sex-specific growth curves for BMI.
- Electronic medical records allow routine calculation and plotting of BMI when height and weight data are entered.

LABORATORY FINDINGS

- Centers for Disease Control and Prevention and AAP recommendations for evaluating obese children (BMI >95%)
  - Cholesterol panel (including low-density lipoprotein cholesterol, high-density lipoprotein cholesterol, and triglycerides)
  - Fasting plasma glucose
- The American Diabetes Association recommends fasting glucose test for children with BMI between 85th and the 95th percentile if:
  - They have a family history of diabetes mellitus or obesity *or*
  - They have signs of insulin resistance, including acanthosis nigricans, polycystic ovary syndrome (PCOS), or hirsutism
- Hemoglobin A_{1C} is sometimes used to screen patients who cannot comply with fasting before laboratory testing.
- Insulin levels
  - Not recommended for evaluating obesity
    - Can be low to high at time of presentation of type 2 diabetes
  - Do not alter medical management
  - Helpful when uncertainty exists as to whether patient has type 1 or type 2 diabetes mellitus
- Liver function tests
  - At baseline
  - Before pharmacologic management for type 2 diabetes
  - Before surgical intervention for obesity
- Other studies
  - Ordered only as indicated by history or physical examination
- Laboratory tests, by indication
  - Thyroid function tests
    - When symptoms of hypothyroidism are present
  - Luteinizing hormone, follicle-stimulating hormone, total and free testosterone; consider pelvic ultrasonography
    - Menstrual irregularity
    - Acne
    - Hirsutism (PCOS)

O

- Genetic consultation, karyotype
  - Short stature
  - Dysmorphic features
  - Cognitive impairment
- When to test for diabetes
  - Patient is obese, with BMI >95th percentile
  - BMI between the 85th–95th percentile with any of the following:
    - Family history of type 2 diabetes
    - Native American, black, Hispanic, Asian, Pacific Islander
    - Signs of:
      - Insulin resistance
      - Acanthosis nigricans
      - Hypertension
      - Dyslipidemia
      - PCOS
- Metabolic syndrome
  - Insulin resistance (decreased ß-cell count)
    - Elevated fasting insulin levels
    - Fasting insulin level >15 mg/dL
    - Peak insulin level >150 mg/dL
  - Dyslipidemia/hypertriglyceridemia
    - Low high-density lipoprotein cholesterol
    - Increased free fatty acids
  - Glucose intolerance or non–insulin-dependent diabetes mellitus
    - Fasting plasma glucose level >126 mg/dL
    - 2-hour plasma glucose level >200 mg/dL (oral glucose tolerance test)

IMAGING

- Plain-film radiography
  - For deformity, hip or knee pain (slipped femoral capital epiphysis or Blount disease)
- Head computed tomography and lumbar puncture to evaluate:
  - Headache
  - Visual changes
  - Papilledema

TREATMENT APPROACH

- Preventing secondary comorbidity and disability is the principal goal in treating overweight children and adolescents.
- Obesity should be approached as a chronic condition that requires permanent lifestyle changes to achieve optimal body weight.

- Prescribing a treatment plan without engaging the child and family can lead to frustration, impairing future attempts at weight control.
- Enhancing the therapeutic relationship can begin with a question to the parent.
  - "Have you ever struggled with your weight?"
    - The answer reveals the family's perception of body weight as an indicator of health and well-being and the parent's empathy for child.
- Readiness to change can be assessed by asking the child and parent 3 questions:
  - "How concerned are you about your weight (your child's weight)?"
  - "Do you think that you can improve your body fitness (your child's body fitness)?"
  - "Do you think that your family can change eating and physical activity patterns?"
- Once the patient and family are ready to begin a treatment plan, the clinician should assist in setting realistic goals.
- Weight maintenance rather than weight loss is usually the first step.
  - The objective is to decrease the rate of weight gain and allow the child to achieve healthier body mass.
  - Learning healthy eating and activity habits improves health over time.
  - Focusing on health and healthy behavior changes allows gradual and long-term change.
  - Fad diets and very–low-calorie regimens are not recommended because they cannot be maintained.
    - Children with acute comorbid conditions, such as sleep apnea, may be managed medically on a very–low-calorie diet, usually in an inpatient treatment program.
- Recommendations for weight maintenance or weight loss are based on:
  - Level of overweight/BMI
  - Age
  - Existence of complications
  - Setting goals for weight maintenance or weight loss may be based on BMI, age, and complications.
- Role of pediatrician
  - Intervene early.
  - Assess the family's readiness to change.
  - Educate the family about medical complications of obesity.
  - Involve the family and caregivers in the treatment program.
  - Aim for permanent dietary and activity change.
  - Avoid short-term diets or exercise programs aimed at rapid weight loss.
  - Teach the family to monitor eating and activity.

- Assist the family in making small, gradual changes.
- Encourage and empathize.
- Avoid criticism.

SPECIFIC TREATMENTS

Pharmacologic approach

- Weight loss
  - No evidence exists that pharmacologic agents for weight loss are safe and effective for children.
- Hyperlipidemia
  - Lipid-lowering medication is considered if behavioral modifications are unsuccessful.
- Metabolic syndrome
  - Evidence for short- and long-term efficacy of pharmacologic treatment of metabolic syndrome in youth remains sparse.
    - Studies of oral hypoglycemics (specifically metformin) in adolescents have demonstrated reductions in blood glucose but have shown little effect on insulin resistance or lipid abnormalities.

Counseling

- May be necessary for the family of a child who is seriously obese (>99th percentile) or has medical complications

Bariatric surgery

- May be considered in severely obese adolescents (BMI >40 kg/m^2) with all of the following:
  - Nearly complete skeletal maturity
  - Significant medical complications
  - Inability to change weight or obesity-related comorbid conditions despite dietary and exercise modifications for 6 months
- After evaluation by a multidisciplinary team, surgery can be performed by surgeons experienced in gastric bypass.
- The major challenge is how to give informed consent or assent about the consequences of both obesity and the alternative of bariatric surgery.
  - The procedure changes the individual's ability to eat and may have unforeseen long-term consequences.
  - On the other hand, obesity may be life threatening.

Dietary modifications

- Drink water, sugar-free beverages, or milk with no more than 1% fat.
- Use cooking spray instead of frying.
- Make cut-up fruits and vegetables accessible.
- Serve appropriate portions and limit seconds to fruits and vegetables.
  - Meat: size of palm
  - Starch: 1/2 cup

- Review school lunch menu with the child to pick healthy options.
- Pack a lunch with 4 oz of lean meat, whole-grain bread, fruit or vegetable, and milk.
- Limit restaurant dining to once per week or less.
- Limit fast food to rarely.
- Eat meals together, and turn off the television while eating.
- Schedule at least 20 minutes for each meal.
  - Eating slowly helps to avoid overeating.
- Eat regular meals.
  - Skipping meals can lead to overeating.
- Remove snack foods, chips, cookies, and desserts from the house.
- Allow occasional treats.
- Make salads with vegetables, not eggs, meat, bacon, or cheese.
  - Toss the family salad to decrease amount of dressing.

Recommendations for increasing physical activity

- Limit television and video games to no more than 1–2 hours per day.
- Engage in active family activities (biking, walking after dinner, swimming, going to zoo/museum).
- Dance to your favorite music.
- Walk with a friend rather than talking on the telephone.
- Walk while you talk on the telephone.
- Engage in team sports.
- Take classes: dance, martial arts, or swimming.
- Strategies for toddlers and preschool-age children
  - Engage in outdoor play every day.
  - Engage in active indoor play, soft balls, jumping, or bouncing balls.
  - Buy active toys rather than computer games or videos.
- Strength training
  - Overweight children often find this rewarding and benefit psychologically and physically.
    - Given their body mass, they may be stronger than peers.
    - It does not require aerobic endurance or agility.

Parenting skills for weight loss

- Find reasons to praise the child's behavior.
- Avoid using food as a reward.
- Establish daily family meal and snack times, as well as physically active family time.
- Determine what food is offered and when.
- Allow child to decide whether to eat.
- Offer only healthy options.
- Remove temptations (snack food in home).
- Walk instead of driving.

O

- Take the stairs.
- Decrease television-viewing time.
- Be a role model in diet and physical activity.
- Be consistent.

Metabolic syndrome

- Treatment is aimed primarily at weight reduction and treating component diagnoses: hypertension, diabetes, and hyperlipidemia.
- Behavioral and dietary modifications are first-line therapy.
- Metformin may be helpful as an adjuvant therapy.

WHEN TO ADMIT

- The morbidly obese patient with BMI >40 kg/m² may need to be hospitalized for a low-calorie weight reduction program.

WHEN TO REFER

- Refer to a pediatric obesity center for acute complications, such as:
  - Pseudotumor cerebri
  - Sleep apnea
  - Obesity hypoventilation syndrome
  - Orthopedic problems

FOLLOW-UP

- A key role for child health professionals is monitoring.
  - BMI should be calculated and plotted at each health care maintenance visit.

COMPLICATIONS

- Obesity is associated with medical comorbid conditions in many organ systems.
  - Some problems are apparent after a relatively short duration of excess body fat.
  - Other complications do not arise for decades.
  - Obesity is responsible for childhood appearance of diseases previously seen only during adulthood, most notably type 2 diabetes mellitus.
- Cardiovascular
  - Hypertension
    - Systolic blood pressure >95th percentile for sex, age, and height
    - Diastolic hypertension increases with BMI.
    - Prevalence of hypertension is 3 times greater in overweight children than in their normal-weight peers.
    - Underdiagnosed in children
      - Blood pressure norms change with height, age, and sex.
      - Technical difficulties, including use of a wrong-size blood pressure cuff, can cause errors.

- Dyslipidemia
  - High-density lipoprotein cholesterol level <40 mmol/L, low-density lipoprotein cholesterol level >130 mmol/L, total cholesterol level >200 mmol/L
- Endocrine
  - Type 2 diabetes
  - Increased insulin resistance
  - PCOS
    - Menstrual irregularities
    - Hirsutism
    - Acne
    - Insulin resistance
    - Hyperandrogenemia
  - Metabolic syndrome (hypertension, dyslipidemia, insulin resistance)
- Gastrointestinal
  - Nonalcoholic steatohepatitis
    - Increased aminotransferase levels
    - May progress to fibrosis or cirrhosis
  - Gallbladder disease
    - Obesity may account for 50% of cases in adolescents.
  - Obstructive sleep apnea
    - Snoring, apnea, restless sleep, behavioral problems
- Orthopedic
  - Slipped capital femoral epiphysis
    - Hip or knee pain, decreased mobility of hip
  - Blount disease
    - Tibia vara; severe bowing of the tibia
  - Osteoarthritis
    - May present in adolescence
- Neuromotor
  - Pseudotumor cerebri
    - Headaches, vision changes, papilledema
- Oncologic
  - Endometrial cancer
  - Breast cancer
  - Colon cancer
  - Increased prevalence with adult obesity
- Chronic inflammation
  - Adiponectin (anti-inflammatory peptide): reduced in obese individuals
    - Low levels correlate with high BMI, as well as elevated levels of plasma triglycerides and free fatty acids.
  - Levels of the proinflammatory peptides tumor necrosis factor-α and interleukin-6 are elevated in obese patients.
    - Interleukin-6 stimulates liver to produce C-reactive protein; this may be a link to coronary disease.

– A linear relationship exists among BMI and C-reactive protein and interleukin-6 levels.
■ Psychiatric
  • Anxiety
  • Low self-esteem
  • Depression
  • Difficult to assess whether depression or low self-esteem is cause of weight gain or if weight gain is cause of depression
  • The effects of obesity on child and adolescent mental health are still not well understood.
    – During early childhood, body weight is not associated with self-esteem.
    – As children approach adolescence, self-esteem is lower in overweight children than in normal-weight peers.
  • Poor emotional and social functioning is self-reported by 12- to14-year-old overweight girls.
  • Adolescent girls concerned about weight also report more depressive symptoms.
    – Depressed adolescents are at increased risk for developing persistent obesity.
  • Overweight youth are likely to report physical but not emotional problems, even though some studies show that they may be socially excluded.
  • Assessing affect and mental health status is advisable.

PROGNOSIS

■ Early childhood obesity often resolves.
  • Optimism is warranted in early years.
■ By adolescence, nutritional and activity patterns are more difficult to change, and families have less influence.
■ Obesity remains an emotionally charged issue, creating more difficulties for the family and clinician than do more purely medical problems.
■ Blood pressure can decrease with as little as 5–10 pounds of weight loss.
■ The age at which the child becomes obese is related to how likely the child is to be obese in adulthood.
  • Children who are obese from 6–11 years
    – 50% of girls and 30% of boys will be obese as adults, compared with 18% of age-matched peers.
  • Obesity during adolescence
    – >60% will maintain obesity into adulthood.
  • Obese adults who became obese during childhood
    – More likely than those who become obese during adulthood to have severe obesity (BMI >40 kg/m^2)
■ Overweight and normal-weight children with 1 obese parent are at twice the risk of adult obesity compared with children without an overweight parent.
  • Overweight 10–14 year olds with ≥1 obese parent: 80% will remain obese as adults.

PREVENTION

■ Prevention of childhood obesity
  • Crucial to public health
  • Requires concerted effort of:
    – Public health officials
    – Government at all levels
    – Schools
    – Health care system
■ Clinicians should educate families about importance of healthy nutrition and physical activity from earliest years.
  • Healthful nutrition begins with breastfeeding.
    – Associated with lower childhood obesity risk
    – Exclusive breastfeeding is recommended for first 4–6 months of life.
  • Consideration of nutrient quality and caloric content
    – Reserve calorie-laden foods with little nutritional value for occasional treats.
    – Plan meals and snacks based on fruits, vegetables, and grains.
    – Include appropriate portion sizes of meat and dairy products
      ■ Should supply fewer calories than fruits, vegetables, and grains
    – Low-fat milk is recommended for most children after age 2 years.
    – Children should be encouraged to drink water to quench thirst.
      ■ Reserve highly sugared beverages for occasional treats.
      ■ Fruit juice in moderation
    – Healthy desserts
      ■ Fruit
      ■ Yogurt
      ■ Cookies made with oatmeal
      ■ Occasional puddings made with milk and eggs
      ■ Ice cream
    – Using lower-fat alternatives is suggested for cardio-vascular health.
    – Attention to portion size is important.
■ Encourage physical activity.
  • Children whose parents are physically active are more likely to be physically active.
  • Clinicians can encourage families to plan opportunities for physical activity as a parental responsibility.
  • Children should engage in ≥60 minutes of physical activity on most, preferably all, days.
  • Children who participate in organized sports should be encouraged to be physically active on days without organized activities.

O

- Pediatricians can reinforce the importance of daily physical activity and to resist reliance on organized sports for all of a child's physical activity.
- Older children and adolescents may benefit from strength training.
- Increased physical activity should be accompanied by decrease in sedentary activities.
  - Limiting television/other recreational screen time to <2 hours per day is recommended.
  - The AAP recommends no television for children <2 years.
- Parents should strive to be role models in their eating and activity habits.
  - Child health professionals can begin to talk to parents about healthy nutrition and activity during the first year of life.
  - Themes can be revisited at annual health care maintenance visits.

■ Monitoring
  - Tracking growth trajectories and explaining patterns to parents is an essential component of primary prevention.
  - Children with increasing BMI percentiles may be at risk for obesity.
    - Health care professionals can help families evaluate nutritional and activity patterns and make adjustments.

Obstructive Uropathy and Vesicoureteral Reflux

DEFINITION

- Obstructive uropathy
  - Impairment of urinary flow that causes:
    - Proliferation and myofibroblastic transformation of interstitial fibroblasts
    - Expansion of extracellular matrix
    - Loss of renal tubular cells
    - Decreased numbers of nephrons
  - These changes may affect the kidney and cause:
    - Sodium wasting
    - Hyperkalemic acidosis
    - Nephrogenic diabetes insipidus
    - Renal insufficiency
    - Renal failure
  - Effects on renal growth, development, and function depend on the timing, severity, and duration of urinary obstruction.
    - Early renal development: dysplasia and arrest of renal development with persistence of fetal architecture
    - Later development: dilatation of collecting system (ie, hydronephrosis)
    - Complete obstruction (such as from urethral atresia) has more detrimental effects on renal development and function than partial obstruction.
- Vesicoureteral reflux (VUR)
  - Occurs when urine in bladder flows in a retrograde manner into upper urinary tracts

EPIDEMIOLOGY

- Obstructive uropathy
  - Leading cause of renal failure in children <2 years
  - Accounts for 17% of cases of kidney transplants in children
  - Incidence of prenatal hydronephrosis: 1:100 to 1:500 (half of all abnormalities detected by prenatal ultrasonography)
  - Prevalence of the causes of prenatal hydronephrosis
    - Transient physiologic–nonpathologic: 50–70%
    - Ureteropelvic junction (UPJ) obstruction: 10–40% (male-to-female ratio of 2:1)
    - VUR: 10–30%
    - Ureterovesical junction (UVJ) obstruction: 5–20% (more common in boys)
    - Multicystic dysplastic kidney: 2–5%
    - Posterior urethral valves (PUVs): 1–5%
    - Other (ureterocele, ectopic ureter, duplex system, urethral atresia, prune belly, polycystic kidney disease, and renal cysts): <1%
      - Ureteroceles: More common in girls (female-to-male ratio of 7:1)
      - Ectopic ureter: Only 15% of cases occur in boys.
- VUR
  - Prevalence
    - No urinary tract infection (UTI) or urologic anomalies: 0.4–1.8% of pediatric population
    - With UTI: 30–50%
    - With prenatal hydronephrosis: 25%
    - With parents who have VUR: 50–67%
    - With sibling who has VUR: 33–50%
  - Race
    - Significantly fewer black persons than white persons
  - Sex
    - Much lower in boys than girls
    - In infants <1 year, proportions of boys and girls are more equivalent.
    - In children with UTI, the ratio of girls to boys is about 4:1
    - In infants evaluated for prenatal hydronephrosis, the ratio of boys to girls is about 1:4.

ETIOLOGY

- VUR
  - May arise from maldevelopment or delayed maturity of the UVJ (primary reflux)
  - May result from distortion of UVJ by changes in bladder caused by other conditions
    - PUVs
    - Neurogenic bladder (secondary reflux)
  - Appears to be heritable

RISK FACTORS

- VUR
  - Association between VUR and renal abnormalities, termed *reflux nephropathy*
    - Renal scarring associated with intrarenal reflux of infected urine (common in older children with primary reflux)
    - Congenital nephropathy associated with VUR but without infection (common in infants with primary reflux)
    - Nephropathy associated with VUR and impaired urinary flow (common in children with secondary reflux)

- Incidence is low in children with mild hydronephrosis detected on prenatal ultrasonography and increases with moderate and severe grades.
- Strong genetic component

SIGNS AND SYMPTOMS

- Obstructive uropathy
  - UTI
  - Abdominal mass
  - Hematuria
  - Urinary stone
  - Poor urinary stream
  - Incontinence
  - Failure to thrive
  - Renal insufficiency or failure
  - Anemia
  - Sudden onset of hypertension
- VUR
  - UTI
    - Fever
    - Vomiting
    - Failure to thrive
    - In older children
      - Flank pain
      - Dysuria
  - Gross hematuria
  - Prenatal hydronephrosis
  - Family history of reflux
  - Hypertension
  - Renal insufficiency or failure

DIFFERENTIAL DIAGNOSIS

Obstructive uropathy (hydronephrosis)

- Unilateral
  - UPJ obstruction
    - Urine flow from the renal pelvis into the proximal ureter is impaired.
    - Intrinsic obstruction results from luminal narrowing of the UPJ, with or without kinking.
    - Extrinsic obstruction is caused by compression of the ureter by anomalous renal vasculature.
      - It is more commonly found in older children and adults.
    - Most common cause of obstructive uropathy in children, second only to transient, physiologic nonpathologic hydronephrosis as the most common cause of antenatal hydronephrosis

- UVJ obstruction, also called *obstructed megaureter*
  - Urine flow from the distal ureter into bladder is impaired.
  - Primary obstruction: due to deficiency of smooth muscle in intravesical ureter
  - Secondary obstruction: results from extrinsic compression of ureter by thick bladder wall in such states as PUVs or neurogenic bladder
  - Accounts for about 8% of children who had symptoms, such as infection, hematuria, or pain, and hydroureteronephrosis on imaging studies
  - Accounts for 23% of newborns with prenatally diagnosed hydronephrosis and is the third most common cause of prenatal hydronephrosis (first: transient, physiologic nonpathologic hydronephrosis; second: UPJ obstruction)
  - Contralateral renal anomalies occur in about 9% of cases.
- Ureterocele
  - Cystic dilatation of the intravesical submucosal ureter, usually associated with stenotic orifice that impairs urinary flow into bladder
- Ectopic ureter
  - Inserts into a site other than the bladder trigone
    - Boys: sites above urinary sphincter
    - Girls: sites above or below sphincter
  - Often obstructive in boys; may not be obstructive in girls
- Polycystic kidney disease
- Extrarenal pelvis
- Unilateral vesicoureteral reflux
- Transient physiologic–nonpathologic
- Bilateral
  - Posterior urethral valves
  - Urethral atresia
  - Prune belly syndrome
  - Megacystis-megaureter syndrome
  - Vesicoureteral reflux
  - Polycystic kidney disease
- Uncommon causes
  - Megacalycosis
  - Renal cyst
  - Urachal cyst
  - Ovarian cyst
  - Hydrocolpos
  - Sacrococcygeal teratoma
  - Bowel duplication
  - Duodenal atresia
  - Anterior meningocele

- Not all children with prenatal hydronephrosis have obstructive uropathy.
  - Most have transient or physiologic hydronephrosis that often resolves during pregnancy or after birth and have no clinical sequelae.

VUR

- Differentiating between UTI and other causes of sepsis may be difficult, particularly in young infants.
- VUR is diagnosed after evaluation for UTI, prenatal hydronephrosis, or family history of reflux.

DIAGNOSTIC APPROACH

- Not all children with prenatal hydronephrosis require extensive radiologic evaluation.
  - If hydronephrosis persists during pregnancy, postnatal ultrasonography (US) after 48 hours is indicated.
  - Earlier US for:
    - Bilateral moderate to severe hydronephrosis
    - Solitary kidney
    - Oligohydramnios
    - Giant hydronephrosis

LABORATORY FINDINGS

- Fetal intervention for obstructive uropathy
  - Obtain serial measurements of urine electrolytes to assess fetal renal function.
  - Increased urine sodium, chloride, and osmolality suggest renal damage or dysplasia.

IMAGING

Obstructive uropathy

- US
  - The first test should be renal and bladder US.
  - Hydronephrosis is almost always present but should not be interpreted as a sign of significant obstruction because US cannot adequately assess renal function and drainage of upper urinary tract.
  - Increased echogenicity and marked parenchymal thinning may portend poor renal function but are not sensitive or specific.
  - US may help differentiate the cause of obstructive uropathy.
  - Presence of dilated ureter on US suggests that obstruction occurs distal to the UPJ.
    - UVJ obstruction
    - Ectopic ureter
    - Ureterocele (visualized as cystic mass inside bladder)
    - PUV (thick wall bladder and dilated posterior urethra)

- Voiding cystourethrography (VCUG)
  - Will identify vesicoureteral reflux, which may cause hydronephrosis itself but is associated with other diagnoses of obstructive uropathy:
    - UPJ obstruction
    - Ureterocele
    - PUV
  - Will help delineate bladder (eg, ureterocele) and urethral (eg, PUV) anomalies
- Radionuclide renography
  - Can assess renal function
  - ^{99m}Technetium dimercaptosuccinic acid (DMSA) renography
    - Most accurate for renal function and renal scarring
  - ^{99m}Tc diethylenetriaminepentaacetic acid and ^{99m}Tc mercuroacetyltriglycine diuretic renography
    - Less accurate for renal function
    - Can assess drainage
    - Quantitatively measure degree of obstruction
- Diuretic renography
  - Done only in children ≥2 months of age (because of tubular function maturation) who have moderate or severe hydronephrosis
- Intravenous pyelography
  - Alternative study to assess renal function and anatomy
  - Use in children is limited because of radiation exposure and presence of bowel gas, which interferes with visualization of urinary tract.

VUR

- US
  - To evaluate for UTI or prenatal hydronephrosis
  - Cannot confirm presence or absence of reflux because severe reflux may be present without significant hydronephrosis
  - Has limited ability to detect renal abnormalities, such as dysplasia and scarring
- VCUG
  - Remains principal method of detecting and quantifying degree of VUR
  - Performed in children with history of moderate or severe hydronephrosis observed on prenatal US
  - Additional indications include the following findings on prenatal US.
    - Dilated ureter
    - Abnormal bladder wall thickness
    - Renal echogenicity
    - Renal parenchymal thinning
    - Decreased amniotic fluid volume

O

- Performed by:
  - Placing a urethral catheter into bladder
  - Instilling contrast agent
  - Obtaining images of bladder and kidneys during filling and voiding
- VUR is diagnosed when contrast instilled into the bladder is detected in ureter or upper urinary tract.
- Helps identify other bladder and urethral anomalies that may cause secondary reflux
  - PUVs
  - Ureterocele
  - Bladder diverticula
  - Neurogenic bladder
- Conventional fluoroscopic VCUG captures images at fixed time points and may miss episodic reflux.
- Especially in infants, a fill-void cycle should be repeated at least once to improve sensitivity.
- Radionuclide cystography
  - Radioisotope is placed in bladder; bladder, kidneys, and ureters are continuously monitored.
  - Continuous imaging causes increased sensitivity in detecting reflux compared with fluoroscopic VCUG.
  - Exposes patient to less radiation than does conventional VCUG
  - Poor resolution of anatomic details (eg, grade of reflux and associated urethra, bladder abnormalities)
  - Used for follow-up studies (after VCUG is done to identify and characterize reflux)
- DMSA scan
  - Accurately assesses renal development
  - Evaluates for renal scarring from UTI
- Intravenous pyelography
  - Once used to assess renal parenchymal abnormalities
  - Replaced by renal scintigraphy as gold standard because of increased sensitivity of DMSA scans in detecting renal scarring
- Renal scintigraphy
  - For children with VUR who have ≥1 episode of UTI and those with at least grade III VUR

CLASSIFICATION

- International Reflux Study classification system for vesicoureteral reflux
  - Grade I
    - Reflux into ureter: distal segment only
    - Reflux into calices: none
  - Grade II
    - Reflux into ureter: without tortuosity
    - Reflux into calices: without distention

- Grade III
  - Reflux into ureter: with minimal tortuosity
  - Reflux into calices: with mild distention
- Grade IV
  - Reflux into ureter: with moderate tortuosity
  - Reflux into calices: with moderate distention
- Grade V
  - Reflux into ureter: with severe tortuosity
  - Reflux into calices: with severe distention

TREATMENT APPROACH

- Goals for treating obstructive uropathy
  - Preserve renal function
  - Prevent associated complications
    - UTI
    - Pain
    - Stone formation

SPECIFIC TREATMENTS

Obstructive uropathy

- UPJ obstruction
  - Surgical correction for patients with:
    - Severely dilated renal pelvis (anteroposterior >2 cm on US)
    - Decreased renal function (relative renal function >40%)
    - Marked obstructed pattern on renography
    - UTI
    - Renal colic
    - Pulmonary compromise from giant hydronephrosis
  - Procedures
    - Removal of stenotic or adynamic UPJ
    - Transposing ureter anterior to lower pole-crossing vessels
  - Patients with moderate to severe hydronephrosis but preserved renal function may be managed without surgery.
- UVJ obstruction
  - Symptomatic patients seeking care for UTI, pain, or nausea and vomiting
    - Removal of distal adynamic segment of ureter with or without ureteral tapering
  - Asymptomatic patients (ie, diagnosed by evaluation of prenatal hydronephrosis)
    - Observation and prophylactic antibiotics allow spontaneous regression of obstruction, do not compromise renal function, and minimize risk of UTI.
  - Infants diagnosed in evaluation for prenatal hydronephrosis
    - Surgical correction

O

- Lower urinary tract obstruction
  - For suspected PUV, catheter drainage is needed until diagnosis is confirmed and surgical correction performed.
  - Before surgery:
    - Stabilize pulmonary status (particularly in newborns diagnosed in utero with oligohydramnios).
    - Correct associated metabolic abnormalities.
    - Treat UTI.
  - Procedures
    - Endoscopic fulguration of PUV relieves bladder outlet obstruction in most patients.
    - Vesicostomy or alternative treatment (eg, ablation with Fogarty balloon) in very small or premature infants because endoscopic instruments are too large
- Ureterocele and ectopic ureter
  - Surgical correction is usually needed.
    - Urgently for symptomatic patients
- Fetal intervention
  - Indicated only for cases in which:
    - Pulmonary or renal dysfunction can be identified.
    - Severe oligohydramnios occurs without associated renal dysplasia, poor renal function, or associated chromosomal anomalies.
  - The goal is to prevent pulmonary hypoplasia and preserve renal function.
  - Procedures
    - Open fetal surgery
    - Percutaneous vesicoamniotic shunt placement
    - Fetoscopic surgery

VUR

- Medical therapy should be instituted, with the goal of preventing following long-term complications.
  - Renal scarring
  - Hypertension
  - Renal insufficiency or failure
- See Prevention for discussion of antibiotic prophylaxis.
- Indications for surgical correction
  - Recurrent UTI during antibiotic prophylaxis
  - Lack of adherence to medical regimen
  - Low probability of spontaneous resolution of reflux (eg, in older children with higher-grade reflux)
  - New renal scar formation during prophylaxis
  - Anatomic abnormalities, such as a paraureteral diverticulum
- Overall rate of surgical correction: 13–20%
- Procedures

  - Transurethral (endoscopic)
    - Much lower morbidity and shorter recovery time than open surgery but lower success rates
  - Laparoscopic
  - Open
    - High success rate (98%), but often requires a few days of hospitalization and subsequent recovery time

WHEN TO ADMIT

- All patients with significant metabolic abnormalities and electrolyte imbalances.
- Patients with urosepsis
- Patients with markedly impaired renal function

WHEN TO REFER

- All patients with obstructive uropathy should be managed in collaboration with pediatric nephrologists and pediatric urologists.
- All patients with VUR should be managed with pediatric nephrologists.
  - Pediatric urologists should be consulted if surgery is indicated.

FOLLOW-UP

- Ureterocele and ectopic ureter
  - Long-term follow-up is needed to evaluate renal function and look for recurrent obstruction.
  - Since hypertension and proteinuria can develop in patients with renal insufficiency or dysplasia, yearly blood pressure and urinalysis are indicated in all patients with obstructive uropathy.
- VUR
  - Monitor children for long-term complications, such as reflux nephropathy
  - About 10% of children with renal scarring will develop hypertension.
  - About 10% of children with reflux nephropathy will develop end-stage renal disease, and 90% will have diminished glomerular filtration rate.
  - Measure blood pressure and urinary protein periodically if renal scarring is present.
  - Monitor pregnant patients with history of VUR and reflux nephropathy because of increased rates of the following.
    - Pyelonephritis
    - Toxemia
    - Preterm delivery
    - Fetal growth retardation
    - Fetal loss
    - Decreased maternal renal function

O

COMPLICATIONS

- Lower urinary tract obstruction
  - Children with PUV and renal insufficiency:
    - Cannot concentrate urine to a specific gravity >1.015, leading to excessive fluid loss
    - May develop renal salt wasting and metabolic acidosis with hyperkalemia
    - May develop severe dehydration and cardiovascular compromise with minor gastrointestinal illness
    - Bladder dysfunction is often associated with PUV despite adequate relief of obstruction.
    - VUR occurs in approximately 30–75% of children with PUV.
- Fetal intervention is associated with a high complication rate.
  - Premature labor
  - Inadequate drainage or migration of shunt
  - Perforation of fetal bowel or bladder
  - Chorioamnionitis
  - Iatrogenic gastroschisis
  - Bleeding

PROGNOSIS

Obstructive uropathy

- UPJ obstruction
  - Hydronephrosis often resolves, but it may take several years.
  - Declining renal function may occur, necessitating surgery.
  - In most cases, renal function is recovered after surgery, suggesting small risk to obstructed kidney from conservative management.
- UVJ obstruction
  - Most symptoms resolve spontaneously.
  - Surgery is indicated in infants who are diagnosed during evaluation for prenatal hydronephrosis and have greatly decreased renal function at onset.
    - Renal function after surgery is preserved but never normalizes.
- Lower urinary tract obstruction
  - After treatment of PUV, postobstructive diuresis may develop with urine output as high as 15 mL/kg per hour.
  - Pay careful attention to fluid balance after relief of distal obstruction.
  - Renal insufficiency and failure can occur in up to 50% of patients with PUV.
  - In some patients with PUV, the ability to hold large urine volumes at high intravesical pressures can lead to:
    - Increased upper tract dilatation
    - Increased pressure
    - Progressive renal compromise

- Early treatment reduces incidence of bladder and renal dysfunction
  - Anticholinergic medications
  - Intermittent catheterization
  - Nighttime drainage
- Fetal intervention
  - Success varies.
  - Normal amniotic fluid volume is restored.
  - Lung development improves.
  - Renal outcome does not significantly improve.

VUR

- Usually resolves spontaneously without surgical intervention
  - Spontaneous resolution rate depends on:
    - Reflux grade: low-grade more likely to resolve than high-grade
      - Grades I and II, 70–80% resolution rate; grade III, 50%; grades IV and V, <30%
    - Laterality
      - Bilateral high-grade VUR tends to resolve less often than unilateral high-grade VUR.
    - Sex
      - Tends to resolve more slowly in girls than boys
    - Mode of presentation
      - High-grade VUR detected after evaluation for prenatal hydronephrosis tends to resolve more quickly than that detected after evaluation for UTIs.
    - In patients with sibling reflux, the rate of resolution is similar to that of probands, with grade the primary determining factor.
- Voiding dysfunction
  - Can impede resolution of reflux
  - Can worsen reflux severity with time
  - Ascertain symptoms for dysfunctional voiding (eg, urinary urgency and incontinence) and begin treating with timed voiding, anticholinergic therapy, or both.
- Constipation
  - Can increase risk of UTI
  - Can delay resolution of VUR
  - Treat aggressively to decrease risk of UTI and improve voiding function
- Fetal intervention
  - Favorable prognosis for good renal function is associated with following laboratory values.
    - Sodium <100 mEq/L
    - Chloride <90 mEq/L
    - Osmolality <210 mOsm/kg
    - ß$_2$-Microglobulin <508 mmol/L

O

PREVENTION

- VUR
  - Screening for reflux in families with VUR is indicated.
  - Goal: identify affected children early and decrease risk of long-term complications
  - Screening US
    - For older siblings or offspring with no history of UTI
  - Screening with radionuclide cystography
    - For siblings or offspring <5 years of age
    - For older siblings with history of UTI or hydronephrosis or evidence of parenchymal thinning on US
  - Predicting which children will and will not develop renal scarring is impossible.
  - Antibiotic prophylaxis
    - Can prevent UTI and prevent VUR complications
      - Age <3 months
        - Amoxicillin, 25 mg/kg once a day
        - Cephalexin, 25 mg/kg once a day
      - Age ≥3 months
        - Trimethoprim, alone or with sulfa, 2 mg/kg once a day
        - Nitrofurantoin, 1–2 mg/kg once a day (not to exceed 100 mg/day)
    - Should be maintained until VUR has resolved spontaneously or after surgical correction
    - Can be used as long as no breakthrough UTIs or compliance issues occur
    - Length of therapy varies depending on parental preference and likelihood of reflux resolution.
    - When reflux resolution seems unlikely, consider stopping antibiotics and correcting the reflux.
    - Most providers use monotherapy; little evidence suggests that alternating antibiotic prophylaxis is more effective than monotherapy.
    - In teenagers with reflux, an antibiotic trial is reasonable, but chance of resolution is somewhat lower.
    - Consider observing children >7–8 years of age with persistent low-grade VUR, but no recent UTIs, while they are no longer receiving antibiotic prophylaxis because their risk of renal scarring is low.

O

Ocular Trauma

DEFINITION

- Accidental injury to the eye is a major public health issue accounting for permanent visual loss and monocular blindness.
- Severe trauma in children can present significant developmental and emotional challenges, especially if a cosmetic defect is present.

EPIDEMIOLOGY

- Prevalence
  - 5% of all eye injuries result in permanent visual loss.
  - Trauma accounts for 40% of all cases of monocular blindness.
- Sex
  - Boys are 3 times more susceptible than girls.

ETIOLOGY

- Common sources of injury
  - Sports-related injuries
    - Baseball (most common)
    - Basketball
    - Tennis
    - Hockey
  - Motor vehicle crashes
  - Falls
  - Projectiles
    - BB guns
    - Knives
    - Rocks
  - Other children
- Nontraumatic causes of subconjunctival hemorrhage
  - In newborns, small, bilateral hemorrhages, presumably from the pressure of uterine contractions
  - Severe coughing, such as that caused by pertussis or forceful vomiting
  - Viral conjunctivitis
    - Can be hemorrhagic
    - Usually associated with chemosis (edema of the conjunctiva) and symptoms of irritation and mild discharge
  - Blood dyscrasias (rarely), such as leukemia
    - Hemorrhage usually bilateral

RISK FACTORS

- Lack of eye protection
  - Most severe injuries occur in children with no eye protection.
  - Mandatory eye protection in organized sports, such as hockey, has significantly reduced eye injuries.

SIGNS AND SYMPTOMS

Physical examination

- If the history is clear and reliable (eg, the child was poked in the eye with a finger), more directed examination is possible.
- External inspection and observation is helpful to characterize the severity of the injury.
- If a full-thickness injury through the eyeball is apparent, further examination is best left to an ophthalmologist.
- If index of suspicion for a serious injury or foreign body is high and the patient is uncooperative, examination under sedation or anesthesia may be necessary.
- Important signs include:
  - Swelling or bruising of lids
  - Lacerations of lids or face
  - Proptosis or enophthalmos
  - Foreign bodies and possible entrance sites
    - If a foreign body is likely, eversion of the upper lid is required to inspect the palpebral conjunctiva properly.
  - Conjunctival hemorrhage
- Obvious globe laceration with prolapse of intraocular contents may be visible by inspection alone.
- If the globe appears intact, palpation of the orbital rim can be performed to check for fracture of orbital or facial bones.

Ocular motility

- Ocular motility should be evaluated to ensure full range of motion in all gaze positions.
  - Limited movement can result from:
    - Orbital hemorrhage or swelling
    - Orbital fractures
    - Cranial nerve palsies
    - Direct muscle trauma
  - Diplopia generally results from limited motility, although young children may not verbalize this symptom.

Pupils

- Round and equally reactive
  - Greatly reduces (but does not eliminate) likelihood of severe, vision-threatening injury
- Irregularity in size or shape
  - Can result from blunt trauma with damage to the pupillary sphincter
  - Can result from a full-thickness laceration of the cornea or sclera

Anterior segment

- Initial assessment of anterior chamber can be performed simply with penlight examination or direct ophthalmoscope.
- Without a slit lamp, it is possible to detect:
  - Conjunctival hemorrhages
  - Corneal or conjunctival lacerations

- Foreign bodies
- Anterior chamber depth
- Iris and pupillary irregularities
■ If a slit lamp is available, the primary care physician should evaluate for smaller conjunctival or corneal lacerations.
- Depth of laceration
- Presence of foreign bodies not visible with penlight
- Presence of erythrocytes or leukocytes in anterior chamber
- Cataract formation or dislocation of lens

Fundus

■ Detailed fundus examination can be difficult in a child without pupillary dilatation.
■ Red reflex should be observed, looking for asymmetry.
- Absence or asymmetry of the red reflex can indicate:
  - Vitreous hemorrhage
  - Cataract formation
  - Hyphema
- Corneal abrasion or irregularity and corneal foreign body can be appreciated as an opacity in the red reflex.

Specific ocular injuries

Eyelid and lacrimal injury

■ The anterior segment must be examined to exclude globe injury.
■ Eyelid injuries (see Figure 51 on page F19)
- Lacerations medial to the lacrimal puncta
  - High risk of disrupting lacrimal drainage system
  - Failure to recognize and treat a canalicular laceration can result in chronic tearing, particularly if the lower canaliculus is involved.
  - Dog-bite injuries often involve the lacrimal system.
- Lacerations of the upper lid that are deep enough to expose orbital fat
  - Risk of damage to the levator muscle
  - Failure to recognize levator involvement can result in posttraumatic ptosis, which may require additional surgery.

Chemical injury

■ After irrigation, more detailed examination should be performed.
■ Examiner should note degree of conjunctival injection.
- Lack of hyperemia, particularly in perilimbal area, may be a sign of ischemia.
- Permanent damage to stem cells can significantly impair the patient's ability to regenerate corneal epithelial loss.
■ The cornea should be examined for clarity.
- Hazy or edematous cornea is a sign of serious injury.
■ The examiner should instill fluorescein to check for corneal abrasions.

Thermal injury

■ Ocular involvement from thermal injury
- Can be isolated
- Is often seen in the setting of severe facial burns
■ Globe injury
- Typically mild because of the protective blink reflex
- Can be severe if the blink reflex is impaired or if loss of consciousness occurs
■ Severe lid involvement can lead to contracture and cicatricial changes, resulting in corneal exposure and ulceration.

Subconjunctival hemorrhage

■ May cause significant discoloration (see Figure 52 on page F19)
- Various color changes may occur while blood is being resorbed.
- Several days to weeks may elapse before hemorrhage has completely disappeared.
■ Surrounding blood often masks conjunctival laceration.
- A small, superficial laceration often does not require repair.
- Examine to ensure that no underlying laceration of sclera or other trauma to the eye has occurred.

Corneal abrasion

■ Extreme pain and sensitivity
- Only in rare situations of neurotrophic disease are corneal abrasions relatively asymptomatic.
- Abrasions may be linear or patchy and can be of any size (see Figures 53 and 54 on page F19).
■ Photophobia
■ Blepharospasm
■ Conjunctival injection
■ Mild lid swelling
- Lids must be opened well enough to gain view of the entire cornea.
- Fine, linear abrasions in the superior cornea may easily be missed and often are a sign of a foreign body lodged in the superior tarsal conjunctiva.

Conjunctival and corneal foreign bodies

■ Conjunctival foreign bodies
- Typically produce irritation and discomfort
- Mild to moderate conjunctival injection
- Lids should be forcefully opened, if necessary, for direct examination of the bulbar conjunctiva.
  - If this area appears normal, attention should be turned to the tarsal conjunctival surfaces (see Figure 55 on page F20).
- Lower-lid eversion can be accomplished readily with gentle inferior traction.

- Upper-lid eversion can be much more difficult, especially if the child is very young or uncooperative.
  - The lashes are grasped and lid stretched minimally.
  - A cotton-tipped applicator shaft is placed horizontally along superior margin of the tarsal plate.
  - The lid is then reflected over applicator for inspection.
- Once conjunctival foreign body has been identified, topical anesthetic should be administered, and a cotton tip used to remove it gently.
- If conjunctival foreign body is not identified, cotton tip may be used to sweep the upper and lower conjunctival fornices for small foreign particles.
- Finally, fluorescein should be administered to check for corneal abrasions.
- Multiple, fine vertical abrasions of superior aspect of the cornea are highly suggestive of a foreign body of the upper tarsal conjunctiva.

- Corneal foreign bodies
  - 2 types
    - Particle resting on the surface of the epithelium
    - Particle that has penetrated epithelium and is embedded in the anterior stroma (more common)
  - Normal blink and secondary movement of the tears usually will expel a nonembedded particle or move it to a conjunctival surface.
  - Lids should be opened to gain full view of the cornea and a light source used.

Hyphema

- The presence of blood in the anterior chamber
  - Results when enough force is transmitted to the globe to cause rupture of blood vessels located within the iris root (see Figure 56 on page F20) and ciliary body
- Can be of varying severity
  - Microhyphema: floating erythrocytes in the aqueous fluid without layering
  - 8-ball hyphema: blood filling the entire anterior chamber
  - Most cases are in between and are described by percentage of the anterior chamber occupied by layered blood.
- Readily identified with a light source and good exposure of the anterior segment

Traumatic iritis

- Iritis, or anterior uveitis: inflammation of the iris and ciliary body
  - Occurs in trauma or in a nontraumatic setting, eg, in association with autoimmune disorders
  - Causes blurry vision, pain, and significant photophobia
- The eye usually is quite injected, and the pupil may not constrict briskly.
- If diagnosis is suspected, referral to an ophthalmologist is indicated.

Traumatic mydriasis

- A mid-dilated pupil noted on examination of a patient after a blunt, traumatic event
  - Can be a result of small ruptures or tears of the iris sphincter muscle
  - The pupil cannot constrict normally.
- Injury may involve only part of sphincter muscle, giving a slightly irregular appearance to the pupil.
- Care must be taken to rule out possibility of a ruptured globe.
- Ophthalmologist often can identify free pigment cells released into the anterior chamber.
- Unless true associated inflammation or iritis exists, treatment usually is not indicated.

Ruptured globe

- Open-globe injuries occur primarily in adults.
- Pediatric open-globe injuries are caused by penetrating injury (79%), blunt trauma (13%), and perforating injury (8%).
  - Penetrating injuries are most common in boys.
  - Blunt trauma is the primary cause of ruptured globe in girls.
- Blunt trauma
  - Motor vehicle crashes
  - Air bag, paintball, and fist injuries
  - External signs
    - An irregular pupil
    - A deep anterior chamber
    - A subconjunctival hemorrhage
    - Conjunctival chemosis
- Anterior segment penetration
  - Lid laceration
  - Conjunctiva laceration
  - Subconjunctival hemorrhage
  - Scleral laceration with uveal prolapse
  - Corneal laceration with iris prolapse
  - Cataract
- Most common rupture locations are at limbus and posterior to the eye muscle insertion.
- Associated clinical findings in an open-globe injury include:
  - Vision loss
  - An afferent pupillary defect
  - Retinal detachment
  - Optic disc edema
- In many cases, diagnosis is evident from initial inspection with a penlight.

O

- Further assessment can include:
  - Dilated ophthalmic examination
  - Intraocular pressure (IOP) measurement
    - In most instances, the IOP is <8 mm Hg.
    - IOP is safest with applanation tonometer or Tono-Pen.
    - A Schiotz tonometer should not be used, because the weight of the tonometer may cause an expulsive hemorrhage.
- Intraocular foreign body should be considered based on the mechanism of injury.
  - The presence of a hyphema or vitreous hemorrhage may preclude visualizing an intraocular foreign body.
- Retinal tear or detachment is commonly associated with intraocular penetration.

Orbital trauma

- Primary care evaluation includes assessment of:
  - Visual acuity
  - Motility
  - Pupils
  - Anterior segment
  - Intraocular pressure
  - Proptosis or enophthalmos should be noted.
- Emergent ophthalmologic evaluation is needed for:
  - Marked decrease in vision
  - Relative afferent pupillary defect
  - Elevation of IOP
- Blunt or penetrating trauma may cause intraorbital hemorrhage.
  - Traumatic orbital hemorrhage in a child is unusual.
  - Iatrogenic hemorrhage is well reported with preoperative peribulbar and retrobulbar anesthetic injections.
- Hemorrhage causes anterior displacement of the globe.
- Blindness may be caused by a marked elevation of the IOP or tension on the optic nerve.
  - To relieve tension on the globe, a lateral canthotomy of the upper and lower lids may be performed at the bedside.
- Blunt trauma to midface and orbital rim may cause a fracture of the orbital wall.
  - Inferior floor is the most common site, with medial wall second.
  - Associated facial fractures are frequent, most commonly a zygoma-malar fracture.
  - Diplopia is common.
- A defect in the orbital floor may allow prolapse of orbital fat, leading to enophthalmos.
  - Vertical restrictive strabismus may be caused by prolapse of inferior rectus into floor defect or bony impingement on muscle.

- Reduced vision can occur secondary to:
  - Retrobulbar hemorrhage
  - Optic neuropathy
  - Optic nerve impingement
  - Retinal detachment
  - Rupture of the globe
- Decreased facial sensation inferior to orbital rim may indicate damage to the infraorbital nerve.
- Midfacial trauma may be associated with traumatic optic neuropathy.
- Neurologic findings with facial trauma may include:
  - Cranial nerve palsies
  - Optic neuropathy
- Examination of traumatic optic neuropathy may demonstrate:
  - Decreased vision
  - An afferent pupillary defect
  - Decreased color vision
- The optic nerve may appear normal or edematous.

Abusive trauma

- Eye injuries may be present in up to 40% of pediatric abusive injury.
- Retinal hemorrhage associated with shaking injury is a primary concern, but many other signs of trauma may involve the eyes.
  - Cranial nerve palsies
  - External lid trauma
  - Anterior and posterior segment injuries
  - Orbital injury
  - Sexually transmitted infections
    - *Chlamydia* and gonorrhea conjunctivitis
    - *Phthirus pubis* on the lashes
  - Münchausen syndrome by proxy has been reported in connection with recurrent conjunctivitis.
- Violent, repetitive, abusive acceleration-deceleration injury may cause:
  - Retinal hemorrhages
  - Retinal schisis
  - Retinal folds
  - Cranial nerve palsy
  - This type of injury typically occurs in children <3 years but has been seen in children as old as 8 years of age.
- Retinal hemorrhages
  - Occur at multiple layers of the retina
    - Vitreous
    - Preretinal
    - Nerve fiber layer
    - Intra- and subretinal layers

O

- Are associated with abusive head trauma
- Nerve fiber layer heme is the most common type.
- Distribution of hemorrhages
  - Primarily around the optic nerve and macula
  - Often distributed to the periphery of the retina
- Retinal heme has been reported in:
  - 60–72% of abusive head trauma
  - 0–20% of nonabusive head trauma
- Bilateral involvement is more common in abusive injury, but unilateral hemorrhages are well reported in known shaking injuries.
- Abusive head trauma is associated with much more severe retinal hemorrhages.
- Brain findings include:
  - Subdural bleeding (93%)
  - Cerebral edema (44%)
  - Subarachnoid bleeding (16%)
  - Parenchymal bleeding (8%)
- Forceful vomiting does not commonly cause retinal hemorrhaging.
- Cardiopulmonary resuscitation has been reported to cause few retinal hemorrhages around the optic nerve.
- Falls from <1.5 meters are not likely to cause serious neurologic trauma.
- Retinal folds associated with severe shaking injury are perimacular along vascular arcades.
  - The presence of perimacular folds most likely indicates a shaking injury, although there are reports of retinal folds with known severe accidental injury.
  - Macular holes and peripheral retinoschisis (separation of the layers of the retina) have been noted.
  - Retinal folds and peripheral retinoschisis are indicative of severe neurologic trauma.
    - The vitreous gel of the eye is tightly adherent to retina at the macula, optic nerve, and periphery in a child.
    - Adherence creates tractional forces on the retina with repetitive acceleration-deceleration injury.
- Shaken baby syndrome
  - Hemorrhages usually resolve within 4 weeks but have been reported to last up to 4 months.
  - Retinal hemorrhages often resolve without serious visual effects unless the macula is involved (see Figure 57 on page F20).
    - Macular holes and macular scar tissue may result in visual loss.
  - Severe visual impairment or blindness may occur with significant neurologic trauma and cortical damage, optic atrophy, or retinal detachment.
  - Abusive head trauma combined with retinal heme offers a poor neurologic prognosis.

- History and associated physical findings aid in establishing the cause of the trauma.
  - Patients often exhibit physical findings inconsistent with variable caregiver histories.
  - If abuse is suspected, then dilated fundus examination by an ophthalmologist is mandatory.

DIFFERENTIAL DIAGNOSIS

- Shaken baby syndrome
- Preseptal edema caused by an orbital hemangioma
- Preseptal ecchymosis caused by neuroblastoma
- Ruptured vascular malformation
- Other causes of retinal hemorrhage confused with shaken baby syndrome include:
  - Zellweger syndrome
  - Glutaric aciduria type 1
  - Hermansky-Pudlak syndrome

DIAGNOSTIC APPROACH

History

- An accurate and detailed history can suggest mechanism and nature of injuries.
  - History can be difficult to obtain if an adult or other reliable observer did not witness the injury.
  - Details obtained from smaller children may not always be reliable.
  - In such instances, the primary care physician must verify that physical findings are consistent with the history.
- Certain historical details are particularly helpful.
  - Is there potential for chemical injury?
    - If so, then treatment must be delivered immediately, before obtaining a full history and performing an examination, to minimize damage from an acid or alkali burn.
    - Use pH indicator paper to determine the nature and extent of acid or alkali injury.
    - A small strip can be quickly placed in the conjunctival sac.
    - Normal pH of the eye is 6.8–7.4.
    - If pH paper is not readily available, then time should not be wasted in obtaining it.
  - Has a severe head injury or other nonocular injury occurred that may require attention?
    - Significant head trauma can been associated with:
      - Globe rupture
      - Traumatic optic neuropathy
      - Cranial nerve palsies
      - Orbital fractures
      - Cortical visual damage

- Is the injury blunt or sharp in nature?
  - A sharp injury is more likely to be penetrating, resulting in a full-thickness laceration through the cornea or sclera.
  - A severe blunt impact can also lead to globe rupture as a result of globe compression and increased intraocular pressure.
- Is there the possibility of a foreign body?
  - Superficial (in the eyelid, cornea, or conjunctiva)
  - Intraocular
  - Intraorbital
  - Injury associated with flying debris, metallic fragments, projectiles, or any broken object is high risk for a retained foreign body.
- Once details surrounding mechanism of injury have been obtained, additional history taking should focus on:
  - Ocular history (eg, presence of amblyopia)
  - Medical history
  - Medications and allergies
  - Date of the last tetanus immunization

Vision testing
- Examination should begin with an age-appropriate assessment of vision.
- Verbal children
  - Acuity is measured with letter charts or with letter matching (such as the HOTV chart) if the child cannot name the letters.
  - Acuity testing should be performed with proper optical correction, if applicable.
  - Care should be taken to ensure that normal eye is fully occluded when testing the injured eye.
  - If the child cannot see the largest target on the chart (usually 20/200 or 20/400), alternative methods are used.
    - Ability to count fingers (recorded as "count fingers at *x* feet")
    - Ability to perceive hand motion (recorded as "hand motion at *x* feet")
    - Ability to perceive light (recorded as "light perception" or "no light perception")
- Preverbal children
  - Assessed by ability to fix and follow a small object or toy
  - Each eye should be tested separately.
  - Decreased vision in the injured eye is suggested by:
    - Inability to follow smoothly with one eye compared with the other
    - Attempts to look around the occlusion of the normal eye

Physical examination
- Pupils
  - Ideally, the reaction of each pupil to light (direct and consensual) is checked with the child fixating at a distant target.
  - The swinging flashlight test is performed to check for the presence of afferent pupillary defect, or Marcus Gunn pupil.
    - Alternately shine the light source into each eye.
    - Both pupils should normally stay constricted as a result of direct and consensual response to light.
    - Paradoxical dilatation of the illuminated pupil indicates presence of an afferent pupillary defect resulting from optic nerve or extensive retinal injury.
- Anterior segment
  - If a slit lamp is available, more detailed and accurate examination is possible in a cooperative child.
  - Primary care physician should evaluate for smaller conjunctival or corneal lacerations.
    - Depth of laceration
    - Foreign bodies that might not be visible with a penlight
    - Presence of erythrocytes or leukocytes in the anterior chamber
    - Cataract formation or dislocation of the lens
  - Once penlight, slit-lamp, or both examinations have been completed, fluorescein solution or strips and cobalt-blue filter or lamp should be used to check for abrasions, lacerations, or foreign bodies that might otherwise go undetected.
- Posterior segment
  - Any child who is thought to have posterior segment injury or unexplained vision loss should have dilated fundus examination by an ophthalmologist with the aid of indirect ophthalmoscope.
- Corneal abrasion
  - Diagnosis of a corneal abrasion may be facilitated by the instillation of a topical anesthetic followed by fluorescein.
  - Use of a cobalt-blue filter will then easily highlight areas of epithelial loss.
- Traumatic iritis
  - Floating leukocytes in the anterior chamber are visualized under the high magnification of a slit lamp, confirming the diagnosis.

IMAGING
- Orbital trauma
  - Radiologic evaluation of the orbit to delineate the size of the floor defect
- Ultrasonography or computed tomography for orbital or intraocular foreign body

- Shaken baby syndrome
  - On computed tomography, severe shaking injury may be associated with:
    - Cerebral edema only
    - Subdural bleeding
    - Normal brain
- Radiologic evaluation of the optic canal for a displaced fracture is paramount after orbital trauma.

TREATMENT APPROACH

- Chemical injury
  - Immediate management to prevent serious complications
  - Treatment should be administered before arrival, either by the caregiver or by emergency medical services.
    - Should be tailored to injury but often includes an antibiotic drop or ointment and artificial lubricants
  - Corneal abrasions associated with chemicals should not be patched, so that tears and natural blinking can eliminate residual chemical.
- Thermal injury
  - Immediate irrigation to cool ocular surface
- Corneal and conjunctival abrasions
  - Treat with artificial lubricants and topical antibiotics
  - Initial treatment of lid injury consists of topical antibiotic ointment.
  - Severe injury may require subsequent skin grafting to prevent lid malposition and exposure.
  - Most abrasions heal quickly, particularly in children.
  - Treatment is aimed at keeping the patient comfortable and preventing infection.
- Hyphema
  - Usually treated with a topical corticosteroid drop to reduce associated inflammation, and a topical cycloplegic agent
  - Initial management involves placing a protective shield over the eye to avoid further injury; shielding may be continued.
  - Bed rest (often advised)
  - If hyphema is worrisome and the child is too young to cooperate with restricted activity, hospitalization may be indicated.
    - Restriction of activity is particularly important in the first 2–5 days after injury, when clotted blood may start to resorb and cause rebleeding of injured vessels.
    - In many instances, rebleeding can be more visually devastating than original injury.
  - Patients should be instructed to limit activities until seen by a specialist.
- Traumatic iritis
  - Topical corticosteroid and cycloplegic agent if inflammation is severe

SPECIFIC TREATMENTS

Eyelid

- Initial treatment consists of topical antibiotic ointment.
- Superficial lacerations to eyelid can be closed.
  - 6-0 nylon suture, removed in 5–7 days
  - 6-0 plain suture if the child might be uncooperative for suture removal
- Severe injury may require subsequent skin grafting to prevent lid malposition and exposure.
- Lacerations involving the lid margin
  - Should be repaired by an experienced surgeon to ensure that the smooth contour of the lid margin is maintained
  - Poor closure or reapproximation can result in a notch along lid margin, with cosmetic and functional consequences.
- Lacrimal injury
  - Requires referral and surgical repair with tube placement in the lacrimal drainage system
  - Removal of the tube several months later
- Laceration of upper lid that exposes orbital fat
  - Surgical exploration is required:
    - To repair any involvement of the levator muscle
    - To close the laceration

Chemical injury

- Eye(s) should be irrigated with up to 2 L of a pH-neutral solution, such as buffered saline.
  - A lid speculum may be used to keep lids open if necessary.
  - Alternatively, irrigating contact lens can be used.
  - Care must be taken to ensure flow of saline is adequate; a steady drip will not be sufficient.
- Once irrigation is completed, pH indicator paper can be used to determine whether the pH of the eye has returned to normal.
  - The conjunctival fornices should be examined to check for residual chemical agent.
  - A cotton-tipped applicator may be used to gently remove any precipitate, and the area should be reirrigated.

Thermal injury

- Immediate irrigation to cool the ocular surface

Traumatic optic neuropathy

- Standard treatment is intravenous corticosteroids for 1–3 days after injury.
  - Dose, time, and efficacy are controversial.

Ruptured globe

- If rupture is suspected:
  - Bed rest
  - Antiemetics, if required
  - Shield placed over eye
- Ophthalmology consultation is required for operative repair.

Foreign body

- Topical anesthetic and cotton-tipped applicator can be used to dislodge the particle gently, with care not to debride epithelium in the process.
- In many instances, removal of an embedded object will require referral to an ophthalmologist.
- Management of intraocular foreign body is based on injury.
  - Copper or iron is toxic to the retina and requires urgent removal.
  - Plastic, graphite, lead, and aluminum are better tolerated in the eye than either copper or iron.
  - If the child can sit at a slit lamp, ophthalmologist may be able to use a fine needle, forceps, or burr to remove the foreign body.
  - Younger or uncooperative children usually require sedation or general anesthesia.
  - Removal by a retina specialist with a vitrectomy is the treatment.

Corneal and conjunctival abrasions

- Antibiotic ointment or drop 2–4 times a day until abrasion has healed
- Nonsteroidal antiinflammatory eyedrops may be used as an adjunct to reduce pain, particularly in older children.
- Pressure patch
  - Antibiotic ointment is instilled with soft oval gauze taped over the eye to keep it shut.
  - Patch and antibiotic are then replaced after 24 hours, or decision is made to discontinue use.
  - Prolonged patching is discouraged for young children because of the possibility of amblyopia or strabismus.
  - Placement of a patch may provide additional patient comfort and may be particularly useful if a child tends to rub the eye excessively.
  - No evidence has been found to suggest the abrasion will heal more quickly.
- Some ophthalmologists believe that allowing natural tears, which contain immunoglobulin A, lysozyme, and other antiinfective agents, to stream over the cornea with normal blinking may result in improved healing and decreased risk of infection.
- Whichever method is used, the patient should be monitored closely, usually within 1 to 2 days.
- Delayed healing may suggest:
  - Foreign body
  - Ulcer
  - A different pathologic process (eg, herpes keratitis)

Orbital trauma

- A large defect or bony muscle impingement may require early surgical treatment, but treatment of a globe injury is primary.

- Most floor fractures do not require immediate surgery.
  - Lid edema, proptosis, and diplopia may resolve in the first week.
  - If diplopia persists or enophthalmos is significant, then repair of the orbital floor defect can be done safely up to 4 weeks after the injury.
- Bone impingement into the optic nerve requires urgent neurosurgical intervention.

WHEN TO ADMIT

- Hyphemas
- Ruptured globe
- Abusive trauma

WHEN TO REFER

- Lacerations
  - Involving the lid margin
  - Medial to the lacrimal puncta
  - Deep lacerations of the upper lid
- Canalicular injury
- Levator muscle injury
- Corneal abrasion
- Removal of corneal foreign bodies
- Hyphema
  - Because of potential vision-threatening complications, all hyphemas, regardless of size, should be referred to an ophthalmologist.
- Traumatic iritis
- Traumatic mydriasis
- Ruptured globe
- Abusive trauma
- Chemical injury
  - Refer to an ophthalmologist within 24 hours, particularly with moderate to severe injuries, which can result in permanent vision loss from corneal scarring, corneal vascularization, and other sequelae.

FOLLOW-UP

- Foreign body
  - Antibiotic drop or ointment typically is prescribed for a few days after removing a surface foreign body, particularly if:
    - The source was organic
    - The disturbance occurred in the corneal epithelium
  - Follow-up
    - Not necessarily indicated for a simple conjunctival foreign body
    - Required in cases of corneal involvement

COMPLICATIONS

- In addition to the obvious visual consequences, severe trauma can present significant developmental and emotional challenges, especially if a cosmetic defect is present.
- Amblyopia can develop after injury in children <8 years of age, placing additional physical and psychological burdens.
- Hyphema
  - Corneal bloodstaining
  - Glaucoma
    - Patients with sickle cell anemia or trait are at greater risk for visual compromise from optic neuropathy or central artery occlusion at lower pressures.
  - Amblyopia
- Traumatic iritis
  - Iris synechiae
  - Glaucoma
  - Cataract formation
- Ruptured globe
  - Spontaneous or induced expulsive hemorrhage
  - Retinal detachment
  - Endophthalmitis
    - Incidence of associated endophthalmitis after open-globe injury has been reported to be 6.8%.
- Corneal and conjunctival abrasions
  - Severe lid involvement can lead to contracture and cicatricial changes, resulting in corneal exposure and ulceration.

PROGNOSIS

- Ruptured globe
  - The visual prognosis is worse with blunt than with penetrating trauma.

PREVENTION

- Eye protection for appropriate activities

O

Odor (Unusual Urine and Body)

DEFINITION

- Unusual odors may be a chief complaint, symptom, or sign and provide clues in diagnosis of many specific conditions.
- Unusual odors may emanate from:
  - Breath
  - Urine
  - Skin
  - Sputum
  - Vomitus
  - Stool
  - Vagina
- *Bromhidrosis* refers to malodorous and offensive sweat.
  - Caused by decomposition of products from the apocrine, eccrine, and sebaceous glands
  - Apocrine bromhidrosis begins after puberty with a characteristic acrid or sweaty odor.
  - Eccrine bromhidrosis results from bacterial interaction with moist keratin.
    - Associated with hyperhidrosis, obesity, intertrigo, and diabetes mellitus
    - Aggravated by hot weather and occurs primarily in the soles, palms, and intertriginous areas
- *Halitosis* is offensive odor emanating from the mouth or air-filled cavities (nose, sinuses, or pharynx).
  - May be physiologic or pathologic and has numerous causes

MECHANISM

- Axillary odor
  - Aerobic diphtheroids act on apocrine secretions.
  - Bacterial decomposition of androsterone is a possible cause.
  - Axillary hair appears to retain and spread odor.
  - Possible explanations for osmidrosis axillae (unusually strong axillary odor)
    - Apocrine androgen metabolism
    - Bacterial alteration of sweat
    - Abnormally large and numerous apocrine glands
- Vaginal odor may be caused by:
  - Vulvar secretions
  - Vaginal wall transudates
  - Exfoliated cells
  - Cervical mucus
  - Fluids from endometrium and uterine tubes
  - Metabolic products of vaginal microflora
  - Odor during menses is usually rated as the most offensive (but normal).
- The rotten fish smell of vaginal discharge is associated with bacterial vaginosis, caused by trimethylamine.
- Mouth odor
  - Halitosis is exacerbated by infrequent eating and drinking, which have a flushing action.
  - Acutely, it may accompany variety of respiratory tract and gastrointestinal infections.
  - When inhalation or ingestion of a toxic substance is suspected, odor may provide a clue to the substance involved.
- Foot odor
  - Eccrine bromhidrosis results from the breakdown of keratin and lipids by diphtheroids.
    - Fatty acid metabolites may be the agents responsible for the odor.
  - Tinea pedis (athlete's foot)
  - Pitted keratolysis
    - White plaques and shallow pits on the plantar surface
    - Various gram-positive bacteria and dermatophytes have been identified.
    - Odor is related to breakdown products (such as thiols and thioesters) of the microorganisms within the stratum corneum.
  - Each of these conditions may be exacerbated by occlusive footwear and a hot, humid climate.
- Metabolic abnormalities
  - Unusual odor of urine, sweat, and other body fluids may be caused by accumulation of odoriferous metabolic precursors or byproducts.
- Foreign body retained in an orifice
  - Focal foul smell can be from retention of a foreign body in:
    - Vagina (eg, tampons, diaphragms)
    - Auditory canals
    - Nostrils
  - May also be related to generalized body odor because odoriferous substances in a retained foreign body can be absorbed and then secreted in sweat

HISTORY

- When approaching the differential diagnosis of unusual odors, a thorough history and physical examination must first be conducted.
- If unusual body odor is the chief symptom, a history of present illness helps.
  - Questions may include:
    - When did you first notice the odor?
    - What does it smell like?
    - Does it smell like anything familiar?
    - What is the quality?

– What is the intensity?

– Does it seem to come from a certain part of the body?

– Does bathing or cleaning make it better?

– Are there any associated symptoms, such as vomiting, weight loss, or lethargy?

– Do other members of the family have similar odors?

– Do any family members have metabolic or infectious diseases?

– Have you seen any insertion of a foreign body in the nose, ear, anus, or vagina?

– Has your child taken any oral or topical medications, vitamins, herbal supplements, or toxins?

– How has the odor affected the child and family?

■ Reporting by the patient of intermittent unusual odor that is never detected by others may indicate temporal lobe epilepsy with olfactory manifestations.

PHYSICAL EXAM

■ The examiner should:

● Note the character of the odor.

– Physicians and patients may vary in their ability to detect certain odors and whether they are offensive.

– If the practitioner notices a clearly offensive body odor, but the patient or parent does not, anosmia should be considered.

● Determine the patient's stage of pubertal development.

● Check for other signs or symptoms during a complete examination with the child unclothed.

● Attempt to localize the odor to a particular body site.

■ Metabolic disorders should be suspected in infants with unusual body odor, especially if the infant appears ill, malnourished, or ketotic.

DIFFERENTIAL DIAGNOSIS

■ The differential diagnosis of unusual odors is extensive.

● Includes numerous systemic, metabolic, toxic, and infectious diseases

● Can become more focused after thorough history and physical examination

Characteristic odors, metabolic disease, associated symptoms

■ Cat urine

● 3-hydroxy-3-methylglutaryl-coenzyme A lyase deficiency

– Malaise, hypoglycemia, hepatomegaly, transaminitis, mild acidosis

■ Sweaty feet, acrid

● Glutaric aciduria type II

– Hypoglycemia, hypotonia, hepatomegaly, respiratory distress

● Isovaleric acidemia

– Vomiting, dehydration, coma, mild to moderate intellectual disability, aversion to protein foods

■ Swimming pool

● Hawkinsinuria (4-hydroxyphenylpyruvate dioxygenase deficiency)

– Failure to thrive, hepatomegaly, anemia, irritability

■ Boiled cabbage

● Hypermethioninemia

– Usually asymptomatic; some develop intellectual disability, dystonia

● Tyrosinemia (odor may be like rancid butter)

– Liver failure

■ Fruity, acetone-like, decomposing apples

● Ketoacidosis (eg, from starvation or insulin deficiency)

– Vomiting, dehydration, altered mental status, lethargy

■ Maple sugar, burnt sugar, caramel

● Maple syrup urine disease (mitochondrial branched-chain α-keto dehydrogenase complex deficiency)

– Severe form

■ Acidosis

■ Feeding difficulty, vomiting

■ Lethargy

■ Seizures

■ Coma leading to death in the first months of life

– Intermediate form

■ Mild acidosis

■ Intellectual disability, developmental delay

■ Ophthalmoplegia

– Intermittent form

■ Episodic ataxia and lethargy that may progress to coma

■ Tomcat urine

● Multiple carboxylase deficiency

– Failure to thrive, hypotonia, vomiting, seizures, rash

■ Dried celery, malt, hops; yeast, beer

● Oasthouse urine disease (methionine malabsorption syndrome)

– Diarrhea, intellectual disability, spasticity, attacks of hyperpnea, fever, edema

■ Musty; similar to a mouse, horse, wolf, or barn

● Phenylketonuria

– Vomiting, progressive intellectual disability, microcephaly, eczema, decreasing pigmentation, seizures, spasticity

■ Dead/rotting fish

● Trimethylaminuria

– Usually asymptomatic, except for odor

Infections that can be identified by their associated odors

- Respiratory and ear, nose, and throat infections
  - Candidiasis: sweet, fruity
  - Diphtheria: sweet
  - Intranasal foreign body: foul, putrid
  - Lung abscess, empyema, fetid bronchitis: putrid breath or sputum
  - *Pseudomonas* infections, otitis externa: foul cerumen
  - Rubella: fresh-plucked feathers
  - Tonsillitis, gingivitis, trench mouth: severe halitosis
  - Tuberculous lymphadenitis (scrofula): stale beer
  - Typhoid fever: fresh-baked brown bread
  - Yellow fever: butcher shop
- Skin infections
  - Candida (skin): heavily sweet
  - Decubitus ulcer: foul
  - Diphtheria (skin): sweet
  - Erythroderma: rancid
  - Hidradenitis suppurativa: lingering, pungent
  - Pitted keratolysis (gram-positive bacteria and dermatophytes): cheesy, sweaty, rotten smell from feet
  - *Pseudomonas* skin infection (burns): musty, fruity, grapelike, wet corn tortillas
  - Syphilis (condyloma latum): foul
  - Tinea capitis: mousy, mouse urine
- Genitourinary infections
  - Bacterial vaginosis: fishy vaginal discharge
  - Genital warts (condyloma acuminatum): foul
  - Urinary tract infection with urea-splitting bacteria: ammoniacal urine
  - Vaginal foreign body, vaginitis: foul vaginal discharge
- Gastrointestinal infections
  - Rotavirus gastroenteritis: full
  - Shigellosis: rancid stool
- Neurologic infections
  - *Cryptococcus* meningitis: alcohol smell to cerebrospinal fluid

Recognizable odors on the breath indicating ingestion of poisonous substances or toxins

- Bitter almond: cyanide (chokecherry, apricot pits), jetberry bush
- Burned rope: marijuana
- Camphor: naphthalene (mothballs)
- Carrots: water hemlock (cicutoxin)
- Coal gas: carbon monoxide
- Disinfectant: phenol, creosote
- Fishy: zinc or aluminum phosphide
- Fruity, acetone or decomposing apples: lacquer, salicylates, chloroform
- Fruity, alcohol: alcohol (ethanol, isopropyl alcohol), phenol, acetone, amyl nitrite (poppers)
- Fruity, pearlike: chloral hydrate, paraldehyde
- Garlic: arsenic; also phosphorus, tellurium, parathion, malathion, dimethyl sulfoxide, selenium
- Glue: toluene, solvents (huffing)
- Rotten eggs: hydrogen sulfide mercaptans, disulfiram, dimethyl sulfate, *N*-acetylcysteine
- Severe bad breath: amphetamines
- Shoe polish: nitrobenzene
- Stale tobacco: nicotine
- Violets: turpentine
- Wintergreen methyl salicylate

Odors that can indicate disease or abnormal conditions

- Breath
  - Musty fish, raw liver, feces, rotten eggs, or newly mown clover (*Fetor hepaticus*) (caused by mercaptans, such as dimethyl sulfide): liver failure
  - Fruity, acetone-like, decomposing apples (caused by ketones): ketoacidosis
  - Sweet: portacaval shunt, portal vein thrombosis
  - Feculent, foul
    - Esophageal diverticulum
    - Intestinal obstruction
- Vomitus
  - Fecal: peritonitis
- Urine
  - Fishy (caused by dimethylamine and trimethylamine): uremia
  - Stale water: acute tubular necrosis
- General
  - Sour or musty bread: pustular psoriasis
  - Putrid: scurvy
- Skin
  - Heavy: psoriasis (pustular)
  - Foul, unpleasant: skin diseases with protein breakdown (pemphigus)
  - Unpleasant, pungent, heavy: trans-3-methyl-2-hexanoic acid, may be elevated in patients with schizophrenia
- Feces: foul
  - Malabsorption
  - Melena (gastrointestinal bleeding)
- Skin and nasal cavity
  - Fetid, putrid: nasal foreign body

O

LABORATORY EVALUATION

- Infants with odor and other findings suggesting underlying metabolic disorder may need appropriate laboratory evaluation based on the suspected metabolic disease.
- In most cases with suspected metabolic disorder, the evaluation begins with, but is not limited to, checking serum glucose, liver enzymes, and liver function tests.

DIAGNOSTIC PROCEDURES

- Gas-liquid chromatography allows more precise identification of odors.
- Artificial noses or bioelectronic noses have been used to detect:
  - Tuberculosis
  - *Helicobacter pylori* infection
  - Urinary tract infections
  - Bacterial vaginosis
  - Diabetes

TREATMENT APPROACH

- Once an odor is identified and evaluated, a proper diagnostic and treatment plan can begin.
- Treatment is based on the underlying condition.

SPECIFIC TREATMENT

- Osmidrosis axillae or axillary apocrine bromhidrosis can be treated by:
  - Topical interventions
  - Surgical excisions
- Conditions associated with foot odor may respond to combination of:
  - Moisture control
  - Topical antibiotics
  - Antifungal agents

WHEN TO REFER

- Infants with odor and other findings suggesting underlying metabolic disorder
  - A specialist in metabolic diseases should be consulted.
  - An appropriate diet should be started while a more thorough metabolic evaluation is being completed.

WHEN TO ADMIT

- Infants with odor and other findings suggesting underlying metabolic disorder and have symptoms/signs of failure to thrive, hypoglycemia, and other complications

O

Osteochondroses

DEFINITION

- Juvenile osteochondroses are related to irregular mineralization resulting from necrosis followed by regeneration of bone tissue.
- Sites of osteochondroses
  - Femoral head
    - Legg-Calve-Perthes disease: aseptic necrosis secondary to interruption in blood supply
  - Tibial tuberosity
    - Osgood-Schlatter disease: avulsion of part of patellar ligament and attached fragments from tuberosity
  - Tibial shaft, proximal tibial physis
    - Rickets: softened metaphyses of long bones from vitamin D deficiency
    - Tibia vara: failure of cartilage to transform to bone at the medial aspect of the epiphysis
  - Tarsal navicular bone
    - Köhler disease: aseptic necrosis secondary to interruption in blood supply
  - Metatarsal heads 2, 3, or 4
    - Freiberg disease: aseptic necrosis leading to susceptibility to functional trauma, such as running and jumping
  - Vertebrae, especially lower thoracic
    - Scheuermann disease: cartilage plates covering vertebral bodies thin from intervertebral disk swelling, leading to narrowed disk spaces, and impeded anterior longitudinal growth, resulting in kyphosis
  - Distal radial epiphysis
    - Madelung disease
  - Lunate
    - Kienbock disease: aseptic necrosis

EPIDEMIOLOGY

- Legg-Calve-Perthes disease
  - Onset in early school-age years
  - Occurs in boys 4 times more frequently than in girls
  - Usually unilateral; in the <10% where both hip joints are involved, involvement is successive not concurrent
  - Surgery or orthotic devices can be used to encourage proper reformation of a spherical femoral head.
- Tibial tuberosity (Osgood-Schlatter disease)
  - Onset is earlier in girls than boys, because ossification of tibial tuberosity occurs earlier.
  - Incidence is higher in boys than in girls.
  - ~25% of cases with bilateral involvement
- Tibia vara (Blount disease)
  - Obesity appears to be a factor in adolescent-onset tibia vara, which is more common in boys of African descent.

- Köhler disease of the tarsal navicular bone
  - Seen primarily in boys between 3 and 7 years of age
- Freiberg disease (aseptic necrosis of the metatarsal head)
  - Girls are affected more often than boys.
- Kienbock disease (aseptic necrosis of lunate bone)
  - Right hand (the usual working hand) is involved more frequently than the left.
  - Boys are affected more frequently than girls.
- Scheuermann disease
  - Common cause of kyphosis in teenagers, occurring in ~5% of this population

ETIOLOGY

- Juvenile osteochondroses are related to irregular mineralization resulting from necrosis followed by regeneration of bone tissue.
- Exact causes and mechanisms are not known.
- Possible contributors include endogenous stress, ischemia, and genetic factors.

RISK FACTORS

- Excessive endogenous mechanical stress appears to play a role.
  - The degree of deformity and disability depends on the duration and degree of stress to which softened fibrous parts are subjected.
  - Excessive stress can lead to disordered cellular or local microvascular growth.
- Inherited tendencies to hypercoagulability may cause vascular thromboses in the osteochondroses.

SIGNS AND SYMPTOMS

- Legg-Calve-Perthes disease
  - Often presents with intermittent limp, especially after exertion
  - May be associated with hip and ipsilateral knee pain
  - The hip may develop adduction flexion contracture, with discomfort on internal rotation.
  - The acute phase generally lasts for 1 or 2 weeks.
  - Followed by the active phase, which can last for 12–40 months, during which no clinical signs or symptoms are evident.
- Osgood-Schlatter disease
  - Local pain and tenderness in the region of the knee, particularly the tuberosity
    - Pain is most severe at the end of active flexion or extension of knee.
  - If present for several months, the tuberosity enlarges, and a bony prominence may be found on its anterior aspect (see Figure 58 on page F20)

- Tibia vara (Blount disease)
  - Consider with bowing of the legs that persists or progresses beyond 2 years of age.
- Köhler disease of the tarsal navicular bone
  - Pain is localized to inner aspect of the midtarsal part of the foot, and the foot is held in a slight varus position.
  - The child walks on the outer side of the foot or in a flat-footed manner.
  - Skin over the navicular bone may be warm, red, and swollen, with tenderness to palpation.
- Freiberg disease (aseptic necrosis of metatarsal head)
  - Pain occurs in the region of the affected metatarsal while the child is walking.
  - Plantar pressure or abrupt release of pressure elicits tenderness in the area of affected metatarsal.
  - Swelling occurs over the dorsum of the involved metatarsophalangeal joint.
  - Plantar flexion becomes limited.
  - The transverse arch of the involved foot becomes flattened.
  - Callus develops on the plantar surface of the foot, overlying the involved metatarsal head.
- Kienbock disease (aseptic necrosis of lunate bone)
  - Pain is experienced on movement of the wrist; in long-standing cases, pain may be present at rest.
  - Swelling over the dorsum of the wrist, with tenderness over the affected bone
- Scheuermann disease
  - Aching pain aggravated by physical exertion in the affected portion of the vertebral column
  - The affected area is tender to palpation.
  - Assuming a stooping position often will increase the pain.
  - Within 1 year or so, kyphosis easily is apparent as a round back deformity.
  - In many cases, the pain is so minor that the complaint is that of poor posture.

DIFFERENTIAL DIAGNOSIS

- See Extremity Pain.

IMAGING

- When indicated, the first diagnostic imaging study in all the cases below is radiography.
  - Legg-Calve-Perthes disease
    - Early in the course of disease, radiography shows widening of hip joint, and occasionally, metaphyseal demineralization.
    - During the active phase, may see increased radiodensity in the femoral head ossification center caused by resorption of dead trabecular bone

- Osgood-Schlatter disease
  - The best view is one with the knee rotated inward, giving a tangential view of the tibial tuberosity.
  - Soft-tissue swelling, opaque patellar ligament, and fragmented tuberosity are seen.
- Köhler disease of the tarsal navicular bone
  - Lateral radiographs of the feet show a very narrowed, wafer-like, irregular navicular ossification center, with increased radiopacity and loss of trabecular markings.
- Freiberg disease (aseptic necrosis of the metatarsal head)
  - A deformed, broadened metatarsal head is seen.
- Kienbock disease (aseptic necrosis of lunate bone)
  - Flattened fragmented lunate bone seen with variable radiodensity
- Scheuermann disease
  - Narrowing of anterior disk spaces is seen, with defects on surfaces of adjacent vertebrae.

TREATMENT APPROACH

- Treatment is aimed at the underlying disease entity.

SPECIFIC TREATMENTS

Legg-Calve-Perthes disease

- During the remolding phase (after active phase of first 1–2 weeks, for next 12–40 months), care is directed toward maintaining the femoral head abducted and internally rotated in relation to the acetabulum.
- Surgery or orthotic devices can be used to encourage proper reformation of a spherical femoral head.

Osgood-Schlatter disease

- Treatment is directed at decreasing stress on the tubercle until the tuberosity fuses with the tibial metaphysis.
- Fusion occurs at approximately 15 years of age in girls and 17 years in boys.
- Management depends on the degree of pain.
  - In most cases, it is sufficient to restrict strenuous activities involving deep-knee bending and jumping.
  - In some instances, casting may be required to completely immobilize the knee.

Rickets

- Treatment with vitamin D will produce radiographic evidence of healing within a few weeks with eventual straightening of bones.

Tibia vara (Blount disease)

- Most children whose Blount disease persists or develops beyond 6 years of age require osteotomy.

Köhler disease of the tarsal navicular bone

- The disease process is self-limiting; surgical intervention is to be avoided.
- The process of revascularization and reconstruction occurs over 1–3 years.
- Orthotic pads can be used to absorb weight and pressure forces until healing occurs.

Freiberg disease (aseptic necrosis of the metatarsal head)

- High heels should not be worn, and long walks should be avoided until symptoms subside.
- Nonsteroidal antiinflammatory drugs can be used for symptomatic relief.

Kienbock disease (aseptic necrosis of lunate bone)

- Treatment includes wrist immobilization.
- On occasion, fusion of the lunate with adjacent wrist bones is required for stabilization and pain relief.

Scheuermann disease

- Most children require only careful observation.
- Treatment is aimed at preventing further deformity, occasionally using casting or bracing.
- Rarely, spinal fusion is necessary when progression is rapid or pain is persistent and severe.
- Rare instances of myopathy have occurred.

WHEN TO ADMIT

- For surgical intervention

WHEN TO REFER

- When uncertain of diagnosis
- When treatment requires orthopedic assessment or intervention

O

Osteomyelitis

DEFINITION

- Infection of bone that can be acute or chronic
- Chronic osteomyelitis may occur if:
  - Infection is indolent.
  - Diagnosis is delayed.
  - Treatment does not completely eradicate infection.
- Chronic multifocal osteomyelitis is a recurring inflammatory disease not typically associated with infection that can mimic bacterial osteomyelitis.

ETIOLOGY

- *Staphylococcus aureus* is most likely to cause hematogenous osteomyelitis in all age groups.
- Other possible pathogens include:
  - Coagulase-negative staphylococci
  - Gram-negative organisms
    - *Haemophilus influenzae* type b is currently very rare but previously occurred frequently in preschool-age children.
  - Other unusual organisms can become pathogens.
- In newborns, other frequent pathogens include:
  - Group B streptococcus (*Streptococcus agalactiae*)
  - Gram-negative bacteria, such as *Escherichia coli*
  - Fungal pathogens, especially *Candida* species, in infants who have been in the neonatal intensive care unit and who have had vascular lines in place
- In older infants or children, the most common pathogens are:
  - *S aureus*
  - Group A streptococcus (*Streptococcus pyogenes*)
  - *Streptococcus pneumoniae* occurs mostly in children <2 years.
  - *Kingella kingae* occurs in young children.
- The most common pathogens in children with hemoglobinopathies are:
  - *Salmonella* species
  - *S aureus*
- Unusual pathogens reflect the source of contamination.
  - *Pseudomonas aeruginosa* commonly follows foot puncture wounds through a sneaker.
  - *Aeromonas* infections may occur after trauma to bare feet while walking in river water.
- Multiple pathogens, including anaerobes, may be present, especially if the wound has been contaminated with dirt.

RISK FACTORS

- Trauma
  - Open fracture
  - Orthopedic surgery, especially placement of a foreign body, such as the insertion of pins or screws into bone
- Adjacent soft-tissue infection
- Hemoglobinopathies
  - Bone infarcts can occur with sickle cell crisis.

SIGNS AND SYMPTOMS

- Chronic osteomyelitis
  - Symptoms may have been present for months.
  - Nonspecific malaise
  - Poor appetite
  - Nonspecific pain may be elicited in the area of the bone.
- Acute osteomyelitis
  - Bone pain and fever
  - Child who had open fracture or bone surgery and develops fever and new pain or drainage at the same site.
  - A child with a fracture, either open or closed, who has new or worsening pain under a cast should have the cast removed and the area evaluated for infection.
- Infection causing bacteremia
  - History of high fever spike before the onset of pain may be described.
  - Signs of bacteremia
    - Chills and high fever
    - Malaise
    - Acute illness
- Vital signs
  - May be normal, especially with chronic infection
  - May be abnormal if child is bacteremic
  - Fever (may be low grade) is often present.
- Local signs
  - Localized pain is almost always present
  - Tenderness is often exquisite; in younger children, a new limp or absence of movement of an arm or leg may be noted.
  - Inflammation, including swelling, redness, and warmth is present over the involved bone; this can be confused with cellulitis.
  - Characteristically, the child is reluctant to move the adjacent joint and, when a lower extremity is involved, may refuse to bear weight.
  - In the young infant, the loss of active movement in an extremity may be confused with a neurologic problem.
  - Erythema is often present over the infected bone, in addition to tenderness to palpation or movement.
    - If associated arthritis occurs, pain on movement of the joint may be prominent.
  - Chronic osteomyelitis can result in a spontaneously draining sinus.
- Gastroenteritis and *Salmonella* infection may present with new fever and bone pain.

DIFFERENTIAL DIAGNOSIS

- Trauma
  - If fever is not prominent, osteomyelitis is likely to be confused with trauma or other conditions not caused by infection.
- Intraabdominal infection, especially in the area of the psoas muscle
  - Hip or femur pain can be confused with intraabdominal infection.
  - Missed appendicitis can result in a phlegmon, causing a limp that can be confused with osteomyelitis of the femur.
- Osteomyelitis, septic arthritis, and juvenile idiopathic arthritis
  - All could be signalled by limp.
  - Careful abdominal examination is necessary in a child who limps.
- Back pain and diskitis
  - Diagnostic considerations must include vertebral body infection, with or without nearby epidural abscess and diskitis.
- Leukemia
  - Bone pain can be a presenting symptom of leukemia.
  - Abnormal blood count with anemia, low leukocyte count, or thrombocytopenia signal possible leukemia.
- Lymphoma or other cancer
  - Can be confused with osteomyelitis caused by cat-scratch disease
- Bone tumors
  - Can cause nonspecific bone pain and lytic bone lesions on radiograph
  - To differentiate from chronic osteomyelitis, biopsy and culture the bone.
- Septic arthritis
  - May coexist with osteomyelitis, especially in infants
  - Requires prompt treatment
- Cellulitis
  - Difficult to differentiate from osteomyelitis because of erythema over the infected bone
- Chronic multifocal osteomyelitis
  - Can only be diagnosed over time by observing recurring disease, usually with cultures that are negative for acute infection

DIAGNOSTIC APPROACH

- Careful examination seeking focal areas of tenderness is necessary in the young child who may not be able to describe pain adequately.
  - Ask about trauma, fracture, or orthopedic surgery.

- Infants with signs and symptoms of septic arthritis of the hip must always be evaluated for accompanying osteomyelitis of the femur.
  - If the child is >1 year of age, infection tends to be held in place by the metaphysis.
  - After infancy, infection is most likely to spread into the diaphysis and down the bone.
- Blood culture and a needle aspirate of the infection site are the most helpful procedures.
  - If history and examination fit the diagnosis and a blood culture is positive, therapy can be started without bone aspiration.
- Evaluation for related arthritis is crucial, given that joint infections can progress rapidly and need adequate drainage to avoid damage to the joint.

LABORATORY FINDINGS

- Complete blood count and smear review
  - The leukocyte count may be elevated in acutely ill children with bacteremia.
  - Very low leukocyte counts occur with sepsis.
  - Anemia, low leukocyte count, or thrombocytopenia in the absence of disseminated intravascular coagulation should raise concern for leukemia or other cancer.
- Erythrocyte sedimentation rate
  - May be normal at first, but almost always becomes elevated in acute osteomyelitis
- C-reactive protein
  - Usually elevated early
- Blood cultures
  - Helpful in identifying the presence of bacteremia and the cause of the infection
  - Positive in 40–50% of cases
  - If infection with tuberculosis is suggested because of history or setting, cultures for acid-fast bacteria should be included and tuberculin skin testing added.
- All tests can produce normal findings, especially early in the infection.

IMAGING

- Radiography
  - Early: no bone changes seen
  - Earliest detectable signs are blurred soft-tissue planes secondary to edema spreading into fatty tissues.
  - Bone changes are apparent 7–10 days or longer after onset of symptoms.
    - Nonspecific periosteal reaction; lytic lesions occur later
    - In chronic osteomyelitis, shows extensive disease, usually along the diaphysis of the bone; bone changes may need to be differentiated from cancer by history and ultimately, cultures and biopsy.

O

- Radiographs should always be obtained to exclude other abnormalities, such as fracture or a malignant lesion.

■ Magnetic resonance imaging (MRI) is better than skeletal scintigraphy (technetium bone scan).

- Provides excellent views of bone and soft-tissue anatomy
- Reveals subperiosteal abscesses that require surgical intervention; frequently produces false-negative results
  - Presence of a subperiosteal abscess is diagnostic for acute osteomyelitis that has broken through the metaphyseal cortex.
- MRI is the imaging technique of choice when pelvic or spine osteomyelitis is suspected.

■ Bone scans

- Not useful in neonates because of low bone mineralization
- Provide limited information regarding soft-tissue involvement, subperiosteal space, and bone marrow edema
- Results may be normal in up to 20% of children during first days of illness.
- Cancer, cellulitis, trauma, and bone infarction can affect specificity.
  - 3-stage scans improve sensitivity
- Require large amounts of radiation but no sedation or general anesthesia
- Can be useful in cases in which multiple sites of osteomyelitis are suspected
- Less sensitive and specific than MRI, and often difficult to interpret

■ Ultrasonography

- Can detect a subperiosteal abscess
- May help guide needle aspiration of an infected bone
- Can help evaluate a nearby joint for an effusion present with an associated arthritis

DIAGNOSTIC PROCEDURES

■ Aspiration

- Confirms diagnosis
- Can determine the necessity for operative decompression if frank pus is obtained
- May alleviate pain caused by pressure from an abscess
- Provides a specimen for pathogen identification by culture and material for immediate Gram stain
- Aspiration of the subperiosteal space and of the metaphysis for culture is indicated to obtain culture identification of the pathogen.
  - When blood cultures are pending
  - Whenever a collection of pus exists

TREATMENT APPROACH

■ Acute osteomyelitis should be aggressively treated to decrease the risk of chronic osteomyelitis.

■ Chronic infection requires surgical drainage or debridement and is more difficult to eradicate.

- Antibiotics for up to 1 year

■ Surgery

- Should be prompt
- Antibiotics should be started as soon as culture material is obtained.

■ Once blood cultures and needle aspiration have been performed, intravenous antibiotics should be given empirically.

■ Antibiotics

- Should be adjusted once cultures and sensitivities are available, narrowing the spectrum to cover the pathogen
- Should be continued for 4–8 weeks, using clinical response and sedimentation rate to guide length of therapy
- Oral antibiotics can be considered to finish the course of therapy, if:
  - An oral agent is available that has good bone penetration.
  - An oral agent has excellent activity against the pathogen.
  - Oral medicine is palatable.
  - The child has a social situation that will guarantee compliance.
- The switch to oral therapy should not occur before clinical response to IV therapy, including:
  - Absence of fever
  - Return to normal function
  - Decrease or normalization of inflammatory markers
- Oral antibiotics often require 2–3 times the usual dose, making gastrointestinal tolerance a requirement.

■ Abscess

- Must be drained surgically when detected or suspected
- Lack of pus should suggest that the site of aspiration may have been inaccurate, or that pus may be present but too thick to pass through even a large-bore needle.

SPECIFIC TREATMENTS

Pharmacologic therapy

■ After the newborn period, in a previously well child thought to have hematogenous osteomyelitis, give a penicillinase-resistant penicillin or first-generation cephalosporin unless:

- The child is severely ill.
- The child has signs of bacteremia and sepsis.
  - If the child has sepsis, vancomycin should be considered because of the increasing incidence of methicillin-resistant *S aureus* (MRSA).

O

■ Therapy should cover all likely pathogens.

- In newborns, initial therapy should always include coverage against Gram-negative enterics.
  - Oxacillin and gentamicin
  - Vancomycin and ceftazidime
    - When concern about MRSA infection exists
    - For coagulase-negative staphylococci
  - Neonates who have been in a neonatal intensive care unit and who have been on antibiotics should be treated most broadly, pending culture results.

■ Antifungal agents are not usual unless blood culture or other epidemiologic data suggest the presence of a fungal infection.

■ Children with sickle cell hemoglobinopathies are at special risk for *Salmonella* species in addition to *S aureus*.

- Treat with cefuroxime or with vancomycin and ceftriaxone or cefotaxime, pending culture results.

■ If pseudomonal infection is suspected or there is contamination with dirt (eg, after a puncture wound of the foot), initial treatment should be either:

- Ceftazidime
- A carboxypenicillin or acylureidopenicillin combined with an aminoglycoside, such as piperacillin-tazobactam and gentamicin or ceftazidime and gentamicin
- Piperacillin-tazobactam is appropriate to treat *S aureus* while cultures are pending.

■ Clindamycin

- Often used in cases of allergy to ß-lactams or to treat MRSA isolates that are sensitive

■ Linezolid

- Should not be used empirically
- May be helpful in patients with ß-lactam allergies and as a drug that can be used orally to treat a serious infection
- Side effect of thrombocytopenia limits its long-term use.

WHEN TO ADMIT

■ Children with acute osteomyelitis require admission to the hospital for rapid evaluation and to initiate treatment.

■ Initial evaluation can begin as an outpatient, before diagnosis is established.

- Complete blood count, blood culture, and radiography
- The physician must follow up closely and consider hospitalization as soon as the diagnosis becomes likely.

WHEN TO REFER

■ Diagnosis requires thorough evaluation and usually includes consultation with radiology and orthopedic surgery.

- Radiologist can help focus the radiologic evaluation effectively.
- Early consulting with orthopedic surgeon helps expedite aspiration of the bone or open drainage.

■ Infectious disease specialists may help:

- To organize the evaluation
- To start therapy
- With follow-up with children who are discharged on home intravenous therapy and who have chronic disease

COMPLICATIONS

■ Chronic osteomyelitis can result in lifelong disability related to recurrences and, rarely, to cancer.

■ Chronic osteomyelitis may result in bone loss and areas of devascularized bone, which separate and create sequestrum or pieces of dead bone in the shaft of the long bones.

- If this occurs, surgery will be required to treat the infection.
- A Brodie abscess has a capsule that can develop in the bone; it appears to be the result of walled-off chronic infection.

O

Otitis Media and Otitis Externa

DEFINITION

- *Otitis media* means "inflammation of the middle ear."
- *Acute otitis media* (AOM) is the presence of inflammatory fluid in the middle-ear space, accompanied by acute onset of local findings, such as erythematous and/or bulging tympanic membrane, distorted landmarks and light reflux, and a tympanic membrane that is not mobile on insufflation.
- *Otitis media with effusion* (OME), or *serous otitis media,* describes inflammatory fluid in the middle-ear space in an asymptomatic child or in a child with mild upper respiratory tract symptoms.
- *Recurrent otitis media* has generally been used to refer to the occurrence of:
  - ≥3 episodes of AOM in 6 months
  - 4 episodes in 1 year
  - Recurrent otitis media should not be confused with chronic otitis media, which may be used to describe OME that:
    - Lasts >3 months
    - Is a suppurative middle-ear process that fails to respond to initial antibiotic therapy
- Otitis externa (OE) is an inflammatory process that involves structures of the outer ear, specifically the external auditory canal.
- Malignant OE is a complicated form of OE that can develop in immunocompromised children and those with severe malnutrition.

EPIDEMIOLOGY

Otitis media

- Age
  - By the age of 1 year, 62% of children have experienced ≥1 episode of AOM.
- Sex
  - More common in boys
- Socioeconomics
  - More common in children of low socioeconomic status
- Race
  - Incidence rates in white and black children are similar.
- Otitis media is the most common reason that children in the US receive antibiotics.
  - >90% of all antibiotic use in the first 2 years of life is attributable to the treatment of otitis media.
  - By the age of 7 years, between 65% and 95% of children will have been treated for ≥1 episode of otitis media.
- Each year in the US, >$3.5 billion is spent on the treatment of otitis media.

Otitis externa

- Common finding in children
- Especially prevalent during the warm-weather months

ETIOLOGY

Otitis media

- Otitis media is an inflammatory process of the upper respiratory tract.
- Usually results from a viral infection
  - As viruses infect the respiratory mucosa, edema can lead to eustachian tube dysfunction.
  - Inflammatory fluid and pathogenic respiratory bacteria that reflux into the middle-ear space do not drain normally.
  - This process leads to formation of an abscess in the middle ear.
- In studies of children with AOM, specimens of middle-ear fluid:
  - Were positive for bacteria approximately 70% of the time
  - The most frequently identified pathogens are:
    - *Streptococcus pneumoniae*
    - *Haemophilus influenzae*
    - *Moraxella catarrhalis*
  - Group A ß-hemolytic streptococcus and *Staphylococcus aureus* (including methicillin-resistant strains) are much less common.
  - Rarely, *Mycoplasma pneumoniae* is detected.
    - Not often enough to affect the empirical selection of an antibiotic for treatment
  - Respiratory viruses, such as respiratory syncytial virus (RSV), influenza viruses, and parainfluenza viruses, are also recovered often from middle-ear aspirates, either in addition to bacteria or in isolation.
    - RSV has a tendency to infect the mucosa of the middle ear.
    - Probably contributes substantially to the development of otitis media in children

OE

- Multifactorial in etiology
- Involves interaction between the host and environmental factors, including:
  - Trauma to the external auditory canal
  - Presence of a foreign body
  - Repeated ear cleansing
  - Prolonged exposure to standing water in the ear canal
    - For example, following swimming or bathing (swimmer's ear)
  - High environmental temperature and humidity
  - Increased sweating
  - Allergy
  - Stress

O

- Inflammation may be:
  - Focal, at the site of trauma or an infected hair follicle
  - Diffuse, as is the case with swimmer's ear
- When inflammation is focal and associated with infection, the organism is often *S aureus*.
  - Can lead to furuncle formation at the site of the inflammation
- The most common organism associated with diffuse inflammation is *Pseudomonas aeruginosa*.
  - Hydrophilic bacterial species
- Infection is often polymicrobial.
- Enteric bacilli and fungi are less common causes.

Malignant OE

- Necrotizing infection of the external auditory canal
- Often begins as minor trauma to the canal
- Usually caused by *P aeruginosa*
- Rapidly spreads to involve:
  - Soft tissue
  - Cartilage
  - Nerves and the temporal bone
- Leads to osteomyelitis of the base of the skull

RISK FACTORS

- Several environmental factors increase the risk for otitis media.
  - Exposure to tobacco smoke
  - Use of a pacifier
  - Formula feeding (not breastfeeding)
  - Feeding in a lying-down position
  - Attendance at child-care centers
    - Particularly those serving large numbers of children
- Children at high risk for AOM include those with:
  - Craniofacial anomalies that alter the normal air and fluid dynamics of the middle-ear space, eg, cleft palate
  - Allergic rhinitis
  - Immunodeficiencies
  - Certain ethnic groups, such as:
    - Native Americans
    - Alaskan Natives
- A mild hereditary predisposition to recurrent otitis media appears to exist.
  - Some of the variation in presentation and incidence is explained by genetic factors.
  - Familial and individual environmental factors account for the remainder.

SIGNS AND SYMPTOMS

Otitis media

- In the classic case of AOM, a young child with a history of a recent upper respiratory tract infection develops acute onset of:
  - New fever
  - Ear discomfort or pain
- Other symptoms include:
  - Otorrhea
  - Distortion of the tympanic membrane (bulging, erythema, opacity, limited mobility)
- In children old enough to localize pain, the affected ear is often obvious.
- In younger children, discomfort may be more generalized, exhibited by unexplained crying or irritability.
- Examination may reveal other signs of upper respiratory infection, such as:
  - Rhinorrhea
  - Cough
  - Conjunctival injection

OE

- Children complain of ear pain.
- May report pain with chewing
  - Because of proximity of the temporomandibular joint to the external auditory canal
- May report difficulty hearing
  - Result of swelling within the external auditory canal and conductive hearing loss
- Examination reveals tenderness with manipulation of the pinna or pressure on the tragus.
- Insertion of otoscope into the external auditory canal can be painful and should be undertaken carefully.
- Within the canal, focal erythema and swelling may be seen at the site of trauma or folliculitis.
- If inflammation is diffuse, swelling of the entire canal renders a boggy appearance.
- Edema and the presence of inflammatory debris may prevent complete visualization of the tympanic membrane.
- The tympanic membrane should appear normal in OE, unless coexistent otitis media is present.

Malignant OE

- Pain is severe.
- Discharge from the external canal is copious.

DIAGNOSTIC APPROACH

- Concern is growing that overdiagnosis of otitis media and liberal use of antibiotics for treatment have contributed to the rapid emergence of antibiotic-resistant bacteria.
  - Particularly penicillin-resistant *S pneumoniae*
- Accurate diagnosis is critical to appropriate management.
- Diagnosis is based on recognition of:
  - Characteristic clinical context
  - Physical findings on pneumatic otoscopic examination
- Diagnosis of AOM is confirmed using pneumatic otoscopy.
  - To perform this technique, the child must either cooperate or be restrained in a comfortable position that allows manipulation of the pinna and insertion of otoscope into the external auditory canal.
  - Cleanse the external auditory canal for clear visualization of the tympanic membrane.
    - Cerumen or foreign bodies should be removed using a cerumen spoon or gentle irrigation with warm water.
  - The largest speculum that will fit into the external auditory canal at a depth of one-third inch to one-half inch should be attached to pneumatic otoscope.
    - Permits visualization of the largest possible area and ensures a relatively airtight seal for insufflation
  - AOM is present when:
    - Distortion (usually bulging) of the tympanic membrane is noted on direct visualization.
    - In some cases, the tympanic membrane may be retracted rather than bulging.
    - Restricted movement of the tympanic membrane, indicative of fluid in the middle ear, is noted with gentle insufflation and exsufflation using the squeeze bulb attached to the otoscope.
  - Erythema of the tympanic membrane alone is not sufficient to diagnose AOM.
    - Possibly the incidental result of fever or crying
  - Occasionally, a child with AOM experiences spontaneous rupture of the tympanic membrane.
    - Leads to marked improvement in ear pain
    - Otorrhea is evident on examination.
- OME may be an incidental finding on physical examination.
  - Decreased mobility of the tympanic membrane
  - Signs of acute inflammation seen in AOM are absent.

LABORATORY FINDINGS

- In AOM, some experts advocate making a specific bacteriologic diagnosis (see Diagnostic Procedures).

DIAGNOSTIC PROCEDURES

- Tympanocentesis or carbon dioxide laser-assisted myringotomy
  - Used to obtain middle-ear fluid for culture and sensitivities
  - Not necessary for routine diagnosis of AOM
  - Useful in specific clinical situations in which identification of the organism to guide therapeutic decisions is a high priority
    - Episodes of AOM that do not respond to empirical antibiotic therapy
    - Children who experience frequent recurrences despite seemingly appropriate therapy
    - Children who are young and particularly toxic in appearance
- Cultures of other areas of the upper respiratory tract are useful for research.
  - Do not assist in the management of individual episodes of AOM
  - Theame organisms usually are recovered from the nasopharynx as from middle-ear fluid.
    - The presence of an organism from nasopharyngeal culture does not prove presence in the middle ear.
- Tympanometry is a technique for documenting tympanic membrane compliance.
  - Can be used to document objectively presence of fluid in the middle-ear space
  - Does not add to information obtained on carefully performed pneumatic otoscopy.
  - Can be useful for monitoring the course of an episode of OME over time

TREATMENT APPROACH

- Otitis media is usually self-limited.
  - As viral illness resolves, eustachian tube function is restored.
  - The middle-ear space drains normally.
- Acute symptoms generally resolve spontaneously within a few days.
- Middle-ear effusions can persist for weeks after an episode of AOM.
  - 60% of middle-ear effusions resolve spontaneously within 3 months.
  - 85% resolve within 6 months.
- Persistence of middle-ear effusions (or OME) after an episode of AOM has raised concern about:
  - Conductive hearing loss that accompanies these effusions
  - Impact on speech and language development, especially in younger children
- Effusions are sterile.
  - In the absence of other acute signs and symptoms, they do not require antibacterial therapy.

SPECIFIC TREATMENTS

Management of AOM

- Whether an episode of AOM should be treated with antibiotics is a matter of ongoing discussion.
  - The 2004 AAP and American Academy of Family Physicians practice guidelines delineate very specific criteria for:
    - Patients who should receive antibiotic therapy
    - Patients who are candidates for observation
  - Clinical experience should be used to determine which course of therapy is most appropriate when patients do not quite fit criteria.
  - The modest benefits of antibiotic therapy must be weighed against the negative impact of widespread antibiotic use and its effect on producing antibiotic-resistant species of organisms, such as *S pneumoniae*.
    - In some areas of the US, 40% of strains of this organism are resistant to penicillin.
- Several guiding principles should be observed when selecting patients to be treated with antibiotics.
  - The diagnosis should be clear.
    - Presence of fever, upper respiratory symptoms, or a middle-ear effusion are not sufficient indications without objective findings on pneumatic otoscopy
    - Antibiotics should not be prescribed without a clear diagnosis.
  - Younger patients may benefit more from empirical antibiotic therapy than older children.
    - Positive effects of antibiotic administration have been more prevalent in children <2 years.
    - Possibly because of their more limited immune response to encapsulated organisms
  - Uniquely susceptible individuals, such as those with immunodeficiencies or those with craniofacial anomalies, are at increased risk of complications or protracted course of illness.
    - These patients warrant a lower threshold for treatment.
  - Observation of a patient off antibiotic therapy for 48–72 hours is now considered an acceptable management option in low-risk patients >6 months of age.
    - If symptoms have not resolved spontaneously within 48–72 hours:
      - Reexamination is indicated.
      - Prescription of antibiotics is appropriate if objective findings of AOM are still present.
- An effective antibiotic with the narrowest spectrum should be chosen.
  - Antibiotics for treatment of this common condition include:
    - Penicillins
    - First-, second- and third-generation cephalosporins
    - Macrolides
    - Carbacephems
  - In the absence of specific microbiological information, selection of empirical antibiotic therapy should be guided by:
    - Knowledge of the most common bacterial pathogens identified in middle-ear aspirates of children
    - Efficacy of the antibacterial agent (based on minimal inhibitory concentration and pharmacokinetic and pharmacodynamic data) against these organisms
  - In population-based studies of children with AOM, the most common organisms isolated were *S pneumoniae*, *H influenzae*, and *M catarrhalis*.
- High-dose amoxicillin is the recommended first-line choice.
  - Inexpensive
  - Good spectrum of activity against target organisms, including strains of *S pneumoniae* with intermediate resistance to penicillin
  - Studies of amoxicillin treatment of AOM show cure rates of 85–94% based on clinical criteria.
  - Treatment should be administered for 10 days.
  - Shorter courses of 5–7 days may be acceptable in low-risk patients (older children with uncomplicated histories).
- If fever, ear pain, and objective findings of AOM persist despite ≥72 hours of therapy, then a change of antibiotic may be warranted.
  - Second-line agents, such as second- or third-generation cephalosporins or amoxicillin plus clavulanate
    - Cover ß-lactamase–producing strains of *H influenzae* and *M catarrhalis*
    - Penicillin-resistant *S pneumoniae*
  - Clindamycin only provides coverage for resistant gram-positive organisms.
    - Alternative agent if otitis is proven to be secondary to a resistant strain of *S pneumoniae*
  - For patients who develop hives or anaphylaxis to ß-lactam antibiotics, azithromycin may be used.
    - This drug has decreased activity against:
      - Penicillin-resistant strains of *S pneumoniae*
      - ß-Lactamase–producing strains of *H influenzae*
- No proven benefit has been found from use of:
  - Antihistamine or decongestant preparations
  - Steroids
  - Nonsteroidal antiinflammatory drugs
- Topical Auralgan otic solution is somewhat effective in reducing acute ear pain.

O

Management of OME

■ OME presents a different therapeutic challenge.

- The goal of therapy is to limit potential long-term detrimental effects on speech and language development.

- Weak associations have been found between OME and abnormal speech and language development in children <4 years.

- Problems with attention and expressive language delay have been found in older children.

- Associations may be the result of environmental influences that predispose patients to both OME and developmental delays.

- The effects of treating OME on these outcomes are not well established.

■ Medical therapies for OME have produced unsatisfactory results.

- Very limited scientific evidence exists.

- A few experts believe that empirical antibiotic therapy either early or later, when the effusion has persisted for ≥3 months, may hasten resolution of the effusion.

    – Most experts strongly discourage this practice, given increasing rates of antibacterial resistance.

- No role exists for:

    – Steroid medications

    – Antihistamine or decongestant preparations

    – Tonsillectomy

    – Adenoidectomy

- The most effective therapy is surgical insertion of tympanostomy tubes.

- Placement of tympanostomy tubes evacuates middle-ear effusion and restores near-normal hearing.

    – The effect on long-term speech and language outcomes is unclear.

    – Laser-assisted myringotomy may soon replace tympanostomy tube placement.

■ Adenoidectomy is used in the management of patients with OME.

- May be effective in a select group of children

- Chronically infected adenoids are thought to serve as a reservoir of pathogenic organisms, leading to tubal edema and malfunction and persistent OME.

- Removal of enlarged adenoids has been shown to improve effusion resolution.

- Adenoidectomy and myringotomy plus ventilation tube insertion is recommended therapy for:

    – Children with severe ear disease

    – Children undergoing replacement of a second set of ventilation tubes

Management of recurrent otitis media

■ Occurrence of ≥3 episodes of AOM within 6 months or of 4 episodes within 1 year satisfies many experts' definition of recurrent otitis media.

- Therapy is controversial.

- Studies have shown that long-term administration of prophylactic antibiotics (usually either amoxicillin or trimethoprim plus sulfamethoxazole) can reduce incidence of subsequent episodes of AOM.

    – The effect is modest.

    – To improve outcome in 1 child, 9 must be treated with daily medication, and prophylactic antibiotics contribute to the development of resistant organisms.

- Use of prophylactic antibiotics is currently not recommended for management of recurrent otitis media.

- Controlling environmental risk factors, such as exposure to tobacco smoke and attendance at large child-care centers, is a more desirable approach.

■ Tympanostomy tube placement or laser-assisted myringotomy should be considered in the management of recurrent otitis media.

- This approach may be justified when recurrent AOM complicates OME and is accompanied by hearing loss.

- Frequent episodes of AOM (without OME) that respond to appropriate antibiotic therapy are not an indication.

- AOM tends to occur less frequently in children who have had tympanostomy tubes placed.

    – Requires administration of anesthesia

    – Tubes may not remain in place for a sufficient duration to have a measurable impact on health of an individual child.

■ Strategies that show promise for prevention of future episodes of otitis media

- Use of conjugated vaccine against *S pneumoniae*

- Widespread use of influenza vaccine in healthy children

- Development of an effective vaccine against RSV

Care of the child with tympanostomy tubes

■ Tympanostomy tube placement is the most common surgical procedure performed in children.

- Examination of the child with tympanostomy tubes should show a patent tube traversing the pars flaccida.

- A tympanic membrane that contains a tympanostomy tube is not intact.

    – Mobility is affected.

    – Pneumatic otoscopy cannot be used as a reliable indicator of AOM.

- Tympanostomy tubes are usually extruded naturally some time after insertion.
  - Some otolaryngologists recommend actively removing tympanostomy tubes that have been in place for ≥2 years to prevent complications, such as chronic perforation or tympanosclerosis.
  - If a tympanostomy tube is visualized in the external canal and is no longer seated within the tympanic membrane, it may be removed with a cerumen spoon under direct visualization.
- Otorrhea is common in children with tympanostomy tubes.
  - Otorrhea associated with other symptoms of upper respiratory infection may indicate the presence of AOM.
    - Treat accordingly.
  - When otorrhea occurs in isolation, it may respond to topical application of an otic solution containing:
    - Neomycin
    - Polymyxin B
    - Hydrocortisone
  - Otorrhea is no more common in children with tympanostomy tubes who swim or submerge their heads in a bathtub than in those who do not.
  - Use of topical antibiotics or earplugs does not reduce incidence of swimming-related otorrhea.
  - Children with tympanostomy tubes who do not dive to depths >6 feet or swim in potentially contaminated water (such as a pond) require no special precautions to swim.
    - Use of earplugs or molds may increase drainage from the ears.

Management of OE

- When OE is accompanied by furuncle formation, incision and drainage may be necessary.
  - Diffuse OE usually responds to 4 times-a-day application of a topical otic solution containing:
    - Neomycin
    - Polymyxin B
    - Hydrocortisone
  - With the patient lying on the unaffected side, 5 drops of this solution are instilled into the affected ear.
  - The patient should remain in position for 5–10 minutes after instillation to ensure that the medication has come in contact with affected skin.
  - Insertion of a cotton wick can prolong this contact.
- OE can be prevented by keeping the external auditory canal dry.
  - Avoid vigorous cleaning of the canal that can lead to superficial trauma.

Management of malignant OE

- Treatment requires administration of intravenous antibiotics.
- Occasionally, surgical intervention is required.

WHEN TO ADMIT

- Admit any patient with severe otitis media who has:
  - Toxic appearance
  - Malignant OE
  - Suppurative complications of otitis media
- Hospitals provide:
  - Institution of prompt, effective intravenous antibiotic therapy
  - Evaluation for possible surgical intervention

WHEN TO REFER

- Otitis media with effusion
  - If, at 3 months, middle-ear effusions are persistent and bilateral, refer for audiologic testing.
- Care of the child with tympanostomy tubes
  - Occasionally, a granuloma may develop at the site of tympanostomy tube insertion.
    - May lead to bleeding from the external auditory canal
    - Patients should be referred to an otolaryngologist for intervention.
- Patients with recurrent or chronic otitis media and persistent otitis media with effusion (present for ≥3 months) should be referred for ear, nose, and throat evaluation.
- Infectious diseases consultation should be obtained in patients with the following conditions.
  - Suppurative complications of otitis media
  - Recurrent or chronic episodes of otitis media unresponsive to standard therapy
  - Patients with unusual or multiple antibiotic resistant organisms isolated from middle ear fluid
  - Patients with chronic suppurative otitis media unresponsive to conventional therapy
  - Patients with malignant OE
- In many of the these conditions, a team approach with both ear, nose, and throat and infectious diseases referrals should be used for optimal management of the patient's condition.

FOLLOW-UP

- Acute otitis media treatment
  - Most children who respond satisfactorily to treatment do not require specific follow-up.
  - As long as a child is asymptomatic, the main reason for follow-up is to document resolution of a middle-ear effusion that may contribute to conductive hearing loss.

O

- Only 50% of middle-ear effusions resolve by 6 weeks after initial presentation.
- Follow-up for an otherwise healthy and asymptomatic child should be scheduled no sooner than 6 weeks post-diagnosis, if at all.
- An effusion that is persistent at 6 weeks does not warrant specific intervention other than perhaps checking for resolution again in 6 more weeks.
- Documented OME
  - Follow-up at 3 months is reasonable, assuming that acute symptoms have not intervened.
  - If hearing is normal, then further observation to allow spontaneous resolution is appropriate.
  - If a conductive hearing loss at a threshold ≥20 dB is documented at 3-month follow-up, consideration should be given to tympanostomy tube placement or laser-assisted myringotomy to drain the effusions and restore hearing.
  - Use of these procedures for OME in otherwise healthy children with normal hearing is not recommended.

COMPLICATIONS

Otitis media

- Conductive hearing loss resulting from chronic middle-ear effusions associated with otitis media may contribute to speech and language delay in some children.
- Overuse of antibiotics to treat otitis media is thought to contribute significantly to the emergence of antibiotic-resistant bacteria.
- Suppurative complications of otitis media are:
  - Mastoiditis
  - Intracranial extension of infection
  - Lateral sinus thrombosis
- Suppurative complications are rare.
  - Occur much less frequently than in the era before routine antibiotic treatment of AOM
  - The incidence of these complications has declined in areas of the world where routine antibiotic treatment of AOM is less common.
  - Factors other than early antibiotic treatment may have contributed to this trend.

- Early signs and symptoms associated with suppurative complications include:
  - Mastoid tenderness
  - Persistent fever associated with chronic tympanic membrane perforation
  - Persistent and severe headache
  - Severe otalgia
  - Retroorbital pain on the side of the affected ear
  - Vertigo
  - Mental status changes
  - Nystagmus
  - Other focal neurologic signs can signal intracranial extension of suppurative otitis media.
    - Facial paralysis
    - Meningismus
    - Papilledema

Malignant OE

- Stenosis of the external auditory canal
- Auricular cartilage deformity
- Tympanic membrane necrosis
- Sensorineural hearing loss

PROGNOSIS

- Most otitis media is self-limited and resolves spontaneously in several days.
- Malignant OE
  - Development of facial paralysis indicates a poor prognosis.

PREVENTION

- Exclusive breastfeeding early in life has a protective effect.
- Immunizations with influenza and pneumococcal vaccines
- Avoiding passive smoke exposure
- Using appropriate feeding positions (not feeding in lying down position)
- Treating allergic rhinitis appropriately
- Treating the underlying cause, such as cleft palate

Parasitic Infections

DEFINITION

- Disease caused by any 1 of a variety of parasites, including protozoa, nematodes, trematodes, and cestodes

EPIDEMIOLOGY

Leishmaniasis

- Endemic areas for cutaneous form
  - Mediterranean basin
  - Middle East, including Iraq
  - Southern Asia
  - Parts of Africa
    - Ethiopia
    - Yemen
    - Kenya
  - Central and South America
  - Texas
- Visceral form
  - Disease involves different age groups depending on parasite species and geographic distribution.
    - India: affects adolescents and young adults
    - Sudan and East Africa: affects young men
    - Mediterranean basin and northern China: affects infants and young children
    - Latin America (rare): affects primary infants and young children

Chagas disease

- Areas from the southern US to southern Argentina
  - Highest prevalence in Brazil, Argentina, and Venezuela
  - In the US, infection is common in immigrants from Central and South America
- Most infections occur in poor, remote rural areas or areas with poor sanitation.
- Prevalence
  - 16–18 million people in endemic areas are infected.
  - An estimated 100,000 chagasic Latin Americans are living in the US.

African trypanosomiasis

- Transmission occurs in areas between the latitudes of 15 degrees north and 20 degrees south, with temperatures between 20°C and 30°C (distribution of the tsetse fly).
- Rare in children because of limited exposure

Giardiasis

- Prevalence
  - 20–30% in developing countries to 2–7% in the developed world
- Incidence in US
  - Approximately 2.5 million new cases annually

- Most cases occur in children in the first 5 years of life.
  - Children attending child care centers
    - Prevalence among children who attend child care centers can be as high as 35%.
  - Internationally adopted children
    - Tend to be older than those in child care centers and to have additional parasitic infections
- Peak incidence is in late summer and early fall.

Amebiasis

- Incidence
  - Worldwide, 40–50 million people develop colitis or extraintestinal disease annually, with 40,000 deaths.
- Prevalence
  - Developing countries have high prevalence rates, up to 50% in certain developing areas.
    - Related to poor hygiene, inadequate water sanitation, and human waste that is used to fertilize crops
- In developed countries
  - Mainly seen in migrants from and travelers to endemic countries

Amoebic meningoencephalitis

- Primary amoebic meningoencephalitis (PAM)
  - Disease in previously healthy children and young adults
  - The responsible organism is found in warm bodies of water.
    - Human-made lakes and ponds
    - Hot springs
    - Thermally polluted streams, rivers, and healing swimming pool waters
- Granulomatous amoebic encephalitis (GAE)
  - Disease in immunocompromised patients
  - The responsible organism is identified in:
    - Soil
    - Various water sources
    - Air conditioners
    - Contact lens fluid

Cryptosporidiosis

- Common in developing countries that have increased crowding and poor sanitation
- Prevalence
  - 1–3% of immunocompetent patients with diarrhea in developed countries
  - 7–10% of immunocompetent patients in developing countries
  - 3 cases per 100,000 in the US and 6 per 100,000 persons in Canada
  - Higher in children than in adults

P

- Cause of outbreaks
  - Contaminated drinking water
  - Contaminated apple cider
  - Playing in contaminated water at a water park
  - Contaminated food (less frequent)
  - Person-to-person transmission at child care centers (attack rates of 30–60%)

Isosporiasis

- Common in tropical/subtropical regions of Central and South America, Africa, and Southeast Asia
- In the US, seen in homosexual men

Cyclosporiasis

- Worldwide
- From ingesting contaminated food or water
- Eating infected fruit, herbs, and vegetables

Toxoplasmosis

- Worldwide distribution
- Highest incidence in countries where consumption of raw meat is common (US and Western countries)
- Common in regions with warm, humid climates, including tropical areas

Malaria

- Incidence
  - 350–500 million clinical episodes of malaria occur every year, resulting in ≥1 million deaths.
- Most cases are in sub-Saharan Africa.
  - Most occur in African children <5 years of age.
- *Plasmodium falciparum*
  - Causes most severe disease
  - Predominant malarial parasite in tropical Africa, Southeast Asia, and Oceania
- *Plasmodium vivax*
  - Predominant in Southeast Asia
  - Causes most malaria infections worldwide
- *Plasmodium malariae*
  - Least common
  - Produces long-lasting infections

Babesiosis

- In Europe
  - Affected patients usually those who have undergone splenectomy
  - Cases have been reported from Yugoslavia, France, Germany, Spain, Sweden, Ireland, Great Britain, and the former Soviet Union.

- In the US
  - Most cases occur in the northeastern part of the country, including islands and coastal areas near Massachusetts, New York, New Jersey, and Rhode Island and areas in Connecticut.
    - Cases from other states have also been reported.
  - Most cases occur between May and August.
  - Most infected patients are immunocompetent.
- Cases also reported in other parts of the world.
  - Taiwan
  - Canary Islands
  - Egypt
  - South Africa
  - Mexico
  - China

Trichuriasis

- Worldwide, but most frequently found in tropical/subtropical areas and areas of poor sanitation
- Infection is common in warm, humid areas.
- In US, most common in Latin immigrant children in rural areas of the southeastern states

Strongyloidiasis

- Worldwide, but particularly common in the tropical/ subtropical regions
- In US, most common in the southeastern states
- Disease is most frequent among white men.

Hookworm infections

- Worldwide

Cutaneous larva migrans

- Most cases occur in tropical/subtropical areas of Africa, Southeast Asia, the Caribbean, and Central and South America.
- In US, most cases occur in the southeast.

Pinworm infections

- Infections are more prevalent in temperate and cold climate regions than in the tropics.

Enterobiasis

- Infections occur across socioeconomic levels but are more common in close, crowded conditions.

Toxocariasis

- Humans acquire infection by ingesting soil contaminated with infective eggs of the parasites, shed by dogs.
- Endemic in areas where dogs are present
  - Estimates suggest that 20% of dogs and 98% of puppies are infected.

P

- Most reported cases of toxocariasis occur in the US.
  - Highest rates of transmission are in the southern US, particularly in rural areas
  - Infection can be acquired in urban areas.
- Most affected patients are children 1–4 years of age.

Lymphatic filariasis

- Hot, humid climates
- Most cases worldwide
  - Sub-Saharan Africa
  - China
  - India
  - Indonesia
- Most affected patients are 15–44 years of age.

Onchocerciasis

- Tropical Africa
- Central and South America
- Arabian peninsula, mainly Yemen

Schistosomiasis

- Each species of *Schistosoma* has a specific geographic distribution.
  - Sub-Saharan Africa: *Schistosoma haematobium, Schistosoma mansoni,* and *Schistosoma intercalatum*
  - Brazil, Venezuela, the Caribbean, and the Arabian peninsula: *S mansoni*
  - Eastern Mediterranean: *S haematobium*
  - China, Indonesia, the Philippines: *Schistosoma japonicum*
  - Cambodia and Laos: *Schistosoma mekongi*
- Persons most commonly infected
  - School-age children
  - Women
  - Persons involved in water-related occupations, such as irrigation, fishing, and farming
  - Most cases among travelers to Africa
    - Particularly if they swim in Lake Malawi and the Zambezi River

Taeniasis and cystercercosis

- *Taenia* species have worldwide distribution, with higher prevalence in areas with the custom of eating undercooked beef or pork.
  - *Taenia saginata*
    - Some new independent states of the former Soviet Union
    - The Near East
    - Central and Eastern Africa
    - Europe
    - Southeast Asia
    - South America

- *Taenia solium*
  - Mexico
  - Central and South America
  - Africa
  - Southeast Asia
- In US, human infections are usually found in immigrants from areas with high disease prevalence or travelers to endemic areas.
- In US, cysticercosis can be acquired from patients or immigrants from endemic area who have adult-stage *T solium* infection in the intestine.

Hydatid disease

- *Echinococcus granulosus,* seen practically worldwide
  - Predominantly in rural livestock-raising areas
    - South and Central America
    - Middle East
    - Some sub-Saharan countries
    - Central Asia
    - Southern Europe
    - Former Soviet Union
  - In US
    - Most human infections are seen in immigrants from areas with high disease prevalence.
    - Sporadic transmission in some states
      - California
      - Arizona
      - New Mexico
      - Utah
      - Alaska
- *Echinococcus multilocularis*
  - Northern and Central Europe
  - Russia
  - Western China
  - Certain areas of North America
  - Northern Africa
  - Incubation period of cyst is 5–15 years; average age at its manifestation is 55 years.
- *Echinococcus vogeli* and *Echinococcus oligarthrus* are seen in Central and South America and have only rarely been associated with human infection.

Diphyllobothriasis

- Infestation occurs worldwide.
- High prevalence where there is a common culinary habit of eating undercooked or raw fish
  - Scandinavia
  - Newly independent states of the former Soviet Union

P

- North America (in US, mostly in the Southeast)
- Latin America
- Asia

Hymenolepiasis

■ Infections most common in children because they are prone to fecal-oral contamination.
■ Prevalence
  - Highest prevalence is among institutionalized school-age children in developing areas of the world.
  - In US, a 4% infection rate has been reported among schoolchildren in the rural Southeast.

ETIOLOGY

Protozoal infections

■ Leishmaniasis
  - Cutaneous, mucocutaneous, and visceral forms
  - Caused by protozoa of the genus *Leishmania,* and transmitted by the sandfly
  - Dogs and rodents are considered reservoir hosts.
■ Chagas disease (American trypanosomiasis)
  - Caused by the flagellated protozoan parasite *Trypanosoma cruzi*
  - Transmitted to humans by blood-sucking insect vectors of the family Reduviidae (*cone-nose, kissing,* or *assassin bug*)
  - Organisms enter the host at the site of bite wound or through intact mucous membranes of the eye or mouth.
  - Parasite can also be transmitted by:
    - Blood transfusion
    - Organ transplantation
    - Transplacentally
    - Ingestion of the vector
    - Vector's excretion
    - In the laboratory from handling blood from infected people or laboratory animals.
■ African trypanosomiasis
  - Caused by *Trypanosoma brucei*
    - 2 subspecies infect humans.
      - *T brucei gambiense* is the cause of West African sleeping sickness.
      - *T brucei rhodesiense* is the cause of East African sleeping sickness.
  - Transmitted by the tsetse fly
■ Giardiasis
  - *Giardia intestinalis* (syn *Giardia duodenalis* or *Giardia lamblia*) is a flagellated binucleated protozoan, intestinal parasite.

- Humans acquire giardiasis directly by ingestion.
  - Ingesting cysts by hand-to-mouth transfer of fecally contaminated material from an infected person
  - Ingesting contaminated water or food
■ Amebiasis
  - Caused by *Entamoeba histolytica*
  - *E histolytica* cysts can be ingested with contaminated food or drink and survive the gastric barrier.
  - Cysts transform into trophozoites that:
    - Lodge in the submucous layer of the cecum and rectosigmoid
    - Transform into cysts, which are passed in the stool
    - Can invade the bowel wall, producing ulcers and causing destruction and tissue necrosis
    - May disseminate to the liver, lungs, pericardium, or the brain through the bloodstream, causing abscesses
■ Amoebic meningoencephalitis
  - Free-living amoebas that cause 2 distinct clinical manifestations
    - PAM: acute, fulminant disease caused by *N aegleria fowleri*
    - GAE: chronic and slowly progressive disease caused by *Acanthamoeba* and *Balamuthia* species
■ Cryptosporidiosis
  - Caused by *Cryptosporidium,* an intracellular coccidian protozoan parasite
  - Humans acquire infection by ingesting thick-walled oocysts.
  - Infection is generally limited to the superficial parts of the small intestine.
  - In immunocompromised patients infection, may:
    - Spread to involve the biliary tree and the pancreas
    - Disseminate to extraintestinal sites, mainly the respiratory tract
  - Causes diarrhea and inflammatory changes in the gastrointestinal (GI) tract
■ Isosporiasis
  - Humans acquire infection by ingestion of sporulated oocysts in contaminated food or water.
  - Oocysts are released into the intestinal lumen.
■ Cyclosporiasis
  - Caused by the coccidian protozoan parasite *Cyclospora cayetanensis*
■ Toxoplasmosis
  - Caused by *Toxoplasma gondii*
  - Cats are definite hosts; humans and other mammals are intermediate hosts.

- Humans acquire infection by ingesting cysts in raw or undercooked meat or oocysts in material contaminated by cat feces.
- Other causes of infection
  - Contamination of drinking water supplies
  - Blood transfusion
  - Stem cell or solid organ transplantation
- Congenital toxoplasmosis
  - Follows a primary infection in the mother during pregnancy
  - Newborns are most frequently infected when maternal infection is acquired during third trimester.
  - In rare instances, the fetus may be infected after *Toxoplasma* reactivation in immunocompromised mothers, including those with HIV.

- Malaria
  - 4 species of plasmodia infect humans.
    - *P falciparum*
    - *P vivax*
    - *P malariae*
    - *Plasmodium ovale*
  - Transmitted from person to person by the bite of the female *Anopheles* mosquito.
  - Infected cells lyse and release waste products and toxic factors into the bloodstream which act to produce fever and rigor
- Babesiosis
  - Caused by a tick bite
  - Results in ischemic damage in different organs, including liver, spleen, heart, and brain

Nematode infections

- Trichinellosis
  - Caused by the roundworm *Trichinella* in infected meat (mainly pork, but also beef and wild game)
- Trichuriasis
  - Caused by *Trichuris trichiura* (whipworm)
  - Humans acquire infection by ingesting eggs.
  - Larvae are released in the intestine and develop over 2–3 weeks into adult worms.
- Strongyloidiasis
  - Caused by:
    - *Strongyloides stercoralis*
    - Less frequently by *Strongyloides fulleborni,* which causes infantile protein-losing enteropathy with high mortality rates
  - Humans acquire infection by skin contact with infective (filariform) larvae in soil or other material contaminated with human feces.

- Disease may range from asymptomatic eosinophilia in healthy people to life-threatening disseminated infection with septic shock in immunocompromised patients.
- Hookworm infections
  - The 2 most common hookworms are *Ancylostoma duodenale* and *Necator americanus.*
  - Humans acquire infection after percutaneous penetration of larvae.
  - *A duodenale* may also be acquired by the oral route or human milk.
- Cutaneous larva migrans
  - Caused by the infective larvae of the cat and dog hookworms *Ancylostoma braziliense* and *Ancylostoma caninum*
  - Infection occurs among individuals with direct skin contact to infective larvae.
- Pinworm infections
  - Disease is caused by the nematode *Enterobius vermicularis.*
  - Humans acquire infection by ingesting eggs from the same host (autoinfection) or from another person.
    - Direct anus-mouth contact
    - Eating contaminated food
    - Contaminated hands and fomites
    - Contaminated clothing, linen, toilet seats, and baths contribute to spread among families and close contacts.
  - Eggs hatch in the intestine into larvae, and adult worms develop over several weeks.
  - Female adult worms travel at night from the GI tract and migrate through the rectum to lay eggs onto the perianal skin.
- Ascariasis
  - Caused by *Ascaris lumbricoides,* the largest roundworm that infects humans
  - Human infection occurs by ingesting eggs from contaminated soil.
  - Larvae hatch in the intestine, penetrate the intestinal wall, and migrate to the right side of the heart, lungs, and bronchial tree; they ascend to the pharynx and are swallowed to mature into adult worms in the small intestine.
- Toxocariasis (visceral larva migrans)
  - Caused by the dog ascarid, *Toxocara canis,* and less frequently by the cat ascarid, *Toxocara cati.*
  - Humans are unusual hosts for *T canis* and *T cati.*
  - The parasite fails to mature in humans and remains alive in the body for months to years.
  - Humans acquire infection by ingesting soil contaminated with infective eggs of the parasites.

P

- Lymphatic filariasis
  - Caused by 3 species of filarial nematodes
    - *Wuchereria bancrofti* (accounts for 90% of cases)
    - *Brugia malayi*
    - *Brugia timori*
  - Humans acquire infection by bites of mosquitoes that contain larvae; larvae travel to the lymphatic vessels, where they mature into adult worms.
  - Female adult worms release microfilariae in the bloodstream.
- Onchocerciasis (river blindness)
  - Caused by the filarial nematode *Onchocerca volvulus*
  - Disease is transmitted by various species of the blackfly *Simulium,* distributed along turbulent waters.
  - Blackflies suck microfilariae from human skin and subcutaneous tissue.
  - Infective larvae develop inside the blackfly and are released in the skin when a human host is bitten.
  - Adult worms develop from larvae inside the skin, subcutaneous tissue, or fascia over approximately 1 year.
    - Adult worms live curled up in nodules under the skin and subcutaneous tissue.
  - Female worms produce microfilariae in the skin; their migration is responsible for skin lesions.

Trematode infections

- Schistosomiasis
  - Caused by the trematode *Schistosoma*
  - Snails are an intermediate host, infected by schistosome eggs.
  - Cercariae are released from snails and penetrate the skin of humans exposed in fresh water.
  - After skin penetration, cercariae become schistosomulae.
  - Schistosomulae travel via blood vessels and lymphatics to the right side of the heart and pulmonary circulation and then the arterial circulation; they are carried to the mesenteric and splanchnic arteries, and finally the portal circulation, where they mature to adult forms.
  - Mature worms migrate to their final habitat in the mesenteric vein (*S mansoni* and *S japonicum*) or the vesical veins (*S haematobium*).
  - Eggs laid by female worms are transported to other organs or traverse the circulation through adjacent tissue to the lumen of the intestine or the urinary bladder.
  - Skin penetration by cercariae induces a delayed-type hypersensitivity reaction leading to dermatitis.
  - Host response to eggs is formation of granulomas and by infiltration of cells around the eggs.

Cestode infections

- Taeniasis and cystercercosis
  - Taeniasis
    - Caused by the adult worm of *T solium* and *T saginata*
    - People are infected by eating undercooked beef (*T saginata*) or pork (*T solium*) that contains cysticerci in the muscle.
    - Inside the intestine, proctoscopics are released from the cysticerci and attach to the intestinal wall with suckers and hooks.
    - The proctoscopics become the head of the tapeworm, which later develop by forming proglottids and maturing into adult tapeworms over 2 months.
  - Cysticercosis
    - Caused by the larval stage of only *T solium*
    - Infection occurs after embryonated eggs are ingested, which can be either from eating food contaminated with human feces or by autoinfection.
    - Inside the human intestine, the oncospheres hatch, penetrate intestinal wall, and migrate via circulation or lymphatic channels to various tissue sites.
    - Cysticerci may develop in any organ, most commonly the brain, subcutaneous tissue, eye, and liver.
- Hydatid disease (echinococcal disease)
  - Caused by the tapeworm of the genus *Echinococcus*
  - Eggs are ingested by the human/intermediate host, and under appropriate conditions, they hatch and release oncospheres in the small intestine.
  - The oncosphere penetrates intestinal mucosa and migrates through circulatory or lymphatic system into various visceral organs, mainly lungs and liver.
  - In the visceral organ, the oncosphere develops into a fluid-filled cyst, enlarges, and differentiates into the metacestode or hydatid cyst.
  - Infection is usually from contamination of the environment (water, cultivated vegetables) and direct contact with infected pet dogs through the fecal-oral route.
    - Fecal-oral transmission occurs mostly in children.
  - Direct human-to-human transmission does not occur.
- Diphyllobothriasis
  - Caused by *Diphyllobothrium* (fish tapeworm or broad tapeworm)
- Hymenolipiasis
  - Caused by *Hymenolepis nana* (dwarf tapeworm)
  - Infection is usually acquired by ingesting food or water contaminated with human or rodent feces.

P

RISK FACTORS

- Giardiasis

  - Hypochlorhydria
  - Previous gastric surgery
  - Reduced gastric acidity
  - Cystic fibrosis
  - Chronic pancreatitis
  - Risk of infection and transmission are highest among:
    - Children age 12–36 months
    - Children not yet toilet trained
    - Young adults with homosexual activity (because of direct contact with infectious cysts)
    - Travelers in former Soviet Union, South/Southeast Asia, tropical Africa, western South America, and Mexico

- Babesiosis

  - Risk factors for severe infection
    - Age >40 years of age
    - Asplenia
    - HIV infection
    - Immunosuppressive therapy, including corticosteroids
    - Disease is particularly overwhelming in patients without a spleen.

- Cryptosporidiosis

  - Risk factors for prolonged/severe course
    - AIDS
    - Immunoglobulin (Ig)A deficiency
    - Hypogammaglobulinemia
    - Immunosuppressive treatment

- Toxoplasmosis

  - Presence of a domestic cat

SIGNS AND SYMPTOMS

Leishmaniasis

- Cutaneous form

  - Skin lesion on an exposed area of the body, mostly the face and extremities
    - Itchy papule surrounded by erythema and induration; progresses to become a nodule
    - May have accompanying satellite lesions and adjacent adenopathy resembling sporothroid nodules
  - Moist cutaneous form
    - Shallow ulcer with raised borders may develop.
    - May progress slowly, leading to an open sore as large as 5 cm in diameter with a granular center
    - Takes 3–12 months to heal and leaves a depressed scar

  - Dry cutaneous form
    - No ulcers form.
    - The papule heals to a scar over a longer period, which may extend to 1 year or more.
  - Diffuse cutaneous leishmaniasis
    - Seen in patients with underlying immune disorders, particularly cellular immunodeficiency
    - The primary lesion is a localized papule with surrounding satellite lesions.
    - Dissemination to multiple nodules on the face and extremities
    - Lesions slowly progress and may last for years.

- Mucosal form

  - Lesions occur months to years after the primary cutaneous lesion heals.
  - Lesions commonly involve nose, mouth, soft palate, and larynx.
    - Usually begins with nasal congestion and ulceration
    - The cartilage of the nose is commonly involved, leading to nasal septal perforation.
    - Formation of granulomas and secondary bacterial infections are common.

- Visceral form (kala-azar, which means *black fever*)

  - Amastigotes spread from macrophages at the site of inoculation to the liver, spleen, bone marrow, and sometimes lymph nodes.
  - Typical manifestations
    - Fever
    - Anorexia
    - Malaise
    - Weight loss
    - Hepatomegaly
    - Splenomegaly (spleen is massively enlarged)
    - Skin hyperpigmentation occurs commonly in Indian patients.
    - Jaundice (less common)
    - Guillain-Barré syndrome (less common)

Chagas disease

- Bite wounds are frequently found at the lateral canthus of the eye, mucocutaneous border of the lips, and exposed areas of face and upper extremities.

- Acute phase

  - Local inflammatory reaction commonly occurs at site of parasite inoculation.
  - Chagoma (erythematous, firm, nodular swelling at the bite site) or Romaña sign (unilateral periorbital edema with conjunctivitis and ipsilateral preauricular lymphadenopathy) may be present when the portal of entry is lateral canthus of the eye.

P

- Generalized infection with fever
- Malaise
- Headache
- Generalized lymphadenopathy
- Hepatosplenomegaly
- Edema
- Some degree of acute myocarditis, generally present in all symptomatic cases; can be fatal
- Meningoencephalitis may follow and is usually associated with high mortality rate.
- In congenital infection, may see:
  - Hepatosplenomegaly
  - Jaundice
  - Skin hemorrhage
  - Neurologic signs, especially in premature infants
- Latent or indeterminate phase
  - 1–3 months after acute disease
  - Asymptomatic
- Chronic phase
  - Chronic heart failure
  - Severe cardiomegaly
  - Ventricular conduction defects
  - Various types of arrhythmia
  - Palpitations
  - Dizziness
  - Syncope
  - Dyspnea
  - Chest pain
  - 8–10% of all patients have a variable degree of changes in motility or severe dilatation of the digestive tract.
    - Extreme enlargement of the colon is slightly more common than the esophagus.
    - Difficulty swallowing
    - Regurgitation
    - Severe constipation
    - Abdominal pain
  - Neurologic symptoms in a minority of patients
    - Paresthesia or anesthesia
    - Convulsions
    - Alteration of homeostatic equilibrium

African trypanosomiasis
- Course differs by form.
  - East African
    - Characterized by acute, severe, rapidly fatal disease with minimal central nervous system (CNS) symptoms

- West African
  - Milder, chronic course associated with lymph node and CNS invasion
- Trypanosomal chancre usually develops a few days after inoculation.
  - Indurated, erythematous, painful lesion that develops at the bite site
  - Usually resolves within 3 weeks
- During dissemination of parasite
  - Fever
  - Headache
  - Generalized malaise
  - Papular skin lesion
  - Generalized lymphadenopathy, especially in the posterior cervical triangle (Winterbottom sign)
  - Mild hepatosplenomegaly
  - Generalized weakness
  - Dyspnea
  - Chest pain
  - Anemia
  - Arthralgia
  - Cachexia
  - Local swelling of the joints, hands, or feet
- As parasite invades CNS (sleeping sickness stage)
  - Severe headache
  - Irritability
  - Personality and behavioral change
  - Gradual loss of cognitive function
  - Alteration in motor function
  - Psychiatric manifestations
  - Sleep disorders
    - Somnolence
    - Inappropriate episodes of sleeping
    - Nocturnal insomnia
  - Signs and symptoms of congestive heart failure

Giardiasis
- Most infections are asymptomatic.
- Symptomatic children may have acute self-limited infection or chronic infection associated with malabsorption.
- Acute symptoms
  - Last 2–4 weeks; may be intermittent
  - Acute watery diarrhea
  - Malaise
  - Abdominal pain, cramps
  - Bloating

P

- Flatulence
- Foul-smelling and fatty stools
- Nausea
- Fatigue
- Chronic symptoms
  - Chronic diarrhea with steatorrhea
  - Marked weight loss
  - Failure to thrive/growth retardation
  - Rash
  - Urticaria
  - Aphthous ulcers
  - Reactive arthritis
  - Iridocyclitis
  - Retinal arteritis

Amebiasis

- Usually asymptomatic
- Symptoms, when present, range from mild to severe.
  - Abdominal pain
  - Diarrhea
  - Bloody stools
  - Weight loss in 50% of patients
  - Fever
- Amoebic liver abscess
  - Most common extraintestinal manifestation of amebiasis
    - Less common in children than in adults
  - Symptoms usually appear within 8–20 weeks (5 months after return from endemic area in 95% of patients)
    - Longer lags have been reported.
  - In the US, most diagnosed patients are from a country where amebiasis is endemic or have traveled to such an area.
    - Pain in the right upper quadrant
    - Fever
    - Anorexia
    - Fatigue
    - Diarrhea (in fewer than one-third of patients)
    - Jaundice is uncommon.

Amoebic meningoencephalitis

- PAM
  - Bifrontal headaches that do not respond to analgesia
  - Fever (temperature 38°C–41°C)
  - Alteration in sense of taste or smell, with or without rhinitis, may be noted early.
  - Emesis
  - Seizures
  - Lethargy

- Nuchal rigidity
- Cerebellar ataxia
- Dysfunction of the third, fourth, and sixth cranial nerves
- GAE
  - Disease of immunocompromised and debilitated individuals; chronic and insidious
  - Hemiparesis
  - Personality changes
  - Seizures
  - Neck stiffness
  - Headaches
  - Fever
  - Sinusitis
  - Otitis media
  - Cutaneous lesions
  - Corneal ulcers

Cryptosporidiosis

- Varies from asymptomatic infection to severe enteritis and fatal dehydration
- Acute diarrhea (frequent, watery, foul-smelling, nonbloody stools)
  - Resolves spontaneously in 1–20 days
  - Occasionally, healthy infants may develop chronic and persistent diarrhea, leading to malnutrition and growth retardation.
- Malaise
- Nausea
- Anorexia
- Fatigue
- Abdominal cramps
- Weight loss
- Fever
- Vomiting
- Clinical manifestations of cryptosporidiosis in patients with AIDS include:
  - Cholecystitis
  - Cholangitis
  - Hepatitis
  - Pancreatitis
  - Respiratory cryptosporidiosis is seen mainly in patients with AIDS; symptoms include:
    - Cough
    - Dyspnea
    - Fever
    - Expectoration
    - Chest pain

- Biliary cryptosporidiosis is exclusively seen in patients with AIDS; symptoms include:
  - Right upper quadrant pain
  - Fever
  - Nausea and vomiting with or without diarrhea

Isosporiasis

- Diarrhea
  - Self-limited and resolves spontaneously in days to weeks
  - Typically watery
- Fever
- Malaise
- Vomiting
- Headache
- Abdominal pain
- Weight loss

Cyclosporiasis

- Profuse, watery diarrhea
  - Intermittent and prolonged
- Fatigue
- Anorexia
- Abdominal cramps and bloating
- Nausea
- Vomiting
- Fever
- Myalgia
- Weight loss

Toxoplasmosis

- Congenital disease
  - Most (70–90%) congenitally infected infants are asymptomatic.
  - Clinical manifestations at birth include:
    - Hepatosplenomegaly
    - Lymphadenopathy
    - Hydrocephalus or microcephaly
    - Seizures and neurologic deficits
    - Chorioretinitis
    - Rash
    - Jaundice
- Acquired disease
  - Usually asymptomatic
  - Cervical lymphadenopathy
  - Fever
  - Myalgia
  - Fatigue

- In some, infectious mononucleosis–like manifestations
  - Sore throat
  - Fever
  - Malaise
  - Adenopathy
  - Splenomegaly
  - Rash
- Disease in immunodeficient patients
  - Localized infections
    - Encephalitis
    - Meningoencephalitis
      - Fever
      - Headache
      - Deterioration in mental status
      - Seizures
      - Hemiparesis
      - Abnormal speech
    - Pneumonitis
    - Myocarditis
    - Pericarditis
    - Hepatitis
- Ocular disease/chorioretinitis
  - Bilateral in congenital form and unilateral in acquired form
  - Nystagmus
  - Blurred vision
  - Photophobia
  - Central vision loss

Malaria

- Attacks occur:
  - Every second day with *P falciparum*, *P vivax*, and *P ovale*
  - Every third day with *P malariae*
  - These classic patterns are rarely observed.
- Combination of influenza-like symptoms
  - Fever
  - Chills
  - Sweats
  - Headaches
  - Nausea and vomiting
  - Body aches
  - General malaise
  - Anemia
  - Enlarged spleen

- Severe malaria
  - Cerebral malaria
    - Abnormal behavior
    - Impairment of consciousness
    - Seizures
    - Coma
    - Other neurologic abnormalities
  - Severe anemia
  - Pulmonary edema
  - Acute respiratory distress syndrome
- Congenital malaria
  - Fever
  - Severe anemia
  - Hepatosplenomegaly

Babesiosis

- Gradual onset of malaise, fatigue, and anorexia
- Followed by fever with:
  - Chills
  - Sweats
  - Myalgia
  - Headache
  - Vomiting
- Less commonly
  - Conjunctival injection
  - Meningismus
  - Altered sensorium
  - Nonproductive cough
- Symptoms may last for several weeks or sometimes months.
- In immunodeficient patients
  - Hemolytic anemia
  - Jaundice
  - Dark urine

Trichinellosis

- 1–7 days after infection
  - Asymptomatic or GI symptoms
    - Nausea
    - Vomiting
    - Diarrhea
    - Constipation
    - Abdominal pain
- Muscle stage (lasts 1–5 weeks or longer)
  - Myalgia; may mimic rheumatic pain
  - Eyelid edema
  - Eosinophilia
  - High and prolonged fever

- Weakness
- Malaise
- Headache
- Subconjunctival hemorrhages, retinal hemorrhages
- Splinter hemorrhages under fingernails
- Facial flushing
- Urticarial or macular rashes
- Hoarseness
- Dyspnea
- Dysphagia

Trichuriasis

- Often present with other helminthic/protozoal infections
- Diarrhea
- Heavy infection symptoms
  - Mucoid bloody stools with abdominal pain and tenesmus (trichuris dysentery syndrome)
  - Rectal prolapse
  - Colonic obstruction and perforation
  - Finger clubbing

Strongyloidiasis

- Usually asymptomatic
- Peripheral eosinophilia may be the only symptom.
- Cutaneous reactions when larvae penetrate skin, especially on feet
  - Edema
  - Rash
  - Severe pruritus
- Pulmonary migration of larvae
  - Dry cough
  - Wheezing
  - Tachypnea
  - Hemoptysis
  - Pneumonitis or Loeffler-like syndrome (acute transient pneumonitis)
- If adult worms are in the GI tract:
  - Abdominal pain
  - Vomiting
  - Diarrhea
  - Malabsorption/failure to thrive
- Larvae in perianal skin
  - Pruritic lesions in the perianal area, buttocks, and upper thighs
- Infants with *S fulleborni* infection may develop swollen belly syndrome.
  - Marked abdominal distention
  - Ascites, pleural effusions

P

■ Hyperinfection in immunocompromised patients

• Gram-negative bacteremia and sepsis

Hookworm infections

■ Symptoms and signs correlate with the stage of infection.

■ Early findings

• Itching

• Focal eruptions with or without edema

• Enlargement of adjacent lymph nodes (ground itch)

• Mild respiratory symptoms, cough

• If severe, Loeffler syndrome may develop.

■ Intestinal phase

• Abdominal pain

• Nausea

• Vomiting

• Increased flatulence

• Diarrhea

• Constipation

• Symptoms of anemia

Cutaneous larva migrans

■ Erythematous pruritic papule at site of skin entry, usually lower extremities

■ Days or weeks later, dermal skin rash (creeping eruption)

• Pruritic, elevated serpiginous tract that elongates several mm/day

• May become vesiculated and secondarily infected by bacteria

■ Rarely, dry cough and Loeffler-like syndrome

Pinworm infections

■ Most infections are asymptomatic.

• However, the most common symptom is perianal itching (pruritus ani), mainly at night.

– Less frequently, pruritus vulvae as a result of aberrant migration to genital tract

■ Other rare manifestations

• Salpingitis

• Urethritis

• Vaginitis

• Pelvic peritonitis

■ Patients with a heavy worm burden

• Abdominal pain

• Nausea

• Vomiting

Ascariasis

■ Usually asymptomatic

■ Loeffler syndrome occurs 1–2 weeks after ingestion of the eggs.

• Fever

• Eosinophilia

• Urticaria

■ Patients with ascariasis

• Abdominal discomfort

• Nausea

• Vomiting

• Diarrhea

• Malnutrition

• Intestinal obstruction

■ Worm migration into the biliary tree

• Biliary colic

• Cholecystitis

• Ascending cholangitis

• Biliary strictures and hepatic abscesses

• Pancreatitis

• Appendicitis

■ Migration may occur through body orifices, such as the mouth, nose, anus, and lacrimal duct.

Toxocariasis

■ Most patients who are lightly infected are asymptomatic.

■ Symptomatic children with toxocariasis usually experience:

• Fever

• Leukocytosis with eosinophilia

• Hypergammaglobulinemia

• Hepatomegaly

• Splenomegaly and lymphadenopathy

■ Allergic manifestations are possible.

• Urticaria

• Rhinorrhea

• Asthma

■ Constitutional symptoms may be present.

• Anorexia

• Weakness

• Failure to gain weight

• Myalgia

• Arthralgia

• Nighttime sweats

■ Neurologic symptoms are less frequent.

• Irritability

• Seizures

- Myocarditis
- Congestive heart failure
- Pleural effusion
- Eosinophilic ascites
- Meningoencephalitis
- Ocular involvement, usually without other systemic involvement
  - Unilateral solitary posterior retinal lesion
  - Granulomatous mass or multiple lesions may be seen
  - Lesions are painless; some are asymptomatic and are found incidentally during routine retinal examination.
  - Strabismus
  - Visual impairment
  - Unilateral loss of vision
  - Leukocoria

Lymphatic filariasis

- Usually asymptomatic
- Most common acute symptoms in the early stages are:
  - Lymphangitis and lymphadenitis
  - Fever
  - Headache
  - Myalgia
  - Pain in the affected extremities
  - Male genital area effects
    - Acute epididymitis
    - Orchitis
    - Funiculitis
- During chronic stage
  - Elephantiasis (lymphedema)
    - Recurrent superimposed bacterial infections
    - The skin over affected extremity becomes thick and warty.
  - Tropical pulmonary eosinophilia in a small proportion of patients
    - Nocturnal paroxysmal respiratory symptoms, such as cough and wheezing

Onchocerciasis

- Dermatitis
  - Intensely pruritic and may develop into an erythematous papular rash
- Subcutaneous nodules
  - Vary from a few millimeters to several centimeters
  - Can be discrete or clustered
  - Tend to occur over bony prominences
  - Secondary bacterial infection may cause acute inflammation or abscess formation.

- Lymphadenitis
- Ocular lesions
- Skin papules and depigmentation in chronic infections
- Hydroceles
- Elephantiasis
- Hanging groins
- Ocular involvement
  - Punctuate keratitis
  - Sclerosing keratitis
  - Iridocyclitis
  - Chorioretinitis
  - Optic neuritis

Schistosomiasis

- Maculopapular eruption may develop at the site of cercarial skin penetration.
  - Few hours or up to 1 week after infection
- Eosinophilia 4–8 weeks after exposure
  - Fever
  - Headache
  - Generalized myalgia
  - Hepatomegaly
  - Bloody diarrhea
  - Splenomegaly (30% of patients)
  - Cough
  - Aseptic meningitis
- If GI tract involvement
  - Colicky pain
  - Diarrhea
  - Occasionally, constipation
  - Blood, either gross or occult, may appear in stools.
  - Colonic or rectal stenosis
- If liver involvement
  - Hepatomegaly
  - Late stages: esophageal varices, bleeding, and splenomegaly
- If genitourinary involvement
  - Microscopic hematuria, early stages
  - Moderate to severe lesions in the urinary tract

Taeniasis

- Often asymptomatic
- Main symptom is intermittent passage of the proglottids.
  - Either with the stool or spontaneously
- Nausea, diarrhea, and abdominal pain or discomfort

Cysticercosis

- In infants, the initial manifestation of neurocysticercosis is generalized seizures.

P

- Cysticercal encephalitis
  - Fever
  - Headache
  - Vomiting
  - Impaired consciousness
  - Reduced visual acuity
  - Seizures
- Extraneural cysticercosis
  - Some patients may notice small palpable nodules that may become inflamed, or patients may experience muscle pain.

Hydatid disease

- Although most infections are acquired during childhood, clinical manifestations do not develop until adulthood because of the slow-growing nature of the cyst.
- Symptoms seen in adults include:
  - Hepatic enlargement/right upper quadrant pain
  - Nausea
  - Vomiting
  - Pulmonary hydatidosis
    - Chronic cough
    - Chest pain
    - Pleuritis
    - Dyspnea

Diphyllobothriasis

- Usually asymptomatic, especially in younger children
- Abdominal pain
- Nausea
- Vomiting
- Diarrhea
- Weight loss
- Fatigue
- Numbness
- Dizziness
- Allergic symptoms
- Intestinal obstruction if worm burden is massive

Hymenolipiasis

- Usually asymptomatic
- Symptoms of heavy infection are:
  - Abdominal pain
  - Nausea
  - Vomiting
  - Diarrhea
  - Anorexia
  - Weakness
  - Irritability
  - Headache

DIAGNOSTIC APPROACH

Leishmaniasis

- Diagnosis is made by identification of parasites in tissue biopsy samples or in aspirate.
- Serologic tests may be helpful in diagnosing visceral and mucosal leishmaniasis but not cutaneous disease.
  - False-positive results may occur with other diseases, such as trypanosomiasis, tuberculosis, leprosy, and malaria.

Chagas disease

- Acute phase
  - Diagnostic test of choice is detection of parasites in a blood specimen.
- Chronic phase
  - Diagnosis is usually made by immunodiagnostic tests or isolation of parasite.

African trypanosomiasis

- Diagnosis is made by microscopic detection of trypomastigotes in specimens from various sites.
  - Chancre fluid
  - Blood
  - Bone marrow
  - Lymph node aspirates
  - Cerebrospinal fluid (CSF)

Giardiasis

- Routine blood tests are not helpful in diagnosing giardiasis.
- The mainstay of diagnosis is demonstrating cysts or trophozoites by direct stool examination for ova and parasites.
  - Cysts are more likely to be seen in formed stools.
  - Frequent loose stools increase yield of identifying trophozoites.
  - 3 stool samples should be collected and examined every other day.
- Duodenal fluid sampling may be warranted.
  - If clinical suspicion is high and stools are negative

Amebiasis

- Stool examination from 3 fresh stool samples from separate days
- Liver amoebic abscesses are usually diagnosed on the basis of:
  - Clinical presentation
  - Recognition of epidemiologic risk factors
  - Serologic testing
  - Noninvasive imaging studies

P

Amoebic meningoencephalitits

■ PAM

- Neuroimaging studies may be normal early in disease but may show signs of increased intracranial pressure later.
- Laboratory studies (including CSF examination and wet mount)

■ GAE

- Neuroimaging
- CSF examination
- Corneal scrapings to look for cysts, and culture

Cryptosporidiosis

■ Diagnosis depends on microscopic identification of oocysts in:

- Stools
  - The laboratory should be alerted to potential diagnosis of cryptosporidiosis to perform specific staining of samples.
- Aspirated fluid
- Tissue samples

Cyclosporiasis

■ Diagnosis is made by microscopic examination of stool specimens.

Toxoplasmosis

■ If suspected, the patient should undergo complete clinical evaluation, including ophthalmologic, neurologic, and auditory examination (see Laboratory Findings and Imaging).

■ After delivery, infants should be evaluated for congenital toxoplasmosis if:

- The mother had a primary infection, *or*
- The mother is HIV infected and has serologic findings suggestive of past infection

■ In patients with ocular involvement, the diagnosis is based on classic eye findings and serologic testing.

■ Clinical and laboratory data should be carefully correlated during patient evaluation and management.

Malaria

■ Most commonly used diagnostic tools

- Microscopic diagnosis
  - Thick smears are more sensitive, but cannot be used to differentiate among species
- Rapid diagnostic tests are based on immunochromatographic techniques.

■ Diagnosis can be difficult in nonendemic areas.

- Health care providers are not familiar with the disease.
- Laboratory workers may fail to detect parasites in blood smears.

Trichinellosis

■ The diagnosis should be suspected in patients with:

- Suggestive clinical history (consumption of inadequately cooked meat, particularly pork)
- Eosinophilia

■ The presence of symptoms in other patients who ate the same food makes the diagnosis stronger.

Strongyloidiasis

■ Diagnosis is made by detecting rhabditiform larvae in stool specimens.

■ When stool samples are not diagnostic, examination of duodenal fluid for larvae should be considered.

Hookworm infections

■ Diagnosed by identifying eggs in stools

- Stool smears are often negative in early stages of infection.

Cutaneous larva migrans

■ Most cases are diagnosed clinically, with no further diagnostic evaluation needed.

Pinworm infections

■ Stool examination for ova and parasites is not helpful in establishing the diagnosis.

■ The test of choice is the use of the cellophane tape swab.

- Alternatively, sterile pinworm collector kits are commercially available.

Ascariasis

■ Diagnosis is made by demonstrating characteristic eggs in stools by direct microscopy.

- Eggs may not appear in the stools until after ≥40 days of infection.

■ Imaging studies may demonstrate worms if there is:

- Intestinal obstruction
- Hepatobiliary or pancreatic ascariasis

Toxocariasis

■ Definitive diagnosis requires demonstration of larvae in tissue sections but is rarely needed.

■ Diagnosis is usually based on clinical findings and serologic testing.

Lymphatic filariasis

■ Diagnosis is made by demonstrating microfilariae on peripheral blood smears obtained between 10PM and 2AM.

- If blood cannot be obtained at night, a dose of diethylcarbamazine (DEC) can be provided to stimulate filaria release, followed by blood draw 1 hour later.

■ If microfilariae cannot be demonstrated on blood smears:

- Fine-needle aspirate or biopsy of the involved lymph node or epididymis may demonstrate worms or microfilariae.

P

- Serologic tests are helpful once microfilariae are no longer detectable.
- Chronic filariasis (lymphedema) is usually diagnosed on clinical grounds.

Onchocerciasis

- Diagnose by identifying microfilariae in direct histologic examination.
- Surgical excision of a skin nodule can be diagnostic and therapeutic.
  - Adult worms are found in these nodules.
- Ocular lesions
  - Diagnosed by slit-lamp examination, which may reveal microfilariae in the cornea or anterior chamber of the eye

Taeniasis

- Diagnosis is made by microscopic identification of eggs or proglottids in stool.
  - May not be possible during the first 3 months of infection

Cysticercosis

- Definitive diagnosis is made by demonstrating the cysticercus in the involved tissue.
- Demonstration of eggs or proglottids in stool specimen may support the diagnosis, but does not prove it.
- For neurocysticercosis, magnetic resonance imaging (MRI) and computed tomography (CT) are the most reliable imaging techniques.

Hydatid disease

- Diagnosis is usually made by a combination of imaging studies and serologic testing.
- History of exposure to possible animal hosts in an endemic area in a patient with a cystic, masslike lesion may help support diagnosis.

Diphyllobothriasis

- Diagnosis is made by microscopic identification of eggs or proglottids in stool.
- Pernicious anemia and vitamin B_{12} deficiency provide clues to diagnosis.

Hymenolipiasis

- Diagnosis is made by demonstrating eggs in stool specimens.

LABORATORY FINDINGS

Leishmaniasis

- Staining for *Leishmania* parasites (intracellular amastigotes, Leishman-Donovan bodies)
  - Wright
  - Giemsa
  - Hematoxylin and eosin

- Culture of tissue or peripheral blood on special media (Novy-MacNeal-Nicolle medium) if available
  - Days to several weeks may be needed.
- Leishmanin skin test (Montenegro test) for diagnosis of cutaneous leishmaniasis
  - Usually positive in the ulcerative phase, which occurs 1–3 months after infection
  - Not helpful for diagnosing visceral disease
  - A positive skin test may indicate an old rather than acute infection.
  - Not approved for use in the US.
- Serologic tests
  - May be helpful for visceral and mucosal leishmaniasis but not cutaneous disease
  - False-positive results may occur with trypanosomiasis, tuberculosis, leprosy, and malaria.
- Laboratory findings
  - Leukopenia
  - Anemia
  - Thrombocytopenia
  - Hypoalbuminemia
  - Hypergammaglobulinemia
  - Reversal of the albumin-globulin ratio may be seen.
- Nucleic acid–based techniques (DNA hybridization and polymerase chain reaction [PCR])
  - To identify parasite sequence in tissue samples and peripheral blood
  - Especially useful in diagnosis of visceral leishmaniasis and in aspirates that are negative for parasites by microscopy
  - PCR is highly sensitive but not routinely available.

Chagas disease

- Acute phase: detection of parasites in blood specimen
  - Thin and thick blood smears stained with Giemsa for parasites
  - Direct wet mount of fresh blood sample or buffy coat for parasites
- Chronic phase: Diagnosis is usually made by immunodiagnostic tests or isolation of the parasite.
  - Available tests
    - Indirect fluorescent antibody (IFA) test
    - Complement fixation
    - Enzyme immunoassay (EIA)
    - In US, IFA and complement fixation tests are available at the Centers for Disease Control and Prevention (CDC).
  - Sensitivity and specificity of these serologic tests are highly variable.
    - 2 different, independently performed methods should be used to confirm the diagnosis of Chagas disease.

- Serologic tests may cross-react with other conditions, such as:
  - Leishmaniasis
  - Malaria
  - Syphilis
  - Infectious mononucleosis
  - Tuberculosis
  - Leprosy
  - Collagen vascular diseases
- Isolation of parasite can be accomplished by:
  - Culture in special media *or*
  - Mouse inoculation *or*
  - Xenodiagnosis
    - Reduviid insects are fed the infected patient's blood, and their gut contents are examined 4 weeks later for the parasites.
  - The animal inoculation method is unreliable and should be performed only after repeated culture attempts have failed to isolate the organism.
- Molecular methods, such as PCR, are available as an investigational diagnostic tool.

African trypanosomiasis

- Giemsa stain and wet preparation to look for trypanosomes
- Concentration technique may be used with body fluid specimen examination to increase sensitivity.
- Isolation of parasite by rat or mice inoculation is a sensitive test.
  - Use is limited to *T brucei rhodesiense*.

Giardiasis

- Staining of fresh stool sample (or sample preserved in polyvinyl alcohol or merthiolate-formalin) with:
  - Iodine *or*
  - Trichrome *or*
  - Giemsa *or*
  - Iron hematoxylin
- Cysts and trophozoites may be identified in saline wet mount.
- If organisms are not found on direct examination of 3 stool specimens, feces should be checked for *Giardia* antigens.
  - Several commercial kits are available that use enzyme-linked immunosorbent assay (ELISA) or IFA.
  - Sensitivity is 95–99% and specificity 95–100% compared with stool microscopy.

Amebiasis

- Serologic testing
  - Infection with *E histolytica* results in development of antibodies; *Entamoeba dispar* infection does not.

- 10–35% of uninfected individuals in endemic areas have antiamoebic antibodies as a result of previous, often undiagnosed, infection with *E histolytica*.
  - Negative serologic result in these populations helps exclude disease.
  - Positive serologic result is not particularly helpful because it does not distinguish between acute infection and past exposure to parasite.
- Fecal and serum antigen detection assays
  - Quick and easy tests
  - Ability to differentiate between strains
  - Greater sensitivity than microscopy
  - Potential for diagnosis in early infection and in endemic areas where serologic testing is less useful
- PCR techniques can detect *E histolytica* in stool specimens.
  - PCR-based techniques are the most sensitive and specific methods.
    - Not widely available

Amoebic meningoencephalitis

- PAM
  - Increased leukocyte count
  - Hyperglycemia
  - Glycosuria
  - CSF examination
    - Pleocytosis with polymorphonuclear neutrophil predominance
    - Increased CSF protein
    - Normal or decreased glucose
    - Motile amoebas may be seen on wet mount; preferably, use unrefrigerated CSF collected within 30 minutes of the evaluation.
  - Culturing amoebas on nonnutrient agar plated with *Escherichia coli* is the definitive way to diagnose.
- GAE
  - Diagnosis is made by finding amoebas in tissue sections, either:
    - Stained with hematoxylin and eosin *or*
    - IFA staining with rabbit antiamoeba sera
  - Cysts of infecting amoebas can be recognized in corneal scrapings that have been stained with calcofluor white.
  - *Acanthamoeba* can also be cultured onto nonnutrient agar with bacteria for identification.

Cryptosporidiosis

- Modified Kinyoun acid-fast stain of ≥3 stool samples
  - Stool samples are usually concentrated by either the sucrose flotation or the formalin acetate method.
- Immunofluorescent staining that uses monoclonal antibodies and ELISA kits can be used to detect oocysts in stool and tissue specimens.

P

Isosporiasis

- Diagnosis is made by finding oocysts in stool using special stains.
  - Kinyoun acid-fast or modified acid-fast stain
  - Alternatively, specific fluorescent techniques may be used.
- Oocysts may also be detected in duodenal fluid aspirates.

Cyclosporiasis

- Staining of samples for oocysts
  - Modified Ziehl-Nelson or Kinyoun acid-fast staining
- Fluorescent microscopy reveals autofluorescence of the cell wall of *Cyclospora* oocysts.

Toxoplasmosis

- The most definite test for diagnosis of toxoplasmosis is isolation of the organism from infected tissue or body fluids by either inoculation into laboratory animals or by tissue culture.
  - However, these techniques are not routinely available.
- The primary method currently used for diagnosis is based on detecting specific antibodies and monitoring immune response.
- Molecular methods involving PCR for detecting *Toxoplasma* DNA in tissue and fluid samples have been used.
- ELISA tests
  - Serum IgG usually becomes positive 4–8 weeks after infection.
    - Remains positive indefinitely
  - Paired sera should be tested simultaneously 3 weeks apart to document an increase in titers of ≥4-fold.
  - Serum IgM levels should also be tested simultaneously with IgG.
  - ELISA IgM tests are more sensitive than the IFA test.
    - IgM test may remain positive for 6 months, and false-positive results can occur.
  - In newborns, serum levels of IgA and IgE for *Toxoplasma* can also be tested.
    - These become negative sooner than IgM test, giving more precise information about the timing of infection.
    - However, anti-*Toxoplasma* IgA and IgE tests are available only at *Toxoplasma* referral laboratories.
- Definitive diagnosis of congenital toxoplasmosis during pregnancy can be made by testing amniotic fluid.
  - Detecting *Toxoplasma* in amniotic fluid by either DNA PCR or tissue culture or mouse inoculation is considered diagnostic.
  - Similarly, fetal blood sampling to isolate *Toxoplasma* from fetal leukocytes and to test for IgM antibody may also be used.

- In infant with suspected toxoplasmosis:
  - Diagnosis is confirmed serologically by demonstrating:
    - Positive IgM or IgA
    - Higher infant IgG titer than the mother, *or*
    - Persistently positive IgG beyond 1 year of age
  - CSF should be analyzed for cells, protein, glucose, *Toxoplasma* antibodies, and PCR.
  - Serum samples should be evaluated for IgG, IgM, IgA, and IgE antibodies for *Toxoplasma*.
- Diagnosis of toxoplasmosis in older children and adults who are immunocompetent relies on identification of a positive IgM titer or a 4-fold increase in IgG titers after 3 weeks.
- Classic histopathologic findings in tissue samples, such as lymph nodes, strongly supports the diagnosis.
  - Identification of proliferating organisms on histology provides a definite diagnosis.
- Isolation of *Toxoplasma* from tissue or body fluid by culture or identification of nucleic acid material by DNA PCR is definitive.
- In immunocompromised patients, including those with HIV infection, serologic testing may not be reliable.

Malaria

- Examine peripheral blood smears.
- Serologic testing (IFA test or ELISA) does not detect current infection.

Pinworm infections

- Cellophane tape swab
  - Adhesive part of tape is applied to skin and then onto a glass slide and examined by light microscopy.
  - Higher diagnostic yield if specimen is obtained at night or early morning
- Commercially available test kits work on the same principle.
- Examination of multiple samples may be needed.

Ascariasis

- Usually a single stool sample is sufficient to confirm the diagnosis.
- Adult worms are sometimes passed in stool and provide a clue to diagnosis.
- Eosinophils and occasionally *Ascaris* larvae may be demonstrated in sputum samples.

Lymphatic filariasis

- Diagnosis is made by demonstrating microfilaria on peripheral blood smears obtained between 10 PM and 2 AM.
  - If blood cannot be obtained at night, a dose of DEC can be provided to stimulate filaria release, followed by blood draw 1 hour later.

- Serologic tests
  - Helpful once microfiliariae are no longer detectable
  - Enzyme immunoassays may cross-react with other helminthic infections.
  - Antifilarial IgG4 antibody detection: good index of the intensity and duration of filarial exposure in endemic areas.
  - Filarial antigen can be detected by monoclonal antibodies.
    - Filaremic patients are more likely to have positive results than those who are not.
- DNA probes/PCR assays have been developed but not routinely available.

Babesiosis

- Diagnosis is made by demonstrating the organism in thick and thin smears prepared for Wright and Giemsa staining.
  - Presence of a cluster of 4 small merozoites ("tetrads") in erythrocytes
  - Multiple parasites may be present in a single cell.
  - Occasional presence of 3 chromatin dots in a single parasite
- Serologic testing if blood smears are nondiagnostic
  - IFA test (available in reference laboratories)
- PCR is more sensitive than blood smear.

Trichinellosis

- Serologic tests are usually used to make the diagnosis.
  - ELISA (most sensitive)
  - IFA test
  - Latex agglutination
    - Only helpful after the second week of infection
  - Testing of paired acute and convalescent serum is diagnostic.
  - Eosinophilia usually appears during second week of the muscle phase and can be as high as 70%.
  - Creatine kinase and lactate dehydrogenase concentrations may be high.
  - Ig levels may be high.
- The definitive diagnostic test is finding larvae in muscle biopsy samples.
  - Only occurs after first week after ingestion

Trichuriasis

- Diagnosed by detecting typical ova on direct stool examination
  - Eggs have a typical barrel shape, 3-layer shell, and transparent bipolar plugs.
  - Eggs can be quantified by Kato-Katz smear.
    - Number of eggs per gram of stool can be used to assess worm burden.

Strongyloidiasis

- Examining multiple specimens and using stool concentration procedures may increase yield.
- In disseminated infection, rhabditiform larvae may be recovered from:
  - Stools
  - Sputum
  - Bronchoalveolar lavage
  - Pleural fluid
  - Peritoneal fluid
  - Spinal fluid
- Serologic testing (available at reference laboratories)
  - Highly sensitive and specific, but false-negative results in immunocompromised patients

Hookworm infections

- Stool concentration techniques may be needed if infection is light.
  - Repeat stool examinations may also be needed.
- Species identification can be accomplished by PCR.

Toxocariasis

- Serologic testing used to confirm diagnosis
  - ELISA is the most frequently used test, with high sensitivity and specificity.
  - Western blot and immunofluorescence tests are also used.
- Total leukocyte count may be as high as 30,000 cells/mm^3, with up to 80% eosinophils.
- Hypergammaglobulinemia with high IgE levels
  - Sometimes 10–15 times normal levels
- Increased isohemagglutinins to A and B blood groups
- During the pulmonary phase, eosinophils may be detected in respiratory secretions.
- With CNS involvement, the CSF may show eosinophils.

Onchocerciasis

- Peripheral eosinophilia is common.

Schistosomiasis

- Nonspecific laboratory tests
  - Peripheral eosinophilia
  - Anemia
  - Hypoalbuminemia
  - Hypergammaglobulinemia
- Diagnosis may be made by demonstrating eggs in stool or urine samples.
  - 3 specimens may be needed.
  - Egg excretion peaks at noon to 3PM.
- Serologic tests (available at reference laboratories)
  - Not useful in differentiating old infection from reinfection

P

Taeniasis

- The egg is indistinguishable microscopically from egg of other tapeworm species, especially *Echinococcus.*
- Species determination is made by microscopic examination of the gravid proglottids and rarely the scolex, if available.

Cysticercosis

- Serologic test of choice for confirming diagnosis is the CDC immunoblot assay with purified *T solium* antigens
  - 100% specificity
  - 50–97% sensitivity
- The other test is EIA.
  - Lower sensitivity and specificity
  - Can cross-react with other helminthic infections, such as echinococcosis and filariasis

Hydatid disease

- Eosinophilia seen in <25% of cases
- Serologic testing (EIA or indirect hemagglutination)
  - More reliable in diagnosing *E multilocularis* than *E granulosus* infection
  - Immunoelectrophoresis or immunoblot assay as specific confirmatory test
  - Both false-positive and false-negative results can occur.
  - Children usually have less antibody response and more frequently have a negative result.
  - Cyst in the liver elicits more antibody response than cyst in the lung.
  - Cyst in the brain, eye, or spleen almost always yields negative serologic findings.
  - Cyst in bone typically elicits a serologic response.

Diphyllobothriasis

- The infected person usually passes a large number of eggs in stool that can be demonstrated without a concentration technique

Hymenolipiasis

- Eggs are apparent in stool specimens
  - Detection of light infection may require a concentration technique and repeated examination.
- Peripheral blood eosinophilia may be present.

IMAGING

- Amoebic meningoencephalitis
  - PAM
    - Neuroimaging studies may be normal early in the disease but may show signs of increased intracranial pressure later.
    - Meningeal enhancement of the basilar region is frequently reported.
    - Severe brain edema is late finding and indicative of poor outcome.
  - GAE
    - Neuroimaging may reveal space-occupying lesions resembling abscesses, tumors, or hemorrhagic infarction.
- Toxoplasmosis
  - In congenital toxoplasmosis
    - CT of the brain should be performed to rule out brain calcification or hydrocephalus.
  - To detect congenital toxoplasmosis during pregnancy:
    - Serial ultrasonographic examinations to assess brain ventricular size or other signs of infection can be performed.
- Ascariasis
  - Imaging studies may demonstrate worms if there is:
    - Intestinal obstruction
    - Hepatobiliary or pancreatic ascariasis
- Hydatid disease
  - Ultrasonography
    - Most widely used, and wide availability
    - Sensitivity is 90–95%.
    - Allows cyst classification based on biological activity (active, transitional, or inactive), which helps guide the choice of treatment
  - CT
    - Higher sensitivity than ultrasonography
    - Better than ultrasonography in detecting extrahepatic cysts and cyst complications
- Cysticercosis
  - MRI
    - Allows good visualization of ocular, ventricular, and subarachnoid cysts
    - Demonstrates degree of edema and inflammation, as well as viability of the cysticercus
  - CT
    - Better than MRI for detection of granuloma or calcification

DIAGNOSTIC PROCEDURES

- Leishmaniasis
  - Skin samples obtained by:
    - Punch biopsy
    - Scraping or needle aspiration of the nonnecrotic edge
  - Other samples
    - Bone marrow aspirate and biopsy
    - Needle aspirate and biopsy of lymph node, liver, or spleen
      - The highest yield for diagnosis is splenic aspirate, but this test is considered too invasive.

- Giardiasis
  - Duodenal fluid sampling
    - Entero-Test, in which the patient swallows a gelatin capsule that contains a string (string test)
    - Examination of fresh specimens for motile trophozoites is diagnostic.
  - Duodenal biopsy is considered the last resort for diagnosis.
    - Rarely required
- Isosporiasis
  - Parasites may be found in biopsy specimens from the small intestine.
- Cutaneous larva migrans
  - If biopsy is performed, then eosinophils will be demonstrated in tissue samples.
    - However, the parasite can rarely be seen.
- Lymphatic filariasis
  - If microfilariae cannot be demonstrated on blood smears, fine-needle aspirate or biopsy of involved lymph node or epididymis may demonstrate worms or microfilariae.
    - Lymph node biopsies may worsen the obstructive manifestations of filariasis and should not be routinely done
- Trichinellosis
  - Muscle biopsy
    - Number of larvae per gram of muscle may be used as guide of severity of infection.
    - Specimens should be either:
      - Fresh and compressed between 2 microscope slides *or*
      - Digested by artificial gastric juice to increase yield
  - PCR testing to detect *Trichinella*-specific DNA in muscle biopsy specimens is used but not readily available.
- Strongyloidiasis
  - Duodenal fluid can be obtained by the Entero-Test or by endoscope.
- Schistosomiasis
  - Rectal or bladder biopsy may be needed (most sensitive) if stool or urine smears are negative.
- Onchocerciasis
  - Identify microfilariae in direct histologic examination of:
    - Skin snips
    - Biopsy samples
    - Lymph node biopsy sample
- Hydatid disease
  - Cyst aspiration or biopsy is usually reserved for cases with an uncertain diagnosis because of potential anaphylaxis reaction or spread of infection.
  - If needed, aspiration is usually performed under ultrasonographic or CT guidance along with benzimidazole treatment to minimize the risk of spreading.

TREATMENT APPROACH

- Leishmaniasis
  - Treatment decisions should be individualized.
  - In general, all patients with visceral and mucosal leishmaniasis should be treated.
  - Most patients with cutaneous leishmaniasis will heal spontaneously, but consider treatment if:
    - Lesion is cosmetically important (eg, on the face)
    - Lesions are multiple
    - Lesions are enlarging
    - Lesions overlie joints
    - May be caused by *Leishmania braziliensis* or other species that may disseminate to nasopharyngeal mucosa
- Chagas disease
  - Provide specific treatment for:
    - Acute and indeterminate phases of infection
    - Congenital infection
    - Reactivation of infection associated with immunosuppression
    - Infection associated with transfusion or organ transplantation
- Giardiasis
  - Treatment not warranted for asymptomatic patients
  - To prevent spread, therapy may be provided to children attending child-care centers.
  - Treatment may be provided to carriers in close contact with patients who have hypogammaglobulinemia or cystic fibrosis.
- Amebiasis
  - *E dispar* and *Entamoeba moshkovskii* infections do not require treatment.
- Amoebic meningoencephalitis
  - Treatment should be in centers where neurologic, neurosurgical, and infectious disease experts are available.
  - Consultation with the CDC is advisable.
- Cryptosporidiosis
  - In immunocompetent patients, supportive care, including hydration and nutritional support, may be adequate.
- Toxoplasmosis
  - Treatment is not indicated in immunocompetent patients unless clinical symptoms are severe or complications occur.
  - Immunocompromised patients with acute infection should be treated even if asymptomatic.
  - Infected pregnant women and neonates, whether symptomatic or not, should be treated as soon as diagnosed.
  - Patients with chorioretinitis are treated when symptoms are present or progressive.

P

- Malaria
  - Malaria must be recognized promptly to treat the patient in time, to prevent cerebral malaria and to prevent further spread of infection in the community.
  - Malaria is a nationally notifiable disease.
    - All cases should be reported to the state health department, which forwards them to the CDC.
  - 3 main factors should be considered.
    - Infecting *Plasmodium* species
    - Clinical status of patient
    - Drug susceptibility of the infecting parasites, determined by geographic area where infection was acquired
  - If malaria is suspected and cannot be confirmed, or if the diagnosis is confirmed but species determination is not possible, then antimalarial treatment effective against *P falciparum* must be initiated immediately.
- Cutaneous larva migrans
  - Disease is usually self-limited, but specific treatment may be needed.
- Toxocariasis
  - Treatment is suggested only for symptomatic patients and those with systemic forms of the disease.
- Cysticercosis
  - Appropriate management depends on:
    - Location of cyst
      - For neurocysticercosis, treatment not generally provided to an asymptomatic patient with a nonviable single parenchymal cyst that is evidently destroyed by the host immune response.
    - Viability of cyst
      - In children with viable cysticercus with minimal or no surrounding inflammatory response, cysticidal agent should be provided to prevent further perilesional damage and to reduce the risk of developing chronic seizures.
    - Host immune response
    - Presence or absence of symptoms

SPECIFIC TREATMENTS

Leishmaniasis

- Drugs of choice are the pentavalent antimonials.
  - Sodium stibogluconate (Pentostam) and meglumine antimonate (Glucantime)
  - Common side effects
    - Nausea
    - Vomiting
    - Myalgia
    - Headache
    - Malaise
    - High hepatic and pancreatic enzymes
  - More severe/dose-dependent side effects
    - Leukopenia
    - Thrombocytopenia
    - Behavioral changes
    - Electrocardiographic abnormalities (ST-segment changes, QT prolongation, and arrhythmias)
    - Cardiac toxicity and sudden death may occur with higher-than-recommended doses.
- Amphotericin B is increasingly used for visceral leishmaniasis.
  - Side effects
    - Infusion-related reactions and nephrotoxicity
  - Liposomal amphoteric in B (AmBisome) is better tolerated and distributes well to the reticuloendothelial system but is expensive.
- Pentamidine isothionate is an alternative treatment.
  - Significant side effects
    - Hypotension
    - Hypoglycemia
    - Nausea
    - Vomiting
    - Headache
    - Electrolyte disturbances (hyperkalemia, hypomagnesemia, and hypocalcemia)
- Topical paromomycin
  - Partially effective in treatment of Old World cutaneous leishmaniasis when risk of mucosal spread is low
- Parenteral paromomycin has been used as adjunctive therapy with antimonial therapy in the treatment of visceral leishmaniasis.
- Miltefosine
  - Oral formula
  - Shows promise in treating cutaneous and visceral leishmaniasis
- Oral fluconazole may speed healing of cutaneous lesions caused by *Leishmania major*.
- Other drugs used with limited efficacy
  - Itraconazole
  - Allopurinol
  - Dapsone
- Local treatments, such as thermotherapy and cryotherapy, are sometimes used for cutaneous leishmaniasis.
  - Unreliable in patients with New World lesions as a result of the risk of mucosal dissemination

Chagas disease

- Benznidazole and nifurtimox
  - Benznidazole is not available generally in the US but may be obtained through a compounding pharmacy.
  - Nifurtimox is available in the US under an investigational new drug protocol from the CDC drug service.
  - Side effects are dose dependent.
    - Hypersensitivity reactions
    - Bone marrow suppression
    - Peripheral neuropathy
- Pacemakers are implanted in patients with symptomatic heart block.
- Balloon dilation of the esophagogastric junction may be performed in patients with megaesophagus.
- Fecaloma and atonic segment of megacolon can be removed surgically.

African trypanosomiasis

- West African form
  - Pentamidine isethionate during hemolymphatic stage
    - In late-stage disease with CNS involvement, the drug of choice is melarsoprol or eflornithine.
- East African form
  - Suramin during hemolymphatic stage
  - Melarsoprol during late disease with CNS involvement
- Suramin and eflornithine are available only as investigational new drugs from the CDC's drug service.
  - Patients should be monitored closely for possible adverse reactions.

Giardiasis

- Metronidazole
  - Cure rate of 80–95%
  - Common side effects
    - Metallic taste in mouth
    - Nausea
    - Headache
    - Dizziness
- Nitazoxanide
  - Shorter course is as effective as a longer course of metronidazole.
  - Has advantage of treating other intestinal parasites, such as *Cryptosporidium*
- Alternative medications:furazolidone and quinacrine
  - Furazolidone well tolerated and results in a cure rate of 72–100%
  - Quinacrine has high cure rate (90–95%) but adverse effects
    - GI upset
    - Nausea

- Vomiting
- Abdominal pain
- Rarely, dermatitis, jaundice, and toxic psychosis
- No longer available in US

Amebiasis

- Antibiotic therapy with metronidazole followed by the intraluminal agents iodoquinol or diloxanide furoate
- If the patient's disease is slow to respond to metronidazole or if the patient has relapse after therapy:
  - Aspiration or a prolonged course of metronidazole, or both, should be considered.
- Asymptomatic *E histolytica* infection should be treated with an intraluminal agent.
  - Because of potential risk of invasive disease and risk of spread to household members

Amoebic meningoencephalitis

- PAM
  - Intravenous or intrathecal amphotericin B
- GAE
  - For encephalitides caused by *Acanthamoeba,* no optimal antimicrobial therapy has been developed.
- Multiple drugs have been used in both PAM and GAE infections with varying degrees of success.
  - Amphotericin B
  - Azithromycin
  - Fluconazole
  - Flucytosine
  - Pentamidine isethionate
  - Sulfa drugs
- Amoebic keratitis
  - Treatable with ≥1 drugs topically
  - Drugs of choice are:
    - Chlorhexidine gluconate (component of germicidal soaps)
    - Polyhexamethylene biguanide (disinfectant and swimming pool cleaner)

Cryptosporidiosis

- Nitazoxanide
  - Treatment for children ≥1 year of age
  - Treatment for adults with diarrhea caused by cryptosporidiosis or giardiasis
- Paromomycin
  - With or without azithromycin has been used in HIV-infected patients
    - Concurrent immune therapy, such as oral administration of human immunoglobulin, hyperimmune bovine colostrum, and bovine transfer factor, has demonstrated some benefit.

P

– Total parenteral nutrition may be needed in HIV-infected patients with chronic diarrhea and weight loss.

■ Fluid and electrolyte management of affected patients is essential.

■ Nutritional supplements containing medium-chain triglycerides may be helpful.

■ Milk and dairy products should be avoided.

Isosporiasis

■ Trimethoprim-sulfamethoxazole (TMP-SMX) for 10 days

  • Should not be provided to infants <2 months because of risk of kernicterus

  • Patients with AIDS may require maintenance courses with TMP-SMX or pyrimethamine-sulfadoxine to prevent relapses.

■ Pyrimethamine

  • May be provided for patients who cannot tolerate TMP-SMX

■ Ciprofloxacin

  • May be effective, but should not be provided to people <18 years of age

Cyclosporiasis

■ TMP-SMX

  • In patients infected with HIV, a prolonged course may be needed.

  • Secondary prophylaxis with TMP-SMX for months may also be needed in these patients.

Toxoplasmosis

■ Pyrimethamine-sulfadiazine

  • Lifelong daily maintenance therapy is needed in patients with AIDS.

  • Supplemental leucovorin (folinic acid) is provided to prevent bone marrow toxic effects.

  • For congenital toxoplasmosis, pyrimethamine and sulfadiazine(with folinic acid supplements) should be continued for a prolonged period, often for 1 year.

■ Clindamycin and pyremethamine

  • For patients who are allergic to sulfa drugs

■ Ocular toxoplasmosis

  • Corticosteroids provided in addition topyrimethamine and sulfadiazine

■ Patients with CNS disease

  • Corticosteroids provided in addition to pyrimethamine and sulfadiazinein selected patients

Malaria

Uncomplicated (nonsevere) malaria

■ See table Chemotherapy for Uncomplicated Malaria for chemotherapy for uncomplicated cases.

Severe malaria

■ Treatment should be parenteral administration of quinidine gluconate, with continuous infusion until:

  • The patient can take oral medicationand

  • Parasite density is <1%

■ Therapy should be combined with doxycycline, tetracycline, or clindamycin.

■ Monitor the patient closely in an intensive care unit.

■ Consult the CDC regarding treatment of severe cases.

Artemisinin derivatives

■ In China and Southeast Asia, artemisinin derivatives, such as artemether and artesunate, are replacing quinine.

  • These agents can be administered orally or rectally.

  • Some concerns about possible neurotoxicity and a high rate of recurrence have been raised.

    – Thus these drugs should be used when malaria resistance to quinine is suspected.

    – Should be administered for a minimum of 3 days and followed up with mefloquine to ensure a cure rate >90%

Supportive measures to optimize management

■ Closely monitor fluid and electrolytes status.

■ Treat the convulsions with phenobarbital or diazepam.

■ Be vigilant about hypoglycemia.

■ Correct anemia with packed red blood cell transfusions

  • The CDC recommends that exchange transfusion be considered when parasite density is >10% or severe complications.

■ Gram-negative sepsis must be suspected whenever patients experience shock.

  • Appropriate antibiotic therapy should be initiated after blood cultures are obtained.

Self-treatment

■ Self-treatment course of atovaquone-proguanil can be provided to travelers who:

  • Do not receive antimalarial drugs for prophylaxis

  • Are on a less-than-effective regimen

  • May be in remote areas when they develop fever

■ Travelers should be advised that self-treatment is not considered a replacement for seeking prompt medical help.

Babesiosis

■ Clindamycin plus or alquinine or atovaquone plus azithromycin for treatment of symptomatic infection

■ Exchange transfusion

  • Consider in fulminant cases with severe hemolysis and high-grade parasitemia. (>10%)

Chemotherapy of Uncomplicated Malaria[a]

	Route	Drug	Dosage
All *Plasmodium* Species Except Chloroquine-Resistant Species	Oral drug of choice	Chloroquine phosphate	10-mg base/kg (max 600-mg base), then 5-mg base/kg 6 hr later, then 5-mg base/kg at 24 and 48 hr
	Parenteral drug of choice	Quinidine gluconate	10-mg/kg loading dose (max 600 mg) in normal saline over 1–2 hr, followed by continuous infusion of 0.02 mg/kg/min until oral therapy can be started
OR		Quinine dihydrochloride for *P falciparum* acquired in areas of chloroquine resistance	20-mg/kg loading dose in 5% dextrose over 4 hr, followed by 10 mg/kg over 2-4 hr every 8 hr (max 1800 mg/day) until oral therapy can be started
	Oral drug of choice	Atovaquone-proguanil	<5 kg: not indicated
			5–8 kg: 2 pediatric tablet once a day × 3 days
			9–10 kg: 3 pediatric tablet once a day × 3 days
			11–20 kg: 1 adult tablet once a day × 3 days
			21–30 kg: 2 adult tablet once a day × 3 days
			31–40 kg: 3 adult tablet once a day × 3 days
			>40 kg: 4 adult tablet once a day × 3 days
OR		Quinine sulfate	30 mg/kg/day in 3 doses × 3–7 days
PLUS		Doxycycline	4 mg/kg daily in 2 doses × 7 days
OR		Quinine sulfate	30 mg/kg daily in 3 doses × 3-7 days
PLUS	Alternatives	Clindamycin	20 mg/kg daily in 3 doses × 7 days
		Mefloquine	15 mg/kg followed 12 hr later by 10 mg/kg
OR		Artesunate	4 mg/kg daily × 3 days
PLUS		Mefloquine prevention of relapses: *P vivax* and *P ovale* only	15 mg/kg followed 12 hr later by 10 mg/kg
		Primaquine phosphate	0.6-mg base/kg × 14 days

[a] Modified in part from: American Academy of Pediatrics. Malaria. In: Pickering LK, Baker CJ, Long SS, McMillan JA, eds. *Red Book: 2006 Report of the Committee on Infectious Diseases.* 27th ed. Elk Grove Village, IL: American Academy of Pediatrics; 2006:435–441.

Trichinellosis

■ Mebendazole and albendazole have comparable efficacy.

• Both drugs are ineffective for larvae in the muscles.

■ Coadministration of corticosteroids (eg, prednisone)

• Indicated in severe cases, especially with cardiac and CNS involvement

Trichuriasis

■ Mebendazole is the drug of choice.

• Alternatives are:

– Albendazole

– Ivermectin

– Nitazoxanide (not yet approved by the US Food and Drug Administration for this indication)

Strongyloidiasis

■ Ivermectin is the drug of choice.

• Alternatives are thiabendazole and albendazole.

– In the past, thiabendazole was the preferred medication.

– Lower cure rates have been reported with the use of thiabendazole or albendazole compared with ivermectin.

■ In immunocompromised patients with hyperinfection or disseminated disease, prolonged or repeat courses of treatment (or both) may be needed.

P

Hookworm infections

- May need to correct malnutrition and anemia, including iron supplementation
- Drugs of choice are:
  - Albendazole
  - Mebendazole
  - Pyrantel pamoate

Cutaneous larva migrans

- Topical thiabendazole should be provided if available.
  - An alternative is albendazole or ivermectin.

Pinworm infections

- Drugs of choice are:
  - Mebendazole
  - Pyrantel pamoate
  - Albendazole
- Reinfection rates are high, and subsequent treatment may be needed.

Ascariasis

- Treat with either:
  - Albendazole, mebendazole, or ivermectin
    - Experience with these 3 drugs is limited in children <2 years of age.
    - Limited data suggest that these drugs are safe.
      - However, risk and benefits of treating ascariasis should be considered in this age group.
- Pyrantel pamoate and nitazoxanide are also effective.
- Patients with suspected intestinal or biliary obstruction:
  - Should be treated with conservative management to alleviate obstruction
    - Followed by albendazole, mebendazole, or ivermectin
- Surgery
  - If medical therapy is not successful in relieving obstruction or if complications exist (eg, volvulus peritonitis or perforation)
  - During laparotomy for obstructive cases, the small bowel should be milked down to the cecum, avoiding incision of bowel wall.
  - Endoscopic retrograde cholangiopancreatography is used to extract worms in hepatobiliary cases.

Toxocariasis

- Albendazole and mebendazole
- Corticosteroids are indicated for patients with severe cardiac and CNS involvement.
- Ocular involvement
  - Anthelmintic therapy, surgery, corticosteroids, or a combination of these
  - DEC is an alternative.

Lymphatic filariasis

- The drug of choice is DEC.
  - Systemic side effects
    - Headache
    - Anorexia
    - Nausea
    - Vomiting
    - Lymphadenitis and transient lymphedema
    - Systemic reactions if heavy load
      - May want to initiate low-dose treatment at first
- A single oral dose of ivermectin has been shown to be effective.
- Combination therapy of single doses of DEC and ivermectin may be more effective than single doses alone.
- Surgical and cosmetic therapy may be needed in some patients with chronic filariasis.
- Decongestive physiotherapy may be helpful in some cases of lymph edema.
- Bacterial superinfections, most commonly caused by *Staphylococcus* and group A *Streptococcus,* should be treated appropriately.

Onchocerciasis

- The drug of choice is ivermectin.
  - Does not kill adult worms, and therapy is not curative
  - Improves dermatitis and prevents ocular lesions
- DEC
  - No longer drug of choice because of high incidence of severe Mazzotti reactions
- Surgery
  - Surgical excision of the lesions (nodulectomy), particularly on the head, can reduce microfilarial load and decrease risk of ocular complications.
- *Wolbachia* endosymbiotic bacteria have emerged as a target for treatment with doxycycline.
  - Doxycycline should not be provided to children <8 years of age.

Schistosomiasis

- Praziquantel is drug of choice.
- Alternative treatments are:
  - Oxamniquine for *S mansoni*
  - Metrifonate for *S haematobium*

Taeniasis and cysticercosis

Taeniasis

- Praziquantel
  - Drug of choice for the treatment of taeniasis from both *T solium* and *T saginata*
  - Highly effective in eradicating the adult stage (intestinal stage) of the tapeworm

- Niclosamide
  - An alternative agent
  - Not available commercially in the US

Cysticercosis

- In general, albendazole is preferred over praziquantel because of its higher cysticidal activity and lower cost.
- An anticonvulsant agent is usually provided to patients with:
  - Seizures
  - Multiple cysts but no history of seizure, because of risk of seizures after treatment starts
- Cysticercal encephalitis
  - The initial goal is to reduce inflammation and cerebral edema with a corticosteroid or an immunosuppressive agent.
  - Treatment with a cysticidal agent should be deferred until clinical signs of encephalitis have subsided and imaging studies demonstrate improvement of brain edema.
  - A small cyst located in the lateral ventricle can be treated effectively with an anthelmintic agent.
  - A ventriculoperitoneal shunt should be placed before treatment begins in patients with hydrocephalus.
  - If the cyst is in the fourth ventricle, is attached to the middle cerebral artery, or is compressing the optic chiasm, surgery should be performed before the cysticidal agent is administered.
  - Patients with subarachnoid cysts or a large cyst in the fissures should be treated for ≥30 days.
- Intraocular subretinal cyst
  - Treatment with albendazole combined with a corticosteroid is effective.
  - An intraocular cyst located in the vitreous chamber should be removed surgically.
  - An ophthalmologic examination should be performed in all cases to rule out intraocular cyst before initiating treatment.
- Symptomatic subcutaneous or muscular lesions
  - Treatment with antiinflammatory medication may be provided.
  - Surgical excision of a solitary subcutaneous or intramuscular cyst may be considered if symptoms persist.

Hydatid disease

- Surgery
  - Most common treatment modality
  - The goal is complete removal of the cyst, which may lead to a cure.
- Nonresectable cysts
  - Treatment with an anthelmintic agent (albendazole [preferred] or mebendazole) usually provides improvement and sometimes a cure.

- Response to treatment depends on the size and location of the cyst.
  - Cysts inside bone generally respond less well to drug therapy.
- PAIR treatment (puncture, aspiration, injection, and reaspiration)
  - Percutaneous drainage of cyst with a needle or catheter, followed by instillation of a protoscolicide agent and reaspiration of cyst content
  - Should be provided only to children >3 years of age
- Long-term treatment with albendazole and mebendazole has been demonstrated to inhibit growth of cyst in alveolar infection.
  - Sometimes leads to a cure

Diphyllobothriasis

- Praziquantel is the drug of choice.
  - An alternative agent, niclosamide, is no longer available in the US.
- Patients with clinical or laboratory evidence of vitamin B_{12} deficiency should be treated with cobalamin injections and oral folic acid.

Hymenolipiasis

- Praziquantel is the drug of choice.
- Close family members, especially siblings, may also need treatment.

WHEN TO ADMIT

- All patients with systemic symptoms caused by primary infection or as a complication of parasitic infection should be hospitalized.

WHEN TO REFER

- If the physician is not well versed in taking care of children with parasitic infections, referral to an infectious disease specialist is prudent.

FOLLOW-UP

- Leishmaniasis
  - Patients receiving antimonials should have complete blood counts and electrocardiographic monitoring at baseline and weekly thereafter.
- African trypanosomiasis
  - Patients taking suramin or eflornithine should be monitored closely for possible adverse reactions.
- Hookworm infections
  - Repeat stool examination should be performed 2 weeks after treatment.
    - If positive, then additional treatment should be considered.

P

- Schistosomiasis
  - Patients treated with praziquantel in the first 4–8 weeks of exposure should be retreated in 1 or 2 months.
  - Reexamination of stool or urine 1 month after treatment should be performed to assess efficacy of treatment.
    - If patients continue to shed eggs, treat again.
- Cysticercosis
  - Patients with neurocysticercosis should be monitored with a brain imaging study after completion of treatment.
- Hymenolipiasis
  - Stool examination should be repeated 2–4 weeks after treatment to document cure.
    - Especially in patients with many worms

COMPLICATIONS

Leishmaniasis

- Cutaneous form
  - Secondary bacterial infection is common.
- Visceral form
  - Secondary bacterial and mycobacterial infections, including tuberculosis
- Patients with thrombocytopenia may develop:
  - Epistaxis
  - Gingival bleeding
  - Other hemorrhagic manifestations
- If patients go untreated
  - Disseminated intravascular coagulation
  - Pulmonary or intestinal superinfections
- Patients infected with HIV and stem cell and solid organ transplant recipients are:
  - At risk of reactivation of latent infection and disseminated disease
- Post–kala-azar dermal leishmaniasis after recovery in patients from visceral disease:
  - Indicates reversal to dermal form
  - Lesions occur predominantly on the face, extremities, and upper trunk.

Trypanosomiasis

- Death from meningitis, heart failure, and other complications

Giardiasis

- *G intestinalis* uncommonly spreads from the duodenum to other organs.
  - Hepatitis
  - Cholangitis
  - Pancreatitis

Amebiasis

- Extension or rupture into lung, pleural space, peritoneum, or pericardium may complicate the course of amoebic hepatic abscess.

Cryptosporidiosis

- The biliary tract is affected in 10–30% of HIV-infected patients.
  - Can lead to sclerosing or acalculous cholangitis

Trichinellosis (severe)

- Fatal myocarditis with subsequent heart failure and cardiac arrhythmias
- Encephalitis
- Meningitis
- Focal neurologic deficits
- Bronchopneumonia
- Nephritis

Amoebiasis

- Fulminant colitis with bowel necrosis leading to perforation and peritonitis
  - Rare, but associated with mortality rate >40%
- Other rare complications
  - Ameboma (a nodular, tumorlike focus of proliferate inflammation in the wall of the colon)
  - Toxic megacolon
  - Local perforation
  - Peritonitis
  - Extraintestinal extension
- Complications of amoebic hepatic abscess
  - Jaundice
  - Extension or rupture into the lung, pleural space, peritoneum, or pericardium

Toxoplasmosis

- Rare complications of primary toxoplasmosis infection
  - Hepatitis
  - Pneumonitis
  - Myocarditis
  - Pericarditis
  - Encephalitis
- Complications of congenital toxoplasmosis infection
  - If untreated, a large proportion of infants may develop late-onset sequelae, such as:
    - Chorioretinitis: Relapses are frequent, and vision loss may occur.
    - Learning disabilities
    - Intellectual disability months to years later

P

- Other complications of congenital ocular involvement
  - Chorioretinal scars
  - Microphthalmia
  - Cataract
  - Retinal detachment

Babesiosis

- Vascular injury may also cause renal insufficiency.

Trichuriasis

- Colitis results from chronic infection.
  - May mimic inflammatory bowel disease
- Colonic obstruction and perforation may occur.
- Chronic infection in children may also be associated with malnutrition, growth retardation, and cognitive abnormalities.

Ocular larva migrans

- Chronic endophthalmitis
- Retinal detachment
- Keratitis
- Uveitis
- Iritis
- Vitreous abscess
- Optic neuritis
- Retinal tracks with larvae

Pinworm infections

- Bacterial superinfection may develop in the perianal region.

Schistosomiasis

- Genitourinary lesions include obstructive lesions that may eventually lead to chronic renal failure or bladder carcinoma.
- Schistosome eggs may occasionally embolize to other organs with subsequent granuloma formation.
  - Skin
  - Lungs
  - Brain
  - Adrenal glands
  - Skeletal muscles
- Neurologic complications
  - Transverse myelitis occurs with either *S mansoni* or *S japonicum* infection.
  - Seizures, either focal or generalized, have been reported in patients infected with *S japonicum*.
  - Focal neurologic deficits may rarely occur.

Cysticercosis

- After treatment initiation, patients may develop a treatment reaction, usually with an inflammatory reaction in the surrounding tissue.
  - Severe headache and vomiting

- Reaction can be minimized by administration of dexamethasone 2–3 days before treatment initiation and during treatment with a cysticidal agent.

Hydatid disease

- Possible complications from surgical procedures or PAIR are spreading of the infection and allergic or anaphylaxis reaction.
  - These can be minimized by perioperative administration of anthelmintic agents against echinococcal cysts.

Lymphatic filariasis

- Hydrocele and chyluria result from obstructed lymph drainage in the genital area and urinary bladder, respectively.
- Other complications of lymphatic obstruction include chylothorax and chylous ascites.

Diphyllobothriasis

- Because *Diphyllobothriasis latum* can compete with the human host for vitamin B_{12}, chronically infected people may develop pernicious anemia as a result of vitamin B_{12} deficiency.

PROGNOSIS

- Chagas disease
  - In the acute phase, children <2 years of age who develop heart failure or meningoencephalitis have a high mortality rate.
  - Patients in the chronic phase with digestive tract involvement generally have a good prognosis.
  - Prognosis is usually poor among chronic-phase patients with heart failure.
- Amoebic meningoencephalitis
  - PAM
    - Even with combined therapy, survival has been the exception.
- Cryptosporidiosis
  - In immunocompromised patients, particularly those infected with HIV
    - Cryptosporidiosis frequently takes a severe and protracted course.
    - Can lead to significant malnutrition and wasting, dehydration, and death
- Strongyloidiasis
  - Patients may remain infected for decades.

PREVENTION

Leishmaniasis

- Travelers to endemic areas should use personal-protection measures to prevent bites by the sandfly.
  - Long-sleeve shirts, pants, and socks
  - Insect repellents

P

- Limit exposure to the fly from dusk to dawn.
- Bed nets

Giardiasis

- Personal hygiene is the most important way to prevent spread.
- In child care centers, strict hand washing and appropriate diaper disposal
- Symptomatic children should be excluded from child care centers.
- *Giardia* cysts are resistant to the usual chlorination levels and are not easily killed in cold water.
  - Cysts can be killed by boiling or heating water to ≥70°C for 10 minutes.
  - Travelers, hikers, and campers should be advised to ensure safe drinking water.
    - Heat or boil water *or*
    - Chemically disinfect *or*
    - Filter (high-quality filtration units are effective)

Amoebic meningoencephalitis

- Effective levels of chlorine in water used in swimming pools and spas
- Avoidance of swimming in warm, stagnant, and possibly feces-contaminated waters
- Compliance with procedures for contact lens care

Cryptosporidiosis

- Effective hand washing and appropriate disposal of infected material
- Contact precautions are suggested for diapered and incontinent children.
- Infected people should not use public recreational water when they have diarrhea and for ≥2 weeks after resolution of symptoms.
- Boiling water intended for drinking for 1 minute kills *Cryptosporidium*.
  - Alternatively, filtration devices with particle-size ratings of 1–5 mcm removes *Cryptosporidium*.

Toxoplasmosis

- General prevention measures
  - Hygienic practices during cat contact
  - Prevention of consuming raw meat
    - Deep freezing and cooking meat, particularly ham and lamb, to an internal temperature of 65.5°C–76.6°C or until no longer pink kills cysts.
    - All fruits and vegetables should be washed thoroughly.
  - Pregnant women and immunocompromised individuals should avoid contact with cats, cat litter, or soil contaminated by cat feces.
    - Stress wearing gloves and hand washing in such settings.

- Cats may be prevented from acquiring infection by restricting their outdoor activities and feeding them commercially prepared cat food.
- Because oocysts are not infective until 36–48 hours or longer after passage, daily cleaning of cat litter boxes is a simple and effective control measure.
- Prophylactic therapy
  - Children with HIV or AIDS with severe immunosuppression and positive *Toxoplasma* IgG antibodies
    - The drug of choice is TMP-SMX.
    - Alternative therapies: dapsone plus pyrimethamine (with supplemental folinic acid) or atovaquone
  - To prevent recurrence of toxoplasmosis in immunosuppressed patients with prior *Toxoplasma* encephalitis:
    - Pyrimethamine plus sulfadiazine plus folinic acid
    - Alternatively, clindamycin plus pyrimethamine plus folinic acid for patients who cannot tolerate sulfa drugs

Malaria

- To prevent recurrence when treating *P vivax* and *P ovale*
  - Antimalarial drugs that target the liver stage (eg, primaquine) should be added.
    - Patients should be checked for glucose-6-phosphate dehydrogenase deficiency before being given primaquine.
- Reducing population of *Anopheles* mosquitoes
- Avoiding bites by parasite-carrying mosquitoes (vector control)
- Providing antimalarial drugsprophylactically
- Detailed guidelines about chemoprophylaxis of malaria for travelers to endemic areas are available (www.cdc.gov/travel/).

Chemoprophylaxis by geographic area

- Begin 1 week before arrival in area, except doxycycline and atovaquone-proguanil, which should be started 1–2 days before arrival, to allow time to develop blood concentrations of the drug/permit evaluation for adverse reactions; medications should be continued after departure from endemic areas.
- Areas with chloroquine-sensitive *Plasmodium* species
  - Chloroquine phosphate: 5-mg base/kg once a week; up to adult dose of 300-mg base
- Areas with chloroquine-resistant *Plasmodium* species
  - Atovaquone-proguanil
    - 5–10 kg: 1-8 tablets once a week
    - 11–20 kg: 1 pediatric tablet/day
    - 21–30 kg: 2 pediatric tablets/day
    - 31–40 kg: 3 pediatric tablets/day
    - >40 kg: 1 adult tablet/day

- *Or* mefloquine
  - 11–20 kg: 0.25 tablet once a week
  - 21–30 kg: 0.5 tablet once a week
  - 31–45 kg: 0.75 tablet once a week
  - >45 kg: 1 tablet once a week
- *Or* doxycycline: 2 mg/kg per day, up to 100 mg/day
- Alternatives: primaquine: 0.6-mg base/kg daily
- *Or* chloroquine phosphate: 5-mg base/kg once/week, up to 300-mg base, *plus*
- Proguanil
  - 2–6 yr: 100 mg once a day
  - 7–10 yr: 150 mg once a day
  - >10 yr: 200 mg once a day

Babesiosis

- Avoid tick-infested areas.
  - Particularly from May to September
- Wear clothing that covers arms, legs, and other exposed areas.
  - Tuck pants into socks or boots.
- Tick and insect repellents that contain *N,N*-diethyl-meta-toluamide (DEET) may be considered.
  - Repeat applications may be needed.
- Tick-toxic agents, such as permethrin, may be sprayed on clothes and shoes but not the skin.
- Inspect bodies of self and children, as well as all clothing, for ticks after possible exposure.
  - Exposed hairy areas, including the scalp and behind the ears, should be thoroughly inspected.
- If a tick is found:
  - Grasp with a tweezers close to the skin and gently pull out straight.
- Pets should be inspected for ticks daily.

Trichinellosis

- Prevent by thorough cooking of pork and game meat.
  - Heat at a temperature of 77°C.
- Freezing is also effective in killing larvae in meat.
  - Freezing at –15°C for 3 weeks (available in home freezers)
  - Freezing pork meat at –23°C for 10 days

Trichuriasis

- Proper disposal of human fecal material may be the most effective control measure.

Strongyloidiasis

- Proper disposal of human fecal material
- Screening
  - Consider in patients with immunodeficiency if history of living in or traveling to endemic areas.
    - Especially those receiving corticosteroids or with human T-lymphotropic virus type 1 infection

- Screening of immigrants or returned travelers from endemic areas should also be considered before initiating immunosuppressive therapy.

Hookworm infections

- Proper disposal of human feces

Pinworm infections

- Hand hygiene is essential.
- Morning bathing is suggested for all infected persons.
- Prevention of autoinfection
  - Avoid scratching the perianal area.
  - Wash the hands before eating.
  - Keep fingernails short.
  - Frequently change and wash underwear, bed linen, and clothing.
  - Shaking of bed linen should be avoided.
  - Treating all family contacts should be considered if there are repeated symptomatic infections.

Ascariasis

- Sanitary disposal of human feces is essential to prevent soil contamination.
  - Particularly near children's play areas
- Mass deworming programs with a single dose of mebendazole or albendazole have been used in some communities endemic for ascariasis.

Toxocariasis

- Correct underlying causes of pica in children.
- Cat and dog feces should be properly disposed of.
- Sandboxes not in use should be covered.
- Anthelmintic therapy for puppies and kittens at 2, 4, 6, and 8 weeks may prevent secretion of eggs in feces and subsequent potential transmission.

Onchocerciasis

- Prevent blackfly bites in endemic areas.
  - Bites during the day
  - Insect repellents and protective clothing are suggested.

Schistosomiasis

- Sanitary disposal of human waste
- Travelers should be advised to avoid contact with fresh water in lakes or streams.
- Artemether, an antimalarial agent, has been suggested for use as a prophylactic agent.
  - Kills schistosomula (the migrating larvae) in the first 21 days in the body
  - When administered every 2 weeks, kills all immature schistosomes
  - Should be avoided in malaria-endemic areas because of risk of emergence of resistance

P

Pectus Excavatum and Pectus Carinatum

DEFINITION

- Pectus excavatum
  - A congenital syndrome characterized by a concave depression of the sternum
  - Phenotypically, the appearance resembles a funnel chest.
  - Concavity often is asymmetric, with the right side usually more depressed than the left.
    - Severity of the concavity can range from a mild depression to a profound indentation.
- Pectus carinatum
  - The second-most common chest wall abnormality
  - Characterized by a protuberance of the sternum that mimics a pigeon's chest

EPIDEMIOLOGY

- Pectus excavatum
  - The most common congenital chest wall deformity
  - Affects approximately 1 in 400 live births
  - Accounts for ~90% of chest wall defects
  - 80% of children with pectus excavatum are boys.
- Pectus carinatum
  - Accounts for <5% of chest wall defects

ETIOLOGY

- Pectus excavatum
  - Results from excessive growth of the costal cartilage, which displaces the sternum posteriorly
  - Defect may be exaggerated by rapid skeletal growth during adolescence.

RISK FACTORS

- For pectus excavatum
  - Family history

SIGNS AND SYMPTOMS

Pectus excavatum

- Typically becomes problematic as children reach early adolescence
  - Embarrassment over cosmetic appearance of the chest
    - Many patients describe having social anxiety, problems with body image, and depression.
  - Respiratory impairment from the defect
- Defect can progress from barely noticeable to extremely prominent in the span of a few years.
  - Severity usually does not increase after age 18.
  - Rapid growth during adolescence tends to make deformity more pronounced.

- Most patients do not exhibit symptoms.
  - Some may have decreased chest excursion and diminished inspirations, causing:
    - Decreased exercise tolerance
    - Easy fatigability
    - Frequent respiratory tract infections
    - Chest pain (unusual)
- Auscultation of the chest may reveal diminished inspiration or a cardiac murmur, especially in the presence of mitral valve prolapse.
- Patients tend to have *pectus posture*:
  - Rounded shoulders
  - Protuberant abdomen
- Pectus excavatum is associated with:
  - Asthma
  - Bronchial atresia
  - Bronchomalacia
  - Down syndrome
  - Marfan syndrome
  - Mitral valve prolapse (≤30%)
  - Noonan syndrome
  - Osteogenesis imperfecta
  - Poland syndrome
  - Rett syndrome
  - Rickets
  - Scoliosis (15%)
  - Turner syndrome
  - Wolff-Parkinson-White syndrome

Pectus carinatum

- Usually a symmetric, midline deformity
- Only infrequently associated with cardiovascular compromise

DIAGNOSTIC APPROACH

- Pectus excavatum
  - Thorough history and physical examination, with attempt to rule out associated disorders that may have been undiagnosed
  - Severity is measured by the Haller index: CT scan–measured transthoracic diameter divided by sternovertebral diameter.
    - An index of >3.5 is considered to be a severe defect.
    - Even indices <2.5 can cause significant cardiopulmonary impairment.
    - Repair usually is considered for defects with an index of >1.5–1.7.

IMAGING

- Pectus excavatum
  - Transthoracic echocardiogram
    - May reveal diminished cardiac output from decreased stroke volume and mitral valve prolapse

DIAGNOSTIC PROCEDURES

- Pectus excavatum
  - Pulmonary function tests tend to demonstrate a restrictive pattern.

TREATMENT APPROACH

- Pectus excavatum
  - Nonoperative measures are aimed at decreasing symptoms, but generally are only minimally effective.
    - Patients can be taught to increase breathing efforts to increase diaphragmatic excursion and oxygen exchange.
    - Improvement in posture can improve air exchange.
      - External braces can help correct posture but have been largely associated with only minimal correction.
    - Some authorities have advocated the use of continuous external vacuum.
  - Repair should be performed in patients with:
    - Cardiopulmonary impairment
    - Pain
    - Concerns about cosmesis resulting in poor body image
  - The best time for repair is uncertain; however children should undergo surgical repair between 12–18 yr of age, when old enough to:
    - Understand the nature, consequences, and magnitude of the surgery
    - Understand the level of pain that might be experienced postoperatively and accept a temporary limitation of activity
  - Although the surgery can be performed later, it should not be delayed too long, to take advantage of the pliable chest wall of the growing adolescent.
- Pectus carinatum
  - Open surgical repair similar to that used for pectus excavatum
- A minimal open repair has been described for both the excavatum and carinatum deformities.

SPECIFIC TREATMENTS

Pectus excavatum

- Two methods of surgical repair
  - Ravitch method (1949)
    - Transverse incision is made over the middle portion of the sternal defect.
    - Dissection is performed below the level of the pectoralis fascia and muscles.
    - Costal cartilage of ribs 1–8, on each side of the sternum, is resected, proceeding from the costochondral junction to the costosternal junction.
    - Transverse osteotomy of the sternum is performed at the level of the third costal cartilage.
    - Lower sternum is then repositioned to correct the deformity, and pectoralis muscles are reattached to the midline.
    - Despite its extensive nature, this repair has been associated with good long-term outcome.
  - Nuss procedure (1987)
    - Less invasive
    - Elevates the sternal depression without cartilage resection
    - Bilateral incisions are made at the anterior axillary line at the level of the greatest depression of the pectus defect.
    - Incision is made in the fourth intercostal space, and a thoracoscope is introduced.
    - Under direct vision, a pectus bar is passed across the chest.
    - Bar then is flipped anteriorly to raise the sternum.
    - Bar remains in place for 2 to 3 years to allow for proper remodeling of the costal cartilage.
    - This process is slower in the older patient because of the decreased rate of growth.
    - Bar is removed as an outpatient procedure.
    - The method has been associated with equivalent cosmetic results and may be more cost effective because it has a shorter operating time.
  - Adequate analgesia typically is the most troublesome problem in the postoperative period.
    - Epidural patient-controlled analgesia catheter greatly reduces pain after the procedure.
    - The epidural catheter usually is required for several days, and is the main reason the patient remains in the hospital.

Pectus carinatum

- Typically, open Ravitch repair method (as for pectus excavatum) is performed to correct deformity.
- Thoracoscopic techniques also are used.
- Some investigators have advocated the use of conservative measures as an alternative to surgical repair, such as:
  - External braces applying constant pressure

WHEN TO REFER

- Pectus excavatum
  - Patients may be referred to pulmonologists and cardiologists to manage the pulmonary and cardiac complications until the defect is corrected surgically at 12–18 years of age.

P

COMPLICATIONS

■ Pectus excavatum

- Complications with the Ravitch repair method include:
  - Impairment of growth of the chest wall
  - Possible constriction of the thorax
- Complications with the Nuss repair method include
  - Displacement of the bar
    - Modifications in technique and increased surgeon experience have led to low rates of bar migration.
  - No cases of cardiac perforation have occurred with the use of thoracoscopy during the procedure.

PROGNOSIS

■ Pectus excavatum

- Long-term outcomes have shown both types of repair to be effective.
- Almost all patients report satisfaction with cosmetic results.

- Pain and decreased exercise intolerance generally improve after surgery.
- Many asymptomatic patients with normal preoperative pulmonary function test and cardiac echo report significant improvement in their exercise tolerance and endurance, although they had not previously reported presurgical limitations.
- Advent of a minimally invasive technique has changed the approach to a patient with this deformity.
  - Children who previously lived with psychological issues because of poor body image or physical limitations (or both) can now undergo a safe and effective operation with minimal morbidity.
  - Number of patients referred for surgical repair is likely to increase.

P

Pertussis (Whooping Cough)

DEFINITION

- A highly contagious, bacterial respiratory infection
  - Caused by *Bordetella pertussis,* an aerobic gram-negative coccobacillus
  - Characterized by paroxysms of intense coughing and a protracted clinical course lasting several weeks

EPIDEMIOLOGY

- Incidence
  - 300,000 pertussis-related deaths annually worldwide
  - Before availability of pertussis vaccines, almost 300,000 cases and 10,000 deaths annually in the US.
  - 11,647 cases were reported in the US in 2003, with an annual incidence of 4.0 cases per 100,000 population.
  - Epidemic peaks occur every 3–5 years.
    - In highly immunized populations as well as in infants who have not received 3 doses of vaccine
  - Overall number of cases is likely underestimated because the infection is often underdiagnosed in adolescents and adults.
- Prevalence
  - A very common cause of prolonged cough in adolescents and adults
    - Accounts for 12–32% of cases of cough lasting 2 weeks or longer
- Age
  - By the late 1980s, infants <1 year of age had the highest age-specific incidence, which declined with increasing age.
  - Since the early 1990s, a marked increase has occurred in reported cases in children aged 10 years and older.
  - Between 2001 and 2003, children aged 10–19 years accounted for 33% of all reported cases; 23% of cases occurred in individuals ≥20 years of age.
  - Between 2001 and 2003 infants <1 year accounted for 23% of all cases.
  - Severe paroxysmal cough ending in the inspiratory *whoop* is most often seen in infants and young children, who experience the most severe manifestations.
  - Annual incidence by age
    - Infants <1 year: 55.2 per 100,000 population
    - Ages 10–19 years: 7.7 per 100,000
    - Adults: 1.1 per 100,000
- Geographic distribution
  - Disease is endemic, with all 50 states reporting cases annually.
- Seasonality
  - Most cases in the US occur between June and October.

ETIOLOGY

- *Bordetella pertussis* is a highly contagious organism.
  - 80–90% secondary attack rates among susceptible household contacts
  - Acquired through direct transmission from close respiratory contact
- Subclinical or mild illness commonly occurs in fully or partially immunized, and naturally immune individuals.
- Immunity
  - Wanes within 3–5 years of vaccination or natural infection
  - Often undetectable at 12 years after vaccination or natural infection
  - Thus neither vaccination nor natural disease provides long-lasting immunity.
- Adults and adolescents with pertussis serve as
  - Important reservoirs for infection
  - Index cases for younger infants and children

SIGNS AND SYMPTOMS

Infants and children

- 3 stages of illness, each lasting at least 2 weeks
- Classic stages are evident most commonly in unimmunized infected young children.
  - In partially or totally immunized children, stages are shortened and may be atypical.
  - Neonates do not have an apparent catarrhal phase.
- Incubation period of 7–10 days
- *Catarrhal* phase
  - Nonspecific upper respiratory tract symptoms with:
    - Rhinorrhea
    - Lacrimation
    - Mild cough
    - Conjunctival injection
- *Paroxysmal* stage
  - Intermittent dry hacking cough
  - Repetitive series of forceful coughs within a single expiration
  - Sudden massive inspiratory respiratory effort often occurs at the end of cough paroxysm, resulting in a high-pitched *whoop.*
  - Between attacks, patient appears comfortable, without apparent distress.
  - Very young infants often lack the characteristic *whoop* and exhibit episodes of:
    - Gagging
    - Gasping
    - Apnea

– Bradycardia

– Cyanosis

■ *Convalescent* stage

- Diminishing severity and frequency of paroxysms

- Continued intermittent coughing for weeks to months, often exacerbated by subsequent intercurrent respiratory illness

■ Physical examination is usually normal, except for evidence of the forcefulness of their cough and posttussive emesis.

- Conjunctival hemorrhage

- Upper body petechial lesions

■ Fever

- Characteristically absent at all stages

- If present, suggests secondary bacterial infection

Adolescents and adults

■ Usually does not have distinct phases.

■ Persistent (>21 days) cough, indistinguishable from other respiratory infections, can be the only symptom.

■ Paroxysmal nature of the cough is present in approximately 70–99% of infected individuals.

■ Other features include:

- Inspiratory whoop

- Posttussive emesis

- Choking

- Sleep disturbed by cough

■ Positive predictors of confirmed pertussis include:

- History of prolonged duration of violent cough (median, 43 days)

- Longer duration of cough illness (median, 56 days)

- Posttussive emesis

■ Adults with pertussis do not have fever

DIFFERENTIAL DIAGNOSIS

In infants

■ Respiratory viral illnesses

■ Infection with *Chlamydia trachomatis* and with other *Bordetella* species

■ Bacterial pneumonia

■ Foreign body aspiration

■ Reactive airway disease

■ Adenovirus

- Can produce clinical syndrome of:

- Prolonged paroxysmal cough

- Posttussive emesis

- Inspiratory whoop

- Presence of associated features commonly found with adenovirus can help distinguish clinically

- Pharyngitis

- Conjunctivitis

■ Respiratory syncytial virus (RSV)

- A common cause of upper and lower respiratory tract infection in neonates and infants

- Dual infection with RSV and *B pertussis* can occur.

- Apnea is a common complication of both infections.

- Predominantly lower respiratory tract signs (wheezing), fever, and ongoing symptoms between cough episodes more suggestive of RSV

■ *Chlamydia trachomatis*

- A common cause of afebrile pneumonia in young infants

- Infants with chlamydial infection usually have:

- Staccato rather than paroxysmal cough

- Lower respiratory tract signs such as tachypnea and rales

- Frequent history of neonatal conjunctivitis

■ *Bordetella parapertussis* and rarely *Bordetella bronchiseptica*

- Characteristically cause a less protracted illness

■ Bacterial pneumonia caused by *Staphylococcus aureus* and *Streptococcus pneumoniae*

- Not difficult to distinguish based on the clinical manifestations

- High temperature

- Ill appearance

- Respiratory distress

- These agents can secondarily complicate pertussis infection.

In the older child, adolescent, and adult

■ Adenoviral infection

■ *Mycoplasma pneumoniae*

- Common cause of prolonged cough and may be difficult to distinguish

- Suggested by presence of systemic symptoms such as:

- Headache

- Sore throat

- Rales on auscultation of the chest

- Chest radiograph that characteristically appears worse than the appearance of the patient would indicate

■ *Chlamydophila pneumoniae*

■ Reactive airway disease

■ Upper respiratory tract infection

■ Concurrent outbreaks have been reported.

DIAGNOSTIC APPROACH

- Definitive diagnosis of pertussis is problematic.
- A complete history is by far the most important aspect of the evaluation of the infant or child with possible pertussis.
- Clinical diagnosis can be supplemented by:
  - Physical examination
  - Laboratory studies
  - Radiographic studies
- Physical examination usually normal
- Diagnosis may be missed if attention is not paid to historical description of coughing paroxysms.
- Cough paroxysms in a young infant should be witnessed by a medical professional before a disposition is planned.

LABORATORY FINDINGS

- Culture
  - Isolation of the organism by culture is the diagnostic standard.
    - Highly dependent on appropriate specimen collection, transport, and isolation technique
  - Culture is obtained from the posterior nasopharynx using a calcium alginate or Dacron-tipped (not cotton-tipped) swab.
  - Specimen should be immediately inoculated onto Regan-Lowe medium and incubated for 7 days.
  - Semisolid transport media is available if specimen cannot be inoculated immediately onto solid media.
  - Even in ideal conditions, sensitivity of culture is suboptimal.
    - Most likely to be positive early in the illness (catarrhal and early paroxysmal phase) in unimmunized children
    - Greatly diminished when obtained late in the illness, in immunized individuals, and in those who have received macrolides or sulfonamides
- Polymerase chain reaction (PCR) testing
  - Nasopharyngeal specimens
  - Appears to be more sensitive than culture, including in individuals who are mildly symptomatic and in those who have been treated with macrolides.
  - Sensitivity highly dependent on the age of the patient; likely a reflection of past immunization and immune responses
    - 60–70% sensitive in infants and young children
    - <10% sensitive in older children and adults
  - PCR also can detect *B parapertussis*.
- Direct fluorescent antibody testing for pertussis antigens
  - Nasopharyngeal specimens
  - Plagued by poor sensitivity when compared with culture
  - Requires experienced laboratories for accuracy
  - Rarely used today

- Serologic testing for detection of antibodies to components of *B pertussis* in acute and convalescent samples
  - The most sensitive mode of diagnosis
  - Used extensively in epidemiologic studies and vaccine trials
  - Not readily available
  - Results are difficult to interpret in immunized individuals
  - Not helpful for the diagnosis of pertussis

IMAGING

- Chest radiography in infants and children
  - Commonly normal
  - May reveal:
    - Perihilar infiltrates
    - Pneumothorax
    - Pneumomediastinum

TREATMENT APPROACH

- Supportive care is the mainstay of management.
- Hospitalization is indicated for most infants <6 months of age
  - To assess for life-threatening events associated with paroxysms, such as:
    - Apnea
    - Bradycardia
    - Hypoxia
- Hospitalization provides:
  - Continuous cardiorespiratory monitoring
  - Vigilant suctioning of the nasopharynx
  - Oxygen therapy if needed
  - Careful attention to feeding and hydration
  - Monitoring and treatment of acute complications
- A macrolide antibiotic is indicated for proven or suspected pertussis to:
  - Eliminate the organism from the nasopharynx
  - Limit spread to others
- If administered early, this therapy can reduce duration and severity of symptoms.
- These agents have little influence on clinical course of pertussis unless use is started early in the catarrhal phase.

SPECIFIC TREATMENTS

Macrolide agents

- Erythromycin traditionally has been antibiotic of choice.
- Newer macrolide agents—clarithromycin and azithromycin—are:
  - As effective in persons aged 6 months and older
  - Better tolerated
  - Associated with fewer and milder adverse effects

P

■ Based on these data, the Centers for Disease Control and Prevention developed guidelines recommending that erythromycin, clarithromycin, and azithromycin be used for the treatment of pertussis in persons aged 1 month and older.

■ Although studies evaluating the safety and efficacy of the newer macrolides for infants younger than 6 months are limited, their use is encouraged based on:

- In vitro effectiveness
- Demonstrated safety in older infants and children
- More convenient dosing schedule

■ Erythromycin therapy is associated with infantile hypertrophic pyloric stenosis.

- Thus azithromycin is the preferred macrolide in infants younger than 1 month.
- Limited data to date have not documented an association between azithromycin and infantile hypertrophic pyloric stenosis.

Antimicrobial treatment and postexposure prophylaxis by age group

■ <1 month

- Azithromycin 10 mg/kg/day as single daily dose for 5 days

■ 1–5 months

- Azithromycin 10 mg/kg/day as single daily dose for 5 days *or*
- Erythromycin 40–50 mg/kg/day in 4 divided doses for 14 days *or*
- Clarithromycin 15 mg/kg/day in two divided doses for 7 days

■ Infants 6 months and older and children

- Azithromycin 10 mg/kg/day as single dose on day 1 then 5 mg/kg/day (maximum 500 mg) on days 2–5 *or*
- Erythromycin 40–50 mg/kg/day (maximum 2 g/day) in 4 divided doses for 14 days *or*
- Clarithromycin 15 mg/kg/day in 2 divided doses (maximum 1 g/day) for 7 days

■ Adults

- Azithromycin 500 mg as single daily dose on day 1, then 250 mg/day on days 2–5 *or*
- Erythromycin 2 g/day in 4 divided doses for 14 days *or*
- Clarithromycin 1 g/day in 2 divided doses for 7 days

■ Treatment of parapertussis is the same as for pertussis.

Care of household and other close contacts

■ A macrolide should be given promptly to all household and close contacts (eg, those in child care).

■ Chemoprophylaxis

- Significantly reduces but does not eliminate risk of pertussis
- Should be given to close contacts regardless of age and immunization status

- Should be given to health care workers with definite or likely exposure

■ Antimicrobial agents that should be used for postexposure prophylaxis are the same as for treatment.

■ Trimethoprim-sulfamethoxazole

- An alternative treatment or prophylactic option for patients who cannot tolerate macrolides
- Contraindicated in infants younger than 2 months

WHEN TO ADMIT

■ Strongly consider in any young infant younger than 6 months suspected of having pertussis

■ When complications such as apnea, bacterial pneumonia, bradycardia, or pulmonary hypertension exist

■ When the infant has an oxygen requirement or when the infection is interfering with feeding

COMPLICATIONS

■ Secondary bacterial pneumonia is the most common complication.

- Occurs in ~5% of all reported cases
- Causes most pertussis-related deaths

■ Infants <6 months have highest rate of hospitalization (69%), secondary bacterial pneumonia (13%), and seizures (2%).

■ Important complications include:

- Apnea
- Bradycardia
- Dehydration
- Pulmonary hypertension
- Pneumothorax
- Central nervous system changes
- Retinal hemorrhages

■ Complications are much more common in infants.

■ In adults, morbidity includes:

- Pneumonia
- Otitis media
- Sinusitis
- Rib fracture
- Pneumothorax
- Pneumomediastinum
- Weight loss
- Urinary incontinence

PROGNOSIS

■ Young infants have the highest incidence of morbidity and mortality.

- 91% of pertussis-related deaths occur in children <6 months

PREVENTION

- AAP recommends universal immunization with pertussis vaccines for children <7 years of age.
  - Vaccination of all children starting in infancy has resulted in >97% decrease in incidence of pertussis in the US.
- Currently available acellular vaccines have been shown to be 75–90% effective and well tolerated.
  - Purified subunit vaccines
  - Combination vaccines with diphtheria and tetanus toxoids (diphtheria-tetanus-acellular pertussis [DTaP])
- AAP recommends that a total of 5 doses of pertussis vaccine be administered to every child before school entry, unless contraindicated.
  - First dose at 2 months of age
  - 2 subsequent doses at intervals of 2 months
  - Fourth dose at 15–18 months
  - Fifth dose at 4–6 years
- Because of the role that adolescents and adults play in transmission, studies have evaluated efficacy and safety of acellular pertussis vaccines in these age groups.
  - Adverse reactions to these vaccines among adolescents and adults have been mild.
  - Although these vaccines appear well tolerated in trials to date, concern exists about the possibility of more severe limb swelling in individuals vaccinated with booster doses of acellular vaccines after primary immunization with the same acellular vaccines.
    - However, limb swelling does not appear to be a problem in those who received whole-cell vaccine as their primary immunization.

- Thus adolescents and adults who previously received acellular vaccines will need to be observed closely when given booster doses to determine the frequency and severity of such reactions.
- AAP recommends that adolescents aged 11–18 years receive acellular pertussis vaccine combined with tetanus and reduced diphtheria toxoid (Tdap).
  - Single dose of Tdap instead of tetanus and diphtheria toxoids (Td) vaccine for booster immunization for adolescents 11–18 years of age.
  - The preferred age for Tdap immunization is 11–12 years.
  - Adolescents 11–18 years of age who have received Td but not Tdap are encouraged to receive a single dose of Tdap.
- An interval of at least 5 years between Td and Tdap is suggested.
- Intervals <5 years can be used, particularly in settings of:
  - Increased risk
  - Complicated disease
  - Danger of transmitting infection to vulnerable contacts

P

Petechiae and Purpura

DEFINITION

- Petechiae
  - Small (1–3 mm), red, nonblanching macular lesions caused by intradermal capillary bleeding
- Purpura
  - Larger, typically raised lesions resulting from bleeding within the skin

EPIDEMIOLOGY

- May occur at any age

MECHANISM

- Petechiae and purpura result from a wide variety of underlying disorders.
  - Petechiae are caused by intradermal capillary bleeding.
  - Purpura result from bleeding within the skin.

HISTORY

- Evaluation begins with a complete history.
  - Can readily eliminate a majority of disorders from the differential diagnosis
- Special attention to:
  - Recent trauma
  - Bleeding history
  - Medication use
  - Symptoms consistent with:
    - Infection
    - Malignancy
    - Autoimmune disorders
    - Rheumatologic disorders

PHYSICAL EXAM

- Petechiae
  - Small (1–3 mm), red, nonblanching macular lesions
- Purpura
  - Larger
  - Typically raised lesions
  - Can vary somewhat in color
    - Based on the age of the lesion as the blood within the skin is metabolized
  - Do not blanch
  - May occur anywhere on the body
- Physical examination should determine:
  - If skin findings are isolated
  - If evidence of a more generalized process is present
- Particular physical findings to evaluate include:
  - Hepatosplenomegaly
  - Lymphadenopathy
  - Arthritis
  - Arthralgias
  - Findings consistent with an acute viral syndrome

DIFFERENTIAL DIAGNOSIS

General

- Neither petechiae nor purpura are pathognomonic of a specific disorder.
- Petechiae and purpura must be evaluated according to:
  - Overall context of the patient
  - Severity and extent of lesions
  - History and age of the patient
- Clinician must entertain a broad differential diagnosis:
  - Hemostasis
  - Infection
  - Autoimmune disorders
  - Trauma
  - Malignancy
  - Other rare causes
- Underlying pathophysiological mechanism may be defined by:
  - Age at presentation
  - Overall appearance
  - Extent of the lesions
- Scant petechiae on the face of an otherwise well-appearing newborn after a vaginal delivery are likely caused by the trauma of passing through the birth canal.
  - Newborn with diffuse petechiae warrants further evaluation.
- If the child appears ill:
  - Sepsis must be strongly considered.
- If the child appears well:
  - Platelet disorder should be considered.
- With petechiae or purpura the possibility of a hemostatic defect is always a concern.
  - For isolated petechiae, the clinician must consider a primary platelet disorder:
    - Low platelet number
    - Platelet dysfunction
  - Purpura may result from a platelet disorder or other coagulation defect.
    - Can be classified as primary or as a secondary phenomenon from an underlying disease
  - Platelet disorders can be classified as disorders of:
    - Platelet production
    - Platelet survival (destruction)
    - Platelet function

- Clinician must consider thrombocytopenia as the proximate cause.
- Normal platelet count is 150,000–450,000/mm^3.
- Low platelet counts
  - >80,000: child will be hemostatically normal as long as platelet function is not altered.
  - 50,000–80,000: increased bleeding with trauma is likely, but spontaneous bleeding would be unusual.
  - 20,000–50,000: a mild bleeding diathesis is expected.
  - <20,000, spontaneous mucosal bleeding can occur.
  - <10,000: spontaneous severe bleeding is a danger.

Infectious causes of petechiae and purpura

- Mechanism by which a variety of viruses cause thrombocytopenia is not clear.
  - May involve:
    - Decreased platelet production
    - Immune-mediated destruction
  - Live-virus vaccinations can cause moderate thrombocytopenia.
    - Varicella
    - Measles
  - Cytomegalovirus has been implicated in thrombocytopenia.
    - Treatment of cytomegalovirus has not affected the outcome of patients monitored for chronic thrombocytopenia.
  - Parvovirus has been associated with:
    - Isolated thrombocytopenia
    - Pancytopenia
  - Dengue fever and other viral hemorrhagic fevers are known to cause thrombocytopenia.
    - Patients may develop petechiae and purpura as a result.
  - Rickettsial diseases such as Rocky Mountain spotted fever may produce a petechial rash.
  - Alterations of the endothelial lining of blood vessels cause:
    - Thrombi formation
    - Platelet destruction
  - Thrombocytopenia and disseminated intravascular coagulation (DIC) may develop.
  - Malaria can cause either mild or profound thrombocytopenia; mechanisms are not well defined.
  - HIV has been associated with thrombocytopenia resulting from bone marrow suppression.
    - Poor production
    - Immune-mediated destruction
- Platelet consumption is common in children with bacteremia and sepsis before frank DIC has developed.

- In an ill-appearing child with petechiae or purpura:
  - Infectious causes must be considered.
  - Appropriate antibiotics administered based on likely pathogens
- Bacterial meningitis must be considered for the febrile child with petechiae or purpura.
- Purpura fulminans has been associated with
  - Viral infections
  - *Streptococcus*
  - *Meningococcus*
- Microscopic thromboses in arterioles result in
  - Purpura
  - Infarction
  - Bleeding within the skin and subcutaneous tissue
- These lesions may coalesce and become necrotic.
  - Patients typically develop full DIC.

Disorders of platelet production: malignancy and bone marrow failure syndrome

- Most patients with petechiae or purpura have a benign process.
  - The greatest concern for clinician and parents is malignancy.
- History must rule out the classic signs and symptoms of malignancy:
  - Fevers
  - Night sweats
  - Weight loss
  - Lymphadenopathy or other masses
  - Pallor
  - Malaise
  - Bone pain
  - Anorexia
- Many of these symptoms overlap with those seen in infectious and autoimmune processes.
- Petechiae or purpura in the setting of hepatosplenomegaly or impressive lymphadenopathy would put leukemia high on the differential diagnosis.
- Other marrow infiltrating malignancies must be considered.
  - Chest radiograph should be obtained immediately.
    - Patients may have occult but massive mediastinal lymphadenopathy.
- Petechiae and purpura may be the presenting signs in patients with bone marrow failure secondary to nonmalignant processes.
  - Abnormal hematopoiesis usually causes *pancytopenia*, defined as alteration of more than one cell line, or even all cell lines.

P

- Bone marrow failure may occur secondary to:
  - Infectious processes
    - Viral
    - Bacterial with sepsis
  - Medication use, notably a variety of antibiotics and anticonvulsants
  - Profound nutritional deficits
  - Rare bone marrow failure syndromes
    - Fanconi anemia
    - Myelodysplastic disease
    - Wiskott-Aldrich syndrome
- Indicated to rule out malignancy and define abnormal hematopoiesis
  - Bone marrow aspiration
  - Biopsy

Disorders of platelet function: primary platelet disorders

- Petechiae and purpura may result from a primary platelet disorder.
- Qualitative disorders result from platelet dysfunction.
  - Absolute platelet number is normal.
  - Platelets lose normal hemostatic function.
  - In most instances, platelet dysfunction is acquired from medication use.
  - Classic example is aspirin, which causes irreversible inhibition of cyclooxygenase within platelets.
  - Other causes of acquired platelet dysfunction
    - Uremia
    - Liver disease
  - Mechanisms of poor platelet function in these settings are not clear.
- von Willebrand disease
  - Typically produces mucocutaneous bleeding
  - Should be considered in patients who have:
    - Petechiae and purpura
    - Normal platelet count
    - No other obvious systemic disease
  - Most common bleeding disorder
    - Affects ~1% of the population.
  - Establish the diagnosis with:
    - Coagulation screening
    - Factor VIII and von Willebrand factor assays
- Variety of rare platelet function disorders
  - Can be considered in patients with:
    - Normal platelet number
    - Bleeding
    - Petechiae or purpura

- Can be diagnosed with:
  - Specialized platelet aggregation studies
  - Morphologic study of platelets
- These disorders are rare.
- Hematology consultation should be made to define disorders such as:
  - Glanzmann thrombasthenia
  - Bernard-Soulier syndrome
  - Hermansky-Pudlak syndrome
  - Chédiak-Higashi syndrome

Disorders of platelet survival (destruction)

- Isolated thrombocytopenia in an otherwise well child may lead to petechiae or purpura as the chief complaint.
- Idiopathic (or immune) thrombocytopenic purpura is a diagnosis of exclusion.
  - Produces profound isolated thrombocytopenia and petechiae or purpura
  - Few other findings on physical examination
  - Laboratory workup should be normal except for thrombocytopenia.
    - No other blood cell line is affected.
  - Microscopic review of the blood reveals platelets that are too few in number but large in size.
    - Indicates that they are young
    - Platelet lifespan is reduced to minutes or hours rather than the normal several days.
  - Incidence is highest in children 2–8 years of age.
  - Formerly, clinicians performed bone marrow aspirates to rule out malignancy or other bone marrow failure syndromes.
    - Most now believe that the diagnosis can be made clinically.
    - Bone marrow studies rarely are indicated.
- Typically, one-third of the total body platelet mass is sequestered within the spleen at any time.
  - Whatever the cause of increased spleen size, mild thrombocytopenia may result.
  - Common causes of hypersplenism include:
    - Liver disease
    - Variety of infections, such as Epstein-Barr virus, malaria
    - Metabolic diseases, such as Gaucher disease
  - Hypersplenism alone does not typically cause platelet counts <50,000.
    - Alternative explanations should be considered for patients with moderate–severe thrombocytopenia.

- Henoch-Schönlein purpura
  - Autoimmune vasculitic syndrome
  - Produces purpura in most patients
    - Classic distribution is on the buttocks and legs.
    - May be more disseminated
  - Other findings in Henoch-Schönlein purpura
    - Arthritis
    - Arthralgias
    - Abdominal pain
    - Renal impairment
- Hemolytic-uremic syndrome
  - Produces a constellation of findings:
    - Thrombocytopenia
    - Hemolytic anemia
    - Renal failure
  - Associated with a variety of infections, most notably *Escherichia coli* 0157:H7
- Thrombotic thrombocytopenic purpura
  - Distinct syndrome rarely seen in children
  - Shares some clinical features with hemolytic-uremic syndrome
  - Findings include:
    - Purpura
    - Thrombocytopenia
    - DIC
    - Hemolytic anemia
    - Elevated lactate dehydrogenase
- Giant vascular malformations may cause intravascular destruction of platelets.
  - Kasabach-Merritt syndrome is classic example of a giant hemangioma causing severe thrombocytopenia secondary to platelet destruction.
  - Lesions usually are readily apparent.
    - Multiple smaller vascular malformations that are more difficult to define may cause platelet destruction.
  - Thrombocytopenia or altered hemostasis may be associated with rare vascular disorders and connective tissue syndromes, such as
    - Hereditary telangiectasias
    - Ehlers-Danlos syndrome
    - Marfan syndrome
    - Osteogenesis imperfecta

LABORATORY EVALUATION

- History and physical examination dictate the appropriate laboratory evaluations.
- At minimum
  - Complete blood count with platelets and differential count
  - Prothrombin time and partial thromboplastin time
- If the history or physical examination is consistent with a malignancy, the following should be obtained immediately:
  - Complete blood count
  - Screening coagulation studies
  - Comprehensive metabolic panel
  - Liver function tests
  - Lactate dehydrogenase
  - Uric acid
  - Manual differential count of the peripheral blood
- Absence of leukemic blasts on a peripheral blood smear does *not* rule out leukemia.
- Diagnosis of leukemia can be made if peripheral blasts are present.
  - Having few or no peripheral blasts seen on routine microscopy is not uncommon for patients with leukemia.
- Isolated profound thrombocytopenia is not likely to result from a malignancy.
- When >1 cell line on a blood count is abnormal, bone marrow process must be considered.
- Laboratory findings consistent with malignancy include:
  - Elevated lactate dehydrogenase
  - Elevated uric acid
  - Abnormal serum electrolytes
    - May result from tumor lysis even before therapy is started

WHEN TO REFER

- Platelet count <100,000/mm³
- Diffuse petechiae or purpura
- Focal petechiae
- Purpura not clearly associated with trauma
- Evidence of >1 cell line abnormality on complete blood count

WHEN TO ADMIT

- Toxic-appearing patient
- Moderate to severe bleeding
- Concern for poor adherence

P

Pharyngitis and Tonsillitis

DEFINITION

- *Pharyngitis* implies inflammation of throat with or without presence of exudate.
- *Tonsillitis, tonsillopharyngitis,* and *pharyngotonsillitis* are used when tonsils are affected.

EPIDEMIOLOGY

- Prevalence
  - Acute pharyngitis is a very common diagnosis in pediatric practice.
    - Exceeded only by otitis media and viral upper respiratory tract infections
    - Most common diagnosis requiring treatment with antibiotics in school-age children
- Seasonality
  - Pharyngitis caused by coxsackievirus A and echovirus is common in late summer or early fall.
- Relative prevalence of infectious agents
  - Adenoviruses account for up to 23% of cases.
  - Epstein-Barr virus (EBV) is a copathogen of group A ß-hemolytic *Streptococcus* (GABHS) in 5–10% of cases.
  - Herpes simplex viruses
    - Studies in a college-aged population showed that herpes simplex virus types 1 and 2 account for 5.7% of pharyngitis cases.
  - GABHS
    - Not fully recognized as a frequent cause of pharyngitis with possibility of subsequent rheumatic fever until the 1940s
    - In children <3 years, GABHS is the cause of tonsillopharyngitis in <3% of cases.
    - In children >3 years, GABHS is the cause of 15–20% of pharyngitis episodes.
    - Ingestion of GABHS-contaminated food has led to outbreaks of pharyngitis.
  - *Corynebacterium diphtheriae*
    - Now rare in North America
      - Still being reported in some developing countries
  - *Haemophilus influenzae* type b (Hib)
    - As many as 20% of sampled tonsils have Hib infection.
      - In recent years, most infants in the US have Hib immunization.
    - Because of immunization, the organism may be less likely to play a role in pathogenesis of acute tonsillitis and pharyngitis.
  - *Arcanobacterium haemolyticum*
    - Causes ~7% of tonsillopharyngitis cases in adolescents and young adults
- *Mycoplasma pneumoniae*
  - In school-age children, as much as 5% of pharyngitis may be caused by this organism.

ETIOLOGY

Viruses

- Pharyngitis and tonsillitis are most commonly caused by viral agents.
  - Associated with upper respiratory tract symptoms, such as conjunctivitis, nasal congestion, and rhinorrhea
- Adenoviruses
  - At least 12 different types have been found to cause pharyngitis in children and adolescents.
  - Cause both nasopharyngitis and tonsillitis
  - Adenovirus type 3 causes the unique clinical illness pharyngoconjunctival fever.
- Enteroviruses
  - Coxsackievirus A and echovirus have been shown to cause pharyngitis.
  - Various strains of coxsackievirus A and B cause herpangina.
- EBV
  - Etiologic agent of infectious mononucleosis
  - Frequently causes a severe exudative pharyngitis
- Other viruses (though pharyngitis is usually not the primary manifestation of the illness) include:
  - Herpes simplex virus
  - Influenza
  - Parainfluenza
  - Respiratory syncytial virus
  - Human metapneumovirus
  - Measles
  - Coronavirus
  - Rhinoviruses

Bacteria

- Many primary care physicians associate pharyngitis and tonsillitis with bacterial origins.
  - However, GABHS and other bacterial agents are highly unlikely causes.
- GABHS is the most frequent bacterial cause.
  - GABHS can be divided into M and T serotypes, which have been associated with:
    - Rash of scarlet fever (GABHS T4)
    - Development of rheumatic fever (GABHS M3 and M18)
  - Pharyngitis caused by GABHS characteristically begins after a 2- to 5-day incubation period.
    - Usually after exposure to another individual who has the infection

- Spread occurs by way of respiratory secretions.
- Fomites have occasionally been shown to be vectors.
  - Shared silverware
  - Household cats (but not dogs)
- Other groups of *Streptococcus* (B, C, F, and G) have been associated with pharyngitis.
- *Neisseria gonorrhoeae*
  - Acquired from oral sex
    - Seek as cause of pharyngitis in sexually active adolescents or sexually abused children.
- Hib
  - Possible involvement of Hib organism in pharyngitis and tonsillitis (controversial)
  - Evidence suggests that it may contribute to infection in some children, especially those with recurrent tonsillitis.
- *Mycoplasma pneumoniae*
  - Causes mild pharyngitis in children
  - Associated with a laryngotracheitis or progressing to bronchitis or pneumonia
- Other bacteria include:
  - *C diphtheriae*
  - *A haemolyticum*
  - *Actinomyces*
  - *Chlamydia trachomatis*
  - *Chlamydia pneumoniae*
  - *Yersinia enterocolitica*
  - *Coxiella burnetii*
  - *Francisella tularensis* (oropharyngeal tularemia)
  - *Mycoplasma hominis*

Fungi

- *Candida* infection
  - Uncommon cause of pharyngitis in the healthy host
  - Can be seen in immunocompromised patients and in those taking corticosteroids

RISK FACTORS

- Exposure to cigarette smoke
  - Smoke itself has not been reported to cause pharyngitis or tonsillitis.
  - A significant association has been found between parental smoking and incidence of tonsillectomy in children.
    - Children of smokers also had a much higher frequency of attacks of acute tonsillitis compared with children in a smoke-free environment.

SIGNS AND SYMPTOMS

- A clinical complaint of sore throat indicates some degree of pharyngitis.

Viral causes

- Nasopharyngitis and tonsillitis caused by adenoviruses can be exudative.
- Pharyngoconjunctival fever
  - Cough
  - Myalgias
  - Conjunctivitis
- Herpangina
  - Typified by pharyngitis associated with small, shallow, ulcerated areas on soft palate and peritonsillar
  - Coxsackievirus A and echovirus
  - Often accompanied by respiratory symptoms
- EBV
  - White, shaggy membrane on tonsils and palatal petechiae
  - In older children, EBV infection is accompanied by:
    - Fever
    - Adenopathy
    - Malaise
    - Swelling of the eyelids
    - Hepatosplenomegaly
- Herpes simplex virus
  - Most oral colonization and covert infection with herpes simplex virus type 1 is asymptomatic.
  - Virus can cause painful gingivostomatitis and pharyngitis in ~1% of infected children.

Bacterial causes

- GABHS
  - Sudden onset of:
    - Fever
    - Sore throat
    - Dysphagia
    - Other associations include headache and abdominal pain.
  - Examination of throat reveals an erythematous pharynx and tonsillar area.
    - Often with exudate present
  - Small petechiae (enanthem) are sometimes seen on uvula and soft palate.
  - Cervical lymph nodes are usually enlarged and tender.
  - Symptoms can last for 4–5 days.
    - Gradually subsiding when no antibiotic therapy is instituted
  - Key findings
    - Red throat or tonsils and/or exudative tonsils
    - Swollen and usually tender anterior cervical nodes
    - Fever
    - Scarlet fever rash

P

- *N gonorrhoeae*
  - Exudative tonsillitis is rarely seen with pharyngitis caused by *N gonorrhoeae*.
- *C diphtheriae*
  - Characteristic gray pseudomembranous exudate over the posterior pharynx and tonsils
- *A haemolyticum*
  - Physical findings are identical to those seen with GABHS infection.
  - Includes a scarlatiniform rash present in ~20% of cases
  - Sore throat may persist until patients are treated with antibiotics.

DIFFERENTIAL DIAGNOSIS

- Sore throats are common in children.
  - May be sole finding in an illness
- Streptococcal infections should be considered in children >3 years who have pharyngitis.
  - Even if no exudate is present
  - Pharyngitis associated with nasal, chest, or cold symptoms is much more likely to be a viral illness.
- In atypical pharyngitis, either in duration or severity, suspect:
  - Infectious mononucleosis
  - 1 of the rarer bacterial causes
    - Including those that are sexually transmitted
- Peritonsillar abscess or cellulitis also may cause a sore throat.
  - Thorough examination will reveal:
    - Swelling extending into the soft palate
    - Deviation of the uvula
    - Change in tonal quality of the voice
- Postnasal drip from viral respiratory tract infection or allergies has been thought to irritate the posterior pharynx.
  - This finding is not well documented.
- Allergies may lead to chronic inflammation of the mucous membranes, which might include the pharynx.
  - Pharyngitis would be infrequent as the sole manifestation.
- Epiglottitis
  - Diagnosis that must not be missed
  - Can be life threatening
  - The child with epiglottitis:
    - Has severe throat pain
    - Rapidly becomes ill
    - Appears to have a toxic condition
    - Experiences respiratory distress accompanied by stridor or a croupy cough
- Kawasaki disease
  - Unknown cause

- Occurs mostly in preschool children who have:
  - Pharyngitis associated with erythema and fissuring of the lips
  - Palmar and pedal edema
  - Erythema
  - An association with staphylococcal toxin has been postulated, as have other viral and bacterial etiologies.
- Oral thrush
  - In otherwise healthy children, severe mouth pain can occur.
  - May be interpreted as a sore throat
- Pharyngitis may be associated with other inflammatory conditions of the mucous membranes.
  - Herpes gingivostomatitis
  - Herpangina
  - Stevens-Johnson syndrome

DIAGNOSTIC APPROACH

- The major step is to establish whether GABHS is the responsible pathogen.
  - Almost all children >3 years need to be examined to rule out GABHS as the cause.
  - Multiple studies have shown that streptococcal pharyngitis cannot be distinguished purely on clinical grounds.

LABORATORY FINDINGS

Rapid streptococcal test and cultures

- Traditional method for determining whether cause of pharyngitis or tonsillitis is viral or GABHS: obtain a throat swab and perform a culture.
  - With availability of rapid streptococcal tests, the process was made simpler.
    - Allows a result to be obtained in minutes rather than waiting 1–2 days
    - Strict federal guidelines for office laboratories require certification for use of these rapid tests.
    - Most clinicians now perform a rapid streptococcal diagnostic test on all patients whose pharyngitis is suggestive of GABHS.
- Various rapid streptococcal tests claim differing levels of specificity and sensitivity.
  - Appear to be specific (95–98%)
  - Sensitivity can be as low as 70–85%.
  - Some cases of GABHS are not detected.
  - Positive rapid streptococcal test result is a sufficient indication to treat the patient.
- Culture should be sent if:
  - Rapid test result is negative, but high index of suspicion exists that GABHS is the causative agent.

P

- Throat culture is not necessary:
  - If little clinical evidence of pharyngitis or tonsillitis can be found in a child with sore throat
  - In patients with manifestations highly suggestive of viral infection
    - Coryza
    - Conjunctivitis
    - Cough
    - Hoarseness
    - Herpangina
    - Stomatitis
    - Sindbis virus
- Some individuals are *Streptococcus* carriers.
  - They may be found to be positive for *Streptococcus* infection during a viral illness.
  - An asymptomatic *Streptococcus* carrier does not need to be treated.
    - When symptoms are present, most physicians treat these individuals.
  - Difficult to ascertain that GABHS is not the cause of illness
  - Performing pre- and post-illness rapid streptococcal tests or cultures on every child who presumably has GABHS pharyngitis is impractical.
    - All those who test positive are treated.

Serologic tests

- If EBV infection is suspected, a heterophile antibody or specific EBV test can be ordered.
  - Ascertain with the reference laboratory whether an immunoglobulin (Ig)G or IgM test has been performed.
    - A positive heterophile test result may confirm only that children were exposed sometime in their life to EBV.
  - Tests of specific IgG and IgM antibody to various components of EBV are available.
    - Usually expensive and slow to produce results
    - Less-than-ideal test to determine cause of acute pharyngitis
- Serologic tests exist to determine recent streptococcal infections.
  - Rarely helpful in evaluating for acute pharyngitis
  - Antistreptolysin-O titer is used more commonly in diagnosing rheumatic fever.
    - Documents recent exposure to streptolysin with production of antibody

Leukocyte count

- Only real value in performing is if infectious mononucleosis is suspected
  - Patients with acute EBV infection tend to have relative lymphocytosis.
    - 10–20% atypical lymphocytes

- The leukocyte count may be a helpful diagnostic study.
  - Combine with heterophile or specific EBV antibody test for children who have severe pharyngitis and are culture negative for GABHS

TREATMENT APPROACH

- Pharyngitis caused by viruses generally is treated symptomatically with:
  - Saline gargles
  - Throat lozenges
  - Analgesics, such as acetaminophen
- When GABHS has been documented, either by positive rapid *Streptococcus* test or by culture, antibiotics are indicated primarily to prevent subsequent development of rheumatic fever.
  - Early antibiotic treatment will shorten duration and severity of symptoms by 24–36 hours.
  - Patients should be kept out of school and avoid close contact with family and friends for only 24 hours.
    - Numerous studies have shown that they become culture negative after just 24 hours of antibiotic therapy.
- Controversy exists over whether to begin antibiotics for presumptive GABHS pharyngitis while waiting for culture results.
  - Rheumatic fever can be prevented even if treatment is started as late as the ninth day of symptoms.
  - The decision to begin therapy immediately rests with the individual physician who knows the circumstances.

SPECIFIC TREATMENTS

Antibiotic therapy
GABHS

- The presence of GABHS mandates early antimicrobial therapy.
  - Start within 9 days of onset of symptoms
- Various antibiotic regimens have been used for GABHS pharyngitis or tonsillitis
  - Standard therapy has been a 10-day oral course of potassium penicillin or amoxicillin given 2 or 3 times a day.
  - Alternatively, intramuscular benzathine penicillin G may be given as a single injection.
    - These injections are often painful not only initially, but also for a few days afterward.
  - Patients allergic to penicillin may be given:
    - Erythromycin or a cephalosporin for 10 days *or*
    - Azithromycin for 5 days
  - Shorter courses of newer antibiotics have been studied and shown to be effective in eradicating GABHS from the pharynx.
    - Their efficacy in preventing rheumatic fever is not clear, although presumed.

P

- Cephalosporins have been shown to be superior to penicillin in eradicating GABHS from pharynx.

Other bacteria

- Gonococcal pharyngitis
  - 1 intramuscular injection of ceftriaxone is recommended.
  - In young children with this diagnosis, sexual abuse must be investigated.
- *A haemolyticum*
  - Clarithromycin
  - Erythromycin
  - Azithromycin
- Other possible bacterial causes of pharyngitis are treated with appropriate antibiotics, once the causative organism has been determined.

Corticosteroids

- Administration of corticosteroids to decrease pain in acute exudative pharyngitis has been studied in adults and found to provide some benefit.
- Use in children is not recommended
  - Except in rare situations, such as infectious mononucleosis infection with imminent airway obstruction

Tonsillectomy

- Parents often raise the question of tonsillectomy after a child has multiple episodes of pharyngitis or tonsillitis.
  - Tonsillectomy is not indicated in children with recurrent pharyngitis except:
    - In cases of documented recurrent, frequent streptococcal infection
    - In those who develop peritonsillar abscess

WHEN TO ADMIT

- Toxic appearance (suspected toxic shock syndrome)
- Peritonsillar abscess
- Retropharyngeal abscess
- Acute rheumatic fever

WHEN TO REFER

- Suspected peritonsillar abscess
- Suspected retropharyngeal abscess
- Recurrent GABHS (5 episodes in 1 year) for tonsillectomy

FOLLOW-UP

- The physician must be aware of the possibility of peritonsillar or retropharyngeal abscess or cellulitis.
  - Should reexamine the throat of any patient who is not improving

COMPLICATIONS

- Most cases of pharyngitis present no unusual complications.
  - Many are viral.
  - Resolve with or without therapy
- Acute tonsillopharyngitis may progress to a peritonsillar abscess.
  - Infection begins with the typical signs and symptoms of pharyngitis, such as:
    - Sore throat
    - Dysphagia
    - Fever
  - Usually in an older child who often has a history of recurrent tonsillitis
  - Systemic symptoms may develop.
    - Malaise
    - Poor appetite
    - Chills
    - Mild dehydration
  - Symptoms progress rapidly to more severe pharyngeal symptoms.
    - Difficulty in swallowing and speaking
    - The child has a toxic appearance.
    - Trismus almost always occurs.
  - The characteristic signs are:
    - Muffled (hot potato) voice, trismus, and major leukocytosis
  - Needle aspiration can be performed only if the abscess is within the superior pole.
    - The success rate of needle aspiration compares favorably with that of incision and drainage in these type cases.
  - Computed tomography and intraoral ultrasonography are quite reliable in distinguishing abscesses from cellulitis alone.
  - Initial antimicrobial therapy is clindamycin *plus* a third-generation cephalosporin, such as:
    - Ceftriaxone
    - Cefotaxime
    - Ceftazidime
  - Routine tonsillectomy along with or after medical management is recommended.
- Other suppurative complications can also develop, such as:
  - Cervical adenitis
  - Acute otitis media
  - Sinusitis
  - Pneumonia

- Hematogenous spread of a bacterial organism is possible, which can result in:
  - Bacteremia
  - Joint, bone, or meningeal infection
- Rheumatic fever is the major complication of streptococcal pharyngitis.
  - Can be life threatening
  - Occurs some time after the acute throat infection
  - The incidence of rheumatic fever is low in North America.
    - Still occurs and has been seen in increasing numbers
- Acute glomerulonephritis is possible after streptococcal throat infections.
  - Much more likely after streptococcal skin infections
- Some evidence has shown association between GABHS infection and obsessive-compulsive disorders and tic behavior in children.
  - This clinical entity is termed *pediatric autoimmune neuropsychiatric disorder associated with group A streptococcal infection* (PANDAS).

- Documentation is largely anecdotal.
  - Includes the observation that these children have high concentrations of antibody to streptococcal antigens
- Small series have noted improvement in obsessive-compulsive disorder behavior or tics when these children are GABHS positive and treated with penicillin.
- Many still question the authenticity of PANDAS.

PREVENTION

- History of parental smoking should be sought.
  - If history exists, advise measures to reduce the child's exposure to cigarette smoke.

P

Phimosis

DEFINITION

- *Phimosis:* unretractile foreskin

EPIDEMIOLOGY

- Prevalence
  - Problems and questions related to the foreskin of young boys are frequently seen in pediatric practices.
  - Most of the referrals made to urologists are for boys with physiologic phimosis.
  - True phimosis is uncommon: ~1 case per 1,000 boys
    - Rate obtained after looking at pathologic specimens after circumcision
    - Individuals with evidence of inflammation were counted as true phimosis.
- Age
  - In children, balanitis occurs most frequently between the ages of 2 and 5 years.

ETIOLOGY

- Pathologic phimosis is believed to have several different causes.
  - Chronic nonspecific inflammatory process
  - Repeated infections that cause scarring and stricture
  - Forcible premature retraction of the foreskin, causing scarring and adhesions
  - Balanitis xerotica obliterans (BXO): a chronic dermatitis
    - Unknown etiology
    - Causes pathologic phimosis
- Balanoposthitis
  - Most common causative organisms are:
    - *Staphylococcus*
    - Coliforms
    - *Pseudomonas*
    - *Candida*
  - Potential cause is *Streptococcus*
    - Can cause a thin purulent discharge in the preputial-glanular sulcus (but not from the urethra)
    - Associated with a red, glistening glans
  - Sexually transmitted infections (gonorrhea and chlamydia) must be considered when purulent discharge from the urethra is present.
    - Presence of sexually transmitted infections in the absence of purulent discharge is extremely unlikely in a prepubertal boy.

RISK FACTORS

- Risks for nonspecific balanitis include:
  - Poor hygiene
  - Trauma
  - Irritation from soaps or detergents

SIGNS AND SYMPTOMS

Phimosis

- Can be either physiologic or pathologic
- At birth, most boys have physiologic phimosis.
  - Inner surface of the foreskin is developmentally fused to the glans penis.
- Over time, desquamation and glanular secretions allow gradual separation of the foreskin.
- Smegma
  - The epithelial debris generated during desquamation
  - Sometimes can be seen under the foreskin as pearls
    - Requires no intervention
- Accumulations are released as the foreskin becomes more retractile.
  - May be mistaken for infection
- Retractability increases yearly.
  - By 1 year of age, 50% of uncircumcised boys have retractile foreskins.
  - By age 3, 90%
  - By age 6–7, 92%
  - By adolescence, 99%
- Lack of clear diagnostic criteria makes it difficult to distinguish pathologic from physiologic phimosis.
  - *Physiologic phimosis* is described as unretractile foreskin that is supple and unscarred.
    - On attempted retraction, foreskin lies flat against the penis and is effaced.
    - Tip opens as a flower (see Figure 59 on page F21).
    - Young boys may exhibit preputial adhesions where part of the foreskin does not completely retract.
    - No visible constricting ring
    - Not pathologic
    - Resolves on its own
  - In *pathologic phimosis,* margin between foreskin and glans is rolled and thickened.
- BXO
  - Histologically resembles lichen sclerosus et atrophicus

Paraphimosis

- Occurs when the foreskin is retracted, is not replaced immediately, and becomes trapped behind corona
  - May happen during cleaning
  - May occur during procedures such as catheterization
- Fibrous ring at the base of the corona causes venous congestion.
  - Leads to:
    - Extreme penile pain
    - Swelling of the glans with a collar of swollen foreskin at the coronal sulcus

Balanitis or balanoposthitis

- Characterized by:
  - Erythema
  - Edema of prepuce that produces purulent discharge from the preputial orifice
    - Edema can involve some of the penile shaft.
- Patients may complain of dysuria.
- Condition usually occurs when the prepuce is wholly or partially retractable.

LABORATORY FINDINGS

- Sexually transmitted infections
  - Appropriate diagnostic tests (DNA probes) should be obtained.

TREATMENT APPROACH

- Treatment approach depends on whether the phimosis is thought to be physiologic or pathologic.
  - Watchful waiting results in resolution of most cases of physiologic phimosis.
  - Treatment alternatives if child is believed to have pathologic phimosis include:
    - Topical corticosteroid cream
    - Surgery
- Choice regarding which patients should be referred and receive therapy may be unclear.
- Little agreement exists in the literature.
- Circumcision should be undertaken for:
  - BXO
  - Phimosis resistant to corticosteroid therapy
  - Voiding problems
  - Recurrent balanitis
  - Urinary tract infections
- Ballooning of the foreskin during micturition is not, by itself, a reason for circumcision.
- Most cases of phimosis probably are physiologic and will resolve spontaneously over time.

- Some urologists question whether true phimosis can exist before age 5 and question whether any treatment need be initiated.
- Others use the age of 3 years as an upper limit and initiate a trial of corticosteroid creams (if no indication for surgery) at that time.
- Argument in favor of treating children who are younger (>3 but <5 or 6):
  - Most noninvasive therapy (topical corticosteroids) is more successful in younger children than older children.
  - Compliance is greater at that age because parents are able to apply the cream.
  - When older children become responsible for cream application, compliance and success decrease.

SPECIFIC TREATMENTS

Phimosis

- Topical corticosteroid creams
  - Multiple studies have investigated the use of topical corticosteroid creams.
  - 4- to 8-week course of therapy has been found to be approximately 85% effective.
  - High-potency corticosteroid creams such as 0.05% betamethasone have been studied the most.
  - Medium-potency topical corticosteroid (clobetasone butyrate 0.05%) has been shown to have similar resolution rates.
    - Lower-strength corticosteroid may be an option.
  - Creams are applied to the tip of the prepuce and down to its junction with the glans.
    - Twice a day for 4–8 weeks
  - Corticosteroids are believed to be therapeutic by
    - Decreasing any potential inflammation between the foreskin and glans
    - Thinning the skin, making it more supple
  - Topical corticosteroid therapy has multiple advantages over more traditional surgical management:
    - Less invasive
    - Avoids risks of surgery: bleeding, deformity, meatal stenosis
    - No anesthesia risks
    - Cost effective—25% the cost of surgery
    - Preservation of prepuce may be desired for social and cultural reasons.
    - Neurologically complex and erogenous tissue
    - Avoids potential emotional problems
      - Some boys who undergo circumcision at an older age may develop severe emotional problems.

P

■ Surgery

- Surgical alternatives include dorsal slit surgery or circumcision
- Dorsal slit procedure involves making a single slit dorsally in the foreskin.
  - Preserves the prepuce
  - Allows easy retraction of the foreskin
  - Surgery is less involved than circumcision.
  - Cosmetic result is not as satisfactory as with circumcision.
  - Can be complicated by scarring
- Circumcision is more commonly used.
- Forced premature retraction of the foreskin is *never* recommended.
  - May lead to significant adhesions and scarring
  - Painful
  - Traumatic

Paraphimosis

■ Paraphimosis is a urologic emergency.

■ Goal of treatment is to replace the foreskin in its normal position.

- In early stages, the foreskin may be replaceable manually without sedation.
- As condition progresses, anesthesia may be required:
  - Penile block
  - Sedation
  - General anesthesia

■ Gentle persistent pressure is used to decrease edema and allow reduction of foreskin.

- Ice packs or a compressive elastic dressing decrease swelling.
- Sometimes, to relieve swelling
  - Incision must be made in the fibrous ring.
  - Multiple punctures must be made in the glans.

Balanoposthitis

■ Local hygienic measures

- Sitz baths
- Gentle cleaning
- 1% hydrocortisone cream

■ If irritation does not resolve, treatment with antimicrobials may be necessary.

■ Circumcision usually is considered only for recurrent episodes.

WHEN TO ADMIT

■ Paraphimosis

- Failure of manual reduction with vascular compromise of the glans

■ Balanoposthitis

- Systemic infection or sepsis
- Inability to urinate
- Vascular compromise of the glans

WHEN TO REFER

■ Phimosis

- Failure of topical corticosteroids
- BXO
- Parents desire circumcision
- Association with urinary tract abnormalities/obstructive uropathy

■ Paraphimosis

- Failure of manual reduction

■ Balanoposthitis

- Recurrent episodes

COMPLICATIONS

■ Paraphimosis

- If no treatment is initiated, ischemia and necrosis of the glans can result.

P

Phobias and Anxiety

DEFINITION

- **Phobia**
  - Extreme and persistent fear of an object, event, or situation that in reality is not dangerous to the individual
  - The feared object, event, or situation would not be of concern to most people.
  - Phobias are divided into 3 categories.
    - Specific phobia
    - Social phobia
    - Agoraphobia (often associated with panic disorder)
- **Specific phobia**
  - Fears related to a single stimulus for ≥6 months
  - Categories of feared stimuli commonly include:
    - Animals
    - Insects
    - Certain situations (eg, health care or dental care procedures)
    - Objects in the natural environment
  - Exposure to the feared stimulus or even thoughts of the feared stimulus result in an immediate anxiety response.
    - Physiologic (tachycardia, sweating)
    - Cognitive (thoughts of being harmed)
    - Emotional reactivity (crying, tantrums)
- **Social phobia**
  - More complex and potentially more disabling diagnosis than a specific phobia
  - Often begins in late childhood or early adolescence
  - Characterized by evident fear of social or performance situations for ≥6 months
  - The child has fears of doing or saying something that will be socially inappropriate and thus humiliating.
  - Typical situations that trigger fears include:
    - Reading aloud in front of class
    - Making a telephone call
    - Joining conversation with peers
    - Going to parties
    - Ordering at restaurants
  - Such children limit contacts.
  - At risk for social immaturity and stigmatization by other children
- **Agoraphobia**
  - Fear of being in places from which:
    - Escape may not be possible
    - Help might not be available
  - Often begins in late adolescence

- May be associated with:
  - Panic disorder
  - Fears of panic
  - Fears of embarrassing happenings
- Individuals often progressively limit outside activities.
- Persistent and disabling if left untreated

EPIDEMIOLOGY

- **Prevalence**
  - In a large-scale population studies of adults, phobias and other anxiety disorders are the most frequent psychiatric disorders occurring in the general population.
- No comparable studies of the frequency of psychiatric disorders in childhood or adolescence have been conducted.
- Most common specific phobias occurring in children and adolescents involve:
  - Animals
  - Insects
  - Objects in the natural environment
    - Storms
    - Water
- Other common phobias of closed spaces (*claustrophobia*) and heights (*acrophobia*) are much less frequent in children.
  - Tend to have their origins in adulthood
- Other common phobias are associated with:
  - Injury
  - Blood
  - Health care
    - Injections
    - Other invasive medical procedures
- **Age**
  - Phobias are common in all age groups.
    - In Rutter's Isle of Wight Study, ~2.5% of children had disabling specific fears or phobias.
    - A more recent community study found specific phobias in 2.6% of children.
    - In a study of children and adolescents with anxiety disorders, except for separation anxiety disorders, specific phobias and social phobias were extremely common.
  - Likely to begin before the age of 7 years

ETIOLOGY

- Various theoretic speculations about the cause of phobias
  - Early theories postulated unconscious conflicts as the source.
  - Others suggest phobias are learned responses in the context of a child's experience.

- In recent years, increased emphasis has been placed on the way in which factors affect the development of childhood anxiety disorders.
  - Genetic influences
  - Temperamental predispositions
  - Parental functioning
  - Practices
- A multidimensional understanding of the cause of such childhood disturbances is crucial to best practices in diagnostic and treatment approaches.

SIGNS AND SYMPTOMS

Relevant history

- A complete history will usually help define possible diagnoses in the primary care setting.
- Further assessment should be prompted by reports of:
  - Fearful behavior
  - Symptoms of anxiety
  - Development of avoidance behavior or compulsions
    - Repetitive, purposeful, intentional behaviors in response to fears or obsessions
- Some important areas to screen include:
  - Onset of symptoms, including review of recent life changes (deaths, births, moves)
  - Specific history of symptoms and associated behaviors
  - Circumstances in which symptoms occur
  - Responses of parents, teachers, peers, and others to symptoms
  - Review of the patient's general pattern of psychosocial development
- Children, and more commonly adolescents, may recognize that their fear is irrational.
  - May invent another reason for avoidance behavior
  - The possibility of a traumatic experience with the phobic object should be explored.
    - Frightening experience
    - Being lost
    - Threatened
    - Abused
- Social anxiety can sometimes produce depressive symptoms that mask anxiety symptoms.
  - Use of a brief screening instrument can help the primary care physician identify anxiety symptoms.
  - Depending on the level of impairment, the primary care physician can decide whether to:
    - Intervene
    - Consult
    - Refer to a mental health specialist

- Practitioners should review available screening instruments to determine which best fits their practice.
- Consultation with mental health care provider can help selection.
- Self-report for Childhood Anxiety Related Emotional Disorders
  - 41 items
  - Takes an average of 5 minutes to complete
  - Can be used with children age ≥8 years
- The Liebowitz Social Anxiety Scale—Child Adolescent Version screens for social anxiety symptoms.
  - 24 items
  - Takes an average of 10–20 minutes to complete
  - Can be used with children age ≥7 years
- Providing results of initial screening and assessment to mental health care specialist is helpful.
  - Especially if the primary care practitioner has an established relationship with the patient
- Children do not typically realize their fears are unreasonable.
- In extreme cases, panic may occur for adolescents.
- The degree to which avoidance or anticipatory anxiety occurs is often a critical factor in parents' seeking help.

Physical

- Thorough physical examination should be completed if physical problems are likely.
- Producing symptoms similar to anxiety
  - Hypoglycemia
  - Hyperthyroidism
  - Pheochromocytoma
- Withdrawal from some abused substances may be associated with episodes of severe anxiety.
- Side effects from prescribed medications may produce similar symptoms.
- Key symptoms of phobias include avoidance of the fear-provoking object or situation and fear often associated with:
  - Sweating
  - Tachycardia
  - Difficulty in breathing
  - Light-headedness or dizziness
- According to the *Diagnostic and Statistical Manual of Mental Disorders, Fourth Edition, Text Revision (DSM-IV-TR)*, children may express anxiety by:
  - Crying
  - Tantrums
  - Clinging
  - Freezing

DIFFERENTIAL DIAGNOSIS

Phobias and development

- Some fears are common and expected at various developmental levels.
  - Stranger anxiety
    - Seen at ~8 months of age
    - Decreases around the middle of 2nd year
  - Toddlers are commonly fearful of being left alone or with babysitters.
  - Preschool children are afraid of the dark.
  - Parents often do not consult physicians about these common fears.
- Many children have fears that meet criteria for a diagnosis of specific phobia, but then disappear without specific intervention.
  - Avoidance behavior associated with a phobia may interfere with:
    - Usual activities
    - Productive social relationships
  - Animal phobias may prevent a child from:
    - Playing with neighbors
    - Attending after-school activities
  - When a particular specific phobia disappears spontaneously, consequences linger.
    - Missed opportunities
    - Embarrassment
    - Interference with social development
- Social phobias commonly occur in adolescence as the importance and impact of peer interactions emerges.
  - Teenagers turn toward peers to help with identity development.
    - This process can be interrupted if adolescent has intense fears about social interactions.

Psychiatric disorders

- As defined by the *DSM-IV-TR*, other psychiatric disorders have overlapping symptoms.
- Separation anxiety disorders
  - Children are afraid of leaving parents or others to whom they are attached.
  - Fear something may happen to parents when they are not present
  - Fear of the dark, animals, or objects
  - Unlike a specific phobia, the added fear of separation from loved ones exists.
  - School phobia or school refusal is a specific manifestation.

- Selective mutism
  - Persistent failure to speak in certain social situations
    - The child will talk in other situations.
  - Rare
  - Usually occurs by 5 years of age
  - Lasts for ≥1 month
  - Typically lasts a few months
  - Disorder can last several years (uncommon).
  - Should not be diagnosed if the child is encountering a significant transition
    - First month of a school term
    - Recent immigration to a new country
  - Should be diagnosed only in a child who has demonstrated ability to speak at the appropriate developmental level in more familiar social situations
  - Social anxiety and social avoidance associated with social phobia may be present in children with selective mutism.
    - In this case, both diagnoses would be appropriate if the child's symptoms meet the criteria for social phobia.
- Generalized anxiety disorders
  - The essential feature is excessive or unrealistic anxiety or worry for ≥6 months.
  - Worries are considered uncontrollable by the patient.
  - Significantly interfere with daily functioning
  - Phobias are often present.
  - Global disorder with fewer focused fears
- Obsessive-compulsive disorder
  - Avoidance behaviors are associated specifically with the content of obsession, rather than a feared stimulus.
    - Dirt
    - Contamination
  - May develop to neutralize or prevent the occurrence of anxiety or worry
    - Repetitive, purposeful, intentional behavior
- Posttraumatic stress disorder
  - Develops subsequent to experiencing a traumatic stressor
  - Symptoms include:
    - Reexperiencing the trauma
      - Flashbacks
      - Witnessing a similar event
      - Frightening dreams
      - Repetitive play in which the child expresses themes or aspects of the trauma
    - Restricted affect

P

- Acute stress disorder may be diagnosed if disturbances related to the trauma persist.
  - Minimum of 2 days
  - Maximum of 4 weeks
  - Occur within 4 weeks of the traumatic event
- Hypochondriasis
  - Distinguishing between specific phobia (blood-infection-injury type) and hypochondriasis depends on the presence or absence of disease conviction.
  - People with hypochondriasis are preoccupied with fears of having a disease.
    - Individuals with a specific phobia fear contracting disease.
    - Do not believe it is already present
  - Vasovagal fainting response is typical for a phobia of the blood-infection-injury type.
    - Not common for hypochondriasis
- Additional psychiatric factors
  - Avoidance behaviors or phobias may be present with:
    - Other anxiety disorders
    - Depressive disorders
    - Substance abuse
    - Psychotic disorders
  - Symptoms of these other disorders are typically the focus of treatment.
  - Tend to produce more distress and impairment of daily functioning than symptoms of phobias

TREATMENT APPROACH

- Treatment of phobias includes:
  - Thorough assessment
  - Initial intervention
  - Short-term follow-up
- If phobia persists:
  - Further assessment
  - Potential consultation
  - Referral to a mental health specialist
- The primary care physician should inform the patient and parents of diagnosis and treatment.
  - Parents need to be partners in treatment.
  - Without intending to do so, parents can reinforce and perpetuate symptoms by allowing the child to avoid the feared stimulus.
  - Family therapy can provide additional treatment opportunities by:
    - Offering education to parents about the diagnosis
    - Strengthening the child's coping skills

- Improving familial support
- Helping the family cope with any recent life transitions
- Addressing best-parenting practices
- When evaluating and treating patient, developmental issues should be considered.
  - Children may exhibit phobic behaviors, such as a fear of the dark.
    - Common
    - Likely to be self-limited
  - Provide a nightlight and use simple cognitive self-control strategies.
    - Relaxation
    - Visualizing a pleasant scene
    - Teaching the child positive self-statements, such as, "I am brave; I can take care of myself in the dark."
  - More likely, the phobia will abate spontaneously over time.
- Systematic desensitization can be difficult to establish because of:
  - Complexity of anxiety-provoking stimuli
  - Social immaturity of patient
- Range of psychotherapeutic interventions may be used to promote socialization and improve social skills
  - Cognitive-behavioral individual therapy
  - Family therapy
  - Group therapy with age-appropriate peers
- In vivo exposure with response prevention
  - Most effective treatment for agoraphobia with and without panic attacks
  - Effectiveness ranges from 60–70%
- Booster sessions for symptoms of panic are usually necessary.
- Anticipatory guidance plays an important role in:
  - Recognizing
  - Diagnosing
  - Treating
- In many instances, the child would rather avoid discussing fears.
- In some cases, parents may not recognize avoidant and anxious behavior as something that should be reported.
- Routine screening for fears that might interrupt or impair normal development should be included when treating children and adolescents in primary care.
- Well-child visits provide a good opportunity for such screening.

SPECIFIC TREATMENTS

Cognitive-behavioral therapy

- Patients typically treated by a mental health specialist with systematic desensitization.
  - Approach includes a combination of progressive exposure to feared stimulus using:
    - Hierarchy of fears (ranked by the patient according to level of anxiety)
    - Relaxation techniques
  - As anxiety occurs in response to actual feared (in vivo) or imagined (in vitro) stimulus, relaxation techniques are invoked and stimuli removed.
  - The feared stimulus will gradually become paired with a relaxed state instead of an anxious state.
- Other behavioral approaches used by mental health specialists can enhance the effectiveness of systematic exposure, including use of:
  - Behavioral contracts
  - Modeling procedures
- Getting a child to participate in deliberate exposure to a feared stimulus is often difficult for parents.
  - Contracts can increase the patient's compliance by using specific contingencies to reinforce positively desired behavior toward the feared stimulus.
  - Contracts can ensure treatment plans are followed consistently outside of the office by patient and family.
  - Modeling includes direct observation of the desired behavior.
    - Not avoiding feared stimulus
  - Demonstrated by practitioner, family members, or peers
  - Initially show a comparable level of fear, which they are able to overcome

Psychopharmacologic therapy

- Psychiatric consultation is typically considered when:
  - The child is in so much distress ability to function is significantly impaired.
  - The condition prevents success with cognitive-behavioral treatment.
- Medications are usually used in combination with behavioral interventions.

- Medications of choice for majority of children and adolescents
  - Anxiolytics
  - Antidepressants

Other therapy

- Social phobia and agoraphobia are difficult to treat.
  - Often require psychological treatment and pharmacotherapy

WHEN TO ADMIT

- If a comorbid condition exists that is threatening the safety of the patient or others, psychiatric admission may be necessary to stabilize the patient.

WHEN TO REFER

- Psychological consultation is indicated if initial treatment does not result in symptom relief.
- May result in a need for further assessment, including referrals for:
  - Cognitive-behavioral psychotherapy
  - Psychiatric consultation
  - Both
- Maintaining collaboration with referral sources helps coordinate treatment planning.

PROGNOSIS

- Most phobias in children and adolescents seem to respond to treatment.
- Lack of controlled studies creates difficulty in attributing remission clearly to treatment.
- Follow-up studies are limited.
  - Those that exist suggest a positive long-term outcome.
  - Adults seeking treatment for phobias and other anxiety disorders often report onset of a phobia or similar symptoms during childhood or adolescence that diminished or disappeared for some time.
- The prognosis for children and adolescents with social phobia is less clear.
  - Experience suggests that these disorders are less likely to remit spontaneously or as a consequence of treatment.
  - Agoraphobia has a more guarded prognosis than social phobia.

P

Pinworm Infestations

DEFINITION

- Pinworm is a condition caused by an infestation with *Enterobius vermicularis*.

EPIDEMIOLOGY

- Prevalence
  - *E vermicularis* infestation is exceptionally common.
    - Adults are often infested.
  - Can be found in at least 30% of children worldwide
  - Finding pinworms in all members of a family is not uncommon.
  - Infestation rates may approach 100% in:
    - Day care centers
    - Boarding schools
    - Institutions
- Socioeconomic factors
  - Good sanitation and advanced socioeconomic status are feeble deterrents.

ETIOLOGY

- *E vermicularis*
  - A white, threadlike worm that lives primarily in the cecum and adjacent bowel
  - Gravid female worm
    - Approximately 1 cm long
    - Migrates to perianal area to deposit up to 10,000 eggs
    - Dies shortly thereafter
  - Infestation would be self-limited were it not for reinfestation.
  - Eggs are:
    - Approximately 50×30 μm
    - Oval
    - Flat on 1 side
    - Thin shelled
    - Become infective in approximately 6 hours
- Eggs are hardy and may survive for weeks in:
  - Dirt
  - House dust
  - Clothing
  - Bed sheets
- Survival is enhanced by:
  - Lower temperature
  - Inhalation or swallowing
- Pets may carry eggs in their fur.

- Once ingested, the eggs hatch in the upper small intestine.
  - Worms mature while migrating to the lower ileum and ascending colon.
  - Cycle from ingestion to deposition of eggs is ~4–6 weeks.
  - Adult worms may live up to 13 weeks.
  - The worm burden within an individual may reach the hundreds.
  - In an infested population, most individuals would be harboring few parasites.

RISK FACTORS

- Inadequate hand washing after contact with perianal area

SIGNS AND SYMPTOMS

- One-third or more of infestations are asymptomatic.
- Signs and symptoms include:
  - Localized perianal pruritus (most commonly reported symptom)
  - Restlessness
  - Fitful sleep
  - Secondary excoriation
  - Sermatitis
  - Genitourinary symptoms
    - Migrating pinworms may enter the vagina or urinary tract in female patients.
  - Granulomatous reaction (rare)
    - Granulomas-containing worms have been an incidental finding in the:
      - Gut
      - Vulva
      - Cervix
      - Fallopian tubes
      - Peritoneum
      - Bladder
  - Appendicitis and eosinophilic colitis (rare)
    - Inflammation associated with the parasite has been found in these conditions.
    - Lack of abdominal symptoms supports the notion of minimal gastrointestinal abnormality with this parasite.

DIAGNOSTIC APPROACH

- Diagnosis is dependent on identifying either adult worms or eggs.
- Eggs are seldom found in feces even using concentration techniques.
- The best way to make a diagnosis is to use the cellophane tape technique.

LABORATORY FINDINGS

- Cellophane tape technique to visualize pinworm eggs
  - When the child awakens in the morning, press the adhesive side of a 2-inch strip of clear cellophane tape against the perianal skin using a tongue depressor.
    - Commercially produced kits are available for this purpose.
  - Tape is then placed on a microscope slide with the adhesive side down.
    - Eggs are naturally transparent.
    - Staining with lactophenol cotton blue enhances detection.
  - A single test should detect at least 50% of infestations.
    - 3 will detect 90%.
    - 5 will detect virtually 100%.

TREATMENT APPROACH

- Eradication is extremely difficult because of:
  - Ubiquity, infectivity, and persistence of the parasite
  - High level of infestation in symptomatic patients
- Vigorous pursuit of a permanent cure may provoke needless turmoil and anxiety in the family.
- The most important aspects of treatment:
  - Humility on the part of the physician
  - Reassurance of the family

SPECIFIC TREATMENTS

Pharmacologic treatment

- Reasonable to treat either a confirmed individual patient or the entire family
  - Single dose of either mebendazole (100 mg for all ages) or albendazole (400 mg for all ages)
    - Extremely effective and has virtually no side effects
  - Pyrantel pamoate administered as a single dose of 11 mg/kg (maximum 1 g)
    - Effective
    - Transient headache and abdominal symptoms have been reported.
- Treatments are effective against adult worms only.
  - Therapy is usually repeated in 2 weeks to eradicate emerging parasites.

General measures

- Clipping the fingernails (a repository for eggs)
- Frequent hand washing
- Daily morning showers
- Tight-fitting cotton underpants
- Bland ointment (eg, petroleum jelly) applied to the perianal region to limit dispersal of eggs
- Cleaning floors in sleeping areas thoroughly, particularly in cases of recurrence
- Washing clothing and bedding at the time of treatment

P

Plagiocephaly

DEFINITION

- *Plagiocephaly* means "oblique head" (Greek origin).
  - Term is used to describe any abnormality in the shape of the head, irrespective of its cause.
- *Posterior deformational plagiocephaly (PDP)* is a condition in which flattening of the occiput occurs as a result of mechanical factors that affect the malleable growing skull in utero or during early infancy.
  - Also referred to as *benign positional molding, posterior plagiocephaly,* and *occipital plagiocephaly*

EPIDEMIOLOGY

- Prevalence
  - Before 1992, when more than 70% of infants were placed in the prone position during sleep, PDP was estimated to be present in 1 in 300 live births.
  - After the *Back to Sleep* campaign was initiated by the AAP, PDP has been on the rise, with a 2004 study showing PDP in almost 1 in 68 infants.
  - More common on the right side because of the right-sided sleep position preference of most infants.
    - Almost 85% of neonates have left occipital anterior presentation during birth, which causes pressure on the infant's right occiput and left forehead by the mother's pelvis and lumbosacral spine.
- Sex
  - More common in boys, probably because male infants have larger heads and because boys tend to be less flexible
- PDP is first noticed by parents and health care providers when the infant is 2–3 months of age.
  - Severity of PDP peaks at 4 months
  - Resolves gradually over time.
    - In two-thirds of cases, PDP resolves by 2–3 years of age.
    - Resolution is observed to be slow in children with limited head rotation and low activity level.

ETIOLOGY

- Abnormalities in skull shape
  - May develop prenatally *or*
  - May develop postnatally during the first 2 years of life
- Whether PDP begins prenatally or is an acquired phenomenon remains controversial.
- Some investigators believe that many infants who develop PDP are born with mild flattening of the occiput that initially goes unnoticed.
  - Worsens as the infant continues to sleep on the flat side in the position of comfort
  - Termed *positional plagiocephaly*

- Deformity present from birth is usually the result of in utero conditions such as:
  - Small maternal pelvis
  - Uterine abnormalities
  - Large baby
  - Multiple gestations
  - Oligohydramnios or polyhydramnios
- Some researchers believe constrictive and restrictive uterine environment leads to conformational changes in the skull and fusion of the sutures.
- Others believe that the uterine environment simply causes severe molding and leads to flattening.

RISK FACTORS

- Primiparity
- Prolonged labor
- Assisted delivery
- Frequently associated with PDP:
  - Supine sleeping position
  - Congenital torticollis
    - Some theories suggest that torticollis develops as a result of PDP.
  - Prolonged periods in car seats and infant carriers
  - Prematurity
    - Infants maintained in 1 position for prolonged periods on ventilator support
  - Neurologic conditions such as hydrocephalus
    - Movement of bones and sutures as a result of volume changes from hydrocephalus
    - Limitations imposed by the draining devices and shunt
  - Position of baby's crib in relation to the room's major light source.
    - Infants usually look toward a light source when in the supine position.

SIGNS AND SYMPTOMS

- PDP is first noticed by parents and health care providers when the infant is 2–3 months of age.
- Severity peaks at 4 months and then resolves gradually over time.
- Infants with PDP exhibit preferential head position and turn the head only to 1 side.
- When head is viewed from above:
  - Frontal prominence is observed on the same side as the occipital flattening.
  - Ear on that side is anterior as compared with the other ear.

- Other craniofacial abnormalities that may be observed on the affected side are:
  - Prominent mandibular sulcus with mandibular tilt
  - Uplifted lower helix
  - Smaller ear
  - Unilateral epicanthal fold
  - Most have 1-sided occipital bald spots.

DIFFERENTIAL DIAGNOSIS

- Distinguishing lambdoid synostosis from PDP in infants with flat posterior plagiocephaly is critical because of differences in management.
  - Rarely, clinically differentiating between them may be difficult.
- Lambdoid synostosis is a rare condition that occurs in ~2% of all cases of craniosynostosis.
  - Head is trapezoid shaped.
  - Ear is displaced inferiorly and posteriorly.
  - Posterior basal skull is tilted, with prominence of mastoid process present on the same side.
  - Facial deformity is absent or minimal.
- PDP
  - Head is shaped like a parallelogram.
  - Significantly greater protrusion of the forehead on the same side of the occipital flattening than with lambdoid synostosis.
  - Ear on flattened side is displaced anteriorly.
  - Facial deformity
- Presence of torticollis must be ruled out in every case of flattened occiput because of its greater association with PDP.
  - Primary care physician should perform both passive and active head rotations and check for tightness of the sternocleidomastoid muscle.
  - Eye on the side of torticollis appears to be incompletely open as a result of the vertical displacement of soft tissues of the cheek.
  - Mothers of infants with torticollis note that they have difficulty feeding the infant from both breasts because the infants have trouble turning their heads.

DIAGNOSTIC APPROACH

- Diagnosis of PDP in infancy is made primarily based on history and physical examination.
- If the infant has a normal, rounded head at birth and after a few weeks or months develops an occipital flattening, then the most likely diagnosis is PDP.

IMAGING

- Imaging studies usually are not required.
- In the past, skull radiographs were used to rule out lambdoid suture synostosis.
  - Ultrasound examination of the lambdoid suture also has been shown to be useful in ruling out lambdoid suture synostosis.
- Three-dimensional CT scans have been shown to be sensitive in diagnosing common and rare causes of posterior plagiocephaly.

TREATMENT APPROACH

- Early recognition and intervention improves outcome.
  - If not treated appropriately, then quality of life may be reduced.
- In most patients, the head shape improves with changes in head position or helmet therapy.
- Definitive treatment guidelines have not been developed.
- Early treatment is successful in most cases of mild to moderate PDP.
- Treatment started after 12 months does not produce significant benefits.

SPECIFIC TREATMENTS

Initial management

- Early treatment is similar to preventive measures.
- Educate parents about changing the infant's head position frequently.

Neck motion exercises

- If the infant is found to have torticollis, parents should be taught neck motion exercises to use with the baby.
  - First exercise is used to stretch the sternocleidomastoid muscle.
    - Place one hand on the infant's upper chest.
    - Rotate infant's neck with the other hand so chin touches the shoulder.
    - Hold infant's head in this position for 10 seconds.
    - Then rotate head to the other side and hold in that position for an additional 10 seconds.
  - Second exercise stretches the trapezius muscle.
    - Infant's head is tilted so that the ear touches the shoulder and is held in that position for 10 seconds.
    - Same process is followed on the other side.
- Parents should perform these neck exercises with every diaper change, with 3 repetitions of each exercise.
  - ~2 additional minutes per diaper change are required for these exercises.
- Infant should be referred for physical therapy for stretching exercises if these exercises fail to improve torticollis within 2–3 months.

P

- If no improvement is evident, or if plagiocephaly worsens after 2 months of repositioning and physical therapy, infant should be referred to a pediatric neurosurgeon or a craniofacial surgeon for further management.

Helmets

- Skull-molding helmets have been used for reshaping affected skull.
- Must be used in the age range of 4–12 months because of the malleability of the infant's skull during this period.
- Ideally, therapy is begun at 4–6 months of age; may be continued until 12–14 months of age.
- Head growth remains normal during helmet therapy; helmet works by symmetrically shaping the cranial growth.
- Use of helmets is more beneficial for:
  - Patients with severe deformity
  - Infants with mild to moderate severity who are resistant to position changes and physical therapy
- No consensus exists on use of helmets.
- Disagreement exists on cost effectiveness of helmets.
- AAP states that helmets are beneficial in the treatment of PDP after position changes and exercise have failed.
- Helmets used for treating PDP are considered to be class II neurologic devices and are regulated by the US Food and Drug Administration.
- Information on the approved orthotics can be obtained at www.fda.gov.

Surgery

- Rarely needed
- May be indicated in severe cases in which infants have been presented late for management, missing the window of opportunity for success with repositioning, physical therapy, or helmet therapy
- Craniotomy
  - Does not provide superior results as far as a cosmetic outcome is considered
- Associated with significant morbidity

WHEN TO ADMIT

- Surgical correction of PDP

WHEN TO REFER

- After position change and physical therapy have failed to correct PDP
- In severe cases
- When the patient who has PDP is >12 months
- When lambdoidal craniosynostosis is a possibility

COMPLICATIONS

- Uncorrected or improperly treated PDP can lead to marked psychosocial developmental sequelae.

PROGNOSIS

- In two-thirds of cases, PDP resolves by 2–3 years of age.
- Resolution is slow in children with limited head rotation and low activity level.
- In most cases, early implementation of repositioning and neck exercises yields considerable response over a 2- to 3-month period.
- The ipsilateral temporomandibular joint is pushed anteriorly in patients with PDP, and the mandible develops asymmetrically.
  - Positional and helmet therapy improve the head shape but not the position of the temporomandibular joint or the asymmetry of the mandible.
- PDP also causes forehead and facial shifts that may lead to asymmetric positioning of eyes and bilateral astigmatism.
  - Fitting corrective glasses on an asymmetric head is difficult.
- Cognitive and psychomotor development has been observed to be mildly delayed in patients with PDP.
  - Whether delays can be corrected with therapy is not known.
  - Whether delays are the cause or the effect of PDP is not known.
  - Long-term follow-up of patients with PDP has shown persistence of developmental delay.

PREVENTION

- In most infants, PDP can be prevented by:
  - Alternating supine head position during sleep
  - Periodically changing position of the crib to require the child to look away from the flattened side to see parents or to look at a light source
- AAP has recommended a certain amount of prone positioning, or *tummy time,* while the infant is awake and being observed.
  - May help prevent development of a flat occiput
  - May also facilitate development of upper shoulder girdle strength necessary for timely attainment of certain motor milestones
  - Theories suggest that prone position prevents PDP by correcting or preventing infants' positional preferences.
- Parents and health care professionals should be educated on different techniques to reduce the risk for development of PDP.
  - Caregivers should be encouraged to change the head position of a sick newborn whenever possible.
  - Caregivers should be encouraged to:
    - Provide care from alternate sides of the crib
    - To reposition the infant from head to foot periodically
- Breastfed infants are less likely to develop PDP because alternate head positioning is promoted.
  - Parents should be advised to use alternate arms during each bottle feeding.

Pneumonia

DEFINITION

- Pneumonia is defined by the presence of infiltrates on a chest radiograph.
- In less-developed parts of the world, evidence of retractions along with tachypnea leads to a clinical diagnosis of pneumonia.

EPIDEMIOLOGY

- Incidence varies according to age:
  - Infants and toddlers are infected more commonly than older children.
  - In children ≤5 years of age, incidence is 30–45 episodes per 1000 children per year.
  - In children aged 5–9 yr, incidence is ~16–20 cases per 1000 children per year.
  - In older children and adolescents, incidence is 6–12 cases per 1000 patients per year.

ETIOLOGY

- Pneumonia results from:
  - Overwhelming load of pathogenic organisms
  - Breach of host defense mechanisms
- Causes vary depending on patient's age.
- In the neonatal period, acute pneumonia is caused by bacteria that may cause sepsis and meningitis.
  - Group B *Streptococcus* (GBS) causes a severe lower respiratory tract infection.
    - Major morbidity and mortality
  - Infections from GBS have been found in infants up to 8 months of age.
    - Approximately 75% develop infection by 2 months of age.
  - Other organisms include:
    - *Escherichia coli*
    - *Klebsiella pneumoniae*
    - Other enteric gram-negative bacteria
  - *Listeria monocytogenes* must be considered.
  - Less frequently, the following may be implicated in episodes of lower pulmonary infections:
    - Nontypeable *Haemophilus influenzae*
    - Other strains of *Streptococcus*
    - *Enterococcus* spp
  - Rarely, anaerobic bacteria may be found.
  - Infection with *Chlamydia trachomatis* leads to pneumonia with significant auscultatory findings.
  - Conjunctivitis frequently precedes or accompanies respiratory infection in infants who have been colonized during delivery.

- Bacterial causes beyond the neonatal period
  - *Streptococcus pneumoniae* is the most important pathogen.
    - Highest number of cases
    - Greatest potential for complications
  - Pneumococcus may be the etiologic agent in 25–38% of cases.
- Other bacterial pathogens associated with acute lower respiratory infections in toddlers and young children include:
  - *H influenzae* type B
  - Nontypeable strains of
    - *H influenzae*
    - *C trachomatis*
    - *Mycoplasma pneumoniae*
    - *Moraxella catarrhalis*
- Cases of severe group A ß-hemolytic streptococcal pneumonia have been reported.
  - Often with marked comorbidity
    - Pleural effusion
    - Empyema
    - Shock
- Among school-aged children and adolescents
  - *M pneumoniae* is the major treatable cause.
  - *Chlamydia pneumoniae* may cause pneumonia.
  - *S pneumoniae* may be the cause.
  - *Legionella pneumophila* may be a rare cause.
- Children <5 yr of age are at risk for viral pneumonias.
  - Respiratory syncytial virus (RSV) infects almost all toddlers by the age of 3 yr.
    - 1% are ill enough to require hospitalization.
  - Other viral etiologies that may be seen in the first years of life include:
    - Parainfluenza virus
    - Influenza
    - Adenovirus
  - Human metapneumovirus has been shown to cause bronchiolitis that may be similar to that caused by RSV.
  - Influenza also may cause significant respiratory illness within all pediatric age groups.
    - Infants are at risk during yearly influenza outbreaks.
  - Multiple pathogens may be found in the same patient.
  - Viral infections, with consequent epithelial loss and inflammation, may lead to secondary bacterial infections.
    - 16–50% of patients may harbor more than one pathogen.

RISK FACTORS

- Exposure to environmental tobacco smoke and air pollutants
  - Associated with >190,000 cases of pneumonia per year in the US among persons in the youngest age groups
- Malnutrition
- Immune deficiency
- Loss of normal cellular components of the immune system (polymorphonuclear leukocytes and alveolar macrophages) caused by either acquired or congenital immune deficits
- Severe developmental delay
- History of prematurity
- Chronic lung disease

SIGNS AND SYMPTOMS

- During the neonatal period, signs and symptoms may be nonspecific.
  - Infants may have:
    - Fever
    - Irritability
    - Altered feeding patterns
    - Cough
    - Tachypnea or apnea
  - Findings on examination may include:
    - Retractions
    - Nasal flaring
    - Grunting
  - Auscultation may reveal:
    - Crackles
    - Decreased breath sounds
    - Occasionally wheezing, especially if the cause is viral
- Among older children
  - Indicators include:
    - Tachypnea
    - Cough
    - Fever
    - Crackles
    - Respiratory distress
  - Complaints of pleuritic chest pain may accompany pneumonia, and help localize attention to the chest.
  - Abdominal pain may be associated with acute lower respiratory tract infections.
  - Milder cases of pneumonia may be associated with findings in the upper respiratory tract:
    - Pharyngitis
    - Hoarseness
    - These symptoms are especially likely in illnesses caused by *Mycoplasma* and *Chlamydia* organisms.

LABORATORY FINDINGS

- Sputum sample
  - If the patient is able to provide a good specimen
    - Producing sputum samples often is difficult for children.
- Nasopharyngeal or throat culture specimens
  - Use for diagnosis of childhood pneumonia is not supported by the Canadian Medical Association or the British Thoracic Society.
- Blood cultures
  - Positive only ~10% of the time
- Serologic testing
  - May be useful
  - Often yields results (based on acute and convalescent titers) only after patient has recovered from acute illness
- Direct antigen testing
  - Currently available for influenza A, influenza B, and RSV
  - To assist in determining viral etiologies
- Because of the effectiveness of therapies against influenza, consideration should be given to obtaining nasal or respiratory secretions for testing.

IMAGING

- Radiographs of the chest
  - Radiographic patterns may be helpful in suggesting whether the infection is bacterial or viral.
  - Bacterial process
    - Lobar involvement
    - Pleural effusions
    - Pneumatoceles
    - Pulmonary abscess
  - Viral etiology
    - Bilateral perihilar infiltrates
    - Increased interstitial markings
  - Mycoplasmal infection
    - Focal or interstitial infiltrates
- Repeat chest radiographs should be obtained in 3–6 wk after diagnosis for documenting resolution.
  - Lack of radiologic resolution may suggest:
    - Congenital lung malformation
    - Foreign body
    - Neoplastic process

DIAGNOSTIC PROCEDURES

- Bronchoalveolar lavage
  - May help define therapeutic choices

- Useful for patients with:
  - Significant respiratory distress
  - Clinical picture that fails to fall into a readily recognized category
- May allow the discontinuation of certain antimicrobial drugs and alleviates risk of adverse reactions and cost associated with these agents.
- Bronchoscopy with lavage
  - Particularly valuable in patients with immune defects
  - May be performed quickly with minimal morbidity in almost any child
  - Should be considered early in the illness, before therapy with multiple antibiotics has been initiated
    - Increases yield of the test
  - May not be available to every practitioner

TREATMENT APPROACH

- For unhospitalized patients
  - Oral antibiotics
- For patients admitted to the hospital
  - Parenteral antibiotics

SPECIFIC TREATMENTS

Antimicrobials

- For young, hospitalized infants, ampicillin *and* either an aminoglycoside or a third-generation cephalosporin
  - Combination provides good coverage for specific organisms frequently seen in the neonatal period:
    - GBS
    - Gram-negative enteric bacteria
    - *Listeria* organisms
- Older infants and toddlers requiring hospitalization may be treated with intravenous cefuroxime or cefotaxime.
  - Many of these illnesses are caused by pneumococci and are increasingly resistant to ß-lactam antibiotics.
  - If illness worsens significantly while patient is receiving either of these antibiotics, consideration should be given to therapy with vancomycin.
  - Treatment failures are uncommon in spite of penicillin-resistant strains of *S pneumoniae*.
- For children with severe illness, additional antibiotic coverage with erythromycin or a newer macrolide may be considered.
  - These antibiotics may be first-line choices for the treatment of pneumonia (*M pneumoniae* and *C pneumoniae*) in school-aged children and adolescents.
- Patients with less severe illness may be treated with the same antibiotics.

Parapneumonia effusions

- Video-assisted thoracoscopic drainage
- Thoracostomy tube placement

Lung abscesses

- Imaging studies show an irregularly shaped cavity with an air-fluid level inside.
  - Prolonged antibiotic therapy will resolve this complication.

WHEN TO ADMIT

- Clinical assessment is most important in determining whether hospitalization is needed.
- Admission is indicated if:
  - Child is <8 wk
  - Child is in significant respiratory distress, indicated by:
    - Grunting
    - Nasal flaring
    - Retractions
  - Hypoxia is present.
  - Child appears toxic.
  - Family cannot adequately assess and care for child.
  - Normal hydration status cannot be maintained.
  - Child cannot be brought back for reassessment after outpatient therapy.
  - Pneumonia is recurrent.

WHEN TO REFER

- Child continues to have fever 48 hours after starting appropriate antibiotic therapy.
- Child develops a pleural effusion.
- Child develops a lung abscess.

COMPLICATIONS

- Infections of the lower respiratory tract have varying morbidity and mortality when comparing illness in developed and developing countries.
- Combined effects of malnutrition and inadequate immunization may cause much more severe respiratory disease for children.
  - Particularly for those without access to advanced therapy to treat underlying infection and subsequent complications
- Many more deaths are caused by pneumonia in the developing world.
- *S pneumoniae*
  - Patients may be gravely ill.
  - Sepsis and meningitis possible

- Overuse of antibiotics has led to development of pneumococci with reduced antibiotic susceptibility.
  - *S pneumoniae* resistant to penicillins and advanced-generation cephalosporins
  - Resistance to other antibiotics may occur.
  - Resistance genes often are plasmid-borne and may be transferred between bacteria.
- Despite appropriate antimicrobial therapy, complications are seen.
  - Parapneumonic effusions may occur in 40–60% of pneumonia cases.
    - Initially result from inflamed pleural surfaces caused by underlying infection
    - Later, fibrin levels increase along with increased numbers of inflammatory cells.
    - May allow previously thin fluid to organize and become a thick rind, compromising lung function
- Lung abscesses are seen intermittently during the evolution of pediatric pneumonia.

PREVENTION

- Routine use of conjugated pneumococcal vaccine has lessened the incidence of *S pneumoniae* infections, including those of the lung parenchyma.

Pneumothorax and Pneumomediastinum

DEFINITION

- Pneumothorax is a collection of air in the potential space between the parietal and visceral layers of the pleura.
- Pneumomediastinum is a condition in which air is present in the mediastinum.

EPIDEMIOLOGY

- Pneumothorax and pneumomediastinum are uncommon events in healthy children.
- Primary spontaneous pneumothorax
  - The incidence of primary spontaneous pneumothorax in children is not known.
  - In adults, the estimated incidence is:
    - 7.4–18 cases per 100,000 population per year among men
    - 1.2–6 cases per 100,000 population per year among women
- Secondary spontaneous pneumothorax
  - The pediatric incidence has not been reported.
  - The adult estimated incidence is:
    - 6.3 cases per 100,000 population per year among men
    - 2 cases per 100,000 population per year among women
- Traumatic pneumothorax
  - In 1 report of children with blunt trauma, 38% had associated pneumothorax, hemothorax, or both.
  - In children with penetrating thoracic trauma, 64% had associated pneumothorax, hemothorax, or both.
- Iatrogenic pneumothorax
  - Rates of pneumothorax caused by mechanical ventilation have decreased in all age groups.
  - The observed rate of iatrogenic pneumothorax in hospitalized children was recently reported as 0.06 per 1000 discharges.
  - Some reports note an incidence of iatrogenic pneumothorax that exceeds that of spontaneous pneumothorax.
- Neonatal pneumothorax
  - Incidence depends on:
    - Gestational age
    - Birth weight
    - Presence of lung disease
  - Spontaneous pneumothorax is present in 1–2% of live births.
    - Most are term infants.
  - Incidence increases with prematurity.
  - Approximately one-half of affected infants have symptoms.
  - A history of delivery-room resuscitation efforts or infant aspiration of meconium or blood often exists.
  - Pneumothoraces are very common in critically ill ventilated neonates.
    - Incidence increases with prematurity.
  - Pneumothorax in an infant with neonatal respiratory distress syndrome has been associated with mortality rates exceeding 60%.
  - Familial cases of spontaneous pneumothorax in neonates have been described.
- Pneumomediastinum
  - Uncommon in the pediatric population
  - Usually self-limited
  - Often go undetected
    - The actual incidence is difficult to ascertain.

ETIOLOGY

- Spontaneous pneumothorax
  - Usually related to underlying lung disease (76–100%)
  - Precipitating factors
    - Foreign body ingestion, particularly children age 6 months to 6 years
    - Exposure to loud music
    - Illicit drug use
      - Attempted jugular or subclavian vessel injection (mainlining)
      - Cavitating septic thromboemboli
      - Forceful exhalation of crack smoke into another individual's respiratory tract (shotgunning)
      - Deep inhalation and Valsalva maneuvers while smoking marijuana
    - Emesis and coughing
- Traumatic pneumothorax
  - Causes of blunt thoracic trauma include:
    - Vehicle-pedestrian injuries
    - Motor-vehicle crashes
    - Falls
    - Child abuse
  - The leading causes of penetrating thoracic trauma are:
    - Gunshot
    - Stab wounds
- Iatrogenic pneumothorax caused by diagnostic or therapeutic interventions, including:
  - Transthoracic needle aspiration
  - Central venous catheter insertion
  - Thoracocentesis
  - Barotrauma or volutrauma related to mechanical ventilation

- Pneumomediastinum
  - The 3 main causes are:
    - Alveolar rupture
    - Perforation or rupture of esophagus, trachea, or main bronchi
    - Dissection of air from the neck or the abdomen
  - The most common cause is bronchospasm related to respiratory tract infection.
  - Often associated with exaggerated Valsalva maneuvers during:
    - Cough
    - Emesis
    - Hiccupping
    - Heavy lifting
    - Straining at stool
    - Illicit drug inhalation
    - Sports activities
  - Has been noted in situations in which external pressure changes occur, such as:
    - Scuba diving
    - Air travel
  - Other causes include:
    - Marked decreases in interstitial pressure, eg, with hyperpnea from diabetic ketoacidosis
    - Barotrauma or volutrauma secondary to mechanical ventilation or manual resuscitative ventilation
    - Foreign body ingestion, especially in children <6 years
  - Trauma
  - Child abuse
  - Blunt thoracic trauma, such as motor-vehicle crashes
  - Isolated facial trauma
  - Tracheobronchial and esophageal rupture

RISK FACTORS

- Primary spontaneous pneumothorax
  - The typical patient is:
    - Tall
    - Thin
    - Male
    - Age 10–30 years
  - Smoking increases the risk of primary spontaneous pneumothorax:
    - 9-fold among women
    - 22-fold among men
  - Risk is increased in various inherited disorders, such as:
    - α_1-Antitrypsin deficiency
    - Marfan syndrome
    - Ehlers-Danlos syndrome

- Pneumomediastinum
  - Asthma

SIGNS AND SYMPTOMS

Pneumothorax

- History
  - Patients often note abrupt ipsilateral pleuritic chest pain, with or without acute dyspnea.
  - Pleuritic pain may be more prevalent in primary spontaneous pneumothorax.
  - Dyspnea is typically severe in secondary spontaneous pneumothorax.
    - Patients have decreased cardiopulmonary reserve at baseline.
  - Symptoms associated with primary spontaneous pneumothorax often resolve within 24 hours.
    - Unlike the progressive course of secondary spontaneous pneumothorax
  - Respiratory symptoms might be vague in young children.
  - Parents may note sudden dyspnea and irritability.
- Physical examination
  - Findings in primary spontaneous pneumothorax are variable and depend on:
    - Pneumothorax size
    - Patient age
  - Most commonly, vital signs demonstrate tachycardia and tachypnea.
  - Patient with pneumothorax occupying <15% of the hemithorax may have a normal physical examination.
  - Hypoxemia caused by small primary spontaneous pneumothorax is uncommon in older children.
    - Most have adequate alveolar reserve to preserve oxygenation.
  - Smaller children are often hypoxemic.
  - Underlying lung function is normal.
  - Hypercarbia does not typically develop in patients with primary spontaneous pneumothorax.
  - Patients with secondary spontaneous pneumothorax often have hypoxemia and hypercarbia.
  - As size pneumothorax increases, characteristic signs include:
    - Diminished or absent breath sounds
    - Hyperresonance to percussion on the involved side
    - Chest asymmetry
  - Neonates may have severe respiratory distress with marked:
    - Tachypnea
    - Grunting
    - Retractions
    - Cyanosis

- Pneumothorax can be rapidly life threatening in infants with:
  - Respiratory distress syndrome
  - Other underlying lung disease
- Such infants may have cardiorespiratory instability and progress to cardiac arrest.
- Detection of pneumothorax by physical examination in infants can be difficult because of small thorax size.
- Shift of the apical heart impulse away from side of the pneumothorax has been reported to be a reliable sign.
- Iatrogenic pneumothorax should be suspected in:
  - Any patient who becomes more dyspneic after medical or surgical procedure known to be associated with the development of pneumothorax
  - Any patient treated with positive pressure ventilation who:
    - Experiences sudden clinical deterioration
    - Demonstrates unexplained increase in peak and plateau pressures or decreased tidal volume
- Tension pneumothorax is life threatening and requires immediate attention.
  - Heralded by:
    - Hypotension
    - Profound hypoxemia
    - Tracheal deviation in the setting of diminished breath sounds

Pneumomediastinum

- History and physical findings
  - Healthy young people do not often have severe symptoms or physical examination findings.
  - Patients may have:
    - Chest pain
    - Cough
    - Dyspnea
    - Dysphonia
    - Dysphagia
    - Neck pain
  - Examination will often reveal subcutaneous cervical emphysema with crepitance.
  - Less commonly, the physician may hear the Hamman sign.
    - Mediastinal crunching sound synchronized with systole

DIFFERENTIAL DIAGNOSIS

- Pneumomediastinum
  - Spontaneous esophageal perforation (Boerhaave syndrome)
  - Mediastinitis
- In young infants, neonatal pneumothorax must be differentiated from congenital lobar emphysema.

DIAGNOSTIC APPROACH

- Pneumomediastinum
  - The term *spontaneous pneumomediastinum* is applied to younger patients with no obvious precipitating event.
  - Care must be taken to evaluate for penetrating injury.
  - Air can enter the mediastinum from penetrating neck or chest wall injury.

IMAGING

Pneumothorax

- Routinely diagnosed by chest radiography
  - Preferably with the patient in an upright position
  - The main radiologic feature is a white visceral pleural line, separated from the parietal pleura by avascular collection of gas (see Figure 60 on page F21).
  - In many instances, no pulmonary vessels are visible beyond the visceral pleural edge.
  - In films in which the patient is in an upright position, the accumulation of gas is primarily in an apicolateral location.
  - In supine views, more pleural gas is needed for definitive diagnosis of pneumothorax.
  - Pleural gas accumulates in a subpulmonic location, outlining:
    - Anterior pleural reflection
    - Costophrenic sulcus (*deep sulcus sign*)
    - Anterolateral border of the mediastinum
- Computed tomography (CT) can detect pneumothoraces that do not appear on radiograph (occult pneumothoraces).
  - Often not practical in the initial workup
  - In young infants, neonatal pneumothorax must be differentiated from congenital lobar emphysema.
    - Can appear as an expanded radiolucent pulmonary segment
    - CT may be required to make this important differentiation; the treatment for congenital lobar emphysema is lobectomy.
    - Aspiration or chest tube placement in a patient with congenital lobar emphysema is associated with substantial risk of death.
- Portable ultrasonography devices may play a role in the future.
  - An application for thoracic ultrasonography for pneumothorax in children has yet to be established.
- Tension pneumothorax
  - Intervention should not be delayed for radiologic imaging to confirm the diagnosis.

P

Pneumomediastinum

- Recognized by air outlining mediastinal structures, such as:
  - Thymus (sail sign)
  - Superior surface of the diaphragm (continuous-diaphragm sign)
- Usually bilateral
- Does not move with decubitus positioning
  - Helps differentiate from anteromedial pneumothorax (see Figure 61 on page F21)
  - Pneumothorax may also be present.

DIAGNOSTIC PROCEDURES

- Pneumothorax
  - Fiberoptic bronchoscopy
    - Assesses the possibility of a bronchial tear
    - Used in trauma patients with a large pneumothorax and persistent air leak into the pleural space despite tube thoracostomy
    - Clinicians must rule out traumatic rupture of the esophagus; mortality approaches 100% if surgical treatment is not prompt.

CLASSIFICATION

- Pneumothoraces are typically classified as:
  - Spontaneous
  - Traumatic
  - Iatrogenic
- Spontaneous pneumothorax
  - Occur in the absence of antecedent thoracic trauma
    - Primary spontaneous pneumothorax
    - Secondary spontaneous pneumothorax
- Primary spontaneous pneumothorax affects patients who do not have:
  - Clinically apparent lung abnormality
  - Underlying condition known to promote pneumothorax
- Secondary spontaneous pneumothorax occurs in the setting of underlying pulmonary disease, such as:
  - Pneumonia
  - Asthma
  - Cystic fibrosis
- Traumatic pneumothorax
  - Trauma to the chest is classified as:
    - Blunt
    - Penetrating
- Pneumomediastinum
  - No apparent consensus exists regarding classification of pneumomediastinum.

TREATMENT APPROACH

- Failure to recognize and properly manage pneumothorax or pneumomediastinum can have serious consequences.
- Primary spontaneous pneumothorax
  - Guidelines for the management of spontaneous pneumothorax in adult patients have been published by the British Thoracic Society and American College of Chest Physicians.
  - No similar guidelines exist for treatment of infants and small children.
  - In the recommended treatment pathways, adult guidelines distinguish between:
    - Small primary spontaneous pneumothorax, defined as <15–20% of the chest volume
    - Large primary spontaneous pneumothorax
  - Guidelines estimate loss of lung volume by:
    - Distance from the lung apex to ipsilateral thoracic cupola at the parietal surface on a standard upright radiograph
      - Usually underestimates volume loss
  - Another way to estimate the size of a pneumothorax: The volume of the lung approximates the ratio of lung diameter to hemithorax cubed.
  - Using this system, a pneumothorax smaller than 15% would be considered small.

SPECIFIC TREATMENTS

Pneumothorax

Primary spontaneous pneumothorax

- Supplemental oxygen and observation in the emergency department for 3–6 hours, followed by repeat chest radiography to exclude progression of pneumothorax, is recommended for adolescents and young adults if:
  - Pneumothorax is small.
  - Severity of acute symptoms is mild with unlabored breathing.
  - Room air saturations are >90%.
- Patients must have careful instructions to:
  - Return for worsening shortness of breath
  - Have follow-up in 12 hours to 2 days with planned chest radiography to document improvement
- Breathless patients should undergo intervention, regardless of pneumothorax size.
- Supplemental oxygen is administered to all patients with pneumothorax.
  - Increases pleural air reabsorption rate 3- to 4-fold above the baseline of 1.25% per day
  - Recommended to hasten resolution
- A 15% pneumothorax is expected to resolve in ~12 days without oxygen therapy.

■ Management of small primary spontaneous pneumothorax

- Children with small primary spontaneous pneumothorax are typically admitted for observation.

- Based on adult guidelines, older children and adolescents with asymptomatic small primary spontaneous pneumothorax who have been observed in the emergency department for 3–6 hours can be discharged home.

  – Closely follow up, as recommended for adult patients.

- Any patient with breathlessness should:

  – Be admitted

  – Undergo intervention to remove the air

■ Management of moderate to large primary spontaneous pneumothorax in adolescents and young adults

- British guidelines recommend simple aspiration as first-line treatment for:

  – All symptomatic primary spontaneous pneumothoraces

  – All pneumothoraces with >2 cm rim of air on chest radiograph (large)

- US guidelines do not generally endorse attempts at simple aspiration over placement of a chest drain.

- Recent publications regarding primary spontaneous pneumothorax in adults show that aspiration is successful in >50% of cases.

  – Failure is more likely if pneumothorax is >40%.

- In British guidelines, patients with successful aspiration of a primary pneumothorax may be observed in the emergency department for similar follow-up.

- The American College of Chest Physicians recommends placement of a chest drain for symptomatic or any large (>3 cm rim) primary spontaneous pneumothorax.

- Patients are then managed with either a:

  – Heimlich valve (one-way valve)

  – Chest tube to water seal or suction

■ Management of large primary spontaneous pneumothorax in children

- Simple aspiration versus chest tube placement for children with large pneumothorax is based on experience of the treating physician.

- Published pediatric series suggest that hospital admission with placement of a pleural catheter or chest tube is usual practice.

Spontaneous secondary pneumothorax in young adults and children

■ Guidelines recommend hospital admission for:

- Treatment of the underlying condition

- Symptomatic treatment, if needed

■ Small pneumothoraces can be treated with oxygen therapy and observed.

■ Large pneumothoraces are drained either by aspiration or by chest tube placement.

Traumatic pneumothorax

■ If tension pneumothorax is suspected, emergency needle aspiration of the second intercostal space in the midclavicular line is required.

■ If the patient improves with needle aspiration, a chest drain should immediately be placed on that side.

■ A substantial number of pneumothoraces not seen on initial chest radiographs are found on subsequent CT or ultrasonography of the chest.

■ Placement of a larger-caliber chest drain for symptomatic or large pneumothorax among trauma victims is customary treatment.

- Many patients require positive pressure ventilation.

- May have an accompanying hemothorax

- Small asymptomatic pneumothorax may be observed if:

  – The patient is not receiving positive pressure.

  – Radiographic evaluation does not reveal chest multitrauma.

Iatrogenic pneumothorax

■ Should be tailored to the patient's clinical circumstance

■ Patients receiving positive pressure ventilation are at risk of extension of pneumothorax.

- Generally require chest tube placement

■ Provide supportive care with close observation for patients not on mechanical support who have a small pneumothorax and limited symptoms.

Chest tube insertion and management

■ Planning

- Before inserting the chest tube, predrainage risk assessment is appropriate.

- Risk of hemorrhage should be corrected when possible.

- Routine platelet count and bleeding times are recommended only for patients with known risk factors.

- When possible, the clinician should obtain informed consent and provide sedation with standard monitoring.

- Risks include:

  – Bleeding

  – Infection

  – Failure of pneumothorax resolution

  – Laceration of the lung

  – Extrathoracic placement with potential injury of abdominal organs

■ Positioning

- The preferred position for chest drain insertion is supine with the ipsilateral arm above the patient's head to expose the axilla.

P

- Alternative positions are:
  - Patient sitting upright leaning over an adjacent table with a pillow
  - Lateral decubitus position
- The safe area is bordered by:
  - Lateral margin of pectoralis major muscle
  - Anterior margin of the latissimus dorsi muscle
  - Line superior to the horizontal level of the nipple
  - Apex below the axilla
- Supine position minimizes risk to underlying structures, such as:
  - Internal mammary arteries
  - Breast tissue
  - Solid organs
- A more posterior position is chosen if pneumothorax is loculated and posterior.
  - Loculated collections are most safely approached under fluoroscopic guidance.
  - A more posterior position is safe.
- The second intercostal space in the midclavicular line may be chosen for apical pneumothorax.
  - The position is uncomfortable.
  - May leave a visible scar

■ Thoracostomy tube size selection
- Smaller tubes are recommended for aspirating air.
  - More comfortable compared with larger tubes, which are recommended for draining blood or a large air leak
- Age-based sizes for thoracostomy tubes recommended for trauma victims by the American Heart Association are:
  - Newborns (2–5 kg): 8–12 French
  - <1 yr (5–11 kg): 14–20 French
  - Children 1–8 yr (12–30 kg): 20–28 French
  - Children >8 yr (>30 kg): 29–36 French
■ Adult guidelines for pneumothorax management recommend relatively smaller tubes for draining air.
- British guidelines recommend a 10–14 French tube for management of pneumothorax in adults.
- The American College of Chest Physicians recommends initial management with a 16–22 French tube in patients not at risk for large air leaks.
■ Insertion techniques
- Small-bore chest tubes are usually inserted with aid of a needle and guidewire using a modified Seldinger technique.
- Blunt dissection is not needed because a dilator is used.
- Blunt dissection of subcutaneous tissue and muscle into pleural cavity is performed for insertion of medium and large chest drains.

- A finger-sized opening allows exploration to ensure that no underlying organs will be damaged.
- Once the tube is past the chest wall, it is directed:
  - Apically to drain air
  - Basally to drain fluid
- The chest tube is sutured in place.
- If an incision has been made:
  - 1 stitch is placed to assist with wound closure after tube removal.
  - 1 stitch is placed to secure drain.
- Chest radiography is done to check placement and resolution of pneumothorax.
■ Management of chest drain
- The chest tube is connected to a closed system with a water seal device.
- If the lung fails to expand quickly:
  - Continuous suction is delivered through a measured column of water until the lung has completely reexpanded.
- The closed system allows detection of air bubbles through water chamber, suggesting continued visceral pleural air leak.
- Air leak may be caused by a leak in the system.
  - Chest tube air holes are outside the chest.
  - Chest tubing connections are not airtight.
- The chest tube should remain in place as long as persistent air leak is present.
- Surgical referral is recommended if:
  - Air leak persists for >4–7 days in patients without preexisting lung disease.
- Earlier referral is recommended if:
  - The lung fails to expand.
  - A large air leak and underlying lung disease are present.
- Chest tubes are removed in a staged manner after pneumothorax is resolved.
- Suction is discontinued.
- The chest tube is placed on a water seal.
- Opinions differ regarding the appropriate length of time for a water seal trial, ranging from 3–24 hours.
- Chest radiography is done to rule out recurrence, and the chest tube may be removed.
- The chest tube should never be clamped unless:
  - The clinician is expert in chest tube management.
  - The patient has constant nursing supervision.

Management of pneumomediastinum

■ Initial therapy for pneumomediastinum is directed at the underlying disease process.

- Observation is standard management because:
  - Mediastinal air decompresses into the cervical fascia.
  - Rarely causes tamponade
- Continued air leakage among patients receiving mechanical ventilation may be decreased by:
  - Efforts to decrease intrathoracic pressures
  - Efforts to decrease tidal volume
- If signs of tamponade occur:
  - A mediastinal tube should be placed via echocardiographic guidance by a skilled specialist.
- High prevalence of asthma-related pneumomediastinum
  - Children for whom the underlying cause of pneumomediastinum is unknown should undergo diagnostic pulmonary function tests after an acute episode.

WHEN TO ADMIT

- Children with symptomatic pneumothorax of any size should be admitted to a hospital for observation or management.
- All infants with pneumomediastinum or pneumothorax should be admitted to a hospital.
- Any trauma victim with pneumothorax or pneumomediastinum should be admitted to a trauma center for evaluation and management.

WHEN TO REFER

- Infants and children with primary or secondary spontaneous pneumothorax or spontaneous pneumomediastinum
  - Refer to either a hospital or an emergency department for evaluation and management.
- All children with spontaneous pneumothorax
  - Refer to a lung specialist for follow-up because of the risk of recurrent pneumothorax.
- Infants and children with traumatic pneumothorax
  - Refer to a trauma center for evaluation and management.
- Infants and children with iatrogenic pneumothorax
  - Should be cared for by physicians with expertise in chest drain insertion and management
- Infants and children with pneumomediastinum and signs of cardiac tamponade
  - Should be evaluated by a cardiologist or surgeon able to place a mediastinal drain

FOLLOW-UP

- Children can be discharged from emergency department with follow-up within 24 hours in emergency department if they have:
  - Asymptomatic small primary spontaneous pneumothorax
  - Been observed for 6 hours in the emergency department
  - Reliable transportation and social circumstances

- All patients should be referred to a lung specialist for follow-up care.

COMPLICATIONS

- Risk of recurrence
  - Children with primary spontaneous pneumothorax have a 17–54% risk of recurrence.
    - The greatest risk of recurrence is within 1 year.
  - Some experts recommend CT to detect pleural blebs after initial pneumothorax to help determine risk of recurrence.
  - At this point, surgical treatment is generally limited to children with recurrent pneumothorax.
  - Surgery usually involves:
    - Repair of the air leak
    - Adhering the visceral pleura to the parietal pleura (pleurodesis)
  - Surgical approach via mini-thoracotomy or video-assisted thoracoscopic surgery (VATS) is based on the surgeon's preference.
  - VATS is associated with:
    - Less postoperative pain
    - Shorter hospital length of stay
- Spontaneous pneumothorax
  - Known complication of asthma
    - Tension pneumothorax is present in almost 30% of patients who die suddenly of asthma.
  - Nearly 3.5% of all patients with cystic fibrosis will experience pneumothorax.
    - Subsequent pneumothoraces are common.
  - Some familial cases without evidence of connective tissue disease occur.
  - Spontaneous pneumothorax is a well-recognized complication of AIDS associated with *Pneumocystis (carinii) jiroveci* pneumonia.
  - Catamenial pneumothorax
    - Condition related to endometriosis with diaphragmatic hernia
    - Should be considered in female patients with spontaneous pneumothorax temporally related to menstruation

PREVENTION

- Primary spontaneous pneumothorax recurrence
  - Smoking cessation should be encouraged.

P

Poisoning

DEFINITION

- Injuries are a leading cause of pediatric morbidity and mortality.
- Poisoning is one important mechanism of injury.

EPIDEMIOLOGY

- Incidence
  - >2 million exposures are reported annually to the American Association of Poison Control Centers (AAPCC).
    - 65% are exposures that involve children and adolescents ≤19 years old.
  - 2.5% of annual childhood and adolescent deaths from unintentional injury are poison related.
  - For children <6 years of age, an average of 24 deaths per year from poisoning (1983–2004), 4% of all poisoning fatalities and a 94% decrease from 1959.
- Prevalence
  - Repeat exposures may occur in 10–40% of childhood poisoning victims.
- Age
  - Of children exposed to poisoning, 80% are <6 years old.
  - 55% of childhood exposures are in boys.
  - 45% of adolescent exposures are in boys.
  - Childhood exposures peak between 1 and 3 years of age.
    - Unusual in children <6 months
    - Unintentional ingestion is unusual after age 5 years.

ETIOLOGY

- Top poison exposure categories
  - <6 years old
    - Cosmetics and personal care products: 13%
    - Cleaning substances: 10%
    - Analgesics: 7%
    - Topical agents: 6%
    - Plants: 6%
    - Cough and cold preparations: 5%
    - Insecticides, pesticides, rodenticides: 4%
    - Vitamins: 3%
    - Gastrointestinal (GI) preparations: 3%
    - Antimicrobial drugs: 3%
    - Other: 40%
  - 6–19 years old
    - Analgesics: 14%
    - Cough and cold preparations: 6%
    - Antidepressants: 5%
    - Cleaning substances: 5%
    - Cosmetics and personal care products: 5%
    - Stimulants and street drugs: 4%
    - Sedative-hypnotic drugs: 4%
    - Antihistamines: 3%
    - Art and craft supplies: 3%
    - Other: 44%
- Top fatal poisoning categories
  - <6 years old
    - Analgesics: 24%
    - Carbon monoxide (CO): 14%
    - Hydrocarbons: 11%
    - Cough, cold, antihistamine preparations: 10%
    - Insecticides, pesticides, rodenticides: 5%
    - Envenomations : 4%
    - Cardiovascular agents: 4%
    - Anticonvulsants: 3%
    - Drugs of abuse: 3%
  - 6–19 years old
    - Analgesics: 26%
    - Drugs of abuse: 26%
    - Antidepressants, antipsychotics: 12%
    - Hydrocarbons: 10%
    - Cough, cold, antihistamine preparations: 4%
    - Alcohols: 3%
    - CO: 3%
    - Cleaning agents and chemicals: 3%
    - Cardiovascular agents: 2%
    - Sedative-hypnotic drugs: 2%

RISK FACTORS

- Behavioral characteristics that increase the risk of ingestion
  - Hyperactivity
  - Impulsive risk-taking behavior
  - Rebelliousness
  - Negativistic attitude
  - Social isolation
  - Poor parenting skills
  - Maternal depression
- Unintentional or intentional (in older children and adolescents) exposures occur at times of:
  - Family disorganization
  - Deviations from normal routines
  - Family stress
- Most exposures occur in the child's own home.
  - Kitchen
    - Cleaning products are often stored in easily accessible locations.
    - Improper storage containers

- Bedroom
  - Medications are left out.
- Bathroom
  - Medications and cosmetics
- Grandparents' home
  - Lower level of vigilance
  - Lack of child-resistant containers
- Children <6 months old are at risk from:
  - Second hand exposure to psychoactive substances
  - Medication error
  - Child abuse and neglect

SIGNS AND SYMPTOMS

- When no specific history of toxic exposure can be found, the diagnosis of poisoning can be challenging.
- Signs and symptoms of poisoning can mimic those of many acute illnesses.
- Physicians should ask about possible exposure to medications, gases or fumes, or other potentially harmful substances around the home in the face of rapid onset of symptoms in:
  - Central nervous system (CNS)
  - GI system
  - Respiratory system
- Physicians should always consider poisoning when faced with a puzzling situation in which the diagnosis is unclear.
- Some toxins, such as opioids or anticholinergic agents, produce a typical constellation of signs and symptoms known as a *toxidrome,* or toxic syndrome.
  - Sympathomimetic
    - Agitation
    - Diaphoresis
    - Fever
    - Mydriasis
    - Tachycardia
  - Opioid
    - Respiratory depression
    - Miosis
    - Coma
    - Bradycardia
  - Anticholinergic
    - Blind as a bat—mydriasis
    - Dry as a bone—dry skin
    - Hot as Hades— fever
    - Red as a beet—red skin
    - Mad as a hatter—central nervous system stimulation
    - Decreased GI motility—decreased bowel sounds
    - Urinary retention—full bladder
  - Cholinergic
    - **D**efecation
    - **U**rination
    - **M**iosis, muscle fasciculations, muscle weakness
    - **B**ronchorrhea, bradycardia, bronchospasm
    - **E**mesis
    - **L**acrimation
    - **S**alivation

DIFFERENTIAL DIAGNOSIS

Analgesics

Acetaminophen

- Available in many formulations and dosages
- Often formulated in combination with other medicines, such as opioids, diphenhydramine, dextromethorphan, and pseudoephedrine
- Acetaminophen-containing products lead to:
  - 7% of all childhood exposures
  - 4% of all adolescent exposures
  - 12% of all childhood and adolescent poisoning fatalities
- Toxicity occurs after overdose or therapeutic error.
  - After an overdose, patients are usually asymptomatic for the first 24 hours, although they may have mild GI distress.
  - Clinical hepatitis develops over the next 2 days and may progress to fulminant hepatic failure.
  - Patients may recover spontaneously.
  - Liver transplantation may be necessary in severe cases.
  - Poison control centers will refer children for evaluation after ingestion of 150 mg/kg.
  - Toxicity in an adult is expected after an ingestion of 15 g.
- The only test necessary in an otherwise healthy patient is an acetaminophen level drawn 4 hours after the exposure.
  - Levels drawn before this time will not reliably predict the need for antidotal therapy.
- Additional laboratory testing may be appropriate in the following scenarios.
  - Overdose of extended-release preparation
  - Mixed overdose
  - Patient seeking care late
  - Underlying chronic disease
  - When otherwise medically indicated

Salicylates

- Available in many formulations, including standard, enteric-coated, extended-release, and chewable tablets
- Salicylate sare formulated together with opioids and over-the-counter cold remedies, antidiarrheal agents, herbal medications, and analgesic ointments.
- Patients ingesting >150 mg/kg are at risk of toxicity.

P

- Methylsalicylate is a liquid formulation used as a topical analgesic (oil of wintergreen).
  - 100% solution contains 1.5 g/mL.
  - Even a single teaspoon of this formulation presents a significant risk for toxicity in a toddler.
- Patients may have respiratory alkalosis, a metabolic acidosis, or a mixed acid-base disturbance; children usually exhibit acidosis.
- Patients demonstrate:
  - Altered mental status
  - Hypovolemic shock
  - Seizures
  - Coma
  - Hyperthermia
  - Hypoglycemia
  - Hypokalemia
  - Noncardiogenic pulmonary edema (sometimes)
- Laboratory evaluation requires assessment of electrolytes, blood gas, and salicylate level.
- Symptoms of acute intoxication are typically seen with salicylate levels >30 mg/dL.
- Severe toxicity is typically found with levels of 80–100 mg/dL.
- Ferric chloride can be used as a quick bedside test to confirm exposure.
  - Urine that contains salicylate turns purple or brown when 1 or 2 drops of 1% ferric chloride are added to 1 mL of urine.
  - This test is positive after taking even 1 aspirin tablet; thus, proof of overdose still requires a salicylate level.
- Salicylate toxicity is likely with elevated salicylate levels, but toxicity does not specifically correlate with salicylate levels.

Antidepressants

Tricyclic antidepressants

- Classic tricyclic antidepressants, such as imipramine or amitriptyline, have largely been replaced by selective serotonin reuptake inhibitors (SSRIs) as first-line agents in the treatment of depression.
- Tricyclic antidepressants are still used to augment SSRIs and to treat such conditions as insomnia or neuropathic pain.
- Ingestion of 1 or 2 pills may be toxic in a toddler.
- Symptoms of toxicity appear within 6 hours of ingestion.
  - Patients who remain asymptomatic throughout this observation period are unlikely to develop toxicity.
- Symptoms include:
  - Hypotension
  - Prolonged QRS and QT intervals on electrocardiography (ECG); right bundle branch block; and wide, complex dysrhythmias
  - Brief generalized seizures occur 1 to 2 hours after ingestion.

- Anticholinergic effects contribute to delirium, coma, and seizures.

SSRIs

- SSRIs, such as fluoxetine, sertraline, and paroxetine, are first-line agents for treatment of depression and anxiety.
- SSRIs have decreased toxicity compared with the classic tricyclic antidepressants.
- The primary adverse effects of SSRIs result from excessive serotonergic stimulation.
- Serotonin syndrome, a rare but potentially lethal condition, includes:
  - Altered mental status
  - Agitation
  - Myoclonus
  - Hyperreflexia
  - Diaphoresis
  - Tremor
  - Diarrhea
  - Incoordination
- If untreated, patients may develop:
  - Lactic acidosis
  - Rhabdomyolysis with renal failure
  - Hepatic dysfunction
  - Disseminated intravascular coagulation
  - Acute respiratory distress syndrome
- Serotonin syndrome most commonly results from therapy with a combination of serotonergic agents or combination of an SSRI with amonoamine oxidase inhibitor.

Antihistamines

- Antihistamines are commonly available in prescription and over-the-counter allergy medications, antinausea medications, and sleep aids.
- Available in both short- and long-acting formulations and found in combination with other medications, such as acetaminophen
- First-generation H1 antagonists (eg, diphenhydramine) typically cause sedation and CNS depression.
- Second-generation H1 antagonists (eg, loratadine) generally have less sedation than the first-generation agents.
  - However, several agents in this class (eg, terfenadine) were withdrawn from the US market because of the high risk of torsades de pointes.
- H2-receptor antagonists, such as ranitidine and cimetidine, primarily act in the GI tract.
- Antihistamine toxicity is marked by either:
  - CNS depression with somnolence or coma
  - CNS excitation with tremor, hyperactivity, hallucinations, or seizures

- Peripherally, antihistamines cause an anticholinergic toxidrome.
- Association of fever and altered mental status may be confused with meningitis or encephalitis.

CO

- CO, an odorless, colorless, tasteless, and nonirritating gas, is a by-product of hydrocarbon combustion and is the leading cause of poisoning deaths in the US.
- Toxic effects of mild CO poisoning can be nonspecific.
  - Headache is the most common.
  - A nonspecific viral syndrome is mimicked with:
    - Malaise
    - Nausea
    - Dizziness
- Severe disease produces CNS and cardiac toxicity.
  - Altered mental status
  - Seizure
  - Syncope
  - Coma
  - Dysrhythmias
  - Myocardial ischemia
- Significant toxicity is often associated with:
  - Metabolic acidosis
  - Increased lactate levels
- Cherry-red skin, although frequently mentioned, is rarely seen.
- Higher carboxyhemoglobin (CO-Hb) levels are associated with more severe disease; no correlation exists between specific symptoms and a particular level.
  - Children develop symptoms at lower CO-Hb levels than adults.
- CO causes lesions in the deep white matter and damage to the thalamus, basal ganglia, hippocampus, and globus pallidus.
- After 2 weeks, delayed effects include:
  - Neurocognitive deficits
  - Personality changes
  - Focal neurologic symptoms
  - Movement disorders
  - Although children can experience delayed effects, adults have a higher risk, particularly if loss of consciousness occurs during the early phase of the exposure.
- When a pregnant woman is exposed to CO, the fetus is at particular risk.
  - Brain damage and fetal death have been reported, generally after severe maternal exposures.

- The best measure of CO exposure is the CO-Hb level.
  - Normal CO-Hb levels are 1–2%; smokers may have levels of 5–10%.
  - Fetal hemoglobin may be assayed as CO-Hb.
    - Infants may have a CO-Hb level of approximately 3%.
  - Standard pulse oximeters cannot differentiate CO-Hb from oxyhemoglobin.
  - Blood gas CO oximetry is necessary to obtain accurate measurements of CO-Hb and methemoglobin.
  - High levels indicate significant exposure.

Cardiovascular medications

- Although childhood poisoning with cardiovascular agents is unusual, small doses may cause serious toxicity.
- Cardiovascular agents may be divided into 4 important classes.
  - Cardiacglycosides
  - ß-Adrenergic blockers (BBs)
  - Calcium-channel blockers (CCBs)
  - α_2-Adrenergic agonists

Cardiac glycosides

- Cardiac glycosides include:
  - Digoxin
  - Digitalis, and related compounds found in such plants as oleander and foxglove
  - Some toad venoms (bufotoxin) (popular as hallucinogens and aphrodisiacs)
- Symptoms associated with acute overdose are typically:
  - Nausea
  - Vomiting
  - Headache
  - Weakness
  - Confusion
  - Changes in vision
  - Palpitations
  - Dizziness
- Severe acute overdose will lead to:
  - Hyperkalemia
  - Bradycardia
  - Hypotension
  - Dysrhythmia
  - Hypercalcemia, hypokalemia, hyperkalemia, or hypomagnesemia can exacerbate cardiac toxicity.
- Chronic overdose is often characterized by:
  - Nausea and vomiting
  - Psychiatric disturbances
  - Drowsiness

P

- Headache
- Hallucinations

BBs and CCBs

- BBs, such as propranolol, atenolol, and metoprolol, are commonly prescribed for treatment of hypertension, angina, dysrhythmias, and headache.
  - β_1-Receptor blockade results in decreased myocardial contractility and conduction.
  - β_2-Receptor blockade increases smooth muscle tone (bronchospasm) and peripheral vascular tone (hypertension).
- After an oral overdose of BBs, symptoms begin within 2 hours; sustained-release formulations may result in delayed onset.
- Manifestations include:
  - Hypotension
  - Bradycardia
  - Wide QRS and PR intervals on ECG
  - Bundle branch block
  - Ventricular dysrhythmias such as ventricular tachycardia and torsades de pointes
  - CNS depression ranging from drowsiness to coma and seizures
  - Bronchospasm in patients with a history of asthma
  - Hyperkalemia
  - Hypoglycemia

a_2-Adrenergic agonists (clonidine)

- Used to treat hypertension and other disorders, such as attention-deficit/hyperactivity disorder and nicotine withdrawal
- Oral and patch formulations are both available.
- Even 1 or 2 clonidine pills may cause toxicity in a toddler.
- Patches contain high doses of clonidine to ensure transdermal delivery, and they are a particular problem when ingested by children.
- Toxic symptoms begin within an hour of ingestion and can last up to 24 hours.
- Clonidine toxicity mimics opioid toxicity, with:
  - Altered mental status
  - Coma
  - Respiratory depression
  - Miosis
- Other symptoms include:
  - Hypotension
  - Bradycardia
  - Dysrhythmias, such as first- and second-degree atrioventricular block

Caustic ingestions

- Caustic agents are broadly categorized as *acids* and *alkalis.*
- Serious caustic exposures are unusual in childhood, but these agents can cause significant injury.
- Acids injures tissue by coagulation necrosis.
  - Even though the resulting eschar may limit the initial depth of injury, esophageal, gastric, or intestinal injuries frequently occur.
  - Significant exposures may cause metabolic acidosis or acute renal failure.
- Alkali ingestions injure tissue rapidly by liquefactive necrosis.
  - Within minutes, tissue edema develops in the oropharynx and esophagus, potentially leading to airway obstruction.
  - Scar tissue from full-thickness burns in the esophagus may progress to strictures over several weeks.
- Caustic ingestions produce:
  - Dysphagia
  - Odynophagia
  - Drooling
  - Stridor
  - Hoarseness
  - Abdominal pain
  - Nausea
  - Vomiting
  - GI hemorrhage and perforation
  - Tissue eschar may sometimes mask findings despite a significant acid ingestion.

Hydrocarbons

- Categorized into 3 classes:
  - Aliphatics (kerosene, gasoline, mineral seal oil, solvent, paint thinners)
  - Aromatics (industrial solvents, such as benzene and toluene)
  - Terpenes (turpentine and pine oils)
- Hydrocarbon aspiration after unintentional exposure to such household products is a leading cause of poison-related death in young children.
- Pulmonary toxicity results from chemical pneumonitis after aspiration.
- Local or diffuse infiltrates, pleural effusions, and pneumatoceles may develop.
- Lipoid pneumonitis may result from ingesting hydrocarbons with high viscosity, such as petroleum jelly.
- Most patients experience coughing after hydrocarbon exposure, but cough does not by itself indicate pulmonary toxicity.
- Within 30 minutes, significant exposures cause:
  - Gasping
  - Choking

P

- Gagging
- Vomiting
- Patients may develop:
  - Cough
  - Tachypnea
  - Rales
  - Rhonchi
  - Wheeze
  - Diminished breath sounds
- In the most severe cases
  - Acute lung injury
  - Hemorrhagic pulmonary edema
  - Respiratory failure
  - Long-term respiratory dysfunction
- Respiratory effects may progress over the first 24 hours and resolve over the next 2–5 days.
  - Associated acute symptoms may include CNS depression and fever.

Insect repellents

Diethyltoluamide

- *N,N*-diethyl-3-methylbenzamide (DEET) provides broad protection against many insects and is available in a variety of formulations.
- Toxicity may occur after acute ingestion or with dermal exposures.
- Systemic toxicity causes:
  - Confusion
  - Ataxia
  - Generalized seizures
  - Encephalopathy
- Severe exposures may result in:
  - Hypotension
  - Bradycardia
- Encephalopathy may result from oral ingestions or chronic cutaneous exposures at high doses.
- Chronic exposures can lead to:
  - Insomnia
  - Muscle cramps
  - Mood changes
  - Rash

Lindane

- Lindane (γ-hexachlorocyclohexane) is an organochlorine insecticide used topically to treat scabies and pediculosis.
- Organochlorines are absorbed from the skin and are distributed into fat.
- Elimination half-life is between 20 hours and 10–20 days.

- Prodrome of headache, dizziness, ataxia, and tremors may be followed within 1–2 hours by self-limited seizures.
- Other complications include:
  - Disseminated intravascular coagulation
  - Anemia
  - Myoglobinuria
- Repeat and chronic exposures may be associated with:
  - Elevated aminotransferase levels
  - Leukopenia
  - Leukocytosis
  - Thrombocytopenia
  - Pancytopenia
  - Aplastic anemia

Iron

- Iron poisoning remains a problem for toddlers.
- Most significant toxicity is related to ingestion of adult iron tablets, not children's liquid or chewable vitamin preparations.
- Iron is a GI irritant that causes:
  - Abdominal pain
  - Nausea
  - Vomiting
  - Diarrhea
- Severe poisoning causes mucosal ulceration and hemorrhagic necrosis, leading to hematemesis, melena, or hematochezia.
- GI fluid losses lead to hypovolemic shock and contribute to positive anion gap metabolic acidosis.
- Absorbed iron leads to the production of free radicals, with adverse effects on cellular metabolism, which exacerbate the acidosis.
- A shock state in combination with iron's direct toxic effects contributes to progressive myocardial dysfunction and acute hepatic injury.
- As hepatocellular damage progresses, coagulation is disrupted, further exacerbating the GI hemorrhage.
- In rare cases, corrosive injury to the GI tract leads to gastric outlet obstruction weeks after the ingestion.
- In general, the higher the dose of iron ingested, the greater the likelihood of toxicity.
- Iron toxicity based on the ingested dose of elemental iron:
  - <20 mg/kg: none or minor
  - 20–40 mg/kg: mild to moderate
  - 40–60 mg/kg: moderate to severe
  - >60 mg/kg: severe
- Iron toxicity based on serum iron level (mg/dL)
  - Serum iron <300: expected toxicity, none or minor
  - Serum iron 300–500: expected toxicity, mild to moderate
  - Serum iron >500: expected toxicity, severe

- Peak serum iron level is best measured 4–6 hours after ingestion.
- GI symptoms alone do not predict severe toxicity but do confirm exposure.

Isoniazid

- Isoniazid (isonicotinyl hydrazine [INH]) is primarily used for prophylaxis and treatment of tuberculosis.
- It can cause hepatic toxicity, peripheral neuropathy, and optic neuritis even at therapeutic doses.
- INH doses of >30 mg/kg are likely to cause acute toxicity.
- Effects occur within 2 hours of ingestion.
- Patients initially experience:
  - Nausea
  - Vomiting
  - Slurred speech
  - Dizziness
  - Tachycardia
  - Urinary retention
  - Hyper- or hyporeflexia
- Significant toxicity causes:
  - Anion gap metabolic acidosis
  - Coma
  - Refractory seizures
  - Seizures

Lead poisoning

- The principal childhood source of lead is from deteriorating paint in pre–1970s-era houses.
- Other sources include:
  - Pica
  - Lead-based plumbing
  - Ceramics
  - Imported goods in lead-soldered cans
  - Folk remedies for colic advocated by some Chinese, South Asian, and Hispanic cultures
- GI absorption is facilitated by deficiencies in essential trace elements, such as iron, calcium, and zinc, which compete for the same absorption sites.
- Most children with a long history of lead exposure and absorption are asymptomatic.
  - A threshold no-effect level for lead has not been defined, and decreased IQ has been observed among children with whole-blood lead (BPb) levels <10 mcg/dL.
  - BPb levels as low as 15–20 mcg/dL have been associated with learning disabilities and mild decreases in IQ.
- Manifestations include:
  - Pallor
  - Hearing impairment
  - Constipation

- Behavioral disturbances
- Loss of developmental milestones
- Declines in school performance
- Encephalopathy is the most significant clinical manifestation of lead toxicity.
  - Subacute encephalopathy may cause:
    - Anorexia
    - Intermittent abdominal pain
    - Nausea
    - Vomiting
    - Constipation
- Children with BPb levels >70 mcg/dL may experience:
  - Coma
  - Intractable seizures
  - Death
- Patients with BPb <70 mcg/dL may exhibit:
  - Ataxia
  - Incoordination
  - Lethargy
  - Irritability
- Peripheral neuropathy is uncommon in children, but wrist and foot drops may occasionally occur with sickle cell disease.

Organophosphates

Pesticides

- Ingestion of the agent directly or through contaminated fruit is the most common route of exposure in children, although these agents are highly lipophilic and are well absorbed through the skin, eyes, and lungs.
- Assistance in identifying individual agents can be obtained from the US National Pesticide Telecommunications Network, 800/858-7378.
- Acute organophosphate poisoning causes cholinergic symptoms.
- CNS symptoms are often the presenting symptoms in younger children.
- The diagnosis is made when patient has a confirmed exposure or history of a suspected exposure and consistent physical findings.
- Hydrocarbon carrier may produce an odor of garlic.
- Symptoms occur within several hours but may be delayed for several days with more fat-soluble compounds.
- The poisoned patient has:
  - Pinpoint pupils
  - Vomiting
  - Changes in mental status
  - Copious secretions

P

- If untreated, combination of bronchial hypersecretion, bronchial constriction, and failure of respiratory musculature leads to respiratory failure, which may be complicated by coma and convulsions.
- Atypical presentations can occur in children.
- Clinical sequelae that have been reported in children include:
  - Mydriasis
  - Tachycardia
  - Hyperglycemia
  - Metabolic acidosis
  - Prolongation of the QT interval with subsequent torsades de pointes
- Intermediate syndrome, uncommon in children, is delayed toxicity that occurs after the resolution of initial cholinergic symptoms.
  - Symptoms (below) present 1–3 days after the cholinergic crisis, are not responsive toatropine, and require supportive care for several weeks.
    - Proximal muscle weakness
    - Cranial nerve deficits
    - Hyporeflexia
  - Increased risk of the intermediate syndrome appears to exist with the more lipophilic agents.
    - These may not have been accessible to antidote.
    - They are released from fat-storage sites into the circulation.
- Delayed symptoms reported up to 3 weeks after exposure
  - Polyneuropathy
  - Ataxia
  - Neuropsychiatric symptoms
  - Peripheral neuropathy
  - Spasticity
  - Most improve with time and do not cause permanent disability.
- Serum levels of both butyrylcholinesterase (pseudocholinesterase) and red blood cell cholinesterase (true cholinesterase) can be measured, but red blood cell cholinesterase is a more sensitive measure of toxicity.
  - Red blood cell cholinesterase testing is not available in most hospital laboratories.
  - Treating a patient for suspected poisoning should not wait for laboratory confirmation.

Nerve agents

- Sarin, soma, tabun, and VX are all agents with very rapid rates of permanent cholinesterase inactivation, leading to the rapid onset of severe cholinergic symptoms.
  - Agents can be dispersed through a blast or aerosolized.
  - Overall, these agents are more dense than air and are concentrated near the ground; thus, children may have an increased exposure risk.

- Sarin, soma, and tabun are volatile liquids with easily inhaled fumes.
  - The volatile fumes of sarin, soma, and tabun are quickly dispersed in the air and degrade within several hours.
- VX is less volatile and more likely to be absorbed through the skin.
- Patients exposed to these agents are not at further risk once they are removed from the site of exposure.
  - VX is more persistent in the environment and may present risk for ongoing exposure.
- More information on organophosphates and other chemical agents with potential for use as chemical weapons can be found at www.bt.cdc.gov/chemical.

Plants

- >750 toxins have been identified in >100 plant species.
- Plants do not require labeling for potential toxins, as is done for pharmaceuticals and household products, and no federal regulations exist on sales of plants or herbs.
- Exposure occurs by contact with the skin or eyes or by ingestion.
- Only a very few patients seek medical attention; even fewer require intervention (see table Toxic Plants).
- The most common plants that result in clinical sequelae are peace lily, holly, philodendron, poinsettia, pokeweed, poison ivy, rubber tree, and nightshade.

Substance abuse

Marijuana

- Made from dried leaves of the plant *Cannabis septiva*
- Extracts of the *Cannabis* plant are available as hashish (dried resin) and hash oil (liquid extract).
- Medical marijuana is available in pill form (Dronabinol).
- The active component is tetrahydrocannabinol, a psychoactive compound.
- When inhaled, the onset of action is 10–30 seconds, and the effects last from 1–4 hours.
- Ingestion results in slower onset of action (30–60 minutes) and more prolonged effects.
- Clinical effects include euphoria, impaired motor coordination and speech, impaired short-term memory, paranoia, and agitation.
- Other effects include dry mouth, conjunctival injection, tachycardia, and urinary retention.
- In rare circumstances, patients may experience hallucinations, delusions, and psychosis.

Lysergic acid diethylamide (LSD)

- LSD is available in several forms, including liquid-impregnated blotter paper, microdots, tiny tablets, windowpane gelatin squares, liquid, powder, and tablets.
- LSD is usually ingested and has rapid GI absorption.

P

Toxic Plants[a]

	Plant	Toxin or Toxic Part	Toxicity and Treatment
Houseplants and Cultivated Flowers	Aloe	Latex contains anthraquinones	Oral irritation, nausea, vomiting, diarrhea
	Anemone	Protoanemonin aglycone	Irritation of mucous membranes and GI system
	Autumn crocus, glory lily	Colchicine	GI, respiratory, renal, CNS toxicity
	Christmas pepper	Capsicum	Strong irritant, stinging or burning of mucous membranes
	Chrysanthemum	Sesquiterpene, lactones, pyrethrins	Skin reactions
	Iris	Resin-like podophyllotoxin	Gastroenteritis
	Jerusalem cherry	Solanine alkaloids	GI, CNS depression
	Lily-of-the-valley, foxglove, oleander	Cardiac glycosides	Irritation of mucous membranes, CV toxicity
	Monkshood, larkspur	Alkaloid aconitine	• Restlessness, salivation, irregular heartbeat • Rx: gastric decontamination
	Narcissus, amaryllis, daffodil	Alkaloid lycorine	Vomiting and diarrhea
	Philodendron, caladium, dumb cane, elephant ear, peace lily, pothos	Oxalates	• Irritation of buccal mucosa, edema, gastroenteritis, hypocalcemia • Rx: rinse mouth with milk; administercalcium
	Snow-on-the-mountain	Unknown acrid principle in milky sap	Irritation of mucous membranes and GI system
Wildflowers and Weeds	Buttercup, morning glory	Protoanemonin; seeds contain lysergic acid monoethylamide	GI irritation, CNS stimulation, hallucinations
	Deadly or black or climbing nightshade, jimson weed, henbane	Atropine, solanine, and related glycoalkaloids	• Anticholinergic • Rx: physostigmine
	Death camus	Veratrum alkaloids	• Nausea, vomiting, hypotension, bradycardia, syncope, paresthesia, weakness • Rx: atropine
	Green or false hellebore	Veratrum alkaloids	• GI irritation, respiratory, CV depression • Rx: atropine
	Horse nettle	Solanine alkaloid	GI, CNS depression
	Jack-in-the-pulpit, wild calla, skunk cabbage	Calcium oxalate crystals	• Irritation and burning of mouth • Rx: rinse with milk and magnesium hydroxide
	May apple	Podophylloresin	May produce peripheral neuropathy, vomiting, colic, diarrhea, drowsiness, impaired vision
	Poison hemlock	Alkaloid coniine	Salivation, nausea, vomiting, diarrhea, sensory disturbances, seizure, coma; death from respiratory paralysis
	Poison ivy, oak, sumac, wood	Urushiol	• Rhus dermatitis—red, itchy and clear blisters that exude serum; if ingested, causes severe mucosal irritation • Rx: topical or oral corticosteroids

P

Toxic Plants[a], *continued*

	Plant	Toxin or Toxic Part	Toxicity and Treatment
Wildflowers and Weeds, *continued*	Pokeweed	Podophyllotoxins	Vomiting, sweating, colic, diarrhea, CNS depression
	Rosary pea	Abrin	Burning sensation of mouth and throat, delayed GI, depression of vasomotor center, CV collapse
	Spurges	Unknown acid principle	Severe mucosal irritation
	Water hemlock	Cicutoxin	• Generalized seizures • Rx: symptomatic to prevent/control seizures
	White snakeroot	Tremetol, may be in milk of poisoned cow	Weakness, vomiting, tremor, and death
Cultivated Flowers and Crops	Castor bean	Ricin, must be chewed to release	Burning sensation of mouth and throat, delayed GI, depression of vasomotor center, hepatic, hemolysis, convulsions, and death
	Potato, tomato	Foliage and sprouts contain solanine alkaloids	GI irritation, headache, CNS depression, dermatitis
	Rhubarb	Leaves contain oxalate crystals and soluble oxalates	• Irritation of mucosa, hypocalcemia with seizures • Rx: rinse mouth with milk, replacecalcium
	Tobacco	Nicotine	Salivation, gastroenteritis, seizures
Trees and Woody Shrubs	Black locust	Toxalbumin	Anorexia, weakness, GI, dilated pupils, irregular and weak pulse
	Cherry, apple, peach, apricot, choke cherry	Leaves, pits, or seeds contain glycosides hydrolyzed to hydrocyanic acid upon chewing	• Dyspnea, paralysis, convulsions, coma, and death • Rx: cyanide antidote kit
	Daphne	Glycoside in which the aglycone is dihydroxycoumarin	Burning and irritation to the skin and GI tract, bloody diarrhea, stupor, weakness, and convulsions
	English holly	Ilexanthin and ilex acid	Vomiting and diarrhea
	Mistletoe	Berries contain lectins, phoratoxin, viscotoxin, polysaccharides	Gastroenteritis and CV collapse
	Mountain laurel, rhododendrons	Grayanotoxin	• Local and GI irritation, respiratory and CV depression • Rx: atropine
	Yew	Alkaloid taxine	Vomiting, colic, hypotension, respiratory depression

Abbreviations: CNS, central nervous system; CV, cardiovascular; GI, gastrointestinal; Rx, treatment.
[a] Adapted from: Rodgers GC, Matyunas NJ. *Handbook of Common Poisonings in Children.* 3rd ed. Elk Grove, IL: American Academy of Pediatrics; 1994.

- Psychedelic effects include existential experiences, intensified perceptions, hallucinations, and paranoia.
- Clinical signs of LSD intoxication are most intense in the early part of the intoxication and include:
  - Tachycardia
  - Palpitations
  - Blurred vision
  - Tremors
  - Incoordination
  - Mydriasis
- Users may experience flashbacks during which an individual re-experiences aspects of the acute intoxication.
  - These episodes are short-lived and self-limited but may provoke anxiety.

Phencyclidine (PCP) and ketamine

- PCP can be used orally or intravenously, smoked, or inhaled.

- Ketamine is a derivative of PCP and is used medically as a dissociative anesthetic.
  - Also a popular recreational agent because of its short duration, low cost, and hallucinatory effects
  - Recreational ketamine is diverted from medical, dental, and veterinary sources and is administered orally, intramuscularly, and intravenously.
- Clinical effects of PCP can last up to 48 hours after a large dose is ingested.
- Ketamine intoxication will typically last for ~8 hours after oral exposure and 90–120 minutes after intramuscular or nasal exposure.
- PCP and ketamine cause a dissociative psychotic reaction demonstrating as changes in body image and feelings of spiritual separation from the body.
  - Users may have difficulty seeing themselves as separate from their environment.
  - PCP users may experience dangerous or violent behavior.
  - The emotional state created by PCP is frequently unpleasant.
- Physical signs of PCP and ketamine intoxication include:
  - Nystagmus
  - Ataxia
  - Sensory impairment
  - Catatonia
  - Tachycardia
  - Hypertension
  - Increased secretions
- Ketamine intoxication is usually less severe and more short-lived than PCP intoxication.
- Both ketamine and PCP also have sympathomimetic effects.
- Supportive care in a quiet environment with minimal loud or noxious stimuli is usually all that is needed.
- Verbal and physical contact with friends or family members may be helpful.
- When agitated, patients should be sedated with appropriate doses of benzodiazepines.
- Prolonged or severe psychosis will require psychiatric evaluation.

Stimulants

- Cocaine, amphetamines, and related compounds are the most commonly used stimulants.
  - All have sympathomimetic effects.
  - Cocaine is a short-acting stimulant with local anesthetic properties.
  - Cocaine can be insufflated (snorted), smoked, or injected.
  - When smoked or used intravenously, cocaine effects begin almost immediately and peak within several minutes.
  - With nasal use, effects begin in a few minutes and peak after 30 minutes.

- Crack is a purified alkaloid form of cocaine that vaporizes instead of burning, allowing it to be smoked.
  - *Freebasing* describes heating a cocaine solution until it vaporizes and then inhaling the fumes.
- Amphetamines are α-methylphenylethylamine and its derivatives.
  - Amphetamines have been used to treat narcolepsy, asthma, and obesity, but their primary current medical indication is for treatment of attention-deficit/hyperactivity disorder (eg, methylphenidate).
  - Amphetamines cause altered perception, stereotypical and psychotic behaviors, and locomotor stimulation.
- Methylenedioxymethamphetamine (MDMA) is an amphetamine derivative commonly known as *ecstasy,* a popular club drug used at raves and rock concerts.
  - MDMA stimulates feelings of enhanced emotion and arousal, and hallucinations can occur at high doses.
  - Acute ingestion causes a functional increase in the serotonin concentration; with chronic use, however, serotonin stores are depleted.
- The clinical effects associated with these agents are related to stimulation of the CNS and cardiovascular system.
  - Severe effects include seizures and intracranial hemorrhage.
  - Cardiac toxicity of stimulants can cause tachycardia, hypertension, myocardial ischemia, and dysrhythmias.
  - Specific sequelae of cocaine use include:
    - Endocarditis
    - Pneumothorax
    - Tactile hallucinations
  - Amphetamines have been reported to cause:
    - Choreoathetoid movements
    - Compulsive behaviors
  - MDMA can cause hyponatremia resulting from the intake of large volumes of water combined with the release of alcohol dehydrogenase.

Inhalants

- Inhalation of volatile hydrocarbons, such as glue, spray paint, or gasoline, is a common form of adolescent substance abuse.
- Typically, patients sniff (inhale directly), huff (soak a rag and inhale from it), or bag (squirt or spray hydrocarbon in a bag and inhale from the bag or place the bag over the head).
- Acute presentation and management of inhalant intoxication differs from the hydrocarbon aspiration syndrome.
- The primary acute effect of hydrocarbon inhalation is altered mental status.
- At high doses, inhalation may cause:
  - Significant CNS depression
  - Coma
  - Respiratory depression

- Halogenated hydrocarbons, such as typewriter correction fluid (trichloromethane) or Freon, are cardiotoxic.
  - Sensitize the heart to catecholamines
  - Can cause malignant dysrhythmias
  - Sudden sniffing death occurs when a patient has been using these agents, experiences a catecholamine surge (eg, when running away from police), and develops sudden ventricular fibrillation.

Sedative-hypnotic agents

- Sedative-hypnotic agents encompass a diverse group of agents, including benzodiazepines, barbiturates, ethanol, and γ-hydroxybutyrate(GHB).
- Benzodiazepines, such as diazepamoralprazolam, are commonly prescribed anxiolytic agents.
  - Flunitrazepam (Rohypnol, or "roofies") is an illicit benzodiazepine common in drug-facilitated sexual assault (date rape); its anxiolytic effects are also used to soften the coming-down phase after cocaine or heroin use.
- Barbiturates, such as phenobarbital, thiopental, or pentobarbital, are commonly used sedative, anesthetic, or anticonvulsant agents.
- Ethanol (ethyl alcohol) is commonly used by teens and preteens and is a contributing factor to injuries related to motor-vehicle collisions, homicide, fire, drowning, and suicide attempts.
  - At high doses, ethanol intoxication progresses to CNS depression, with coma and death resulting from respiratory suppression.
  - Ethanol is frequently ingested with other drugs.
- GHB was introduced as an anesthetic agent and gained popularity with bodybuilders as a reputed facilitator of growth hormone release.
  - It is currently a schedule-3 drug prescribed for narcolepsy and other sleep disorders.
  - Available in either pill or powder form
  - May cause agitation or sedation, vomiting, bradycardia, hypotension, coma, and seizures
- Sedative-hypnotic agents are usually identified on urine drug screens.
  - Benzodiazepines can be detected from 1–30 days after ingestion, depending on the individual agent.
  - Barbiturates may be detected up to 4 days after ingestion, although phenobarbital may be detected in urine up to 4 weeks later.
  - Blood alcohol concentrations are routinely available.
  - Standard urine drug assays do not screen for GHB.
- The hallmark of sedative-hypnotic intoxication is CNS depression with or without respiratory depression.
  - Respiratory depression can be seen with barbiturate intoxication but is unusual after benzodiazepine intoxication alone.
  - Any combination of agents, including ethanol, increases the risk of respiratory depression.

Opioids

- Morphine, meperidine, codeine, hydrocodone, oxycodone, and propoxyphene are commonly used analgesic agents.
- Heroin is primarily used for its psychoactive effects; methadone is prescribed to treat heroin addiction.
- Different formulations of these agents are available for oral, intravenous, intramuscular, and subcutaneous administration.
  - These agents can also be insufflated or smoked.
  - Intravenous administration (morphine, meperidine, and heroin) leads to rapid onset of effect and carries the highest risk for adverse effects.
- Management of intoxication is based on history of exposure and the presence of clinical symptoms.
- Classic opioid toxidrome includes:
  - Respiratory depression
  - CNS depression
  - Miosis

Toxic alcohols

Methanol and ethylene glycol

- Found in many commercial products, including antifreeze, windshield washing fluid or de-icer, and picnic stove fuel
- Ethylene glycol has a sweet taste and is found in antifreeze, inks, pesticides, adhesives, cosmetics, and paints.
- Metabolites of methanol and ethylene glycol are toxic.
- Methanol intoxication causes:
  - Nausea
  - Headache
  - Decreased vision with mydriasis
  - Weakness
- Symptoms, if untreated, may progress to:
  - Blindness
  - Coma
  - Death
- Ethylene glycol intoxication produces neurologic symptoms.
  - Drunkenness
  - Coma
  - Tachypnea
  - Pulmonary edema
- Ethylene glycol toxicity may cause acute renal failure with precipitated oxalate crystals.
- Antifreeze often contains fluorescein as an additive to help mechanics locate radiator leaks; thus, a Wood lamp examination of the urine for fluorescence is sometimes suggested to help identify ethylene glycol.
  - This test lacks sensitivity.

Isopropyl alcohol (isopropanol)

- Found in common household products, such as rubbing alcohol.

- May be ingested intentionally as a substitute for ethanol

- Unmetabolized isopropanol causes clinical toxicity; as little as 20 mL can cause symptoms.

- GI toxicity causes nausea and vomiting and can progress to hemorrhagic gastritis.

- CNS findings include ataxia, muscle weakness, areflexia, lethargy, and coma.

- Isopropanol ingestion can cause myocardial depression with tachycardia and hypotension, renal tubular acidosis, and tracheobronchitis.

- Patients have increased serum osmolality and ketonuria but do not have metabolic acidosis.

- The clinical presentation is not usually severe and is rarely fatal.

Warfarin-like rodenticides

- The most common rodenticides (rat poisons) are coumarin anticoagulants that cause the rodent to bleed to death.

- Signs of coagulopathy become apparent when active factor levels fall below 30% and may not occur until days after ingestion.

- Superwarfarins are more lipophilic and occupy hepatic binding sites with a higher affinity.

- Warfarin ingestion may produce symptoms for approximately 1 week; superwarfarins may cause effects that persist for months.

- Single toddler exposures to standard warfarin or superwarfarin rodenticides do not typically lead to toxicity.

- Toxicity has been reported in children who repeatedly ingest superwarfarins or in large suicidal ingestions by adolescents or adults.

- Prothrombin time will remain normal for 1–2 days until factor levels have decreased; therefore, testing immediately after exposure is not very helpful.

DIAGNOSTIC APPROACH

- Telephone triage is an important first step in managing potentially toxic exposures.

  - Many exposures can be managed over the telephone, although home therapy of serious poisonings is limited.

- Determine:

  - Name and type of agent
  - Quantity involved
  - Weight of the child
  - Presence or absence of symptoms

- Symptoms alone may indicate toxicity even though, by history, neither the agent nor the dose would have predicted it.

- In the case of nontoxic exposures, reassurance is appropriate.

- Prompt decontamination may reduce subsequent symptoms and need for further treatment.

  - Skin and eyes may be washed in the home or office, if appropriate.

  - Activated charcoal is available in some areas for home administration, but its use has not gained widespread acceptance.

- All calls regarding potentially toxic exposures should be referred to trained poison information specialists at local and regional poison control centers.

  - A list of regional poison centers can be found at the Web site of the AAPCC.

  - The AAPCC toll-free telephone number is 800/222-1222.

- All patients with altered mental status should be evaluated for hypoglycemia.

- Intoxication or poisoning is only one cause of altered mental status.

  - Other important causes are trauma and CNS infection.

  - Trauma is especially important to consider because intoxication is common before trauma.

  - When the cause of altered mental status is unclear, cranial computed tomography should be considered.

  - Lumbar puncture may be performed in cases of altered mental status, especially in the presence of fever.

- Screening tests that are generally appropriate, especially for adolescent patients include:

  - ECG for agents, such as tricyclic antidepressants, that have characteristic ECG findings

  - Pregnancy testing in adolescent girls, because suicidal adolescents often have an acute stressor (such as pregnancy)

  - Acetaminophen levels should be assessed after a suicidal ingestion

    - Acetaminophen is widely available

    - Most patients are asymptomatic after acetaminophen ingestion.

    - A limited window exists for antidotal therapy.

TREATMENT APPROACH

Resuscitation

- Some poisons cause toxicity that requires immediate attention.

  - Airway obstruction
  - Difficulty breathing
  - Dysrhythmias
  - Hypotension
  - Seizures

- Resuscitation generally proceeds according to the recommendations of pediatric advanced life support and advanced cardiac life support.

- Patients with airway obstruction or respiratory failure require urgent airway management and may require assisted ventilation or endotracheal intubation.
- Antidotes are described in detail in the Antidote Table.
- Patients with respiratory depression should receive an empirical trial ofnaloxone.
  - Both diagnostic and therapeutic for opioid (or clonidine) intoxication
  - May preclude the need for intubation
  - Escalating the dosing scheme allows administration of sufficient naloxone to reverse respiratory depression without precipitating withdrawal in a long-term user.
  - For patients with a prolonged opioid effect that outlasts the effect of a single dose of naloxone, it can be administered as a continuous infusion.
  - Naloxone administration may precipitate seizures as part of withdrawal in newborns born to opioid-dependent mothers.
  - Seizures are not a typical part of the withdrawal syndrome in long-term users.
- Hypotension
  - Should be treated with a saline bolus and infusion
  - If unresponsive to fluid alone, may require use of a vasopressor
  - Use of dopamine is common, but it acts indirectly by releasing epinephrine and norepinephrine, which are stored in the nerve terminal.
    - When these stores are depleted, a direct-acting agent, such as norepinephrine, may be useful.
- Empirical use of the benzodiazepine antagonist flumazenil to treat CNS depression after an overdose of an unknown agent is controversial.
  - Flumazenil administration is appropriate in a known acute benzodiazepine exposure associated with significant CNS or respiratory depression.
  - Flumazenil may precipitate withdrawal seizures in the patient with benzodiazepine dependence.
  - It may induce dysrhythmias or seizures in patients exposed totricyclic antidepressants.
  - If the duration of flumazenil effect is shorter than that of the toxin, then repeat doses or a continuous intravenous infusion of flumazenil may be required.
- Seizures require urgent intervention.
  - Benzodiazepines, specifically lorazepam or diazepam, are the preferred agents for the initial treatment of most toxin-induced seizures.
  - Seizures related to INH or the *Gyromitra* species of mushrooms (false morel) should be treated with pyridoxine (vitamin B_6).
  - Seizures related to hypoglycemia should be treated with dextrose.

- Agitation is a common manifestation of altered mental status and places the patient at risk of injury, hyperthermia, and rhabdomyolysis.
  - Benzodiazepines are the preferred sedative agents, and dose should be titrated to effect.
  - Extremely agitated patients may require high doses.

Decontamination

- Considered in 2 large categories:
  - Surface decontamination of the skin and eyes
  - GI decontamination

Surface decontamination

- Skin exposures require thorough washing with soap followed by copious rinsing.
- Eye exposures require copious irrigation with water or saline.
- Decontamination must occur before other interventions, even resuscitation, with agents in which significant dermal absorption occurs.
  - Remove and secure clothing.
  - Health care workers must be appropriately protected.
  - Prehospital approach to managing chemical incidents includes decontamination at the site, although decontamination facilities are being built at many health care facilities.
  - Information can be found at the Web site of the Centers for Disease Control and Prevention.

GI decontamination

- *GI decontamination* refers to any procedure that removes toxin or reduces absorption from the GI tract and includes:
  - Emetic agents
  - Lavage
  - Activated charcoal
  - Cathartic agents
- Emetic agents
  - Both the AAP and American Academy of Clinical Toxicology currently recommend against the use of syrup of ipecac for poison management, even at home.
- *Gastric lavage* describes the procedure of irrigating the stomach with a large volume of fluid through a large-bore tube passed through the mouth into the stomach.
  - Should be performed when:
    - Risk of toxicity is great.
    - Likelihood of recovering the toxin is high.
    - Other treatment modalities are unavailable.
  - Certain agents, such as anticholinergic agents or opioids, may delay gastric emptying and slow GI transit time.
    - May remain in the stomach for >1 hour
    - May be available for removal by lavage
  - Contraindicated after the ingestion of hydrocarbons, acids, or alkaline agents

P

Antidote Table[a]

Substance	Antidote	Dose	Comments
Acetaminophen	N-acetylcysteine	• IV: 150 mg/kg over 15 min, then 50 mg/kg over 4 hr, then 100 mg/kg over 16 hr • PO: 140 mg/kg load, then 70 mg/kg/dose every 4 hr for 17 doses	• AE: vomiting (PO); anaphylactoid reaction (IV). • IV protocol requires large volumes of free water, which may cause hyponatremia and seizures in children.
Anticholinergic agents (eg, atropine)	Physostigmine	• P: 0.5 mg IV slowly • A: 2 mg IV slowly	• May repeat dose after 15 min. • AE: cholinergic symptoms occur with excessive dosing.
Benzodiazepines	Flumazenil	• P: 0.01 mg/kg IV slowly every min (max 1 mg) • A: 0.1–0.2 mg IV slowly every min (max 1 mg)	• Titrate to effect or maximal dose. May not reverse respiratory depression. If positive response is of short duration, may be administered as a continuous infusion. • AE: withdrawal symptoms in dependent or chronic use; seizures or dysrhythmias in cyclic antidepressant overdose.
ß-Adrenergic antagonists	Glucagon	• P: 0.1 mg/kg IV slowly • A: 3–5 mg IV slowly	• If positive response is of short duration, may be administered as a continuous infusion. • AE: vomiting, hyperglycemia, hypocalcemia.
	Insulin and dextrose	• Insulin0.5 U/kg/hr IV, with • Dextrose 1 g/kg/hr	AE: hypo- or hyperglycemia, hypokalemia.
	Amrinone	750 mcg/kg over 3–5 min slowly (max 3 mg/kg)	• May use other phosphodiesterase inhibitors with equal efficacy (eg, milrinone). • AE: hypotension.
Carbon monoxide	Oxygen (100%)	100% oxygen by nonrebreather	Treat until normal CO level or until hyperbaric oxygen initiated.
	Oxygen (hyperbaric)	100% oxygen at 2–3 atmosphere for 20 min	AE: pneumothorax, perforated tympanic membrane.
Calcium-channel blockers	Calcium chloride (10%)	• P: 20 mg/kg (0.2 mL/kg) IV slowly, via central line • A: 1–2 g (10–20 mL) IV slowly	May use glucagon, insulin, and dextrose as adjunctive treatment in CCB as in BB toxicity.
	Calcium gluconate (10%)	• P: 60 mg/kg (0.6 mL/kg) • A: 3–6 g (30–60 mL) IV	AE: hypercalcemia, phlebitis, nausea, vomiting, flushing, confusion, angina.
Cyanide	Amyl nitrate	One ampule by inhalation for 30 seconds every 3 min until IV access	AE: methemoglobinemia (see caution for sodium nitrite below).
	Sodium nitrite (3%)	• P: 0.33 mL (10 mg) IV (for Hb at 12) • A: 10 mL IV over 10 min	• Dose varies according to weight and Hb level. See package insert. • AE: methemoglobinemia. • Use with caution in unconfirmed or unlikely cyanide poisoning (eg, in the setting of smoke inhalation), because induced methemoglobinemia may exacerbate hypoxemia from other causes.
	Sodium thiosulfate (25%)	• P: 1.6 mL/kg IV (for Hb at 12) • A: 50 mL IV over 3 min	• Dose varies according to weight and Hb count. See package insert. • AE: hypotension, CNS toxicity.

Antidote Table^a, continued

Digoxin	Digoxin-specific antibody fragments (Digibind)	• For known ingested dose: number of vials = mg ingested × 1.5 • For known serum digoxin concentration (SDC, ng/mL): number of vials = SDC × weight (kg)/100 • For unknown SDC or dose acute overdose: 10–20 vials • For chronic overdose: P: 2 vials; A: 5 vials	• Each 40-mg vial binds 0.6 mg digoxin. • AE: hypokalemia, worsening CHF.
Ethylene glycol and methanol	Ethanol (10%)	800 mg/kg (8 mL/kg) IV over 20–60 min, then 80-130 mg/kg/hr (0.8-1.3 mL/kg/hr) IV	Titrate to serum ethanol 100 mg/dL. Increase dose during dialysis and in chronic alcoholics. Oral dosing may be used in select cases.
	Fomepizole (4-methylpyrazole)	15 mg/kg over 30 min IV, then 10 mg/kg/dose every 12 hr × 4 doses, then 15 mg/kg/dose every 12 hr	• Continue therapy until serum methanol or ethylene glycol level <20 mg/dL. Increase dose during dialysis. • AE: headache, nausea, dizziness, bradycardia, eosinophilia, transient increase of liver enzyme levels
Heparin	Protamine sulfate	Use 1 mg protamine for every 100 units of heparin to be neutralized.	AE: hypotension, bradycardia, hemorrhage. Use with caution with known fish allergy.
Iron	Deferoxamine	5–15 mg/kg/hr IV (max 6 g/24 hr)	• Titrate dose slowly to avoid hypotension. Continue therapy until *vin rose* urine color clears, symptoms clinically resolve, or maximal dose attained. • Deferoxamine challenge no longer suggested. • AE: flushing, hypotension, acute respiratory distress syndrome.
Isoniazid	Pyridoxine (vitamin B$_6$)	• Known INH dose: 1 g per g of INH ingested IV slowly • Unknown INH dose: 5 g IV over 10 min	• Administer 1 g every 23 min. • AE: CNS toxicity—headache, seizure, peripheral neurotoxicity.
Lead	Succimer (DMSA)	10 mg/kg/dose PO every 8 hr × 5 days, then 10 mg/kg/dose twice daily × 14 days	AE: rash, neutropenia, increased LFTs, GI upset.
	Dimercaprol (BAL)	• 75 mg/m²/dose IM every 4 hr • Max: 450 mg/m²/dose/24 hr	• Pretreatment with diphenhydramine suggested. Contraindicated with peanut allergy, hepatic insufficiency. • AE: G6PD hemolytic crisis, nausea, vomiting, histamine release.
	CaNa$_2$ EDTA	1–1.5 g/m²/day continuous IV infusion × 5 days	• In cases of encephalopathy, administer after dimercaprol to prevent increased CNS lead levels. • AE: phlebitis.
Methanol	See Ethylene glycol		
Methemoglobinemia	Methylene blue (1%)	1–2 mg/kg IV over 5 min	• Repeat doses as needed. • AE: dyspnea, chest pain, and hemolysis.

P

continued

Antidote Table[a], *continued*

Opioids	Naloxone	0.5–2 mg IV/IM/SC/ET (max 10 mg)	• Higher dose may be required for certain agents. Can repeat dose every 2–3 min until response or max dose. If no response to total 10-mg dose, unlikely opioid intoxication. If positive response is of short duration, may be administered as a continuous infusion. In setting of possible opioid dependence, consider initial dose of 0.05 mg to avoid withdrawal. • AE: opioid withdrawal (piloerection, agitation, vomiting).
Cholinergic agents (eg, malathion)	Atropine	• P: 0.02 mg/kg IV initial dose (minimum 0.1 mg) • A: 0.5–1 mg IV initial dose	• Double dose every 3–5 min. Titrate to reduced bronchorrhea or improved oxygen saturation. May require total doses 5 or 10 times the initial dose or higher. • AE: anticholinergic toxicity.
	Pralidoxime	• P: 25–50 mg/kg over 30–60 min, then 20 mg/kg/hr • A: 1–2 g IV over 15–30 min, then 0.5 g/hr	Pralidoxime should be administered in addition to atropine. Continue therapy for 24–72 hr.
Oral antidiabetic agents	Octreotide	• P: 1–2 mcg/kg SC/IV every 6–12 hr • A: 50–100 mcg SC/IV, then 50 mcg every 12 hr	• Continue therapy until euglycemic. May require several days of therapy. • AE: bradycardia, dysrhythmias, GI upset, hyperglycemia.
	Dextrose	• Neonate: 0.2 g/kg IV (use $D_{10}W$, 2 mL/kg) • P: 0.5–1 g/kg IV (use $D_{25}W$, 2–4 mL/kg) • A: 25–50 g IV (use $D_{50}W$)	AE: hyperglycemia, extravasation may cause local tissue reaction.
Tricyclic antidepressants	Sodium bicarbonate	1–2 mEq/kg IV bolus, then titrate to pH ~7.5 with additional doses or with continuous infusion	AE: volume overload, hypernatremia, metabolic alkalosis.
Warfarin	Vitamin K	• P: 1–5 mg SC/IM/IV/PO, every 6–8 hr PRN • A: 10 mg SC/IM/IV/PO, every 6–8 hr PRN	Much larger doses may be required. Continue therapy until INR within normal limits.

Abbreviations: AE, Adverse effects; BB, ß-adrenergic blocker; CCB, calcium-channel blocker; CHF, congestive heart failure; CNS, central nervous system; CO, carbon monoxide; $D_{10}W$, 10% dextrose and water; ET, endotracheally; G6PD, glucose-6-phosphate dehydrogenase; GI, gastrointestinal; Hb, hemoglobin; INH, isoniaizid; IM, intramuscular; INR, international normalized ratio of prothrombin time; IV, intravenous; LFT, liver function tests; max, maximum; PO, oral; PRN, as needed; SC, subcutaneous; SDC, serum digoxin concentration.
[a] Pediatric (P) and adult (A) doses are the same unless specifically noted.

- The most likely complication is vomiting, with aspiration of stomach contents.
  - Risk is highest in patients with a depressed level of consciousness and a diminished gag reflex.
  - Risk can be reduced by intubating the patient with a cuffed endotracheal tube.
- Unusual complications include esophageal or gastric perforation, dysrhythmias, hypothermia, and fluid and electrolyte abnormalities.

- Activated charcoal is a mainstay in poison management.
  - Adsorbs toxins in the GI tract to prevent absorption into the bloodstream
  - Effectively binds most large molecules, such as acetaminophen, aspirin, and phenobarbital
  - Does not adsorb small molecules, such as lithium or iron
  - Can be administered in single or multiple doses
  - The most common side effect is vomiting.
  - If the patient has a depressed level of consciousness, then the airway must be protected.

- Only contraindication is GI tract obstruction or perforation
- Should not be provided after acid or alkali exposures, because the charcoal will obscure endoscopic view of the esophagus and stomach
- Cathartic agents are used to enhance elimination from the GI tract.
  - Evidence supporting this therapy is not strong.
  - Such agents as magnesium citrate and magnesium sulfate are rarely used because of associated fluid and electrolyte abnormalities.
  - Sorbitol is the most frequently used and is typically administered with activated charcoal.
    - Fluid and electrolyte abnormalities are uncommon unless multiple doses are administered.
    - Only 1 combination dose of sorbitol and charcoal is suggested, even for cases in which multiple doses of activated charcoal are planned.
- *Whole-bowel irrigation* (WBI) is flushing the entire GI tract with an isoosmotic electrolyte solution, polyethylene glycol.
  - Frequently used to prepare the bowel for surgery
  - Large volumes (liters) of polyethylene glycol are infused until the effluent turns clear.
  - Not associated with fluid and electrolyte abnormalities, but patients sometimes experience GI discomfort and bloating
  - May be particularly helpful for agents that cannot be adsorbed with activated charcoal, such as iron or lithium, and for extended-release medications

Enhanced elimination

- Ion trapping, particularly urinary alkalinization, enhances drug clearance.
  - Most often used for salicylate poisoning
  - May enhance elimination of phenobarbital, chlorpropamide, and myoglobin
  - In theory, elimination of weak bases, such as phencyclidine and amphetamines, should be enhanced in acidic urine; however, urinary acidification has greater risk than benefit and is not used therapeutically.
- Hemodialysis provides definitive therapy for a limited number of agents, including:
  - Ethylene glycol
  - Lithium
  - Methanol
  - Salicylate
- Charcoal hemoperfusion is generally suggested for theophylline and sometimes for carbamazepine poisonings.
  - However, specialized charcoal cartridges have been difficult to obtain recently, and these poisonings are being treated with new high-efficiency, high-flux hemodialysis techniques.

Supportive care

- Continuation of care given in resuscitation, with ongoing attention paid to cardiorespiratory and neurologic status

SPECIFIC TREATMENTS

Analgesics

Acetaminophen

- N-acetylcysteine (NAC) is the specific antidote.
  - The decision to initiate NAC therapy requires using the Rumack-Matthew nomogram (see Figure 62 on page F21).
  - If a level on samples drawn 4 hours or later is above the possible toxicity line, then the patient should receive NAC.
  - This treatment approach is also applicable to patients who overdose with an extended-release preparation of acetaminophen.
- The oral formulation of NAC may still be available for use in some locations.
  - The sulfurous smell and foul taste of oral NAC frequently lead to nausea and vomiting.
- Intravenous NAC is reconstituted in 5% dextrose in water and administered according to a complex regimen that delivers a large volume of free water to the patient.
  - Intravenous NAC should be administered in consultation with a toxicologist familiar with its use.
  - The incidence of adverse reactions to intravenous NAC administration, primarily anaphylactoid reactions, may be as high as 20%.
    - These side effects are not completely mitigated by lowering the infusion rate but are usually amenable to therapy, after which treatment can be restarted.
  - Sick patients show altered mental status and hypovolemic shock.
  - Hepatotoxicity is unlikely if NAC is administered within 8–10 hours of the time of ingestion.
    - After this time, efficacy may be reduced, especially when patients wait before seeking care.
    - If a patient arrives ≥4 hours after ingestion and a level will not be available within the 8-hour window, then NAC should be administered pending results.
    - Although efficacy is reduced after 8 hours, NAC should still be administered, even to patients who seek care very late after the time of ingestion.
  - Reports have been issued of children developing hyponatremia and seizures secondary to intravenous NAC.
- If patients progress to fulminant hepatic failure, they may require liver transplantation.
  - Spontaneous recovery is not associated with long-term clinical or pathological sequelae.
- If a patient's acetaminophen levels are assessed on samples

P

drawn ≥4 hours after ingestion and the level is below the possible toxicity line of the nomogram, then the patient is medically clear.

■ If the level is above the line and the patient begins NAC therapy within 8–10 hours, then the patient is medically clear at the end of treatment.

Salicylates

■ Decisions regarding therapy are based on clinical evidence of toxicity.

■ Need for intubation is unusual; hypoventilation after intubation may worsen acidosis.

■ Fluid resuscitation is critical.

■ Patients may require treatment for hypoglycemia.

■ Several doses of activated charcoal are useful to prevent the absorption of ingested salicylate and may interrupt enterohepatic circulation.

■ Rarely, salicylate tablets form a conglomeration in the stomach that requires surgical removal.

■ In the case of methylsalicylate, patients may require skin decontamination to prevent ongoing dermal absorption.

■ The first intervention to enhance salicylate elimination is to alkalinize the urine.

  ● Optimal elimination occurs at a urine pH >8.

■ Any patient with clinical evidence of salicylate toxicity is a candidate for alkalinization unless administering large volumes of fluid is contraindicated.

■ Hemodialysis is used to eliminate salicylate and correct acidosis.

  ● Indications for hemodialysis include:
    – Persistent CNS toxicity
    – Severe, worsening, or intractable acidosis
    – Extremely high salicylate levels (usually >100 mg/dL)
    – Any condition that precludes the administration of a high-volume bicarbonate infusion, such as pulmonary edema, renal insufficiency, or congestive heart failure

■ Any patient with evidence of significant toxicity requires hospital admission for further evaluation and management.

  ● If no evidence of toxicity is found after 4–6 hours of observation, then the patient is medically clear.

Antidepressants

Tricyclic antidepressants

■ Gastric lavage should only be performed when adequate airway protection is ensured because of the high risk of coma, seizures, and dysrhythmias in tricyclic antidepressant overdose.

■ Reversal agents, such as flumazenil and physostigmine, are contraindicated in the setting of known or possible tricyclic antidepressant overdose.

■ Initial management of patients with significant cardiovascular or CNS toxicity follows the principles in Treatment Approach (Resuscitation).

■ Specific therapy for tricyclic antidepressant–related wide complex ventricular dysrhythmias and hypotension is hypertonic sodium bicarbonate administration.

  ● Increase the serum pH to approximately 7.5.

  ● A more alkaline pH lowers the concentration of free drug by stimulating protein binding; increased serum sodium overcomes sodium-channel blockade.

  ● Adverse effects include volume overload, hypernatremia, and severe metabolic alkalosis.

■ For persistent wide-complex tachycardias or torsades de pointes, limited evidence supports the use of magnesium.

■ Benzodiazepines are suggested for seizures.

  ● Barbiturates and propofol may be considered as adjuncts for seizures refractory to benzodiazepines.

  ● Phenytoin should not be used because it blocks sodium channels and exacerbates tricyclic antidepressant cardiotoxicity.

■ Medical admission will be required for patients with signs of cardiovascular or neurologic toxicity.

SSRIs

■ The main focus of therapy is to decrease muscle rigidity and its sequelae, myoglobinuria and renal failure.

■ Initial therapy to achieve muscle relaxation is benzodiazepines.

■ Adjunctive therapy may be provided with cyproheptadine, a histamine and serotonin antagonist.

■ Severe hyperthermia should be treated with aggressive cooling.

■ If muscle rigidity is severe and unresponsive to conventional measures, then neuromuscular blockade can be used after the patient is intubated.

■ Asymptomatic patients do not require medical admission.

■ Patients with symptoms of serotonin syndrome should be admitted to the hospital for further evaluation and management.

Antihistamines

■ Most patients with antihistamine toxicity do well with supportive care alone.

■ For large ingestions or ingestions of sustained-release formulations:

  ● Gastric lavage or
  ● WBI

■ Administration of activated charcoal is appropriate.

■ Significant agitation or seizures should be treated with benzodiazepines.

- Physostigmine, a carbamate with cholinergic properties, is an antidote for patients with anticholinergic toxicity and is appropriate for use in a pure antihistamine overdose with moderate to severe symptoms.
  - Adverse effects of physostigmine include seizures and ventricular dysrhythmias.
  - Physostigmine is contraindicated for patients with evidence of cardiotoxicity or for treatment of overdoses of cardiotoxic agents, such as tricyclic antidepressants.
  - Physostigmine therapy should not be administered as nonspecific therapy for unknown coma or agitation.
- Patients who remain asymptomatic after 4–6 hours may be medically cleared.
- Symptoms may sometimes be delayed after a large ingestion, and patients may require a longer period of observation.

Carbon monoxide

- All exposed patients should initially receive 100% oxygen until an accurate estimate of exposure can be determined or a CO-Hb level can be measured, or both.
- A pH and blood lactate should be obtained concurrently; lactate seems to correlate to some extent with severity.
- Hyperbaric oxygen therapy is the preferred treatment for serious CO poisoning.
  - Increases concentration of dissolved oxygen to displace CO from binding sites on hemoglobin, myoglobin, and cytochrome oxidase
  - Improves the delivery of oxygen to tissues
  - Reduces lipid peroxidation
  - Limited data suggest it reduces the incidence of delayed neurologic and neuropsychiatric effects, particularly if administered within 6 hours, although data are conflicting.
  - Seems to be safe for pregnant women and may benefit the fetus
  - Hyperbaric chambers can be located through the Undersea and Hyperbaric Medical Society Web site (www.uhms.org/).
- Potential candidates for hyperbaric oxygen therapy include patients with:
  - Significant CNS, cardiovascular, or neuropsychiatric symptoms
  - Persistent metabolic acidosis or other symptoms that do not respond to standard 100% oxygen therapy
  - CO-Hb levels >25%
  - Pregnant women or children with CO-Hb levels >15%
- In general, symptomatic patients require hospitalization for further evaluation and management.
- Patients with relatively low CO-Hb levels and mild symptoms, especially when symptoms resolve after a short course of oxygen therapy, do not require hospitalization.
- Identifying and ameliorating the source of CO is imperative.

- Contact other potentially exposed persons who may require evaluation.

Cardiovascular medications

Cardiac glycosides

- Activated charcoal and steroid binding resins, such as cholestyramine, will adsorb cardiac glycosides in the GI tract and may interrupt their enterohepatic circulation.
- Hyperkalemia should be aggressively treated with bicarbonate, insulin, and glucose.
  - Calcium administration is contraindicated for the treatment of hyperkalemia, as it can exacerbate glycoside toxicity.
- Magnesium sulfate should be used in patients with hypomagnesemia.
- Kayexalate can also be administered.
- Significant toxicity is treated with digoxin-specific antibody antigen-binding fragments.
  - In the acute setting, Digibind therapy is used to treat:
    - Significant dysrhythmia
    - Serum digoxin levels >15 ng/mL at any time or >10 ng/mL 6 hours after ingestion
    - Serum potassium level >5 mEq/L
    - Hypotension
    - Second- or third-degree heart block
    - Digoxin dose >10 mg in a teenager or adult or >4 mg in a child
  - Digibind causes a marked increase in the measured serum digoxin level; thus, posttreatment levels do not reliably indicate a response to therapy.
- Adjunctive therapy includes:
  - Atropine for bradycardia
  - Phenytoin and lidocaine for ventricular dysrhythmias
- Cardioversion should be avoided because the ensuing sympathetic discharge can be fatal.
- Classes Ia, Ic, II, and IV antidysrhythmics are contraindicated because they decrease atrioventricular conduction and worsen bradycardia and other dysrhythmias.

BBs and CCBs

- For both BB and CCB ingestions (see also Antidote Table):
  - Activated charcoal can be administered.
  - WBI should be considered for ingestions of sustained-release preparations.
  - Glucagon is considered the specific antidote for significant cardiovascular symptoms related to BB overdose.
    - It may also be useful for CCB ingestions.
  - High-dose insulin and glucose is another therapeutic option.
    - Insulin may increase myocardial glucose utilization or alter myocardial calcium handling.
  - Calcium chloride may be useful.

- Amrinone, a phosphodiesterase inhibitor, may be useful for refractory hypotension.
  - By inhibiting the breakdown of cyclic adenosine monophosphate, amrinone, as does glucagon, increases inotropy.
- In both CCB and BB overdose, adjunctive therapy for severe refractory bradycardia includes:
  - Atropine
  - Epinephrine
  - Isoproterenol
  - Cardiac pacing
- Patients may require therapy for hyperglycemia, hyperkalemia, or seizures.
- All symptomatic patients with a history of a BB or CCB overdose should be admitted to an intensive care unit.
- Patients who are asymptomatic 6 hours after ingestion may be discharged unless they ingested a sustained-release formulation.

α_2-adrenergic agonists (clonidine)

- Naloxone should be administered in cases of respiratory depression; high doses may be required (see Antidote Table).
  - May also be useful in cases of CNS depression or hypotension
- When naloxone is effective but clonidine toxicity outlasts naloxone's effect, continuous infusion of naloxone is indicated.
- Decontamination with activated charcoal is appropriate.
- WBI may be indicated for children who have ingested clonidine patches.
- Atropine may have modest effects on bradycardia, and fluids and pressors are indicated for hypotension.
- All symptomatic patients should be admitted to the hospital.
- Patients may be discharged if they are asymptomatic 4 hours after ingestion.

Caustic ingestions

- Gastric lavage is contraindicated because of the risk of esophageal or gastric perforation.
- Activated charcoal absorbs caustic chemicals poorly and may interfere with endoscopy.
- Plain-film radiography of the chest and abdomen is helpful to rule out pneumomediastinum, pneumoperitoneum, and aspiration pneumonitis.
- Esophagoscopy defines the extent of injury and should be performed in symptomatic patients.
- If any suspicion of perforation exists:
  - Surgical consultation should be obtained.
  - Broad-spectrum antibiotics should be administered.
- In large-volume acid ingestions, nasogastric suction performed within 30 minutes of exposure may prevent the passage of acid into the small intestine.

- Neutralization of acids and bases should be avoided because of the excessive heat and the risk of emesis.
- Repeat esophagraphy will be required 3–4 weeks after caustic ingestion to check for strictures.

Hydrocarbons

- Contaminated clothing should be disposed of properly.
- Skin should be washed with soap and water to limit continuing exposure.
- GI decontamination plays only a limited role; toxicity is related more to pulmonary exposure than to GI absorption.
- Most patients experience nausea and vomiting after hydrocarbon exposure and do not require further gastric emptying.
  - Gastric emptying is contraindicated after most hydrocarbon ingestions; risk of aspiration increases with any gastric-emptying procedure.
  - Gastric emptying (although controversial) may be considered in 2 cases.
    - When the patient has swallowed a large volume of hydrocarbon but has not already vomited
    - When the swallowed hydrocarbon can have systemic toxicity or is the carrier for another toxin, characterized by the mnemonic CHAMP (camphor, halogenated hydrocarbons, aromatic hydrocarbons, heavy metals, and pesticides)
- Symptomatic patients have radiographic evidence of aspiration as early as 30 minutes after exposure.
  - Asymptomatic patients occasionally develop radiographic changes, but importance of these changes is unclear.
- Management of pulmonary toxicity includes:
  - Supplemental oxygen
  - Humidified air
  - Intravenous fluids
  - Nebulized β_2-agonists may be useful.
- Severely ill patients may require:
  - Continuous positive airway pressure
  - Mechanical ventilation with positive end-expiratory pressure
  - Extracorporeal membrane oxygenation
- Corticosteroids are not beneficial.
- Leukocytosis and fever are associated with hydrocarbon aspiration, and at least early in the course, do not signify infection.
- Patients with persistent respiratory symptoms should be hospitalized.
- Patients should be observed for 6 hours if:
  - They are symptomatic.
  - Symptoms have resolved and radiographic findings are normal.

- If they are asymptomatic at the end of the observation period, then they may be medically cleared.

Insect repellents

- Treatment entails avoidance and decontamination with soap and water.

Iron

- Asymptomatic patients do not require gastric emptying.
- Patients experiencing toxicity vomit spontaneously, and no additional benefit exists to gastric emptying.
- Gastric lavage has a limited role after significant ingestion or when pills are radiologically evident in the stomach.
  - Gastric lavage is often unsuccessful at removing pills from the stomach and cannot remove pills that have passed into the lower GI tract.
  - WBI may be more effective than other treatments at removing these residual pills.
  - In rare cases, surgery may be necessary to remove iron pills.
- Radiographs detect residual iron pills in <3% of all ingestions, but their does not exclude a toxic overdose.
  - Chewable and liquid iron formulations do not appear on abdominal radiographs.
- Significant iron poisoning is associated with both increased serum glucose level and an increased leukocyte count; however, normal values do not rule out significant exposure.
- Total iron-binding capacity greater than the serum iron level was once thought to be protective in poisoning.
  - However, total iron-binding capacity is factitiously increased in the setting of iron poisoning.
  - Deferoxamine also interferes with the accurate measurement of total iron-binding capacity.
- Patients with significant poisoning are often in shock, with positive anion gap metabolic acidosis.
  - These patients need immediate and vigorous resuscitation.
  - Decisions regarding treatment will usually have to be made on clinical grounds alone.
- Chelation therapy with deferoxamine should be considered for any symptomatic child who:
  - Is in shock *or*
  - Has an altered mental status *or*
  - Is experiencing protracted vomiting or GI bleeding
- Serum iron levels >500 mcg/dL or abdominal radiographs suggesting a serious ingestion may also be an indication for chelation.
- Desferrioxamine, the deferoxamine-iron chelate, is excreted in the urine and imparts a dark brown or *vin rose* color to the urine.
  - This color change is only a qualitative measure of desferrioxamine and is an unreliable marker of iron elimination.

- Chelation therapy should continue until the child is clinically improved and the metabolic acidosis is resolved, but duration of therapy >24 hours may present an increased risk of toxicity.
- Patients who remain asymptomatic without treatment for 6 hours after ingestion are medically clear.

INH

- If an asymptomatic patient seeks care soon after a significant exposure, then gastric lavage is appropriate.
- Activated charcoal may be provided.
- To prevent seizures, prophylactic pyridoxine should be administered to patients who seek care within 2 hours of ingestion.
- Seizure therapy
  - Can begin with typical anticonvulsants, such as benzodiazepines or phenobarbital
  - Phenytoin is not useful in treating INH-related seizures.
- Definitive therapy requires administration of pyridoxine, the specific antidote for INH toxicity.
- If intravenous pyridoxine is unavailable, crushed tablets can be given by nasogastric tube.
- Hemodialysis may be considered for patients with massive toxic ingestions.
- Patients who remain asymptomatic for 6 hours can be medically cleared.

Lead poisoning

- In all cases of suspected lead poisoning:
  - Any sources of lead exposure should be identified and abated.
  - Parents should be counseled regarding optimal nutrition.
- Symptomatic children are typically hospitalized to remove them from the source of lead and to administer chelation therapy.
  - Oral intake should be restricted.
  - Intravenous fluid resuscitation should be started if the use of ethylenediaminetetraacetic acid (EDTA) is anticipated.
  - If abdominal radiography finds radiopaque material, then WBI with polyethylene glycol should be initiated.
- BPb levels <45 mcg/dL
  - Patients do not require chelation therapy.
- Asymptomatic children with BPb between 45 and 70 mcg/dL
  - Chelate with oral succimer *or*
  - Intravenous $CaNa_2$ EDTA
- Children with BPb >70 mcg/dL
  - Chelate in the hospital with intramuscular dimercaprol (also known as *British anti-lewisite*) *and*
  - Intravenous $CaNa_2$ EDTA
- After initial chelation therapy, decision to repeat treatment depends on symptoms and follow-up BPb levels.

P

- Encephalopathy
  - Treated with the same 2-drug regimen but for a longer course
- 3 lead chelating agents are available in the US:
  - Dimercaprol
  - CaNa$_2$ EDTA
  - Succimer (dimercaptosuccinic acid [DMSA])
- A fourth agent, D-penicillamine, is not approved by the US Food and Drug Administration, but its use may be necessary in the unusual event of adverse reactions to both DMSA and CaNa$_2$ EDTA.

Organophosphates

Pesticides

- For a suspected or confirmed organophosphate exposure, decontamination should follow the principles above.
  - Rescuers and health care workers are at risk of exposure if the patient has not been appropriately decontaminated.
  - Contaminated clothing must be safely discarded.
  - For ocular exposures, the eyes should be copiously irrigated.
- After ingestions, gastric lavage may be appropriate.
  - Activated charcoal can be administered.
  - Lavage fluid is contaminated and must be safely discarded.
- The immediate life-threatening problem is bronchorrhea (copious airway secretions).
  - A patient in severe respiratory distress should be intubated.
  - The goal of therapy is to dry the airway secretions with atropine.
    - High-dose, continuous infusions of atropine may be required.
  - Succinylcholine should not be used for rapid-sequence intubation because it requires the inactivated cholinesterase for its metabolism.
  - Tachycardia, which may be related to either atropine administration or hypoxia, is not a contraindication to use of higher doses.
- The organophosphate-acetylcholinesterase enzyme complex ages over time, leading to irreversible inactivation of the enzyme.
  - 2-Pralidoxime, also known as 2-PAM, can hydrolyze the bond and reactivate the cholinesterase when administered before complete aging.
  - Because this agent does not cross the blood-brain barrier, reversal of neurologic symptoms requires atropine.
  - The efficacy of pralidoxime varies with the different organophosphate compounds, but it should be administered in all cases of severe toxicity.

- All patients with organophosphate toxicity require admission.
- Time to full recovery depends on the agent and can range from a few hours to several weeks.

Nerve agents

- Treatment for these agents is the same as that outlined for organophosphate pesticides above.
- The US Food and Drug Administration has approved an atropine autoinjector for children that is available for prehospital use.

Plants

- Only a very few patients seek medical attention; even fewer require intervention (see table Toxic Plants).
- Prevent plant exposures through education.
  - Parents must learn the names of plants they purchase, be familiar with plants that are toxic, and keep them safely away from children.

Substance abuse

Marijuana

- Compared with other hallucinogens, the effects of marijuana are usually mild and self-limited and require minimal medical intervention.

PCP and ketamine

- Supportive care in a quiet environment with minimal loud or noxious stimuli is usually all that is needed.
- Verbal and physical contact with friends or family members may be helpful.
- When agitated, patients should be sedated with appropriate doses of benzodiazepines.
- Prolonged or severe psychosis will require psychiatric evaluation.

Stimulants

- Treatment of stimulant intoxication requires good supportive care.
  - Benzodiazepine sedation is the most effective treatment for agitation, chest pain, hypertension, hyperthermia, and seizures.
  - Rhabdomyolysis is a common complication of stimulant use and may require:
    - Aggressive intravenous hydration
    - Urinary alkalinization
    - Hemodialysis (rarely)
  - Hyperthermia requires aggressive cooling.
- Patients who respond appropriately to sedation and remain asymptomatic for a 4- to 6-hour period of observation are medically clear.
- Cocaine-associated chest pain is usually short-lived and benign; approximately 6% of patients will have acute myocardial infarction.

- Most cases occur in the absence of underlying heart disease and can occur in adolescence.
- Management of myocardial ischemia and dysrhythmias may require the use of benzodiazepines, nitroglycerin, phentolamine, aspirin, morphine, and CCBs.
- Wide-complex tachycardias associated with cocaine may respond to bicarbonate.
- If patients display persistent signs of cardiac involvement (eg, chest pain, ECG changes, abnormal cardiac enzymes), admit to a chest pain observation unit.
- Patients are medically clear if they have normal levels of troponin I, no new ischemic ECG changes, and no cardiovascular complications during a 12-hour observation period.

Sedative-hypnotic agents

- Medical interventions should be focused on drug-specific side effects.
- Flumazenil, a specific benzodiazepine antagonist, is appropriate in the setting of a known benzodiazepine exposure associated with significant CNS depression, respiratory depression, or both.
  - Empiric use of flumazenil to treat respiratory or CNS depression after overdose of an unknown agent is not suggested.
  - Flumazenil should not be administered to patients with possible long-term benzodiazepine use because of the high risk of inducing withdrawal.
- Patients with suspected sedative-hypnotic intoxication should be admitted for monitoring of respiratory and neurologic status.
  - Barbiturate and benzodiazepine use may require prolonged hospitalization as a result of prolonged duration of effect.
  - Patients with uncomplicated ethanol ingestion can usually be observed and discharged after observation in an emergency department setting.
  - GHB and Rohypnol usually have short durations of action and can typically be managed in the emergency department.

Opioids

- Patients with respiratory or CNS depression related to known or presumed opioid intoxication should receive naloxone (see Antidote Table).
- Opioid metabolites are excreted in the urine and can be detected on a urine drug screen up to 4 days after acute use and longer after long-term use.
- Patients who are awake and alert after opioid use do not require further medical evaluation.
- Patients whose status is reversed by a single dose of naloxone should be observed for at least several hours in case of recurrence of symptoms.

- Patients with significant opioid symptoms who have received high doses or a continuous infusion of naloxone require hospitalization.

Toxic alcohols

Methanol and ethylene glycol

- These agents have rapid absorption from the GI tract, so gastric lavage and activated charcoal have limited utility.
  - May be useful for patients who seek care soon after large-volume ingestions
  - Maintaining the pH near normal with sodium bicarbonate will reduce availability and enhance the elimination of some toxic metabolites.
- Fomepizole is available for the treatment of methanol and ethylene glycol intoxication.
  - If the patient ingested ethanol along with methanol or ethylene glycol, onset of toxicity may be delayed.
  - Folate enhances the metabolism of formic acid and is adjunctive therapy for methanol poisoning.
  - Thiamine and pyridoxine shunt ethylene glycol metabolism toward less toxic metabolites and are adjunctive therapy for ethylene glycol poisoning.
- Definitive therapy requires hemodialysis to remove both the toxic alcohols and their metabolites.
  - Indications are severe acidosis, visual or mental status changes, or high serum concentrations (methanol or ethylene glycol >25 mg/dL).

Isopropyl alcohol (isopropanol)

- These patients require supportive care and symptomatic therapy.
- In severe cases, hemodialysis may be necessary for:
  - Persistent hypotension
  - Plasma levels >400 mg/dL
  - Prolonged coma
  - Underlying renal or hepatic disease that limits the metabolism and excretion
- Any patient with suspected or confirmed significant toxic alcohol ingestion and any symptomatic patient should be hospitalized.
- Patients with no symptoms who are treated early have an excellent prognosis.
- Patients with seizures, coma, or pH <7.20 have a poor prognosis.
- Asymptomatic patients who ingested small volumes of isopropanol can be medically cleared after several hours of observation.

Warfarin-like rodenticides

- Ingestions >0.0125 mg/kg of brodifacoum should be treated with charcoal and decontamination.

P

- Blood products (fresh-frozen plasma, packed red blood cells, whole blood) should be administered for significant bleeding, such as intracranial hemorrhage.
- Symptomatic patients should receive vitamin K (see Antidote Table).
  - Oral administration of vitamin K is preferred to intravenous administration, which has been associated with anaphylactoid reactions.
- An asymptomatic patient whose samples have abnormal laboratory values should be monitored and provided oral vitamin K.
- Asymptomatic patients with an international normalized ratio of prothrombin time <3.0 should not receive vitamin K and may be monitored as outpatients.

WHEN TO ADMIT

- Altered mental status, dehydration, electrolyte abnormalities, respiratory distress, and acid-base abnormalities after exposure to poisons
- After exposure to delayed onset toxins/drugs, when the amount of toxin/drug exposed to is not known
- Exposure to cardiotoxic drugs for monitoring

WHEN TO REFER

- A poison center should be consulted when one is not familiar with the management of patient exposed to particular drugs/toxins.

FOLLOW-UP

- Poisoning and injury prevention should be discussed with parents within a few days of a poison exposure call.
  - Experience suggests that addressing prevention at the time of the initial call is less effective than doing so later.
  - Recent exposure focuses the mind of the parents, providing a valuable opportunity to impart advice on poison prevention.

PREVENTION

- Effective prevention strategies are directed toward the environment of all children and require parental cooperation.
- Primary care physicians must educate parents and caregivers in the importance of:
  - Safe storage practices for household products and prescription drugs
  - Use of child-resistant closures

- The AAP recommends anticipatory guidance about poisoning prevention, beginning with the 6-month well-child visit.
- All parents should be given the telephone number of the local or regional poison control center and should be advised to keep the number posted by the telephone for immediate use.
- Toxic substances (medications, psychoactive substances, alcohol, household chemicals and products) must be:
  - Inaccessible to children
  - Stored in locked cabinets or boxes
  - Kept in their original containers
  - Discarded in a manner that prevents access by the child
- Parents should be advised to exercise particular care with agents that can be fatal to a toddler in small doses.
  - Antihistamines
  - Benzocaine
  - BBs (sustained release)
  - CCBs (sustained release)
  - Camphor
  - Clonidine
  - Diphenoxylate-atropine (Lomotil)
  - Ethylene glycol
  - Methanol
  - Methylsalicylate (oil of wintergreen)
  - Opioids (methadone, codeine, OxyContin)
  - Phenothiazine
  - Quinine, chloroquine
  - Sulfonylurea antidiabetic agents
  - Theophylline
  - Tricyclic antidepressants
- Other highly toxic substances
  - Acetonitrile (artificial fingernail remover)
  - Ammonium fluoride (wheel cleaner, rust-removal agent)
  - Selenious acid (gun bluing compound)
  - Brodifacoum (superwarfarin rat poison)

P

Polyuria

DEFINITION

- Clinical definition: urine production >2 L/m^2 per 24 hr
- Functional definition: inappropriately high urine output relative to circulating volume and osmolarity

MECHANISM

- Polyuria can be a manifestation of:
  - Excessive persistent fluid intake (primary polydipsia)
  - Osmotic (solute) diuresis, as in uncontrolled diabetes mellitus
- Polyuria in diabetes insipidus
  - Central diabetes insipidus results from a deficiency in vasopressin secretion.
    - Secretion of vasopressin by the posterior lobe of the pituitary gland is inadequate to maintain normal serum osmolality, resulting in diuresis of varying degrees of severity.
    - Vasopressin deficiency is associated with certain congenital malformations
      - Septooptic dysplasia
      - Holoprosencephaly
    - Can result from central nervous system (CNS) injury or tumor resection
    - Familial vasopressin deficiency is rare, accounting for approximately 5% of all cases.
    - Nearly one-half of cases result from a primary brain tumor.
    - Approximately 18% of cases result from histiocytosis or other infiltrative processes.
    - Approximately 25% of cases are idiopathic.
  - Nephrogenic diabetes insipidus is the result of reduced renal sensitivity to circulating vasopressin.
    - Renal disorders, both congenital and acquired, may be associated with polyuria because of complete or partial inability of the renal tubule to concentrate urine despite normal or elevated circulating levels of vasopressin.

HISTORY

- A detailed history often reveals the cause of polyuria.
  - Age at onset
  - Pattern of fluid intake
  - Rate of onset
  - Feeding history
    - To identify infants who have water intoxication
- Urine output >5 mL/kg per hr in a child should raise concerns.
- Polyuria often is associated with:
  - Polydipsia
  - Frequent urination

- Nocturia
  - New onset of nocturia often is the first manifestation of loss of concentrating ability.
- Differentiating polyuria from other conditions depends on total urine output.
  - If the exact daily urinary volume is unknown, a detailed history of fluid intake and urinary habits is helpful.
- With an older child, parents may notice increased fluid intake rather than polyuria.

PHYSICAL EXAM

- Infants with polyuria do not have independent access to fluids and may fall into negative water balance, resulting in:
  - Weight loss
  - Dehydration
  - Electrolyte disturbances

DIFFERENTIAL DIAGNOSIS

Systems involved in maintenance of serum osmolality and water balance

- In reaching a diagnosis in a patient who has polyuria, the clinician must consider systems involved in maintaining normal serum osmolality and water balance.

Neurogenic vasopressin deficiency

- Familial
- Idiopathic
- Congenital malformations
  - Septooptic dysplasia
  - Holoprosencephaly
  - Encephalocele
- Acquired
  - Head trauma
  - Vascular event
    - Thrombosis
    - Hemorrhage
  - Postinfection
    - Meningitis
    - Encephalitis
    - Congenital cytomegalovirus
    - Toxoplasmosis
  - Tumor
    - Craniopharyngioma
    - Germinoma
    - Optic glioma
  - Systemic infiltrative diseases
    - Histiocytosis
    - Syphilis

P

- Tuberculosis
- Sarcoidosis
- Guillain-Barré syndrome
- Autoimmune disorders

Renal vasopressin insensitivity

- Familial nephrogenic diabetes insipidus
  - V2-receptor gene defect (X-linked)
  - Aquaporin-2 gene defect (autosomal recessive)
- Renal tubular defects
  - Cystinosis
  - Distal renal tubular acidosis
  - Bartter syndrome
  - Renal Fanconi syndrome
  - Arthrogryposis-renal tubular dysfunction-cholestasis (ARC) syndrome
- Renal structural defect
  - Renal dysplasia
  - Familial juvenile nephronophthisis–medullary cystic disease
  - Oligomeganephronia
- Acquired
  - Postobstructive
    - Chronic pyelonephritis
    - Obstructive uropathy
  - Drug-induced
    - Lithium
    - Amphotericin B
  - Associated with systemic disease
    - Sickle cell disease
    - Sarcoidosis
    - Amyloidosis
  - Metabolic
    - Hypercalcemia
    - Hypokalemia

Excessive fluid intake

- Primary polydipsia
- Water intoxication

Osmotic diuresis

- Diet-induced
- Drug-induced
- Diabetes mellitus (type 1 or 2)

Diabetes insipidus

- Characterized by:
  - Polyuria
  - Polydipsia

- Dilute urine
- Dehydration
- Hypernatremia

- Hypernatremia and dehydration may cause irritability in young children.
- Familial forms of both central and nephrogenic diabetes insipidus exist.
  - In most familial nephrogenic diabetes insipidus, severe polyuria occurs within the first weeks of life.
  - Growth failure is common with both nephrogenic and central diabetes insipidus.

Central diabetes insipidus

- When a diagnosis of central diabetes insipidus has been made, studies must be undertaken to ascertain the cause.
  - Although many cases are idiopathic, thorough evaluation for an underlying organic lesion must be conducted.
  - Once vasopressin deficiency has been identified, full investigation of other pituitary functions, visual field examination, and magnetic resonance imaging of the brain will likely be the next steps in evaluation.
- Autosomal-dominant form typically does not occur until 5–10 years of age.
- DIDMOAD syndrome typically presents in early childhood.
  - Diabetes insipidus, diabetes mellitus, optic atrophy, and deafness
- After head trauma or surgery, patients may have a period of antidiuresis after transient polyuria, followed by persistent central diabetes insipidus (triple-phase response).
- In recent years, fewer cases of diabetes insipidus have been diagnosed as idiopathic; more have been diagnosed as secondary to CNS infection or intracranial birth defects.
  - Autoantibodies to hypothalamic vasopressin cells have been detected in some children previously thought to have idiopathic diabetes insipidus.
  - Approximately 50% of the patients who have histiocytosis also have vasopressin cell autoantibodies.
- In adolescents with acquired lymphocytic or granulomatous hypophysitis, hyperprolactinemia and other anterior pituitary dysfunction may accompany diabetes insipidus.
- The underlying lesion may not be evident at the initial evaluation.

Nephrogenic diabetes insipidus

- Inherited forms of nephrogenic diabetes insipidus are rare.
- Symptoms of profound polyuria typically occur within the first weeks of life.
  - Vomiting
  - Fever
  - Failure to thrive

- Hypernatremic dehydration
  - Recurrent hypernatremic dehydration may lead to CNS damage or even death.
  - Breastfed infants may show signs later than those who are bottle fed because of the lower osmotic load in human milk.
- Older children and adults may be able to adjust oral fluid intake to maintain serum osmolality.
- A rare form of autosomal-recessive nephrogenic diabetes insipidus has been described in patients with mutations in the gene for the water-channel protein aquaporin-2.
- Other renal tubular defects in which vasopressin resistance has been observed must be considered.
- An association between nephrogenic diabetes insipidus and the ARC syndrome has been recognized.
  - Affected children are prone to severe growth impairment, intellectual disability, and deafness.
- The most commonly reported risk factors for reversible vasopressin insensitivity in 1 study were:
  - Lithium
    - Longer duration of treatment with lithium correlated with increased risk of irreversible diabetes insipidus.
  - Antibiotics
  - Antifungals
  - Antineoplastic agents
  - Antivirals
- Metabolic disturbances can result in reversible vasopressin resistance.
- Hypercalcemia and hypokalemia each may be associated with nephropathy in which tubular ability to conserve water is lost.
- Certain systemic disorders may cause renal tubular dysfunction and result in polyuria.
  - Sickle cell disease
  - Sarcoidosis
  - Amyloidosis

Excess water intake

- Polyuria may be a consequence rather than a cause of excessive fluid intake.
- Primary polydipsia, or compulsive water drinking, is a rare cause in childhood.
  - Most common in older children or adults who have emotional disturbances
  - Approximately 80% of cases are believed to occur in girls and women.
  - Onset is gradual.
  - Some investigators believe the disorder to be caused by a primary psychiatric disturbance.

- One study in adults showed evidence of a defect in water excretion, osmoregulation of water intake, and vasopressin secretion.
- Water intoxication is another cause of polyuria.
  - Incidence has increased over the past 20 years.
  - Particularly common among infants in impoverished circumstances in which caretakers feed diluted formula or water
  - Life-threatening hyponatremia may ensue without prompt treatment.

Osmotic diuresis

- May cause polyuria with renal water loss
- Glycosuria often is found to be the cause of sudden onset of polyuria in children with uncontrolled diabetes mellitus.
  - In both type 1 and type 2 diabetes mellitus, diminished carbohydrate utilization results in hyperglycemia and glycosuria.
  - When present in urine at high concentrations, glucose acts as an osmotic diuretic, resulting in polyuria.
- Chronic hyperglycemia can cause a form of partial nephrogenic diabetes insipidus.
- Treatment with large volumes of dextrose-containing intravenous fluids can result in hyperglycemia and polyuria.
- In contrast, renal glycosuria is characterized by a defect in renal tubular reabsorption of glucose, resulting in glycosuria without hyperglycemia or polyuria.
- Osmotic diuresis also may be provoked by:
  - Mannitol
  - Radiologic contrast agents
  - High-protein feedings (in which urea acts as the osmotic agent)
  - Release of bilateral urinary tract obstruction

LABORATORY EVALUATION

- Baseline values
  - Serum sodium level (mEq/L)
    - Normal: 135–145
    - Central diabetes insipidus: normal or elevated
    - Nephrogenic diabetes insipidus: normal or elevated
    - Psychogenic polydipsia: low normal
  - Serum osmolality (mOsm/kg)
    - Normal: 280–290
    - Central diabetes insipidus: normal or elevated
    - Nephrogenic diabetes insipidus: normal or elevated
    - Psychogenic polydipsia: <280
  - Urine osmolality (mOsm/kg)
    - Normal: 50–1200
    - Central diabetes insipidus: <200

P

– Nephrogenic diabetes insipidus: <300

– Psychogenic polydipsia: <200

- Plasma vasopressin

  – Central diabetes insipidus: low

  – Nephrogenic diabetes insipidus: normal or elevated

  – Psychogenic polydipsia: low

■ Urine osmolality is best interpreted with a concomitant serum sample.

- A hyperosmolar state suggests vasopressin deficiency or insensitivity, provided that the serum glucose concentration is normal.

- Low serum osmolality with hyponatremia suggests either primary polydipsia or water intoxication.

- Serum sodium usually is normal in diabetes insipidus as long as free access to fluids exists and thirst mechanism is intact.

- Hypernatremia is commonly seen in infants with diabetes insipidus or when a central lesion exists that also impairs thirst.

■ Blood chemistries will detect causes of nephrogenic diabetes insipidus, such as hypercalcemia and renal impairment.

■ 24-hour measurement of fluid intake and output

- Useful for confirming polyuria before ordering laboratory tests

■ Urinary specific gravity on a first-voided morning specimen can be affected by the presence of glycosuria, proteinuria, or radiocontrast material.

- Both types of diabetes insipidus and primary polydipsia result in relatively dilute urine.

- Disorders resulting in renal tubular damage, such as sickle cell disease, are more likely to have isosthenuria with specific gravities of approximately 1.010.

■ Urinalysis with microscopy performed on a first-voided morning specimen also provides valuable information.

- Protein, casts, or formed blood elements in the urine suggest a renal disorder.

- Glycosuria with ketonuria strongly suggests diabetes mellitus.

■ Other baseline studies include:

- Serum electrolytes

- Glucose

- Urea

- Phosphate

- Creatinine

- Calcium

- Osmolality

- Liver function tests

- Complete blood count

IMAGING

■ When central diabetes insipidus has been diagnosed, studies must be undertaken to ascertain the cause.

- Magnetic resonance imaging of the pituitary and hypothalamus to assess for:

  – Pituitary masses

  – Craniopharyngioma

  – Pinealoma

  – Pituitary stalk abnormalities

DIAGNOSTIC PROCEDURES

Water deprivation test

■ In children with low urine specific gravity, polyuria, and no glycosuria, the next step in evaluation is referral to a specialist for a formal water deprivation test to determine if a defect exists in vasopressin production or renal responsiveness.

■ Should be undertaken with great caution in younger children

■ Should not be performed in newborns

■ Should follow a 24-hour period of free access to fluids

■ Because of the possibility of volume depletion, the study should be carried out during the day, when supervision is optimal.

■ At baseline, the clinician should:

- Record vital signs and weight.

- Obtain blood and urine for:

  – Osmolality

  – Urine specific gravity

  – Serum sodium concentration

  – Serum urea nitrogen level

  – Hematocrit

■ Blood also should be obtained at the beginning and conclusion of fluid restriction to determine plasma antidiuretic hormone (ADH) levels.

- These may be helpful if the response to the water restriction test is equivocal.

■ Fluid intake is restricted for up to 8 hours, during which the patient must be supervised closely to avoid surreptitious drinking.

- In patients with very low urine osmolality who are strongly suspected of having nephrogenic diabetes insipidus, the response to exogenous ADH can be determined without the need for prior fluid restriction.

■ The patient should be weighed and have vital signs recorded every 2 hours for the first 4 hours, then hourly.

■ Blood and urine should be collected after 4 hours, then every 2 hours, for measurement of:

- Osmolality

- Serum sodium

- Urine specific gravity

- The test should be terminated when one of the following end points is reached.
  - The patient has lost ≥5% of body weight.
  - Urine specific gravity is >1.020.
  - Urine osmolality exceeds 600 mOsm/kg.
  - Plasma osmolality exceeds 300 mOsm/kg.
  - Serum sodium exceeds 147 mEq/L.
- At the conclusion of the test:
  - Weight and vital signs are recorded.
  - Blood and urine are collected for measurement of:
    - Osmolality
    - Serum sodium
    - Urine specific gravity
- In healthy children, and in most children with primary polydipsia:
  - Weight remains constant.
  - Urine specific gravity increases.
  - Urine volume decreases.
- Concentrating ability
  - Often impaired in primary polydipsia
  - Maximal urine osmolality of 500–600 mOsm/kg, compared with >800 mOsm/kg in healthy individuals
- Diabetes insipidus should be suspected in the setting of:
  - Continued diuresis
  - Dehydration
  - Weight loss
  - Hyperosmolarity
- A small increase in urine osmolality may occur in both forms of diabetes insipidus from either partial vasopressin deficiency (central) or partial vasopressin resistance (nephrogenic).
- Administration of exogenous ADH may help differentiate between the 2 disorders.
  - In an older child, the test can be performed after water deprivation test or at a subsequent visit.
  - Extreme caution is required with infants or small children because of the danger of fluid overload and hyponatremia.
  - Patient is given free access to water after administration of desmopressin acetate, a synthetic derivative of vasopressin.
  - Intake, output, and urine specific gravity are recorded every 30–60 minutes.

Interpretation of water deprivation test

- Clinical situation: normal
  - Plasma vasopressin: increased
  - Urine osmolality: >800
  - Urine specific gravity after vasopressin: increased

- Clinical situation: central diabetes insipidus
  - Plasma vasopressin: Low
  - Urine osmolality: <300
  - Urine specific gravity after vasopressin: increased
- Clinical situation: nephrogenic diabetes insipidus
  - Plasma vasopressin: high
  - Urine osmolality: <200
  - Urine specific gravity after vasopressin: unchanged
- Clinical situation: psychogenic polydipsia
  - Plasma vasopressin: unchanged
  - Urine osmolality: 500–600
  - Urine specific gravity after vasopressin: unchanged/increased

TREATMENT APPROACH

- Management of polyuria depends largely on the underlying diagnosis and must be individualized.
- Patients often are found to have a chronic disease that requires close, long-term surveillance.

SPECIFIC TREATMENT

Central diabetes insipidus

- In a severely ill patient, aqueous vasopressin, 0.1–0.2 units/kg, subcutaneously every 4–6 hours
  - Vasopressin may also be given by continuous intravenous infusion.
  - Reported starting doses vary from 0.5–4.6 mU/kg per hour; doses should be increased or decreased as needed.
- Once the child's condition has stabilized, management consists of desmopressin acetate.
  - Desmopressin can be administered orally in tablet form or instilled intranasally.
  - Should be given at the lowest dose that produces antidiuretic effect
  - Intranasally
    - Total daily dose may range from 5 mcg in infants to 40 mcg in older children, divided into 2 or 3 doses as needed.
    - Children receiving dose multiples of 10 mcg may use nasal spray; those on smaller or intermediate doses must use a rhinal tube.
  - Orally
    - Therapeutic doses of oral desmopressin generally are 15–20 times larger than intranasal doses.
    - Greater variability exists in the effective dose.
    - Response to treatment must be monitored closely if the route of administration is changed.
- Treatment of small children and infants with central diabetes insipidus can be difficult, with rapid changes in serum osmolality potentially leading to complications.

P

- Parents must carefully monitor fluid intake and output in younger children.
- Because young infants are fed liquids exclusively and have high fluid requirements, vasopressin can greatly increase risk of severe hyponatremia.
  - These children are best managed with fluid therapy alone.
    - Small doses of desmopressin may be required:
      - If adequate fluid intake is difficult to maintain
      - If caloric intake is inadequate because of excessive fluid consumption
  - The risk of hyponatremia can be reduced by allowing escape from the antidiuretic effect for 1 hour before the next dose.
- A child with adipsia or hypodipsia is best managed by fixing the desmopressin dose and fluid intake.
- Daily weights and frequent sodium levels are useful in assessing fluid status at home.

Nephrogenic diabetes insipidus

- Children with nephrogenic diabetes insipidus should be allowed free access to fluids.
- Parents of infants who have this disorder need to offer frequent water feedings to allow infants to maintain osmotic homeostasis.
- A low-salt diet has been helpful in reducing urine output.
- Thiazide diuretics can reduce polyuria further by reducing amount of urine delivered to the distal tubule.
  - Both indomethacin and amiloride, when given concurrently with a thiazide, have been found effective at reducing urine output.

Primary polydipsia

- Once a neurogenic lesion has been ruled out, medical therapy is not indicated.
- Psychotherapy may be useful in addressing the emotional problem causing the polydipsia.

Hyponatremia

- Can result from several factors, including:
  - Excessive ingestion of hypotonic fluids *and/or*
  - Exogenous administration of vasopressin derivatives
- Patients with asymptomatic hyponatremia can be treated safely with:
  - Fluid restriction *or*
  - Isotonic saline, if a fluid deficit is present
- Symptomatic or severe hyponatremia (serum sodium <115 mEq/L) is an emergency.
  - Should be treated with hypertonic saline to increase the serum sodium level at a rate of 1 mEq/L per hour for 3–4 hours, limiting the increase in sodium to no greater than 10 mEq/L over 24 hours.
  - Rapid increases in serum sodium may lead to central pontine myelinosis.

- The primary care physician should take a cautious approach and limit initial therapeutic increase in sodium to 125 mEq/L with subsequent small incremental elevations in serum sodium concentrations.

Osmotic diuresis

- Osmotic diuresis induced by drugs or diet generally is self-limited.
- In diabetes mellitus, polyuria secondary to hyperglycemia and glycosuria resolves with treatment of the underlying condition.

WHEN TO REFER

- Hypotonic polyuria (confirmed by 24-hour urine and urine osmolality <300 mOsm)
- Need to perform water deprivation test
- Polyuria after neurosurgery
- Polyuria and polydipsia secondary to diabetes mellitus
- Structural renal diseases leading to polyuria should be referred to a pediatric nephrologist.
- Children with vasopressin deficiency are best referred to an endocrinologist or neurologist so that the cause of the diabetes insipidus can be determined.

WHEN TO ADMIT

- Polyuria and dehydration
- Diabetic ketoacidosis
- Severe hyponatremia or hypernatremia
- Suspected diabetes insipidus in an infant

FOLLOW-UP

- Patients with diabetes insipidus should be closely observed, after diagnosis, until an appropriate dose of desmopressin acetate is determined.

COMPLICATIONS

- Hypernatremia in patients with diabetes insipidus
- Hyponatremia in patients with psychogenic polydipsia
- Central pontine myelinosis if hyponatremia is corrected rapidly

P

Postoperative Care

BACKGROUND

Ambulatory surgery

- Routinely performed outpatient surgical procedures include:
  - General surgery
    - Femoral, inguinal, and umbilical herniorrhaphies
    - Lymph node and other diagnostic biopsies
    - Central line insertion
    - Fistulotomy
  - Genitourinary surgery
    - Orchiopexy, hydrocele
    - Circumcision
    - Hypospadias repair
  - Otorhinolaryngeal surgery
    - Myringotomy and tube placement
    - Adenoidectomy
    - Tonsillectomy
    - Bronchoscopy
  - Ophthalmologic surgery
    - Strabismus
    - Examination under anesthesia
  - Orthopedic surgery
    - Tendon lengthening
    - Spica changes
    - Fracture reductions
- Complications
  - Incidence of serious postoperative complications in healthy children undergoing ambulatory surgery is relatively low (<1%).
  - Some minor postoperative problems occur commonly.
    - Can be classified as early or late, depending on time of onset
    - Often, family will call on primary care physician, rather than surgeon or anesthesiologist, to diagnose and treat these problems.
    - Primary care physician must be aware of existence of and recommended treatment for these complications.

Postoperative nausea and vomiting

- Postoperative nausea and vomiting (PONV) are the most frequent complications of general anesthesia.
- Most common cause of:
  - Delayed discharge from postanesthesia care unit (PACU, formerly called the recovery room)
  - Unanticipated hospitalization after outpatient surgery
- Cause is multifactorial, with following factors playing an important role:
  - Predisposition
    - History of postoperative vomiting
    - Susceptibility to motion sickness
  - Anesthetic drugs or techniques used
  - Procedure being performed
  - Skill of the anesthesiologist providing anesthetic
  - Motion
- Certain surgical procedures are associated with a >50% incidence of postoperative vomiting.
  - Strabismus surgery
  - Middle ear surgery
  - Orchiopexy
  - Umbilical hernia repair
- Perioperative use of *any* opioidis associated with a high incidence of PONV.
  - Even when general anesthetic drugs associated with a lower incidence of nausea, such as propofol, are used
- The complex act of vomiting
  - Involves coordination of the respiratory, gastrointestinal, and abdominal musculature controlled by emetic center
  - Stimuli from several areas within the central nervous system can affect the emetic center, including:
    - Afferents from the pharynx, gastrointestinal tract, and mediastinum
    - Afferents from the higher cortical centers (including the visual center and the vestibular portion of the eighth cranial nerve)
    - Chemoreceptor trigger zone in the area postrema of the ventral lateral nucleus
      - Area postrema of the brain is rich in dopamine, opioid, and serotonin receptors
      - Blockade of these receptors is an important mechanism of action of the most commonly used antiemetics.

Emergence phenomena after general anesthesia

- Emergence from general anesthesia in healthy patients is often accompanied by transient symmetrical neurologic changes.
  - Sustained and nonsustained ankle clonus
  - Bilateral hyperreflexia
  - Babinski reflex
  - Decerebrate posturing
  - These reflexes can often be detected within minutes of discontinuing general anesthetic and may persist for hours.
- The discovery of focal neurologic deficits in a postoperative patient is never normal.

- Such neurologic deficits:
  - Should point to a possible central or peripheral nervous system injury
  - Require investigation
- During emergence from general anesthesia, children are prone to:
  - Disorientation
  - Hallucinations
  - Uncontrollable physical activity at times
  - This hyperexcitable, hyperactive state is sometimes referred to as *emergence delirium*.
  - Occurs most commonly if a patient awakens in pain after receiving a potent vapor anesthetic
    - Halothane
    - Sevoflurane
    - Isoflurane
    - Desflurane
  - Other causes include:
    - Sensory deprivation (eye bandages, eye lubricant)
    - Residual anesthetic
    - Awakening in a strange, *unfriendly* environment (the PACU)
    - Perioperative use of ketamine
- Occasionally, some lingering evidence of behavioral perturbations may persist for 12–24 hours.
- Some children who have undergone general anesthesia and surgery may experience:
  - Sleep disturbances
  - Nightmares (terrors)
  - Separation anxiety
  - Aggression toward authority
  - Loss of nighttime bladder control on the night after surgery

Intubation-related complications

- On awakening from general anesthetic, children who have undergone the following will report sore throat:
  - Endotracheal intubation
  - Airway manipulation or instrumentation (laryngeal mask airway)

Postintubation croup

- Also known as *postextubation subglottic edema*
- Children are more prone to develop croup after intubation than are adults because of differences in airway anatomy.
  - Narrower laryngeal and tracheal lumens that are more easily compromised by mucosal edema
  - Narrowest portion of the younger child's airway is at the level of cricoid cartilage, not at the level of the larynx.

- Endotracheal tube can easily pass through the vocal cords and become wedged in the subglottic area.
  - Internal tracheal mucosal injury can occur.
- Other contributing factors to development of croup are:
  - Traumatic or repeated intubations
  - Coughing (bucking) on the tube
  - Changing the patient's position after intubation
  - Providing general anesthesia to children who have a current or recent upper respiratory tract infection
  - Children who have Down syndrome may be at increased risk because of increased incidence of occult subglottic narrowing.
- The incidence of postintubation croup has been reduced to 1% (from 6%) of all endotracheally intubated children through:
  - Use of sterile, implant-tested endotracheal tubes
  - Routine intraoperative use of humidification of administered gases
  - Use of appropriately sized (air leak pressure of <30 cm of water), uncuffed endotracheal tubes in children <5

Succinylcholine

- Succinylcholine is a short-acting, depolarizing muscle relaxant.
- Used to facilitate intubation of the trachea in children
- Carries risk of fatal hyperkalemia in children with undiagnosed Duchenne muscular dystrophy
- It was commonly used in the past, but now used less frequently in favor of relatively fast-onset, nondepolarizing muscle relaxants such as rocuronium.
  - Use reserved for patients:
    - Who have no known risk of malignant hyperthermia or hyperkalemia
    - Who need true rapid sequence intubation because of:
      - Intestinal obstruction
      - Increased gastric contents from a recent meal

Early postoperative surgical problems

Fever

- Postoperative fever is generally caused by the 4 Ws (see table Common Causes of Postoperative Fever).
  - Wind (lungs): atelectasis
  - Wound (operative site): infection
  - Water (urinary tract): urinary tract infection
  - Walker (legs): deep vein thrombosis
- In most patients, fever in the early postoperative period is so common that it can be regarded as a normal response to:
  - Operative trauma
  - General anesthesia

Common Causes of Postoperative Fever

Site	Etiology	Time	Incidence	Sign or Symptoms	Diagnosis	Therapy
Wind (lungs)	Atelectasis	24–48 hr	Very common	Cough, shortness of breath, retractions	Examination, chest radiography	Cough, deep breathing, incentive spirometer
Wound (operative site)	Infection	<24 hr–7 days	Rare	Pain, erythema, induration	Examination wound cultures	Antibiotics, open wound
Water (urinary tract)	Urinary tract infection	3–5 days	Very rare	Dysuria, hematuria	Examination urinalysis, culture	Remove indwelling catheter, antibiotics
Walker (legs)	Deep-vein thrombosis	>3 days	Extremely rare	Swelling, heaviness of lower extremities, superficial venous congestion, palpable cord	Examination, duplex Doppler, venography	Bed rest, elevation, heparin (Coumadin), thrombolytics

- Pyrexia (rectal temperature greater than 101.2°F [38.5°C]) within 24 hours of operation and general anesthesia is common.
- Fever is usually caused by atelectasis, which has many causes.
  - Ciliary motion within the tracheal-bronchial tree is depressed by:
    - Endotracheal intubation
    - Inhalational general anesthetics
    - Use of nonhumidified gases
    - This interferes with normal pulmonary clearance mechanisms.
  - Atelectasis occurs when these factors are combined with:
    - Small tidal volume breathing
    - Somnolence
    - Splinting caused by pain
    - Cough suppression caused by pain or opioid analgesics
- Other causes of postoperative pyrexia are rare, and include:
  - Urinary tract infections
    - Do not usually produce symptoms in the immediate postoperative period
    - Are a cause of late postoperative fever, usually occurring 3–5 days after operation
    - Children generally are symptomatic and complain of dysuria.
    - Infants may have hematuria.
  - Dehydration
  - Infected intravenous access sites
  - Thyroid storm
  - Pheochromocytoma
  - Malignant hyperthermia
    - Fever associated with malignant hyperthermia usually starts intraoperatively.

Wound infection

- Rarely a cause of fever
  - A retrospective analysis of the postoperative course of 256 febrile children at the Hospital for Sick Children in Toronto, Canada, found:
    - Only 4 had infections that required treatment, and all 4 had significant and obvious associated signs of infection.
      - Local tenderness
      - Crepitance, or erythema at the incision site
      - Tachypnea
      - Cough
      - Dysuria
      - Headache
- The postoperative day on which a wound infection becomes apparent and local signs of sepsis produced by the infection vary according to the organism and the concomitant use of antibiotics (see table Postoperative Wound Infections).
- As a general rule, the earlier the onset of wound sepsis, the more destructive and life-threatening the infection will be.
- Most wound infections do not usually become apparent until the fifth to tenth postoperative day.
  - Rare exceptions are infections caused by beta-streptococcus, *Clostridium difficile, Clostridium perfringens (welchii)*.
    - Produce life-threatening wound infections that can become apparent within 24–48 hours of surgery
    - In most instances, children with these infections:
      - Develop high, spiking fevers (temperatures of 102.2°F–105.8°F [39 C–41°C])
      - Become irrational
      - Develop jaundice
      - Have a surgical incision site that is red, warm, and intensely painful on palpation
      - Have vesicle formation, wound crepitance, and an exudate may be present

P

Postoperative Wound Infections

Onset (Postoperative Day)	Usual Pathogens	Wound Appearance	Other Signs
1–3	*Clostridium welchii*	Brawny, hemorrhagic, cool	High standard fever (temperature 39–40°C)
		Occasional gaseous crepitance	Irrational behavior
		Putrid *dishwasher* exudate	Leukocytosis (>15,000 leukocytes/mm^3)
		Intense local pain	Occasional jaundice
2–3	*Streptococcus*	Erythematous, warm, tender	High, spiking fever (temperature 39–40°C)
		Occasionally, hemorrhagic with blebs	Irrational at times
		Serous exudate	Leukocytosis (white blood cell count >15,000 mm^3)
			Rare jaundice
3–5	*Staphylococcus*	Erythematous, warm, tender	High, spiking fever (temperatures of 38–40°C)
		Purulent exudate	Irrational behavior at times
			Leukocytosis (12,000–20,000 leukocytes/mm^3)
>5	Gram-negative rods	Erythematous, warm, tender	Sustained low-grade to moderate fever (temperature 38–40°C)
		Purulent exudate	Rational behavior
			Leukocytosis (10,000–16,000 leukocytes/mm^3)
>5	Symbiotic (usually anaerobes plus gram-negative rods)	Erythematous, warm, tender	Moderate to high fever (temperature 38–40°C)
		Focal necrosis	Leukocytosis (>15,000 leukocytes/mm^3)
		Purulent, putrid exudate	Occasional jaundice Mentation variable

Drainage

- A small amount of serosanguineous drainage in the post-operative dressing is normal.
  - Not a cause for alarm
- Superficial hematoma just below incision site
  - May cause serosanguineous discharge from the operative site 2–3 days after the operation
  - Recognized by characteristic ecchymoses and fluctuance
- Serous drainage from a wound may be caused by:
  - Creation of a large dead space during the operative procedure
    - Usually drain 4–7 days after surgery
  - Liquefaction of adipose tissue
    - Characterized by yellow drainage
    - Occurs 2–3 weeks after surgery

Postoperative bleeding

- Persistent bleeding is defined as:
  - Bleeding and bloody ooze that continues for more than 6–8 hours after the operation *or*
  - Need to change a blood-soaked wound dressing more than twice in the first 6–8 hours after surgery
- Almost always indicates inadequate hemostasis
- Is usually due to a superficial skin arterial bleeding site
- Coagulopathy might also be responsible.

Posttonsillectomy hemorrhage

- Incidence is estimated to be 5–10%.
- 1–3% of patients who have tonsillectomy require additional operation.

- Bleeding that occurs after tonsillectomy may occur either early or late.
  - Early: in the first 24 hours, but usually after hospital discharge
    - Due to failure of hemostasis and may be due to coagulopathy
  - Late: 5–14 days after surgery
    - Results from dislodgement of the scab from the operative bed
  - Either form may be severe and life-threatening.
- Hemorrhage is frequently associated with:
  - History of poor postoperative fluid intake *and*
  - Volume contraction resulting from blood loss

Miscellaneous early postoperative problems

Urinary retention

- In contrast to adults, urinary retention is rare in pediatric surgical outpatients.
- Most children who undergo surgery through the inguinal canal void within 8 hours of the operation.
  - Regardless of intraoperative anesthetic technique or postoperative analgesic regimen
    - Parenteral and enteralopioids *and/or*
    - Regional anesthesia (caudal epidural blockade or ilioinguinal-iliohypogastric nerve blocks)
  - This finding is significant.
    - Theoretically, opioids and regional anesthetics, particularly caudal epidural blockade, may interfere with the neural mechanisms responsible for emptying of the bladder.
    - Many investigators who argued against the routine use of caudal anesthesia and/or opioids for the treatment of postoperative surgical pain based their opinions on the theoretical risk of urinary retention.

Scrotal swelling

- Scrotal swelling and concomitant discoloration of the scrotum commonly occur after:
  - Inguinal herniorrhaphy *and/or*
  - Hydrocelectomy
- Initially, this process:
  - Can produce swelling alone
  - May progress to bluish discoloration as bleeding and clot lysis occur
- Usually the result of bleeding from the cut edge of the peritoneal sac
  - Derived from either a hernia or hydrocele
- The swelling and color change should resolve in 4–6 weeks.

Late postoperative surgical problems

Pyrexia

- Pyrexia 48 hours or more after outpatient surgery:
  - Is unusual
  - May indicate a serious wound infection (see tables Common Causes of Postoperative Fever and Postoperative Wound Infections)
- In patients who develop fevers more than 5 days after a surgical procedure:
  - Primary care physicians should suspect an anaerobic infection or a mixed (symbiotic) infection of anaerobic and gram-negative rods.

Wound infection

- Gram-positive infections
  - The most common causes of wound infection
  - Wound infections caused by *Staphylococcus aureus* or *Staphylococcus epidermidis*
    - Usually characterized by a milky white, purulent drainage
    - Usually occur 3–5 days after surgery (see table Postoperative Wound Infections)
  - Usually produce high, spiking fevers (temperatures of 102.2°F–104°F [39°C–40°C])
  - Leukocytosis (white blood cell count of >12,000/mm^3)
    - After Gram stain and culture, treat patient with a penicillinase-resistant antibiotic such as oxacillin.
- Enteric, encapsulated, gram-negative organisms such as *Escherichia coli*
  - Usually associated with:
    - Erythema
    - Tenderness
    - Possibly, purulent discharge
  - Usually occur >5 days after surgery
  - Enteric organisms such as *E coli* are sensitive to:
    - Penicillin
    - Cephalosporins
    - Aminoglycosides
- Anaerobic infection or a mixed (symbiotic) infection of anaerobic and gram-negative rods caused by:
  - Gram-positive cocci of *Clostridium perfringens*; infection causes:
    - Exquisite pain
    - Brown discoloration
    - A wound that is crepitant to palpation
    - Gas may be seen in the subcutaneous tissues on a plain radiograph.

P

- Gram-negative rods of the *Bacteroides* species (usually *Bacteroides fragilis*)
  - Wound infections caused by *Bacteroides* are usually purulent and malodorous.
- Both of these anaerobic infections are life threatening.

Venous thromboembolism

- Not as common in children as in adults
- Occurs in children during postoperative period
- Incidence increases in adolescence.
- Primary care physician should be alert to following symptoms, which may indicate deep-vein thrombosis:
  - Extremity pain
  - Swelling
  - Discoloration
  - Patient should be referred for immediate evaluation.
- Patients at highest risk are those who are immobilized after surgery and have at least 1 of the following other risk factors:
  - Major lower extremity orthopedic surgery
  - Spinal cord injury
  - Major trauma or trauma to the lower extremities
  - Previous history of deep-vein thrombosis or venous thromboembolism or pulmonary embolism
  - Pregnancy
  - Oral contraceptive use
  - Inflammatory bowel disease
  - Nephrotic syndrome
  - Burns
  - Obesity
  - Central venous catheter in the lower extremity
  - Known acquired or inherited thrombophilia
  - Acute infection
- Pulmonary embolism
  - Patients who develop venous thromboembolism are at risk.
  - Mortality rate is as high as 20%.
  - Symptoms include:
    - Dyspnea
    - Chest pain
    - Cough
    - Hemoptysis
    - Fever

Practical aspects of the postsurgical wound

- Wound healing represents a highly dynamic, integrated series of cellular physiological and biochemical events.
- Morphological events that make up the healing of closed wounds include:
  - Inflammation
  - Epithelialization
  - Cellular influx
  - Fibroplasia
- The inflammatory phase begins immediately.
  - During its early stages, white blood cells:
    - Migrate into the wound
    - Engulf and remove cellular debris and tissue fragments
  - This phase sets the stage for subsequent events in the healing process.
- After dead material is removed, the epidermis and dermis immediately adjacent to the wound edges begin to thicken within 24 hours after injury.
- Within 48 hours, entire wound surface is reepithelialized.
  - During this critical period, wound should be kept dressed and dry.
- Between days 2 and 3, an influx of fibroblasts into the wound occurs deep in the epithelium.
- By the fourth or fifth day, fibroblasts begin to lay down collagen fibers, which continues for several months.
  - Remodeling of collagen takes place for >1 year.
- From surgeon's point of view, all morphological events of wound healing lead to a single important conclusion: Wounds become stronger with time.
  - Closing the wound with suture material only serves to hasten the process.
  - Normally, a simple wound will attain 50% of the strength of surrounding uninjured tissue by 28 days.

Scar formation

- Hypertrophic scars
  - Predisposition of black people and white people of Mediterranean descent
  - Tend to resolve with time
  - As a rule, not associated with prolonged itchiness
- Keloid formation
  - Tumors characterized by massive formation of scar tissue in and beneath the skin after any trauma, including surgery.
  - Keloids grow well beyond the borders of the incision unlike hypertrophic scar formation.
  - Keloids tend to recur after excision.
  - Children have a greater tendency to form and re-form keloids than adults do.
- All skin wounds and surgical skin incision sites will scar.
  - Regardless of the expertise of the surgeon or use of plastic surgical techniques in closing the skin
  - Notion that plastic surgery is scarless is a myth.
- Scar tissue will permanently pigment when exposed to intense sunlight during the first 6 months of its formation.
  - Will usually become red to dark brown-black

GOALS

- Guidelines to select appropriate procedures and patients for outpatient surgery and anesthesia are continually evolving.
  - In general, procedure itself should not involve:
    - Excessive bleeding
    - Open entry into a major body cavity
  - Patient should not require any special postoperative nursing care.
  - Patient must have a responsible adult at home available to provide care until recovery is complete.
- Postoperative pain management
  - Physician's obligation to manage pain and relieve patient suffering is:
    - Crucial element of the professional commitment to patient care
    - Not merely a lofty ideal
  - Effective pain management produces a myriad of patient benefits, including:
    - Reduced morbidity and mortality
    - Early mobilization
    - More rapid recovery
    - Return to work, school, and play

GENERAL APPROACH

PONV

Contribution of anesthetic technique to PONV

- Certain anesthetic agents and techniques produce more vomiting than others.
- Effects of the following general anesthetic inhalational agents are controversial:
  - Sevoflurane
  - Isoflurane
  - Nitrous oxide
  - Some studies report significantly more vomiting when these anesthetics are used, whereas others do not.
- Newer inhalation agents, such as desflurane, claim to be associated with less PONV.
- Gas anesthetics have repeatedly been shown to cause more PONV than intravenous techniques.
- Regional anesthetic techniques that use local anesthetics either centrally (eg, epidural) or peripherally (peripheral nerve block) produce less vomiting than general anesthetic techniques.
  - Rarely feasible without concomitant general anesthesia in children
- Propofol
  - New intravenous general anesthetic agent
  - Produces significantly less vomiting and nausea than others when given alone

- Opioids have been consistently shown to cause nausea and vomiting.
  - Morphine
  - Meperidine
  - Fentanyl
  - Codeine
  - Oxycodone
  - Hydromorphone
  - Individual patients may find 1 opioid drug more nauseating than another.
  - Changing from 1 drug to another may decrease amount of nausea and vomiting.
  - Avoiding opioids perioperatively may solve only part of the puzzle.
    - However, pain control is essential in children who undergo surgery.
    - Opioids are the most common analgesic drugs used for this purpose.
- Use of nonsteroidal antiinflammatory drugs (NSAIDs)
  - Ketorolac is a powerful NSAID.
    - Almost as potent as morphine as an analgesic
    - Does not produce nausea, vomiting, or respiratory depression
  - NSAIDs affect platelet aggregation and adhesiveness.
  - Use limited in many patients who are at risk for postoperative bleeding (especially after tonsillectomy)
  - Have been shown to impair osteoblastic activity
  - Many orthopedic surgeons forbid use of NSAIDs during and after operations in which new bone formation is important (fractures, spine fusions).
  - Extent to which this effect is clinically important is controversial.

Contribution of postoperative oral intake to PONV

- Many anesthesiologists prefer to restrict patients from taking anything by mouth until they are ready and willing to drink and eat.
  - This restriction means that child leaves the hospital while still fasting.
  - Children must say they are thirsty, or better still hungry, and specifically ask for something to drink or eat before any food or liquid is offered.
  - Even in the youngest patients, risk of dehydration is low, particularly if intravenous fluids were appropriately administered perioperatively.
  - In current practice, virtually all children undergoing surgery and anesthesia receive intravenous fluids that contain salt and sugar in the operating room and PACU.
    - If fluids sufficient to supply maintenance and replacement requirements were given during this period, postoperative fast will be readily tolerated.

P

- As anesthesiologists are abandoning stringent, prolonged preoperative fasts, they are increasingly appreciating benefits postoperatively.
  - Unfortunately, many institutions continue to require that patients drink and ambulate before discharge.
  - This restriction contributes to incidence of unanticipated hospital admission after outpatient surgery because of vomiting.

Emergence phenomena after anesthesia

- Before discharge from the PACU, the following should be completely resolved:
  - Disorientation
  - Hyperactivity
  - Excitability
  - Hallucinatory visual disturbances

Early postoperative surgical problems

Fever

- Most patients with low-grade postoperative fevers require only physical examination to differentiate between a septic and nonseptic process.
- Extensive (and expensive) diagnostic workups are rarely indicated.

Drainage

- Only persistent bleeding requires immediate surgical attention.
- Small hematomas directly below a wound, umbilicus, or scrotum usually spontaneously drain or resorb.
  - A nonexpanding hematoma will usually resolve within 4–6 weeks after surgery.
  - If wound hematoma is associated with pain, child should be examined by the operating surgeon.
- Regardless of size, hematomas and seromas:
  - Are excellent culture media for bacteria
  - Increase the likelihood of wound infection
- Hematomas and seromas should be closely watched for.
  - Usually characterized by the triad of:
    - Pain
    - Wound dehiscence
    - Persistent drainage

Miscellaneous early postoperative problems

Urinary retention

- Many surgeons, anesthesiologists, and ambulatory care administrators have insisted that children void before discharge after outpatient procedures that require anesthesia.
  - Many patients cannot void on command, particularly in the PACU or hospital.
  - The knowledge that all patients void within 24 hours of operation and virtually all spontaneously void within 10 hours of a procedure strongly suggests that voiding before discharge is unnecessary.

Late postoperative surgical problems

Pyrexia

- Pyrexia 48 hours or more after outpatient surgery requires evaluation and examination by the patient's primary care physician or surgeon.
  - The wound is examined for signs of inflammation, such as:
    - Warmth
    - Tenderness
    - Erythema
    - Swelling
  - If any of these signs or symptoms are present, the operating surgeon should be informed.

Wound infection

- Gram-positive infections
  - After Gram stain and culture, patient is treated with a penicillinase-resistant antibiotic such as oxacillin.
- Enteric, encapsulated, gram-negative organisms such as *E coli* are sensitive to:
  - Penicillin
  - Cephalosporins
  - Aminoglycosides

Scar formation

- Overall management of the abnormal scar should be determined by:
  - Anatomic position of the wound
  - Age of the patient
  - Any underlying associated diseases
- Advise patients and their families that when exposing the surgical incision site to the sun, the incision site should be:
  - Completely covered *or*
  - Protected with zinc oxide or a sunblock with a sun-protection factor number >30 for 6 months after surgery

SPECIFIC INTERVENTIONS

PONV

Treatment

- Several techniques are available to treat or prevent PONV, including:
  - Altering the anesthetic technique (eg, avoiding perioperative use of opioids)
  - Using antiemetics perioperatively (either prophylactically or as treatment) (see table Dosage Guidelines for Commonly Used Antiemetics)
    - Droperidol
    - Phenothiazines
    - Ondansetron

Dosage Guidelines for Commonly Used Antiemetics[a]

Pharmacological Group (Generic)		Brand Name	Dosage (mg/kg)	Adverse effects
Phenothazines	Chlorpromazine	Thorazine	IV, PO: 0.5–1.0 every 6–8 hr	Drowsiness, hypotension, arrhythmias, extrapyramidal symptoms; potentiates effects of opioids, sedatives
	Prochlorperazine	Compazine	PO, PR: 0.1 every 6–8 hr (maximum dose 10 mg)	
Butryophenones	Droperidol	Inapsine	IV: 0.01–0.03 every 6-8 hr	Drowsiness, hypotension, arrhythmias; droperidol has black box warning: prolongs QT interval, extrapyramidal symptoms; lowers seizure threshold; potentiates effects of opioids, sedatives
	Haloperidol	Haldol	IV: 0.01 every 8–12 hr	
Antihistamines	Promethazine	Phenergan	IV: 0.25–0.5 every 6 hr	Drowsiness, hypotension, arrhythmias; contraindicated in patients taking MAO inhibitors; Phenergan contraindicated in children <2 years old because of cases of fatal respiratory depression[a]
	Diphenhydramine	Benadryl	0.5–1.0 every 4–6 hr (maximum dose 50 mg)	
Benzamides	Metoclopramide	Reglan	IV, PO: 0.05–0.1 every 6 hr	Adverse effects include extrapyramidal symptoms
Anticholinergic	Scopolamine	Hyoscine transdermal scopolamine	IV, PO: 0.005 every 4–6 hr apply behind ear 4 hr before needed; lasts 72 hr	Adverse effects include dry mouth, blurred vision, fever, tachycardia, constipation, urinary retention, drowsiness, amnesia
Antiserotonin	Ondansetron	Zofran, Zofran ODT	IV, PO: 0.15 every 8 hr, (maximum dose 4 mg)	Adverse effects include bronchospasm, tachycardia, headaches, lightheadedness, may prolong QT interval

Abbreviations: MAO, monoamine oxidase; IV, intravenous; ODT, oral dissolving tablet; PO, orally.
[a] FDA MedWatch (www.fda.gov/Safety/MedWatch/SafetyInformation/SafetyAlertsforHumanMedicalProducts/ucm52554.htm).

- – Antihistamines
- • Limiting oral intake postoperatively
- ■ Treatment of PONV is the same as that used for viral gastroenteritis.
  - • Cooling-off period of 2–4 hours followed by sips of clear fluids that contain sugar and salt
  - • Oral rehydration solution
  - • Each sip is separated by several minutes.
  - • Giving fluids or solids prematurely only aggravates the problem.

Antiemetics

- ■ Antiemetics can be used either prophylactically or to treat the problem once it develops.
- ■ The most common antiemetics are those that block receptors within the vomiting center.
- ■ Four major neurotransmitter systems play a role in mediating the emetic response:
  - • Dopaminergic
  - • Histaminic
  - • Cholinergic
  - • Serotonergic

- ■ Antiemetic drugs may act at more than 1 receptor.
  - • Tend to have a more prominent action at 1 or 2 receptors
- ■ The most commonly used antiemetics, in order of use, include:
  - • Benzamides
  - • Metoclopramide
  - • Trimethobenzamide hydrochloride
  - • Serotonin antagonists
    - – Ondansetron
    - – Dolasetron
  - • Phenothiazines
    - – Prochlorperazine
    - – Promethazine (Phenergan)
  - • Butyrophenones
    - – Droperidol
    - – Haloperidol
  - • Antihistamines
    - – Hydroxyzine
    - – Diphenhydramine

P

- Anticholinergics
  - Scopolamine
  - Atropine
- Most of these antiemetic classes (except serotonin antagonists) produce sedation.
  - Can interfere with rapid return to baseline function and hospital discharge
- Promethazine
  - Identified as a contributing cause in a significant number of deaths in children <2 years to whom it had been administered for vomiting:
    - Occurring either in the postoperative period after hospital discharge or
    - Because of gastroenteritis
  - In 2004 the US Food and Drug Administration mandated a black box warning.
    - Original warning seemed to apply only to brand name suppository formulations.
    - Warning was clarified in 2006 to make sure that both health care professionals and parents understood that the warning applies to all formulations: *"Medications containing promethazine hydrochloride (HCl) should not be used for children less than 2 years of age because of the potential for fatal respiratory depression. This includes promethazine HCl in any form: syrup, suppository, tablet, or injectable. Cases of respiratory depression including fatalities have been reported with use of promethazine HCl in children less than 2 years of age. Caution should also be exercised when administering promethazine HCl in any form to pediatric patients 2 years of age and older."*
    - This warning is especially germane in children postoperatively who may be receiving opioids that may cause respiratory depression.
- Ondansetron oral dissolving tablet
  - New dose form
  - Found to be an effective and acceptable formulation in:
    - Children undergoing adenotonsillectomy
    - Infants and children with gastroenteritis treated in an emergency department
  - Like all serotonin antagonists, it is more expensive than older antiemetics.
  - Has advantages of:
    - Oral dosing
    - Lack of side effects, such as sedation or extrapyramidal reactions seen with metoclopramide
- Effective dose and cost of serotonin antagonists
  - Can be reduced by the coadministration of intravenous dexamethasone in the perioperative period
  - Has also been shown to prolong the duration of antiemetic effect

Prolonged nausea and vomiting

- Nausea and vomiting that persists beyond 12–24 hours is unusual.
  - Requires evaluation to determine the state of hydration
  - Intravenous rehydration and consideration of alternative conditions may be necessary.
- In rare instances, excessive postoperative air swallowing may lead to acute gastric dilation in young children.
  - Recognition of the characteristic distended abdomen and gastric splash, if present, should be followed by nasogastric decompression.

Concomitant medications

- Postoperative vomiting may interfere with resumption of long-term oral medication regimens.
- All long-term administered oral medications should be taken on the morning of surgery, except:
  - Monoamine oxidase inhibitors
  - Oral hypoglycemics
  - Diuretics
- Ability of patients to take medications preoperatively has reduced stress associated with deciding when to restart oral medications postoperatively.
- Most drugs administered in the long term have half-lives of elimination >12 hours.
  - Anticonvulsants
  - Bronchodilators
  - Digitalis
- Missing a dose of these drugs for 1 or 2 half-lives (12–24 hours) will have minimal, if any, effect on blood levels.
  - This situation assumes that therapeutic blood levels existed before surgery began.
- If vomiting persists beyond 24 hours, parenteral drug administration may be required.

Emergence phenomena after general anesthesia

- PACU treatment for these phenomena may include:
  - Small doses of analgesics (eg, fentanyl)
  - Flumazenil, if midazolam was administered
- In some instances, atropine may be responsible for this reaction.
  - It will be accompanied by other features of anticholinergic syndrome.
    - Flushed cheeks
    - Mydriasis
    - Low-grade fever
  - This reaction may be treated by administration of physostigmine, ananticholinesterase that:
    - Crosses blood-brain barrier
    - Reverses central nervous system effects of atropine
    - Potentiates action of acetylcholine at nerve terminals

- Prevalence of such anticholinergic reactions has been reduced since the replacement of halothane with sevoflurane as the primary gas for mask anesthetic induction in children.
  - Sevoflurane does not cause the bradycardia seen with halothane.
  - Makes routine use of atropine unnecessary in pediatric anesthetic practice, except to counteract the muscarinic effects of anticholinesterase administration for reversal of nondepolarizing muscle relaxant
- Children who are extremely anxious during induction of anesthesia:
  - Are more at risk of developing postoperative negative behavioral changes compared with children who appear calm during the induction process
  - Benefit from premedication with a benzodiazepine (midazolam) before induction of anesthesia
  - Kain et al have clearly demonstrated that oral premedication with midazolam is more effective at reducing preoperative anxiety and postoperative, delayed alterations in behavior than either:
    - Parental presence
    - Extensive preoperative behavioral program
- Ketamine is associated with sleep disturbances after administration.
  - Incidence of nightmares after ketamine administration is lower in children than in adults.
    - Reported to occur in 5–10% of patients who receive it
    - Incidence is mitigated by concomitant administration of benzodiazepine, usually midazolam.
  - Regardless of cause, sleep disturbance is time limited.
    - Rarely persists beyond 48 hours after surgery and general anesthesia
    - If it becomes overwhelming, can be treated with oral diazepam
    - In most cases, 1 dose given at bedtime cures the problem completely.

Intubation-related complications

- Once cough, gag, and swallowing reflexes have returned to baseline, intubation-related discomfort can be alleviated with:
  - Fruit-flavored ice pops
  - Ice chips
  - Common throat lozenges or sprays
- Analgesics are rarely required.
  - If needed, acetaminophen will usually suffice.

Postintubation croup

- Treatment of postintubation croup is the same as for viral laryngotracheitis.
- Humidification is effective in most cases.

- Nebulized racemic epinephrine therapy is rarely necessary.
  - If needed, patient should not be discharged from PACU to home.
  - Must be admitted for overnight observation because of potential for rebound edema formation.
- Efficacy of corticosteroids in treating postintubation croup has been controversial.
  - Most studies have shown them to be effective.
- Most anesthesiologists will prescribe dexamethasone for this problem.
  - No controlled, prospective trials have validated its use for this purpose.

Succinylcholine-induced myalgia

- Succinylcholine administration normally will result in:
  - Some damage to the muscle cell
  - Leakage of intracellular potassium
  - Increased blood levels of:
    - Creatinine phosphokinase
    - Myoglobin
  - Myalgia
    - As intense and debilitating as myalgia produced by an influenza infection
    - Treatment is supportive.
    - Pain usually resolves over several days.
  - Magnitude can be avoided by pretreating the patient with small doses of:
    - A nondepolarizing muscle relaxant
    - Calcium

Early postoperative surgical problems

Fever

- Early ambulation, deep breathing, and coughing
  - Can be extremely helpful in alleviating or preventing atelectasis and postoperative fever
  - Important medical advantage of ambulatory surgery
    - Patients are more likely to be up and about when they are at home rather than in the hospital.

Wound infection

- Beta-streptococcus, *C difficile*, *C perfringens (welchii)*:
  - Produce life-threatening wound infections that can become apparent within 24–48 hours of surgery
  - Patients require immediate hospitalization and treatment.

Postoperative bleeding

- Direct digital pressure applied to the wound will slow or stop flow of blood until bleeding site can be investigated and controlled by the operating surgeon or designee.

P

Drainage

- If a hematoma progressively expands, it may require operative exploration to:
  - Evacuate the clot
  - Control any ongoing bleeding

Posttonsillectomy hemorrhage

- Requires immediate emergency evaluation
- Rehydration with isotonic fluid is always required.
- Transfusion, although unlikely, may be required even if:
  - A subsequent operation is performed and
  - Control of bleeding is achieved

Miscellaneous early postoperative problems

Urinary retention

- To minimize bladder distention, children and adolescents should be encouraged to urinate:
  - Immediately before coming to the operating room
  - As soon as possible postoperatively
- In some practices, primary care physicians do not routinely require patients to void before postoperative discharge from the PACU; exceptions to this rule include patients who report lower abdominal distention and discomfort, who are initially treated with:
  - Ambulation, in the case of the older child or adolescent
  - Gentle pressure on the lower abdomen, in the case of infants
  - If these measures do not lead to voiding and amelioration of symptoms, bladder catheterization should be performed.
    - The need for bladder catheterization is rare.
    - Patients requiring bladder catheterization should then be observed for ability to urinate spontaneously.
    - If bladder function does not return:
      - Patient should be admitted to the hospital.
      - Specimen of urine should be sent for urinalysis and culture.
      - Patient's surgeon should decide whether a bladder catheter should be reinserted.
- In the experience of some practitioners, urination after outpatient surgery requires a *less is more* attitude.
  - The more attention the physician pays to this issue, the more problems are created.

Scrotal swelling

- An urgent consultation with the patient's surgeon is needed if the following occur:
  - Fever
  - Erythema
  - Tenderness
  - Progressive enlargement of the hemiscrotum

- In many instances, such patients require:
  - Additional exploratory surgery
  - Operative evacuation of the hematoma via a suprainguinal or transscrotal approach

Late postoperative surgical problems

Pyrexia

- Pyrexia 48 hours or more after outpatient surgery
  - If the wound appears to be the source of the fever and infection, the wound:
    - Can be probed with a sterile swab (Q-Tip)
    - A Gram stain and culture obtained
  - If pus is present, the wound should be:
    - Opened
    - Copiously irrigated
    - Debrided
  - Regardless of the presence of pus, a culture swab should always be sent for Gram stain and culture.
- In patients who develop fevers >5 days after a surgical procedure
  - Primary care physicians should suspect an anaerobic infection or a mixed (symbiotic) infection of anaerobic and gram-negative rods.
  - Skin surrounding the wound should be examined closely for the presence of:
    - Crepitus and vesicle formation
    - Purulent and putrid discharge
    - Focal necrosis
    - All of these conditions indicate the development of:
      - Gas gangrene *or*
      - Necrotizing fasciitis
- These anaerobic types of infections can be caused by:
  - Gram-positive cocci of *Clostridium* perfringens
  - Gram-negative rods of the *Bacteroides* species (usually *Bacteroides fragilis*)
    - Both of these anaerobic infections are life threatening and require:
      - Immediate hospitalization
      - Resuscitation
      - Operational evaluation and intervention
- If surgical incision site does not appear to be responsible for development of fever
  - Thorough history and physical examination should be performed.
    - Particular attention should be devoted to the lungs and intravenous administration sites.
    - Atelectasis often follows general anesthesia and surgery.

- Infected intravenous insertion sites, phlebitis, or thrombophlebitis, especially in the female adolescent taking birth control pills, also can occur.
- Additionally, routine causes of pyrexia in children can occur in the postoperative patient and include:
  - Upper respiratory tract infections
  - Gastroenteritis
  - Otitis media

Wound infection

- Treatment of a serious wound infection is straightforward.
  - Inpatient hospitalization
  - Opening the wound along its entire length
  - Drainage
  - Wide debridement of necrotic tissue
  - High-dose intravenous antibiotics
    - Penicillin
    - Clindamycin
    - Metronidazole
    - Cefotetan
  - In selected cases, hyperbaric oxygen therapy
  - These wounds are not closed.
    - Are allowed to close spontaneously by contracture.
  - If only cellulitis is detected, wound should not be opened.
    - Patient should be given intravenous antibiotic therapy.
  - Lymphangitis, characterized by its characteristic red streaks and tender regional adenopathy, should also be treated with intravenous antibiotics in the hospital.

Venous thromboembolism

- Patients at risk for venous thromboembolism should receive prophylactic measures, which may include:
  - Compression stockings
  - Pneumatic sequential compression devices
  - Or both (until ambulatory)
- Patients with 3 or more risk factors may be treated with pharmacologic prophylaxis:
  - Subcutaneous heparin *or*
  - Low–molecular-weight heparin

Practical aspects of the postsurgical wound

- Wound dressings are not required after 48 hours.
- Wound contamination with stool and urine should be cleansed with water or saline.

- Overlying dressing should be replaced.
- Detergent soaps and peroxide should be avoided.
- By postoperative day 4, wound may be washed with:
  - Warm water
  - Bland soap (eg, Ivory, Dove, Neutrogena)
- Most wounds are closed using absorbable suture material, which:
  - Maintains tensile strength for 60–90 days
  - Supplies an appreciable amount of wound strength to allow normal healing process to take place
  - Does not require suture removal
- Closing wounds with absorbable suture material allows child to return to activity at an earlier time.
- Adolescents with uncomplicated inguinal hernia repair may return to:
  - Nonstrenuous activity 7–10 days postoperatively
  - Full activity by 4–6 weeks
- Whenever possible, toddlers are kept off tricycles and bicycles for 7–10 days.
- Infants should be treated as if no operation was performed.
  - Full bath by the fourth postoperative day
  - No restrictions for carrying the infant

Scar formation

- Keloid formation
  - A thorough family history may be a predictor of this pathological process.
  - An abnormal scar should be observed for a minimum of 6 months postoperatively.
  - If it does not resolve
    - Trial excision should be attempted staying within the confines of the lesion to see what response is obtained.
  - If it recurs
    - Should be reexcised and 1% triamcinolone injected beneath the scar, which will produce some keloid resolution
- Hypertrophic scar
  - Should be treated with pressure

P

Posttraumatic Stress Disorder

DEFINITION

- Posttraumatic stress disorder (PTSD) is a psychiatric disorder that can develop in response to being the direct victim of or witnessing traumatic events.
  - Child abuse
  - Domestic, community, or school violence
  - Vehicular or other accidents
  - Fires
  - Natural disasters
  - Terrorism
  - War
  - Traumatic medical conditions
- To receive a diagnosis of PTSD:
  - The child must have experienced a traumatic event that qualifies as a serious traumatic stressor.
    - The American Psychiatric Association *Diagnostic and Statistical Manual (DSM-IV)* requires specific criteria for a PTSD-level stressor: It threatens the child's or significant others' life or physical integrity.
    - For children, more leeway exists in defining PTSD-level traumas.
  - In reaction to the traumatic exposure, the child must have experienced subjective fear, helplessness, or horror.

EPIDEMIOLOGY

- Most children are remarkably resilient in the face of trauma.
  - Do not go on to develop PTSD
- Prevalence
  - Has been estimated based on studies of various types of stressful events
  - Rates vary considerably by type of event.
    - Other characteristics related to prevalence
      - Demographics
      - Family characteristics
      - Research methods
  - Few nationally representative studies
    - Early studies of adolescents and young adults reported overall lifetime PTSD rates of 9.2%.
    - Some rates reported separately
      - 2.8% of boys
      - 10.3% of girls
    - A more recent study of adolescents (age 12–17 years) reported different rates than previous studies.
      - Slightly higher rates for boys (3.7%)
      - Lower rates for girls (6.3%)
  - Among inner-city children
    - As many as 90% of inner-city adolescents report significant exposure to traumatic events.

- Rates of PTSD vary after different types of traumatic events.
  - Exposure to acute physical injury (23%)
  - Natural disasters (24–39%)
  - Community violence (27%)
- Many children may not meet the full criteria for PTSD.
  - Show heightened posttraumatic stress symptoms after exposure to various events, including:
    - Family violence (15%)
    - Natural disasters (24%)

RISK FACTORS

- Risk factors for PTSD and other mental health difficulties after traumatic exposure include:
  - Female sex
  - More frequent or intense exposure to traumatic event
  - Preexisting anxiety disorder
  - Lack of parental or other support
  - Parental psychopathology
  - Parental PTSD related to the index trauma
  - Past trauma exposure

SIGNS AND SYMPTOMS

Components of PTSD

- The 3 core symptom clusters of PTSD are reexperiencing, avoidance or numbing, and hyperarousal.
- To meet full PTSD criteria, the patient must have at least:
  - 1 reexperiencing symptom
  - 3 avoidance or numbing symptoms
  - 2 hyperarousal symptoms
  - These symptoms must all:
    - Be present for at least 1 month *and*
    - Cause functional impairment in social, school, family, health, other important area of daily living
- Children who do not meet these criteria are still considered to have significant PTSD symptoms.

Reexperiencing symptoms

- Reexperiencing symptoms occur when upsetting feelings are experienced after memories or reminders of traumatic event recur.
  - Example: The child saw her father shot to death.
    - Began reliving the shooting whenever a thunderstorm occurred
    - The sound of thunder reminded the child of the sound of the gunshots that killed her father.

- Symptoms may be idiosyncratic and hard for parents and primary care physicians (PCPs) to identify.
  - Example: The child screamed and hit his grandmother whenever she sang what she thought was his favorite lullaby.
    - It gradually emerged that the boy's mother had sung this song to him before she was hit by a car and killed.
    - The song was not a reminder of comfort and happy times with his mother, but rather a traumatic reminder of the night she died.
- Symptoms include:
  - Recurrent and distressing memories or thoughts of the event
  - Repetitive play
  - Recurrent distressing or frightening dreams
  - Nonspecific scary dreams in younger children
  - Feeling as though traumatic event is occurring again in the present (flashbacks, rare in younger children)
  - Intense psychological distress when reminded of the trauma
  - Physiologic reactions to trauma reminders, including:
    - Upset stomach
    - Headaches
    - School refusal

Avoidance or numbing symptoms

- Children's trauma reminders are accompanied by strong, upsetting feelings.
- Children may develop avoidance coping strategies to escape upsetting feelings.
  - Will try to avoid talking about the traumatic experience
  - Will avoid thinking about it
  - Will avoid places, people, and situations that serve as trauma reminders
  - For some children, these avoidant strategies become generalized.
    - Avoid place where the traumatic event happened and all similar places.
      - A child who was beaten up on the way to school becomes avoidant of going to school at all.
      - A child who was sexually abused in the bathroom at home is now afraid of all bathrooms.
  - Children who deal with fear through avoidance are:
    - Reinforcing their fears
    - Not extinguishing them
  - As avoidance strategies become ineffective:
    - Some children may become emotionally numb to escape the overwhelming fear they feel.

- Symptoms include:
  - Efforts to avoid thoughts, feelings, or talking about traumatic event
  - Avoiding activities, places, people, or situations that serve as trauma reminders
  - Inability to remember an important aspect of the trauma
  - Loss of interest or participation in significant activities
  - Detachment or estrangement from others
  - Restricted affect
  - In older children and teens, a sense of a foreshortened future

Hyperarousal symptoms

- Includes hyperarousal symptoms not present before the traumatic event
- In children who have experienced chronic trauma, it may be difficult to:
  - Assess the onset of these symptoms
  - Distinguish them from other syndromes such as attention-deficit/hyperactivity disorder
- Symptoms include:
  - Difficulty falling or staying asleep
  - Irritability
  - Temper outbursts
  - Trouble concentrating
  - Hypervigilance
  - Increased startle response
  - In young children, development of new fears not previously present

DIFFERENTIAL DIAGNOSIS

- Subclinical PTSD
  - Children with significant PTSD symptoms without meeting strict psychiatric criteria of the disorder often have comparable functional impairment to those with the full disorder.
  - Many exposed children may experience subclinical PTSD.
    - With or without symptoms that interfere with their functioning or cause impairment in other domains, such as:
      - Behavioral dysfunction
      - Aggression
      - Hypersexuality
      - Social incompetence
      - Anger
      - Explosiveness
      - Relationship conflicts or problems
- PTSD is not the only, or even most common, outcome for children to experience after trauma exposure.

P

- PTSD most typically co-occurs with other difficulties, such as:
  - Depression
  - Anxiety
  - Behavioral problems
  - The PCP may have to include other assessments or instruments to evaluate these potential comorbidities.
- In some cases, parents may initially identify other clinical concerns that may relate to child's recent exposure to traumatic events.
  - Children may develop problems in the absence of PTSD symptoms.
  - Substance abuse, self-injury, and serious behavior problems are common sequelae of traumatic experiences.
    - Particularly in child physical abuse and domestic violence
- Childhood traumatic grief
  - A condition that PCPs should be prepared to recognize and refer for specialized intervention
  - Occurs in a minority of children who lose significant others to death under traumatic (frightening, unexpected) circumstances
    - The child gets stuck on traumatic circumstances of the death.
    - The child cannot move through typical stages of grieving.
    - The child may seem less sad than children who are mourning in a more usual fashion because the affected child develops PTSD symptoms of avoidance and numbing, and the child may:
      - Not talk about the deceased
      - Avoid visiting the cemetery
      - Seem detached from parents and friends
      - Become easily angered and irritable when others want to reminisce about the deceased
  - Parents may become angry because they interpret this behavior to mean the child:
    - Is not mourning loss of the deceased
    - Does not seem to care about the death
  - PCP can help the child and family by:
    - Recognizing the signs and presentation of childhood traumatic grief
    - Educating the family about this condition

DIAGNOSTIC APPROACH

Role of the pediatrician

- PTSD is often underrecognized in:
  - Young children who have difficulty reporting certain PTSD symptoms
  - Those who have experienced traumas associated with shame, secrecy, or stigma
    - Sexual abuse

- Domestic violence
- Bullying
- Reliance on parental reports of the child's symptoms greatly improves diagnosis.
  - Parents may not wish to provide accurate reports of the child's trauma exposure or symptoms.
    - Traumatized themselves
    - Perpetrators of the child's traumatic experience
- Many traumatized children do not spontaneously report traumatic experiences or trauma symptoms.
- PCPs may be in the best position to:
  - Identify these children
  - Influence developmental trajectory positively
- PCPs should be:
  - Aware of the high prevalence of child trauma exposure
  - Willing and able to assess children for presence of PTSD symptoms in the primary care setting

Assessing trauma exposure

- PCPs who have a favorable relationship with patients will feel comfortable asking the child about possible exposure to a variety of different types of traumas at well-child care appointments.
- Children and parents should be asked these questions in private, rather than together.
  - Many types of trauma are believed by children or parents to be:
    - Stigmatizing
    - Shameful
    - Things that should be kept secret within the family
  - Children may be less likely to disclose such information in the presence of a parent than when alone with the PCP.
    - Reporting requirements in the case of child maltreatment should be followed if the child discloses maltreatment in this context.
  - Some general questions designed to elicit information about the child's potential exposure to traumatic events:
    - Has any significant change occurred in the child's life or functioning since the last visit?
    - Since the last time the child was seen, has something really scary or upsetting happened to the child or someone in the child's family?
    - Has any significant change occurred in the child's behavioral or emotional functioning?
    - Has anyone reported or observed any sudden changes in the child's behavior or mood?

- Monitor children's potential exposure to specific traumatic events or experiences.
  - Key domains that should be included in an interview
    - Severe crashes or injury-causing events
      - Vehicular
      - Falls
      - Fires
    - Medical trauma, illness, or related procedures
      - Long hospitalization
      - Painful procedures
    - Natural disasters
      - Storm
      - Hurricane
      - Blizzard
      - Earthquake
      - Flood
      - Hit by lightning
    - Physical violence
      - Toward child or other
      - Threatened or happened
      - Bullying
    - Domestic violence
      - Adults fighting, attacking, shooting, stabbing, beating each other up at home
    - Sexual abuse
      - Unwanted touches in private parts
      - Taking pictures
      - Internet abuse
    - Physical abuse at home
      - Beating, punching, hitting by parent or older sibling
    - Traumatic death
      - Knew of or observed someone die
      - Ask about circumstances: was death sudden, shocking, terrifying, gory?
    - Other scary, frightening events
      - Kidnapping
      - Terrorism
  - Self-report instruments are available for inquiring about trauma exposure.
    - Commonly used exposure instruments include:
      - Trauma Exposure Structured Interview for Children
        - Can be administered as a self-report instrument
      - UCLA PTSD Index for *DSM-IV*

Assessing PTSD symptoms

Physician assessment

- When assessing the child for the presence of PTSD symptoms, symptoms should be anchored to a specific stressor.
  - The child should be asked whether any specific experienced events were upsetting or scary.
  - If the child reports that any of these events were distressing, the clinician should:
    - Determine which was most traumatic from the child's perspective
    - Assess child for presence of PTSD symptoms

Self-report screening methods

- In most PCP practices, time demands will preclude PCPs from conducting personal interviews to assess PTSD symptoms for all children.
  - A child self-report PTSD screening measure can be used in office settings.
- 9-item Abbreviated UCLA PTSD Index (see Figure 63 on page F22)
  - Has been used in school settings after disasters, with good results
  - Score of 20 highly correlates with a diagnosis of PTSD.
    - Children with scores ≥20 should be referred for evaluation.
  - Clinical judgment should be used to determine whether children with scores between 10 and 19 should also be referred for evaluation, especially if they have clinically meaningful symptoms of PTSD.
- Trauma Symptom Checklist for Children
  - Alternative self-report method for evaluating severity of posttraumatic symptoms
  - Developed to evaluate children's responses to unspecified traumatic events in an array of symptom domains by using several scales
    - Posttraumatic stress
    - Anger
    - Anxiety
    - Depression
    - Sexual concerns
    - Preoccupation
    - Dissociation
  - Includes several scales relevant to the assessment of post-traumatic stress symptoms and other symptoms related to PTSD.
  - Standardized on a large sample of racially and socioeconomically diverse children from urban and suburban settings.

P

- Provides norms according to age and sex, as well as clinical cutoff scores
- The child is asked to indicate how often each item happens by using a 4-point scale.
  - 0 = never
  - 1 = sometimes
  - 2 = lots of times
  - 3 = almost all the time
- Posttraumatic stress subscale consists of 10 items reflecting posttraumatic stress symptoms
  - Intrusive recollections of traumatic events
  - Sensory reexperiencing and nightmares
  - Dissociative avoidance
  - Fears
  - This particular subscale has high internal consistency and good criterion validity.

TREATMENT APPROACH

- The PCP is in a unique position to promote an initial response to a child who may have been exposed to traumatic events and who exhibits symptoms of PTSD.
  - Opportunities to observe the child during routine physical examinations provide both observational and physical evidence that may be relevant to identification of traumatic exposure and symptoms.
  - These impressions may be confirmed through parental interview when questions about the child's experiences and timing of any recent or sudden reactions to these events can be ascertained.
- Children exposed to traumatic life events who have several risk factors for PTSD may need:
  - More prompt mental health referrals
  - Closer PCP follow-up
  - Both
- Effective treatment is available for children who have significant PTSD symptoms.
  - With optimal interventions, most children are able to recover in as few as 12 treatment sessions.

SPECIFIC TREATMENTS

- Mental health therapies with evidence of effectiveness for PTSD; may be considered for subclinical problems
  - Parent-Child Interaction Therapy
    - Use with physically abused children
  - Abuse-Focused Cognitive-Behavioral Therapy
    - Use with children exposed to domestic violence by using parent-child psychotherapy

- Cognitive Behavioral Intervention for Trauma in Schools project tools
  - Use with adolescents exposed to community violence

WHEN TO REFER

- Children who do not meet full PTSD criteria (ie, do not have ≥3 PTSD symptoms and ≥1 in each cluster)
  - Still considered to have significant PTSD symptoms and should still be referred for mental health evaluation and treatment
  - Even if the child has only a few PTSD symptoms, if they are of sufficient severity to cause functional impairment, they may warrant a referral for further evaluation.
- Abbreviated UCLA PTSD Index scores
  - Score ≥20: The child should be referred for evaluation.
  - Scores between 10 and 19: Clinical judgment should be used to determine need for referral for evaluation; child should be referred if:
    - Child has clinically meaningful symptoms of PTSD *and*
    - Symptoms are accompanied by functional impairment
      - The child or parent reports that the child is having difficulty getting along with people at school or at home, or child has trouble sleeping, eating, or concentrating.
  - Score <10: The child should be referred for further mental health if:
    - The parent or PCP has concerns based on child's clinical symptoms or history after exposure to a traumatic event, because avoidant children are likely to underreport PTSD symptoms.

FOLLOW-UP

- PCPs may be well placed to:
  - Follow up on high-risk children
  - Monitor them for later emergence of mental health difficulties

COMPLICATIONS

- Left untreated, childhood trauma and PTSD are associated with serious and long-lasting negative outcomes.
  - Impairments in:
    - Learning
    - Memory
    - Academic performance
  - Increased risk for:
    - Depression
    - Suicide attempts
    - Completed suicide in adolescence and adulthood

P

- Substance abuse
- Self-injury
- Risky sexual behaviors
- Impaired physical health and immunity
- Increased health care use in adulthood

PROGNOSIS

- If children are identified and treated with optimal interventions, PTSD symptoms generally:
  - Remit relatively quickly
  - Remit cost effectively
  - Do not return
- Most tested treatment for PTSD leads to reduction of:
  - Depression
  - Anxiety
  - Shame
  - Behavioral difficulties

PREVENTION

- Work toward preventing PTSD by noting when children appear to be at risk for traumatic exposure or experiences.
  - Potential high-risk scenarios that may be reported by the family include:
    - Sudden and frequent moves
    - Major disruptions in caregiving environment or caregiver functioning or status
    - Reports of increased frustration or physical force during child management or disciplinary interactions
    - Exposure to or knowledge of age-inappropriate sexual activities
    - Child reactions to a caregiver that have changed suddenly
    - Exposure to drugs and alcohol
    - Spending a lot of time with nonbiologically related men
  - Offer advice regarding steps that may minimize a child's exposure to high-risk situations.
  - Encourage parents to monitor and promote child safety, both in and out of the home.

P

Preoperative Assessment

BACKGROUND

- Ambulatory or same-day surgery provides significant medical, psychological, and economic benefits to children and their families.
- Much of the preoperative and postoperative patient care that in the past was provided in the hospital by the surgeon and anesthesiologist is now being performed by the child's primary care physician (PCP).
  - Preoperative evaluation and decisions about medical interventions to minimize perioperative risks often are performed by the PCP because most anesthetics are given on an outpatient basis.
  - The PCP's knowledge of the child's medical history and established relationship with the family means he or she is in the best position to:
    - Determine the state of the child's health
    - Help the family prepare psychologically for surgery
- The child is reevaluated by the anesthesia and surgical teams on the morning of the procedure to determine whether an acute illness has developed.
- Compliance with preoperative medication administration and *nil per os* (NPO) status is determined at that time.

GOALS

- Goal of preanesthetic evaluation is to determine risk of anesthetizing a particular child in his or her current medical condition for a specific procedure
- Factors to consider include:
  - Probability of an adverse event and its associated estimated risk
  - Benefits of the procedure
  - Consequences associated with either proceeding with or delaying the procedure
- All 3 variables—risk, benefit, and consequence—must be considered in the decision to administer an anesthetic:
  - Optimal improvement in underlying disease
  - Effect of any intercurrent processes on overall physiology
  - The risk of adverse perianesthetic events common in children

GENERAL APPROACH

American Society of Anesthesiologists Physical Status Classification

- Summarizes patient's physical condition and may provide means of assessing relative risk of anesthesia
- Class 1: extremely suitable for anesthesia
  - Normal healthy person
    - No underlying medical condition
- Class 2: generally good
  - Mild systemic disease without functional limitations
    - Mild asthma
    - Anemia
    - Controlled seizures
    - Controlled diabetes mellitus
- Class 3: intermediate
  - Severe systemic disease
    - Moderate to severe asthma
    - Poorly controlled seizures
    - Pneumonia
    - Tracheostomy without ventilatory support
    - Poorly controlled diabetes
    - Moderate obesity
    - History of prematurity
    - Cancer
    - Stable organ dysfunction (moderate renal or liver insufficiency)
- Class 4: poor risk
  - Severe systemic disease that is a constant threat to life
    - Severe bronchopulmonary dysplasia (BPD)
    - Sepsis
    - Morbid obesity
    - Advanced organ insufficiency: cardiac, pulmonary (eg, tracheostomy with ventilatory support), hepatic, renal, adrenal disease
- Class 5: extremely poor risk
  - Moribund patient, not expected to survive without procedure
    - Septic shock
    - Severe organ failure
    - Severe trauma

Trends and statistical information in adverse events

- Pediatric Perioperative Cardiac Arrest (POCA) Registry identifies trends in adverse events that occur in children receiving anesthetics and provides data on perioperative risk.
  - Infants and those children with severe systemic disease are at highest risk for perianesthetic mortality.
  - Most common cardiovascular causes of arrest
    - Hemorrhagic hypovolemia
    - Metabolic consequences of massive blood transfusions
- Closed pediatric anesthesia malpractice claims registry allows evaluation of risk of adverse perioperative events.
  - Procedures most commonly cited
    - Dental, ear, nose, throat, maxillofacial procedures (36%)
    - Abdominal procedures (17%)

- Suggests procedures related to the airways are associated with increased risk
- Incidence of adverse events is 75 per 1000 anesthetics
  - Most common events result from:
    - Respiratory causes during the procedure
    - For younger children, respiratory adverse events in the recovery period as well
    - Vomiting during the recovery period

Child's preprocedure anxiety

- Preprocedural sedation, usually by an oral or rectal route, often is effective in modulating anxiety.
- Omitting premedication in an anxious child will result in a traumatic induction, leading to
  - Postoperative maladaptive behaviors
  - Enuresis
  - Night terrors
  - Violent behavior
- Children requiring repeated invasive procedures can develop a posttraumatic stress–like syndrome.

Preoperative fasting guidelines

- Guidelines for type of ingested material (in hours)
  - Clear liquids: 2
  - Breast milk: 4
  - Infant formula: 6
  - Nonhuman milk: 6
  - Light meal: 6
- Many pediatric anesthesiologists require a fast of 8 hours after solid food for elective surgery.
- Children are encouraged to drink clear liquids to minimize:
  - Anxiety
  - Hypovolemia
  - Possible hypoglycemia that may result from a prolonged preoperative fast
- Institution's pediatric anesthesiology division should be consulted to determine specific practice protocols for fasting.

Preoperative laboratory tests

- Routine laboratory tests are rarely indicated in an otherwise healthy child scheduled for outpatient surgery.
- Hemoglobin (Hgb)
  - Routine determination of hematocrit and Hgb are not necessary if previous results during well-child care have been normal.
  - Selective determination should be used in children:
    - With chronic medical illnesses
    - About to undergo procedures with potential for significant blood loss

- Infants <6 months should have preoperative Hgb level measured because the physiological nadir of red blood cell production may cause level to decrease as low as 7 g/dL.
- In ex-premature infants, Hgb levels <10 g/dL have been associated with an increased incidence of postoperative apnea.
- Children of African or African-American ethnicity who have not had Hgb and hematocrit determination after 6 months of age should have these measurements and a sickle cell screening test.
- Coagulation status
  - Required by most surgeons in children undergoing procedures with an increased risk of intra- or postoperative bleeding, even when no history of bleeding disorder in patient or family
    - Tonsillectomy or adenoidectomy
    - Intracranial procedures
  - Studies typically include:
    - Prothrombin time
    - Partial thromboplastin time
    - Platelet count
- Electrolytes
  - Routine preoperative testing is not indicated, even for hospitalized patients.
  - Child with cardiovascular diseaseand undergoing digoxin therapy should have
    - Serum sodium
    - Potassium
    - Digoxin
  - Serum electrolytes should be evaluated if patient:
    - Has renal insufficiency
    - Is taking diuretics
    - Is taking angiotensin-converting enzyme inhibitors
    - Is taking other medications that increase likelihood of abnormal result
    - Is limited to enteral (nasogastric or gastrostomy tube) feedings or parenteral nutrition
- Pregnancy testing
  - Routine pregnancy screening of all menarcheal girls is performed in many institutions.
    - Many question cost-effectiveness of this practice.
  - Pregnancy testing on the day of surgery using point-of-care urine testing is recommended.
    - If positive, the procedure is canceled, the patient is notified, and a pediatric social worker is consulted to help the young woman.
- Other tests
  - Chest radiograph in patients with history of chronic aspiration or lower airway disease

P

- Electrocardiogram (ECG) is warranted in a child with:
  - Obstructive sleep apnea syndrome
  - BPD
  - Congenital heart disease
  - Severe scoliosis
- Children being treated with anticonvulsants should have serum levels checked to ensure that anticonvulsants are in the therapeutic range.
- Pulmonary function tests
  - May be useful in predicting whether children with pulmonary or thoracic cage abnormalities (eg, scoliosis) are at increased risk for anesthetic complications and postoperative respiratory insufficiency.
  - Most common tests
    - Pulse oximetry
    - Forced vital capacity (FVC)
    - Forced expiratory volume in 1 second (FEV_1)
    - Ratios of the 2 measurements (absolute values of FEV_1/FVC), as predictor of need for postoperative mechanical ventilation
    - Reliable results usually cannot be obtained in children <6 years of age.

SPECIFIC INTERVENTIONS

Preanesthetic history and exam

- Focus on fundamental systems that may have physiological consequences during anesthetic use
- Most departments of anesthesiology provide a standardized form.
- When this form is not provided, the PCP should provide a history and physical exam with all abnormalities identified:
  - Pulmonary (including airways anatomy)
  - Cardiovascular
  - Endocrine
  - Hematologic
  - Neuromuscular
  - When applicable:
    - Premature birth and neonatal course
    - Oncologic disease
    - Exposure to chemotherapeutic agents
    - History of corticosteroid use
    - History of congenital anomalies and corrective procedures
    - Autism and other behavioral-communicative disorders
  - Weight
  - Blood pressure
  - Room-air oxygen saturation or saturation with baseline oxygen supplementation

- Allergies (drugs and latex)
- Cardiac murmur history
- Previous subspecialty encounters: findings, recommendations, and interventions
- Medications
- Extent of neuromuscular disease (eg, hypotonia)

- Airways exam is essential to allow appropriate advanced preparation for special techniques to secure the airways.
  - Adequacy of mouth opening
  - Neck mobility
  - Loose teeth
- Parents should be questioned about any neurologic symptoms, such as:
  - Long-tract signs
    - Hyperreflexia
    - Positive Babinski response
    - Clonus
  - Hand weakness
  - Bladder and bowel dysfunction
  - History of torticollis or neck pain
- Under no circumstances should the words "cleared for surgery" be written on a prescription form after completion of a preoperative history and physical exam.

Respiratory tract risk assessment

- Risk factors for perianesthetic respiratory events
  - Age <5 years
  - Copious secretions
  - Plan for endotracheal intubation required for procedure
  - History of reactive airway disease
  - History of prematurity
  - Parental smoking history
  - Upper respiratory infection within the previous 4 weeks
  - Wet cough
  - Wheezing

Assessment of infections

- Upper respiratory infection (URI) mandates careful risk, benefit, and consequence analysis.
  - If URI is active or recent, patient is more likely to experience laryngospasm, oxygen desaturation, bronchospasm, severe coughing, and breath holding during anesthetic induction and emergence.
  - Incidence of perioperative respiratory events is increased 7 times in children with URI and 11 times if intubated.
  - Risk of airways complications remains high for up to 6 weeks after URI, probably as a result of altered airways reactivity.

- Children with URIs undergoing elective cardiac surgery
  - 4-fold increased incidence of airways complications at induction of anesthesia
  - 2-fold increased incidence of postoperative respiratory complications
  - 5-fold increase in postoperative bacterial infections, as well as extended stay in intensive care unit (ICU)
- Respiratory events associated with a mild to moderate URI commonly are managed with:
  - Additional oxygen supplementation
  - Prolonged postanesthesia care unit stay
  - Inhaled beta-agonists
  - Corticosteroids
- Small percentage of patients require unplanned hospitalization for stridor, pneumonia, or other complications.
- Usually, no significant increase in respiratory complications among children anesthetized *during* an acute URI, which has led some researchers to advocate *not* canceling surgery for these children.
- Delay surgery 4–6 weeks after resolution of symptoms if:
  - Temperature >101.3°F (38.5°C)
  - Purulent nasal discharge
  - Lower respiratory symptoms (eg, productive cough, crackles, wheezes, or positive chest radiograph findings)
- An additional screening tool is the child's room-air oxygen saturation.
  - If child with a URI (and no chronic lung disease) has room-air oxygen saturation of less than 96% at sea level, then the case will be rescheduled.
- Parents should be told that increased adverse perioperative respiratory events occur in children exposed to cigarette smoke at home.

Asthma

- Many anesthetic procedures can produce bronchospasm, which is frightening, challenging to treat, and sometimes catastrophic.
  - Ventilation is difficult, if not impossible, and may result in:
    - Hypercapnia
    - Acidosis
    - Hypoxia
    - Cardiovascular collapse
    - Death
- To prevent, asthma medical therapy should be escalated preoperatively, even in asymptomatic patients or patients with well-controlled asthma.
  - Short courses of corticosteroids are extremely effective in preventing perioperative wheezing, even in patients who have severe asthma.

- Children who take asthma medications only as needed should begin use of their inhaled beta-agonists or oral medications 3–5 days preoperatively.
- Children taking medications on a long-term basis (oral or inhaled) should have corticosteroids added in doses normally used for an acute exacerbation.
- The child with severe asthma who takes bronchodilators and corticosteroids regularly requires:
  - Intensification in frequency of nebulizer treatments
  - Added bronchodilators
  - Increased corticosteroids
  - On occasion, all of these measures
- Asthma therapy should never be deescalated or stopped before surgery.
- Optimization of child's condition should be documented by achieving maximal peak flow rate for that child.
- Children taking theophylline (uncommon) should have serum levels measured preoperatively to optimize drug administration and avoid possible toxic effects.
- Despite fasting, all oral medications may be taken with small amounts of water on the morning of surgery.
- Children with asthma are not candidates for procedures performed at freestanding facilities if they:
  - Have been hospitalized for asthma within previous 3 months
  - Had an exacerbation in the previous month
  - Have a room-air oxygen saturation of ≤96%
- *Elective* surgery should never be performed in a child who is wheezing actively or who has had a recent asthma attack.

Premature infants and risk of postoperative apnea

- Nonanemic premature infants who have postconceptual age (gestational age added to age after birth) >56 weeks have less than a 1% risk of developing postoperative apnea.
- Hemoglobin concentration <10 g/dL increases the risk.
- Postoperative apnea may resolve spontaneously.
  - Considered serious because cerebral arterial desaturation can occur after only 5 seconds of apnea
- All at-risk patients (those with a postconceptual age <60 weeks), regardless of anesthetic technique, should be admitted to monitored, high-surveillance inpatient units for 24 hours after anesthesia and surgery.
- Infants born prematurely who were intubated and received ventilatory assistance as neonates are at increased risk for subglottic stenosis.
  - Negative history does not exclude the diagnosis.
  - History of croup or stridor is an important warning sign.

P

BPD

■ Evaluate pulmonary status and optimize conditions before anesthesia and surgery to minimize perioperative risks of:

- Bronchospasm
- Atelectasis
- Pneumonia
- Respiratory/cardiac failure

■ These children may benefit from:

- Bronchodilators
- Antibiotics
- Diuretics
- Nutritional support
- Corticosteroid therapy

■ Respiratory infections or bronchospasm in children who have BPD must be treated thoroughly before elective surgery.

■ If severe BPD and bronchospasm are present, preoperative treatment with increased inspired oxygen tension may decrease pulmonary vasoreactivity and improve cardiovascular function.

■ Possibility of associated right-ventricular dysfunction should always be considered and, when indicated, evaluated with ECG and echocardiography.

■ Children taking diuretics (eg, furosemide and spironolactone) on a long-term basis require a preoperative measurement of serum electrolytes.

■ Many infants with BPD receive frequent courses of corticosteroids, and perioperative corticosteroid coverage may be required.

■ Children with BPD may require continuous postoperative monitoring and ventilatory assistance for an extended period (24–48 hours).

- Risks of general anesthesia and intubation can sometimes be avoided with judicious use of either a laryngeal mask airway or a regional anesthetic.
- Parents must be cautioned that either approach might be unsuccessful and intubation still required.

Obstructive sleep apnea syndrome (OSAS)

■ OSAS can be consequence of abnormal upper airways anatomy, upper airways dysfunction, or both

■ With adenotonsillectomy, 10–30% incidence of perioperative complications that can include:

- Laryngospasm
- Pulmonary edema
- Postoperative airways obstruction
- Respiratory arrest

■ Risk factors for these complications include:

- Age <3 years
- Severe OSAS on polysomnography
- Infants born prematurely

- Right-ventricle hypertrophy
- Pulmonary hypertension
- Recent URI
- Signs of respiratory distress
- Trisomy 21
- Craniofacial anomalies
- Neuromuscular disease
- Failure to thrive
- Obesity

■ Oxygen saturation nadir <80% during sleep study has been noted to increase a child's probability of postoperative complications to 50%.

■ Children undergoing urgent, as opposed to elective, tonsillectomy have a 2-fold increased risk of postoperative complications.

■ Children <3 years have high rate of postadenotonsillectomy airways obstruction and respiratory complications

- Should be admitted overnight for observation and cardio-respiratory monitor and continuous pulse oximetry

■ Details of the sleep study, if performed, should be reviewed, but due to study expense and the unavailability of pediatric sleep centers, many children undergoing adenotonsillectomy have the diagnosis of OSAS made on clinical grounds.

■ Postoperatively, children with OSAS, especially those <3 years, should be admitted to the pediatric ICU or other highly monitored location

- Incidence of obstructive events and pulmonary complications may increase in first 24 hours after surgery.

Cystic fibrosis

■ In patients with cystic fibrosis, anesthesia usually is required for:

- Otolaryngology procedures (eg, sinus surgery)
- Central line placement
- Bronchoscopy
- Esophagoscopy
- Laparotomy for intestinal obstruction
- Placement of enteral feeding devices

■ Incidence of postoperative complications is 10–22%.

■ Inicidence of perioperative mortality is 1–5%.

■ Adolescents with severe pulmonary dysfunction are at risk for massive hemoptysis (25% will experience recurrent massive hemoptysis).

■ Most complications are pulmonary; general anesthesia may have at least short-term deleterious effects on pulmonary function.

■ Primary focus

- Determine severity of pulmonary disease.
- Use all methods possible to optimize it in consultation with pediatric pulmonologist.

- Pulmonary function tests will demonstrate:
  - Hyperinflation
  - Lower airways obstruction
  - Responsiveness to bronchodilators
- Chest radiographs/computed tomography studies document degree of disease heterogeneity.
  - Useful in determining risk of pneumothorax during positive pressure ventilation
- Preoperative room air pulse oximetry further helps to quantify the degree of underlying pulmonary dysfunction.
  - Patients with cystic fibrosis who are chronically hypoxemic are at risk for pulmonary hypertension and cor pulmonale.
  - An echocardiographic evaluation should be performed in this subset of patients.
- Recent sputum culture to detect any acute pulmonary infections that need preoperative antibiotics or contact precautions
- Chest physiotherapy and mucolytics are useful in improving sputum clearance.
- Preoperative nutritional support and optimization of pancreatic enzyme supplementation mitigates effects of growth failure and hypoalbuminemia.
- Correction of electrolyte and coagulation abnormalities with oral agents is useful in decreasing need for acute interventions.

Preexisting cardiovascular disease, risk assessment

- Disqualification for procedures performed at freestanding ambulatory surgical facilities:
  - Current use of cardiac medications
  - Prolonged QT syndrome
  - Residual cardiac disease

Heart murmurs

- Innocent murmurs, frequently episodic and associated with a normally split second heart sound, normal exercise tolerance, and a normal ECG, include:
  - Still's murmur
    - Most common in late preschool
    - Exacerbated by fever, exercise, and anemia
    - Low pitch vibratory
    - Increased by exercise
    - Decreased by standing
  - Pulmonary murmur
    - Most common during middle to late childhood
    - Can appear during febrile illnesses, anemia, and pregnancy
    - Blowing midsystolic
    - Increased by expiration
    - Decreased by standing

  - Supraclavicular bruit
    - Harsh systolic ejection
    - Increased by pressure
    - Decreased by shoulder extension
- All murmurs of questionable status should be evaluated by a pediatric cardiologist.
- All pathologic findings should be communicated directly to the pediatric anesthesiologist.
- Children with congenital heart disease (whether repaired or not) should have a cardiac evaluation within 1 year before surgery, even if asymptomatic.

Williams syndrome

- High risk for perioperative complications
- Thorough history noting change in exercise tolerance, dyspnea, angina, and syncope
- Complete cardiologic evaluation, including an ECG, should be performed before the administration of each anesthetic, looking for:
  - Evidence of outflow tract obstruction
  - Coronary artery anomalies
  - Segmental wall motion abnormalities suggestive of myocardial ischemia
  - Anesthetic induction must be performed with great care, avoiding extremes in heart rate and blood pressure.

Prolonged QT syndrome

- Patients at increased risk for torsade de pointes
- Perform preoperative ECG (looking for a QT_c >470 ms in male patients and >480 ms in female patients) if there is history of any of the following manifestations:
  - Syncope
  - Seizures
  - Sudden cardiac death after an increase in sympathetic activity (in the form of exercise, auditory stimulus, or emotional stress)
  - Family history of sudden death
  - Long-term administration of one of the drugs listed in the table Drugs That Prolong the QT Interval or Induce Torsades de Pointes
    - Children with long QT syndrome should have electrolytes measured to ensure that serum levels of potassium, calcium, and magnesium are normal.

Subacute bacterial endocarditis prophylaxis

- Antibiotic prophylaxis to prevent bacterial endocarditis is recommended if undergoing any procedure with a risk of bacteremia (eg, dental, sinus, airways) or when the surgical site is contaminated.
  - Unrepaired cyanotic congenital heart defect (CHD), including palliative shunts and conduits

P

Drugs That Prolong the QT Interval or Induce Torsades de Pointes

Generic Name	Brand Name	Category[a]
Albuterol[b,c]	Ventolin, Proventil	3
Amantadine	Symmetrel	2
Amiodarone	Pacerone, Cordarone	1
Amphetamine/dextroamphetamine	Adderall	3
Atomoxetine[c]	Strattera[c]	3
Azithromycin	Zithromax	2
Chloral hydrate	Noctec	2
Chloroquine	Arelan	1
Chlorpromazine	Thorazine	1
Clarithromycin	Biaxin	1
Clozapine	Clozaril	2
Dextroamphetamine	Dexedrine	3
Disopyramide	Norpace	1
Dobutamine[b]	Dobutrex[b]	3
Dolasetron[b]	Anzemet[b]	2
Dopamine[b]	Intropin[b]	3
Droperidol	Inapsine	1
Ephedrine	Rumatuss	3
Epinephrine	Primatene, Bronkaid	3
Erythromycin[c]	Erythrocin[c], EES[c]	1
Felbamate[c]	Felbatol[c]	2
Flecainide	Tambocor	2
Foscarnet	Foscavir	2
Fosphenytoin[c]	Cerebyx[c]	2
Gemifloxacin	Factive	2
Granisetron[b,c]	Kytril[b,c]	2
Halofantrine	Halfan	1
Haloperidol	Haldol	1
Isoproterenol	Isupres, Medihaler-Iso	3
Isradipine	Dynacirc	2
Levalbuterol[c]	Xopenex[c]	3
Levofloxacin	Levaquin	2
Lithium	Lithobid, Eskalith	2
Metaproterenol	Alupent, Metaprel	3

Generic Name	Brand Name	Category[a]
Methadone	Dolophine, Methadose	1
Methylphenidate[c]	Ritalin[c], Concerta[c]	3
Milodrine	ProAmatine	3
Moxifloxacin	Avelox	2
Nicardipine	Cardene	2
Norepinephrine	Levophed	3
Octreotide	Sandostatin	2
Ofloxacin	Floxin	2
Ondansetron[b,c]	Zofran[b,c]	2
Pentamidine	Pentam, NebuPent	1
Phenylephrine	Neosynephrine	3
Pimozide	Orap	1
Procainamide	Pronestyl	1
Pseudoephedrine	PediaCare, Sudafed	3
Quetiapine	Seroquel	2
Quinidine	Quinaglute, Cardioquin	1
Risperidone[c]	Risperdal[c]	2
Salmeterol	Serevent	3
Sotalol	Betapace	1
Tacrolimus	Prograf	2
Telithromycin	Ketek	2
Terbutaline	Brethine	3
Thioridazine	Mellaril	1
Tizanidine	Zanaflex	2
Venlafaxine	Effexor	2
Ziprasidone	Geodon	2

[a] Category 1: Drugs that are generally accepted by authorities to have a risk of prolonging the QT interval and causing torsades de pointes.
Category 2: Drugs that may prolong the QT interval but at this time lack substantial evidence for causing torsades de pointes.
Category 3: Drugs to be avoided for use in patients with diagnosed or suspected congenital long QT syndrome (in addition to drugs in categories 1 and 2).
[b] Drugs that are commonly used in the perioperative period.
[c] Drugs that are commonly used in children.
A continuously updated and complete list of drugs that prolong QT may be found at www.azcert.org/medical-pros/drug-lists/drug-lists.cfm.

P

- Completely repaired CHD with prosthetic material or device (placed by surgery or by catheter intervention) within 6 months of procedure
- Repaired CHD with residual defects or adjacent to the site of a prosthetic patch or prosthetic device (which inhibit endothelialization)
- Cardiac transplantation recipients who develop cardiac valvopathy
- Prosthetic cardiac valves
- Previous infective endocarditis

- Oral endotracheal intubation by itself is not an indication for subacute bacterial endocarditis (SBE) prophylaxis, but nasotracheal intubation requires it.
- Hemodynamically insignificant lesions (eg, bicuspid aortic valve, mitral valve prolapse) no longer require prophylaxis for any procedure.
- CHD repaired with prosthetic material require prophylaxis only for the first 6 months after repair.
- Patients with prosthetic valves or those palliated with shunts or conduits require prophylaxis.
- In most circumstances, prophylactic antibiotics can be administered orally 1 hour before the procedure, with a minimal amount of water.
  - When necessary, give antibiotic intravenously, when started after induction of anesthesia.
  - Starting an IV catheter in an awake child is unnecessary solely to administer antibiotics for SBE prophylaxis.

Endocrine disorders

Diabetes mellitus
- Avoid hyperglycemia complications
  - Increases in perioperative morbidity and mortality
  - Delayed wound healing
  - White blood cell dysfunction
  - Increased infectious complications
- Perioperative evaluation includes evaluation of insulin regimen, adequacy of metabolic control, and any end-organ dysfunction.
  - Normal electrolyte levels
  - No evidence of ketonuria
  - HbA_{1C} level should be within endocrinologist's acceptable range.
    - HbA_{1C} level is a dynamic reflection of mean blood glucose level during the previous 8–12 weeks.
- Unfavorable systemic manifestations include:
  - Renal microangiopathy
  - Coronary artery disease
  - Hypertension
  - Retinopathy
  - Peripheral neuropathies

- Delayed gastric emptying
- Limited joint mobility

- Involvement of the cervical spine and temporomandibular joints can result in difficulties with laryngoscopy and intubation of patients with diabetes.
- Most diabetic patients can undergo minor surgical procedures with insulin administered subcutaneously, as outlined below for procedures less than 2 hours, by type of insulin:
  - Mixed insulin
    - Day before procedure: usual intermediate or long-acting
    - Day of procedure: 50% intermediate or long
  - Short-acting insulin
    - Day before: usual short-acting
    - Day of: no short-acting
  - Glargine (lantus)
    - Day before: usual short-acting or take none
    - Day of: Take none
  - Insulin pump
    - Day before: normal rate
    - Day of: normal rate
- Diabetic patients should be the first case of the day.
- Blood glucose levels should be measured on arrival to preoperative preparation area.
  - If blood glucose level is >250 mg/dL, then subcutaneous regular insulin or an insulin pump bolus should be administered according to a sliding scale to decrease to 150 mg/dL.
- For major procedures, or if brittle diabetes, give continuous infusion of insulin, along with infusion of glucose to maintain a blood glucose level of 150–200 mg/dL.
- Many institutions prohibit use of the patient's insulin pump intraoperatively with conversion to a continuous intravenous infusion.
- Hourly blood glucose measurements are performed throughout the procedure, and additional glucose or insulin is titrated as appropriate.

Congenital adrenal hyperplasia
- Focus of preoperative evaluation for patients with congenital adrenal hyperplasiais to:
  - Characterize exact nature of enzymatic deficiency
  - Understand whether both glucocorticoid and mineralocorticoid arms of steroidogenesis are involved
- State of hydration, blood pressure, and electrolytes are evaluated to determine adequacy of baseline supplementation.
- Usual maintenance hydrocortisone dose is inadequate to cover physiological stresses.
  - Patients scheduled for major surgery are given 100 mg/m^2 hydrocortisone in 4 divided IV doses for the first 24 hours, then tapered slowly.

P

- Some endocrinologists prefer a continuous infusion of hydrocortisone during surgery.

Secondary adrenal insufficiency

- Due to exposure to exogenous corticosteroids
- Asthmatic children who received a single 5-day course of high-dose systemic corticosteroids have normal adrenal function by 10 days after treatment.
- Children who have received at least 3 courses of high-dose burst (5 days) systemic corticosteroids within the previous year in addition to their maintenance inhaled corticosteroids have no evidence of adrenal dysfunction 30 days after the last burst.
- Patients receiving prolonged therapy for >3 weeks, evening doses, and continuous dosing (versus alternate-day dosing) are more likely to have adrenal insufficiency, which may take more up to a year to resolve.
- Fluticasone at doses >500 µg/day causes adrenal suppression in 20% of children.
  - Children receiving high doses of fluticasone may undergo a cosyntropin stimulation test to determine risk for adrenal suppression.
    - If they do not have this test, the best course is to administer *stress-dose* corticosteroids perioperatively.
  - Intranasal corticosteroids can cause adrenal suppression in children.
- Situations requiring stress-dose corticosteroid coverage:
  - <10 days after a burst (5 days) of corticosteroids
  - <30 days after completion of the last of multiple short courses of corticosteroids
  - <1 year after completing a prolonged course of steroids (>3 mo)
  - Previously treated with fluticasone >500 µg/dL
  - Daily parenteral or enteral corticosteroids for >3 weeks
  - Evening doses of corticosteroids
  - Impaired response to cosyntropin stimulation test
- Stress-dose corticosteroid recommendations by degree of surgical stress
  - Minor: <1 hr (eg, hernia)
    - Hydrocortisone 25 mg/m² IV
    - Methylprednisolone 5 mg/ m² IV
  - Moderate (extremity surgery)
    - Hydrocortisone 50 mg/m² IV
    - Methylprednisolone 10 mg/m² IV or usual oral dose and reduced parenteral dose
  - Major (laparotomy)
    - Hydrocortisone 25 mg/m² IV every 6 hr
    - Methylprednisolone 5 mg/m² IV 6 hr
      - At start of surgery through the operative day

- May return to maintenance corticosteroid administration on the first postoperative day if the patient is stable
- Wean over 1–3 days.

Thyroid disease

- Hypothyroidism
  - Patients with undertreated hypothyroidism have multisystem disease that can have profound anesthetic implications.
    - Cardiac dysfunction
      - Myocardial depression
      - Bradycardia
      - Torsade de pointes
      - Hypotension
      - 2nd-degree baroreceptor dysfunction
      - Decreased intravascular volume
    - Respiratory
      - Blunted ventilatory response to hypoxia and hypercapnia
    - Pharmacologic
      - Increased sensitivity to depressant effects of anesthetic agents
      - Hypothermia
      - Reduced metabolic rate
      - Adrenal insufficiency
      - Delayed gastric emptying
  - Primary objective in preoperative evaluation is to confirm that the patient is euthyroid.
    - If thyroxine (T_4) level is low and thyroid-stimulating hormone level is elevated, *elective* surgical procedures should be postponed for at least 2 weeks to allow for adequate thyroxine supplementation.
  - Children recently diagnosed with hypothyroidism and those with unexpected bradycardia should undergo a cardiologic evaluation to determine extent of myocardial involvement.
  - T_4 supplementation in the perioperative period should be managed in collaboration with a pediatric endocrinologist.
  - 8 AM cortisol level is useful in establishing whether the child has occult adrenal dysfunction.
  - Children should take their levothyroxine on the morning of surgery.
- Hyperthyroidism
  - During perioperative period, undertreated patients with hyperthyroidism can have thyroid storm with malignant hyperthermia-like symptoms.

- Corticosteroids improve outcomes in patients with thyroid storm; antithyroid medications, potassium iodide, ß-blockers are useful in the management of these children.
  - ß-Blockers should be titrated to restore heart rate to age-appropriate norms.
- Children with hyperthyroidism should have clinical and chemical evidence of euthyroid state before elective procedures.
  - Elective procedures may need to be delayed until euthyroid state is established.
- Children with goiters should undergo sufficient imaging to delineate extent of airways compromise.

Hematologic conditions

- Previously undiagnosed anemia could indicate serious underlying disorder that requires additional evaluation before surgery:
  - Sickle cell anemia
  - Blood dyscrasia
- Any significant anemia (hemoglobin <9 g/dL) should be determined preoperatively.
- Presence of a mild anemiashould not delay urgent surgery.
- Anemia from nutritional causes (eg, iron deficiency) often requires relatively brief period of therapy for improvement.
- For elective surgery, consultation with anesthesia and surgical teams may be required.

Inherited coagulopathies

- Von Willebrand disease (vWD)
  - Patients with type 1 vWD can undergo minor surgical procedures with preoperative DDAVP administered IV 30 minutes before the procedure.
  - 10% of patients with type 1 vWD do not respond to DDAVP.
    - Advance determination of quality of response is fundamental to the preoperative evaluation.
  - Type 1 nonresponders, and patients with type 2 and type 3 vWD, require preoperative administration of plasma-derived human factor VIII concentrate (Humate-P)
  - All patients with vWD undergoing major surgical procedures require factor replacement preoperatively.
- Hemophilia A, B, and C
  - Perioperative management depends on the planned procedures.
  - Patients undergoing major surgical procedures require factor VIII and factor IX levels approximating 100% of normal from 30 minutes before procedure, through the first postoperative week.
  - Patients undergoing minor procedures can be covered with factor levels that are 50% of normal after second postoperative day.

- Some patients with mild hemophilia A have a sufficient response to DDAVP to provide adequate protection for minor procedures.
- Need for fresh-frozen plasma transfusion in hemophilia type C patients should be determined by a pediatric hematologist.
- Platelet abnormalities that usually require perioperative platelet transfusions include:
  - Wiskott-Aldrich syndrome
  - Diamond-Blackfan syndrome
  - Thrombocytopenia absent radii
  - Glanzmann thrombasthenia
  - Bernard-Soulier syndrome

Oncologic disease

- Treatments often have the potential to cause profound perianesthetic complications.
- Most recent ECG report should be included in preoperative evaluation.

Cerebral palsy

- Preoperative evaluation for patients with cerebral palsy should include:
  - Assessment of room-air oxygen saturation
  - Degree of underlying reactive airway disease
  - Presence of snoring and other obstructive symptoms suggestive of inadequate airways tone
- Preoperative evaluation and preparative regimen is often directed toward ensuring pulmonary status is optimal.
- Chest radiographs may be helpful in the child who has had previous episodes of significant pulmonary consolidation.

Genetic disease

- Airways obstruction and hypoxemia are preeminent concerns resulting from:
  - Abnormalities of upper airways and trachea
  - Altered chest wall mechanics and respiratory drive
  - Reduction in the pulmonary bed from hypoplasia or destruction as the result of gastroesophageal reflux.
- Hypertension and dysrhythmias, cardiomyopathies, and structural heart disease are common.
- ~60% of the 10,000 genetic diseases have central or peripheral nervous system abnormalities.
- Presence of neuromuscular diseases will often dictate specific drug use and technique for airways management.

Down syndrome

- Perioperative evaluation focuses on numerous anomalies associated with Down syndrome that have perianesthetic implications.
- With craniofacial and upper airways anomalies, airways obstruction often persists after adenotonsillectomy because of mid-face hypoplasia.

- Smaller tracheal diameter usually require endotracheal tube that is 1–2 sizes smaller.
- 40–50% have congenital heart disease
  - Often requires surgical correction
  - Postoperative conduction defects or valvular dysfunction (or both)
  - Need for SBE prophylaxis
  - Pulmonary hypertension and pulmonary vascular disease result.
- See Upper airways obstruction and endothelial cell dysfunction.
- Much higher risk for developing pulmonary hypertension in setting of chronic upper airways obstruction
- Perioperative complications occur in 8–10% of patients with Down syndrome undergoing noncardiac surgery:
  - Severe bradycardia
  - Airways obstruction
  - Difficult intubation
  - Postintubation croup
  - Bronchospasm
  - Incidence of OSAS as high as 57%
    - Some recommend screening with polysomnography for OSAS age 3–4 years.
- Cervical spine instability
  - Can lead to catastrophic neurologic injuries in perianesthetic period
  - Atlantoaxial instability (in approximately 15%)
    - Screened with lateral flexion and extension views of the cervical spine, odontoid views, and measurements of the neural canal width
    - Atlantoaxial distance interval >4–5 mm in any lateral view is abnormal.
- Parents should be asked about recent changes in neuromuscular functions indicative of cord impingement:
  - Loss of bowel or bladder control
  - Sensory deficits
  - Motor changes
- Even in the absence of symptoms, children who have Down syndrome and are ≥2–3 years should have lateral flexion and extension radiographs of the cervical spine before anesthesia to identify patients at risk for subluxation.
  - If radiographs reveal an atlantodens interval of greater than 5 mm (usually maximal in the flexion view), refer for orthopedic or neurosurgical consultation before elective surgery.
- Children <3 years may be at risk
  - Neck radiographs not helpful in diagnosis because of the lack of ossification
  - Anesthesiologist should use neck-protection strategies.

Connective tissue disorders

- Often treated with aspirin or other NSAIDs
  - Should be stopped 1 week preoperatively
  - If agents cannot be stopped, evaluate the extent of platelet impairment by measuring bleeding time.
- Associated dysphagia and esophageal dysmotility can predispose patients to pulmonary aspiration of gastric and esophageal contents.
- Extensive fibrosis of temporomandibular or cricoarytenoid joint can complicate airways management and endotracheal intubation.
- Pulmonary infiltration and fibrosis may complicate intraoperative care by causing hypoxemia.
- Hematologic abnormalities, including anemia of chronic disease, may complicate management.
- History should focus on the extent of disease, the type of treatment, and the child's response to therapy.
- Laboratory assessment may include:
  - ECG
  - Chest radiograph
  - Electrolytes
  - Blood urea nitrogen
  - Creatinine
  - Hemoglobin, hematocrit, and platelet levels
  - Peripheral blood smear
- Patient who has quiescent disease and who has regular follow-up may need nothing other than hematocrit determination.

Skin diseases

- Skin diseases associated with skin fragility
  - Epidermolysis bullosa (EB)
  - Ectodermal dysplasia
- Use of all tape and dressings such as Tegaderm may be forbidden, because removal may cause denuding of the skin, pain, and infection.
- In EB, conventional methods of intubation such as direct laryngoscopy or use of airways adjuncts, such as laryngeal mask airways or oral airways, may be associated with blister formation in the pharynx, tongue, or supraglottic area.
- Scarring on skin of hands and feet may restricts options for venous access.
- Involvement of face, neck, and mouth may result in decreased mouth opening, neck mobility, supraglottic airway narrowing, or any combination.
- Anesthesia team needs advanced notice for face-to-face preoperative evaluation and consultation with patient's dermatologist and PCP, followed by discussion with the family of risks and methods for skin protection and airways management.

Medications

- Dosage should be adjusted to ensure adequate therapeutic levels perioperatively.
- Administration ordinarily is continued at usual doses up to and including day of surgery, except monoamine oxidase (MAO) inhibitors and tricyclic antidepressants.
  - Discontinue use of these agents 2–3 weeks before the scheduled operation.
    - If discontinuation cannot be done without risk, preoperative consultation with anesthesiologist is necessary.
- Selective serotonin reuptake inhibitors
  - Should not be stopped to prepare for surgery
  - Withdrawal can precipitate anxiety, agitation, and diaphoresis.
- Anesthesiologist must be informed because interactions with drugs administered perioperatively can lead to unexpected adverse effects.
- Discontinue psychotropic drugs in perioperative period:
  - Lithium
  - MAO inhibitors
  - Tricyclic antidepressants (eg, amitriptyline)
  - Clozapine
  - Cessation of medications requires involvement of the patient's mental health professional.
- Drugs for attention-deficit/hyperactivity disorder (eg, Strattera, Concerta, and Adderall) may continue preoperatively, but reports of tachycardia and arrhythmias mandate vigilance.
- Herbal or homeopathic medications may lead to unexpected anesthetic reactions; many anesthesiologists advise stopping 2 weeks before surgical procedure
  - Echinacea: purple coneflower root
    - Allergic reactions; decreased effectiveness of immunosuppressants; potential for immunosuppression with long-term use
    - No data on whether to discontinue
  - Ephedra: ma huang
    - Risk of myocardial ischemia and stroke; ventricular arrhythmias with halothane
    - Life-threatening interaction with MAO inhibitors
    - Discontinue ≥24 hours before surgery
  - Garlic
    - Potential to increase risk of bleeding, especially when combined with other medications that inhibit platelet aggregation
    - Discontinue ≥7 days before surgery

- Ginkgo: duck foot tree, maidenhair tree, silver apricot
  - Potential to increase risk of bleeding, especially when combined with other medications that inhibit platelet aggregation
  - Discontinue ≥36 hours before surgery
- Ginseng
  - Hypoglycemia
  - Potential to increase risk of bleeding
  - Potential to decrease anticoagulation effect of warfarin
  - Discontinue ≥7 days before surgery
- Kava: awa, intoxicating pepper, kawa
  - Potential to increase sedative effect of anesthetics
  - Potential for addiction, tolerance, and withdrawal after abstinence unstudied
  - Discontinue ≥24 hours before surgery
- St John's wort: amber, goat weed, hardhay, Hypericum, klamathe weed
  - Induction of cytochrome P450 enzymes, affecting cyclosporine, warfarin, corticosteroids, protease inhibitors, and possible benzodiazepines, calcium channel blockers, and many other drugs; decreased serum digoxin levels
  - Discontinue ≥5 days before surgery
- Valerian: all-heal, garden heliotrope, vandal toot
  - Potential to increase sedative effect of anesthetics
  - Benzodiazepine-like acute withdrawal
  - Potential to increase anesthetic requirements with long-term use

Syndromes that may cause difficult intubation

- Beckwith-Wiedemann
  - Macroglossia
- Down syndrome
  - Macroglossia
  - Midface hypoplasia
  - Tracheal narrowing
  - May have atlantoaxial instability that may exhibit only under general anesthesia/neuromuscular blockade
  - Can result in damage to the cervical spinal cord
- Pierre Robin sequence
  - Micrognathia
  - Cleft palate
  - Glossoptosis
- Treacher Collins
  - Hypoplasia of the maxilla and mandible

P

- Hemifacial microsomia (Goldenhar)
  - Unilateral or bilateral mandibular hypoplasia
  - Macrostomia
- Apert
  - Craniosynostosis
  - Midface hypoplasia
- Freeman-Sheldon ("whistling face")
  - Microstomia
  - Facial anomalies
- Mucopolysaccharidoses
  - Redundant facial, pharyngeal, and supraglottic soft tissue
  - Neck immobility
- Klippel-Feil
  - Cervical vertebral fusion
  - Neck immobility
- Crouzon
  - Craniosynostosis
  - Midface hypoplasia
- Stickler
  - Mandibular hypoplasia
  - Joint stiffness
- Pfeiffer
  - Craniosynostosis
  - Mid-face hypoplasia
- Some dwarfing syndromes

Prevention of malignant hyperthermia crisis

- Malignant hypothermia (MH) is an inherited disorder of muscle calcium channels, triggered in affected individuals by exposure to inhalational anesthetic agents or succinylcholine.
- Most patients who are MH susceptible have normal history and physical examinations.
- MH crisis is a cascade of hypermetabolism, electrolyte derangements, arrhythmias, skeletal muscle damage, and hyperthermia, which progresses to death if untreated.
  - Prevalence is 1 in 15,000 general anesthetics in children.
  - Incidence increases if succinylcholine is given in addition to volatile anesthetics.
  - Appropriately treated, mortality is estimated at less than 10%.
- Standard test to screen for MH susceptibility is in vitro caffeine-halothane contracture test; uses a muscle biopsy specimen.
  - Indications for performing:
    - Documented episode of hyperthermia
    - Acidosis
    - Rhabdomyolysis induced by a triggering agent
    - Episode of masseter muscle spasm after exposure to a triggering agent
    - Availability of testable relatives of an MH-susceptible patient
    - Patient at least 5 years of age and 20 kg
- Dantrolene, a muscle relaxant that reduces the release of calcium from muscle sarcoplasmic reticulum, significantly improves outcomes.

Preparticipation Physical Evaluation

BACKGROUND

- >6 million high school students participate in sports each year.
- Preparticipation Examination Task Force
  - Formed in the early 1990s by the American Academy of Family Physicians, AAP, American Medical Society for Sports Medicine, American Orthopaedic Society for Sports Medicine, and American Osteopathic Academy of Sports Medicine
  - Preparticipation physical evaluation (PPE) guidelines were updated in 1997, 2002, and 2004.
    - Are the basis for current PPE
    - Are one of the most commonly performed examinations
- PPE has evolved to allow physicians to provide consistent, high-quality examinations nationwide.

GOALS

- Primary goals of PPE are to:
  - Detect conditions that might predispose athlete to injury
    - Musculoskeletal history and physical examination are the best ways to discover orthopedic problems.
  - Detect conditions that might be life-threatening or disabling
    - Sudden cardiac death in young athletes is rare, but a history of syncope or chest pain with exercise or family history of sudden death under age 50 should be evaluated.
    - Topics that must be discussed and emphasized include:
      - Concussion
      - Heat injury
      - Use of nutritional supplements
  - Meet legal or insurance requirements
- Secondary goals are to:
  - Determine general health
  - Counsel athletes on health-related issues
  - Assess fitness level
- The purpose of PPE is not to disqualify athletes.
  - <2% are actually disqualified based on an evaluation's results.
- Identifying athletes who may need further diagnostic testing, counseling, or rehabilitation is primary goal of PPE, but many other expectations exist.
  - Parental expectations
    - May sometimes expect PPE to be a comprehensive evaluation of athlete's health, including areas that may be considered unrelated to sports participation (eg, teenage sexuality, substance abuse, immunizations)
    - Often think of PPE as comprehensive and the only medical evaluation a child or adolescent needs
  - Physicians often view PPE as a cursory examination intended only to detect conditions that might limit or impair athletic endeavors.
- Because parents and physicians may view PPE differently:
  - Parents must be advised about the intent of PPE.
  - The scope and purpose of PPE must be made clear to parents.
- Ideally, all steps in PPE should be performed by a single physician, even if mass screening is taking place.

GENERAL APPROACH

- PPE typically is conducted by 1 of 3 methods.
  - Locker-room method
    - Athletes traditionally line up single file; the physician examines each athlete individually.
    - Requires few personnel and can be performed with little preparation
    - Affords little privacy for athletes, is usually so noisy that the physician has a hard time auscultating the heart and lungs, and is often too brief
  - Station method
    - Divides examination into several components
      - Physicians, nurses, athletic trainers, and coaches each assigned to a single task
    - Ideally suited for screening large numbers of athletes
    - The benefits are relative efficiency and good ability to identify abnormalities.
      - Affords less rapport with athletes and offers no privacy
    - Athletes have little opportunity to ask questions regarding their health or other medical or personal issues.
  - Office-based method
    - Has the advantage of an established physician-patient relationship
      - The athlete's medical history is known, and continuity of care is fostered.
    - Disadvantages include lack of consistency among physicians, potential for physician unfamiliarity with the sport and its disqualifying conditions, and lack of cost effectiveness.
    - Routine laboratory studies and radiographs are not generally performed.
      - Based on information obtained during history and physical examination, the physician may think that further studies are indicated.
- Timing
  - PPE should be performed:
    - Early enough before the sport's season begins to ensure that athletes with medical problems can be thoroughly evaluated and treated
    - Not so early that intervening injuries are likely to occur

- The best time for evaluation is 4–6 weeks before the first scheduled practice.
  - Allows enough time for thorough evaluations, consultations, and rehabilitation of any identified musculoskeletal injuries
- Current AAP guidelines suggest that PPE should be performed every year.
  - Other sources suggest that PPE be conducted before the beginning of each new level of competition (ie, junior high, high school), with annual updates of history and targeted physical examinations of areas of concern.
- Most state high school athletic associations require annual evaluations.
  - A recent survey found that 65% of states require annual examination for all athletes competing in high school sports.

- History
  - History identifies most potential problems for young athletes.
  - Despite best screening of athletes with intent of preventing sudden death, only a few who die would have been detected through history and physical examination.
    - The key to identifying such problems is the questionnaire that systematically screens for conditions that might cause problems or lead to sudden death during athletic activity.
  - The table Medical History Questions lists some of the most important questions to ask during the examination.
  - PPE forms provided by state high school athletic associations often do not incorporate all the screening questions recommended by the Preparticipation Examination Task Force.
  - Athletes typically complete history forms without input from parents.
    - A study showed that only 40% of PPE forms matched when filled out independently by parent and child.
    - The athlete and his or her parents should complete the form together to obtain a thorough and accurate history.
    - Some issues may arise (particularly when the practice is the medical home) in which adolescent privacy on certain topics should be respected.

- Sports are classified based on the likelihood of collision injury and strenuousness of the exercise.
  - These classifications are used to guide physicians on risk of injury and degree of cardiopulmonary fitness required to engage in the sport successfully.
  - The AAP has established classification guidelines by intensity (see table Sports Classification by Intensity) and level of contact.
    - Contact or collision
      - Basketball
      - Boxing
      - Diving
      - Field hockey
      - Football (flag, tackle)
      - Ice hockey
      - Lacrosse
      - Martial arts
      - Rodeo
      - Rugby
      - Ski jumping
      - Soccer
      - Team handball
      - Water polo
      - Wrestling
    - Limited contact
      - Baseball
      - Bicycling
      - Cheerleading
      - Canoeing and kayaking (white water)
      - Fencing
      - Field events (high jump, pole vault)
      - Floor hockey
      - Gymnastics
      - Handball
      - Horseback riding
      - Racquetball
      - Skating (ice, in-line, roller)
      - Skiing (downhill, water)
      - Softball
      - Squash
      - Ultimate frisbee
      - Volleyball
      - Windsurfing and surfing
    - Noncontact
      - Archery
      - Badminton
      - Bodybuilding
      - Canoeing and kayaking (flat water)
      - Crew rowing
      - Curling
      - Dancing
      - Field events (discus, javelin, shot put)
      - Golf
      - Orienteering
      - Power lifting
      - Race walking
      - Riflery
      - Rope jumping

Medical History Questions

	Question	Reason
1.	Injury or illness since last checkup?	Targets potential physical examination concerns
2.	Chronic illnesses, hospitalizations, or surgeries?	Identifies potential counseling or rehabilitation issues
3.	Any medications or supplements of any type?	Identifies drugs that may inhibit or interfere with sports participation
4.	Allergies to medications, insects, or food?	Alerts physicians and trainers for potential allergic reactions
5.	Dizziness, passed out, chest pain with exercise; history of sudden death in a close relative <50 years of age?	Identifies potential causes of sudden death caused by cardiovascular problems
6.	Have you ever passed out or nearly passed out during exercise? Have you ever passed out or nearly passed out after exercise? Have you ever had discomfort, pain, or pressure in your chest during exercise? Does your heart race or skip beats during exercise? Does anyone in your family have Marfan syndrome?	Targets cardiovascular concerns
7.	Ever been restricted from sports by physician?	Identifies potential disqualifying problems
8.	Any skin problems?	Identifies potential transmittable disease during contact
9.	Concussion, knocked out, unconsciousness, memory loss, seizure, or severe or frequent headache?	Targets neurologic concerns
10.	Stinger, burner, pinched nerve, numbness or tingling in extremities?	Targets neurologic concerns
11.	Problems while exercising in the heat?	Targets heat illness concerns
12.	Asthma, allergies, wheezing, difficulty breathing, or chest pain?	Identifies potential for exercise-induced asthma
13.	Special equipment or devices not usually used in your sport?	Identifies potential concerns for physician follow-up
14.	Glasses, contacts, or vision or eye problems?	Identifies ophthalmologic concerns
15.	Strain, sprain, fracture, joint pain, or swelling?	Identifies potential musculoskeletal problems
16.	Concerns about weight: Do you lose weight regularly for your sport?	Identifies potential disordered eating
17.	Feel stressed out?	Clue to ask follow-up questions regarding drug use, eating problems, sexuality, and home and school problems
18.	Recent immunizations (tetanus, measles, hepatitis B, chickenpox)?	Health maintenance issues
19.	Girls only: menstrual history?	Identifies oligomenorrhea and amenorrhea and potential risk for poor nutrition, stress fractures
20.	Do you wear protective braces, splints?	Identifies injuries that have not been fully rehabilitated

- Running
- Sailing
- Scuba diving
- Strength training
- Swimming
- Table tennis
- Tennis
- Track
- Weight lifting

- Clearance to play
  - Few athletes are disqualified from activity on the basis of conditions identified during PPE.
    - The table Medical Conditions and Sports Participation lists the most current recommendations regarding medical conditions and contraindications to participation.
    - Working with athletes to find safe, enjoyable sports in which they can participate is important.
    - If possible, and depending on the condition detected, sports participation should not be eliminated altogether.

Sports Classification by Intensity[a]

High-to-Moderate Intensity High-to-Moderate Dynamic High-to-Moderate Static Demands	High-to-Moderate Intensity High-to-Moderate Dynamic Low Static Demands	High-to-Moderate Intensity High-to-Moderate Static Low Dynamic Demands	Low Intensity Low Dynamic Low Static Demands
• Boxing • Crew rowing • Cross-country skiing • Cycling • Downhill skiing • Fencing • Football • Ice hockey • Rugby • Running (sprint) • Speed skating • Water polo • Wrestling	• Badminton • Baseball • Basketball • Field hockey • Lacrosse • Orienteering • Table tennis • Race walking • Racquetball • Soccer • Squash • Swimming • Tennis • Volleyball	• Archery • Auto racing • Diving • Equestrian • Field events (jumping, throwing) • Gymnastics • Karate or judo • Motorcycling • Rodeo • Sailing • Ski jumping • Water skiing • Weight lifting	• Bowling • Cricket • Curling • Golf • Rifle shooting

Adapted from: Rice SG, American Academy of Pediatrics Council on Sports Medicine and Fitness. Medical conditions affecting sports participation. *Pediatrics*. 2008;121(4):841–848.

PHYSICAL EXAMINATION

General

■ 2 key components of physical examination (cardiovascular and musculoskeletal) identify most athletes who warrant further evaluation or disqualification.

Cardiovascular examination

■ See table Cardiovascular Screening in Athletes.

■ Should include evaluation of peripheral pulses, murmurs, and blood pressure

• All diastolic murmurs and grade 3/6 systolic murmurs warrant further evaluation.

• Hypertrophic cardiomyopathy

– One of the most important conditions to detect

– May produce a systolic murmur that cannot be distinguished from an innocent murmur; the murmur of hypertrophic cardiomyopathy:

■ Increases in intensity with a Valsalva maneuver (decreased ventricular filling, increased obstruction)

■ Decreases with squatting (increased ventricular filling, decreased obstruction)

■ Increases in intensity when the athlete moves from squatting to standing position

• Blood pressures obtained during PPE often are high.

– This may be the result of using a blood pressure cuff that is too small, particularly in large adolescents.

■ Sometimes the athlete's blood pressure truly is high when an age-based table of norms is consulted.

– Hypertension rarely is severe enough to disqualify an athlete from participation, but it must be identified and monitored by the athlete's regular physician.

– Weight-training activities should be restricted in patients who have severe hypertension.

• Sudden cardiac death

– Rare in young athletes; however, history of syncope, chest pain with exercise, or family history of sudden death <50 should be evaluated.

– Recent research showed that screening for sudden cardiac death that included standardized history, physical examination, and electrocardiography may have helped prevent sudden death caused by cardiomyopathy.

Musculoskeletal examination

■ Musculoskeletal examination typically accounts for 50% of abnormal physical findings on PPE.

■ Should focus on previously injured or symptomatic areas

■ 92% of orthopedic injuries are detected by history alone.

■ Some authorities suggest a sport-specific approach to the physical examination.

• Emphasizes the areas that are most commonly affected or injured in each specific sport

■ Special considerations for examination of injured or symptomatic joints include:

• Inspection for visual deformity, muscle mass, asymmetry, and swelling

Medical Conditions and Sports Participation[a]

Condition	Participate?	Explanation
Atlantoaxial instability (instability of the joint between cervical vertebrae 1 and 2)	Qualified yes	Athlete needs evaluation[b] to assess risk of spinal cord injury during sports participation.
Bleeding disorder	Qualified yes	Athlete needs evaluation.
Carditis (inflammation of the heart)	No	Carditis may result in sudden death with exertion.
Hypertension (high blood pressure)	Qualified yes	Persons with significant essential (unexplained) hypertension should avoid weight and power lifting, bodybuilding, and strength training. Those with secondary hypertension (hypertension caused by a previously identified disease) or severe essential hypertension need evaluation.
Congenital heart disease (structural heart defects present at birth)	Qualified yes	Persons with mild forms may participate fully; those with moderate or severe forms or who have undergone surgery need evaluation.
Dysrhythmia (irregular heart rhythm)	Qualified yes	Athlete needs evaluation because some types require therapy or make certain sports dangerous, or both.
Mitral valve prolapse (abnormal heart valve)	Qualified yes	Persons with symptoms (chest pain, symptoms of possible dysrhythmia) or evidence of mitral regurgitation (leaking) on physical examination need evaluation. All others may participate fully.
Heart murmur	Qualified yes	If the murmur is innocent (does not indicate heart disease), then full participation is permitted; otherwise the athlete needs evaluation (see Congenital heart disease and Mitral valve prolapse above).
Cerebral palsy	Qualified yes	Athlete needs evaluation.
Diabetes mellitus	Yes	All sports can be played with proper attention to diet, hydration, and insulin therapy. Particular attention is needed for activities that last 30 minutes or more.
Diarrhea	Qualified no	Unless disease is mild, no participation is permitted, because diarrhea may increase the risk of dehydration and heat illness. See Fever below.
Eating disorders, anorexia nervosa, bulimia nervosa	Qualified yes	These patients need both medical and psychiatric assessment before participation.
Eyes: functionally one-eyed athlete, loss of an eye, detached retina, previous eye surgery or serious eye injury	Qualified yes	A functionally one-eyed athlete has a best-corrected visual acuity of <20/40 in the worse eye. These athletes would experience significant disability if the better eye were seriously injured, as would those with loss of an eye. Some athletes who have previously undergone eye surgery or had a serious eye injury may have an increased risk of injury because of weakened eye tissue. Availability of eye guards approved by the American Society of Testing Materials and other protective equipment may allow participation in most sports, but this determination must be judged on an individual basis.
Fever	No	Fever can increase cardiopulmonary effort, reduce maximal exercise capacity, make heat illness more likely, and increase orthostatic hypotension during exercise. Fever may rarely accompany myocarditis or other infections that may make exercise dangerous.
History of heat illness	Qualified yes	Because of the increased likelihood of recurrence, the athlete needs individual assessment to determine the presence of predisposing conditions and to arrange a prevention strategy.

P

Medical Conditions and Sports Participation[a], *continued*

Condition	Participate?	Explanation
HIV infection	Yes	Because of the apparent minimal risk to others, all sports may be played that the state of health allows. In all athletes, skin lesions should be properly covered, and athletic personnel should use universal precautions when handling blood or body fluids with visible blood.
Kidney: absence of one	Qualified yes	Athlete needs individual assessment for contact or collision and limited contact sports.
Liver: enlarged	Qualified yes	If the liver is acutely enlarged, then participation should be avoided because of risk of rupture. If the liver is chronically enlarged, then individual assessment is needed before collision or contact or limited contact sports are played.
Malignancy	Qualified yes	Athlete needs individual assessment.
Musculoskeletal disorders	Qualified yes	Athlete needs individual assessment.
History of serious head or spine trauma, severe or repeated, concussions, or craniotomy	Qualified yes	Athlete needs individual assessment for collision or contact or limited contact sports and for noncontact sports if deficits exist in judgment or cognition. Recent research supports a conservative approach to management of concussions.
Convulsive disorder (well controlled)	Yes	Risk of convulsion during participation is minimal.
Convulsive disorder (poorly controlled)	Qualified yes	Athlete needs individual assessment for collision or contact or limited-contact sports. Avoid the following noncontact sports: archery, rifle shooting, swimming, weight or power lifting, strength training, or sports involving heights. In these sports, occurrence of a convulsion may be a risk to self or others.
Obesity	Qualified yes	Because of the risk of heat illness, obese persons need careful acclimatization and hydration.
Organ transplant recipient	Qualified yes	Athlete needs individual assessment.
Ovary: absence	Yes	Risk of severe injury to the remaining ovary is minimal.
Respiratory, pulmonary compromise (including cystic fibrosis)	Qualified yes	Athlete needs individual assessment, but generally, all sports may be played if oxygenation remains satisfactory during a graded exercise test. Patients with cystic fibrosis need acclimatization and good hydration to reduce the risk of heat illness.
Asthma	Yes	With proper medication and education, only athletes with the most severe asthma will have to modify their participation.
Acute upper respiratory infection	Qualified yes	Upper respiratory obstruction may affect pulmonary function. Athlete needs individual assessment for all but mild diseases. See Fever previously listed.
Sickle cell disease	Qualified yes	Athlete needs individual assessment. In general, if status of the illness permits, then all but high-exertion, collision or contact sports may be played. Overheating, dehydration, and chilling must be prevented.
Sickle cell trait	Yes	Individuals with sickle cell trait do not likely have an increased risk of sudden death or other medical problems during athletic participation except under the most extreme condition of heat and humidity and possibly high altitude. These individuals, as with all athletes, should be carefully conditioned, acclimatized, and hydrated to reduce any possible risk.

Medical Conditions and Sports Participation[a,] *continued*

Condition	Participate?	Explanation
Skin: boils, herpes simplex, impetigo, scabies, molluscum contagiosum	Qualified yes	Because the patient is contagious, participation in gymnastics with mats, martial arts, wrestling, or other collision or contact or limited-contact sports is not allowed. Herpes simplex virus is probably not transmitted via mats.
Spleen: enlarged	Qualified yes	Persons with acutely enlarged spleens should avoid all sports because of risk of rupture. Those with chronically enlarged spleens need individual assessment before playing collision or contact or limited contact sports.
Testicle: absent or undescended	Yes	Certain sports may require a protective cup.

[a] Adapted from: Rice SG, American Academy of Pediatrics Council on Sports Medicine and Fitness. Medical conditions affecting sports participation. *Pediatrics*. 2008;121(4):841–848.

[b] *Needs evaluation* means that a physician with appropriate knowledge and experience should assess the safety of a given sport for an athlete with the listed medical condition. Unless otherwise noted, this term is used because of the variability of the severity of the disease, the risk of injury among the specific sport, or both.

- Palpation for localized areas of tenderness, warmth, and effusion
- Assessment of range of motion (eg, an athlete with hip pain should be tested for loss of internal rotation and abduction, which can be seen in slipped capital femoral epiphysis and Legg-Calvé-Perthes disease)
- Evaluation of neurovascular status by evaluating muscle strength, sensation, reflexes, and pulses of involved limb (eg, an athlete with history of burners should undergo complete neurovascular testing of the neck and upper extremities)
- Evaluation of joint stability (eg, an athlete with knee pain should undergo tests for valgus and varus stress, Lachman test, and posterior drawer test)

Laboratory studies

- Have not been shown to be cost effective or warranted in young asymptomatic athletes
- Routine urinalysis and hematocrit for all athletes have been largely abandoned.
  - Do not identify athletes who require disqualification
  - Have a high rate of false-positive results
- Electrocardiography, echocardiography, and stress testing are not suggested as screening tests in asymptomatic individuals because of the high rate of false-positive findings and high cost.

Special considerations

- Nutritional supplements
  - Sports supplements have become a billion-dollar industry.
    - Athletes as young as age 11 are taking performance-enhancing supplements.

- PPE is the ideal time to question athletes briefly about supplement use.
- Sports supplements contain impurities; when taken inappropriately, they may result in adverse side effects.
  - Muscle cramps
  - Dehydration
  - Abdominal bloating
  - Tachycardia
  - Arrhythmia
  - Death
- Supplement use should be discouraged; young athletes should be told about their possible ill effects.
- Obesity
  - Up to 30% of children are obese.
    - Many are seeking to participate in sports.
  - Obesity is not a contraindication to sports participation unless a comorbid finding, such as severe hypertension, is present.
  - Obese children are at increased risk of heat injury and should be counseled accordingly.
  - Sports participation with emphasis on activities that improve fitness should be encouraged for the obese child.
- Concussion
  - History of concussion should be addressed during PPE.
  - 2 grades of severity: simple and complicated
    - Complicated concussion may include:
      - Amnesia
      - Seizure
      - Prolonged symptoms
      - Loss of consciousness

P

Cardiovascular Screening in Athletes[a]

Condition	Cardiovascular Examination	Abnormality
Hypertension	Blood pressure	Varies with age—general guideline is >135/85 mm Hg in adolescents
Coarctation of aorta	Femoral pulses	Decreased intensity of pulse
Hypertrophic cardiomyopathy	Auscultation with provocative maneuvers (standing, supine, Valsalva maneuver)	Systolic ejection murmur that intensifies with standing or Valsalva maneuver
Marfan syndrome	Auscultation	Aortic (decrescendo diastolic murmur) or mitral insufficiency (holosystolic murmur)

[a] Adapted from: Maron BJ, Thompson PO, Puffer JC. Cardiovascular preparticipation screening of competitive athletes: a statement for health professionals from the Sudden Death Committee (clinical cardiology) and Congenital Cardiac Defects Committee (cardiovascular disease in the young), American Heart Association. *Circulation.* 1996;94:850–856.

- Neuropsychological testing is suggested with repeat or complicated concussion.
- Patients must meet 3 criteria to return to play after concussion.
  - Asymptomatic at rest
  - Asymptomatic with exercise
  - No neurocognitive deficits (eg, memory loss, concentration problems, fatigue, fogginess, confusion)

- Medical home
  - Adolescents are the most underserved population in health care today.
    - In many instances, their only contact with medical system is PPE.
    - All young athletes should be referred to their pediatric primary care physician for routine care and for follow-up of any ongoing medical conditions.

P

Preseptal and Orbital Cellulitis

DEFINITION

- Infection of tissues anterior to the orbital septum is described as a *preseptal* or *periorbital* infection.
  - The terms *preseptal* and *periorbital* may be used interchangeably.
- Preseptal cellulitis, or periorbital cellulitis, is often considered as a diagnosis.
  - However, the term is an inadequate diagnostic label unless accompanied by a modifier that indicates the probable pathogenesis.
- Orbital cellulitis is infection of the soft tissues of the orbit posterior to the orbital septum.

ETIOLOGY

- Preseptal cellulitis infections after trauma
  - Result from secondary bacterial infection of local skin trauma, including
    - Insect bites
    - Spread of infection from a focus of impetigo
  - The traumatic injury may be modest or inapparent.
  - Can be caused by any of the following organisms:
    - *Staphylococcus aureus*
    - *Streptococcus pyogenes*
    - *Mycobacterium tuberculosis*
      - In countries where *M tuberculosis* is endemic, this etiology should be considered in patients who present with a swollen lid.
    - *Bacillus anthracis*
    - *Nocardia brasiliensis*
    - *Pasteurella multocida*
    - Ringworm (caused by *Trichophyton* species)
- Bacteremic periorbital cellulitis
  - *Haemophilus influenzae*
  - *Streptococcus pneumoniae*
- Preseptal (periorbital) cellulitis caused by inflammatory edema of sinusitis
  - Complication of paranasal sinusitis
  - Results in swelling around the eye
  - Infecting organisms are the same as those that cause uncomplicated acute sinusitis.
    - *S pneumoniae*
    - Nontypeable *H influenzae*
    - *Moraxella catarrhalis*
- Orbital infections
  - Least common cause of swollen eye
  - Most orbital infections involve formation of a subperiosteal abscess that, in young children, results from ethmoiditis and ethmoid osteitis.
  - In the adolescent, subperiosteal abscess can be a complication of frontal sinusitis and osteitis.
  - Rarely, orbital cellulitis evolves without formation of subperiosteal abscess.
    - Direct spread from ethmoid sinus to the orbit via natural bony dehiscences in the bones that form the medial wall of the orbit

RISK FACTORS

- Infections can spread to the eye from contiguous structures.
- Venous system provides opportunities for spread of infection from 1 anatomic site to another.
  - Predisposes patient to involvement of:
    - Cavernous sinus
    - Meninges
    - Brain
- Infection originating in the mucosa of the paranasal sinuses can spread to involve the bone (osteitis with or without subperiosteal abscess) and the intraorbital contents.
- Preseptal cellulitis infections after trauma
  - Localized infection of the eyelid or adjacent structure
  - Conjunctivitis
  - Hordeolum
  - Dacryoadenitis
  - Dacryocystitis
  - Trauma
  - Acute sinusitis
- Bacteremic periorbital cellulitis
  - Viral upper respiratory infection (URI)
- Preseptal (periorbital) cellulitis caused by inflammatory edema of sinusitis
  - Sinusitis
- Orbital infections
  - Subperiosteal abscess
  - Orbital abscess
  - Orbital cellulitis
  - Cavernous sinus thrombosis
  - Traumatic inoculation
  - Endophthalmitis
  - In young children, ethmoiditis and ethmoid osteitis
  - In adolescents, frontal sinusitis and osteitis
  - Patients with diabetes and immunocompromised children are at higher risk of fungal orbital cellulitis (especially *Mucor* species).

SIGNS AND SYMPTOMS

Preseptal cellulitis infections after trauma

- Loosely bound periorbital soft tissues permit impressive swelling to accompany minor infection.

- Overlying skin can be bright red with subtle textural changes.
- Intense swelling can lead to shininess (see Figure 64 on page F22).
- Ulceration and vesicle formation in the presence of ringworm
- Some patients have fever.
- Many are afebrile despite dramatic local findings.
- Peripheral leukocyte count is variable.

Bacteremic periorbital cellulitis

- Age <18 months
- History of viral URI for several days
- Sudden increase in temperature (to >39°C)
- Acute onset and rapid progression of eyelid swelling
  - Swelling usually begins in the inner canthus of the upper and lower eyelid.
  - Can obscure the eyeball within 12 hours
- Markedly discolored and erythematous periorbital tissues
- If swelling has been rapidly progressive, the area may have violaceous discoloration.
- The child's resistance to examination commonly leads to an erroneous impression of tenderness.
- Retraction or separation of the eyelids reveals that:
  - The globe is normally placed.
  - Extraocular eye movements are intact.
- The young age of patients, high fever, and rapid progression of findings differentiate bacteremic preseptal cellulitis from other causes of swelling around the eye (see Figure 65 on page F23).
- Bacteremic cellulitis rarely arises from the paranasal sinus cavities.
  - Typeable *H influenzae* organisms are rarely recovered from maxillary sinus aspirates.
  - Typeable *H influenzae* organisms are rarely recovered from abscess material in patients who have serious local complications of paranasal sinus disease (eg, subperiosteal abscess)
  - *S pneumoniae* can cause subperiosteal abscess in patients with acute sinusitis.
    - Such patients are not usually bacteremic.

Preseptal (periorbital) cellulitis caused by inflammatory edema of sinusitis

- Several complications of paranasal sinusitis can result in swelling around the eye.
- The most common and least serious complication is often called *inflammatory edema* or *sympathetic effusion*.
- Typical patient is:
  - ≥2 years old
  - Has had viral URI for several days when swelling is noted
- History of intermittent early-morning periorbital swelling that resolves after a few hours often is present.

- On the day of presentation, eyelid swelling does not typically resolve, but progresses gradually.
- Striking degrees of erythema can also be present.
- Eye pain and tenderness are variable.
- Eyelids can be very swollen and difficult to evert, requiring the assistance of an ophthalmologist.
- When the ethmoid sinuses are completely congested, venous drainage is physically impeded (see Figure 66 on page F23).
  - Resulting in soft-tissue swelling of the eyelids, maximal at the medial aspect of the lids
  - Infection is confined within the paranasal sinuses.
- No displacement of the globe or impairment of extraocular eye movements
- Fever, if present, is usually low grade.
- Peripheral leukocyte count is unremarkable.
- Blood culture results are always negative.
- If a tissue aspiration is performed, culture of specimen has negative result.
- Sinus radiographs show ipsilateral ethmoiditis or pansinusitis.
- The following differentiate inflammatory edema from bacteremic periorbital cellulitis:
  - Age of the child
  - Gradual evolution of lid swelling
  - Modest temperature elevation

True orbital disease secondary to sinusitis

- Orbital infection is the least common cause of a swollen eye.
- Sudden onset of erythema and swelling around the eye (see Figure 67 on page F23)
- Preceded by several days of a viral URI
- Eye pain can precede swelling.
  - Is often dramatic
- Presence of fever, systemic signs, and toxicity is variable.
- Orbital infection is suggested by:
  - Proptosis (with the globe displaced usually anteriorly and downward)
  - Impairment of extraocular eye movements (most often upward gaze)
  - Chemosis (edema of the bulbar conjunctiva) or
  - Loss of visual acuity or decreased pupillary reaction (late in the evolution of the infection)

DIFFERENTIAL DIAGNOSIS

- Young age, high fever, and rapid progression of findings differentiate bacteremic preseptal cellulitis from other causes of swelling around the eye.
- Blunt trauma (resulting in a "black eye")
  - History provides the key to diagnosis.
  - Eyelid swelling continues to increase for 48 hours and then resolves over several days.

- Tumors that characteristically involve the eye include:
  - Hemangioma of the lid
  - Ocular tumors, such as:
    - Retinoblastoma
    - Choroidal melanoma
  - Orbital neoplasms, such as:
    - Neuroblastoma
    - Rhabdomyosarcoma
    - Langerhans cell histiocytosis
  - Tumors usually cause gradual onset of proptosis in the absence of inflammation.
- Orbital pseudotumor
  - Autoimmune inflammation of orbital tissues, which exhibits:
    - Eyelid swelling
    - Red eye
    - Pain
    - Decreased ocular motility
- Hypoproteinemia and congestive heart failure cause eyelid swelling as a result of local edema.
  - Characteristic findings are bilateral, boggy, nontender, nondiscolored soft-tissue swelling.
- Allergic inflammation
  - Includes angioneurotic edema or contact hypersensitivity
    - Superficially, these problems can resemble findings in acute infection.
    - However, presence of pruritus and absence of tenderness are helpful distinguishing characteristics of allergic inflammation.

DIAGNOSTIC APPROACH

- The child with a swollen eye is commonly seen in primary care.
- Approach to diagnosis (see Figure 68 on page F24) depends on physical examination.
- By far, preseptal infections are most common.
- Infections behind the septum that cause eyelid swelling include:
  - Subperiosteal abscess
  - Orbital abscess
  - Orbital cellulitis
  - Cavernous sinus thrombosis
  - Panophthalmitis
  - Endophthalmitis
  - Although all of these entities can be labeled as orbital cellulitis, a systematic approach allows a more specific diagnosis, thereby directing management.

LABORATORY FINDINGS

- Preseptal cellulitis infections after trauma
  - Peripheral leukocyte count is variable.
- Bacteremic periorbital cellulitis
  - A precise bacteriologic diagnosis is made by recovery of the organism from blood culture.
- Preseptal (periorbital) cellulitis caused by inflammatory edema of sinusitis
  - Peripheral leukocyte count is unremarkable.
  - Blood culture results are always negative.

IMAGING

- Bacteremic periorbital cellulitis
  - Radiographs of the paranasal sinuses are often abnormal.
    - Abnormalities almost certainly reflect the viral respiratory syndrome that precedes and probably predisposes the patient to the bacteremic event rather than a clinically significant sinusitis.
- If retraction of the lids is not possible, orbital computed tomography (CT) may be necessary.
- Orbital infections
- Imaging studies:
  - Are usually performed if orbital disease is suspected.
  - Help determine cause of the clinical findings (see Figure 69 on page F24)
    - Subperiosteal abscess
    - Orbital abscess
    - Orbital cellulitis
- On occasion, CT results can be misleading.
  - They may suggest abscess when inflammatory edema is present.

DIAGNOSTIC PROCEDURES

- Preseptal cellulitis infections after trauma
  - Patients with bacterial cellulitis of traumatized areas rarely have bacteremia.
  - The precise bacteriologic diagnosis is made through culture of exudate from the wound.
  - If there is no drainage, tissue aspiration is carefully attempted.
    - Perform only if it can be done safely (ie, at a distance far enough from the orbit that no potential damage to the eye can occur).
    - Tuberculin syringe with a 25-gauge needle can be used for aspiration.
    - Usually, only a minuscule amount of infected material can be aspirated.

- – Small volume of nonbacteriostatic saline (0.2 mL) is drawn into the syringe before the procedure.
  - ▪ Not injected into skin
  - ▪ Used to expel small volume of tissue fluid onto chocolate agar for culture
- Bacteremic periorbital cellulitis
  - If tissue aspiration is performed, culture of specimen may have a positive result.
  - Lumbar puncture should be performed unless the clinical picture precludes meningitis.
- Preseptal (periorbital) cellulitis caused by inflammatory edema of sinusitis
  - If tissue aspiration is performed, specimen culture is negative.

CLASSIFICATION

- Preseptal
  - Infections: due to local trauma or spread from local infectious site
- Bacteremic
  - Inflammatory: due to inflammatory swelling secondary to sinusitis
- Orbital

TREATMENT APPROACH

- Practitioners frequently need to manage the child whose chief symptom is a swollen eye.
  - Some are trivial or self-limited disorders.
  - Others are sight- or life-threatening problems.
- If orbital disease is suspected, the clinical course is the ultimate guide to management.

SPECIFIC TREATMENTS

Preseptal cellulitis infections after trauma

- Oral antibiotic therapy may be initiated in children who:
  - Are >5 years
  - Are afebrile
  - Have mild cellulitis
  - Have reliable caregivers

Bacteremic periorbital cellulitis

- Requires parenteral therapy
- *S pneumoniae* is the most likely cause in a child who has received both the *H influenzae* type B and pneumococcal conjugate vaccine series.
- Infection is usually bacteremic in the age group in which the meninges are susceptible to inoculation.
  - Use an advanced-generation cephalosporin, such as:
    - – Cefotaxime (150 mg/kg per day, divided into 8-hour doses) or ceftriaxone (100 mg/kg per day, divided into 12-hour doses)

- Lumbar puncture should be performed unless the clinical picture precludes meningitis.
  - If cerebrospinal fluid pleocytosis is present, add:
    - – Vancomycin (60 mg/kg/day divided into doses every 6 hours) *or*
    - – Rifampin (20 mg/kg once daily, not to exceed 600 mg/day)
- If evidence of local infection has resolved and meningitis is not present:
  - A 10-day course of oral antimicrobial therapy is prescribed.

Preseptal (periorbital) cellulitis caused by inflammatory edema of sinusitis

- Antibiotic therapy can be given orally if at the time of the first examination:
  - Eyelid swelling is modest *and*
  - The child does not appear toxic *and*
  - The parents will adhere to management
  - Otherwise, admission to the hospital and parenteral treatment should be undertaken.
- The only source of bacteriologic information is that obtainable by maxillary sinus aspiration.
  - Usually not performed
- Appropriate agents for outpatient therapy have activity against ß-lactamase–producing organisms.
  - Amoxicillin–potassium clavulanate
  - Cefuroxime axetil
  - Cefpodoxime proxetil
- Parenteral agents include:
  - Cefuroxime
  - Ampicillin-sulbactam
    - – This combination is an attractive choice.
    - – Not approved for children <12 years
  - After several days, once the affected eye has returned to near normal, a 14-day course of an oral antimicrobial agent is substituted.
- The use of topically applied intranasal decongestants (eg, oxymetazoline) has not been systematically evaluated.
  - Such agents may be helpful during the first 48 hours.

Orbital infections

Antimicrobial therapy

- Usually, patients with these symptoms are managed successfully with antimicrobial therapy alone.
- Empirical antimicrobial therapy should be chosen to provide activity against:
  - *S aureus and*
  - *S pyogenes and*

P

- Anaerobic bacteria of the upper respiratory tract
  - Anaerobic cocci
  - *Bacteroides* species
  - *Prevotella* species
  - *Fusobacterium* species
  - *Veillonella* species
- In addition to the usual pathogens associated with acute sinusitis
  - *S pneumoniae*
  - *H influenzae*
  - *M catarrhalis*
- Appropriate selections include:
  - Cefuroxime (150 mg/kg per day divided into doses every 8 hours) *or*
  - Ampicillin-sulbactam (200 mg/kg per day divided into doses every 6 hours).
  - Clindamycin (40 mg/kg per day divided into doses every 6 hours) *or* metronidazole (30–35 mg/kg per day divided into doses every 8–12 hours) can be added if cefuroxime is used and anaerobic infection is likely
- If surgery is performed
  - Gram stain of material drained from the sinuses or the abscess guides consideration of additional drugs or a change to the regimen.
  - When final results of culture are available, antibiotic therapy may be changed, if appropriate.
  - Intravenous therapy is maintained until the infected eye appears nearly normal.
    - At that time, 3 weeks of oral antibiotic therapy can be substituted.

Surgical drainage

- Presence of a large, well-defined abscess with complete ophthalmoplegia or impairment of vision prompts operative drainage of the paranasal sinuses and the abscess.
- Several studies have reported successful drainage of subperiosteal abscess via endoscopy.
  - Performed through an intranasal approach
    - Avoids external incision
  - In many cases, a well-defined abscess is not seen.
  - Instead, inflammatory tissue is interposed between the:
    - Lateral border of ethmoid sinus *and*
    - Swollen medial rectus muscle
    - On occasion, CT results can be misleading, suggesting abscess when inflammatory edema is present.

WHEN TO ADMIT

- Hospitalize a child with a swollen eye:
  - For parenteral therapy when bacteremic periorbital cellulitis is diagnosed
  - For parenteral therapy when diagnosis of likely bacterial cellulitis is made and
    - Oral therapy has failed *or*
    - The child is febrile *or*
    - The child is <5 years
  - For parenteral therapy and consultation with an ophthalmologist when diagnosis is dacryocystitis
  - When oral therapy has failed
  - If eye is swollen shut and parenteral antibiotics and close observation are required for the management of inflammatory edema (sympathetic effusion)
  - If proptosis, impairment of extraocular movements, diminished pupil reaction, or loss of visual acuity occurs:
    - These signs herald subperiosteal abscess, orbital abscess, orbital cellulitis, and cavernous sinus thrombosis.
    - Presence indicates the need for parenteral antibiotics and the likely need for surgical intervention.

WHEN TO REFER

- Refer a child with a swollen eye to an ophthalmologist in the following instances:
  - When visual acuity is lost
  - When any eyelid swelling occurs in an immunocompromised child or child with diabetes, referral should be immediate.
    - The situation may require urgent treatment.
  - If conjunctivitis is diagnosed, referral is appropriate if clinical findings do not begin to improve after 5 days.
    - Circumstance suggests a diagnosis of either adenovirus or herpes simplex infection.
  - When a chalazion is large and causes local irritation, incision and drainage of the chalazion may be required.
  - When dacryoadenitis has not begun to resolve after 5 days
  - All patients with suspected or proven orbital cellulitis

COMPLICATIONS

- Preseptal (periorbital) cellulitis caused by inflammatory edema of sinusitis
  - Inflammatory edema is part of a continuum.
  - More serious complications result from spread of infection outside the paranasal sinuses into the orbit.
  - Rarely, infection progresses despite initial optimal management of sympathetic effusions.

P

Prevention of Dental Caries

BACKGROUND

- Dental caries is characterized by progressive destruction of tooth structure by localized bacterial activity.
  - One of the most common bacterial infections afflicting children and adolescents
  - Related to critical interrelationships among:
    - Teeth
    - Dietary carbohydrate
    - Saliva
    - Specific oral bacteria
  - The decay process is initiated by demineralization of the outer tooth surface.
    - Result of organic acids formed during bacterial fermentation of dietary carbohydrates
    - Saliva functions as a remineralizing and buffering solution to counter the effect of demineralization.
    - Carious lesions form if bacterial-derived demineralization exceeds saliva's remineralization and buffering capacity.
  - Incipient lesions first appear as opaque white spots.
    - With progressive loss of tooth mineral, cavitation occurs.

Mechanism

Microbial factors

- *Mutans streptococci*
  - Primary etiologic agent in human dental caries

Salivary factors

- Saliva is the primary host defense against dental caries.
  - Severe caries observed in desalivated experimental animals and xerostomic humans
  - Salivary hypofunction may be a consequence (in part) of diverse factors.
    - Radiotherapy when the salivary glands are within the radiation ports
    - Long-term administration of anticholinergic or parasympatholytic drugs
    - Salivary gland disease (eg, Sjögren syndrome)
- The relationship between salivary gland hypofunction and dental caries involves several factors.
  - Physical flow of saliva augmented by activity of the oral musculature removes a large number of bacteria from teeth.
  - Salivary proteins and enzymes (lysozyme, lactoferrin, and lactoperoxidase) work with other salivary components to:
    - Kill bacteria
    - Interfere with bacterial replication
    - Interfere with the acidogenic potential of cariogenic bacteria

- Other features of saliva
  - Interferes with bacterial attachment through molecular interactions
  - Protects the tooth surface from demineralization
  - Buffers acid through salivary bicarbonate, phosphate, and histidine-rich peptides
  - Remineralizes teeth

Dietary factors

- Most dietary sugars, carbohydrates, and starches are:
  - Readily metabolized to organic acids by *M streptococci*
  - Termed *cariogenic substrates*
- Frequent and prolonged oral exposure to sugars, carbohydrates, and starches facilitates dental caries activity.
- Cariogenic potential
  - Determined not by how much sugar a person eats, but how the sugar is eaten
    - The cariogenic potential of apple juice consumed over a long period (eg, from a bottle all night) differs greatly from that of the same volume of apple juice consumed at a single meal.
    - Sugar from foods retained orally for a long time (eg, a raisin or caramel) is more cariogenic than sugar in foods retained orally for a short time (eg, a liquid that is immediately swallowed).

GOALS

- Promote practice of proper oral hygiene
- Prevent development of dental caries
- Reduce intraoral levels of *M streptococci*
- Refer patients with salivary hypofunction to a pediatric dentist
- Decrease the frequency of cariogenic substrate ingestion
- Refer patients chronically exposed to sweetened medication elixirs to a pediatric dentist

GENERAL APPROACH

- Pediatricians play an important role in the prevention and early diagnosis of dental caries.
  - Routinely question parents about feeding behaviors.
  - Make recommendations that promote dental health.
- Examine the child's dentition as part of routine physical examination.
  - Required equipment
    - An intraoral light
    - Pediatric tongue blade
  - Begin with the distal maxillary molar.
  - Continue with the inspection of each tooth from right to left.
  - Repeat the procedure from the patient's left to right in the mandibular arch.

- Dental caries
  - Frequently appears as a darker-stained area
  - Usually begins in the pits and fissures on the biting surfaces of the molar teeth
  - Contact surfaces between the molar teeth are the second most common area.
    - These areas are difficult to examine.
    - Dentists usually depend on intraoral radiographs.
- Carious lesions
  - Often detected on the front surface of the primary incisor teeth near the gingiva
  - Routinely found in children with severe early childhood dental caries
  - Retracting the lips is necessary to inspect adequately the entire surface of primary incisor teeth.
- Refer to a dentist any child with:
  - Evidence of cavitation
  - Stained fissures
  - Areas of enamel decalcification
- Every child should be evaluated by a dentist by 12 months of age.

SPECIFIC INTERVENTIONS

Fluoride

Water fluoridation

- The recommended optimal level of water fluoridation is 0.7–1.2 ppm fluoride, depending on the amount of water intake.
- Fluoridation of public water supplies has proven to be the most effective, convenient, and economical measure available to prevent dental caries.

Fluoride supplements

- Dramatic reduction in dental caries was demonstrated in populations drinking fluoridated water.
  - Led to recommendations to administer fluoride as dietary supplement for people who did not receive it in drinking water
  - However, fluoride acts topically to prevent dental caries through salivary remineralization of demineralized enamel.
  - This action works best by frequent exposure to relatively low levels of fluoride, as occurs with drinking fluoridated water.
- New fluoride supplementation recommendations have been developed because of:
  - Realization that systemic fluoride ingestion is not the major mechanism of action of fluoride in dental caries prevention
  - Reports of increased dental fluorosis (hypomineralization of enamel)

- Before prescribing fluoride supplements, assess child's exposure to other fluoride sources (eg, toothpaste, fluoridated commercial beverages).
  - Risk of fluorosis increases with increased exposure to fluoride.
- Supplements should be sucked or chewed to enhance the topical action of the fluoride in the supplements.
- Recommended fluoride dose by age and concentration of fluoride in drinking water (ppmF)
  - Birth–6 months
    - <0.3 ppmF: 0
    - 0.3–0.6 ppmF: 0
    - >0.6 ppmF: 0
  - 6 mo–3 years
    - <0.3 ppmF: 0.25 mg
    - 0.3–0.6 ppmF: 0
    - >0.6 ppmF: 0
  - 3–6 years
    - <0.3 ppmF: 0.5 mg
    - 0.3–0.6 ppmF: 0.25
    - >0.6 ppmF: 0
  - 6–16 years
    - <0.3 ppmF: 1.0 mg
    - 0.3–0.6 ppmF: 0.5
    - >0.6 ppmF: 0

Fluoride dentifrice (toothpaste)

- Highly effective in preventing dental decay
- Toothbrushing with a pea-size amount of dentifrice on a toothbrush should be encouraged as soon as teeth begin to emerge.
- Before 6 years of age, children tend to swallow rather than expectorate dentifrice.
  - Nearly all ingested fluoride is absorbed, primarily from the small intestine.

Fluoride rinses

- Those containing 0.05% fluoride are highly effective in reducing dental decay.
- Available without a prescription
- Should be recommended for children ≥6 years of age who are at risk for dental decay because of such conditions as:
  - Compromised salivary flow rates
  - Orthodontic therapy
  - Extensive dental caries
- Not recommended for children <6 years because they cannot expectorate properly
  - Results in excessive fluoride ingestion

Fluoride varnish

- Can be painted on teeth
- Now available in the US
- Contains high concentrations of fluoride (up to 22,600 ppm) suspended in a viscous delivery medium
- Can be applied to teeth of high-risk children by trained personnel in various settings, including the medical office
- Does not require trays or oral suction equipment
  - Unlike foams, rinses, and gels

Dental fluorosis

- Hypomineralization of enamel that occurs when higher than optimal levels of fluoride are ingested during period of enamel formation
  - May vary from very mild to severe
  - Very mild to mild cases appear as chalky whitening of the enamel.
  - Severe fluorosis exhibits as mottled enamel that is pitted and brown.
  - Recent reports have shown a trend toward a higher prevalence of dental fluorosis relative to historical data from earlier studies.
  - Increase was found to correlate with ingestion of fluoride from sources other than drinking water, including:
    - Fluoride supplements
    - Fluoridated toothpaste
    - Commercial beverages containing fluoridated water
- New fluoride supplementation schedule (see above, endorsed by Council on Dental Therapeutics of the American Dental Association)
  - Not recommended prenatally or during the first 6 months of life
  - Not recommended for breastfed infants residing in optimally fluoridated communities
  - Dose level based on the patient's age and fluoride content of the water supply
  - Recommended supplement dose should be considered a maximum.
    - Other sources of ingested fluoride (eg, toothpastes, commercial beverages) should also be taken into account.
- Fluoride level of a water supply can usually be obtained by calling the local water board.
  - Fluoride analysis is indicated when a private water supply is used.
    - The patient's parent should use a plastic container for the water specimen (a glass container may impair the accuracy of the fluoride assay).
    - Send the sample to an appropriate laboratory.

- No fluoride prescription should be written for >120 mg of fluoride, to prevent poisoning from ingestion.
  - Even if a child ingested the entire supply, probably only mild gastric upset would ensue.
    - However, in such an event, a poison control center should be contacted immediately.
- Toothpaste can also provide a topical form of fluoride supplement for children who swallow the toothpaste after brushing.
  - For children who cannot spit, maximal recommended fluoride dose may be ingested simply by brushing a child's teeth once or twice a day.
  - To reduce the risk of dental fluorosis from toothpaste ingestion, a small amount of toothpaste (pea size) should be used in brushing a young child's teeth.
  - Parents should dispense the toothpaste.
  - Young children should not have access to toothpaste.

Oral hygiene

- Thorough daily brushing and flossing of the teeth helps prevent dental caries.
  - Mechanical cleaning disturbs the attachment of dental plaque biofilm to the tooth surface.
- Parents should verify that the child's teeth are clean before bedtime.
  - Buffering capacity and antimicrobial action of saliva decrease during sleep with diminished secretion of saliva.
- Parents should receive professional instruction regarding oral hygiene techniques for children.
  - Information can be obtained from the American Dental Association (see Resources).
- Clinical studies demonstrate that most children ≤8 years do not have the hand-eye coordination required for adequate oral hygiene.
  - Parents must assume responsibility for oral hygiene.
    - Degree of parental involvement should reflect the child's level of competency.

Sealants

- Sealants are plastic coatings that are applied professionally to the occlusal (biting) surfaces of the posterior teeth.
- The use of sealants has been shown to be effective in preventing pit and fissure caries.
  - Excellent oral hygiene and optimal fluoride exposure have minimal effect in preventing dental caries in the pits and fissures on the occlusal surfaces of the posterior teeth.
- A survey conducted by the National Institute of Dental Research indicated that relatively few school children in the US have sealants on their teeth.
  - Although efficacious, use of sealants is not routine in prevention of dental caries.

Diet

- Decreasing the frequency of cariogenic substrate ingestion prevents dental caries.
  - Encourage avoidance of between-meal snacks that contain cariogenic substrates.
  - Use of gum, candy, and soft drinks containing sugar substitutes (mannitol, sorbitol, xylitol, and aspartame [with precautions]) is an effective approach for the child with a sweet tooth.
    - Chewing sugarless gum has been proven clinically to enhance salivary flow rate and, in turn, neutralize plaque biofilm pH.
- Infants should be weaned from the bottle by 1 year of age to eliminate risk for early childhood dental caries (also known as *nursing bottle dental caries*) (see Figure 70 on page F24).
  - Bedtime and naptime nursing bottles should contain only water.

Prevention of Obesity

BACKGROUND

Obesity and its comorbidities

- Childhood obesity has emerged as a major health problem that increases the risk for chronic illness.
- Obesity is rapidly overtaking smoking as the largest preventable cause of disease in the US.
  - It has the potential to make the current generation of US children the first to have a shorter life expectancy than their parents.
- Obesity prevention, intervention, and treatment must be part of primary care.
- Obesity comorbidities include:
  - Dyslipidemia
  - Type 2 diabetes
  - Nonalcoholic steatohepatitis
  - Polycystic ovarian syndrome
  - Sleep apnea
  - Uniquely pediatric comorbidities occur as a result of injury to open growth plates in the hip and knee.
    - Slipped capital femoral epiphysis
    - Blount disease
  - Comorbidities of obesity add to the burden of chronic disease in children and the health care system.
- Secondary depression and self-esteem issues are becoming increasingly common.
- The number of children who are overweight has increased from 4% in 1962 to 16% in 2002.

Body mass index (BMI)

- A measure that correlates with body fat
  - Calculated as wt/ht^2
  - Used to screen populations for obesity and to categorize individuals to target obesity prevention, intervention, or treatment
  - In adults
    - BMI of 25–29 is overweight.
    - BMI of ≥30 is obese.
    - Increased BMI in adults is correlated with increases in obesity-related comorbidities.
  - In children
    - Percentage of body fat changes throughout development.
    - BMI *percentile* must be used as a measure.
    - BMI in 85th–94th percentile is overweight; BMI >95th percentile is obese.
    - BMI >99th percentile has been associated with cardiovascular risk factors:
      - High blood pressure
      - Elevated insulin
      - Lipid abnormalities
      - Severe adult obesity

Causes of obesity

- The causes of the obesity epidemic are multifactorial and complex.
- These factors play out at the individual, family, community, and population level and account for the global shift in obesity demographics.
- Genetic predisposition
  - The contribution of genetic effects to obesity suggests a strong genetic predisposition toward weight gain.
    - Parental obesity increases the risk that a child will become an obese adult.
    - Infants of mothers who are obese or have diabetes during pregnancy have an increased risk for childhood and adult obesity.
  - The explanation of gene–environment interaction involves *epigenetic mechanisms*, "a set of reversible heritable changes that occur without a change in DNA sequence."
- A shifting nutrition and activity environment plays a role in both population risk and individual risk of obesity.
- Nutrition- and activity-related behaviors act at the interface between the individual and family and the environment.
  - The concept of the *thrifty genotype*: the transition of a population that evolved under conditions of periodic food scarcity to a state of abundant food and increased inactivity
    - This concept may partially explain the differential susceptibility of ethnic populations.
    - Populations in developing countries who are transitioning to a Western lifestyle also are experiencing a rapid rise of childhood obesity.
    - Minority and disadvantaged children are disproportionately affected by obesity.
    - Lower physical activity levels have been associated with factors that differentially affect disadvantaged populations.
  - Changes in the secular environment have increased calories available to children and families.
    - Portion sizes of commercially available foods began to increase above recommended dietary guidelines in the 1970s.
    - The availability and consumption of snack foods can lead to excess calorie consumption.
    - Consumption of >1 soda per day by children as young as 2 years was correlated with obesity.
    - Eating out has been cited as one of the factors important in the development of the obesity epidemic.
      - The proportion of foods that children consumed from restaurants and fast-food outlets increased by nearly 300% between 1977 and 1996.
      - Fast-food consumption is a significant risk factor for obesity.

- Obesity correlates with the number of hours of television viewing.
  - After-school time is a particularly vulnerable time for children in terms of television exposure.
  - Food advertising may play a role in increases in high-energy food consumption.
- Inactivity has been associated with obesity.
  - In a review of obesity prevention trials moderate to vigorous physical activity was significantly correlated with obesity prevention in children.

GOALS

- Calculation of BMI and classification of weight status at least once a year is an essential component of well child care.
- Pediatricians must be prepared to:
  - Prevent, identify, and treat obesity
  - Treat obesity-related comorbidities
  - Deal with obesity-related emergencies that occur in obese children
    - Hyperosmolar hyperglycemia
    - Pseudotumor cerebri
    - Pulmonary emboli
    - Cardiomyopathy

GENERAL APPROACH

- Early infant weight gain is independently associated with being overweight in childhood.
  - Infants who gain excess weight in the first 4 months of life are likely to be overweight at the age of 7 years.
  - Weight increase between birth and 12 months of age as a ratio of birth weight is independently associated with becoming overweight at 6 years of age.
    - This early weight gain combined with protein intake at 9–12 months of age was able to explain 50% of the variance in boys' BMIs at 6 years.
- Prolonged breastfeeding has been associated with a reduced risk of becoming overweight.
  - In an evidence-based review of breastfeeding studies, breastfeeding was associated with reduction in:
    - Risk of obesity and type 2 diabetes in the children
    - Risk of type 2 diabetes in mothers

Age-appropriate obesity prevention guide

- Age: newborn or infant
  - Nutrition information
    - Promote breastfeeding
    - Teach parents to recognize hunger and satiety cues.
    - Assess family's eating habits and nutrition environment.
    - Limit juice.

- Appropriate activities
  - Encourage face-to-face play time to lay groundwork for shared activity.
  - Take daily walk in stroller to establish outdoor time.
  - Use safe toys.
  - Limit television viewing.
- Age: toddler
  - Nutrition information
    - Remind parents of appropriate portion sizes.
    - "Parents provide (correct portions), child decides (what to eat)"
    - Encourage structured meals and snack time with family.
    - Model desired eating behavior.
    - Address picky eating, food refusal, and grazing if problematic.
    - Discuss safe eating to prevent choking.
    - No sugar-sweetened beverages.
  - Appropriate activities
    - Encourage free play in safe indoor and outdoor environment.
    - Spare use of strollers.
    - Limit television and computer time.
    - No television or computer in the bedroom.
    - Review age-appropriate motor skill development.
- Age: preschool
  - Nutrition information
    - Parents, not children, should be deciding on food choices.
    - Limit eating out.
    - Review growth charts, with goal of keeping on the chart.
    - Help parents identify and assess all the different nutritional environments in their child's day (ie, child care, school, extended family, friends).
    - No sugar-sweetened beverages.
    - Be aware of food marketing that targets children.
    - Help parents maintain structured meals and snacks.
    - Help parents address child's behavior around demands for food if a problem.
  - Appropriate activities
    - Encourage free play.
    - Encourage outdoor play.
    - Encourage participation, not competition.
    - No more than 2 hr/day television or computer time.
    - Encourage family time that is physically active.

P

- Age: school age
  - Nutrition information
    - Check nutritional choices at school, after-school care, extra-curricular activities; may need to pack food from home.
    - Advocate for change if necessary.
    - Address weekend, vacation, and summer nutritional challenges.
    - Minimize junk food.
    - No sugared beverages.
    - Nutrition decisions are health decisions.
    - Do not bring food into the house that you do not want your child to eat.
    - Monitor after-school eating.
  - Appropriate activities
    - Balance free play and entry-level sport participation (fundamental skill development with minimal competition and flexible rules).
    - Focus on fun activities.
    - Limit television and computer time.
    - No television or computer in bedroom.
    - Do not mix television watching and eating.
    - Help child find other indoor activity options.
- Age: early adolescent
  - Nutrition information
    - Encourage family meals.
    - Discuss the importance of breakfast (breakfast skipping is common at this age).
    - Help child and family with healthy after-school snack.
    - Help child make decisions around social eating.
    - No sugar-sweetened beverages.
  - Appropriate activities
    - Help schedule physical activity around homework and social demands.
    - Encourage extracurricular activities to avoid sedentary time after school.
    - Limit television and computer time.
    - Social-skill building, if needed, can help encourage participation in peer activities.
- Age: middle adolescent
  - Nutrition information
    - Review growth chart with adolescent.
    - Help teen self-assessment eating and nutritional choices.
    - Encourage breakfast.
    - Discourage meal skipping.
    - Discuss social eating, healthy choices.
    - Limit fast food.
    - No sugared beverages.

- Appropriate activities
  - Find ways to help teen keep participating in physical activity.
  - Encourage lifestyle activities.
  - Limit television and computer time; find alternatives such as volunteering, hobbies, clubs.
- Age: late adolescent and young adult
  - Nutrition information
    - Encourage self-monitoring.
    - Discuss structure and time management of meals, activity, and sleep.
    - Go over health priorities.
    - Provide nutrition information on fast food.
    - Screen for binge eating.
  - Appropriate activities
    - Maintain activity of daily living.
    - Limit television and computer time.
    - Encourage lifestyle sports and activities.
    - Take advantage of community and school recreation facilities.

Relying on families

- Obesity prevention and treatment are family based.
  - Children's eating habits and preferences can be predicted by their mothers' behaviors.
  - Maternal preferences predict child preferences for milk type and amount, which predicts the intake of calcium and cholesterol in the child's diet.
  - Early parental behavior influences a child's eating behavior through at least 5 mechanisms:
    - Availability and accessibility of foods
    - Meal structure
    - Adult food modeling
    - Food socialization practices
    - Food-related parenting styles
- Parental modeling appears to be consistently correlated with child eating behaviors and attitudes.
  - Attempts by parents to control what children eat or to use food to control other behaviors often is not effective and may have the opposite effect from that which is desired.
  - The authoritative parenting style that sets limits in a supportive rather than punitive way has been linked with improved health outcomes and preventing obesity.
- Engaging parents and families to partner in obesity prevention and treatment is a core skill for pediatricians.
- Techniques such as motivational interviewing show promise as feasible office-based interventions.

SPECIFIC INTERVENTIONS

Assessment

■ The most current methods for preventing childhood obesity, recommended by an expert panel and endorsed by the AAP, are as follows:

■ All children should have BMI measured and weight status classified at least yearly.

  ● Children with a BMI in the 99th percentile should be identified for additional study.

■ At each well-child visit for all children:

  ● Measure height and weight.

  ● Calculate and classify BMI.

  ● Assess self-efficacy readiness to change lifestyle behaviors.

  ● Assess diet, including attention to the following behaviors that may be targets for change:

    – Frequency of eating outside the home

    – Excessive consumption of sweetened beverages, including juice

    – Consumption of excess portion sizes

    – Frequency of breakfast

    – Excessive snack-food consumption

    – Low fruit and vegetable consumption

    – Meal frequency and snack patterns and portions

  ● Assess activity, including the following:

    – Environmental support and barriers to physical activity

    – Whether child is meeting a recommendation of 60 minutes of moderate exercise every day

    – Level of sedentary behavior, including whether television and computer time is <2 hours a day in children older than 2 years as recommended

  ● Take a focused family history for obesity, type 2 diabetes, and cardiovascular disease, including hypertension and early deaths from cardiovascular disease or stroke.

  ● Assess risk for current or future obesity-related comorbidities.

  ● Perform a complete physical examination that includes pulse and blood pressure, as well as signs of obesity-related comorbidities.

  ● Order the following laboratory tests:

    – BMI in 85th–94th percentile with no risk factors

      ▪ Lipid profile

    – BMI in 85th–94th percentile with risk factors for obesity-related conditions

      ▪ Aspartate aminotransferase

      ▪ Alanine aminotransferase

      ▪ Fasting glucose

    – BMI >95th percentile

      ▪ Fasting lipid profile

      ▪ Aspartate aminotransferase

      ▪ Alanine aminotransferase

      ▪ Fasting glucose

      ▪ Blood urea and nitrogen with creatinine

Prevention of obesity

■ For children ages 2–18 years with a BMI >5th percentile and <84th percentile, counsel as follows:

  ● Diet

    – Limit sugar-sweetened beverages.

    – Encourage recommended fruits and vegetables.

  ● Activity

    – Limit television and computer time to 1–2 hours per day.

    – Allow no television or computer in bedroom.

    – Engage in moderate physical activity daily.

  ● Behavior

    – Eat breakfast daily.

    – Limit eating out.

    – Encourage family meals.

    – Limit portion sizes.

■ Actively engage families with parental obesity or maternal diabetes

  ● Child is at increased risk of developing obesity.

■ Encourage authoritative parenting style.

  ● Discourage *restrictive* parenting style.

■ Encourage parents to model:

  ● Healthy diets and portion sizes

  ● Physical activity

  ● Limited television time

■ Encourage a diet rich in calcium, high in fiber, and balanced macronutrients.

■ Limit consumption of energy-dense foods.

■ Ask parents and children about physical activity at school and child care.

Treatment of obesity

■ For children who have a BMI >85th percentile, treatment consists of 4 stages, depending on the status of the child.

■ Stage 1: Prevention Plus

  ● Goal: weight maintenance

  ● Monthly follow-up appointments

  ● Nutrition

    – ≥5 servings of fruits and vegetables per day

    – Maximum of 2 hours of television or computer time per day; no television in the bedroom

P

- 1 hour or more of physical activity daily
- No sugar-sweetened beverages
- Behavior
  - Eat breakfast daily.
  - Limit eating out.
  - Eat family meals 5–6 days a week.
  - Allow children to self-regulate eating at meals, and avoid overly restrictive behavior.
- If no improvement is seen after 3–6 months, then the physician should move to Stage 2.

■ Stage 2: Structured Weight Management Protocol
- Goal: weight maintenance that results in decreasing BMI as height increases
- Stress the following:
  - Develop a plan for use of a low-energy, dense, balanced macronutrient diet.
  - Increase structured daily meals and snacks.
  - Supervised active play at least 60 minutes a day
  - Television and computer time <1 hour per day
  - Increased monitoring of these behaviors, encouraging parents to do so as well.
  - Weight loss is not to exceed 1 pound per month in children aged 2–11 years; 2 pounds per week in children older than 11 years.
- If no improvement in BMI or weight after 3–6 months, move to Stage 3.

■ Stage 3
- Multidisciplinary intervention by an obesity care team

■ Stage 4
- Tertiary care intervention

Screening and treatment of comorbidities
■ Type 2 diabetes
- History
  - Maternal diabetes during pregnancy
  - Small for gestational age
  - Intrauterine growth restriction
  - Family history of diabetes
- Review of systems
  - Polyuria
  - Polydipsia
  - Nocturia
  - Recurrent vaginal, bladder, or other infections
  - Recent weight loss
- Physical examination
  - Acanthosis nigricans

- Laboratory assessment
  - Elevated fasting glucose
  - Glycosuria
  - Positive glucose tolerance test
  - Hyperinsulinemia

■ Nonalcoholic steatohepatitis
- History
  - No specific history; some cases have other family members affected
- Review of systems
  - Possible nausea and right upper quadrant discomfort
- Physical examination
  - Hepatomegaly
- Laboratory and imaging assessments
  - Elevated serum aminotransferases
  - Echogenicity of liver on ultrasound
- Treatment
  - Referral to pediatric gastroenterologist for evaluation and definitive diagnosis
  - Weight loss

■ Hypertension
- History
  - Family history of hypertension or other obesity-related comorbidity
- Review of systems
  - Usually asymptomatic
- Physical examination
  - Elevated systolic or diastolic blood pressure
- Laboratory assessments
  - Evaluation for other causes of hypertension as indicated
- Treatment
  - Referral to pediatric hypertension specialist
  - Dietary treatment
  - Pharmacologic treatment

■ Dyslipidemia
- History
  - Family history of lipid disorders
  - Cardiovascular disease
- Review of systems
  - Asymptomatic
  - Other obesity comorbidities, particularly signs of metabolic syndrome
- Physical examination
  - No specific signs
  - Acanthosis nigricans may indicate metabolic syndrome

- Laboratory assessment
  - Lipid panel
- Treatment
  - Referral to lipid specialist
  - Dietary management
- Sleep apnea
  - History
    - Family history of sleep apnea
  - Review of systems
    - Snoring
    - Snoring with apnea
    - Daytime tiredness
    - Napping
    - Poor concentration in school
    - Enuresis
  - Physical examination
    - Large tonsils or adenoids
  - Imaging assessment
    - Nighttime polysomnography
  - Treatment
    - Referral to pediatric pulmonologist
    - Weight loss
- Slipped capital femoral epiphysis
  - History
    - Knee or hip pain
  - Review of systems
    - Knee or hip pain
    - Limp
  - Physical examination
    - Limp
    - Knee or hip pain
  - Imaging
    - Hip and knee films
  - Treatment
    - Immediate referral to pediatric orthopedist

- Blount disease
  - History
    - Bowing of legs
  - Review of systems
    - Bowing (tibia vera)
    - Knee pain
    - Limp
  - Physical examination
    - Bowed legs
    - Knee pain
    - Limp
  - Imaging
    - Knee films
  - Treatment
    - Referral to pediatric orthopedist
- Depression
  - History
    - Family history of depression
    - History of abuse
    - Psychological trauma
    - Teasing
    - Low self-esteem
  - Review of systems
    - Loss of interest
    - Anger
    - Irritability
    - Sadness
    - Suicidal ideation
  - Physical examination
    - No signs
    - May have sad, irritable appearance with lack of self-care
  - Laboratory or imaging assessments
    - None
  - Treatment
    - Mental health referral for counseling or pharmacologic treatment

P

Prevention of Smoking

BACKGROUND

- Cigarette smoking is the leading cause of premature death in the US.
- It is categorized as a pediatric disease because it generally starts before adulthood.
- Passive smoking may be the major preventable cause of death in infants and young children.
- The evidence that passive smoking is a cause of death, disease, and disability is extensive.
  - Absorption of tobacco smoke by children is a function of the number of cigarettes smoked around the child and the proximity of the smokers.
  - A dose–response relationship has been noted between exposure and health effects.
  - Passive smoking increases the risk in children for:
    - Respiratory disease, ranging from the common cold to pneumonia and cystic fibrosis exacerbations
    - Acute and chronic otitis media
    - Difficulty with breastfeeding
    - Atopic eczema and skin infections
    - Meningitis
    - Birth defects
    - Decrease in linear growth of 1–2 cm
    - Cataracts
    - Colic
    - Febrile seizures
    - Dental caries
  - Parental smoking increases the risk that a child will become an adult active smoker.

GOALS

- National health priorities include reducing:
  - Smoking prevalence
  - Youth smoking
  - Childhood exposure to passive smoke
- Because of their regular contact with young children and their families, pediatricians and family physicians have a unique opportunity to intervene against both active and passive smoking.
  - Pediatricians must energetically support public health efforts to promote a tobacco-free environment for all children.
  - Pediatricians and family physicians are the only health care professionals who routinely come into contact with nonsmokers who are at high risk of becoming smokers (ie, preadolescents).
  - They may also be the only medical professionals in routine contact with parents of young children, given that young men and women may have few physician visits for check-ups.

GENERAL APPROACH

- Despite considerable effort, attempts to promote smoking cessation in the pediatric office setting have not been shown to be effective or practical.
- Although bupropion and nicotine-replacement therapy (gum, patch, lozenge, spray) increase quit rates with motivated adult quitters, pharmacotherapy for adolescent smokers has not demonstrated effectiveness overall.
- Reasons for unsuccessful interventions include:
  - Incomplete interventions, lacking either sufficient pharmacotherapy or the right type of counseling
  - Pediatricians' lack of formal training in cessation counseling and discomfort with the process
  - Lack of reimbursement for cessation in the pediatric setting
  - Complexities that arise when the pediatrician recommends over-the-counter pharmaceuticals for a parent rather than the patient (even though the patient is suffering from passive smoking)
- Future clinical efforts should involve:
  - Focus on motivated quitters
  - Availability of cessation experts
  - Reimbursement from medical insurance for comprehensive nicotine addiction treatment
    - Brief motivational counseling that addresses individual psychosocial barriers to successful abstinence
    - Pharmacotherapy (eg, nicotine replacement therapy for the physiological effects of nicotine withdrawal)

SPECIFIC INTERVENTIONS

Clinical interventions

- Ask about smoking.
  - Use a nonaccusatory manner.
  - Communicate that smoking is addictive and harms both the smoker and those around the smoker.
  - Indicate that help is being offered to stop the habit.
- Make informational brochures and smoking cessation programs available.
- Consider nicotine replacement therapy.
- Congratulate nonsmokers (including quitters).
- Record smoking status routinely.
- Notice red flags.
  - Visits for recurrent otitis or hospitalizations for asthma (effects of passive smoking)
  - Preteens who are poor
  - White girls with relatives or friends who smoke
    - Focusing on preadolescent girls for prevention may be the best place to break the cycle of active and passive smoking.

- Suggest steps for smoking parents who are unwilling or unable to quit:
  - Reduce exposure to passive smoking.
  - Forbid smoking inside the home.
  - If these options are not possible, smoke as far away from the child as possible.
- Refer interested parents or teens to a qualified cessation expert or a quit line.

Population-level interventions

- Interventions to increase the unit price for tobacco products
  - Reduce the number of people who start using tobacco
  - Increase the number who quit

- Mass media campaigns
  - Reduce initiation of tobacco use when combined with other actions (eg, increasing the excise tax)
  - May decrease consumption of tobacco products and increase tobacco use cessation
- Providing counseling and support to patients by telephone (as part of a multicomponent cessation strategy)
  - Increases the number of adult smokers who succeed
- Pediatricians can help with community-level efforts by connecting with their local tobacco-control coalitions.

P

Preventive Cardiology

BACKGROUND

Risk factors for heart disease and atherosclerosis

- Multiple factors should be considered when assessing a child's global risk for premature cardiovascular disease.
  - For more on general aspects of screening, see Hypertension, Heart Failure, and Congenital and Acquired Heart Disease.
- This topic addresses 3 items that should be a part of routine pediatric preventive cardiology assessment for all children and adolescents.
  - Atherosclerosis
  - Obesity
  - Smoking
- Epidemiologic evidence indicates that atherosclerosis is not an inevitable consequence of aging.
  - Rather, it is an acquired disease with well-described risk factors.
  - Evidence of emerging risk factors in children
- Atherosclerosis continues to be a leading cause of death and disability in the US.
- The known risk factors for atherosclerosis include:
  - Hypertension
  - Smoking
  - Elevated low-density lipoprotein cholesterol (LDL-C) level
  - Decreased high-density lipoprotein cholesterol (HDL-C) level
  - Diabetes mellitus
  - Advancing age
  - Male sex
  - A family history of premature heart disease
  - Hypertriglyceridemia
  - Sedentary lifestyle
  - Obesity

Hypercholesterolemia

- Hypercholesterolemia is a primary target in the prevention of atherosclerosis.
- Total cholesterol measures the cholesterol contained in several lipid particles, including:
  - LDL-C, one of the atherogenic lipoproteins; the focus of screening algorithms
  - HDL-C, considered protective against the development of coronary heart disease
  - VLDL-C, very–low-density lipoprotein cholesterol
- Both genetic and environmental factors play a role in the development of hypercholesterolemia.
  - Plasma cholesterol levels are influenced by the quantity and quality of dietary fat intake and the individual's ability to synthesize and degrade cholesterol.

- Severe or familial hypercholesterolemia secondary to a defect in the LDL receptor occurs in approximately 1 in 500 individuals.
- Children with this defect commonly have LDL-C values between 200 and 300 mg/dL.
  - This is 2–3 times higher than the acceptable limits of normal.
  - These children inherit the receptor defect and have a strong predilection for atherosclerotic heart disease as young adults.
- >600 different mutations of the LDL receptor have been described.
  - Approximately 50% of men with 1 of these mutations will have myocardial infarction by age 50 years.
  - Between 75% and 85% will have myocardial infarction by age 60 years.
- Causes of secondary hypercholesterolemia
  - Exogenous
    - Drugs
    - Corticosteroids
    - Isotretinoin (Accutane)
    - Thiazides
    - Anticonvulsants
    - ß-Blockers
    - Anabolic steroids
    - Certain oral contraceptives
    - Alcohol
    - Obesity
  - Endocrine and metabolic
    - Hypothyroidism
    - Diabetes mellitus
    - Lipodystrophy
    - Pregnancy
    - Idiopathic hypercalcemia
  - Storage diseases
    - Glycogen storage diseases
    - Sphingolipidoses
  - Obstructive liver diseases
    - Biliary atresia
    - Biliary cirrhosis
    - Alagille syndrome
  - Chronic renal diseases
    - Nephrotic syndrome
  - Others
    - Anorexia nervosa
    - Progeria
    - Collagen disease
    - Klinefelter syndrome

Obesity and physical activity

- Obesity increases the risk for heart disease through its association with abnormalities, such as:
  - Dyslipidemia
  - Hypertension
  - Insulin resistance
  - Glucose intolerance
  - There may be other undefined mechanisms.
- The magnitude of the effect of childhood obesity on cardiac risk is not precisely known.
  - The US Preventive Services Task Force concluded that evidence was insufficient to recommend for or against screening of overweight children and adolescents.
  - Body mass index (BMI)and the thickness of the subcutaneous fat as measured by a skin-fold test are correlated with the degree of coronary atherosclerosis in young adults.
- Adiposity in childhood is strongly associated with adiposity in adulthood.
- BMI is considered an appropriate measure of obesity.

Smoking

- The evidence that cigarette smoking is a risk factor for cardiovascular disease is overwhelming.
- Studies as early as 1940 documented a relationship between tobacco use and coronary artery disease.
- Tobacco use adversely affects lipid levels and is associated with:
  - Decreased exercise capacity
  - Increased platelet aggregation
  - Increased incidence of respiratory illness
  - Increased incidence of low–birth-weight deliveries
  - Increased infant mortality
- Passive smoking is linked with changes in risk factors for coronary artery disease in children.
  - Associated with reduced HDL-C in nonsmoking children, as well as those with high-risk lipid profiles
  - In 2006 the US Surgeon General issued an update on findings and recommendations to eliminate secondhand or passive smoke exposure for children.
- Adolescents are more likely than any other age group to smoke or use tobacco.
  - In 2002 the National Youth Tobacco Survey estimated that:
    - 13% of middle school students were current users of tobacco products.
    - 28% of high school students used tobacco.
  - In 2003 the National Youth Risk Behavior Survey showed a decline in reported current tobacco use among high school students.
    - The estimate was still 22%.

- The risk of smoking initiation increases from ages 12–16 years.
  - Most initiate and become addicted during this critical period.
  - Addiction can occur after smoking as few as 100 cigarettes.
  - Most youth do not become nicotine dependent until after 2–3 years of smoking.
- Children whose parents or siblings smoke are at an increased risk of beginning to smoke.
- Other factors that may predict smoking include:
  - Peer influence
  - Less-educated parents
  - Independence and rebelliousness
  - Decreased concerns about the health risks associated with smoking
- Identifying these factors and addressing them openly is helpful in counseling.

GOALS

- Identify and treat potential atherosclerotic cardiac risk factors in children.
- Providers can educate children and families on preventive strategies.
- A goal of primary care is to prevent disease and to prevent the development of risk factors in children.
  - The long-term hope is that early interventions will ultimately decrease the burden of atherosclerotic heart disease in adult life.
- The relatively new concept of primordial prevention challenges health care providers to work to prevent risk factors.
  - Address the social and environmental factors that maintain them.
  - It is particularly important to address:
    - Obesity
    - Smoking
    - Sedentary lifestyle

GENERAL APPROACH

Guidelines

- Optimal methods of heart disease prevention have generated controversy on such fundamental issues as:
  - What age to begin screening
  - Who should be screened
  - How to treat individuals with elevated cholesterol levels
- The most recent report by the US Preventive Services Task Force found good evidence that children with dyslipidemia become adults with dyslipidemia.

P

- The study concluded that the evidence was insufficient to recommend for or against screening of lipid disorders in children and adolescents.
- The pediatric National Cholesterol Education Program (NCEP) guidelines will undoubtedly be revised, as have the adult guidelines.
- A revision by the AAP in 2008 has suggested lowering the treatment age to 8 years and adding 3-hydroxy-3-methylglutaryl coenzyme A (HMG CoA) reductase inhibitors, specifically pravastatin, to the arsenal of medications.
  - This change has not been endorsed by the NCEP or American Heart Association (AHA).
  - Controversy surrounds the lack of long-term data and potential impact of 40–50 years of exposure.
- For now, pediatricians should use the basic strategy proposed by the NCEP and endorsed by the AAP and AHA.

Risk factors and screening

- Although many risk factors for heart disease remain beyond the control of the individual, some can be modified.
  - Hyperlipidemia
  - Level of physical activity
- At least 1 factor—smoking—is completely avoidable.
- Several risk factors for coronary heart disease are now easily identified during childhood.
- The process of atherosclerosis and the habits that influence the risk of heart disease begin early in life.
- Scientifically based recommendations to begin prevention in childhood have been developed.
- Schedule for integrated cardiovascular health promotion in children
  - Age 0–2 years
    - Family history
      - Early heart disease (age ≤55 years)
    - Cholesterol
      - Parent's total cholesterol ≥240 mg/dL
    - Obesity
      - Plot height and weight on growth charts.
      - Parental obesity present
    - Blood pressure (BP)
      - Family history of hypertension
    - Diet
      - Diet history
      - Early foods influence future food preferences.
    - Physical activity
      - Parent physical activity
      - Discourage television and video viewing.

  - Smoking
    - Parental or household smoking?
    - If yes, counsel to quit and refer to smoking cessation.
  - Age 2–6 years
    - Family history
      - Update family history
      - Early heart disease (age ≤55 years)
      - Parent's total cholesterol ≥240 mg/dL
    - Cholesterol
      - Fasting lipids screening
      - Total cholesterol screening
    - Obesity
      - Plot height, weight, and BMI (kg/m^2) on growth charts
      - BMI percentiles
    - BP
      - Start routine BP measurement at 3 years of age (determine if >90th or 95th percentile for sex, age, and height).
    - Diet
      - Diet history
      - Low-saturated-fat diet including 1% or nonfat milk
      - Moderate salt intake
    - Physical activity
      - Encourage active child-parent play.
      - Limit sedentary behaviors, such as television and video viewing.
    - Smoking
      - Parental or household smoking?
      - If yes, counsel to quit and refer to smoking cessation.
      - Antismoking counseling
        o Includes immediate physical, social, and physiological effects of smoking, risk of addiction, counter-arguing techniques, and resisting social and environmental pressures to smoke.
  - Age 6–10 years
    - Family history
      - Update family history
      - Early heart disease (age ≤55 years)
      - Parent's total cholesterol ≥240 mg/dL
    - Cholesterol
      - Fasting lipids screening
      - Total cholesterol screening
    - Obesity
      - Plot height, weight and BMI (kg/m^2) on growth charts
      - BMI percentiles

- BP
  - BP measurement
  - BP percentiles
- Diet
  - Diet history
  - Low-saturated-fat diet including 1% or nonfat milk
  - Moderate salt intake
- Physical activity
  - Physical activity history
  - Lifestyle and family activities
  - Limit sedentary behaviors, such as television and video viewing.
- Smoking
  - Parental/household smoking?
  - If yes, counsel to quit; referral to smoking cessation.
  - Antismoking counseling
    - o Includes immediate physical, social, and physiological effects of smoking, risk of addiction, counter-arguing techniques, and resisting social and environmental pressures to smoke.

- Age >10 years
  - Family history
    - Update family history
    - Early heart disease (age ≤55 years)
    - Parent's total cholesterol ≥240 mg/dL
  - Cholesterol
    - Fasting lipids screening
    - Total cholesterol screening
  - Obesity
    - Plot height, weight and BMI (kg/m²) on growth charts
    - BMI percentiles
  - BP
    - BP measurement
    - BP percentiles
  - Diet
    - Diet history
    - Low-saturated-fat diet including 1% or nonfat milk
    - Moderate salt intake
  - Physical activity
    - Physical activity history
    - Lifestyle and family activities
    - Daily moderate to vigorous activity
    - Limit sedentary behaviors
  - Smoking
    - Parental or household smoking?
    - Assess child smoking.

- If yes for either, counsel to quit and refer to smoking cessation
- Antismoking counseling
  - o Includes immediate physical, social, and physiological effects of smoking, risk of addiction, counter-arguing techniques, and resisting social and environmental pressures to smoke.
- The risks of smoking should be a part of routine preventive care discussions.

SPECIFIC INTERVENTIONS

NCEP recommendations

- The NCEP suggests 2 separate approaches to managing hypercholesterolemia in children.
  - A broad, population-based approach
  - An individualized patient approach
- Universal screening of all children is not recommended.

Population-based approach

- The panel suggests that all children >2 years follow the Step 1 diet.
  - No more than 30% of total calories should come from fat.
  - <10% of total calories should come from saturated fat.
  - Total cholesterol consumption should be <300 mg per day.
  - The diet should contain a variety of foods.
  - Diet should be adequate to support growth and maintain an ideal body weight for height and age.
- Characteristics of the AHA Step 1 and Step 2 diets
  - Calories: Step 1 + 2: Adequate for normal growth
  - Total fat: Step 1 + 2: ≤30% of calories
  - Saturated fat
    - Step 1: <10% of calories
    - Step 2: ≤7%
  - Polyunsaturated fat: Step 1 + 2: Up to 10% of calories
  - Monounsaturated fat: Step 1 + 2: Remainder of fat calories
  - Carbohydrates: Step 1 + 2: Approximately 55% of calories
  - Protein: Step 1 + 2: Approximately 15–20% of calories
  - Cholesterol
    - Step 1: <300 mg/dL
    - Step 2: <200 mg/dL

Individualized screening

- In addition to the population-wide diet recommendations, the NCEP guidelines suggest:
- Assessing risk and performing cholesterol testing in children:
  - >2 years of age with a positive family history
  - Who have a parent with hypercholesterolemia (total cholesterol ≥240 mg/dL)

- Whose parent or grandparent has or had premature coronary heart disease, ie, onset of disease at <56 years
- Conditions that suggest heart disease include:
  - A history of documented myocardial infarction
  - Angina pectoris
  - Peripheral vascular disease
  - Cerebrovascular disease
  - Sudden cardiac death
  - Coronary atherosclerosis as determined by angiography
  - A history of balloon angioplasty or coronary artery bypass graft surgery
- Children whose parental history is unknown or unobtainable may be screened to identify those in need of nutritional advice, especially if they have other risk factors.
- Parents with unknown cholesterol levels should be encouraged to obtain a full lipoprotein analysis.
- Cholesterol levels may need to be determined for children at higher risk for coronary heart disease independent of family history.
  - Those who smoke
  - Those who are obese
  - Those with diets rich in saturated fats and cholesterol
  - Those with diabetes mellitus
- For children with a family history of premature heart disease, guidelines suggest obtaining a fasting lipid profile that includes:
  - Total cholesterol
  - LDL-C
  - HDL-C
  - Triglycerides
- Initial screening for children with a family history of hypercholesterolemia and no history of early heart disease should be done by measuring total cholesterol only.

Risk stratification and treatment

- The AHA and AAP recently proposed a risk stratification and treatment algorithm for children at increased risk for premature coronary heart disease.
- Children identified as needing special consideration for more careful attention to cardiovascular risk factors:
  - Homozygous or heterozygous familial hypercholesterolemia
  - Diabetes mellitus (type 1 or 2)
  - Chronic kidney disease or end-stage renal disease
  - Kawasaki disease
  - Congenital heart disease
  - Chronic inflammatory disease
  - Post–cardiac transplantation
  - Cancer treatment survivors

High-risk stratification

- Tier I: High risk
  - Rationale: Exhibit coronary artery disease at <30 years of age: clinical or pathologic evidence
    - Disease process or condition
      - Homozygous familial hypercholesterolemia
      - Diabetes mellitus, type 1
      - Chronic kidney disease or end-stage renal disease
      - Postorthotopic heart transplantation
      - Kawasaki disease with current coronary aneurysms
- Tier II: Moderate risk
  - Rationale: Accelerated atherosclerosis: pathophysiologic evidence
  - Disease process or condition
    - Heterozygous familial hypercholesterolemia
    - Kawasaki disease with regressed coronary aneurysms
    - Diabetes mellitus, type 2
    - Chronic inflammatory disease
- Tier III: At risk
  - Rationale: High-risk setting for accelerated atherosclerosis: epidemiologic evidence
  - Disease process or condition
    - Cancer treatment survivors
    - Congenital heart disease
    - Kawasaki disease without detected coronary aneurysms

Algorithm for screening, with tier-specific test value cutoffs

- High-risk pediatric populations
  - Step 1: Risk stratification by disease process
  - Step 2: Assess all cardiovascular risk factors.
    - If ≥2 comorbidities exist, assign the patient to the next higher risk tier for subsequent management.
  - Step 3: Define tier-specific intervention cut points or treatment goals.
  - Step 4: Initial therapy
    - Tier I: Initial management is therapeutic lifestyle change plus disease-specific management.
    - Tiers II and III: Initial management is therapeutic lifestyle change.
  - Step 5
    - Tiers II and III: If goals are not met after initial management, consider medication.

Tiers I, II, and III treatment recommendations

- Growth and diet
  - Nutritionist evaluation and diet education for all; see Step 1 diet recommendations

- Calculate BMI percentile for sex and height.
  - Step 1, if initial BMI >95th percentile
    - Age-appropriate reduced-calorie training for child and family
    - Specific diet and weight follow-up every 2–4 weeks for 6 months; repeat BMI calculation at 6 months
    - Activity counseling
  - Step 2, if follow-up BMI is:
    - >85th percentile for tier I *or*
    - >90th percentile for tier II *or*
    - >95th percentile for tier III
    - Weight-loss program referral plus exercise training program appropriate for cardiac status
- BP (tiers I, II, and III)
  - BP measurement or interpretation for age, sex, and height
    - Step 1, if systolic BP or diastolic BP is:
      - Equal to the 90th to 95th percentile *or*
      - >120/80 mmHg on 3 separate occasions within 1 month
      - Recommend decreased calorie intake, increased activity for 6 months
  - Step 2, if initial systolic BP or diastolic BP is:
    - >95th percentile (confirmed within 1 week) or
    - 6-month follow-up systolic BP or diastolic BP is >the 95th percentile
    - Initiate pharmacologic therapy per Fourth Task Force recommendations.
- Lipids
  - Step 1, if initial LDL-C level ≥130 mg/dL (tier II) or >160 mg/dL (tier III)
    - Nutritionist training for Step 2 diet along with avoidance of trans fats for 6 months
  - Step 2, if repeat LDL-C level ≥130 mg/dL in tier II or >160 mg/dL in tier III and the child is 10 years of age
    - Initiate statin therapy with LDL-C goal of 130 mg/dL.
- Triglycerides
  - Step 1, if initial triglyceride level >150 to 400 mg/dL
    - Nutritionist training for low simple carbohydrate, low-fat diet
    - If elevated triglycerides are associated with excess weight, refer to a nutritionist for weight loss management: energy balance training plus activity recommendations.
  - Step 2, if triglyceride level >700 to 1000 mg/dL, initial or follow-up
    - Consider fibrate or niacin if the child is >10 years of age.
    - Weight loss is recommended when triglyceride elevation is associated with overweight or obesity.

- Glucose (tiers I, II, and III, except for patients with diabetes mellitus)
  - Step 1, if fasting glucose level is 100–126 mg/dL
    - Recommend a reduced-calorie diet and increased activity aimed at 5–10% decrease in weight over 6 months.
  - Step 2, if repeat fasting glucose level is 100–126 mg/dL
    - Recommend insulin-sensitizing medication as per an endocrinologist.
  - If the casual glucose is >200 mg/dL or fasting glucose level is >126 mg/dL, diabetes mellitus can be diagnosed.
    - Endocrine referral for evaluation and management
  - Maintain hemoglobin A_{1C} at <7%.
- Smoking (tiers I, II, and III)
  - Step 1: Obtain parental smoking history at every visit and child smoking history beginning at age 10 years. Provide active antismoking counseling for all; a smoke-free home is strongly recommended at each encounter.
  - Step 2: Provide smoking cessation referral for any history of cigarette smoking.
- Activity (tiers I, II, and III)
  - For children in all tiers, participation in activity is at the discretion of the physician.
  - For specific cardiac diagnoses, such as Kawasaki disease and congenital heart disease, activity guidelines are referenced.
    - Step 1: Obtain specific activity history for each child, focusing on time spent in active play and screen time (television + computer + video games).
      - ≥1 hour of active play per day
      - Screen time limited to <2 hours per day
      - Encourage activity at every encounter.
    - Step 2: After 6 months, if goals are not met, consider referral for exercise testing and recommendations from an exercise specialist.

Tier I specific treatment recommendations

- Rigorous age-appropriate education in diet, activity, and smoking cessation for all
  - Specific therapy as needed to achieve BP, LDL-C, glucose, and HbA_{1C} goals as indicated for each tier, as outlined in the algorithm (see Figure 71 on page F25)
    - Timing should be individualized for each patient and diagnosis.
  - Homozygous familial hypercholesterolemia
    - LDL management: scheduled apheresis every 1–2 weeks beginning at diagnosis to maximally lower LDL-C, plus statin and cholesterol absorption inhibitor
    - Treatment per cardiologist or lipid specialist; specific therapeutic goals for LDL-C are not meaningful with this diagnosis.

P

- Assess BMI, BP, and fasting glucose: Step 1 management for 6 months
- If tier I goals are not achieved, proceed to Step 2.
- Diabetes mellitus, type 1
  - Intensive glucose management per an endocrinologist, with frequent glucose monitoring or insulin titration to maintain plasma glucose level <200 mg/dL and HbA_{1C} <7%
  - Assess BMI and fasting lipids: Step 1 management of weight, lipids for 6 months
  - If goals are not achieved, proceed to Step 2; statin therapy if >10 years of age to achieve tier I treatment goals
  - Initial BP above the 90th percentile: Step 1 management plus no added salt, increased activity for 6 months
  - BP consistently above the 95th percentile for age, sex, and height: Initiate angiotensin-converting enzyme inhibitor therapy with BP goal to be <90th percentile or <130/80 mm Hg, whichever is lower.
- Chronic kidney disease or end-stage renal disease
  - Optimization of renal failure management with dialysis or transplantation as per nephrologist
  - Assess BMI, BP, lipids, fasting glucose: Step 1 management for 6 months
  - If goals are not achieved, proceed to Step 2; statin treatment if >10 years of age to achieve tier I treatment goals.
- After heart transplantation
  - Optimization of antirejection therapy, treatment for cytomegalovirus, routine evaluation by angiography or perfusion imaging per transplant physician
  - Assess BMI, BP, lipids, fasting glucose: initiate Step 2 therapy, including statins, immediately in all patients >1 year of age to achieve tier I treatment goals.
- Kawasaki disease with coronary aneurysms
  - Antithrombotic therapy, activity restriction, ongoing myocardial perfusion evaluation as per cardiologist
  - Assess BMI, BP, lipids, fasting glucose: Step 1 management for 6 months
  - If goals are not achieved, proceed to Step 2; statin treatment if >10 years of age to achieve tier I treatment goals.
- Most of the information regarding the risk of heart disease in adults is based on fasting LDL-C values.
  - Recommendations in children are also based on fasting LDL-C values.
  - Treatment values are based on percentile ranks of children in the US that exceed the upper norms.
    - Values >95th percentile for children and are considered *high*.
      - Total cholesterol level >200 mg/dL and LDL-C >130 mg/dL

- Values <75th percentile are considered *acceptable*.
  - Total cholesterol level <170 mg/dL and LDL-C <110 mg/dL
- Values between these limits are considered *borderline*.
- A lipid profile, including an assessment of LDL-C, should be ordered if:
  - The initial fasting total cholesterol level is high.
  - After an initial borderline value, the average of the first and second test values is >170 mg/dL.
- The final evaluation should be based on the average of at least 2 LDL-C measurements.
  - Treatment should follow the general strategy described.
  - Individualized approach: algorithm for assessing and managing hyperlipidemia based on LDL cholesterol.
    - Acceptable (LDL-C <110 mg/dL): Repeat cholesterol testing in 5 years, and advise the family to follow the Step 1 diet.
    - Borderline (LDL-C 110–129 mg/dL): Advise the family to follow the Step 1 diet, provide advice regarding other risk factors, and reevaluate the child in 1 year.
    - High (LDL-C ≥130 mg/dL): Before recommending dietary or medical treatment, obtain a history detailing the use of drugs, such as isotretinoin (Accutane), steroids, and alcohol, to identify any secondary cause of hypercholesterolemia. In addition, screen for other secondary causes of elevated cholesterol, such as liver, thyroid, and renal disease.

- The initial dietary treatment is to follow a Step 1 diet.
  - This diet is safe and efficacious for managing children with borderline to high LDL-C levels.
  - The child must consume adequate calories while decreasing fat intake.
  - Current dietary guidelines suggest that all children should consume enough calories to reach or maintain desirable weight.
  - Weight reduction in overweight and obese children is often helpful in correcting cholesterol profiles.
  - In contrast to adults, some children with hypercholesterolemia are not overweight.
    - In children who are not overweight, caloric restriction is not the primary treatment for hypercholesterolemia.
  - For children whose LDL-C level remains >130 mg/dL after at least 3 months of careful adherence to the Step 1 diet, the Step 2 diet is advised.
    - No more than approximately 30% of calories from total fat (similar to the Step 1 diet)
    - <7% of calories (compared with 10% in the Step 1 diet) from saturated fat

- Adherence to the Step 2 diet is often improved by having the family meet with a registered dietitian trained in managing hyperlipidemia in children.
- For children >10 years whose LDL-C level remains >190 mg/dL after 6–12 months of dietary therapy:
  – Consider drug treatment with bile acid–binding resins.
    ▪ Cholestyramine
    ▪ Colestipol
  – Drug therapy should also be considered for those who maintain an LDL-C level >160 mg/dL and have a family history of premature cardiovascular disease.
- Commercially available dietary products are available in supermarkets.
  – Special margarines with plant sterols and stanols to reduce LDL-C absorption
  – The 2005 AHA/AAP Dietary Recommendations caution against using these spreads
    ▪ Given the possible decrease in absorption of fat-soluble vitamins and ß-carotene
- Other medications, such as HMG CoA-reductase inhibitors (or statins), are not recommended routinely for children.
  – Except in consultation with a lipid specialist
  – For children in designated high-risk groups (see above) who are nonresponsive to diet/exercise intervention
  – A revision by the AAP in 2008 suggested lowering the treatment age to 8 years and added statins, specifically pravastatin, to the arsenal of medications. This change has not been endorsed by the NCEP or AHA. Controversy surrounds the lack of long-term data and potential impact of 40–50 years of exposure.
- The cholesterol screening and dietary treatment guidelines can be initiated safely by a primary care practitioner interested in nutrition and the prevention of heart disease.
  - Initiation includes:
    – A review of family history
    – Evaluation for secondary causes of hyperlipidemia
    – Dietary counseling
    – Identification of children with risk factors for coronary heart disease should lead to screening of other family members.
      ▪ Many risk factors tend to cluster in families.
  - Evaluation by a lipid specialist with continued general support from the primary care pediatrician is recommended.
    – When the child has severe hypercholesterolemia that is:
      ▪ Unresponsive to dietary treatment.
      ▪ From a family with early onset of heart disease

Obesity and physical activity

- A common and reasonable approach in defining obesity in children is based on the use of age and sex percentiles of body mass index.
  - BMI = kg/m^2, where body weight is measured in kilograms and height is measured in meters.
  - Children with a BMI >95th percentile are considered *obese*.
  - Those with a BMI between the 85th and 95th percentile are considered *overweight*.
  - The Centers for Disease Control and Prevention (CDC) in 2000 adopted different terms to avoid negative labeling of children.
    – *Risk of overweight* is used for children between the 85th and 95th percentile.
    – *Overweight* is used for those above the 95th percentile.
- Current recommendations from the AHA and AAP suggest that:
  - Pediatricians should feel confident in assessing and charting BMI, beginning at 2 years of age.
  - Pediatricians should counsel parents to address the at-risk child's eating and activity patterns.
- BMI can be easily calculated and charted for all children.
  - Charting materials for BMI by age and sex should be a part of every primary care pediatrician's practice.
  - Free materials from the CDC can be found online.
- Overweight children (BMI >95th percentile) should be further screened for:
  - Hypertension
  - Orthopedic symptoms
  - Hypoventilation
  - Abnormalities of lipids and glucose metabolism
- The magnitude of the abnormalities is an important consideration; additional specialty evaluations should be recommended in individual situations.
- No single treatment program for overweight children has been proven to be uniformly successful.
- A combination of diet and exercise therapy with behavioral modification and family counseling is often needed and is the first-line approach.
- AHA pediatric dietary strategies for individuals >2 years of age.
  - Balance dietary calories with physical activity to maintain normal growth.
  - Perform 60 minutes of moderate to vigorous play or physical activity daily.
  - Eat vegetables and fruits daily; limit juice intake.
  - Use vegetable oils and soft margarines low in saturated fat and trans fatty acids instead of butter or most other animal fats in the diet.

P

- Eat whole-grain breads and cereals rather than refined grain products.
- Reduce the intake of sugar-sweetened beverages and foods.
- Use nonfat (skim) or low-fat milk and dairy products daily.
- Eat more fish, especially oily fish, broiled or baked.
- Reduce salt intake, including salt from processed foods.

■ The importance of physical activity in preventing or ameliorating cardiac risk factors (obesity, hyperlipidemia, hypertension) has been increasingly recognized.

- In adults, higher levels of physical activity have been associated with decreased rates of heart disease, above and beyond changes in known cardiac risk factors.

■ Health care professionals should encourage children to make physical activity a part of their daily routine.

- A Cochrane Review found that many diet and exercise interventions improve eating behaviors and physical activity levels, but are not effective in preventing weight gain.
- Studies also suggest that children are more likely to be physically active if their parents are active.

Proteinuria

DEFINITION

- In adults, *proteinuria* is defined as a urinary protein excretion >150 mg/day.
- In children, *proteinuria* is defined as protein excretion >4 mg/m^2/hr.
  - Finding proteinuria in a single urine specimen in children and adolescents is relatively common.
  - Persistent proteinuria is called *fixed proteinuria*.

EPIDEMIOLOGY

- Prevalence
  - Generally 5–15%
- Age
  - Incidence increases with age
  - Peaks in adolescence
  - Subsequently declines, reaching nadir in adulthood
- Sex
  - For boys, peaks at age 16
  - For girls, peaks at age 13
- Postural or orthostatic proteinuria
  - Accounts for 60% of all cases of asymptomatic proteinuria in children
  - Higher incidence in adolescents
- Transient proteinuria
  - Found in as many as 30–50% of children with proteinuria
- Persistent or fixed asymptomatic proteinuria
  - Prevalence may be as high as 6% in school-aged children.

MECHANISM

- The glomerular filtration barrier, composed of podocytes and vascular endothelium separated by the glomerular basement membrane, prevents passage of macromolecules from blood into urine:
  - Based on both molecular size and electrical charge
  - Size barrier for filtration consists of pores with diameter ~40 Å in the slit diaphragm located between foot processes
    - Approximately the size of albumin (69 kDa)
  - Glomerular capillary wall contains heparan sulfate and proteoglycans:
    - Negatively charged
    - Repel macromolecules with the same electrical charge, such as albumin
- Most inflammatory glomerular diseases lead to proteinuria by:
  - Morphologic alteration of the size barrier
  - Loss of negative charges
- Glomerular hemodynamics affect protein movement across glomerular capillary walls:
  - Glomerular plasma flow rate
  - Hydrostatic forces
  - Oncotic forces
- Reduction in the number of functioning nephrons leads to proteinuria:
  - Hyperfiltration in the remaining nephrons
- Low–molecular-weight proteins (<40 kDa), such as β_2-microglobulin, retinol-binding protein, and α_1-microglobulin
  - Freely filter through the glomerulus
  - Subsequently reabsorbed by the proximal tubule
  - Tubular injury results in:
    - Inability to reabsorb these proteins
    - Their loss in the urine
- Tamm-Horsfall mucoprotein (uromodulin)
  - Major constituent of urinary casts
  - Formed by the cells of the thick ascending loop of Henle

HISTORY

- First steps in evaluating a child with proteinuria
  - Thorough history
  - Physical examination, looking for indicators of renal disease
- Basic evaluation of proteinuria
  - Presence or absence of symptoms
  - Amount of protein loss
  - Presence or absence of associated findings such as
    - Hematuria
    - Hypertension
    - Azotemia
  - Other urinary or systemic abnormalities
- Warning signs of proteinuria
  - Persistent, fixed, nonorthostatic proteinuria
  - Proteinuria associated with other urinary abnormalities, such as hematuria
  - Proteinuria associated with renal insufficiency, anemia, or hypertension
  - Family history of renal disease, deafness, or autoimmune conditions
  - Proteinuria associated with comorbidities such as:
    - Prematurity
    - Congenital anomalies of other organ systems
    - Hypertension
    - Diabetes
    - Obesity
- Postural or orthostatic proteinuria
  - Children with this type usually are asymptomatic.
    - Proteinuria usually is found on a routine urinalysis.

P

- When upright, they may spill abnormal amounts of protein in the urine.
- When supine, they have normal urinary protein excretion.
  - After they are recumbent for a few hours (asleep overnight), proteinuria decreases to normal range or disappears.
- Transient proteinuria
  - Can accompany:
    - Fever
    - Exercise
    - Stress
    - Dehydration
    - Congestive heart failure
    - Seizures
  - Usually does not exceed 2+ on the dipstick test
- Symptomatic proteinuria
  - Patients with a combination of nephritis and nephrotic syndrome pose a clinical challenge even to the most experienced nephrologist.
  - History should include questions about:
    - Recent illnesses
    - Fever
    - Rash
    - Arthralgias
    - Change in urine output and color
    - Symptoms of chronic disease
      - Weight loss
      - Fatigue
    - Duration and severity of symptoms
  - Pay attention to
    - History of urinary tract infections
    - Family history of
      - Urinary reflux
      - Hypertension
      - Deafness

PHYSICAL EXAM

- Measurements of growth parameters
- Blood pressure
- Identification of edema, ascites, and pallor

DIFFERENTIAL DIAGNOSIS

Nonpathological proteinuria

- Results from adjustment of the kidney to extraneous physiological conditions
  - Growth
  - Exercise

- Fever
- Systemic illness
- Level of proteinuria
  - Generally <1 g/day
  - Not associated with edema
- Postural or orthostatic proteinuria
  - Cause is unknown.
  - No edema, hypertension, or hematuria
  - Normal creatinine clearance and complements
- Transient proteinuria
  - Proteinuria associated with vigorous exercise rarely exceeds 2+ on dipstick test.
  - Seems related to intensity rather than duration of exercise
  - May be explained by:
    - Increased glomerular filtration barrier permeability
    - Partial inhibition of tubular reabsorption of protein
  - Effect of exercise increases with age.
  - Considered benign if proteinuria resolves after 48 hours of rest

Pathological proteinuria

Persistent or fixed asymptomatic proteinuria

- Glomerular causes
  - Nephrotic syndrome
  - Idiopathic
  - Minimal change disease
  - Mesangial proliferation
  - Focal segmented glomerulosclerosis
  - Membranous nephropathy
  - Glomerulonephritis
  - Postinfectious
  - Immunoglobulin A nephropathy
  - Systemic disease
  - Systemic lupus erythematosus
  - Vasculitis
  - Tumor
  - Subacute bacterial endocarditis
  - Infection (HIV, hepatitis)
  - Drugs or toxins
  - Obesity
- Tubular causes
  - Genetic
  - Polycystic kidney disease
  - Cystinosis
  - Wilson disease
  - Lowe syndrome
  - Galactosemia

- Renal tubular acidosis
- Interstitial nephritis
- Acute tubular necrosis
- Interstitial nephritis
- Heavy metal poisoning
- Glomerular proteinuria
  - More common of the 2 forms
  - Associated with increased permeability of glomerular filtration barrier
  - May be selective (plasma proteins with molecular weights up to and including albumin), as in minimal change disease
  - May be nonselective (albumin and large–molecular-weight proteins, such as immunoglobulin G), as in most forms of glomerulonephritis
- *Tubular proteinuria* results from decreased tubular protein reabsorption caused by tubular dysfunction.

Symptomatic proteinuria

- When defined as a nephrotic syndrome, often associated with:
  - Gravity-dependent edema
  - Hypoalbuminemia
  - Hyperlipidemia
- Some children with nephrotic-range proteinuria and hypo-albuminemia remain completely asymptomatic.
- Edema in nephrotic syndrome results from several factors acting in concert, including:
  - Increased distal nephron sodium reabsorption
  - Increased capillary permeability
  - Low plasma oncotic pressure associated with hypo-albuminemic states
- May be associated with other abnormalities, including:
  - Hematuria
  - Hypertension
  - Azotemia, as seen in glomerulonephritis

LABORATORY EVALUATION

- Diagnosis of proteinuria depends on laboratory assessment of the level of protein in the urine.
  - Presence of persistent proteinuria on repeat testing indicates renal disease until proven otherwise.
  - Presence of proteinuria should be confirmed by a urine protein/creatinine (P/Cr) ratio on a first morning urine sample.
  - Once confirmed, proteinuria should be quantified by a 24-hour urine collection for measurement of protein and creatinine to determine adequacy of the sample.

Dipstick test

- Most commonly performed urine screening method for protein

- Tetrabromophenol on the reagent strip reacts with the amino group of the protein and changes the color of the strip.
- Test reports findings as:
  - Negative
  - Trace
  - 1+ (30 mg/dL)
  - 2+ (100 mg/dL)
  - 3+ (300 mg/dL)
  - 4+ (2000 mg/dL)
- Primarily detects albumin
- Less sensitive to low–molecular-weight proteins and γ-globulins
- Result of ≥1+ in a specimen with a specific gravity of <1.015 indicates abnormal protein loss.
- False-negative results may be caused by highly dilute urine.
- False-positive results may be caused by:
  - Concentrated urine
  - Extremely alkaline urine
  - Prolonged immersion of the strip
  - Hematuria, pyuria, or bacteriuria
  - Presence of detergents and contaminating antiseptics
    - Chlorhexidine
    - Benzalkonium chloride
  - Presence of antibiotics
    - Penicillins
    - Cephalosporins
    - Sulfonamides
    - Tolbutamide
  - Presence of radiographic contrast materials
- An alternative office procedure is precipitation with sulfosalicylic acid.
  - Provides a more accurate estimate of the total urinary proteins
    - Includes those of low molecular weight
  - To prevent false-positives, should be performed on the first urine voided in the morning.
  - Results should be confirmed by urinalysis.

Timed urine sample

- Traditional and most accurate method
- Measures protein in a timed sample collected over a 24-hr period
- Patient is instructed to void right after waking in the morning and discard this first urine.
- All subsequent urines are collected.
- Last sample added to the collection should be 24 hr after the first sample.

P

- In adults, a protein excretion of <150 mg in 24 hr is considered normal.
- In children, excretion rates are categorized as:
  - Normal: <4 mg/m^2/hr
  - Abnormal: 4–40 mg/m^2/hr
  - Nephrotic-range proteinuria: >40 mg/m^2/hr
- Sample adequacy can be determined by measuring the creatinine excretion in the sample.
- Steady-state daily creatinine excretion is:
  - 20 mg/kg/day in children 1–12 years of age
  - 22–25 mg/kg in older children
- Weaknesses of this method
  - Cumbersome
  - Can be impractical in children
  - Frequent errors from under- and over-collection

Urine protein-creatinine ratio

- Measurement of the P/Cr ratio in an untimed (spot) urine sample
- Reliable for classification of proteinuria
- Easier than 24-hr urine collection
- Studies in adults and children have shown strong correlation between untimed urine P/Cr ratio and 24-hr urine collection.
  - Nephrotic-range proteinuria: ratio >3.5:1
  - Normal
    - Ratio <0.2:1 in patients ages ≥2 yr
    - Ratio <0.5:1 in children aged 6–24 months

Postural or orthostatic proteinuria

- Children with low-grade asymptomatic proteinuria should be assessed.
- Orthostatic test for postural proteinuria includes 2 separate collections:
  - Supine position
  - Upright position
- At bedtime, the child goes to bed without voiding.
- 30 minutes later the child is asked to void.
- Urine is discarded and time is noted as the start of the collection in supine position.
- Child is then given a large glass of water or another fluid and allowed to sleep.
- All urine passed during the night, including the first specimen voided the next morning, is collected in a jar (specimen 1)
  - Time of the first morning voiding is recorded.
- Child goes about daily activities.
- All urine is collected in a second jar (specimen 2) for approximately the next 12 hr.
- This collection is the upright collection and ends at bedtime when time is again recorded.

- In patients with orthostatic proteinuria
  - Sample obtained in the supine position will be free of protein or will contain a normal amount of protein.
  - Sample obtained in upright position will contain an abnormal amount of protein.
- Children with orthostatic proteinuria generally excrete <1 g of protein in 24 hr.
- Diagnosis of postural proteinuria can be made by assessing first morning urine.
  - Presumptive diagnosis of orthostatic proteinuria can be made if sample has:
    - No protein
    - P/Cr ratio <0.2:1

Persistent or fixed asymptomatic proteinuria

- Patients with a positive dipstick test (≥1+) should undergo a more accurate test.
  - P/Cr ratio
  - Quantitative measurement of protein excretion
- Orthostatic proteinuria should be excluded by repeat measurements on a first morning void.
- In the absence of other abnormalities, patients are diagnosed as having *fixed proteinuria* with
  - ≥2 positive semiquantitative or quantitative tests, 1–2 weeks apart

Other tests

- Level of kidney function can be determined by
  - Serum electrolytes
  - Blood urea nitrogen
  - Creatinine
- Determination of the severity of metabolic changes that occur as a result of urine protein loss guided by
  - Serum albumin
  - Cholesterol
  - Triglycerides
- Based on the child's history, the following testing may be indicated:
  - Complement levels
  - Anti–streptolysin O titers
  - Hepatitis serologic testing
  - HIV testing
- Children should be routinely screened by a standard dipstick test on 2 occasions:
  - Before starting school
  - In early adolescence
- Subsequent testing should be performed as needed.

P

- Assessment of total protein is appropriate in children to identify both albuminuria and low–molecular-weight proteinuria.
  - Under most circumstances, spot urine samples should be used to detect and monitor proteinuria in children.
  - Obtaining 24-hr timed urine collections usually is unnecessary.
  - First morning specimens are preferred.
  - Random specimens are acceptable if a first morning sample is unavailable.
  - Patients with a positive dipstick test of ≥1+ should undergo confirmation by assessment of the P/Cr ratio within 3 months.

IMAGING

- Renal ultrasound
  - Normal in postural or orthostatic proteinuria, but not usually performed in the evaluation process
  - Should be performed when structural abnormalities are a possibility

DIAGNOSTIC PROCEDURES

- Indications for renal biopsy
  - Fixed, asymptomatic, isolated proteinuria >1 g/day
  - Persistent proteinuria <1 g/day *plus*:
    - Hematuria and casts
    - Renal insufficiency
    - Low complement levels
    - Hypertension
    - Systemic symptoms such as recurrent rashes, joint pains, or fever
    - Family history of kidney disease or autoimmune disease
  - Corticosteroid-resistant nephrotic syndrome

TREATMENT APPROACH

- Medications that reduce proteinuria may provide important long-term benefits for patients with chronic kidney disease.

SPECIFIC TREATMENT

- Orthostatic proteinuria
  - Child should be monitored with annual office visits and check of urine P/Cr ratio.
- Isolated fixed proteinuria <1 g/day detected (urine P/Cr ratio <1:1)
  - Twice-yearly visits with determination of urine P/Cr ratio are sufficient.
  - Patient should be assessed for hematuria and hypertension.
  - Restrictions on lifestyle and physical activity are not necessary.
  - Children should receive the recommended daily allowance of protein for their age.

- If proteinuria persists for >1 yr, renal biopsy should be considered.

WHEN TO REFER

- Patient should be referred to a pediatric nephrologist if any abnormalities are found during the initial workup.
- Other indicators
  - Persistent, fixed, nonorthostatic proteinuria
  - Proteinuria associated with other urinary abnormalities, such as hematuria
  - Proteinuria associated with renal insufficiency, anemia, or hypertension
  - Family history of renal disease, deafness, or autoimmune condition
  - Proteinuria associated with comorbidities such as:
    - Prematurity
    - Congenital anomalies of other organ systems
    - Hypertension
    - Diabetes
    - Obesity

WHEN TO ADMIT

- Anasarca
- Proteinuria associated with significant renal insufficiency
- Proteinuria associated with significant hypertension

FOLLOW-UP

- Postural or orthostatic proteinuria
  - Long-term follow-up studies in adults have documented the benign nature of orthostatic proteinuria.
  - Rare cases of glomerulosclerosis have been identified later in life in patients who initially were found to have proteinuria with an orthostatic component.
    - Long-term follow-up of children is necessary if the proteinuria does not resolve.
    - Signs to anticipate include:
      - Appearance of hematuria
      - Hypertension
      - Increase in serum creatinine concentration
      - Proteinuria >1 g/day

COMPLICATIONS

- Proteinuria may indicate:
  - Renal injury
  - Progressive renal disease
- Proteinuria is an established independent risk factor for cardiovascular disease.
  - Large losses of protein through the urine lead to hypercholesterolemia and hypertriglyceridemia.

P

Pruritus

DEFINITION

- Pruritus, or itch, is the subjective perception of a cutaneous disturbance that is relieved by scratching or rubbing.
- Usually not brought to the primary care physician's attention unless it is generalized, chronic, or associated with an eruption.
  - In such instances, pruritus must be treated with great respect.
    - Severe itching can be physically incapacitating.

MECHANISM

- Because itch is a subjective sensation, objective evaluation to delineate its pathophysiologic characteristics has been difficult.
- Current thinking implicates nonspecific itch receptors.
  - Thought to be free, fine nerve endings at the dermoepidermal junction
  - The exact mediators and their release triggers are unknown.
- Experimental triggers that have produced itch include:
  - Mast cell histamine
  - Physical pressure
  - Heat
  - Electric shock
- Researchers believe that nerve impulses from the intra-epithelial mechanoinsensitive C fibers:
  - Ascend to the lamina I in the dorsal horn of the spinal cord
  - Travel along the contralateral spinothalamic tract to the thalamus
  - Are then transferred to multiple areas of the cortex
  - Are interpreted as itch
- Subsequent desire to scratch arises in the motor cortex.
- Area 3a in the sensorimotor cortex and the anterior cingulate cortex have been identified as activated when histamine-induced itch and scratch are traced.
- Itch is not a mild form of pain.
  - The pathways are different.
  - Aspirin alone does not relieve itch.

HISTORY

- Most common cutaneous diseases associated with generalized pruritus can be diagnosed based on history and physical examination.
- The answers to the following questions may help diagnose infestation:
  - Are any individual pruritic papules found with a central punctum?
  - Are they on exposed or nonexposed areas?
  - Does anyone else in the family have similar lesions?

- Atopic dermatitis
  - Family history of allergy, asthma, or eczema in a child
  - Chronic eczematous dermatitis over:
    - Extensor surfaces in infancy
    - Flexural areas in childhood
- Acute urticaria
  - Usually from exposure to a drug or other ingestant
  - Cause of contact allergic dermatitis or contact irritant dermatitis may be revealed through thorough history and environmental sleuthing.
  - The cause of 90% of acute urticaria cases remains unknown.
- Certain circumstances alter interpretation: eg, the itch threshold in and around areas of active dermatitis, can be lowered with:
  - Psychic stress
  - Decreased skin hydration
  - Increased skin temperature
  - Night time

PHYSICAL EXAM

- Contact dermatitis
  - Recognizable because of a linear array of:
    - Papulovesicular erythematous lesions
    - Sharp borders that conform to the shape of the contactant
- Acute urticaria
  - Produces intensely pruritic, erythematous, and edematous plaques and papules

DIFFERENTIAL DIAGNOSIS

- In children, generalized pruritus is more commonly associated with local cutaneous disease than systemic disease.
- The major differential diagnoses of generalized pruritus with skin lesions in children are:
  - Infestation
    - Scabies
    - Pediculosis
    - Insect bites
  - Atopic dermatitis
  - Miliaria
  - Contact dermatitis
  - Acute or chronic urticaria
- Children may itch with cutaneous diseases, such as:
  - Psoriasis
  - Lichen planus
  - Linear IgA bullous disease of childhood

- The child who has pruritus, from whatever cause, is at risk for:
  - Psychological damage
  - Infection secondary to impetiginization
  - Scarification
- Systemic causes of pruritus in the child who has pruritus but no skin lesions are:
  - Hyperthyroidism and hypothyroidism
  - Leukemia or lymphoma
  - Chronic renal failure
  - Obstructive biliary disease
  - Xerosis (generalized dry skin)

LABORATORY EVALUATION

- For the child who has pruritus with no primary skin disorder assess for possible systemic causes
  - Complete blood count with differential
  - Urinalysis
  - Complete chemistry panel
  - Thyroid-stimulating hormone test
- With urticaria, if the patient has not used any new drug or food, and if the hives persist despite regular use of antihistamines for several days, rule out occult streptococcal, mycoplasmal, and viral infections by performing:
  - Throat culture and a complete blood count with differential
  - Screens for mycoplasmal disease and infectious mononucleosis

IMAGING

- Chest radiography for the child with pruritus and no primary skin disorder

DIAGNOSTIC PROCEDURES

- Skin biopsy, in rare instances of undiagnosed but persistent lesions

TREATMENT APPROACH

- To relieve itching and prevent scarring (both mental and physical), the scratch-itch cycle must be broken.
  - Itching provokes scratching.
  - When the scratching stops, the itching returns.
- To control itching, the following steps can be helpful:
  - Keep fingernails short to prevent damage from scratching.
  - Keep the child fully clothed except when applying medications.
  - Apply bland emollient creams frequently, especially after bathing.
  - Apply cool compresses to relieve intense pruritus and to remove crusts and debris.

- Apply topical steroids for short periods (generally <2 weeks) to control inflammation.
- Increase the dose of antihistamine until the scratching stops or marked drowsiness occurs.
  - Then reduce the dose to a level that controls scratching but does not cause drowsiness.
- Advise the family to avoid stress, heat, and irritants.
- See the patient frequently to provide support.
- If the child is old enough to understand, explain why these methods are being used.

SPECIFIC TREATMENT

Atopic dermatitis

- Hydration and emollients are the mainstay of therapy.
- Mid- and low-potency topical steroids for inflammation
- Antibiotics for secondary infection
- Cool compresses to bring the scratch-itch cycle under control
- Topical immunomodulators (tacrolimus and pimecrolimus)
  - Short courses (<8 weeks) may be helpful in relieving atopic itch on:
    - Facial skin
    - Thin areas, such as the axillae
  - These medications should not be prescribed for long-term therapy.
- Antihistamine in a tolerable (nonsoporific) dose may relieve itch.
  - Should be given approximately 1 hour before bedtime
    - The itch threshold is lower at night.
  - Hydroxyzine seems to be the most effective agent.
  - Data about the use of nonsedating antihistamines for controlling itch are not consistent.

Heat rash

- Pinpoint crystalline or erythematous papules in areas of occlusion and sweating (miliaria crystallina and miliaria rubra)
  - Controlled by simple measures, such as:
    - Dusting powders
    - Avoidance of tight clothing
    - Reduced exposure to high ambient temperatures

Contact dermatitis

- For use of antihistamines, topical steroids, and compresses, see Atopic Dermatitis.

Topical capsaicin and pramoxine

- May be indicated for localized use in some cases
- Potential for systemic absorption limits prolonged or widespread use.

P

Ultraviolet B light therapy

- May be helpful for generalized pruritus, such as occurs in:
  - Biliary cirrhosis
  - Severe chronic atopic dermatitis

WHEN TO REFER

- Pruritus with uncommon disease (eg, psoriasis, bullae)
- Chronic pruritus without cutaneous disease (to evaluate for systemic cause)
- Pruritus uncontrolled by usual topical steroids and antihistamines

COMPLICATIONS

- Scratching or rubbing can:
  - Produce extensive disfigurement
    - Linear excoriations
    - Lichenified plaques
  - Predispose the patient to cutaneous infections
  - Cause social isolation
    - The child may be viewed as being contagious or unclean.

P

Psoriasis

DEFINITION

- T cell–mediated chronic inflammatory disease, clinically characterized by well-demarcated, erythematous plaques with overlying silvery-white scale
- *Plaque-type psoriasis*
  - Most common type
  - Scalp, elbows, knees, and lumbosacral regions are the most commonly affected areas, often with bilateral symmetry.
  - Scalp is the most frequently involved site in children.
  - Facial psoriatic lesions, especially around the eyes, are more common in affected children and may be the only involved site.

EPIDEMIOLOGY

- Incidence
  - Unknown, but common among children
- Age
  - 10% of affected children experience onset of disease before age 10 years and 2% before the age of 2 years
  - Can occur during infancy
- Gender
  - Female-male ratio approaching 2:1, although this finding is controversial
- Race
  - Childhood-onset psoriasis occurs more frequently in the white population compared with the black, Asian, and Native-American populations.
- Psoriatic arthritis
  - Rare in children
  - Most severe form, arthritis mutilans, very rare in children

ETIOLOGY

- Both genetic and environmental factors play a role.
- Associated with a family history of psoriasis in 1st-degree relatives, as well as with certain human leukocyte antigen (HLA) subtypes such as HLA-Cw6, -A3, -Cw1, -DR-7, and -DR-8
  - Chromosome 6, the site of HLA I and II complexes, is thought to carry a gene important in determining genetic susceptibility to psoriasis.
- Environmental triggers that likely precipitate or exacerbate childhood psoriasis
  - Streptococcal infections
  - Upper respiratory infections
  - Trauma
  - Psychological stress

SIGNS AND SYMPTOMS

- Plaque psoriasis
  - Large erythematous plaques with overlying silvery-white or grayish scale
    - Scalp
    - Face
    - Elbows
    - Knees
    - Lumbosacral area gluteal cleft
    - Umbilicus
- Inverse psoriasis
  - Bright-red glazed erythema with no scale
    - Diaper area
    - Axillae
    - Groin
    - Postauricular area
- Pustular psoriasis
  - Widespread bright red erythema studded with 1- to 2-mm pustules
  - Deep-seated 2- to 4-mm pustules in areas of erythema and scaling
  - Widespread, especially in:
    - Flexural areas
    - Genitals
    - Finger web spaces
    - Palms
    - Soles
- Erythrodermic psoriasis
  - Bright red erythema with massive exfoliation
  - Widespread
- Guttate psoriasis
  - Can be the first manifestation of psoriasis
  - Characteristics of lesions
    - 2–10 mm
    - Widespread
    - Symmetrically distributed
    - Round or oval erythematous papules and plaques with silvery-white scale
    - Often have a predilection for the trunk and proximal extremities
- Nail involvement, common with psoriasis
  - Nail pitting (most characteristic finding)—multiple, small, irregularly spaced depressions in the nail plate
  - Other nail findings
    - Discoloration
    - Onycholysis (separation of the nail from the nail bed)

- Longitudinal striations
- Subungual hyperkeratosis
- Presentation of psoriatic arthritis in children
  - Similar to that seen in rheumatoid arthritis, but with no rheumatoid factor or systemic symptoms
  - Bluish discoloration over affected joints
  - Preferentially affects the distal interphalangeal and proximal interphalangeal joints of the hands and feet but also can affect the knees and ankles

DIFFERENTIAL DIAGNOSIS

- Psoriatic diaper rash and other forms of inverse psoriasis
  - Seborrheic dermatitis
  - Langerhans cell histiocytosis
  - Candidal intertrigo
  - Contact dermatitis
- Plaque psoriasis—must be differentiated from other papulosquamous disorders
  - Atopic dermatitis (AD)
    - Psoriatic plaques tend to be more clearly demarcated from surrounding uninvolved skin and usually are less pruritic than AD lesions.
    - AD lesions lack the characteristic silvery-white scale of psoriasis.
    - Psoriasis tends to localize to the extensors, whereas AD preferentially affects flexural areas.
    - Some children exhibit overlap between psoriasis and AD.
  - Pityriasis rubra pilaris
    - Lesions have a classic salmon color.
    - Focal areas of sparing
    - Follicular accentuation
- Pustular psoriasis
  - May be confused with disseminated candidiasis or staphylococcal scalded-skin syndrome.
  - To differentiate:
    - Skin biopsy
    - Gram stain
    - Culture of the contents of several pustules
  - Noninfectious pustular eruptions, such as pustular drug eruptions, may also mimic pustular psoriasis.
  - The history of a recently started medication and a skin biopsy can sometimes help differentiate between pustular psoriasis and a pustular drug eruption.

- Scalp psoriasis
  - May be mistaken for tinea capitis or seborrheic dermatitis
  - Potassium hydroxide preparation and a fungal culture of the scale is important to rule out tinea capitis because the treatment for scalp psoriasis (topical corticosteroids) can exacerbate tinea capitis.
- Guttate psoriasis
  - Pityriasis rosea
  - Pityriasis lichenoides
- Nail changes of psoriasis can be seen in other conditions:
  - Alopecia areata
  - Onychomycosis

DIAGNOSTIC APPROACH

- Issues to investigate when evaluating a child for suspected psoriasis
  - Family history of psoriasis
  - Recent history of streptococcal throat or perianal infection
  - Frequency and duration of eruptions
  - Koebner phenomenon
    - Tendency for lesions to appear on traumatized skin (eg, sunburned, scratched, tattooed)
  - Nail changes (eg, nail pitting)
    - Evaluation for characteristic nail changes can help lead to the diagnosis when it is otherwise not apparent.
  - Behavior of lesions in response to sunlight or tanning bed
  - Joint pains
  - Previous treatment modalities and their efficacy

LABORATORY FINDINGS

- Bacterial culture of oropharynx and perianal area; antistreptolysin titer
  - Rules out streptococcal infection, especially in guttate psoriasis
- Potassium hydroxide preparation of scale
  - Rules out fungal infection, especially in scalp psoriasis and annular lesions

DIAGNOSTIC PROCEDURES

- Skin biopsy
  - Confirm clinical diagnosis of psoriasis, especially in atypical presentations

TREATMENT APPROACH

- Psychosocial impact of the disease on the child and the child's family is a critical consideration.
  - Adverse effect on quality of life
  - Educate the child, siblings, and parents, as well as teachers and classmates, about the nature of psoriasis.

- Give affected families information about available psoriasis support groups.
- Psychological counseling should be sought to equip patients with effective coping skills.

■ Identify and eliminate potential triggers/exacerbating factors:
- Streptococcal infection
- Medications
  - Lithium
  - ß-Blockers
  - Interferon
  - Systemic corticosteroids
- Stress
- Skin trauma (piercings, sunburn)

■ Topical corticosteroids are most common treatment.

■ Less commonly used topical therapies
- Salicylic acid
- Topical retinoids
- Topical calcineurin inhibitors

■ Bland emollients are an essential part of the skin care regimen.
- Moisturization and application of emollients lessens the dryness and scaling associated with psoriasis.
- In some cases, emollients alone may be sufficient to improve mild psoriasis.
- In most patients, emollients should be used as adjunctive therapy to antiinflammatory topical medications.

■ Oral retinoids, such as acitretin, should be 1st-line systemic agent for severe, recalcitrant cases of childhood psoriasis.

SPECIFIC TREATMENTS

Topical agents

■ Emollients
- Petroleum jelly
- Aquaphor
- Theraplex emollient

■ Corticosteroids by class
- Class 1 (ultrapotent)
  - Clobetasol propionate 0.05%
  - Betamethasone dipropionate 0.05%
  - Reserved for unresponsive, thick psoriatic plaques
  - Continuous treatment should not last >2 weeks.
- Class 2 and 3 (medium to high potency)
  - Fluocinonide 0.05%
  - Betamethasone valerate 0.1%
  - Triamcinolone ointment 0.1%

- Class 4/5 (medium potency)
  - Hydrocortisone valerate 0.2%
  - Mometasone cream
- Class 6/7 (low potency)
  - Hydrocortisone (all concentrations)
    ■ Hydrocortisone 2.5% can be used for facial psoriasis, but is ineffective in many children.
  - Desonide 0.05%
- Side effects of corticosteroids
  - Possible cutaneous side effects: atrophy, striae, telangiectasia
  - Possible systemic side effects: hypothalamic-pituitary-adrenal axis suppression, growth impairment, cataracts, glaucoma
  - Avoid use of high-potency preparations on face and intertriginous areas.
- Ointment is the preferred vehicle when treating psoriasis:
  - Occlusive effect
  - Increased potency
  - Useful for dry, scaly lesions
- Gels
  - Readily absorbed
  - Useful in hairy areas
  - Can cause dryness and irritation
- Creams
  - Rub in well
  - Are aesthetically pleasing
  - May be less potent than ointment form of same drug
- Foams, solutions, and oils can be used in the scalp.

■ Calcipotriol (Dovonex)
- Can be used twice a day
  - As monotherapy in limited disease
  - As an adjunct to topical corticosteroids in more severe disease
- Ointment form
  - Suitable for use on any affected area
  - More likely to cause burning and irritation on the face or groin
- Available in liquid form for use on the scalp
- Causes irritation

■ Coal tar preparations
- Liquor carbonis detergens in combination with emollients or corticosteroids
- Liquid form in bath

P

- Side effects
  - Irritation, staining, unpleasant odor, folliculitis
  - Increased risk of irritation on face and intertriginous areas
- Anthralin (for stubborn plaques)
  - Anthralin 1% is applied for 5 minutes, with increasing contact time with subsequent treatments as tolerated.
  - Causes irritation and staining of skin, bathtub/sink
- Calcineurin inhibitors
  - Tacrolimus ointment (Protopic) 0.03% or 0.1%
  - Pimecrolimus cream (Elidel) 1%
  - Side effects
    - Occasional burning or itching with first few applications
    - US Food and Drug Administration black-box warning (theoretical malignancy risk based on oral forms)
- Retinoids
  - Tazarotene cream or gel (Tazorac)
  - Issues
    - No data on efficacy in children
    - Dryness, local irritation
    - Pregnancy category X
- Topical application of oils
  - Nighttime application, such as Derma-Smoothe Oil (fluocinolone), or nonsteroid oils, such as olive, mineral, or soybean oil, can be a useful adjunct in treating scalp psoriasis in older children.
  - Can be applied to the scalp at night to loosen adherent scale and then shampooed out in the morning
  - Some black patients prefer oilier scalp preparations, such as lotions, ointments, or oils, rather than the foams or gels, because the former preparations also lubricate the hair and prevent brittleness and breakage.
- For scalp lesions
  - Liquid or foam corticosteroid preparations (may cause stinging)
    - Clobetasol foam
    - Clobetasol solution
    - Fluocinonide solution
  - Corticosteroid, tar, zinc, or salicylic acid shampoos
    - Clobex shampoo (clobetasol)
    - T-Sal shampoo
  - Parents should be warned that these might cause dryness of the hair and scalp.

Phototherapy
- Psoralen plus ultraviolet A
  - Should not be used in preadolescent children
  - Issues
    - Cataracts
    - Skin aging
    - Skin cancer
    - Expensive
    - Inconvenient
- Ultraviolet B (UVB)
  - Narrow-band UVB (311–313 nm) can clear plaques with lower amounts of UV light
  - Issues
    - Temporary erythema
    - Expensive
    - Inconvenient
    - Skin aging
    - Skin cancer
    - Very difficult for younger patients

Systemic agents
- Methotrexate
  - Indications
    - Recalcitrant widespread psoriasis
    - Erythrodermic psoriasis
    - Pustular psoriasis
    - Psoriatic arthritis
  - Side effects
    - Bone marrow toxicity
    - Hepatotoxicity
    - Nausea
    - Vomiting
    - Must monitor patient's complete blood count and liver function tests
      - Liver biopsy often performed after a cumulative dose of 1.5–2 g.
- Cyclosporine
  - Indications
    - Recalcitrant widespread psoriasis
    - Erythrodermic psoriasis
    - Pustular psoriasis
  - Side effects
    - Renal and hepatic toxicity
    - Hypertension
    - Hypertrichosis
    - Immunosuppression

- Oral retinoids
  - Indications
    - Erythrodermic psoriasis
    - Pustular psoriasis
  - Side effects
    - Cheilitis
    - Xerosis
    - Skin fragility
    - Hypertriglyceridemia
    - Skeletal abnormalities
    - Teratogenicity (avoid in adolescent girls)
- Systemic retinoids
  - Children with generalized pustular psoriasis have been successfully treated with etretinate.
  - Side effects
    - Pruritus
    - Cheilitis
    - Skin fragility
    - If chronic use
      - Ossification of interosseous ligaments and tendons
      - Skeletal hyperostosis
      - Premature epiphyseal closure (may affect growth)
- Etanercept
  - Indications
    - Severe generalized, recalcitrant psoriasis in older children
    - Psoriatic arthritis
  - Side effects
    - Injection site reactions
    - Live vaccination should be avoided
    - Caution if congestive heart failure, multiple sclerosis, tuberculosis risk factors

WHEN TO ADMIT
- Widespread pustular psoriasis
- Erythrodermic psoriasis

WHEN TO REFER
- Unresponsive to 1st- or 2nd-line therapy
- Widespread disease
- Pustular psoriasis
- Erythrodermic psoriasis
- Worsening joint pains (refer to rheumatologist)

COMPLICATIONS
- Possible complications of erythrodermic psoriasis include:
  - Electrolyte imbalances
  - Cardiovascular compromise
  - Sepsis
  - Considered a dermatologic emergency

P

Psychosocial Screening

BACKGROUND

- 5–20% of US children have significant functional impairments and psychiatric disorders.
  - Defined by the 4th edition of *Diagnostic Statistical Manual of Mental Disorders* (*DSM-IV*) and the text revision edition (*DSM-IV-TR*)
  - The majority of cases are not detected by primary care physicians because of:
    - Time limitations at visit
    - Hesitancy among practitioners to attach labels that may stigmatize
    - Absence of widely available and easily implemented screening procedures
    - Lack of adequate training on psychiatric issues
    - Limited resources for referral and treatment, eg, insurance barriers
- A significant number of children and adolescents consider suicide.
- Psychiatric diagnoses do not always take into account important developmental and functional assessments.
- Psychosocial dysfunction can be grouped into 3 main categories:
  - Normal variation
    - Allows for different temperaments, personalities, and developmental paths among healthy children
  - Problems
    - A range of issues that may not meet formal criteria for a psychiatric disorder (eg, anxious reaction to divorce)
  - Disorders
    - Specific conditions that meet the *DSM-IV* criteria
- Psychosocial issues have multiple secondary consequences.
  - Risk factor for unintentional injuries (common cause of death)
    - Fires, falls from windows, drowning, and car accidents are more common among children with psychosocial stressors.
  - School failure
  - Family conflict
  - Juvenile justice interaction

GOALS

- To provide screening methods in harmony with primary care for early, efficient, and effective recognition of developing psychosocial problems.
  - Problems are recognized:
    - Through parental complaints of overt behavioral problems
    - Through school referral
    - In the primary care setting
      - In this setting, less obvious dysfunction is often identified (eg, dysfunction stemming from divorce or depression)
- Built-in screening tests can be initiated according to age and risk factors.
  - For example, family history of attention-deficit/hyperactivity disorder (ADHD) or a cluster of positive answers to school dysfunction questions may elicit an ADHD screening questionnaire.

GENERAL APPROACH

- Psychosocial challenges are heterogeneous.
- The average primary care visit is limited in time but includes increasing psychosocial demands.
- Pediatricians should broadly screen for psychosocial dysfunction rather than focusing on psychiatric diagnoses.
  - They should play an active role in detection and treatment of psychosocial problems through routine screening practices with structured instruments.
  - General psychosocial screening increases the referral rate from 1–2% to 4%.
- Once information from assessments is gathered, the presenting symptom should be categorized as:
  - Needs no further action
  - Requires intervention
- Innovative practices may be able to provide adequate treatment despite current health care insurance limits on intervention.
- Many issues can be addressed by primary care with comanagement by mental health professionals or school personnel.
- Some pediatricians have mental health professionals in their practices to provide follow-up, consultation, and ongoing services.
- An office social worker can provide referral services.
  - Provide family and group treatment in the pediatric office setting
  - Provide:
    - Preventive measures in cases of recent divorce or other risks
    - Support for parents raising children with ADHD
    - Treatment for adolescents using substances or dealing with depression, if trained
- More serious problems require:
  - Outside referral for evaluation by a specialist
  - Possibly, ongoing treatment
- The most severe cases often require emergency referral.

SPECIFIC INTERVENTIONS

Interviewing patients

- Pay careful attention to developmental aspects of the child's environment.
  - Family
  - Friends
  - School
  - Play
  - Mood
- Face-to-face interviewing, in which high-risk issues are discussed with the patient and parents, offers many advantages.
- At intake, ask parents for a family history of psychiatric disorder (eg, depression, substance use).
  - Factors in the family that put a child at risk
    - Depression
    - Anxiety
    - Substance use
    - ADHD
- At annual visits, ask about parental discord and marital stability.
- For newborns, assess:
  - Parental coping
  - Family support
  - Maternal depression
    - Has profound emotional and cognitive impact on infant
    - Treatment can greatly help the entire family.
- For toddlers, ask about autonomy and the ability to separate.
- For early school-age children, ask about social functioning.
- For adolescents
  - Ask parents about the teen's autonomy.
  - Ask the adolescent about mood and substance use.

Screening tools

- Parent questionnaires
  - Achenbach Child Behavior Checklist
    - Most studied and best validated instrument
    - Requires approximately 20 minutes
  - Pediatric Symptom Checklist (PSC)
    - A less cumbersome alternative
    - Takes 3–5 minutes
    - Parents can complete the checklist in the waiting room and have it scored by the receptionist or clinical assistant.
    - Pediatrician can quickly recognize and evaluate significant issues.
    - Hampered by parents' limitations in correctly assessing their child's intrapsychic state

  - Strength and Difficulties Questionnaire
    - Assesses specifically for emotional difficulties
    - Completed by parents and teachers of children age 4–16 years
    - Similar to the PSC but is perhaps slightly more complicated to score
- Patient questionnaires
  - Human Figure Drawing Screening Device
    - For young children
    - Detects occult anxiety and depression
  - Teenscreen (paper or computer) for depression and suicidality
  - Beck Depression Inventory
    - $\geq 20\%$ of teenagers have scores that raise concerns.
- Specific screening for Asperger syndrome or autism (young children only)
  - Modified Checklist for Autism in Toddlers
  - Parents Evaluation of Developmental Status

Assessing severity of dysfunction

- Symptoms
  - Number
  - Frequency
  - Duration
  - Places where experienced
- Functioning
  - Family
  - Friends
  - School
  - Activities
  - Self-esteem
- Burden of suffering
  - Intensity
  - Duration
  - Limitations on family activities
  - Danger to self and others
  - Intrusion into developmental tasks or daily activities

Risk factors

- Risk factors for psychosocial problems include:
  - Poor health or chronic medical conditions of child
  - Impaired parenting
  - Poverty
  - Unsafe or inadequate home environment
- See table Children's Well-being: Risk and Protective Factors.

P

Children's Well-being: Risk and Protective Factors

	Protective Factors That Decrease the Impact of Stress	Risks Factors That Increase the Impact of Stress
Health	Good health	Chronic disease, ill health
Temperament	Example: pleasant mood	Example: negative mood, irritable
Cognitive status	Normal IQ (particularly verbal)	Learning disability or low IQ
Emotional health	Good mental health function	Preexisting emotional disorder
Sociability	Good peer relations	Poor peer relations
Child reaction to stress	Perceives stress as limited; does not blame self	Perceives continued threat; blames self
Quality of attachment	High quality, high continuity; securely attached	Low quality, discontinuous; ambivalent, insecurely attached
Parent competence	Competent	Incompetent
Family resources	Adequate economic resources	Poverty or discrimination
Quality, stability, safety of environment	Adequate, stable, safe	Inadequate, unstable, unsafe
Family relationships	Good communication; little conflict	Poor communication; excessive conflict
Emotional and physical health of caregivers	Caregivers in good emotional and physical health	Mental illness or physical illness in caregivers
Availability or access to community resources	High access	Low access

Brief evaluation

- Clinicians should be consistent with their screening instruments.
- If the patient has a definite psychosocial complaint, attempt to elaborate the symptoms.
- Consider risk factors and developmental concerns.
- Try to assess the child's daily functioning using the following guidelines.
  - Observe younger children while directing questions to the parents.
  - For school-age children, use confirmatory questions, if possible, without the parents being present.
- For adolescents, perform a separate interview with the patient alone.
  - Assess substance use and depression.
  - Inquire about sexual activity.
  - Consider parental abuse, depression, and substance use.
  - Review relevant risk factors and potentially protective factors.
  - Assess safety, eg, potential accident, suicidal ideation, and risk-taking behaviors.
- Complete the severity estimate using the Achenbach Child Behavior Checklist and PSC, ranking the current issue as mild, moderate, or severe.

P

Puberty: Normal and Abnormal

DEFINITION

- Normal puberty
  - Series of complex hormonal changes that begins at 8–13 years of age in girls and 9–14 years of age in boys
- Delayed puberty
  - Girls
    - No breast development by age 13 years
    - Delay >4–5 years from onset of puberty to menarche
  - Boys
    - No testicular enlargement by age 14 years
    - Maturation arrest
- Precocious puberty
  - Appearance of secondary sexual characteristics before 8 years of age in girls and 9 years in boys
  - Trends toward earlier onset of puberty in girls have led the Lawson Wilkins Pediatric Endocrine Society to publish recommendations that the cutoff age for precocious puberty should be decreased to 7 years in white girls and 6 years in black girls unless:
    - The tempo of puberty is abnormal.
    - The bone age is advanced >2 years.
    - The predicted height is <150 cm (59 inches).
    - Focal neurologic deficits are present.
    - Headaches are present.
    - The family's or child's emotional state is adversely affected.
  - The recommendations remain controversial.
- Variations of puberty
  - Premature thelarche
    - Isolated premature breast development
  - Premature adrenarche
    - Isolated premature development of sexual hair

EPIDEMIOLOGY

Normal puberty

- Onset of pubertal milestones (years) in girls
  - Thelarche
    - Non-Hispanic whites: 11.05
    - Non-Hispanic blacks: 10.25
    - Mexican Americans: 10.70
  - Sexual hair development
    - Non-Hispanic whites: 10.96
    - Non-Hispanic blacks: 10.25
    - Mexican Americans: 11.17
  - Menarche
    - Non-Hispanic whites: 12.52
    - Non-Hispanic blacks: 12.06
    - Mexican Americans: 12.09

- Association between increasing levels of adiposity and earlier sexual maturation in girls: causal nature is unclear
- Overall age at menarche has decreased by 2.3 months between National Health and Nutrition Examination Survey (NHANES) III (1988–1994) and NHANES IV (1999–2002).
  - NHANES IV had more girls with body mass index >85th or 95th percentile and had different racial and ethnic composition.
  - Changes within racial and ethnic groups were much smaller, indicating that overall decrease in age at menarche may result from changes in population distribution of race and ethnicity and relative weight.
- Onset of pubertal milestones (years) in boys
  - Testicular enlargement
    - Non-Hispanic whites: 11.08
    - Non-Hispanic blacks: 10.79
    - Mexican Americans: 11.09
  - Sexual hair development
    - Non-Hispanic whites: 11.81
    - Non-Hispanic blacks: 11.48
    - Mexican Americans: 12.2
  - Peak height velocity for boys is typically 2 years later than for girls and usually occurs during mid to late puberty.

Abnormal puberty

- Delayed puberty
  - Identified much more frequently in boys
- Precocious puberty
  - Significantly more common in girls than boys
  - Girls adopted from developing countries may be at particular risk.
  - Internationally adopted girls show a trend toward early and rapidly progressing puberty that may be related to increased metabolic activity exhibited if catch-up growth occurs after adoption.
- Gynecomastia
  - Occurs in about 40% of healthy boys
  - Mean age of occurrence: 14–15.5 years

MECHANISM

Normal puberty

- The hypothalamus secretes pulses of gonadotropin-releasing hormone (GnRH), which stimulates pituitary gonadotropin production of luteinizing hormone and follicle-stimulating hormone.
- The previously very sensitive hypothalamic-pituitary-gonadal feedback loop becomes less sensitive to the negative effect of gonadal steroids.
- Thus gonadotropin levels increase and stimulate secretion of more sex steroids (testosterone or estradiol, depending on sex), leading to physical changes of puberty.

P

- Hypothalamic-pituitary-gonadal axis is active during fetal life and infancy until it enters an inactive state during prepubertal years.
- Factors influencing pubertal timing
  - Genetic factors (50–80% of the variation)
  - Environmental influences, especially nutritional status
  - Leptin
    - Secreted by adipocytes and regulates appetite
    - May play permissive role in regulating timing of puberty
- Adrenarche
  - Increase in secretion of adrenal androgens during puberty
  - Associated with development of:
    - Pubic hair
    - Axillary hair
    - Body odor
    - Acne
  - The mechanism that triggers maturation of adrenal cortex at puberty remains poorly understood.

Abnormal puberty

- Delayed puberty
  - Constitutional delay is a slow maturation with appropriate hormonal levels and delayed bone age.
    - Frequently familial
    - Accounts for the majority of cases of pubertal delay
    - Identified more frequently in boys
  - Delayed puberty secondary to underlying chronic systemic disease
  - Deficiency of gonadotropin-releasing hormone secretion by the hypothalamus
    - Either genetic or acquired
  - Deficiency of gonadotropin secretion by the pituitary
    - Either genetic or acquired
  - Gonadal dysfunction
    - Either genetic or acquired
  - Adrenal and gonadal enzyme deficiencies
  - Malnutrition
  - Excessive exercise
- Precocious puberty
  - Central precocious puberty results from early stimulation of the hypothalamic-pituitary axis, with resultant gonadotropin secretion and sex-steroid secretion.
    - Idiopathic
    - Central nervous system abnormalities
    - Severe hypothyroidism
  - Peripheral precocious puberty results from sex-steroid secretion independent of pituitary gonadotropin secretion.
    - Gonadal tumors or cysts

- Adrenal hyperplasia or tumor
- Ectopic gonadotropin-secreting tumors
- Genetic disorders
- Exogenous sex steroids

- Gynecomastia
  - May result from increase in ratio of estrogen to androgen
- Premature thelarche
  - Occurs in girls between 6 months and 3 years of age
  - Breast development
    - Usually moderate
    - Often regresses
    - Seen without other signs of precocious puberty
  - Estrogen or gonadotropic levels do not increase significantly.
  - Statural and skeletal maturation accelerate only mildly, if at all.
  - Does not progress to complete precocious puberty
- Premature adrenarche
  - Usually occurs between 5 and 7–8 years of age
  - Development of sexual hair frequently accompanied by:
    - Mild growth spurt (with slight bone age advancement)
    - Signs of increased adrenal androgens
      - Increase in levels of plasma dehydroepiandrosterone and its sulfate to early pubertal range
  - In girls, no signs of increased estrogen secretion

HISTORY

- History related to possibly abnormal puberty should include thorough review of:
  - Child's medical history, with emphasis on growth, development, significant illnesses, and signs and symptoms related to the endocrine and central nervous systems
  - Exposure to medications and other exogenous agents that can affect puberty
  - Family history of pubertal onset and progression

PHYSICAL EXAM

- Physical examination related to possibly abnormal puberty should include careful:
  - Measurement of growth parameters, with calculation of growth velocity
  - Determination of Tanner staging
  - Attention to the endocrine and central nervous systems

DIFFERENTIAL DIAGNOSIS

Delayed puberty

- Constitutional delay

- Deficiency of gonadotropin-releasing hormone secretion by the hypothalamus
  - Genetic and molecular causes
    - Isolated deficiency
    - Kallmann syndrome
    - Laurence-Moon-Bardet-Biedl syndrome
    - Präder-Willi syndrome
  - Acquired causes
    - Infection
    - Neoplasm
    - Infiltrative disease
    - Trauma
- Deficiency of gonadotropin secretion by the pituitary
  - Genetic
    - Panhypopituitarism (including transcription factor mutations in *PROP1, HESX1,* and *LHX3*)
    - Isolated deficiency
    - Fertile eunuch (normal follicle-stimulating hormone level, low luteinizing hormone level)
    - Leptin or leptin-receptor deficiency
  - Acquired
    - Infection
    - Tumor
    - Excess prolactin secretion, adenoma
    - Trauma
- Gonadal disorders
  - Genetic and molecular
    - Turner syndrome (45, X or structural X abnormalities or mosaicism)
    - Klinefelter syndrome (47, XXY)
    - Noonan syndrome
    - Syndromes of complete androgen insensitivity (no sexual hair)
    - del Castillo syndrome (Sertoli cells only)
    - Pure gonadal dysgenesis
    - Myotonic dystrophy
    - Receptor mutations
  - Acquired
    - Gonorrhea (male)
    - Virus (mumps, coxsackie)
    - Tuberculosis (male)
    - After radiation or chemotherapy
    - Torsion
    - Surgery
    - Congenital anorchia (vanishing testes syndrome)
    - Autoimmune
- Adrenal and gonadal steroid enzyme deficiencies

- Malnutrition
- Excessive exercise
- Chronic systemic diseases
  - Congenital heart disease
  - Chronic pulmonary disease
  - Inflammatory bowel disease, celiac disease
  - Chronic renal failure and renal tubular acidosis
  - Hypothyroidism
  - Poorly controlled diabetes mellitus
  - Sickle cell anemia, thalassemia
  - Collagen-vascular disease
  - Anorexia nervosa
  - HIV infection

Isosexual precocious puberty
- Central (with pituitary gonadotropin secretion)
  - Idiopathic
  - Central nervous system abnormalities
  - Diagnosis is made only after a search for a pathologic cause is negative.
    - Congenital anomalies (hydrocephalus)
    - Tumors (hypothalamic, pineal, other)
    - Hamartoma
    - Postinflammatory condition
    - Trauma
    - Neurofibromatosis
    - Tuberous sclerosis
    - Hypothyroidism (severe)
- Peripheral
  - Exogenous sex steroids
    - Both testes are small.
  - Gonadal tumors or cysts
  - Adrenal hyperplasia or tumor
    - Both testes are small.
  - Ectopic gonadotropin–secreting tumors (chorioepithelioma, hepatoblastoma, teratoma)
    - Both testes are of pubertal size.
  - Familial Leydig cell hyperplasia, receptor mutation
  - McCune-Albright syndrome, G-protein mutation

Heterosexual precocious puberty
- Girls
  - Congenital adrenal hyperplasia
  - Androgen-secreting tumors
    - Adrenal
    - Ovarian
    - Teratoma
  - Exogenous androgens

P

- Boys
  - Estrogen-producing tumors
    - Adrenal
    - Teratoma
    - Hepatoma
    - Testicular
  - Exogenous estrogens
  - Increased peripheral conversion of androgens to estrogens

Gynecomastia

- Klinefelter syndrome
- Partial androgen insensitivity syndrome
- Hyperprolactinemia
- Liver disorders
- Adrenal carcinoma
- Biosynthetic defects in testosterone production
- Androgen receptor defects
- Increased activity of peripheral aromatase
- Certain drugs
  - Estrogen-like effect
    - Diethylstilbestrol
    - Oral contraceptive pills
    - Digitalis
    - Estrogen-containing cosmetics
  - Increase estrogen formation
    - Gonadotropins
    - Clomiphene
  - Inhibit testosterone action
    - Ketoconazole
    - Spironolactone
    - Cimetidine
    - Isoniazid
    - Methyldopa
    - Captopril
    - Tricyclic antidepressants
    - Diazepam
    - Marijuana
    - Phenothiazine

Adrenarche

- An abnormal androgen source (eg, tumor or late-onset congenital adrenal hyperplasia) must be excluded.
- May occur in children with mild neurologic problems

LABORATORY EVALUATION

- Evaluation for delayed puberty
  - Initial screening tests
    - Luteinizing hormone, follicle-stimulating hormone

    - Testosterone or estrogen, depending on sex
    - Thyroid-stimulating hormone, thyroid hormone
    - If systemic disease is thought to exist:
      - Complete blood count
      - Erythrocyte sedimentation rate, C-reactive protein
      - Comprehensive panel
      - Insulin-like growth factor 1, insulin-like growth factor binding protein 3
      - Urinalysis
      - Celiac disease panel (anti-endomesial IgA antibody or tissue transglutaminase immunoglobulin A and total immunoglobulin A level)
      - Inflammatory bowel disease panel
      - Prolactin
  - Other tests (if indicated)
    - Karyotype
    - GnRH or GnRH analogue stimulation test
- Evaluation for precocious puberty
  - Initial screening tests
    - Luteinizing hormone, follicle-stimulating hormone
    - Estradiol, testosterone
    - Dehydroepiandrosterone sulfate
    - 17-Hydroxyprogesterone
    - Thyroid-stimulating hormone, thyroid hormone
  - Secondary tests (if indicated)
    - Serum ß-human chorionic gonadotropin
    - GnRH
  - Measurement of serum gonadotropin levels before and after injection of GnRH usually distinguishes central and peripheral precocious puberty.
- Gynecomastia
  - Initial screening blood work
    - Testosterone
    - Estradiol
    - Luteinizing hormone
    - Follicle-stimulating hormone
    - Liver function tests
    - Prolactin
    - ß-Human chorionic gonadotropin level

IMAGING

- Evaluation for delayed puberty and precocious puberty can include, if indicated:
  - Bone age
  - Brain magnetic resonance imaging
  - Pelvic ultrasonography

SPECIFIC TREATMENT

Delayed puberty

- Treatment is directed toward the cause when possible.
- In all cases, provide strong psychological support to the adolescent and sometimes to the family.
- Gonadal failure or gonadotropin deficiency
  - Treatment focuses on replacing the appropriate sex steroid.
- Constitutional delay
  - Waiting may be the best course.
  - Boys
    - A short course of low-dose injectable testosterone (eg, 50–100 mg monthly for 4 doses) if delayed development affects psychological well-being
  - Girls
    - Cosmetic treatment (eg, padded bra)
    - Estrogen therapy necessary only occasionally
- GnRH or gonadotropin deficiency
  - Fertility may be induced with GnRH or gonadotropin therapy.

Isosexual precocity

- Suppression or removal of underlying cause
- Idiopathic central precocious puberty
  - GnRH analogues lead to pituitary desensitization and reduce gonadotropin secretion to prepubertal levels.
  - Available intramuscularly (depot), subcutaneously, and intranasally.
  - Depot leuprolide is used most commonly in US.
    - Usually given every 3–4 weeks
    - Longer-acting forms given every 12 weeks are available.
    - Has been used for years, is effective, and has minimal side effects
- Gonadotropin-independent precocious puberty
  - Testolactone and other aromatase inhibitors (anastrozole, letrozole)
  - Spironolactone (androgen receptor inhibitor)
  - Ketoconazole (steroidogenesis inhibitor)
- McCune-Albright syndrome
  - Tamoxifen (estrogen receptor inhibitor)

Heterosexual precocious puberty

- Removal of sex hormone source (exogenous or tumor)
- Suppression with glucocorticoid replacement therapy (congenital adrenal hyperplasia)

Gynecomastia

- Treatment in most cases is reassurance.
- For unresolved or rapidly developing cases:
  - Medical therapy
    - Clomiphene (antiestrogen)
    - Tamoxifen (estrogen antagonist)
    - Testolactone (peripheral aromatase inhibitor)
    - Danazol (synthetic derivative of testosterone)
    - No randomized, controlled trials have assessed these drugs.
  - Surgical intervention remains the mainstay of treatment.

Isolated premature thelarche and adrenarche

- No treatment is required.

WHEN TO REFER

- Delayed puberty
  - No breast development in girls by 13 years of age
  - No menarche 4–5 years after onset of breast development in girls
  - No testicular enlargement in boys by 14 years of age
  - Maturational arrest
  - Hormonal abnormalities identified by initial screening tests
  - Parental or physician discomfort
- Precocious puberty
  - Signs of puberty before 6–8 years of age in girls
  - Signs of puberty before age 9 in boys
  - Rapidly progressive puberty (eg, stage 3 breast when first noted)
- Heterosexual precocious puberty
  - Hormonal abnormalities identified by initial screening tests
  - Parental or physician discomfort
- Gynecomastia
  - Does not resolve after 2 years
  - Develops rapidly

FOLLOW-UP

- Premature thelarche and premature adrenarche
  - Careful follow-up physical exams are necessary to ensure they do not represent early stages of complete sexual precocity.

PROGNOSIS

- Precocious puberty
  - Can significantly reduce adult height
  - Sometimes adversely affects the child's and family's emotional state
- Adrenarche
  - May be a marker of future polycystic ovary syndrome
- Gynecomastia
  - Usually resolves within 2 years

P

Pyloric Stenosis

DEFINITION

- Pyloric stenosis (PS) is a condition characterized by abnormal thickening of the antropyloric muscles.

EPIDEMIOLOGY

- Prevalence
  - One of the most common conditions requiring surgery in infants
  - Seen in 100–300 per 100,000 live births
- Incidence
  - Early population-based studies reported an increase in the incidence of PS.
    - More recent reports indicate that the incidence seems to have leveled.
- Sex
  - Boys are affected 4 times more than girls.
  - The commonly held belief that PS primarily afflicts first-born male infants has not been confirmed.
- Race, ethnicity
  - Incidence in white infants exceeds that in black, Native American, or Asian infants.
- Familial association
  - Develops in 5% of boys and 2.5% of girls whose fathers had PS
  - Develops in 19% of boys and 7% of girls whose mothers were affected
  - Concordance is:
    - 0.25–0.44 in monozygotic twins
    - 0.05–0.1 in dizygotic twins

ETIOLOGY

- Obstruction of the intervening lumen of the pyloric channel causes progressively worsening vomiting, resulting in dehydration.
- The mechanism for hypertrophied pyloric muscle and gastric outlet obstruction is not known.
- Uncoordinated gastric peristalsis and pyloric relaxation have been speculated to lead to gastric contractions against a closed pylorus, resulting in work hypertrophy of the pyloric muscle.
- Theories that have been proposed to explain hypertrophy of the pyloric muscle include:
  - Alterations in gastrin production
  - Changes in breastfeeding practice
  - Variations in infant milk formulas
- Impaired neuronal function has been implicated in the development of PS caused by reduction in:
  - Smooth-muscle vasoactive amines
  - Neurons and nerve fibers
  - Interstitial pacemaker cells of Cajal

- Investigators have proposed that deficiency of nitric oxide, a ubiquitous mediator of smooth-muscle relaxation, may be associated with the development of PS.
  - Nitric oxide synthase is selectively depleted in the pyloric muscle of patients with PS.
  - Studies of neuronal nitric oxide synthase gene polymorphisms suggest that this gene represents a susceptibility locus for PS.
- Whether PS is acquired or congenital disorder is still unclear.
  - Onset of clinical symptoms between 2 and 8 weeks of life supports an acquired condition.
  - A genetic basis is supported by:
    - Male predilection
    - Familial cases
    - PS among twins
    - An increased frequency of coexisting malformations

RISK FACTORS

- Prenatal exposure to macrolides
- Postnatal exposure to systemic erythromycin, particularly within the first 2 weeks of life
- Postnatal prostaglandins
- Most infants with PS are otherwise healthy and genetically normal.
- PS has been reported with a greater frequency in infants with:
  - Hiatal and inguinal hernias
  - Malrotation
  - Junctional epidermolysis bullosa
  - Hirschsprung disease
  - Ovarian cysts
  - Ichthyosis
  - Smith-Lemli-Opitz syndrome
  - Deletions of the long arm of chromosome 11
- PS is believed to be associated with the variable transmission of an inheritable trait.
  - Transmission of the PS trait is more frequent from the mother than the father.

SIGNS AND SYMPTOMS

- Typical presentation is projectile, nonbilious vomiting in a full-term male infant between 3 and 6 weeks of age.
- Common age of symptom manifestation is 3–6 weeks.
  - Has been reported in newborns and older infants
- Vomiting
  - Initially, the infant vomits a small amount of food immediately after feeding and continues to gain weight.
  - After a few weeks, vomiting becomes more frequent and projectile, and occurs after every feeding.
  - Initially, the vomitus is nonbilious; over time, it may become brownish in color.

- The infant continues to be hungry immediately after vomiting.
- The infant may subsequently develop gastritis.
- Infants are usually active and alert.
- Lethargy ensues only after significant dehydration.
- Physical examination reveals weight loss and dehydration.
- The enlarged pylorus may be felt as a firm, mobile, ovoid-shaped mass—the so-called olive.
  - If the infant is relaxed, the mass can be felt in approximately 80–90% of cases.
  - The infant's feet should be elevated.
  - The knees should be placed in the flexed position to relax the abdominal muscles.
  - 2 or 3 fingertips are placed in the right upper quadrant, gently advanced into the deeper tissues below the liver edge, and then slowly swept toward the umbilicus.
    - The mass can be felt to roll under the fingertips during this sweeping motion.
  - The mass is rarely palpable in an agitated, crying infant with a contracted abdominal wall.
  - The mass can be best felt immediately after an episode of projectile emesis.
    - At this time, the pylorus is fully contracted and at its firmest consistency.
  - If the mass is not felt with the infant in the supine position, palpation while the infant is lying prone may be successful.
  - Occasionally, the primary care physician may need to:
    - Pass a nasogastric tube
    - Empty the stomach
    - Feed the infant small quantities of dextrose in water to help relax the abdominal wall
- Gastric contractions, which move across the upper abdomen from left to right, may be seen in some infants.
  - Best observed with a bright light directed across the abdomen from the patient's side
  - The examiner should stand at the foot of the examining table.

DIFFERENTIAL DIAGNOSIS

- Other causes of gastric outlet obstruction should be considered in the differential diagnosis of an infant with nonbilious emesis.
  - Foregut stenosis
  - Gastric duplications
  - Antral webs
  - Pylorospasm
  - Annular pancreas
  - Malrotation
  - Many of these causes can be excluded by ultrasonography or an upper gastrointestinal (GI) tract series.
- When a diagnosis of PS cannot be established in an infant with persistent emesis and a normal ultrasonogram and upper GI tract series, the following possibilities should be considered.
  - Poor feeding regimen
  - Gastroesophageal reflux
  - Sepsis
  - Intracranial disease
  - Renal disorder
  - Adrenal insufficiency
- Salt-losing congenital hyperplasia
  - Prompt diagnosis and immediate therapy are crucial.
  - This condition should be suspected in an infant with:
    - Abnormal genitalia
    - Hyponatremia
    - Hyperkalemia
- When the workup is inconclusive, reevaluating in 1 week to 10 days is reasonable.

DIAGNOSTIC APPROACH

- Palpation of a mass on physical examination alone should aid in making an accurate diagnosis in most patients.
- Once the mass is felt unequivocally, the diagnosis of PS is established and no further diagnostic maneuvers are necessary.
- A large volume of fluid aspirated from the stomach of a fasting infant who has a history of projectile vomiting strengthens the possibility of PS.

LABORATORY FINDINGS

- Persistent vomiting caused by gastric outlet obstruction results in the continuous loss of gastric hydrochloric acid.
- Dehydration causes an increase in aldosterone production, leading to increased renal excretion of potassium.
- The potassium excretion results in a hypochloremic, hypokalemic metabolic alkalosis.
- Depletion of chloride in the blood leads to an exchange of hydrogen and potassium for sodium in the distal tubule, resulting in a paradoxical aciduria.
- A spectrum of electrolyte abnormalities may be seen:
  - Hypoglycemia may be present and may cause seizures.
  - Unconjugated hyperbilirubinemia is common.
    - Correlates with a decrease in hepatic glucuronosyl transferase activity
    - Resolves after treatment

P

IMAGING

- Ultrasonography
  - Sensitivity approaches 100%
  - The most useful technique to confirm the diagnosis in cases in which:
    - PS is suspected clinically
    - Hypertrophied pylorus cannot be palpated
  - Measurement of pyloric wall thickness, diameter, and pyloric channel length accurately establishes the diagnosis of PS.
    - Pyloric muscle wall thickness ≥3.7 mm and a channel length ≥17 mm have been shown to have ≥90% positive predictive value (see Figure 72 on page F26).
    - Diagnostic criteria for wall thickness may be reduced to 3 mm in infants <30 days.
- Upper GI tract contrast study
  - May be performed in infants in whom ultrasonography is not diagnostic
  - Characteristic upper GI tract findings in infants with PS include:
    - An elongated and narrowed pyloric channel (string sign)
    - The shoulders of the hypertrophied pylorus bulging into the intestinal lumen (see Figure 73 on page F26)
- Palpation of a mass on physical examination alone should aid in making an accurate diagnosis in most patients.
- Increasing reliance is now placed on noninvasive, highly accurate, and relatively inexpensive radiologic tests, such as ultrasonography.

TREATMENT APPROACH

- Management of PS consists of hydration and pyloromyotomy.

SPECIFIC TREATMENTS

Preoperative management

- In the past, infants often had overwhelming malnutrition and electrolyte abnormalities.
- In the current era of early diagnosis, infants infrequently progress to this severe state.
- Anatomic correction of PS is not a surgical emergency.
- Although PS is a form of intestinal obstruction, gangrene and intestinal perforation do not occur.
- Infants should not undergo surgery until fluid and electrolyte deficits have been corrected.
- If infants undergo surgery with uncorrected alkalosis, the profound effect that surgical stress has on the urinary excretion of sodium may intensify the electrolyte abnormalities.
- Fluid replacement should include deficit correction and daily maintenance fluids.
  - Continuous maintenance infusion of 5% dextrose in 0.45 normal saline

- Addition of 20 mEq/L potassium chloride once urine output is established
- Repeated boluses of isotonic sodium chloride at 20 mL/kg until a serum chloride level of 100 mEq/L is achieved.
- Nasogastric decompression should be performed during fluid and electrolyte resuscitation.

Surgical management

- Surgical myotomy is a reliable and safe procedure.
- Once the volume and electrolyte status is corrected, the infant is ready for surgery.
- Ramstedt pyloromyotomy through a right upper quadrant transverse incision has been the traditional treatment for hypertrophic PS.
- New alternative methods include:
  - Laparoscopy
    - Shorter mean operative time
    - No increase in complications or costs
  - Circumumbilical approach
  - Earlier data suggested that the circumumbilical approach is associated with greater mean operative time and cost.
  - The only randomized trial shows no difference between the 2 approaches.

Postoperative management

- Postoperative vomiting occurs is most infants.
  - Will usually subside by the 2nd to 5th feeding
- Parental education regarding postoperative vomiting is important before surgery.
- Infants should be fed full-strength formula or breast milk every 3–4 hours starting 6 hours after surgery.
- In case of emesis, infants can be refed the amount vomited 1 hour later, with resumption of the feeding schedule thereafter.
  - This early refeeding has resulted in a reduction in the postoperative hospital stay.
- Discharge criteria
- Infants are usually discharged 24–48 hours after surgery.
- Feeding tolerance must be reassessed before discharge.

Medical management

- Medical management alone has been largely discarded during the last several decades.
- May be considered as an alternative to pyloromyotomy, particularly in children with major concurrent primary disease
- The anticholinergic agent atropine sulfate has been used with success.
  - Prolongs the duration of hospital stay
  - Studies comparing predominantly oral atropine sulfate with surgical myotomy have reported similar success rates.

WHEN TO ADMIT

- All infants need to be hospitalized to correct electrolyte imbalance and for surgery.

WHEN TO REFER

- All infants with PS should be referred to a surgeon for surgery.

COMPLICATIONS

- Intraoperative and early postoperative complications
  - General
    - Morbidity and mortality from surgical repair
      - Have decreased from 50% to <1%
    - Negligible risk of:
      - Intestinal perforation
      - Hemorrhage
      - Wound dehiscence
      - Postoperative infection
  - Hypoglycemia
    - Reactive hypoglycemia
      - Reported in infants who have a wide variety of medical and surgical conditions
      - May cause respiratory arrest and death
      - Constant infusion of dextrose results in hyperinsulinemia.
        o May result in severe hypoglycemia if suddenly terminated before adequate oral feeding is established.
      - Particularly likely if liver glycogen stores have been depleted, as has been shown in infants with PS
  - Death
    - Mortality is <0.1%.
    - Potential causes of death include:
      - Delayed diagnosis
      - Inadequate preoperative rehydration
      - Pulmonary aspiration
      - Unrecognized perforation
      - Hypoglycemia
      - Persistent obstruction
      - Hemorrhage
      - Presence of other associated congenital anomalies
  - Late complications
    - Postoperative obstruction
      - Radiographic evaluation is necessary if vomiting persists beyond 5–7 days.
      - Excessive vomiting may be caused by:
        - Persistent stenosis
        - Gastroesophageal reflux
        - Gastric outlet obstruction
        - Small-bowel obstruction attributable to adhesions
      - Upper GI tract contrast series is difficult to interpret but may be helpful.
      - Narrowing and elongation of the pyloric channel
        - Usually persist for weeks to months after a successful operation, even in infants who have minimal or no postoperative vomiting
      - Subsequent operation may be indicated in the rare event of persistent pyloric obstruction.

PROGNOSIS

- The long-term outcome for patients treated for PS is excellent.
- Rapid gastric emptying and duodenogastric reflux have been identified in some patients who had undergone pyloromyotomy 5–7 years earlier.
  - Other studies have shown no differences between previous patients with PS and controls after long-term follow-up.

P

Rape

DEFINITION

- *Rape* is a legal term or condition, not a medical diagnosis.
- Every state has statutory definitions of sexual assault and rape.
  - Clinicians should be familiar with the statutes in their local jurisdictions.
- In general, *rape* refers to sexual intercourse:
  - With force or threat of force
  - Without a person's consent
- Sexual intercourse may include:
  - Penile-oral penetration
  - Penile-vaginal penetration
  - Penile-anal penetration
- Threat may be:
  - Overtly physical
  - Verbal
  - Implicit
    - Result of age and power differentials between individuals
- Rape entails an assault acted out sexually, rather than a sexual act per se.
- *Male rape* refers to same-sex rape.
- Statutory rape is defined as sexual activity of an adult with an adolescent under the age of legal consent.

EPIDEMIOLOGY

- Prevalence
  - Estimates of unreported rape range from 40–90%.
    - Many victims never report the crime.
- Age
  - Between 40–60% of all rape victims are <18 years of age.
    - Most are adolescents.
    - Female adolescents aged 16–19 are 4 times more likely to be sexually assaulted than women in all other age groups.
    - Worldwide, estimates indicate that between one-third and two-thirds of rape victims are ≤15 years of age.
    - Exact statistics on adolescent rape are not available.
  - 90% of adolescent rape victims are assaulted by someone they know.
    - >50% of these cases occur on a date.
- Sex
  - Most rape victims are women.
  - 5–10% are men.
- Legal statistics
  - Approximately one-half of all reported rapes in the US eventually lead to arrests.
  - Approximately two-thirds of those arrested are prosecuted.
  - Approximately one-half of those prosecuted are found guilty.

- In other words, for every 100 reported rapes, only 16 perpetrators are convicted.
  - Male adolescents constitute a large proportion of convicted rape assailants.
    - 40% of convicted rapists are 16–20 years of age.
    - 25% are 20–24 years of age.
- Stranger rape
  - 15–55% of reported rapes are committed by unknown individuals.
- Date rape
  - Estimates of the incidence of date rape are unclear.
  - One survey of middle and high school students reported a history of unwanted sexual activity on dates in:
    - Nearly 20% of the girls
    - >10% of the boys
  - Surveys of college students report history of date rape by:
    - ~25% of female students
    - 6% of male students
  - None of the college students in these surveys reported the sexual assault to authorities.

ETIOLOGY

Types of rape

Known assailant

- In most reported pediatric rape cases, victim knows the assailant.
  - Parent
  - Stepparent
  - Adult relative
  - Family friend
  - Neighbor
  - Acquaintance
  - Classmate
- Victim–assailant relationship may cause conflicting family or social loyalties.
  - Makes victims less likely to report the rape
- Rape victims who know their assailants are prone to:
  - Self-doubt
  - Self-blame
- When rape is reported, information may be received with skepticism and disbelief.
  - Even by professionals to whom victim turns for help

Stranger rape

- More likely to entail:
  - Threats
  - Use of violence
  - Fear of immediate danger

- Associated with a higher incidence of:
  - Reporting
  - Subsequent conviction of the assailant
- Most likely to occur in areas of:
  - Poverty
  - High crime

Date rape

- In cases of young female adolescents (ages 10–15) and older men, questions arise about:
  - Statutory rape
  - Consent
  - Refusal skills
  - Exploitation
- Least likely type of rape to be reported
- More likely to occur on weekends between 10 PM–1 AM
- Occurs in automobiles or at home of assailant
- May not be reported if the rape was facilitated by the administration of pharmaceuticals *(date rape drugs)* that cause anterograde amnesia
  - γ-Hydroxybutyric acid
  - Flunitrazepam (Rohypnol)
  - Ketamine hydrochloride (Ketamine)
- Important issues for victims include:
  - Long-term issues of trust
  - Self-blame
  - Vulnerability
- Female date rape victim may:
  - Not trust her judgment concerning men
  - Blame herself, erroneously believing that
    - She did not resist clearly.
    - She did not resist convincingly enough.
  - Be ashamed that she ended up in a situation that resulted in rape
- Thoughts of guilt may be reinforced by response and degree of support provided by parents, guardians, friends.
- Secrecy applies to discussing the incident in general, making it difficult to obtain catharsis, verbal support, emotional support.

Gang rape

- Typically involves a group of young men raping a solitary female victim
  - May be associated with:
    - Ritualistic behavior
    - Displaced rage on the part of the assailants
- Issues of sexualized rites of passage apply to:
  - Stereotypical adolescent gangs
  - College fraternities

- Victims of college campus gang rapes are more likely to drop out of college than pursue legal recourse.
  - Avoids confrontation with perpetrators at long-term expense of victims

Male rape

- Remains understudied
- Male rape in institutionalized settings often is attributed to:
  - Displaced heterosexual behavior
  - Undifferentiated sexual orientation
  - Aggressive dominance of a weaker partner
- Male rape outside institutions often occurs through coercion by an individual perceived as an authority figure.
- Relevant issues for the male rape victim
  - Loss of control
  - Depression
  - Anxiety
  - Sleep disturbances
  - Suicidal ideation
- Conflicted sexual identity is common after rape among all male rape victims, whether homosexual or not.
- Male rape victims often are controlled by:
  - Entrapment
  - Intimidation
  - Physical force
  - Combination
- Intimidation is accomplished by:
  - Threats of physical harm
  - Brandishing a weapon
- Male victims often perceive the rape as a life-threatening event.
  - Perception may result in long-term psychological problems.
- Boys and men remain reluctant to report rape.
  - Precludes them from benefits of social support, intervention

Male perpetrators

- Tend to fall into 1 of 3 categories:
  - Anger is the primary dynamic.
  - Power or conquest is the central issue.
  - Sadistic person who finds anger and control erotic.
- Anger-driven rapist
  - Act tends to be impulsive, with the intent of hurting, humiliating, degrading.
  - Physical brutality is common.
  - Rape functions as the outlet for anger, with sex as a weapon.

R

- Power-oriented rapist
  - Engages in premeditated, obsessive, or stalking behavior
  - Rape compensates for social and sexual incompetence or inadequacy.
  - Aggression is less likely to be violent than a means of domination.
  - Both anger- and power-driven rapists have:
    - Serious deficits in social skills
    - Inability to interpret and respond to social cues
- Sadistic rapist
  - Eroticism and violence are enmeshed.
  - Victims typically subjected to premeditated, deliberate acts of cruelty and dehumanization
  - Sadistic perpetrator finds gratification in victim's pain and powerlessness.
- Some rapists are dysfunctional sexually at time of the rape.
  - Most rapists are sexually active with available, consensual partners outside the rape.
- Perpetrators usually appear ordinary by most standards.
  - Most do not have symptoms of:
    - Major psychiatric illnesses such as psychoses
    - Intellectual disability
  - Characteristics noted more commonly among convicted rapists than in general population:
    - Antisocial
    - Schizoid
    - Paranoid
    - Narcissistic
- Alcohol and drug use have been associated with rape.
  - Alcohol intoxication sometimes seems to have the dual effect of:
    - Diminishing perpetrator's sense of responsibility
    - Increasing victim's culpability
  - Perpetrator's act of rape is excused because he was drinking and not responsible for his actions.
  - Victim intoxication is consistently coupled with the process of *unfounding,* or disproving, rape charges.
  - For date rape victims, having been seen drinking with the perpetrator before the attack has serious implications in relation to public, social, and legal responses to the charges.

RISK FACTORS

- Survivors of prior sexual abuse are at particular risk of revictimization.
- Risk for rape is increased in adolescents who engage in high-risk behaviors, including:
  - Running away
  - Using drugs and alcohol

- Date rape
  - Incidence appears highly correlated with one or both parties drinking or using other drugs.
- Male rape
  - Specific subgroups of young men are at particular risk for sexual abuse:
    - Those in institutionalized settings, such as the criminal justice system
    - Street youth who may engage in prostitution
    - Young male homosexuals who may be runaways
    - Youths who have a parental history of physical or sexual abuse
- Parents who were abused themselves may become abusers as adults.

SIGNS AND SYMPTOMS

History

- History taking necessarily entails asking personal and potentially awkward questions.
  - Patient should be assured of privacy and offered respectful compassion.
  - History should include time, date, and location of both event and examination.
  - Recalling the event may be emotionally traumatic.
  - Beginning with relevant, but relatively neutral, medical history sometimes is useful.
  - Include important information such as:
    - Medical history
    - Physical and behavioral symptoms
    - Menstrual history, including
      - Age of menarche
      - Date of last menstrual period
      - Frequency of menses
    - Sexual activity, if relevant
    - Previous pregnancies, miscarriages, and abortions
    - Use of contraceptives
    - Use of feminine hygiene products
  - Additional history should include:
    - Parental response
    - Fear of parental reaction
    - Risk of running away
    - Past and current suicidal ideation
- Next, focus on event itself.
  - Questions should be asked calmly, with sensitivity and patience.
  - Victim's own words should be recorded whenever possible.

R

- Medical chart is a legal document.
  - Will be subjected to the same scrutiny as any other form of evidence
  - Only historical facts, without embellishment or interpretation, should be recorded.
- Patient should be asked about:
  - Use of intoxicating substances before or during event
  - Any loss of consciousness
  - Use of weapons or restraints during the assault
- Patient should be asked to describe in detail:
  - Location of event
  - Appearance of perpetrator
  - Type of sexual contact
  - Positions used
  - Use of force by perpetrator or by victim
  - Removal of clothing and manner in which it was removed
  - Any measures patient took to cleanse or relieve himself or herself
    - Bathing
    - Douching
    - Changing clothes
    - Urinating
    - Defecating
- Physician should also ask about:
  - Whether assailant used condom or any other means of contraception
  - Presence of clinical symptoms in:
    - Musculoskeletal system
    - Gastrointestinal system
    - Genitourinary system

Physical examination

- Complete physical examination from head to toe is warranted, collecting specimens for forensic and laboratory evaluation.
  - Particular focus should be placed on the evaluation of oral cavity, genitals, anus.
  - 40–60% of sexual assault victims will have no visible physical injuries.
  - Inspection of the entire body may provide corroborative evidence necessary to convict perpetrator.
  - Follow-up examinations may reveal emerging bruising or injuries in areas initially noted to have tenderness or swelling, but no visible bruising.
- Note patient's:
  - Physical appearance
  - Emotional state

- If patient is wearing same clothing worn at time of the event:
  - Condition should be noted.
  - Each piece should be saved in a separate, labeled bag.
- Applying a fluorescent lamp to the clothing and skin may illuminate presence of dried semen.
  - Semen fluoresces best at wavelengths of 420 and 450 nm, when viewed through orange goggles.
  - Specialized alternate light sources that emit wavelengths at 420 and 450 nm, such as a Bluemaxx, should be used.
    - Improves detection of dried semen
    - Many other substances will fluoresce as well.
    - Presence of semen cannot be confirmed with this method.
  - Specimens should be marked for later analysis for presence of seminal vesicle–specific antigen.
- Topical survey of the body
  - Document any evidence of recent trauma or bruising.
  - Photographs may be useful during subsequent litigation.
  - Use a diagram to indicate locations of visible injuries.
  - Clinician should use fluorescent lamp to:
    - Identify fluorescent areas on the skin
    - Obtain swabs of these areas
- Give particular attention to the examination of the head and neck.
  - Compression injuries of the neck are common if force is used.
  - This type of injury may lead to obstruction of venous return from the head, causing development of:
    - Neck bruising
    - Petechial hemorrhages in eyelids and conjunctiva
  - Inner surface of lips may have tiny abrasions from forced pressure applied to the mouth to prevent the victim from screaming.
  - Common injuries to mouth include:
    - Torn frenulums
    - Palate petechiae
- Breasts may show bite marks or bruises.
  - Swab all bite marks to collect genetic markers (ABO group)
  - Photo-document injuries
    - Bite impression may be matched to a potential perpetrator.
- Perform Tanner staging to determine the victim's level of sexual maturation.
  - Breasts and pubic hair in female patients
  - Genitalia and pubic hair in male patients

Genital examination: female patient

- After initial physical examination, patient can be draped and placed in lithotomy position.

R

- Supine frog-leg position may be a suitable alternative if:
  - Patient seems too anxious.
  - Speculum examination is not required to investigate for source of undiagnosed internal bleeding.
- Speculum examination is not necessary for younger adolescents or children, unless active vaginal bleeding is present.
- In rare instances of active vaginal bleeding:
  - It may be necessary to perform the pelvic examination with the patient under sedation or general anesthesia.
- Pelvic examination should begin with inspection of thighs and perineum for evidence of:
  - Trauma
  - Bruising
  - Semen
  - Blood
- Take appropriate forensic evidence at this time.
  - Recommended procedures for collecting forensic data
    - Forensic evidence kit
      - Complete forms for authorization and release of evidence, history, and physical examination
      - Individual envelopes to be completed if indicated by history provided
    - Additional tests to strongly consider
      - Pregnancy test
      - Syphilis screening
      - HIV test
      - Cultures for gonorrhea (oral, urethral, vaginal, and anal)
      - Cultures for *Chlamydia* (urethral, vaginal, and anal)
      - Wet mount for detection of *Trichomonas* and spermatozoa
- General inspection of the external genitalia should be performed, documenting any:
  - Erythema
  - Edema
  - Ecchymosis
  - Abrasions
- In some cultures, an intact hymen is an important indicator of virginity.
  - Patient and parents will be concerned with its structural integrity.
  - An intact hymen does not rule out the diagnosis of rape.
  - Document any acute injuries to the hymen such as:
    - Bruising
    - Petechiae
    - Acute transactions

- Describe any active bleeding and the location using clock-face orientation.
- Entire rim of hymen must be visualized.
  - Proper labial traction along with saline-moistened cotton swab rolled around the edges of the hymen is necessary.
- Use of light source or application of aqueous toluidine blue (1%) to posterior fourchette may help locate and identify acute tears.
- Many experts use colposcopy, which provides light source, magnification, photodocumentation of exam.
- Colposcopy or photodocumentation with a camera is essential.
  - Images can later be evaluated by expert review.
- Older female adolescents should be able to undergo speculum examination of the internal genitals.
  - Will allow a clear view of:
    - Vaginal walls
    - Fornices
    - Cervix

Genital examination: male patient

- Examine thoroughly for the presence of infection or trauma:
  - Testes
  - Epididymis
  - Vas deferens
  - Penile shaft
  - Foreskin
  - Glans penis

Anal examination

- History of sodomy in both male and female victims indicates need to conduct thorough anal inspection.
- Clinician should document any:
  - Erythema
  - Ecchymosis
  - Abrasions
  - Rectal bleeding
- Aqueous toluidine blue (1%) may be applied to help visualize acute microtrauma to the perianal area.

DIAGNOSTIC APPROACH

- Purpose of the initial medical evaluation is 4-fold:
  - Treatment of injury and infection
  - Prevention of pregnancy
  - Collection of evidence
  - Psychological assessment with referral for follow-up counseling

General concepts

- Many metropolitan areas have treatment centers with trained interdisciplinary teams available for adolescent and child victims of rape.
  - These treatment centers are ideal sites for an initial evaluation.
  - An interdisciplinary approach is beneficial for several reasons, including ability to:
    - Provide support to the child and family simultaneously
    - Serve as a resource for future services
- Most pediatric rape victims do not use such specialized facilities.
  - May receive medical evaluations at:
    - Emergency departments
    - Private medical offices
  - To minimize physical and psychological trauma of the evaluation
    - Eliminate need for repeat evaluations
    - Maximize probability of collecting forensic evidence
  - The most skilled professional available should perform the initial evaluation.
  - Gender of examiner is less important than his or her:
    - Comfort with adolescents and children
    - Skill at conducting examination
    - Level of compassion
- Rape evaluation can be long and tedious, but should never be rushed.
  - Young person is coping with:
    - Personal outrage
    - Physical pain
    - Psychological pain
  - Patient is expected to tolerate and cooperate with uncomfortable procedures.
    - May feel similar to acts of intrusion and aggression experienced previously
  - Approach to evaluation should be calm, gentle, private.
- Rape protocols, if available, are helpful.
  - Minimize chance for error or omission in evidence-collection process
  - Most jurisdictions have printed standardized forms for the evidence-procurement process.
    - Available in each state's forensic evidence kit
    - Clinician should become familiar with these forms before examining victim.
- Clinician should avoid making inappropriate assumptions about victim based on her psychological state.
  - Many victims are in a state of shock or denial immediately after event.

- How a patient responds in emergency department depends on numerous factors, including developmental maturity.
- Physically mature appearance, but cognitive function at the level of a preadolescent, is not uncommon for a 13-year-old child.
- Patient's psychological state should not alter the physician's approach to care.
- Clinician should not attempt to minimize victim's sense of personal guilt, shame, anxiety.
- Clinician should offer immediate reassurance.
- Before proceeding with evaluation, take a few minutes to
  - Empathize with patient
  - Acknowledge patient's feelings
- Establishment of patient safety is crucial.
  - Particularly in cases in which acute trauma may compromise pediatric patient's existing coping skills
- Clinician should never leave patient alone.
- Take whatever time is necessary at the beginning of the evaluation to explain the process.
  - Allow for questions:
    - Particularly for those who never had previous sexual relationships or prior gynecologic examination
    - More experienced patients may still be anxious and fearful of anticipated pain and discomfort.
  - Whenever possible, clinician should allow patient some control over proceedings.
  - Patient should set pace of examination.
  - Patient should be the one who signals when to begin procedures.
  - If victim becomes visibly agitated, clinician should stop and allow patient to regain composure.
  - At no point, should physician continue to examine a child or adolescent against the patient's will.
- When applicable, make reference to prior experience with similar-aged rape survivors.
  - May establish that the patient is not the only child or adolescent to whom this ordeal has happened
  - Establishes that physician:
    - Is familiar with such circumstances
    - Has some practical knowledge with which to anticipate patient's concerns
- Physician should obtain a detailed and relevant history, followed by a thorough general physical examination (see History).
- Some aspects of evaluation will change depending on temporal proximity of evaluation to event.
  - Modifications are necessary if evaluation is conducted later than 72 hours after the assault.

R

Summarizing examination

- When the physical examination is complete, give patient time to dress and regain composure.
- It is important to discuss:
  - Physical findings
  - Treatment options
  - Plans for follow-up
- Most patients will benefit from knowing their genital anatomy is normal.
- Several studies have demonstrated that >90% of anogenital examination after rape are normal.

Psychological assessment

- Psychosocial and emotional implications of rape in children and adolescents are complex.
  - Circumstance is tempered further by:
    - Young person's stage of development
    - Family's response
  - Young adolescents just beginning to grapple with their own sexuality may believe they deserved to be raped because they have begun to experience sexual urges.
  - Female child who sees her mother respond with tearful distress may feel guilt because of rape and emotional trauma inflicted on the mother.
- How young person copes with rape is related to how society responds to victims.
  - Unlike most crimes, rape often is blamed on victim rather than on perpetrator, particularly in adolescents.
  - Following no other crime is the victim subject to such scrutiny in regard to:
    - Prior reputation
    - Appearance
    - Behavior
  - Justification for rape may include:
    - Running away
    - Sexual activity
    - Hitchhiking
  - This justification places further blame on an already-troubled young victim.
  - Providers of care must avoid compounding such punitive dynamics.

Response to rape

- Immediate response to rape by the victim
  - May vary considerably, ranging from
    - Distraught histrionics *to*
    - Near-mute withdrawal
  - Most victims have intense levels of fear and anxiety.
  - Post-rape acute phase is characterized by varying levels of:
    - Cognitive disorganization

- Shock
- Disbelief
  - As occurs in any crisis, many adolescents regress to previous stages of development.
  - An adolescent rape victim who was previously self-assured and appropriately independent may become clinging and dependent on parent or health professional.
- Immediate response by the family
  - Unlike other crime victims, the victim of rape rarely contacts the police immediately.
  - Typically, victim contacts an intermediary (friend or family member) first.
  - Most family and friends need guidance to know how best to support victim.
  - Disclosure of rape usually is traumatic for the family, as well as the victim.
  - Parents may blame themselves inappropriately.
  - Parental activities or neglect may have contributed to the rape.
  - Familial responses to a child's rape range from:
    - Denial and disbelief *to*
    - Shame and outrage
  - No guarantee exists that a family is prepared to respond appropriately to a raped child's needs.
  - In some cases, a victim's mother's financial dependence on a perpetrator may confound reactions.
  - During the initial evaluation session, health care professionals must spend time with the family members and friends of the victim to determine:
    - Their psychological response
    - Their ability to support the victim

LABORATORY FINDINGS

- Recovery of laboratory and forensic data probably is the most controversial aspect of evaluation, especially when recovery of semen and sperm is involved.
  - Finding of male ejaculate is neither predictive nor essential for criminal conviction.
    - In one study, physical evidence of rape was found in only 23% of all of the cases that resulted in felony convictions.
  - Forensic evidence identified in younger victims is more often obtained from
    - Child's clothing
    - Bed linens
- Newest developments in forensic science have occurred in the laboratory analysis of semen, including
  - Demonstration of quantifiable levels of acid phosphatase
  - Positive monoclonal antibody test
  - MH5 enzyme-linked immunosorbent assay (specific for seminal vesicle antigen) in vaginal fluids

TREATMENT APPROACH

Legal issues

- All states have laws that require physicians to report cases involving violent assault, including rape.
  - To report statutory rape, the clinician should be familiar with state's laws regarding:
    - Reporting sexual abuse
    - Legal age of consent
  - Reporting concerns include the possibility that reporting statutory rape can raise barriers preventing adolescents from obtaining appropriate medical care.
  - Clinicians have expressed the desire to use their clinical judgment in reporting cases of sexual activity that fall within the definition of statutory rape.
  - Some states require parental notification of a minor's sexual assault.
    - In those states, this statute overrides issues of confidentiality.
- Most states permit a minor to receive treatment for sexual assault without parental consent.
  - All clinicians must be familiar with local statutes.
  - Health care providers should seek additional guidance from legal counsel, such as:
    - Their state attorney general's office
- Consent for treatment of rape is different from consent for collection of evidence.
  - An adolescent patient above the legal age of consent has the ability to:
    - Consent to a medical evaluation and treatment
    - Refuse collection of forensic evidence
    - Consent to both
  - Many victims are reluctant to give permission because they fear:
    - Social isolation
    - Possible retribution by perpetrator
  - Adolescent victims should be informed that to pursue prosecution in the future, evidence must be collected at this time.
  - Physician must ask adolescent patient for permission to:
    - Complete a full evidentiary examination
    - Release evidence to the police
  - Exceptions are cases identified by state law to be child sexual abuse.
    - Require mandatory reporting to child welfare agency, law enforcement, or both
    - Do not require consent from patient or family to report
- From a medical-legal perspective, physicians must realize that responsibility is limited to the documentation of evidence.
  - Determining whether rape really occurred is a court decision.

- Physician will be of most help to the victim and the authorities by:
  - Presuming victim is telling the truth
  - Thoroughly conducting evaluation
  - Keeping accurate medical records

WHEN TO ADMIT

- Rape victim with significant physical and/or psychological trauma
- If there is concern regarding return of rape victim to unsafe environment

FOLLOW-UP

- After the initial evaluation is complete, arrangements should be made for follow-up care for:
  - Medical issues
  - Assessment of the victim's ability to cope with the rape
  - Counseling concerning the rape
- All rape victims and families should be seen as soon as possible by a mental health professional who is:
  - Trained to work with adolescents
  - Knowledgeable about the emotional sequelae of rape

COMPLICATIONS

Sexually transmitted infection

- Most patients are concerned about risk of acquiring a sexually transmitted infection (STI) as a result of the rape.
  - Risk is related directly to:
    - Health status of the assailant
    - Health status of the victim
    - Site of the assault
    - Infectivity of the disease in question
  - Overall risk of contracting an STI from a single encounter is small.
  - Repeat assaults, or assaults by more than one assailant, increase risk of infection.
  - Many adolescent victims of rape engage in high-risk behaviors that put them at increased risk of having a preexisting STI.
  - As many as 50% of sexual assault survivors do not return for follow-up appointments.
  - Centers for Disease Control and Prevention recommends using prophylactic antibiotics for treating potential sexually acquired infections.
  - Prophylactic hepatitis B vaccination against possible exposure is recommended.
- Regardless of antibiotics given, clinician must emphasize that:
  - Incubation periods for STIs vary.
  - High possibility exists that infection may be present even if not detected.

R

- STI may be missed or treated inadequately at the time of evaluation examination.
- Baseline studies should be obtained at initial evaluation.
- Medical follow-up is crucial.
- After 2 weeks patient should be reexamined for presence of an STI.
- Serial testing should be performed after the assault in most cases for:
  - Syphilis
  - Human papillomavirus
  - HIV infection

Pregnancy

- Occurrence of pregnancy after rape is strongly influenced by:
  - Whether female patient is in fertile interval of her menstrual cycle
  - Possible sexual dysfunction of the assailant
    - Failure to maintain an erection
    - Failure to ejaculate
  - Many adolescents have irregular menstrual cycles.
  - Occurrence of ovulation for any particular cycle may be in question.
- If assault occurred within 5 days of evaluation:
  - Give pregnancy test to rule out presence of existing pregnancy.
  - Offer emergency contraception.
- Two types of emergency contraceptive are available.
  - Plan B is a progestin-only emergency contraceptive that reduces risk of pregnancy by 89%.
    - Low risk of side effects of nausea or vomiting
  - Second type contains both progestin and estrogen.
    - Most brands of daily oral contraception pill contain both progestin and estrogen.
    - Reduces the risk of pregnancy by 75%
    - Offer antiemetics because of frequent side effects of nausea and vomiting.
- Suspect pregnancy when menses do not occur within 4 weeks of rape.
  - At this point, the patient should return for a repeat evaluation.

Short- and long-term psychological sequelae

- Multiple factors will determine how a child or adolescent responds to the rape, such as:
  - Level of social support
  - Coping styles
  - Strengths
  - Developmental variables
  - Cognitive functions

- Response of any given individual cannot be predicted.
- Psychosocial sequelae of rape often vary according to the type of rape involved.
- Children and adolescents who have been rape victims consistently have:
  - Lower levels of self-esteem after rape than general population
  - Higher levels of precocious sexualization than nontraumatized children
- Confusion may exist about normal adult sexual behavior.
  - Sometimes leads to inappropriate sexual, acting-out behaviors
- Some children experience developmental arrests at the time of trauma.
  - Not necessarily readily apparent
- Child and adolescent studies are too scarce to be considered definitive.
  - Earlier and more traumatic rapes correspond with greater chances of developmental and functional impairment.
- Behavioral concerns frequently associated with adolescent rape sequelae include:
  - School phobias
  - Generalized fearfulness
  - Withdrawal
  - Onset of truancy
  - Suicidal ideations
- Increased lifetime risks of major depression and suicide attempts are associated with women in aftermath of rape.
- For male rape victims existing research is less clear.
  - Male sexual trauma in childhood may be associated with sexually abusive behavior toward other boys during adolescence.
- Not all children and adolescents who have been raped will have psychiatric sequelae.
- All of those who have been raped should be assessed and monitored for serious sequelae.
- In cases in which sexual acting out follows rape, careful clinical attention is required to issues such as:
  - Posttraumatic stress disorder
  - Depression
- Self-medication with various substances is an ongoing clinical hazard after rape.
  - Deserves consideration as a red flag for health care providers working with at-risk patients.

PROGNOSIS

- Date rape
  - Parents' and friends' understanding and support of the victim is a significant prognostic factor for recovery.

R

Rash

DEFINITION

- Change in the skin due to a variety of possible conditions, which can have a wide variety of appearances

EPIDEMIOLOGY

- 10–20% of visits by children to outpatient facilities are associated with a dermatologic problem.

HISTORY

- Diagnosis of skin lesions relies heavily on physical examination and the recognition of types of lesions, but an appropriate, problem-oriented history is first step in diagnosis.
- Sample questions to ask the patient
  - *When did the rash begin? Has it gotten better or worse? Has it occurred in the past?*
    - Such conditions as atopic dermatitis are chronic and recurrent.
    - Others, such as viral exanthems (eg, erythema infectiosum), are acute and self-limited.
  - *Are there associated symptoms?*
    - Generalized erythematous macular eruption associated with fever, nasal congestion, and cough suggests presence of a viral exanthem.
    - Fever, petechiae, and purpura in an ill-appearing child may indicate serious bacterial infection, such as meningococcemia.
    - Atopic dermatitis, contact dermatitis, and scabies characteristically produce pruritus.
  - *Are any medications being taken?*
    - Wheals in a child receiving an oral antibiotic might represent urticaria due to drug allergy.
    - Lithium can worsen acne.
    - Minocycline may cause hyperpigmentation.
    - Neomycin (used in certain topical antibiotic preparations), diphenhydramine (used to reduce pruritus), and certain anesthetics (used to reduce pain or pruritus), applied topically, may induce contact dermatitis.
  - *Are there factors that worsen or precipitate the rash?*
    - Malar rash of systemic lupus erythematosus is worsened by sun exposure.
    - For many with atopic dermatitis, reduced humidity during colder months is associated with exacerbation of disease.
  - *What treatment has been tried, and what was its effect?*
    - Example: Treatment for head lice may fail if product is applied incorrectly or left on the scalp for an insufficient period.
    - Repeating a therapy is unwise if it was used correctly but proved ineffective.
  - *Is there a family history of skin disease or other health problems?*
    - Children with atopic dermatitis often have history of atopic disease, including atopic dermatitis, allergic rhinitis, or asthma.
    - If a child has multiple café-au-lait macules (see Figure 74 on page F26) and a diagnosis of neuro-fibromatosis type 1 is considered, determination of affected first-degree relatives is vital.
    - Whether other family members are similarly affected is relevant if cutaneous infections or infestations suspected.
    - Impetigo, tinea capitis, scabies, and head lice are frequently transmitted within families.
  - For adolescents, in particular, the social history may be relevant.
    - *Do you work after school?*
      - Occupational exposure to greases or oils (eg, in a fast-food restaurant or car repair shop) may worsen acne.
    - *Have you ever been involved in a sexual relationship?*
      - Secondary syphilis and disseminated gonococcal infection, for example, have cutaneous manifestations.
      - Molluscum contagiosum, pubic lice, and scabies may be transmitted through sexual contact.

PHYSICAL EXAM

- Recognizing and describing skin lesions accurately are essential to diagnosis.
- Identify the primary lesion, the earliest and most characteristic of the disease.
- Note the distribution, arrangement, and color of primary lesions, along with any secondary changes.
- Types of primary lesions
  - Flat lesions include macules and patches.
    - Macule: small, circumscribed area of color change without elevation or depression
    - Patch: large macule
  - Elevated lesions may be solid or fluid filled.
    - Solid lesions
      - Papules (<0.5 cm in diameter)
      - Nodules (≥0.5 cm in diameter)
      - Wheals: pink, rounded, or flat-topped elevation caused by edema in the skin)
      - Plaques: plateau-shaped structures often formed by the coalescence of papules
    - Elevated fluid-filled lesions
      - Vesicles (<0.5 cm in diameter and filled with serous fluid)
      - Bullae (≥0.5 cm in diameter and filled with serous fluid)

- Pustules (<0.5 cm in diameter and filled with purulent material)
- Cysts (≥0.5 cm in diameter that represent sacs containing fluid or semisolid material)

- Depressed lesions
  - Erosions: superficial loss of epidermis with a moist base
  - Ulcers: a deeper lesion extending into or below the dermis

- Distribution
  - Certain disorders have unique patterns of distribution; noting the parts of the body involved helps with diagnosis.
    - Seborrheic dermatitis commonly involves the scalp, eyebrows, and nasolabial folds.
    - Psoriasis (see Figure 75 on page F26) affects the scalp and areas that are traumatized (elbows and knees).
    - Acne is limited to the face, back, and chest.
  - Lesions may appear in lines.
    - Vesicles in contact dermatitis from poison ivy (see Figure 76 on page F26)
  - Groups or clusters of lesions
    - Vesicles in herpes simplex virus infection (see Figure 77 on page F26)
  - Lesions that follow a dermatome
    - Vesicles in herpes zoster (see Figure 78 on page F27)
  - Lesions forming an annulus or ring
    - Papules in granuloma annulare
    - Patch in erythema migrans

- Color
  - Skin colored
  - Erythematous (pink or red)
    - If erythrocytes are within vessels (as occurs in urticaria, for example), compression of the skin forces the cells into deeper vessels, and blanching occurs.
    - If cells are outside vessels, as in forms of vasculitis, blanching will not occur.
      - Petechiae
      - Purpura
      - Ecchymoses
  - Hyperpigmented (tan, brown, or black)
  - Hypopigmented (pigment is decreased but not entirely absent)
  - Depigmented (all pigment is absent, as in vitiligo)
  - Violaceous

- Secondary changes
  - Crusting (dried fluid)
    - Commonly seen after the rupture of vesicles or bullae (eg, honey-colored crust of impetigo)

- Scaling
  - Fungal infections (eg, tinea corporis) (see Figure 79 on page F27)
  - Psoriasis
- Atrophy
  - Surface depression from absence of dermis or subcutaneous fat
  - Appears thin and wrinkled
- Lichenification
  - Thickening of the skin from chronic rubbing or scratching (eg, as in atopic dermatitis).

DIFFERENTIAL DIAGNOSIS

- The diagnostic approach is best based on the morphology of the patient's lesions.
  - Appropriate history and accurate description of what is seen usually overcomes obstacles to diagnosis.
  - Once primary lesions are identified, along with distribution, arrangement, color, and secondary changes, observations should be captured in 1 or 2 sentences to assist in differential diagnosis.

Elevated lesions in neonates

- Papules
  - Common
    - Erythematous
      - Erythema toxicum
      - Miliaria rubra
      - Acne (see Figure 80 on page F27)
      - Candidiasis
      - Scabies
    - White
      - Milia
    - Yellow
      - Sebaceous gland hypertrophy
    - Skin colored
      - Epidermal nevus
      - Skin tags
  - Uncommon
    - Yellow
      - Mastocytosis
      - Juvenile xanthogranuloma
- Nodules
  - Common
    - Erythematous
      - Hemangioma

- Uncommon
  - Skin colored
    - Condylomata accuminata
    - Dermoid cyst
  - Yellow
    - Mastocytosis
- Plaques
  - Common
    - Skin colored or yellow
      - Nevus sebaceous
    - Skin colored
      - Epidermal nevus
- Vesicles or bullae (see Figure 81 on page F27)
  - Common
    - Erythema toxicum
    - Miliaria crystallina
    - Sucking blisters
    - Bullous impetigo
    - Herpes simplex virus infection
  - Uncommon
    - Incontinentia pigmenti
    - Aplasia cutis congenita
    - Varicella (see Figure 82 on page F27)
    - Epidermolysis bullosa
    - Bullous ichthyosiform erythroderma
- Pustules
  - Common
    - Erythema toxicum
    - Transient neonatal pustular melanosis
    - Miliaria pustulosa
    - Herpes simplex virus infection
    - Folliculitis (see Figure 83 on page F27)
    - Acne
    - Candidiasis
    - Scabies
  - Uncommon
    - Acropustulosis of infancy

Flat lesions in neonates

- Macules
  - Common
    - Hypopigmented
      - Prehemangioma
      - Postinflammatory hypopigmentation

  - Hyperpigmented
    - Transient neonatal pustular melanosis
    - Café-au-lait macule
    - Postinflammatory hyperpigmentation
    - Congenital melanocytic nevus
  - Uncommon
    - Hypopigmented
      - Ash-leaf macule
- Patches
  - Common
    - Erythematous
      - Salmon patch (nevus simplex)
      - Hemangioma (early)
      - Port wine stain (see Figure 84 on page F28)
      - Atopic dermatitis
      - Seborrheic dermatitis
      - Diaper dermatitis (irritant or seborrheic)
    - Hyperpigmented
      - Mongolian spot
      - Lentigo
  - Uncommon
    - Erythematous
      - Acrodermatitis enteropathica (see Figure 85 on page F28)
    - Hyperpigmented
      - Linear and whorled hypermelanosis
    - Hypopigmented
      - Hypomelanosis of Ito
      - Nevus depigmentosus

Depressed lesions in neonates

- Erosions
  - Common
    - Bullous impetigo
    - Neonatal herpes simplex virus infection
    - Staphylococcal scalded-skin syndrome
  - Uncommon
    - Aplasia cutis congenital
    - Acrodermatitis enteropathica
    - Epidermolysis bullosa
    - Bullous ichthyosiform erythroderma

Elevated lesions in older infants, children, and adolescents

- Papules without scaling
  - Common
    - Erythematous
      - Viral exanthems (many exanthems have a papular as well as macular component)
      - Scarlet fever
      - Insect bites
      - Scabies
      - Urticaria (see Figure 86 on page F28)
      - Papular urticaria
      - Acne
      - Early lesions of guttate psoriasis
      - Erythema multiforme
    - Skin colored
      - Keratosis pilaris
      - Molluscum contagiosum
      - Flat warts
    - Hyperpigmented
      - Nevus (intradermal)
  - Uncommon
    - Yellow
      - Mastocytosis
- Plaques without scaling
  - Common
    - Skin colored
      - Nevus sebaceous
      - Epidermal nevus
    - Hyperpigmented
      - Congenital melanocytic nevus
- Papules or plaques with scaling (papulosquamous disease)
  - Common
    - Tinea corporis
    - Pityriasis rosea
    - Chronic atopic or contact dermatitis
    - Psoriasis
  - Uncommon
    - Dermatomyositis
    - Lupus erythematosus
    - Lichen planus
- Nodules
  - Common
    - Erythematous
      - Pyogenic granuloma

- Skin colored
  - Wart
  - Callus
  - Corn
  - Epidermal cyst
  - Granuloma annulare
- Uncommon
  - Erythematous
    - Angiofibroma
  - Skin colored
    - Neurofibroma (see Figure 87 on page F28)
  - Yellow
    - Mastocytosis
- Vesicles or bullae
  - Common
    - Contact dermatitis
    - Bullous impetigo
    - Varicella
    - Herpes simplex virus infection
    - Hand, foot, and mouth disease
    - Erythema multiforme
  - Uncommon
    - Polymorphous light eruption
    - Linear immunoglobulin A dermatosis
- Pustules
  - Common
    - Folliculitis
    - Scabies
    - Acne
    - Perioral dermatitis
  - Uncommon
    - Associated with systemic bacterial infection (eg, disseminated gonococcal infection)

Flat lesions in older infants, children, and adolescents

- Macules
  - Common
    - Erythematous
      - Viral exanthems
      - Drug eruptions
    - Hypopigmented
      - Pityriasis alba (postinflammatory hypopigmentation)
      - Tinea versicolor
      - Vitiligo
      - Halo nevus

- Hyperpigmented
  - Freckles
  - Postinflammatory hyperpigmentation
  - Tinea versicolor
  - Café-au-lait macules
  - Melanocytic nevus
- Uncommon
  - Hypopigmented
    - Lichen sclerosus et atrophicus
    - Scleroderma
    - Ash-leaf macule
    - Piebaldism
- Patches
  - Common
    - Erythematous
      - Salmon patch (nevus simplex)
      - Port wine stain
      - Atopic dermatitis
    - Hyperpigmented
      - Mongolian spot
      - Becker nevus
      - Lentigo
  - Uncommon
    - Erythematous
      - Toxic shock syndrome (diffuse macular erythema)
    - Hyperpigmented
      - Linear and whorled hypermelanosis
      - Incontinentia pigmenti

Depressed lesions in older infants, children, and adolescents
- Erosions
  - Common
    - Bullous impetigo
    - Herpes simplex virus infection
    - Staphylococcal scalded-skin syndrome
  - Uncommon
    - Epidermolysis bullosa

Hair loss in older infants, children, and adolescents
- Congenital
  - Localized
    - Nevus sebaceous
    - Epidermal nevus
    - Aplasia cutis congenita
  - Diffuse
    - Hair shaft abnormalities
    - Hypothyroidism
- Acquired
  - Localized
    - Friction alopecia
    - Tinea capitis
    - Traction alopecia
    - Trichotillomania
    - Alopecia areata
    - Psoriasis
    - Secondary syphilis
    - Scleroderma
  - Diffuse
    - Telogen effluvium
    - Chemotherapy
    - Hypothyroidism
    - Acrodermatitis enteropathica

R

Recurrent Infections

DEFINITION

- Normal pattern of infections in childhood
  - Healthy children experience 6–8 upper respiratory tract infections per year in the first few years of life.
  - Up to 15 infections per year can still be within the normal range.
  - The high frequency of infections results from immunologic immaturity and frequent exposure to respiratory pathogens.
    - Attendance in child care and exposure to secondhand smoke may increase the number of infections.
- Recurrent infections may be a sign of an underlying, possibly immunologic, disorder.
  - This is much less common than "normal" childhood infections.
  - Early identification of these children is critical.
  - Prompt intervention can decrease morbidity and mortality.

EPIDEMIOLOGY

- In the normal host, infections are:
  - Self-limited
  - Occur more frequently in the winter
  - Associated with periods of wellness between infection
  - The average duration of a viral illness is 7–10 days.
    - A toddler may be sick for up to 100 days or almost one third of the year.
- Primary immunodeficiencies
  - Prevalence (excluding selective immunoglobulin A [IgA] deficiency)
    - 1 in 10,000 cases
  - Sex
    - Boys are affected more commonly than girls because many of these syndromes are X-linked.

MECHANISM

- Defects in anatomic, physiologic, and inflammatory host defense barriers can lead to recurrent infections.
  - Increased susceptibility of young children to otitis media results from an age-related dysfunction of the eustachian tubes, rarely associated with underlying immunodeficiency.
  - Recurrent meningitis may occur as the result of an occult cerebral spinal fluid leak.
  - Recurrent pneumonia may result from foreign body aspiration, tracheoesophageal fistula, gastroesophageal reflux, impaired function of mucociliary transport (eg, cystic fibrosis), and immotile cilia syndromes.
  - Reactive airway disease can produce recurrent respiratory symptoms in association with pulmonary infiltrates.
  - Recurrent infections can occur as a result of alteration in the normal microbial flora associated with antibiotic use and circulatory disorders.

- Secondary immunodeficiencies
  - More common than primary
  - Acquired or a consequence of a nonimmunologic process, including:
    - Infection
    - Cancer
    - Medication (cytotoxic, immunosuppressive)
    - Malnutrition
    - Splenic dysfunction
    - Metabolic disorders
    - Organ transplants
    - Rheumatologic diseases
    - New therapies, such as anticytokines or implantation of foreign materials (eg, heart valves, catheters)
- Primary immunodeficiencies
  - Far less common than secondary
  - Caused by intrinsic defects in the immune system that are genetically determined
  - Classified by the component of the immune system that is affected: humoral, cellular, complement, or phagocytic

HISTORY

- A complete history should be obtained for all children being evaluated for recurrent infections.
- Document characteristics of previous infections
  - Types of pathogens and infections
  - Duration of illnesses
  - Need for hospitalization
- Detailed family history is important.
  - Many of the primary immunodeficiencies are hereditary.
- History of risk factors for HIV infection
  - Personal for adolescents
  - Parental when congenital transmission is a possibility
  - Drug use
  - Prostitution
  - Blood-product transfusion
  - Multiple sexual partners
  - History of sexually transmitted infection
  - Homosexual behavior
- Obtain a complete review of systems.
  - Pay attention to known associated features of immunodeficiency syndromes.
    - Failure to thrive
    - Intractable diarrhea and malabsorption
    - Rheumatologic conditions
    - Hepatosplenomegaly
    - Lymphadenopathy

– Absence of lymph tissue

– Thrombocytopenia

– Eczema

– Oculocutaneous albinism

- Immunization history
  - Failure to make protective antibodies in response to immunizations can be indicative of immunodeficiency.
- Infections associated with an underlying immune disorder may present in various ways.
  - Increased frequency of common infections
  - Repeated serious bacterial infections
- Immunodeficiency may cause a common infection to:
  - Have increased severity
  - Have prolonged duration
  - Fail to respond to appropriate treatment
- Immunodeficiency may cause a common infection to present at an uncommon age.
  - Thrush or candidal diaper dermatitis in children >1 year suggests a defect in T-cell immunity.
- Immunodeficiency may produce an infection with an opportunistic pathogen.
  - *Pneumocystis carinii*
  - *Cryptococcus neoformans*
- Immunodeficiency may become apparent as an infection after the administration of a live virus vaccine (rare).

PHYSICAL EXAM

- A complete physical examination should be performed.
- Children with immunodeficiency appear chronically ill.
- Growth parameters should be obtained to determine the presence of failure to thrive.
  - Height
  - Weight
  - Head circumference
- Physical signs that may indicate underlying immunodeficiency
  - Absence of tonsils
  - Presence of generalized lymphadenopathy and hepatosplenomegaly
  - Skin lesions
    – Eczema
    – Abscesses
    – Seborrhea
  - Mucous membrane involvement
    – Telangiectasias
    – Mucositis
- Look for signs of recurrent infection.
  - Dull, retracted tympanic membranes

- Look for evidence of ongoing infection.
  - Thrush
- Note any specific or abnormal signs that may be associated with a particular immunodeficiency syndrome.
  - Oculocutaneous albinism in Chédiak-Higashi syndrome
- Signs associated with primary immunodeficiencies
  - Intractable diarrhea and malabsorption
    – Severe combined immunodeficiency (SCID), X-linked agammaglobulinemia (XLA), common variable immunodeficiency
  - Rheumatologic conditions
    – Common variable immunodeficiency, IgA deficiency, XLA
  - Hepatosplenomegaly, lymphadenopathy
    – Hyper-IgM syndrome
  - Absence of lymph tissue
    – XLA
  - Thrombocytopenia
    – Wiskott-Aldrich syndrome
  - Eczema
    – Wiskott-Aldrich syndrome, chronic granulomatous disease, hyper-IgE syndrome (Job syndrome)
  - Oculocutaneous albinism
    – Chédiak-Higashi syndrome

DIFFERENTIAL DIAGNOSIS

Secondary immunodeficiency

- Infection
  - HIV
  - Congenital rubella
- Cancer
  - Leukemia
  - Lymphoma
- Medication
  - Cytotoxic
  - Immunosuppressive
  - Corticosteroids
- Malnutrition
- Splenic dysfunction
  - Splenectomy
  - Sickle cell disease
  - Congenital asplenia
- Metabolic disorders
  - Uremia
  - Malnutrition
  - Protein-losing enteropathy

R

- Diabetes
- Galactosemia
- Chromosomal
  - Down syndrome
  - Bloom syndrome
- Improvements in medical care
  - Organ transplants
  - Rheumatologic diseases
  - Cancer
  - Anticytokine therapies
    - Anti–tumor necrosis factor-a for rheumatoid diseases and Crohn disease have been associated with an increased susceptibility to tuberculosis and histoplasmosis.
  - Implants
    - Heart valves
    - Catheters

Primary immunodeficiency

- Evaluation of the child for a primary immunodeficiency should be considered after nonimmunologic and secondary immunodeficiency syndromes have been ruled out.
- Most children are symptomatic within the first few years of life, except in:
  - Common variable immunodeficiency
  - Deficiencies of the terminal complement components
- Primary immunodeficiency is classified by the component of the immune system that is affected:
  - Humoral (see table Humoral Immunodeficiencies)
    - The antibody-mediated arm of the immune system
    - Comprises 50–70% of symptomatic primary immunodeficiencies
    - Children are susceptible to recurrent sinopulmonary infections with encapsulated bacteria.
      - *Streptococcus pneumonia*
      - *Haemophilus influenzae*
  - Combined defects in cellular and humoral immunity (see table Combined Immunodeficiencies)
    - The second largest group of primary immunodeficiencies
    - In addition to bacterial infections, affected children are characteristically more susceptible to fungal, mycobacterial, and viral infections.
    - May experience recurrent or persistent candidiasis
      - Thrush
      - Diaper candidiasis
    - Common viral infections of childhood may cause severe or recurrent disease in affected children.
      - Varicella, for example
  - Complement
    - Least common among the primary immunodeficiencies

- Occurs in older children and in adolescents
  - May experience recurrent meningococcal infection: meningitis or meningococcemia
  - Children may also have gonococcal arthritis.
- Phagocytic
  - Absence of a particular cell type
    - Congenital neutropenia
    - Cyclical neutropenia
  - Defects in chemotaxis
    - Leukocyte adhesion disorder
  - Defects in effector function
    - Chronic granulomatous disease
  - Children typically experience:
    - Recurrent skin infections
    - Abscesses
    - Sinopulmonary infections
    - Poor wound healing
    - Delayed umbilical cord separation
    - Gingivitis
    - Eczema

LABORATORY EVALUATION

- Laboratory evaluation should be guided by the type of infections the child is experiencing.
- Initial screening tests usually include:
  - Complete blood count and differential
  - Serum Ig levels (IgG, IgA, and IgM)
  - HIV serology, as indicated by the history and physical findings
- Tests of humoral immunity
  - B-cell count
  - IgG subclass determinations
  - Antibody titers against protein (diphtheria, tetanus toxoid) and polysaccharide *(Pneumococcus, Haemophilus)* antigens
    - Antibody levels must be interpreted with respect to age-appropriate values.
    - High or low levels can be significant.
- Tests of cellular immunity
  - Delayed-type hypersensitivity skin test (skin testing may not be reliable <1 year of age)
  - Lymphocyte count
    - Total lymphocyte count is obtained by multiplying the total leukocyte count by the percentage of lymphocytes.
    - A value <1500 cells/μL is considered lymphopenia.
- Phagocytic (macrophage or neutrophil)
  - Complete blood count
    - Neutrophil count may be abnormal.

R

Humoral Immunodeficiencies

Syndrome	Clinical Features	Associated Features
X-linked agammaglobulinemia	Susceptibility to encapsulated bacterial pathogens	Asymmetric arthritis, dermato-myositis, malabsorption, absence of tonsils, adenoids, and lymph nodes
	Sinopulmonary and gastrointestinal infections, sepsis, meningitis	
	Enhanced susceptibility to enterovirus and rotavirus	
	Symptomatic polio infection following live polio vaccination	
Transient hypogamma-globulinemia of infancy	Recurrent sinopulmonary infections; generally improves by 3–4 yr of age	May develop IgA deficiency
Hyper-IgM syndrome	X-linked	Low levels of IgG, IgA, and IgE
	Recurrent bacterial infections including encapsulated pathogens	Neutropenia, thrombocytopenia, T-cell defects
	Infections associated with T-cell defects (eg, *Pneumocystis [carinii] jiroveci*) also seen	
Common variable immunodeficiency	Sinopulmonary infections	Most common in second and third decade
	Bronchiectasis	Noncaseating granulomas, malabsorption, autoimmune disease
	Giardiasis	
IgA deficiency	Very common (1 in 400 individuals) but usually asymptomatic	Systemic lupus erythematosus, rheumatoid arthritis, chronic diarrhea
	Recurrent pulmonary infections leading to bronchiectasis	Allergic reactions to γ-globulin preparations
		IgG subclass deficiency in some
Specific antibody deficiency with normal immunoglobulins	Recurrent bacterial infections of the respiratory tract	
IgG-subclass deficiency	Normal immunoglobulin levels but with impaired antibody responses to polysaccharide antigens	
	Clinical significance not well delineated	

- IgE level
  - Elevated in hyper-IgE syndrome (Job syndrome)
- Nitroblue tetrazolium test
- Flow cytometric respiratory burst assay
- Complement
  - CH_{50} assay
  - Screening assay for components of classic complement pathway

IMAGING

- Radiologic studies are used primarily in the diagnosis or management of associated infections.
  - The absence of a thymic shadow can be indicative of DiGeorge syndrome or SCID.

TREATMENT APPROACH

- Pending a complete immunologic evaluation, children who are thought to have immunodeficiency syndromes should not receive live attenuated vaccines, such as varicella, rotavirus, and measles/mumps/rubella, to avoid the possibility of vaccine-associated infection.
  - Vaccine recommendations for specific immunodeficiencies can be found in *Red Book: Report of the Committee on Infectious Diseases.*
- Treatment of primary immunodeficiency is condition specific.

SPECIFIC TREATMENT

Intravenous immunoglobulin (IVIG)

- Patients with humoral and combined immunodeficiencies may benefit from IVIG as replacement therapy.

R

Combined Immunodeficiencies

Syndrome	Clinical Features	Associated Features
DiGeorge syndrome	Clinically variable Increased incidence of viral and fungal infections	Hypocalcemia, hypoparathyroidism, congenital heart disease, abnormal facies
Severe combined immunodeficiency (SCID)	Both B-cell and T-cell deficiencies present Includes a variety of disorders that have multiple modes of inheritance Presents early in life (within first 3 mo of age) with recurrent or severe infections with all types of pathogens	Failure to thrive, diarrhea Most common (50%) form is X-linked Thymic hypoplasia Cartilage-hair hypoplasia with certain forms of SCID At increased risk for graft-versus-host disease with red blood cell transfusions
Ataxia telangiectasia	Recurrent sinopulmonary infections	Truncal ataxia, mental retardation, thymic hypoplasia, telangiectasia of skin and conjunctiva, glucose intolerance, increased risk for malignancy
Wiskott-Aldrich syndrome	Recurrent sinopulmonary infections	Eczema, thrombocytopenia, increased risk for malignancy

- Initial regimen is 300–400 mg/kg every 3–4 weeks.
- Should be adjusted on the basis of the patient's response
- The trough concentration of antibody should be ≥500 mg/dL.
- Replacement IVIG is not indicated for all types of humoral deficiency.
  - Patients with IgA deficiency may develop anaphylaxis to certain brands of IVIG that contain small amounts of IgA.

Other therapies

- Bone marrow transplantation
  - SCID
  - Wiskott-Aldrich syndrome
  - DiGeorge syndrome
- Enzyme replacement
  - Certain forms of SCID (adenosine deaminase deficiency)
- Cytokine therapy
  - Interleukin-2 deficiency
- Interferon-γ treatment
  - Decreases the number of infections in patients with chronic granulomatous disease
- Blood transfusion
  - When needed, should be with cytomegalovirus-negative, irradiated cells to prevent graft-versus-host disease

WHEN TO REFER

- Referral to an immunologist or infectious disease specialist should be considered in the following cases.
  - Recurrent serious bacterial infections
    - Sepsis

- Pneumonia
- Meningitis
- Serious bacterial infection in the context of failure to thrive
- Infection with an opportunistic pathogen
  - *Pneumocystis*
  - *Cryptococcus*
- Vaccine-associated infection
- Unusual age for infection
  - Zoster
  - Thrush
- Unusual severity or chronicity for a given infection
- Family history of immunodeficiency

WHEN TO ADMIT

- All patients with severe infections, infections with an unusual organism, or infections requiring intravenous antibiotics
- Patients suspected of having severe immunodeficiencies, such as SCID or Wiskott-Aldrich syndrome

PROGNOSIS

- Prognosis depends on the type of immunodeficiency and promptness of diagnosis and management of these conditions.

PREVENTION

- The genetic basis for many of the primary immunodeficiencies is now known, and prenatal screening is increasingly available.

R

Red Eye/Pink Eye

DEFINITION

- Red eye, pink eye, or conjunctivitis
  - A nonspecific finding that indicates conjunctival inflammation
  - A variety of disease processes can cause conjunctival inflammation.
  - In most children, it is a benign, self-limiting condition.

MECHANISM

- Neonatal infections can be acquired from:
  - Vaginal microorganisms during birth
    - Vaginal delivery
    - Cesarean delivery, if amniotic membranes rupture before delivery
  - Hand-to-eye contamination from hospital workers.
  - Infectious causes of neonatal conjunctivitis usually develop at least 48 hours after birth (see table Causes of Neonatal Conjunctivitis).
    - *Chlamydia trachomatis*
    - *Neisseria gonorrhoeae*
    - Group B *Streptococcus*
    - *Staphylococcus aureus*
    - *Escherichia coli*
    - *Haemophilus influenzae*
    - Herpes simplex virus (HSV) type 2
- Before the use of topical prophylaxis, ophthalmia neonatorum was a devastating disease associated with high morbidity.
  - Routine topical prophylaxis with silver nitrate, tetracycline ointment, or erythromycin ointment has dramatically reduced its incidence.
- Nasolacrimal duct (NLD) obstruction
  - At birth, tear produchistion by the lacrimal gland is minimal.
  - Normal tearing develops several days to 2 weeks after birth.
  - Normally, the process of nasolacrimal canalization is completed by the end of the 9th month of gestation.
  - When canalization is incomplete, failure most often occurs at the distal end of the NLD at the Hasner valve.
    - Outflow obstruction at the Hasner valve is the most common cause of NLD obstruction.
  - Other, less common anatomic variations within the nasolacrimal system can cause obstruction of tear outflow.
    - Agenesis of the canaliculus
    - Crowding of the NLD opening by the inferior turbinate
- The most common bacteria causing conjunctivitis in children include:
  - *H influenzae*
  - *Streptococcus pneumoniae*

Causes of Neonatal Conjunctivitis

Cause	Time of Onset	Presentation	Conjunctival Scraping	Treatment
Silver nitrate toxicity	Within 24 hr	Watery discharge	Negative gram-negative Giemsa; few PMN	None needed
Neisseria gonorrhea	2–4 days	Lid swelling, purulent discharge; corneal involvement can lead to corneal ulcer and perforation	Gram-negative intracellular diplococci and culture	Topical erythromycin and IV cefotaxime; treat even if asymptomatic
Other bacteria (staphylococci, streptococci)	4–7 days	Purulent discharge, with or without lid swelling	Gram-positive for specific bacteria and culture	Topical erythromycin or trimethoprim–polymyxin B eyedrops, or moxifloxacin
Chlamydia	4–10 days	Variable severity of lid swelling and serous or purulent discharge	Giemsa stain, basophilic, cytoplasmic inclusion bodies, positive direct immuno-fluorescent assay and culture	Initial IV erythromycin, then 50 mg/kg/day by mouth for 14 days; treat even if asymptomatic
Haemophilus	5–10 days	Serous or serosanguineous discharge, hemorrhagic conjunctivitis common; lid swelling with petechiae and bluish lid skin indicate preseptal cellulitis	Gram-negative *Coccobacillus* and culture	Topical trimethoprim-polymyxin B eyedrops and IV cefotaxime
Herpes simplex virus type 2	6 days to 2 wks	Usually unilateral, serous discharge with keratitis, positive corneal staining	Gram stain, multinucleated giant cells, Papanicolaou-stained intra-nuclear inclusion bodies, and herpes culture	Topical trifluorothymidine (Viroptic®) and IV acyclovir

Abbreviations: IV, intravenous; PMN, polymorphonucleocytes.

R

- *Moraxella catarrhalis*
- *Staphylococcus*

HISTORY

- A history of friends or family members with conjunctivitis usually indicates a contagious origin.
  - Viral conjunctivitis is usually caused by an adenovirus and is extremely contagious.
- Ask about itching.
  - Hallmark sign of allergic conjunctivitis
- Eye discharge
  - 1 or both eyes
- Watery
  - Allergic or viral conjunctivitis
- Purulent
  - Bacterial infections
- Infectious conjunctivitis usually begins in one eye, then spreads to the second eye after a few days.
- If only 1 eye is affected, consider:
  - Foreign body
  - Corneal ulcer
  - Herpes simplex keratitis

PHYSICAL EXAM

- The pediatric patient should receive an ocular examination using the mnemonic I-ARM.
  - **I**nspection
  - **A**cuity
  - **R**ed reflex
    - The red reflex test should also be performed on older children with conjunctivitis because an abnormal red reflex may indicate a serious disease process.
    - Benign pediatric conjunctivitis almost never interferes with vision.
  - **M**otility

- Note whether conjunctivitis is unilateral or bilateral.
  - Unilateral conjunctivitis may be caused by
    - Foreign body
    - Corneal ulcer
    - Herpes simplex keratitis
- Note whether there is any discharge.
  - Minimal
    - Blepharitis
  - Watery
    - Allergic reaction
    - Viral conjunctivitis
  - Purulent
    - Bacterial conjunctivitis
- Note presence of preauricular lymph adenopathy.
  - Indicative of viral conjunctivitis
- Distinguishing features of conjunctivitis in children (see table Distinguishing Features of Conjunctivitis in Children)
  - Blepharitis
    - Minimal discharge
    - Minimal itching (real irritation, not itching)
    - *Staphylococcus* on culture common
  - Allergic reaction
    - Watery discharge
    - Marked itching
    - Eosinophils on conjunctival scraping
  - Bacterial
    - Purulent discharge
    - Minimal itching
    - Children with a bacterial conjunctivitis often complain that their eyelids stick together in the morning.
    - Most often, one eye is initially involved, with subsequent involvement of the other.

Distinguishing Features of Conjunctivitis in Children

Feature	Blepharitis	Allergic Reaction	Bacterial	Viral
Discharge	Minimal	Watery	Purulent	Watery
Itching	Minimal (real irritation, not itching)	Marked	Minimal	Minimal
Preauricular lymph adenopathy	Absent	Absent	Absent	Common
Laboratory test results	Staphylococcus on culture common	Eosinophils on conjunctival scraping	Bacteria on Gram stain; PMN response	Lymphocytes and monocytes

Abbreviation: PMN, polymorphonuclear neutrophil.

- The bulbar conjunctiva is diffusely injected, and a mucopurulent exudate is present in the inferior conjunctival fornix.
- Viral
  - Watery discharge
  - Minimal itching
  - Commonly preauricular lymph adenopathy
  - Patients often begin with infection in one eye that then spreads to the other.
  - Eyelids may be swollen, and they may produce reactive ptosis, severe conjunctival hyperemia, and hemorrhagic conjunctivitis.
  - The cornea may be involved; such patients are sensitive to light.
  - Tearing, redness, and the sensation of having a foreign body lodged in the eye are the extreme (termed *catarrhal conjunctivitis*).
- Neonatal conjunctivitis
  - As for all newborns, the ophthalmic examination should start with the red reflex test.
    - The red reflex should be normal, if the abnormality is isolated to the conjunctiva and does not involve the cornea or intraocular structures.
    - Conditions that have an abnormal red reflex test finding and require immediate consultation with an ophthalmologist
      - Endophthalmitis
      - Congenital glaucoma
      - Corneal infections
  - An urgent consultation is indicated if the neonatal patient has marked lid swelling or unilateral conjunctivitis that does not improve over 1 or 2 days.
    - This condition may be HSV-2 keratitis.

DIFFERENTIAL DIAGNOSIS

Conjunctivitis

Neonatal conjunctivitis

- Other causes of a red, teary eye in a newborn include:
  - Congenital herpes keratitis
  - Congenital glaucoma, characterized by clear tears, large cornea, hazy cornea due to corneal edema
  - Dacryocystitis, an infection of the nasolacrimal sac that causes swelling in medial canthal area of lower lid

Gonococcal conjunctivitis

- Occurs approximately 48 hours after birth
- It may appear even earlier if rupture of the amniotic membranes occurs several hours before delivery.

- Typically bilateral, purulent conjunctivitis with copious discharge and lid edema
  - *N gonorrhoeae* is one of the few bacteria that can penetrate intact corneal epithelium, causing corneal ulceration and even corneal perforation.
  - Diagnosis is usually made by identifying gram-negative intracellular diplococci on conjunctival scrapings and verifying by culture.

Chlamydial conjunctivitis

- Typically bilateral and mild to moderate in severity
- Approximately 4–10 days after birth
- Eyelid swelling and a tarsal conjunctival pseudomembrane may be present.
  - A conjunctival pseudomembrane is an accumulation of debris, not a true vascular tissue.
- The diagnosis is confirmed by conjunctival scrapings identifying cytoplasmic inclusion bodies in corneal epithelial cells (Giemsa stain) or by indirect immunofluorescence assay or culture.

Viral conjunctivitis

- Pharyngoconjunctival fever consists of an upper respiratory infection (pharyngitis and fever) with bilateral conjunctivitis.
  - Most commonly associated with adenovirus type 3 and type 7
  - Pharyngoconjunctival fever produces:
    - A severe, watery conjunctival discharge
    - Hyperemic conjunctivitis
    - Chemosis (conjunctival edema)
    - Preauricular lymph adenopathy
    - Quite often, a foreign-body sensation that results from corneal involvement
  - Disease is highly contagious and lasts approximately 2–3 weeks.
- Epidemic keratoconjunctivitis (EKC)
  - EKC is caused by adenovirus types 8, 19, and 37.
  - It occurs most often in older children and adolescents.
  - In contrast to pharyngoconjunctival fever, EKC is isolated to the eyes.
  - The virus causes a severe bilateral conjunctivitis with:
    - Conjunctival hyperemia
    - Watery discharge
    - Eyelid swelling
    - A reactive ptosis
    - Petechial conjunctival hemorrhages are common.
    - Pseudomembrane may be found along the conjunctiva.
    - Preauricular adenopathy may be present.
  - In many instances, one eye is involved first, and the second eye becomes affected several days later.

R

- Approximately one-third of patients develop corneal inflammation (keratitis) with subepithelial infiltrates 7–10 days after onset of the conjunctivitis.
- Keratitis is a hypersensitive reaction to the virus, not a true viral infection.
- Corneal infiltrates cause severe photophobia and irritation.

Hemorrhagic conjunctivitis (conjunctivitis with subconjunctival hemorrhage)

- Common causes include:
  - Infection with *H influenzae*, adenovirus, or picornavirus
  - *H influenzae* hemorrhagic conjunctivitis is associated with a purplish discoloration of the eyelids, caused by multiple tiny subcutaneous hemorrhages.
  - Spontaneous subconjunctival hemorrhage is a painless rupture of a small conjunctival vessel.
    - Usually no known reason
    - Conjunctiva surrounding the hemorrhage will be normal.
    - No tearing or exudate is present.
    - Hemorrhage resolves without treatment.
    - A systemic workup is not usually necessary unless:
      - Hemorrhage becomes recurrent.
      - History of prior bleeding or bruising exists.

Phlyctenular conjunctivitis

- A delayed hypersensitivity reaction to bacterial protein usually associated with staphylococcal blepharitis
- Creamy white or yellowish elevated nodules with a surrounding erythematous base
- Usually located at 3 and 9 o'clock around the limbus
- When tuberculosis was prevalent, it was a major cause of phlyctenulosis.

Seasonal allergic conjunctivitis

- Seasonal allergic (hay fever) conjunctivitis is common and affects approximately 10% of the general population.
  - The hallmark is itching and tearing.
  - Seasona lallergic rhinitis often accompanies seasonal allergic conjunctivitis, which is a type-1 hypersensitivity reaction.
  - Conjunctival scrapings or biopsy samples reveal mast cells and eosinophils.
  - Serum quantitative immunoglobulin E levels are usually high.
  - Skin tests may be positive for environmental allergens.
  - Allergic conjunctivitis is most common in the spring, when pollen levels are high.
  - Many cases occur during the winter, when forced-air heating is turned on and filters have not been cleaned or replaced.

- Diagnosis usually can be made through clinical signs and symptoms.
  - A family history of allergies, atopic disease, or asthma may be found.

Vernal conjunctivitis

- Severe allergic condition characterized by:
  - Severe itching
  - Tearing
  - Mucus production
  - Giant papillae of the upper tarsal conjunctiva
  - Most commonly affects young boys from the Mediterranean basin and from Central and South America
  - Patients often have reactive ptosis and squint in bright light.
    - The result of secondary keratitis caused by the giant papillae scraping the cornea
      - Papillae may be found around the limbus (junction of the sclera and cornea) with characteristic white centers (Horner-Trantas dots representing an accumulation of inflammatory cells, predominantly eosinophils).
      - Conjunctival scrapings of the papillae show many eosinophils.
- Full-blown vernal conjunctivitis is a vision-threatening disease; however, with the advent of topical mast cell stabilizers and antihistamines, this outcome is now rare.

Giant papillary conjunctivitis

- Large papillae develop underneath the superior tarsal conjunctiva as a result of wearing soft contact lenses.
  - Similar to vernal conjunctivitis
  - Reaction results from sensitization of the conjunctiva to allergic materials present on the surface of the contact lens or in contact lens solutions.

Atopic conjunctivitis

- Atopic conjunctivitis is a form of allergic conjunctivitis associated with eczema.
- Serum immunoglobulin E concentrations are often high in these patients.
- Patients with atopic dermatitis often have associated conjunctivitis, with itching, burning, and mucus discharge.

Conjunctivitis associated with systemic disease

- Stevens-Johnson syndrome (erythema multiforme major)
  - Most likely a type-III hypersensitivity reaction associated with mycoplasmal and HSV infections and with many drugs, especially antibiotics and anticonvulsants
  - Patients have fever, malaise, headache, loss of appetite, and nausea.
  - Generalized erythematous papular rash
  - The skin is friable, and traction on it can produce tears.
  - Mucous membranes are most severely affected, including nose, mouth, vagina, anus, and conjunctiva.

- Eye involvement consists of conjunctival injection and the formation of bullae that can rupture and lead to scarring.
- Conjunctival scarring can distort eyelids and turn lashes toward the cornea, causing corneal damage.

Herpes infections

- **HSV-2**
  - Usually associated with keratitis
  - Herpes keratoconjunctivitis may be associated with systemic disease and encephalitis, although it can occur as an isolated eye infection.
  - Onset is usually between 1 and 2 weeks after birth.
  - Serous discharge with moderate conjunctival injection
  - Almost always occurs in only 1 eye
  - Breakdown of the normal epithelial barrier can result in a secondary bacterial corneal ulcer.
  - Early stages of keratitis are detected by corneal fluorescein staining with a geographic or dendritic pattern.
  - Diagnosis is confirmed by viral cultures.
    - May take up to 7–10 days to become positive
- **Recurrent ocular HSV**
  - After initial cutaneous facial infection or infection of mucus membranes, HSV gains access to the sensory nerve endings and travels up the axons to the trigeminal ganglion.
  - The virus remains sequestered and protected within the ganglion.
  - Recurrent ocular herpes infections occurs when virus from the ganglion travels down the sensory nerve and infects the cornea or eyelids.
  - Cutaneous eyelid disease consists of a vesicular reaction similar to primary herpes simplex.
  - Corneal disease from recurrent HSV affects the corneal surface epithelium.
    - Active virus replication causes punctate, dendritic, or geographic epithelial defects.
  - The dendritic pattern is a classic sign of herpes keratitis (corneal infection).
  - Recurrent herpes keratitis is almost always unilateral.
  - Cornea becomes anesthetized as a result of sensory nerve damage.
  - With recurrent herpes, the cornea can scar, and a secondary inflammatory reaction can occur in response to the viral antigen.
- **Herpes zoster and varicella-zoster virus**
  - Chickenpox, or varicella-zoster virus, rarely affects the eye, even when vesicular lesions occur on the eyelid or eyelid margin.
  - Some physicians administer topical trifluorothymidine if the conjunctiva becomes involved.

- In immunocompromised patients, herpes zoster can present a high risk.
  - These patients especially should be treated with antiviral therapy.
- Secondary, or recurrent, herpes zoster ophthalmicus affects patients >50 years or immunocompromised patients.
  - This severe ocular inflammation can affect all layers of the eye.

NLD obstruction and aminotocele

- **NLD obstruction**
  - A watery eye and an increased tear lake
  - Eyelash matting
  - Mucus in the medial canthal area
  - Congenital NLD obstruction is common and occurs in 1–5% of the population.
    - Approximately a third are bilateral.
  - If left untreated, NLD blockage spontaneously opens by 6 months of age in almost one-half of cases.
    - The incidence of spontaneous resolution after 13 months of age decreases to only 15%.
- **Amniotocele (dacryocystocele)**
  - Swelling of the nasal lacrimal sac from an accumulation of fluid within the sac as a result of punctal and NLD obstruction
  - A few days after birth, a bluish swelling appears in the medial canthal area, representing fluid that is sequestered within a distended nasolacrimal sac.

Congenital glaucoma

- *Primary congenital glaucoma* refers to increased intraocular pressure occurring at birth or shortly thereafter.
  - Normal intraocular pressure in infants is approximately 10–15 mm Hg.
  - Intraocular pressure in infants with congenital glaucoma is often >30 mm Hg.
- Congenital glaucoma differs from adult glaucoma by causing enlargement of the eye in addition to damaging the optic nerve.
  - The eye enlarges because, in infants, the eye wall is elastic and stretches.
  - Normal corneas at birth are approximately 10.5 mm in diameter.
  - Corneal diameters >12 mm are considered abnormally large (megalocornea).
  - As the cornea enlarges, breaks of the basement membrane of the corneal endothelium (Haab striae) occur, resulting in corneal edema that reduces vision and can lead to amblyopia.
  - After 3 years of age, the eye wall becomes fairly rigid, and ocular enlargement resulting from glaucoma does not occur.

R

- Features of congenital glaucoma include:
  - Tearing
  - Photophobia
  - Blepharospasm
  - Large cornea
  - Corneal clouding
  - Edema
  - Bilateral in approximately 70% of cases
- The classic findings of congenital glaucoma are not always present.
  - Signs of ocular enlargement and corneal edema may be subtle.
- In cases with tearing, diagnosis of congenital glaucoma may be misdiagnosed as NLD obstruction.
  - In contrast to NLD obstruction, however, the tearing associated with congenital glaucoma is caused by corneal edema.
  - Can be seen as a dull red reflex with an ophthalmoscope
- Primary ocular HSV-1
  - Most adults have been exposed to HSV-1, and unless immunocompromised, have circulating antibodies to the virus.
  - Only 1% of the population will exhibit clinical HSV-1 infection.
  - Most infections are asymptomatic.
  - Primary ocular herpes represents the first exposure to HSV-1.
    - Occurs initially as a skin eruption with multiple vesicular lesions
    - Virus can be cultured from vesicle fluid.

Blepharitis

- Blepharitis, or eyelid inflammation, is one of the most common causes of pink eye in children.
- The 2 most common types of blepharitis are staphylococcal blepharitis and meibomian gland dysfunction.
  - Both types of blepharitis are treated with lid hygiene (lid scrubs with baby shampoo) and topical antibiotics.
- Complaints of itching and burning
- Children often awake with eyelids stuck together with crusting.
- The eyes are irritated, but true itching is not present.
- Crusting and scales at the base of the eyelashes
- The eyelid margins are thickened and hyperemic.
- Vascularization of the eyelid margin
- Lashes may become misdirected, broken, or absent (madarosis).
- Sties, or external hordeolums, are common.
  - An external hordeolum is an abscess of the gland of Zeis on the anterior eyelid margin.

- In contrast to a chalazion, which is deeper and an inflammation of the meibomian gland that results from breakdown of the fatty secretions
- Blepharitis may be associated with corneal changes that cause severe photophobia.

Meibomian gland dysfunction

- Meibomian glands are sebaceous glands with orifices at the eyelid margins.
- Secretions consist of sterol esters and waxes that provide a covering to the tear film, thereby preventing evaporation
- Dysfunction or blockage of the meibomian gland orifice by desquamated epithelial cells results in stagnation of the lipids and causes a secondary local inflammation.
- Microbial lipases from *Propionibacterium acnes* and other bacteria contribute to producing irritating fatty acids that increase the inflammatory response.
- Obstruction of the meibomian gland orifices may result in a chalazion or sty.
  - Chalazion appears as a lump near the upper or lower eyelid margin.
    - Swelling can occur externally as a lump on the skin or internally as a lump underneath the conjunctiva.
    - Chalazion is not an infection, but a granulomatous inflammation that results from the irritating lipids within the meibomian gland.

Molluscum contagiosum

- Molluscum contagiosum is a viral disease of the skin caused by a DNA virus of the poxvirus group often occurring on the eyelids.
- Lesions are small, round, discrete bumps with a central pit.
- Presumed to be contagious and are transmitted by direct touch
- When present on the eyelid margin, they can cause a conjunctival reaction and a follicular conjunctivitis.

Kawasaki disease

- Kawasaki disease is a systemic vasculitis occurring in children usually <8 years.
- Onset of fever, present for >5 days, along with 4 of the following 5 criteria:
  - Nonpurulent conjunctivitis
  - Oral mucus membrane injection or swelling (or both)
  - Erythema and edema of the hands and feet
  - Polymorphous rash
  - Cervical lymphadenopathy
- Vasculitis may involve coronary arteries and cause a coronary aneurysm or a thrombosis that may lead to sudden death.
- The cause of Kawasaki disease is unknown.

Graft-versus-host disease

- Approximately 40% of patients who receive a bone marrow transplant will have graft-versus-host disease.
  - Donor T lymphocytes attack the recipient cells, primarily affecting the skin, liver, intestine, oral mucosa, conjunctiva, lacrimal gland, vaginal mucosa, and esophageal mucosa.
  - Ocular effects of graft-versus-host disease consist of conjunctivitis, dry eye, corneal epithelial erosions, and corneal ulcerations.

Conjunctival nevi

- Congenital or acquired lesions of the conjunctiva are usually located near the corneal limbus.
- They appear as pink or inflamed conjunctiva.
- Nevi come from melanocytes, but they have varying amounts of pigmentation.
- 30% of patients have minimal pigmentation.
- The most common types include junctional, compound, and subepithelial nevi.
- All types have low malignant potential and usually become noticeable in the 1st decade of life through puberty.

LABORATORY EVALUATION

- The initial work-up for presumed infectious neonatal conjunctivitis includes conjunctival cultures on:
  - Chocolate agar
  - Thayer-Martin agar
  - Blood agar
- Conjunctival scrapings should be obtained and examined.
  - Gram stain
  - Giemsa stain
  - Indirect immunofluorescent antibody assay for *Chlamydia*
- If herpes keratitis is suspected (unilateral conjunctivitis with corneal fluorescein staining) then a corneal scraping for herpes culture should be obtained.
- A serologic test for concurrent congenital syphilis infection is advised for venereal-transmitted neonatal conjunctivitis.
- Fluorescein staining of the corneal epithelium is indicated if a corneal abrasion is the suspected cause of the pink eye.
  - Fluorescein staining indicates a defect of the corneal epithelium most commonly caused by a traumatic abrasion, less frequently, an infectious process.
  - Bacterial corneal ulcer
  - Herpes simplex keratitis
- Blepharitis
  - *Staphylococcus* is common on culture.
- Allergic reaction
  - Eosinophils likely on conjunctival scraping

- Bacterial conjunctivitis
  - Polymorphonuclear neutrophils are present.
  - Bacteria on Gram stain
- Viral conjunctivitis
  - Lymphocytes and monocytes are present.

TREATMENT APPROACH

- Neonatal conjunctivitis
  - Treatment of presumed infectious neonatal conjunctivitis before receiving laboratory results includes the use of topical erythromycin ointment and intravenous (IV) cephalosporin, such as cefotaxime.
    - Ceftriaxone is usually avoided in neonates because it may result in hyperbilirubinemia.
  - Antibiotic treatment should be provided immediately after samples are taken for culture.
  - Topical trifluorothymidine (Viroptic) and IV acyclovir should be provided if herpes is suspected.
  - Once laboratory results are known, therapy is tailored to treat the identified organism.
- NLD obstruction
  - Optimal timing for initial NLD probing is controversial.
  - Some experts advocate probing even when the patient is only a few months of age.
  - Most pediatric ophthalmologists suggest waiting until the child is ≥6 months of age.
    - Almost one-half the cases will have spontaneously resolved by then.
  - Other experts suggest waiting until the child is 1 or 2 years of age for probing.
    - Evidence indicates that delaying probing until 1.5–2 years of age means that a single probing will be less successful.
  - Performing initial probing when the patient is between 6 months and 1 year of age allows time for most cases to resolve spontaneously, but it also offers the highest opportunity for success.
  - Probing should be performed on an urgent basis in the case of amniotocele.
  - Probing should be performed in the office without anesthesia.
  - Medical management during the observational period is a combination of nasolacrimal sac massage and intermittent topical antibiotics.
    - Initial massage is directed inferiorly to push the tears in the normal direction, out the NLD.
    - Subsequent massage is directed superiorly so that any tears that did not exit are cleared from the punctum.
    - Occasionally, inferior pressure itself will open a mild NLD obstruction.

R

- Topical antibiotic eyedrops or ointments may be provided if signs of infection are present, eg, mucopurulent discharge.
    - For example, moxifloxacin (Vigamox) or trimethoprim-polymyxin B
    - Drops should be prescribed only when evidence of a true infection exists.
- Congenital glaucoma
    - Treatment is based on decreasing the intraocular pressure.
        - Prevent optic nerve damage
        - Prevent progressive expansion of the eye
        - Reduce corneal edema
    - Medications used to lower intraocular pressures include:
        - ß-Adrenergic inhibitors, such as timolol
        - Carbonic-anhydrase inhibitors, such as acetazolamide an be administered topically or systemically.
        - Adrenergic agonists, such as apraclonidine
    - Medical treatment is not effective in most cases of congenital glaucoma, which is almost always treated with surgery directed at opening the outflow channels at the trabecular meshwork.
- Bacterial conjunctivitis
    - In general, cultures and Gram stain are not routinely performed for mild to moderate conjunctivitis.
    - Patients are treated with antibiotic eyedrops, including the quinolones.
        - Moxifloxacin
        - Levofloxacin
        - Gatifloxacin
        - Ofloxacin
    - Other antibiotic eyedrops include:
        - Sulfacetamide
        - Trimethoprim sulfate
        - Trimethoprim-polymyxin B (Polytrim)
        - Gentamicin
        - Tobramycin
    - Erythromycin ointment may also be applied.
    - An ophthalmology referral should be considered for severe conjunctivitis or chronic conjunctivitis that does not improve after 7 days of treatment.

SPECIFIC TREATMENT

Gonococcal conjunctivitis

- Treatment for gonococcal conjunctivitis is topical erythromycin ointment and IV cefotaxime.
- Parents may also need to be evaluated for possible treatment.

Chlamydial conjunctivitis

- The first-line treatment is topical erythromycin ointment.
- Along with oral erythromycin to remove Chlamydia organisms from the nasopharynx at 1–3 months of age
    - To decrease the risk of subsequent Chlamydia pneumonia
    - Because pneumonitis can occur after neonatal conjunctivitis, parents should be warned of this possibility.
        - Parents harbor the infection and should be treated with oral erythromycin or tetracycline even if they do not have any symptoms.

HSV-2

- If herpes neonatal conjunctivitis is suspected, the treatment of choice is topical trifluorothymidine (trifluridine) combined with IV acyclovir.
- Topical antibiotics should be used to prevent a secondary bacterial infection.

NLD obstruction

- NLD probing is a simple but delicate procedure.
- A small steel wire is passed through the nasolacrimal system, through the Hasner valve, and into the nose.
    - In some cases, the inferior turbinate is infractured to relieve crowding.
- The success rate for NLD probing is >90% when performed before 1.5 years of age.
- In cases in which NLD probing fails, intubation with silicone tubes is indicated to establish a patent system.
    - In general, tubes are used only when the probing procedure fails.
- Amniotocele
- Treatment for a noninfected amniotocele is local massage.
- If decompression does not occur within a few days, then infection (ie, dacryocystitis) is almost certain.
- Because of this likelihood, probing the NLD to open the obstruction may be performed.
- An infected amniotocele is red, warm, and large, approximately 1 cm in diameter.
- Treatment of the infection consists of IV antibiotics (cephalosporin).
- Urgent NLD probing should be performed to relieve the obstruction and drain the abscess.
- Although a cutaneous incision into the sac to decompress the abscess may be performed, this procedure leaves a scar and may produce an external fistula.
- NLD probing does not leave a scar and avoids fistulae.
- Probing has the advantage of directly addressing the primary cause of the abscess by opening the NLD obstruction.
- If the abscess is not drained, then an infected amniotocele can result in cellulitis and even sepsis.

Congenital glaucoma

- The 2 most frequently used procedures are goniotomy and trabeculotomy ab externum.
  - Goniotomy
    - A microscopic knife is used to lyse the abnormal trabecular meshwork to open up the angle.
  - Trabeculotomy ab externum
    - A microscopic probe is placed in the Schlemm canal and then swept through the trabecular meshwork and into the anterior chamber to open up the angle.
  - The success rate of these procedures for congenital glaucoma is approximately 60–70%.
  - If the first procedure fails, a second one may be performed.
  - When these procedures are not successful, a trabeculectomy is usually performed.
    - Trabeculectomy is a filtering procedure in which aqueous fluid is filtered through a small hole in the eye to the subconjunctival space.
- If all these procedures fail, congenital glaucoma can sometimes be managed by ciliary body destructive procedures, such as cryotherapy and laser surgery.
  - Eliminate the ciliary body epithelium that produces aqueous fluid
  - These end-stage procedures have a high failure rate.
- The prognosis for congenital glaucoma is fair, with approximately 70% of patients maintaining good, long-term visual acuity.
  - Unfortunately, patients with unfavorable outcomes often become blind.
  - The most important cause of visual loss is attributed to optic nerve damage, which is not reversible.
  - Other causes include chronic corneal edema with corneal scarring, refractive errors, and, importantly, dense irreversible amblyopia.
- Juvenile glaucoma is more amenable to medical treatment.
  - In many cases, however, juvenile glaucoma must also be treated with surgical techniques.

EKC

- EKC is caused by adenovirus types 8, 19, and 37; the treatment of adenovirus conjunctivitis is prevention of further transmission.
- The clinician must thoroughly wash everything before seeing another patient, if a patient seems to have adenoviral conjunctivitis.
- A patient with this disease will be contagious for up to 2 weeks and should observe isolation precautions during this time.
- Patients with adenoviral conjunctivitis should be referred to an ophthalmologist because of the possibility of corneal involvement.

- No effective antiviral treatment for EKC exists.
  - Cold compresses and topical nonsteroidal antiinflammatory drugs may reduce symptoms.
- A scraping for viral antigen quick preparation is indicated.
- Because of the contagious nature of the adenoviral conjunctivitis, if results are positive, then patients should not return to school for 1–2 weeks.
- Corticosteroids are discouraged except for the treatment of keratitis and should be administered only by an ophthalmologist.

Primary ocular HSV-1

- The use of antiviral medications is controversial.
- Oral acyclovir may be used for severe skin involvement.
- Systemic or topical acyclovir may speed recovery if provided within 1 or 2 days of onset.
- Topical antibiotics applied to the skin may be useful for preventing secondary bacterial infection.
- Over several days to 2 weeks, the skin lesions heal, with or without treatment, usually without much scarring.
- The cornea is involved in 30% of patients with primary ocular HSV-1 infection.
- Topical ophthalmic antiviral medications, such as trifluorothymidine, may be provided to prevent secondary corneal involvement.
- Primary ocular HSV rarely causes intraocular inflammation or uveitis.

Recurrent ocular HSV

- The treatment for acute recurrent herpes keratitis is topical antiviral therapy.
  - Usually with trifluorothymidine (trifluridine).
- Systemic treatment with oral acyclovir has proven to be effective, especially in cases of multiple recurrences or in immunocompromised children.
  - Treatment must sometimes last 6 months to 1 year to prevent recurrence.
  - Topical corticosteroids are not indicated for active herpes keratitis because they will decrease the body's immune response.
  - The clinician needs to be careful about unilateral pink eye because some of these cases may be herpes keratitis.
  - Topical corticosteroids in conjunction with antiviral therapy may be used by ophthalmologists to reduce corneal scarring.

Blepharitis

- Treatment of staphylococcal blepharitis includes eyelid hygiene and topical antibiotic ointment, usually erythromycin.
- In severe cases, systemic erythromycin may be indicated.
- Eyelid cultures are not routinely performed because most eyelids normally are colonized with *Staphylococcus* organisms.

R

- Eyelid hygiene includes lid scrubs with baby shampoo once or twice a day.
  - Prevention of recurrent blepharitis consists of ongoing lid hygiene.

Phlyctenular conjunctivitis

- Treatment consists of treating the blepharitis (lid scrubs and topical antibiotics) and the use of topical corticosteroids.
  - If topical corticosteroids are to be administered, then treatment should be monitored by an ophthalmologist.
- When tuberculosis was prevalent, it was a major cause of phlyctenulosis.
  - Patients with phlyctenular conjunctivitis who are at risk should be evaluated for tuberculosis.

Meibomian gland dysfunction

- Chalazia may resolve without treatment.
- Applying hot soaks several times a day helps the drainage of lipid material.
- If the chalazion does not resolve over several weeks of treatment, then incision and drainage may be necessary.
- An external hordeolum is an acute infection of an accessory gland, which can be treated with:
  - Erythromycin ointment
  - Hot soaks
  - Eyewashes with baby shampoo
- Chalazia may be prevented by eyelid hygiene with eye wipes or a baby shampoo eyewash each day.

Molluscum contagiosum

- Lesions can be treated by excising the central core.
- Rarely, through the use of cryotherapy or application of chemical caustics, such as trichloroacetic acid or aqueous phenol

Seasonal allergic conjunctivitis

- Treatment has greatly improved with the advent of combination mast cell stabilizer–antihistamine eyedrops, such as olopatadine.
  - Mast cell stabilizers require 2–3 days of continued use to reduce symptoms
  - Because they do not inhibit activity of already-circulating histamines, combination mast cell stabilizer–antihistamine eyedrops have a double effect.
  - They provide immediate relief because they directly block histamine receptors and prevent the release of histamine by mast cells.
  - Patients with chronic allergic conjunctivitis can use the eyedrops every day, year round.
  - Side effects are rare.
- In cases of severe allergic conjunctivitis, an oral antihistamine may be added to the eyedrops.

- Topical corticosteroids are reserved for severe allergic conjunctivitis not responsive to other treatment.
  - They are only used for a few days.
  - If corticosteroids are used, then an ophthalmologist should monitor the patient for potential side effects of glaucoma and cataracts.
  - Fluorometholone, a mild topical corticosteroid, is a good choice because it does not penetrate the cornea, thus reducing the likelihood of glaucoma and cataracts.

Vernal conjunctivitis

- Treatment is based on avoiding allergens and using combination mast cell stabilizer–antihistamine eyedrops, such as olopatadine.
  - Patients need to use the eyedrops daily during the allergy season.
  - In temperate climates, patients with vernal conjunctivitis may need treatment year round.
- An oral antihistamine can be added to the use of the eye drops if necessary.
- In some instances, severe episodes of inflammation can be controlled only with intermittent short courses of topical corticosteroids.
  - They should be administered and supervised by an ophthalmologist.

Giant papillary conjunctivitis

- Treatment consists of:
  - Using mast cell stabilizers
  - Discontinuing contact lens wear
  - Changing to a regimen of frequent contact lens replacement
- Prognosis is good.

Atopic conjunctivitis

- Treatment of eye symptoms includes:
  - Use of cold compresses
  - Topical vasoconstrictors
  - Topical antihistamines
  - Topical mast cell stabilizers
  - Topical corticosteroids should be used only for short periods while being monitored by an ophthalmologist.

Stevens-Johnson syndrome

- Therapy remains controversial.
- Topical corticosteroids may be administered early, before advanced disease leads to conjunctival scarring.
  - Their use may prevent severe ocular sequelae.
  - Once conjunctival scarring occurs, however, no effective treatment exists.
  - Patients with Stevens-Johnson syndrome should be referred immediately to an ophthalmologist for consultation.

R

Graft-versus-host disease

- Treatment with topical artificial tears, short courses of topical corticosteroids, and, in severe cases, cyclosporine may improve symptoms.
  - These patients should be referred to an ophthalmologist for careful follow-up.

Conjunctival nevi

- Treatment is controversial, but growth or change in pigmentation of the nevus may be an indication for surgical removal.
- Malignant melanoma is rare in children.

WHEN TO REFER

- Severe neonatal conjunctivitis
- Conjunctivitis with poor red reflex
- Conjunctivitis not improving after 1 week of treatment
- Recurrent conjunctivitis, unilateral or bilateral
- Conjunctivitis with positive corneal fluorescein staining
- Conjunctivitis with decreased visual acuity (20/50 or worse)
- Unilateral conjunctivitis in a contact lens user
- Neonatal swollen nasolacrimal sac (amniotocele)
- Tearing with a poor red reflex
- Tearing with large eye (buphthalmos)
- Patients with conjunctivitis associated with contact lens use should be immediately referred to an ophthalmologist.

WHEN TO ADMIT

- Patients with suspected Stevens-Johnson syndrome
- Neonates with gonococcal conjunctivitis

FOLLOW-UP

- Patients with corneal involvement need to be closely followed for development of corneal scars.
- Patients with congenital glaucoma need to be monitored for pressure changes, as well as visual acuity, by the pediatric ophthalmologist.

COMPLICATIONS

- Corneal scarring due to keratitis
- Loss of vision in patients with congenital glaucoma

PREVENTION

- The best agent to use to prevent neonatal conjunctivitis is controversial.
  - The efficacies of erythromycin ointment, tetracycline ointment, and silver nitrate are approximately the same.
  - The use of povidone iodine as prophylaxis has also been advocated.
    - Effective coverage of a broad spectrum of bacteria
    - Coverage for such viruses as HSV and HIV
    - Little chemical irritation reaction

R

Renal Failure, Acute

DEFINITION

- Acute renal failure is a syndrome of sudden diminution or cessation of kidney function.
- Definitions vary according to specific patient populations and the outcome measure.
  - For example, increase in creatinine level versus need for renal replacement therapy
  - Given that most acute renal failure definitions are based on a serum creatinine increase:
    - Lack of a uniform definition may result in lack of recognition of significant kidney injury and delay in treatment.
    - Creatinine-based acute renal failure definitions are problematic for infants and small children.
      - Normal serum creatinine level is 0.2–0.4 mg/dL.
      - A serum creatinine change of 0.1 mg/dL represents a 25–50% change for small children.
- A graded acute renal failure classification system is needed to assess best the state of kidney injury in patients with a renal insult.
  - Identifies patients at risk for significant kidney insult and metabolic disturbance
  - One system uses the RIFLE criteria to classify degree of kidney insult by changes in serum creatinine and duration of decreased urine output.
    - **R**isk
    - **I**njury
    - **F**ailure
    - **L**oss
    - **E**nd-stage renal disease
  - The change in terminology from *acute renal failure* to *acute kidney injury* (AKI) focuses attention on early recognition of kidney insult and interventions to prevent or mitigate effects of significant renal failure.
- Clinicians still rely on historical definitions based on urine output to characterize degree of acute renal failure.
  - Until RIFLE or other AKI classification systems undergo systematic validation
  - The following definitions are used here for decreased urine output.
    - *Anuria:* <100 mL/m² daily
    - *Oliguria:* <300 mL/m² daily
    - *Nonoliguric state:* sufficient urine volume to allow administration of necessary fluids, nutrition, blood products, and medication without resulting volume overload
    - *Oligoanuric state:* insufficient urine volume to allow administration of necessary fluids, nutrition, blood products, and medication without resulting volume overload

ETIOLOGY

- The causes of AKI in children have changed from primary kidney diseases to secondary effects of other systemic illnesses or their treatment.
- In studies of acutely ill hospitalized patients, the most common causes of AKI in children are:
  - Congenital heart disease
  - Sepsis
  - Nephrotoxic medicines
- Classification of AKI should focus on determining the cause and site of kidney insult.
  - Factors leading to diminished kidney function are often grouped as:
    - Prerenal
      - Causes that diminish kidney perfusion without producing actual parenchymal injury
    - Renal (parenchymal)
    - Postrenal *or*
    - A combination of these mechanisms
  - In children, hypovolemia is the most common clinical situation in which diminished kidney function occurs.
    - Usually results from dehydration associated with acute gastrointestinal losses
    - Hypovolemia may also occur in shock as the result of:
      - Hemorrhage
      - Burns
      - Sepsis
      - Trauma
  - Less common causes of prerenal AKI are those that diminish renal blood flow in the absence of hypovolemia, such as:
    - Congestive heart failure
    - Kidney vascular obstruction from thrombosis or embolism
    - Liver failure
    - Increased kidney vascular resistance, occasionally after anesthesia or surgery
  - Although oliguria or AKI (or both) occur in prerenal syndrome, normal compensatory kidney tubular function usually persists.
    - Characterized by high urinary osmolality and low urinary sodium concentrations as the result of kidney water and sodium conservation.
- AKI from glomerular injury results most commonly from any of the glomerulonephritides or microangiopathy of hemolytic-uremic syndrome.
  - Tubular injury is frequently the result of prolonged ischemia or exposure to a variety of nephrotoxins.

R

- Renal ischemia may be seen in:
  - Hypotensive episodes
  - Severe dehydration
  - Sudden hemorrhage
  - Sepsis
- Tubular toxins may be endogenous (eg, hemoglobin, myoglobin) or exogenous (eg, such medications as aminoglycoside antibiotics).
  - Various chemicals (eg, carbon tetrachloride, diethylene glycol, heavy metals) may cause acute parenchymal kidney failure.
  - Drugs can produce acute kidney failure by inducing a hypersensitivity reaction (drug-induced interstitial nephritis).
- Diffuse pyelonephritis may result in AKI, particularly in infants.
- Kidney cortical necrosis associated with infection, hemorrhage, or dehydration can produce significant irreversible injury to both glomeruli and tubules.
- AKI from intrinsic parenchymal injury may result from:
  - Glomerular disorders
  - Tubular disorders
  - Interstitial disorders

SIGNS AND SYMPTOMS

- Many children with AKI have markedly diminished urine output.
- Complete anuria is unusual and leads to consideration of a catastrophic renovascular event or urinary obstruction.
- In the child with anuria or oliguria, fluid retention can produce:
  - Edema
  - Water intoxication
  - Vascular overload with congestive heart failure
  - Pulmonary edema
  - Hypertension
  - Or any combination
- In many instances, fluid overload is iatrogenic.
  - Results from attempts to increase urinary output by increasing fluid intake
- Early detection of fluid retention is determined best by short-term weight gain on serial measurements and carefully recorded intakes and outputs.
- In contrast, nonoliguric AKI may be clinically covert.
  - Usually suspected only after laboratory tests reveal an elevation in serum creatinine level or an electrolyte imbalance

DIFFERENTIAL DIAGNOSIS

- The processes contributing to kidney functional impairment can frequently be identified from the patient's history.
- Reduction in urine production is not included in the definition of AKI.
  - Kidney failure occurs not only in anuric states but also in patients with oliguric or nonoliguric states.
  - Some kidney insults are frequently associated with oligoanuric AKI.
    - Various glomerulonephritides
    - Hemolytic-uremic syndrome
  - Others will more often cause nonoliguric kidney failure.
    - Aminoglycoside toxicity
  - Determining the type of insult provides clinician with insights into:
    - Possible manifestations of kidney failure
    - Probable duration of AKI
    - Overall prognosis
  - History often helps distinguish between an episode of AKI in an otherwise healthy child and acute deterioration of kidney function in a child with preexisting undiagnosed chronic kidney disease.
  - A history of the following would lead the practitioner to suspect undiagnosed kidney disease.
    - Urinary abnormalities
    - Fatigue
    - Pallor
    - Slowed linear growth
    - Poor school performance
    - Anorexia extending over a period
- AKI may be heralded by seizures precipitated by:
  - Hypocalcemia
  - Hypertensive encephalopathy
  - Uremia
  - Water intoxication
  - It is not unusual for a child to first have a sudden onset of seizures and other signs of central nervous system dysfunction, only to be found to have AKI.

LABORATORY FINDINGS

- Abbreviations used in this section: *U*, urine; *Na*, sodium; *Cr*, creatinine; *S*, serum.
- Clinical tests to differentiate functional from parenchymal oliguric AKI
  - Sodium conservation
    - Urine sodium concentration (U_{Na})
      - Functional AKI: <20 mEq/L
      - Parenchymal AKI: >40 mEq/L
      - Discrimination: poor

R

– Fractional excretion of sodium (FE_{Na}):
$FE_{Na} = (U_{Na} \times S_{Cr}) / (S_{Na} \times U_{Cr}) \times 100$

- Functional AKI: <1
- Parenchymal AKI: >1
- Discrimination: good
- Children with nonoliguric acute tubular necrosis can have FE_{Na} <1%.
- The FE_{Na} test is only helpful for oliguric acute tubular necrosis.
- The threshold for FE_{Na} in neonates is 3% and not 1%.

• Water conservation

– Urine osmolality (Uosm)

- Functional AKI: >500 mOsm/L
- Parenchymal AKI: >350 mOsm/L
- Discrimination: Poor

– Urine/serum osmolality ratio (Uosm/Sosm)

- Functional AKI: >2
- Parenchymal AKI: <1.1
- Discrimination: fair

– Response to diagnostic challenge with intravenous mannitol and furosemide

- Functional AKI: urine flow increase
- Parenchymal AKI: no change
- Discrimination: good

■ Biochemical disturbances that contribute to clinical findings in AKI are complex and interrelated.

• Inherent to diagnosis of acute renal failure is accumulation of nitrogenous waste products characterized by increases in blood urea nitrogen and creatinine levels.

• If hypotonic fluids have been used in excess to hydrate the patient, dilutional hyponatremia and anemia may affect central nervous system and cardiac function adversely.

• Hyperkalemia is often the result of injudicious potassium administration or inadequate renal potassium excretion.

• In AKI, metabolic acidosis develops as result of the kidney's failure to excrete hydrogen ions and reabsorb bicarbonate.

– Any state associated with increased catabolism may accentuate degree of acidosis as a result of increased production of organic and inorganic acid radicals.

- Shock
- Fever
- Poor caloric intake
- Extensive tissue damage

– Acidosis promotes further hyperkalemia resulting from:

- Movement of intracellular potassium into extracellular space as the body attempts to accommodate the higher hydrogen ion concentration

– Respiratory compensation for an underlying metabolic acidosis may cause low carbon dioxide pressure resulting from tachypnea or Kussmaul breathing.

• Failure of phosphate excretion can lead to hyperphosphatemia.

– The hypocalcemia associated with hyperphosphatemia may exhibit clinically as:

- Tremors
- Tetany
- Seizures

TREATMENT APPROACH

■ Acute kidney injury management should begin before consulting with a nephrologist and before initiating renal replacement therapy.

• Maintenance of adequate urine volumes and prevention and treatment of metabolic derangements are the goals of therapy in children with acute renal failure.

• The essential first measure to maintain urine output in critically ill patients is:

– Preservation or restoration of renal perfusion with appropriate fluid resuscitation and inotropic agents

SPECIFIC TREATMENTS

Goal-directed fluid therapy

■ Represents use of physiologic end points to guide initiation and termination of fluid resuscitation of patients in shock

• Heart rate
• Central venous pressure
• Mean arterial pressure

■ Goal-directed fluid therapy leads to better survival in adults with shock.

■ Adult patients who receive early goal-directed fluid therapy in the emergency center:

• Received more fluid in emergency center but received less fluid and have better survival in the intensive care unit compared with patients who receive standard therapy

■ The concept that worsening fluid overload is associated with worse outcomes in critically ill pediatric patients who require renal replacement therapy was the focus of a recent pediatric study.

• The Prospective Pediatric Continuous Renal Replacement Therapy Registry Group demonstrated that worsening fluid overload is an independent risk factor for mortality.

• Earlier initiation at lesser fluid overload degrees may:

– Allow more expeditious optimal nutrition and blood product provision without further fluid or waste product accumulation

– Prevent worsening volume overload and, in particular, pulmonary edema

Medication dosing

- Most pediatric drug dosing is based on intensive care unit admission weight.
  - Worsening fluid overload might increase volume of distribution of inotropes, antimicrobials, and chemotherapeutic agents, resulting in underdosing.
- Medication dosing should be altered for specific drugs that are primarily eliminated by the kidneys.
  - Drug dose or interval (or both) may need to be altered on the basis of the level of kidney dysfunction.
  - Drug concentrations can be wholly or partially reduced by dialysis in patients who receive intermittent or continuous renal replacement therapy.
  - Factors associated with enhanced dialytic elimination include low volume of distribution and low protein binding.

Treatment in hyperkalemia in pediatric patients

- Calcium gluconate (10%)
  - Dose: 0.5 mL/kg IV over 2–4 min
  - Effect: rapid but transient
  - Monitor the electrocardiogram for bradycardia during injection; may be repeated but is not likely to be effective.
- Sodium bicarbonate (7.5%)
  - Dose: 2.5 mEq/kg (approximately 3 mL/kg) IV by slow push
  - Effect: rapid but transient
  - Repetition is not recommended.
- Glucose (50%)
  - Dose: 1 mL/kg IV by slow push
  - Effect: Within 1–2 hr
  - Attempt to increase blood glucose level to 250 mg/dL; may be maintained by infusion of 30% glucose at rate equal to insensible fluid loss.
- Insulin (regular)
  - Dose: 0.1 U/kg IV
  - Effect: rapid
  - Give only with hypertonic glucose infusion (30%).
- Sodium polystyrene sulfonate (Kayexalate)
  - Dose: 1 g/kg PO or PR
  - Effect: 3–6 hr
  - Side effects: gastric irritation (nausea and vomiting), diarrhea, or fecal impaction
  - Oral administration is more effective than rectal administration.
  - Enemas should be retained >60 minutes and removed by a cleansing enema.
  - May cause hypokalemia: use cautiously in patients who tolerate sodium loads poorly
  - Chelates Ca^+ and Mg^+

WHEN TO ADMIT

- When AKI is unexplained, rapidly progressive, or oliguric or anuric
- In the presence of severe or potentially dangerous fluid or metabolic abnormalities (eg, hyperkalemia, hypocalcemia, acidosis, clinical fluid overload, dehydration)
- For renal biopsy

WHEN TO REFER

- For guidance on diagnostic evaluation
- Management of complex fluid, mineral, electrolyte, and blood pressure abnormalities
- Evaluation of dialysis options and preparation for and implementation of dialysis or continuous renal replacement therapy (CRRT)
- Disease-specific management

COMPLICATIONS

- Hyperkalemia is a potentially life-threatening complication of AKI.
  - Can be especially severe in disease states associated with cellular damage and the consequent release of intracellular potassium
    - Hemolysis
    - Burns
    - Trauma
    - Infections
- Hyperkalemia produces a state of increased neuromuscular excitability, including a vulnerability to cardiac arrhythmias.
- Unfortunately, hyperkalemia produces no consistent physical signs.
  - Diagnosis depends on measurement of serum potassium *and*
  - If indicated, assessment of electrocardiogram for evidence of altered cardiac electrical activity

PROGNOSIS

- In the past decade, survival rates stratified by the renal replacement therapy modality have been stable.
  - Survival rates for patients receiving hemodialysis are higher than those receiving peritoneal dialysis or CRRT.
    - Hemodialysis: 73–89%
    - Peritoneal dialysis: 49–64%
    - CRRT: 34–42%
  - Better survival in patients who receive hemodialysis likely results from improved hemodynamic stability.
    - No prospective pediatric study that controls for patients illness severity has compared survival across modalities.

R

– Improvements in pediatric specific technology and CRRT techniques have led to:
  ■ Preferential use of CRRT in pediatric patients with AKI
  ■ Decreased morbidity in patients who require CRRT
■ The 3- to 5-year patient survival of an AKI episode is 57%.
  • Approximately 60% of patients demonstrate evidence of chronic kidney injury.

PREVENTION

■ Routine evaluation of all pediatric AKI survivors may help prevent the long-term sequelae of AKI.
  • Chronic kidney disease
  • Hypertension
  • Microalbuminuria

Renal Tubular Acidosis

DEFINITION

- Renal tubular acidosis (RTA) is impaired capacity of the kidney to excrete the usual daily load of acid arising from metabolism.
  - Renal excretory function, as estimated by creatinine clearance, is relatively intact.
  - Metabolic acidosis results from a defect affecting tubular mechanisms for acid excretion, with intact glomerular filtration.
  - Not caused by underexcretion of acid due to kidney failure or increase in acid production (eg, in diabetic ketoacidosis, lactic acidosis, or total parenteral nutrition)
- Consequence of mismatch between the usual rate of acid production and renal acid excretion
- Principal cause of hyperchloremic metabolic acidosis in an infant or child ingesting a typical diet who does not have gastroenteritis or chronic kidney disease

ETIOLOGY

- Possible explanation for impaired growth in children with RTA
  - Metabolic acidosis suppresses pulse amplitude of growth hormone secretion in rats.
  - The principal mediator on target organs of growth hormone is insulinlike growth factor 1 (IGF-1), which is also suppressed by acidosis.
  - Consequent antianabolic effect results in decreased net protein synthesis.
  - Expression of IGF-1 receptor in epiphyseal growth plate of long bones and of hepatic growth hormone receptor is suppressed by acidosis.
  - Metabolic acidosis impairs conversion of 25-hydroxy vitamin D_3 to its biologically active form, 1,25-dihydroxy vitamin D_3.
  - Increase in 1,25-dihydroxy vitamin D_3 by dietary phosphorous restriction may be reversed by metabolic acidosis.
  - Impaired phosphate reabsorption of the Fanconi syndrome contributes to rickets and short stature.
  - Buffering of hydrogen ions (H^+) by bone causes release of calcium (Ca^{2+}) and consequent hypercalciuria, which may contribute to osteopenia and short stature in certain forms of RTA.
  - Metabolic acidosis inhibits osteoblasts and bone turnover.
  - Growth impairment is multifactorial, and some children with Fanconi syndrome continue to lag in growth despite correction of metabolic acidosis.
- Mechanisms of acid excretion
  - The role of the kidneys in maintaining pH homeostasis principally involves 2 discrete processes in handling of bicarbonate (HCO_3^-).
    - Reclamation
      - Absorb filtered HCO_3^- in proximal segments of nephron
    - Regeneration of HCO_3^-
      - Excrete H^+ in form of ammonium (NH_4^+) and dihydrogenphosphate ($H_2PO_4^-$) in collecting duct and, in the process, generate new HCO_3^-
    - These processes are the basis for the physiologic classification of RTA into 2 main types.
      - Reclamation type
        - Traditionally referred to as proximal RTA or type 2 RTA
      - Regeneration type
- Mechanisms of ammonium excretion
  - All forms of RTA are due to inability of the kidneys to maintain the plasma HCO_3^- concentration at a physiologic level in the face of the usual rate of acid production.
  - A common feature is a low rate of NH_4^+ excretion.
  - NH_4^+ excretion involves the proximal and distal segments of nephrons.
  - 4 steps are involved, each of which is implicated in the pathogenesis of forms of RTA.
    - Ammoniagenesis occurs in the proximal tubule.
      - Impaired by hyperkalemia occurring in mineralo-corticoid deficiency or unresponsive states
    - Absorption in the thick ascending limb of the loop of Henle by occupying the K^+ site on the apical $Na^+–K^+– 2Cl^-$ cotransporter
      - Also impaired by hyperkalemia because K^+ more effectively competes with NH_4^+ for same binding site on transporter
    - Interstitial accumulation of NH_3; depends on an intact countercurrent system for concentration of solute in renal medulla
      - Impaired transport of NH_4^+ affects this step, as does inflammation and scarring of inner medulla (distorts the architecture of countercurrent multiplier system responsible for increasing concentration of solutes and NH_3).
      - The countercurrent system is also affected by nephrocalcinosis, which occurs in regeneration-type RTA and is typically accompanied by a low rate of citrate excretion.
    - Diffusion of NH_3, which has accumulated to relatively high concentration in the medullary interstitium, into the lumen of the collecting duct
      - Consequence of 2 different defects affecting iontrapping of NH_4^+—either H^+ secretory defect or voltage defect

SIGNS AND SYMPTOMS

- Rarely presents as isolated idiopathic hypercalciuria or passage of a kidney stone in a child with incomplete RTA, which may be accompanied by a family history of nephrolithiasis in association with hypocitraturia

- For some children in at-risk families, hypocitraturia may be the only indication of so-called incomplete RTA.

- Family history should be explored with questions about other affected family members in preceding generations or affected siblings of the individual with suspected RTA.

- With apparent de novo RTA, consanguinity may play role.

- Apparent isolated nephrolithiasis in other family members may be significant.

- A history of sudden unexplained death in a neonate suggests the possibility of a salt-losing condition that may be associated with RTA.

- Failure to thrive during infancy is often a presenting feature of RTA.

DIFFERENTIAL DIAGNOSIS

- The clinician is more likely to encounter secondary forms of RTA that result from drugs, toxins, or acquired medullary tubulointerstitial disease.

- Other instances of RTA are associated with:
  - Another heredofamilial disorder, such as cystinosis, *or*
  - Other causes of Fanconi syndrome

- The transient form of RTA may occur in young infants with delayed maturity of renal tubular function.

- RTA, in association with hyponatremia and hyperkalemia, can also present as acute life-threatening event in some infants with profound salt-losing condition and hypovolemia.
  - Pseudohypoaldosteronism type 1
  - Congenital adrenal hyperplasia with insufficient mineralocorticoid production

- Reclamation-type RTA may be an isolated defect and, in some infants, simply a transient immaturity of function that eventually resolves.

- Heredofamilial RTA syndromes in children are due to mutations of genes encoding ion transporters or channels that play a key role in the kidney's contribution to acid-base balance.
  - Rare primary monogenic disorders that have classical Mendelian patterns of inheritance
  - Pseudohypoaldosteronism type 1
  - Congenital adrenal hyperplasia with insufficient mineralocorticoid production

DIAGNOSTIC APPROACH

- RTA should be considered in any infant or young child with any of the following conditions.
  - Failure to thrive
  - Recurrent vomiting
  - Short stature
  - Rickets
  - Nephrocalcinosis
  - Hypotonia
  - Muscle weakness
  - Sensorineural hearing loss
  - Recurrent episodes of dehydration
  - Kidney stones
  - Gastroenteritis with incomplete recovery from metabolic acidosis

LABORATORY FINDINGS

- In the absence of blood gas analysis confirming acidemia, consider RTA if:
  - Venous blood carbon dioxide (CO_2) content is <20 mEq/L in an infant or young child.
  - The child has hyperchloremia.
  - The anion gap is normal.
  - Urine pH is not <5.5.

- Once a renal cause for hyperchloremic metabolic acidosis is established, estimate urinary NH_4^+ by measuring Na^+, K^+, and Cl^- in a random urine specimen and calculating the urinary anion gap (UAG).
  - On a typical diet, Cl^- is the main anion accompanying urinary NH_4^+, and the concentration of Cl^- exceeds the sum of Na^+ and K^+.
  - Because urinary NH_4^+ is not directly measured, the UAG is negative or close to zero.
  - With regeneration-type RTA, the rates of NH_4^+ excretion and Cl^- excretion are low; its concentration is usually less than the sum of $[Na^+] + [K^+]$; and in this instance, UAG is positive.
  - This estimate is less reliable if urine pH is relatively alkaline, exceeding 6.7, at which HCO_3^- becomes significant component of unmeasured anions.
  - The UAG is normal in reclamation-type RTA during the acidemia that ensues after stopping alkali treatment.
  - The UAG estimate in such patients is not reliable during alkali treatment because of massive HCO_3^- wasting.

- Urine osmolal gap (UOG): another surrogate measure for urinary NH_4^+
  - Actual NH_4^+ is approximately half the UOG because concentrations of NH_4^+ and Cl^- are approximately equal.

- Use a pH meter to determine urine pH.

- Provocative test of capacity to acidify urine: administer furosemide and, later, measure urine pH.
  - Administer fludrocortisone (Florinef) about 1 hour before infusion of furosemide.
  - Failure to acidify urine to pH <5.5 suggests defect of H^+ secretion.

■ Traditional way to assess rate of H^+ secretion in collecting duct: measure urine-to-blood PCO_2 gradient by intravenous administration of $NaHCO_3$ load in a clinical research center.

  ● In the ambulatory setting, achieve a similar effect by aggressive treatment of regeneration-type RTA with bicarbonate precursor (eg, oral sodium or potassium citrate).

  ● If the urine-to-blood PCO_2 gradient is <20 mm Hg, then an H^+ secretory defect is likely.

  ● Promptly aspirate the voided urine specimen into a syringe, eliminating dead space, to minimize loss of CO_2.

  ● Administering a single dose of acetazoleamide also loads distal H^+ secretory sites with HCO_3^-.

■ The renal HCO_3^- threshold in a child suspected of having reclamation-type RTA may be estimated over several days after beginning treatment with alkali.

  ● Monitor urine pH and blood HCO_3^-.

  ● The threshold is a level of blood HCO_3^- at which urine pH increases markedly, indicating bicarbonaturia, approaching 10–15% of filtered load.

■ If the serum K^+ concentration is low or normal, diagnostic possibilities include reclamation-type or nonhyperkalemic regeneration-type RTA.

■ If urine glucose is positive, further testing is done to establish Fanconi syndrome in association with reclamation defect.

■ Empiric treatment with citrate solution may confirm the diagnosis of reclamation defect if the dose required to correct the serum HCO_3^- approaches 10–15 mEq/kg/day, well above the endogenous rate of acid production.

  ● An increased dose may be required in some infants with regeneration-type RTA as a transient phenomenon during the first few years of life.

■ In young infants, obtaining reliable 24-hour urine collection to estimate calcium excretion is impossible without an indwelling catheter.

  ● Collect multiple random specimens throughout the day.

■ Age range and calcium-to-creatinine ratio (mol/mol, mg/mg), 95th percentiles

  ● 1 month–1 year: 2.2, 0.81

  ● 1–2 years: 1.5, 0.56

  ● 2–3 years: 1.4, 0.50

  ● 3–5 years: 1.1, 0.41

  ● 5–7 years: 0.8, 0.30

  ● 7–10 years: 0.7, 0.25

■ If the serum K^+ concentration is high, suggesting hyperkalemic regeneration-type RTA, an impaired capacity to secrete K^+ may be confirmed by:

  ● Measurement of K^+ and osmolality in plasma

  ● Random urine specimen

  ● Calculation of the transtubular potassium gradient (TTKG)

    – In the setting of hyperkalemia, TTKG should be ≥8 if the distal tubule responds to mineralocorticoid.

  – A value <8 suggests insufficient production of aldosterone or lack of responsiveness of the mineralocorticoid receptor aldosterone.

■ Pseudohypoaldosteronism type 1 is suggested by increased level of plasma aldosterone and renin.

■ If aldosterone and renin are suppressed and blood pressure is increased, the rare familial hyperkalemic hypertension syndrome (pseudohypoaldosteronism type 2) is possible.

■ If blood pressure is normal or low and aldosterone is low in clinical setting of salt-wasting, consider congenital adrenal hyperplasia.

■ If aldosterone is high, consider the severe, potentially fatal neonatal presentation of pseudohypoaldosteronism type 1.

IMAGING

■ Ultrasonography

  ● Medullary nephrocalcinosis confirms nonhyperkalemic regeneration-type RTA because this type is also associated with hypercalciuria and hypocitraturia.

CLASSIFICATION

■ Conventional classification

  ● Type 1: classic distal RTA

  ● Type 2: proximal RTA

  ● Type 3: hybrid of 1 and 2

  ● Type 4: distal defect that results in high levels of potassium in the blood

■ Physiologic classification: now in use because it is physiologically accurate

  ● 2 basic processes of HCO_3^- absorption are the basis.

    – Reclamation type

      ■ Type 2 proximal (conventional classification)

      ■ Most reclamation-type disorders are accompanied by other defects localized to the proximal tubule, such as Fanconi syndrome (impaired absorption of amino acids, glucose, and phosphate).

      ■ May be a transient isolated defect in infancy that resolves in time

    – Regeneration type, including classic distal type 1 RTA—there are 2 types:

      ■ Nonhyperkalemic

      ■ Hyperkalemic (acidification intact: pseudohypoaldosteronism Ia, Ib, II; acidification impaired: medullary tubulointerstitial disease)

    – Hybrid of reclamation and regeneration: old type 3

TREATMENT APPROACH

■ Aims of treatment

  ● Correct metabolic acidosis

  ● Correct growth impairment

R

- Mitigate osteopenia
- Prevent chronic kidney failure caused by progression of nephrocalcinosis (in the instance of a primary H^+ secretory defect)

■ Appropriate treatment with alkali restores growth to the expected trajectory, but the requirement to sustain growth was 2- to 5-fold greater than the expected rate of endogenous acid production.

SPECIFIC TREATMENTS

Citrate solution

■ Mainstay of treatment in most children

■ Hypokalemia and K^+ depletion are characteristic of non-hyperkalemic regeneration-type RTA; thus, potassium citrate preparation is optimal (eg, Polycitra-K).

■ The solution contains:
- 2 mEq/mL of K^+ and 2 mEq/mL of HCO_3^- precursor as citrate
- Citric acid (to make it taste better)
- pH of approximately 5 before further dilution
- Solution is hyperosmolar; must first be diluted 4- or 5-fold with water or formula before oral administration.

■ Potassium citrate is available as a capsule (Urocit-K) in 2 dose forms, providing 5 mEq or 10 mEq of K^+.
- Slowly released from wax matrix; the capsule must be swallowed whole and not opened or crushed.

■ Monitor serum potassium, especially if the glomerular filtration rate is reduced or the patient is receiving angiotensin-converting enzyme inhibitor or angiotensin-receptor blocker.

■ Polycitra (not Polycitra-K) provides 1 mEq of K^+/mL and 1 mEq of Na^+/mL and requires dilution before administration.
- Avoid K^+-containing solutions in hyperkalemic forms of RTA.

■ Sodium-containing solutions (eg, Bicitra)
- May be used for buffer repletion in hyperkalemic regeneration-type RTA
- Provide 1 mEq of Na^+/mL and thus has lower osmolality than Polycitra K or Polycitra
- Requires dilution to lower strength for safety and palatability
- Total daily dose should be divided into 3 or 4 doses to minimize amplitude of fluctuations of serum HCO_3^- level that may occur with less frequent administration.
- Metabolic acidosis inhibits growth hormone secretion, so administer a somewhat larger dose of citrate solution at bedtime to coincide with the nocturnal peak of growth hormone release.

■ $NaHCO_3$ may be used, but rapid buildup of CO_2 in the stomach after ingestion may cause gastric distention.
- This approach may be a preferable means of buffer repletion in infants who refuse citrate solutions.
- 1-quarter teaspoon of baking soda powder ($NaHCO_3$) provides 13 mEq each of Na^+ and HCO_3^- and should be diluted in water or infant formula.
- Tablets of $NaHCO_3$ are available, which may be crushed.

■ Adequate treatment of nonhyperkalemic RTA with citrate should lessen hypercalciuria.
- Nephrocalcinosis, once established, is not reversible.
- The aim of treatment is to prevent its further progression to end-stage kidney disease.

■ Given the risk of hypokalemia, severe K^+ depletion, muscle weakness, and even paralysis, treating hypercalciuria with thiazide should be done only with frequent monitoring of serum K^+ and provision of an adequate dose of potassium citrate.

■ Adequate treatment with potassium citrate should correct metabolic acidosis, reduce urinary calcium excretion, and obviate the need for a thiazide.

■ Correction of acidosis does not ameliorate hearing impairment of autosomal-recessive forms of proton-pump defects of type A intercalated cells.

■ Monitor growth and serum electrolytes periodically.

■ Maintain serum HCO_3^- near the upper limit of range between 25 and 29 mEq/L.

■ Draw blood just before the next dose of alkali.

WHEN TO ADMIT

■ Hypovolemia (often caused by diarrhea or vomiting illness)

■ Hypokalemia with serum K^+ <2.5 mEq/L accompanied by muscle weakness

■ If adherence with the medication regimen or intercurrent illness interferes with taking medication, hospitalization may be needed for parenteral administration of HCO_3^- to treat severe metabolic acidosis.

■ Kidney stone

WHEN TO REFER

■ Comprehensive evaluation of suspected RTA entails studies in a kidney function laboratory; referral to a nephrologist is appropriate.

■ The role of primary care physician is to:
- Be aware of the possibility of RTA
- Take some initial steps in patient's workup, such as calculation of UAG or UOG

■ More detailed studies and explanations to the parents are best accomplished by a pediatric kidney disease specialist.

- Genetic counseling is needed for parents with a child who has monogenic RTA disorder, in anticipation of possible future pregnancies.
- Because commercially available gene testing is not yet available, the consultant nephrologist may have access to a research laboratory capable of sequencing DNA.

FOLLOW-UP

- Once a child is established on an effective treatment regimen and is clinically stable, periodic follow-up by the primary care physician may be done in collaboration with a nephrologist.

COMPLICATIONS

- RTA associated with episodic hypokalemia may be accompanied by profound muscle weakness and, in some instances, recurrent paralysis.
- Most children with RTA (especially those with nephrocalcinosis) have impairment of urinary concentrating mechanism and consequent obligatory polyuria.
- Superimposed dehydrating illness (eg, diarrhea or protracted vomiting) can culminate in profound hypovolemia.
  - This susceptibility warrants prompt hospitalization and fluid administration before signs of severe dehydration emerge.

- Susceptibility to hypokalemia in children with regeneration-type RTA calls for regular monitoring of serum K^+.
  - If low, increase the dose of potassium-containing citrate solution.
  - If profound hypokalemia exists with a serum K^+ concentration <2.5 mEq/L accompanied by muscle weakness, prompt hospitalization is needed.
- Newborns with a salt-losing tendency should be monitored closely.
  - If the disorder was not recognized before discharge from nursery, the following signs call for urgent readmission and vigorous volume repletion.
    - Emergence of vomiting
    - Feeding difficulty
    - Listlessness
    - Hypotonia
    - Hyperventilation
    - Pallor
    - Signs of dehydration
- In the absence of virilization, congenital adrenal hyperplasia in a male infant may not be recognized at birth.
  - Infant may be discharged from nursery only to develop profound salt wasting and hypovolemic shock 1–2 weeks later.

R

Rheumatic Fever

DEFINITION

- Acute rheumatic fever is a systemic connective tissue disorder.

EPIDEMIOLOGY

- Incidence
  - Annual incidence is low, even at large teaching medical centers.
  - During 3 years of pediatric training, a resident physician may not see many children with acute rheumatic fever.
- Prevalence
  - ~2–3% in epidemics of streptococcal pharyngitis
  - ~0.2–0.3% after sporadic streptococcal upper respiratory tract infection
  - In patients who have already had ≥1 attacks of rheumatic fever.
    - Recurrence rate of carditis increases to ~15% after subsequent streptococcal infection.
- Age
  - Most first cases occur between 5 and 15 years of age.
  - Uncommon in patients <5 years
  - Extremely rare in patients <3 years
  - In infancy, acute rheumatic fever is usually associated with:
    - Severe carditis
    - Congestive heart failure
  - In preschool-age children
    - Polyarthritis caused by rheumatic fever is unusual.
    - Rheumatoid arthritis and other inflammatory diseases of the joint are more likely.
  - In early childhood chorea is uncommon
    - Most of the cases occur in patients >8 years.
- Socioeconomic distribution
  - Most studies have noted a strong association with poverty.
  - Major social risk factors that predispose patients to rheumatic fever
    - Crowding
      - Increases likelihood of transmission of group A ß-hemolytic *Streptococcus*
    - Lack of medical attention
    - Precludes timely treatment of streptococcal pharyngitis
    - Late attention to signs and symptoms of acute rheumatic fever
- Sex
  - No sex predisposition in the incidence of arthritis or carditis in childhood
  - Sex differences exist in the type of valvular lesions that develop with carditis.
    - Boys have a higher incidence of aortic regurgitation.
    - In young adults, mitral stenosis is more common in women.
  - Chorea is more common in girls.
- Geographic distribution
  - In the US and Europe, acute rheumatic fever has declined in the past 5 decades.
  - In underdeveloped countries, rheumatic fever remains a common childhood illness.
  - Apparent resurgence of acute rheumatic fever in certain areas of the US both urban and suburban, was reported between:
    - 1984–1988
    - 1997–1998
    - No evidence indicates that this trend has continued.
  - Contribution to prevalence of the disease in the US includes immigration from:
    - Caribbean Islands
    - South America
    - Southeast Asia

ETIOLOGY

- Immunologic reaction to group A ß-hemolytic streptococci infection is the established cause of rheumatic fever.

RISK FACTORS

- Tendency for rheumatic fever to occur in >1 family member has long been recognized.
  - The observation is noted when family members are not concurrently living in the same household.
  - No genetic factors have been clearly established.

SIGNS AND SYMPTOMS

Major clinical manifestations

- The sequence of manifestations of rheumatic fever is noteworthy.
  - Polyarthritis, when it occurs, is usually present before onset of carditis.
  - Carditis may be present without preceding joint symptoms.
    - Most often, apical systolic murmur of mitral valvulitis occurs within 2 weeks of onset of arthritis.
  - Diastolic murmur of isolated aortic valvulitis takes longer to appear.
    - May not be heard for 6–8 weeks after the joint signs and symptoms appear
  - Chorea may develop during the convalescent phase of carditis.
    - A longer latent period usually occurs.
    - Classically, chorea appears as an independent manifestation of rheumatic fever long after initial streptococcal infection.

– Majority of cases begin 2 months after streptococcal infection, with episodes occurring up to 6 months afterward.

- Chorea and carditis may coexist.
- Chorea and polyarthritis rarely appear concurrently, presumably because of the difference in latent periods

Polyarthritis

■ Most common manifestation at the onset of rheumatic fever

- Usually involves large joints of lower extremities, particularly ankles or knees

■ May result in joint pain while walking

- Often initially considered to be secondary to trauma

■ Other large joints become involved in a migratory fashion, eg, wrists and elbows.

■ The affected joint characteristically is:

- Warm
- Reddened
- Minimally swollen

■ Involved joints are:

- Exquisitely sensitive to touch
- Painful on motion

■ Suggestive of but not specific for rheumatic fever

- Arthralgias, or aching in joints without objective signs of inflammation

■ Fever is almost always present.

- Temperatures are usually <102°F (38.8°C).

Carditis

■ Inflammation of cardiac tissue is characteristically expressed as valvulitis.

- Pancarditis involving myocardium and pericardium may be present in severe cases.

■ Murmurs audible in rheumatic carditis are the result of mitral or aortic valvulitis, or both.

- Mitral involvement is by far the most common.

■ Auscultatory diagnosis of valvulitis often includes presence of an apical mid-diastolic murmur.

■ Pericarditis

- Typically silent
- Occasionally, friction rub or distant heart sounds are noted.
- Isolated pericarditis without associated auscultatory findings of mitral or aortic involvement is not consistent with diagnosis of acute rheumatic fever.

■ Viral inflammation of the heart by coxsackievirus type B or Kawasaki disease may be associated with myocarditis and pericarditis.

- These entities do not cause valvulitis.

■ Auscultation of heart and evaluation of murmurs are influenced by fever and tachycardia.

- The patient should be reexamined frequently after:
  – Diagnosis of acute rheumatic fever
  – Normalization of temperature with aspirin therapy
- A changing functional murmur in an anxious or febrile child does not indicate the presence of carditis.

■ Carditis is clinically diagnosed by the presence of valvulitis with characteristic murmurs.

- May be arbitrarily designated as mild, moderate, or severe
- Such categorization is useful in:
  – Approach to management
  – Establishing prognosis for development of rheumatic heart disease

■ Mild carditis

- Characteristically defined by the presence of prominent, high-pitched, apical systolic murmur typical of mitral insufficiency
- Heart murmur of mild carditis is usually of grade 2 or 3 intensity (on a scale of 1–6).
  – Occupies all or most of systole
- Mid-diastolic rumble at the apex is not present.

■ Moderate carditis

- Defined as:
  – Long systolic and prominent mid-diastolic apical murmurs, reflecting greater severity of mitral valvulitis
  – Basilar diastolic murmur of aortic valvulitis
  – Combination of mitral and aortic valvulitis
- Aortic diastolic murmur
  – High pitched, decrescendo in character
  – Heard best during end expiration with diaphragm of stethoscope placed firmly at the third left intercostal space

■ Severe carditis

- Defined by the presence of:
  – Pericarditis
  – Congestive heart failure
  – Mitral or aortic valvulitis
- Quality of heart sounds may be poor because of:
  – Pericardial effusion
  – Low cardiac output
- Murmurs may become more intense as cardiac compensation improves.

Chorea

■ The clinical picture of Sydenham chorea includes poor neuromuscular coordination.

- Sometimes first detected by a change or sloppiness in handwriting

R

- A wide variety of jerky, involuntary movements may occur for 6–8 weeks when most cases of chorea are active.
- Neurologic examination may give evidence of specific deficiencies, particularly in the trunk and upper extremity control of movements.

■ When chorea occurs as an isolated manifestation, the patient is usually afebrile.
  - The sedimentation rate is normal.
  - Long interval after the initiating streptococcal infection
    – Antistreptolysin O titer is typically normal or only mildly elevated.
  - Murmur of mild mitral insufficiency may be noted.

Erythema marginatum

■ Transient pink rash with irregular, deeper-colored serpiginous borders
  - Seen on the smooth, hairless surfaces of the inner aspect of the upper arms and thighs or trunk
■ Infrequently encountered in recent decades

Subcutaneous nodules

■ Characteristically pea-sized
■ Usually located on the extensor surfaces of:
  - Fingers
  - Toes
  - Elbows
  - Other joints
  - Occiput (less frequently)
■ Usually reflect longstanding or smoldering illness after severe carditis
■ Nodules may persist for weeks or months.
■ Subcutaneous nodules are rarely found in children with rheumatic fever in present era.

Minor clinical manifestations

■ Nonspecific fever
■ Nonspecific arthralgia
  - Defined as joint discomfort without objective signs of joint inflammation
■ Elevated acute-phase reactant, such as erythrocyte sedimentation rate (ESR), ranges from 60–120 mm/hour initially.
■ In chorea, the sedimentation rate is normal due to long interval beyond the antecedent streptococcal infection.
■ C-reactive protein is elevated in a variety of other diseases.
  - Helpful in diagnosing cases with borderline findings
■ Streptococcal pharyngitis presumptively precedes an attack of rheumatic fever.
  - Some patients fail to report such a history.

■ Scarlet fever will occasionally be followed by signs of polyarthritis or carditis.
  - Suppurative streptococcal disease, such as skin infection, is not a precursor of rheumatic fever.
■ Polyarthritis and carditis usually occur 3–5 weeks after infection.
■ Streptococcal antibody titer peaks before onset of clinical symptoms, then decreases gradually.
■ Occasionally, children have abdominal pain after streptococcal infection for which medical or surgical evaluation is sought.
  - This symptom may occasionally precede signs of joint or cardiac involvement.

DIFFERENTIAL DIAGNOSIS

■ Throat cultures may be misleading in the evaluation of patients suspected of having rheumatic fever.
  - Streptococcal infection antedates the common manifestations of polyarthritis and carditis by periods varying from 3–8 weeks.
  - ≤50% of patients with rheumatic fever continue to harbor streptococci during the course of their illness.

DIAGNOSTIC APPROACH

■ No pathognomonic clinical findings and specific laboratory tests are available to confirm diagnosis of rheumatic fever.
  - The diagnosis must be somewhat arbitrary and empirical.
  - The tendency to label any low-grade febrile illness with arthralgia for which no obvious cause can be found as rheumatic fever should be avoided.
■ A list of major and minor criteria for the evaluation and diagnosis of rheumatic fever and rheumatic heart disease was published >50 years ago by Dr T. Duckett Jones.
  - These guidelines have been accepted as diagnostic criteria throughout the world.
  - The most recent review of the Jones criteria by the American Heart Association was designated in a 1992 update and was reviewed in 2002.
■ Jones criteria for the diagnosis of an initial episode of rheumatic fever
  - Evidence of antecedent group A streptococcal infections, 2 major manifestations, or 1 major and 2 minor manifestations indicates high probability of acute rheumatic fever.
  - The 5 major manifestations, in descending order of frequency, are:
    – Polyarthritis
    – Carditis
    – Chorea
    – Erythema marginatum
    – Subcutaneous nodules

- Minor manifestations are:
  - Clinical findings
    - Arthralgia
    - Fever
  - Laboratory findings
    - Elevated acute-phase reactants: ESR, C-reactive protein level
    - Prolonged PR interval
- Supporting evidence of antecedent group A streptococcal infections
  - Positive throat culture or rapid streptococcal antigen test
  - Elevated or rising streptococcal antibody titer
- 2 major manifestations involving skin, especially nodules that were most often seen only after multiple attacks of rheumatic fever, have been extremely uncommon during the late 1900s in the US.
- Minor manifestations include 2 laboratory findings.
  - Elevated acute-phase reactants: ESR and C-reactive protein level
  - Electrocardiographic (ECG) evidence of prolongation of the PR interval
- Fever may be present early in the course of polyarthritis or carditis.
  - Usually temperature <102°F (38.8°C)
- Arthralgia
  - Another minor manifestation
  - Nonspecific
  - May affect any joint without objective signs of inflammation
  - Should not be considered a minor manifestation if arthritis is counted as a major manifestation
- The Jones criteria should be viewed as a guide to a probable diagnosis of rheumatic fever.
  - Final diagnosis must remain a clinical judgment.
- Institution of prophylactic regimens requires prolonged administration of antistreptococcal agents, an important responsibility on the physician who diagnoses rheumatic fever.

LABORATORY FINDINGS

- Under current guidelines, laboratory confirmation of recent streptococcal infection should be part of the diagnostic evaluation.
  - Absence of evidence of streptococcal infection should make the clinician suspicious of the diagnosis of rheumatic fever.
  - Exception: cases in which indolent carditis or chorea are the major manifestations

- Minor clinical manifestations
  - Elevated acute-phase reactant is an invaluable though non-specific laboratory sign of inflammation.
    - ESR
- Most reliable evidence of a preceding streptococcal infection
  - Obtained by demonstration of antibody response to ≥1 of the streptococcal antigens
  - ASLO titer
    - Most common
    - Reaches maximal levels 3–5 weeks after infection
    - Gradually declines to preinfection levels 6–12 months later
    - Elevated in ~85% of patients with rheumatic fever
    - Titers are never extremely low.
  - Serologic evidence of an antecedent streptococcal infection increases to 95% if other streptococcal antibody tests are performed.
    - Antihyaluronidase
    - Antideoxyribonuclease B
    - Antistreptokinase

IMAGING

- Ultrasonography
  - 2-dimensional echocardiography for documentation and quantification of pericardial effusion
  - Interpretation of valvular regurgitation by Doppler ultrasonography should not constitute the basis of a diagnosis of carditis without auscultatory evidence of significant mitral or aortic involvement.
  - Doppler studies in healthy individuals frequently show a small degree of regurgitation across the mitral valve.
  - Trivial aortic valve regurgitation may be noted occasionally.
- Radiographic studies
  - In mild carditis, heart size on chest radiography is usually normal.
  - In moderate carditis, may show mild cardiac enlargement
  - In severe carditis, shows obvious cardiomegaly
    - May reveal pulmonary vascular congestion compatible with left-sided heart failure and pulmonary edema
    - Appearance may be consistent with rheumatic pneumonia.

DIAGNOSTIC PROCEDURES

- ECG of minor clinical manifestations
  - Prolongation of the PR interval (first-degree heart block) on ECG is considered to be a vagal effect and supports the diagnosis of rheumatic fever.
    - Most commonly noted when polyarthritis is apparent
    - Not necessarily associated with carditis

R

- ECG is almost always otherwise normal regardless of cardiac involvement.
- PR interval prolongation is the common manifestation.
  - Occasionally, second- or third-degree heart block occurs.
  - Indicates further heightening of vagal tone
  - Perhaps more pronounced in the rheumatic state than in other acute illnesses
- First- or second-degree heart block is not a:
  - Major criterion for carditis
  - Harbinger of potential rheumatic heart disease
  - Threat to progress to complete heart block
  - Cause of symptoms

TREATMENT APPROACH

- Therapeutic management of acute rheumatic fever includes the use of:
  - Antistreptococcal antibiotics
  - Antiinflammatory agents

SPECIFIC TREATMENTS

Chorea

- A protective environment is recommended while the process is active.
- Occasionally, mild sedation is indicated.
- Agents that may help in the treatment of more severe movement disorders
  - Clonazepam (Klonopin)
  - Haloperidol (Haldol)

Antistreptococcal therapy

- Eradication of group A ß-hemolytic streptococcal infection by antibiotic treatment is the foremost principle in management of acute rheumatic fever.
  - Prescribed even in the absence of a positive throat culture
- Antibiotic treatment must always be immediately followed by institution of a prophylactic program to prevent reinfection.
- Penicillin is the drug of choice, prescribed initially at a dose and duration to maintain therapeutic blood levels for 10 days.
- Several treatment schedules are outlined by the American Heart Association.
  - Intramuscular administration of long-acting repository benzathine penicillin G (Bicillin) is preferred.
    - Ensures therapeutic levels for a sufficient length of time
    - A single injection of 1.2 million U for children 5–15 years of age is recommended.
    - Follow by prophylactic injections of 1.2 million U every 3–4 weeks.

- Alternative methods
  - Oral penicillin, 200,000 or 250,000 units (penicillin G or penicillin V), given 3 or 4 times a day for a full 10 days, followed by same dose twice daily thereafter, *or*
  - Combination of oral and intramuscular penicillin
- For patients sensitive to penicillin, erythromycin may be used for antistreptococcal therapy.
- Sulfonamide drugs are not effective for streptococcal eradication.
  - Bacteriostatic rather than bactericidal
  - Can be used in rheumatic prophylaxis programs to prevent reinfection
  - Rarely used in the present era

Antiinflammatory therapy

- Salicylates are indicated in the presence of acute, painful arthritis during the febrile phase of acute rheumatic fever.
  - Duration of therapy usually ranges from 4–8 weeks.
  - Average initial dose should be ~50–75 mg/kg/day, given in 4 divided doses.
  - Extremely high doses are not required.
- Aspirin is used for symptomatic relief only and is usually associated with:
  - Rapid and significant improvement in objective arthritis signs and symptoms
  - Almost immediate defervescence
- Specific blood levels do not need to be reached or maintained if clinical signs have disappeared.
- No evidence exists that salicylate administration affects the clinical course or later manifestations of cardiac involvement.
- Administration of steroid hormones is indicated for severe cardiac involvement characterized by pancarditis with congestive heart failure.
  - Most commonly prednisone
- When myocarditis appears to be fulminant, steroid therapy has been shown to significantly improve survival.
  - No evidence of long-term palliative effects on chronic rheumatic valvular disease is available.
- Duration of steroid treatment may be extended to 1–3 months in severe cases.
  - Varying schedules of tapering dose
  - Possible addition of salicylate therapy
- Specific therapeutic measures to control congestive heart failure may be useful.
  - Diuretics
  - Digitalis
- Furosemide (Lasix) is used for the management of pulmonary congestion with left-ventricular failure.

- Digitalis (digoxin) should be administered cautiously.
  - The threshold for toxicity may be reduced in the presence of inflammatory myocarditis.
  - Withholding digitalis for 1 or 2 days until steroid therapy has begun to suppress the myocarditis may be prudent.
  - Serum potassium levels should be monitored because steroids and furosemide both decrease body potassium.
    - Predispose patient to digitalis intoxication
- Enalapril is sometimes used in patients with mitral valve insufficiency.

Limitation of activity

- The role of bed rest in the treatment of rheumatic fever has been deemphasized in recent years.
- For children with arthritis
  - Ambulation can be permitted when pain and joint tenderness improve.
- Patients with stable, mild cardiac involvement can be allowed to ambulate when they feel well enough.
- Patients with more severe carditis
  - Length of restricted activity is individualized according to the severity of cardiac involvement.

WHEN TO ADMIT

- All children with acute rheumatic fever should be hospitalized.
- Hospitalizing a youngster who has arthritis or carditis may be advisable for:
  - Observation
  - Appropriate documentation of poststreptococcal illness
  - Initiation of treatment
- Hospitalization emphasizes to the parents:
  - Seriousness of the disease
  - Importance of prophylaxis to prevent recurrence
- Specific association of Sydenham chorea with rheumatic fever
  - Hospitalizing a child with this manifestation should not be mandatory if:
    - Abnormal neuromuscular activity is mild.
    - Unlikely to cause self-inflicted injury

WHEN TO REFER

- All children with acute rheumatic fever should be referred to a cardiologist for evaluation and management.

FOLLOW-UP

- An issue that arises is the amount of physical activity permitted.
  - Children with mild mitral regurgitation with normal heart size should be allowed to engage in all athletic activities, except for the most strenuous, competitive sports.
- Children with more severe mitral regurgitation or aortic insufficiency with cardiomegaly should have:
  - Some restriction of their activities
  - Continuing appropriate regimen
- If symptoms of fatigue or exercise intolerance persist despite medical management, a full diagnostic evaluation should be performed.
  - Surgical intervention with valvuloplasty or valve replacement should be considered.

COMPLICATIONS

- The major long-term consequence is the potential for inflammatory cardiac valvar involvement, leading to chronic heart disease.
- Ultimate development of rheumatic heart disease after a first attack of rheumatic fever can be correlated with severity of acute carditis.
  - A 10-year follow-up study of treatments begun in 1951 showed that patients developed chronic rheumatic heart disease (mitral insufficiency or stenosis or aortic regurgitation, or any combination).
    - ~30% of patients who had mild carditis
    - 50% of those who had moderate carditis
    - 75% with severe carditis
- Most children who develop rheumatic heart disease after a single attack of rheumatic fever have mitral regurgitation.
- Others either have both mitral and aortic regurgitation or aortic regurgitation alone.
- Mitral stenosis evolves slowly.
  - Usually after repeated episodes of acute rheumatic fever
  - Sometimes evolves unexpectedly
    - Many years after initial mild mitral valvulitis
    - Perhaps previously undiagnosed
  - Isolated mitral stenosis is:
    - Unusual before early adulthood
    - Rare in developed nations
- Contraception and pregnancy
  - Patients who have severe rheumatic heart disease are at high risk of cardiac complications during pregnancy and delivery.
    - Mitral stenosis has an especially high-risk profile.
    - Mild rheumatic heart disease is well tolerated during pregnancy.
  - Adolescent girls with rheumatic heart disease should be counseled with regard to contraceptive methods.
    - Oral medication with a low level of estrogen can be prescribed.
    - Give instructions on use of the diaphragm.
    - An intrauterine device should be avoided, because of risk of bacteremia.

R

- Added cardiovascular burden during pregnancy
  - Thorough obstetrical care should be provided from the first trimester through delivery.
  - Prophylaxis against streptococcal infection should be continued.
  - Psychosocial support may be needed.
    - Especially for pregnant teenagers with significant rheumatic heart disease who face medical complications during pregnancy
  - If early termination is sought, therapeutic abortion should be performed in the hospital.

PROGNOSIS

- In the months and years following an attack:
  - Auscultatory findings frequently change from those heard during the acute episode.
  - Apical systolic murmurs heard initially may diminish or completely disappear.
  - Aortic diastolic murmur will almost always persist during the follow-up period.
- An initial diagnosis of carditis does not necessarily imply progression to permanent heart damage.
- In children labeled as having history of acute rheumatic fever:
  - An additional appellation of rheumatic heart disease must be reevaluated continually.
- Even patients with severe carditis in the acute phase will show improvement in weeks and months after the recuperative period.
  - >50% of murmurs of mild or moderate mitral insufficiency will disappear completely.
- Other manifestations are self-limiting with no late sequelae.
- Arthritis clears without joint dysfunction or deformity.
- Chorea leaves no neuromuscular impediment.
- Recurrence of rheumatic fever
  - Striking tendency to recur
  - Before the introduction of preventive measures, most patients who had initial attack of rheumatic fever had ≥1 recurrences.
  - Recurrence rate is highest during first 3 years after initial attack.
  - Diminishes with time after the original episode
  - Recurrence is rare in adulthood.

PREVENTION

Rheumatic fever

- The incidence of first attack can be reduced by adequate penicillin treatment in all cases of streptococcal pharyngitis.

- Numerous community primary prevention programs have demonstrated the efficacy of identifying streptococcal infection by:
  - Performing throat cultures on susceptible children
  - Early treatment
- Application of secondary prevention in the form of antistreptococcal prophylaxis after the first attack has significantly reduced:
  - Recurrence rate
  - Additive effects of repeated bouts of carditis

Recurrence

- Preventing recurrent attacks that carry risk of recrudescent heart involvement and further cardiac damage is the most important concern.
- Continuous antimicrobial prophylaxis should be given in all children who have a history of rheumatic fever, including those who present with chorea.
- Prophylaxis may be discontinued if:
  - The patient is 18 years of age
  - A patient who initially had cardiac involvement has no auscultatory evidence of heart disease
- Prophylaxis should be maintained into adulthood if there is:
  - Chronic mitral valve disease
  - Aortic valvular disease
- Prophylaxis can be discontinued after 5 years:
  - In children who had no cardiac involvement during the initial attack
- The rationale for antibiotic prophylaxis in a patient with known rheumatic fever is protection against recurrence of rheumatic fever through prevention of group A streptococcal infection.
- The most effective method for reducing streptococcal infections and rheumatic fever recurrence
  - Intramuscular injections of long-acting penicillin (benzathine penicillin G, 1.2 million U)
- Preventive regimen most effective when given every 3–4 weeks.
  - In residual cardiac involvement, this approach is recommended
    - Every 3 week regimen is recommended for the first 6–12 months.
    - Continue every 3–4 weeks for at least a 1- or 2-year period
    - Followed by oral prophylaxis
- Parenteral therapy is most effective method of prophylaxis.
  - Strict adherence to a program of daily oral medication is especially difficult for children and adolescents.

- Transient discomfort at the injection site (anterior thigh or buttock) may be relieved by:
  - Hot bath
  - Aspirin on the evening of injection
- Alternative methods of prophylaxis include
  - Oral administration of penicillin G
    - 200,000 or 250,000 U, twice a day
  - Sulfisoxazole
    - Gantrisin, 0.5 g twice a day
- For the patient sensitive to both penicillin and sulfisoxazole:
  - Consider daily prophylaxis with another agent.
  - Successful oral prophylaxis is hard to maintain.
    - If used, its value and need for compliance should be reinforced constantly.
  - Rheumatic fever recurrence is less likely after 2–5 years.
- Patients with chronic rheumatic heart disease
  - Oral regimen can be substituted for intramuscular penicillin.
  - Oral prophylaxis can be instituted immediately for patients who did not have carditis during the acute attack.
  - Under these circumstances, recurrences with carditis are extremely rare.

Bacterial endocarditis

- Individuals who have a history of rheumatic fever without evidence of significant murmurs on follow-up examination:
  - Are not susceptible to bacterial endocarditis.
  - Do not have damaged heart valves
- Recent guidelines from the American Heart Association report that patients with heart disease
  - More likely to get infective endocarditis from frequent exposure to random bacteremic events associated with daily activities
  - Less likely to get infective endocarditis from bacteremia following dental or surgical procedures
- Latest guidelines for prevention of infective endocarditis recommend antibiotic prophylaxis for patients with:
  - Prosthetic cardiac valves
  - Previous infective endocarditis
  - Certain types of repaired and unrepaired congenital heart diseases
- Antibiotic prophylaxis before dental or surgical procedures is no longer recommended for patients with mitral or aortic valve disease following rheumatic fever.
- Recommendations for prevention of recurrent episodes of rheumatic fever have not changed.

R

Rocky Mountain Spotted Fever

DEFINITION

■ Rocky Mountain spotted fever (RMSF) is an acute infectious disease.

EPIDEMIOLOGY

■ Incidence
  ● Increased slightly during the past several years
    – >500 cases per year in the 1990s
    – >1000 cases per year since 2000
■ Geographic distribution
  ● First reported in patients from the Rocky Mountain region
  ● Incidence is now greatest east of the Mississippi River, with most cases reported from southeastern and south-central US.
  ● From 1994–2003, 54% of the cases of RMSF reported in the US were in:
    – North Carolina
    – Tennessee
    – Oklahoma
    – South Carolina
    – Arkansas
  ● Disease occurs predominantly in the US but has been reported in other areas in the Western Hemisphere, specifically:
    – Canada
    – Central America
    – South America
■ Age
  ● Two-thirds of cases occur in children <15 years.
  ● Peak ages of infection from 5–9 years
  ● 15% of deaths occur in children <10 years.
■ Sex
  ● Occurs more frequently in boys than girls
■ Race
  ● Higher incidence in white people than people of other races
■ Seasonality
  ● Can occur at any time of the year
  ● 90% of cases occur from April to September.

ETIOLOGY

■ Caused by *Rickettsia* that multiply in endothelial cells
■ May produce cellular injury by various mechanisms, including:
  ● Cell wall penetration
  ● Disturbance of intracellular metabolism
  ● Production of toxic metabolites
  ● Use of metabolites required by the host cell
■ Perivascular mononuclear cell infiltration caused by the reproducing organism results in:
  ● Necrosis of endothelial cell walls
  ● Increase in vascular permeability
  ● Fibrin extravasation
  ● Thrombosis of small blood vessels
■ Resulting cell damage in multiple locations is responsible for the clinical picture.
■ The major pathologic lesion in RMSF, vasculitis, makes RMSF a multisystem disease.
  ● Skeletal muscle
  ● Brain
  ● Lungs
  ● Kidneys
  ● Testes
  ● Adrenal glands
  ● Liver
  ● Heart
■ Ticks serve as a vector for the infectious agent *Rickettsia rickettsii*.
  ● Transmission to humans occurs when:
    – The tick takes a blood meal.
    – Abraded skin is contaminated by tick feces or a crushed tick and may occur when ticks are removed.
  ● Usually, tick attachment lasting 12–24 hours is needed to transfer disease.
  ● 2 specific ticks serve as major carriers.
    – Wood tick, *Dermacentor andersoni*: more important vector in the western US
    – Dog tick, *Dermacentor variabilis*: usual vector in the eastern US
  ● Ticks acquire the rickettsiae by feeding on infected wild mammals, such as:
    – Squirrels
    – Opossums
    – Rabbits
    – Dogs
    – Mice
  ● Dog ticks infected with *R rickettsii* have been found in urban areas.
    – Suggests this tick's ubiquitous nature
    – Places individuals at risk without travel to endemic areas
  ● The brown dog tick, *Rhipicephalus sanguineus*, is implicated in causing outbreak of *R rickettsii* infection in Arizona.
■ Exposure to a tick is not elicited in every case.
  ● Only 60% of patients with RMSF can recall a specific tick exposure or encounter.
  ● Tick bite is painless.
  ● Leaves no local lesion or regional lymphadenopathy

RISK FACTORS

- In adults, occupational or recreational exposure to ticks increases the risk of infection.
- The clinician should question the patient specifically about prior activities that increase risk of exposure.
  - Removal of a tick from a pet
  - Camping or picnicking in high-risk area
- Overall risk to patients, even when in high-risk areas, is low.
  - Approximately only 1–3% of the tick population carries *R rickettsii* at any given time.

SIGNS AND SYMPTOMS

- Characterized by:
  - Fever
  - Headache
  - Myalgia
  - Distinctive exanthem
- After inoculation with rickettsiae
  - Incubation period ranges from 2–12 days.
  - The usual period is 5–7 days.
  - Shorter incubation periods are associated with more serious disease.
- The prodromal period lasts 2–3 days, predominated by:
  - Low-grade fever
  - Chills
  - Muscle aches
- Muscle pain is most common in the calf region in younger patients.
- Headache is an early symptom.
  - Infants and toddlers may express pain from headache or myalgias as crying or fussiness.
- Other frequent symptoms include:
  - Malaise
  - Anorexia
  - Vomiting
  - Photophobia
- The prodrome is followed by accentuation of symptoms.
  - Especially fever
    - Temperatures often as high as ≥104°F (40°C)
    - The lowest temperatures, although still elevated, are recorded in the mornings.
  - Lethargy and mental obtundation become prominent.
  - Symptoms seen at this stage are not diagnostic.
- Rash is the most distinctive sign.
  - Usually appears 3–5 days after onset of fever
  - Begins peripherally on:
    - Wrists
    - Ankles
    - Hands
    - Feet
  - Initially, the lesions are:
    - Macular
    - Discrete
    - Erythematous
    - Blanch on pressure
  - Rash rapidly spreads centrally, involving:
    - Arms
    - Legs
    - Axillae
    - Buttocks
    - Trunk
    - Neck
    - Face
  - Lesions deepen in color, becoming:
    - Dusky red
    - Maculopapular
    - Petechial
      - True petechiae may not form until day 6 of illness.
      - 35–60% of patients never develop petechiae.
      - Petechial lesions may coalesce and form large ecchymotic areas.
      - In severe cases and when treatment is delayed, these ecchymotic areas may ulcerate.
      - Distal regions (eg, fingers and toes) may become gangrenous in as many as 4% of cases.
  - As many as 15% of patients do not develop rash, or develop a fine rash that may be difficult to appreciate in patients with darker skin tones.
  - Rash does not occur until day 4 of the illness.
  - Petechiae may be a much later finding.
  - Some patients never develop a discernible exanthem.
- Tachycardia and an elevated pulse rate are noted early and are proportional to the degree of hyperpyrexia.
- A sudden increase in pulse rate or a decrease in blood pressure may indicate:
  - Peripheral circulatory collapse
  - Severe bleeding
  - Myocardial failure
- Photophobia is associated with conjunctival ecchymosis involving both bulbar and palpebral conjunctivae.
- Other manifestations include:
  - Abdominal pain
  - Retinal hemorrhages
  - Vomiting
  - Hepatomegaly

R

- Splenomegaly with generalized abdominal tenderness
- Lethargy
- Obtunded state of consciousness
- Jaundice is not usually seen except in the most critically ill patients, with disseminated intravascular coagulation (DIC).

■ Diminished urinary output caused by:
  - Fever
  - Poor fluid intake from nausea
  - Vomiting
  - Mild azotemia caused by fluid losses should respond to rehydration.

■ The patient may exhibit nuchal rigidity, resulting from vasculitic reaction in the meninges.

■ Neurologic manifestations include:
  - Disorientation
  - Confusion
  - Seizures
  - Coma
  - Central deafness
  - Cortical blindness
  - Sixth nerve palsies

■ Causes of neurologic effects include:
  - Vasculitis
  - Hemorrhage from coagulopathies
  - Secondary metabolic changes caused by circulatory collapse

DIFFERENTIAL DIAGNOSIS

■ Neurologic and abdominal symptoms early in RMSF may mask its diagnosis.

■ Illnesses to be considered and differentiated from RMSF, especially after the rash appears, include:
  - Rubeola (measles)
  - Meningococcemia
  - Henoch-Schönlein purpura
  - Kawasaki disease
  - Immune thrombocytopenic purpura
  - Leukemia
  - Typhus
  - Ehrlichiosis
  - Infectious mononucleosis

■ Meningococcemia
  - Petechial rash of meningococcemia differs from that of RMSF in:
    - Distribution
    - Rapid extension
    - Coalescence of lesions into larger hemorrhagic, purpuric areas

- Prostration develops rapidly if the patient remains untreated.
  - Often apparent on admission to the hospital
- Helpful points in differentiating meningococcemia from RMSF
  - Absence of myalgia
  - Extremely abrupt onset
- Leukocyte count may be elevated in meningococcemia.
- The sickest patients are frequently leukopenic.
- Other presentations include:
  - Meningitis with pleocytosis
  - Low glucose levels
  - Organisms in the cerebrospinal fluid (CSF)
- Distinguishing between these entities clinically is not often possible.
  - Treatment for both diseases in an ill patient is warranted.

■ Ehrlichiosis
  - Rickettsial disease with clinical similarity to RMSF
  - Rash occurs with less frequency.
    - >60% of children with ehrlichiosis have been noted to have rash.
    - Variable in location and appearance
    - May be petechial
    - Can be confused with rickettsial exanthems
  - Early diagnosis and treatment of with doxycycline reduces morbidity.

■ Rubeola (measles)
  - Characterized by a macular rash
    - Infrequently becoming hemorrhagic
  - Begins on the face and neck
  - Preceded by:
    - An enanthem
    - Koplik spots on the buccal mucosa
  - Coryza and cough in the prodromal stage of illness are not consistent with RMSF.
  - A history of adequate immunization with rubeola vaccine greatly diminishes this possibility.

■ Henoch-Schönlein purpura
  - May produce a petechial or purpuric rash, frequently concentrated on lower extremities and buttocks
  - Cutaneous lesions may be multiform.
  - May occur on other parts of the body
  - Arthralgia with periarticular swelling and accompanying signs and symptoms of upper respiratory tract inflammation, intense abdominal pain, or nephritis

■ Kawasaki disease
  - Fever
  - Puffy hands and feet

- Rash
  - Typically does not begin peripherally and spread centrally or become petechial in 1–2 days
- Conjunctival injection
- Usually, Kawasaki disease is not seriously considered until the following occur.
  - 5 days of fever
  - Enlarged cervical node
  - Pharyngeal hyperemia
  - Dry cracked lips
  - Strawberry tongue
  - Marked irritability
- Leukocyte and erythrocyte sedimentation rates are usually elevated significantly.
- Kawasaki disease usually occurs in the winter and spring months
- Children with Kawasaki disease do not give a history of tick exposures.
- Elevated platelet count begins during the second week of illness.
- Other illnesses that produce petechiae and lack distinctive distribution of rash
  - Immune thrombocytopenic purpura
    - Seen as a petechial rash in an otherwise healthy patient
  - Patients with leukemia who initially have fever and petechiae would be expected to:
    - Be anemic
    - Have lymphadenopathy
    - Have hepatosplenomegaly
  - Patients with infectious mononucleosis with petechial eruption usually have:
    - Lymphadenopathy
    - Hepatosplenomegaly
    - Gradual onset
  - Typhus is a rickettsial infection to be excluded.
  - Murine typhus produces a milder disease.
    - Rash is macular, not petechial.
  - Epidemic typhus may produce a petechial rash that typically begins proximally and extends peripherally.
    - Does not usually involve the palms or soles
    - History of tick bite is absent.

DIAGNOSTIC APPROACH

- The diagnosis is made clinically.
- Clinical diagnosis and treatment are typically required before laboratory confirmation.
- The disease still has a significant risk of morbidity and mortality when treatment is delayed.

LABORATORY FINDINGS

- Available laboratory tests to confirm the presence of *R rickettsii* include:
  - Increase in antibody titer detected by immunofluorescence or latex agglutination
  - Polymerase chain reaction testing
  - Immunofluorescence of skin biopsy
  - Isolation of organism from clinical specimen
- Immunofluorescent staining of the skin biopsy specimen
  - May identify *R rickettsii*
  - May provide early proof of RMSF
  - Not readily available to most clinicians
  - Appropriate antibiotic therapy started 3 days before biopsy has resulted in negative immunofluorescence.
    - When appropriate treatment has been initiated before biopsy, clinical criteria justify a full course of antibiotic therapy.
- Polymerase chain reaction testing provides a specific diagnostic tool for early diagnosis.
  - Expensive
  - Not commonly available
- Complement fixation and immunofluorescent antibody studies in serum will identify patients with RMSF.
  - Test results do not become positive until 7–10 days after the onset of illness, or later if antibiotic therapy has begun early.
  - Titers should be performed during the acute illness.
  - Repeat 3 weeks later.
  - 4-fold increase in titer in the convalescent sera is diagnostic for infection.
- Weil-Felix reaction is at best a nonspecific test for RMSF.
  - Agglutination of *Proteus vulgaris* by the patient's serum
  - Acute and convalescent sera must be compared.
  - Proteus agglutinins may appear by the end of the first week of illness.
  - Availability of more specific and sensitive tests makes this test obsolete.
- Rickettsiae can be isolated from body fluid or tissue specimens when grown in laboratory animals or chick embryos.
  - The high rate of disease transmission to laboratory technicians makes such techniques feasible only in laboratories engaged in *Rickettsia*-related research in which all workers are immunized.
  - Culture identification of rickettsiae is not available in most clinical settings.
- Blood leukocyte counts and differential counts are usually within normal limits, but neutrophils often predominate.
  - Neutrophil predominance may help distinguish RMSF from ehrlichiosis.

R

- Most patients with ehrlichiosis have lymphopenic leukopenia.
- Thrombocytopenia is a complication seen in the later stages of the disease.
  - May be the result of platelet adherence to damaged endothelium
- Up to 20% of patients may have hyponatremia.
  - Possibly caused by increased vascular permeability of the kidney to sodium
  - Nonspecific finding; does not exclude other diagnoses, such as ehrlichiosis
  - The remainder of electrolyte profile is usually normal.
  - Hypochloremia is seen in some.
  - Up to 25% of patients will display increased blood urea nitrogen levels and increased liver enzymes.
  - With the development of DIC, abnormalities can occur.
    - Prothrombin time
    - Partial thromboplastin time
    - Fibrinogen
    - Fibrin split products
- Patients with neurologic manifestations may have normal CSF cell counts.
  - Most have normal CSF glucose and protein levels.
  - CSF analysis might reveal:
    - Neutrophilic or lymphocytic pleocytosis
    - Elevated protein
  - Nonspecific findings; may not help distinguish RMSF from meningococcal disease or ehrlichiosis
- Long-term morbidity from neurologic complications, though rare, are still significant.
  - Hematuria and anemia may occur.
  - Transfusion or renal dialysis is rarely required.

DIAGNOSTIC PROCEDURES

- Skin biopsy

TREATMENT APPROACH

- Treatment should never be withheld or delayed due to:
  - Absence of rash
  - Lack of exposure to ticks
  - Desire to await confirmatory laboratory study results
  - Patient location where RMSF is uncommon
  - Pediatrician discomfort using doxycycline in a child <8 years
- Treatment for RMSF mandated until the diagnosis can be excluded if:
  - Triad of fever, headache, and myalgia
  - Combined with a history of tick bite or removal within the previous 2 weeks

- If a pediatrician strongly suspects RMSF because of patient's clinical history and physical findings, therapy should be initiated immediately.
  - Can be administered concurrently with treatment for meningococcemia

SPECIFIC TREATMENTS

Pharmacotherapy

- Doxycycline
  - Drug of choice for all ages
  - Given and continued for ≥3 days after clinical improvement and defervescence
  - Usual length of therapy is 7–10 days.
  - Intravenous therapy should be given to all ill patients.
  - Transition to oral therapy when the patient's condition has improved.
  - Effective against ehrlichiosis, which may mimic RMSF
  - Has a broad therapeutic index
  - Levels do not need to be monitored as required with other RMSF medications, such as chloramphenicol.
- Tetracycline
  - Shown to be effective against RMSF
  - Can lead to increased dental staining compared with doxycycline in children <9 years
  - No more effective than doxycycline
  - Tetracycline is less commonly used in children.
- Chloramphenicol
  - No longer the drug of choice for RMSF
  - Data have shown it may be more effective than doxycycline.
  - The toxic effects of this drug (aplastic anemia) make it an undesirable treatment option.
  - May be given to patients who cannot tolerate doxycycline or tetracycline
- Combination therapy
  - Initiating treatment for meningococcal disease, as well as RMSF and ehrlichiosis, in an ill patient may be necessary.
  - When this situation arises, doxycycline will treat both ehrlichiosis and RMSF.
  - Can be used in conjunction with a third-generation cephalosporin to treat meningococcal infection

Hospitalization

- Desirable initially for most patients, both to:
  - Confirm diagnosis
  - Observe effect of therapy
- Therapy should be continued until the patient has improved and has been afebrile for 72 hours.
  - Generally occurs after 7–10 days of therapy

- Supportive therapy
  - Includes maintenance of hydration and nutrition with appropriate intravenous fluids and oral feedings (if tolerated).
  - Management of DIC may include therapeutic maneuvers, such as administering:
    - Fresh-frozen plasma
    - Fresh platelets
    - Packed red blood cells
    - Vitamin K
  - Seizures may require the use of anticonvulsant medications.

WHEN TO ADMIT

- Most patients need to be admitted and kept hospitalized until they show clinical improvement.
- Hemodynamic instability
- Dehydration
- Requires intensive monitoring
- RMSF with its complications

WHEN TO REFER

- Uncertain diagnosis
- Clinical suspicion of disease

COMPLICATIONS

- Vascular necrosis and thrombosis may result in local gangrene and loss of tissue.
- DIC may develop (uncommon).
  - Patients with this complication have the greatest risk of dying.
- Myocardial failure may result from myocarditis and arrhythmias.
- Edema may be generalized as a result of:
  - Increase in capillary permeability caused by the vasculitis
  - Heart failure
  - Iatrogenic fluid overload
  - Any combination
- Long-term morbidity from neurologic complications is rare but still significant.
- Hematuria and anemia may occur.
  - Transfusions or renal dialysis are rarely required.

PROGNOSIS

- Mortality of approximately 2–4% in recognized cases
  - Patients who escaped clinical detection have been identified by serologic evidence.
    - Disease may occur in a mild or subclinical form.

- Rocky Mountain spotless fever has also been described.
  - Suggestion that patients who have spotless *or* almost spotless fever have a significantly higher mortality as a result of delayed diagnosis and treatment
- RMSF can be considered a potentially fatal illness.
  - Younger patients are likely to be less severely affected than older patients.
- Early diagnosis and prompt therapy lessen disease severity.
  - Under such circumstances, death would be extremely unusual.
  - In most patients, early clinical diagnosis and adequate therapy shorten the duration of illness appreciably.
- Recovery from the illness is accompanied by immunity to *R rickettsii*.

PREVENTION

- Repellents have been shown to be effective against ticks.
  - *N,N*-Diethyl-meta-toluamide (DEET) skin repellents
  - Permethrin-containing repellents used on clothes
- Systemic reactions to DEET are possible when the repellents contain a high concentration of the chemical.
- The best preventive measure is avoidance of tick exposure.
- When exposure is likely, daily searches for ticks should be performed.
  - In tick-infested areas, twice-daily searches are advised.
  - Careful inspection at bath time is an excellent way to discover ticks.
- Ticks may be removed by gentle traction with forceps or tweezers.
  - Care must be taken not to crush them.
  - Skin should be disinfected both before and after tick exposure to remove feces that may carry *R rickettsii*.
  - The tick should never be covered in:
    - Petroleum jelly
    - Nail polish remover
    - Alcohol
  - No one should attempt to burn the tick to coax it to detach itself.
    - These attempts may lead the tick to defecate or aerosolize infected body fluids.
- Antimicrobial prophylaxis is not indicated after a tick bite.
  - The chance of a tick carrying the disease, even in an endemic area, are low.
  - No demonstrable benefit of prophylaxis has been found.

R

Screening for Anemia

BACKGROUND

- Anemia may be defined by laboratory values (low hemoglobin) or physiologic consequences (inadequate oxygen-carrying capacity).
  - Both are equally important.
- Prevalence of iron-deficiency anemia
  - Varies, but may be as high as 2.9%
  - Has decreased over the past several decades, primarily because of:
    - Improved dietary recommendations
    - Use of iron-fortified formulas
- Sickle cell anemia
  - Affects approximately 1 of every 600 African-American children
  - Early detection with rapid institution of penicillin prophylaxis has dramatically reduced incidence of fatal pneumococcal sepsis in newborns and young children.
  - Screening is now required for all 50 states and District of Columbia.
  - Many states also report variant hemoglobins identified incidentally during the screening process.

GOALS

- Screening programs are directed primarily at detecting disease in otherwise asymptomatic children.
- Adequate iron stores are critical for normal neurocognitive development, and inadequate levels should be detected and treated as early as possible.
  - Iron deficiency is the major impetus behind public health recommendations for anemia-screening programs.
  - Screening for anemia is the most reliable and cost-effective method for detecting occult iron deficiency.

GENERAL APPROACH

- Screening for anemia in infants and young children begins shortly after birth via newborn hemoglobinopathy screening programs.
  - Many of the variant hemoglobins are benign, particularly when patients are heterozygous.
  - Newborn screening improves sensitivity of detection for α-thalassemia.
  - Some forms of ß-thalassemia may not be detectable until after hemoglobin switching from fetal forms has been completed at 6–12 months of age.
- The AAP recommends next screening at 9–12 months.
- The AAP recommends additional screening between 15 months and 5 years for children at risk.
  - Preterm or low-birth-weight infants
  - Infants receiving unfortified formula
  - Infants receiving cow's milk before age 12 months
  - Breastfed infants not getting iron supplementation after age 6 months
  - Children consuming >24 ounces of cow's milk per day
  - Children with special health care needs
- The AAP recommends screening at least once during adolescence for males.
- The AAP recommends annual screening for menstruating females.
- Further information about the morphologic characteristics of the patient's erythrocytes should also be obtained.
- Important information that is relevant to the anemic patient
  - A history of:
    - Neonatal jaundice
    - Ethnicity
    - Dietary intake
  - Family history of:
    - Splenectomy
    - Cholecystectomy
    - Iron therapy
    - Blood transfusions

SPECIFIC INTERVENTIONS

Anemia screening

- Screening is accomplished by determining the whole-blood hemoglobin concentration using blood obtained by skin puncture of the finger or heel.
  - The sample may be analyzed using a small portable spectrophotometer or a bench-top particle counter.
    - Either method is quick and reliable, with minimal quality control and maintenance required.
  - Hemoglobin concentration is compared with reference values for age-matched normal children.
    - Levels that are less than the lower reference limit (2 standard deviations below the mean) are defined as anemic.
- Positive screening tests for anemia must be confirmed and correlated with the clinical presentation.
  - Confirmation is usually performed by submitting a venous blood sample anticoagulated with ethylenediamine tetraacetic acid to the hematology laboratory for:
    - Complete blood count
    - Microscopic examination of a Wright-stained peripheral blood smear.
- Other studies that may be helpful in determining iron status:
  - Serum ferritin (most reliable indicator of iron status/stores in the absence of an underlying inflammatory illness)
  - Serum iron

- Iron-binding capacity
  - Best obtained in the fasting state, since findings may be misleading if the patient has recently eaten an iron-rich meal
- Lead level
  - Younger children may be more prone to lead intoxication secondary to pica associated with iron deficiency.

Differential diagnoses

- Iron-deficiency anemia will generally have microcytic-hypochromic indices:
  - Low mean corpuscular volume
  - Low mean corpuscular hemoglobin concentration
  - High red-cell distribution width
  - May be associated with thrombocytosis
    - Thrombocytopenia may be observed in severe iron deficiency.
- Types of anemia that should be included in the differential diagnosis of microcytic anemia:
  - Thalassemia
  - Sickle-thalassemia syndromes
  - Some hemoglobinopathies (C and E)
  - Severe lead intoxication
  - Anemia of chronic disease
  - Hereditary spherocytosis

- For additional information on differential diagnoses, see Anemia and Pallor.

Management

- Mild microcytic anemia (ie, hemoglobin level 8–10 g/dL)
  - Empiric treatment with iron supplementation (3–4 mg elemental iron/kg daily) is appropriate.
  - Reticulocyte count should increase within 1 week of beginning iron therapy.
  - The hemoglobin level should increase by at least 1 g/dL within a month.
    - Treatment should continue for an additional 2 months in patients who respond.
  - Appropriate dietary counseling is important to prevent recurrence.
  - For patients who fail to respond:
    - Additional laboratory evaluation is indicated.
    - Referral to a hematologist should be considered.
    - An evaluation should be undertaken to identify sources of occult blood loss.
      - Particularly in older children who are not consuming significant amounts of cow's milk.
- If anemia is more severe, then confirmatory laboratory evaluation should be done when empiric iron therapy is begun.

S

Screening for Drugs

BACKGROUND

General

- Adolescent substance abuse is a major public health problem that contributes to potentially preventable morbidity and mortality.
- Up to 1 in 10 adolescents should receive a full diagnostic evaluation for substance abuse.
  - At least half are likely to require treatment.
- Earlier identification can prevent many adverse consequences.
- Very high-risk children (who abuse nicotine, alcohol, marijuana, and other substances) are very likely to suffer from:
  - School failure
  - Sexually transmitted infections, such as HIV infection
  - Teenage pregnancy
  - Delinquency
  - Suicide
  - Homicide

Drug use

- Cigarettes
  - 8th graders
    - 10% report having smoked in the previous 30 days.
    - 5% smoked daily.
  - 12th graders
    - 26.7% report smoking in the previous 30 days
    - >16.9% smoked daily.
  - 75% of adolescents who smoke will become lifetime smokers and face longer exposure to nicotine toxicity.
  - Nicotine alone accounts for more substance-related deaths than all other drugs (including alcohol) together.
  - Adolescents who abuse nicotine and alcohol are more likely to abuse marijuana and other illicit substances.
- Alcohol
  - 8th graders—in the previous 30 days:
    - 19.5% used alcohol.
    - 6.7% had been drunk.
  - 12th graders—in the previous 30 days
    - Nearly 50% used alcohol.
    - 30.3% had been drunk.
  - 3.9% of high school seniors report being drunk daily.
  - In youth 15–24 years of age, half of all motor vehicle accidents are alcohol related.
- Marijuana
  - 21.3% of high school seniors have smoked marijuana in the previous 30 days.
  - 6% smoked marijuana daily.
- Other illicit drugs
  - 11.3% of high school seniors report using some type of other illicit drug.

- Isolated use of drugs other than marijuana and alcohol is uncommon.

Drug abuse

- Excluding nicotine, 7% of 12- to 17-year-olds have a substance use disorder.
- The highest age-specific prevalence occurs during adolescence.
- Rates of current dependence on alcohol and other drugs peak between 16 and 19 years of age.
- Alcohol and marijuana are most commonly abused substances among adolescents.
- Of adolescents with substance use disorders:
  - 41% have alcohol use disorder.
  - 11% have alcohol or marijuana use disorder.
  - 5% have alcohol use disorder with another substance use disorder (other than marijuana).
  - 3% have marijuana use disorder with another substance use disorder (other than alcohol).

Gateway hypothesis

- Progression of substance use from cigarettes and alcohol to marijuana or from marijuana to cocaine and possibly heroin
- Only 12.8% of persons who have smoked marijuana once or twice have tried cocaine.
  - Of those who have smoked >300 times, over 71% have tried cocaine.
- The extent to which nicotine use predisposes to marijuana use or marijuana use predisposes to cocaine use is unclear, but compelling associations exist.
- Age of onset of substance use is also associated with transition between stages.
  - Heroin users typically report first smoking cigarettes at 12.6 years.
  - Cocaine users report beginning cigarettes at 14 years.
  - Marijuana users report beginning cigarettes at 14.6 years.
  - Alcohol-only users report beginning at 15.8 years.
- Early-onset substance abuse disorders
  - The earlier the age of onset, the more likely substance use is to develop into a lifetime disorder.
- Early-onset (adolescent) substance use disorders differ from disorders developing later.
  - Increased degree of disruptive behaviors or delinquency
  - Increased degree of novelty or sensation seeking
  - Decreased dependence on external incentives (eg, doing well in school, performing a job well)
- Late-onset substance abuse disorders
  - Tend to be associated with decreased antisocial behavior and increased reward dependence compared with early-onset disorders

Risk factors

- Behavioral impulsivity, conduct problems, and difficulties in functioning that arise before first use of the substance
- Aggression
  - Sometimes accompanies behavioral impulsivity and develops during the preschool or early school-age period
  - More highly associated with oppositional defiant disorder, which, in turn, is highly associated with early-onset conduct disorder
- Disruptive behavior disorders, such as conduct disorder, strongly predict transition from substance use to abuse.
- Untreated attention-deficit/hyperactivity disorder
  - Increases risk of substance use by about 2 times the general risk
  - If comorbid with conduct disorder, increases risk for substance use disorder by up to 4 times the general risk
- Low levels of parental monitoring
- Parental substance abuse
- Peers who also use substances
- Poverty and neglect

Substance abuse versus substance dependence

- Abuse
  - Maladaptive pattern of substance use leading to clinically significant impairment or distress
  - Symptoms
    - Recurrent substance use resulting in failure to fulfill major role obligations at work, school, or home
    - Recurrent substance use in situations in which it is physically hazardous
    - Recurrent substance-related legal problems
    - Continued substance use despite persistent or recurrent social or interpersonal problems caused or exacerbated by the substance
- Dependence
  - Symptoms indicating tolerance or withdrawal or loss of function due to substance use
    - Tolerance: need for increased amounts of substance to achieve intoxication or desired effect *and* markedly diminished effect with continued use of the same amount of substance
    - Withdrawal: characteristic withdrawal syndrome for the substance *and* use of the same (or a closely related) substance to relieve or avoid withdrawal symptoms
    - Use of substance in larger amounts or for a longer period than expected
    - Persistent desire or unsuccessful effort to reduce or control substance use
    - Much time spent in activities necessary to obtain or use the substance or recover from its effects

  - Surrender of or decrease in important social, occupational, or recreational activities due to substance use
  - Continued use of substance despite knowledge of persistent or recurrent physical or psychological problems probably caused or exacerbated by the substance

GOALS

- After suspecting or detecting substance use, determine whether substance use disorder is present.
  - Substance use alone does not imply substance use disorder.
  - Infrequent substance use may be a normative part of adolescent development.
- Patterns of use in adolescents differ from those in adults (eg, availability, freedom, supervision).
- Some youth can meet 1 or 2 criteria of substance dependence but no criteria for abuse.
  - These diagnostic orphans appear similar to youth with substance abuse diagnoses and make up about one-third of youth who use alcohol regularly.
  - Because of the high prevalence of these diagnostic orphans, ask youth about symptoms of both substance abuse and dependence.
  - Allow the diagnosis to depend largely on the maladaptive significance of substance use.

GENERAL APPROACH

- To identify substance use disorder, pay attention to surrounding behaviors.
  - Disruptive or defiant behavior
  - School failure or truancy
  - Depression or suicidal thoughts
  - Early-onset sexual behavior
  - Sexually transmitted infection
  - Pregnancy
  - Legal problems
- Encourage parents to remain involved in their adolescents' lives so that they may identify and seek help for these problem behaviors.
- Increased parental monitoring and involvement help protect against development of substance abuse.
- The adolescent's self-report of substance-related problems is key to accurate diagnosis and treatment.
  - Create an environment in which the adolescent can talk about alcohol or drug use by defining adolescent confidentiality.
  - Confidentiality involves a safety exclusion: only information that indicates adolescent is a danger to self or others will be revealed to the parent or guardian.
  - By including substance use in this exclusion to confidentiality, any talk of drug use will be muted because of fear of parental knowledge.

S

- Thus do not readily divulge normative substance experimentation to caretakers.
- Decide each case on the basis of the particular risks involved.
- Helping an adolescent self-identify his or her own substance problems is usually the best-case scenario.
  - Family intervention is usually required for effective treatment.
- Assess the adolescent's functioning through several viewpoints.
  - Parents
  - Other health care providers
  - Adolescent's school, if possible

SPECIFIC INTERVENTIONS

Screening

- Standardized instruments
  - The screening instruments that are most sensitive ask about substance use and substance-related problems.
  - The following self-report instruments concentrate on substance-related problems (adaptive significance of substance use symptoms).
    - Substance Abuse Subtle Screening Inventory
    - Personal Experience Inventory
    - Problem Oriented Screening Instrument for Teenagers
    - Rutgers Alcohol Problem Index
  - Structured interviews
    - Assess both symptoms and relationship between substance use and other domains of functioning.
    - Examples
      - Comprehensive Addiction Severity Index
      - Global Appraisal of Individual Needs
    - Both give diagnoses of substance abuse according to the *Diagnostic and Statistical Manual of Mental Disorders*.
    - Both assess:
      - Substance use
      - Substance-related problems
      - Family relationships
      - Peer relationships
      - Legal status
      - Psychiatric problems
      - Leisure activities
  - CRAFFT screening tool
    - Validated for adolescents
    - Consists of 6 items to identify adolescents with problematic substance use
    - Positive answers to ≥2 items suggest that intervention is necessary.

- Urine drug screens
  - Sequence of urine drug screens and clinical interviewing of parents and youth are usually necessary to diagnose adolescent substance abuse.
  - The meaning of a positive urine drug screen varies greatly according to the context in which it is obtained.
    - Hospitalization for medical problem
      - A urine drug screen positive for marijuana more likely indicates use rather than abuse, but use or abuse can be determined only after clinical interview with the adolescent, parent, or teacher or other representative from school.
    - Random positive finding from a urine drug screen for cocaine or heroin
      - Increases suspicion of substance use disorder
    - High index of suspicion of substance abuse
      - Youth who has been truant, verbally aggressive toward parents, not fulfilling obligations at home, staying out late
      - The presence of any substance suggests that the youth has substance use disorder.
  - Youths who refuse to give urine samples or claim they cannot urinate often fear the consequences and are likely to be hiding substance use.
  - To determine severity of use, warn adolescent before urine drug screen.
    - If substance use is infrequent, the adolescent should be able to produce clean urine.
    - A positive drug screen after advance warning indicates a more severe problem.
  - The gold standard is supervised urine collection, but this method can be complicated and overly invasive.
    - Less invasive method: plastic thermometer, which indicates the urine's temperature
  - Test urine for creatinine level.
    - Youth may hydrate themselves or use diuretic substances to reduce drug concentration in urine.
    - Low urine creatinine suggests significant substance use.
  - Urine drugs screens vary in sensitivity.
    - Marijuana: may last 7 to 28 days in urine
      - Duration depends on frequency of marijuana use.
    - Alcohol: lasts only 12 hours in urine
      - Difficult to detect or monitor with this method
      - Alcohol breathalyzers are generally more sensitive than urine tests and can be used readily.
    - Cocaine: lasts up to 48
    - Heroin: lasts up to 72 hours
    - Tests for substances not included on regular drug panels can be costly.
      - Methylenedioxymethamphetamine (MDMA or ecstasy)

- Lysergic acid diethylamide (LSD or acid)
- Ketamine (special K)
- Phencyclidine (PCP or angel dust)

Management

- Referral
  - When substance use disorder is diagnosed or suspected, make an appropriate referral.
  - Referral depends on the severity of the problem.
    - Arrest for driving under the influence: substance abuse treatment center
    - Unclear extent of abuse: private mental health practitioner
  - Adherence to referral varies by the adolescent's relationship with the referring clinician and the clinician's relationship with the adolescent's parents or guardian.
  - Likelihood of a successful referral is lower without development of some understanding with the adolescent and family.
  - Indications for referral
    - Ongoing substance use despite monitoring
    - Prior parent or authority attempts to get the patient to abstain from or control substance use
    - Progression of substance use to substances of greater risk (eg, alcohol to cocaine)
    - Meeting criteria for substance abuse or dependence (by parent, adolescent, or teacher or other authority figure's report)
    - High index of suspicion due to unexplained adaptive impairment or unexplained decline in adaptive function
    - Patient substance use and high index of suspicion due to substance use disorder in parent, sibling, or peer
    - Patient substance use and high index of suspicion due to patient psychiatric comorbidity or delinquent behaviors
    - Dangerous behavior by patient with substance use (eg, self-mutilation, suicidal thoughts, driving under the influence)
- Motivational interviewing in primary care
  - Increases awareness of substance-related problems
  - Emphasizes supporting personal-change goals with a nonjudgmental attitude toward the adolescent's substance use
  - Develops the clinician's empathy with the adolescent and forges an alliance that is less confrontational than most other approaches
  - Effects change by encouraging the adolescent to contemplate discrepancy between personal goals and actions (ie, substance use)
  - Holds great promise in adolescents because of emphasis on personal choice and support of adolescent's developing autonomy

- Outpatient specialty treatments
  - Family therapy
    - Family therapies that include the adolescent have the most empirical support.
    - Seeks to reduce familial contributions to development or maintenance of adolescent substance abuse behaviors
    - Experienced family therapists can help families find the right kind of professional guidance for the problem.
    - Empirically validated family therapies include:
      - Functional family therapy (positive relabeling, consistently clear communication, and development of supportive recovery environment)
      - Family system therapy
  - Behavioral therapy
    - Role playing, response rehearsal, homework assignments, diary keeping
    - Reduces substance use (measured by urine drug screen, adolescent self-reports, and collateral reports) compared with supportive therapy
  - Cognitive-behavioral therapy
    - Short- and long-term benefits for adolescents with substance use disorder
  - 12-step facilitation therapies
    - Most common available treatments in most areas
    - Least empirical support compared with other methods
    - May integrate aspects of evidence-based treatments
- Inpatient or residential treatments
  - Can stop the vicious cycle of substance abuse, particularly when negative reinforcement (eg, withdrawal from opiates or alcohol or, to a lesser extent, marijuana) maintains dependence
  - Can range from a few weeks to ≥1 year
  - Can help establish alternative reinforcers to substance use that may generalize to the outside world
  - Associated with long-term benefits in behavior
    - Reductions in substance use and criminal recidivism
    - Increased adaptive functioning
  - Associated with high levels of attrition (30–40% within the first month; up to 80% within the first year)
  - Direct relationship between length of treatment and outcome
  - Substance abuse treatment can be effective even when mandated.
    - Mandated community support groups reduce criminal recidivism among incarcerated delinquents with drug-related crimes.
    - Voluntary treatment is associated with the best outcomes.

S

Screening for Lead Poisoning

BACKGROUND

- Lead adversely affects:
  - Attention
  - Vigilance
  - Language development
  - Transfer of information from short-term to long-term memory
  - Aggression
  - Antisocial or delinquent behaviors
- Negative effects are seen at levels >10 mcg/dL, but lower levels may also produce negative effects.
- An estimated 310,000 children in the US between 1 and 5 years of age have elevated blood lead levels.
  - Levels peak between 1 and 3 years of age.
  - Levels vary inversely with family income.
    - An impoverished home and Medicaid enrollment are closely linked to increased exposure.
    - All children in Medicaid are required by federal regulation to be tested for blood lead levels at 1 and 2 years of age.
- Lead-contaminated interior or exterior household paint that is peeling or chipping is the most common, concentrated source of exposure.
  - The older a house, the more likely it is to contain lead-based paint.
  - The less affluent the family, the more likely the paint is to be in disrepair.
  - Housing built before 1950 poses the greatest danger.
    - 50% of these houses are in California, Illinois, Massachusetts, Missouri, New York, Ohio, and Pennsylvania.
- Other sources of lead exposure
  - Water
  - Food
  - Soil
  - Toys
  - Ceramics
  - Parents whose clothing becomes contaminated with lead at work
    - Battery production or repair
    - Making pottery
    - Smelting
    - Printing
    - Paint contracting
    - Working on a firing range
    - Brass foundry
    - Work on the demolition or renovation of outdoor structures
  - Hobbies
    - Making lead fishing sinkers or bullets
    - Collecting lead figurines
    - Spending time at indoor firing ranges
    - Making pottery
  - Home remedies (in certain Latin American and Southeast Asian cultures): azarcon or greta
  - Cosmetics (kohl)
  - Lead plumbing, especially in areas with older water supplies

GOALS

- Prevention of severe toxicity and deaths, eg, due to accidental ingestion of lead-containing necklaces and metallic charms
- Reduction of low-level effects through community abatement and clinical screening
  - Screening serves to detect lead levels.
  - Each 10-mcg/dL increase in blood lead results in a loss of 2–3 points in IQ.

GENERAL APPROACH

- Centers for Disease Control and Prevention (CDC) Guidance defines national standards for screening programs.
  - The CDC recommends use of venous or capillary blood lead level as the examination of choice.
    - Capillary specimens collected by finger-stick are acceptable, but values ≥10 mcg/dL must be confirmed with a venous sample.
  - Uses 10 mcg/dL as the cutoff point for defining an elevated lead level
  - Allowable error (per Clinical Laboratory Improvement Amendments) is ±4 mcg/dL or 10% of the value, whichever is greater.
  - At low levels, the allowable laboratory error can result in misclassification that might affect management.
- The CDC advises state health officials to develop screening programs based on risk characteristics of their local communities.
- The CDC advises that professionals use blood lead tests to screen:
  - 1- and 2-year-olds (and 3- to 6-year-olds who have not been screened previously) who meet ≥1 of these criteria:
    - The child lives in a ZIP code where ≥27% of housing stock built before 1950 or ≥12% of children have blood lead levels ≥10 mcg/dL.
    - The child receives services from public assistance programs, eg, Medicaid or the Special Supplemental Nutrition Program for Women, Infants, and Children (WIC).
  - If at the 2-year screen the blood lead level is again <10 mcg/dL and the child's potential exposures have not increased, further screening is not necessary.

- In communities where universal screening is recommended, children whose blood lead screening test result at age 1 year is <10 mcg/dL should be rescreened at age 2 years.
- Screening by questionnaire to evaluate risk
  - Part of the CDC guidelines, but limited by variable sensitivity and specificity
  - Still used by some states and localities as part of an overall lead-screening strategy, often with modifications in the specific questions used based on locale
- In addition to state- or local-level guidelines, health care professionals should watch for children who should be screened because of exposure to less usual sources of lead from parental occupations or hobbies.
- If parents or health care professionals suspect lead exposure, promptly test for blood lead, regardless of:
  - Patient age
  - General health department recommendations
  - Responses to screening questionnaires
- Health care providers must participate in and comply with the recommended program.
  - Compliance needs to be improved, especially for at-risk children.
- The CDC Web site has the latest, most accurate screening questions by region.

SPECIFIC INTERVENTIONS

CDC recommended test schedule for follow-up of positive screens

- Follow-up testing based on initial screening result (using confirmatory venous sample)
  - 10–19 mcg/dL: confirmation test at 3 months
  - 20–44 mcg/dL: confirmation test at 1 week to 1 month
  - 45–59 mcg/dL: confirmation test at 48 hours
  - 60–69 mcg/dL: confirmation test at 24 hours
  - >70 mcg/dL: confirmation test immediately/emergency

Management by blood level results

- Blood lead values 10–19 mcg/dL (confirmed)
  - Parents should be counseled on ways to diminish ongoing exposure.
    - Lead-based paint abatement performed by a properly licensed contractor and, if possible, supervision of the local health department
    - Relocate children and pregnant women to another site while abatement is being performed.
    - Have thorough cleanup of dust before allowing children to reinhabit the home.
  - If levels are between 10 and 14 mcg/dL: retest every 3 months.

- If levels are between 15 and 19 mcg/dL: retest every 2 months.
  - Lead values >10 mcg/dL may prompt a home inspection.
- Blood lead values 20–44 mcg/dL require both medical and environmental intervention.
  - Medical evaluation: detailed medical, nutritional, developmental, and environmental history, and complete physical examination
    - Evaluation should focus on identifying signs and symptoms of lead poisoning (although very unusual at these levels).
    - Assess development to determine the need for early intervention services (although risk of demonstrable delays is unlikely).
    - Concerns about inattention and hyperactivity should prompt referral for early intervention services.
  - Nutritional assessment
    - To identify patterns that result in increased absorption of lead from the gastrointestinal tract, eg, iron deficiency, low calcium intake, or infrequent meals
    - Many children are eligible for support from WIC and should be referred.
    - If the child is iron deficient, then iron supplements should be prescribed.
    - Increasing calcium intake is not proven but generally recommended, especially when calcium intake is low.
    - Increasing meal frequency may decrease lead absorption, but should be done in the context of a diet not excessive in calories.
  - Laboratory evaluation of iron status, including:
    - Hematocrit
    - Mean corpuscular volume
    - Either a ferritin level or iron and iron binding capacity levels
  - Environmental inspection and, when indicated, environmental intervention to diminish or curtail further exposure to lead
    - Case management can ensure that needed counseling and medical, nutritional, and environmental interventions are provided quickly and effectively.
  - Home inspections, usually performed by local public health departments, are often a lengthy process, but abatement of hazards and subsequent dust control are cornerstones of treatment.
- Blood lead values ≥45 mcg/dL
  - Remove from sources of lead.
  - Initiate chelation therapy.

S

How to avoid lead hazards in the home

- Cover leaded paint that is chipping or peeling.
- Move cribs, playpens, furniture, and play areas away from chipping or peeling paint.
- Wet-mop floors and wet-clean windowsills and window wells with a high-phosphate detergent.
- Avoid dry dusting or sweeping.
- Wash children's hands, toys, and pacifiers regularly.
- Use cold water for cooking; run tap water for 2–3 minutes every morning before using.
- Repair deteriorated windowpanes in house and on porches.
- Replace old windows.
- Remove paint in old homes (only by trained contractors).
- Postabatement cleanup, preferably by professional house-cleaners, is essential.
- Relocate the family to lead-safe housing.

Scrotal Swelling and Pain

DEFINITION

- *Scrotal swelling* is usually classified as:
  - Painful versus painless
  - Acute versus chronic
- *Testicular torsion* is the twisting of the spermatic cord, with resulting compromise of the blood supply to the testis.
  - The appendix testis is a vestige of the müllerian duct system that hangs from the upper pole of the testis and is susceptible to torsion.
- *Epididymitis* is inflammation of the epididymis.
- *Orchitis* is inflammation of the testis.
- *Inguinal hernias* and *hydroceles* fall along a continuum, both caused by persistent patency of the processus vaginalis.
- *Varicoceles* are dilatations of the spermatic veins or pampiniform plexus
- *Spermatoceles* and *epididymal* cysts are sperm-filled cystic lesions attached to the upper pole of the testis

EPIDEMIOLOGY

- Prevalence
  - Inguinal hernias and hydroceles are the most common causes of scrotal swelling.
  - Testicular torsion occurs in 1:4000 boys.
  - Varicoceles are present in 15% of male adolescents and adults.
- Age
  - Hernias can occur at any age but are more common in premature infants.
  - Testicular torsion most commonly occurs between the ages of 12 and 18 years.
  - Idiopathic scrotal edema affects children <14 years.
  - Acute inflammation of the epididymis or testis, including mumps orchitis, can occur at any age but is uncommon before adolescence.
  - Varicoceles are usually asymptomatic and are usually detected between 10 and 15 years of age.

MECHANISM

- Acute scrotal swelling with pain
  - Torsion of the testicle
    - Twisting of the spermatic cord, with resulting compromise of the blood supply to the testis
  - Torsion of the appendix testis
    - When the appendix testis torses, inflammation and swelling of the testis and epididymis ensue, causing testicular pain and scrotal erythema.
  - Acute epididymitis-orchitis
    - Results from an anomaly of the urinary tract, either congenital or acquired

- Renal duplications and posterior urethral valves are among the more common anomalies.
- With intermittent catheterization, the condition can occur from retrograde passage of bacteria back from ejaculatory ducts at the level of the prostate to the testis and epididymis.
  - Henoch-Schönlein purpura
    - Systemic vasculitis that can cause abdominal and joint pain
    - May involve the scrotal wall in a minority of cases
  - Trauma
    - Zipper entrapment of scrotal skin
    - Severe blunt or straddle trauma affecting the scrotal contents
  - Scrotal skin disease
    - Insect bites, folliculitis, and allergic dermatitis may cause erythema and edema of the scrotal wall.
- Scrotal swelling without pain
  - Hernias and hydroceles
    - Most are caused by persistent patency of the processus vaginalis (peritoneal out-pouching that accompanies the testis during its abdominal-scrotal descent).
    - Layers of the processus vaginalis condense late in gestation or early postnatally.
    - Obliteration of the processus vaginalis only around the testis leads to an indirect inguinal hernia with protrusion of fluid (or other contents) through the internal ring to the end of the pouch and potentially to the scrotum.
    - Communicating hydrocele occurs when fluid travels through a processus vaginalis into the tunica vaginalis around the testis.
    - Scrotal hydrocele occurs after complete obliteration proximally with patency distally.
    - Hydroceles of the cord occur when the processus vaginalis obliterates proximally and distally, leaving a patent area in the midportion with retained fluid.
  - Varicoceles
    - A predilection for the left side exists, reflecting anatomy of the left gonadal vein entering the left renal vein at a right angle.
    - The right gonadal vein enters the vena cava directly at an angle, precluding reflux of venous blood.

HISTORY

- Take the history from both child (when possible) and parent.

History

- Determine the following.
  - Whether swelling or pain is recurrent and acute or chronic
  - Exact timing of the onset of symptoms, particularly in the presence of acute pain and swelling

- Nature of the pain
  - Sharp
  - Dull
  - Constant
  - Intermittent
  - Constant, with intermittent increases in intensity
  - Associated with nausea or vomiting
- Location of pain
  - Scrotum, specifically the testis
  - Radiation into abdomen or from abdomen into the scrotum
- Laterality of swelling and pain
- Activity or positions that alleviate or aggravate pain and swelling
- Nature of swelling
  - Changes in size during a single day *or*
  - Is constant *or*
  - Increases or decreases with time
- Recent trauma, sexual activity, use of medications, presence of rashes, and weight loss

Specific conditions

- Acute scrotal swelling with pain
  - Torsion of the testicle
    - Acute onset of constant, severe scrotal pain aggravated by physical activity
    - If periods of respite from pain occur, then intermittent torsion and detorsion should be considered.
    - Nausea and vomiting may occur.
    - Possible history of incidental antecedent scrotal trauma, but pain usually occurs during rest or sleep
    - Neonatal testicular torsion
    - Can exhibit at delivery as a nontender hard scrotal mass
  - Torsion of the appendix testis
    - Onset of pain and swelling is commonly acute but can be progressive, usually occurring during rest.
    - Pain can be severe, but nausea and vomiting are less common than with testicular torsion.
  - Acute epididymitis-orchitis
    - History can reveal acute or more protracted onset of pain.
    - The patient may have fever or dysuria.
    - Epididymal inflammation may arise after scrotal trauma.
    - In the adolescent patient, a history of sexual activity or urethral discharge helps guide antibiotic treatment.
  - Henoch-Schönlein purpura
    - Onset may be insidious or acute, producing a variable degree of erythema and edema.

- In more severe cases, the process may involve the testis and epididymis, mimicking testicular torsion.
  - Focal fat necrosis
    - Can exhibit with scrotal pain and swelling, usually after trauma in an obese boy
  - Trauma
    - History (eg, injury from zipper entrapment of scrotal skin) can be definitive.
  - Mumps orchitis
    - Rarely occurs in isolation; pain and swelling usually occur within a week after parotitis.
  - Scrotal skin disease
    - History may be of limited utility.
- Scrotal swelling without pain
  - Inguinal hernias and hydroceles
    - Hernia
      - Swelling expands with increases in intraabdominal pressure (eg, crying, bowel movements, coughing).
      - The parent or child often reports the swelling to be smallest in the morning and largest late in the day.
    - Hydrocele
      - Whether the hydrocele is acute or whether the scrotum has been chronically enlarged is often unclear.
      - The patient may have a history of trauma to the scrotum that stimulates production of serous fluid.
      - When the scrotum changes size during the day, suspect a communicating hydrocele.
  - Tumors
    - Usually present as a hard, painless mass (or vague heavy feeling) in the testicle detected by the child, parent, or examining physician
  - Varicoceles
    - Dilated veins are usually asymptomatic and are detected by the patient or the physician during routine physical examination.
    - Some patients report heaviness or a dragging feeling.
  - Spermatoceles and epididymal cysts
    - Painless and round, they usually remain stable in size but can sometimes enlarge.

PHYSICAL EXAM

- Palpate the abdomen and groin to determine whether an intraabdominal process extends into the scrotum.
- Inspect the scrotum to look for laterality of the process and scrotal erythema.
- Palpate the scrotum to determine the presence of:
  - Cremasteric reflexes
  - Testicular position
  - Tenderness

- Localization of the swelling to the scrotum
- Presence of proximal extension into the cord
■ Acute scrotal swelling with pain
  - Torsion of the testicle
    - Scrotal erythema
    - Swelling of the involved hemiscrotum
    - Higher-than-normal position of the testis within the scrotum
    - Palpation may show a horizontal rather than normal vertical orientation of the testicle.
    - Evaluation of the cremasteric reflex should begin on the contralateral side; palpate the apparently unaffected testis to confirm normal size and position.
      ■ Unilateral loss of the cremasteric reflex on the side of the swelling and pain highly correlates with the presence of torsion.
    - The testis should then be palpated.
      ■ Despite the pain this maneuver may cause, it helps differentiate torsion from epididymitis.
      ■ With torsion, exquisite pain is elicited on palpation from the testis, as well as from the epididymis and distal spermatic cord.
      ■ Actual point of torsion of the spermatic cord can sometimes be palpated.
    - Associated hydrocele may be palpated and confirmed by transillumination.
    - Tense or large hydrocele often makes examination difficult.
  - Torsion of the appendix testis
    - May demonstrate hemiscrotal erythema and swelling
    - A blue-dot sign, the necrotic appendage visible through the scrotal skin, can help make the diagnosis.
    - A normal cremasteric reflex is present bilaterally, and the testis is normally positioned within the scrotum.
    - Testicular discomfort, if present, is typically mild, but point tenderness may be elicited from uppermost pole of the testis near the head of the epididymis—the location of the appendages.
    - On palpation, examiner may feel a 3- to 5-mm tender indurated mass on the upper pole.
  - Acute epididymitis-orchitis
    - Scrotal erythema and swelling are present, along with an intact cremasteric reflex.
    - Palpation during early phase of the inflammatory process demonstrates tenderness limited to the epididymis.
    - In the later phase, tenderness and inflammation include both epididymis and testis, and the distinction between the 2 structures may be difficult to appreciate.
    - The Prehn sign (relief of pain with testicular elevation) may be positive.

- Focal fat necrosis
  - Examination shows pain and swelling limited to the scrotum and not the testis.
  - Examination can be limited by discomfort and degree of obesity.
- Trauma
  - Examination must include both hemiscrotums and surrounding structures (penis, perineum), assessing for swelling, ecchymosis, and bleeding.
  - Palpation may be limited by the degree of swelling or blood in the scrotum.
  - Tenderness may be limited to testis or epididymis, depending on extent of trauma.
- Mumps orchitis
  - Tender testis
- Scrotal skin disease
  - Redness and edema limited to scrotum, with normal testicle and spermatic cord
■ Scrotal swelling without pain
  - Inguinal hernias and hydroceles
    - Feel for the testis first and keep it in mind during the rest of the examination.
    - Avoid confusing testis with contents of an incarcerated hernia.
    - Hernia
      ■ A bulge in the inguinal region with fluid that can be gently reduced back into the abdomen is diagnostic of an inguinal hernia.
      ■ In the cooperative child who can increase his intra-abdominal pressure, this procedure may be repeatedly shown, particularly with the child standing.
      ■ Presence of thickened spermatic cord or silk-stocking sign (the feel of the layers of the processus vaginalis being rubbed against each other) suggests patency of the processus vaginalis or a hernia.
    - Hydrocele
      ■ When fluid is limited to the testis and spermatic cord can be palpated above the fluid, a hydrocele is present.
      ■ Hydrocele of the spermatic cord feels distinct from the testis and is round or ovoid, possibly mimicking the presence of an additional testis.
      ■ Hydroceles (communicating, scrotal, or of the cord) are rarely associated with tenderness on palpation
  - Tumors
    - On palpation, mass is harder than the substance of the testis, but this distinction may be difficult to discern.
    - Mass may bulge from surface of the testis.
  - Varicoceles
    - Perform physical examination with the patient in the supine and standing positions.

S

– Varicocele is usually decompressed in the supine position and present in the standing position.

– Inspection may reveal dilated veins (grade 3 of 3).

– Increased blood pooling in veins can sometimes be prompted by a Valsalva maneuver (grade 2 of 3).

- Spermatoceles and epididymal cysts

– Separate from the testis and can be transilluminated

DIFFERENTIAL DIAGNOSIS

Acute scrotal swelling with pain

- Torsion of spermatic cord
- Torsion of appendix testis
- Acute epididymitis-orchitis
- Mumps orchitis
- Henoch-Schönlein purpura
- Trauma
- Insect bite
- Thrombosis of spermatic vein
- Fat necrosis
- Hernia
- Folliculitis
- Dermatitis, acute

Scrotal swelling without pain

- Tumor
- Idiopathic scrotal edema
- Hydrocele
- Henoch-Schönlein purpura
- Hernia

Chronic scrotal swelling

- Hydrocele
- Hernia
- Varicocele
- Spermatocele
- Sebaceous cyst
- Tumor

LABORATORY EVALUATION

- Laboratory tests are of limited value.
- The leukocyte count may be elevated in the setting of infection.
- Urinalysis may help distinguish orchitis from torsion of the spermatic cord or testicular appendage when leukocytes or nitrites are present.
- Acute scrotal swelling with pain
  - Torsion of the testicle
    - Urinalysis is unremarkable.
    - Although the leukocytes count may be mildly elevated, it is not discriminating.

- Acute epididymitis-orchitis
  - Urinalysis may prove positive for leukocytes and nitrite but is often unremarkable among adolescents.
  - The leukocyte count is usually elevated.
- Scrotal swelling without pain
  - Inguinal hernias and hydroceles
    - Laboratory tests are useful only for incarcerated inguinal hernias, with an elevated leukocyte count and possible acidosis.
  - Tumors
    - Preoperative tumor markers (α-fetoprotein, ß-human chorionic gonadotropin) should be measured and used for postoperative monitoring.

IMAGING

- Ultrasonography can determine whether the scrotal swelling:
  - Is fluid filled or solid
  - Arises from abdomen and extends into groin
  - Is limited to the scrotum
  - Arises from the testis or spermatic cord structures
- Ultrasonography with Doppler can assess the flow of blood into the testis, helping to differentiate torsion of the testis from an inflammatory process.
  - Benefits
    - Does not use ionizing radiation
    - Takes less time to perform than nuclear scanning
  - Drawbacks
    - Limited by user variability
    - Requires placing a probe over a sensitive area
- Nuclear scintigraphy using ^{99m}technetium-pertechnetate evaluates blood flow to the testis.
  - Absence of flow results in a cold spot and suggests torsion.
  - Inflammation results in increased flow to the same area.
  - Benefits
    - Not limited by user variability associated with ultrasonography
    - Does not require placing a probe over a tender area
  - Drawbacks
    - Uses ionizing radiation
    - Takes longer to perform than ultrasonography, thus limiting utility when time is of the essence
  - Sensitivity and specificity of the 2 modalities are similar.
- Acute scrotal swelling with pain
  - Torsion of the testicle
    - Imaging by Doppler ultrasonography or nuclear scintigraphy should be done if the diagnosis of testicular torsion is in question.

– Perform imaging only when it will not delay surgical exploration if torsion exists, adding to the risk of testicular loss.

- Torsion of the appendix testis

  – If an inflammatory process resulting from torsion of the appendage makes differentiation from true spermatic cord torsion impossible, imaging may be helpful.

  – Scrotal Doppler ultrasonography or nuclear scintigraphy will show normal or increased flow to ipsilateral testis.

- Acute epididymitis-orchitis

  – Ultrasonography and nuclear scintigraphy show normal symmetric blood flow or increased blood flow to an enlarged epididymis or testis.

  – Voiding cystourethrography has been a routine part of the evaluation, but its yield is low with a normal ultrasound and a sterile urine.

- Henoch-Schönlein purpura

  – Concurrent Henoch-Schönlein purpura and testicular torsion has been reported; therefore, if torsion is a consideration, imaging with Doppler ultrasonography or nuclear scintigraphy is indicated to evaluate testicular blood flow.

- Trauma

  – Scrotal ultrasonography can document the integrity of the testis and of the tunica albuginea and the adequacy of blood flow.

■ Scrotal swelling without pain

- Inguinal hernias and hydroceles

  – Ultrasonography can delineate scrotal contents, especially when a large or tense hydrocele limits physical examination.

  – Ultrasonography can determine cystic or solid nature of a tense scrotal mass (eg, hydrocele, tumor) or spermatic cord mass (eg, hydrocele of the cord, paratesticular tumor).

- Tumors

  – Scrotal ultrasonography is used to delineate the mass.

- Varicoceles

  – Testicular size, most accurately assessed by ultrasonography, should be measured; significant loss of testicular volume is an indication for surgery.

TREATMENT APPROACH

■ Surgical intervention is indicated not only when testicular torsion is strongly suspected, but also in equivocal cases in which torsion cannot be convincingly excluded.

SPECIFIC TREATMENT

Acute scrotal swelling with pain

■ Torsion of the testicle

- Surgical intervention is indicated not only when testicular torsion is strongly suspected, but also in equivocal cases when torsion cannot be convincingly excluded.

- The likelihood of salvaging the testis is highest when surgery is done shortly after onset of pain.

  – The chance of a successful outcome dissipates rapidly with time.

- With surgery, first explore the affected testis, and, when torsion is present, detorse the cord.

- Explore the contralateral testis (will have the same defect in anatomy) and fix it in place to avert a future torsion.

- Reinspect the affected gonad and determine the possibility of salvage.

- If the testis can be saved, fix it in the scrotum.

■ Neonatal testicular torsion

- At exploration, anchor contralateral testis and remove nonviable testis.

■ Torsion of appendix testis

- Management is nonsurgical.

- The patient should rest and use nonsteroidal pain relievers and cold compresses for several days to reduce inflammation, swelling, and pain.

- Surgical intervention is indicated only when acute testicular torsion cannot be excluded.

  – In these cases, the infarcted appendage is removed at surgical exploration.

■ Acute epididymitis-orchitis

- Treat with antibiotics based on the results of the urine culture and sensitivities.

  – In sexually active adolescents, antibiotic coverage must include gonococcal and nongonococcal sexually transmitted infections.

- Antiinflammatory agents, scrotal elevation, and rest should be prescribed.

■ Focal fat necrosis

- Treat with rest and antiinflammatory agents.

■ Trauma

- Testicular or spermatic cord contusions: Manage symptomatically.

- Testicular rupture requires surgical exploration, evacuation of the hematoma, debridement, and repair (when possible).

■ Mumps orchitis

- Treatment is symptomatic.

Scrotal swelling without pain

■ Inguinal hernias and hydroceles

- Repair on diagnosis to prevent incarceration.

  – The risk of incarceration increases with time and is more likely in the young child or infant.

- Repair communicating hydroceles on diagnosis to avert progression.

S

- Perform surgery inguinally; isolate the sac from the cord structures and ligate it at the level of the internal ring.
- Inspect the contralateral ring using diagnostic laparoscopy through the isolated ipsilateral sac.
  - If the internal ring is open, proceed with contralateral surgical correction.
- If the hydrocele is painful, then surgery should proceed sooner.
- Tumors
  - Perform radical orchiectomy through an inguinal approach.
  - If the mass is not suspicious for cancer, a possible approach is to enucleate the mass and proceed with orchiectomy only if the frozen section is positive.
- Varicoceles
  - Indications for surgery
    - Significant loss of testicular volume
    - Abnormal semen analysis (older adolescent patients)
    - Pain
  - Corrective measures (all aimed at occluding direct venous return through the internal spermatic vein to improve the likelihood of normal fertility)
    - Open surgery
    - Laparoscopic surgery
    - Radiologic ablative techniques
- Spermatoceles and epididymal cysts
  - Management typically is observation.
  - Surgery may be indicated when pain or significant enlargement is present.

WHEN TO REFER

- Acute painful scrotal swelling
- Acute hydrocele
- Hernia
- Scrotal trauma
- Cellulitis of scrotum
- Varicocele
- Testicular mass
- Paratesticular mass

WHEN TO ADMIT

- Acute painful scrotal swelling with suspected testicular torsion
- Acute hydrocele
- Scrotal trauma with suspected ruptured testicle
- Testicular mass

COMPLICATIONS

- Torsion of the testicles
  - Subsequent atrophy may still result after surgery because of vascular insult.
  - Fertility may be compromised.
- Spermatoceles and epidydimal cysts
  - Postoperative scarring can obstruct the epidydimal ductal system and lead to infertility.

PROGNOSIS

- Acute scrotal swelling with pain
  - Torsion of the testicle
    - Spermatogenesis may be compromised after 4–6 hours of ischemia.
    - Testicular salvage is time dependent, with universal loss of the testis after 24 hours of torsion.
  - Neonatal testicular torsion
    - Neonatal testicular torsion can exhibit at delivery as a nontender hard scrotal mass.
      - Salvage in these cases is rare.
    - Torsion may occur after delivery and then is more typical of torsion in the older patient, with greater potential for salvage if intervention is rapid.
  - Mumps orchitis
    - Infertility may occur when the condition results in atrophy of both testicles.
- Scrotal swelling without pain
  - Inguinal hernias and hydroceles
    - Most hydroceles resolve spontaneously by 1 year and should be repaired if they persist beyond this age.
  - Varicoceles
    - After corrective measures, most testes increase in size to equal that of the contralateral testis.

Seborrheic Dermatitis

DEFINITION

- Seborrheic dermatitis (SD) is a common, usually asymptomatic, dermatosis of unknown cause seen primarily in infants but also in adolescents and adults.
- Psoriasiform SD, also known as sebopsoriasis or seborrhiasis, produces features of both SD and psoriasis and may represent a bridge between the 2 conditions.

EPIDEMIOLOGY

- Incidence
  - 2–5% of the general population
- Age
  - In 50% of affected infants, symptoms begin before 5 weeks of age.
- SD is occasionally seen in infants who are infected with HIV.
  - Increased incidence in this group has not been documented.

ETIOLOGY

- The cause of SD remains unknown.
- Different pathogenic mechanisms have been proposed.
  - Early evidence that Pitysporum ovale may play a role in the evolution of SD
  - Recent data supports a causal link between Malassezia yeast and SD.
    - Demonstrated clinical improvement of SD when interventions reduce *Malassezia* counts on the body
    - Separate research has shown that antifungal agents effectively treat SD.
    - No difference has been found in *Malassezia* carriage rates in patients with and without SD.
    - Immunomodulatory factors of the host may influence manifestation of SD, not actual colonization counts.
    - *Malassezia* may serve as the primary trigger in an inflammatory reaction, ultimately resulting in SD.
  - Studies have revealed an increase in both:
    - Lymphocyte transformation response
    - Leukocyte migration inhibition
  - This differing immunogenic host theory may explain the increase prevalence of SD in patients with AIDS.
  - Other research postulates that lesions of SD are induced by:
    - Toxin production
    - Lipase activity of *Malassezia*
  - SD lesions tend to occur on locations corresponding with the highest sebaceous gland concentration.
    - Scalp
    - Face
    - Eyebrows
    - Nasolabial folds
    - Axillary folds
    - Inguinal folds
  - Experts have proposed that the following may result in SD.
    - Abnormality in the sebaceous gland
    - Increased sensitivity to circulating maternal or endogenous hormones
  - Patients with SD have normal sebaceous secretion and hormonal levels.

RISK FACTORS

- No evidence suggests genetic predisposition.

SIGNS AND SYMPTOMS

- Most commonly characterized as greasy, scaly dermatitis
- Less often characterized as psoriasiform SD
- Rarely characterized as erythrodermic SD
- SD in infancy is characterized by:
  - Diffuse, red, crusted, and yellow scaling plaques on the vertex of the scalp (see Figure 88 on page F29)
  - Similar lesions also may be found in:
    - Retroauricular creases
    - Eyebrows
    - Nasolabial folds (see Figure 89 on page F29)
  - Lesions appear as shiny red patches with foul-smelling scale in the folds in:
    - Axillary and inguinal folds
    - Neck
    - Diaper area
- Posterior lymphadenopathy has been shown to be significantly associated with SD in patients with a negative fungal culture.
  - Asymptomatic
  - Distributed symmetrically
  - Similar in adolescents
    - Patients may note a greasy, scaling, pruritic eruption on the scalp.
    - Except for lack of inguinal area involvement, distribution of the lesions is the same as that for infants.
  - HIV-positive children age 2–5 years may exhibit SD with lesions similar to those seen in adolescents and adults.
    - Distinctly unusual in immunocompetent children
    - Appears to be a manifestation of HIV infection
- Psoriasiform SD
  - Psoriasiform plaques
    - Annular, red-brown plaques having a silvery scale
    - May be present among classic greasy, yellow, scaling lesions of SD
  - Patients may or may not have pitted nails as seen with classic psoriasis.

- Erythrodermic SD is rare and causes widespread exfoliative erythroderma.
- Diffuse desquamation usually begins in the flexures and then spreads.
- Patients may have signs and symptoms of systemic involvement.
  - Fever
  - Chills
  - Lymphadenopathy
  - Peripheral edema
  - Dehydration
- Involvement may be the presentation of Leiner disease.

DIFFERENTIAL DIAGNOSIS

- Atopic dermatitis
  - Usually distinguished by the presence of:
    - Extreme pruritus
    - Extensoral distribution in infancy
    - Flexural distribution in older children (tending to spare the scalp and to involve hands and feet)
    - Family history in 70% of affected persons
  - SD may occur concomitantly with atopic dermatitis.
- Psoriasis
  - Common inherited papulosquamous skin disorder
  - Characterized by well-demarcated, annular, thick, red-brown, scaling plaques usually present on:
    - Trunk
    - Extensor areas on the arms
    - Knees
    - Elbows
    - Diaper area
    - Scalp
  - Characterized by nail pitting
  - Usually lacks specific distribution and the greasy component of SD
  - Some cases of SD may overlap with psoriasis.
  - Extensive cases of SD become persistent.
  - When the family history of psoriasis is positive, patients should be referred to a dermatologist for:
    - Biopsy
    - Long-term follow-up care
- Dermatophyte infection of the scalp (tinea capitis)
  - Symptoms may include:
    - Scaling
    - Pruritus
    - Redness of the scalp
  - Usually results in alopecia

- Performing a fungal culture by swabbing the affected area vigorously will yield a positive result.
- Tinea corporis appears as annular, red, scaly plaques with central clearing.
- Cultures from the skin may be obtained in a similar fashion to the scalp.
- Potassium hydroxide preparation of scales from body lesions will demonstrate septate hyphae.
- Diaper dermatitis, or irritant diaper rash
  - Characterized by:
    - Involvement primarily of the convex surfaces by red, scaling plaques
    - Inguinal folds are spared (see Figure 90 on page F29).
  - In candidal diaper dermatitis, similar red, scaling plaques involve the skin folds.
    - Satellite pustules in areas not covered by the diaper may be found (see Figure 91 on page F29).
  - SD in the diaper area involves the skin folds.
    - No satellite lesions
- Histiocytosis X
  - Refers to a group of Langerhans cell histiocytoses
    - Letterer-Siwe disease (diffuse disseminated histiocytosis)
    - Hand-Schüller-Christian disease
    - Eosinophilic granuloma (chronic multifocal or focal histiocytosis)
  - Letterer-Siwe disease may be confused with SD.
    - The pattern of distribution is similar.
  - Letterer-Siwe disease is also characterized by:
    - Axillary, inguinal, and oral mucosal erosions
    - Purpura
    - Petechiae
    - Hepatosplenomegaly
  - Skin biopsy will distinguish these disorders easily.
    - Recommended in cases of SD unresponsive to treatment
- Leiner disease
  - Sometimes referred to as *erythrodermic SD*
  - Inherited immunologic disorder
  - Characterized by:
    - Generalized SD
    - Persistent diarrhea
    - Failure to thrive
    - Recurrent gram-negative infections
  - Diagnosis is made by demonstrating deficient yeast opsonic activity in the patient's serum.
- Other immunodeficiencies and metabolic disorders may occur in an erythrodermic SD pattern.

TREATMENT APPROACH

- Effective treatment for SD may involve:
  - A wide range of keratolytic agents
  - Low-potency corticosteroids
  - Antifungal therapies

SPECIFIC TREATMENTS

- The choice of medication is tailored to the age of the patient.

Infants

- A more conservative approach is suggested when treating infantile SD (cradle cap).
  - Apply mineral oil or white petrolatum to the scalp.
  - Follow with a nonmedicated shampoo.
- If unresponsive, second-line agents include
  - 1–2% salicylic acid in liquid or petrolatum form
  - Follow with a keratolytic shampoo.
    - Sebulex
    - Neutrogena
    - T/Sal P & S
  - Salicylic acid solution or petrolatum should be applied for only 10 minutes, then shampooed out carefully.
    - Avoid the face and particularly eyes because severe contact irritation may occur.
  - Follow with a topical low-potency corticosteroid.
    - 1–2.5% hydrocortisone, Synalar solution
    - Derma-Smoothe
  - Corticosteroid solution should be applied sparingly and left on for several hours.
    - This regimen may be repeated up to twice daily as needed and then tapered.
    - Dramatic improvement occurs usually within 1 week.
- Topical antifungals, specifically the azoles, are effective.
- More recently, use of topical macrolactam immunomodulators has been successful.
- Tacrolimus has antifungal properties that contribute to its therapeutic effectiveness.
- Low-potency topical corticosteroid cream (1% hydrocortisone cream) can be used twice a day to treat lesions occurring on the:
  - Face
  - Intertriginous areas
  - Diaper area
- A midpotency corticosteroid, such as 0.1% Kenalog cream, may be used on the body twice a day.
- A mid-potency or strong halogenated corticosteroid should not be used on the:
  - Face
  - Intertriginous areas
  - Diaper area

- Topical ketoconazole (Nizoral)
  - Has been used to treat adult SD
  - Has been found to be beneficial in treating infantile SD
- Lesions in the diaper and intertriginous areas may become superinfected with *Candida* species.
  - Requires topical antifungal creams twice a day in addition to a topical corticosteroid

Children and adolescents

- Topical corticosteroids
- Keratolytic shampoos applied to the scalp
- Topical and oral ketoconazole may be used in severe cases.
- Psoriasiform SD of the scalp is treated as described for cradle cap.
- Psoriasiform lesions on the face and trunk respond to:
  - Topical corticosteroid ointments
  - Emollients
- If lesions persist into childhood, use:
  - Modified Goeckerman regimen consisting of application of a tar preparation
  - Followed by outdoor exposure to sunlight and topical corticosteroids
- Generalized erythrodermic SD may require:
  - Systemic corticosteroids
  - Antibiotics to control superinfection
- Hospitalization for intravenous antibiotic administration may be required.

WHEN TO ADMIT

- Generalized erythrodermic SD may require systemic corticosteroids and antibiotics to control superinfection.
- Hospitalization for intravenous antibiotic administration may be required.

WHEN TO REFER

- Patients who do not respond to standard accepted therapy
- To rule out such conditions as psoriasis and histiocytosis

COMPLICATIONS

- Infants with SD may be:
  - At increased risk of atopic dermatitis
  - At risk of psoriasis (less often)

PROGNOSIS

- Usually excellent
- Most cases resolve within the first 6 months of life.
- Adolescent-onset and HIV-related SD may be more persistent.
  - Usually responds readily to topical therapy

S

Seizure Disorders

DEFINITION

- Seizures are caused by abnormal discharges of neurons.
- A seizure should be considered a symptom of systemic or central nervous system dysfunction.
- Types of seizures
  - Generalized seizures
    - Absence seizures
    - Myoclonic seizures
    - Atonic seizures (also known as *astatic seizures* or *drop attacks*)
    - Generalized tonic-clonic seizures (also known as *grand mal seizures*)
    - Infantile spasms (also known as *West syndrome*)
    - Lennox-Gastaut syndrome
    - Juvenile myoclonic epilepsy
  - Partial seizures
    - Simple partial seizures
    - Complex partial seizures
    - Benign partial epilepsy of childhood (also known as *rolandic epilepsy*, *sylvian seizures*, and *centrotemporal epilepsy*)
    - Epilepsia partialis continua
  - Unclassified seizures
    - Neonatal seizures
    - Febrile seizures
    - Pseudoseizures

EPIDEMIOLOGY

- Prevalence
  - Seizures occur in approximately 1% of all children up to the age of 14 years.
  - Greatest in first year of life (~120 cases per 100,000 population)
  - Thereafter, 40–50 cases per 100,000 population until puberty
  - ~10 cases per 100,000 population in the early and mid teens
  - ~15% of children who have epilepsy have intractable seizures.
    - ~50% of these may be appropriate candidates for epilepsy surgery.
- Absence seizures
  - Age of onset: 3–8 years
  - Rarely occur before 2 years or after 15 years of age
  - Girls are affected more commonly than boys.
  - 15–44% of first-degree relatives have a history of absence seizures, paroxysmal electroenceophalography (EEG) abnormalities, or both.
- Infantile spasms
  - Peak age of onset: 3–7 months
  - Estimated 0.24–0.60 per 1000 infants

- Boys are more likely to be affected than girls.
- Children with tuberous sclerosis account for up to 25% of patients who have symptomatic infantile spasms.
- Infants in whom no etiologic factor is found tend to be older at onset than symptomatic infants.
- Lennox-Gastaut syndrome
  - Age of onset: 3–5 years
  - Boys are affected slightly more frequently than girls.
- Juvenile myoclonic epilepsy
  - Age of onset: 12–18 years
  - Represents 7% of all epilepsy cases
- Benign partial epilepsy of childhood
  - Age of onset: 5–8 years
  - Boys are more often affected than girls.
- Febrile seizures
  - Age of onset: 3 months to 5 years
  - Median age of occurrence: 18–22 months
  - ~2–5% of children will experience a febrile convulsion.
  - Boys are more susceptible than girls.
- Pseudoseizures
  - Can occur in early childhood but are more frequent in adolescence, especially girls

ETIOLOGY

Neonatal seizures

- Hypoxia-ischemia
  - Most common cause of seizures in both premature and full-term infants
  - These seizures usually begin within the first 24 hours of life and may be difficult to control for several days.
- Intracranial hemorrhage
  - Seen mainly in premature infants within the first 3 days of life
  - Generalized tonic seizures may be associated with severe hemorrhage involving the brain parenchyma.
- Metabolic disturbances
  - Hypoglycemia
  - Hypocalcemia
  - Hyponatremia
  - Hypernatremia
  - Local anesthetic intoxication
  - Pyridoxine dependence
  - Variety of inborn errors of metabolism
- Bacterial and viral intracranial infections
  - Most common bacterial causes are group B streptococci and *Escherichia coli*.
  - Prenatal nonbacterial causes include toxoplasmosis and infections with rubella, herpes simplex virus, coxsackievirus type B, and cytomegalovirus.

- Malformations of the brain
  - Cortical dysgenesis, such as lissencephaly, pachygyria, and polymicrogyria

Childhood seizures

- A cause is identifiable in <20% of children with seizures.
- If a child has no abnormalities by history or examination at the time of seizure onset, then a cause is rarely identified.
- The more abnormal the child's neurodevelopmental status, the more likely a cause will be identified or may already have been determined before seizure onset. These include:
  - Brain malformations
  - Genetic disorders
  - Disorders of metabolism
  - Traumatic or previous infectious injury of the brain
  - Neoplasm
- Children with infantile spasms and Lennox-Gastaut syndrome are more likely to have an identifiable cause.
- Idiopathic generalized epilepsies (eg, childhood absence epilepsy and juvenile myoclonic epilepsy) are more likely to be related to genetic factors.

Cause, by type of seizure

- Infantile spasms
  - Divided into symptomatic and cryptogenic groups based on the presence of a predisposing etiologic factor
  - Symptomatic spasms occur in infants with abnormal neurologic development before onset of spasms.
  - Causes of symptomatic spasms include:
    - Structural abnormalities of the brain
    - Hypoxic-ischemic insults
    - Central nervous system (CNS) infections or hemorrhages
    - Inborn errors of metabolism
- Simple partial seizures
  - Caused by focal epileptiform discharges, but a focal structural lesion may not be found in most patients
  - Identifiable causes include:
    - Prenatal and perinatal insults
    - CNS malformations and tumors
    - Inborn errors of metabolism (rare)
- Complex partial seizure
  - Causes include:
    - Perinatal insults
    - Head trauma
    - Encephalitis
    - Status epilepticus (possibly)
    - Indolent tumors (eg, hamartomas and low-grade gliomas)

- Specific types of neonatal seizure
  - Subtle seizure
    - Abnormal movements may arise from regions of brain from which abnormal electrical activity cannot be detected with surface electrodes.
    - Subtle seizures usually occur in infants with severe CNS insults.
  - Clonic seizure
    - Can result from focal CNS lesions, such as cerebral infarction
    - Can also occur with metabolic disturbances
  - Tonic seizure
    - May be a brain stem phenomenon rather than seizures
  - Myoclonic seizure
    - Infants with myoclonic seizures tend to have severely abnormal dysgenetic brains or metabolic defects.
- Febrile seizures
  - Triggered by any illness that causes fever (eg, otitis media and upper respiratory tract infections)
  - The rate of febrile seizures with shigellosis, salmonellosis, and roseola is high, possibly because of a direct effect of causative organism on the CNS or to a neurotoxin they produce.

RISK FACTORS

- Genetic risk factors
  - The fact that some genetic syndromes (eg, Angelman syndrome and Rett syndrome) predispose a child to seizures raises interest in the role of different genes in the susceptibility to seizures.
  - The following types of seizure have a potentially genetic component.
    - Juvenile myoclonic seizures (a locus on the short arm of chromosome 6 has been identified)
    - Complex partial seizure (secondary etiologic role)
    - Benign partial epilepsy of childhood
    - Febrile seizures
      - Familial clustering of febrile seizures occurs.
      - Mutations of the *SCN1A* gene have been found in some families.
- Other risk factors
  - Lennox-Gastaut syndrome
    - Many patients have neurologic deficits before onset (intellectual disability and cerebral palsy).
    - Neurologic deficits may be related to hypoxic or other insults to the brain or abnormal brain development.
    - Patients may have a history of infantile spasms.
  - Juvenile myoclonic epilepsy may be precipitated by:
    - Sleep deprivation
    - Stress

S

- Alcohol
- Hormonal changes
- Epilepsia partialis continua
- Focal encephalitis and tumor

■ Risk factors for neonatal seizures

- Hypoglycemic seizures
  - Infants small for gestational age
  - Postterm infants
  - Infants of diabetic mothers
- Hypocalcemic seizures (which occur when calcium levels decrease to <7 mg/dL during the first 2–3 days of life)
  - Low–birth-weight infants
  - Infants of diabetic mothers
  - History of hypoxia
  - Hypocalcemic seizures that occur later are usually related to a low-calcium and high-phosphate intake.

SIGNS AND SYMPTOMS

Absence seizures

■ Generalized, nonconvulsive seizures characterized by interruption of activity, staring, and unresponsiveness

■ Usually last 5–15 seconds

■ Start without warning and end abruptly with resumption of the child's preictal activity

■ The child may be unaware that the episode occurred.

■ Unresponsiveness is sometimes accompanied by:

- Eyelid fluttering
- Upward rotation of the eyes
- Mild clonic movements or automatisms (eg, lip smacking, grimacing, or swallowing)

Myoclonic seizures

■ Brief, sudden muscle contractions that may involve only part of the body or may be generalized

■ May occur in clusters, especially when child is falling asleep or shortly after awakening

■ Usually, no alteration in consciousness is associated with jerks.

Atonic seizures

■ Sudden decrease in muscle tone that may cause head nodding or mild flexing of the legs

- More significant decreases in muscle tone may cause the patient to slump to the floor.

■ Usually, no alteration in consciousness is detectable with these seizures.

Generalized tonic-clonic seizures

■ Tonic phase

- Sustained contraction of muscles that causes patient

to fall to the ground, usually in opisthotonus

- Extensor posturing usually occurs with tonic contraction of the diaphragm and intercostal muscles
  - Halts respirations and, in turn, produces cyanosis
- Lasts <1 minute and is followed by the clonic phase

■ Clonic phase

- Consists of bilateral rhythmic jerking
- Jerks may be accompanied by expiratory grunts produced by diaphragmatic contractions against a closed glottis.
- Frequency of jerks decreases as the seizure progresses, although intensity may increase.
- The tongue may be bitten, and bowel and bladder incontinence may occur.
- Usually stops within several minutes
- May be followed by vomiting, confusion, and lethargy, with gradual recovery of consciousness during minutes to hours

Infantile spasms

■ Sudden contraction of neck, trunk, and extremity muscles

■ Spasms may be flexor, extensor, or mixed flexor-extensor.

■ Spasms last only a few seconds each but often occur in clusters of up to 100 individual spasms.

■ A typical episode involves dropping of the head along with abduction of the shoulders and flexion of the lower extremities.

■ The infant may cry during or after the spasm.

■ Pallor, flushing, grimacing, laughter, and nystagmus sometimes occur.

■ Episodes are common on awakening from sleep, during drowsiness, and with feedings but are rare during sleep.

Lennox-Gastaut syndrome

■ Severe epileptic encephalopathy characterized by a variety of generalized seizures

- Tonic seizures cause sudden, sustained contraction of the muscle groups.
- Atypical absence seizures consist of a brief period of staring and immobility.
  - Onset and recovery of atypical absence seizures are less abrupt than in typical absence.
- Episodes may be associated with mild tonic motor manifestations, automatisms, or loss of postural tone.
- Atonic seizures occur and may be preceded by myoclonic jerks.
- Tonic-clonic seizures and partial seizures may occur.

Juvenile myoclonic epilepsy

■ Primary generalized epilepsy characterized by myoclonic jerks that affect mainly the upper extremities and less commonly the lower extremities.

- Jerks usually occur shortly after awakening.

- Patients may report clumsiness or difficulty holding objects early in the morning.
- Myoclonic jerks almost always precede the onset of generalized tonic-clonic seizures by months to years.

Complex partial seizures

- Result in impaired consciousness
- May begin as a simple partial seizure that progresses to impairment of consciousness
- Initial portion of a seizure that occurs before consciousness is lost is called the aura.
- Aura may consist of:
  - Auditory, olfactory, or visual illusions or hallucinations
  - Affective symptoms, such as fear or other unpleasant feelings
- Anger and rage are very rare as seizure manifestations but may occur during postictal confusion if the patient is restrained.

Simple partial seizures

- Seizure activity with focal or limited manifestations and preserved consciousness
- Symptoms may be motor, sensory, or cognitive.
- Motor seizures may be restricted to a body part (eg, face or a limb) or may involve the entire side.
- If seizure discharge spreads to structures involved in consciousness, the seizure will become a complex partial seizure.
- Seizure activity may spread to opposite side of the brain, causing a generalized seizure.
- Partial or secondary generalized seizure may be followed by Todd paralysis, weakness of the limbs most involved in seizure.
- Partial sensory seizures are most often displayed by paresthesias lasting <1–2 minutes.
- Seizure discharges from 1 occipital lobe may cause scintillating colored spots or scotomata in the visual field contralateral to the discharge.
- Seizures with more complex visual hallucinations often progress to complex partial seizures with diminished consciousness.
- Auditory seizures are manifested by hearing noises and, less commonly, by having elaborate but usually nonverbal auditory hallucinations (eg, hearing music).
- Common auras include:
  - Déjà vu (feeling that an experience has occurred before)
  - Jamais vu (feeling that a previously experienced sensation is unfamiliar and strange)
  - Rising epigastric sensation
- Staring and automatisms occur when consciousness is clouded.

- Automatisms include:
  - Chewing, lip smacking, swallowing, and hissing
  - Picking at clothes, searching, or ambulating
- Automatisms are usually followed by postictal amnesia; the child may become tired and go to sleep.

Benign partial epilepsy of childhood

- Seizures typically occur during sleep.
  - Occasionally occur during wakefulness
- The child awakens with 1 side of the face twitching.
- Oropharyngeal muscles are also often involved, causing the child to make unintelligible gurgling sounds.
- The ipsilateral upper extremity may be involved, but the lower extremity involved only rarely.
- The seizure episode rarely becomes generalized.
- Consciousness is often retained during seizure, although the child may not be able to speak.
- Most seizure episodes last <2 minutes.

Epilepsia partialis continua

- Twitching is continuous and limited to 1 side of the body.
- Twitching frequently involves only a few muscles and occurs most often in hand or foot.
- Consciousness is preserved, but seizure activity might weaken the extremity involved.
- Seizure activity may persist for hours to months.

Febrile seizures

- Occur in children with fever but no evidence of intracranial infection or acute neurologic illness
- Simple febrile seizures are generalized tonic-clonic convulsions that last <15 minutes and do not recur within 24 hours.
- Complex febrile seizures are less common and are focal or prolonged beyond 15 minutes or recur within 24 hours.

Pseudoseizures

- Uncommon
- Movements are usually not clonic but may be quivering or random thrashing.
- Episodes may be dramatic, with screaming and shouting.
- Episodes may vary greatly in same patient.
- Usually, no postictal period occurs.

DIFFERENTIAL DIAGNOSIS

- Seizures must be differentiated from other paroxysmal disorders in childhood.
  - Syncope
  - Breath-holding spells
  - Staring related to inattention
  - Paroxysmal vertigo
  - Cardiac arrhythmias
  - Stereotypic behaviors

S

- Complex partial seizures
  - Differentiate from absence seizures, which are also characterized by staring and unresponsiveness.
    - Absence seizures have abrupt onset and termination compared with complex partial seizures, which have a more gradual onset and termination.
    - Absence seizures last <30 seconds and are not associated with postictal confusion.
    - Automatisms can occur if absence episodes are prolonged, but are often just a continuation of motor activity present before onset of seizure.
- Neonatal seizures
  - Clonic seizures
    - Differentiate from benign neonatal sleep myoclonus, which consists of small-amplitude clonic activity that may wax and wane in various parts of the body.
  - Myoclonic seizures
    - Differentiate from benign myoclonic jerks that occur during sleep in neonates
  - Febrile seizure
    - If child is <1 year of age or has not rapidly returned to normal, lumbar puncture should be strongly considered to evaluate for meningitis.
- Pseudoseizures
  - Differentiate from epileptic seizures.
    - Movements are usually not clonic but may be quivering or random thrashing movements.
    - Usually not associated with incontinence, injury, or tongue biting

DIAGNOSTIC APPROACH

- Neonatal seizures
  - Because electrical seizures may not have clinical correlates, EEG should be done for all infants at risk for seizures to identify these clinically silent electrical seizures.
- Pseudoseizures
  - Detailed history and observation of an episode may be all that is needed to diagnose pseudoseizures.

LABORATORY FINDINGS

- Laboratory tests usually performed at the time of the initial seizure include measurement of:
  - Serum electrolytes
  - Calcium
  - Magnesium
  - Blood glucose
- In some cases, history or examination may indicate that more extensive laboratory evaluation is required.

IMAGING

- Plain radiography
  - Radiographs of the skull can detect calcifications that may be seen in some syndromes, but they rarely help in evaluating children who have epilepsy.
- Computed tomography (CT) and magnetic resonance imaging (MRI)
  - Have replaced skull radiography in evaluation of seizures
  - Detect structural abnormalities
  - MRI is more sensitive than CT in detecting:
    - Low-grade tumors
    - Changes in myelination
    - Heterotopic gray matter
  - MRI is not warranted in every child who has epilepsy; however, it should be done in children with focal neurologic abnormalities on examination or intractable epilepsy.
- Positron emission tomography and single-photon emission CT
  - Useful in localizing metabolic alterations with seizure activity and seizure foci
  - Clinically relevant only in individuals with intractable epilepsy being evaluated for epilepsy surgery

DIAGNOSTIC PROCEDURES

- EEG
  - Measures physiologic function of the brain
  - Important in evaluating a child with seizures because it helps define the seizure type
  - Epileptiform EEG may support diagnosis, but a normal tracing does not exclude epilepsy.
  - Other abnormalities, such as slowing and background disorganization, are much less specific.
  - Repeat tracings increase the likelihood of detecting epileptiform discharges in patients who have seizures.
  - Such procedures as hyperventilation, photic stimulation, and sleep should be used when obtaining EEG recordings.
  - Nasopharyngeal and sphenoidal electrodes may be used to detect mesial temporal discharges, but they rarely add to information obtained by special scalp electrode placements.
  - Video EEG monitoring helps correlate clinical symptoms with electrical seizure activity and may be useful when clinical manifestations are atypical or pseudoseizures are in question.
  - EEG abnormalities must be interpreted in view of the clinical symptoms.
- EEG findings, by seizure type
  - Absence seizures
    - Classic EEG finding: bilaterally synchronous 3-Hz spike-and-wave discharges
    - Hyperventilation may be used to precipitate electrical discharge and clinical seizure.

- Photic stimulation during EEG induces seizure discharge in some patients.
- Generalized tonic-clonic seizures
  - Associated with bilaterally synchronous electrical discharges on EEG
  - EEG may demonstrate focal discharge that may spread to both hemispheres or may show only bilateral synchronous discharges.
- Infantile spasms
  - The EEG pattern is hypsarrhythmia, characterized by high-voltage slow waves with irregularly interspersed multifocal spike-and-sharp waves.
  - Hypsarrhythmia may precede the onset of clinical manifestations, or it may occur later or not at all.
  - Over time, hypsarrhythmia usually evolves into other focal or generalized abnormalities; in some cases, the EEG may normalize.
- Lennox-Gastaut syndrome
  - EEG typically shows an irregular, high-voltage, slow (2.5 Hz or slower) spike-wave pattern.
  - Discharges are bilaterally synchronous.
- Juvenile myoclonic seizures
  - Ictal EEG typically shows generalized, symmetrical polyspike and waves at 4–6 Hz.
  - Photic stimulation precipitates the electrical discharges in some patients.
- Benign partial epilepsy of childhood
  - Typical EEG findings are midtemporal or centrotemporal spike discharges occurring unilaterally or independently bilaterally, often frequent in light sleep and sometimes induced by hyperventilation.
  - Neuroradiologic studies show no abnormalities to correlate with the EEG focus.
- Neonatal seizures
  - Subtle seizures: EEG recordings do not always show correlation of electrical seizure discharges with the clinical seizure activity.
  - Clonic seizures: EEG shows multifocal independent areas of electrical discharge.
  - Tonic seizures: often have no electrographic correlate and are usually associated with severe EEG background abnormalities
  - Myoclonic seizures: EEG usually abnormal; may show a burst suppression pattern but might not change during the myoclonic event
- Febrile seizures
  - EEG is generally not helpful in evaluating children who have febrile seizures.
  - EEG within 1 week of the seizure often shows posterior slowing.
  - Paroxysmal activity is seen in EEGs of 35–45% of patients who are followed up for several years.
  - EEG abnormalities do not predict recurrence of febrile seizures or development of epilepsy.
- Pseudoseizures
  - Capturing pseudoseizures during video EEG monitoring establishes the diagnosis in patients in whom the distinction cannot be made clinically.

TREATMENT APPROACH

- ■ Seizures in neonates
  - Electrographic seizures may continue after clinical seizures are controlled.
    - If frequent or prolonged, may merit further anticonvulsant therapy
  - Seizures related to acute injuries (eg, asphyxia, stroke, or acute CNS infections other than herpes) are self-limited and stop after several days.
    - Continuing treatment past neonatal period will not change the chance of recurrence.
    - Such seizures are usually treated short term.
    - Infants are often not sent home on anticonvulsants or receive continued anticonvulsant therapy for only a few weeks.
  - Seizures related to brain malformations or inborn errors of metabolism may be much more persistent.
    - Duration of treatment depends on the infant's clinical course.
- ■ Seizures in children beyond the neonatal period
  - Diagnosing the seizure type correctly is the critical first step in treatment, because some seizure disorders respond to certain medications.
  - Select the drug with the fewest adverse effects.
  - Give medication at a dose that will result in a low therapeutic blood level; increase the dose until seizures are controlled or adverse effects become unacceptable.
  - Add a second medication if the initial medication is not fully effective.
  - Consider discontinuing the first medication if seizures are fully controlled with the second medication.
  - Strive for monotherapy if possible—polytherapy often does not improve seizure control but may significantly increase toxicity.
  - Closely monitor for potential cognitive and behavioral adverse effects of antiepileptic medications.
  - To devise the optimal dosing regimen, consider pharmacokinetics of various antiepileptic medications.
  - Determine dosing frequency according to half-life (time in which the serum level decreases to 50% of initial value).
    - The dosing interval should be no longer than half-life of the medication.

- Most antiepileptic agents may be administered twice a day, some only once daily.
- Evaluate the efficacy of an antiepileptic medication only after 5 half-lives have elapsed because this period is required for medication to reach a steady state.
- In antiepileptic medications that induce hepatic enzymes (eg, phenobarbital, phenytoin, carbamazepine), half-life decreases during first weeks of treatment.
- If breakthrough seizures occur at times of low (trough) serum drug levels, or if toxic effects occur at times of peak serum drug levels, increase frequency of dosing.
- Patients requiring higher antiepileptic medication levels usually need more frequent dosing to avoid toxic effects.
- Serum drug levels can guide adjustment of doses of antiepileptic medications.
  - Obtain a baseline level:
    - When the patient has been taking an appropriate dose long enough to have stable levels
    - To verify adherence, breakthrough seizures, and toxic effect
    - When other medications have been added or deleted from patient's regimen
  - The timing of the sample relative to the last dose received is important in interpretation of levels, especially in drugs with short half-lives.

SPECIFIC TREATMENTS

Treatment, by type of seizure

- Absence seizure
  - Monotherapy with ethosuximide, valproate, or lamotrigine usually controls absence seizures effectively.
  - Valproate and lamotrigine are the drugs of choice if the patient also has tonic-clonic seizures.
  - Any 2 of these medications may be used together when absence seizures are not completely controlled with 1.
  - Benzodiazepines are effective, but adverse effects on behavior make them second-line agents.
  - Phenytoin, phenobarbital, and carbamazepine are usually ineffective for treating absence seizures and may exacerbate them.
- Generalized tonic-clonic seizure
  - Valproate, lamotrigine, phenobarbital, topiramate, and zonisamide
  - Secondary generalized seizures may be effectively treated with these, as well as with carbamazepine, oxcarbazepine, and phenytoin.
  - One of the newest anticonvulsants, levetiracetam, may be effective in both types of generalized seizures.
- Infantile spasm
  - Resistant to treatment with most anticonvulsants

- Cryptogenic group
  - The treatment used most often in cryptogenic group is adrenocorticotropic hormone (ACTH).
  - ACTH in a long-acting form is administered as a single daily intramuscular dose of 20–40 IU.
  - Adverse effects of ACTH and steroids are significant and include Cushing syndrome, hypertension, susceptibility to infections, hyperglycemia, gastrointestinal bleeding, and electrolyte disturbance.
- Symptomatic group
  - Alternative anticonvulsants may be tried before ACTH.
- Benzodiazepines are effective.
- Nitrazepam seems to be more effective than clonazepam or diazepam.
- Both valproic acid and topiramate are effective therapy in some infants.
- Zonisamide can be effective against infantile spasms.
- Lennox-Gastaut syndrome
  - The goal of treatment is to achieve reasonable seizure control with as few medications as possible to minimize adverse effects.
  - Valproate is the drug of choice.
  - Lamotrigine, topiramate, and felbamate significantly reduce the frequency of atonic and generalized tonic-clonic seizures.
  - Benzodiazepines control atonic, myoclonic, and atypical absence seizures.
    - With increasing doses, the frequency of adverse effects also increases.
    - Development of tolerance is a problem.
  - Ethosuximide can help control atypical absence episodes.
  - Phenytoin can be used for tonic seizures.
  - A ketogenic diet has been beneficial in seizure control.
    - Adherence may be a problem because of the nature of the diet.
- Juvenile myoclonic seizures
  - Valproate will control myoclonic jerks, absence seizures, and generalized tonic-clonic seizures in >80% of patients but is often avoided in females of childbearing age.
  - Lamotrigine is effective in most patients.
  - Topiramate, zonisamide, and levetiracetam may be effective.
  - Phenytoin is not effective.
  - Carbamazepine may exacerbate seizures.
- Simple partial seizures
  - Most anticonvulsants are equally effective, but these seizures are sometimes hard to control.
- Complex partial seizures
  - Carbamazepine, oxcarbazepine, and valproate are preferred over phenytoin, phenobarbital, and primidone.

S

- Carbamazepine is the drug of choice in children because of its efficacy and relatively mild adverse effects.
- If seizures are not controlled with carbamazepine, adding acetazolamide may improve seizure control.
- For some, oxcarbazepine is less sedating.
- In infants and very young children, phenobarbital may be tried first.

■ Benign partial epilepsy of childhood
  - For infrequent episodes, no treatment may be needed.
  - If episodes frighten the child and treatment is initiated, carbamazepine has been the drug of choice.
  - Most anticonvulsants are effective.
  - Some children are prone to absence seizures, and carbamazepine may exacerbate absences.

■ Epilepsia partialis continua
  - Most anticonvulsants have some efficacy, but medical control of epilepsia partialis continua is generally difficult to achieve.

■ Neonatal seizures
  - Ensure adequate ventilation and perfusion.
  - Obtain blood for glucose, calcium, magnesium, and electrolyte studies; check a Dextrostix for an immediate determination of glucose.
  - Correct any associated metabolic abnormality.
  - Hypoglycemia: If glucose level is low (<40 mg/dL), immediately give 10% dextrose intravenously in a dose of 2 mL/kg.
    – Maintain blood glucose levels above 40 mg/dL by continuous intravenous infusion.
    – Monitor the levels in both full-term and premature infants.
  - Hypocalcemia: Correct by administering 5% calcium gluconate solution, 4 mL/kg, intravenously at a rate of 1 mL/min to maintain serum calcium levels above 7 mg/dL while monitoring cardiac rate and rhythm.
  - Hypomagnesemia: Correct serum magnesium levels to 1 mmol/L with 50% magnesium sulfate solution, 0.2 mL/kg intramuscularly.
  - For continued seizure activity, administer anticonvulsants.
  - Give phenobarbital in a loading dose of 20 mg/kg intravenously over 10 minutes
    – Additional doses of 5 or 10 mg/kg can be given, up to a total of 40 mg/kg.
  - Give phenytoin or fosphenytoin in a loading dose of 20 mg/kg intravenously while monitoring cardiac rhythm.
  - Give lorazepam in doses of 0.1 mg/kg intravenously for persistent seizures.
    – Respiratory status should be monitored.

■ Febrile seizures
  - Usually, seizure activity has stopped by the time the child is evaluated.

- If the seizure continues, administer lorazepam or diazepam.
- Bring down temperature by using rectal antipyretics, removing blankets and clothing, and sponging.
- Educate the family about the benign nature of seizures, use of antipyretics, and first aid for seizures.

■ Pseudoseizures
  - Treatment is directed toward the psychosocial issues involved.

Specific antiepileptic medications

■ Phenobarbital
  - With its long half-life, it requires dosing only once or twice a day.
  - Relatively safe in terms of serious toxic effects, so monitoring of parameters other than serum levels is not necessary
  - Major disadvantage: effect on behavior and cognitive function
    – Maintaining serum levels at the minimum for seizure control may help decrease these adverse effects.
  - Phenobarbital administration will decrease serum levels of carbamazepine and valproate.
  - Administration of valproate will increase phenobarbital levels.
    – Phenobarbital doses should be decreased by 25–50% to prevent toxic effects when prescribed concomitantly with valproate.
  - Properties
    – Indications: neonatal, febrile, partial, secondary generalized, primary generalized, akinetic seizures
    – Half-life: 36–120 hours
    – Usual daily dose: 3–5 mg/kg (weight <25 kg), 2–3 mg/kg (weight 25–50 kg), 1–2 mg/kg (weight >50 kg)
    – Therapeutic levels: 10–40 µg/mL
    – Adverse effects: sedation, inattention, hyperactivity, irritability, cognitive impairment, rare hypersensitivity reactions

■ Phenytoin
  - Now used infrequently for long-term therapy because alternatives with fewer adverse effects and more steady pharmacokinetics are available.
  - Changes in dose should be monitored via serum levels.
  - Only small dose changes should be made when serum levels are close to or within the therapeutic range.
  - Valproic acid may decrease the total serum phenytoin levels, but the free phenytoin level transiently increases and then returns to original level; thus, no adjustment in dose is necessary.
  - Phenytoin may decrease carbamazepine levels and increase phenobarbital levels.
  - Properties
    – Indications: partial, secondary generalized seizures

S

- Half-life: 7–42 hours (nonlinear kinetics)
- Usual daily dose: 5–7 mg/kg
- Therapeutic levels: 10–20 µg/mL (occasionally lower)
- Adverse effects: rashes, hirsutism, gingival hyperplasia, coarse features, psychomotor slowing, neuropathy, folate deficiency, myelosuppression, drug-induced lupus

- Carbamazepine
  - Widely used because it has relatively few effects on cognitive function
  - May positively affect behavior
  - Complete blood cell count should be obtained before carbamazepine therapy is initiated and should be repeated after 2–3 weeks.
  - The dose may need to be changed during treatment because this drug tends to induce its own metabolic breakdown.
  - Phenobarbital, phenytoin, primidone, and clonazepam decrease carbamazepine serum levels.
  - Properties
    - Indications: partial, secondary generalized seizures
    - Half-life: 18–55 hours initially; 3–23 hours on chronic therapy
    - Usual daily dose: 2–5 mg/kg initially; 5–25 mg/kg
    - Therapeutic levels: 4–12 µg/mL
    - Adverse effects: allergic rashes, nausea, diplopia, blurry vision, dizziness, hypersensitivity, hepatitis, aplastic anemia

- Valproic acid
  - Broad spectrum of efficacy and only minimal cognitive adverse effects
  - Rarely, has been associated with fatal hepatotoxicity
    - Most cases occur during the first 3 months of treatment.
    - Patients at greatest risk for hepatotoxicity are children <2 years who receive valproic acid as part of antiepileptic polytherapy.
    - Valproic acid should be administered cautiously to patients with preexisting hepatic dysfunction.
    - Liver function should be monitored in patients taking valproic acid, especially those in the high-risk group.
  - Valproic acid increases the level of phenobarbital; therefore, the phenobarbital dose must be decreased by 25–50% if valproic acid is added.
  - Carbamazepine, phenobarbital, and phenytoin decrease valproic acid serum levels.
  - Properties
    - Indications: primary generalized, absence, myoclonic, akinetic, and febrile seizures; infantile spasms; Lennox-Gastaut syndrome; partial seizures
    - Half-life: 6–16 hours
    - Usual daily dose: 10–30 mg/kg on monotherapy; may need more in polytherapy

- Therapeutic levels: 50–100 µg/mL (150 µg/mL if tolerated)
- Adverse effects: nausea, tremor, weight gain, hair loss, thrombocytopenia, hepatic failure, pancreatitis

- Ethosuximide
  - Limited spectrum of efficacy
  - Because pancytopenia has been associated with long-term administration, periodic blood cell counts may be necessary.
  - Does not interact significantly with other antiepileptic medications
  - Properties
    - Indications: absence, myoclonic, akinetic seizures
    - Half-life: 15–68 hours
    - Usual daily dose: 15–40 mg/kg
    - Therapeutic levels: 40–100 µg/mL
    - Adverse effects: nausea, abdominal discomfort, hiccups, drowsiness, behavioral problems, dystonias, myelosuppression, drug-induced lupus

- Primidone
  - Not a commonly used antiepileptic agent because it has no specific advantage over other agents and tends to be more sedating
  - Because one third of primidone is metabolized to phenobarbital, phenobarbital levels should be monitored.
  - Phenobarbital levels may be 1.3–2 times higher than primidone levels.
  - Valproate increases primidone serum levels.
  - Phenytoin and carbamazepine increase the phenobarbital/primidone ratio.
  - Properties
    - Indications: partial, secondary generalized, primary generalized seizures
    - Half-life: 3–20 hours
    - Usual daily dose: 1–2 mg/kg initially; 5–10 mg/kg
    - Therapeutic levels: 5–12 µg/mL
    - Adverse effects: sedation, irritability, psychomotor slowing, rare hematologic and hypersensitivity reactions

- Clonazepam
  - A benzodiazepine
  - Not a first-line antiepileptic medication because of adverse effects
  - Causes increased secretions, which may be a problem in children with reactive airways or cerebral palsy and associated compromised swallowing mechanisms
  - May lead to swallowing dysfunction in higher levels
  - Because withdrawal of drug may cause irritability, myoclonus, and increased seizures, it should be withdrawn slowly.
  - Usually reserved for myoclonic seizures that are refractory to ethosuximide and valproic acid

- Properties
  - Indications: absence and primary generalized seizures, infantile spasms
  - Half-life: 20–36 hours
  - Usual daily dose: 0.01–0.2 mg/kg
  - Therapeutic levels: 0.01–0.07 µg/mL
  - Adverse effects: sedation, hyperactivity, inattention, aggressiveness, tolerance, ataxia, withdrawal seizures
- Other benzodiazepines
  - Clorazepate
    - Least sedating of the benzodiazepines
    - Sometimes used adjunctively for resistant seizures
  - Diazepam and lorazepam may be used.
  - All benzodiazepines are associated with tachyphylaxis and some sedation and withdrawal seizures.
    - Rotating from one to another may help retain the efficacy of these medications.
  - Their most significant role in epilepsy is in intermittent use, as in status epilepticus, for which intravenous lorazepam is the drug of choice.
  - Rectal preparation of diazepam may be administered safely during prolonged seizure outside a hospital setting.
  - These drugs may be used:
    - To stop flurries of seizures in patients predisposed to them
    - Sometimes for nocturnal seizures
- Acetazolamide
  - Effective adjunctive therapy
  - Antiepileptic properties are not well understood.
  - Can be used in combination with valproic acid for treatment of absence, myoclonic, and akinetic seizures
  - Adding acetazolamide to carbamazepine may improve control of partial seizures.
  - Acetazolamide metabolism is not affected significantly by other medications.
  - Properties
    - Indications: absence, myoclonic, akinetic, partial seizures
    - Half-life: 10–12 hours
    - Usual daily dose: 10–20 mg/kg
    - Therapeutic levels: 10–14 µg/mL
    - Adverse effects: diuresis, paresthesias, sedation, carbon dioxide retention, rashes
- Felbamate
  - 1 year after felbamate was approved and widely used because of its lack of associated sedation, >20 cases of aplastic anemia among persons taking it were reported.
    - Incidence of and predisposing factors to this problem have not been fully determined.
    - Use decreased significantly after these reports and associated warning.

- Only 1 additional case has been reported in the past 12 years, and no cases have been reported in children <13 years of age.
- Should be used only in patients whose epilepsy is so severe that benefits from use outweigh risk of aplastic anemia
- Interacts with phenytoin, carbamazepine, and valproate ; therefore, these medications must be reduced by 25–50% when felbamate is added
- Felbamate levels are lowered by medications that induce liver enzymes; consequently, felbamate doses may need to be increased.
- Properties
  - Indications: partial seizures (in patients >12 years), Lennox-Gastaut syndrome
  - Half-life: 20 hours (in monotherapy)
  - Usual daily dose: 15–45 mg/kg (maximum of 3600 mg)
  - Adverse effects: anorexia, weight loss, nausea, insomnia, headache, fatigue, aplastic anemia
- Gabapentin
  - Approved for adjunctive therapy in patients ≥3 years
  - Gabapentin significantly reduces seizure frequency in patients refractory to conventional anticonvulsants but is not as effective an anticonvulsant as most other agents.
  - Currently used more for neuritic pain than for seizure control
  - Does not interact with other drugs and is 100% excreted renally, offering an advantage to patients with liver failure
  - Properties
    - Indications: partial seizures, with or without secondary generalized seizures in patients >12 years
    - Half-life: 5–7 hours
    - Usual daily dose: total daily dose 900–1800 mg
    - Adverse effects: somnolence, dizziness, ataxia, fatigue
- Lamotrigine
  - Approved for treating partial seizures in patients >16 years and as add-on therapy in patients ≥3 years with Lennox-Gastaut syndrome
  - Reduces frequency of both partial and generalized seizures
  - Has no effect on metabolism of other antiepileptic drugs; however, phenobarbital, phenytoin, and carbamazepine decrease the half-life of lamotrigine
  - Valproic acid increases the half-life of lamotrigine by 2- or 3-fold; therefore, doses of lamotrigine should be lower when given with valproic acid.
  - The range of therapeutic plasma concentrations is wide (1 to ≥12 µg/mL), making monitoring of serum levels less useful.
  - Properties
    - Indications: partial, primary generalized, absence, atypical absence, atonic, myoclonic seizures

- Half-life: 7–45 hours
- Usual daily dose: total 5–15 mg/kg without valproic acid, 1–5 mg/kg with valproic acid ;muststart at very low doses and titrate slowly over 2–3 months
- Therapeutic levels: 0.01–0.07 μg/mL
- Adverse effects: rash, including Stevens-Johnson syndrome; vomiting

■ Topiramate
  ● Approved for
    - Initial monotherapy for partial seizures and primary generalized tonic-clonic seizures in patients ≥10 years
    - Adjunctive therapy in patients ≥2 years for partial and primary generalized tonic-clonic seizures and for Lennox-Gastaut syndrome
  ● Minimal effect on metabolism of other antiepileptic drugs
    - However, concomitant therapy with phenytoin or carbamazepine will decrease topiramate levels.
  ● Properties
    - Indications: partial, primary generalized, tonic, atonic, and atypical absence seizures; infantile spasms
    - Half-life: 20–30 hours
    - Usual daily dose: 1–9 mg/kg
    - Adverse effects: somnolence, anorexia, fatigue, difficulty with concentration, nervousness, kidney stones, oligohidrosis

■ Tiagabine
  ● Adjunctive therapy of partial seizures in adults
  ● Effective as adjunctive or monotherapy for partial seizures in some children
  ● Enzyme inducers (eg, carbamazepine, phenytoin, and phenobarbital) decrease tiagabine levels.
  ● Therapeutic plasma concentrations for tiagabine have not been established.
  ● Used only infrequently for seizure control in children because other anticonvulsants are more effective
  ● Properties
    - Indications: partial seizures
    - Half-life: 3–9 hours
    - Usual daily dose: 0.25–1.5 mg/kg (maximum of 56 mg)
    - Adverse effects: dizziness, somnolence, headache, depression

■ Levetiracetam
  ● Approved for adjunctive therapy for partial seizures in patients ≥4 years
  ● May be effective in treating primary generalized seizures
  ● Lack of significant adverse effects and significant drug interactions is leading to increasing use.
  ● Half-life of 6–8 hours means that it must be given ≥2 times a day.

  ● Properties
    - Indications: partial, secondary generalized seizures
    - Half-life: 6–8 hours
    - Usual daily dose: start at 10–20 mg/kg/day, increase every 2 weeks; top dose 60 mg/kg or 3000 mg
    - Adverse effects: somnolence, irritability, hostility

■ Oxcarbazepine
  ● Approved for initial monotherapy and adjunctive therapy for partial seizures in patients ≥4 years
  ● Rapidly becoming a drug of first choice for partial seizures
  ● Well tolerated in infants and young children
  ● Properties
    - Indications: partial, secondary generalized seizures
    - Half-life: 4–9 hours
    - Usual daily dose: 10–50 mg/kg; start at 10 mg/kg up to 600 mg divided into 2 daily doses
    - Adverse effects: somnolence, nausea, dizziness, rash, hyponatremia

■ Zonisamide
  ● Approved as adjunctive therapy in adults with partial seizures
  ● Few studies have evaluated its use in children in the US.
  ● In Japan, where it has been available longer, zonisamide is used widely in children with both partial and primary generalized epilepsy and infantile spasms.
  ● Half-life of 24–60 hours allows once-a-day dosing.
  ● Properties
    - Indications: partial, primary generalized seizures; infantile spasms
    - Half-life: 24–60 hours
    - Usual daily dose: start at 1–2 mg/kg and may work up to 10 mg/kg; top adult dose is 600 mg
    - Adverse effects: somnolence, dizziness, kidney stones, oligohidrosis

Other treatments

■ Ketogenic diet
  ● Effective alternative treatment for some children
  ● Half of patients with intractable epilepsy showed decrease in seizure frequency of 50%; some were seizure free at 1 year.
  ● To achieve ketosis, the patient is given a high-fat, low-protein, and low-carbohydrate diet, sometimes with calorie restriction.
    - The patient is usually admitted to hospital for initiation of the diet, which allows monitoring for hypoglycemia and other complications.
    - During hospitalization, a dietitian teaches the parents about the diet, giving them sample menus and explaining how to measure foods.

S

- Initial use of 24 hours of fasting to initiate the diet is no longer adhered to.
- Strict adherence to diet is required for success.
- Complications of diet include constipation, renal stones, fatigue, and metabolic acidosis.

- Vagal nerve stimulation
  - A vagal nerve stimulation device is surgically implanted subcutaneously in the anterior chest wall to stimulate the left vagus nerve.
  - Most studies report approximately 50% improvement of seizure frequency in one half of children, with a few becoming seizure free.
  - Stimulation is associated with alertness, a benefit to many children with intractable epilepsy who have often been experiencing sedation from their anticonvulsant therapy.
  - Adverse effects: generally uncommon and mild
    - Infection
    - Hoarseness
    - Neck pain
    - Insomnia
    - Emergence of behavioral abnormalities (which may be related to increasing alertness)

- Addressing psychosocial issues
  - Parents and patients may have many fears and need reassurance.
    - Explain the terms *epilepsy* and *seizure* disorder.
    - Help parents understand that diagnosis of epilepsy does not mean that the child has intellectual disability or a psychiatric disorder.
    - Give guidelines on what to do when child has a seizure, including positioning on the side and putting nothing in the mouth.
    - Emphasize to parents that death from a seizure is rare.
  - Discuss activities of patients with seizures.
    - Activities should be restricted as little as possible.
    - A child with a seizure disorder should not swim alone or go bike riding without a helmet (as for all children).
    - Contact sports are permissible when epilepsy is controlled.
    - The decision about climbing up to certain heights should be based on how well the child's seizures are controlled.
    - Older children who are not supervised when bathing should be encouraged to take showers rather than baths to minimize risk of drowning if a seizure occurs.

WHEN TO ADMIT

- Seizures are uncontrolled or prolonged
- Video EEG monitoring is needed
- Rapidly changing anticonvulsant medication is needed
- Ketogenic diet is initiated

WHEN TO REFER

- Type of seizure is unclear
- Seizures are refractory to medication
- Patients with medically intractable partial seizures should be evaluated at a comprehensive epilepsy center to determine candidacy for surgical intervention, which results in complete seizure control in up to 90% of patients.

FOLLOW-UP

- Discontinuation of antiepileptic therapy
  - After seizures have been controlled for 2 years, discontinuing antiepileptic medications should be considered.
  - ~75% of children seizure free for >2 years remained seizure free after antiepileptic medications were discontinued.
  - In children with idiopathic epilepsy and normal EEG, the prognosis for remaining seizure free after discontinuation of medications is good, except in juvenile myoclonic epilepsy.
    - If EEG shows slowing, risk of seizure recurrence is higher.
  - Risk of recurrence is not increased if medication is tapered over ≥6 weeks.
  - 50% of recurrences occur within 6 months and 60–80% within 2 years.

- Intractable seizures
  - When seizures continue despite anticonvulsant therapy, 3 possibilities should be considered before deciding that seizures are intractable to anticonvulsant therapy.
    - Seizures may be occurring when the child has lower blood levels of medication because of incomplete adherence or because dosing intervals are too long.
    - Medication may not be appropriate to the seizure type.
      - Primary generalized seizures will often not respond and may even worsen if treated with medications indicated for partial or secondary generalized seizures (eg, carbamazepine, phenytoin).
    - Repeated events may represent an nonepileptiform paroxysmal disorder rather than electrical seizure.
      - Pseudoseizures can be especially difficult to differentiate from seizures because they tend to occur in persons with epilepsy.
  - If the child is having electrographic seizures that continue despite appropriate amounts of correct medications, then the child has intractable seizures.

COMPLICATIONS

- Learning and behavioral problems
  - Children with epilepsy and without intellectual disability tend to have more learning problems, especially reading and attention deficit, than children without epilepsy.

S

- Behavioral problems may be identified in ≤50% of children with epilepsy, and this number may increase with added adverse effects of medication and burden of a chronic disorder.
- The risk of subsequent epilepsy in children with febrile seizures is <5%.
- Factors associated with subsequent afebrile partial seizures include:
  - Focal seizures
  - Prolonged seizures
  - Repeated episodes of seizures with the same febrile illness
- Factors associated with development of afebrile, generalized seizures include:
  - >3 febrile seizures
  - Family history of afebrile seizures
  - Age >3 years at the time of the first febrile seizure

PROGNOSIS

- Risk of seizure recurrence is important when deciding whether to initiate antiepileptic therapy.
- Some types of seizures (eg, absence, myoclonic, and akinetic seizures and infantile spasms) have a recurrence rate of almost 100%.
  - Seizures have usually recurred by the time the child is seen by a primary care physician.
  - These seizures require treatment.
  - Children with generalized tonic-clonic or partial seizures have a recurrence risk of ~40%.
  - Factors that increase risk of recurrence include:
    - Partial complex seizure
    - Abnormal neurologic examination
    - Focal epileptiform abnormalities on EEG
- The best prognosis is in children with a generalized seizure, normal neurologic examination, and a nonepileptiform EEG.
- >50% of recurrences occur within 6 months, up to 69% within 1 year, and 88% within 2 years.
- If epilepsy surgery is performed soon after intractability of seizures has been established, some of the secondary physiologic and psychosocial effects of growing up with epilepsy may be prevented, and children are more likely to be able to live up to their potential in adult life.
- Infantile spasms
  - Prognosis remains grave.
  - Average mortality is ~20%.
    - Aspiration pneumonia related to severe developmental abnormalities is a common cause of death.
  - ~80% of survivors are intellectually disabled.

- Spasms usually remit by a few years of age, but 55–60% of patients subsequently develop other forms of seizures.
- Prognosis is more favorable for infants whose neurologic development was normal before onset of spasms.
- Lennox-Gastaut syndrome
  - Otherwise healthy preschool-age children with normal background and fast polyspike-and-wave changes on EEG have a much better prognosis for seizure control and cognitive development.
- Juvenile myoclonic seizures
  - The rate of seizure recurrence among patients who discontinue therapy is high.
  - Lifelong condition that requires continuous treatment
- Benign partial epilepsy of childhood
  - Remits when child is ~9–12 years of age (no later than 17 years of age)
  - Remission is long lasting.
  - No associated developmental or neurologic impairment, other than some increased incidence of attention deficit
- Febrile seizure
  - One third of children who have a febrile seizure will have another one with another febrile illness.
  - The younger the child is at the time of the first episode, the greater the risk of recurrence.
  - Approximately 50% of recurrences occur within 6 months of the initial seizure; 75% occur within 1 year.

PREVENTION

- Febrile seizures
  - Oral diazepam (0.33 mg/kg of body weight administered every 8 hours during febrile illness) reduces the risk of recurrent febrile seizures.
  - Administering phenobarbital at onset of a febrile illness does not prevent seizure activity because therapeutic blood levels are not achieved soon enough.
  - Prophylactic treatment with anticonvulsant agents should be considered if:
    - Neurologic development is abnormal.
    - Seizure is complex febrile.
    - The child is <1 year of age.
  - Administering phenobarbital in doses that achieve blood levels of 15 µg/mL reduces recurrence of febrile seizures.
  - Valproate appears to be effective in prophylaxis.
  - Phenytoin and carbamazepine do not prevent recurrences.
  - Adverse effects of anticonvulsant therapy must be weighed against possible benefits.

Self-Stimulating Behaviors

DEFINITION

- Self-stimulating behaviors include:
  - Head banging and rocking
    - Rhythmic movements of the head and sometimes the entire body against a solid object
  - Thumb sucking and nail biting
  - Masturbation
  - Hair pulling and twisting
    - Trichotillomania (pulling out the hair)

EPIDEMIOLOGY

- Prevalence
  - Most common behaviors described in preschool children
    - Masturbation: almost universal
    - Thumb/finger sucking: 25–40%
    - Nail biting: 23%
    - Head banging and rocking: 3–20%
    - Hair pulling and twisting: uncommon
- Age
  - Self-stimulating behaviors typically appear before 12 months of age and peak at age 2.5 years.
  - Subsequently, the behaviors decline rapidly.
  - Thumb sucking
    - Continues in 10–20% of American children beyond 6 years of age
  - Nail biting
    - As many as 40% of all children >6 years bite their nails at some time.
    - 20% of college students continue to bite their nails.
  - Masturbation
    - Typically begins at around 2 months of age
    - Peaks at 4 years of age and again in adolescence
  - Hair pulling and twisting
    - A hairball (trichobezoar) in the stomach has been reported in preschoolers, school-age children, adolescents, and adults.
- Sex
  - Head banging and rocking
    - Male-to-female ratio of approximately 3:1
  - Hair pulling and twisting
    - Trichobezoar is more common in girls than in boys.

MECHANISM

- Research has suggested that commonalities exist among such behaviors.
  - Sometimes classified as *stereotypies*

- An interaction of the stage of neuromotor development with environmental influences (eg, restrictive car seats and cribs)
  - Homeostatic mechanism that serves to regulate stimulation from the environment
- Head banging and rocking
  - Appear to be linked to maturational patterns
    - They correlate closely with teething and other transitions of growth and development.
    - Possibly a mechanism for increasing or reducing arousal and maintaining homeostasis
  - Rocking is thought to be a soothing, pleasurable experience.
    - Every infant encounters rocking in utero.
    - Most infants encounter it from the neonatal period onward.
    - Pleasure from movement is repeated throughout life.
- Thumb sucking
  - Pleasurable sensations are associated with the double tactile experience of sucking and being sucked.
  - The feelings of security and comfort that these experiences evoke tend to reinforce this type of behavior.
- Nail biting
  - An extension or permutation of the habit of thumb sucking
  - Some experts consider this behavior a form of more overt self-aggression.
  - Others define nail biting simply as a variation of thumb sucking because this behavior is also seen typically during times of stress.
- Masturbation
  - Generally initiated as a response to the learned pleasure associated with touching of the genitalia first experienced in infancy during normal body exploration
  - May vary from direct manual genital stimulation to movement of the thighs against each other
    - Rhythmic swaying or thrusting motions of the child while straddling a hobby horse, pillow, stuffed animal, or other objects are common methods of masturbation.
  - Infants and children are capable of a physiologic orgasmic response similar to that experienced by the adult except for the absence of ejaculation in the male child.
    - Occasionally, orgasmic response has been incorrectly thought to represent a convulsive disorder in the preschool child.

HISTORY

- Head banging and rocking
  - Most common at bedtime or at times of fatigue or stress
  - May vary in duration from several minutes to hours
  - Often continues even when the child is asleep

S

- Occasionally, a family history of such behavior can be found.
  - Only 20% of siblings of children who rock exhibit similar or other rhythmic pattern disturbances.
- Individual constitutional patterns in childhood account for wide variability in the amount of stimulation any particular child requires.
- Marked rhythmic movements are commonly found in children with:
  - Hearing or sight impairment
  - Emotional disturbance
  - Severe intellectual disability
- Movements may represent a compensatory reaction for lack of stimuli or the inability to integrate stimuli.
- A child who has no disability but who is inactive because of physical illness generally shows a need for motor release.
  - Often characterized by bed rocking or other rhythmic body movements
  - Generally disappears once normal mobility is restored
- Studies indicate no connection between rocking behavior and parental divorce or separation.
  - However, the question of inadequate stimulation should be raised.
  - The presence of family turmoil and stress should be investigated.
- Thumb sucking and nail biting
  - Family history appears to exist in most cases.
    - This habit is so common that an apparent association may be of no significance.
  - No apparent correlation has been found with:
    - Number of children in the family
    - Birth order
    - Type of feeding or feeding schedule
    - Age or race of the parents
  - A significant association exists with the time of weaning.
    - The later the weaning takes place, the less likely the chance of thumb sucking.
    - Underlying causes of tension should also be investigated.
  - Many families substitute artificial pacifiers as a more socially acceptable means of oral pleasure.
    - Children often spontaneously suck a security blanket, doll, or stuffed animal.
  - Thumb sucking usually occurs:
    - With stress or boredom or at bedtime, when young children use it to help them fall asleep
- Hair pulling and twisting
  - Often indicates the presence of psychological stress

PHYSICAL EXAM

- Head banging and rocking
  - Most children will be predominantly within normal limits on physical and neurologic examination.
  - Psychosocial growth and development are apparently not disturbed.
- Thumb sucking and nail biting
  - Increased probability of dental malocclusion
  - Increased incidence of digital cutaneous infections
- Hair pulling and twisting (trichotillomania)
  - The scalp is the most common area affected.
  - The eyebrows and eyelashes are the next most likely sites.
  - Trichobezoar in the stomach if the child ingests the hair
    - Serious problem that often results in hospitalization for surgical removal of the accumulated matted hair
  - Trichotillomania is classified by the *Diagnostic and Statistical Manual of Mental Disorders* as a disorder of impulse control.
    - May best be grouped with the obsessive-compulsive disorder spectrum because of the common pathological compulsion of excessive grooming
  - Focused type
    - The activity is associated with tension before and relief after the hair is pulled.
    - Time is set aside to pull the hair.
  - Sedentary type
    - The patient is generally unaware of the behavior during the hair pulling or twisting itself.
    - The patient recognizes the action as senseless and undesirable.
  - Local irritation from a dermatologic condition
    - Rarely the cause of this disorder, but the possibility should be investigated

DIFFERENTIAL DIAGNOSIS

- Masturbation
  - Exclude:
    - Local genital irritation
    - *Candida* infection
    - Pinworms
- Obsessive-compulsive disorder
  - The clinician should investigate and refer appropriately if the patient engages in excessive:
    - Thumb sucking
    - Nail biting
    - Cuticle picking or biting
    - Hair pulling

- Infantile autism or childhood schizophrenia
  - Body twirling or spinning
  - Hand or arm flapping
- Special problems in severely intellectually disabled or emotionally disturbed children
  - Excessive rocking behavior
  - Severe self-mutilating behaviors (Lesch-Nyhan syndrome, Cornelia de Lange syndrome)
    - Compulsive self-biting
    - Severe head banging
    - Skin gouging
  - Präder-Willi syndrome
    - Severe skin picking
  - These behaviors are part of a symptom complex in a severe disorder, in contrast to generally isolated behavior in normal children.
  - The cause is generally linked to the basic disorder and may also reflect the lack, or disordered integration, of sensory stimuli.

DIAGNOSTIC PROCEDURES

- Electroencephalography
  - Not indicated in head banging and rocking because the findings are generally not helpful

TREATMENT APPROACH

- Most of these behaviors are self-limited to the preschool period and are usually viewed as normal, common, and expected behaviors.
- These habits generally do not signify psychological maladjustment.
- They often require little intervention other than reassuring parents and suggesting adequate stimulation of their child.

SPECIFIC TREATMENT

Head banging and rocking

- Treatment is generally directed toward assuring the parents that:
  - Head banging cannot cause brain injury.
  - The child will show no adverse neurologic effects in later life.
  - Children who engage in head-banging behavior usually grow up as completely normal, coordinated children.
- Padding the crib and securing the bed to prevent rolling may help during the limited rocking behavior.
- Sedation in the form of diphenhydramine may prove effective.
- Psychotropic medication is generally unnecessary and is thus discouraged.

- Rarely, if ever, do fractures of the skull or cerebral hemorrhages result from head banging.
  - Soft-tissue swelling and scalp contusions have been reported.
  - A protective helmet may be advised in severe cases.

Thumb sucking and nail biting

- Parents
  - Clarify with them the nature of these habits.
  - Advise parents to avoid punishment, shaming the child, threats, or anger.
  - Encouragement instead of restrictions helps engage children in their own program to decrease or eliminate the behavior.
- Simple behavioral therapy (based on positive reinforcement) is often sufficient to alleviate the habit.
  - The choice of reinforcement reward should be the child's.
- Bitter-tasting commercial preparations
  - May be applied to the fingers as a reminder
  - These preparations are generally inadequate unless supplemented by consistent positive reinforcement.
  - A combination of aversive taste treatment and a reward system appears to be effective in treating chronic thumb sucking.
- Hypnosis is often successful and poses no danger.
- Psychotropic medications are of little value.

Masturbation

- Counsel parents about masturbatory practices and emphasize that masturbation is:
  - Normal
  - Harmless
  - Almost universal in children
  - A healthy practice that helps the child to derive pleasure from his/her own body
- Dispel persistent myths concerning the belief that masturbation may cause:
  - Intellectual disability
  - Physical deformity
  - Blindness
  - Poor physical and mental health
  - Facial pimples
  - Hair on the palms of the hand
  - Homosexuality
  - Sexual perversions
- Encourage parents to avoid punishing or shaming their child for a normal behavior.

S

- If parents observe masturbatory activity in their child:
  - They may want to suggest to the child the inappropriateness of manipulating their genitalia in public places or in front of others.
  - Parents can inform the child that certain practices, such as using the toilet and masturbating, are best carried out in private.
- Counseling and advice given by the practitioner may be met with covert or overt resistance by parents or school authorities.
  - The pediatrician should be well prepared to educate persons responsible for the growth and development of children.

Hair pulling and twisting
- Treatment is usually indicated.
- Dynamic therapy with little evidence of effectiveness
- Behavioral therapy
- Psychopharmacologic measures in patients unresponsive to nonmedication treatment
  - Clomipramine
  - Selective serotonin reuptake inhibitors
- Hypnosis or psychotherapy

Special problems in disturbed children
- All stimulatory behaviors require treatment for the underlying disorder.
- Special behavioral treatment is needed beyond the scope and expertise of the primary care physician.
- When severe, institutionalization is often required, and methods of treatment include:
  - Aversive behavior modification techniques
  - Use of arm and neck restraints
  - Head helmets
  - Psychotropic medications
  - Psychotherapeutic behavioral programs

WHEN TO REFER
- Persistence of head banging or rocking beyond the age of 3 years
- Preoccupation with self-stimulating behavior to the point that it interferes with healthy social and emotional interaction
- Presence of accompanying symptoms, such as decreased socialization or other behavioral problems
- Presence of tissue damage

FOLLOW-UP
- Weekly visits to the physician for the first month of treatment are important to reinforce the change in behavior.

PROGNOSIS
- Thumb sucking and nail biting
  - Only 4% develop motor stereotypies.
  - The probability of malocclusion in children who suck their thumbs appears to be directly related to the age at which the habit is discontinued.
    - Children who cease the habit when they are >6 years of age generally exhibit some degree of malocclusion when examined at 12 years of age.
    - Thumb sucking that persists into school age can bring on teasing from peers and criticism from teachers and family, leaving the child with decreased self-esteem and increased psychological distress.
- Masturbation
  - Masturbation will continue as a lifelong pleasurable experience unless suppressed by parents or other adults.
- Hair pulling and twistinga
  - Obvious cosmetic damage often results in ridicule by peers and shame for the child.

Septic Arthritis

DEFINITION

- Pyogenic, or septic, arthritis refers to a bacterial infection of the joint space.
- Can lead to permanent deformity and disability, particularly in the young child
- Complications can be minimized by prompt diagnosis and aggressive treatment.

EPIDEMIOLOGY

- Age
  - Most commonly affects young children and infants
  - Can occur at any age

ETIOLOGY

- Hematogenous seeding of the synovial membrane is the most common cause in children.
- Infection also can occur by:
  - Direct inoculation of bacteria into the joint after:
    - Penetrating wound
    - Intraarticular injection
    - Joint surgery
  - Contiguous spread from an adjoining osteomyelitis
    - Occurs most often in infancy
    - Transphyseal blood vessels allow early spread of bacteria from the metaphysis of the bone across the growth plate to the epiphysis and into the joint cavity.
- Potential organisms include:
  - *Staphylococcus aureus*
    - Organism most commonly responsible for septic arthritis across all age groups
  - Group A *Streptococcus*
    - After *S aureus*, the next most common cause of septic arthritis in children >5 years
  - *Neisseria gonorrhoeae*
    - Monoarticular gonococcal arthritis can occur after genital infection.
      - Consider it in the sexually active teenager.
    - Gonococcal septic arthritis is a result of hematogenous seeding of the joint.
    - Can follow the bacteremia of untreated disseminated gonococcal disease
  - *Kingella kingae*
    - First described in Israel, has been identified with increasing frequency in the US.
    - More common in children <5 years
- In neonates, septic arthritis can also be caused by:
  - Gram-negative organisms
  - Coagulase-negative staphylococci
  - *Streptococcus agalactiae* (group B)

- In older infants and young children, *Haemophilus influenzae* type b was once common.
  - Vaccination against *H influenzae* has made it extremely rare as a cause of bacterial infection in children in the US.

SIGNS AND SYMPTOMS

- Joints of the lower extremities are the most common sites of septic arthritis.
  - The knee is the most affected joint.
  - Rarely, and usually with prolonged bacteremia, ≥1 joint can become infected.
- Common signs
  - Pain with joint motion or refusal to move an infected joint (most characteristic finding)
  - Swelling
  - Erythema
  - Tenderness
  - Redness of the skin over the joint
    - Can be difficult to detect in a deep joint, such as the hip
  - Limp or refusal to bear weight when a lower-extremity joint is involved
  - Limited range of motion when an upper-extremity joint is involved
    - May result in concerns about a neurologic problem, a pseudoparalysis
- Older children and teenagers can usually localize the pain.
  - Pain can be referred to an unaffected joint.
- Signs of acute illness most often accompany the onset of septic arthritis.
  - Fever
  - Malaise
  - Poor appetite
  - Irritability
- In the neonate, systemic signs may be less apparent.
  - Localized signs are usually prominent.
    - Failure to move an infected joint
    - Severe pain associated with passive movement of the affected extremity
    - Significant pain on manipulation of the hip joint during diaper changes

DIFFERENTIAL DIAGNOSIS

- Rheumatologic
  - Typically involves multiple joints
  - Presentation is often subacute and chronic.
  - Includes juvenile idiopathic arthritis (JIA)
    - Formerly called *juvenile rheumatoid arthritis*
    - A diagnosis of exclusion

– When children with JIA have high fever and single joint involvement, the diagnosis can be more confusing.

– In many instances, the diagnosis is made only over time, when:

■ Fevers persist.

■ Other joints become involved.

■ The single joint fails to have a pathogen isolated and fails to respond to therapy for a pyogenic infection.

– The diagnosis of JIA can remain unclear for weeks to months until the course clarifies the chronicity of the disease.

■ Reactive or postinfectious arthritis

● An immunologically induced inflammatory response to a distant infection

● Often follows a prior obvious infection

● Children can be very ill from an associated bacteremia.

● In adolescents and older children, can be associated with uveitis and conjunctivitis

■ Leukemia

● Children with leukemia can have:

– Fever

– Bone pain

● Examining the bone marrow is often required to confirm the diagnosis.

■ Isolated neuropathy

● Can cause decreased movement of a joint, but will not be associated with pain or fever

■ *Mycobacterium tuberculosis*

● A history of exposure can direct the diagnosis.

● Culturing of the joint fluid must be done on special media.

● If suspected, place a tuberculin skin test and order a chest radiograph.

■ Lyme disease

● The child with *Borrelia burgdorferi* will often have a history of erythema migrans.

● Serologic testing can help confirm the diagnosis.

● Knowing the frequency of this pathogen in the pediatrician's area of practice is important.

DIAGNOSTIC APPROACH

■ Characteristic signs help suggest the diagnosis.

● The child holds the infected joint very still to decrease pain.

● The joint is held immobile by muscle spasm in a position that:

– Maximizes capsular volume

– Minimizes intraarticular pressure

● Preferred positions

– For the hip, a combination of moderate flexion, abduction, and external rotation

– For the knee, gentle flexion

– For the shoulder, adduction against the trunk

■ The child may appear entirely well and in no distress as long as the affected joint is allowed to remain undisturbed.

■ If the child holds a joint still and has a fever, a septic joint is assumed.

LABORATORY FINDINGS

■ Erythrocyte sedimentation rate is typically elevated.

● May be normal early in the course of infection

■ C-reactive protein level is increased.

● A more sensitive test during initial illness because it increases earlier than the sedimentation rate

■ Blood cultures should always be obtained.

● Blood cultures are positive in ≥40% of children with septic arthritis.

■ Examination of joint fluid in pyogenic arthritis

● Appearance

– Generally cloudy or purulent

● Cell count

– Leukoctye count >50,000 cells/mcL

– There is a predominance of polymorphonuclear cells.

● Gram stain/fluid culture

– Cultures are positive in 50–60% of cases caused by bacterial infection.

– Attention to culture technique and special media is required to isolate *N gonorrhoeae* and *M tuberculosis*.

■ Examination of joint fluid in JIA

● Can also contain many neutrophils

– In general, levels are lower than with bacterial infection.

■ A joint effusion with a low leukocyte count and normal glucose suggests that:

● The arthritis may be caused by a sympathetic effusion from:

– An adjacent osteomyelitis *or*

– An aseptic arthritis caused by a reactive arthritis, JIA, or other rheumatologic disease

■ Serologic testing can help to confirm a diagnosis of Lyme disease.

IMAGING

■ Plain films should be obtained to look for early changes and to exclude other bone abnormalities.

● Early changes include:

– Swelling of the soft tissue

– Edematous infiltration into the fatty tissue planes

- Ultrasonography can:
  - Define the presence of a joint effusion
  - Detect the capsular distention that accompanies septic arthritis of the hip
  - Assist the operator in accurate needle placement during diagnostic aspiration
- Magnetic resonance imaging may be helpful in defining adjacent bony involvement and soft-tissue abscesses, especially in areas of complex anatomy, such as:
  - Hip
  - Sacroiliac joint
  - Pelvic bones

DIAGNOSTIC PROCEDURES

- Joint aspiration with a large-bore needle is the most important diagnostic maneuver.
  - Should be performed by an orthopaedic surgeon skilled in care of pediatric patients
  - Fluoroscopy, or possibly ultrasonography, may be used to confirm entrance into the relatively inaccessible hip and shoulder joints.
  - Failure to obtain pus from a joint that appears clinically to be infected can be caused by the thickness of pus in the joint.
- Open drainage of the joint may be necessary to confirm diagnosis and treat infection.

TREATMENT APPROACH

- Septic arthritis is an urgent situation and requires consultation among the:
  - Primary physician
  - Orthopaedic surgeon
  - Radiologist
  - Infectious diseases specialist
- Empirical therapy with antimicrobial agents that are appropriate for the likely pathogen should be started urgently after aspiration of the joint.
- Length of treatment is a minimum of 3–4 weeks.
  - Treatment should continue until the clinical response is complete.
  - Treatment will be longer if:
    - Concurrent osteomyelitis is present.
    - Most of the course is oral therapy.

SPECIFIC TREATMENTS

Parenteral antibiotic therapy

- Most infections are caused by *S aureus*.
  - An effective antistaphylococcal antimicrobial is almost always part of initial treatment.

- The following is usually sufficient initially.
  - Penicillinase-resistant penicillin (ie, nafcillin or oxacillin) *or*
  - First-generation cephalosporin
- Broader coverage in which vancomycin should be considered as initial therapy instead of a ß-lactam is appropriate
  - For a child with signs of bacteremia and sepsis
  - For a child who lives in an area with a high incidence of methicillin-resistant *S aureus*
- Once a pathogen is identified, therapy should be narrowed to treat the specific organism.
- In a severely ill or immunocompromised child or an adolescent who is thought to be abusing an intravenous drug as the cause of a bacteremia
  - Antibiotics selected empirically should be effective against:
    - *S aureus*
    - Enteric Gram-negative bacilli
    - *Pseudomonas*
  - Broad-spectrum penicillin, such as ceftazidime, and an aminoglycoside with vancomycin might be empirical therapy, pending final joint and blood cultures.
- Adolescent with possible gonococcal joint infection
  - Should be treated for staphylococci and gonococci until diagnosis is clarified
  - Cefuroxime or ceftriaxone, perhaps with vancomycin, might be selected, depending on the specifics of the case.
- Neonate
  - A first-generation cephalosporin should *not* be used in a neonate as empirical therapy because of:
    - Poor cerebrospinal fluid penetration
    - The concern for a bacteremia seeding the central nervous system
  - A safer approach would be to:
    - Start empirical therapy with high doses of a penicillin that is effective for treating *S aureus*
      - *Example:* oxacillin
    - Combine with an antibiotic to treat gram-negative enterics
      - Ceftazidime
      - An aminoglycoside
- Parenteral antibiotic therapy is continued:
  - At least until child is doing well *and*
  - Signs of acute infection have resolved

Oral antibiotic therapy

- Oral therapy can sometimes be used to finish treatment when an organism:
  - Has been identified by blood or joint fluid culture *and*
  - An effective oral agent is available

S

- Oral antibiotics can be used only if:
  - The organism is susceptible to the oral antibiotic.
  - The child's social situation guarantees reliably that the antibiotics will be given as directed.
  - The antibiotic does not cause a gastrointestinal disturbance that might interfere with absorption or compliance.
- The antibiotic must achieve therapeutic levels in bone and joint.
- Laboratory tests (eg, erythrocyte sedimentation rate and C-reactive protein level) should be normalized before switching to an oral agent.

Surgical treatment

- Surgical referral may be required to:
  - Aspirate the joint
  - Reach diagnosis at times
  - Treat the infection
- All children with septic arthritis of the hip should be seen emergently by an orthopaedic surgeon.
  - They require immediate drainage of the joint.
  - Delay in draining a major joint, such as the hip joint, is associated with worse outcomes.
  - Open debridement may be required.
- Other infected joints less often require open debridement but should also be evaluated for surgical treatment.
- Repeated aspirations of a joint may be necessary if fluid reaccumulates.

WHEN TO ADMIT

- All children thought to have bacterial infection of a major joint should be hospitalized.

WHEN TO REFER

- Children being evaluated for bone or joint infection should be evaluated by an:
  - Orthopaedic surgeon *and/or*
  - Infectious disease specialist

COMPLICATIONS

- Pyogenic arthritis constitutes a clinical emergency.
  - Complications of untreated infection include:
    - Dissolution of articular cartilage
    - Necrosis of the underlying epiphysis
    - Destruction of the adjacent growth plate
    - Dislocation of the joint itself
- Possible neuropathies
  - Septic arthritis of the shoulder: brachial plexus neuropathy
  - Septic arthritis of the hip: neuropathies of femoral and sciatic nerves
  - These neuropathies occurring without infection should not be associated with pain or fever.
- Complications can be minimized by:
  - Prompt diagnosis
  - Aggressive treatment

PROGNOSIS

- Consequences of bacterial arthritis can be severe.
  - Direct destructive effect of infection
    - The host's inflammatory response can add to the damage.
  - By increasing intraarticular pressure, intracapsular infection can obstruct blood flow.
    - May lead to necrosis of the epiphysis and underlying growth plate
  - Untreated joint infection can result in joint instability through destruction of the ligamentous fibers of the capsule.
  - These factors are of special concern for the hip joint in children.

Sexually Transmitted Infections

DEFINITION

- Sexually transmitted organisms
  - *Campylobacter* species
  - *Chlamydia trachomatis*
  - Cytomegalovirus
  - *Entamoeba histolytica*
  - *Giardia lamblia*
  - Hepatitis A and B virus
  - Herpes simplex virus types 1 and 2 (HSV-1 and HSV-2)
  - Human immunodeficiency virus (HIV)
  - Human papillomavirus (HPV)
  - Molluscum contagiosum (papovavirus)
  - *Mycoplasma genitalium*
  - *Mycoplasma hominis*
  - *Neisseria gonorrhoeae*
  - *Phthirus pubis* (pubic lice)
  - *Salmonella* species
  - *Sarcoptes scabiei* (mites)
  - *Shigella* species
  - *Treponema pallidum*
  - *Trichomonas vaginalis*
  - *Ureaplasma urealyticum*

EPIDEMIOLOGY

- Prevalence
  - 15- to 24-year-olds represent only one-quarter of sexually active individuals in the US, but almost one-half of all sexually transmitted infections (STIs) occur in this age group.
- Specific agents
  - *C trachomatis*
    - Appears to cause 35–50% of symptomatic nongonococcal urethritis among heterosexual men
  - *N gonorrhoeae*
    - Overall prevalence, 0.4% (range, up to 2.4%); >95% of patients are asymptomatic.
    - Among young adult women: overall rate of infection, 0.4% (range, up to 1.9%); almost 87% of patients are asymptomatic.
  - HPV
    - Most prevalent STI in the US.
    - Infection rates in adolescents and young adults are high.
    - Prevalence of cervical HPV infection among adolescents age 12–21 years is approximately 51–64%.
    - Approximately 45–55% of adolescent girls may become infected over 3 years of observation.
  - HSV
    - Infection with HSV-1 has accounted for an increasing proportion of genital herpes infections.
    - Prevalence of HSV-2 infection in young people has decreased dramatically in the past decade (with a smaller decline for HSV-1).
- STIs/syndromes associated with STIs
  - Syphilis
    - Rates of primary and secondary syphilis decreased by 90% from 1990–2000, then increased (in men only) from 2000–2004.
    - For the first time in a decade, rate of syphilis among women did not continue to decrease from 2003 to 2004.
    - Syphilis remains a significant problem in the southern US and in some urban areas.
    - Rates have increased since 2000 among men who have sex with men.
  - Enteric infections
    - Proctitis and proctocolitis are limited mostly to adolescent boys who practice anal receptive intercourse.

ETIOLOGY

- Causes of syndromes associated with STI
  - Pelvic inflammatory disease (PID)
    - Often results from undetected or inadequately treated STIs of the lower genital tract (endocervix)
    - Sexually transmitted organisms, especially *N gonorrhoeae* and *C trachomatis*, are implicated in many cases.
    - Microorganisms that comprise vaginal flora (eg, anaerobes, *Gardnerella vaginalis*, *Haemophilus influenzae*, enteric gram-negative rods, *Streptococcus agalactiae*) have also been associated with PID.
    - Cytomegalovirus, *Mycoplasma hominis*, *Ureaplasma urealyticum*, and *Mycoplasma genitalium* might be associated with some cases of PID.
  - Perihepatitis (Fitz-Hugh–Curtis syndrome)
    - *C trachomatis* infections can cause a picture similar to this condition.
  - Epididymitis
    - Among sexually active adolescents, acute epididymitis is most frequently caused by *N gonorrhoeae* or *C trachomatis*.
    - Sexually transmitted enteric organisms (eg, *Escherichia coli*) may be the causative agent in male adolescents who practice anal insertive intercourse.
  - Enteric infections
    - A variety of organisms can cause enteritis in HIV-infected patients.
    - Proctitis
      - *N gonorrhoeae*, *C trachomatis* (including lymphogranuloma venereum [LGV] serovars), *T pallidum*, and HSV are the most common sexually transmitted pathogens involved.

- Proctolitis
  - Pathogenic organisms include *Campylobacter* species; *Shigella* species; *E histolytica*; and, rarely, LGV serovars of *C trachomatis*.
- Enteritis
  - In otherwise healthy patients, *G lamblia* is most frequently implicated.
- Vaginitis
  - *T vaginalis* is an important cause of vaginitis among sexually active adolescents.
- Cervicitis
  - Causes include:
    - *C trachomatis* and *N gonorrhoeae*
    - *Trichomonas* species and HSV, especially HSV-2
    - *M genitalium*
    - Bacterial vaginosis
    - Douching
  - In most cases of cervicitis, no etiologic agent is identified.
- Genital HSV infection
  - Most cases of recurrent genital herpes are caused by HSV-2.
  - HSV-1 might become more common as a cause of first-episode genital herpes.

RISK FACTORS

- Why adolescents are at risk for sexually transmitted infections
  - Sense of invulnerability ("It can't happen to me.")
  - Lack of information ("If I don't feel sick, I can't be sick.")
  - Inconsistent and improper use of condoms
  - Poor communication skills with partners and physicians
  - Barriers to care (legal obstacles, concerns about confidentiality)
  - Inability to adhere to treatment regimens
  - Sexual networks with high prevalence of infection
  - Physiologic changes associated with puberty
- STIs/syndromes associated with STIs
  - *Chlamydia*
    - Oral contraceptives, a popular method of contraception among adolescents, may increase the risk for chlamydial infection
    - Injections of contraceptive depot medroxyprogesterone acetate (Depo-Provera) may increase the risk for chlamydia.
  - PID
    - Oral contraceptives may protect against development of symptomatic PID.
    - Among all sexually active girls and women, those <19 years of age are at greatest risk for PID.
    - Risk is 1:8 for sexually active 15-year-olds and 1:16 for 16-year-olds, but only 1:80 for 24-year-olds.

- The major risk factor for PID is a prior episode; adolescent girls who experience illness early in their reproductive life cycle are at great risk for having further significant problems.
- When eliciting history from a patient who has lower abdominal pain, keep in mind factors that place an individual at risk for infection.
  - Failure to use barrier methods of contraception
  - Douching
  - Presence of an intrauterine device
  - Multiple partners
  - Recent change in partner
  - History of other STIs or PID
- Latent syphilis
  - Sex partner documented to have primary, secondary, or early latent syphilis
- Enteric infections
  - Proctitis and proctocolitis are limited mostly to adolescent boys who practice anal receptive intercourse.
  - Enteritis occurs among persons whose sexual practices include oral-anal contact.
- Vaginitis
  - Bacterial vaginosis is associated with:
    - Multiple sex partners
    - New sex partner
    - Douching
  - Male sex partners of women who have bacterial vaginosis more often have *G vaginalis* recovered from urethra than do controls.
  - Nongonococcal, nonchlamydial pathogens associated with PID are recovered more often from endometrium of women who have bacterial vaginosis than from those who do not.

SIGNS AND SYMPTOMS

Signs and symptoms, by sex

- Boys
  - Dysuria, discharge, urethral itching (urethritis)
  - Scrotal pain, swelling (epididymitis)
  - Rectal discharge, tenesmus, anorectal pain (proctitis, proctocolitis, colitis)
- Girls
  - Mucopurulent cervicitis
  - Vaginitis (vaginal discharge)
  - Dysuria, urgency, frequency
  - Right upper quadrant abdominal pain
  - PID (low abdominal pain)
  - Bleeding between periods (cervicitis) or a heavier, more prolonged period (PID)

- Both sexes
  - Dermatitis
  - Genital ulcers (single or multiple)
  - Genital warts
  - Hepatitis A virus or hepatitis B virus infection
  - Lymphadenopathy, especially inguinal or generalized (associated with HIV)
  - Persistent pharyngitis
  - Septic arthritis

Specific agents

- *C trachomatis*
  - Symptoms generally develop 1–3 weeks after infection.
  - Male adolescents may report:
    - Only mild dysuria or itching at terminal urethra
    - May have scanty, mucoid discharge that is easily ignored and may disappear without treatment
  - Dysuria can be the primary manifestation of infection.
  - Female patients may report spotting between periods as a result of cervicitis.
  - If infection has spread to the upper genital tract, female patients may report low abdominal pain or right upper quadrant pain (Fitz-Hugh–Curtis syndrome).
  - Infections in teenage girls and teenage boys are often asymptomatic.
  - At pelvic examination, clues to infection are:
    - Presence of mucopurulent discharge from the cervical os (known as mucopus)
    - Cervical erythema
    - Friability
- *N gonorrhoeae*
  - Produces symptoms similar to those of *C trachomatis*
  - Symptomatic men tend to have more pronounced symptoms.
    - More severe dysuria
    - Greater amount of and more purulent discharge
  - Pharyngitis and proctitis
  - The organism may become blood borne and can lead to the so-called arthritis-dermatitis syndrome, disseminated gonococcal infection (DGI).
    - Strains of *N gonorrhoeae* that lead to DGI characteristically tend to cause few genital symptoms.
    - Patients develop fever (although not always) and may have anorexia, malaise, or both.
    - Skin lesions then appear, generally distributed on extremities (arms more often than legs).
    - Lesions appear as erythematous macules <5 mm in diameter; they become pustular and occasionally hemorrhagic or necrotic.

- Lesions are most often noticed near the small joints of the hands and feet.
- Tenosynovitis tends to occur over extensor and flexor tendons of the hands and feet.
- Once tenosynovitis and dermatitis clear, patients develop polyarthralgia but usually seek care only when an oligoarthritis develops.
  - The knee is the joint most commonly infected.
  - Followed by the elbow, ankle, and small joints of the hands and feet

- HPV
  - Visible warts usually develop within 6 weeks to 8 months after infection, but the incubation period may be longer.
  - Typical pedunculated warts with keratotic and irregular surfaces are easy to recognize.
    - Warts may also be flat and more difficult to detect.
    - Use of a handheld magnifying glass or colposcope is extremely helpful.
  - Among male adolescents, warts are usually seen on the penile shaft, prepuce, frenulum, corona, and glans but may also be present on the skin of the scrotum and anus.
  - Among female adolescents, the posterior vaginal introitus, labia minora, and vestibule are most common sites of infection, but warts can be seen anywhere on the external or internal genitalia.
  - Perianal warts can be seen even in women who have not had anal intercourse.
  - Subclinical disease is most likely to occur on the cervix; this relatively large transformation zone of the maturing adolescent cervix affords a hospitable site of infection.
- HSV
  - In primary infection, symptoms usually occur 2–20 days after sexual exposure.
  - Because primary infection represents the first episode of infection with a particular virus type, systemic symptoms, such as fever, malaise, and headache are common.
  - ~50% of patients have tender inguinal lymphadenopathy.
  - Burning or itching occurs at the site of inoculation, followed by erythema and development of discrete vesicles.
  - Vesicles first contain clear fluid but rapidly form pustules with an erythematous base.
  - Patients typically may have 15–30 vesicles, each full of infectious viral particles.
  - Female adolescents: Lesions are located on the vulva, cervix, clitoris, or perineum.
  - Male adolescents: Lesions may occur on the penile shaft, glans, or prepuce.
  - Infection can involve the urethra, leading to dysuria or urinary retention.

S

- Vesicles can be seen on the thighs, buttocks, groin, or perianal region as a result of autoinoculation or anal receptive perianal region.
- After 2–4 days, pustules break open and coalesce to form wet ulcers (usually prompting patients to seek health care).
- New lesions still may be developing at this point (with a peak at 7–11 days), but within 20 days, all lesions have crusted over, and pain and other symptoms have disappeared.

STIs/syndromes associated with STIs

■ PID

- Suggestive of PID:
  - Presence of a new vaginal discharge (or a change in odor, color, or amount)
  - Abnormal menstrual bleeding (increased or prolonged; occurring at the wrong time in the cycle)
  - Dyspareunia
- Other symptoms include:
  - Dysuria
  - Dysmenorrhea (usually more severe than normal)
  - Nausea
  - Vomiting
  - Diarrhea
  - Fever (<50% of patients)
  - Malaise
- If infection involves capsule of the liver, right upper quadrant tenderness may be elicited.
- With extensive infection, signs of peritonitis, particularly rebound tenderness, are present.
- Palpation of an adnexal mass suggests a coexisting tuboovarian abscess.
- Mucopus visible in the cervical os strongly suggests infection, but its absence does not rule out diagnosis.

■ Syphilis

- The typical chancre of syphilis develops at the site of intimate sexual contact approximately 2–3 weeks after exposure
- The lesion varies in size from a few millimeters to a few centimeters; is clean based and painless; and has sharply demarcated, indurated borders.
- Multiple ulcers may be present.
- Lymphadenopathy is usually present, often bilaterally.
- Because the ulcer is painless, its appearance in the vagina or rectum or even in the mouth is likely to go unnoticed.
- While the ulcer is present, the exudate overlying it is highly infectious.
- Secondary syphilis
  - The rash of secondary syphilis appears 4–10 weeks after chancre appears in an untreated patient.
  - Rash and chancre may coexist.
  - Constitutional symptoms, such as fever, malaise, sore throat, and generalized lymphadenopathy, may be present.
  - Rash is typically papulosquamous but can be macular or pustular.
  - Initially, rash involves trunk and flexor surfaces of arms but then spreads to the entire body, including palms, soles, and mucous membranes.
  - Annular papules can appear on the face, and rash can resemble impetigo or eczema.
  - In some cases, moist, fissured papules or raised, thickened papules (condyloma lata) are seen; both are highly infectious.
  - Loss of scalp or eyebrow hair can be associated with secondary syphilis.
  - Rash disappears spontaneously 3–12 weeks after appearance; at this point, the patient is classified as having latent syphilis.

■ Perihepatitis (Fitz-Hugh–Curtis syndrome)

- Violin-string adhesions between liver and anterior abdominal wall, localized peritonitis of liver's anterior surface, upper abdominal pain and tenderness
- Onset of upper abdominal pain usually follows the onset of lower abdominal pain, but can precede it.
- Pain generally occurs on the patient's right side and can radiate to the shoulder.

■ Epididymitis

- Acute or subacute onset of unilateral scrotal pain
- Adolescent boys may report testicular pain.
- Preceding symptoms may include urethral discharge and dysuria, but these symptoms may be so mild that they are easily ignored.
- Fever may be present.
- At physical examination, tenderness may occur on palpation of the epididymis, but the testicle may also be slightly tender.
- Hydrocele may be present, and the spermatic cord may be swollen and tender.

■ Enteric infections

- Symptoms of proctitis and proctolitis include anorectal pain, tenesmus, constipation, and anal discharge.
- Patients with proctocolitis or enteritis have diarrhea.
- Enteritis: Symptoms are usually limited to abdominal pain and diarrhea; other symptoms of proctitis and proctocolitis are absent.

■ Cervicitis

- Characterized by purulent or mucopurulent discharge from endocervical os or by significant endocervical bleeding (or both) that is induced when a swab is introduced into the os

DIFFERENTIAL DIAGNOSIS

Anatomic area

- Urinary tract
  - Cystitis
  - Pyelonephritis
  - Urethritis
  - Other
- Gastrointestinal tract
  - Appendicitis
  - Constipation
  - Diverticulitis
  - Gastroenteritis
  - Inflammatory bowel disease
  - Irritable bowel syndrome
  - Other
- Reproductive tract
  - Acute PID
  - Cervicitis
  - Dysmenorrhea (primary or secondary)
  - Ectopic pregnancy
  - Endometriosis
  - Endometritis
  - Mittelschmerz
  - Ovarian cyst (torsion, rupture)
  - Pregnancy (intrauterine, ectopic)
  - Ruptured follicle
  - Septic abortion
  - Threatened abortion
  - Torsion of adnexa
  - Tuboovarian abscess

Specific agents

- *C trachomatis*
  - Profuse, purulent discharge should raise the possibility of *N gonorrhoeae* co-infection or of this being the single causative agent.
  - Unless a thorough history is obtained, combination of dysuria and right upper quadrant or right flank pain might lead to the erroneous diagnosis of pyelonephritis.
  - Lower abdominal pain suggests the possibility of PID.
  - Vaginal discharge is more likely to indicate presence of another infection.

STIs/syndromes associated with STIs

- PID
  - Most symptoms of PID occur in patients with diseases of the urinary tract (eg, pyelonephritis) or gastrointestinal tract (eg, appendicitis).

- Clinical diagnosis of PID has a positive predictive value for salpingitis of 65–90%.
  - Positive predictive value is higher for adolescents and in clinical settings with high prevalence of such STIs as chlamydia or gonorrhea.
- Signs and symptoms can be nonspecific, and the only sure method of diagnosis, laparoscopy, is not routinely performed for diagnostic purposes in the US.
- To avoid misdiagnosis, primary care physicians must:
  - Maintain a high index of suspicion
  - Obtain an extensive history
  - Perform a thorough physical examination
- More elaborate diagnostic evaluation is often needed because incorrect diagnosis and management might cause unnecessary morbidity.
- Additional criteria to enhance specificity of minimal criteria and support a diagnosis of PID include:
  - Oral temperature >101°F (38.3°C)
  - Abnormal cervical or vaginal mucopurulent discharge
  - Abundant leukocytes on saline microscopy of vaginal secretions
  - Increased erythrocyte sedimentation rate
  - Increased C-reactive protein level
  - Laboratory documentation of cervical infection with *N gonorrhoeae* or *C trachomatis*
- Other diagnoses to consider include:
  - Cervicitis
  - Dysmenorrhea (primary or secondary)
  - Ectopic pregnancy
  - Endometriosis
  - Endometritis
  - Mittelschmerz
  - Ovarian cyst (torsion, rupture)
  - Pregnancy (intrauterine, ectopic)
  - Ruptured follicle
  - Septic abortion
  - Threatened abortion
  - Torsion of adnexa
  - Tuboovarian abscess
- Latent syphilis
  - Early latent syphilis cannot be reliably distinguished from late latent syphilis solely on the basis of nontreponemal titers.
  - All patients with latent syphilis should have thorough examination of all accessible mucosal surfaces to evaluate for internal mucosal lesions.
    - Oral cavity
    - Perineum in women

S

- Perianal area
- Underneath foreskin in uncircumcised men
- Epididymitis
  - In adolescents, rule out testicular torsion.
- Cervicitis
  - Women with cervicitis should be carefully evaluated for:
    - PID
    - Presence of trichomonas and bacterial vaginosis
    - Chlamydia
    - Gonorrhea

DIAGNOSTIC APPROACH

- When an adolescent seeks care for symptoms and clinical findings that might be caused by an STI, the physician must proceed with appropriate diagnostic tests or therapy, even though the history may appear to exclude such a cause.
- Most sexually active teenagers will be truthful when:
  - Questioned respectfully without parent or guardian present
  - Given appropriate guarantees about confidentiality
- Increasingly widespread availability and use of nucleic acid amplification tests (NAAT) to diagnose *C trachomatis* and *N gonorrhoeae* infections represent major advances.
  - Benefits of these tests
    - More sensitive than culture and previous generations of nonculture tests
    - Do not require recovery of viable organisms
    - Can be performed on urine specimens
  - By eliminating or reducing need for invasive testing, NAAT may expand number of at-risk youth who are screened.
  - Self-collection of vaginal specimens will also enhance detection efforts.

LABORATORY FINDINGS

Specific agents

- *C trachomatis*
  - Gram stain of cervical tissue will reveal presence of 10–30 polymorphonuclear white blood cells (WBCs) per oil-immersion field.
  - Culture of urethral or cervical samples was previously the gold standard for detecting infection.
  - NAAT are considerably more sensitive than culture or older nonculture techniques.
    - Sensitivity of culture for chlamydia is 54–85% from endocervical specimens, versus 88–100% by using various NAAT.
    - Older nonculture tests, such as DNA probes or enzyme-linked immunoabsorbent assays, are only 54–84% sensitive.

- Chlamydia culture remains the only diagnostic test for chlamydia infection admissible in a court of law (eg, in cases of child sexual abuse).
- *N gonorrhoeae*
  - Organism can be grown from:
    - Urethral or cervical discharge
    - Swabs of the vagina, cervix, urethra, pharynx, or rectum
    - Urine sediment (in many cases)
  - In the past, diagnosis rested on culture or classic findings of WBCs and gram-negative intracellular diplococci in Gram stains of discharge or material obtained from a urethral swab.
  - Even under ideal conditions, the organism can be difficult to grow, and physicians relying on culture should be familiar with yield from the laboratory they use.
  - In men, typical Gram stain from a urethral discharge is diagnostic.
  - For samples taken from women, sorting out gram-negative organisms that truly are intracellular versus those that may be overlying or near cells is more difficult.
    - When ≥8 pairs of such diplococci are seen in ≥2 polymorphonuclear leukocytes, culture will be positive 96% of the time.
  - *N gonorrhoeae* infections can now be diagnosed by NAAT.
    - At least as sensitive as culture results
    - Eliminate pelvic examination or swabbing urethral meatus to obtain specimens
    - Allow use of a urine specimen or vaginal swab
- HSV
  - Cultures of intact vesicles are generally positive, as are cultures of the cervix.
  - Recurrence rates for genital HSV-1 and HSV-2 differ significantly; culture should be obtained whenever a patient presents with new-onset genital herpes.

STIs/syndromes associated with STIs

- PID
  - Acute-phase reactants lack the necessary sensitivity and specificity to help diagnose PID.
  - Although 60–80% of patients have an increased WBC count, sedimentation rate, or C-reactive protein level, so do 20–50% of patients with abdominal pain without PID.
- Syphilis
  - When chancre is present, dark-field examination of nonbloody exudate should be performed by expert in dark-field microscopy.
    - If test is done on 3 successive days, the likelihood of obtaining a positive result from an infected individual is extremely high.
    - If results of all 3 tests are negative, reconsider diagnosis of primary syphilis.

S

- If dark-field examination is unavailable, obtain serologic test for syphilis.
- If the examiner is relatively certain that chancre is one of primary syphilis, request a fluorescent treponemal antibody absorption test.
  - The sensitivities of the VDRL (Venereal Disease Research Laboratory) flocculation test, rapid plasma reagin (RPR) test, and microhemagglutination assay for antibody to *T pallidum* at this point in the disease process are relatively low.
- Perihepatitis (Fitz-Hugh–Curtis syndrome)
  - <50% of patients have mildly increased liver enzyme levels.
- Epididymitis
  - Supportive laboratory evidence includes:
    - Positive leukocyte esterase test on first-catch urine specimen (the first 20 mL of urine voided) or presence of >10 WBCs per high-power field if first-catch urine specimen is spun down and sediment examined *or*
    - Gram stain of urethral secretions showing >5 WBCs per oil-immersion field
      - If Gram stain also shows WBCs containing intracellular gram-negative diplococci, *N gonorrhoeae* should be considered the causative agent.
- Enteric infections
  - Proctolitis: Fecal leukocytes may be detected on stool examination, depending on the pathogen.

DIAGNOSTIC PROCEDURES

- Patients with proctitis (the distal 10–12 cm of the rectum) should be examined with anoscopy and evaluated for *C trachomatis* (including LGV serovars), *N gonorrhoeae*, herpes simplex virus, and *T pallidum* infection.
- Patients with anal warts and warts on the rectal mucosa can benefit from inspection of the rectal mucosa by digital examination or anoscopy.
- Primary and secondary syphilis
  - After the newborn period (≥1 month), examine the cerebrospinal fluid (CSF) of children with syphilis to detect asymptomatic neurosyphilis.
  - Review birth and maternal medical records to assess whether the child has congenital or acquired syphilis.
- Latent syphilis
  - After the newborn period, examine the CSF of children with syphilis to exclude neurosyphilis.
  - Review birth and maternal records to assess whether the child has congenital or acquired syphilis.

TREATMENT APPROACH

- Empiric treatment of PID should be initiated in sexually active young women and others at risk for STIs if:
  - They are experiencing pelvic or lower abdominal pain.
  - No cause for illness other than PID can be identified.

- ≥1 of the following minimal criteria are present on pelvic examination.
  - Cervical motion tenderness *or*
  - Uterine tenderness *or*
  - Adnexal tenderness
- Requiring that all 3 of the minimal criteria listed previously be present before initiating antibiotic treatment might result in insufficient sensitivity for diagnosing PID.

SPECIFIC TREATMENTS

C trachomatis

- Co-infection with *C trachomatis* often occurs among patients who have gonococcal infection; therefore, presumptive treatment of such patients for chlamydia is appropriate.
- The following recommended treatment regimens and alternative regimens cure infection and usually relieve symptoms.
- Recommended regimens
  - Azithromycin 1 g orally in a single dose *or*
  - Doxycycline 100 mg orally twice a day for 7 days
- Alternative regimens
  - Erythromycin base 500 mg orally 4 times a day for 7 days *or*
  - Erythromycin ethylsuccinate 800 mg orally 4 times a day for 7 days *or*
  - Ofloxacin 300 mg orally twice a day for 7 days *or*
  - Levofloxacin 500 mg orally once daily for 7 days
- Other considerations
  - Azithromycin
    - Used to treat patients with questionable adherence to multiday dosing
    - In populations with erratic health-care-seeking behavior, poor compliance with treatment, or unpredictable follow-up, may be more cost effective because it offers single-dose, directly observed therapy
  - Doxycycline
    - Costs less than azithromycin
    - No greater risk of adverse events
  - Erythromycin
    - Might be less efficacious than both azithromycin and doxycycline, mainly because gastrointestinal side effects frequently discourage patients from compliance
  - Ofloxacin and levofloxacin
    - Effective but more expensive
    - No advantage with regard to dose regimen
  - Other quinolones
    - Not reliably effective against chlamydial infection *or*
    - Have not been adequately evaluated

S

- To maximize adherence to recommended therapies, dispense medications for chlamydial infections on site; the first dose should be directly observed.

N gonorrhoeae

Dual therapy for gonococcal and chlamydial infection

- Patients infected with *N gonorrhoeae* often are co-infected with *C trachomatis*.
- Patients treated for gonococcal infection should be treated routinely with regimen effective against uncomplicated genital *C trachomatis* infection.
- Most gonococci in the US are susceptible to doxycycline and azithromycin; thus, routine co-treatment might hinder development of antimicrobial-resistant *N gonorrhoeae*.

Quinolone-resistant N gonorrhoeae

- Prevalence of fluoroquinolone resistance among *N gonorrhoeae* isolates in the US has increased and become widespread.
- The Centers for Disease Control and Prevention (CDC) "no longer recommends the use of fluoroquinolones for the treatment of gonococcal infections and associated conditions such as pelvic inflammatory disease."

Uncomplicated gonococcal infections of the cervix, urethra, and rectum

- Recommended regimens
  - Ceftriaxone 125 mg IM in a single dose *or*
  - Cefixime 400 mg orally in a single dose *plus*
  - Treatment for chlamydia if *C trachomatis* infection is not ruled out
  - Ceftriaxone is safe and effective for treating uncomplicated gonorrhea at all anatomic sites.
  - Cefixime offers the advantage of oral administration.
  - May not be available in many areas; the CDC or state health departments can provide updates on its availability.
- Alternative regimens
  - Spectinomycin 2 g IM in a single dose *or*
  - Single-dose cephalosporin regimens
  - Spectinomycin is expensive and must be injected but is effective.
  - Useful for treating patients who cannot tolerate cephalosporins and quinolones
  - Single-dose cephalosporin regimens that are safe and highly effective against uncomplicated urogenital and anorectal gonococcal infections include:
    – Ceftizoxime 500 mg IM
    – Cefoxitin 2 g IM with probenecid 1 g orally
    – Cefotaxime 500 mg IM
  - None of the injectable cephalosporins offer any advantage over ceftriaxone.

Uncomplicated gonococcal infections of the pharynx

- More difficult to eradicate than infections at urogenital and anorectal sites
- Few antimicrobial regimens can reliably cure such infections >90% of the time.
- Although chlamydial co-infection of pharynx is unusual, co-infection at genital sites sometimes occurs.
- Therefore, treatment for both gonorrhea and chlamydia is suggested.
- Recommended regimens
  - Ceftriaxone 125 mg IM in a single dose *plus*
  - Treatment for chlamydia if *C trachomatis* infection is not ruled out

DGI

- Hospitalization is recommended for initial therapy in:
  - Patients who cannot be relied on to adhere to treatment
  - Patients in whom the diagnosis is uncertain
  - Patients with purulent synovial effusions or other complications
- Examine patients for clinical evidence of endocarditis and meningitis.
- For patients who are receiving therapy for DGI, presumptively treat for concurrent *C trachomatis* infection unless appropriate testing excludes this infection.
- Recommended regimen
  - Ceftriaxone 1 g IM or IV every 24 hour
- Alternative regimens
  - Cefotaxime 1 g IV every 8 hours *or*
  - Ceftizoxime 1 g IV every 8 hours *or*
  - Spectinomycin 2 g IM every 12 hours
- Continue all regimens for 24–48 hours after improvement begins, at which time therapy may be switched to 1 of the following regimens to complete at least 1 week of antimicrobial therapy
  - Cefixime 400 mg orally twice a day *or*
  - Cefixime suspension 400 mg twice daily orally (200 mg/5mL) *or*
  - Cefpodoxime 400 mg orally twice daily
- Fluoroquinolones may be an alternative treatment option if antimicrobial susceptibility can be documented by culture.

HPV (genital warts)

- Treatment is primarily directed toward symptomatic warts.
- Clinicians who treat genital warts should determine which technique is most suitable to their practice and become familiar with that technique.
- Clinicians should be knowledgeable about ≥1 physician-applied and 1 patient-applied regimen.
- The primary goal of treating visible genital warts is wart removal.

- In most patients, treatment can induce wart-free periods.
- Factors that might influence selection of treatment include:
  - Wart size
  - Wart number
  - Anatomic site of wart
  - Wart morphology
  - Patient preference
  - Cost of treatment
  - Convenience
  - Adverse effects
  - Provider experience
- Warts located on moist surfaces and in intertriginous areas tend to respond better to topical treatment than do warts on drier surfaces.

Recommended regimens for external genital warts

- Patient-applied options
  - Podofilox 0.5% solution or gel
    - Patients should apply podofilox solution with a cotton swab, or podofilox gel with a finger, to visible genital warts twice a day for 3 days, followed by 4 days of no therapy.
    - Repeat cycle as necessary for a total of 4 cycles.
    - The total wart area treated should not exceed 10 cm, and the total volume of podofilox should not exceed 0.5 mL per day.
    - If possible, the primary care physician should apply initial treatment to show proper technique and identify which warts should be treated.
    - The safety of podofilox during pregnancy has not been established.
  - Imiquimod 5% cream
    - Patients should apply imiquimod cream once daily at bedtime, 3 times a week for up to 16 weeks.
    - Wash the treatment area with mild soap and water 6–10 hours after the application.
    - The safety of imiquimod during pregnancy has not been established.
- Physician-administered options
  - Cryotherapy with liquid nitrogen or cryoprobe
    - Repeat applications every 1–2 weeks.
  - Podophyllin resin 10–25% in compound tincture of benzoin
    - Apply a small amount to each wart; allow to air dry.
    - Repeat treatment weekly if necessary.
  - Trichloroacetic acid (TCA) or bichloroacetic acid (BCA) 80–90%
    - Apply a small amount only to warts and allow to dry, at which time a white frosting develops.

- Powder with talc, sodium bicarbonate (ie, baking soda), or liquid soap to remove unreacted acid if an excess amount is applied.
    - Repeat weekly if necessary.
  - Surgical removal by tangential scissor excision, tangential shave excision, curettage, or electrosurgery
- Alternative treatments
  - Intralesional interferon *or*
  - Laser surgery
- Other considerations
  - Podofilox 0.5% solution or gel
    - Relatively inexpensive
    - Easy to use
    - Safe
    - Self-applied by patients
    - Most patients experience mild or moderate pain or local irritation after treatment.
  - Imiquimod
    - Local inflammatory reactions (redness and irritation) are common and usually mild to moderate.
  - Cryotherapy
    - Clinicians must be trained in proper use because over treatment or under treatment can result in complications or low efficacy.
    - Pain after application of the liquid nitrogen, followed by necrosis and sometimes blistering, is not unusual.
    - Local anesthesia (topical or injected) might facilitate treatment if warts are present in many areas or if the area of warts is large.
  - Podophyllin resin
    - Over application or failure to air dry can result in local irritation caused by spread of the compound to adjacent areas.
  - TCA and BCA can spread rapidly if applied excessively, damaging adjacent normal tissue.
    - If pain is intense, then acid can be neutralized with soap or sodium bicarbonate (ie, baking soda).
  - Because of shortcomings of available treatments, some clinics use combination therapy (≥2 modalities on the same wart at the same time).
    - No data support use of >1 therapy at a time to improve the efficacy of treatment.
    - Combining modalities may increase complications.

Recommended regimens for cervical warts

- For exophytic cervical warts, high-grade squamous intra-epithelial lesions must be excluded before treatment is begun.
- Management of exophytic cervical warts should include consultation with an expert.

Recommended regimens for vaginal warts

- Cryotherapy with liquid nitrogen
  - Use of a cryoprobe in the vagina is not recommended because of risk for vaginal perforation and fistula formation.
- TCA or BCA 80–90% applied to warts
  - Apply a small amount only to warts and allow to dry, at which time a white frosting develops.
  - Powder with talc or baking soda or liquid soap preparations to remove unreacted acid if an excess amount is applied.
  - Repeat weekly if necessary.

Recommended regimens for urethral meatus warts

- Cryotherapy with liquid nitrogen
- Podophyllin 10–25% in compound tincture of benzoin
  - The treatment area must be dry before contact with normal mucosa.
  - Can be applied weekly if necessary
  - The safety of podophyllin during pregnancy has not been established.
- Although data on podofilox and imiquimod for treating distal meatal warts are limited, some specialists recommend their use in some patients.

Recommended regimen for anal warts

- Cryotherapy with liquid nitrogen
- TCA or BCA 80–90% applied to warts
  - Apply a small amount only to warts and allow to dry, at which time a white frosting develops.
  - Powder with talc or baking soda or with liquid soap preparations to remove unreacted acid if an excess amount is applied.
  - Repeat weekly if necessary.
- Surgical removal
- Manage warts on the rectal mucosa in consultation with a specialist.

HSV

- Genital HSV infection
  - Recommended regimens
    - Acyclovir 400 mg orally 3 times a day for 7–10 days *or*
    - Acyclovir 200 mg orally 5 times a day for 7–10 days *or*
    - Famciclovir 250 mg orally 3 times a day for 7–10 days *or*
    - Valacyclovir 1 g orally twice a day for 7–10 days
    - Treatment may be extended if healing is incomplete after 10 days of therapy.
- Established HSV-2 infection
  - Antiviral therapy for recurrent disease can be administered:
    - Continuously as suppressive therapy to reduce the frequency of recurrences *or*

- Episodically to ameliorate or shorten the duration of lesions
  - Suppressive therapy (valacyclovir 500 mg daily) decreases HSV-2 transmission in disease-discordant heterosexual couples in which the source partner has a history of genital HSV-2 infection.
  - Suppressive therapy probably reduces transmission in persons with multiple partners (including men who have sex with men) and those who are HSV-2 seropositive without history of genital herpes.
  - Recommended regimens for daily suppressive treatment
    - Acyclovir 400 mg orally twice a day *or*
    - Famciclovir 250 mg orally twice a day *or*
    - Valacyclovir 500 mg orally once a day *or*
    - Valacyclovir 1.0 g orally once a day
  - Valacyclovir 500 mg once a day may be less effective than other valacyclovir or acyclovir regimens in patients with very frequent recurrences (≥10 episodes per year).
- Episodic therapy for recurrent genital herpes
  - Initiate within 1 day of lesion onset or during the prodrome that precedes some outbreaks.
  - Provide the patient with a supply of drug or prescription for medication with instructions to initiate treatment as soon as symptoms begin.
  - Recommended regimens
    - Acyclovir 400 mg orally 3 times a day for 5 days *or*
    - Acyclovir 800 mg orally twice a day for 5 days *or*
    - Acyclovir 800 mg orally 3 times a day for 2 days *or*
    - Famciclovir 125 mg orally twice a day for 5 days *or*
    - Famciclovir 1.0 g orally twice daily for 1 day *or*
    - Valacyclovir 500 mg orally twice a day for 3 days *or*
    - Valacyclovir 1.0 g once a day for 5 days

M genitalium

- Treatment is more effective with azithromycin than with tetracyclines.

PID

- When selecting a treatment regimen, consider availability, cost, patient acceptance, and antimicrobial susceptibility.
- Parenteral treatment
  - For mild to moderate PID, parenteral therapy and oral therapy appear to have similar clinical efficacy.
  - Clinical experience should guide decisions on transition to oral therapy, which usually can begin within 24 hours of clinical improvement.
  - Recommended parenteral regimen A
    - Cefotetan 2 g IV every 12 hours *or*
    - Cefoxitin 2 g IV every 6 hours *plus*
    - Doxycycline 100 mg orally or IV every 12 hours

S

- Other considerations
  - Doxycycline should be administered orally when possible, even when the patient is hospitalized.
  - Discontinue parenteral therapy 24 hours after the patient improves clinically.
  - Oral therapy with doxycycline (100 mg twice a day) should continue for a total of 14 days.
  - For tuboovarian abscess, many primary care physicians use clindamycin or metronidazole with doxycycline for continued therapy, rather than doxycycline alone, because they provide more effective anaerobic coverage.
  - Other second- or third-generation cephalosporins (eg, ceftizoxime, cefotaxime, ceftriaxone) might be effective therapy for PID and might replace cefotetan or cefoxitin; however, they are less active than cefotetan or cefoxitin against anaerobic bacteria.
- Recommended parenteral regimen B
  - Clindamycin 900 mg IV every 8 hours *plus*
  - Gentamicin loading dose IV or IM (2 mg/kg of body weight) followed by a maintenance dose (1.5 mg/kg) every 8 hours; single daily dosing may be substituted.
  - Other considerations
    - Although a single daily dose of gentamicin has not been evaluated for treatment of PID, it is efficacious in analogous situations.
    - Discontinue parenteral therapy 24 hours after the patient improves clinically.
    - Continuing oral therapy should consist of doxycycline 100 mg orally twice a day or clindamycin 450 mg orally 4 times a day to complete a total of 14 days of therapy.
    - For tuboovarian abscess, many primary care physicians use clindamycin for continued therapy rather than doxycycline because clindamycin provides more effective anaerobic coverage.
- Alternative parenteral regimens
  - Ampicillin/sulbactam 3 g IV every 6 hours *plus*
  - Doxycycline 100 mg orally or IV every 12 hours
- Oral treatment
  - Recommended oral regimen
    - Ceftriaxone 250 mg IM in a single dose *plus*
    - Doxycycline 100 mg orally twice a day for 14 days, *with or without*
    - Metronidazole 500 mg orally twice a day for 14 days *or*
    - Cefoxitin 2 g IM in a single dose and probenecid, 1 g orally administered concurrently *plus*
    - Doxycycline 100 mg orally twice a day for 14 days, *with or without*
    - Metronidazole 500 mg orally twice a day for 14 days *or*
    - Other parenteral third-generation cephalosporin (eg, ceftizoxime or cefotaxime) *plus*

- Doxycycline 100 mg orally twice a day for 14 days, *with or without*
- Metronidazole 500 mg orally twice a day for 14 days
- Other considerations
  - The optimal choice of cephalosporin is unclear.
  - Cefoxitin has better anaerobic coverage; ceftriaxone has better coverage against *N gonorrhoeae*.
  - Metronidazole will effectively treat bacterial vaginosis, which is frequently associated with PID.
  - No data have been published on use of oral cephalosporins for treating PID.
  - Limited data suggest that oral metronidazole plus doxycycline after primary parenteral therapy is safe and effective.
- Alternative regimens
  - If parenteral cephalosporin therapy is not feasible, consider:
    - Fluoroquinolones (levofloxacin 500 mg orally once daily *or*
    - Ofloxacin 400 mg orally twice daily for 14 days), *with or without*
    - Metronidazole (500 mg orally twice daily for 14 days) if the community prevalence and individual risk of gonorrhea are low
  - Perform tests for gonorrhea before instituting therapy.
  - Manage the patient as follows if the test is positive.
    - If NAAT are positive, a parenteral cephalosporin is recommended.
    - If culture for gonorrhea is positive, base treatment on results of antimicrobial susceptibility.
    - If the isolate is quinolone-resistant *N gonorrhoeae* or antimicrobial susceptibility cannot be assessed, a parenteral cephalosporin is recommended.
  - Although data are limited, amoxicillin/clavulanic acid and doxycycline or azithromycin with metronidazole has shown short-term clinical cure.

Syphilis

- Primary and secondary syphilis
  - Parenteral penicillin G is the preferred drug for treating all stages of syphilis.
  - Preparation or preparations used (ie, benzathine, aqueous procaine, aqueous crystalline), dose, and length of treatment all depend on stage and clinical manifestations of disease.
  - Recommended regimen for children
    - Evaluate children with acquired primary or secondary syphilis (including consultation with child-protection services) and treat them by using the following pediatric regimen.
      - Benzathine penicillin G 50,000 units/kg IM, up to adult dose of 2.4 million units in a single dose.

S

- A child or adolescent weighing ≥48 kg would receive the adult dose.
- Latent syphilis
  - Treatment usually does not affect transmission and is intended to prevent late complications.
  - Although clinical experience supports the effectiveness of penicillin in achieving this goal, limited evidence is available for guidance in choosing specific regimens.
  - Recommended regimen for adults (nonallergic patients who have normal CSF examination, if performed)
    - Early latent syphilis
      - Benzathine penicillin G 2.4 million units IM in a single dose
    - Late latent syphilis or latent syphilis of unknown duration
      - Benzathine penicillin G 7.2 million units total, administered as 3 doses of 2.4 million units IM each at 1-week intervals
  - Recommended regimens for children
    - Treat older children with acquired latent syphilis using the following pediatric regimens.
    - These regimens are for penicillin-nonallergic children with acquired syphilis who have normal CSF examination results.
    - Early latent syphilis
      - Benzathine penicillin G 50,000 units/kg IM, up to adult dose of 2.4 million units, in a single dose (a child or adolescent who weighs ≥48 kg would receive the adult dose)
    - Late latent syphilis or latent syphilis of unknown duration:
      - Benzathine penicillin G 50,000 units/kg IM, up to adult dose of 2.4 million units, administered as 3 doses at 1-week intervals (total 150,000 units/kg up to the adult dose of 7.2 million units)

Perihepatitis (Fitz-Hugh–Curtis syndrome)

- Treatment for PID eliminates perihepatitis.

Epididymitis

- All patients should receive ceftriaxone plus doxycycline for initial treatment.
- Additional therapy may include a quinolone if:
  - Acute epididymitis is not caused by gonorrhea (results from culture or NAAT are negative) *or*
  - Infection is most likely caused by enteric organisms.
- Recommended regimens
  - For acute epididymitis most likely caused by gonococcal or chlamydial infection:
    - Ceftriaxone 250 mg IM in single dose *plus*
    - Doxycycline 100 mg orally twice a day for 10 days

- For acute epididymitis most likely caused by enteric organisms, or with negative culture or NAAT, or for patients allergic to cephalosporins or tetracyclines or both:
  - Ofloxacin 300 mg orally twice a day for 10 days *or*
  - Levofloxacin 500 mg orally once daily for 10 days

Enteric infections

- If anorectal exudate is found on examination, or if polymorphonuclear leukocytes are found on Gram-stained smear of anorectal secretions, the following may be prescribed pending results of additional laboratory tests.
- Recommended regimen
  - Ceftriaxone 125 mg IM (or another agent effective against rectal and genital gonorrhea) *plus*
  - Doxycycline 100 mg orally twice a day for 7 days
- Patients with suspected or documented herpes proctitis should be managed as for genital herpes.
- If painful perianal ulcers are present or mucosal ulcers are detected on anoscopy, then presumptive therapy should include a regimen for treating genital herpes.
- If LGV proctitis and proctocolitis are present, administer doxycycline (100 mg orally twice daily for 3 weeks).

Vaginitis

- Treatment of symptomatic women who have bacterial vaginosis is warranted.
- Asymptomatic women who are scheduled to undergo abortion or hysterectomy should also be treated.

Cervicitis

- Adolescents with cervicitis should be presumptively treated for C trachomatis, especially if follow-up is uncertain or if the clinician does not have access to NAAT.
- Appropriate therapy for gonorrhea should be provided if the prevalence of infection in patient population is >5%.

WHEN TO ADMIT

- PID
  - In the past, some experts suggested that all patients with PID be hospitalized so that bed rest and supervised treatment with parenteral antibiotics might be initiated.
  - However, in women with mild or moderate PID, outpatient therapy can provide short- and long-term clinical outcomes similar to inpatient therapy.
  - Limited data support use of outpatient therapy in women with more severe disease.
  - The decision to hospitalize should be based on the discretion of primary care physician.
  - The following criteria for hospitalization are suggested.
    - Surgical emergencies, such as appendicitis, cannot be excluded.
    - The patient is pregnant.

- The patient does not respond clinically to oral antimicrobial therapy.
- The patient cannot follow or tolerate an outpatient oral regimen.
- The patient has severe illness, nausea and vomiting, or high fever.
- The patient has a tuboovarian abscess.
- Many practitioners have preferred to hospitalize adolescents with suspected acute PID, but no evidence supports this approach.
  - Adolescents with mild to moderate acute PID have similar outcomes with outpatient or inpatient therapy.
  - Clinical response to outpatient therapy is similar among adolescents and older women.
  - The decision to hospitalize an adolescent should be based on the same criteria as for older women.
- Most clinicians favor at least 24 hours of direct inpatient observation for patients who have tuboovarian abscesses.
- Epididymitis
  - Consider hospitalization if:
    - Pain is particularly severe.
    - The patient is febrile.
    - Nonadherence is of concern.

WHEN TO REFER

- If the clinician is inexperienced in the diagnosis or management of:
  - PID
  - DGI
  - Syphilis (or positive VDRL or RPR test)
  - Anogenital warts
  - Genital herpes
  - Abnormal Papanicolaou (Pap) smears

FOLLOW-UP

Specific agents

- *C trachomatis*
  - Except for pregnant women, patients do not need to be retested for chlamydia after completing treatment unless:
    - Adherence is in question.
    - Symptoms persist.
    - Reinfection is suspected.
  - False-negative results might occur because of small numbers of chlamydial organisms.
    - NAAT done <3 weeks after completion of therapy for patients treated successfully might yield false-positive results because of continued presence of dead organisms.
  - Rates of infection are high among women retested several months after treatment (presumably because of reinfection by an untreated sex partner).
    - Infection from a new partner with chlamydia is also possible.
  - Repeat infections confer increased risk for PID and other complications compared with initial infection.
  - Consider advising all women with chlamydial infection to be retested approximately 3 months after treatment.
  - Retest all women treated for *C trachomatis* whenever they next seek medical care in the next 3–12 months, regardless of whether the woman believes her sex partner or partners were treated.
- *N gonorrhoeae*
  - Test of cure is not indicated for patients with uncomplicated gonorrhea treated with any of the recommended or alternative regimens.
  - Patients with symptoms that persist after treatment should be evaluated with culture for *N gonorrhoeae*, and any gonococci isolated should be tested for antimicrobial susceptibility.
  - Persistent urethritis, cervicitis, or proctitis also might be caused by *C trachomatis* or other organisms.
- HPV
  - Careful follow-up is essential to monitor results and prevent regrowth between too-widely-spaced treatment intervals.
  - Because identifying external warts may be difficult, follow-up evaluation 3 months after treatment may be useful for patients.
  - Earlier follow-up visits also may be useful to:
    - Document wart-free status
    - Monitor for or treat complications of therapy
    - Provide opportunity for patient education and counseling
  - Traditionally, follow-up visits are not usually recommended for patients using self-administered treatments, but they may be useful several weeks into therapy to:
    - Determine whether treatment is being applied correctly
    - Measure response to treatment
  - The benefit of treating subclinical HPV infection in absence of cervical dysplasia is unclear.
  - Examination and treatment of sex partners is of uncertain benefit.
  - The treatment modality should be changed if the patient has not improved substantially.
  - Most genital warts respond within 3 months of therapy.
  - Response to treatment and side effects should be evaluated throughout therapy.
  - After visible genital warts have cleared, follow-up evaluation may be helpful.

S

- Caution patients to watch for recurrences, which occur most frequently during the first 3 months.
- Counsel women about the need for regular Pap screening as recommended for women without genital warts.

■ HSV

- Lesions generally heal without scarring.
- Safety and efficacy have been documented among patients receiving daily therapy with:
  - Acyclovir for as long as 6 years
  - Valacyclovir or famciclovir for 1 year
- The frequency of recurrences diminishes over time in many patients, and the patient's psychological adjustment to disease might change.
- Periodically (eg, once a year), clinicians should discuss the need to continue suppressive therapy with the patient.

STIs/syndromes associated with STIs

■ PID

- If outpatient therapy is attempted, ensure careful follow-up at 48 hours and establish mechanism for hospitalizing the patient before that time if symptoms worsen.

■ Syphilis

- Follow-up with repeat clinical evaluation and serologic testing should occur at 6 and 12 months.
- More frequent evaluation is warranted if findings at follow-up are uncertain.
- Criteria for reevaluation or retreatment include:
  - Persistence or recurrence of clinical signs and symptoms
  - Sustained ≥4-fold increase in titers
  - Failure of nontreponemal tests to decrease 4-fold within 6 months after treatment for primary or secondary syphilis
- All patients with syphilis should be screened for HIV infection.

■ Primary and secondary syphilis

- Treatment failure can occur with any regimen.
- Assessing response to treatment is often difficult; no definitive criteria for cure or failure have been established.
- Nontreponemal test titers may decline more slowly for patients who previously had syphilis.
- Patients should be reexamined clinically and serologically 6 and 12 months after treatment; more frequent evaluation may be prudent if follow-up is uncertain.
- Patients probably have treatment failure or were reinfected and should be retreated and reevaluated for HIV infection if:
  - They have signs or symptoms that persist or recur.
  - They have a sustained 4-fold increase in nontreponemal test titer (ie, compared with the maximum or baseline titer at time of treatment).

- Treatment failure usually cannot be reliably distinguished from reinfection with *T pallidum*; lumbar puncture should be performed.
- Failure of nontreponemal test titers to decline 4-fold within 6 months after therapy for primary or secondary syphilis might indicate probable treatment failure.
- Persons whose titers remain serofast should be reevaluated for HIV infection.
  - Optimal management of such patients is unclear.
  - At a minimum, they should have additional clinical and serologic follow-up.
  - HIV-infected patients should be evaluated more frequently (ie, at 3-month intervals instead of 6-month intervals).
- If additional follow-up cannot be ensured, retreatment is recommended.
- Because treatment failure might be the result of unrecognized central nervous system infection, many specialists recommend CSF examination in such situations.
- When patients are retreated, most experts recommend:
  - Weekly injections of benzathine penicillin G 2.4 million units IM for 3 weeks *unless*
  - CSF examination indicates that neurosyphilis is present.

■ Latent syphilis

- Patients who are seroreactive but do not have any physical findings of infection are classified as having latent syphilis.
- Patients who are known to have seroconverted within the previous 12 months are classified as having early latent syphilis, as are those who, within the previous year:
  - Have had unequivocal symptoms of primary or secondary syphilis
  - Have had a sex partner documented to have primary, secondary, or early latent syphilis
  - Have reactive treponemal and nontreponemal tests with the only possible exposure occurring within the previous year
- Repeat quantitative nontreponemal serologic tests at 6, 12, and 24 months.
- Patients with normal CSF examination should be retreated for latent syphilis if:
  - Titers increase 4-fold.
  - An initially high titer (≥1:32) fails to decrease ≥4-fold (ie, 2 dilutions) within 12–24 months.
  - Signs or symptoms attributable to syphilis develop.

■ Epididymitis

- Adolescents treated as outpatients should be followed up within 48–72 hours of initiating treatment.
- Failure to improve should prompt reevaluation of the diagnosis and the treatment.

- Sex partners of adolescents with epididymitis suspected of being or confirmed to be caused by chlamydia or gonorrhea should be evaluated and treated if their contact with index patient occurred <60 days before onset of the patient's symptoms.

COMPLICATIONS

■ Long-term sequelae of STIs
  - Cervical cancer
  - Infertility
  - Ectopic pregnancy
  - Chronic pelvic pain
  - AIDS

■ Ample evidence exists that STIs increase an individual's risk for acquiring HIV infection.

■ Specific agents
  - *C trachomatis*
    - Infection with chlamydia is not an independent risk factor for development of cervical dysplasia, but it may play some role.
    - An untreated infected woman can pass the organism to her infant through colonization during birth.
  - *N gonorrhoeae*
    - Gonorrhea may produce epididymitis and PID.
    - In addition and in contrast to chlamydia, the gonococcal organism can become blood borne and can lead to so-called arthritis-dermatitis syndrome, or DGI.
  - HPV
    - HPV infection has been associated with >90% of cervical dysplasia worldwide.
    - Complications rarely occur if treatments for warts are used properly.
    - Persistent hypo- or hyperpigmentation is common with ablative modalities.
    - Depressed or hypertrophic scars are rare but can occur, especially if the patient has had insufficient time to heal between treatments.
    - Treatment can result rarely in disabling chronic pain syndromes (eg, vulvodynia or analdynia, hyperesthesia of the treatment site) or, in the case of rectal warts, painful defecation or fistulas.
    - A limited number of case reports of severe systemic effects from podophyllin resin and interferon have been documented.
      - To prevent the possibility of complications associated with systemic absorption and toxicity, 2 important guidelines should be followed.
      - Application should be limited to <0.5 mL of podophyllin or an area <10 cm of warts per session.
      - No open lesions or wounds should exist in the area to which the treatment is to be applied.

- HSV
  - HSV infections of the male and female genital tract are particularly distressing to patients because of the potential for recurrence after initial episode, especially if caused by infection with HSV-2.
  - After the infection resolves, the virus remains latent in the sacral ganglia and may reactivate at any time.
  - Vesicles usually occur near the initial infection site but tend to be fewer in number.
  - Just before recurrence, the patient may experience burning or itching at the site of infection.
  - Healing takes place within 1–2 weeks.
  - Recurrences may occur in association with stress, local trauma, fever, or menstruation and tend to be shorter and less symptomatic.
  - In the year after a first documented episode of genital HSV-2 infection, 90% of individuals will have ≥1 recurrence, about one-third will have ≥6, and one-fifth will have ≥10.
  - The risk of recurrence depends on many factors.
    - Male adolescents are somewhat more likely to have recurrent disease, as are those whose infection was caused by HSV-2.
    - Once a second episode occurs, the patient is likely to have multiple recurrences.
  - Some patients with recurrent disease may benefit from therapy if it begins during the prodrome or within 1 day lesion onset.
  - Those with ≥6 recurrences per year have a 75% reduction in recurrences with daily suppressive therapy.
  - Patient-initiated administration of a single-day course of famciclovir also shortens the duration of recurrences.
  - Valacyclovir reduces asymptomatic virus shedding and reduces the risk of infection in couples who are serodiscordant for HSV-2.
  - Most cases of recurrent genital herpes are caused by HSV-2, although HSV-1 might become more common as a cause of first episode genital herpes.
  - Most patients with symptomatic, first-episode genital HSV-2 infection will have recurrent episodes of genital lesions; recurrences are less frequent after initial genital HSV-1 infection.
  - Intermittent asymptomatic shedding occurs in persons with genital HSV-2 infection, even in those with long-standing or clinically silent infection.

■ STIs/syndromes associated with STIs
  - PID
    - In the short term, PID can lead to such problems as tuboovarian abscess.
    - In the long run, the following are attributable to PID, even when an acute episode has been managed appropriately.

S

- Tubal factor infertility
- Chronic pelvic pain
- Increased risk for ectopic pregnancy
- Failure to see improvement should raise concerns about the accuracy of diagnosis or presence of complications.
- Repeat pelvic examination to look for a tuboovarian abscess if one has not already been detected.
- Approximately 10–20% of patients with PID develop tuboovarian abscess; 3–15% of these abscesses rupture.
- Risk for infertility and ectopic pregnancy increases with the number of episodes of PID and with the severity of infection.
  - Women >25 years at time of diagnosis are less likely to develop either complication.
- Syphilis
  - Evaluate all patients with latent syphilis for evidence of tertiary disease (eg, aortitis, gumma) and syphilitic ocular disease (eg, iritis, uveitis).
  - Patients with syphilis who demonstrate any of the following should have a prompt CSF examination.
    - Neurologic or ophthalmic signs or symptoms
    - Evidence of active tertiary syphilis (eg, aortitis, gumma)
    - Treatment failure
    - HIV infection with late latent syphilis or syphilis of unknown duration
  - Some specialists recommend examining CSF in all patients who have latent syphilis and a nontreponemal serologic test of at least 1:32 or if the patient is HIV infected with a CD4 count ≤350 cells/mm^3.
    - The likelihood of neurosyphilis in this circumstance is unknown.
  - If CSF examination demonstrates abnormalities consistent with neurosyphilis, then the patient should be treated.

PREVENTION

- Specific agents
  - *C trachomatis*
    - Screening programs reduce the incidence of PID.
    - Treatment of infected patients prevents transmission to sex partners.
    - For infected pregnant women, treatment usually prevents transmission of C trachomatis to infants during birth.
    - Treatment of sex partners helps prevent reinfection of the index patient and infection of other partners.
    - To minimize further transmission of infection, instruct patients treated for chlamydia to abstain from sexual intercourse for 7 days after single-dose therapy or until completion of a 7-day regimen.

- Instruct patients to abstain from sexual intercourse until all sex partners are treated to minimize the risk for reinfection.
- HPV
  - Pap screening
    - Evidence links HPV with the development of dysplastic and malignant changes in the cervix.
    - Routine Pap smear screening to detect precancerous lesions is extremely important.
    - Because most HPV infections among adolescents resolve spontaneously, Pap smear screening in adolescents may lead to additional diagnostic testing that can be psychologically upsetting, unnecessary, and expensive.
    - American Cancer Society recommends that Pap smear screening begin within 3 years of initiation of voluntary sexual intercourse or age 21, whichever comes first.
    - Some experts suggest initiating earlier screening for adolescents who:
      o Have many sexual partners
      o Are immunosuppressed
      o Are at risk for nonadherence to follow-up advice
    - These experts recommend initial screening of teenagers who have been sexually abused (with penetration) whenever feasible by someone skilled in examining this population.
    - Immunosuppressed women should be screened every 6 months in the first year and then yearly as long as the result is normal.
    - Use of HPV DNA typing has become an important adjunct to the management of abnormal Pap smear screening findings in adult women.
      o Use may be limited in teenagers because HPV infection is so common among sexually active adolescents yet tends to be self-limited (ie, rarely progresses to cervical cancer).
      o Current guidelines from the American Society for Colposcopy and Cervical Pathology do not include the use of HPV DNA typing for the management of adolescents (age ≤20 years) with atypical squamous cells of undetermined significance or low-grade squamous intraepithelial cells on Pap smear screening.
  - HPV vaccine
    - The US Food and Drug Administration recently approved a 3-dose (0, 2, and 6 months) quadrivalent HPV vaccine containing virus-like particles of types 6, 11, 16, and 18.

- The Advisory Committee on Immunization Practices recommends:
  - Administration to girls age 11 and 12 as a priority
  - Vaccine can be offered to girls as young as 9 years of age.
  - Recommended for those age 13–26 years who have not been vaccinated or have not received all 3 doses
- Protective effect appears to last for 2.5–3.5 years; whether a booster dose will be needed is unknown at this time.
- Sex partners
  - Examination of sex partners is not necessary for management of genital warts because no data indicate that reinfection plays a role in recurrences.
  - Providing treatment solely to prevent future transmission cannot be recommended because the value of treatment in reducing infectivity is unknown.
  - Sex partners of patients with genital warts might benefit from counseling and examination to assess the presence of genital warts and other sexually transmitted infections.

- Female sex partners of patients with genital warts should be reminded that cytologic screening for cervical cancer is recommended for all sexually active women.
- Herpes genitalis
  - Glycoprotein vaccine to prevent HSV-2 infection has a protective effect at 5 months but not at 1 year for persons receiving the vaccine.
- STIs/syndromes associated with STIs
  - Syphilis
    - Because all syphilis symptoms may not be present in everyone infected, most adolescents with syphilis will be identified only through routine serologic screening.
    - Testing at-risk youth is important.
    - Clinicians should strongly consider screening any sexually active adolescent with a generalized eruption (eg, that seen with pityriasis rosea) for syphilis.

S

Shock

DEFINITION

- Shock can be considered a progressive process of compensated, decompensated, and irreversible states.
- Shock, especially septic shock and hypovolemic shock caused by diarrhea or blood loss, is a common cause of pediatric morbidity and mortality.
- Refractory shock
  - Persists despite aggressive fluid management, use of pressors, and maintenance of normal glucose and calcium levels, and thyroid and adrenal status
- Septic shock
  - Classified by perfusion status
  - Shock can be defined by:
    - Clinical signs and symptoms
    - Hemodynamic variables
    - Parameters of oxygen delivery

EPIDEMIOLOGY

- Prevalence
  - Severe sepsis is one of the most common causes of death in infants and children in the world.
  - In 1995 sepsis was the 4th leading cause of death in infants and the 2nd leading cause of death in children ages 1 to 14 years.
  - Diarrhea leading to dehydration severe enough to produce shock is no longer a common cause of death in the US.
    - Remains a world health problem
  - Septic shock is the most common and best-studied cause of cardiovascular collapse.
    - Causes of bacterial septic shock have changed since vaccination against *Haemophilus influenzae* type b was instituted in 1988.
    - Meningococci and streptococci are the most frequently encountered causes of sepsis.
  - Presence of shock increases morbidity and mortality when it complicates other childhood diseases.
    - Investigators at the University of Pittsburgh evaluated 1766 children with respiratory disease who required transport to a tertiary facility.
      - Shock complicated the respiratory failure presentation in 25% (440) of the children, and this group had a mortality rate of 38%.
      - In the group of children transferred for respiratory failure only, without shock present, the mortality rate was only 3%.
- Incidence
  - Meningitis and sepsis
    - 1.3:100,000 in the US
    - 15:100,000 in Ireland

- Cost
  - In an analysis of data from 1997 hospitalizations, children with severe sepsis had an average hospital stay of 31 days, at a cost of $40,600 per case.
  - In a 2005 report, the national annual cost of caring for children with severe sepsis alone is estimated at $2.3 billion.

ETIOLOGY

- In all shock states, oxygen delivery and blood flow to vital organs is decreased or cellular oxygen needs are increased, and metabolic demands are not met, resulting in multiple organ failure.
- Shock is the result of inadequate perfusion of oxygen and nutrients (eg, glucose) to vital organs.
  - Perfusion is a clinical representation of the combined effects of cardiac output and systemic vascular resistance.
  - Delivery of oxygen to tissue is the product of content of oxygen in blood and cardiac output.
- In young children, the pulse rate is a reasonable proxy of cardiac output, and capillary refill rate is a reliable indicator of perfusion.
  - Cardiac output is the product of heart rate and stroke volume, which is expressed in liters of blood flow per minute.
  - Hypotension (loss of peripheral vascular tone) is sensed by baroreceptors, which act through mediators to increase both heart rate and stroke volume.
- In older children and adults, stroke volume depends on contractility (inotropy) and preload (venous return to the right heart).
  - Contractility of the myocardium is depressed by acidosis, hypoglycemia, and hypocalcemia.
  - Epinephrine and other catecholamines act as inotropic agents, increasing contractility.
- Preload is the vascular volume presented to the heart during diastole, which stretches cardiac muscle, to enable optimal contraction during systole.
  - Clinically, the central venous pressure or a pulmonary capillary wedge pressure and left atrial pressure represent preload to right and left ventricles, respectively.
  - A patient with hypovolemia is said to have a low preload.
  - If blood volume is restored, preload increases and stroke volume is increased (see "point a" in Figure 92 on page F30).
- Hypovolemic shock
  - Shock from loss of blood volume caused by trauma, diarrhea, burns, and third-spacing (as in peritonitis)
  - Most common form of shock in children
  - Loss of fluid leads to low intravascular volume.
  - Preload to the heart is decreased.

- In hypovolemic shock caused by trauma or diarrhea:
  - Pulses would be thready, heart rate would be high, and the capillary refill rate is >2 seconds.
  - Physiologically, patient has a low vascular volume, heart rate is high in an effort to restore blood flow, and systemic vascular resistance is elevated; thus, the skin is cool and poorly perfused.
- Cardiogenic shock
  - Can be caused by mechanical obstruction or muscle (pump) failure
  - In obstructive cardiogenic shock, air and fluid in the pericardium or pleural spaces (rarely) can:
    - Impede venous return to the heart
    - Decrease systolic ejection
  - Massive pulmonary embolus
    - Rare in children
    - Can obstruct flow from the right to the left side of the heart
  - Cardiac output is also compromised in:
    - Coarctation of the aorta
    - Hypoplastic left heart syndrome
    - Left ventricular outflow tract stenosis
  - High volumes may stretch the heart muscle, and diastolic or systolic function (or both) may be altered.
  - Preload is high, but contractility (inotropy) is greatly diminished (see "point b" in Figure 92 on page F30).
- Septic shock
  - The most frequently encountered bacterial causes of sepsis (except in the immunocompromised) are:
    - Meningococci
    - Streptococci
  - Children with sepsis may exhibit symptoms of hyperdynamic, vasodilated shock (see "point c" in Figure 92 on page F30).
  - Physiologically, cardiac output is high, peripheral vasculature is vasodilated, venous return (preload) to the heart is diminished, and systemic vascular resistance is low.
  - Symptoms result not from low cardiac output, but rather from maldistribution of blood flow.
- Distributive shock
  - Global disorder in vasomotor control is present.
  - Causes maldistribution of blood flow and oxygen to tissue
  - The 2 types most likely to be encountered in primary care are:
    - Anaphylaxis
    - Spinal cord injury
  - Cardiac output may be normal or increased.

- Patients lose sympathetic control of the vascular system, which reduces peripheral vascular tone, resulting in pooling of blood in the periphery.
- This leads to decreased venous return to the heart.

RISK FACTORS

- Infants and children at risk of severe septic shock include:
  - Those with septic shock and purpura
  - Those with known or suggested adrenal abnormalities
  - Those who have received a therapeutic course of steroids within 6 months
- Shock in infants
  - Cardiac
  - Hypoplastic left heart syndrome
  - Coarctation of the aorta
  - Myocarditis
  - Arrhythmia
  - Infectious
    - Family history
    - In a study of Danish families, risk of death was increased 5-fold in children whose parent had died of a severe infection before the age of 50 years.
  - Bacterial meningitis
  - Urinary tract sepsis
  - Herpes (meningitis and sepsis)
  - Streptococcal sepsis
  - Metabolic
  - Hypoglycemia
  - Inborn errors of metabolism
  - Traumatic
  - Child abuse
  - Occult central nervous system hemorrhage
  - Surgical
  - Bowel obstruction
  - Occult blood loss
- Causes of hypovolemic shock
  - Gastrointestinal losses
  - Excess urine output, diuretic administration
  - Mannitol administration
  - Hypoalbuminemia
  - Burns
  - Third-space fluid losses
    - Peritonitis
    - Edema
  - Traumatic blood loss
- Causes of obstructive cardiogenic shock
  - Tamponade (air, blood, or effusion)

S

- Coarctation of the aorta
- Aortic valve stenosis or atresia
- Pump failure
  - Arrhythmia
  - Hypoplastic left heart syndrome
  - Decreased contractility acquired in sepsis syndrome or shock of any cause
  - Myocardiopathy
  - Myocarditis
  - Anomalous coronary artery
  - Cardiac contusion
  - Glycogen storage disease

SIGNS AND SYMPTOMS

- Hyperthermia or hypothermia
- Altered mental status
  - Lethargy
  - Confusion
  - Coma (implies significant brain hypoperfusion)
- Oliguria
  - Defined as urine output <0.5 mL/kg/h
  - Caveats
    - Many children have multiple caretakers during a typical day.
    - Frequency and volume of urination may not be accurately recounted.
- Patients with high obligatory urine losses:
  - Those with high-output renal failure
  - Those with hyperglycemia (diabetes mellitus)
  - Those receiving diuretics
  - Those who have received mannitol
- Altered perfusion diagnosed by capillary refill (>2 seconds) before the onset of hypotension
  - Brisk in warm shock (vasodilated)
  - Delayed in cold shock (vasoconstricted)
- Cold shock
  - Patient is cold to the touch, with capillary refill rate >2 seconds.
  - Patient has increased peripheral vascular resistance.
- Warm shock
  - Patient is warm to the touch.
  - Patient has a rapid blush of capillary refill.
  - Patient has a vasodilated, low peripheral resistance shock.
- Fluid refractory dopamine-resistant shock
  - Persistence of symptoms with >60 mL/kg in the first hour of fluid therapy and dopamine infusion of 10 mcg/kg min

- Catecholamine-resistant shock
  - Shock persists despite addition of epinephrine or norepinephrine, or both.
- Hypovolemic shock
  - Increased thirst
  - Increased heart rate
  - Retention of fluid by concentrating urine
  - Large volumes of fluid loss result in:
    - Diminished mental status
    - Tachycardia
    - Poorly perfused skin with prolonged capillary refill; oliguria; and, eventually, hypotension
  - Mild dehydration: 5%
    - Dry skin, mild tachycardia, concentrated urine
  - Moderate dehydration: 10%
    - Lethargy, poor perfusion
  - Severe dehydration: 15%
    - Obtundation, tachycardia, hypotension, very poor perfusion to skin
- Hemorrhagic shock
  - Physical findings correlate to the volume of blood loss.
  - 15% loss: minimal tachycardia, normal respiratory rate, blood pressure, and capillary refill
  - 15–30% loss: tachycardia, tachypnea, decreased pulse pressure, normal systolic pressure, prolonged capillary refill, anxiety
  - 30–40% loss: hypotension, decreased urine output, mental status changes
  - >40% loss: hypotension, loss of consciousness
- Cardiogenic shock
  - Low cardiac output resulting in the clinical signs of:
    - Altered mental status
    - Tachycardia
    - Decreased capillary refill rate
    - Evidence of venous congestion (hepatomegaly, rales)
    - Children with pericardial effusion may have muffled heart sounds.
- Decompensated phase of shock
  - Tachycardia
  - Hypotension occurs as the child's compensatory mechanisms are exhausted.
  - Vital signs and leukocyte count by age group are shown in the table Vital Signs and White Blood Counts by Age.

Differential Diagnosis

- Infants
  - A broader differential diagnosis should be considered for infants <6 weeks.

Vital Signs and White Blood Counts by Age[a]

Age Group	Heart Rate—Tachycardia	Heart Rate—Bradycardia	Respiratory Rate	Systolic Blood Pressure	Leukocyte count × 10/mm
0 days to 1 wk	>180	<100	>50	<65	>34
1 wk to 1 mo	>180	<100	>40	<75	>19.5 or <5
1 mo to 1 yr	>180	<90	>34	<100	>17.5 or <5
2–5 yr	>140	NA	>22	<94	>15.5 or <6
6–12 yr	>130	NA	>18	<105	>13.5 or <4.5
13–<18 yr	>110	NA	>14	<117	>11 or <4.5

[a] From: Goldstein B, Giroir B, Randolph A. International pediatric sepsis consensus conference: definitions for sepsis and organ dysfunction in pediatrics. *Pediatr Crit Care Med*. 2005;6(1):2–8.

- Early discharge of newborns shortly after birth requires attention to both acquired and congenital or inherited conditions.
- Toddlers
  - Shock in toddlers usually has a determinable, apparent cause.
  - Clinician should be aware of the propensities that are unique to this age group, especially:
    - Poisoning
    - Ingestion of medications
    - Inhaling and swallowing of foreign bodies
    - Trauma resulting from falls
    - Playground and household accidents
    - Child abuse
- Adolescents
  - May not be forthright in volunteering an accurate history
  - Risk-taking behavior of the teen years should be taken into consideration.
  - Poisoning after attempted suicide or experimentation with drugs and alcohol may not be reported.
  - Antipsychotic medications can cause cardiovascular collapse and arrhythmias.
  - Ingestion of antihypertensive agents and opiates in the home should be considered.
- In all age groups, note:
  - History of travel
  - Possibility of *Salmonella* infection
    - Recent exposure to pets
  - Exposure to organophosphates
    - Indicated by weakness at presentation
- Hemolytic-uremic syndrome is implicated by:
  - Recent ingestion of meat
  - Early onset of central nervous system symptoms with bloody diarrhea

- Hypovolemic shock
  - Shock from loss of blood volume caused by trauma, diarrhea, burns, and third-spacing (as in peritonitis)
  - Most common form of shock in children
  - Loss of fluid leads to low intravascular volume.
  - Preload to the heart is decreased.
  - In hypovolemic shock caused by trauma or diarrhea:
    - Pulse is thready, heart rate is high, and the capillary refill rate is >2 seconds.
    - Physiologically, the patient has a low vascular volume, heart rate is high in an effort to restore blood flow, and systemic vascular resistance is elevated; thus, the skin is cool and poorly perfused.
- Cardiogenic shock
  - Can be caused by mechanical obstruction or muscle (pump) failure
  - In obstructive cardiogenic shock, air and fluid in the pericardium or pleural spaces (rarely) can:
    - Impede venous return to the heart
    - Decrease systolic ejection
  - Massive pulmonary embolus
    - Rare in children
    - Can obstruct flow from the right to the left side of the heart
  - Cardiac output is also compromised in:
    - Coarctation of the aorta
    - Hypoplastic left heart syndrome
    - Left ventricular outflow tract stenosis
  - High volumes may stretch the heart muscle, and either or both diastolic and systolic function may be altered.
  - Preload is high, but contractility (inotropy) is greatly diminished (see "point b" in Figure 92 on page F30).

S

- Septic shock
  - The most frequently encountered bacterial causes of sepsis (except in the immunocompromised) are:
    - Meningococci
    - Streptococci
  - Children with sepsis may exhibit symptoms of hyperdynamic, vasodilated shock (see "point c" in Figure 92 on page F30).
  - Physiologically, cardiac output is high, peripheral vasculature is vasodilated, venous return (preload) to the heart is diminished, and systemic vascular resistance is low.
  - Symptoms result not from low cardiac output, but rather from maldistribution of blood flow.
  - Children and adults have developmental differences in hemodynamic response.
    - In adults, death is caused by a pressor- and volume-resistant state characterized as vasomotor paralysis.
    - Myocardial dysfunction is common in adults.
    - Cardiac output is maintained by tachycardia and ventricular dilatation.
    - In pediatric septic shock, low cardiac output, not vasodilatation, is associated with mortality.
    - In children, oxygen delivery is the major determinant of oxygen consumption.
    - In adults, oxygen used by tissues (oxygen extraction) is more important.
  - Survival correlates to the restoration of:
    - Cardiac output
    - Oxygen delivery
- Distributive shock
  - Global disorder in vasomotor control is present.
  - Causes maldistribution of blood flow and oxygen to tissue
  - The 2 types most likely to be encountered in primary care are:
    - Anaphylaxis
    - Spinal cord injury
  - Cardiac output may be normal or increased.
  - Patients lose sympathetic control of the vascular system, which reduces peripheral vascular tone, resulting in pooling of blood in the periphery.
  - This leads to decreased venous return to the heart.

DIAGNOSTIC APPROACH

- In the primary care setting, the diagnosis is based on clinical signs and symptoms.
- Shock in the pediatric setting is a relatively common emergency.
- Early stages of shock are easy to recognize.
- The primary care physician can dramatically reduce morbidity and mortality by:
  - Recognizing and treating shock early in the community setting
  - Following consensus guidelines and algorithms
- Infants in shock present unique diagnostic challenges.
  - Algorithmic approaches to shock diagnosis developed for children and adults may not be appropriate.
- Shock can be diagnosed in the early compensated state by easily detectable clinical signs:
  - Altered mental status
  - Tachycardia
  - Decreased capillary refill rate
  - Changes in blood pressure and urine output
  - Intervention in this state has the highest likelihood of success.
- Children with sepsis may exhibit symptoms of hyperdynamic, vasodilated shock (see "point c" in Figure 92 on page F30).
  - Cardiac output is high.
  - Peripheral vasculature is vasodilated.
  - Venous return (preload) to the heart is diminished.
  - Systemic vascular resistance is low.
  - Symptoms result not from low cardiac output, but rather from maldistribution of blood flow.
  - On physical examination, the patient:
    - Has brisk capillary refill
    - Is warm to the touch
    - Has bounding pulses, tachycardia, and a hyperdynamic precordium
- Heart rate
  - Infants cannot increase stroke volume as readily as adults.
    - Increase in heart rate is a compensatory mechanism to increase blood flow to vital organs.
    - An infant in shock whose heart rate is 2 standard deviations above normal is attempting to increase cardiac output.
  - The return of pulse rate and blood pressure to normal values is a valuable indicator of therapeutic success.
  - After the patient is stabilized, an accurate history may help selection of appropriate treatments and guide referral.

LABORATORY FINDINGS

- In a patient with cardiovascular symptoms, confirm inadequate perfusion:
  - Unexplained metabolic acidosis (base deficit >3.0 mEq/L)
  - Increased arterial lactate level (2 times upper limit of normal)

TREATMENT APPROACH

- Early treatment with fluids and pressor therapy for shock remains the same regardless of the cause.

- The clinician should be confident in treating the hemodynamic abnormalities first and establishing the cause later.
- Early treatment does not require:
  - Sophisticated monitors
  - Central venous catheters
  - Invasive monitoring
- The 3 basic principles that should guide therapy are:
  - Prompt recognition of a patient in shock
  - Rapid restoration of systemic and regional perfusion to prevent ongoing shock and cellular injury
  - Prevention of the development of end-organ failure
- Treatment of shock, especially in primary care settings, is based on:
  - Restoring adequate circulating blood volume
  - Achieving adequate delivery of glucose and oxygen to all tissues
  - Monitoring and documenting the patient's response to each intervention is essential.
  - Early volume resuscitation and vasopressor therapy are always indicated in the treatment of shock.
  - A common error is to give too little fluid too slowly.
  - Gauge the patient's response to fluid administration.
- Patients are critically ill and in catecholamine-resistant shock if they:
  - Remain tachycardic
  - Have poor capillary refill
  - Have inadequate urine output (<0.5 mL/kg/h) after 60 mL/kg of fluid and the addition of 2 vasopressors
  - Placement of a central venous catheter is recommended at this point.
  - Patients in this decompensated state will require referral to a tertiary pediatric intensive care unit for further diagnosis and treatment.
- Hypotension and tachycardia are indicative of severe shock in a decompensating patient.
- Restoration of blood pressure and reduction of heart rate indicate therapeutic success.
- Severe septic shock
  - Some patients may develop a hypoadrenal response characterized by refractory shock.
  - By definition, these patients are unresponsive to:
    - Volume resuscitation
    - Addition of 2 catecholamine drugs
    - Normalization of:
      - Acid-base status
      - Glucose level
      - Calcium homeostasis

SPECIFIC TREATMENTS

Guidelines for treatment of shock

- Guidelines for diagnosis, care, and treatment of infants and children are simple to understand and follow (see Figure 93 on page F31).
  - Timely recognition and treatment are critical.
- American College of Critical Care Medicine Clinical Practice Parameters for Hemodynamic Support of Pediatric and Neonatal Shock
  - 5 minutes:
    - First, secure airway and ventilation.
    - Children have low lung volumes and are at risk for hypoxemia.
    - Establish venous access within 5 minutes of recognition of shock.
    - An intraosseous device or peripheral intravenous device suffices for this purpose; central access is not part of the first response.
    - Begin monitoring the child.
  - 15 minutes:
    - Administer intravenous fluids.
    - Fluid needs can exceed 60 mL/kg of body weight.
    - The volume of each fluid bolus should be 20 mL/kg.
  - 30 minutes (15 minutes after fluid therapy begins):
    - For children who do not immediately respond to fluid administration (15 minutes from beginning of fluid therapy), begin infusion of dopamine, a first-line catecholamine, at a dose of 5–20 mcg/kg/min.
      - Infants <6 months may not respond as well to dopamine.
    - Children who do not respond to dopamine infusion up to 20 mcg/kg/min and fluid resuscitation have dopamine-fluid refractory shock.
    - Institute epinephrine (for cold shock) or norepinephrine (for warm shock) infusions.
    - Monitor and restore the following to normal levels:
      - Glucose
      - Serum hemoglobin or hematocrit
      - Acid-base homeostasis
      - Ionized calcium
  - 60 minutes:
    - Children who do not respond to fluid and an infusion of 2 catecholamine agents within 60 minutes have catecholamine-resistant shock.
    - Adrenal insufficiency should be considered.
    - Refer to a tertiary care pediatric intensive care unit if children do not respond to:
      - Fluid administration
      - Dopamine and epinephrine or norepinephrine infusions

S

- These children require diagnostic evaluation for cardiac function and will require:
  - Central venous access
  - Echocardiography
  - Mixed venous oxygen saturation monitoring

Management of shock

- Fluid replacement
- No conclusive data are found in the literature proving superiority of one fluid.
  - Commonly used solutions are:
    - Normal saline (20–80 mL/kg)
    - Lactated Ringer solution
    - 5% albumin (20–80 mL/kg)
- Glucose replacement
  - Children consume glucose at a faster rate than adolescents and adults.
  - In infants and toddlers, glucose levels should be considered a vital sign.
  - Blood glucose needs to be added to maintain adequate blood glucose levels.
  - Glucose replacement is crucial, especially in very young patients.
  - Glucose level should be maintained at >60 mg/dL.
- Oxygen
  - All patients in shock should immediately be given 100% oxygen.
  - Oxygenation should be monitored continuously with a pulse oximeter.
    - Values should be documented in the patient's record.
    - Normal oxygen saturation on a pulse oximeter does not imply adequate tissue delivery.
  - Maintain hemoglobin (the carrying vehicle for oxygen) at a normal level.
  - In septic shock, adequate oxygen delivery is associated with improved survival.
  - Blood transfusions may be necessary to ensure adequate oxygen delivery.
    - Despite concerns over the adverse effect of transfusion, hemoglobin or hematocrit must be monitored.
    - Maintaining the hemoglobin at least 10-g percentage is reasonable.
  - If circulation is compromised and cardiac output decreases, oxygen delivery to tissues will be compromised.
    - Oxygen delivery is the product of oxygen content and cardiac output.
  - Oxygen content = 1.36 × the percentage of saturation × hemoglobin (in grams), expressed as milliliters of oxygen per 100 mL of blood.

- In healthy children, oxygen consumption is 25% of oxygen delivery.
- In shock states, oxygen consumption may increase simultaneously with inadequate cardiac output, leading to inadequate tissue oxygenation.
- In lung disease or hypoventilation:
  - Hemoglobin is desaturated.
  - Oxygen delivery is compromised further.
- Arterial lactic acidosis (normal level is <2 mmol/L) or an increasing base deficit (>3 mEq) document inadequate perfusion.
- The effects of restoring the pH to >7.25 are important.
  - Myocardial contractility is enhanced.
  - Sensitivity to catecholamines is improved.
  - Potassium is returned to the intracellular space.
- Sodium bicarbonate may be required to:
  - Improve blood pH to >7.25
  - Bring serum bicarbonate levels to >15 mEq/dL
- Any remaining base deficit may be corrected by using the following guide:
  - 0.3 × body weight in kilograms × base deficit = milliequivalents of sodium bicarbonate
- Hypocalcemia is common.
  - Total calcium measurements do not correlate with measurements of the biologically important ionized calcium.
  - Restoring ionized calcium to normal levels improves myocardial contractility.
- Platelet counts
  - Unless bleeding is evident, platelet counts of 20,000 to 50,000 cells/mm³ are tolerated well.
  - Prothrombin time and partial thromboplastin time should be maintained at approximately 1.3 times normal values.
  - Fresh frozen plasma, administered at 10 mL/kg, is a reasonable method of:
    - Repairing volume deficit
    - Replenishing coagulation factors
  - Rapid infusion of fresh frozen plasma can contribute to hypotension resulting from the presence of vasoactive kinins.
- Therapeutic end points are:
  - Capillary refill rate <2 seconds
  - Normal peripheral pulses
  - Warm limbs
  - Urine output >1 mL/kg/hr
  - A decreasing lactic acid level or improved base deficit
  - Normalization of mental status

Anaphylactic shock

- The inciting agent should be removed if possible.
- These patients uniformly respond well to:
  - Volume administration
  - Epinephrine infusion
  - Antihistamines that include an H_2-receptor blocker
  - Steroid therapy

Catecholamine-resistant shock

- In patients whose shock state is refractory to volume restoration, dopamine or dobutamine, and addition of epinephrine or norepinephrine
  - Empirically initiating stress-dose steroids (hydrocortisone at stress doses of 50–100 mg/m²/day would be reasonable).
- If time and condition allow:
  - A baseline serum cortisol level
  - A 250 microgram dose of corticotropin
  - Repeat cortisol level measurement at 30 minutes.
    - The response (or absence of) will determine the presence of a hypoadrenal state and the need for continued steroid administration.
  - A baseline serum cortisol <18 mcg/dL and a poststimulation increment <9 mcg/dL indicate a hypoadrenal state.
  - If a stimulation test cannot be done, continuation of steroid therapy for 3–5 days should be based on clinical response.

Vasopressor drugs

- Drugs of choice in the early treatment of shock are:
  - Dopamine (5–20 mcg/kg/min)
    - In the majority of cases of shock, dopamine with adequate fluid replacement saves the patient.
  - Norepinephrine (0.01–0.2 mcg/kg/min)
  - Epinephrine (0.01–0.2 mcg/kg/min)
  - Dobutamine(5–20 mcg/kg/min)
- A vasoactive drug should be infused continuously with a calibrated infusion pump.
- Continuous heart rate and blood pressure monitoring is required.
- Catecholamines do not replace adequate, aggressive, and early fluid administration as the initial treatment of shock.
- Catecholamines are classified by their relative effects on the α- or ß-receptor.
  - The α-receptor produces vasoconstriction, which accounts for its salutary effect in raising blood pressure.
  - ß-Agonists have 2 receptor sites.
  - $ß_1$-Agonist receptors stimulate heart rate and cardiac muscle contractility.
    - Toxicity is reflected in cardiac tachyarrhythmias and ischemia.
  - $ß_2$-Agonist receptors are present in bronchial and arteriole smooth muscles.
    - These muscles relax when stimulated.
  - These agents stimulate adenyl cyclase activity.
  - One of the effects is increased entry of potassium into cells.
- Dopamine
  - The drug of choice
  - Administered at 5–20 mcg/kg/min, titrated to effect
  - The α-adrenergic effects predominate with:
    - Vasoconstriction
    - Reduced peripheral perfusion
  - Patients who do not respond to fluid resuscitation of 60 mL/kg and dopamine at 20 mcg/kg/min:
    - Are in a state called *dopamine fluid resistant shock*
    - Require addition of epinephrine (cold shock) or norepinephrine (warm shock)
  - Infants <6 months may not respond well to dopamine; epinephrine (0.01–0.2 mcg/kg/min) may be more effective.
  - In some circumstances, especially shock after hypoxemic-ischemic injury,epinephrine or dobutamine may be preferred because dopamine may:
    - Precipitate tachyarrhythmias
    - Increase myocardial oxygen consumption
- Dobutamine (5–20 mcg/kg/min)
  - Children who are thought to have low cardiac output may benefit from dobutamine.
  - Dobutamine differs from dopamine because of:
    - Enhanced inotropic effect
    - Less chronotropic effect
    - Less effect on systemic vascular resistance
- Hydrocortisone (2 mg/kg/dose)
  - Indicated in limited circumstances
  - Stress-dose steroids at 1–2 mg/kg hydrocortisone are indicated in:
    - Children with anaphylaxis
    - Those with known or suggested adrenal abnormalities
    - Children who have received a therapeutic course of steroids for chronic illness in the previous 6 months
  - Children in refractory septic shock may respond to hydrocortisone.
- Other vasodilator drugs, such as nitroprusside, milrinone (0.3–0.7 mcg/kg/min), and nitroglycerine, may be beneficial in reducing afterload when the patient has high peripheral vascular resistance and low cardiac output.
  - Should only be used in selected situations and in tertiary care settings
  - Optimizes myocardial contractility
  - Improves cardiac output

S

- Requires sophisticated monitoring, including:
  - Pulmonary arterial oximetry
  - Cardiac output measurement
  - Pulmonary vascular pressure catheters

Experimental therapies

- Trials of activated protein C and granulocyte-macrophage colony stimulating factor have been unsuccessful or have not affected outcomes for pediatric patients.
- Extracorporeal membrane oxygenation has not been explored adequately in children in shock and should be performed only at the few centers capable of supporting this technology.
- Survival in cases of septic shock has not been improved in trials of:
  - Ibuprofen
  - Antibody to endotoxin
  - Antibody to tumor necrosis factor-α

FOLLOW-UP

- Monitoring the child in shock includes:
  - Measurement of the capillary refill rate
  - Documentation of mental status
  - Pulse oximetry
  - Continuous electrocardiography
  - Blood pressure (measured with a cuff)
  - Temperature measurement
  - Urine output measurement
  - Glucose and ionized calcium level
  - Serum hemoglobin level or hematocrit
- Hepatomegaly is a reliable indicator of volume overload and cardiac compromise.
- Successful resuscitation is recognized by:
  - Return of pulse rate to normal
  - Improvement in mental status
  - Return of capillary refill
  - Improvement in acid-base status

COMPLICATIONS

Organ failure in septic shock

- Cardiovascular dysfunction despite administration of isotonic intravenous fluid bolus ≥40 mL/kg in 1 h
  - Decrease in blood pressure (hypotension): <5th percentile for age or systolic blood pressure >2 standard deviations below normal for age*or*
  - Need for vasoactive drug to maintain blood pressure in normal range (dopamine >5 mcg/kg/min or dobutamine, epinephrine, or norepinephrine at any dose) *or*
  - 2 of the following:
    - Unexplained metabolic acidosis: base deficit >5.0 mEq/L

- Increased arterial lactate: >2 times upper limit of normal
- Oliguria: Urine output <0.5 mL/kg/h
- Prolonged capillary refill: >5 seconds
- Core to peripheral temperature gap: >3°C

- Respiratory
  - PaO_2/FiO_2 ratio: <300 in absence of cyanotic heart disease or preexisting lung disease*or*
  - $PaCO_2$: >65 torr or 20 mm Hg over baseline $PaCO_2$ *or*
  - Proven need or >50% FiO_2 to maintain saturation ≥92% *or*
  - Need for nonelective invasive or noninvasive mechanical ventilation

- Neurologic
  - Glasgow Coma Score ≤11 *or*
  - Acute change in mental status with a decrease in Glasgow Coma Score ≥3 points from abnormal baseline

- Hematologic
  - Platelet count: <80,000 cells/mm^{3}or a decrease of 50% in platelet count from highest value recorded over the past 3 days (for patients with chronic hematologic disease or cancer) *or*
  - International normalized ratio: >2

- Renal
  - Serum creatinine: ≥2 times upper limit of normal for age *or*
  - 2-fold increase in baseline creatinine level

- Hepatic
  - Total bilirubin level: ≥4 mg/dL (not applicable for newborn) *or*
  - Alanine aminotransferase levels: 2 times upper limit of normal for age

Acute respiratory distress syndrome (ARDS)

- A common form of hypoxemic respiratory failure that occurs 24–48 hours after presentation in shock
- The child becomes dyspneic and hypoxemic.
  - PaO_2/FiO_2 ratio: <200
- Physical examination reveals rales and tachypnea.
- Chest radiography reveals diffuse infiltrates.
- These changes may be delayed for ≥24 hours.
- Interstitial edema that appears to be caused by a capillary leak syndrome
- ARDS is life threatening, and patients should be referred to a tertiary intensive care unit.
  - The following may be required.
    - Mechanical ventilation
    - Positive end-expiratory pressure
    - Right heart catheters
    - High-frequency oscillatory ventilation
    - Extracorporeal membrane support

Myocardial depression

- Commonly encountered in septic shock
- Inadequate perfusion, increased work, and distension in the presence of inflammatory mediators affect contractility.
- May lead to a decrease in cardiac output

Renal failure

- Renal failure, especially acute tubular necrosis, is a common complication.
- Suggested when the urine output is <0.5 mL/kg/hr, despite adequate restoration of blood volume.
- A serum creatinine level more than twice normal for age is diagnostic.
- Aggressive use of dialysis and hemofiltration has minimized morbidity resulting from this complication.
- Unrecognized renal failure will increase mortality resulting from shock.
- Serum levels of drugs in the blood become uncertain.
- Doses of antibiotics, sedatives, and analgesics must be monitored carefully, following blood levels in serum whenever possible.
- Fluid therapy must be titrated carefully to insensible fluid loss replacement; otherwise, congestive heart failure will result.
- Anuria or oliguria complicating shock requires referral or consultation with a nephrologist or intensivist.
- Diuretics may increase mortality in acute renal failure.

Hypoxemia and ischemia

- The central nervous system is most susceptible.
- A child may suffer significant neurologic impairment, although other organs are spared.
- Early central nervous system signs of shock include:
  - Delirium
  - Irritability
  - Confusion
  - Coma
- Signs of increased intracranial pressure are usually delayed 24–72 hours after a hypoxemic-ischemic insult.
- Presence of increased intracranial pressure accompanying the acute presentation of shock implies a traumatic or metabolic etiology.
- A Glasgow Coma Score <11 or a decrease of 3 points from baseline is diagnostic of central nervous system compromise.

Impaired liver function

- May become impaired as a result of inadequate perfusion
- Bilirubin levels >4 mg/dL and alanine aminotransferase levels greater than twice normal are diagnostic of hepatic failure.
- Clotting factors may be diminished.
- In septic shock, liver perfusion may be adequate, but bacteria or toxins may damage hepatic cells.
- Liver failure is usually transient.

PROGNOSIS

- The most important predictor of outcome is appropriate resuscitation and reversal of shock within 75 minutes of recognition.
- Mortality rates
  - Higher in patients with infection caused by:
    - *Staphylococcus aureus*
    - *Pseudomonas aeruginosa*
    - *Candida* species
    - *Streptococcus pyogenes*
  - Lower in patients with infection caused by:
    - Coagulase-negative *Staphylococcus*
    - *Acinetobacter* species
  - Invasive meningococcal disease
    - Mortality remains high despite modern advances in critical care.
    - Most common in children <4 years
    - Characteristics of cases rapidly progressing to death include:
      - Young age
      - Absence of meningitis
      - Thrombocytopenia
      - Leukopenia
      - Multiorgan failure
      - Severity of petechiae
- If organ failure develops, the child can enter a phase of refractory shock, with increased morbidity and mortality.
- A study of children who were treated following the American College of Critical Care Medicine *Pediatric Advanced Life Support* (ACCM-PALS) practice parameters for hemodynamic support:
  - Demonstrated increased survival and decreased morbidity in infants and children in shock treated by community physicians compared with a group where these algorithms were not followed.
- In a 9-year study, community physicians successfully achieved shock reversal within 75 minutes of recognition in 24 of 91 children.
  - Survival increased to 96%.
  - >9-fold increase in the odds of survival
  - Each additional hour of persistent shock was associated with >2-fold increase in the odds of death.
  - Shock resuscitation was consistent with ACCM-PALS guidelines in 30% of patients.
  - When practice was consistent with these guidelines, mortality was only 8% compared with 38% in the children treated without following the guidelines.
  - These data parallel and corroborate findings in adults.

S

Short Stature

DEFINITION

- The accepted medical definition of when a child is too short may be at variance with when parents worry about their child's height.
- The normal range for height encompasses 2 standard deviations above and below the mean (between the 97th and the 3rd percentiles).
  - The 3rd percentile may be difficult to appreciate, since the lowest curve on many growth charts is the 5th percentile.
- A single point on a growth chart often does not define a worrisome growth pattern.
  - Previous growth data should be plotted whenever available.
  - Any suggestion of growth deceleration should be reviewed.
- Standard growth charts do not incorporate pubertal stage.
  - Short children who start puberty relatively late may appear to fall further behind even though they are growing at a normal rate.

MECHANISM

- Constitutional growth delay (CGD)
  - Children grow below but parallel to the 3rd percentile line.
  - Birth weight is normal, but between 6 and 24 months, linear growth and weight track downward to the 3rd percentile or below.
  - After age 3 years, children follow their own curve parallel to the low end of the growth chart.
  - Children with CGD typically have a delayed onset of puberty/growth spurt.
- Familial short stature (FSS)
  - The child is growing at a normal rate below the 3rd percentile.
  - ≥1 parents are quite short.
  - Tend to have puberty at a normal age and to achieve an adult height within 2–3 inches of their adult target height
- Other causes of short stature
  - Certain syndromes
  - Being born small for gestational age (SGA)
  - Chronic illness
  - Nutritional disorders
  - Medications
  - Endocrine disorders
  - Idiopathic short stature (ISS): no known cause

HISTORY

- The growth curve is most helpful for evaluation.
  - If the growth rate has been normal for the previous ≥2 years, the child most likely has CGD or FSS and is unlikely to have a defined, treatable cause.
- A single point that falls off the established curve is often a measurement error and should be rechecked.
- A history of stimulant medications or glucocorticoid use might be key information.
- Decreased energy level and poor appetite
  - Could indicate a chronic, growth-limiting illness
  - Many short, healthy children are picky eaters.
- Abnormal stool history could indicate:
  - Malabsorption
  - Celiac disease
  - Inflammatory bowel disease
- Family history
  - May suggest FSS in a healthy child who is short but growing at normal rate
    - Height of parents and grandparents
    - Growth percentiles of siblings
  - Two-thirds of children with CGD have a family history of a parent who was a late maturer.
    - Mother's menarche after age 14 years
    - Father who continued to grow after high school

PHYSICAL EXAM

- Usually, there are no physical findings that point to a specific diagnosis.
- In children with decreased subcutaneous fat stores, weight is more affected than height.
  - May not be getting enough calories
  - May have bowel disease or another chronic illness
- A short child who is relatively pudgy (particularly if excess rippled fat is present over the trunk) may have growth hormone (GH) deficiency.
- Dysmorphic features may suggest a syndrome associated with short stature.
  - In girls, look for Turner syndrome.
    - High-arched palate
    - Cubitus valgus
    - Fingernails that bend upward
- An enlarged thyroid may be the only clue to hypothyroidism.
- Pubertal staging should be done on any short child ≥10 years of age.
  - A short, healthy 14-year-old boy (and less often, a short, healthy 13-year-old girl) who is still prepubertal is most likely to have CGD.
  - A child with a flattened growth curve at 13–16 years and who is in the late stages of puberty has completed or has nearly completed growing (nothing can increase the individual's adult height).

DIFFERENTIAL DIAGNOSIS

- Most common causes of short stature
  - CGD
  - FSS
- Syndromes with short stature
  - Often associated with being born SGA
  - Turner syndrome
    - Should be considered in any girl with height well below the 3rd percentile
    - Common features
      - Lymphedema as a newborn
      - Frequent ear infections beyond 2 years of age
      - Narrow, high-arched palate
      - Cubitus valgus
      - Upturned fingernails
      - Webbed neck present in only about 40%
      - Congenital heart disease in about 15%
        - Coarctation of the aorta and bicuspid aortic valve are the most common.
  - Russell-Silver syndrome
    - SGA
    - Triangular face with down-turned mouth
  - Noonan syndrome
    - Typical facial features
      - Flat nasal bridge
      - Hypertelorism
      - Ptosis
    - Webbed neck
    - Cryptorchidism
    - Pulmonic stenosis
  - Other syndromes with short stature
    - De Lange
    - Rubinstein-Taybi
    - Seckel
- Chronic illnesses and nutritional disorders
  - Should be considered in short children whose weight is further below the curve than their height, or whose BMI is <10% for age
  - Inadequate caloric intake
    - Not commonly the result of poverty in the US, because high-calorie foods are cheap
    - Overly restricted diet to avoid gaining weight or to lower cholesterol
      - Anorexia nervosa is the extreme example.
  - Inflammatory bowel disease
    - Growth attenuation may start before gastrointestinal (GI) symptoms are apparent.
  - Celiac disease
    - May have few, if any, GI symptoms
  - Renal disease
    - Renal tubular acidosis
    - Chronic renal failure
  - Liver disease
- Medication-related poor growth
  - Long-term oral glucocorticoid therapy
    - Much less impact from inhaled corticosteroids for asthma
  - Stimulant medications
- Endocrine disorders
  - Height is often more affected than weight.
  - GH deficiency
    - Not a common cause of short stature
    - Should be suspected in children below the 3rd percentile who are falling further behind over time
    - A suggestive physical finding is an increase in truncal subcutaneous fat.
    - Most cases are congenital, with fall-off in growth starting late in the first or in the second year of life.
    - Acquired GH deficiency is less common and raises the possibility of a pituitary tumor.
    - Partial GH deficiency is difficult to distinguish from CGD and FSS.
  - Hypothyroidism
    - Acquired hypothyroidism needs to be excluded in any child with growth deceleration, even if height is above the 3rd percentile.
  - Cushing syndrome
    - Endogenous Cushing syndrome is extremely rare.
    - Iatrogenic Cushing syndrome is more common.
    - Key findings include:
      - Rapid truncal, rather than generalized, weight gain
      - Slowing of linear growth
      - Moon facies
      - Abdominal striae
      - Increased skin pigmentation
- ISS
  - Moderately to severely short children who do not meet the criteria for CGD and FSS, often with subnormal rate of growth
  - After extensive testing, no cause for poor growth is found.

S

LABORATORY EVALUATION

- Resist the temptation to order multiple laboratory tests for a child who is only mildly short (at or above the 3rd percentile) and whose growth rate appears to be normal.
  - Clinically significant abnormal test results are rarely found to explain short stature.
- Screening tests before a visit with a specialist might be appropriate if:
  - Height is well below 3rd percentile.
  - There is growth deceleration that cannot be explained by medication is well documented.
- A specialist can order any needed test at first consultation.
- Insulinlike growth factor-1 (IGF-1) is the best screening test if GH deficiency is suspected.
  - However, many children with CGD have borderline low IGF-1 levels for their age.
  - A random GH level is of no value because of the pulsatile nature of GH secretion.
- Thyroid testing
  - Limit to free thyroxine (T_4) and thyroid-stimulating hormone (TSH).
    - Will pick up both primary and secondary hypothyroidism
  - Borderline TSH (5.5- to 10-mcU/mL range) with normal free T_4 is usually a normal variation and will not explain poor growth.
- Complete blood count and erythrocyte sedimentation rate are mainly useful in the occasional child in whom inflammatory bowel disease is suspected.
- Microcytic anemia may be a clue to occult GI blood loss.
- Tests to screen for celiac disease
  - Tissue transglutaminase immunoglobulin A (IgA) antibody or antiendomyseal antibody
  - Antigliadin IgG and IgA are much less specific and not worth the extra cost.
- A comprehensive metabolic profile will rule out rare causes of short stature
  - Electrolyte disturbances
  - Kidney disease
  - Liver disease

IMAGING

- A bone age film is the only radiographic examination that should be considered.
  - Not very useful as a diagnostic test, since most children who are short (aside from genetic short stature) have a bone age delay of ≥1 year
  - A consultant may order bone age film in a child >7 years of age to make a height prediction if either CGD or FSS is suspected.

TREATMENT APPROACH

- In healthy children at or above the 3rd percentile and growing at normal rate, the chances of finding a treatable cause for shortness are small.
  - The child should have growth carefully measured and plotted at each visit to make sure it is not dropping below the 3rd percentile.
  - If the parents insist on seeing a specialist, they should be told that their child will not likely need or be eligible for coverage of GH therapy.
- A child who is in the normal range but crossing percentiles
  - Between 6 and 24 months, such shifts are common, especially in CGD.
  - If the child crosses 1 percentile channel (eg, from the 25th to the 10th percentile) over ≥3 years, and history and examination are normal, a cause will not likely be found.
  - Children who cross >1 percentile channel in <3 years have a greater chance of having a definable cause for short stature.
    - The most common cause is the use of stimulant medication for attention-deficit/hyperactivity disorder.
- Parents of children short enough to be referred can be told that screening tests and a period of observation are needed before a decision can be made regarding the need for GH therapy.
- Such children are best referred between the ages of 3 and 6 years.
  - Children who are pubertal or on the verge of puberty do not usually benefit from GH therapy.

SPECIFIC TREATMENT

Human GH

- Children with a history of intrauterine growth retardation (born SGA) who have not caught up to the normal range by age ≥2 years:
  - The US Food and Drug Administration has approved use of GH without the need for GH testing.
- GH treatment
  - Children within normal range in height with a drop-off in linear growth >1 percentile channel over ≤3 years or who have shown documented growth arrest for 1 year
  - Children with short stature who have not started puberty by age 14 years (occurs mostly in boys with CGD)
    - When the boy is anxious to start his growth spurt sooner rather than later, treatment with a brief course of testosterone injections is appropriate.
  - The US Food and Drug Administration has approved GH for children at or below the 1st percentile with an anticipated adult height (based on bone age) below the normal range.
- Some insurance companies refuse to cover GH to treat ISS, arguing that no medical condition exists.

WHEN TO REFER

- Children below the 3rd percentile, particularly if height is falling further below the normal range over time

- Children who were born SGA (intrauterine growth restriction) who have not caught up to the normal range by ≥2 years

- Children within the normal range for height who have dropped off >1 percentile channel over the past ≤3 years or who have documented growth arrest for 1 year.

- Children with short stature who have not started puberty by age 14 years

- Dysmorphic children with short stature should be referred to a geneticist for a specific diagnosis.

- For children reporting poor self-esteem because they are short, referral to a psychologist may be more helpful than to an endocrinologist.

- If weight gain is persistently poor, referral to a GI or nutrition specialist should be considered.

FOLLOW-UP

- Follow-up of patients with short stature is important before the diagnosis, to establish the growth velocity, and after the therapy, to monitor its success.

COMPLICATIONS

- Some children with short stature develop significant psychosocial problems, such as poor self-esteem.

PROGNOSIS

- Children with CGD usually end up with heights in the lower half of the normal range.

- Children with FSS tend to achieve adult height within 2–3 inches of their adult target height.
  - Target height is calculated by averaging the heights of the parents and adding 2.5 inches for boys and subtracting 2.5 inches for girls.

- Children with ISS respond variably to GH, with a modest average improvement in adult height.

PREVENTION

- Measuring length and height at each clinic visit, and plotting them on growth curves, can lead to earlier identification of children with short stature.

- Appropriate evaluation and therapy can be instituted sooner for better outcomes.

Sinusitis

DEFINITION

- Sinusitis is infection of the paranasal sinuses.

EPIDEMIOLOGY

- Prevalence
  - Infection of the paranasal sinuses in children occurs frequently.
  - 5–13% of viral upper respiratory tract infections in children are complicated by acute bacterial sinusitis.
- Incidence
  - On average, children develop 5–10 upper respiratory tract infections yearly.

ETIOLOGY

- Respiratory viruses that contribute to the development of sinusitis
  - Adenoviruses
  - Influenza viruses
  - Parainfluenza viruses
  - Rhinoviruses
- The most common bacterial pathogens associated with acute sinusitis are:
  - *Streptococcus pneumoniae*
  - *Haemophilus influenzae*
  - *Moraxella catarrhalis*
  - *Staphylococcus aureus* and anaerobes are prevalent in chronic sinusitis
  - *Streptococcus pyogenes* (group A *Streptococcus*) may be associated with both acute and chronic disease.
- Inflammation and edema of the respiratory mucosa lead to obstruction of the ostium.
  - Pressure changes in the sinus that result from occlusion or from blowing and sniffing through the nose allow bacteria to invade the normally sterile sinus cavity.
- The ostia of the maxillary sinuses are located in the upper part of the chamber, where cilia must battle gravity to clear secretions.
  - This circumstance probably contributes to the high frequency of infection in these sinuses.

RISK FACTORS

- Sinusitis occurs most frequently after a viral upper respiratory tract infection or nasal allergy.
- Conditions that can predispose the sinuses to infection
  - Occlusion of the ostia
  - Impairment of ciliary motility
  - Alterations in the consistency of mucus secretions
    - Alone or in combination

- Several anatomic and physiologic conditions can predispose a child to paranasal sinusitis.
  - Anatomic
    - Nasal malformations
    - Nasal trauma
    - Tumors and polyps
    - Cleft palate
    - Foreign bodies
    - Dental infection
    - Cyanotic congenital heart disease
  - Physiologic barotrauma
  - Abnormalities of local defense mechanisms
    - Allergy
    - Cystic fibrosis
    - Immotile-cilia syndrome and Kartagener syndrome
  - Abnormalities of systemic defense mechanisms
    - Immunodeficiency
      - Primary or secondary

SIGNS AND SYMPTOMS

- Cough and nasal discharge are the most common clinical manifestations of acute sinusitis.
  - The cough occurs during the day but may be worse at night when the child is supine.
  - Nasal discharge may be clear or purulent.
- Parents of young children may report fetid breath.
- Headache and facial pain are uncommon symptoms in children with acute sinusitis.
- Painless swelling of the periorbital tissues without erythema is an occasional symptom.
  - May be confused with periorbital cellulitis in its early stage
- A less common presentation of acute sinusitis is an unusually severe upper respiratory tract infection.
  - Most uncomplicated upper respiratory tract infections improve after 5–7 days.
    - Symptoms that persist without improvement for >10 but <30 days suggest bacterial superinfection.
  - In most cases of viral upper respiratory infection, fever precedes the onset of watery nasal discharge and is associated with constitutional symptoms.
  - Thickening of nasal secretions occurs later in the course, before resolution.
    - A high fever and purulent discharge that coexist for ≥3 days suggests acute sinusitis.
- Cough and nasal discharge persisting for >30 days occurs with both subacute or chronic sinusitis.

- During physical examination, carefully inspect the nasal mucosa.
  - It will usually be erythematous and swollen.
  - It may be pale and boggy.
- Mucopurulent material can sometimes be seen in the nose or draining into the nasopharynx.
- Palpation or percussion of the sinuses may elicit tenderness.

DIFFERENTIAL DIAGNOSIS

- The presence of a foreign body in the nose must be ruled out.

DIAGNOSTIC APPROACH

- The distinction between viral infections and acute bacterial sinusitis is based on the persistence and severity of upper respiratory symptoms.

LABORATORY FINDINGS

- Nasopharyngeal culture results correlate poorly with sinus culture results.

IMAGING

- Sinus radiographs can help confirm the diagnosis of sinusitis.
  - Routine use to confirm the diagnosis of uncomplicated sinusitis is not recommended in young children.
  - Sinus radiographs are more specific and therefore more helpful in children >6 years of age.
- Cysts and polyps also may be seen on sinus radiographs.
- Computed tomography (CT) of the sinuses should be reserved for patients with:
  - Frequent recurrences or persistent symptoms that are not improving
  - Complicated sinusitis accompanied by orbital or intracranial complications
  - Need for consideration of sinus surgery

DIAGNOSTIC PROCEDURES

- Transnasal aspiration of the maxillary sinuses can be performed by an otolaryngologist for diagnostic purposes in specific situations.
- Bacteria are present in a sinus aspirate 75% of the time when:
  - Clinical signs and symptoms suggest acute sinusitis.
  - Maxillary sinus radiographs show:
    - Air-fluid levels
    - Complete opacification
    - Mucosal thickening of at least 4–5 mm
- Sinus aspiration and lavage are indicated only in children who:
  - Fail to respond to conventional antibiotic therapy
  - Are immunosuppressed
  - Have an illness that is severe or life threatening

TREATMENT APPROACH

- Treatment of sinusitis in children involves:
  - Antibiotic therapy
  - Symptomatic relief measures
  - Drainage, if necessary
  - The following are recommended to help drain the sinuses:
    - Decongestants
    - Antihistamines
    - Saline nose drops
  - No proof of the efficacy of these agents exists.
  - The AAP does not recommend the use of antihistamines and decongestants in children <6 years of age because of possible side effects and occasional adverse effects due to accidental overdosing.
- Amoxicillin is an appropriate initial choice for treating uncomplicated sinusitis.
  - It is most appropriate in geographic areas where the prevalence of ß-lactamase–producing strains of *H influenzae* and *M catarrhalis* is low.
- Intranasal steroids may provide some benefit, particularly in the second week of therapy.
  - Further research is necessary to define their role in management.

SPECIFIC TREATMENTS

Amoxicillin

- Amoxicillin is the drug of choice for treatment of uncomplicated sinusitis.
- For children who do not respond to amoxicillin, broader coverage should be considered with amoxicillin plus:
  - A clavulanate *or*
  - A carbacephem *or*
  - A macrolide *or*
  - A 3rd-generation cephalosporin
- These alternatives should also be considered for the child who has:
  - Recently been treated with amoxicillin
  - Frontal or sphenoid sinusitis
  - Complicated ethmoid sinusitis
  - Very protracted symptoms
- Patients who are allergic to amoxicillin may be treated with:
  - A carbacephem *or*
  - A macrolide *or*
  - A 3rd-generation cephalosporin

WHEN TO ADMIT

- In unusually severe cases, hospitalization and parenteral antibiotics may be required.

S

WHEN TO REFER

■ Otolaryngologic consultation is appropriate in cases where hospitalization is needed.

■ Surgery may be required in cases of medically recalcitrant severe chronic sinusitis in children.

■ Patients with recurrent sinusitis or chronic sinusitis associated with immunodeficiencies should be referred to otolaryngologists and/or infectious disease consultants.

FOLLOW-UP

■ For the child who has recurrent sinusitis and no underlying disorder:
  ● Some experts have recommended antibiotic prophylaxis.
    – No scientific studies support this practice.
    – May lead to the rapid development of antibiotic resistance

COMPLICATIONS

■ Complications of sinusitis are most often due to local extension of the disease.
  ● Orbital cellulitis is the most common serious complication of sinusitis.
    – In many cases, it lacks the common symptoms of sinusitis.
    – The eyelids appear intensely red and swollen.
    – Fever, malaise, and an increased leukocyte count are present.
    – To distinguish this condition from preseptal (periorbital) cellulitis, evaluate the child for:
      ■ Orbital pain
      ■ Proptosis
      ■ Limitation of eye movement (ophthalmoplegia)
      ■ Diminished visual acuity
    – CT may be needed to differentiate the 2 conditions.
    – This complication has been reported most frequently in male adolescents.
■ Intracranial infection is the second most common complication of sinusitis.
  ● Subdural empyema (most common)
    – Low-grade fever
    – Malaise
    – Frontal headache

– Then, as the disease progresses:
  ■ Vomiting
  ■ Decreased level of consciousness
– Infection can occur by direct extension through necrotic bone or by bacterial spread through the venous system.
– Peak age of incidence of this complication is between 10 and 20 years, but it can develop in younger children.

■ If a patient is thought to have an intracranial abscess:
  ● Head CT with contrast should be obtained.
  ● Lumbar puncture should be avoided until intracranial mass effect has been ruled out.
  ● Treatment with high-dose parenteral antibiotics should be started immediately.
  ● To drain the abscess and to debride necrotic bone:
    – Neurosurgery should be consulted.
  ● Steroids and hypertonic agents (mannitol or glycerol) may be necessary to control intracranial hypertension.

■ Other, less common complications of sinusitis in children include:
  ● Meningitis
  ● Osteomyelitis of the frontal bone (Pott puffy tumor)
  ● Epidural abscess
  ● Cavernous sinus thrombosis

PROGNOSIS

■ Clinical improvement should be expected within 48 hours after treatment is initiated.

■ A minimum of 10 days of antibiotic therapy usually is adequate.
  ● If symptoms fail to resolve completely within 10 days, patients should be treated for an additional 7 days beyond the resolution of symptoms.

PREVENTION

■ If the patient is known to have allergic rhinitis, environmental controls, anti-allergic medications, and/or referral to an allergist may help prevent recurrent sinusitis.

■ Chronic prophylactic antibiotic use did not prove to be successful in preventing recurrent sinusitis.

S

Spina Bifida

DEFINITION

- *Neural tube defects* are congenital defects of the head and spine. They include:
  - Head
    - Anencephaly
    - Cranial meningocele
    - Encephalocele
  - Spine
    - Spina bifida occulta
    - Occult spinal dysraphism (OSD)
    - Meningocele
    - Meningomyelocele
- *Spina bifida* refers to defects in the caudal region of the spine.

EPIDEMIOLOGY

- Prevalence
  - Neural tube defects: 1–2 cases per 1,000 live births in the US
    - Second most common major congenital defect
  - Meningomyelocele (or myelomenigocele): 0.4–0.8 cases per 1000
  - Greater among:
    - Girls
    - Children of lower socioeconomic status
    - Families of English, Irish, or Welsh extraction
  - Has been declining for the last several decades due to:
    - Improved nutrition
    - Fortification of food with folic acid
    - Establishment of prenatal diagnosis with elective termination

ETIOLOGY

- The cause of neural tube defects is unknown.
  - The primary mechanism seems to be faulty closure of the neural groove by day 28 of gestation.
  - Most recent etiologic hypothesis
    - Neural tube defects result from the interaction of many genes (polygenic expression).
    - Can be modified by factors in the embryonic (maternal) environment
- Meningomyelocele may be associated with certain chromosomal aberrations, including:
  - Trisomy 13
  - Trisomy 18
  - Cri du chat syndrome
- 4 major malformations account for findings of meningomyelocele.
  - Soft-tissue malformation
  - Brain malformation
    - Vertebral body malformation
    - Spinal cord malformation
- Soft-tissue malformation
  - Failure of skin and other soft tissues to close leaves the spinal cord open to infection.
  - Lipomas that occasionally accompany the defect may grow larger, possibly:
    - Compressing the spinal cord
    - Causing progressive neurologic symptoms
- Brain malformation
  - Chiari type II deformity
    - Pons and medulla are distorted and elongated.
    - Cerebellar vermis is displaced inferiorly into the spinal canal.
- Most neural tube defects are isolated findings, but some may be associated with other malformations:
  - Tracheoesophageal fistula
  - Diaphragmatic hernia
  - Imperforate anus
  - Cryptorchism
  - Inguinal hernias
  - Renal anomalies
  - Cleft palate
  - Ventricular septal defect

RISK FACTORS

- Increased risk for neural tube defects
  - Maternal exposure to:
    - Hyperthermia
    - Valproic acid (Depakene, Depakote)
    - Carbamazepine (Tegretol)
    - Isotretinoin (Accutane)
    - Ethanol
  - Mothers who have:
    - Diabetes
    - Obesity
    - Maternal malnutrition
    - Folic acid deficiency
- Family member with the disease
  - Assuming overall incidence of 1 per 1000
    - For a second affected child, from the same parent incidence is 2–3 per 100.
    - For a third affected child, the incidence is 10 per 100.
  - Adult with meningomyelocele
    - 2–3% chance of having a child with a neural tube defect

S

SIGNS AND SYMPTOMS

History

- Affected newborns may have a family history of neural tube defects or spontaneous abortions (miscarriages).
- Historical facts worth noting in the newborn period include:
  - Length of gestation
  - Type of delivery
  - Complications with and length of labor
  - Maternal nutrition
  - Environmental exposures
  - Current family functioning, including social support and stress
  - Parental expectations and understanding of malformation
- For older children, obtain information about current and past therapies for:
  - Neurologic conditions
  - Orthopedic conditions
  - Urologic conditions
  - Ophthalmologic conditions
  - Dermatologic conditions
  - Gastrointestinal conditions
- Educational and social functioning
- Child's knowledge of condition
- Sexual function
- Understanding of sexuality
- Assess the child's:
  - Growth
  - Development
  - Mobility
  - Independence in activities of daily living
    - Personal hygiene
    - Ability to self-feed
    - Self-help skills
- Determine any onset of new neurologic symptoms, such as:
  - Pain
  - Fatigue
  - Weakness
  - Changes in bowel and bladder function
  - Tripping
  - Clumsiness
- These symptoms usually indicate treatable conditions, such as:
  - Tethered spinal cord
  - Diastematomyelia
  - Syringomyelia
  - Ventricular shunt malfunction

- Up to 50% of children who have meningomyelocele have allergies to latex.
- Seek history of reactions to products made of latex, such as:
  - Balloons
  - Bandages
  - Balls
- Contact with latex-containing products should be restricted from the first day of life.
- All operative procedures should be performed in a latex-free environment.

Findings

- Spina bifida occulta
  - Common, benign condition
  - Spinal cord and soft tissues are normal.
  - Vertebral arches are incomplete.
- OSD
  - The underlying spinal cord is at risk for deterioration.
  - The infant is born with a visible abnormality on the lower back, which may be:
    - Birthmark (eg, hemangioma)
    - Tuft of hair
    - Dermal sinus
    - Lipoma
    - Atypical dimple
  - Many healthy infants are born with a small, midline sacral dimple.
  - Dimples associated with OSD are:
    - Not in the middle
    - Above the sacral region
    - Large
    - Without visible base
  - Spinal cord may be connected to the surface through a sinus that increases the risk for meningitis.
  - The cord itself may be:
    - Tethered to surrounding tissue
    - Split (diastematomyelia or diplomyelia)
- Meningocele
  - Meninges protrude through abnormal vertebral arches and soft tissue.
    - The spinal cord is normal.
  - On rare occasions, may appear as an anterior mass in:
    - Pelvis
    - Abdomen
    - Thorax
- Meningomyelocele
  - The malformed spinal cord and nerve roots protrude through abnormal vertebral arches and soft tissue.

S

Physical examination

- Backs of all children should be examined for signs that may indicate OSD.
  - Pigmented spots
  - Hairy patches
  - Sinuses that extend into spine
- These children are at high risk for:
  - Meningitis
  - Neurologic deterioration secondary to:
    - Diastematomyelia
    - Lipoma
    - Tethering of spinal cord
- Children with meningomyelocele should have a complete physical examination that emphasizes:
  - Neurologic function
  - Orthopedic function
  - Gastrointestinal function
- Neurologic examination should include determination of:
  - Motor function
  - Sensory functional levels
- Assisting in the evaluation of lesions at S2–S4
  - Rectal examination
  - Assessment of the anal wink
- Assess upper extremity:
  - Strength
  - Function
- Aids to evaluation of shunt function
  - Palpation of the anterior fontanelle
  - Ophthalmoscopic visualization of the eyegrounds
  - Assessment of the cranial nerves, especially extraocular movements
  - Palpation of shunt valve and tubing
- Orthopedic examination should include assessment of:
  - Posture
    - Scoliosis
    - Lordosis
    - Kyphosis
  - Joint mobility
  - Stability
- Erythema and swelling of joint or bone in an area that lacks sensation means fracture until proved otherwise.
- Skin should be examined for evidence of:
  - Erythema
  - Ulcers in insensate areas

- Formal and informal developmental assessment
  - Verbal
  - Performance
  - Sensory integration
  - Educational measures
  - Fine-motor
  - Gross-motor
  - Language
  - Social-adaptive skills
- Determine the child's learning profile before school entry.
  - Helps the school provide appropriate interventions that will optimize the child's learning
  - Formal psychoeducational testing is a critical part of the evaluation.
    - Identify academic strengths and weaknesses.
    - Test before an individualized education plan is developed.

LABORATORY FINDINGS

- Serum blood urea nitrogen and creatinine levels should be obtained as a baseline assessment of renal function.
- As the child grows, urinalysis and urine cultures should be performed as indicated.

IMAGING

- Infants with abnormal findings on the back should have evaluation of underlying soft tissue and spinal cord using:
  - Ultrasonography
  - Magnetic resonance imaging (MRI)
  - Ultrasonography or computed tomography (CT), or both, of the head
- Monitor kidneys with:
  - Routine renal ultrasonography
  - Voiding cystourethrography
  - Renal scans
  - Urodynamics
- Periodic CT of the head to detect asymptomatic ventricular enlargement
- Condition of the spine and joints should be monitored by plain radiography.
- Special studies that may be indicated include:
  - MRI of the spine and posterior fossa, including evaluation of cerebrospinal flow in the posterior fossa
  - $_{99m}$technetium dimercaptosuccinic acid renal scan to evaluate kidney structure and function, including damage from recurrent infections

S

- A child with signs and symptoms of ventricular shunt malfunction or other neurologic deterioration should undergo:
  - CT of the head
  - Shunt series (to evaluate the integrity of the tubing)

TREATMENT APPROACH

- 2 overriding goals
  - Prevent dysfunctions (eg, neurologic defects) from becoming disabilities (eg, cannot walk).
  - Prevent disabilities from becoming handicaps.
- Achieving these goals requires:
  - Comprehensive, coordinated care
  - Routine care, such as:
    - Immunizations
    - Anticipatory guidance
- The newborn and family should be evaluated by a team, consisting of:
  - Pediatrician
  - Nurse
  - Social worker
  - Neurosurgeon
  - Orthopedist
  - Physical therapist
  - Urologist
- Long-term management goals
  - Optimize the child's activities and participation in society.
- To optimize health and well being, all of these children should have:
  - Healthy diets
  - Regular physical activities
- Should have access to:
  - Appropriate recreation
  - Leisure activities

SPECIFIC TREATMENTS

Initial actions

- Once the neonate has received supportive care, central nervous system infection must be prevented.
- For infants with an open lesion:
  - As soon as possible, give parenteral antibiotics that provide coverage against:
    - Gram-negative bacilli
    - *Staphylococcus aureus*
- Surgery to close the open defect, typically within the first 72 hours of life

- Ventriculoperitoneal shunt placement to reduce hydrocephalus, guided by ultrasonography or CT
  - No universally accepted criteria exist to determine the need or the timing of shunt placement.
- Daily measurement of head circumference
- Genetic counseling and social support should be provided to the family.

Orthopedic treatment

- Goals include:
  - Optimal alignment
  - Maximal range of motion
  - Stability of spine and extremities
  - Maximal function and comfort, while protecting the skin
- Deformities, such as clubfoot and joint contractures, should be managed with
  - Range-of-motion exercises
  - Splinting
  - Casting
- May include surgery for:
  - Joint contractures
  - Scoliosis
  - Kyphosis
- 1 or both hips may become dislocated.
  - Surgical treatment may not be indicated if:
    - Dislocation is bilateral.
    - The child has complete paraplegia.
- Prevention of contractures and dislocations may require:
  - Regular passive range-of-motion exercises
  - Splints
  - Body jackets
  - Casts
- Various exercises and orthoses (braces) may be used to enhance locomotion.
  - Between 18 and 24 months, start using:
    - Parapodium—a standing brace that allows the child to be in an upright position with hands unencumbered
    - Reciprocal gait orthosis
  - Crutches or walkers in conjunction with more standard bracing may be used.
  - Early use of wheeled mobility is encouraged, especially for children with quadriceps paralysis.
  - Adaptive equipment, such as carts and hand-pedaled tricycles, can enhance function and self-esteem.

Urologic treatment

- Goals include:
  - Protecting the kidneys and ureters by:
    - Emptying the bladder
    - Lowering intravesicular pressure
    - Preventing urinary tract infections
    - Treating reflux
  - Achieving continence
- Urologic system should be evaluated by:
  - Urine culture
  - Renal ultrasonography
- Clean intermittent catheterization
  - Safer than urinary diversion via ileal loops
  - More acceptable
  - Results in better renal function
- Vesicostomy may be indicated in the infant with:
  - Vesicoureteral reflux
  - Hydronephrosis
- Most families can perform clean intermittent catheterization when the child is 4–5 years of age.
  - Many children this age can perform the procedure themselves.
  - Clean intermittent catheterization has been used in children <3 years of age to manage:
    - Vesicoureteral reflux with or without hydronephrosis
    - Frequent urinary tract infections
- Drugs that relax the detrusor muscle or increase sphincter tone can enhance continence.
  - Imipramine hydrochloride
  - Oxybutynin chloride
  - Pseudoephedrine
- In older children in whom catheterization does not provide continence:
  - Use a surgical procedure, such as bladder augmentation.
  - Create a continent stoma with clean intermittent catheterization.
- Prevent renal damage by:
  - Obtaining regular urine cultures to detect urinary tract infection
  - Administering prophylactic antibiotics in children who have frequent infections
- Prophylaxis—use the following in less than the therapeutic dose:
  - Trimethoprim-sulfamethoxazole
  - Sulfisoxazole
  - Nitrofurantoin
  - Cephalexin

Neurosurgery

- Goals include monitoring for signs and symptoms of:
  - Ventricular shunt dysfunction
  - Occurrence of spinal cord problems, such as tethering
  - Assessment of functioning
    - Decrease in school performance may indicate chronic shunt malfunction.
- Occasionally, cranial imaging (ultrasonography in infants and CT in older children) is performed.
  - The optimal frequency of these studies has not been determined.
- Surgical treatment to correct OSD should be performed early.
  - Even in asymptomatic infants
  - Prevents progressive neurologic damage

Reproductive issues

- Impotence in the male patient may be managed:
  - Surgically
    - Penile implants
    - Vacuum pumps
    - Injection or insertion of prostaglandin
  - With such medications as sildenafil (Viagra)
- Women have normal fertility.
  - Should use precautions to prevent pregnancy and sexually transmitted infections
  - Precocious puberty is common in young women who have meningomyelocele with hydrocephalus, because of disorder of the hypothalamus.
  - Precocious puberty can be treated with leuprolide (Lupron).
  - Pregnant women may need to have cesarean delivery because of hip contractures.
  - Frequent neurologic evaluations throughout pregnancy are recommended.
    - Intervertebral disks may become herniated, with neurologic sequelae.

Fecal continence

- Often difficult to achieve:
  - Bowel continence after 4 years of age
  - Avoidance of severe constipation
- Use the following singly or in combination to attain this goal.
  - High-fiber diet
  - Stool softeners
  - Regular toileting
  - Regular stimulants
  - Biofeedback in children who have rectal sensation

S

- Regular enemas, using 20 mL/kg of normal saline
- Suppositories
- Small-volume enemas (Enemeez)
■ Several surgical procedures (antegrade colonic enema) have been developed to help children achieve fecal continence.
  - Show promise for a select group for whom more conventional constipation-relieving techniques have failed
  - Original surgical procedure (Malone)
    - Removes appendix
    - Opens its distal end
    - Uses it to create a channel between the colon and the abdominal wall
  - In a related procedure (cecostomy)
    - An opening is made in the cecum, either surgically or in the radiology suite.
    - A gastrostomy button is placed into the cecum.
  - In a newer antegrade colonic enema procedure
    - An opening is placed into the descending colon.
  - After all of these procedures, irrigation fluids are flushed into the colon, washing out stool.
  - These procedures are used on a regular basis.

Psychosocial support

■ A child with a disability has the same psychosocial needs as a healthy child.
■ The clinician should help the family achieve shift to independent function.
■ If a child has a learning disability, the school should provide:
  - Remediation
    - Additional instructional time
    - Different instructional approaches
    - Fixing an area of weakness
    - Building strength in a particular area to facilitate potential learning
  - Compensation
    - Alternative approaches (eg, assistive technology) to offset, or counterbalance, a learning disability
■ Children, especially teens are at increased risk for:
  - Depression
  - Anxiety
  - Both
■ These conditions should be considered causes of:
  - Changes in physical functioning
  - Problems at school

Alternative medicine

■ Alternative therapies include:
  - Cutaneous electrical field stimulation
  - Therapeutic electrical stimulation

- Transrectal electrostimulation
- Bladder stimulation
- Biofeedback
- Acupuncture
■ These methods have been tried with varying success.
■ Little evidence-based research exists to support their use.
■ Families often turn to alternative therapies, including herbal medications, because:
  - Many conventional therapies are ineffective in treating the symptoms of spina bifida.
  - No cure exists.
■ Inquire about the use of these treatments.
  - Be aware of their nature, possible interactions with medications, and potential for harm.

WHEN TO ADMIT

■ When the child is acutely ill and cannot be managed at home
■ When the child requires surgical intervention

WHEN TO REFER

■ Infants born with meningomyelocele should be referred to a tertiary medical center that specializes in the care of these children.
  - Ideally before delivery
■ All infants born with meningomyelocele should be monitored during childhood by a multidisciplinary team that includes experts in:
  - Child development
  - Neurosurgery
  - Orthopedics
  - Urology
  - Orthotics
  - Social work
  - Nursing
  - Physical and occupational therapies
  - Plastic surgery
■ Early on, refer to:
  - Ophthalmologist
    - At least 1 visit by an ophthalmologist during infancy because of risk of strabismus leading to amblyopia
  - Geneticist
  - Early intervention program

FOLLOW-UP

■ Head circumference, height, and weight should be monitored.
■ Some clinicians recommend substituting arm span for height because growth below the waist is disproportionately slow.

- As the child grows, the primary care physician should:
  - Coordinate the child's care
  - Be the child's advocate
- In most instances, children may benefit from services.
  - Services are mandated under the Individuals with Disabilities Education Act. They include:
    - Formal early-intervention programs
    - Special education services
    - Physical and occupational therapies
- Opportunities for interactions with people and objects (toys) should be provided.
- The child should be encouraged to develop the best social interaction and self-help skills possible, including development of independence in hygiene and eating.

COMPLICATIONS

Hydrocephalus

- Abnormality is often associated with progressive hydrocephalus, which may lead to:
  - Laryngeal nerve palsy
  - Difficulty in swallowing
  - Hypoventilation
  - Apnea
  - Sudden death
- Central precocious puberty develops in many girls with hydrocephalus.
- 25–60% develop evidence of hydrocephalus within the first year of life.
- The higher (ie, the more cephalad) the spinal lesion is, the greater the likelihood of developing hydrocephalus.
- Subtle abnormalities of cranial nerve nuclei occur in many affected children.
- Seizures occur in 15–20% of children and adolescents.
  - ~25% have seizures at birth.

Shunt malfunction

- Sudden shunt malfunction may produce life-threatening elevations of intracranial pressure, requiring emergency intervention.
  - Signs and symptoms of acute shunt malfunction include:
    - Headache
    - Lethargy
    - Irritability
    - Paralysis of upward gaze
    - Sixth cranial nerve palsy
    - Bulging fontanelle (in infants)
    - Vomiting

- Progression may rapidly ensue to:
  - Loss of consciousness
  - Abnormal pupillary reflexes
  - Papilledema
  - Deterioration of vital signs
  - Death

Intellectual development

- Most children have normal overall IQ scores.
- Most have selective cognitive disabilities, including:
  - Nonverbal learning disabilities
  - Impairment of executive functions
- Even children with very low performance scores may have surprising verbal fluency, sometimes referred to as *cocktail party syndrome.*
- Specific cognitive testing often reveals deficiencies of:
  - Selective visual attention
  - Visual-spatial perception
  - Tactile perception
  - Auditory concentration
  - Higher-order functioning (eg, organizational skills)
- Children with hydrocephalus and higher spinal lesions are more likely to have these deficits.
- Manifestations seen in school include:
  - Short attention span
  - Distractibility
  - Perseveration
  - Poor comprehension
  - Poor handwriting
  - Disorganization
  - Poor memory
  - Faulty problem-solving and decision-making skills
  - Reduced social skills
  - Emotional instability
  - Impulsivity
  - Irritability
  - Difficulty with subjects requiring visual-motor integration and visual-perceptual integration, eg, arithmetic

Surgical complications

- Surgery to cover the cord may:
  - Result in loss of neurologic function
  - Lead to scar tissue that tethers the cord and results in further neurologic deterioration as the child grows

S

■ ≤50% may have allergies to latex, including anaphylaxis, during surgery.
  • Contact with products made from latex should be avoided.
    – All surgical procedures should occur in latex-free settings.
    – Catheterization should be performed with nonlatex catheters.
    – Gloves worn during care should be of nonlatex material.
    – Toys that contain significant amounts of latex should be avoided.
    – Products that contact the skin, such as adhesive or Ace bandages, should be latex-free.

Complications of vertebral malformations

■ Caused by abnormal segmentation or formation, including:
  • Absent vertebrae
  • Fused vertebrae
  • Hemivertebrae
  • Butterfly vertebrae
  • Bony or ligamentous spurs that lead to diastematomyelia (occasionally)
■ Of children who have thoracic lesions:
  • 10% are born with kyphosis.
  • Rate increases to 33% by adolescence
■ Children with lumbar lesions have a 5% occurrence of kyphosis by adolescence.
■ In addition to cosmetic deformity, severe kyphosis can lead to:
  • Back pain
  • Pulmonary and cardiac dysfunction
  • Recurrent skin ulceration
  • Interference with walking
■ Occurrence of scoliosis is related to the level of the lesion.
■ Curves ≥30 degrees appear in:
  • 81% of adolescents with thoracic lesions
  • 23% of those with lower lumbar lesions
■ Consequences of scoliosis are similar to those of kyphosis.
■ Lordosis is much less common.

Complications of spinal cord malformation

■ Results in:
  • Loss of sensation, making child vulnerable to burns, abrasions
  • Loss of motor function
■ Decubitus ulcers, especially among adolescents and adults who spend extensive time in wheelchairs
  • Skin lesions may become infected, leading to osteomyelitis.

■ Loss of motor function leads to decreased movement in utero.
  • May lead to deformities seen at birth, such as clubfoot (talipes equinovarus), dislocated hips
■ Loss of efferent nerve stimuli to urinary bladder and sphincter results in neurogenic voiding dysfunction in virtually all patients.
  • Bladder dysfunction may be classified as:
    – Failure to store urine
      ■ Hypotonic urinary outlet
      ■ Spastic, hypertonic bladder
    – Failure to empty completely
      ■ Spastic urinary sphincter
      ■ Hypotonic bladder
  • The combination of spastic outlet and hypertonic bladder is especially serious.
    – Reflux and hydronephrosis occur frequently with this combination.
  • Urinary tract infections lead to:
    – Fibrosis of the bladder
    – Chronic renal damage, a significant source of morbidity and mortality
  • Repeated urinary infections in the presence of reflux lead to renal failure.
■ Altered sexual function, especially in men
  • ~25% of men with meningomyelocele cannot have erections.
  • Of those who can, most have retrograde ejaculation and decreased fertility.
■ Women have:
  • Decreased sensation
  • Decreased lubrication in response to sexual stimulation
  • Most can experience orgasm and have normal fertility.
■ Children usually have neurogenic bowel.
  • Most children have intact internal rectal sphincter function.
  • Many have intact rectal sensation.
  • Abnormal migration of neural cells in utero can lead to diminished peristalsis.
  • Constipation or obstipation with overflow soiling are caused by:
    – Abnormal rectal function
    – Poor peristalsis
    – Limited mobility
    – Ingestion of a low-fiber diet because of difficulty swallowing or fear of incontinence

- Loss of motor function in the lower extremities leads to loss of mobility.
  - Degree of mobility is related closely to the level of the lesion.
  - Children with intact quadriceps (L2–L4) are much more likely to be ambulatory through adolescence than are those with higher-level lesions.
  - Joint contractures develop in children who have:
    - Imbalance of forces around a joint
    - No function
  - A child with a thoracic-level lesion who has no hip function is at risk for hip flexion contractures from sitting all day in a wheelchair.
  - Loss of mobility and innervation increases risk for:
    - Osteoporosis
    - Pathologic fractures in the lower extremities
    - Unnoticed fractures

Psychosocial complications

- The birth of a child with meningomyelocele is potentially devastating.
- Most parents go through the phases characteristic of people undergoing a loss.
- Some families may go through part of the grief process several times during the child's life, particularly at significant milestones.
- Parents must share in:
  - Grieving
  - Difficult medical decisions
- Parents will require support from medical professionals.
- Most children with meningomyelocele have multiple medical problems.
  - Require money, time, patience, understanding
  - Such demands stress parents and can lead to isolation of one parent from the other.
  - Stresses may affect siblings, who can develop behavioral problems.
- Children may have difficulty at home if parents cannot:
  - Provide affection
  - Set consistent limits

- These children may have difficulty:
  - With peers who see them as "cripples" rather than as children with disabilities
  - Performing academically
- They may:
  - Lose interest in school because of frequent negative reinforcement
  - Have no adult role models
  - Lose self-esteem

PREVENTION

- Periconceptual folate supplementation has been shown to decrease:
  - Primary occurrence of neural tube defects
  - Recurrence of these defects in families
- The AAP and Centers for Disease Control and Prevention recommend that all women of child-bearing age receive 0.4 mg of folic acid daily.
  - Women who have a first-degree relative with a neural tube defect should receive 4.0 mg of folic acid daily.
- Open neural tube defects may be diagnosed prenatally.
  - Measurement of α-fetoprotein levels in maternal serum between 14 and 16 weeks of gestation *and*
  - Confirmation of diagnosis via high-resolution ultrasonography
  - Amniocentesis is recommended for women with elevated serum α-fetoprotein levels to confirm diagnosis.
- Prenatal detection of a neural tube defect allows the family to:
  - Consider termination
  - Plan peri- and postnatal care, including the decision to deliver by cesarean section
- Prenatal surgery to cover the open lesion on the back during the second trimester may decrease the severity of:
  - Hydrocephalus
  - Chiari malformation
  - Major risks of this procedure include premature delivery and maternal complications (bleeding and infection).
  - A multicenter controlled clinical trial is underway in the US to evaluate the effects of prenatal surgery (www.spinabifidamoms.com).

S

Spinal Deformities

DEFINITION

- Scoliosis is a side-to-side curve of the spine.
  - Most cases are idiopathic scoliosis.
  - Less common types include:
    - Congenital: absent or fused spinal segments
    - Metabolic: juvenile osteoporosis
    - Neuromuscular: poliomyelitis, cerebral palsy
- Larsen syndrome is an autosomal-dominant osteochondrodysplasia.
- Dysraphism is failure of closure of the primary neural tube.
- Kyphosis is an acquired dorsal hump.
- Spondylolysis is a defect in the continuity of the pars inter-articularis of the posterior portion of L4 or L5.
- Spondylolisthesis is a forward slippage of one vertebra on the vertebra below.

EPIDEMIOLOGY

Congenital malformations

- Congenital scoliosis
  - The overall incidence of congenital anomalies of the spine is unknown.
  - One estimate of thoracic spine congenital deformity is 0.5 per 1000 persons.
- Goldenhar syndrome: ocular-auricular-vertebral spectrum (OAVS)
  - Rare; prevalence is estimated to be ~1 in 45,000 live births.
  - Male infants are affected more often than females.
  - The right side of the face or body (or both) is generally more commonly and severely affected than the left.
- VACTERL complex (see description in Etiology)
  - Estimated incidence: 1 in 25,000 live births with ≥3 components of the spectrum

Acquired abnormalities

- Scoliosis
  - Most cases are idiopathic; ~75% of all cases
  - Idiopathic scoliosis can appear at any age.
  - The majority of cases begin in adolescence.
  - More prevalent in girls
  - Right thoracic or right thoracolumbar pattern is prevalent
- Adolescent idiopathic scoliosis
  - 2% of adolescents have a scoliosis (>10 degrees).
- Spondylolysis and spondylolisthesis
  - Gymnasts and other athletes who repeatedly hyperextend the spine have a higher incidence of spondylolysis than the general population.
  - In adolescence and adulthood, incidence is estimated at 5%.
- Infections of the spine
  - Exceedingly rare

ETIOLOGY

Spinal cord and vertebral embryonic development

- Factors that adversely affect normal differentiation of the musculoskeletal system during the embryonic period are:
  - Genetic abnormalities
  - Teratogen exposure
- Errors in the embryologic sequence of the spine cause several congenital defects of spinal column and cord.
  - Range in severity
    - From isolated hemivertebrae to:
    - More complex errors of vertebral formation and segmentation associated with defects of the neural tube or spinal cord
  - Structural spinal curves, such as congenital scoliosis or kyphosis, develop when errors:
    - Result in asymmetric vertebral formation
    - Produce asymmetric vertebral growth potential
- In patients with high thoracic and cervical curves, frequent occurrences include malformations of:
  - Head and neck, especially internal and external auditory apparatuses
  - Maxillae
  - Mandibles

Congenital malformations

- Congenital scoliosis
  - Due to:
    - Failure of formation
    - Failure of segmentation
  - Produced by deformities in the coronal plane
- Congenital kyphosis
  - Due to:
    - Lack of segmentation of vertebral bodies anteriorly
    - Lack of formation of a vertebral body
  - Produced by deformities in the sagittal plane
- Larsen syndrome
  - Recently shown to be caused by missense mutations or small in-frame deletions in the *FLNB* gene
- Morquio syndrome (mucopolysaccharidosis [MPS] type IV)–odontoid dysplasia with atlantoaxial subluxation
  - MPS IV-A results from mutations in the gene-encoding galactosamine-6-sulfatase, located at *16q24.3.*
  - MPS IV-B (a milder variant) is due to ß-galactosidase deficiency.
  - Clinical features result from accumulation of keratan sulfate and chondroitin-6-sulfate.

- Klippel-Feil syndrome–association of:
  - Short neck
  - Low posterior hairline
  - Restriction in neck motion caused by the congenital fusion of cervical vertebrae
  - Common associated anomalies include:
    - Renal anomalies
    - Congenital elevation of the scapulae (ie, Sprengel deformity)
    - Impaired hearing
    - Congenital heart disease
- VATER syndrome
  - **V**ertebral defects
  - Imperforate **a**nus
  - **T**racheoesophageal fistula
  - **R**adial andrenal dysplasia
- VACTERL complex—VATER syndrome with:
  - Congenital **c**ardiac lesions
  - **R**ib and **l**imb lesions

Acquired abnormalities

- Scoliosis
  - Nonstructural scoliosis results from:
    - Posture habit
    - Splinting because of pain
    - Muscle spasm
    - Hysteria
- Kyphosis
  - Can be secondary to:
    - Spinal tumor
    - Radiation
    - Infection
    - Surgery
  - Most common cause of acquired kyphosis
    - Osteochondrosis known as *Scheuermann disease*
    - Occurs in 5% of the population
  - Glucocorticoid-induced osteoporosis
    - Caused by:
      - Supraphysiologic levels of endogenous glucocorticoids (Cushing disease)
      - Exogenously administered glucocorticoids
    - Can provoke kyphosis
    - Excess glucocorticoids often act to suppress bone formation and increase bone resorption, leading to:
      - Trabecular bone loss
      - Vertebral body collapse

- Pathologic fractures
- Increased propensity toward kyphotic spinal malalignment
- Spondylolysis
  - Often due to stress fracture/trauma in a genetically susceptible host
- Spondylolisthesis
  - Spondylolysis may lead to forward slippage of the vertebral body.

RISK FACTORS

- Scoliosis
  - Increased risk when there is an affected family member
- Adolescent idiopathic scoliosis
  - Key risk factors for curve progression are combinations of:
    - Remaining spinal growth (skeletal immaturity)
    - Curve magnitude at a given time
- Spondylolysis and spondylolisthesis
  - Spondylolysis is fairly common in young athletes with low back pain.
  - The propensity for spondylolysis to become spondylolisthesis with forward slippage is increased during growth spurts.

SIGNS AND SYMPTOMS

Postural

- Back pain in children is often a sign of an underlying disorder.
- Postural abnormalities may or may not indicate an underlying spine disorder.
- The challenge to the physician is to determine whether the child's posture is caused by:
  - Underlying skeletal deformity
  - A habit that has altered—exaggerates, increases, or decreases—normal spinal curves
- Abnormal curvatures and protrusions merit careful investigation.
- Thoracic spine normally has some kyphosis.
- Lumbar spine normally has slight lordosis.
- If either condition is excessive, progressive, or painful, then concern is appropriate.
- Scoliosis is always abnormal.

Congenital malformations

- When the newborn is held prone in the examiner's palm, the infant's back falls into slight flexion, allowing detection of:
  - Meningomyelocele
  - Scoliosis
  - Kyphosis
  - Dorsolumbar hyperflexion

S

- Lumbar spinal deformity may be indicated by:
  - Hair tuft
  - Dimple
  - Discoloration
  - Palpable spina bifida lamina defect

Congenital scoliosis

- Vertebral anomalies are present at birth.
- Clinical deformity develops with spinal growth.
  - May not become apparent until later childhood
  - Sometimes related to cardiac or urologic abnormalities

Congenital kyphosis

- More severe deformities are usually recognized in neonate.
  - Rapidly progress thereafter
- Less obvious deformities may not appear until several years later.

Spina bifida

- Spina bifida can be mild and of no clinical significance (occulta).
- Can be severe (vera), with meningeal protrusion (meningocele) or protrusion of both meninges and neural elements (myelomeningocele) posteriorly
  - When the protrusion includes bony elements, it may transfix the spinal cord.
  - Transfixing spur is called *diastematomyelia.*
  - Most of the lesions occur in the lower lumbar and upper sacral areas.
  - Few spinal defects are at a higher level.

Larsen syndrome

- Characteristic pattern of spinal deformity consisting of:
  - Vertebral anomalies
  - Spondylolysis
  - Scoliosis
- Cervical spine is the most severely involved.
- Most consistent patterns of deformity represented by:
  - Dysraphism
  - Hypoplasia
- Scoliosis is the most common deformity seen in the thoracic spine.
- Dysraphism, scoliosis, and spondylolysis are common in the lumbar spine.
- Dysraphism is the most common anomaly in the sacrum.
- Joint, facial and palate abnormalities occur in some patients.
  - Tracheomalacia is also seen.

Goldenhar syndrome: OAVS

- Abnormalities include
  - Ocular
  - Auricular
  - Vertebral
- The terms *Goldenhar syndrome* and *OAVS* are used interchangeably to describe this myriad of congenital anomalies.
- Wide phenotypic variation
- Multiple malformations have been seen in small numbers of patients with OAVS, including congenital diseases of heart, brain, and kidneys.

Morquio syndrome (MPS type IV)—odontoid dysplasia with atlantoaxial subluxation

- The disorder consists of 2 forms with similar clinical findings and autosomal recessive inheritance.
  - MPS IV-A
  - MPS IV-B
- In both forms, mental symptoms are absent or only mildly present.
- Neurologic symptoms may result from compression of spinal cord or medulla.
- Skeletal changes include:
  - Joint laxity
  - Short stature
  - Pectus carinatum
  - Shortened vertebrae
  - Genu valgum
  - Pes planus
  - Enlarged joints
- Corneal clouding is present in 50% of cases.
- The neck is short.

VACTERL complex

- The categorical breakdown of anomalies in a large series was as follows.
  - Vertebral (25%)
  - Anal, esophageal (or other gastrointestinal) atresia (15%)
  - Cardiac (33%)
  - Tracheoesophageal fistula (95%)
  - Urinary (renal dysplasia, urethral valves) (17%)
  - Skeletal (16%)

Acquired abnormalities

Adolescent idiopathic scoliosis

- Usually painless and is discovered on routine physical examinations or at school scoliosis screening programs
  - Incidence of pain in children with idiopathic scoliosis is no different than in the general population.
    - ~30% report back pain at some time.

- Pain:
  - Mary arise during a phase of rapid progression of scoliosis
  - Might be related to underlying neurologic disorder
- The physician should be concerned about pain that arouses the child from sleep.
  - Unlike usually benign pain that delays falling asleep
- Constant pain is reason for concern.

Kyphosis

- The most common site is the lower thoracic vertebrae.
  - Can occur in any site in the vertebral column
- The initial event is bulging of intervertebral disks in direction of contiguous vertebral bodies.
  - Exerts pressure against cartilage plates
  - Causes thinning of plates
- Interferes with endochondral bone formation on the growth surface of plates
  - Causes gaps that are basis for herniation of disk into the bodies
  - Isolates apophyseal ossification center from vertebral body
- Disk space narrows, more so anteriorly
  - Causes increased pressure on anterior portions of contiguous vertebral bodies
  - Impedes their longitudinal growth anteriorly
  - Results in attendant kyphosis
- An aching pain aggravated by physical exertion is present in the affected part of the vertebral column.
  - The affected area is tender to palpation.
  - Having the patient assume a stooping position often causes pain to increase.
  - Once backache has been present for 1 year or so, kyphosis is easily apparent as a round-back deformity.
- In many instances, pain is so minor that the patient first complains to the physician about pain caused by poor posture; then kyphosis is noted.

Spondylolisthesis

- Horizontal slippage usually involves the L5 vertebral body moving anteriorly in relationship to S1.
  - Can occur anywhere in the vertebral column
- Spondylolysis often causes back pain before spondylolisthesis develops.
  - Flattening of normal lumbar lordosis with posterior tilting of pelvis is noted in spondylolysis.
  - Defect in the arch dissociates vertebra from its inferior facet and posterior ligamentous restraints.
    - Separation may allow slow forward slippage of vertebra on the vertebra below.
- Low back pain is the most common symptom.

- Some cases are diagnosed because the patient has:
  - Abnormal gait
  - Postural deformity
- Only 10–15% of patients ever develop symptoms.

Infections of the spine

- Bone destruction, initially in the anterior portion of the vertebrae, leads to collapse caused by:
  - Acute pyogenic osteomyelitis
  - Tuberculosis (Pott disease)
- Disk space inflammation, or diskitis, can appear as:
  - Fever of unknown origin accompanied by a limp
  - Low back pain
  - Refusal to walk
- The majority of younger patients do not have evidence of bacterial infection.
- Children >8 years of age occasionally have staphylococcal infections of the spine.

DIFFERENTIAL DIAGNOSIS

Classification of spinal deformity

- Idiopathic
  - Infantile
  - Juvenile
  - Adolescent
- Neuromuscular
  - Neuropathic
    - Upper motor neuron lesions
      - Cerebral palsy
      - Spinocerebellar degenerations
      - Syringomyelia
      - Spinal cord tumor
      - Spinal cord trauma
    - Lower motor neuron lesion
      - Poliomyelitis
      - Other viral myelitis
      - Trauma
      - Spinal muscular atrophy
      - Meningomyelocele (paralytic)
    - Dysautonomia (Riley-Day syndrome)
  - Myopathic
    - Arthrogryposis
    - Muscular dystrophy
    - Fiber-type disproportion
    - Congenital hypotonia
    - Myotonia dystrophica

S

- Congenital
  - Congenital scoliosis
    - Failure of formation
      - Wedge
      - Hemivertebra
    - Failure of segmentation
      - Unilateral bar
      - Bilateral bar
  - Congenital kyphosis
    - Failure of formation
    - Failure of segmentation
    - Mixed
  - Congenital lordosis
  - Associated with neural tissue defect
    - Meningomyelocele
    - Meningocele
    - Spinal dysraphism (diastematomyelia)
- Neurofibromatosis
- Mesenchymal
  - Marfan syndrome
  - Ehlers-Danlos syndrome
- Traumatic
  - Fracture or dislocation
  - After irradiation
  - After laminectomy
- Soft-tissue contractures
  - After thoracoplasty
  - Burns
- Osteochondrodystrophies
  - Achondroplasias
  - Spondyloepiphyseal dysplasia
  - Diastrophic dwarfism
  - MPS
- Scheuermann disease
- Infection
- Tumor
- Rheumatoid disease
- Metabolic
  - Rickets
  - Juvenile osteoporosis
  - Osteogenesis imperfecta
- Lumbosacral anomalies
- Hysterical

- Functional
  - Postural
  - Secondary to short limb
  - Secondary to pain

DIAGNOSTIC APPROACH

Congenital malformations

Goldenhar syndrome: OAVS

- No clear standard for diagnosis
- Authorities generally agree that the spectrum includes ≥2 of the following abnormalities.
  - Ear malformations
    - Including microtia and accessory tragi
  - Low-set ears, hemifacial microsomia
    - Including micrognathia
  - Coloboma
  - Vertebral anomalies
    - Fused or cervical hemivertebrae
- Multiple accessory tragi in a preauricular-mandibular distribution
  - 1 of the more constant findings
  - Important diagnostic clue to recognizing the syndrome

Acquired abnormalities

Adolescent idiopathic scoliosis

- Discovered at:
  - Routine physical examinations
  - School scoliosis screening programs
- Perform an Adams forward-bend test to screen for scoliosis.
  - Child bends forward until:
    - Spine is horizontal with the neck relaxed.
    - Knees fully extended
    - Feet together
    - Upper limbs dependent
    - Palms opposed
- When the patient bends forward, the site and direction of the scoliosis are indicated by prominence of:
  - 1 scapula
  - 1 side of the rib cage
  - Lumbar paraspinous muscles
- Truncal rotation (prominence) may be quantified with inclinometer or scoliometer.
  - Center over the apical spinous process (at the maximal degree of rotation and prominence).
- Seven degrees of rotation corresponds with 20 of coronal deviation.

LABORATORY FINDINGS

- Infections of the spine
  - Blood cultures are indicated in all cases.

IMAGING

- Infantile idiopathic scoliosis
  - Rib vertebral angle difference is defined as the difference in angulation of the left and right ribs on the apical vertebra as measured on an anteroposterior radiograph.
- Kyphosis
  - Radiography
    - Reveal narrowing of anterior disk space and defects on surfaces of adjacent vertebrae at sites where disk tissue has penetrated vertebral bodies
    - Schmorl nodule: prolapsed disk tissue that, in time, becomes walled off by osseous tissue and forms a bulbous mass of extruded tissue appearing as area of lucency in the affected body
- Spondylolysis and spondylolisthesis
  - Single-photon emission computed tomography is an important aid in diagnosis.
  - Oblique radiography reveals the pars interventricularis defect.
  - Standing lateral radiography demonstrates spondylolisthesis.
- Infections of the spine
  - Narrowing of disk space is the usual radiographic finding.
  - Bone scanning with ^{99m}technetium is helpful in assessing and localizing inflammatory spine lesions.

TREATMENT APPROACH

- Several groups have reported exciting advances in spinal surgery techniques to correct acquired and congenital deformities.
- Growing rods
  - Revived technique
  - Research is showing it a viable option for preserving near-normal growth of the spine.
- New techniques have been described recently, including:
  - Vertebral stapling that produces asymmetric and corrective growth of the concavity of a deformity
  - Vertical expandable prosthetic titanium rib instrumentation
    - Indirectly corrects spine deformity
    - Protects spine growth remaining to treat an associated thoracic insufficiency syndrome

SPECIFIC TREATMENTS

Congenital malformations

Congenital scoliosis

- Management requires frequent clinical and radiographic follow-up to detect progression.
- When located near the middle of the spine:
  - Segments of spine above and below compensate by curving in opposite directions.
  - The result is a balanced spine and a straight back.
  - Treatment is unnecessary.
- When asymmetrical vertebra is at the base of the spine (lumbar, sacral, or lumbosacral):
  - The compensatory curve that develops above is insufficient.
  - Curvature progresses as the patient grows.
  - Requires surgical correction before adolescence
- When deformity occurs in the cervical spine:
  - *Wryneck* deformity results.
  - Thoracolumbar compensatory curvature severely distorts posture.
  - Unilateral surgical fusions are required to minimize deformity.

Congenital kyphosis

- When necessary, the treatment is fusion.

Spina bifida

- Severe forms require prompt neurosurgical correction.
- Exercises to maintain the neck's functional range of motion are indicated.
- Surgery is contraindicated in mild cases.
  - Danger of injuring the cervical spinal cord

Morquio syndrome (MPS type IV)— odontoid dysplasia with atlantoaxial subluxation

- Surgery to stabilize upper cervical spine
  - Perform before development of cervical myelopathy.
  - Use posterior spinal fusion
  - Can be lifesaving

Acquired abnormalities

Juvenile idiopathic scoliosis

- If the scoliosis is in the thoracic region, surgery is required in >95% of cases.

Adolescent idiopathic scoliosis

- Treatment is undertaken to prevent sequelae of untreated severe scoliosis.
  - Pulmonary restriction
  - Significant back pain
  - Cosmetic deformity

S

- Exercises are of no benefit in retarding or reversing progress of scoliosis.
- Curvature
  - >40°: requires surgical fusion regardless of the patient's age.
  - 20–40°: should not require treatment if skeletal maturation is complete; bracing is often recommended in the growing child
  - <20°: should be observed for possible progression; does not require treatment

Kyphosis

- Treatment is aimed at preventing further deformity by casting or bracing.
- In rare instances of rapid progression or very severe pain, spinal fusion is necessary.
- The majority of youngsters require careful observation, with intervention only if progression of deformity occurs.

Spondylolysis and spondylolisthesis

- In the absence of symptoms, requires no treatment or activity restriction
- Treatment is typically aimed at alleviation of back pain.
  - Can usually be accomplished with activity restrictions or a period of bracing
  - Activities that hyperextend the lumbar spine should be avoided.
  - Exercises to reduce lumbar lordosis relieve the pain of spondylolysis.
- Once slippage occurs, surgical spinal fusion is necessary.

Infections of the spine

- Bone destruction
  - Vigorous antibiotic therapy and immobilization are indicated.
- The majority of younger patients require only immobilization.
- Indications for using antibiotics include:
  - Positive blood culture results
  - Recurrences of back pain accompanied by systemic signs, such as:
    - Fever
    - Leukocytosis with a left shift in the leukocyte count
    - Elevated erythrocyte sedimentation rate
    - Bone erosion
    - Clinical advancement of disease despite immobilization

WHEN TO REFER

- Adolescent idiopathic scoliosis
  - Refer to a pediatric orthopedist when 7 of rotation corresponds with 20 of coronal deviation.

COMPLICATIONS

Congenital malformations

- Congenital kyphosis
  - Progressive deformity in the thoracic spine can result in paraplegia.
  - Associated with failure of the formation of the vertebral body
- Morquio syndrome (MPS type IV)—odontoid dysplasia with atlantoaxial subluxation
  - Odontoid process in the cervical region is often dysplastic and fails to ossify, leading to:
    - Atlantoaxial instability
    - C1–C2 subluxation
  - Insidious onset of cervical cord compression, beginning with fatigue and progressing to weakness, can occur.
  - Acute cord compression and respiratory arrest may occur after minor falls.

Acquired abnormalities

- Infantile idiopathic scoliosis
  - The vast majority of these curves are self-limiting.
  - Those that progress can be difficult to manage.
    - Usually double structural curves
  - In cases in which the rib vertebral angle difference is >20°, progression is likely.

PROGNOSIS

Congenital malformations

- Congenital scoliosis
  - Curve progression is strongly related to the type of vertebral abnormality.
  - The poorest prognosis is for unilateral unsegmented bars with contralateral hemivertebrae.
    - Up to 10°/year progression
  - Less severe progression in cases of hemivertebrae (seen in 40% of cases) or double hemivertebrae
    - 1–2.5°/year and 2–5°/year, respectively
  - Least severe progression in patients with block and wedge vertebrae
- Congenital kyphosis
  - After progression begins, it does not cease until end of growth.
- Spina bifida
  - The physician should assess defect level accurately because it affects prognosis.
    - All thoracic lesions are associated with paraparesis.
    - Lesions below L4 are associated with normal ambulation.
    - Prognosis with lesions between L1 and L4 is mixed.

- Juvenile idiopathic scoliosis
  - Often progressive
    - Estimated at ~70%
  - Potential for trunk deformity with cardiac and pulmonary compromise exists.
    - Especially in scoliosis with onset before 5 years of age
  - Curves >30° are almost always progressive.
    - Rate of 1–3°/year before 10 years of age
    - Rate of 4.5–11°/year after 10 years of age

Acquired abnormalities

- Adolescent idiopathic scoliosis
  - 5% of those with disease have a progression of the curve to >30°.
    - Progression of scoliosis is dependent on:
      - Growth velocity
      - Magnitude of the curve at first visit
    - Progression is most notable with a growth velocity of >2 cm/year.
      - Between 9 and 13 years
      - At bone ages between 9 and 14 years
      - Between 0.5 and 2 years before menarche
    - Main progression occurs at the time of most rapid skeletal growth.
      - 11–13 years for girls
      - 13–15 years for boys
    - Primary thoracic curve scoliosis progresses more than primary lumbar curve scoliosis.
- Kyphosis
  - In some children, the condition can progress to cause severe deformity and dysfunction.
  - In others, it stabilizes and the deformity may disappear.
- Spondylolysis and spondylolisthesis
  - Progression is estimated to occur in 5–7% of patients with spondylolisthesis.
    - Most likely to occur during the adolescent growth spurt

S

Splenomegaly

DEFINITION

- Splenomegaly is enlargement of the spleen resulting from abnormalities of the lymphoid, reticuloendothelial, or vascular components of the spleen.

EPIDEMIOLOGY

- Prevalence
  - A soft spleen is normally palpable in 15–30% of neonates.
  - By 1 year of age, 10% of healthy children have a palpable spleen.
  - After 10 years of age, 1% of children have palpable spleens.
- Sex
  - No sex-based differences in spleen size have been found.

MECHANISM

- The spleen has many functions:
  - Hematopoietic
    - The spleen is a major hematopoietic organ during fetal life and can resume extramedullary hematopoiesis in children and adults with bone marrow failure.
  - Phagocytic
  - Immunologic
    - The spleen is a major lymphoreticular organ that acts as a filter for infectious organisms in the blood.
    - Removes senescent and abnormal erythrocytes
    - Removes particulate material
    - Acts as a site of immunoglobulin M and properdin production
  - Reservoir for blood-borne elements, including:
    - Platelets, reticulocytes, and plasma proteins (in particular, factor VIII)
- Splenomegaly may be caused by:
  - Systemic infections
    - In infectious processes, splenomegaly results from hypertrophy of lymphatic and reticuloendothelial elements.
  - An increase in the normal splenic process, eg, hemolytic anemia
  - Infiltration from storage diseases or cancer
  - Congestion from splenic or portal vein obstruction
  - Inflammatory diseases
- Splenomegaly associated with hemolytic states results from:
  - Engorgement of the splenic sinusoids by abnormal erythrocytes
  - Increased phagocytic activity (work hypertrophy) of the reticuloendothelial elements.

HISTORY

- In most cases, the cause of splenomegaly can be determined by history and physical examination.
- Family history may be relevant.

- In infants, ask about birth history and the early neonatal period.
  - A history of umbilical vein catheterization or omphalitis in the neonatal period may suggest a diagnosis of portal vein thrombosis.
- In a newborn with unexplained jaundice, consider congenital hemolytic anemia, especially if there is a family history of:
  - Anemia
  - Jaundice
  - Splenomegaly
  - Splenectomy
- A viral cause (Epstein-Barr virus, cytomegalovirus) should be considered in a child with a history of:
  - Fever
  - Pharyngitis
  - Malaise
- Malaria or histoplasmosis may be the cause if the patient has recently traveled to areas endemic for these diseases.
- An underlying inflammatory, infectious, or malignant process should be suspected in the patient with:
  - Fever
  - Night sweats
  - Malaise
  - Weight loss
  - Rash
  - Arthralgia
  - Bone pain

PHYSICAL EXAM

- Spleen length is correlated with age, height, weight, and body surface area in a nonlinear fashion, similar to the liver.
- Wide interobserver variability exists in the ability to detect an enlarged spleen on examination.
  - Not generally associated with clinical experience
- The spleen:
  - Moves downward with inspiration
  - Enlarges diagonally across the midline toward the right ileac fossa.
- An enlarged spleen may extend into the pelvis.
- Palpation and percussion are important techniques in the physical examination of the child with suspected splenomegaly.
- Palpation
  - Begin in the right lower quadrant.
  - Move across the abdomen toward the left upper quadrant.
  - The normal palpable spleen is:
    - Soft
    - Smooth

- Nontender
- <1–2 cm below the left costal margin
- A pathologically enlarged spleen:
  - Is usually firm
  - Has an abnormal surface
  - Is often associated with signs and symptoms of an underlying disease
- Spleen may be tender if it has enlarged quickly.
  - Splenic sequestration
  - Splenic trauma with subcapsular hemorrhage
- When portal hypertension causes splenomegaly, dilatation of the superficial abdominal veins can be seen.
- Consider an autoimmune disorder when the following are present:
  - Rash
  - Arthritis
  - Mucosal ulcerations
  - Splenomegaly
- A palpable spleen may be normal.
  - However, the concomitant finding of hepatomegaly is usually pathologic, and further investigation is warranted.
- A palpable spleen may be encountered as a result of thin abdominal musculature.
- Percussion
  - Percussion cannot confirm splenic enlargement but can raise suspicion.
  - Percuss the left lower anterior chest wall between lung resonance above and the costal margin below.
    - This is known as the *Traube space.*
  - An enlarged spleen replaces the tympany of the stomach and colon with the dullness of a solid organ.
  - If tympany is prominent, especially laterally, then splenomegaly is not likely.
  - A change from tympany to dullness on inspiration when percussing at the lower interspace in the left anterior axillary line suggests splenic enlargement.

DIFFERENTIAL DIAGNOSIS

Infection

- Viral infection
  - The most common cause of splenomegaly in children
  - Splenic enlargement is usually transient and mild to moderate in severity.
  - Common viral infections include:
    - Epstein-Barr virus (infectious mononucleosis)
      - Splenomegaly occurs in 50–75% of cases of infectious mononucleosis.

  - Cytomegalovirus
  - HIV
- Bacterial infection
  - Acute bacterial infections
  - Subacute bacterial endocarditis
  - Congenital syphilis
  - Tuberculosis
  - Other chronic bacterial infections
  - Septicemia from meningococcus or pneumococcus may also be associated with splenomegaly.
- Parasitic infection
  - Toxoplasmosis
  - Malaria
  - Leishmaniasis
- Fungal infection
  - Candidiasis
  - Histoplasmosis
    - Progressive disseminated histoplasmosis can occur in healthy children <2 years.
    - Results from exposure to the fungus in endemic areas of the US (Mississippi, Ohio, and Missouri River valleys)
    - Early symptoms are fever, failure to thrive, and hepatosplenomegaly.
  - Coccidioidomycosis

Hematologic disorders

- Splenic enlargement as a result of extramedullary hematopoiesis
  - Occurs in diseases associated with increased demand on the bone marrow for cell production, eg, thalassemia major
- Acute splenic sequestration crisis is a medical emergency that requires prompt recognition and treatment.
  - It is a leading cause of death in children with sickle cell anemia.
  - A rapidly enlarging spleen with:
    - Falling hematocrit
    - Pallor
    - Dyspnea
    - Weakness
    - Left-sided abdominal pain
- Hemolytic anemias—congenital and acquired
  - Red cell membrane defects
    - Hereditary spherocytosis
    - Hereditary elliptocytosis
  - Red cell hemoglobin defects
    - Sickle cell disease and related syndromes
    - Thalassemia

S

- Red cell enzyme defects
  - Pyruvate kinase deficiency
  - Glucose-6-phospate dehydrogenase deficiency
  - Others
- Autoimmune hemolytic anemia
■ Extramedullary hematopoiesis
- Occurs in diseases associated with increased demand on the bone marrow for cell production.
  - Thalassemia major
  - Osteopetrosis
  - Myelofibrosis

Infiltrative disorders

■ In malignant infiltration, the spleen is firm, massively enlarged, and crosses the midline of the body.
■ The spleen is commonly infiltrated in:
- Leukemias and lymphomas
- Lipidoses
- Mucopolysaccharidosis
  - Phagocytic reticuloendothelial elements of the spleen accumulate large amounts of lipid and mucopolysaccharide, respectively.
- Langerhans cell histiocytosis
- Metastatic neoplasia of the spleen is rare and is usually caused by neuroblastoma.

Congestive splenomegaly (Banti syndrome)

■ Splenomegaly may occur from obstruction of the hepatic, portal, or splenic veins.
■ Common causes include:
- Portal vein thrombosis
- Cirrhosis
- Congestive heart failure
- Umbilical vein catheterization or septic omphalitis in neonates may also result in obliteration of the portal, hepatic, or splenic veins.
■ Congestive splenomegaly is the most common cause of hypersplenism (splenomegaly), peripheral blood cytopenias from excessive splenic function, and increased bone marrow production of the affected blood cells.

Inflammatory diseases

■ Splenomegaly is the result of increased numbers of reticuloendothelial cells that remove antibody-coated cells and proteins in inflammatory diseases, such as:
- Systemic lupus erythematosus
- Rheumatoid arthritis (Still disease)
- Serum sickness
- Sarcoidosis
- Immune thrombocytopenias and neutropenias

■ Lymphoid hyperplasia may occur as a result of accelerated antibody production in the spleen.

Primary splenic disorders

■ Splenoptosis (wandering spleen)
- Splenoptosis, or wandering spleen, is a congenital fusion anomaly of dorsal mesogastrium.
- Results in a spleen of normal size that moves freely within the peritoneal cavity
- A patient with splenoptosis usually has an asymptomatic abdominal mass.
■ Cysts
- Splenic cysts may mimic splenomegaly.
- 2 types of splenic cysts have been identified:
  - Congenital (epidermoid)
  - Acquired (pseudocyst) from trauma or infarction
- Cysts are generally asymptomatic, and their presence is usually confirmed by radiologic studies.
■ Hemangiomas and lymphangiomas
■ Subcapsular hemorrhage
- Abdominal trauma may cause subcapsular hemorrhage of the spleen.
- Abdominal pain
■ Accessory spleen may also mimic splenomegaly.
- Found in 10–15% of individuals

LABORATORY EVALUATION

■ The initial laboratory testing of a child with splenomegaly should include:
- Complete blood count
- Leukocyte differential
- Reticulocyte count
- Examination of the peripheral blood smear
■ Further laboratory investigations should be directed at the suspected diagnosis, based on findings from:
- History
- Physical examination
- Initial laboratory tests

IMAGING

■ Imaging of the spleen can be an important adjunct to the physical examination in defining pathologic changes in this organ.
■ Radiologic confirmation of a mass in the left upper quadrant should be performed if any question exists about the nature of the mass.
- Retroperitoneal tumors may be mistaken for an enlarged spleen, eg, neuroblastoma or Wilms tumor.

S

- Ultrasonography
  - Used to quantify splenic enlargement
  - Differentiates the spleen from other left upper-quadrant abdominal masses
  - Contrast-enhanced sonography is a novel technique that allows real-time assessment.
- Radioactive (technetium-99m) sulfur colloid scintigraphy
  - Used to assess splenic function
- Computed tomography
  - Used to evaluate splenic trauma and focal splenic pathology
- Magnetic resonance imaging
  - Can further clarify abnormalities in size and shape
  - Can define parenchymal disease

TREATMENT APPROACH

- Treatment of splenomegaly should be aimed at the underlying disease entity.
  - Patients who have bacterial infections should receive appropriate antibiotic therapy.
  - Viral causes of splenomegaly require supportive care.

SPECIFIC TREATMENT

Infectious mononucleosis

- Patients should refrain from contact or collision sports until illness has completely resolved clinically and the spleen has returned to a normal size.
  - Generally, this is at least 4 weeks from the onset of illness.
  - Sonographic evaluation of spleen size may be necessary to determine when the patient can resume full athletic activity.

Splenectomy

- May be indicated to help control or stage some diseases that cause splenomegaly
  - Hereditary spherocytosis
  - Autoimmune thrombocytopenia or hemolysis
  - Lymphoma, Hodgkin disease
- Splenectomy may also be indicated to treat chronic, severe hypersplenism.

- Laparoscopic splenectomy is being performed more commonly in children.
  - The procedure is safe and hospital stay is shorter compared with open splenectomy.

WHEN TO REFER

- Splenomegaly with concomitant hepatomegaly
- Palpation of a hard spleen
- Suspicion of cancer or other infiltrative disorders
- Evidence of hemolytic anemias

WHEN TO ADMIT

- Admission may be required when there is:
  - Splenic sequestration in sickle cell disease
  - Injury to the spleen from abdominal trauma
  - Possible cancer

FOLLOW-UP

- All children without spleens:
  - Are at risk for fulminant bacteremia, particularly from:
    - *Streptococcus pneumoniae*
    - *Haemophilus influenzae*
    - *Neisseria meningitides*
  - Should receive appropriate immunizations
  - Daily antimicrobial prophylaxis against pneumococcal infections (in addition to immunization) is recommended:
    - In children <5 years of age and
    - For ≥1 year after splenectomy

Complications

- Rupture of the enlarged and friable spleen is possible if the child participates in contact sports.
- Hypersplenism can cause cytopenias and severe anemia.

Prognosis

- Prognosis depends on underlying cause.
  - Splenomegaly caused by Epstein-Barr virus or cytomegalovirus infection usually resolves by 4 weeks.

S

Sports Injuries

DEFINITION

- Sports medicine is a discipline in itself; an introduction to some of the more common problems is presented here.
- Types of sports injuries include:
  - Heat injury
    - Heat cramps
    - Heat exhaustion
    - Heatstroke
  - Drug use in athletes
  - Injuries to bone and soft tissue
    - Overuse syndromes
    - Stress fracture
    - Metaphyseal and diaphyseal stress injuries
    - Osgood-Schlatter disease
    - Sinding-Larsen-Johansson disease
    - Calcaneal apophysitis
    - Little League shoulder
    - Physeal widening of the distal radius
    - Panner disease
    - Osteochondritis dissecans of the capitellum
    - Tendonoses
    - Rotator cuff tendonitis
  - Acute trauma
    - Ankle sprains
    - Collateral ligament injuries of the knee
    - Meniscal tears
    - Quadriceps contusion
    - Avulsion fracture of the pelvis
    - Muscle strain
    - Patellar dislocation
    - Shoulder dislocation
    - Chondromalacia patella
    - Patellofemoral pain syndrome
    - Winter sports injury

EPIDEMIOLOGY

Drug use in athletes

- Anabolic steroid use has been reported to be as high as 5–11% among high school boys and 2.5% among high school girls.

Injuries to bone and soft tissue

- Metaphyseal and diaphyseal stress injuries
  - Most occur in later adolescence (age 16–19 years); some occur at younger ages.
  - Distribution of male and female patients is typically equal.
- Osgood-Schlatter disease
  - Patients are typically 10–15 years of age at onset.

- Boys are more commonly affected than girls; however, female gymnasts are particularly prone to this problem.
- Sinding-Larsen-Johansson disease
  - Affected youngsters are typically 10–13 years of age.
- Calcaneal apophysitis
  - The patient is typically 9–14 years of age, with a substantial peak occurring at 10 and 11 years of age.
  - Most (60–80%) cases are bilateral.
- Tendonoses
  - The most common tendonitis in young athletes is that of the Achilles tendon.

Acute trauma

- Ankle sprains
  - The most common musculoskeletal injury in sports
  - Approximately 97% involve the lateral ankle ligaments.
- Anterior cruciate ligament (ACL) injuries
  - As adolescents become skeletally mature, the incidence of ACL injuries increases rapidly.
  - The incidence of injuries to young female athletes, particularly in soccer, basketball, and gymnastics, is increasing rapidly.
- Meniscal tears
  - For patients >10 years of age, the incidence of tearing of normal menisci rises.
- Muscle strain
  - Muscle strains are not as common in young athletes as they are in older ones.
- Patellofemoral pain syndrome
  - The typical patient is a teenage girl >12 years of age.
- Winter sports injury
  - Children are more likely to experience upper-extremity injuries.
  - Lower-extremity injuries are more frequent in adolescents and adults.
  - Children <10 years incur more fractures and catastrophic injuries (head injuries) with individual recreational activities than they do with organized sports.

ETIOLOGY

- Organized sports account for only about one-third of sports injuries.
- The remainder occur in physical education classes and in recreational sports.

Heat injury

- Heat exhaustion is probably caused by ineffective cardiovascular and autonomic responses to heat.

Injuries to bone and soft tissue

- Overuse syndromes
  - Characterized by injury to bone, cartilage, or soft tissue caused by repetitive submaximal physical stress
  - In contrast to acute injury, tissue breakdown in overuse injuries occurs gradually, and the body continually remodels these tissues so that they recuperate fully.
  - When imbalance occurs between rate of breakdown of connective tissues and the body's ability to remodel them, stress injuries occur.
- Stress fracture
  - Repetitive loading of relatively rigid musculoskeletal tissue leads to work hardening.
  - Unless remodeling occurs, the bone becomes brittle and eventually breaks.
- Metaphyseal and diaphyseal stress injuries
  - Metaphyseal and diaphyseal stress fractures in young athletes most commonly involve the fibula, metatarsals, tibia, femur, and ulna, but virtually any bone can be affected.
- Osgood-Schlatter disease
  - The tubercle of the proximal tibia is the insertion site of the patellar tendon.
  - The quadriceps is the strongest muscle group, and tensions it generates through the patellar tendon are enormous.
  - Stresses applied at interface between tendon and apophysis disrupt normal transition from ossified and unossified tubercle into the tendon.
- Sinding-Larsen-Johansson disease
  - Due to chronic repetitive stress to the inferior pole of the patella
  - In response, the patellar periosteum creates a bony reaction.
- Calcaneal apophyisitis
  - Occurs at the apophyseal insertion of the Achilles tendon into the calcaneus
- Little League shoulder
  - Actually, physiolysis of the proximal humerus
  - Due to a widening of the proximal humeral physeal plate
- Physeal widening of the distal radius
  - Physeal stress injury of the distal radius
- Osteochondritis dissecans of the capitellum
  - The disorder is a repetitive stress phenomenon, not due to an inflammatory process.
    - As the ball is released during the pitching motion, a valgus movement occurs at the elbow.
    - Tension occurs on the medial side of the elbow, and compressive forces are created across the radial capitellar articulation.

- The capitellum has an end arterial blood supply, which may be responsible for its susceptibility to developing avascular necrosis.
- Tendonoses
  - Due to overuse injury to a tendon
  - In adults, divided into 3 stages
    - Inflammation of the paratenon
    - Inflammation of the tendon itself
    - Degenerative change of the tendon that ultimately results in rupture
  - In children, typically only the earliest stage of inflammation is seen.
- Rotator cuff tendonitis
  - The rotator cuff is a convergence of the tendons of the subscapularis, supraspinatus, infraspinatus, and teres minor muscles.
  - Due to stress to the shoulder, especially when the arm extends overhead
  - The inherent laxity of the glenohumeral capsule is likely to be a significant factor in younger athletes.

Acute trauma

- Ankle sprains
  - Inversion and external rotation of the foot results in sequential tearing of the anterior talofibular ligament, calcaneal fibular ligament, and finally the posterior talofibular ligament.
  - Other areas are sometimes involved: the anterior talofibular ligament, syndesmosis complex, and deltoid ligament.
- ACL injuries
  - The ACL is a key stabilizer of the knee joint, particularly to rotational movements, and is frequently injured in sports that involve cutting and twisting.
  - Alternatively, the knee may be struck from the lateral side, injuring the medial collateral ligament and then the ACL.
- Meniscal tears
  - In youths ≤10 years of age, most meniscal tears are related to the discoid menisci.
  - For patients >10 years, tearing occurs in association with significant ligament injury, such as a tear of the ACL.
    - Tear without a substantial injury is rare in teens.
- Patellar dislocation
  - Often result of a trivial injury
  - History of injury can vary from a minor twisting episode to a significant direct blow to the knee.
- Shoulder dislocation
  - Dislocations of glenohumeral joint can occur.
    - From relatively minor trauma in predisposed individuals
    - As a result of major trauma in the average person

S

- Chondromalacia patella
  - Softening of the articular surface of the patella, which can occur in mild to severe grades, ranging from edema of the cartilage to complete ulceration of the articular surface
- Patellofemoral pain syndrome
  - Although the cause of this problem is not clear, abnormality of patellar tracking may be responsible.
  - Abnormal stresses in the patellofemoral articulation or surrounding soft tissues are probably responsible.

RISK FACTORS

In general

- Wrestling and football have the highest significant injury rates per participant in high school, followed by softball, gymnastics, track and field, and soccer.
- Tennis and swimming produce the fewest injuries.
- Frequency of injury is not always the best measure of a sport's risk.
  - Trampoline accounts for a disproportionately large number of injuries that cause paralysis.
- Risk of injury is much greater among senior high school students than among junior high and younger participants.
- Inexperienced coaches with high expectations of young athletes and poor understanding of training may contribute to injury.

Heat injury

- Heat cramps, heat exhaustion, and heatstroke are increasingly common in athletes who:
  - Do not drink adequate fluids
  - Are not acclimatized to local heat and humidity
  - Are poorly conditioned
- Heatstroke
  - Most often seen in long-distance runners
  - Second-most common cause of death in football players
  - Most common when temperature >95°F (35°C) and humidity >50%

Drug use in athletes

- Anabolic steroid use is most common among football players and track participants.

Injuries to bone and soft tissue

- Overuse syndromes
  - Training errors
  - Increased recreational time
  - Increased intensity and duration of competition
  - Increasing standards of competition
  - Inadequate preseason conditioning
  - Suboptimal facilities and equipment
  - Overly enthusiastic coaches and parents
  - Participation in multiple sports
  - Lengthy seasons
- Stress fracture
  - Commonly occurs with long-distance running
- Little League shoulder
  - Almost exclusive to Little League baseball players
  - Typically affects pitchers, but sometimes occurs in players who do a lot of throwing from other positions
- Physeal widening of the distal radius
  - Almost exclusively in young female gymnasts
- Osteochondritis dissecans of the capitellum
  - Most common in baseball pitchers
  - Any pitching style that releases the ball lateral to the body's midsagittal plane accentuates valgus moment at the elbow.
  - Side-arm pitches, many curve-ball techniques, and others can increase compression loads across the lateral side of the elbow.
- Rotator cuff tendonitis
  - In young athletes, inherent laxity of the glenohumeral capsule (ligament complex) is likely to be a significant factor.
  - Sporting activities that stress the shoulder joint with the arm extended overhead are particularly prone to precipitate symptoms.
    - Overhead throwing in baseball
    - Swimming
    - Tennis serves
    - Gymnastics

Acute trauma

- ACL injuries
  - Girls: soccer, basketball, and gymnastics
  - Boys: football, soccer, and basketball
- Quadriceps contusion
  - Common in contact sports, such as football, soccer, and lacrosse
- Patellar dislocation
  - Predisposition to dislocation of the patella as a result of genetic variability in knee extensor mechanism
  - Variations leading to easy dislocation include:
    - Shallow sulcus in the distal femur
    - Lateral translation of the insertion of the patellar tendon into the tibia
    - Relative underdevelopment of the vastus medialis muscle
    - Tightness of the lateral retinaculum

- Patellofemoral pain syndrome
  - May result from training errors
    - Sudden increase in mileage
    - Running on hard surfaces
    - Poor preseason conditioning
    - Inadequate footwear
- Winter sports injury
  - Downhill snow skiing: knee contusions, ACL sprains, spiral fracture of tibia
  - Cross-country snow skiing: medial collateral ligament sprain, acute ankle inversion strain, acromioclavicular joint separation, skier's toe, hypothermia
  - Snowboarding: wrist, ankle, and knee injuries
  - Snowmobiling: multisystem trauma with head injury
  - Sledding: head and face, extremity, abdominal injuries
  - Water skiing: lower-extremity and trunk injuries
  - Wakeboarding: head and face injuries

SIGNS AND SYMPTOMS

Heat injury

- Heat cramps
  - Usually involve the arms, abdomen, or legs
  - Affected individuals usually have been sweating profusely.
- Heat exhaustion
  - Patients feel weak, faint, dizzy, and nauseous.
  - They may vomit and appear pale.
  - Syncope sometimes occurs.
  - Patients may sweat profusely, or if severely dehydrated, the skin may feel warm and dry.
  - Body temperature is often normal.
- Heatstroke
  - High rectal temperature
  - Hot and dry skin
  - Signs of central nervous system dysfunction, such as irritability, combativeness, and disorientation, which may progress to obtundation
  - Tachycardia and hypotension are often present.

Drug use in athletes

- Anabolic steroid use
  - Clues to excessive use include:
    - Jaundice
    - Increased acne
    - Behavioral changes (aggressiveness, irritability, marked mood swings)
    - Gynecomastia
    - Testicular atrophy
    - Hirsutism and deepening of the voice (in women)
- Anabolic steroid withdrawal
  - Mood changes
  - Irritability
  - Hot flashes
  - Nausea
  - Myalgia
  - Malaise
  - Tachycardia
  - Hypertension

Injuries to bone and soft tissue

- Stress fracture
  - Progressive discomfort with activities
- Metaphyseal and diaphyseal stress injuries
  - Gradual onset of symptoms
  - Eventually, pain may preclude running.
- Osgood-Schlatter disease
  - Pain is well localized to the tibial tubercle; it typically increases with activity.
  - Significant pain, tenderness, and swelling of the tubercle on the presenting side and, usually, some degree of findings on the contralateral side
  - Many patients have a history of heel pain compatible with Sever disease (calcaneal apophysitis).
  - No signs or symptoms of intraarticular problems of the knee joint itself
- Sinding-Larsen-Johansson disease
  - Well-localized pain at the inferior pole of the patella
  - No signs or symptoms of internal derangement of the knee joint itself
  - On physical examination, point tenderness at the inferior edge of the patella and typically no other abnormal findings
- Calcaneal apophysitis
  - Complain of heel, ankle, or foot pain
  - On physical examination, discomfort is typically well localized at the region of the calcaneal apophysis.
  - Pain is typically medial or posterior, although occasionally may be on the lateral side.
  - Tenderness rarely occurs distal near the origin of the plantar fascia.
  - No swelling, warmth, or limitation of motion
  - Occasionally, because of concurrent tendonitis, some tenderness can occur along the course of the Achilles tendon itself.

S

- Little League shoulder
  - Pain in the shoulder related to overhead throwing
  - Many of the signs and symptoms are the same as for rotator cuff tendonitis, but the patient with Little League shoulder typically has more pain in the deltoid region as opposed to the subacromial region.
- Physeal widening of the distal radius
  - Progressive pain in the wrists
  - Most often the pain is bilateral, but it may be more prominent on one side.
  - On physical examination, point tenderness is often present, and a prominence may be noted on the dorsum of the distal radial physis.
- Osteochondritis dissecans of the capitellum
  - Aching pain in the lateral side of the elbow
  - With time, patients can lose range of motion.
  - Osteochondral fragments can displace acutely, resulting in a loose body sensation, a locked elbow, significant synovitis and pain, or any combination.
- Tendonoses (specifically Achilles tendonitis, the most common tendonoses in children)
  - Symptoms are typically located 2–6 cm above the insertion of the Achilles tendon into the calcaneus.
  - Lack of flexibility in the gastrocnemius muscle group may be found on physical examination.
- Rotator cuff tendonitis
  - Pain with overhead activities
  - In many instances, the athlete will report the arm becoming heavy or tired, or feeling dead.

Acute trauma

- Ankle sprains
  - Persistent anterolateral ankle pain can occur after even mild ankle sprains.
- ACL injuries
  - Patients report an acute "pop" and moderate to severe pain, causing them to fall to the ground.
  - The knee may not swell immediately, but typically it does swell within the first few hours because of the development of hemarthrosis.
  - Tenderness is sometimes not marked, and athletes will attempt to return to their sporting competition, only to discover that the knee is not stable, which may worsen the injury.
- Quadriceps contusion
  - Minor hematomas do not limit knee movement.
  - Large ones limit knee movement.

- Avulsion fracture of the pelvis
  - Acute onset of pain following a sudden athletic movement, such as:
    - An explosive start for a sprint
    - An extreme pike maneuver (hips flexed and knees extended) in gymnastics
    - A combination twisting movement and direct blow to the iliac crest
  - Focal tenderness to palpation over the affected apophysis
  - Pain with resisted strength testing of the corresponding muscle insertion or origin
- Muscle strain
  - Slipped capital femoral epiphysis is the most common disorder of the hip in adolescents.
    - Although classically exhibiting with hip pain, discomfort may be referred to the thigh or knee joint.
  - Hamstring strain causes pain at the musculotendinous junction, which is at the junction of the middle and distal thirds of the posterior thigh.
- Patellar dislocation
  - The patellae typically dislocates to the lateral side.
- Patellofemoral pain syndrome
  - Typical onset is insidious and without a specific history of trauma.
  - No history of erythema, warmth, induration, or true effusion
  - Slightly puffy knee in some patients
  - No mechanical complaints of catching or locking
  - Popping may be present, but the popping is usually painful.
  - On physical examination:
    - Tenderness along the medial and lateral sides of the patellofemoral articulation
    - Mild discomfort over the anterior portion of the joint line, but typically no tenderness over the middle or posterior portion of the tibial femoral articulation
    - The joint has full range of motion with no crepitation.
    - Stable knee

DIFFERENTIAL DIAGNOSIS

Injuries to bone and soft tissue

- Osgood-Schlatter disease
  - Tumor or infection can mimic Osgood-Schlatter disease.
- Sinding-Larsen-Johansson disease
  - Irregular ossification at the inferior pole of the patella may be mistaken for a fracture.
- Calcaneal apophysitis
  - Significant irregularity of the ossifying calcaneal apophysis is a normal finding in children and should not be confused with evidence of a fracture.

- Need to rule out other osseous processes, such as tumor or infection.
- Little League shoulder
  - Rotator cuff tendonitis: Many of the signs and symptoms are the same.
  - Impending pathologic fracture from a simple bone cyst in the upper humerus
- Physeal widening of the distal radius should be distinguished from:
  - Carpal laxity with dorsal wrist capsular impingement
  - Posterior interosseous neuroma
  - Avascular necrosis of the lunate
- Rotator cuff tendonitis
  - Need to rule out other bony abnormalities

Acute trauma

- Collateral ligament injuries of the knee
  - Consider concurrent injury to the cruciate ligaments, menisci, and articular surfaces.
  - Lateral knee and ligament injuries are uncommon in young athletes; they should raise suspicion of another explanation for the patient's signs and symptoms, and referral is wise.
- ACL injuries
  - A high index of suspicion should be maintained for ACL injury, and it must be ruled out before a young athlete who has a knee injury returns to practice or competition.
- Quadriceps contusion
  - Differentiating a large quadriceps hematoma from a malignant tumor (eg, Ewing sarcoma and osteosarcoma) becomes challenging, since those tumors have a propensity to occur in teenagers and may bleed internally.
- Muscle strain
  - Muscle strains are not as common in young athletes as they are in older ones.
  - An unknown musculoskeletal malady is often misdiagnosed as strain.
  - Particularly around the hip and thigh area, the examiner should be careful not to miss a slipped capital femoral epiphysis, an avulsion fracture, an infection, or a tumor as causes of pain.
  - More proximal hamstring tenderness should raise suspicion of an occult injury to the ischial apophysis.
- Patellar dislocation
  - Should not be labeled as knee dislocation, which denotes displacement of the articulation between the tibia and femur.
    - The latter is a high-energy injury and has high associated morbidity, including, occasionally, loss of limb.

- Shoulder dislocation
  - Pathologic collagen disorders, such as Marfan syndrome, need to be considered.
    - Physical findings consistent with Marfan syndrome include tall, thin body habitus; arachnodactyly; pectus excavation; heart murmur; dislocated lens; and myopia.

Anterior knee pain

- Can arise from many disorders, including:
  - Osgood-Schlatter disease
  - Sinding-Larsen-Johansson disease
  - Patellar tendonitis
  - Patellar instability
  - Chondromalacia patella
  - Patellofemoral pain syndrome
- Less common disorders
  - Quadriceps tendonitis
  - Bipartite patella
  - Osteochondritis dissecans of the femur or patella
  - Iliotibial band tendonitis
  - Popliteus tendonitis
  - Inflamed plica
  - Prepatellar bursitis
  - Synovial flat pin impingement syndrome
  - Osteomyelitis
  - Septic arthritis
  - Inflammatory arthritis
  - Tumors

IMAGING

Injuries to bone and soft tissue

- Metaphyseal and diaphyseal stress injuries
  - Magnetic resonance imaging (MRI) may be the most sensitive study for stress fractures.
  - Only about 10% of radiographs are abnormal at symptom onset.
  - Bone scan may detect an early stress fracture of the metaphysis or diaphysis.
    - Bone scan findings must be correlated to clinical symptoms.
    - Up to 50% of adolescents with stress fractures will show multiple areas of stress response on bone scan, many of which do not correlate to areas of symptoms.
- Osgood-Schlatter disease
  - A lateral radiograph of the knee can show irregularity of the tibial tubercle.

S

- Sinding-Larsen-Johansson disease
  - Lateral radiograph of the knee may show irregular ossification at the inferior pole of the patella.
- Calcaneal apophysitis
  - Because of concurrent tendonitis, some tenderness can occur along the course of the Achilles tendon itself; no classic radiographic change of calcaneal apophysitis.
  - In bilateral cases, radiographs are necessary only if some atypical component of the history and physical examination raises concern about some other diagnosis.
- Physeal widening of the distal radius
  - Anteroposterior and lateral radiographs show physeal widening.
  - Comparison films of the other side are almost always obtained, although both sides may be involved.
  - Typically, some asymmetry is noted.
- Osteochondritis dissecans of the capitellum
  - Plain-film radiographs often show a lesion of the capitellum.
    - Sclerotic region or simply radiolucency may be present.
    - Tangential views may be necessary to see the lesion.
  - Computed tomography (CT) and/or MRI are sometimes helpful.
- Tendonoses
  - Radiography and MRI are rarely indicated.
- Rotator cuff tendonitis
  - Plain-film radiographs are not diagnostic of rotator cuff tendonitis but are often obtained to rule out other bony abnormalities.
  - MRI can be diagnostic for rotator cuff tendonitis but is often not necessary.

Acute trauma

- Ankle sprains
  - The decision to obtain radiographs is based on several factors.
    - Patient age
    - History of injury
    - Physical findings
    - Ability to bear weight
    - Progress since injury
  - A typical fracture of the distal fibular physis has a Salter-Harris type I fracture pattern without displacement, which results in a normal radiograph of bone, showing only soft-tissue swelling.
  - Diagnosis is made clinically; radiography excludes displacement of fracture or presence of other fractures.
- Collateral ligament injuries of the knee
  - Plain-film radiographs may not be diagnostic.

- Stress radiography or MRI is occasionally needed to make this diagnosis.
- Meniscal tears
  - If a meniscal tear is suspected, referral or MRI is appropriate.
  - Arthrograms are obtained much less commonly than before.
- Avulsion fracture of the pelvis
  - Diagnosis can often be confirmed with plain-film radiographs.
  - Special oblique views and, occasionally, CT or MRI are helpful.
- Patellar dislocation
  - Unless patellar dislocation or subluxation is a trivial event that incites little joint pain, radiographs should be obtained to assess for osteochondral fragments.
- Shoulder dislocation
  - Unless the episode is minor, radiographs confirm reduction and rule out an associated fracture.
- Anterior knee pain
  - Diagnostic imaging, including MRI, often does not reveal source of pain.
  - These studies are sometimes indicated to rule out other definable abnormalities.
- Patellofemoral pain syndrome
  - Plain-film radiographs are usually negative; further diagnostic evaluation is not indicated.

DIAGNOSTIC PROCEDURES

Overuse syndromes

- Rotator cuff tendonitis
  - Positive impingement test: pain when bringing the shoulder fully overhead
  - Examination should include:
    - A thorough examination of the neck and shoulder
    - Range-of-motion limitation, muscle atrophy, and focal tenderness in the subacromion region, both anteriorly and laterally
    - Tenderness along the biceps tendon
    - Supraspinatus strength
    - Glenohumeral laxity

Acute trauma

- ACL injuries
  - Lachman examination
    - Performing this examination competently requires experience.
    - The patient lies supine and the knee is gently flexed to approximately 30 degrees.

S

– The patient must relax quadriceps and hamstrings enough to allow the examiner to attempt to slide the proximal tibia anteriorly.

– Although the amount of tibial movement is important, the key factor is the end point.

■ If the test is negative (ie, ligament is intact), a distinct end point or cessation of forward movement should be felt.

■ The end point should feel similar to holding 2 ends of a short piece of rope and quickly pulling the ends apart until movement suddenly stops.

– Comparison with the uninjured knee can be helpful.

– Success depends on:

■ Size of patient's leg

■ Ability of patient to relax

■ Size of examiner's hands

– If doubt exists, the knee should be reevaluated later or the patient referred to an orthopedist.

CLASSIFICATION

Acute trauma

■ Severity grading of sprains

● Grade I (mild)

– Stretching of the ligament with minimal microscopic injury

– Clinical presentation: mild swelling, limp

– Typical recuperation time: 0–2 weeks

● Grade II (minor)

– Partial disruption of the ligament

– Clinical presentation: modest swelling, diffuse tenderness, difficulty in weight bearing

– Typical recuperation time: 1–4 weeks

● Grade III (severe)

– Complete disruption of the ligament

– Clinical presentation: extensive swelling and bleeding, instability, and disability

– Typical recuperation time: 4–12 weeks

SPECIFIC TREATMENTS

Heat injury

■ Heat cramps

● Rest in a cool environment

● Stretching

● Fluids

■ Heat exhaustion

● Provide cool fluids and place the athlete in a cool environment.

● Cool compresses and fanning

● If the affected athlete cannot tolerate oral fluids, consider administering intravenous fluids.

■ Heatstroke

● Apply ice water–soaked towels or wet sheets with fans (if ice is not available).

● The patient should be taken to the emergency department immediately.

Injuries to bone and soft tissue

■ Overuse syndromes

● Metaphyseal and diaphyseal stress injuries

– Managed by rest

– Crutches often necessary

– Casts and immobilization sometimes needed

– Surgical intervention required occasionally

■ Suspected stress fracture of proximal femur is probably best managed by an orthopedic surgeon.

■ Screw stabilization for slipped epiphysis or stress fracture may be needed.

■ Stress fractures of the fifth metatarsal tend to be recurrent and are often best managed with an intramedullary screw.

■ Osgood-Schlatter disease

● Symptoms are often relieved with:

– Application of an ice pack

– Intermittent use of oral nonsteroidal antiinflammatory drugs (NSAIDs)

– Application of compression band

– Activity modifications as indicated by symptoms

– Hamstring stretching

● Casts are not routinely used because immobilization may weaken ligament insertions

● Brief periods of rigid immobilization may be necessary for acute exacerbations.

■ Sinding-Larsen-Johansson disease

● Treatment with ice, NSAIDs, and activity modification

● Immobilization and surgery are rarely necessary.

■ Calcaneal apophysitis

● Ice, NSAIDs, and activity modification are dictated by symptoms.

● Shoe inserts that provide padding beneath the heel can be helpful; a three-eighths–inch silicone or felt pad works best.

● Casts or Cam walkers (a removable rigid walking splint) are occasionally necessary for severe cases.

● Surgery is not indicated.

■ Little League shoulder

● Managed by rest of the shoulder

- Physeal widening of the distal radius
  - The treatment goal is resolution of symptoms and normalization of radiographs.
- Panner disease
  - Treatment simply involves rest.
- Osteochondritis dissecans of the capitellum
  - May heal with prolonged rest, but surgery is often necessary to remove an unstable or displaced bone fragment
- Tendonoses
  - In young athletes, treatment is entirely nonoperative.
  - If analysis of lower-extremity mechanics during gait suggests hyperpronation, custom foot orthoses can be helpful.
  - Ice, stretching, and NSAIDs
  - Training modifications and heel lifts
  - Immobilization rarely is necessary.

Acute trauma

- The fundamental principles of treatment for many musculoskeletal injuries go by the acronym RICE (**r**est, **i**ce, **c**ompression, and **e**levation).
  - Rest
    - Especially important for the first 24–72 hours after significant injury
    - For lower-extremity injuries, crutches should be used to avoid weight bearing.
  - Ice
    - May be applied for 20 minutes every 2–4 waking hours
    - Use a wet cloth between ice and skin to decrease chance of cold injury.
    - Continue using ice until swelling disappears completely.
  - Compression
    - Applied with an elastic bandage
  - Elevation
    - Place the injured extremity above the level of the heart to aid in reducing edema.
- Ankle sprains
  - Treatment options are complicated and are chosen on the basis of:
    - Severity of injury (see Classification)
    - Demands of the athlete
    - Experience of the health care team
  - Minor sprains
    - Apply RICE principles and periodically reevaluate.
    - At reevaluation, if pain is minimal, test the ankle for stability.
    - Observe athlete in functional tasks (eg, running, cutting, and twisting).

- If tasks are performed well without significant pain, the individual may return to competition.
- Ideally, tape or splint the ankle to lessen risk of reinjury, and consider a preventive physical therapy program.
- Moderate sprains
  - For the less serious athlete, use an expectant approach.
    - Crutches
    - Elastic bandage wrap
    - Gradual progression of weight bearing
    - Cast or Cam walker
    - Return to sports only after symptoms resolve
  - For the serious athlete, referral to a physical therapist is often helpful.
- Severe sprains
  - Should be managed by someone with advanced skills in dealing with musculoskeletal problems (eg, an experienced primary care physician or orthopedic surgeon)
  - A period of immobilization to reduce bleeding and swelling is often helpful.
  - Myriad rehabilitation protocols can be used successfully.
  - Assessment for chronic laxity and tarsal coalitions should be made.
- Persistent anterolateral ankle pain can occur after even mild ankle sprains; initial treatment includes:
  - NSAIDs
  - Ankle supports
  - Physical therapy modalities
  - Steroid injection
- Collateral ligament injuries of the knee
  - First, use RICE principles.
  - Depending on the severity of the injury, mobilize knee as the swelling and tenderness diminish.
  - Assess strength as range of motion returns.
  - For moderate and severe sprains, consider using a dual, upright, hinged, functional knee orthosis.
- ACL injuries
  - Most reconstructive techniques involve drilling holes through the proximal tibia and distal femur to insert grafts along the anatomic course of the ACL.
    - For the skeletally immature individual, this procedure raises some concerns about potential injury to the physis.
- Meniscal tears
  - Symptomatic discoid lateral menisci require surgical intervention.
    - Preserves as much of a normal functioning rim of meniscal cartilage as possible
    - Alleviates the mechanical snapping that ultimately leads to degenerative changes of the articular surfaces

- If a normal meniscus is torn, general principles of surgical treatment are preservation of meniscal tissue and reconstruction of the unstable joint.
- Quadriceps contusion
  - Initial treatment of quadriceps hematoma involves RICE and crutches.
  - As pain and swelling diminish, begin active knee flexion exercises.
- Avulsion fracture of the pelvis
  - Crutches and rest for the first few weeks
  - Stretching may inhibit healing and should be avoided until it is pain free.
- Muscle strain
  - For hamstring strain, RICE and crutches
- Patellar dislocation
  - Manipulative reduction can often be achieved.
    - Place the patient in a prone position, which facilitates hip extension and relaxes the hamstrings.
    - Gently extend the knee; as the knee extends, the patella should reduce without forced manipulation.
  - Significant patellar dislocation
    - Immobilize the knee.
    - Use RICE principles.
- Shoulder dislocation
  - Traditional treatment: 3 weeks of immobilization, followed by a rigorous physical therapy program
- Chondromalacia patella
  - In mild cases, pain from chondromalacia patella will abate with:
    - Intermittent NSAID use
    - Quadriceps-strengthening program
    - Judicious activity modification
- Patellofemoral pain syndrome
  - Education, reassurance, and symptom management are the cornerstones of treatment.
  - Stretching and strengthening quadriceps muscles often reduce anterior knee pain.
  - Principles are to strengthen the vastus medialis and improve patellar tracking.
  - Taping or supportive knee sleeves sometimes provide relief.
  - Intermittent and judicious use of NSAIDs may help.
  - In some cases, adjustment of expectations and activities is necessary.
  - In refractory cases, referral to a musculoskeletal specialist may become appropriate.
  - Surgery is occasionally performed, although the exact indications and preferred techniques are controversial.

WHEN TO ADMIT

- Fractures requiring open reduction
- Internal organ injuries
- Possible or definite traumatic brain injury

WHEN TO REFER

- When the diagnosis of the musculoskeletal injury is uncertain
- When the patient is not responding to initial treatment
- When injuries involve the growth plate in which future growth may be compromised
- When uncertainty exists in the safety of the young athlete to return to a competitive sports environment

FOLLOW-UP

Injuries to bone and soft tissue

- Metaphyseal and diaphyseal stress injuries
  - A well-designed plan of alternative training, gradual resumption of participation in sports, and monitoring for recurrent symptoms is necessary.
- Physeal widening of the distal radius
  - Once the athlete returns to gymnastics, clinical and radiographic monitoring are required.

Acute trauma

- Ankle sprains
  - For moderate strains in a serious athlete, a variety of physical therapy modalities can help reduce the swelling.
  - Range of motion is begun early, and strengthening is emphasized.
  - As the ankle becomes comfortable, the proprioception training phase of rehabilitation begins.
  - Lace-up and Velcro ankle supports may be used.
  - For some, taping may be an option.
  - In all cases, functional criteria for return to sports, prevention of reinjury, and reassessment of progress are key components.
- Collateral ligament injuries of the knee
  - A physical therapist or athletic trainer can help design an adequate rehabilitation program.
- Quadriceps contusion
  - Monitoring for reinjury is essential.
- Avulsion fracture of the pelvis
  - The athlete should be gradually returned to activity and monitored for recurrence of symptoms.
- Muscle strain
  - Once the patient is comfortable, a gradual stretching and strengthening program is initiated.
  - The athlete is returned to activities as tolerated and monitored for recurrent symptoms.

S

- Patellar dislocation
  - As pain and swelling subside, a rehabilitation program is initiated that emphasizes strengthening of the quadriceps muscles, particularly the vastus medialis.
    - Hamstrings are stretched.
    - A lower-extremity rehabilitation program is undertaken.
  - A patellar-stabilizing knee sleeve is used during the initial phases of return to activity.
- Shoulder dislocation
  - After 3 weeks of immobilization, a rigorous physical therapy program begins.
    - Directed at strengthening the rotator cuff muscles
    - The principle is to strengthen these dynamic stabilizers of the joint to help compensate for laxity of the shoulder joint capsule (ligaments).
    - The patient's program is advanced, and an experienced therapist monitors progress.
    - Recurrent instability despite a therapy program is generally an indication for surgical stabilization.
    - Support is growing for earlier surgical intervention, particularly with less invasive arthroscopic techniques.
- Chondromalacia patella
  - Although a therapy program can be helpful, the patient must have a clear understanding that the goal is to reduce symptoms.
  - Completely eliminating symptoms may not be possible.
  - Surgical intervention to alter the patella's articular surface is sometimes indicated.

PROGNOSIS

Injuries to bone and soft tissue

- Metaphyseal and diaphyseal stress injuries
  - Healing time ranges from 4–12 weeks.
- Osgood-Schlatter disease
  - In most patients, will run its course with time
  - Symptoms can last 1–4 years.
  - In about 3% of patients, a persistent ossicle will form that can remain symptomatic and may ultimately require surgical excision.
  - Fracture of the tibial tubercle has been reported in patients with Osgood-Schlatter disease.
    - Incidence is not known, but it appears to be low.
    - Remaining active in sports is not absolutely contraindicated.
- Sinding-Larsen-Johansson disease
  - This entity is self-limited and typically lasts 3–12 months.
  - In general, athletes may participate in sports as tolerated.

- Calcaneal apophysitis
  - Almost always resolves with time
  - Complications are extremely rare.
- Little League shoulder
  - If symptoms are minimal, the patient can often be allowed to bat and play in an infield position that involves minimal throwing.
  - Clinical and radiographic resolution can take up to 6 months.
  - Carefully planned resumption of pitching can then begin, but monitoring for recurrence of symptoms is necessary.
- Physeal widening of the distal radius
  - Goal of treatment is resolution of symptoms and normalization of radiographs, which usually takes ≥3 months.
- Osteochondritis dissecans of the capitellum
  - Can result in permanent arthrosis of the elbow joint
- Tendonoses
  - Gradual reintroduction of sporting activities

Acute trauma

- Collateral ligament injuries of the knee
  - Most medial collateral ligament injuries heal satisfactorily.
- ACL injuries
  - In contrast to collateral ligaments of the knee, healing potential of the ACL is limited because of its susceptible vascular supply.
  - As a result, most ACL injuries do not heal well, and primary surgical repairs (as opposed to reconstructive surgery) are not effective.
  - Left without ACL stability, most knees in young, active patients eventually become symptomatically unstable, and reinjury will occur.
  - In older and less active individuals, nonoperative management of these injuries plays a role; however, most ACL injuries in young athletes should be reconstructed.
  - Leaving the knee unstable makes it vulnerable to injury to the joint capsule, other ligaments, and menisci.
- Meniscal tears
  - Young patients have the potential to heal.
  - Pattern and location of tear determine whether meniscus may heal on its own or will require arthroscopic partial removal or repair.
- Quadriceps contusion
  - Full return of motion is the minimal requirement for return to contact sports, at which time a padded guard should be used.
- Avulsion fracture of the pelvis
  - Most do not displace significantly; almost all heal with time and rest.

- Muscle strain
  - Mild injuries heal fairly rapidly, whereas severe strains can lead to large areas of scar tissue that are prone to reinjury.
  - Reduction of tenderness can take days to weeks, depending on the initial severity of the injury.
  - Reinjury is a problem with hamstring strains.
- Patellar dislocation
  - Recurrent patellar instability, particularly in those with a familial history, may require reconstruction.

PREVENTION

- 4 basic principles of injury-prevention measures
  - Passive strategies are more effective than those requiring repeated actions.
  - Specific advice is more effective than generalized information.
  - Injury control must also include postinjury care and rehabilitation.
  - Attention should focus on common problems for which effective interventions are available.
- Although many sports injuries are random events, nearly two-thirds of all injuries might be reduced by improvements in:
  - Conditioning
  - Equipment
  - Compliance with rules
  - Coaching and supervision
  - Rehabilitation of existing injuries
  - Efforts to prevent reinjury

- Many schools now use certified athletic trainers for prevention of and rehabilitation from sports injuries.
- Heat injury
  - Most authorities suggest that adult-sized athletes drink 0.5 L of fluids per hour during persistent activity.
  - Water is usually adequate.
  - Thirst is not a reliable indicator of fluid requirements during vigorous exercise.
  - Salt tablets should not be provided because most athletes receive abundant salt in their diets.
- Injuries to bone and soft tissue
  - Overuse syndromes
    - Prevention involves the education of young athletes, parents, coaches, and the entire health care team, from trainers to physicians.
    - Understanding these principles is crucial to returning an athlete to sports successfully after experiencing overuse conditions.
    - Failure to change underlying problems leads to reinjury.
  - Osteochondritis dissecans of the capitellum
    - The most important lesson about this condition is the opportunity for prevention.
    - Junior baseball programs typically have rules limiting duration of pitching.
      - Typically, the limit is 3 innings per game and up to 6 innings per week.
    - Young athletes, parents, and coaches need to be educated about this condition so that excessive pitching does not occur at other times.

S

Staphylococcal Toxic Shock Syndrome

DEFINITION

- Staphylococcal toxic shock syndrome (TSS) is a distinct clinical entity characterized by:
  - Fever
  - Diffuse, nonexudative mucous membrane inflammation
  - Vomiting and profuse diarrhea
  - Generalized myalgia
  - Scarlatiniform erythroderma
  - Hypotension
  - Shock associated with multiple organ failure—renal, myocardial, pulmonary, hepatic, hematologic, and central nervous system

EPIDEMIOLOGY

- Incidence
  - 0.53 cases per 100,000 population; rate varies by geographic region
- Prevalence
  - >90% of adults, but fewer children, have antibodies against TSS toxin type 1
  - Occurs in 3 per 100,000 population following all types of surgery
  - Occurs in 16.5 per 100,000 following ear, nose, and throat surgery
- Association with menstruation
  - TSS was first described in association with menstruation and tampon use, but a public health information campaign resulted in a shift to predominantly nonmenstrual cases.
  - Incidence of nonmenstrual cases now exceeds that of menstrual cases.
- Nonmenstrual cases
  - 18.3% were reported after surgical procedures.
  - 11.5% were postpartum or postabortion.
  - 23% were associated with nonsurgical cutaneous lesions.

ETIOLOGY

- Patients who develop staphylococcal TSS are colonized or infected with specific strains of *Staphylococcus aureus*.
- The syndrome is thought to be a superantigen-mediated disease.
  - Superantigens are proteins that can activate the immune system by bypassing steps in the usual antigen-mediated immune response sequence and thus cause an amplified immune response.

RISK FACTORS

- The following superantigens are the major toxins associated with staphylococcal TSS.
  - TSS toxin type 1, a staphylococcal exotoxin
  - Staphylococcal exotoxins A, B, C, D, E, and H

- Absence of antibodies to these superantigens appears to be a major risk factor for staphylococcal TSS
- Their absence explains in part why not all patients exposed to virulent strains develop TSS.

SIGNS AND SYMPTOMS

- Patients are usually healthy before the onset of symptoms.
- Prodrome
  - Occasionally a prodrome may occur in the week before acute illness.
    - Low-grade fever
    - Malaise
    - Myalgia
    - Vomiting
- Acute onset
  - Spiking fever (temperature, 102.2°F–105.8°F [39 C–41°C])
  - Chills
  - Severe gastrointestinal symptoms (abdominal cramps; nausea; vomiting; and profuse, watery, nonbloody diarrhea)
  - Headache
  - Myalgia
  - Sore throat
- 24–72 hours
  - Diffuse, blanching, macular erythroderma (sunburn-like) or scarlatiniform rash that:
    - May be faint or evanescent
    - Is not pruritic but is occasionally petechial
  - Bilateral conjunctival hyperemia without discharge
  - Photophobia
  - Oropharyngeal inflammation, sometimes with an associated strawberry tongue or buccal ulcerations
  - Vaginal erythema with minimal clear watery discharge (in cases associated with menstruation)
  - Orthostatic dizziness or syncope or both (due to orthostatic hypotension)
    - Hypotension: systolic blood pressure 90 mm Hg for adults or <5th percentile by age for children <16 years of age, orthostatic drop in diastolic blood pressure 15 mm Hg from lying to sitting, or orthostatic syncope
- Illness peak (day 2 or 3) (multisystem involvement: ≥3 of the following systems)
  - Central nervous system dysfunction
    - Headache
    - Confusion
    - Disorientation
    - Hallucinations
    - Paresthesias of the hands and feet
    - Stiff, tender neck

- Musculoskeletal
  - Exquisite muscle tenderness
  - Severe myalgias
  - Arthralgias
  - Joint effusions
  - Nonpitting edema over the wrists and ankles
  - Synovitis of the small joints of the hands and feet
- Abdominal
  - Abdominal musculature tenderness
  - Absent or hypoactive bowel sounds
- Renal
  - Azotemia and diminished creatinine clearance (indicating renal involvement)
  - Oliguria
- Pulmonary
  - Shock lung or adult-type respiratory distress syndrome
- Hematologic
  - Progressive normochromic normocytic anemia
  - Thrombocytopenia
  - Leukocytosis
- Cardiac
  - Arrhythmias or prolonged shock, possibly leading to eventual myocardial failure

DIFFERENTIAL DIAGNOSIS

- Staphylococcal TSS must be distinguished from other serious or potentially life-threatening disease.
  - Staphylococcal TSS
    - Hypotension
    - Diffuse erythroderma, Nikolsky sign
    - Red lips
    - Erythematous oral cavity
    - Nonpurulent conjunctivitis
    - Erythematous, edematous hands and feet
    - Desquamation of hands and feet; can be generalized
    - Diarrhea, renal, hepatic, central nervous system, hematologic abnormalities
    - Clinical: culture of S aureus from nasopharynx, vagina, or wound
  - Staphylococcal scalded-skin syndrome
    - No hypotension
    - Erythroderma, bullae, Nikolsky sign
    - Purulent conjunctivitis
    - Hands and feet relatively spared or grossly involved
    - Gross desquamation
    - Clinical: culture of S aureus from nasopharynx or wound, skin biopsy

- Stevens-Johnson syndrome
  - No hypotension
  - Erythema multiforme
  - Bleeding, fissured lips
  - Bullous enanthem of the oral cavity
  - Purulent conjunctivitis
  - Involvement of hands and feet
  - Desquamation involves only individual lesions
  - Respiratory and gastrointestinal tract involvement
  - Clinical: skin biopsy
- Kawasaki disease
  - No hypotension
  - Polymorphous rash
  - Red, fissured lips
  - Erythematous, strawberry tongue
  - Nonpurulent conjunctivitis
  - Erythematous, edematous hands and feet
  - Desquamation of fingertips
  - Coronary aneurysms, generalized vasculitis
  - Clinical: no diagnostic test
- Streptococcal scarlet fever
  - No hypotension
  - Diffuse erythroderma, circumoral pallor, Pastia lines
  - Strawberry tongue
  - Hands and feet relatively spared
  - Fine, flaky desquamation
  - Rheumatic fever, glomerulonephritis
  - Clinical: culture of group A streptococci from pharynx, serology
- Measles
  - No hypotension
  - Morbilliform rash
  - Koplik spots
  - Conjunctivitis
  - Involvement of hands and feet
  - Fine desquamation
  - Respiratory tract involvement
  - Clinical: serology
- Leptospirosis
  - Hypotension, sometimes
  - Erythematous, macular, petechial, purpuric
  - Pharyngitis
  - Conjunctivitis
  - Hands and feet relatively spared
  - Central nervous system, renal, hepatic involvement
  - Clinical: serology

S

- Drug-related toxic epidermal necrolysis
  - Hypotension, sometimes
  - Painful erythroderma, bullae, Nikolsky sign
  - Conjunctivitis
  - Involvement of hands and feet
  - Gross desquamation
  - Clinical: serology
- Streptococcal TSS
  - Hypotension
  - Diffuse erythroderma, maculopapular rash
  - Cracked lips
  - Erythematous oral cavity
  - Injected eyes
  - Confusion, abdominal pain and vomiting, hyperesthesia
  - Clinical: culture of group A streptococci

DIAGNOSTIC APPROACH

- Although no laboratory test is available to confirm the diagnosis of staphylococcal TSS, obtain the following cultures.
  - Blood
  - Throat
  - Vagina
  - Nares
  - Rectum
  - Other appropriate sites

LABORATORY FINDINGS

- Initial laboratory findings
  - Leukocytosis, with a striking increase in the percentage of immature neutrophils
  - Progressive anemia
  - Thrombocytopenia, accompanied by:
    - Prolongation of prothrombin time
    - Prolongation of partial thromboplastin time
    - Appearance of increased fibrin split products
  - Hypoproteinemia and hypoalbuminemia
  - Metabolic acidosis, possibly complicated by hyponatremia and hypokalemia as a result of accompanying persistent vomiting and diarrhea
  - Dangerously low serum concentrations of calcium (tetany is rare)
  - Elevated blood urea nitrogen and creatinine levels (at least twice the upper limit of normal [early in the illness])
    - Urinary sediment with pyuria (>5 leukocytes/high-power field) in the absence of urinary tract infection
    - Peak abnormal values occur after 5–7 days and then usually return rapidly to normal.
  - Hypophosphatemia (first days of illness)

- Elevated creatine phosphokinase level (at least twice the upper limit of normal) with occasional myoglobinemia
- Total bilirubin, serum aspartate aminotransferase, or serum alanine aminotransferase levels at least twice the upper limit of normal
- Platelet count <100,000 cels/mm^3

TREATMENT APPROACH

- Initial steps in management
  - Consider other possible diagnoses.
  - Remove potentially infected foreign bodies (eg, tampons).
  - Drain and irrigate infected sites.
  - Give an intravenous antistaphylococcal ß-lactamase–resistant antimicrobial agent at maximal dose for weight and age.
  - Consider methylprednisolone for severe cases.
  - Treat aggressively and monitor for the following.
    - Hypovolemia and inadequate tissue perfusion
    - Adult-type respiratory distress syndrome
    - Myocardial dysfunction
    - Acute renal failure
    - Cerebral edema
    - Hypocalcemia, hypophosphatemia
    - Metabolic acidosis
    - Disseminated intravascular coagulation
    - Fluid and electrolyte abnormalities
- The first and major resuscitative goal is:
  - Administer large volumes (2–4 times normal daily maintenance) of crystalloid (lactated Ringer solution) or colloid (fresh-frozen plasma or albumin) solutions to restore normal intravascular volume and correct hypotension.
    - Treatment of hypotension may require vasopressor therapy (eg, dopamine or dobutamine).
      - Much of the administered fluid is sequestered outside the intravascular space, sometimes leading to marked edema.
    - Have a central venous pressure line or a Swan-Ganz catheter in place to monitor left-ventricular end-diastolic pressure (prevent congestive heart failure due to overly vigorous fluid resuscitation).
- Patients who develop adult-type respiratory distress syndrome or shock lung require endotracheal intubation and ventilatory assistance with positive end-expiratory pressure and high oxygen flow rates. The following can occur in such patients:
  - Renal failure
  - Severe electrolyte and acid-base abnormalities
  - Ventricular ectopy
  - Refractory ventricular arrhythmias
  - Disseminated intravascular coagulation

S

SPECIFIC TREATMENTS

Antibiotics

- High-dose ß-lactamase–resistant antistaphylococcal antibiotics are recommended to eradicate the organism and prevent recurrences.
- Nafcillin, oxacillin, and first-generation cephalosporins are the first-line agents for *S aureus*.
- Vancomycin should not be used routinely as initial empirical therapy.
  - Methicillin-resistant *S aureus* causes <1% of cases of staphylococcal TSS.
  - Methicillin-resistant *S aureus* recently emerged as a community pathogen and thus raised an important issue of initial empirical antibiotic therapy in these patients.
  - Clindamycin plus a ß-lactamase–resistant antistaphylococcal agent may help by decreasing the synthesis of TSS toxin type 1.
  - Duration of antimicrobial therapy:
    - ≥10–14 days, to eradicate the organism and prevent recurrences
    - Total duration is based on the usual duration established for the underlying focus of infection.

Intravenous immunoglobulin

- May be an effective adjunctive therapy for diseases associated with superantigens
  - Usual dose: 400 mg/kg over 4–8 hours as a single dose
  - A higher dose may be required for staphylococcal TSS to achieve protective titers and clinical efficacy.

High-dose corticosteroids

- May be of possible benefit for shock syndromes, but should not be administered routinely to patients with TSS because they:
  - May result in a shorter time to defervescence and clinical stability
  - Make no difference in overall risk for death

Nonsteroidal anti-inflammatory drugs

- Contraindicated because they may increase progression to TSS by enhancing production of tumor necrosis factor

WHEN TO ADMIT

- Nearly all patients with staphylococcal TSS should be hospitalized.
- For significant hypotension (and probable coexistence of multiple organ system failure), pursue the steps outlined in Management while arranging transport to a tertiary care facility.
  - There, continued management largely will be supportive and dictated by the degree of organ dysfunction.

WHEN TO REFER

- All patients must be managed in consultation with infectious disease and critical care specialists.
  - The pediatrician plays a key role in coordinating the care.

COMPLICATIONS

- Adult-type respiratory distress syndrome
- Multi-organ failure
- Death

PROGNOSIS

- Most patients with staphylococcal TSS recover within 7–10 days.
- Fatigue and weakness for as long as 3 months may occur in the recovery phase.
- The case fatality rate is 2–5%.
- Convalescence is characterized by a desquamation of the palms and soles within 1–2 weeks after the onset of illness.
- Some patients also experience hair and nail loss.
- Although most patients with TSS do not experience pulmonary compromise, mortality is increased if early or prolonged adult-type respiratory distress syndrome becomes apparent.
- Nongenital TSS seems to carry a worse prognosis than vaginal disease, probably because of delayed diagnosis and the more serious nature of the primary infection.
- Refractory hypotension is associated with mortality rates of up to 50%.

PREVENTION

- The incidence of recurrent staphylococcal TSS may be as high as 28% if the patient does not receive antistaphylococcal antibiotics and does not produce antibody to toxin.
- The criteria for recurrent disease are less stringent than those required for defining an initial episode.
- Recurrent vaginal TSS occurs, but much less frequently than genital vaginal disease.
- Persistent neuropsychological symptoms, such as fatigue, depression, and memory loss, have been described in up to 50% of patients who recover from nonvaginal TSS.

S

Stomatitis

DEFINITION

- Inflammation of the oral mucosa, characterized by multiple ulcerations inside the mouth
  - Frequently painful
  - May lead to decreased oral intake and dehydration

EPIDEMIOLOGY

- Recurrent aphthous stomatitis (RAS) is the most common form of painful oral ulcers.
  - Prevalence
    - 37% of surveyed school-age children reported a history of RAS.
  - Age
    - Peak age of onset is the second decade of life.
    - Bouts may recur throughout adulthood.
- Viral infection is the most common infectious cause of stomatitis.
  - In 1 study, 33% of 5- to 17-year-old participants reported a history of recurrent herpes labialis.
  - Herpangina (acute febrile illness associated with the development of lesions in the posterior oropharynx) and hand-foot-mouth disease (HFMD) are quite frequent in young children.
    - Outbreaks of acute stomatitis caused by herpangina are most likely to occur in the summer and early fall.
    - HFMD is most likely to occur in the spring and summer.
- Stomatitis as the only presenting feature of a systemic disorder does occur, but it is rare.
  - Approximately 15% of patients with aphthous ulcers and other symptoms have a systemic disorder.
- Periodic fever accompanied by aphthous stomatitis, pharyngitis, and (cervical) adenopathy (PFAPA) syndrome is a relatively new entity.
  - Multiple case series have been reported in the medical literature.

ETIOLOGY

- Stomatitis can be a disease entity unto itself, such as RAS, or it may be a symptom of an underlying condition.
- RAS is a benign condition characterized by painful oral ulcers that recur at irregular intervals.
  - In otherwise healthy individuals, most cases are idiopathic.
  - Exact cause of RAS is not known.
- Medical interventions may lead to stomatitis.
  - Chemotherapy agents and radiation disrupt the mucosal barrier of the mouth, allowing ulceration, desquamation, and secondary infection by both acquired and endogenous flora.
- Medications that can lead to oral dryness and the development of aphthous stomatitis
  - Cyclooxygenase-2 inhibitors
  - Nonsteroidal anti-inflammatory drugs
  - Sertraline

RISK FACTORS

- Suggested triggers include:
  - Stress
  - Genetics
  - Hormonal and immunologic influences
  - Trauma
  - Smoking
- Viruses
  - Herpes simplex
  - Varicella-zoster
  - Various subtypes of coxsackie
    - Herpangina
    - Coxsackie A16 is the most common cause of HFMD, but other enteroviral subtypes have been implicated as causative agents.
  - Rubeola
  - Epstein-Barr virus
  - HIV
- Trauma
  - Secondary to biting one's own mucosa
  - Friction from dental appliances
  - Riga-Fede syndrome (rare)
    - Formation of ulcerative lesions of the lower lip, lingual frenulum, and ventral tongue secondary to repeated rubbing of the teeth against these mucosal surfaces
    - Age of onset: 6–8 months
    - Coincides with the age of primary tooth eruption
- Irritant exposure
  - Excessive heat
  - Cold
  - Acidic or basic substances
  - Smokeless tobacco
    - Leads to oral lesions in older school-age children
  - Misuse of commercial mouthwash with high alcohol content
- Allergic contact stomatitis
  - Incites an allergic delayed-type hypersensitivity reaction
  - Preservatives and oral flavorings (eg, cinnamon, menthol, peppermint) may cause a reaction.

- Metals (eg, nickel found in dental instruments) may elicit an oral allergic reaction.
- Systemic disorders
- Bacteria
  - *Borrelia vincentii* and *Fusobacterium dentium* are bacterial causes of oral inflammation known as *necrotizing ulcerative gingivitis.*
  - Syphilis
  - Gonorrhea
  - Tuberculosis
- Fungi
  - Infrequently cause stomatitis in otherwise healthy children
  - *Candida albicans*
    - Infection is common in the newborn.
  - Histoplasmosis
    - Can develop in otherwise healthy children and produce mucosal ulceration along with other systemic manifestations

SIGNS AND SYMPTOMS

- RAS
  - Oral lesions are the only physical examination finding.
    - Assess for ≥1 painful ulcers on the buccal, labial, and lingual surfaces, as well as on the floor of the mouth.
  - 3 clinically distinct types of RAS
    - Minor variety
      - Small, round craters, <5 mm in diameter and surrounded by an erythematous halo
      - Heal in 1–2 weeks
    - Major variety
      - Lesions >5 mm that often scar
      - May last 6 weeks
    - Herpetiform variety
      - Herpes-like appearance of multiple, small clusters of pinpoint lesions
      - Resolve in 7–10 days
      - Not caused by the herpes virus
  - Children with RAS are otherwise healthy.
- Herpes simplex virus type 1
  - Fever, malaise, sore throat, and cervical adenopathy are present.
  - Vesicles can develop anywhere on the oral mucosa, most typically in the anterior oropharynx on the lips, tongue, and buccal mucosa
  - Gingiva may be swollen and erythematous.
  - The perioral area may also display vesicles and small ulcers that coalesce and continue to appear for the next week.

- Oral pain is present.
  - May result in anorexia and dehydration
- Spontaneous resolution in 7–10 days
- Coxsackievirus
  - Herpangina
  - Ulcers surrounded by erythematous halos located in the posterior oropharynx
  - Spontaneous resolution in 3–5 days
  - HFMD
    - Along with lesions of the posterior oropharynx, blanching red macules or vesicles appear on the palms, soles, and buttocks.
    - Erythematous halos may surround the macules.
    - Resolve spontaneously within a week
  - Fever, malaise, dysphagia, and anorexia accompany coxsackie infections and can lead to dehydration in children.
- Necrotizing ulcerative gingivitis
  - Painful, erythematous, and friable gingiva
  - Necrotic tissue accumulates as a pseudomembrane over the gingival surface.
  - Foul breath
  - Fever, malaise, anorexia, and dehydration may be present.
- Candidal mucositis
  - White, curdlike patches on many of the surfaces of the oral mucosa
    - If white patch is scraped and removed, an ulceration will be present at the base.
  - Diaper dermatitis may also be present.
- Contact stomatitis
  - Can present in 4 general ways
    - Red lesions with general mouth erythema
    - White lesions and leukoplakia
    - Erosions and ulcerations
    - No obvious lesions accompanied by mouth pain and burning
  - The manifestation of stomatitis in the multitude of potential underlying multisystem diseases will vary depending on the diagnosis.
  - Immunocompromised patients may:
    - Experience more frequent and severe episodes of oral ulceration
    - Take longer for episodes to resolve
  - Appearance of individual aphthae in stomatitis secondary to a benign or self-limiting condition may be indistinguishable from that associated with a serious underlying systemic disease.

S

- Important to identify other symptoms and use physical examination findings to determine the appropriate etiology
- PFAPA syndrome
  - Recurrent fevers every 4–6 weeks with onset in the first 6 years of life
  - General malaise, anorexia, headache, abdominal pain, and arthralgias are present.
  - Symptoms typically resolve within 1 week.
  - The child has complete resolution of symptoms between recurrences.

DIFFERENTIAL DIAGNOSIS

- RAS infection
  - Viruses
    - Herpes simplex type 1
    - Varicella-zoster, coxsackie
    - Other enteroviruses
    - Rubeola
    - Epstein-Barr virus
    - HIV
  - Bacteria
    - *B vincentii*
    - *F dentium*
    - Syphilis
    - Gonorrhea
    - Tuberculosis
  - Fungi
    - *Candida*
    - Histoplasmosis
- Irritant contact stomatitis
- Allergic contact stomatitis
- Iatrogenically induced stomatitis
- Systemic disorders
  - Behçet syndrome
  - Inflammatory bowel disease
  - Celiac disease
  - Diabetes mellitus
  - Systemic lupus erythematosus
  - Scleroderma
  - Dermatomyositis
  - Wegener granulomatosis
  - PFAPA syndrome
  - Cyclic neutropenia
  - Nutritional deficiencies
  - Dermatologic disorders

LABORATORY FINDINGS

- In most cases, laboratory evaluation is not helpful in diagnosis or management.
- Measure serum electrolytes in patients with severe dehydration during the rehydration process.
- If frequently recurring or persistent oral aphthae are present, along with genital lesions or other systemic findings, an evaluation for the underlying cause may include:
  - Complete blood count
  - Erythrocyte sedimentation rate
  - Serum levels of:
    - Iron
    - Folate
    - Vitamin B_{12}
    - Zinc
  - Depending on the history, screening for the following may be necessary:
    - Antinuclear antibodies
    - HIV
    - Celiac disease

TREATMENT APPROACH

- Goals of treatment
  - Relieving pain
  - Preventing dehydration
- By maximizing pain relief, the child will be able to remain hydrated and consume a soft diet.

SPECIFIC TREATMENTS

Pain relief

- Systemic ibuprofen, acetaminophen, or opiates
- Application of topical substances
  - Swish and then spit *or*
  - Paint the substance on the sores with a cotton-tip swab.
  - Topical agents that have been studied minimally for safety and efficacy include:
    - Saline rinses
    - Diphenhydramine–aluminum hydroxide with magnesium hydroxide–viscous lidocaine compounded in various combinations
    - Benzocaine
    - Kaolin
    - Pectin
  - Most of these agents, if used too aggressively, can lead to overdose and adverse side effects.

S

- Topical anesthetic preparations in particular must be used cautiously.
  - Risk of aspiration, loss of protective airway reflexes, and systemic toxicity caused by absorption through inflamed oral mucosa
- In the immunocompromised child or child with stomatitis secondary to cancer treatment:
  - Use topical and systemic analgesics for pain relief.
    - Topical sucralfate and capsaicin have been found to relieve pain of chemotherapy- or radiation-induced mucositis.
    - These agents are not routinely used for children with benign, self-limiting conditions.
  - Monitor for secondary infection.

Antimicrobial treatment

- Antimicrobials are of limited value.
  - In patients with necrotizing ulcerative gingivitis, the following may be required:
    - Chlorhexidine mouth rinses
    - Systemic antibiotics, such as penicillin
- Oral acyclovir is of limited therapeutic benefit in the otherwise healthy child with herpes stomatitis.
  - Topical acyclovir is ineffective.

PFAPA syndrome

- Typically responds well to short course of oral steroids (1–2 mg/kg per day for 5 days) if prescribed at the onset of symptoms

WHEN TO ADMIT

- Hospitalization may be required for intravenous rehydration therapy in a child who cannot eat and drink because of severe pain from mouth lesions.

WHEN TO REFER

- Referral to an oral surgeon or otolaryngologist should be considered when:
  - Underlying cause of the stomatitis is uncertain *or*
  - If oral lesions persist for >2 weeks
  - Biopsy of the lesion may be necessary.
    - Especially for a child who uses smokeless tobacco
- Children with stomatitis plus multiple symptoms and abnormal physical examination findings may require specialty expertise to establish the definitive diagnosis and administer appropriate treatment.
  - Allergist-immunologist
  - Rheumatologist
  - Dermatologist
  - Gastroenterologist
  - Ophthalmologist

PREVENTION

- Most causes of stomatitis cannot be prevented.
- In general, promote:
  - Avoidance of tobacco products and any possible irritants
  - Good oral hygiene to reduce the risk of dental caries and gingivitis
- Minimize exposure to the proposed triggers for RAS.
- On the basis of studies in adults, continuous oral acyclovir is a therapeutic option for preventing recurrences in a child with frequent herpetic flares.
- Children with cancer may benefit from a preventive protocol that includes:
  - Frequent plaque biofilm removal and teeth brushing
  - Chlorhexidine or saline rinses
  - Nystatin

S

Strabismus

DEFINITION

- *Strabismus* is the condition of ocular misalignment.
  - Esotropia: eye turned in
  - Exotropia: eye turned out
  - Vertical strabismus: eye turned up or down
    - Hypertropia: deviation upward
    - Hypotropia: deviation downward
- Comitant strabismus: deviation the same in all fields of gaze
- Incomitant strabismus: limited eye movement and different deviation in different fields of gaze
- A *phoria* is a tendency for the eyes to drift apart, but alignment is maintained by binocular fusion.
- A *tropia* is a manifest deviation of the eyes, without binocular fusion.
- Infantile (congenital) esotropia: a large esotropia with onset before 6 months of age
- Pseudoesotropia: The eyes are straight, but a wide nasal bridge and epicanthal folds give the appearance of esotropia.
- Accommodative esotropia: an acquired deviation (most often at 1–5 years) usually associated with farsightedness
- Sensory esotropia: an esodeviation caused by unilateral blindness
- Convergence insufficiency: an exotropia at near fixation, but straight eyes with distance fixation

MECHANISM

- Comitant strabismus
  - Not usually associated with neurologic disease
- Incomitant strabismus involves limited eye movement from:
  - Restriction
    - Periocular scarring
    - Tight extraocular muscles
  - Neuromuscular paresis
    - Cranial nerve palsies: third, fourth, sixth

PHYSICAL EXAM

Infantile estropia

- The patient may show a strong fixation preference for one eye, indicating amblyopia.
- The patient may alternate fixation.
- Amblyopia occurs in approximately 50% of children with infantile esotropia.
- Some limitation of abduction often is found in voluntary version testing.
  - However, the doll's head maneuver reveals normal abduction and normal lateral rectus function.
- Associated motor anomalies are often related to infantile esotropia.
  - Develop late, at age 1 or 2 years, often several months after the esotropia has been surgically corrected

- Vertical strabismus (inferior oblique overaction in 70% and dissociated vertical deviation in 75%)
- Nystagmus
  - Unusual in children with congenital esotropia
  - Latent nystagmus is found in approximately 50% of cases.
    - Becomes evident during standard vision testing when one eye is covered.
    - The best visual potential in children with latent nystagmus is obtained by testing with both eyes open (binocular vision) to avoid inducing nystagmus.

Pseudoestropia

- Pseudoesotropia is common and should be distinguished from infantile esotropia.
  - The infant has a wide nasal bridge and wide, prominent epicanthal folds, giving the appearance of esotropia.
  - However, the eyes actually are orthotropic.
  - Hirschberg corneal light reflex test can document proper eye alignment.
  - Follow-up is important in patients with pseudoesotropia, because a small percentage will develop true esotropia.

Accommodative esotropia

- Esotropia is seen mostly at near fixation or when the child is tired.
  - The child may squint or close 1 eye.
  - The deviation initially is small and intermittent.
- Over time—sometimes only a few weeks—the deviation may increase to become constant, and amblyopia may develop.

Intermittent exotropia

- Initially, an exotropia may be present only when the patient is fatigued or ill.
- Covering 1 eye will produce the exotropia; thus, this form of strabismus is best detected by the cover test.
- Symptoms include:
  - Blurred vision
  - Asthenopia (vague visual discomfort, such as eyestrain or brow ache)
  - Visual fatigue
  - Photophobia with squinting is thought to be a mechanism for eliminating diplopia or confusion.
- The natural history is variable.
  - Approximately 70% of patients show increasing frequency of exotropia and progressive loss of fusion.
  - 20% stay the same.
  - A small percentage improve over time.
  - During the exophoric phase, patients have bifoveal fusion with excellent stereo acuity.
    - When exotropia (developed strabismus) is present, most patients demonstrate suppression.

– Patients with late-onset intermittent exotropia (after 5 or 6 years of age) sometimes experience diplopia.

– Significant amblyopia is rare in patients with intermittent exotropia.

Convergence insufficiency

■ A type of intermittent exotropia characterized by an exotropia at near fixation but straight eyes with distance fixation

■ Appropriate near convergence is insufficient.

Fourth nerve palsy

■ A superior oblique palsy (fourth nerve palsy) is the most common cause of a vertical deviation.

■ The superior oblique muscle is a depressor and intortor (twists the eye nasally).

■ A weak superior oblique muscle will cause:

• Strabismus consisting of hypertropia (vertical strabismus)

• Extorsion (temporal twisting of the eye)

■ The hypertropia is worse when the patient's head tilts to the side of the weak superior oblique muscle.

■ The hypertropia diminishes with head tilt to the side opposite the palsy.

■ Patients with a superior oblique paresis usually exhibit a compensatory head tilt to the opposite side of the paresis to help keep their eyes aligned.

■ A family photo album should be examined to estimate onset of the head tilt.

■ Patients with congenital superior oblique paresis typically have good stereopsis and exhibit the hyper-deviation intermittently when fatigued.

■ Most have the ability to suppress so as not to experience diplopia when the deviation is apparent.

■ Facial asymmetry

• A subtle finding in most children with a congenital superior oblique palsy

• The dependent side of the face is more shallow and atrophied, possibly as the result of the effects of gravity on facial development.

■ Even though the paresis present at birth, symptoms may develop in late childhood or even adulthood.

■ Over time, the fusional control weakens and results in a deviation that becomes apparent later in life.

Sixth nerve palsy

■ Results in limited abduction and an esotropia that is worse on the side of the palsy

■ Neonates can have a transient sixth nerve palsy, often associated with a facial palsy.

• Resolves spontaneously by 4–8 weeks

■ Approximately one half of sixth nerve palsies resolve over a 6-month observational period.

Third nerve palsy

■ Involves all extraocular muscles (ie, medial rectus, superior rectus, inferior rectus, inferior oblique muscles) except the lateral rectus (sixth cranial nerve) and the superior oblique (fourth cranial nerve)

• Because both major vertical muscles are weak, the eye does not move up or down and is exotropic because of the weak medial rectus muscle.

• The levator muscle of the upper eyelid is also innervated by the third cranial nerve, and ptosis is usually present.

• The pupil is large and nonreactive in complete third nerve palsy.

Brown syndrome

■ Clinical findings include:

• Limited elevation in adduction

• An exodeviation in attempted upgaze

• An ipsilateral hypotropia that increases in upgaze

■ Most patients with Brown syndrome have good binocular vision with a compensatory chin elevation and slight face turn away from the affected eye.

Double elevator palsy

■ Congenital limitation of elevation of 1 eye

■ The term *double elevator* implies paresis of the superior rectus muscle and inferior oblique muscle.

• However, in 70% of cases, the deficient elevation results from a tight inferior rectus muscle.

■ May be mistaken for Brown syndrome

• The limited elevation in Brown syndrome is worse in adduction than in abduction.

DIFFERENTIAL DIAGNOSIS

Differential diagnosis of infantile esotropia

■ Duane syndrome

• Caused by a congenital hypoplasia of the sixth nerve nucleus with misdirection of the medial rectus nerve, innervating both the medial rectus and the lateral rectus muscles

• Because both the medial and the lateral rectus muscles are innervated by the nerve to the medial rectus muscle, both muscles fire and contract simultaneously on attempted adduction.

• This co-contraction of the medial and lateral rectus muscles causes globe retraction and lid fissure narrowing on attempted adduction.

• Most children with Duane syndrome adopt a compensatory face turn to keep their eyes straight.

■ Congenital fibrosis syndrome of extraocular muscles

• Rare

• Congenital fibrosis of the extraocular muscles usually is inherited as an autosomal-dominant trait.

S

- Cause unknown
- Associated with fibrotic replacement of extraocular muscle tissue
- Clinical features may be classified into 5 groups.
  - Generalized fibrosis syndrome
  - Fibrosis of inferior rectus with blepharophimosis
  - Strabismus fixus
  - Vertical retraction syndrome
  - Unilateral fibrosis blepharoptosis and enophthalmos
- Because of the tight fibrotic muscles, ductions are limited.
- The medial rectus muscle is affected most commonly, producing an esotropia.
- The fibrosis can be generalized and can affect virtually all of the rectus muscles.
- Congenital sixth nerve palsy
- Möbius syndrome associated with sixth nerve paresis
  - Rare
  - Characterized by:
    - Facial palsy
    - Sixth nerve palsy, often with a partial third nerve palsy
    - Distal limb abnormalities such as syndactyly or even amputation defects
  - Craniofacial anomalies can occur.
    - Micrognathia
    - Tongue abnormalities
    - Facial or oral clefts
  - Ocular motility abnormalities include:
    - Failure of the eyes to abduct
    - Presence of lid retraction on adduction (also typical in some patients with Duane syndrome)
  - The facial palsy usually spares the lower face, although orbicularis function is weak.
  - Skeletal abnormalities also include pectoralis muscle deficits.
  - Inheritance pattern is variable and may be familial, but most cases are sporadic.
- Infantile myasthenia gravis
- These disorders all have limited abduction, and they can therefore be differentiated from infantile esotropia, in which the ductions should be full.
- Esotropia in an infant may also be an important sign of vision loss.
  - Disorders, such as congenital cataracts and retinoblastoma, often first exhibit as infantile esotropia.

Differential diagnosis of acquired esotropia

- Includes any neurologic cause of a sixth nerve palsy, including:
  - Intracranial tumors
  - Meningitis
  - Mastoiditis (Gradenigo syndrome)
  - Hydrocephalus
  - Arnold-Chiari malformation
  - Myasthenia gravis
  - Viral illness

Differential diagnosis of an incomitant strabismus

- Fourth nerve palsy
  - Congenital superior oblique palsy
    - The most common cause of vertical strabismus
    - The child has a compensatory head tilt, often misdiagnosed as torticollis.
  - Acquired superior oblique paresis
    - Trauma—tends to be bilateral
    - Vascular disease
    - Multiple sclerosis
    - Intracranial neoplasm
    - Herpes zoster ophthalmicus
    - Diabetes with mononeuropathy
- Sixth nerve palsy (see above)
- Duane syndrome (see above)
- Möbius syndrome (see above)
- Third nerve palsy
  - Congenital
  - Trauma
  - Intracranial tumor
  - Viral illness
  - Posterior communicating aneurysm
- Brown syndrome
  - Inability to elevate eye in adduction
  - Acquired Brown syndrome
    - Inflammation around the superior oblique tendon, often from chronic sinusitis
  - Congenital Brown syndrome
    - Congenitally tight superior oblique tendon complex
  - Clinical findings include:
    - Limited elevation in adduction
    - Exodeviation with attempted upward gaze
    - Ipsilateral hypotropia that increases with upward gaze
  - Most patients with Brown syndrome have good binocular vision with a compensatory chin elevation and slight face turn away from the affected eye.
- Double elevator palsy
  - May be mistaken for Brown syndrome, but limited elevation in Brown syndrome is worse in adduction than abduction
- Congenital fibrosis syndrome (see above)

IMAGING

- If no specific cause of an acquired superior oblique paresis can be found, then a neurologic workup, including neuroimaging, should be performed.

SPECIFIC TREATMENT

Infantile esotropia

- Best treated with early surgery
  - Surgery usually is performed when the patient is between 6 months and 2 years of age.
  - Peripheral fusion can be achieved if the eyes are aligned before 2 years of age.
  - Surgery should be considered as early as 3 months of age if the following criteria are met.
    - Large-angle esotropia (≥40 prism diopters)
    - Constant or increasing deviation documented by 2 visits 1 month apart
    - Infant able to tolerate anesthesia
- Approximately half of children with congenital esotropia will require multiple surgeries.
- Excellent fusion with high-grade stereopsis and good alignment can be obtained when surgery is performed before the child is 6 months old.

Acquired esotropia

- Immediate referral is important.
  - To provide early treatment to establish binocular vision
  - To rule out ocular or neurologic disease

Accommodative esotropia

- Unlike children with congenital esotropia, patients with acquired accommodative esotropia have had straight eyes during early visual development; thus, they retain relatively good fusion potential.
  - The earlier the eyes are straightened, the better the chances will be for recovering fusion.
- Accommodative estropia is usually associated with farsightedness.
- The first line of treatment is to prescribe spectacles.
  - If spectacles do not correct the esotropia, then surgery will be needed.
- Patients who are corrected to proper alignment with glasses for distance viewing, but whose eyes still cross at near viewing, can be prescribed bifocal glasses.
  - In most cases, these children will need spectacles after surgery to maintain good alignment.
- Early treatment is critical to achieving best results.

Sensory esotropia

- An esodeviation caused by unilateral blindness
- Loss of vision may cause an eye to drift.
  - If the visual loss occurs before 2 years of age, then patients develop esotropia.
  - If the vision loss occurs after 2 years of age, then patients develop exotropia.
- Requires urgent intervention
- Treatment
  - Recession-resection procedure of the blind eye
  - Surgery is not performed on the eye with good vision.

Intermittent exotropia

- Treatment is elective.
  - Eye muscle surgery is the treatment of choice for most forms of intermittent exotropia.
    - Usually requires strabismus surgery if the deviation is poorly controlled
- Indications for surgery include:
  - Increasing exotropia
  - Exotropia is present >50% of the time.
  - Poor fusion control of the exotropia
- Nonsurgical treatments include:
  - Part-time occlusion of the dominant eye
  - Correction for myopia
  - Eye exercises
- Nonsurgical interventions act as temporary treatments at best, except in patients with a special type of exotropia known as convergence insufficiency.
  - The one form of strabismus that is best treated with eye exercises instead of surgery

Duane syndrome

- Strabismus surgery
  - Effective for correcting the compensatory face turn
  - Improves abduction slightly, but does not result in full abduction capabilities

Brown syndrome

- The management of true congenital Brown syndrome is conservative unless the vertical deviation in primary position is significant.
- In most cases, waiting until the child's vision is mature before performing surgery is advised because an induced strabismus after surgery is not uncommon and can lead to the loss of binocular vision.

S

- Acquired Brown syndrome
  - Usual treatment is treating sinusitis, if present, and providing oral nonsteroidal antiinflammatory drugs
  - Surgery usually is not usually indicated for acquired inflammatory Brown syndrome.

Congenital fibrosis syndrome

- Treatment is surgical recession of the fibrotic muscle.
- These cases can be technically difficult because exposure of the muscle is limited, especially in cases with a fibrotic medial rectus muscle.

WHEN TO REFER

- Acquired strabismus
- Diplopia
- Limited eye movements (incomitant strabismus)
- Ptosis or other neurologic signs
- Poor vision or abnormal red reflex

Strange Behavior

DEFINITION

- Pervasive developmental disorder (PDD) is a neuropsychiatric disorder that is usually identified in the first 5 years of life.

- In separation anxiety disorder (SAD), the child experiences excessive anxiety of a magnitude that leads to disruptions in social or academic function when separated from home or from those to whom the child is attached.

- Posttraumatic stress disorder (PTSD) requires exposure to an extreme traumatic stressor involving direct personal experience of an event that included actual or threatened death or serious injury to make the diagnosis.

- Pica is the persistent eating of nonnutritive substances.

- Rumination disorder is characterized by repeated regurgitation and rechewing of food.

- Feeding disorder of infancy or early childhood involves persistent failure to eat adequately.

- Gender identity is the child's sense of being male or female.

- A transitional object is the first possession used by the child as a defense against anxiety, which arises in the course of separation and individuation from the mother or primary caretaker.

- Oppositional defiant disorder (ODD) is characterized by recurrent, severe pattern of negativistic, defiant, disobedient, and hostile behaviors toward authority figures lasting >6 months.

- Conduct disorder is characterized by repetitive and persistent pattern of behavior in which basic rights of others and social rules and norms are violated.

- Pathological dissociation is defined as disruption of integrated functions of consciousness, memory, identity, or perception of environment.

- Depersonalization is a subjective sense of being unreal, strange, or unfamiliar to oneself.

- Major depressive disorder is the presence of a single major depressive episode, with ≥5 or more symptoms lasting for ≥2 weeks and occuring daily.

- Manic episode is a distinct period of abnormally and persistently elevated, expansive, or irritable mood lasting for at least 1 week.

- Psychosis currently implies serious disturbance in an individual's reality testing, as evidenced by hallucinations, delusions, and disturbances in the form of thinking.

EPIDEMIOLOGY

- Transitional objects and imaginary companions
  - Existence of transitional objects and imaginary companions is common in early childhood.
  - In 1 study:
    - 65% of children between 3 and 5 of age years had imaginary playmates.
    - 75% of children had transitional objects.

- Attention-deficit/hyperactivity disorder (ADHD)
  - Most prevalent and important psychiatric disorder of middle childhood years
  - Current prevalence estimates in the school-age population are between 3% and 5%.
- ODD
  - Occurs frequently in children with ADHD
- Dissociative disorders
  - Prevalence in children and adolescents is unknown.
  - 85–100% of adults who have dissociative identity disorder have documented histories of severe childhood abuse.
- Psychotic disorders
  - Very uncommon in prepubertal children
- Schizophrenia
  - In adolescence, frequency increases dramatically.
- Eating disorders
  - Anorexia nervosa and bulimia nervosa are common psychiatric disorders of childhood.
  - Commonly occur in adolescence
  - Prevalence has increased markedly over the last 50 years.
  - Much more common in girls, with onset typically in later adolescence
  - Most typically girls are white and upper middle-class
  - Seen mostly in Western industrialized nations

MECHANISM

- Pathological dissociation
  - Major risk factors
    - Childhood trauma
    - Early sexual abuse
  - Dissociation is a defensive coping mechanism that functions to protect the child against extreme pain and vulnerability in severe childhood abuse.
- Eating disorders
  - In puberty, the need for the young girl to integrate realities of menstruation, breast development, and the broadening of hips can result in:
    - Transient perturbations of body image
    - Abnormal eating behaviors

HISTORY

Infancy and early childhood (birth to 5 years)
PDD

- Specific deviance noted in the domains of:
  - Language
  - Communication
  - Personal-social domains

- Includes related abnormalities in stereotypic and repetitive behaviors
■ Communication impairments seen in children with PDD include:
  - Abnormalities in verbal and nonverbal communication
  - Delay in spoken and gestural language
  - Use of echolalia
■ About two-thirds of children with PDD are mentally retarded.
■ Cognitive delay is not intrinsic to the diagnosis.
■ Social abnormalities seen in PDD are present in the first year of life.
■ Children who have PDD have little interest in
  - Human faces
  - Interactions with others
■ Deficit in social interaction can be identified in the 1st year of life by astute and experienced observer.
■ Frequent signs include bizarre, restricted, and repetitive stereotypic behaviors, such as:
  - Flapping
  - Spinning
  - Head banging
■ Asperger disorder
  - Subcategory of PDD
  - Differs from classical presentation of PDD
  - Language and cognitive functioning are preserved.
  - Social abnormalities and stereotypic behaviors are present.

Reactive attachment disorder of infancy or early childhood

■ Abnormalities of social relatedness are the hallmark.
■ Abnormalities are rooted in grossly pathological care of the child in the earliest years of life.
■ Children can display inhibited type of reactive attachment disorder in which they appear:
  - Withdrawn
  - Hypervigilant
  - Resistant to all attempts to establish relatedness or comfort
■ In the disinhibited type, children show:
  - Indiscriminate sociability
  - Excessive sociability
  - Superficial sociability
■ In both cases, failure to develop age-appropriate attachment behaviors is obvious.
■ In extreme cases, children may fail to thrive with:
  - Severe growth and cognitive delays
  - Developmental deviances are related to failure of caretaking and attachment.

SAD

■ The child often refuses to go to school.
■ Unwilling to travel independently
■ Unwilling to be separated from the parent for brief, developmentally appropriate activities, such as:
  - Play dates
  - Sleepovers
  - Camping
■ Child with SAD will often:
  - Shadow the parent
  - Refuse to be on a different floor of the house
  - Refuse to sleep alone
■ Common traits are excessive worries, including:
  - Generating frightening fantasies about misfortune occurring to the parent

PTSD

■ Well established in adults, adolescents, and children
■ Formidable challenge to diagnose in children <5 years
■ *Diagnostic and Statistical Manual of Mental Disorders, 4th edition (DSM-IV)* criteria require:
  - Verbal descriptions of thoughts and experiences, which are difficult to obtain from children whose language skills are limited
■ Clinical observations of the posttraumatic symptoms of early childhood
  - Strongly visualized or repetitively perceived memories of the traumatic event can either take form of the well-known flashback or be less intrusive.
  - Posttraumatic play
    - Compulsive
    - Repetitive
    - Grim
    - Incorporates a portion of the trauma, known as play reenactment
    - Much less imaginative and more rigid than normal play
    - Does not relieve anxiety or trauma-specific fears
    - Does not change attitudes about people and life; characterized by excessive pessimism and hopelessness about the future
■ Preliminary investigation to explore whether *DSM-IV* PTSD criteria accurately describe the symptoms of young, traumatized children found that it did not.
  - Authors suggest more objective, behaviorally anchored, and developmentally sensitive criteria, including assessment of:
    - Posttraumatic play
    - Sleep disturbances
    - Emergence of new aggressive and separation anxiety symptoms

Feeding and eating disorders of infancy and early childhood

- The *DSM-IV* recognizes 3 feeding disorders in early childhood.
  - Pica
  - Rumination disorder
  - Feeding disorder of infancy or early childhood
- Pica is frequently seen in association with:
  - Mental retardation
  - Developmental disorders
- Rumination disorder
  - Frequently seen in mentally retarded infants and children
- Failure to thrive
  - Failure to gain weight or significant weight loss over ≥1 month
  - Must not result from a medical condition
  - Often associated with:
    - Parental psychopathological abnormality
    - Child neglect
    - Abuse

Cross-gender behavior and gender identity disorder (GID)

- Emerges in early childhood
- Usually consolidated by age 3–4 years
- Children with clinically significant GID exhibit a persistent, pervasive desire to be of the opposite sex.
- In the *DSM-IV*, GID is defined as having 2 important components.
  - Strong, persistent cross-gender identification and persistent discomfort with child's own sex
  - Sense of inappropriateness in assigned gender role
- Boys with GID will assert that:
  - Their genitalia are disgusting.
  - They wish them to disappear.
- Rejection of stereotypical toys, games, and activities is common.

Transitional objects and imaginary companions

- Soft object or stuffed animal
- Emerges at age 4-12 months
- Persists well into early childhood

Middle childhood years (5 years to puberty)

ADHD

- According to the *DSM-IV*, core symptoms require onset of inattention and hyperactivity-impulsivity by age 7 years, occurring in ≥2 settings.
- Symptoms must be more severe and frequent than those seen in a normal child at a comparable development level.
- Tend to emerge once the child enters school because of taxing of limited attention and impulse control available

- Highly structured setting
- Significant demands
- Lack of one-to-one adult-to-child supervision

ODD

- Symptoms are seen invariably in the home.
- Frequently focused on one particular authority figure
- Behaviors must be particularly frequent, severe, and persistent to prevent inappropriate labeling of children exhibiting developmentally normal oppositionalism as having ODD.

Conduct disorder

- Mild antisocial behaviors can be developmentally normal in certain settings, such as:
  - A preschooler who cannot play by the rules in structured games
- In the school-age child and adolescent, conduct disorder symptoms are grossly developmentally deviant and include:
  - Aggressivity
  - Deceitfulness
  - Theft
  - Serious rule violations
  - Property destruction
- Children and adolescents who have conduct disorder are at high risk for developing antisocial personality disorder in adulthood.

Dissociative disorders

- DSM-IV includes 4 diagnoses within the category of dissociative disorders.
  - The most familiar is dissociative identity disorder, also known as multiple personality disorder.
- Core of these disorders is the presence of pathological dissociation.
  - Can be transient or chronic
  - Onset can be acute or gradual.
  - Capacity for dissociation develops in childhood and is a normal process used in imaginative play.
  - This normal process declines markedly by late adolescence.
  - The key differences between the normal dissociation of a daydreaming child or a child in the throes of fantasy play and the pathological dissociation seen in the dissociative disorders are:
    - Amnesia for complex behaviors
    - Extreme forms of depersonalization
    - These symptoms rarely occur in healthy children or in children who have psychiatric disorders other than dissociative disorders.

Adolescence

Major depressive disorder and bipolar disorder

- Signs and symptoms

S

- Depressed mood for most of the day
- Markedly diminished interest or pleasure in almost all activities
- Significant weight loss or gain caused by a decrease or increase in appetite
- Insomnia or hypersomnia
- Psychomotor agitation or retardation
- Fatigue or loss of energy
- Feelings of excessive worthlessness or guilt
- Diminished ability to concentrate
- Recurrent thoughts of death or suicide
- Adolescents with bipolar disorder characteristically have occurrence of a major depressive episode before a first manic episode.
  - Characteristics of a manic episode
    - Grandiosity
    - Decreased sleep requirement
    - Pressured speech
    - Racing thoughts
    - Agitation
    - High-risk behaviors
      - Spending sprees
      - Sexual promiscuity
      - Gambling
- Both major depressive disorder and bipolar disorder typically occur in adolescence.
- Milder forms of depressive and manic disorders exist and can be seen in adolescence.
- Prepubertal manic and depressive disorders
  - Have been diagnosed more frequently in recent years
  - Are associated with a more severe course

Schizophrenia and other psychotic disorders

- Before 1980, all serious forms of childhood psychiatric disturbance were labeled schizophrenia.
- The label of psychosis has been significantly narrowed in a climate of growing understanding that perception of reality differs in:
  - Various developmental phases
  - Diverse cultural contexts
- In adolescents, schizophrenic symptoms closely parallel those seen in adult-onset schizophrenia.
- The *DSM-IV* identifies characteristic symptoms of schizophrenia as:
  - Delusions
  - Hallucinations
  - Disorganized speech
  - Grossly disorganized behavior

- So-called negative symptoms
  - Avolition
  - Alogia
  - Affective flattening
- These symptoms are accompanied by significant occupational and social dysfunction.

Eating disorders

- 2 classic eating disorders: anorexia nervosa and bulimia nervosa
- Signs and symptoms are typically seen by pediatrician before any mental health intervention is sought.
- In the eating disorders, both thinking and behavior are disturbed.
- Anorexia nervosa produces:
  - Intense fear of gaining weight or becoming fat, even when patient is underweight
  - Disturbance in the way in which body weight is experienced
- The patient refuses to maintain body weight above a minimally normal level.
  - Specified in *DSM-IV* as 85% of expected body weight
- 2 forms of behavior are used by patients with anorexia nervosa to inhibit weight gain.
  - Restricting food intake
  - Cycle of binge eating followed by purging
- Methods of purging may include:
  - Self-induced vomiting
  - Excessive use of laxatives
  - Excessive exercise
  - Use of diuretic medications and enemas
- Patients with bulimia nervosa:
  - Are typically within a normal weight range
  - Often have had a prior period of anorexia nervosa
- Bulimia nervosa is characterized by recurrent episodes of binge eating.
  - During a discrete period, an excessive amount of food intake occurs, accompanied by a feeling of total lack of control.
  - The binge is then followed by purging behavior.

DIFFERENTIAL DIAGNOSIS

- SAD
  - Must be distinguished from the developmentally appropriate anxiety of early childhood during the rapprochement phase.
    - In the second year of life, the child shows normal separation and stranger anxiety.

S

- Cultural variations on acceptable child-from-parent separation must always be considered.
  - Traditional cultures place great emphasis on family interdependence.
- Pica
  - The clinician should recognize that this practice is sanctioned in certain cultures.
  - In this context, it would not be appropriately viewed as a pathological behavior.
- Feeding and eating disorders of infancy and early childhood
  - Developmental disorders and extreme difficulties in temperament
    - May lead to feeding difficulties
    - Must be distinguished from feeding disorders for proper management
- Cross-gender behavior and GID
  - Must be distinguished from developmentally normal failure to conform to stereotypical gender role behavior, such as:
    - Tomboyism of some latency age girls
    - Cultural variants such as effeminate style of the bohemian artist or dandy
  - Normal variants are usually distinguished easily from true GID by:
    - Lack of severe disgust with the individual's anatomy and assigned gender role
    - Absence of a strong identification with the other sex
- Transitional objects and imaginary companions
  - Normal developmental element of early childhood should be distinguished from the transitional phenomena and imaginary companions of the severely disturbed child.
    - These experiences are not always easy to distinguish in early childhood.
  - Children with a history of severe physical or sexual abuse may develop symptoms of
    - Pathological dissociation
    - Psychosis, including auditory hallucinations or imaginary companions
  - Unlike the benign imaginary companions of a normal child, the hallucinatory experiences of the dissociative or psychotic child are:
    - Threatening
    - Frightening
    - Aggressive toward others
  - The child feels little control over the experience.
  - The child often cannot distinguish between reality and this frightening product of the imagination.
  - Assessment by an experienced child psychiatrist is required if doubt exists.

- ADHD
  - Normal exuberance of early childhood is most commonly confused with ADHD.
- ODD
  - To prevent inappropriate labeling of developmentally normal oppositionalism as ODD, behaviors must be particularly:
    - Frequent
    - Severe
    - Persistent
- Conduct disorder
  - Mild antisocial behaviors can be developmentally normal in certain settings, such as:
    - A preschooler who cannot play by the rules in structured games
- Dissociative disorders
  - Aspects of normal adolescent development in the psychological and cognitive area can gain clinical attention and can be mistaken for an abnormality.
  - Tendency toward egocentric, grandiose thinking and abstract theorizing is pronounced during adolescence.
  - Obsessive, ruminative focus on the body or on the person's own thinking process can be mistaken for:
    - Anxiety disorders
    - A hypomanic episode
    - Oppositional behavior
- Schizophrenia
  - Severe symptoms can be contrasted with disturbances in reality testing seen in various phases of normal development.
  - Transient hallucinatory experiences, often tactile or visual in nature, are commonly seen in:
    - Early childhood
    - In older children during times of stress
  - Magical, animistic thinking is common and developmentally normal in preschool and early school-age children.
  - Imaginary companions and transitional objects imbued with lifelike qualities by the child are normal in early childhood.
  - All such normal phenomena should gradually disappear by the end of middle childhood.
- Eating disorders
  - Distinguishing factors that identify eating disorders from the transient, developmentally normal process
    - Severity of weight loss
    - Persistence of a disturbed body image
    - Loss of menses in anorexia nervosa is necessary to make the diagnosis.

S

TREATMENT APPROACH

- The first 2 decades of life comprise the most complex and dynamic links among
  - Mind
  - Body
  - Development
- Behaviors and thoughts that at one phase are entirely normal can be a harbinger of a serious pathology when they emerge in a different stage of development and with subtle differences in presentation.
- Organic illness during childhood or adolescence may:
  - Cause regressions or deviances in thinking and behavior
  - Blur the clinician's understanding of the patient
- Nuances of different cultural and belief systems can be interpreted as pathological thinking and behavior to the culturally naive observer.
- Successful collaboration between child psychiatry and pediatrics is crucial in diagnosis and treatment of children.

Infancy and early childhood (birth to 5 years)

- Psychiatric assessment of children is unique and most challenging in the first 5 years of life.
  - Accurate evaluation of a psychopathological abnormality requires a firm grasp of normal development.
  - To identify abnormalities, combine:
    - Keen observation
    - Skilled and informed probing
  - In assessment of infants and preschoolers, break down observations into 4 categories (Gesell).
    - Motor skills
    - Language abilities
    - Personal-social abilities
    - Adaptive functioning
      - Manipulation of objects
      - Alertness
      - Hand-eye coordination
  - The Bayley scale breaks down infant assessment into useful subdivisions focusing on:
    - Social communication
    - Object constancy
    - Capacity for discrimination
  - Abnormalities in any can direct more serious consideration of major types of psychopathological abnormality.

Middle childhood years (5 years to puberty)

- Phase of middle childhood begins:
  - Elementary school
  - Formal learning and participation in a structured peer group
  - Interaction in the world beyond the family
  - Period during which disruptive behavior disorders emerge and gain clinical attention
- Industriousness is called for in acquisition of:
  - Academic skills
  - Social competence with peers
  - Successful relationships with authority figures outside the family
- One-to-one supervision by an adult gives way to:
  - Structured classroom setting
  - Formal rules of behavior within a distracting group of peers
- Several psychiatric disorders emerge or are more readily identifiable in this developmental stage and social setting.
- Accurate understanding of symptoms gathered from a combination of:
  - Skilled interview
  - Supporting information from parents, teachers, and other relevant reporters

Adolescence

- Adolescence is a developmental phase unique to human beings.
- Hormonal and neurologic changes develop slowly over many years, culminating during puberty.
- With biological changes come psychological and social changes, including:
  - Preoccupation with the body
  - Development of sexuality
  - Social anxiety
  - Increased importance of the peer group over parents and other adult figures
  - Development of more abstract cognitive abilities
- These developments result in unfamiliar changes in thinking and behavior.
  - May at times be mistaken for psychopathology
- Several major psychiatric disorders occur typically in adolescence.

Special considerations
Extreme temperment in childhood

- 9 categories have been identified that define temperament.
  - Activity level
  - Rhythmicity or regularity
  - Approach or withdrawal behavior
  - Adaptability to new situations
  - Threshold of responsiveness
  - Intensity of reaction
  - Quality of mood
  - Distractibility
  - Attention span

- 3 distinct temperamental styles.
  - Easy temperament
    - Regular, easily adaptable child
    - Displays a predominantly positive mood and only mild intensity
  - Difficult temperament
    - Behaviorally opposite of easy temperament
    - Characterized by biological irregularity, withdrawal in reaction to novel stimuli, slow adaptability to change, predominantly negative mood, high intensity
  - Slow-to-warm-up temperament, also known as shy
    - Slow adapters
    - Significant withdrawal responses, low intensity, and frequent negative mood
- The difficult child and the slow-to-warm-up child are developmentally and psychologically normal.
  - Because of their difficulty to manage, may be labeled as behaviorally disordered by caretakers and brought to pediatric attention.
  - Extremely negative temperamental features have not been found to be equivalent to psychiatric disorders in childhood.
    - Can predict poor psychiatric functioning in adolescence
    - Particularly in the context of poor caretaker-child interaction and dysfunctional behavioral control among adult family members

Medically ill child

- The pediatrician is a primary observer of the child in the role of patient.
- The pediatrician needs to understand emotional and developmental reactions to pain and illness exhibited by children.
- Cognitive-developmental theory define a predictable sequence of stages by which cognitive concepts are acquired throughout childhood.
  - Sensorimotor stage, infancy to 2 years
    - Things exist only insofar as the child can act on them.
    - The ultimate cognitive outcome is the achievement of object permanence.
  - Preoperational stage, age 2–7 years
    - Symbolic thought and representations, including language, develop.
    - Thinking is not logical.
    - Egocentric and animistic
  - Concrete operational stage, ages 7–puberty
    - Logical thinking takes hold
  - The formal operational stage begins at puberty.
    - Formal abstract thinking is the predominant mode of thought.
    - Not all individuals reach the formal operational stage, even in adulthood.

- In cognitive-developmental theory, a systematic and predictable sequence exists by which concepts of illness are acquired.
- Children who are ill often exhibit strange behavior that can be understood by:
  - Appreciation of child's cognitive level
  - The fact that children often regress to an earlier level of cognitive functioning under stress
- Symptoms that existed previously and were overcome by the child may recur and persist during the course of the illness, such as:
  - Enuresis
  - Soiling
  - Sleep difficulties
  - Separation anxiety
- Elements specific to the plight of the child with a medical illness may predispose the child to unusual thinking and behavior.
- The experience of being nursed and change in parental emotional climate can cause great anxiety and may even be traumatic.
- Being forced into a passive role and being treated by the parent and medical staff as a much younger child can be upsetting to the child who has acquired independent functioning and detachment from parents.
- The resulting anxiety can create a difficult, even intractable, patient.

WHEN TO REFER

- When a high index of suspicion exists for a psychiatric disorder:
  - Refer to a child and adolescent psychiatrist for a full diagnostic assessment
- Clinical situations in which immediate referral should be made
  - Suicidal ideation or intent
  - Violence or serious recent history of violence
  - Thought disorder and other psychotic symptoms
  - Suspicion of serious substance abuse
  - Pediatric depression
  - Assessment for initiation or continuation of treatment with psychotropic medication

WHEN TO ADMIT

- Suicidal ideation
- Violent behavior

PROGNOSIS

- Psychotic disorders
  - When present in prepubertal children, harbingers of a poor prognosis

S

Streptococcal Toxic Shock Syndrome

DEFINITION

- Streptococcal toxic shock syndrome (STSS)
  - A syndrome caused by group A streptococci (GAS) that involves severe invasive diseases, including:
    - Necrotizing fasciitis
    - Necrotizing myositis
    - Bacteremia
    - Sepsis with vascular collapse, hypotension, and multiorgan failure

EPIDEMIOLOGY

- Incidence
  - Severe invasive GAS infections: 1.5–7.0 cases per 100,000 population annually
- Patients with STSS have epidemiologic features that distinguish them from patients with other invasive GAS infections:
  - Younger age
  - Alcohol abuse
  - Fewer underlying illnesses
- Outbreaks of severe invasive GAS infections have occurred in some closed environments:
  - Military bases
  - Nursing homes
  - Hospitals
- Overall fatality rate of invasive GAS diseases
  - Children: 5–10%
  - Adults: 30–80%
- Case fatality rate associated with STSS remains high in both pediatric and adult populations.

ETIOLOGY

- Most cases of STSS are caused by GAS strains that produce bacterial superantigens known as the *streptococcal pyrogenic exotoxins*.

RISK FACTORS

- Clinical risk factors
  - History of soft-tissue injury
    - Animal or insect bite
    - Blunt or penetrating trauma
    - Surgical wounds
    - Subcutaneous injections of insulin or illicit drugs
  - Varicella infection (15–30% of invasive GAS diseases are associated with varicella)
  - Invasive GAS infections
    - Pneumonia
    - Meningitis
    - Peritonitis
    - Osteomyelitis
    - Bacteremia
    - Septic arthritis
  - Inconsequential scratch or abrasion
  - STSS occurs without readily identifiable focus of infection in 21% of cases.
  - Relative risks of invasive GAS infections among household contacts of patients with invasive GAS infections are 19–200 times the baseline risk in general population
- Biochemical risk factor
  - Major human host defense against invasive GAS infection is phagocytosis and killing by polymorphonuclear leucocytes.
  - Thus, a critical somatic GAS virulence factor is an antiphagocytic surface constituent known as M protein.
  - Strains of GAS isolated from patients with STSS are not of a single M type, but M1 and M3 infections are associated with invasive diseases and STSS.

SIGNS AND SYMPTOMS

- Sudden severe pain
  - Most common initial symptom of STSS
  - Usually involves an extremity
- Fever
  - Hypothermia may be present in patients with shock.
- Rapid-onset hypotension
  - Systolic blood pressure ≤90 mm Hg in adults or below 5th percentile for age in children
  - Nearly one-half of patients with STSS may have normal blood pressure at admission but soon develop hypotension.
  - Hypotension is significant risk factor for death.
- Rapidly accelerated renal failure
- Acute respiratory distress syndrome
- Necrotizing fasciitis in up to 70% of patients
  - Life-threatening soft tissue infection primarily involving the superficial fascia with relative sparing of skin and muscles, both of which may be infected secondarily
  - Ominous signs of necrotizing fasciitis
    - Progression of soft tissue swelling to the formation of violaceous or hemorrhagic vesicles, then bullae
    - Line of demarcation becomes sharply defined.
    - Dead skin begins to separate at margins or breaks in center, revealing extensive necrosis of subcutaneous tissue.
  - Crepitus on physical examination, which is pathognomonic for necrotizing soft-tissue infections, is seen in only one-third of cases.

- Myositis: up to 70% of patients
  - Early signs
    - Severe pain
    - Swelling
    - Erythema
    - Fever
  - Pain often out of proportion to clinical findings, possibly related to muscle compartment syndrome
- Pharyngitis and local soft tissue infection (eg, cellulitis, abscess)
- Soft tissue swelling and erythema: 80% of patients
- Confusion: 55% of patients
- Preceding influenza-like syndrome (20% of patients), characterized by:
  - Fever
  - Chills
  - Myalgia
  - Nausea
  - Vomiting
  - Diarrhea
- Diffuse scarlatina-like erythema: 10% of patients
- Coma or combativeness
- Erythematous, tender, swollen area that resembles cellulitis, with disproportionately severe pain at the site of involvement

DIFFERENTIAL DIAGNOSIS

- Pain of STSS usually involves an extremity but also may mimic the following:
  - Peritonitis
  - Pelvic inflammatory disease
  - Acute chest syndrome
- Necrotizing fasciitis and myositis are difficult to diagnose.
  - Some patients with STSS may have both.
  - Emergent surgical exploration should be done to establish and distinguish GAS infection from other soft tissue infections.

LABORATORY FINDINGS

- Case definition includes the following laboratory findings:
  - Isolation of group A ß-hemolytic streptococci
    - From normally sterile site (eg, blood, cerebrospinal fluid, peritoneal fluid, tissue biopsy specimen)
    - From nonsterile site (eg, throat, sputum, vagina)
  - Clinical signs of severity, ≥2 of the following signs:
    - Renal impairment (creatinine ≥2 mg/dL for adults or twice the upper limit or more of normal for age)
    - Coagulopathy (platelets ≤100,000/μL or disseminated intravascular coagulation)

- Hepatic involvement (alanine aminotransferase, aspartate aminotransferase, or total bilirubin levels twice the upper limit of normal or more for age)
- Other possible laboratory findings include:
  - Hypoalbuminemia
  - Hypocalcemia
  - Lactic acidosis
  - Hyperglycemia
  - Thrombocytopenia
- When serum creatinine kinase level is increased, a good correlation exists with necrotizing fasciitis or myositis.
- Mild leucocytosis may be seen initially, but the mean percentage of immature neutrophils can reach 40–50%.
- Culture
  - Blood cultures are positive for GAS in 60% of cases.
- Gram stain
  - Subcutaneous fluid may be aspirated from the affected limb for Gram stain and culture.
  - Subject all tissues from initial surgical debridement to Gram staining and culturing for aerobic and anaerobic microorganisms
- Rapid antigen detection tests for GAS
  - Approved only for pharyngeal swab specimens
  - May be able to identify GAS from necrotic tissue
  - In necrotizing soft-tissue infections in children, GAS is identified as a single organism in only 25% of cases; the remaining cases are polymicrobial.

IMAGING

- Imaging studies are only adjuncts in evaluations of STSS and necrotizing soft tissue infections and should not be relied on to exclude the diagnosis.
- Diagnosis of invasive GAS infection, including STSS, is still primarily clinical.
- Radiography
  - May depict soft tissue air at affected area (50% of cases)
- Computed tomography and magnetic resonance imaging
  - Help diagnose necrotizing fasciitis and myositis and delineate extent of infection
  - Features of necrotizing fasciitis
    - Deep fascial thickening
    - Enhancement
    - Presence of fluid and gas in the fascial planes
  - Features of myositis
    - General homogenous enlargement of the muscle
    - Low attenuation values
    - Edema or presence of intramuscular gas

S

SPECIFIC TREATMENTS

Severe invasive GAS infection

- Hemodynamic stabilization
- Specific antibiotic therapy
- Prompt and aggressive surgical exploration
- Fasciotomy
- Debridement of suspected deep-seated infection
- Surgical exploration and incisional biopsy, to provide both definitive diagnosis and treatment

Suspected STSS

- Empiric broad-spectrum antibiotic therapy with drugs that cover gram-positive, gram-negative, and anaerobic organisms
  - Combination of ampicillin, penicillin, aminoglycosides, and clindamycin
  - Combination of expanded-spectrum penicillin or cephalosporins, clindamycin, and aminoglycosides
- Patients allergic to penicillin may receive vancomycin in place of ampicillin or penicillin.
- Antibiotic regimen can be changed once the causative organism is identified.

Treatments

- Penicillin
  - Less efficacious in overwhelming GAS infections when large numbers of organisms are present (so-called Eagle effect).
  - Fails to halt GAS infection because of physiologic state of organism
  - Less efficacious against slowly growing organisms
- Clindamycin
  - Administering clindamycin in addition to penicillin seems advisable in patients with overwhelming invasive GAS infection.
  - Should not be used alone, because strains of GAS with clindamycin resistance have been reported
- Intravenous immunoglobulin
  - May be provided as adjunctive therapy for patients with STSS, because it:
    - Decreases mortality rates
    - Is associated with significant improvement of organ dysfunction after therapy
    - Leads to significant increase in plasma-neutralizing activity against superantigens
- Hyperbaric oxygen
  - Patient is enclosed in a chamber and breathes 100% oxygen at pressure >1 atmosphere absolute.
  - Results of clinical studies of necrotizing fasciitis have been inconsistent.
  - May improve patent survival and decrease the number of debridements required to achieve wound control.

WHEN TO ADMIT

- All patients with STSS need to be admitted.

WHEN TO REFER

- All patients with STSS should be managed in consultation with infectious diseases specialists.

COMPLICATIONS

- Renal dysfunction
  - May occur before or after hypotension
  - Progresses or persists in all patients for 48–72 hours despite treatment
  - Many patients require dialysis.
  - In survivors, serum creatinine values return to normal within 4–6 weeks.

PROGNOSIS

- High fatality rate is associated with invasive GAS infections:
  - Necrotizing fasciitis: 22%
  - STSS: 45%
  - Case-fatality rate among patients with neither STSS nor necrotizing fasciitis: 10%
- Survival is possible with:
  - Early surgical debridement
  - Reexploration at 24–36 hours
  - Intensive supportive care
    - Extent of debridement is determined by radiographic findings and physical findings at surgery.
- Recurrent STSS episodes have not been reported.

PREVENTION

- Protective humoral immunity
  - Immunity to cell-associated and soluble GAS virulence factors is important in preventing invasive disease.
  - Patients with invasive GAS disease have significantly lower serum levels of protective antibodies against M protein and superantigens compared with serum samples from noninvasive cases.
  - Lack of immunity against GAS virulence factors contributes to susceptibility to invasive infection.
- Opportunities for preventing STSS are few.
  - Varicella vaccination
    - Because of association between invasive GAS infections, including STSS and varicella infection, in healthy children, routine childhood immunization against varicella is suggested.
    - Children who receive varicella vaccine are less likely to be hospitalized for varicella-related invasive GAS infections.

S

- Nonsteroidal antiinflammatory drugs (NSAIDs)
  - Relationship between NSAID use and necrotizing fasciitis has been reported.
  - NSAIDs can impair granulocytic function and enhance production of cytokines.
  - A causal relationship between NSAID use and severe invasive GAS infections has not been established.
- Infection-control practices
  - To prevent nosocomial GAS infections, improve infection-control practices for:
    - Surgical and obstetric procedures
    - Placement and care of intravascular devices
- Household spread
  - GAS can easily spread through household.
  - Family members, usually children, are identified with pharyngitis or with carriage of same strain of GAS that caused invasive disease.
  - Secondary cases of invasive GAS infections, including STSS within same household, have been reported.
  - Although risk of subsequent invasive GAS disease among household contacts is higher than in general population, such infections are rare.
  - No studies on effectiveness of chemoprophylaxis in preventing invasive GAS disease among household contacts of patients with invasive GAS infections
    - Routine chemoprophylaxis and routine use of cultures among household contacts is not warranted.
  - Health care providers should:
    - Inform members of the household about clinical manifestations of pharyngeal and invasive GAS infections.
    - Emphasize importance of seeking immediate medical attention if they develop such symptoms, particularly within 30 days after index case is diagnosed.
- Chemoprophylaxis among household members
  - Those age ≥65 years
  - Those with:
    - HIV infection
    - Concurrent varicella infection
    - Diabetes mellitus
    - Cancer
    - Chronic cardiac or pulmonary diseases
    - Injection drug use
    - Alcoholism
    - Known immunodeficiency disorder
    - Corticosteroid use
- Because the source of GAS in households may not be the person with invasive infection, prescribe chemoprophylaxis for both the elderly or high-risk household member *and* all members in household.
- If available, use antibiotic susceptibility data to select most appropriate chemoprophylactic agent.
- Everyone receiving chemoprophylaxis should watch for sign and symptoms of invasive GAS disease for 30 days after diagnosis of invasive disease in index case.
- Chemoprophylactic regimens:
  - Single dose of benzathine penicillin G (600,000 units intramuscularly for persons weighing <27 kg *or* 1,200,000 units intramuscularly for persons weighing ≥27 kg) *and* oral rifampin 20 mg/kg/day (maximum daily dose, 600 mg) in 2 divided doses for 4 days
  - Clindamycin 20 mg/kg/day (maximum daily dose, 900 mg) in 3 divided doses for 10 days
  - Azithromycin 12 mg/kg/day (maximum daily dose, 500 mg) once a day for 5 days
- Other agents
  - Limited evidence that first- and second-generation cephalosporins eradicate pharyngeal colonization of GAS
  - Consider these agents for patients allergic to penicillin whose allergic reactions are not anaphylactic.
  - Rifampin is not recommended for pregnant women because of its teratogenic effect.
- Postpartum or postsurgical invasive GAS infections
  - Implement enhanced surveillance by infection control personnel.
  - Store all GAS isolates from suspected cases and compare them by serotyping or molecular techniques.
  - Suspect that health care worker may be source of cluster if ≥2 cases of invasive GAS infection by same GAS type occur within 6 months.
  - Screen health care workers who are epidemiologically linked to case patients by obtaining cultures from throat, anus, vagina, and skin lesions.
  - Prescribe one of the three regimens above to health care workers who are colonized with GAS.
  - Perform follow-up culture 7–10 days after completion of therapy.

S

Stridor

DEFINITION

- Stridor is a high-pitched, monophonic noise caused by turbulent airflow through a partially obstructed extrathoracic airway, heard predominately on inspiration.

MECHANISM

- During the normal respiratory cycle, rhythmic expansion and contraction of the thorax leads to dynamic changes in thoracic pressures.
  - Result: Air flows into and out of the lungs.
- During expiration, the volume of the thoracic cavity decreases.
  - Result: Positive pressures within the thorax are created.
- Airways located within the thorax are directly subjected to these positive pressures.
  - Result: These airways are more prone to obstruction during expiration, leading to turbulent airflow and wheezing.
- On inspiration, the thoracic cavity expands.
  - Result: Negative intrathoracic pressures occur and patency of intrathoracic airways improves.
- This portion of the airway is susceptible to obstruction, and thus stridor, during inspiration because:
  - Intraluminal airway pressure decreases to allow inflow of air.
  - Extrathoracic airways (nose, nasopharynx, oropharynx, and larynx) may collapse from transmitted negative intrathoracic pressures.

HISTORY

- Age at initial presentation and a description of the events surrounding symptom onset can provide important clues to the underlying diagnosis.
- Viral croup
  - Stridor preceded by fever, upper respiratory symptoms, and a barky or seal-like cough
  - No stridor between episodes
  - The patient may have history of similar episodes in the past.
  - Stridor caused by viral croup improves within days.
- Laryngomalacia
  - Suspected if stridor begins in the first few weeks of life and presents only during specific phases of alertness, such as eating, sleeping, or excitement
  - Laryngomalacia is the most common cause of congenital stridor in infancy.
  - Stridor caused by laryngomalacia is typically intermittent and worsens over the first several months of life.
    - With age, episodes become less severe and less frequent; symptoms usually completely resolve by the first birthday.
- Subglottic stenosis or granulation tissue
  - Stridor that develops shortly after a prolonged intubation
  - May be continuous
  - Often seen in premature infants who required mechanical ventilation during the neonatal period
- Retropharyngeal abscess
  - Fever
  - Difficulty swallowing
- Hemangioma
  - Worsening stridor
  - History of cutaneous hemangiomas
- Bilateral vocal cord paralysis
  - History of injury to both recurrent laryngeal nerves
  - Arnold-Chiari malformation or increased intracranial pressure
- Foreign body
  - Sudden onset
  - History of choking or placing small objects in the mouth
- Vocal cord cyst
  - Hoarse voice
  - Chronic irritation to vocal cords or airway instrumentation
- Recurrent respiratory papillomatosis
  - Usually associated with stridor or hoarseness 2–3 years after birth
  - Infection is acquired through vertical transmission in the birth canal from maternal cervical human papillomavirus infection.
- Laryngeal web
  - Develops shortly after birth (congenital)
  - Develops after airway instrumentation (acquired)
- Onset of stridor in an older child or adolescent with no previous history should prompt a more thorough evaluation.

PHYSICAL EXAM

- Assess position.
  - Extension of the neck is often seen with serious infection, such as epiglottitis or retropharyngeal abscess.
- Look for drooling.
  - Suggests a mass effect or edema in the posterior pharynx, causing dysphagia in addition to stridor.
- Keep the patient calm and maintain the airway.
- Examine the oropharynx to detect:
  - Retropharyngeal bulge
  - Lateral displacement of the uvula and swelling of a tonsillar pillar from an underlying infection

- Externally examine the neck for:
  - Presence of suprasternal retractions when obstruction is severe
  - Displacement of the larynx, a mass obstructing the airway, or signs of trauma
- Note the quality of the voice.
  - Hoarseness, aphonia, or a weak cry suggest vocal cord disease.
- Physical examination findings
  - Laryngomalacia
    - Predominately inspiratory
    - May be positional
  - Viral croup
    - Predominately inspiratory
    - No change with position
  - Subglottic stenosis
    - Predominately inspiratory, but often biphasic
  - Foreign body
    - Predominately inspiratory if obstruction is extrathoracic
    - Retropharyngeal abscess
    - Often present with stertor
    - Presence of drooling
  - Hemangioma
    - Cutaneous hemangiomas may be present.

DIFFERENTIAL DIAGNOSIS

- Causes of stridor
  - Laryngomalacia
  - Viral croup
  - Subglottic stenosis
  - Foreign body
  - Retropharyngeal abscess
  - Hemangioma
  - Bilateral vocal cord paralysis
  - Vocal cord cyst
  - Laryngeal papillomatosis
  - Laryngeal web
- Because the extrathoracic airways extend from the nose to the proximal trachea, high-pitched laryngeal stridor must be differentiated from other abnormal inspiratory noises.
  - Stertor
    - Noisy, rumbling-type noise similar to snoring
    - Heard with partial airway obstruction in the oropharynx or nasopharynx

- For stridor that worsens or persists, coexisting or alternate diagnoses should be considered.
  - Laryngopharyngeal acid reflux may aggravate the underlying condition.
  - Mild stridor caused by a subglottic hemangioma may initially be attributed to a more common problem (eg, laryngomalacia).
    - Similar to laryngomalacia, obstruction from a hemangioma tends to worsen after initial presentation as the lesion enlarges.
    - Unlike with laryngomalacia, natural resolution of the hemangioma, and thus the stridor, may take several years rather than months.
- History of a hoarse voice or cry suggests glottic disease and might result from chronic irritation of the vocal cords.
- Other clues that suggest more ominous conditions include:
  - Constant stridor
  - Failure to thrive
  - Difficulty swallowing
  - Severe and sudden onset of symptoms

LABORATORY EVALUATION

- Although laboratory testing has limited value for stridor, *Bordetella pertussis* infection can sometimes cause stridor and can be diagnosed by:
  - Polymerase chain reaction
  - Culture of pharyngeal secretions

IMAGING

- Radiographic findings
  - A simple radiograph of the neck can identify obstructive lesions in the retropharynx, glottis, and subglottic area.
  - Viral croup
    - Steeple sign on neck radiograph
  - Subglottic stenosis
    - Subglottic narrowing on neck radiograph
  - Foreign body
    - May be visualized on radiograph if radio-opaque
  - Retropharyngeal abscess
    - Retropharyngeal mass on lateral neck radiograph
  - Hemangioma
    - Subglottic obstruction on neck radiograph

DIAGNOSTIC PROCEDURES

- Pulmonary function testing
  - Not often necessary, but can confirm suspicion of an extrathoracic obstruction

- Flexible laryngoscopy
  - Direct visualization of the airway (including the posterior pharynx and glottis) by flexible laryngoscopy often provides definitive information.
  - Usually well tolerated, and most often with topical anesthesia alone
  - For laryngomalacia:
    - Laryngoscopy merely confirms presence of laryngomalacia while excluding other causes of airway obstruction.
    - For severe laryngomalacia, laryngoscopy can also identify specific structural obstruction that might be amenable to surgical correction.
    - Severe laryngomalacia might obscure the view of the subglottic area such that a more distal lesion would not be visible.
      - Direct visualization of the subglottic region and proximal trachea may be indicated to exclude a second lesion.
  - Direct laryngoscopy and bronchoscopy under sedation or general anesthesia can help diagnose and quantify the severity of subglottic stenosis or identify other subglottic lesions that cause obstruction.
- Findings on diagnostic tests
  - Laryngomalacia
    - Obstruction of glottic space by collapsing supraglottic structures on laryngoscopy
  - Subglottic stenosis
    - Flat inspiratory and expiratory loop on spirometry
    - Subglottic narrowing on direct laryngoscopy
  - Hemangioma
    - Seen on direct laryngoscopy
  - Bilateral vocal cord paralysis
    - No movement of vocal cords during laryngoscopy
  - Vocal cord cyst
    - Visible on laryngoscopy
  - Laryngeal papillomatosis
    - Visible on laryngoscopy
  - Laryngeal web
    - Visible on laryngoscopy

TREATMENT APPROACH

- Ensure airway patency before reaching a differential diagnosis.
  - Stridor reflects obstruction of a large centralized airway.
  - Stridor can range in severity from mild to life threatening.
- For most cases of stridor:
  - Obtain a succinct, focused history.
  - Perform physical examination.
  - Perform directed diagnostic tests.

- For the child with signs of severe respiratory compromise—distressed appearance, severe retractions, nasal flaring, pallor or cyanosis, altered mental status—initially focus on:
  - Maintaining the airway
  - If possible, relieving the obstruction
  - Intubation
    - Attempted only by personnel skilled at airway management
    - Performed in as controlled a setting as possible
    - If potentially difficult, surgical support should be present in case tracheostomy is required.

SPECIFIC TREATMENT

Laryngomalacia

- Most cases can be managed with observation alone, with particular attention to adequate caloric intake and weight gain.

Viral croup

- Most cases of croup can be managed with close observation alone.

More severe obstruction (nasal flaring, retractions)

- Racemic epinephrine may temporarily relieve symptoms of obstruction.
- Dexamethasone may temporarily alleviate inflammation.

WHEN TO REFER

- Progressive or continuous stridor
- Poor weight gain or growth associated with persistent stridor
- Repeated hospitalization
- Presence of cutaneous hemangiomas in association with persistent stridor
- Severe episodes of stridor causing hypoxemia or cyanosis
- Laryngomalacia requiring surgical management to relieve the obstruction caused by redundant epiglottic folds or arytenoid tissue

WHEN TO ADMIT

- Respiratory distress or hypoxemia
- Inability to eat or drink
- Altered mental status or signs of fatigue
- Stridor associated with signs of increased intracranial pressure

S

Stuttering

DEFINITION

- Speech disorder marked by involuntary interruptions or breaks in speech fluency
- Breaks/disfluencies include:
  - Part-word repetitions (eg, "pi-pi-picture," "mo-mother")
  - Single-syllable or single-word repetition (eg, "but-but," "he-he-he")
  - Prolongations of speech sounds (eg, "winnnter," "annnnd")
  - Blocks or abnormal pauses (eg, "be...because")
- Developmental stuttering causes the following reactions.
  - Fear and avoidance of speech
  - Chronic and worsening stuttering
- Acquired stuttering
  - Appears suddenly
  - Appears long after speech and language skills have been developed

EPIDEMIOLOGY

- Prevalence
  - 4–5% of children demonstrate persistent or chronic stuttering at some point.
  - Lifetime prevalence: approximately 5% of general population
  - Point prevalence estimate is 1%.
- Age
  - Typically emerges in early preschool years (2–5 years of age)
  - Onset rarely observed after puberty
- Sex
  - More prevalent in boys
  - First-grade children: 3:1 male/female ratio
  - Fifth-grade children: 5:1 male/female ratio

ETIOLOGY

- Developmental stuttering
  - Specific causes are still unknown.
  - Some evidence of a genetic component
    - Genes on chromosomes 1, 13, 16, and 18 are associated with stuttering.
  - Relation to child's efforts to learn to talk
    - Physical, cognitive, emotional, or motor effort
    - Early stuttering begins between the ages of 2 and 5 years, when the child is rapidly mastering speech and language skills.
  - Demands and capacities model
    - Internal or external demands for fluency exceed the child's capacity for speech at that point.
    - Environmental demands include parental pressures and self-imposed pressures.

- Acquired stuttering is neurogenic or psychogenic in origin.
  - Neurogenic stuttering
    - Due to brain damage; however, no consistent pattern in type of damage has been found

RISK FACTORS

- Family history of stuttering
- Presence of other speech or language disorders
- Male sex
- Child's temperament

SIGNS AND SYMPTOMS

- Age 2–6 years
  - Sound and syllable repetitions, produced with some tension and effort
  - Some reactions to the stuttering; mild tension may be observed
  - Child's initial reactions are surprise and frustration.
  - Reactions when stuttering continues include:
    - Fear of being stuck
    - Children as young as 2 years may hide or twist their faces or show other signs of struggle.
  - Stuttering is considered severe when all of the criteria below are seen.
    - Stuttering is very frequent (≥10% of the syllables spoken).
    - Repetitions are rapid and uneven.
    - Sound prolongation or blocking lasts ≥1 second.
    - The child appears to struggle in an attempt to say a word.
    - Fear or avoidance of speaking is evident.
- Age 6–10 years
  - Syllable repetitions
  - More tension and struggles at point of stutter
    - Tongue protrusions
    - Jaw tremors
    - Grimaces and other involuntary behaviors may become habituated.
  - Blocks appear.
  - Child pushes to get unstuck.
- Early teens and adolescents
  - Blocks (eg, getting stuck)
  - Sound prolongations ("...mmmmouse pad")
  - Frequent use of escape/avoidance behaviors to hide the stuttering
  - Some fear of or avoidance of specific words, speaking situations, or both
  - Feelings of shame and embarrassment are evident, and that individual may begin to have a significant negative self-concept.

DIFFERENTIAL DIAGNOSIS

- All children exhibit some disfluency
- Disfluencies often increase when the child is excited or tired.
- Normally disfluent speech
  - Repetitions are usually brief (typically ≤1 second).
  - Repetitions occur infrequently (≤1 in 10 syllables).
  - No signs of struggle in speaking
  - Repetitions of a word or phrase are normal and often associated with searching for a word.
- Early stuttering
  - Occurs on initial sound or syllable of an utterance
  - Repetitions are common but produced with more tension and effort.

DIAGNOSTIC APPROACH

- At onset, stuttering is variable and often difficult to diagnose.
  - Many young children are hesitant to talk with unfamiliar people, particularly in a medical setting.
  - Physician may not hear a sample of speech.
  - All speakers are disfluent sometimes, and young children are even more likely to be so.
- Obtaining information about disfluent speech by questioning the parents or caregivers may be necessary.
- Critical clinical questions to ask
  - Which of these children will naturally recover?
  - Which will require intervention services from speech-language pathologists?

TREATMENT APPROACH

- Speech pathologists commonly practice early intervention with young children.
- Many therapy approaches are based on play and use parental participation to facilitate the transfer of treatment effect to the child's daily speaking.

SPECIFIC TREATMENTS

- Parents should be advised to reduce communication time pressure by:
  - Pausing briefly before speaking
  - Avoiding bringing attention to disfluencies
  - Giving the child their full attention
  - Allowing the child plenty of time to say what he or she wants to say
- Physician can assist teenagers who stutter by:
  - Showing an understanding for the difficulties they encounter
  - Urging them not to let the stuttering prevent them from engaging in activities they would otherwise attempt
- The Lidcombe Program (developed in Australia, used in the US and elsewhere) is a highly systematic direct intervention approach.

- Efficacy has been well documented.

WHEN TO REFER

- Mild stuttering: refer to a speech-language pathologist if:
  - The child has stuttered for ≥3 months.
  - Stuttering continues after the parents have tried to follow suggestions for patient listening.
- Severe stuttering: refer to a speech-language pathologist as soon as possible.
  - Treatment may last ≥1 year.
- The speech-language pathologist should have:
  - A certificate of clinical competence from the American Speech-Language-Hearing Association
  - License by state board of examiners in speech-language abnormalities
  - Experience working with childhood stuttering (preferred)

COMPLICATIONS

- As a child who stutters enters school, stuttering can make reading aloud difficult and interfere with academic performance or learning.
  - Many stuttering children will not ask or answer questions of a teacher.
- Psychosocial impact
  - Teasing
  - Embarrassment (usually increases in adolescence)
  - Teens may avoid speaking or participating in specific speaking and social situations.
  - Adults who formerly stuttered often report feeling embarrassed and guilty about their use of tactics to avoid or conceal the problem.

PROGNOSIS

- 80% experience recovery from stuttering.
- Developmental stuttering
  - When treated appropriately, especially in beginning stages, the prognosis is generally good.
  - The key to success is early identification and intervention.
  - Behaviors seen in advanced stuttering (severe struggling and fear of talking) can usually be prevented.
  - If therapy starts when stuttering consists primarily of easy, effortless repetitions, chances for success are much better than when the stuttering has become complicated by struggle and avoidance behaviors.
  - Even adults who have stuttered for years can learn to decrease severity of stuttering and improve attitudes about speaking.
- Acquired stuttering
  - Prognosis is uncertain because of variability in type of neurologic damage or trauma.

Sudden Infant Death Syndrome

DEFINITION

- The National Institute of Child Health and Human Development defines sudden infant death syndrome (SIDS) as sudden death of an infant <1 year of age, which remains unexplained after a thorough case investigation, including:
  - Performance of a complete autopsy
  - Examination of the death scene
  - Review of the clinical history

EPIDEMIOLOGY

- Prevalence
  - Leading cause of death of infants between 1 month and 1 year of age in the US
- Incidence
  - Accounts for ~200 deaths per year in the US
- Racial disparity
  - 2.5-fold higher rate in black infants than in white infants in 2001
  - This disparity may be partially attributed to the increased prevalence of prone positioning in black infants.
- Age distribution
  - Rare in the first month of life
  - Peaks between 2 and 3 months of age
  - Decreases thereafter
  - ~90% of SIDS deaths occur in the first 6 months of life.

ETIOLOGY

- The leading hypothesis is that certain infants, for reasons yet unknown, have a maldevelopment or delay in maturation of the brainstem neural network responsible for arousal and the physiologic responses to life-threatening challenges during sleep.
  - When the physiologic stability of such infants becomes compromised during sleep, they may not arouse sufficiently to avoid fatal noxious insult or condition.
- Possible theories
  - Rebreathing and associated hypoxia and hypercarbia provide a noxious stimulus.
  - Hyperthermia, perhaps in combination with asphyxia, is the stimulus.

RISK FACTORS

- Prone or side sleep position
  - The prone position increases risk for SIDS, particularly if the infant is unaccustomed to it.
    - Secondary caregivers (grandparents, babysitters, child care providers, relatives) are more likely to place infants prone.
  - Now that a large number of infants are placed to sleep on their backs, contribution of the side sleep position to SIDS risk has increased.
    - The side sleep position is unstable.
    - A large proportion of infants placed on the side will roll to prone.
- Sleeping on a soft surface, such as pillows, quilts, comforters, sheepskins, and porous mattresses
  - A strong association has been found between prone sleep position and soft bedding surface, indicating that these 2 factors together are very hazardous.
  - Soft surfaces have been implicated in infant deaths occurring on adult beds.
- Maternal smoking during pregnancy
  - Postnatal exposure to tobacco smoke has emerged as a separate risk factor, although separating this variable from maternal smoking prenatally is difficult.
- Overheating
  - Increased risk of SIDS has been associated with increased layers of clothing or blankets on infant and warmer room temperatures.
  - The increased risk of overheating is particularly evident when infants sleep prone but is less clear when they sleep supine.
  - It is unclear whether overheating is an independent factor or merely a reflection of use of more clothing, quilts, and other potentially asphyxiating materials in the sleeping environment during cold weather.
- Late or no prenatal care
- Young maternal age
- Preterm birth or low birth weight (or both)
  - Risk increases with decreasing gestational age or birth weight.
  - Increased risk cannot be explained by greater likelihood of apnea of prematurity among preterm SIDS victims while they are in hospital after birth.
  - Whether other complications of prematurity can explain increased risk is unclear.
  - The association of sleep position and SIDS is the same for infants born preterm as for those born at term.
  - Strategies designed to reduce risk in full-term infants should be applied to infants born preterm after they are no longer in an intensive care setting.
- Male sex
- Race
  - SIDS rates are consistently 2–3 times the national average in African-American and Native American infants.

- Bed sharing
  - Risk of sudden unexpected death with bed sharing seems to be particularly high when:
    - Multiple people share the bed.
    - The infant is <11 weeks of age.
    - Bed sharing occurs on a couch.
    - Bed sharing occurs for the whole night.
  - Likelihood of bed sharing may be increased when the bed sharer has consumed alcohol or is overtired.
  - Bed sharing is particularly hazardous with mothers who smoke, but bed sharing with nonsmoking mothers is a risk factor among infants <11 weeks.
  - Breastfeeding in bed has not been shown to carry a risk if the baby is returned to the crib after feeding.
    - Because breastfeeding has many benefits, parents should be encouraged to bring infant into bed for breastfeeding and for bonding.
- A family in which an infant has previously died of SIDS has a 2–6% risk of a second SIDS death.

DIFFERENTIAL DIAGNOSIS

- Illnesses that should be considered in the differential diagnosis include:
  - Sepsis
  - Pneumonia
  - Myocarditis
  - Cardiomyopathy
  - Congenital heart defect
  - Arrhythmia
  - Prolonged QT syndrome
  - Trauma (accidental or nonaccidental)
  - Suffocation
  - Adrenal hypoplasia
  - Inherited metabolic disorders, such as fatty acid oxidation disorders
- The large majority of SIDS cases have no evidence suggesting parental psychiatric disease or neglect of the infant.
  - The proportion of SIDS deaths attributable to homicide probably is <10%.
- Suffocation, either accidental or nonaccidental, is difficult to distinguish on autopsy from SIDS.
  - Since 1999, some deaths that would previously have been classified as SIDS are now being classified as suffocation.

DIAGNOSTIC APPROACH

- SIDS is a diagnosis of exclusion.
- Other conditions must be ruled out by autopsy, death scene investigation, and review of the clinical history.

TREATMENT APPROACH

- SIDS risk reduction has centered on eliminating risk factors that have been shown epidemiologically to be associated with SIDS.

SPECIFIC TREATMENTS

- The AAP has made the following recommendations for SIDS risk reduction.
  - Infants should be placed in a supine position for every sleep.
    - Side sleeping is not advised.
  - A firm sleep surface should be used.
  - Firm crib mattress
  - Well-fitted sheet
  - Soft materials or objects, such as pillows, quilts, comforters, sheepskins, and stuffed toys, should be kept out of the infant's sleeping environment.
  - Loose bedding, such as blankets and sheets, should be avoided.
  - Smoking during pregnancy or in the infant's environment is strongly discouraged.
  - A separate but proximate sleeping environment is recommended; the infant should sleep in the same room, in a crib or bassinet, next to the parent's bed.
- Offering a pacifier at nap time and bedtime should be considered.
  - It does not need to be reinserted once the infant falls asleep and should not be forced if the infant refuses it.
  - Introduction of the pacifier should be delayed in breastfeeding infants until 1 month of age to ensure that breastfeeding is fully established.
- Overheating should be avoided.
- Commercial devices marketed to reduce risk of SIDS should be avoided.
- Home monitors should not be used as a strategy to reduce risk of SIDS.

FOLLOW-UP

- Loss of an infant to SIDS is devastating for the family, friends, and health care providers.
  - Uncertainty as to how the infant died adds an additional and difficult element to the grief process.
- Physician can play an active role by:
  - Ensuring that an autopsy is performed in all cases of sudden unexpected death
  - Discussing results of the autopsy with parents
  - Providing emotional support to the entire family, including age-appropriate support for surviving siblings
- The family should be directed to local counseling and support groups.

S

COMPLICATIONS

- With the increased rate of supine sleeping, the incidence of plagiocephaly without synostosis has increased.
  - Infants with plagiocephaly are:
    - More likely not to have had head position altered when put down to sleep
    - More likely to have spent little awake time in the prone position ("tummy time")
    - Less likely to have been held in the upright position while awake
- Development of positional plagiocephaly can be avoided by:
  - Altering supine head position during sleep
  - Encouraging upright cuddle time
  - Avoiding excessive time in car seats, infant carriers, and bouncers, all of which place pressure on the occiput
  - Encouraging tummy time when the infant is awake and observed
    - Awake tummy time will also enhance upper body motor development.
- A perception exists that sleeping supine may increase the risk of:
  - Gastroesophageal reflux
  - Choking
  - Aspiration
- However, evidence indicates that infants who vomit are at greater risk of choking when they are prone.
- The incidence of aspiration or vomiting has not increased with increased supine sleeping.

PREVENTION

- Sleeping in a non-prone position
  - The rate of prone sleeping decreased from 70% in 1992 to 13% in 2004.
  - The rate of SIDS decreased from 1.2 deaths per 1000 live births to 0.57 deaths per 1000 live births in 2002.
  - Similar decreases in SIDS have been experienced in other countries that have initiated similar educational campaigns.
- Use of pacifiers
  - By a yet unidentified mechanism, pacifiers appear to reduce the risk of SIDS when used at sleep time.
  - 2 recent meta-analyses demonstrate a strong protective effect.
  - Several studies have shown a negative correlation between pacifier use and breastfeeding duration.
    - Early pacifier use may interfere with establishment of good breastfeeding practices.
    - Thus, in breastfed infants, pacifiers should not be offered for the first month of life until breastfeeding has been well established and incidence of SIDS is low.

S

Syncope

DEFINITION

- Syncope: a transient sudden loss of consciousness and postural tone
- Presyncope: the presence of sensory and postural impairment without actual loss of consciousness

EPIDEMIOLOGY

- Prevalence
  - Syncope affects 3.5% of the general adult population.
  - Almost one-third of these adults will have recurrent syncope.
  - Corresponding numbers for children are not known, but recurrence appears to be less common in childhood.
- Age
  - Both neurocardiogenic syncope and orthostatic hypotension affect adolescents more commonly than adults or children of any other age.
    - Also common from 6 months to 3 years, when breath-holding spells are prevalent
    - Children with the pallid type of breath-holding spell have an increased risk of neurally mediated syncope (NMS) as adults.

MECHANISM

- Two causes account for almost 80% of all cases of benign syncope.
  - Neurocardiogenic (vasovagal) syncope
  - Orthostatic hypotension
- Neurocardiogenic or vasovagal syncope
  - The most common cause of benign syncope
  - Also known as *common faint, church faint, reflex syncope,* and *NMS*
  - Classified into 3 types
    - Postural syncope
      - The most common type of NMS
      - Associated with the upright position
      - Typically develops while the person is standing or walking
    - Central syncope
      - Occurs in response to strong emotional stimuli, such as pain, anticipated pain, or the sight of blood
      - In susceptible individuals, emotional stimulation activates ill-defined areas in the central nervous system that trigger sympathetic inhibition and parasympathetic activation.
    - Situational syncope
      - Occurs after specific stimulation of sensory or visceral afferents, resulting in hypotension and then syncope
        - Syncope evoked by the hypersensitivity of carotid baroreceptors
        - Micturition syncope
        - Defecation syncope
        - Hair-grooming syncope
        - Swallow syncope
        - Cough syncope
        - Weight-lifter's syncope
      - Much less common in teenagers than in adults
- Orthostatic hypotension is the decrease in blood pressure after assuming the upright position.
  - The autonomic nervous system provides the principal responses to changes in position.
  - If mechanisms that balance cardiac output and cerebral perfusion cannot maintain the blood pressure on standing, then the decrease in the pressure in the carotid sinus leads to reduced afferent traffic in the carotid sinus and thus to an increase in the heart rate.
  - The compensatory increase in heart rate is inadequate in patients with orthostatic hypotension.
  - Symptoms of weakness and light-headedness develop, typically within seconds of standing.
  - Sinus tachycardia of orthostatic hypotension sets this type of syncope apart from NMS, during which bradycardia is a prominent sign.
- The origin of syncope that is not benign can be:
  - Cardiac
    - Structural lesions
    - Dysrhythmias
      - Bradyrhythmias
      - Tachyrhythmias
  - Neurologic
  - Metabolic
  - Psychiatric

HISTORY

- Detailed inquiry into exact circumstances surrounding the event
  - Time of day
  - Presence of upper respiratory infection
  - Time since last meal
  - Posture during syncope and time spent in this posture before syncope
  - Presence of prodromal symptoms
  - Duration of loss of consciousness
    - Consciousness usually is regained quickly in the case of vasovagal syncope (a few seconds to 1 or 2 minutes).
    - A seizure may last longer, and the postictal state may be characterized by prolonged confusion and fatigue.

- Bystander testimony
  - In orthostatic hypotension, symptoms occur within seconds of standing; in NMS, symptoms characteristically appear after being upright for at least a few minutes.
- Any headache or prolonged disorientation after syncope
- Circumstances precipitating the event
  - The prodrome of a seizure may consist of an aura; a cardiac event often occurs without warning or is induced by exercise.
  - NMS is most often brought about by pain or prolonged standing, especially in warm environments.
- Degree of unconsciousness
  - Was the child completely unconscious?
  - Was some degree of responsiveness present, suggesting hysteria or malingering?
    - A truly unconscious person will not respond if the eyelashes are lightly brushed.
    - A hysterical person will respond, albeit often with just a mild flickering of the lids.
  - In NMS of childhood, loss of consciousness typically is preceded by:
    - Light-headedness, nausea, yawning, feeling of being hot, sounds seeming distant
- The presence of seizure-like movements
  - However, generalized tonic-clonic movements may be seen in any form of syncope.
- Significant diseases in the medical history include:
  - Congenital heart disease
  - Seizure disorder
  - Endocrine abnormality, such as diabetes
- Migraine
  - The primary care physician should always ask about migraine when a syncopal episode that does not fit the typical pattern of NMS, particularly if dizziness occurs in the sitting position and no other provoking factors can be elicited.
  - History of flashing lights, severe headache preceding syncope, and family history of migraines usually help clinch the diagnosis of migraine.
- Recurrent syncopal episodes are unusual and may require more extensive testing.
- The family history
  - Seizure disorders and cardiac disease leading to syncope may be inherited in an autosomal-dominant fashion.
    - Marfan syndrome
    - Hypertrophic cardiomyopathy
    - Prolonged QT syndrome
  - Breath-holding spells also can have a familial pattern.
- Occasionally, a cause is not identifiable.

PHYSICAL EXAM

- Level of consciousness
  - A child who is not alert and oriented:
    - Has not had a benign syncopal episode
    - Needs immediate evaluation for potentially life-threatening causes
  - In most children who are fully alert after a syncopal episode, physical examination is normal.
- Heart
  - Cardiac murmur may point to an obstructive lesion, such as aortic or pulmonic stenosis.
  - Listening to the heart in both the supine and upright positions is important.
    - A mild obstructive gradient in hypertrophic cardiomyopathy may become audible only when the patient is upright.
  - Heart rate and blood pressure
    - Obtain in both the supine and upright positions to ascertain the presence of orthostatic intolerance.

DIFFERENTIAL DIAGNOSIS

Behavioral or psychiatric causes

- Breath-holding spells
  - Two types of breath-holding spells typically occur in children between 6 months and 3 years.
    - Cyanotic
      - Cyanosis and apnea are precipitated after a child is upset and begins to cry.
      - Stiffening of the body and loss of consciousness may soon follow.
      - The pathophysiologic basis is unclear, but crying during expiration may cause increased intrathoracic pressure, which leads to low cardiac output.
      - Hypoxia combined with decreased cerebral blood flow leads to loss of consciousness.
      - The event is brief, and afterward, the child becomes fully conscious.
    - Pallid
      - Pallid breath-holding spells (pallid infantile syncope) are less common and usually begin with sudden pain.
      - The child suddenly becomes pale and limp and loses consciousness.
      - The pathophysiologic basis is increased vagal tone causing apparent asystole.
      - Ordinarily lasts only seconds to minutes, and the child awakens to full consciousness
- Hyperventilation
  - Benign
  - Frequent among adolescents, especially in the presence of anxiety

S

- It results in the washing out of carbon dioxide, and hypocapnia causes reduced cerebral blood flow, dizziness, and syncope.
- Classically, hyperventilation is associated with numbness and parasthesias of the hands and feet.

■ Psychiatric syncope
- The child is likely to be unusually calm.
- No autonomic effects, such as change in heart rate or blood pressure, are noted during episodes.
- Episodes tend to be recurrent and frequent and to occur in front of an audience.
- Recovery of consciousness often is prolonged, and usually no injury is sustained.

Cardiac causes

■ Syncope can result from low cardiac output secondary to either a dysrhythmia or a structural problem.

■ The abnormal rhythm underlying the syncope may be either too slow or too fast.

■ Bradyrhythmias
- Sick sinus syndrome is extremely rare in a child with a normal heart.
- Usually seen after extensive surgery in the atria with the Senning and Mustard operations for transposition of the great arteries
- Patients who have undergone the Fontan procedure for a single ventricle may be at risk secondary to atriotomies and dilated atria.
- Atrioventricular (AV) block
  - Very slow heart rates from AV block can lead to syncopal episodes termed *Stokes-Adams attacks*.
  - Congenital AV block in the presence of a structurally normal heart is most commonly associated with a mother who has a history of systemic lupus erythematosus.
  - Structural heart disease most commonly associated with congenital AV block or risk of acquired AV block is corrected transposition of the great arteries.
  - AV block is also occasionally acquired after cardiac surgery or Lyme disease.

■ Tachyrhythmias
- Supraventricular tachycardia
  - Majority of children with supraventricular tachycardia have a structurally normal heart
    - In those children, palpitations and dizziness are more common symptoms of supraventricular tachycardia than syncope.
  - With a structural abnormality resulting in reduced hemodynamic reserve (eg, a single ventricle), syncope may be a presenting feature.

- In patients with congenital heart defects, Wolff-Parkinson-White syndrome is seen most often in children with disorders of the AV fibrous valve annuli, such as Ebstein disease and corrected transposition of the great arteries.
- Ventricular tachycardia (VT)
  - Rare in children, but can cause sudden death
  - Early identification of underlying conditions that predispose to VT can be life saving.
  - Prolonged QT syndrome
    - Patients are at risk of sudden death secondary to a polymorphic VT termed *torsades de pointes.*
    - Prolongation of the QT interval may be part of a congenital syndrome.
    - Two syndromes that result in prolonged QT interval are caused by mutations in genes encoding cardiac ion channels
      - Romano-Ward syndrome: autosomal dominant
      - Jervell and Lange-Nielsen syndrome: autosomal recessive, associated with congenital neural deafness
    - May be caused by an electrolyte imbalance, such as
      - Hypokalemia
      - Hypocalcemia
    - May be caused by a variety of drugs, including:
      - Tricyclic antidepressants
      - Certain macrolide antibiotics
      - Antiarrhythmic medications
  - VT also can occur in children as a complication of myocarditis or in adolescents with Tetralogy of Fallot who have undergone surgical repair in infancy.

■ Pacemaker malfunction
- Syncope in a child with a pacemaker should prompt immediate interrogation of the device for either a malfunction or inappropriate programming.

■ Structural heart disease
- Acute reduction in cardiac output can result in reduced cerebral perfusion and syncope.
- With certain heart conditions, patients may be able to maintain adequate cardiac output at rest but experience syncopal episodes with exercise.
- Aortic stenosis
  - Mechanisms that may contribute to syncope in children with severe aortic stenosis include:
    - Impediment to the forward flow of blood from marked left ventricular hypertrophy
    - Stimulation of the ventricular mechanoreceptors, resulting in systemic vasodilatation
    - Subendocardial ischemia causing a ventricular arrhythmia

- Hypertrophic cardiomyopathy
  - Syncope with exercise may be an important presenting sign.
  - Most affected patients have no left ventricular obstruction at rest.
    - With exercise, they can develop a dynamic gradient with an acute reduction in cardiac output.
    - These patients also may develop VT from subendocardial ischemia.
  - The electrocardiogram often is abnormal.
  - The echocardiogram is diagnostic.
- Tetralogy of Fallot
  - Children with unrepaired tetralogy of Fallot may have syncopal episodes in association with hypercyanotic tet spells.
  - Syncope is often precipitated by crying, straining with a bowel movement, or awakening from sleep.
- Pulmonary hypertension
  - With exertion, children with pulmonary hypertension may experience syncope from an inability to maintain transpulmonary flow.
- Marfan syndrome
- Coronary artery abnormalities
  - A patient with syncope who is demonstrated to have a coronary artery aberrant either in its origin or course should be presumed at risk for sudden death.
  - Typically, syncope occurs with exercise.
  - Acquired abnormalities of the coronary arteries include:
    - Coronary artery aneurysms
    - Stenosis caused by Kawasaki disease in early childhood.
  - Cocaine
    - Can cause acute coronary vasoconstriction and ventricular arrhythmias, with consequent syncope

Postural orthostasis tachycardia syndrome

- Diagnosis requires either
  - Orthostatic heart rate acceleration >120 bpm
  - Absolute increase ≥30 bpm in the absence of significant orthostatic hypotension
- Two forms have been identified, both more common in young women.
  - Peripheral variety (more common)
    - Persistent tachycardia, associated with fatigue, exercise intolerance, and palpitations, is present while the patient is upright.
    - Onset may occur after a viral illness, trauma, or surgery.
  - ß-Hypersensitivity (or central) form
    - Often associated with migraines, tremor, and excessive sweating

Neurologic causes

- Seizures
  - Typically, generalized seizures are preceded by a prodrome that includes tonic-clonic activity with loss of consciousness and a period of confusion and lethargy after recovery.
  - Atypical seizures can be difficult to differentiate from the benign forms of syncope.
  - Loss of consciousness in the recumbent position is more likely to occur from seizure, especially if the heart is normal.
  - Pallor is seen more often in benign syncope, and flushing is more common with seizures.
  - Bowel incontinence points toward a seizure disorder.
- Migraine
  - Migraine should be considered in a child who has a syncopal episode that does not fit the pattern of typical NMS.
  - A history of flashing lights, severe headache preceding the episode of syncope, and a family history of migraines usually help clinch the diagnosis.
- Head trauma
  - Brief loss of consciousness with head trauma is not uncommon and is termed *concussion*.
- Narcolepsy

Metabolic causes

- Hypoglycemia can cause syncope, most commonly in a child who has diabetes and is on medication.
  - Presyncopal symptoms may be present: weakness, hunger, confusion
  - This syncope typically is not brief.
- Dehydration
- Severe anemia
- Pregnancy should always be considered when a woman of childbearing age faints.
  - Pregnancy-associated fainting results from increased estrogen and progesterone levels that cause decreased peripheral vascular resistance and hypotension.

Drug-induced syncope

- Diuretics
- Vasodilators

LABORATORY EVALUATION

- The complete blood count should be checked if anemia is suspected as the cause for syncope.
- Serum glucose should be checked if hypoglycemia is considered to be a cause of syncope.

IMAGING

- Echocardiography
  - When suspicion exists based either on history (eg, syncope with exercise) or on examination of a structural cardiac lesion
  - Usually can demonstrate the origin and course of the coronary arteries adequately

DIAGNOSTIC PROCEDURES

- Electrocardiography
  - The only test indicated in most patients with a history typical of benign syncope
  - May reveal the presence of AV block or dysrhythmia
  - Abnormally large left ventricular forces, especially with left ventricular strain, may be the only evidence of hypertrophic cardiomyopathy in a patient with normal findings on physical examination.
  - Corrected QT interval should be measured in all children with syncope or seizures to ensure that prolonged QT syndrome is not missed.
- Monitors
  - Holter monitor
    - 24-hour electrocardiographic monitoring test
    - Used if a cardiac dysrhythmia is strongly suspected because of:
      - Prominent palpitations that occurred before the episode
      - History of cardiac surgery that may predispose a child to abnormal rhythms
  - Event monitor
    - Patients can keep the monitor for 1 month and use it when symptoms are occurring.
- Electrophysiologic testing and cardiac catheterization
  - Must be considered for any patient who has had syncope during active exercise and no abnormality on physical examination, electrocardiogram, and echocardiogram.
- Tilt-table testing
  - Creates an orthostatic stress
  - Can provoke symptoms in patients with NMS and orthostatic hypotension
  - A means of provoking vasodepressor syncope in susceptible individuals after other more serious causes have been ruled out
  - Procedure
    - The patient is placed supine on a table that has a footboard.
    - The table is then tilted up 60–80 degrees for 30–60 minutes.
    - Patients are monitored closely for a syncopal episode.
  - Sensitivity and specificity
    - Sensitivity ranges from 30–80%, depending on the laboratory.
    - Some centers use low-dose intravenous isoproterenol infusions to increase sensitivity.
    - The specificity of a negative test without isoproterenol ranges from 80–100%.
  - The utility of head-upright tilt-table testing in children is still controversial.
  - Indications for the use of this test include:
    - ≥3 syncopal episodes during a 12-month period with no evidence of heart disease
    - Syncope during exertion in which heart disease has been ruled out after an exhaustive workup
    - Recurrent syncopal episodes thought to be hysterical in nature

TREATMENT APPROACH

- The management of cardiac, neurologic, metabolic, and behavioral/psychiatric syncope depends on the cause.
- For most patients with NMS or orthostatic hypotension:
  - Reassurance
  - Education regarding the cause of the syncope and how to avoid aggravating factors, such as extreme heat or standing still for long periods
  - Patients should be instructed to sit down or lie down at the onset of any prodromal symptoms to avoid injury.

SPECIFIC TREATMENT

Isometric exercises

- In a small randomized trial of adults, intense gripping of hands and tensing of the arms for 2 minutes at the onset of tilt-induced symptoms increased systolic blood pressure.
  - Syncope occurred in 37% of these patients, compared with 89% in those who did not perform the maneuver.
- "Tilt training"
  - Controversial, but may be helpful to some patients
  - Patients are instructed to stand with their backs against a wall, initially for short periods, and slowly increasing the duration to approximately 30 minutes per day.

Volume expansion

- A reduced frequency of syncope in adolescents with neurocardiogenic syncope was reported after they drank 2 liters of water in the morning.
- Fludrocortisone is a synthetic mineralocorticoid that causes salt retention and expansion of the central blood volume.
  - One randomized trial in adolescents showed similar results to atenolol, but no placebo was studied.

ß-Blockers

- Have been used for many years as therapy for neuro-cardiogenic syncope
- Studies of their effectiveness have been at best equivocal.

Investigational agents

- Mitodrine
  - A direct α_1-receptor agonist that has been shown to reduce episodes in adults with severely symptomatic neurocardiogenic syncope
- Selective serotonin reuptake inhibitors
  - Serotonin may have a role in regulating the sympathetic nervous system activity.
  - Selective serotonin reuptake inhibitors have been considered for treatment of NMS.
- Paroxetine
  - In a trial in adults, has been shown to be superior to placebo
- Cardiac pacing
  - Currently has a very limited role in the management of syncope
  - Has been used for children in whom asystole is the prominent symptom in recurrent syncope caused by vagal hypertonia, including some patients with deglutition syncope

WHEN TO REFER

- Patient history of cardiac disease
- Family history of sudden death, cardiac disease, or deafness
- Recurrent episodes
- Recumbent episode
- Exertional syncope
- Prolonged loss of consciousness
- Associated chest pain or palpitations
- On medications that can alter cardiac conduction

FOLLOW-UP

- All patients with syncope need a close follow-up to monitor the frequency of syncopal episodes and also to monitor the response to therapy.

COMPLICATIONS

- Injury due to fall

PREVENTION

- Prognosis for syncope depends on its cause.

S

Tics

DEFINITION

- *Tics* are recurring, nonrhythmic, sudden, rapid, stereotyped, involuntary movements or vocalizations.
- Tics may be classified as motor or vocal and as simple or complex.
  - The most common *simple motor tics* are:
    - Eye blinking
    - Neck twisting
    - Shoulder shrugging
    - Grimacing
  - The most common *simple vocal tics* are:
    - Coughing
    - Throat clearing
    - Sniffing
    - Grunting
  - *Complex motor tics* include more sustained, orchestrated, or seemingly purposeful gestures.
    - Touching, stomping on, or sniffing objects
    - Jumping
    - Sustained dystonic movements
    - Copropraxia (obscene gestures)
    - Echokinesis (automatic imitation of another person's movements)
  - *Complex vocal tics* include:
    - Sudden changes in volume or prosody
    - Syllables, words, or stock phrases spoken out of context
    - Palilalia (repeating one's own words)
    - Echolalia (repeating the words of others)
    - Coprolalia (uttering obscenities)

EPIDEMIOLOGY

- Tic disorders exist on a clinical spectrum ranging from:
  - Transient, isolated, inconsequential tics to
  - More persistent multiple motor and vocal tics that interfere with daily functioning
- Isolated and transitory tics are common.
  - Occur in as many as 24% of first- and second-graders
- The childhood prevalence of Tourette syndrome (TS) is thought to be 2 to 185 per 10,000 persons.
  - Much higher than previously believed
  - Many milder, uncomplicated cases do not come to clinical attention.
  - Boys are affected more than girls by TS.
    - A ratio as high as 9:1 to 14:1
- The most common age at onset for tics is 6 or 7 years.

MECHANISM

- Tics are a neurobiological disorder.
  - They are not caused, but only worsened, by psychological factors.
- The cause of tics is unknown.
  - Areas of research include:
    - Basal ganglia
    - Cortico-striatal-thalmo-cortical circuitry
    - Genetics
    - Immunology
  - Current research is considering a multifactorial cause for TS.
    - Genetic vulnerability
    - Environmental and perinatal risk factors
    - Disturbances in the prefrontal cortex and basal ganglia
- Developmental basis
  - Tics are common in middle childhood.
  - Usually begin to disappear by early adolescence, pointing to maturation in the neuromuscular apparatus
- Sex
  - Boys are more affected than girls.
    - This supports the motor developmental view.
    - Boys are more active in terms of motor movement than girls at all ages, especially in middle childhood.
    - Androgens are implicated for the following reasons.
      - Postnatal exposure to androgens may elicit TS.
      - Antiandrogen therapy may improve tics.
      - Androgen-dependent alterations in prenatal brain development may be associated with TS.

HISTORY

- Obtain history on potential prenatal and perinatal risk factors.
  - Maternal smoking
  - Vomiting and stress during pregnancy
  - Drugs
  - Fetal nutrition
  - Low birth weight
  - Exposure to androgens

PHYSICAL EXAM

- Assess tics, considering how to distinguish them from other neurologic disorders.
  - Evaluate for:
    - Stereotyped nature
    - Variability over time
    - Transient suppressibility
    - Accompanying premonitory urges
    - Lack of other neurologic symptoms

- The usual initial motor tics are blinking or facial grimacing, followed by rostral-caudal involvement.
- The most common initial vocal tics are:
  - Sniffing
  - Coughing
  - Throat clearing
  - Symptoms are often initially mistaken for allergies or otolaryngologic or respiratory symptoms.
    - With tics, other characteristics of such disorders are absent.
- Tics wax and wane in intensity and frequency.
  - One tic disappears, and a new one takes its place.
- Stress or excitement often exacerbates tics.
- Children are generally unaware of their tics.
  - Premonitory urges are often reported in more severe cases or in older children.
- Tics are often transiently suppressible with effort.
  - This usually results in an increased urge to perform the tic.
  - Many patients describe their tics as neither fully voluntary nor involuntary.
    - Some consider the effort to suppress tics in social situations as burdensome as the tic.

DIFFERENTIAL DIAGNOSIS

- Anxiety, stress, and excitement make existing tics worse and may even precipitate them.
  - Children with anxiety disorders are overrepresented in clinical samples.
    - Little is known about the psychological status of most children in the general population who have tics because they are rarely seen in clinics.
    - However, evidence exists for increased autonomic lability in individuals with TS.
- Psychiatric disorders should be distinguished from psychological or stress factors because of severity.
  - Studies point to a relationship between tics and:
    - Attention-deficit/hyperactivity disorder (ADHD)
    - Obsessive-compulsive disorder (OCD) with symptoms
      - Premonitory urges
      - Intrusive thoughts
      - Compulsive actions
- Many cases of tics are genetic in origin.
- Drugs that may produce or exacerbate tics include:
  - Amphetamines and other dopaminergic drugs
  - Cocaine and other stimulants
  - Sympathomimetics
  - Caffeine

- Serotonin uptake inhibitors and other antidepressants
- Anabolic steroids
- Neuroleptics
- Distinguish tics from chorea.
  - Centripetal location
  - Repetitive form
  - Normal muscle tone
  - Lack of postural impersistence
- Distinguish true tics from stereotypies or self-stimulating behaviors, such as rocking. head banging, flapping, or spinning.
  - Tics are characterized by:
    - Later onset
    - Lower complexity
    - Fluctuating intensity and locus
    - Intrusive, bothersome, disruptive, and involuntary nature
  - In contrast, stereotypies are bothersome to parents but not to the child.
    - The child finds them pleasurable and resists adult attempts to interrupt them.
  - Self-stimulating movements
    - Mostly occur at times of boredom or excitement
    - Rarely disrupt coordinated movements
    - Persist without much change in form or location
- The *Diagnostic and Statistical Manual of Mental Disorder,* fourth edition, distinguishes 4 arbitrary subtypes of tic disorder.
  - Transient
    - Duration >4 weeks but <1 year
  - Chronic
    - ≥1 year
  - Tourette disorder (also known as TS)
    - ≥1 year in duration with any remission, lasting <3 months
  - Tic disorder not otherwise specified
    - Minimum duration of 4 weeks *or*
    - Frequency of many times a day *and*
    - Present most every day
- Whether these 4 classifications reflect varying severity of the same disorder is unknown.
- Most recent research has been restricted to TS and suggests that these subtypes are probably related.

TREATMENT APPROACH

- Most tics in children are mild and short lived and do not require treatment.

T

- The possible role of any medications the child is receiving should be considered because their removal or reduction may be the required treatment.
  - Stimulants
  - Sympathomimetics
  - Selective serotonin uptake inhibitors (SSRIs) and other antidepressants
  - Neuroleptics
  - Androgenic steroids
  - Any drug that interferes with dopamine
- Once a tic has persisted for several months, treatment may be considered, if the tic is:
  - Conspicuous
  - Disabling
  - Distressing to the child
- No treatment for tics can be said to be simple, entirely effective, or free of side effects.
- Pharmacotherapy
  - Only physicians thoroughly familiar and experienced with the drugs indicated in children with tics should undertake pharmacotherapy.
  - The first consideration is deciding which symptom to target.
    - Tics
    - Comorbid conditions, such as OCD or ADHD, are often a greater source of impairment.
  - Because of frequent side effects (especially sedation), medication should be administered only when the tics are seriously disruptive, stigmatizing, or painful.
    - Start with a low dose.
    - Titrate the dose upward gradually.
    - Avoid sedation and cognitive blunting.
  - Set realistic goals in terms of reducing tics to tolerable levels.
    - Attempts to suppress tics completely often result in overmedication.
  - Discontinuing anti-tic medications should be done gradually.
    - Abrupt discontinuation may produce bothersome acute rebound or withdrawal-related exacerbation of tics that may persist for several weeks.

SPECIFIC TREATMENT

Behavioral interventions

- A variety of behavioral techniques (eg, relaxation, massed practice, avoidance learning) have been tried for tic disorders.
- Habit-reversal therapy has empirical support.
  - It is best carried out by a psychologist who is experienced in the technique and used to working with children.

- Anxiety reducing and supportive interventions
  - Relaxation training and biofeedback are not of proven value in treating tics.
  - Psychotherapy (specifically focused on stressful interpersonal difficulties), work with parents, and other means of addressing environmental stresses may be helpful.
    - Stress and high expressed emotion can exacerbate tics.
  - These procedures should not be considered specific; they are ancillary and holistic in meeting therapeutic objectives.
- Acceptance interventions
  - Explain to parents, teachers, and peers that the tics are a physical disability and the child cannot help them.
  - Acceptance of both the child and tics is the kindest, safest, and simplest way to deal with them.
    - Criticizing and belittling the child are likely to make tics worse and prolong their course.
  - Peer problems can be a major difficulty for children with tics and TS.
    - Collaboration with school staff to reduce peer teasing and stigmatization is a major therapeutic task.

Pharmacotherapy for tics

- Various medications are effective in partially suppressing tics but are not curative.
- First choice: α-adrenergic agonists
  - Clonidine
  - Guanfacine
  - Preferred first-choice agents because they are longer acting, less sedating, and more effective for attentional problems
  - These agents are relatively benign; their principal dose-related side effects are sedation and hypotension.
- Next line of agents: dopamine-blocking neuroleptics (antipsychotic drugs)
  - They appear to be effective because tics are executed through the basal ganglia.
  - There is apparent relative overactivity in the dopaminergic nigrostriatal systems that inhibits cholinergic basal ganglia systems.
  - Haloperidol, pimozide, or fluphenazine are preferred.
  - Even at relatively low doses, neuroleptics may produce:
    - Acute dystonic reactions
    - Sedation
    - Cognitive blunting
    - Medication-induced separation anxiety
    - Parkinsonism
    - Akathisia (restless legs)
  - If moderate doses are not effective, then higher doses, which increase the risk of side effects, are not likely to be either.

- Higher doses make weaning the patient from the drug difficult without rebound exacerbation.
- In many patients, typical antipsychotics are now being replaced by atypical antipsychotics, such as:
  - Risperidone, olanzapine, and ziprasidone
  - However, atypical neuroleptics have the same other adverse effects as typical neuroleptics.
    - Acute dystonic or extrapyramidal reactions
    - Hyperphagia and weight gain, with potentially serious metabolic consequences (risperidone and olanzapine)
- When neither a-adrenergic agents nor neuroleptics are effective, a variety of second-line drugs or augmentation strategies may be tried with caution.
  - Clonazepam should only be used in unusual instances.
    - Side effects: cognitive blunting, sedation, irritability, disinhibition
    - Can lead to dependence and withdrawal symptoms

Pharmacotherapy for comorbid conditions

- These conditions include ADHD, OCD, anxiety, or depression.
- Stimulants may increase tics or precipitate new tics.
- ADHD is often more disabling than the child's tics.
  - A cautious trial of a stimulant may be necessary, beginning with very low doses and increasing gradually.
  - Alternatives to the stimulants are:
    - α-Adrenergic agents (clonidine or guanfacine)
    - Atomoxetine (may also increase tics)
  - Second-line drugs are older tricyclic antidepressants.
    - Initiate electrocardiographic monitoring.
  - Most children with tics and ADHD can tolerate methylphenidate.
    - The combination of methylphenidate and clonidine is better than either agent alone.
- SSRIs are effective in children with OCD and tics.
  - Evidence suggests that monotherapy with SSRIs is less effective in the presence of tics.
  - Augmentation with a low dose of a neuroleptic often boosts the treatment response.
  - In rare cases, SSRIs can exacerbate or even precipitate tics, akathisia, or other movement abnormalities, or can increase suicidal thinking.

WHEN TO REFER

- Criteria for referring children who have tics to a mental health specialist
  - Presence of tics associated with additional evidence of a psychiatric disorder, such as ADHD, generalized anxiety, or OCD
  - Presence of chronic or recurrent tics that seem to have a clear relationship to stress, particularly if there is reason to believe that psychosocial interventions may be helpful
  - Presence of chronic, disabling, or discomforting tics for which differential diagnosis or treatment is needed
  - When the primary physician knows little about tics and wants an expert opinion
  - When psychoactive drugs, such as antipsychotics (neuroleptics) or clonidine, may be indicated
    - Psychiatrists routinely use these medications and are well informed about risks, side effects, dose levels, and newer drugs.
- Referral may be only for consultation, not necessarily for continued management.
- The preferred mental health specialist is a well-trained child or adolescent psychiatrist.
  - Broad biopsychosocial perspective
  - Knowledge of neuropsychiatry and pharmacotherapy
  - Capacity to work closely with behavioral psychologists
  - The child psychiatrist should also be alert to the possibilities of rare neurologically induced tics.
    - Will order any appropriate neuroimaging studies and neurologic consultations
- Referral should be made to a child psychologist experienced in behavioral types of treatment when:
  - The tic is disabling and no further diagnostic workup is required
  - Pharmacotherapy is not an option or is already in place, but further relief is necessary

WHEN TO ADMIT

- Never in the first instance (for tics alone)
- Occasionally, for complex assessments to initiate treatments or to taper a child from high doses of multiple medications

COMPLICATIONS

- Children with tics and especially TS can experience related problems of self-image when adult criticism and peer rejection result.
- Persistent tics are associated with an increased risk of comorbid ADHD.
  - Predates the tics or any accompanying OCD
  - Children with combined ADHD and tics have the greatest social and academic difficulties.
  - ADHD severity is a better predictor of poor adjustment than tic severity.
  - Chronic tics are often associated with learning impairment independent of ADHD.

T

- Individuals with TS are also at risk for:
  - Other anxiety disorders
  - Depression
  - Fine-motor difficulties
  - Uneven cognitive profile
    - Performance IQ scores are lower than verbal IQ scores.
  - ADHD is common and is seen in 50% of patients with TS.
  - OCD is found in up to 50% of patients with TS.
    - Most common compulsions and obsessions are around:
      - Symmetry
      - Evening up
      - Sex
      - Aggression
- OCD may develop during adolescence or late in TS.
- OCD can be a persistent source of distress despite the improvement in tic severity with age.
- Occasionally, severe complex motor tics result in injury or self-mutilation.

PROGNOSIS

- Most tics last only a few weeks.
  - Tics may flit from one muscle group to another.
  - Tics change their form at irregular intervals.
- Even the chronic tics of TS are likely to disappear in later adolescence.
  - Tic severity peaks at age 10 to 12 years.
  - Although most tics improve by late adolescence, OCD or ADHD symptoms may persist.
- Prevalence of tics drops sharply after age 13 years.
  - Tics that persist into later adolescence are more likely to become chronic.
- Tic severity in adulthood is inversely proportional to:
  - Caudate volume in childhood.
  - Childhood performance on a dominant hand fine-motor skill test

T

BACKGROUND

- Tonsillectomy is surgical removal of the tonsils.
- Adenoidectomy is surgical removal of the adenoids.
- Tonsillectomy and adenoidectomy are 2 of the most common surgical procedures performed on children worldwide.
- A consensus is just beginning to emerge regarding the proper indications for these procedures.
- Obstructive sleep apnea syndrome (OSAS)
  - Prolonged partial upper airway obstruction and/or intermittent complete obstruction (obstructive apnea) disrupts normal ventilation and sleep patterns.
  - Poor-quality sleep leads to:
    - Emotional problems
    - Increased school difficulties, including deficits in memory, vocabulary, and learning
  - Severe and untreated airway obstruction may contribute to:
    - Growth failure
    - Development of cor pulmonale
  - Enlargement of adenoids and tonsils is a common cause of OSAS.
  - OSAS can also be found in children with:
    - Obesity
    - Genetic syndromes
    - Neuromuscular disorders
    - Abnormalities of the oropharynx
  - Signs include:
    - Nighttime snoring
    - Respiratory pauses
    - Snorts
    - Gasps
  - ~10% of the population has benign primary snoring; only ~2% of children have true obstructive sleep apnea.
  - Additional diagnostic testing is needed in the habitually snoring child before proceeding with surgical intervention.
- Tonsillitis
  - Many children with recurrent tonsillitis are referred for tonsillectomy.
  - The criteria for recommending surgery are controversial.
  - The Cochrane Database of Systematic Reviews states:
    - Effectiveness of tonsillectomy has not been formally evaluated.
    - Further trials addressing relevant outcome measures are required.
  - The American Academy of Otolaryngology supports surgery in patients with ≥3 infections of tonsils or adenoids per year.

- Pittsburgh criteria: selection of patients with recurrent tonsillitis for tonsillectomy with or without adenoidectomy (document ≥1 of the following):
  - Tonsillar exudate
  - Positive cultures
  - Tender cervical lymphadenopathy (>2 cm)
  - Temperature >38.3°C (101°F)
  - *Plus* antibiotics for proven or possible streptococcal infection

GOALS

- Elimination of OSAS
  - Almost all patients with OSAS will have clinical resolution of symptoms and normalization of polysomnography after adenotonsillectomy.
  - Patients with the following conditions are less likely to have complete resolution of sleep abnormalities after an adenotonsillectomy and warrant restudy postoperatively.
    - Obesity
    - Neuromuscular weakness
    - Craniofacial anomalies
    - Severe OSAS
  - Some patients have significant improvement after adenotonsillectomy despite negative polysomnograms.
    - May respond to treatment with montelukast or nasal steroids
    - More controlled trials are needed to delineate adequate criteria for recommending surgery in patients with negative polysomnograms.
- Reduction of throat infections and elimination of tonsillitis
  - However, most experts recommend surgery only for patients with recurrent pharyngitis who meet stringent Pittsburgh criteria because of costs and complications of surgery.
  - In 1 study, children who had tonsillectomy consistently had fewer throat infections, particularly in episodes rated moderate or severe.
    - Despite better outcomes in the surgical group, rates of infection in the control group in subsequent years were relatively low, favoring observation over surgical intervention.
    - A complication rate of 14% occurred in the surgical group: all were self-limited and readily managed.
  - More recent research analyzed the adenotonsillectomy for patients with less severe criteria.
    - Differences between the surgical group and controls were statistically but not clinically significant.
      - Moderate inclusion criteria did not justify the risks of surgery, including morbidity (7.9% complication rate) and cost.

T

- In another study in which a wait-and-see approach was proposed for patients who do not meet stringent Pittsburgh criteria:
  - 4% complication rate
  - 1% required surgery for hemorrhage.
  - 2.6% had severe nausea or dehydration.
  - Did not justify minimal reductions in the frequency of tonsillitis
- Adenoidectomy
  - Adenoidectomy (but not tonsillectomy) appears to be effective in decreasing the rate of pressure-equalization tube reinsertion.
  - Has a limited role in treatment of chronic otitis media with effusion for children >4 years, particularly with those with:
    - Nasal obstruction
    - Recurrent sinusitis
    - Chronic sinusitis
  - Does not reduce the incidence of recurrent acute otitis media when performed in conjunction with insertion of pressure-equalization tubes for children <4 years.
- Improved quality of life
  - Polysomnography and parental questionnaires show significant resolution of the following symptoms after adenotonsillectomy.
    - Sleep disturbance
    - Growth
    - Breathing problems
    - Emotional problems
    - Hyperactivity
    - Aggression
    - Swallowing disorders
    - Speech problems
    - Parental anxiety or concerns
    - Activity limitations
    - Somatization behaviors

GENERAL APPROACH

- Clear indications for tonsillectomy; these conditions are uncommon:
  - Recurrent peritonsillar abscess
  - Infectious mononucleosis with immunodeficiency
  - Cancer: suspect in cases of
    - Lymphadenopathy >3 cm
    - Splenomegaly with asymmetric tonsillar hypertrophy
  - Hemorrhagic tonsillitis
- Indications for adenoidectomy are not well studied.
  - Chronic otitis media with effusion if pressure-equalization tubes have to be reinserted

- Significant nasal obstruction
- Recurrent sinusitis
- Chronic adenoiditis
- Speech or orthognathic issues

- Referring all children who have snoring as the only symptom of OSAS for further testing is impractical.
  - ~40% of children with a combination of snoring and other symptoms (mouth breathing, adenoid facies, hyponasal speech, tonsillar enlargement) have OSAS and should be referred for further testing.
  - High-risk patients are those with:
    - Cardiac disease
    - Peritonsillar abscess
    - Craniofacial anomalies
    - Trisomy 21 syndrome
    - Cerebral palsy
    - Neuromuscular disease
    - Chronic lung disease
    - Sickle cell disease
    - Central hypoventilation syndromes
    - Genetic, metabolic, or storage diseases
  - Strong consideration of further testing is recommended in snoring children who are struggling academically or being evaluated for hyperactivity.
  - The gold-standard test used to diagnose OSAS accurately is the nocturnal polysomnogram.
    - Polysomnography is useful to identify those at risk for adverse outcomes who require surgery, those for whom surgery is unnecessary, and those at risk from complications.
    - Overnight pulse oximetry, unsupervised home study, and nap studies are diagnostic but not sensitive enough to rule out OSAS.
      - Thus, when these test results are negative, the patient should be referred for polysomnography.
      - If positive, the patient should be referred for surgery.
- Nonsurgical treatment options for OSAS
  - Continuous positive airway pressure
  - Weight loss if patient is obese
  - Referral to sleep specialist
- Contraindications for tonsillectomy and adenoidectomy include:
  - Cleft palate or submucous cleft palate
    - Risk for velopharyngeal insufficiency
    - Evaluate for the presence of a bifid uvula or a notched hard palate as clues to making this diagnosis preoperatively.
  - Severe bleeding disorders should be given special consideration.

SPECIFIC INTERVENTIONS

Tonsillectomy and adenoidectomy

- Techniques for adenoidectomy
  - Blunt curettage with a ring curette
  - Vaporization using an electrocautery device
- Various techniques for tonsillectomy have evolved over the last several years.
  - Objectives
    - A surgical approach that can be performed with fewer complications in an ambulatory surgery setting
    - Less postoperative pain
- Dissection and snare tonsillectomy
  - Traditional technique
  - Blunt dissection of the tonsillar capsule from the adherent pharyngeal constrictor muscle
    - From the superior to the inferior pole of the tonsil
    - Causes stretching and avulsion of the small tonsillar arteries, leading to arterial spasm and subsequent hemostasis
  - Proven to be safe, but abandoned because of the relatively large amount of intraoperative blood loss
- Electrocautery
  - Currently the most common technique for tonsillectomy
  - Dissection is conducted in a manner similar to the dissection and snare technique.
  - Minimal additional safety precautions are required.
  - Equipment is relatively inexpensive and widely available.
  - Technique is safe and rapid, with little or no blood loss.
  - Disadvantages
    - Increased postoperative pain from thermal injury to underlying constrictor muscle
    - Delayed return to normal diet
- Surgical lasers
  - Used in tonsillectomy for the past 2 decades
  - The oropharynx and tonsils are easily accessible with laser handpieces used in either:
    - Illumination mode (thermocoagulation)
    - Contact mode (vaporization)
  - Advantages include:
    - Less superior pharyngeal constrictor muscle injury
    - Better hemostasis
    - Less pain than with the more popular electrocautery technique
  - Disadvantage
    - Requires special and extensive precautions to avoid injury to the patient or operating room staff by reflected or misdirected laser light

- Extracapsular tonsillectomy
  - Uses traditional or powered instrumentation (frequently a microdebrider) to remove 90–95% of the tonsil tissue medial to the tonsillar capsule
  - Decreased injury to the pharyngeal constrictor muscle yielding decreased postoperative pain
- Harmonic scalpel tonsillectomy
  - Uses ultrasonography to disrupt and coagulate tissues
  - Operates at a lower temperature than laser or electrocautery
- Radiofrequency tonsillectomy
  - Radiofrequency energy is applied directly to tissues to generate heat and vaporize tonsillar tissue
  - Compared with electrocautery or dissection tonsillectomy
    - Less postoperative pain
    - Faster return to normal diet

COMPLICATIONS

- Life-threatening situations are rare (see table Posttonsillectomy and Adenoidectomy Complications) and generally result from catastrophic hemorrhagic and respiratory complications.
- Mortality rates after tonsillectomy are difficult to estimate because death is such a rare outcome.
  - Death usually results from aspiration of blood into the lungs, not from exsanguination.
  - If the patient can be intubated and the airway protected during an acute and catastrophic bleeding event, risk of mortality is decreased.
  - Recent improvements in outcomes are probably attributed to advances in anesthesia, monitoring equipment, medications, and preparation for hemorrhagic consequences.
- Patients at high risk for postoperative complications who require special attention to maintaining airway include:
  - Infants
  - Those with:
    - Craniofacial disorders
    - Trisomy 21 syndrome
    - Cerebral palsy
    - Neuromuscular disorders
    - Chronic lung disease
    - Sickle cell disease
    - Central hypoventilation syndromes
    - Obesity
    - Genetic or metabolic storage diseases

T

Posttonsillectomy and Adenoidectomy Complications

Complication	Onset	Presentation	Treatment
Immediate hemorrhage	<24 hr	Oral bleeding Hemoptysis Hematemesis	Exploration and ligation of blood vessel
Delayed hemorrhage	5–14 days	Oral bleeding Hemoptysis Hematemesis	Ice pack to neck and iced liquids Elevation of head and neck $AgNO_3$ cautery Blood vessel ligation Coagulopathy workup
Immediate airway compromise	Extubation—2 hr	Cyanosis Stridor	Rule out pulmonary edema Rule out aspiration Rule out laryngospasm
Delayed airway compromise	2–24 hr	Shortness of breath Stridor	Intravenous or oral steroid Nasopharyngeal airway
Dehydration	1–6 days	Lethargy Tachycardia Anuria	Intravenous rehydration Pain control Parent education

Abbreviation: $AgNO_3$, silver nitrate.

T

Torticollis

DEFINITION

- The word *torticollis* originates from 2 Latin words: *tortus*, which means *twisted,* and *collum,* meaning *neck.*
- The classic clinical picture of torticollis is of the head tilted to one side and rotated in such a way that the chin and face point to the contralateral side.
- Torticollis can be broadly classified as 1 of 2 types.
  - Congenital
  - Acquired
- Facial asymmetry is often observed in congenital torticollis but not in acquired torticollis.
  - This finding can be useful in clinically distinguishing between the 2 forms.

MECHANISM

Congenital torticollis

- Muscular torticollis is the most common form of congenital torticollis.
- Occurs clinically in the first 8 weeks of life
  - Not obvious at birth, but begins to become apparent at approximately 2 weeks of age
- Several theories have been proposed to explain the cause of this disorder.
  - Difficult delivery may result in stretching of the neck, with rupture and hemorrhage within the sternocleidomastoid muscle (SCM).
    - Subsequent muscle ischemia results from increased pressure from blood trapped within the fascial compartment, producing progressive muscle fibrosis and contracture, with eventual clinical torticollis.
    - This theory is supported by the fact that approximately 40% of patients with congenital torticollis have had a difficult birth, including forceps delivery and breech presentation.
    - Against the theory are the facts that:
      - Congenital torticollis has also been reported in children after uncomplicated births.
      - Specimens of SCM in patients with torticollis some-times show no evidence of trauma or hemorrhage.
  - Torticollis may result from an intrauterine position that occludes venous drainage from the SCM, leading to vascular congestion, ischemia, muscle damage, and fibrosis.
    - This theory is supported in that 75% of congenital muscular torticollis cases are right sided because of intrauterine, left occiput–anterior positioning.
    - Approximately 20% of patients who have congenital torticollis also have other musculoskeletal anomalies.
      - Congenital hip dysplasias
      - Talipes equinovarus
      - Metatarsus adductus

- Possible variations in congenital torticollis
  - A sternomastoid tumor or pseudotumor is palpable as a characteristically nontender, soft, and mobile mass in or next to the inferior aspect of the SCM.
    - The mass enlarges in the first few weeks of life, reaching its maximal size at 1 month of age.
    - Then, it begins to shrink until it disappears by 4–6 months.
    - The mass is replaced by a fibrous band, leading to contracture.
    - Normal growth and range of motion of the neck are prevented.
    - Facial asymmetry results from uneven growth forces.
  - A second form of congenital torticollis involves thickening and tightness of the SCM itself.
- Congenital postural torticollis occurs without the presence of a palpable mass or tightness of the SCM.

Acquired torticollis

- Most cases of torticollis in older children are primarily muscular in origin.
  - Cervical muscle or ligament injury arising from trauma can cause a head tilt and unilateral neck tenderness.
  - The condition can also occur on awakening as a result of awkward positioning of the neck during sleep.
- Benign paroxysmal torticollis
  - Disease of infancy with an unknown cause
  - A familial pattern has been described.
  - Manifestations of the condition begin in the first year of life.
    - Recurrent episodes of head tilt are associated with:
      - Emesis
      - Pallor
      - Agitation
      - Ataxia
      - Malaise
      - Behavioral changes
    - Attacks may last from several hours to several days.
    - Spontaneous and complete remission usually occurs by 5 years of age.
    - Some patients develop migraines or benign paroxysmal vertigo.

HISTORY

- Obtain a thorough and detailed history.
- Particular attention should be given to:
  - Duration of symptoms
  - Previous trauma
  - Presence of fever
  - Other systemic manifestations
- In younger patients, the birth history is essential.

PHYSICAL EXAM

- Physical examination should not be limited to the head and neck.
  - Include all organ systems.
- Such findings as craniofacial asymmetry suggest a congenital torticollis of long duration.
- Webs or cysts in the neck should raise the suspicion of pterygium colli or remnant cysts.
- Patients with acquired torticollis as a result of trauma often have a tender SCM.
- Point tenderness over the cervical spine may suggest an underlying fracture or subluxation.
- Cervical vertebral osteomyelitis should be suspected in patients who have point tenderness in association with unexplained fever.

DIFFERENTIAL DIAGNOSIS

Congenital

- Muscular torticollis
- Postural torticollis
- Cervical spine anomalies
- Hemivertebra
- Atlantooccipital fusion
- Klippel-Feil syndrome
- Sprengel deformity
- Pterygium colli
- Sternocleidomastoid cysts
- Cystic hygroma
- Bronchial cleft cyst
- Unilateral absence of sternocleidomastoid
- Occipital condylar dysplasia

Acquired

- Muscular
- Cervical muscle injury
- Psychogenic torticollis
- Benign paroxysmal torticollis
- Vertebral
- Atlantoaxial subluxation
  - Laxity of the transverse cervical ligaments results in atlantoaxial instability in up to 15% of patients with Down syndrome.
- Atlantooccipital subluxation
- C2–C3 subluxation
- Rotary subluxation
- Cervical fractures
- Cervical vertebral osteomyelitis
- Rheumatoid arthritis

- Inflammatory reactions around the spine produce hyperemia and edema, which lead to laxity of the supporting ligaments and a predisposition to spontaneous subluxations and torticollis.
- Acute cervical disk calcification caused by trauma or respiratory infection
- Eosinophilic granuloma

Infectious

- Infections of the head and neck (Grisel syndrome)
- Upper respiratory infection
- Retropharyngeal abscess
- Cervical lymphadenitis
- Cervical vertebral osteomyelitis
- Dental infections

Neurologic

- Ocular torticollis caused by:
  - Paralysis of the extraocular muscles
  - Strabismus
  - Nystagmus
  - Refractive errors
- Spasmus nutans, including acquired nystagmus, head nodding, torticollis
  - No known cause
  - Signs and symptoms usually develop within the first 2 years of life.
  - May persist for months to years, but the clinical course often is benign and self-limited
- Dystonic torticollis may follow administration of phenothiazines, carbamazepine, or phenytoin.
  - The presence of other extrapyramidal signs can often be used to distinguish patients who have dystonic reactions.
- Wilson disease
- Syringomyelia
- Labyrinthine torticollis
- Accessory nerve palsy
- Brachial plexus palsy
- Arnold-Chiari malformation
- Neoplasms, including cervical cord tumors, cerebellar tumors
  - Ataxia is often a cardinal feature.
- Soft-tissue tumor
- Histiocytosis X (Langerhans cell histiocytosis)
- Infantile desmoid fibromatosis

Other

- Sandifer syndrome is an abnormal posturing that includes torticollis and opisthotonos.
  - Believed to be a protective mechanism adopted by some patients with one of several conditions, including gastroesophageal reflux, esophagitis, or hiatal hernia

- Dermatogenic torticollis is a painful, stiff neck that results from extensive local skin lesions.
- Spurious torticollis is stiffness of the neck resulting from dental malformations and caries.

LABORATORY EVALUATION

- Helpful adjuncts to diagnose torticollis caused by infection or inflammation
  - Peripheral leukocytosis
  - Increased sedimentation rate

IMAGING

- Imaging of the cervical spine should be obtained:
  - In all neonates with torticollis
  - In older children with findings that suggest vertebral involvement
  - In older children with persistent torticollis
- Ultrasonography is the imaging modality of choice for initial evaluation.
- Patients with neurologic deficits should undergo prompt computed tomography or magnetic resonance imaging of the head and neck.
- Several congenital cervical spine anomalies can occur in conjunction with torticollis.
  - Most of these anomalies can be diagnosed by radiographic studies of the cervical spine.
    - Pterygium colli, a congenital web of the skin of the neck extending from the acromial process to the mastoid, can be restrictive and result in torticollis.
    - Congenital remnant cysts within the body of the SCM are a less common cause of torticollis.
    - Unilateral absence of 1 SCM results in unopposed action of the other muscle and produces a contralateral torticollis.

TREATMENT APPROACH

- Congenital muscular torticollis responds well to prompt conservative treatment during the first year of life.
- The treatment of acquired torticollis arising from other specific diseases should be directed at the cause.
- Any child with severe neck pain or tenderness over the vertebra requires immediate cervical immobilization until radiography can be performed to exclude the possibility of vertebral fracture or subluxation.

SPECIFIC TREATMENT

Congenital torticollis

- Medical management includes passive and active stretching of the neck.
  - Gentle (passive) stretching can be performed daily by parents or a physical therapist.
  - Active stretching

  - Manipulate the infant's environment in such a way that objects of interest are located on the side of the room opposite to the torticollis to induce the infant to turn the neck in the desired direction.
- Surgical correction is essential if:
  - Deformity persists beyond the first year of life.
  - Range of motion is restricted >30%.
  - Residual craniofacial deformity exists.
- Craniofacial asymmetry is best reversed early, when the child's growth potential is at its maximum.
- The surgical procedure that has the best results involves:
  - Bipolar tenotomy of the affected SCM
  - Followed by casting or bracing to maintain the corrected posture

Acquired torticollis

- Acquired muscular or ligamentous torticollis should be managed with:
  - Local heat
  - Massage
  - Analgesics
  - Muscle relaxants
  - Soft cervical collar
- Symptoms usually resolve in 7–10 days.
- Patients with acquired muscular or ligamentous torticollis experience only mild discomfort.
- For drug-induced dystonic reaction:
  - Discontinue the offending drug.
  - Administer intravenous diphenhydramine.

WHEN TO REFER

- Presence of craniofacial asymmetry
- Radiographic evidence of cervical spine abnormality
- >30% restriction in range of motion
- Persistence beyond the first year of life

WHEN TO ADMIT

- Presence of neurologic deficits
- Severe neck pain
- Point tenderness over the vertebrae

FOLLOW-UP

- Congenital torticollis should be followed carefully for development or worsening of craniofacial deformities.

COMPLICATIONS

- If not treated appropriately, patients with congenital torticollis may develop craniofacial deformities or worsen existing craniofacial deformities.

Tuberculosis

DEFINITION

- Tuberculosis (TB)
  - Serious disease caused by *Mycobacterium tuberculosis*
  - Distinguished from latent TB infection (LTBI)
  - Common clinical presentations
    - Pneumonia
    - Intrathoracic or peripheral lymphadenopathy
    - Meningitis
    - Disseminated TB
    - Bone and joint disease
- Latent TB infection
  - Occurs when the organism is in a metabolically dormant state and replicating slowly within granulomata in the lung and other tissues
- Tuberculosis exposure
  - A person is defined as exposed to TB if he or she has spent time in close proximity to a potentially contagious patient with TB disease.
  - The exposed individual may or may not be infected.

EPIDEMIOLOGY

- Prevalence
  - TB disproportionately affects young children because of:
    - Increased risk of progression to disease once infected by *M tuberculosis*
    - Increased likelihood of disseminated disease
  - Case rates of TB per 100,000 US children (2006 report)
    - Children age 0–14 years: 1.3
    - Children age <5 years: 2.4
      - Foreign-born: 21.9
      - US-born: 2.1
      - Hispanic or Latino: 5.5
      - Asian: 5.2
      - Black or African American: 4.5
      - White: 0.2
  - Among US children with TB in 2006
    - 485 were <5 yrs of age; 322 were ages 5–14.
    - 48% were Hispanic (most from Mexico).
    - 31% were black.
    - 25% of TB cases in children occurred in the foreign-born group.
      - 15% were <5 years of age
      - 40% were 5–14 yrs of age.
    - 36% of cases were reported from California, Texas, and New York.
    - 73% had pulmonary TB (with or without extrapulmonary TB).

- Because LTBI is not a reportable condition in most states, the number of children who have LTBI is unknown.

ETIOLOGY

- TB is caused by a member of the *M tuberculosis* complex, which includes *M tuberculosis* and *Mycobacterium bovis*.

RISK FACTORS

- Children at highest risk for TB
  - Children of color
  - Children born in countries with a high prevalence of TB or into families from these countries
  - Children who live with or in contact with adults who are at risk for TB
  - Children <4 years
- If several family members have positive tuberculin skin test results, then likelihood that patient's disease is TB increases.
- Ingestion of foreign unpasteurized milk and milk products, such as Mexican-style soft cheeses (queso fresco), raises possibility of infection with *M bovis*.
- Patients infected with HIV or who have another immuno-compromising conditions are more likely than others to have:
  - TB *or*
  - Atypical or extrapulmonary presentation of TB

SIGNS AND SYMPTOMS

- US children diagnosed with TB disease
  - Often are asymptomatic, *but*
  - Have radiographic evidence of disease, eg, infiltrate or intrathoracic adenopathy
- Common symptoms of TB
  - Weight loss or failure to gain weight
  - Anorexia
  - Fever
  - Cough
  - Decreased energy, playfulness, or activity
- Symptoms of extrapulmonary TB
  - Lymph node enlargement
  - Headache
  - Personality changes
  - Focal neurologic changes
  - Musculoskeletal pain
- TB can produce fulminant or indolent symptoms, but symptoms typically are more chronic when caused by TB than when caused by bacterial or viral infections.
  - Cough often is noted for weeks rather than days.
  - Lymph node swelling develops over weeks, with gradual and modest changes in the overlying skin.

- Occasionally, symptoms such as cough and fever actually have begun to improve by the time of diagnosis.

DIFFERENTIAL DIAGNOSIS

Forms of Tuberculosis

- Pulmonary infiltrate
  - Community-acquired pneumonia (eg, bacterial pneumonia, including lung abscess and necrotizing pneumonia; viral pneumonia)
  - Atelectasis caused by reactive airways disease or other processes
  - Other granulomatous diseases (eg, coccidiomycosis, histoplasmosis)
- Intrathoracic lymphadenopathy
  - Infections caused by fungus, virus, or bacteria
  - Nontuberculous mycobacterial infections
  - Malignancies
  - Round pneumonia
  - Other granulomatous diseases (eg, coccidiomycosis, histoplasmosis)
- Subacute peripheral adenopathy
  - Scrofula caused by nontuberculous mycobacteria
  - Cat-scratch disease
  - Toxoplasmosis
  - Partially treated pyogenic infection
- Viral, bacterial, fungal, and chemical meningitis
- Differential diagnosis for tuberculin skin test (TST) results
  - Truly positive
    - Caused by infection with *M tuberculosis* complex
  - Falsely positive
    - Cross-reaction with nontuberculous mycobacteria (eg, *Mycobacterium avium* complex and *Mycobacterium scrofulaceum*); often, but not always, smaller than reactions caused by *M tuberculosis*
    - Cross-reaction with recent or multiple vaccinations with bacille Calmette-Guérin (BCG) (see below)
  - Allergic-type reactions—peak within 24 hours of TST placement and should be gone within 48–72 hours
    - Induration that peaks >24 hours after TST placement is due to a delayed-type hypersensitivity, the mechanism of a true-positive TST reaction.
      - Irritation from a circular Band-Aid or tape
      - Injection with a substance other than purified protein derivative (PPD)
  - Falsely negative
    - Recent infection with *M tuberculosis* (delayed-type hypersensitivity reaction takes 2–8 weeks after infection to develop)
    - Infancy

- Improper storage of the PPD skin test material (eg, not refrigerated, prolonged storage in syringe)
- Improper placement (eg, subcutaneous placement, pressure by gauze or a Band-Aid leading to the absorption of PPD solution)
- Vaccination with a live virus vaccine within the previous 6 weeks
- Generalized or specific anergy associated with extensive or disseminated TB or as seen in immunocompromised patients, especially those infected with HIV

Prior BCG vaccination

- Sometimes causes a small, transient TST reaction as a result of cross-reactivity among antigens
- Clinicians are advised to discount history of BCG vaccination when interpreting TST.
- The following factors decrease the likelihood that the skin test reaction is caused by BCG:
  - TST reaction (induration) >10 mm
  - Previous receipt of a single rather than multiple BCG vaccines
  - BCG given in the first month of life
  - A long period since the BCG dose
  - Receipt of no other recent TST
- New blood tests may further clarify the impact of BCG on TST reactions and allow for more accurate TST cutoff points in individuals who have received BCG.

DIAGNOSTIC APPROACH

- TB diagnosis in a child usually is a clinical diagnosis, influenced by:
  - Probability of exposure to a person with infectious TB
  - TST results
  - Clinical symptoms and signs
  - Results of imaging tests
- All of these factors are weighed, along with the risk to the child of not treating TB, when considering whether to begin treatment.
- Universal skin testing for TB is not recommended.
- Annual assessment for TB risk factors and testing of children with defined risk factors are the standard of care.
- Testing asymptomatic children without known risk factors for TB is no longer performed.
- Use the TST to diagnose LTBI and support the diagnosis of TB disease.
- Because of the poor sensitivity and specificity of the TST in low-incidence populations, administer it only to the following children:
  - Those who have clinical disease that raises concern for TB
  - Those at high risk for progression to TB disease

- Those who have new risk factors for TB exposure since their last TST
- Most children with US-born parents never require a TST.
- If a child has a positive TST result, the evaluation includes:
  - Chest radiograph
    - A 2-view chest radiograph (frontal and lateral views) is particularly helpful in differentiating intrathoracic lymphadenopathy from other hilar structures.
    - National guidelines suggest obtaining 2-view radiographs on all children when resources permit.
    - If resources are limited, children >6 years of age should be screened with 1-view chest radiographs.
  - Focused history
  - Physical examination
- Pertinent medical history
  - Previous TB skin test results
  - Previous TB treatment
  - Results of any previous chest radiographs
  - Factors that would complicate TB therapy, including underlying liver disease and use of potentially hepato-toxic drugs
- If the family does not know anyone with TB disease, ask family members if they:
  - Have close contact with an adolescent or adult with chronic cough, fever, or unexplained weight loss
  - Have household contact with an individual with a positive TST result (especially a newly positive result)
- Because >50% of adult patients with TB disease are born outside the US (primarily in Latin America, Asia, Africa, and Eastern Europe), contacts from these areas should be solicited.
- Ask family members:
  - Where children were born
  - Where they have traveled
  - How long they stayed
  - With whom they stayed when traveling in TB-endemic areas
- Immediately perform a TST on any family member who has not recently had such a test (and has never had a positive result in the past).
- To prevent possible continued transmission of TB, obtain chest radiographs of adults with a previous or newly positive TST result or suspicious TB-like symptoms.
- Physical exam
  - Assess vital signs
  - Assess growth parameters
  - Examine conjunctiva
  - Check neck flexion
  - Palpate lymph nodes

- Auscultate heart and lungs
- Palpate abdomen and flank
- Palpate spine and bone
- Briefly examine skin
- Conduct neurologic exam (depending on concerns for TB of the central nervous system).
- Limitations of physical exam
  - LTBI: no examination abnormalities that suggest TB disease
  - Even children with pulmonary TB may have no findings at physical exam.
  - Findings on chest radiograph often are more useful than those found by physical exam or history.

LABORATORY FINDINGS

- Routine testing for children suspected of having TB includes:
  - HIV serologic testing
  - Mycobacterial cultures
- Sputum specimens are challenging to collect from young children, but they can be collected by 3 methods:
  - Gastric aspiration (procedure is described below)
    - Aspirates typically are collected on 3 consecutive mornings after an overnight fast.
    - Yields of 30–50%; highest in the youngest infants and from the initial sample collected
    - If the patient is not otherwise ill enough to require inpatient management, then gastric aspirates can be collected in the outpatient setting.
  - Sputum induction
    - In older children, attempt sputum induction with hypertonic saline.
    - Inducing sputum in infants is difficult.
  - Bronchoalveolar lavage
    - Used primarily when diagnoses other than TB are being strongly considered
    - Yield in children: 10–21%
    - Yields are lower than for gastric lavage in children.
- Other tests
  - Cerebrospinal fluid (CSF): 50–75% yield in diagnosis of TB meningitis
  - Acid-fast bacillus (AFB) smear: even lower yield, but can be improved by centrifugation of large volumes of CSF
  - Polymerase chain reaction: disappointing, but may play a role as an adjunct diagnostic method
  - AFB smear and culture of other tissues, as indicated for:
    - Lymph node tissue
    - Abscess drainage
    - Bone or synovial fluid
    - Urine

- Blood
- Bone marrow
- Other tissue
- Submit specimens for AFB smear and culture in a sterile cup (rather than on a swab) and without formalin preservative.

■ Regardless of the culture method or specimen, culture for *M tuberculosis* in children has suboptimal yields.

■ Families should understand that:
- AFB smears usually are not positive from specimens from children.
- Cultures must be incubated for several weeks before results are available.
- Yield from cultures is <50% in most situations.

■ Consider other laboratory evaluations based on individual circumstances.

■ Measure liver transaminase levels in patients with:
- TB-HIV coinfection
- Severe TB disease
- Symptoms or signs of hepatitis
- Known underlying liver disease

■ The QuantiFERON-TB Gold test
- In vitro diagnostic test for detecting interferon gamma (IFN-γ) when a patient's whole blood is incubated with specific TB proteins and controls.
- Detection of IFN-γ indicates a T-cell response by the patient's lymphocytes and probable infection with *M tuberculosis*
- Few data support its applicability to children, although studies are underway.

■ Gastric aspirate procedure for culture of *M tuberculosis*
- Health care workers present during gastric aspirate procedures of a patient with suspected or confirmed infectious TB disease should wear at least N-95 disposable respirators.
- Collect all supplies and have everything ready:
  - N-95 respirators
  - Papoose board or sheet
  - No. 10-French or larger nasogastric or suction tube
  - 30-mL syringe with appropriate connector for tube
  - Pen
  - Sterile water
  - Specimen cup or laboratory-preprepared tube containing bicarbonate for bedside neutralization
  - Requisition and label
  - Helper
- Child should not take anything by mouth for at least 6 hours before the procedure.

- Immobilize the child with a sheet, with or without a papoose board.
- Measure the distance from the nose to the stomach.
- Insert a No. 10-French nasogastric tube through the nose into the stomach.
- Puff in the child's face as the tube enters the throat to elicit a swallow reflex.
- Gently aspirate the tube with an appropriately fitted 30- to 60-mL syringe.
- If no significant yield, then advance and withdraw the tube slightly while aspirating.
- If yield is still <5–10 mL, then place any collected mucus into a container.
- Check tube position by auscultating the stomach while pushing air from the syringe into tube.
- Instill 20 mL of sterile water into the stomach and quickly aspirate again.
- If yield is <5–10 mL, roll the child on the side and advance the tube, aspirating continuously to find the pool of mucus in the stomach.
- As tube is withdrawn, continuously aspirate the syringe.
- Place any yield, including any spontaneously vomited emesis, in the specimen container.
- Label the specimen and order AFB smear and culture.
- Promptly transport the specimen to the laboratory for processing (tell the laboratory if the specimen has already been neutralized).

IMAGING

■ Radiography
- Perform in children with:
  - Positive TST result
  - Suspicion of pulmonary or extrapulmonary TB
- For the best-quality radiograph, the child should be in full inspiration and should not be rotated.
- Guidelines suggest obtaining 2-view radiographs on all children when resources permit. If resources are limited, children >6 years can be screened with 1-view chest radiographs.
  - Lateral view helps distinguish other central shadows from intrathoracic lymph nodes, which are spherical and often can be seen on both views.
- Films should be interpreted by a clinician or radiologist experienced in pediatric TB.
- Findings on chest radiographs
  - Enlarged intrathoracic lymph nodes and infiltrate are the most common abnormalities.
  - Intrathoracic adenopathy: present in up to 85% of children <3 years of age

T

- Hilar, mediastinal, paratracheal, and subcarinal nodes may be seen, most often on the right side.
- Isolated adenopathy should be treated as TB disease.
- An infiltrate may be seen in any lung field and is seen in multiple lobes in one-quarter of children.
- Older children, especially adolescents, may have radiographic findings that are consistent with adult reactivation (postprimary) TB, including:
  - Upper lobe disease with fibronodular infiltrates
  - Volume loss
  - Hilar retraction
  - Cavities
- Segmental lesion (infection spread to other parenchymal locations) when the material is limited to one bronchus
- Diffuse bronchopneumonia (when the organism spreads throughout the lung)
- Disseminated disease (distribution of *M tuberculosis* via hematogenous dissemination that causes disease to the lung and other organs) causes lesions with small, round, millet-like radiographic appearance.
  - These disseminated processes do not always appear radiographically in the classic disseminated pattern.
- Larger, patchy, reticulonodular lesions may be present and are difficult to distinguish from other diffuse lung infections.
- Pleural effusion and empyema are less common in children with TB compared with adults.
- Signs of healed *M tuberculosis*
  - Isolated, dense nodules with calcification
  - Nonenlarged calcified lymph nodes
  - Isolated pleural thickening
- Peribronchial cuffing or thickening is commonly associated with reactive airway disease and viral infection and, in isolation, is not consistent with TB.
- Computed tomography
  - Not indicated in evaluation of an asymptomatic child with a normal chest radiograph and a positive TST result
  - Can be helpful when the radiograph is equivocal and it is necessary to look for other causes of lung disease

DIAGNOSTIC PROCEDURES

- Tuberculin skin testing
  - The only recommended TST is intradermal instillation of 5 TU (0.1 mL) PPD by the Mantoux method.
  - The skin test should be placed and interpreted by a trained health care professional.
  - The definition of a positive TST result depends on risk factors for infection and the likelihood of TB disease.

- TST results are considered positive under the following circumstances:
  - ≥5-mm induration
    - Child is immunosuppressed (receiving immunosuppressive therapy) or immunocompromised, including HIV infection.
    - Child is a recent contact of a person with TB or suspected TB disease.
    - Radiograph or clinical evidence suggests TB disease.
    - Fibrotic changes on chest radiograph are consistent with prior TB infection.
  - ≥10 mm induration
    - Child is <4 years of age.
    - Child has preexisting medical conditions (eg, lymphoma, Hodgkin disease, diabetes mellitus, chronic renal failure, malnutrition).
    - Child or parent was born in a country with a high prevalence of TB.
    - Child has frequent exposure to high-risk adults (HIV infected, homeless, residents of nursing homes, institutionalized, incarcerated, users of illicit drugs, migrant farm workers).
    - Child has traveled to a high-prevalence country.
    - Child is a resident of California.
  - ≥15-mm induration
    - Child is ≥4 years of age and has no risk factors.

TREATMENT APPROACH

- Asymptomatic presentations of TB disease are treated with multidrug therapy because they will progress in most children if not treated.
- Providers are legally mandated to report persons suspected of having or confirmed to have TB to the local health department.
- Manage children with TB disease in a dedicated TB clinic or by the most experienced pediatric TB clinician available.
- In areas where this treatment is not feasible, seek close and ongoing consultation with an experienced clinician.

SPECIFIC TREATMENTS

Tuberculosis

- Four-drug empiric regimen
  - Isoniazid (INH), rifampin, pyrazinamide, and ethambutol
  - Recommended for individuals who
    - Are at higher risk for having INH-resistant TB, including exposure to an individual from an area of high prevalence of drug-resistant TB
    - Have known drug-resistant TB
    - Previously received treatment for TB

- Directly observed therapy (DOT) by a health care professional (not parents) is recommended for treatment of TB in children and adolescents.
- Corticosteroids
  - Beneficial in central nervous system disease, particularly stage 2 and 3 (altered mental status)
  - Sometimes used for any child with symptomatic TB meningitis
  - Frequently used for TB pericarditis
  - Two reports support the use of corticosteroids in children with symptomatic airways compression caused by lymphatic disease.
- Prednisone
  - Generally used at a dose of 1–2 mg/kg/day given for 4–8 weeks, then tapered over several weeks
- Treatment regimens for TB in children
  - Pulmonary TB
    - Minimal duration of therapy: 6 months
    - Initial regimen: Isoniazid, rifampin, pyrazinamide, and ethambutol daily for 2 weeks to 2 months (3-drug therapy only if no risk of resistance)
    - 4-drug initial therapy is provided if any risk exists of drug resistance.
    - If a cavitary lesion was present on the chest radiograph and sputum culture is positive after 2 months of treatment, extend total treatment duration to 9 months rather than 6 months.
  - Extrapulmonary (meningitis, bone or joint, disseminated)
    - Minimal duration of therapy: 9–12 months
    - Initial regimen: Isoniazid, rifampin, pyrazinamide, and ethambutol daily for 2 weeks to 2 months (3-drug therapy only if no risk of resistance)
    - Some clinicians use an injectable drug (eg, amikacin, kanamycin) for initial treatment of disseminated or meningeal disease.
    - Strongly consider corticosteroid therapy for some types of extrapulmonary disease (eg, meningitis, pericarditis).
  - Other extrapulmonary (cervical adenopathy)
    - Minimal duration of therapy: 6 months
    - Initial regimen: isoniazid, rifampin, pyrazinamide, and ethambutol daily for 2 weeks to 2 months (3-drug therapy only if no risk of resistance)
    - 4-drug initial therapy is provided if any risk exists of drug resistance.
    - If a cavitary lesion was present on the chest radiograph and sputum culture is positive after 2 months of treatment, extend total treatment duration to 9 months rather than 6 months.

Latent tuberculosis infection

- INH
  - Patients should receive INH monotherapy daily for 9 months unless they have a medical contraindication (including infection with a known INH-resistant strain).
  - Dosing is 270 daily doses (or twice a week administered by DOT) within a 12-month period.
  - Available as 100-mg and 300-mg scored tablets and as a liquid suspended in sorbitol. The tablet can be crushed and mixed with or layered into a strong-flavored semisoft food in a spoon.
  - Doses by weight (10–15 mg/kg per day; maximal dose, 300 mg)
    - Daily dose for weight 3–5 kg (6.6–11 lbs)
      - 50 mg
        - 100-mg tablets: ½
    - Daily dose for weight 5–7.5 kg (11–16.4 lbs)
      - 75 mg
        - 100-mg tablets: ¾ *or*
        - 300-mg tablets: ¼
    - Daily dose for weight 7.5–10 kg (16.5–22 lbs)
      - 100 mg
        - 100-mg tablets: 1
    - Daily dose for weight 10–15 kg (22–33 lbs)
      - 150 mg
        - 300-mg tablets: ½
    - Daily dose for weight 15–20 kg (33–44 lbs)
      - 200 mg
        - 100-mg tablets: 2
    - Daily dose for weight >20 kg (>44 lbs)
      - 300 mg
        - 100-mg tablets: 3 *or*
        - 300-mg tablets: 1
  - When a prolonged break occurs after a short initial treatment period, restart therapy.
  - Short lapses are tolerated, especially if the regimen is well underway.
  - If therapy is interrupted for >2 months, reevaluate child for possible TB disease before restarting INH.
  - Vitamin-B_6 (pyridoxine) supplementation is indicated only for
    - Exclusively breastfed infants
    - Children and adolescents on milk- and meat-deficient diets
    - Children who experience paresthesias while receiving INH therapy
    - Children with HIV infection

T

- Examine children monthly and question them about symptoms of toxicity.
- Most side effects of INH can be overcome with adjustments of timing or symptomatic management.
- Patients receiving antiepileptic drugs (particularly phenytoin and carbamazepine) should have these drug levels monitored.

■ Rifampin

- Occasionally used as an alternative for a patient who is intolerant to INH or is known to be infected by an INH-resistant TB strain
- Given for 180 daily doses
- May accelerate the metabolism or have other interactions with several important classes of drugs:
  - Anticonvulsants
  - Antiarrhythmics
  - Antifungals
  - Barbiturates
  - ß-Blockers
  - Calcium channel blockers
  - Antibiotics
  - Corticosteroids
  - Oral contraceptives
  - Oral hypoglycemics
  - Drugs used to treat HIV infection

WHEN TO ADMIT

■ For culture collection if local resources are not available for outpatient culture collection

■ Patients with increased work of breathing, meningitis, or complicating simultaneous conditions

■ Patients who require diagnostic evaluation

■ Few children require admission to the hospital based on clinical severity of TB disease.

WHEN TO REFER

■ All patients suspected of having active TB should be reported to the local health department according to state statute (eg, within 1 working day).

■ In many jurisdictions, young children with LTBI should be reported to the local health department, according to local regulations.

■ Ideally, an experienced pediatric TB clinician should manage children with TB disease. If local resources are not available, then close and ongoing consultation with a pediatric TB expert should be established.

FOLLOW-UP

■ Monitor patients monthly during therapy.

■ For children from whom sputum can be obtained, follow-up sputum to document culture conversion

■ Twice-weekly dosing by DOT can be used after induction phase of daily treatment if child is tolerating the regimen well and has shown considerable clinical improvement.

- Number of doses actually observed should be counted when considering whether a patient has completed therapy.
- Patients receiving daily doses for the first 2 months typically will receive 40 observed doses
  - Monday through Friday for ~8 weeks
  - Followed by 36 twice-weekly doses in the following 18 weeks

■ Routine laboratory evaluation is not necessary, unless:

- Patient has symptoms of toxicity or underlying liver disease.
- Patient is taking other medications that might interfere with the TB drugs or cause similar toxicities.

■ Obtain end-of-therapy chest radiograph.

- Most children do not have a normal radiograph at the end of therapy, but significant improvement is expected.

■ Follow-up regimen for pulmonary TB

- Stop ethambutol as soon as the patient or reliable source case isolate is found to be drug susceptible.
- Document a follow-up chest radiograph 2 months into therapy.
- If isolate is sensitive and patient is clinically well and radiographically improving or stable, then change to isoniazid and rifampin at 2 months to complete a 6-month course; twice-weekly therapy can be provided by directly observed therapy.
- Document chest radiograph at end of treatment—frequently not quite normal.

■ Follow-up regimen for extrapulmonary TB (meningitis, bone or joint, disseminated)

- 7–10 months of isoniazid and rifampin, either daily or twice a week by directly observed therapy

■ Follow-up regimen for other extrapulmonary TB (cervical adenopathy)

- Same as for pulmonary TB disease, except no need to follow chest radiographs if initially normal

■ Unless an alternative diagnosis is established, most often, once TB therapy is begun, course should be completed.

T

COMPLICATIONS

- INH
  - The liquid formulation causes cramping and diarrhea in more than one-half of children because of its osmotic load.
  - INH-related transient increase of transaminases has been noted in children, with effects increasing with increasing age.
    - INH rarely causes clinical hepatotoxicity in children.
  - Routine monitoring of liver transaminases is not indicated for asymptomatic children who do not have underlying liver disease and who are not receiving other hepatotoxic drugs.
  - Thoroughly educate families about recognizing symptoms of hepatotoxicity (eg, anorexia, malaise, abdominal pain, vomiting) and instruct them to stop therapy and return to clinic if these symptoms arise.
  - Lack of association with other viral symptoms and lack of improvement after a few days should suggest possibility of hepatotoxicity rather than an intercurrent illness.

PREVENTION

- Identify children at risk for exposure to TB
  - Aggressively evaluate and treat children exposed to potentially contagious adolescents and adults with TB (young children usually are not contagious)
  - Treat LTBI
  - Promptly treat contagious TB patients

- Targeted testing
  - Skin testing only for children who are at high risk of contracting TB infection or developing TB disease if infected
    - Results in fewer unnecessary skin tests
    - Avoids evaluation and treatment of children with false-positive TST results
  - At each well-child visit, screen child with a risk-factor questionnaire (modify based on local risks).
  - Conduct skin testing only if a new risk factor has been identified since the last TST.
- Tuberculosis exposure
  - Contagious TB requires prompt and thorough evaluation to determine whether the child already has evidence of LTBI or TB disease.
  - Children <5 years and all immunocompromised individuals with significant exposure should receive window prophylaxis after TB disease has been ruled out by a normal chest radiograph and negative physical examination.
    - Window prophylaxis: treatment with INH until a repeat TST (given 8–10 weeks after their last exposure) is performed and is negative.

T

Umbilical Anomalies

DEFINITION

- Aberrations in configuration, formation, or position of the umbilical cord, including minor anomalies, can offer helpful clues to underlying disease in the young child.

EPIDEMIOLOGY

- Prevalence
  - Meckel diverticulum
    - Present in 2.5% of newborns in the US
  - Vascular abnormalities
    - Variations in the pattern of 2 arteries and 1 vein occur in 0.7% of all births.
    - The most common variation is the presence of only 1 artery (single umbilical artery) and 1 vein.
      - In 25–50% of cases, it is associated with various anomalies, including malformations of central nervous system, genitourinary tract, spine, and extremities.
      - Absence of the left umbilical artery is more commonly associated with fetal anomalies.
      - Associated aneuploidies include trisomy 13, trisomy 18, and triploidy.
    - A persistent right umbilical vein has been reported to occur in 1 in 400 births; this is a benign finding.
  - Umbilical hernia
    - Extremely common; could be considered a variation of normal
    - Varies with race and age
    - More common in African-American infants (32%) than in white infants (4%)
      - Decreases to 12% and 2%, respectively, at 1 year
    - More common in low–birth-weight babies
    - Boys and girls are equally affected.

ETIOLOGY

- The umbilical cord appears within the first 6 weeks of gestation.
- It is derived from the fusion of 3 separate embryonic structures.
  - The primitive or primary yolk sac, which contains:
    - Allantois and a portion of the vitelline duct, transient structures that ultimately form the central portion of the embryonic gut
    - Urinary bladder
    - Umbilical blood vessels
  - The secondary yolk sac
    - Remainder of the vitelline duct
  - The mesenchyme of the connecting body stalk of the embryo
    - Tissue that produces Wharton jelly, which is the packing substance that holds the cord together

- Many of the structures that form the umbilical cord are present for only brief periods during embryogenesis.
- After fusion is complete, these unified structures become covered by amnion and ultimately are surrounded by amniotic fluid.
- Anomalies may result when these structures fail to undergo normal regression and persist into postnatal life.

SIGNS AND SYMPTOMS

Failure of closure and regression of the vitelline duct

- Failure of closure and total regression by the 7th week of gestation may lead to:
  - Meckel diverticulum
    - Outpouching of gut without attachment to anterior abdominal wall
    - Well-known cause of clandestine lower intestinal bleeding from the presence of ectopic gastric mucosa within the diverticulum
    - Can occur anywhere from the ileocecal valve to a point ≥3 feet proximal to the valve
    - Resembles supernumerary vermiform appendix
    - Presence may be signaled by symptoms and signs of acute appendicitis.
  - Vitelline cyst or enterocystoma
    - A connection between the midgut and umbilicus without communication with either structure
  - Enteric or vitelline fistula
    - Formed from a communicating connection between the midgut and the umbilicus
  - Urachal sinus, cyst, or fistula
    - Results from a connection between the bladder and the urachus
- Presence of these anomalies may be indicated by:
  - Signs of infection and lower midline abdominal mass caused by infection of a vitelline cyst
  - Discharge of feces and urine can lead to erosive dermatitis (from enteric and urachal fistulas)
  - Urinary tract infections resulting from urachal fistulas
- Persistence of a fibrous band of tissue attached to the gut results from incomplete involution.
  - May serve as the lead point for a volvulus or the cause of intestinal obstruction

Vascular abnormalities of the umbilical cord

- Blood vessels are the most important structures in the umbilical cord.
  - The pattern of anomalies in infants with aberrant cord vessels often depends on which vessels are present and which are missing.
    - 3 patterns have been described.

- Single umbilical artery of allantoic origin, associated with growth restriction, anomalies of central nervous system, such as anencephaly and spina bifida, and abnormalities of the lower genitourinary tract

- Single artery of vitelline origin, associated with sirenomelia, sacral agenesis, reduction defects of lower extremities, anal atresia (features of VACTERL [vertebral, anal atresia, cardiac, trachea, esophageal, renal, and limb defects]), and trisomy 18

- 3 vessels, including a single umbilical artery (of either allantoic or vitelline origin); a left umbilical vein; and a persistent and aberrant right umbilical vein, described in some children with Noonan syndrome and *47,XXY* karyotype

Umbilical hernia

- Usually no associated medical sequelae

  - Incarceration, strangulation, rupture, or skin breakdown occurred in <5% of 590 children in 1 study.

  - Other studies have revealed even lower rates of complication.

- Most close spontaneously without medical intervention.

  - The major indication for surgical treatment is cosmetic, and surgery should only be considered in carefully selected individuals.

- Although most umbilical hernias occur as isolated findings in otherwise healthy children, they can be associated with a variety of known conditions, many of which feature increased abdominal girth or hypotonia.

  - Common autosomal trisomies
  - Mucopolysaccharidoses
  - Inborn errors of metabolism associated with organomegaly
  - Dysmorphic syndromes, such as Beckwith-Wiedemann syndrome

Umbilical granulomas

- At birth, the normal umbilical cord contains only umbilical vessels surrounded by protective Wharton jelly.

- Within the first 2 weeks after birth, the umbilical stump normally dries and separates from the abdomen; the umbilicus is completely covered by skin in 3 to 4 weeks.

- Delayed healing with accumulation of excessive amounts of granulation tissue produces an umbilical granuloma, a small, reddened mass.

- The lesion may be associated with infection at its base or with a foreign body, such as talcum, but recedes rapidly after repeated topical applications of silver nitrate.

- Persistence of embryonic remnants may be suggested by:

  - Persistence of a granulomatous-appearing lesion after treatment
  - Presence of erosive dermatitis at the site
  - Egress of gas, feces, or urine from the site

Umbilical polyps

- External remnants of the umbilical cord may superficially resemble umbilical granulomas

- May be sinuses of the vitelline duct or urachus

- Differ from granulomas

  - Larger
  - Bright red
  - Not responsive to treatment with silver nitrate

DIFFERENTIAL DIAGNOSIS

- Variations may be linked to specific dysmorphic syndromes.

  - Aarskog-Scott syndrome: prominent, protruding, pouting
  - Achondroplasia: low placement
  - Bladder exstrophy: low placement
  - Cloacal exstrophy: low placement
  - Cornelia de Lange syndrome: hypoplasia
  - Rieger syndrome: prominent, broad, redundant periumbilical skin
  - Robinow syndrome: high placement, broad, scar is poorly epithelialized

- Conditions associated with umbilical hernias

  - Chromosomal anomalies

    - Trisomy 21
    - Trisomy 18
    - Deletion 9p
    - Duplication 3q

  - Metabolic disorders

    - Hypothyroidism
    - Mucolipidosis III (pseudo-Hurler syndrome)
    - Mucopolysaccharidoses
    - Type 1 (Hurler syndrome)
    - Type 2 (Hunter syndrome)
    - Type 4 (Morquio syndrome)
    - Type 6 (Maroteaux-Lamy syndrome)

  - Dysmorphic syndromes

    - Aarskog syndrome
    - Beckwith-Wiedemann syndrome
    - Fetal hydantoin syndrome
    - Marfan syndrome
    - Opitz syndrome
    - Weaver syndrome

U

LABORATORY FINDINGS

- Presence of urachal fistula can be documented by the presence of methylene blue dye in urine after dye has been instilled at the umbilicus.
- Diagnosis of umbilical polyps depends on histologic examination.

IMAGING

- Gastrointestinal radionuclide scans using ^{99m}technetium pertechnetate
  - To detect embryonic umbilical remnants lined with gastric mucosa

- Sonography or computed tomography
  - Helpful in delineating vitelline cysts that exhibit as abdominal masses after onset of infection

TREATMENT APPROACH

- Treatment of all symptomatic internal umbilical cord remnants is surgical excision and repair.

U

Urinalysis and Urine Culture

BACKGROUND

- Examination of the urine is a simple and efficient office procedure that may detect or evaluate for renal, urinary tract, and systemic disorders.
  - A first-morning, midstream, clean-catch specimen is most reliable.
  - Usually only needed in symptomatic children to aid in diagnosis
  - Important in evaluating the child with renal symptoms
    - Should be considered in patients with vague signs and symptoms, because some renal disorders may exhibit in such nonspecific ways
  - Less useful as a screening procedure in asymptomatic patients than in patients with symptoms

GOALS

- Several principles need to be considered in screening for abnormalities in the urine.
  - A screening test should be reliable and accurate.
  - Screening should be done for conditions that can be diagnosed with certainty and benefit from early diagnosis and treatment.
  - A screening test should be cost effective for the individual and the general population.
- Early discovery of a symptom-free child who has renal disease may prove to be beneficial.
  - The cost-effectiveness to society of mass screening in young children remains unproven.
- Current data do not support the current practice of routine screening urinalysis.
  - High degree of sensitivity
  - Lack of specificity (ability to minimize false-positive results)
  - The low prevalence of end-stage renal disease in children limits the positive predictive value of screening for hematuria or proteinuria.

GENERAL APPROACH

- Recommendations for urine screening have evolved over time.
  - The majority of pediatricians conduct screening urinalyses frequently.
  - The AAP and Bright Futures practice guidelines recommend:
    - Complete urinalysis at 5 years of age
    - Annual urinalysis for sexually active adolescents
  - Bright Futures also recommends that complete urinalysis be performed at least once during adolescence even if the individual is not sexually active.
    - This policy is currently under review by the AAP and may be changed in the near future.

- Findings that can help diagnose and manage a pathologic condition
  - Presence of heavy proteinuria
    - Nephrotic syndrome or other significant renal disease
  - Hematuria
    - Glomerulonephritis
  - Glucosuria
    - Diabetes mellitus
  - Leukocyte esterase or nitrites
    - Urinary tract infection (UTI)
- When to refer
  - Persistent proteinuria (first morning void)
  - Gross hematuria of unknown cause
  - Persistent hematuria associated with proteinuria or hypertension
  - Hematuria suggested to be of lower urinary tract origin, accompanied by elevated serum glucose level
  - Physician discomfort with diagnosis and management
  - Family reassurance

SPECIFIC INTERVENTIONS

Proteinuria

- Detected most easily by the dipstick method
- The presence of protein causes a change in indicator color from yellow to blue-green.
  - Proportional to the amount of protein present
    - Albumin causes the color to change more readily than do other proteins.
  - Does not usually detect the small quantity of protein that healthy persons normally excrete.
- Sensitivity of detecting proteinuria with a urine dipstick ranges from 83.9–95.1%.
- Specificity ranges from 93.8–95.5%.
- False-positive findings can occur in:
  - Alkaline urine
    - pH >6.5
  - Urine contaminated by skin antiseptics, including chlorhexidine or benzalkonium chloride
- Urine concentration also affects dipstick results and should be taken into consideration.
- Results are considered to be persistent if:
  - Dipstick is positive (≥1+) for ≥2 of 3 random urine specimens collected ≥1 week apart
  - Quantifying proteinuria using the protein-to-creatinine ratio on a random urine sample is recommended.
    - A ratio ≥0.2 mg protein per mg creatinine is considered abnormal for children ≥2 years.

– This method is suggested because accurately obtaining a 24-hour urine collection in children can be difficult.

■ The prevalence rate in the symptom-free pediatric population depends on the definition of proteinuria used.

- Prevalence increases with age and is greater in girls than it is in boys.

- The prevalence of proteinuria can range from <1% in 6-year-old boys to as high as 6% in adolescent girls using less stringent criteria.

- If more strict criteria are used (2+ on each dipstick with ≥2 performed), prevalence decreases considerably.

  – 0.2–0.45% in boys

  – 1–1.6% in girls

■ More than 50–75% of symptom-free patients found to have protein in a single urinalysis will have normal urine on repeat testing.

- Of those having several positive random urinalysis results, ≥60% will have orthostatic proteinuria.

  – Not considered to be a harbinger of clinically significant renal disease

- Regular follow-up is important.

  – Changes in the pattern of protein excretion

  – Appearance of hematuria

- Follow-up care

  – Spontaneous resolution occurs in >40% of cases within 4 years.

  – Identifiable renal disease is present in 1 per 1000 children screened.

- Asymptomatic children who have proteinuria without hematuria are not likely to have overt renal disease.

- Patients with hematuria and proteinuria have high rates of significant parenchymal renal disease.

■ Isolated cases of significant renal disease can sometimes exhibit solely with proteinuria in the asymptomatic child.

- Significant glomerular changes which progress with time to chronic renal impairment

  – Focal segmental glomerulosclerosis

  – Immunoglobulin A (IgA) nephropathy

  – Mesangial proliferative glomerulonephritis

  – Membranous glomerulonephritis

  – Pyelonephritic scarring

- Most children with significant renal disease will have other signs and symptoms.

  – These symptoms cause them to seek medical care and thus can be identified even in the absence of urine screening.

■ High sensitivity and low specificity of screening for proteinuria in asymptomatic children can produce undue anxiety in patients and parents.

- Can direct the practitioner to perform more invasive testing

  – Often provides no new information

  – May detract from the overall well-being of the population

  – May be costly

- Currently, less enthusiasm is found for mass screening for proteinuria in symptom-free children.

  – Satisfactory compromise for the health of children is to screen a first morning urine at 5 years of age.

    ■ First morning urine avoids the identification of children with orthostatic proteinuria.

■ In the case of persistent proteinuria:

- Meticulous examination of fresh urinary sediment should precede any additional laboratory evaluation.

Hematuria

■ Not all discolored urine indicates hematuria.

- Urine can be discolored by many substances.

- The presence of blood should be confirmed by dipstick for symptoms of gross hematuria.

  – Dipstick is highly sensitive.

    ■ Reacts to hemoglobin levels as low as 0.015–0.062 mg/dL

  – Sensitivity of the dipstick for blood is 85–100%.

  – Specificity is 86.3–99.3%.

- False-positive tests for blood in the urine may result from:

  – Presence of oxidizing cleansing agents

    ■ Povidone-iodine or hypochlorite

  – Microbial peroxidases

- False-negative tests may be caused by the presence of large amounts of a reducing agent.

■ A positive dipstick result for blood:

- Does not discriminate between hemoglobin and myoglobin from muscle

  – Differentiation requires spectrophotometric analysis.

- Does not differentiate hemoglobinuria from hematuria or whether the blood originates from the upper or lower urinary tract

  – Microscopic examination of the centrifuged urine sediment

  – Dipstick-positive, red, or cola-colored urine without red blood cells (RBCs) on microscopic examination is diagnostic of free hemoglobin or myoglobin in the urine.

- In presence of RBC casts, proteinuria, brown or tea-colored urine, and dysmorphic RBCs, glomerular bleeding (upper tract) is suggested.
- Red or pink urine or clots usually indicate lower urinary tract bleeding.
- The prevalence of microscopic hematuria in an ambulatory setting
  - 2–6% when a single urinalysis is abnormal
  - Approximately 1% when >1 urinalysis is positive
    - Persists >6 months in <0.5% of these cases
  - The annual incidence of new cases is 0.4%.
    - Defined as at least 5 RBCs/high-power field
  - No consistent trends exist for age, sex, and race dependence of hematuria.
- Few children whose hematuria was detected in screening programs are found to have significant renal or urologic disease.
- Hematuria persisting for >6 months is more likely to be associated with renal disease if patient has:
  - ≥1 episode of gross hematuria or proteinuria
  - Family history of hematuria in a first-degree relative
  - The most likely diagnoses in these cases are:
    - IgA nephropathy thin basement membrane disease
    - Alport syndrome (hereditary nephritis)
- In a review of studies of screened, symptomless microhematuria
  - IgA nephropathy was found in 2–21% of biopsies.
    - Other glomerular lesions were much less frequent.
  - The most common nonglomerular finding was asymptomatic UTI (4.8–6.0%).
    - Less common were ureteropelvic junction obstruction and reflux nephropathy.
- In more recent follow-up studies of children referred for isolated hematuria, the most common underlying diagnosis (11–16%) was hypercalciuria.
- Screening for hematuria is limited by low specificity.
  - Potential value exists in identifying patients at risk for renal disease in patients with:
    - Symptoms
    - Gross hematuria, especially if recurrent
    - Proteinuria
    - A positive family history
- Persistent isolated microscopic hematuria
  - A careful examination of fresh urinary sediment and microscopic analysis should precede any additional laboratory evaluation for asymptomatic children.
    - The great majority of these children will not have clinically significant disease.
    - Continued observation without work-up is appropriate.

Glucosuria

- Can be detected by glucose oxidase-impregnated dipsticks
  - Glucose is not detectable in the urine when the plasma glucose level is <180 mg/dL.
  - Seen most commonly when the filtered load of glucose is increased as a result of hyperglycemia in diabetes mellitus
    - Less often, a defect can be found in proximal tubular reabsorption that may be selective, or may be part of a more generalized proximal tubular dysfunction.
    - Measurement of blood glucose will help differentiate among these conditions.
  - Observed in the latter stages of tubular destruction seen in a variety of chronic kidney diseases
    - Urinalysis usually also shows proteinuria, and the urinary sediment may contain renal tubular cells and casts.
- Urine screening reveals a prevalence of glycosuria that is <0.1%.
  - Up to 10–50 previously undetected cases of diabetes mellitus per 100,000 children could be identified.
    - New-onset diabetes mellitus is much more likely to produce classic symptoms of polyuria and polydipsia. (See Diabetes Mellitus.)
  - Rarely cases of renal glucosuria, Fanconi syndrome, and other tubular dysfunction may be identified.
    - The cost-effectiveness of screening asymptomatic patients for glucosuria is low.
      - Not recommended for routine visits

Bacteriuria

- Defined as growth of >100,000 colony-forming units/mL in ≥2 consecutive urine specimens in a child who has no other symptoms of infection at a regular checkup
- Prevalence of asymptomatic bacteriuria in school-age children is:
  - 1–2% in girls
  - 0–0.1% in boys
- In a child with symptoms consistent with a UTI, the presence of leukocyte esterase or nitrites generated by gram-negative organisms from nitrates will increase suspicion for bacteriuria.
- Nitrites are extremely specific to bacteriuria.
  - Specificity of 98%
  - Sensitivity of 50%
- Leukocyte esterase is much more sensitive.
  - Specificity of only 78%
  - Sensitivity of 84%
- When either leukocyte esterase or nitrite is positive:
  - Sensitivity is 88%.
  - Specificity is 93%.

U

- When both leukocyte esterase and nitrites are positive:
  - Sensitivity is 72%.
  - Specificity is 96%.
- Dipstick detection of leukocyte esterase or nitrites is variable depending on the method of collection and the age of patient.
  - In 1 study:
    - The sensitivity of bag-collected urine was 85%.
    - Catheter-collected urine samples had a sensitivity of 71% in non–toilet-trained children.
    - The specificity of bag-collected urine was 62%.
    - The specificity of catheter-collected urine was 97%.
  - The sensitivities of the 2 methods are decreased by approximately 20% in infants <90 days.
- When investigating a possible UTI with urinalysis:
  - The AAP has provided guidelines on the use of bagged urine specimens for analysis.
    - A negative result can be trusted, and no further invasive collection of urine is needed.
    - The following bagged urine sample results require that another urine sample be obtained via more invasive measures for urine culture before starting antibiotic therapy.
      - Positive leukocyte esterase or nitrites
      - A positive Gram stain
      - >5 leukocytes per high-power field

- Asymptomatic or covert bacteriuria in school-age girls
  - Nontreatment does not influence episodes of:
    - Symptomatic UTI
    - Renal growth
    - Renal function in normal or scarred kidneys
  - Treatment of asymptomatic bacteriuria may be associated with:
    - A greater risk for pyelonephritis because of development of more pathogenic and resistant organisms
  - Antibiotic treatment does not prevent further renal scarring once it has occurred or restore poor renal growth.
- Child with signs and symptoms consistent with UTI
  - Physician should have a low threshold for obtaining a diagnostic urinalysis.
  - Positive results should be confirmed by urine culture and treated.
- Screening of asymptomatic patients for asymptomatic bacteriuria is not recommended.
  - If asymptomatic bacteriuria is discovered, it should not be treated.
- Persistent bacteriuria should be more thoroughly evaluated.
  - Obtain a careful history for renal and urinary tract symptoms.
  - Assess growth and blood pressure.
  - Consider obtaining renal ultrasonography.

Urinary Tract Infections

DEFINITION

- Urinary tract infection (UTI) is a common childhood infectious disease.

EPIDEMIOLOGY

- Incidence
  - ~2–8% of children experience at least 1 UTI episode by 10 years of age.
- Age
  - Highest incidence in children <1 year of age
  - ~30% of children <12 months of age are affected by recurrent infections.
  - 85% of recurrences occur within 6 months after the primary episode.
  - Febrile UTI (pyelonephritis) is more common in children <12 months.
  - Cystitis mostly occurs in older children.
- Sex
  - Boys constitute the majority of infants ≤6 months of age.
  - Girls more commonly have UTIs beyond 6 months of age.
  - In school-age children, symptomatic UTI is 5 times more common in girls than boys.
  - Recurrence rates do not differ significantly between boys and girls.

ETIOLOGY

Community-acquired infections

- *Escherichia coli*
  - Occurs naturally in feces
  - Responsible for >75% cases of community-acquired UTI
- *Enterococcus*
- *Klebsiella*
- Coagulase-negative *Staphylococcus*
- *Proteus*
- Other commonly occurring pathogens
  - Each accounts for ~3–5% of cases.
- Genotypic analysis of pathogens causing second-time UTIs
  - 65% of recurrences caused by same pathogen as the first episode of UTI
  - Anatomic abnormalities of urinary tract significantly more frequently among patients with:
    - Non–*E coli* UTI
    - Infections caused by nonvirulent *E coli* strains

Non–community-acquired and unusual infections

- Non–*E coli* organisms should be considered possible causes of UTI in sexually active adolescents.
  - *Neisseria gonorrhoeae*
  - *Chlamydia trachomatis*
- Common pathogens causing nosocomial infections
  - Multidrug-resistant *E coli* strains
  - Non–*E coli* pathogens, eg, *Candida*
- The majority of nosocomial infections are associated with:
  - Urinary tract instrumentation
  - Catheterization
- Thus critically ill children are especially prone to UTI.
- Fungal infections are significant in:
  - Immunocompromised patients
  - Diabetic patients
- Fungal overgrowth may complicate antibiotic treatment of immunologically normal children with:
  - Abnormal urinary tract emptying
  - Indwelling urinary catheters
- Viral uropathogens are relatively uncommon, except for adenovirus infections in patients with acute hemorrhagic cystitis.
- Adenovirus, polyomavirus, cytomegalovirus
  - Can cause UTI and hemorrhagic cystitis in immuno-compromised patients
  - Especially those undergoing solid organ or bone marrow transplantation
- Protozoan infections of the urinary tract are important in many parts of the world.
  - Uncommon in the United States
- Urinary infections with *Mycobacterium tuberculosis* occur rarely in secondary tuberculosis.
  - Should be considered when sterile pyuria is found in a suspect clinical setting
  - Prevalence of tuberculosis is increasing in the US.

Bacterial virulence factors

- Uropathogenicity of the bacteria depends on:
  - Presence of virulence genes, which determines their adhesive capacity
  - Resistance to host defense mechanisms
  - Ability to cause tissue damage by toxin production
- These factors influence:
  - Severity of symptoms, such as fever and dysuria
  - Long-term effects of UTI, such as renal cell damage and scarring

RISK FACTORS

- Constipation
- Encopresis
- Not circumcised
- Bladder dysfunction (detrusor instability)

U

SIGNS AND SYMPTOMS

History

- Clinical presentation of UTI depends on:
  - Age of the child
  - Virulence of underlying pathogen
  - Inflammatory response of the host
- Symptoms most often associated with UTI
  - Dysuria
  - Frequency
  - Urgency
  - Lower back pain
- Symptoms of UTI are variable and nonspecific in young children, especially infants.
- Bacteremic UTI can be clinically indistinguishable from other types of infection in very young children.
- Small children usually cannot:
  - Localize pain
  - Report precise symptoms
- By 4 years, their capability improves to report more specific symptoms.
  - Abdominal pain
  - Pain at micturition
- Fever is the most prominent and often the only clearly recognized sign of UTI in children.
- With some caveats, fever can be used as a rough estimate of the level of UTI.
  - Body temperature <38°C suggests cystitis.
  - Temperature ≥38.5°C is most often is associated with upper UTI.

Physical examination

- Findings of UTI vary depending on severity of the infection.
- In infants, findings are nonspecific and rarely suggestive of a definitive diagnosis.
- In addition to fever, other findings suggestive of septicemia can be seen in young infants, including:
  - Irritability
  - Abnormal crying
  - Peripheral cyanosis
  - Hypothermia
  - Long capillary filling time
- Tenderness on palpation of the abdomen in the suprapubic region can be found with cystitis.
- Costovertebral angle tenderness is elicited with pyelonephritis in older children.
- An absence of typical findings does not rule out the possibility of UTI.

- Examination of the urethral meatus should be included in the examination of every child with suspected UTI.
- In some cases, dysuria can be caused by local inflammation or irritation of external genitalia.
  - External genitalia in girls should be examined carefully.
  - Labial adhesions are often associated with UTI.

DIFFERENTIAL DIAGNOSIS

- UTI should be included in the sepsis workup of seriously ill infants and younger children.
- UTI should always be considered as a possible cause of unexplained fever.
- Fever can be an inconsistent finding.
  - In newborn infants, normal body temperature does not exclude the possibility of upper UTI.
  - Fever exists in only ~10–40% of UTI cases in children <2 years of age.
  - In these cases, other symptoms should be considered as indications for urine screening, such as:
    - Vomiting
    - Irritability
    - Abnormal crying
    - Lethargy
    - Failure to thrive
    - Feeding problems

DIAGNOSTIC APPROACH

- UTI should be suspected in infants and young children with unexplained fever.
- Thoroughly assess:
  - Degree of toxicity
  - Dehydration
  - Ability to retain oral intake
- If child is critically ill, a urine specimen should be obtained by:
  - Catheterization
  - Suprapubic percutaneous aspiration
- If the urinalysis suggests UTI, repeat urine collection by:
  - Catheterization
  - Suprapubic aspiration
- Correct diagnosis is crucial for successful treatment and follow-up of childhood UTI.
  - Incorrect diagnosis of UTI may lead to:
    - Missing a potentially harmful urinary tract abnormality
    - Unnecessary studies, costs, and stress
- UTI must be always confirmed by adequate urine collection and culture.

LABORATORY FINDINGS

Urine collection

■ Adequate urine collection is essential for correct diagnosis.

- To prevent contamination, all samples should be carefully collected, stored, and analyzed.
  - Sample collection at home is discouraged because of the high risk of contamination.
  - Urine samples should be kept at 4°C until cultured.

■ Toilet-trained children and adolescents

- A midstream urine sample is preferred for culture.
- Before micturation, the periurethral area and surrounding skin should be washed and dried properly.

■ Incontinent children

- A urine bag or absorbent pad may be suitable for urine collection.
- Urine contamination rates are similar for bag and pad (75% of positive cultures).
- Contamination is significantly higher than for clean-catch urine, catheterization, or suprapubic aspiration.
- A negative culture result from urine collected by bag or pad excludes UTI.
- A positive culture result from a urine bag or urine pad sample should always be verified by:
  - Catheterization
  - Suprapubic aspiration

■ Guidelines for suprapubic percutaneous aspiration

- Indications
  - Verification of UTI in newborns and infants
  - Sepsis workup in critically ill children
- Equipment
  - 21- to 25-gauge needle
  - 5- to 10-mL syringe
  - EMLA cream
  - Sterile gloves
  - Portable ultrasonography equipment
- Technique
  - Put a small amount of EMLA cream on a circle area (~3 cm) ~2–3 cm above symphysis midline.
  - Wait about 30 minutes.
  - Set the child in a supine position.
  - Clean the patient's skin with antiseptic solution.
  - Insert the needle percutaneously at ~1 fingerbreadth above the symphysis pubis.
  - Advance slowly with continuous suction.
  - Usually urine is obtained at a depth of 2–3 cm.

- Complications
  - Generally safe and reliable
  - Occasionally transient hematuria (2–3%)
  - Intestinal puncture not harmful

Urine culture

■ Diagnosis is confirmed by the growth of a single pathogen on urinary culture.

■ The bacteria level considered significant depends on the method used for urine collection.

- For voided samples (clean-catch urine, urine bag, and absorbent pad)
  - Bacterial count ≥100,000 colony-forming units (CFU)/mL is considered significant.
- Contamination risk for catheterization and suprapubic aspirate is considerably lower.
  - Any bacterial growth in suprapubic aspirate or a bacterial count ≥50,000 CFU/mL in a catheter sample is indicative of UTI.

■ If signs and symptoms strongly suggest UTI:

- Lower bacteria counts (≥10,000 CFU/mL), particularly in the presence of pyuria, may be considered diagnostic.

■ Urine cultures showing growth of ≥1 pathogen should be considered contaminated; a repeat sample is required before starting any treatment.

Urinalysis

■ Urinalysis by itself is not sufficient to diagnose UTI.

- Normal urinalysis does not rule out UTI.
- If UTI is suspected, urine culture should always be sent despite normal urinalysis.

■ Results of urine culture are not generally available on the same day the sample is collected.

■ Urinalysis showing leukocytouria can support the diagnosis of UTI.

- Leukocytes may be present in urine (pyuria) for several reasons besides UTI.
- Pyuria is defined as ≥10 leukocytes/mcL in an uncentrifuged urinary specimen.
  - A count <10 leukocytes/mcL is almost invariably associated with a sterile urine culture.
  - A count ≥10 leukocytes/mcL is found in 90% of patients with bacterial growth ≥50,000 CFU/mL.
- The dipstick leukocyte esterase test can be used for detecting urinary leukocytes.
  - This method has a low sensitivity in detecting:
    - ≥10 leukocytes/mcL (~53%)
    - ≥20 leukocytes/mcL (~67%)

■ UTI can be an important cause of microscopic hematuria.

- The presence of erythrocytes in urine does not have diagnostic or prognostic value.

U

- The combination of cell count and Gram stain can be:
  - More sensitive (87.7%)
  - More specific (99.2%)
- The combination of leukocyte esterase test and nitrite can improve:
  - Sensitivity (78.7%)
  - Specificity (98.3%)
- The nitrite test is usually positive if bacterial counts are high enough (>10 CFU/mL).
  - A positive nitrite test result usually requires bladder time ≥4 hours.

Determining location of UTI

- Reliable differentiation of upper UTI from lower UTI can be difficult.
- Pyelonephritis is suggested by:
  - Temperature ≥38.5°C
  - Increased C-reactive protein level (≥40 mg/L)
  - Leukocytosis
  - Infants may have afebrile bacteremic UTI.
- Several biomarkers are currently being evaluated as possible indicators of upper UTI.
  - Procalcitonin
    - Recently proposed as a possible indicator of pyelonephritis
    - Increased serum procalcitonin levels correlate significantly with renal parenchymal involvement in children with febrile UTI.
    - This method is not currently routinely available.
  - No correlation between level of UTI and serum electrolyte, creatinine, and blood urea nitrogen concentrations has been reported.
  - These parameters should be measured to assess level of hydration or other attendant complications in:
    - Children <12 months of age
    - Patients with febrile UTI
    - Patients with associated symptoms, such as vomiting or diarrhea

IMAGING

General

- Imaging studies of the urinary tract are recommended for children with first-time UTI to exclude:
  - Obstructive disorders
  - Vesicoureteral reflux (VUR)
  - Severe loss of renal parenchyma
  - Significant bladder abnormalities

- Imaging studies used in UTI include:
  - Renal ultrasonography (RUS)
  - Voiding cystourethrography (VCUG)
  - ^{99m}Technetium dimercaptosuccinic acid (DMSA) scan

Indications for imaging studies in children

- Ultrasonography
  - First-time UTI: age <2 years
  - Febrile UTI: all ages
  - Non–*E coli* UTI: all ages
  - Second episode of afebrile cystitis: age >2 years
- VCUG
  - First-time UTI: age <2 years
  - If ultrasonogram or DMSA scan (or both) is abnormal and suggestive of VUR: all ages
  - Consider if family history of VUR
  - Consider if recurrent pyelonephritis
- DMSA scan
  - Abnormal ultrasonogram (parenchymal thinning, suggestive of renal dysplasia or hypoplasia)
  - High-grade VUR
  - Consider before VCUG if febrile UTI and age >2 years
  - Consider if recurrent UTIs
- The AAP recommends that children <2 years with first-time UTI should be studied by:
  - Ultrasonography in the acute phase
  - Cystography or renal cortical scan thereafter as soon as possible
- Infants and children who do not demonstrate the expected clinical response within 2 days of antimicrobial therapy should promptly undergo:
  - Ultrasonography
- At the earliest convenient time, perform either:
  - VCUG *or*
  - Radionuclide scan
- Infants and young children who have the expected response to antimicrobials should have:
  - Ultrasonography
  - At the earliest convenient time, either:
    - VCUG *or*
    - Radionuclide scan
- The optimal time for VCUG is ~2–6 weeks after the infection.
- Recommendations about imaging studies after UTI in older children are:
  - More variable
  - Dependent on clinical presentation

U

- The probability of factors predisposing patient to renal damage is relatively low in children >2 years.
  - Imaging studies are recommended in this age group in the following scenarios.
    - Recurrent UTI
    - Non–*E coli* infection
    - Positive family history

RUS

- Least invasive, most widely available imaging modality
- Can be performed during the acute phase of UTI
- Can detect:
  - Dilated collecting system
  - Thinning of kidney parenchyma
  - Size of kidneys
  - Thickness and size of urinary bladder
- May not be able to detect:
  - VUR
  - Smaller renal scars
- Reliability is highly dependent on the experience of the ultrasonographer.
- Recent studies have suggested that results may have little or no influence on treatment, because of routine prenatal ultrasonography.
  - The need for ultrasonography after UTI has been questioned.
  - Widespread use of maternal-fetal ultrasonography in industrialized countries has possibly lessened the need for ultrasonography later in childhood.
  - Several studies have shown that a significant kidney or urinary tract abnormality may be missed despite prenatal RUS in 5–6% of children with first-time febrile UTI.

VCUG

- Traditionally used to diagnose VUR because VUR:
  - Predisposes patients to pyelonephritis and recurrent infections
  - May be associated with renal scarring
  - The incidence of VUR is highest in children <2 years of age.
- VCUG can be performed using:
  - Radiocontrast medium
  - Radiolabeled nuclides
- Contrast VCUG is usually preferred in boys.
  - More reliable than other methods in detecting urethral valves
  - Recommended as a baseline study in all children with first-time UTI
  - Allows more exact grading of reflux
- Isotope VCUG is recommended for follow-up studies.

- Cystography requires catheterization.
  - Relatively invasive and stressful, especially in older children
- Spontaneous resolution of VUR occurs in a high proportion of children.
  - Isotope VCUG is recommended every 1–3 years until resolution of VUR is documented.
- Some authors have suggested that VCUG be performed only on selected patients with abnormalities on DMSA scan.
  - This approach would reduce the number of VCUGs performed by ~50% without adding any major risk for the patient.
- VCUG should be performed only if:
  - Positive family history of VUR exists.
  - Urinary tract dilation is detected prenatally.
  - History is found of recurrent pyelonephritis.

DMSA scan

- One of the most reliable methods to differentiate pyelonephritis from lower UTI
- Radionuclide is taken up by renal tubular cells and provides information on:
  - Functional anatomy
  - Scarring of renal parenchyma
- More often abnormal in patients with documented reflux than in children without VUR
- Only 55–85% of children with febrile UTI have changes on radionuclide studies, such as DMSA scan.
  - Suggested as a gold standard for diagnosing pyelonephritis

CLASSIFICATION

- International classification of VUR
  - Grade I: involves only ureters
  - Grade II: involves ureters and intrarenal collecting systems
  - Grade III: mild ureteral and pelvic dilatation; no or slight obliteration of caliceal fornices
  - Grade IV: moderate ureteral and pelvic dilatation; clear obliteration of caliceal fornices
  - Grade V: gross dilatation of ureters and renal pelvis and calyces

TREATMENT APPROACH

- Initial antibiotics should be administered parenterally if the child with suspected UTI is:
  - Septic
  - Dehydrated
  - Unable to retain oral intake
- Antibiotic therapy should be initiated parenterally or orally in a child who:
  - May not appear ill
  - Has a urine culture confirming the presence of UTI

U

- Reevaluate infants and children who do not demonstrate expected clinical response within 2 days of antimicrobial therapy.
- Infants and young children should complete a 7- to 14-day antimicrobial course.
- After antimicrobial therapy and sterilization of urine:
  - Infants and young children should receive prophylactic antimicrobial doses until the imaging studies are completed.

SPECIFIC TREATMENTS

General

- Successful treatment includes:
  - Early recognition
  - Early, appropriate treatment
- Before initiating treatment, adequate samples of urine should be collected for:
  - Culture
  - Antibiotic sensitivities of organisms
- If the patient is septic or dehydrated:
  - Adequate rehydration should coincide with antibiotic therapy.
- Route of antibiotic administration (oral or parenteral) depends on:
  - Age
  - Clinical condition of patient

Pyelonephritis

- Infants <1 year are:
  - Hospitalized
  - Treated with parenteral antibiotics for ≥3 days
  - Followed by oral antibiotic therapy for 11 days (total of 14 days)
- Research has shown that oral antibiotics are as effective as parenteral antibiotics, even in young children with febrile UTI.
  - If the child does not appear septic and can tolerate oral medications:
    - Initial treatment with oral antibiotic might be appropriate.
    - Follow-up is essential to ensure complete recovery.

Cystitis

- Oral therapy alone is usually adequate to treat cystitis.
- First-line therapy for outpatient treatment of UTI
  - Trimethoprim-sulfamethoxazole (TMP-SMX)
  - Amoxicillin
- Other choices include:
  - Amoxicillin-clavulanate
  - First-generation cephalosporins, such as cephalexin
- 5 days of treatment with appropriate antibiotics is adequate.

Asymptomatic bacteriuria (ABU)

- Studies on infants and school-age girls have shown that untreated ABU does not increase the risk for:
  - Pyelonephritis
  - Renal damage
- Children treated with antibiotics for ABU can have a higher incidence of pyelonephritis than untreated children.
- Researchers have suggested that pathogens causing ABU have low virulence and may protect against overgrowth of uropathogenic bacteria.
- Current recommendations
  - Should not be treated with antibiotics in:
    - Children who use intermittent catheterization
    - Children with neurologic bladder dysfunction
  - These children frequently have ABU.
    - Asymptomatic
    - Often do not have leukocyturia

Antibiotic dosing

- Parenteral therapy
  - Ampicillin
    - 100 mg/kg/day divided every 6 hr
  - Amikacin
    - 15–22.5 mg/kg/day divided every 8 hr
  - Ampicillin-sulbactam
    - 100–200 mg/kg/day ampicillin divided every 6 hr
  - Cefepime
    - 100–150 mg/kg/day divided every 8 hr
  - Cefotaxime
    - 100–150 mg/kg/day divided every 8 hr
  - Ceftazidime
    - 100–150 mg/kg/day divided every 8 hr
  - Gentamicin
    - 5–7.5 mg/kg/day divided every 8 hr
  - TMP-SMX
    - 6–12 mg/kg/day TMP with 30–60 mg/kg/day SMX divided every 12 hr
- Enteral therapy
  - Amoxicillin
    - 30–40 mg/kg/day divided every 12 hr
  - Amoxicillin-clavulanate
    - 30 mg/kg/day divided every 12 hr
  - Cefixime
    - 8–16 mg/kg/day once daily or divided every 12 hr
  - Cephalexin
    - 40–50 mg/kg/day divided every 6–8 hr

- Cefpodoxime
  - 10 mg/kg/day divided every 12 hr
- Methenamine mandelate
  - 40–50 mg/kg/day divided every 8–12 hr
- Nitrofurantoin
  - 5–7 mg/kg/day divided every 6 hr
- Sulfisoxazole
  - 150 mg/kg/day divided every 6 hr
- TMP-SMX
  - 6–12 mg/kg/day TMP with 30–60 mg/kg SMX divided every 8–12 hr

WHEN TO ADMIT

- Suspected urosepsis
- Infant <3 months of age with UTI
- Suspected UTI in a dehydrated patient or a patient who cannot retain oral fluids.
- Patients whose symptoms worsen or do not improve despite oral treatment

WHEN TO REFER

- Abnormal findings on imaging
- Frequently relapsing UTI
- Suspicion of voiding dysfunction

FOLLOW-UP

- After the first UTI, prophylactic antibiotics are started and continued until imaging studies are performed.
- Patients with VUR need to be continued on prophylactic antibiotics and should have regular follow-up and repeat VCUG to determine the status of VUR.

COMPLICATIONS

- Association of anatomic abnormalities in the kidneys or in the urinary tract is increased in children with UTI.
  - Risk is higher in children with non–*E coli* UTI versus those with *E coli*–associated UTI.
- Renal scarring
  - Isotope uptake studies (DMSA scans) have shown that the renal parenchyma is affected in ~55–75% of children with febrile UTI.
  - ~ 20–40% of these children will develop permanent renal parenchymal damage (renal scarring).
  - In some cases, renal disease may be congenital rather than acquired and not dependent on UTI.
  - In an analysis of 1221 children with first-time UTI, the incidence of permanent renal damage was:
    - 86% in boys
    - 30% in girls

- The mean age of boys at the time of UTI was significantly lower compared with girls.
- VUR was present in:
  - 67% of boys (higher incidence of congenital renal disease and damage to the kidney parenchyma)
  - 19% of girls (renal damage is acquired and results from UTI)
- Infants (mean age 4 months) with high-grade VUR without UTI have fewer scars than patients with VUR with a history of UTI.
- It may be difficult to determine the exact cause of renal dysfunction in children with high-grade VUR, UTI, and renal damage.
- Contributing factors include congenital factors, reflux, and infection.
- Risk factors for renal parenchymal damage include:
  - Gross VUR
  - Young age at the time of first infection
  - Delayed initiation of treatment
  - Recurrent infections
- Incidence of complications after UTI can be dramatically reduced by:
  - Thorough radiologic investigation of young children with UTI
  - Appropriate treatment
  - Follow-up
- Long-term effects of UTI
  - Risk of permanent renal damage
    - May increase risk of hypertension
    - May ultimately cause varying degrees of renal failure
  - Increased risk of preeclampsia during pregnancy
  - Risk for end-stage kidney disease is relatively small in children with UTI.
  - According to theNorth American Pediatric Renal Trials and Collaborative Studies:
    - Pyelonephritis or interstitial nephritis accounts for renal failure in only 1.8% of all patients who require renal transplantation.
    - Obstructive uropathy accounts for renal failure in 16.1%.
    - Renal hypoplasia or dysplasia accounts for renal failure in 16%.
    - Reflux nephropathy accounts for renal failure in 5.2%.
  - Anatomic abnormality with or without UTI is a more important threat for kidney function than UTI itself.
  - Hypertension has been shown to be a significant long-term complication of childhood febrile UTI associated with renal scarring.
    - Exact risk ranges from 6–23%.

U

– Lower incidences of hypertension may be the result of increased awareness of risk factors related to childhood UTI.

– Remains an important long-term complication of childhood UTI

– Incidence may be decreased by careful attention to risk factors and early treatment.

- Bacteriuria and symptomatic UTI are significantly more frequent in pregnant women with history of childhood UTI.

- UTI may contribute to increased risk to preeclampsia (hypertension and proteinuria).

  – May be harmful to the fetus

  – Can cause premature labor

PREVENTION

Prophylaxis

■ Recommended for all children after their first UTI until imaging studies are performed

■ Thereafter, prophylaxis should be considered for children with an increased risk of UTI.

- Children with higher grades of VUR (higher than grade II)

- Children with obstructive uropathy and a history of UTI

- Children with recurrent UTIs (>2 per year)

■ The most common prophylactic regimen is:

- Co-trimoxazole (TMP-SMX [2 mg/kg TMP with 10 mg/kg/day SMX once every night])

- Nitrofurantoin (1–2 mg/kg/day) as a single daily bedtime dose

■ Duration of prophylaxis depends on indication.

■ In children with VUR, prophylaxis is usually continued until:

- Reflux has resolved spontaneously.

- Reflux has been surgically corrected.

- The child has been free of symptoms and bacteriuria for ≥1 year.

■ Dosing

- Amoxicillin

  – 10–15 mg/kg once daily at bedtime

- Amoxicillin-clavulanate

  – 25 mg/kg once daily at bedtime

- Cephalexin

  – 12–15 mg/kg once daily at bedtime

- Nitrofurantoin

  – 1–2 mg/kg once daily at bedtime

- Sulfisoxazole

  – 50 mg/kg once daily at bedtime

- TMP-SMX

  – 2 mg/kg TMP with 10 mg/kg/day SMX once every night

Supplemental therapy

■ Constipation and encopresis are known to be risk factors for UTI.

- Anticipated in children with recurrent UTI

■ Treatment of these problems is important to prevent recurrent UTI by:

- Dietary modification

- Medication

■ The role of circumcision in preventing UTI has been studied.

- Relative risk of UTI in uncircumcised male infants compared with circumcised male infants is increased from 4-fold to as much as 10-fold during the first year of life.

- Absolute risk of UTI in an uncircumcised male infant is low (at most, ~1%).

- Currently, data are not sufficient to recommend routine neonatal circumcision.

Vaginal Bleeding

DEFINITION

- Assessing vaginal bleeding depends largely on the pubertal status of the patient.

MECHANISM

- In prepubertal girls, vaginal bleeding probably reflects a localized problem in the vagina or uterus.
- In pubertal girls and young women, bleeding can be caused by:
  - Disorders affecting the hypothalamic-pituitary-ovarian axis
  - Complications of pregnancy
  - Local causes

HISTORY

- Most causes of vaginal bleeding or abnormal uterine bleeding can be ruled out by history and physical examination.
- Maternal support during the initial history taking can be useful.
  - Many mothers track the menstrual periods of their daughters in the early years and are acutely aware of:
    - Quantity of bleeding based on the amount of feminine products purchased and stained laundry
    - Evidence of fatigue
    - General activity level and behavior
  - Mothers can also provide detailed family medical histories for:
    - First-degree female relatives
    - Their daughters
- Key aspects of the history may be difficult to obtain, ie, sexual intercourse or sexual abuse.
- The patient should be interviewed alone regarding:
  - Sexual activity
    - Occasionally, a small amount of bleeding or spotting may follow sexual intercourse.
  - Sexually transmitted infections and associated symptoms, such as:
    - Cramping
    - Vaginal discharge
    - Dyspareunia
  - Abuse
  - Stress
  - Weight changes and eating habits
  - Participation in sports and other activities
  - Chronic illnesses
  - Other bleeding problems
  - Medication use (particularly contraceptives)
  - Substance use

- Menstrual pattern
  - Is there bleeding between normal periods?
  - Have previously regular menses become more frequent or heavier?
    - A teenager whose prior menses have been regular might begin to have infrequent but heavy menstrual bleeding.
  - Likelihood of a coagulopathy or another pathologic condition is increased by:
    - Heavy bleeding at menarche
    - Significant anemia
    - Need for hospitalization to control the bleeding
- In general, normal periods in adult women are:
  - 28 days apart (measured from the first day of one period to the first day of the next)
  - Range of 21–45 days
  - Flow of 3–7 days
  - Flow >1 week is considered excessive.
  - A similar cycle pattern is observed in adolescent girls.
    - Cycle length is more variable especially in the first few years after menarche.
  - Some women will have spotting around the time of ovulation.
- Normal blood loss during menses
  - 30–40 mL
  - Upper limit of 80 mL
  - Quantity of blood loss is difficult to assess by history unless bleeding is scant.
  - The patient should describe the number of pads or tampons used.
- Changes related to hormonal contraceptive use
  - Bleeding between periods is common during the first 2 or 3 cycles of oral contraceptive use.
  - Teenagers who forget to take 1 or 2 oral contraceptive pills may experience bleeding.
  - Depot medroxyprogesterone acetate (Depo-Provera) injections
    - Associated with frequent and irregular periods of xcess bleeding, particularly in the first months after beginning use
- Complete family history
  - Important to determine whether other family members have any kind of bleeding problem
  - Family history is a better predictor of coagulopathy than menstrual history.

PHYSICAL EXAM

- Make sure that the bleeding is vaginal in origin.
  - A prolapsed urethra can mimic vaginal bleeding.

Prepubertal girls

- Any suggestion of sexual abuse
  - Careful, nonthreatening questioning of the child or care-taker may reveal necessity for a referral to child protective services for a forensic interview and examination.
  - Bruises
  - Hymenal tears
  - Other signs of trauma
- Nighttime pruritus
  - May indicate a pinworm infestation
  - The Scotch tape slide test to look for pinworm eggs can help establish Enterobius vermicularis infestation.
- Petechiae or numerous bruises
  - Possible coagulopathy
- Foreign body in the vagina
  - Should always be considered, even if no history of such exists
- Excoriation, erythema, or a rash in the perineal area
  - Vaginitis is a distinct possibility.
  - Microscopic examination of vaginal discharge demonstrates large numbers of leukocytes.
  - Diarrhea in the weeks preceding onset of the bleeding suggests vaginitis caused by *Shigella* organisms.
  - Group A ß-hemolytic streptococcus can also cause vaginitis.

Pubertal girls

- Normal findings help rule out many causes of vaginal bleeding or abnormal uterine bleeding.
  - Height
  - Weight
  - Blood pressure
  - Thorough palpation of the thyroid gland
  - Pelvic examination
  - Fundoscopic and visual fields examinations to exclude prolactinoma
- Endocrine disorders are indicated by:
  - Increased facial hair
    - Polycystic ovaries
    - Adrenal tumor
  - Cold intolerance
    - Hypothyroidism
  - Polyuria
    - Pituitary tumor
  - Nipple discharge
    - Hyperprolactinemia
  - Headache
    - Pituitary tumor

- Acne
  - Polycystic ovaries
  - Adrenal tumor
- Striae
  - Cushing disease
- Enlarged clitoris
  - Androgen-secreting tumor
  - Late-onset 21-hydroxylase deficiency
- Vulvar or vaginal bruising or lacerations
  - Probable sexual abuse
- Lack of adnexal or cervical motion tenderness
  - Excludes pelvic inflammatory disease
- Ovaries of normal size
  - Ovarian tumors or cysts are unlikely
- Uterus size
  - Minimal enlargement consistent with early pregnancy may not be noted by an inexperienced examiner.
  - Endometrial polyps or submucosal leiomyomas (unusual in women <20 years) cannot be palpated by the examiner on the usual pelvic examination.
- Crampy lower abdominal pain
  - Possible ectopic pregnancy
  - Incomplete or spontaneous abortion
    - History of 1 or 2 missed periods
    - Prior menstrual period lighter than normal
    - Tissue present in the vaginal canal or history of passing tissue
    - Other symptoms of pregnancy (breast tenderness or nausea)
- Foul-smelling and bloody discharge
  - Foreign body or retained tampon is likely.
  - Necrotic tumors can result in similar bleeding patterns
- Pruritus or dysuria
  - Vaginitis (*Trichomonas vaginalis*)
  - Cervicitis (*Neisseria gonorrhoeae* or *Chlamydia trachomatis* infection)

DIFFERENTIAL DIAGNOSIS

- Pubertal girls and young women
  - Most teenagers who seek evaluation for genital bleeding in the first few years after menarche will have dysfunctional uterine bleeding (DUB).
    - DUB is abnormal bleeding not resulting from uterine disease, medications, systemic illness, or pregnancy.
    - DUB is considered a diagnosis of exclusion.
    - Disorders affecting the hypothalamic-pituitary-ovarian axis can mimic DUB.

- Systemic disease
  - Renal failure
  - Hepatic failure
  - Cancer
  - Sexually transmitted infection
- Conditions of the reproductive tract
  - Vagina
    - Vaginitis
    - Trauma
    - Foreign body
    - Congenital anomaly (septum)
    - Neoplasia
  - Cervix
    - Cervicitis, erosion
    - Cervical polyp
    - Neoplasia
  - Uterus
    - Endometritis
    - Endometrial polyp
    - Submucosal leiomyoma
    - Arteriovenous malformation
    - Congenital anomaly
    - Neoplasia
  - Pelvis
    - Endometriosis
    - Pelvic inflammatory disease
- Pregnancy complications
  - Spontaneous abortion
  - Ectopic pregnancy
  - Retained gestational products
  - Trophoblastic disease
- Endocrine disorders
  - Hypothalamus, pituitary
    - Immature hypothalamic-pituitary-ovarian axis
    - Hyperprolactinemia
    - Anorexia nervosa, malnutrition
    - Excessive exercise
    - Emotional stress
    - Chronic illness
  - Adrenal
    - Congenital adrenal hyperplasia
    - Cushing disease
    - Adrenal insufficiency
    - Neoplasm
  - Thyroid
    - Hypothyroidism
    - Hyperthyroidism
  - Ovary
    - Polycystic ovary syndrome
    - Luteal phase abnormality
    - Premature ovarian failure
    - Neoplasia (hormone secreting)
- Coagulation disorders
  - von Willebrand disease
  - Immune thrombocytopenia
- Other causes
  - Disorders of platelet function (Glanzmann thrombasthenia, Bernard-Soulier syndrome)
  - Leukemia
- Iatrogenic
  - Hormonal medications
  - Anticoagulants
  - Neuroleptics
  - Intrauterine contraceptive device

LABORATORY EVALUATION

- For most cases of vaginal bleeding, relatively few laboratory tests are needed.
- Complete blood count with indices
  - Provides an objective measurement of the amount and duration of bleeding
  - Determines whether significant blood loss resulting in anemia has occurred
  - Guides the treatment approach for patients with an otherwise negative evaluation
- Urinalysis
- Urine pregnancy test
  - Quantitative serum pregnancy test also should be obtained if ectopic pregnancy is suspected.
- Cultures in sexually active patients or where there is concern for sexual abuse
  - *N gonorrhoeae*
  - *C trachomatis*
  - *Trichomonas*
  - Bacterial vaginosis
- Coagulation tests (prothrombin time, partial thromboplastin time, von Willebrand panel) if the patient has:
  - Profuse hemorrhage
  - Menorrhagia at menarche
  - Family history of bleeding disorders
  - Unexplained heavy vaginal bleeding

V

- If hormonal therapy is contemplated:
  - Thyroid-stimulating hormone function tests
  - Prolactin
  - Luteinizing hormone and follicle-stimulating hormone
  - Coagulation tests
- Patients with any evidence of hyperandrogenism:
  - Free and total testosterone
  - Dehydroepiandrosterone sulfate

IMAGING

- Pelvic sonography when:
  - Ectopic pregnancy is suspected.
  - The patient has a pelvic mass on bimanual examination.
  - Pelvic examination is difficult.

DIAGNOSTIC PROCEDURES

- Endometrial biopsy: rarely indicated
- Dilation and curettage: rarely indicated
- Transvaginal ultrasonography: pelvic mass on bimanual examination

TREATMENT APPROACH

- Most cases of vaginal bleeding in adolescent girls are caused by DUB.
  - In other instances, the clinician must manage the bleeding without knowing the cause.
    - Treatment decisions can be guided using:
      - The patient's clinical symptoms
      - Results of basic laboratory testing
- If treatment of the presumed cause does not end the bleeding, referral for a more thorough examination is indicated.

SPECIFIC TREATMENT

Infants

- After birth, estrogen levels in the infant decrease.
  - The result is a physiologic vaginal discharge that can be blood tinged or frankly bloody.
    - No treatment, except reassurance, is necessary.
    - The discharge usually disappears within 10 days.

Foreign bodies or vulvitis

- Removal of the foreign body
  - Foreign bodies can often be washed out with a soft, flexible catheter.
  - Sharp objects should be removed carefully, under direct visualization.
  - Referral to a gynecologist may be required if the patient is uncooperative.

- After removing a foreign body, bleeding should subside within 10 days.
  - If not, referral to a gynecologist is indicated.
    - The entire foreign body may not have been removed.
    - A tumor, not readily visualized by the primary care physician, may be the actual cause of the bleeding.
- Proper perineal hygiene
  - Occasionally, systemic antibiotics may be necessary.

Sexually transmitted infections

- Usually treated with antibiotics

Complications of pregnancy

- Threatened or spontaneous abortion can be managed in the outpatient setting.
  - A clinician experienced in the management of early pregnancy should be consulted.
  - For patients with bleeding disorders, consultation with a hematologist may be required.

DUB: hormonal therapy

- Indicated in:
  - Teenagers who have moderate bleeding (enough to cause a decrease in hematocrit level to <34%)
  - Girls who have menses every 1–3 weeks
  - The primary care physician may prefer the guidance of a more experienced clinician.
- Combined oral contraceptives (COCs) or progestin alone
  - COCs are easier to use (1 pill is taken daily every day of the month).
  - If the patient has a condition in which COCs are contraindicated or this method is rejected by the patient or her parents:
    - Medroxyprogesterone, 10 mg orally, can be given daily for 10–14 days.
    - Begin treatment on the first day of each month (calendar method) or on the 14th day of the menstrual cycle (day 1 being the first day of bleeding).
  - Assure the parents that:
    - COCs are, in this instance, being used as treatment.
    - COCs are the most convenient way to package and deliver hormonal treatment.
    - Short-term use of COCs for 3–6 months is anticipated.
    - Close follow-up will be given during the treatment period.
  - Such an approach will often:
    - Alleviate concerns about hormonal treatment
    - Prevent rejection of these methods by the family

DUB: mild bleeding

- No anemia
  - Does not greatly upset the patient and her parents
    - Can be managed expectantly with no immediate, specific therapy
- Mild anemia
  - Hemoglobin value 11–12 g/dL
  - Treated with iron supplementation
- Some problems will resolve in 3 or 4 cycles.
  - If the patient is sexually active, COCs can be prescribed to treat the bleeding, as well as to provide contraception.
- Nonsteroidal antiinflammatory drugs
  - Can also be used for their demonstrated antiprostaglandin effects
    - Ibuprofen
    - Naproxen

DUB: severe prolonged heavy bleeding

- Severe prolonged heavy bleeding accompanied by a decrease in hemoglobin to ≤10 g/dL must be treated more aggressively.
  - An adolescent medicine or gynecologic consult should be sought.
  - Clotting studies should be obtained.
  - Hospitalization should be strongly considered.
- COCs (1 tablet taken twice daily for 3–4 days) will generally stop the bleeding.
  - LoOvral every 4 hours may be necessary initially until the bleeding stops.
    - Then every 6 hours for 24 hours
    - Then every 8 hours for 4 days
    - Then twice daily to complete 3 weeks of hormonal therapy
  - Some clinicians prefer to use conjugated estrogens (25 mg IV every 4 hours).
  - Antiemetic medications may be required to counteract the side effects of the high levels of estrogen contained in this regimen.
  - Withdrawal bleeding will occur 2–4 days after completion of this initial course of therapy.
  - Patients with significant bleeding should avoid the placebo pills contained in the COC pill packs and continue continuous COCs until hemoglobin and hematocrit levels begin to normalize.
- Iron and folic acid supplementation
  - Should be included as a part of the therapeutic plan

- Blood transfusion
  - Need depends on the hemodynamic stability of the patient.
- Endometrial biopsy
  - Rarely indicated
- Dilation and curettage
  - Rarely indicated

WHEN TO REFER

- The patient is experiencing severe bleeding or initial attempts to control the bleeding by the primary care physician have failed.
- Vaginal bleeding appears to be secondary to a chronic illness that the primary care physician cannot manage.
- The primary care physician feels uncomfortable performing a pelvic examination.
- Long-term hormonal therapy is required.
- Evidence exists for:
  - Anatomical abnormality
  - Complicated endocrine disorder
  - Coagulopathy, especially if causing severe bleeding
  - Cancer
  - Sexual abuse

WHEN TO ADMIT

- Severe prolonged heavy bleeding accompanied by a decrease in hemoglobin to ≤10 g/dL
- Hemodynamic instability

FOLLOW-UP

- All patients with abnormal vaginal bleeding should be instructed to maintain a menstrual calendar to facilitate follow-up management.
- Patients with mild bleeding should be reevaluated in 6–8 weeks.
- Patients with severe bleeding require long-term, close follow-up.
- Even when measures succeed in controlling the vaginal bleeding, an appreciable number of patients will continue to have menstrual abnormalities.

COMPLICATIONS

- Anemia

V

Vaginal Discharge

DEFINITION

- Vaginal discharge is fluid produced by glands in the vaginal wall and cervix that drains from the opening of the vagina.

MECHANISM

- Newborns
  - In utero, the vaginal epithelium is stimulated by maternal hormones that cross the placenta into the fetal circulation.
  - After delivery, these hormone levels decrease rapidly, and there may be a thick, grayish-white, mucoid discharge from the neonate's vagina.
  - In many instances, the discharge is blood-tinged or even grossly bloody.
- Prepubertal girls
- The genital area of prepubertal girls is susceptible to infection.
  - Labial folds are smaller and lack pubic hair.
  - Distance between the vagina and the anus is relatively short.
  - Low levels of circulating estrogen render the vaginal mucosa relatively thin and susceptible to irritation or infection.
  - Alkaline pH (approximately 7.0) of the vaginal secretions is hospitable to bacteria and allows fecal flora to establish themselves.
- Nonspecific vaginitis
  - No clear causative agent for the discharge can be established.
  - Accounts for 25–75% of cases of vulvovaginitis
- Sexually transmitted organisms
  - *Neisseria gonorrhoeae, Chlamydia trachomatis,* or *Trichomonas vaginalis* cause vaginal infections in prepubertal girls.
  - *N gonorrhoeae* clearly causes vaginal discharge; evidence that *C trachomatis* alone does so is limited.
- Foreign body
  - Typically, the child has placed an object, such as toilet paper, a coin, or a small toy, in her vagina.
  - Accounts for <5% of cases of vaginal discharge
- Pubertal and postpubertal adolescents
  - With the onset of puberty, circulating estrogen and progesterone levels increase, stimulating vaginal mucus production and an increase in the turnover of vaginal epithelial cells.
  - Bartholin and sebaceous glands are also stimulated.
    - Generally, the clear mucoid discharge that results will not cause problems.
  - Amount of secretion can increase midway through a normal menstrual cycle or with sexual excitement.
  - Discharge is particularly prominent at the onset of puberty (physiological leukorrhea).

- Sexually transmitted organisms
  - *N gonorrhoeae, C trachomatis,* and *T vaginalis* are all known to cause vaginal infections in sexually active adolescents.
  - Herpesvirus infections of the vulvovaginal area or cervix (or both) are associated with vaginal discharge.
- Bacterial vaginosis
  - Associated with multiple sex partners, douching, smoking, and the presence of sexually transmitted infections
  - Vaginosis is not considered a sexually transmitted infection.

HISTORY

- Prepubertal girls
- Inquire about hygiene.
  - Wiping from the anus toward the vagina brings intestinal flora to the vaginal introitus.
  - Use of chemicals, such as bubble baths, deodorants, or strong laundry detergents, can irritate the vulva and vagina.
- Parents should be asked about recent or concomitant illness.
  - *Streptococcus pyogenes* infection (with or without scarlet fever)
  - *Shigella flexneri* infection, occurring coincident with or after an episode of diarrhea
  - Systemic illnesses, such as varicella
  - Rectal infestations with *Enterobius vermicularis* (pinworms) can lead to vaginitis if the eggs are deposited around or in the vagina.
  - *Candida vulvovaginitis* is an uncommon cause of vaginal discharge in prepubertal girls unless the child:
    - Has recently taken antibiotics
    - Has diabetes mellitus
    - Is immunocompromised
- Pubertal and postpubertal adolescents
  - In addition to the above, inquire about sexual activity.
    - Many teenagers fear admitting to sexual intercourse.
      - Negative response to queries about sexual activity should not rule out consideration of a sexually transmitted organism as the cause.
    - Sexual abuse should be considered.
  - Presence of a foreign body (eg, a retained tampon or condom)
  - Use of spermicides or douching can cause vaginitis.

PHYSICAL EXAM

- Prepubertal girls
  - Physical examination should include:
    - Entire genital and anal area
    - Vulva, urethral meatus, and vaginal introitus

- Infections in prepubertal girls usually involve the vulva as opposed to only the vagina.
- Presence of bruises, lacerations, or scrapes in the genital area is suggestive of sexual abuse.
- Excoriations around anus or vagina suggest itching caused by pinworms.
- A rash that spares skin folds is consistent with an irritative cause.
- A rash that is predominantly within the skin folds suggests candidiasis.
- Positioning options for examination
  - Sitting on the mother's lap with legs spread so that they dangle outside mother's legs
  - Lying supine in the frog-leg position
  - Lying face down in the knee-chest position
- If a foreign body is thought to be present but not visualized
  - Irrigating the vagina with a soft, flexible catheter and tepid saline solution will often flush out bits of toilet paper or small objects.

DIFFERENTIAL DIAGNOSIS

- Causes of vaginal discharge in prepubertal girls
  - Nonspecific vaginitis (the most common cause)
  - Irritative agents (bubble baths, sand); the vulva is often involved as well. Nonabsorbent occlusive clothing (nylon undergarments, tights, bathing suits) also irritate the vulva, leading to skin breakdown and infection.
  - Poor perineal hygiene
  - Foreign body
  - Associated systemic illness (group A streptococci, varicella)
  - Other respiratory pathogens (eg, *Haemophilus influenzae*)
  - Enteric infections
  - *Escherichia coli* with foreign body
  - *Shigella* organisms
  - *Yersinia* organisms
  - *E vermicularis* (pinworm)
  - Sexually transmitted infections (strong presumption of sexual abuse in prepubertal girls)
  - *N gonorrhoeae*
  - *T vaginalis*
  - *C trachomatis* (whether this organism alone can cause discharge is unclear. *C trachomatis* is often isolated in conjunction with *N gonorrheae*.)
  - Primary vulvar skin disease
  - Tumor, polyps (rare)
- Major causes of vaginal discharge in pubertal girls

- *Candida albicans*
  - Discharge: thick, white, curdlike, cheesy
  - Odor: none usually
  - pH: 4.5 (obtained from midvagina with nitrazine paper)
  - Dysuria: frequent
  - Pruritus: 4+
  - Other clues: Vulva affected; associated with use of some oral contraceptives and, in some women, with antibiotic use
- *T vaginalis*
  - Discharge: frothy; yellow green or gray
  - Odor: foul-smelling
  - pH: 5.2–5.5
  - Dysuria: frequent
  - Pruritus: yes
  - Other clues: Low abdominal pain; "strawberry" cervix; punctate vaginal hemorrhages
- Bacterial vaginosis
  - Discharge: homogeneous, thin, white discharge that smoothly coats the vaginal walls
  - Odor: a fishy odor of vaginal discharge before or after addition of 10% KOH (ie, the whiff test)
  - pH: >4.5
  - Dysuria: no
  - Pruritus: slight
  - Other clues: Occurs in association with anaerobes and *Gardnerella vaginalis*
- Herpesvirus (occasionally associated with vaginal discharge)
  - Pain or a burning sensation is felt in the genital area
  - Vulva is reddened.
    - Groups of small vesicles are noted on the vulva, in the vagina, or on the cervix
    - If the vesicles have ruptured, only small ulcerations may be present.
  - Inguinal adenopathy, fever, and malaise are usually present if this attack is the first one.

LABORATORY EVALUATION

- Slide preparation
  - If sufficient vaginal discharge is present, several drops of the secretion should be placed on 2 glass slides.
  - If discharge is scant, a saline-moistened cotton swab can be introduced into the vagina to obtain samples.
  - First slide
    - Add several drops of normal saline solution.

V

- Second slide
  - Add several drops of 10% potassium hydroxide and gently heat to dissolve epithelial cells, allowing visualization of hyphae.
- If indicated, culture for *N gonorrhoeae* and *C trachomatis*.
- Cellophane tape with its sticky side applied to the perianal area and then onto a glass slide may reveal the typical eggs of *E vermicularis*.
- Typical findings
  - *C albicans*
    - Hyphae on potassium hydroxide examination
  - *T vaginalis*
    - Motile trichomonads on wet preparation; avoid drying specimen
  - Bacterial vaginosis
    - Clue cells on wet preparation (bacteria-coated epithelial cells)

TREATMENT APPROACH

- In the newborn, no treatment is needed, and the discharge usually resolves by 10 days of age.
- Prepubertal girls
  - If the history or physical examination suggests an irritative origin:
    - Discontinue the offending agent.
    - Have the child wear cotton underpants.
    - Sitz baths will provide temporary relief until natural healing takes place.
  - Removal of a foreign body will result in rapid improvement and cessation of the discharge.
  - Pinworm infestations should be treated in the usual manner (mebendazole, pyrantel pamoate, or albendazole).
  - Infections caused by poor personal hygiene will respond to general measures, coupled with instructions about proper perineal hygiene.
  - If discharge is associated with another infection (such as *S pyogenes* or *Shigella* organisms), treat the underlying infection.
  - When the organism causing the vaginal discharge is found to be sexually transmitted, more comprehensive evaluation and treatment are required.
    - A report to Child Protective Services should be made.
- Pubertal and postpubertal adolescents
  - Persistent discharge unresponsive to therapy may indicate:
    - Noncompliance with treatment
    - Reinfected by an untreated sexual partner

- In the absence of *N gonorrhoeae*, *C trachomatis*, and *T vaginalis* or causes described above, recommend:
  - Trial of sitz baths
  - Use of cotton as opposed to nylon underwear
  - Careful attention to perineal hygiene
- Candidal infections can be especially difficult to treat and may recur.
  - Predisposing factors include:
    - Oral contraceptive use
    - Broad-spectrum antibiotic use
    - Diabetes mellitus

SPECIFIC TREATMENT

Prepubertal girls

- Nonspecific vaginitis
  - Usually responds to thorough perineal hygiene, sitz baths, and mild soaps
  - Patients should:
    - Wear white cotton underpants and loose-fitting pants or skirts
    - Avoid nylon tights and tight pants
    - Avoid sitting for long periods in nylon bathing suits
    - Wipe only from front to back
  - For persistent cases, treat in standard childhood doses for 10–14 days with:
    - Amoxicillin
    - Amoxicillin-clavulanate
    - Cephalosporin
    - Clindamycin
  - Alternatively, a 1- to 2-month daily low-dose antibiotic may be helpful.
  - If unsuccessful, then antibiotic or estrogen creams may be used.
    - Mupirocin
    - Gentamicin
    - Metronidazole
    - Clindamycin

Pubertal and postpubertal adolescents

- Vulvovaginal candidiasis (*C albicans*)
  - Topical therapy for 7–14 days or
  - Oral fluconazole, 150 mg repeated 72 hours after the first dose
  - If more intensive treatment is warranted
    - Oral fluconazole, 150 mg once weekly for 6 months after initial treatment of 1 dose every 3 days for 3 doses
  - A variety of month-long antifungal treatments have been successful; however, intravaginal treatment over a long period is inconvenient.

- Long-term ketoconazole has been used to suppress recurrent infection, but hepatotoxicity is a concern.
- Male sexual partners should be treated if they have any signs or symptoms of penile candidal involvement.

■ *T vaginalis*

- Metronidazole 2 g orally in a single dose
  - Alternatively, this medication can be given as 500 mg twice daily for 7 days.
  - Some strains of *T vaginalis* have decreased susceptibility to metronidazole.
  - Repeated failures should be treated with 2 g once daily for 3–5 days.
  - The patient should be told to avoid alcohol until 24 hours after completion of therapy.
- Sexual partners must be treated.

■ Bacterial vaginosis

- Metronidazole 500 mg orally twice daily for 7 days or
- Metronidazole gel 0.75% one full applicator (5 g) intravaginally once daily for 5 days or
- Clindamycin cream 2%, one full applicator (5 g) intra-vaginally every night at bedtime for 7 days or
- Alternative regimens that include:
  - Metronidazole 2 g orally in a single dose
  - Clindamycin 300 mg orally twice daily for 7 days
  - Clindamycin ovules 100 g intravaginally every night at bedtime for 3 days

WHEN TO REFER

■ If the clinician is uncomfortable with evaluating genital symptoms in prepubertal girls

■ If the clinician lacks experience in performing pelvic examinations

■ If the evaluation yields evidence of sexual abuse

■ If discharge persists despite seemingly appropriate therapy

PREVENTION

■ Proper perineal hygiene
- Keeping the area clean
- Wiping from front to back

■ Patients should be advised:
- To wear white cotton underpants and loose-fitting pants or skirts
- To avoid nylon tights and tight pants
- To avoid sitting for long periods in nylon bathing suits

Verrucae (Warts)

DEFINITION

- Verrucae (warts) are virally induced tumors of the skin.

EPIDEMIOLOGY

- Cutaneous warts
  - Affect up to 10% of children between 2 and 12 years of age
  - Rank among the top 3 dermatoses in this age group
  - No sex predilection
- Genital warts
  - Uncommon in children before puberty
  - One of the most common sexually transmitted infections in adolescents and adults

ETIOLOGY

- Warts are caused by human papillomavirus (HPV).
  - Infects epidermal cells
  - Causes focal epidermal proliferation
  - Expressed clinically as a verrucous papule
- >100 types of HPV have been characterized.
- Specific types have been associated with specific warts.
  - HPV types 1, 2, and 4: plantar warts
  - HPV-2 and HPV-7: common warts
  - HPV-3 and HPV-10: flat warts
  - HPV types 1, 6, and 11: benign genital warts
  - HPV types 6, 7, 11, 16, and 32: laryngeal papillomas
  - HPV types 16, 18, 31, 33, 35, 39, 45, 51, 52, 56, 58, 59, and 68: genital warts with malignant potential
- HPV typing holds promise in helping identify:
  - Premalignant warts
  - Sources of transmission
- HPV types 6, 11, 16, and 18 cause:
  - 70% of cervical cancers
  - 90% of genital warts
- Presumably inoculated into the skin from an external source
  - Neither source nor event of inoculation is elicitable.
- Asking about and searching for warts on other areas of the body is reasonable.
  - Patients who have warts on their lips often have them on their fingers.
  - Warts are transmissible.
  - Other family members may have them.
- Genital warts in children can raise the question of sexual abuse.
  - A complete social history and thorough physical examination is indicated.

- On the basis of HPV typing, anogenital and laryngeal HPV infection in most infants appears to be acquired by:
  - Nonsexual transmission from the mother's vaginal tract during delivery
  - Evidence exists pointing to possibility of in utero transmission of HPV.
- A study demonstrating a high incidence of HPV-2 in anogenital warts in prepubertal children suggested that common means of acquisition may be innocent auto- or heteroinoculation from cutaneous warts.

RISK FACTORS

- Patients with systemic defects in cell-mediated immunity are more susceptible to warts.
  - Often recalcitrant to treatment
- Cellular immune responses in the skin are impaired with atopic dermatitis.
  - These patients have more difficulty with warts and other viral infections of the skin.

SIGNS AND SYMPTOMS

- Clinical appearance of warts varies, depending on the type and location.
- Common wart, or verruca vulgaris
  - Easily recognized as a superficial, light-colored papule
  - Coarse, roughened surface
- Warts are often studded with black specks.
  - Actually small, superficial dermal capillaries
- Warts are sometimes found in a linear array, presumably as a result of autoinoculation through scratching.
- Not all warts appear as verrucous papules.
  - Variants include:
    - Flat (planar) warts
    - Plantar warts
    - Periungual warts
    - Anogenital warts

DIFFERENTIAL DIAGNOSIS

- The distinctive clinical appearance of the common wart usually presents no problem in diagnosis.
- Epidermal nevi
  - Hamartomas that may be confused with warts
  - They are:
    - Softer
    - More pigmented
    - More persistent
    - Much less common

- Flat (planar) warts appear as small, flesh-colored papules (see Figure 94 on page F32).
  - Flat warts have sharp borders and a finely verrucous surface.
  - When located on the face, warts may be confused with the closed comedones (whiteheads) seen in acne.
    - Closed comedones are smooth, dome-shaped lesions.
- Plantar warts
  - Named for their appearance on the plantar surface of the foot (see Figure 95 on page F32)
  - Often confused with calluses and corns
    - Corns are much less common in children.
  - Large plantar warts are often composed of confluent smaller warts.
    - Form a mosaic wart surrounded by satellite lesions
  - Differ from corns by having a verrucous surface that interrupts skin markings and often punctuated with black specks
    - In some cases, the 2 entities can only be distinguished by paring down the surface.
      - Wart tissue still has a roughened texture and remains the same size as it is pared.
      - Corn tissue is smooth, and it becomes smaller in diameter as it is pared.
- Periungual warts
  - Occur around the nail fold and should not pose diagnostic difficulty
  - Warts under free edge of the nail
    - Can cause nail plate to separate from nail bed
    - May be confused with fungal infection
    - On close inspection, the verrucous nature of the wart usually can be appreciated.
- Anogenital warts (condylomata acuminata)
  - Sometimes, but not always, acquired by sexual contact
  - Can usually be identified as verrucous papules (see Figure 96 on page F32)
  - Sometimes small or flat and more difficult to see
  - May be confused with the less common condylomata lata found in secondary syphilis
    - Condylomata acuminata is drier and more verrucous.
  - Condylomata lata are flat and moist.
  - If doubt exists, a serologic test for syphilis should settle the issue.

DIAGNOSTIC APPROACH

- Warts are almost always diagnosed clinically.
- If doubt exists, skin biopsy can provide histologic confirmation.

DIAGNOSTIC PROCEDURES

- Anogenital warts: Acetowhitening technique can aid in the diagnosis.
  - A compress containing 5% acetic acid is applied for several minutes to the suspected area.
  - Reexamine, ideally under magnification.
  - With this technique, warty tissue turns white and is visualized more easily.

TREATMENT APPROACH

- Among schoolchildren:
  - Warts are often a focus for teasing and insensitive remarks.
  - Children usually ask that their warts be treated because of social pressure.
  - Successful therapy gives patients the opportunity to feel better about themselves and their appearance.
- Warts commonly regress spontaneously.
  - Time required varies considerably.
  - In some patients, therapy may only serve to appease the patient while nature takes its course.
- In some patients, the destructive techniques may:
  - Initiate an inflammatory reaction
  - Expose the viral antigen to the body's immune system, which rejects the wart
- Whenever warts are treated, the physician must guard against doing harm by being overzealous.
  - Surgical excision is usually discouraged.
  - Radiotherapy is contraindicated.
- The goal of therapy is to shorten the time required for the wart to disappear.

SPECIFIC TREATMENTS

Cryotherapy

- Tissue is frozen by applying liquid nitrogen (–195°C).
  - Swab
  - Canister delivery system
- Freezing should extend beyond wart to include a 1- to 2-mm rim of normal skin.
- To destroy affected tissue more effectively, the wart may be refrozen after initial thaw.
- Patients must be advised:
  - The frozen area will be sore for several days.
  - A blister may form.
  - Several weeks are usually needed for the wart to turn dark and drop off.
- Cryotherapy is a favorite office therapy for common warts.
- For small warts, a single treatment is often successful.
- Large warts frequently need to be refrozen about every 3 weeks.

- Scars may result, but are uncommon.
- Skin may become hypopigmented.
- In freezing warts on the fingers:
  - Care must be taken to avoid freezing too deeply.
  - Underlying structures, such as digital nerves, can be damaged.
- Over-the-counter freezing treatments
  - May not be as effective as liquid nitrogen

Keratolytic (acid) therapy

- Slower and involves more patient participation than freezing
  - Less immediately painful
  - Least likely to cause scarring
- Variety of acids are available for treating warts.
- Convenient outpatient medication incorporates 17% salicylic acid in a polyacrylic or flexible collodion vehicle (Occlusal-HP, Duofilm).
  - Dries rapidly to prevent spread of acid onto surrounding skin
  - Patients are instructed to:
    - Apply medication at bedtime
    - Cover area with thick tape
  - Superficial necrotic tissue should be pared daily using a pumice stone.
- Thick palmar or plantar warts often require stronger acid, such as a 40% salicylic acid plaster.
  - These products can be bought over the counter (Mediplast and Duofilm patches).
  - Patients need instruction in application.
  - A plaster is cut to match size of the wart.
  - The adhesive, medicated side is applied to the wart and held in place with tape.
  - The plaster is changed every 24 hours and the macerated wart pared daily using a callus grater.
- Flat warts are often treated successfully with:
  - Nightly applications to the affected area with:
    - Topical adapalene (Differin)
    - Tretinoin (Retin-A)
    - Imiquimod (Aldara)
  - Products act as peeling agents.
  - Painful irritation may necessitate less frequent use.
- Home acid therapies usually require ≥1 month of continuous use to be effective.
  - If no progress has been made after several months, other treatments should be considered.
  - For deeply seeded warts, paring after a combination of acid and cryotherapy usually provides successful treatment.

- Caustic acids, such as trichloroacetic acid at concentrations of 30–100%, are reserved for office treatment of palmar or plantar warts.
  - Must be carefully applied
  - Can cause destruction of normal tissue
- Cantharidin is a protein phosphatase inhibitor produced by the Spanish fly, Lytta vesicatoria.
  - Penetrates the epidermis
  - Causes acantholysis
  - Results in vesiculation
  - Destroys infected keratinocytes
  - Can be used for almost all nongenital warts
  - Reapplication may be required at 1- to 3-week intervals.
  - Painless when initially applied
  - Causes little risk of scarring
  - Occasionally, a ring wart will develop at the edge of the treated site.
- All of these treatments are nonspecific.
- In some instances, different modalities are used in sequence.

Imiquimod

- Imiquimod (Aldara) 5% cream
  - Immunomodulator that augments cellular immunity by inducing a variety of cytokines
  - Can be self-administered daily or every other day
  - Should be left on overnight
  - Controlled, multicenter trials have evaluated its role in treating genital warts; trials will soon be under way for common warts.
  - Smaller studies and case reports are suggesting its potential as an alternative treatment.
    - Used alone or in combination with other modalities, such as cryotherapy and salicylic acid
- Mechanism of action may make it especially useful in treating nongenital warts in immunosuppressed patients.

Electrodesiccation and laser therapy

- Electrodesiccation can be preceded or followed by curettage.
  - The advantage is the patient leaves the office without visible evidence of the wart.
  - Cure rate is probably no higher than with cryotherapy.
  - Disadvantages are:
    - The procedure requires local anesthesia.
    - Scarring is more likely.
- Carbon dioxide laser can be used to destroy large or refractory warts.
  - Risk of scarring is significant.
- Pulsed dye laser destroys vascular component of the wart.
  - May become another alternative
  - Less risk of scarring

- Used for some recalcitrant warts, particularly:
  - Palmar
  - Plantar
  - Periungual
  - Anogenital

Other treatments

- A recent study showed that duct tape occlusion therapy was significantly more effective than cryotherapy in treating non-genital warts.
- Efficacy of oral cimetidine in the treatment of warts is still controversial.
  - May be useful in the treatment of flat warts
  - Use in other types of warts is under investigation.
- Immunotherapy
  - Involves sensitization to antigens, such as:
    - *Candida*
    - Mumps
    - *Trichophyton*
  - Used by dermatologists when topical therapies fail
  - Studies have demonstrated response rates ranging from:
    - 54–74% in treated warts
    - 34–78% in untreated, distant warts

Genital warts

- Condylomata in children are usually asymptomatic.
  - May be treated to:
    - Curtail spread
    - Allay parental concerns
  - Some forms of therapy may be painful.
  - Recurrence rates may be as high as 50%.
  - Weighing the risks versus benefits is wise before treating genital warts in children.
- 2 therapeutic options for condyloma have been approved by the US Food and Drug Administration in adults; case reports with children have shown promise.
  - Imiquimod
  - Podophyllotoxin
- Podophyllin
  - Available in 10–25% solutions in alcohol or benzoin
  - Exclusively for office use
  - Painless when applied
  - Can be toxic if used over large areas
  - Must be washed off within 6 to 8 hours of application
  - Marketed as purified 0.5% podophyllotoxin (Condylox) solution or gel
  - Can be very irritating for some patients

- Other options include:
  - Cryotherapy
  - Lasers
  - Caustic acids
  - Cimetidine

WHEN TO REFER

- Patients with persistent warts may benefit from an evaluation by a dermatologist.

COMPLICATIONS

- Major complications are those caused by overzealous therapy, resulting in:
  - Short-term discomfort
  - Scarring
- The annoyance of a wart (usually temporary) must be balanced against the inconvenience of a scar.
  - Lifelong
  - May be unsightly
  - Sometimes tender, particularly if present on a pressure-bearing surface

PROGNOSIS

- Most warts eventually involute spontaneously.
  - Probably through immunologic rejection
- The time required for involution varies greatly.
  - Predicting when it might occur for an individual patient is impossible.
- The therapies discussed in Specific Treatments result in clearing in most cases.

PREVENTION

- Gardasil
  - Vaccine for HPV types 6, 11, 16, and 18
  - Approved by the US Food and Drug Administration in June 2006
  - For use in female patients 9–26 years
  - Administered 3 times over a 6-month period
  - Whether it should be mandatory or remain voluntary is being addressed at the state level.

SUGGESTED RESOURCES

- What is a Pediatric Dermatologist? (fact sheet), AAP (www.aap.org/family/PedDermatologistfacts.pdf).

V

Violence Prevention

BACKGROUND

- Most peer violence in the US results from conflicts among:
  - Friends
  - Acquaintances
  - Intimate partners
- Stranger violence ranges from 6–40% among all instances of personal violence.
- Primary prevention
  - Preventing a child from becoming a victim
  - Helping the child learn nonviolent problem-solving skills and attitudes
    - Developing these skills and attitudes begins in infancy.
  - Effective, nonviolent discipline is key to developing resilient children who can resist being drawn into violence.
- Violence is learned.
  - Parents can help reduce the risk of serious violence through attention to the child's environment.
    - Decreased exposure to media violence
    - Decreased exposure to domestic violence
    - Decreased access to firearms
    - All of these measures effectively reduce serious violence.
  - Parents can encourage a nonviolent attitude by:
    - Resisting toys that promote violence (eg, toy guns, violent video games, and toys that encourage racial or ethnic stereotypes)
  - Although many factors place children at high risk for violence, countervailing resilience factors help reduce the risk.
- Witnessing violence
  - Domestic violence
    - One of the greatest risks of violence for infants and toddlers comes from the family through domestic violence and child abuse.
  - Television (TV) violence
    - US children spend more time watching TV than any other activity except sleep.
    - Violence is pervasive on TV: the average child will see >10,000 TV deaths before completing high school.
    - Violence on TV is generally viewed as socially acceptable behavior.
    - The American Psychological Association has concluded that exposure to TV violence is a major risk factor for children.
    - Children who view TV violence are more likely to experience violence as victims or aggressors and are much less likely to intervene in tense situations, as bystanders, to reduce the likelihood of violence.
  - Violence in urban minority communities
    - A pattern of violence that has been observed is known as the *code of the streets* or the *sucker phenomenon*.
- Individuals who cannot defend themselves are likely prey to multiple and repeated attacks.
- Parents may adopt protective strategies that keep their children out of harm's way in the first place, often by enrolling them in supervised after-school programs or keeping them safely in the house, watching TV.
- Bullying
  - Repeated infliction of harm on younger, smaller, or less powerful peers
  - A nearly universal problem for school-age children
  - Bullies are usually larger and stronger (among boys) or more socially powerful (among girls) than are their victims.
  - Targets of bullies are physically and emotionally weaker and cannot strike back, either physically or verbally.
  - Negative behaviors often happen outside of school supervision: before school, after school, or at recess.
    - Classroom teachers are often unaware of the problem.
    - Usually cannot solve it without significant support from their administrators
  - Bullying has severe adverse consequences for both bully and victim.
    - Victim outcomes—a bullied child may be:
      - Physically hurt
      - Unable to concentrate on his/her studies
      - Lacking in self-esteem
    - Several perpetrators in school shootings in the US were victims of bullies, and their lethal outbursts may have resulted from the effects of being bullied.

GOALS

- Overall goal: reduce death and disability for children in the US resulting from violence
- Primary prevention: anticipatory guidance for young children
  - During infancy and early childhood, patterns of behavior and family interactions are established.
  - Discuss with the parents:
    - Reduction in exposure to violence, including:
      - Domestic violence
      - TV violence
  - Teach appropriate, nonviolent methods of discipline.
    - Alternatives to corporal punishment
    - Awareness of the effects of TV violence during early childhood
  - Such interventions are effective.
- Secondary prevention: older children and adolescents
  - Identification, counseling, and referral of high-risk patients should be a standard of care.
- Advocacy
  - Advocate for school policies and state and federal legislation to reduce the risk of violence for children.

GENERAL APPROACH

Young children

- The overall goal is to ameliorate risk factors and reinforce factors that protect the child from harm.
- Anticipatory guidance for parents should include:
  - Reduction in exposure to violence, including both domestic violence and television violence.
  - Teaching appropriate, nonviolent methods of discipline (violence-free parenting).
- Because patients and families see their physicians often during this period, opportunities for brief, focused interventions are numerous.

School-age children

- As children get older, the external influences of their behavior become more important.
  - TV has an enormous effect.
  - Children begin to deal with playground fights and bullying.
    - Bullying has also been identified as an important precursor to other forms of violence.
    - "Stop Bullying Now" is a comprehensive set of resources for parents, schools, and communities, developed by the federal government.
- Despite a general reduction in traumatic injury and death, child and adolescent deaths caused by firearms continue to increase.
  - Individual families can be counseled that the safest home for children is one without handguns.
  - Any guns present in the home should be locked and unloaded.

Adolescents

- The overall goal is to reduce the risk of violence.
  - Screen all adolescents to identify those at high risk.
  - Prevent reinjury to injured adolescents.
  - Refer high-risk or traumatized adolescents for appropriate treatment.
- Identify and reinforce teen resilience factors.
  - Attachment to school, family, community, and pro-social peer groups all exert strong protective effects.
  - Programs that provide opportunities to belong to a pro-social group and develop mastery protect young adults from health-risk behaviors, including fighting.

SPECIFIC INTERVENTIONS

Infants and young children

- Violence-free parenting: effective parenting without corporal punishment
  - Describe and endorse specific effective behavioral techniques to help discipline children.
  - Toddlers gain power over their world by being able to understand what is happening and predict what will happen next.
    - Maintaining a schedule, eg, bedtimes, naptimes, mealtimes, bath time, and playtime, provides a feeling of mastery for the child.
  - Pay attention to the child.
    - The best attention is parental praise for good behavior.
    - In the absence of this positive reinforcement, toddlers may feel ignored and misbehave simply to grab parental attention.
    - A misperception is that children who are praised will become self-centered; this is not true.
      - Parents can be told very simply to tell their child, "I love it when you…."
  - There will be times when a child's misbehavior necessitates negative consequences.
    - An effective, simple negative reinforcement technique is the time out.
    - Time-out periods should be used:
      - Judiciously in the background of positive reinforcement
      - Consistently whenever the child has behavior patterns that need to be stopped
    - Children should be placed in time-out for approximately 1 minute per year of age.
    - Parents should explain clearly why the time-out was deserved and ignore the child during the time-out.
    - Longer explanations and discussions should be deferred until things have calmed down.

School-age children

- Interventions to deal with bullying
  - Antibullying programs have been shown to be effective in Scandinavia and the US.
  - Identify where and when bullying usually occurs.
  - Control bullying on 3 levels.
    - In the school building and grounds:
      - Ensure a safe physical environment.
      - Coordinate classroom activities.
    - In the classroom
      - Teacher-led discussions on roles of bullies, victims, and bystanders
      - Establish that bullying behavior will not be tolerated.
    - With individual students
      - Help to generate rules to prevent bullying.
      - Report bullying behavior.
      - Encourage resistance of attempts by bullies to ostracize their victims.
  - When bullies are identified:
    - The child should receive a stern message from the principal.
    - The principal should speak with the child's parents.

– A social worker or guidance counselor is assigned to work with the child on setting appropriate and enforceable behavioral limits at home.

Adolescents

■ Screening for violence: general screen to identify adolescents at risk

- Ask about drug use and fighting.

  – Ask, "How many fights have you been in the past 12 months?"

  – Teens who are in school and report neither drug use nor fighting are at low risk of violence-related injuries.

  ■ Teens at low risk deserve acknowledgment of their success at avoiding this problem.

  ■ Note that courage is often needed to walk away from a fight.

  – Teens who are in school and are passing courses but report either fighting or drug use are at medium risk.

  ■ Risk is approximately 3 times that of low-risk students.

  ■ These teens need to hear that risks are real and individual: "You are strong and healthy. However, I am worried about your telling me that you have been in several fights this year."

  ■ Basic information concerning techniques for defusing tense situations should be discussed.

  – Teens who are failing school, already dropped out of school, or report both fighting and drug use are at high-risk.

  ■ Risk is approximately 7-fold increase for future violence-related injury.

  ■ Refer to appropriate community-based intervention services.

  ■ Emphasize the importance of follow-up to both the teen and parents.

■ Obtain a violence history, particularly from teens you suspect are at risk, using the acronym FISTS:

- **F**: Fighting

  – When was your last pushing or shoving fight? How many fights have you been in the last month? In the last year?

  – Teens who have been in ≥1 physical fight in the preceding 12 months are at increased risk of violence-related injury.

- **I**: Injuries

  – Have you ever been injured in a fight? Has anyone you know been injured in a fight? Has anyone you know been injured or killed?

  – Multiple or serious previous injuries may indicate an increased risk of future injury.

- **S**: Sexual violence

  – What happens when you and your boyfriend or girlfriend have an argument? Have you ever been forced to have sex against your will?

  – Teen dating violence is both a serious problem in itself and a harbinger of future domestic violence.

- **T**: Threats

  – Have you ever been threatened with a knife? With a gun?

  – Previous threats with a weapon indicate that the patient is at future risk of weapons-related injury.

- **S**: Self-defense

  – How do you avoid getting in fights? Do you carry a weapon for self-defense?

  – Young people who have learned to de-escalate situations of conflict (or to avoid them altogether) deserve praise and encouragement.

  – Teens who arm themselves in self-defense are at extremely high risk.

■ After a fight: secondary prevention

- Patients who have been hurt in a fight are at high risk for further violence, either as the victim of another violence-related injury or by attempting to exact revenge on the assailants.

- The immediate need is for crisis intervention. Ask:

  – "Is the fight over? Do you feel safe leaving here? If the fight is ongoing, is there someone who can mediate?"

  – If the situation is volatile, the patient and family should be referred to social services or, occasionally, the police.

  ■ Police intervention is warranted whenever the patient is in danger or reveals specific plans to harm another person.

■ Parents and patients should be advised of the risk of serious injury and that successful injury prevention involves learning how to de-escalate conflicts.

■ After a serious injury, the following steps have been advocated:

- Have the child tell you about the problem, allowing narrative to flow freely, avoiding judgments.

  – This approach allows feelings of revenge to be expressed and offers an opportunity to learn patient's perspective before offering advice.

- Evaluate the youth's other risks: Does he or she carry a weapon? Does he or she use alcohol or other drugs? Is the youth involved in a gang?

- Discuss the known risk factors for violence, including the fact that most violent injuries occur between friends or acquaintances and often involve alcohol or drugs.

- Develop a plan to stay safe after leaving the hospital or clinic. Does he or she have a relative with whom to stay who lives out of the neighborhood? Do the police need to be involved?

- Discuss conflict-avoidance strategies. This discussion can start with the particular incident involved and may need to be continued on subsequent visits.

- Refer to others, including a psychologist or social worker. Referral may involve reaching out to church members, recreation departments, or mentoring programs.

Vision Screening

BACKGROUND

- Amblyopia is permanent uncorrectable vision loss caused by long-standing visual image disturbance.
  - Major threat to vision
  - Preventable when detected early
- During development, the visual cortex must receive focused images from both eyes to learn how to see.
  - Conditions that interfere with the normal visual image during this time can lead to amblyopia if not identified and corrected.
    - Strabismus
    - Certain refractive errors
    - Cataracts
- Prevalence
  - Approximately 5% of preschool-age children have amblyopia.
  - Up to 10% have other vision problems, such as refractive error.
    - The prevalence of refractive error increases with age.
    - Refractive error affects over 20% of high school–age children.

GOALS

- Goals of vision screening
  - To identify deficits in vision or conditions that might threaten vision or impair function
  - To detect amblyogenic conditions before 5 years of age
    - The likelihood of successfully treating amblyopia decreases with age.
    - Amblyopia can be prevented with early identification and treatment.
  - To ensure that appropriate diagnostic and therapeutic referrals are made so that conditions threatening vision are ameliorated
- Few data are available about the accuracy of vision screening in the primary care setting.
  - A proportion of children will fail vision screening but have a normal ophthalmologic evaluation.
  - False-positive results are a feature of all screening programs and should not discourage practitioners from screening.
  - Vision screening examinations will detect the overwhelming proportion of children who have treatable vision problems.
  - Once identified, these cases must be detected and treated properly.
- Screening for vision problems is justified.
  - Vision problems are common.
  - Vision problems pose a threat to a child's well-being.
  - Vision problems are likely to go undetected without screening.
  - Screening tests can identify children who have or are at risk for vision problems.
  - Efficacious treatments for vision problems are available.
  - Early diagnosis and treatment can have positive outcomes for many vision problems, including:
    - Congenital cataracts
    - Strabismus
    - Amblyopia

GENERAL APPROACH

- Appropriate vision screening techniques and procedures vary by age.
  - Infants and toddlers (<3 years)
  - Preschool children (3–5 years)
  - School-age children and adolescents
- Performing vision screening
  - Some elements of vision screening can be done during the physical examination.
    - This is particularly true with infants and toddlers.
  - In older children, vision can be tested by ancillary personnel.
    - Nonprofessional personnel can be trained to conduct vision screens.
  - Children who have developmental disabilities are often at increased risk for vision problems.
    - May require special expertise for assessment
- Equipment and location for vision screening
  - The necessary equipment for vision screening (ie, Snellen chart) is readily available.
  - Vision testing requires a well-lit environment and ≥10 feet of available space for nonmachine testing.
    - Vision testing machines require less space but are expensive.
  - Vision screening in the practice setting is appropriate.
    - Continuity of care is more likely in this setting.
- Children should be screened during well-child visits.
  - Record and communicate the results of the screening to parents.
  - Make sure that follow-up and referral appointments are made and kept.
  - Rates of screening follow-up are suboptimal.
  - Many children whose visual testing is abnormal never receive evaluation by an eye care specialist.

SPECIFIC INTERVENTIONS

Infants and toddlers

- Physical examination
  - Eye examination is part of the newborn assessment.
  - Eyes should be assessed at every visit.

- Inspect the eyes for structural abnormalities.
- Evaluate the red reflex with an ophthalmoscope for:
  - Absence
  - Asymmetrical appearance
- After an infant can fixate on an object (usually by 3 months), corneal light reflections should be tested with the Hirschberg test.
  - Use a penlight held in midline 12 inches in front of the eye.
  - Asymmetry of the light's reflection on the 2 corneas suggests strabismus.
  - Assess ocular motility by having the child follow a brightly colored object.
- Perform a cover-uncover test to observe movement of each eye when the other is covered and then uncovered.
  - If movement is present, it can suggest:
    - Unilateral visual defect
    - Ocular muscle weakness in the eye that moves

- Formal screening
  - New technology is available for screening young children.
    - Photorefractive screening (photoscreening)
    - Autorefraction
  - The validity and reliability of these devices in the primary care setting are unknown.

- Special circumstances
  - The following infants should be evaluated by an ophthalmologist.
    - Preterm infants at risk for retinopathy of prematurity
    - Infants with a family history of congenital eye problems
    - Infants with problems that place their eyes at risk
      - Genetic (eg, trisomy 21)
      - Acquired (eg, cerebral palsy)
- Parents may report a history of asymmetry that cannot be demonstrated at the visit.
  - Some problems of muscle imbalance occur only when the child is fatigued.
  - Pay attention to such history and refer to a specialist if symptoms persist.
  - Positive family history of the following should prompt consideration of referral.
    - Amblyopia
    - Lazy eye
    - Crossed eyes

Preschool children
- Physical examination at every visit:
  - Inspection
  - Bilateral red reflex

- Corneal light reflection
- Ocular motility
- Formal screening
  - Testing for visual acuity should be attempted beginning at 3 years.
    - An interpretable result should be achieved by 4 years.
  - A child who is uncooperative or inconsistent in responses should return for a repeat test.
    - Repeated failure to achieve an interpretable test result may indicate a visual problem.
  - At this age, simpler tests of acuity that do not rely on knowledge of letters are the most acceptable.
    - The Lea chart requires the child to identify 4 symbols.
    - Tests are available for testing from a distance of 10 and 20 feet.
      - At 10 feet, children are less likely to become distracted by other activities in the immediate environment.
- Testing for binocular vision (stereoacuity) is not a substitute for assessing visual acuity but is a useful adjunct.
  - Will sometimes identify a child whose vision problems have been missed on physical examination and acuity testing
  - Acceptable tests for this age group
    - The Random Dot E Test
    - The Stereo Fly Test
- Special circumstances
  - Children at high risk for poor vision should be referred if satisfactory results cannot be obtained on screening.

School-age children and adolescents
- Physical examination
  - At every visit
    - Inspection
    - Bilateral red reflex
    - Corneal light reflex
    - Ocular motility tests
- Formal screening
  - The Snellen letters on a wall chart are appropriate for visual acuity screening.
  - A child will usually accept testing on a vision testing machine that combines acuity testing with tests of binocular vision.
- Special circumstances
  - School difficulties may be a presenting symptom of visual problems.
  - The prevention of amblyopia becomes less of a concern with increasing age.
  - Children should continue to be tested at well-child visits.

Referral

- The child should be referred to an eye care specialist if the following are suspected or found:
  - Strabismus
  - Amblyopia
  - Structural abnormality of the eye or its movements
  - Asymmetry or abnormality of the red reflex
  - Asymmetry of the corneal reflection
  - Aversion to the occlusion of one eye
  - Any movement of the eyes on the cover-uncover test
- Refer preschool children who:
  - Fail a visual acuity test in either or both eyes at the 20/40 level
  - Have a 2-line discrepancy between the eyes, eg, 20/20 and 20/40
- Refer any child who cannot be tested successfully by age 4 years after repeated attempts.
- School-age children and adolescents who fail to pass at the 20/30 level in either or both eyes
- Children with developmental disabilities who cannot be tested successfully
- Children of any age who fail a test of binocular vision

Vomiting

DEFINITION

- Vomiting is a common symptom of acute and chronic illness in childhood.
- Vomiting is a coordinated, active process, usually preceded by nausea in association with increased salivation, gastric atony, and reflux of duodenal contents into the stomach that results from nonperistaltic contractions of the small bowel.
- Vomiting should be distinguished from regurgitation, a passive reflux of gastric contents into the esophagus and mouth through a relaxed lower esophageal sphincter.
  - In infancy, regurgitation, or spitting up, is very common.
    - Most often a developmental event
    - Has no sequelae and gradually resolves
  - Pathologic gastroesophageal reflux is defined by the association of regurgitation with severe complications, including:
    - Esophagitis with or without anemia secondary to blood loss or stricture
    - Recurrent apnea
    - Aspiration pneumonia
    - Failure to thrive

MECHANISM

- Retching immediately precedes actual vomiting.
  - Coordinated contraction of abdominal and intercostal muscles, as well as the diaphragm and simultaneous closure of the glottis
- Increased intragastric pressure from contraction of the abdominal wall musculature, lowering of the diaphragm, and pyloric contraction are associated with elevation and relaxation of the cardia, and vomiting occurs.
- The process of vomiting is coordinated in the medullary vomiting center, which may be inflluenced:
  - Directly by visceral afferent stimuli
  - Indirectly through the chemoreceptor trigger zone
- The chemoreceptor trigger zone is the site of action of many of drugs that cause nausea and vomiting, including apomorphine and digitalis.
- Stimulation of the vestibular system (as with motion sickness) can activate the vomiting center and perhaps the chemoreceptor trigger zone.
- Higher central nervous system centers may also influence the medullary vomiting center.
- Understanding the role of neurotransmitters as mediators of the initiation of vomiting has led to a range of new antiemetics.
- The area postrema, which is a major lower brainstem center for coordination of drug-induced vomiting, is rich in enkephalins, 5-hydroxytryptamine (HT) receptors, and dopamine receptors.
- Enkephalins and 5-HT both stimulate release of dopamine.

- Dopamine and 5-HT antagonists have been successful in the treatment of chemotherapy-induced nausea and vomiting.
- Antihistamines and anticholinergics prevent motion sickness by acting at histamine (H_1) and muscarinic cholinergic receptors in the nucleus ambiguus in the lower brainstem and in the lateral vestibular nucleus in the midpons.

HISTORY

- Bilious vomiting usually occurs only with ileus or intestinal tract obstruction below the ampulla of Vater in the second portion of the duodenum.
  - Especially when associated with the first vomitus
  - In newborns, bilious vomiting can be associated with necrotizing enterocolitis, especially when there is blood in the stool.
  - In older children who vomit persistently, reflux of bile from the duodenum into the stomach may lead to bilious vomiting without gastrointestinal tract obstruction.
  - When a previously well newborn develops sudden-onset of bilious vomiting, especially within the first few days of life:
    - Consider a malrotation with secondary midgut volvulus, a surgical emergency requiring early diagnosis and surgical intervention.
- Projectile vomiting commonly occurs with pyloric stenosis.
  - When this condition persists, however, gastric atony may eliminate the projectile character.
  - A succussion splash may be present, as in other causes of gastric outlet obstruction.
    - The splashing sound present when a patient who has fluid in a hollow organ is shaken on physical examination
  - Vomiting associated with increased intracranial pressure may be projectile and may take place in the absence of nausea or retching.
- Persistent vomiting in a newborn or young infant who has no evidence of infection usually suggests:
  - Congenital gastrointestinal anomaly
  - Inborn error of metabolism
  - Central nervous system abnormality, eg, hydrocephalus or subdural effusion
    - If history and physical examination do not suggest a cause, then evaluating all 3 possibilities simultaneously is best.
  - Beyond the first week of life but within the first 2 months, pyloric stenosis is the most common cause of persistent vomiting.
  - Persistent or recurrent vomiting without other symptoms may be the major manifestation of an emotional disorder.
    - A complete psychosocial history is an important part of the evaluation.
- With a history of acute vomiting and somnolence, the clinician should always consider:
  - Drug overdose, especially aspirin toxicity

- Meningoencephalitis
- Inborn errors of mitochondrial fatty acid oxidation
- Reye syndrome

■ Cyclic vomiting is characterized by repeated episodes of vomiting.

- Sometimes associated with abdominal pain
- Uncontrollable vomiting and retching are typical of an attack.
- Patients are well between episodes.
- Approximately 10% of these children have an identifiable disorder as the probable cause.
  - Gastrointestinal
  - Extraintestinal (renal, metabolic, neurologic)
  - Abdominal migraine is a common cause of cyclic vomiting.
    - Paroxysmal onset of repetitious attacks is often relieved with sleep.
    - Strong family history of migraine
    - May be accompanied by typical migraine headache
  - Abdominal epilepsy is a much less common cause of cyclic vomiting.

PHYSICAL EXAM

■ Physical examination should begin with measurement of weight, length/height, heart rate, blood pressure and orthostatic changes in blood pressure.

■ Determine the hydration status of the child.

■ Observe the shape of the abdomen

- Distention may be associated with ascites, paralytic ileus, and abdominal masses.

■ Visible peristalsis and gastric splash are associated with gastric outlet obstruction in infants.

■ Acute abdominal signs, such as generalized tenderness and rigidity, suggest surgical abdomen.

DIFFERENTIAL DIAGNOSIS

Causes of emesis, by usual age of earliest occurrence

■ Infancy/early childhood

- Gastrointestinal
  - Congenital
    - Regurgitation—gastroesophageal reflux (developmental or pathologic)
    - Atresia—stenosis (tracheoesophageal fistula, antral web, intestinal atresia, annular pancreas)
    - Duplication
    - Volvulus (secondary to an error in rotation and fixation or to Meckel diverticulum)
    - Congenital bands
    - Meconium ileus (cystic fibrosis), meconium plug

    - Hirschsprung disease
  - Acquired
    - Acute infectious gastroenteritis
    - Pyloric stenosis
    - Intussusception
    - Incarcerated hernia—inguinal, internal secondary to old adhesions
    - Food allergy, cow's milk protein intolerance, eosinophilic gastroenteritis
    - Disaccharidase deficiency
    - Celiac disease—risk is inherited, but clinical manifestations occur only after introduction of gluten in diet; occasionally, vomiting is prominent with minimal or no diarrhea
    - Postviral gastroparesis
    - Adynamic ileus—the mediator for many nongastrointestinal causes of vomiting
    - Neonatal necrotizing enterocolitis
    - Chronic granulomatous disease with gastric outlet obstruction

- Nongastrointestinal
  - Infectious—otitis, urinary tract infection, pneumonia, upper respiratory tract infection, sepsis, meningitis
  - Metabolic—aminoaciduria and organic aciduria, galactosemia, fructosemia, adrenogenital syndrome, renal tubular acidosis, hyperammonemia, disorders of fatty acid oxidation (eg, medium-chain acyl-coenzyme A dehydrogenase deficiency), mitochondrial disease, Reye syndrome
  - Central nervous system—trauma, tumor, infection, diencephalic syndrome, rumination, autonomic responses (pain, shock)
  - Medications— anticholinergics, aspirin, alcohol, idiosyncratic reaction (eg, codeine)

■ Childhood/adolescence—most of the above remain considerations, with additional possible causes.

- Gastrointestinal
  - Appendicitis
  - Food poisoning (staphylococcal, clostridial)
  - Peptic disease—ulcer, gastritis, duodenitis
  - Trauma—duodenal hematoma, traumatic pancreatitis, perforated bowel
  - Pancreatitis—mumps, trauma, cystic fibrosis, hyperparathyroidism, hyperlipidemia, organic acidemias
  - Gallbladder—cholelithiasis, choledochal cyst
  - Crohn disease
  - Adhesions—congenital or secondary to abdominal surgery
  - Idiopathic intestinal pseudoobstruction
  - Superior mesenteric artery syndrome

V

- Nongastrointestinal
  - Central nervous system—cyclic vomiting, migraine, anorexia nervosa, bulimia
  - Motion sickness
  - Metabolic— diabetic ketoacidosis, acute intermittent porphyria
  - Pregnancy—must always be considered in the differential diagnosis of vomiting in a postpubertal girl

LABORATORY EVALUATION

- With persistent vomiting, the clinician should expect to see a metabolic alkalosis.
- Metabolic acidosis raises concerns about underlying metabolic disorder or drug intoxication.

IMAGING

- Evaluation of the gastrointestinal tract usually includes an upper gastrointestinal contrast roentgenographic study.
- In an infant between 2 and 12 weeks of age, the first study is often ultrasonography of the abdomen for pyloric stenosis.
- Magnetic resonance imaging is more sensitive than computed tomography of the head if brain tumor is a consideration in an infant.
  - Further workup for metabolic or neurologic disease should be considered, as appropriate.
- If a midgut malrotation is suspected:
  - Plain-film radiography of the abdomen may show a paucity of gas distal to the upper small intestine.
  - If a midgut volvulus is suspected, an upper gastrointestinal roentgenographic series should be done at once.
    - Should be performed with controlled introduction of barium through a nasogastric tube after gastric aspiration
  - A barium enema investigation of cecal position is less reliable when evaluating a patient for malrotation.
    - Lack of complete correlation of developmental rotation of the cecum with that of the duodenum

DIAGNOSTIC PROCEDURES

- The following tests are all useful in establishing a diagnosis of gastroesophageal reflux.
  - Esophageal pH monitoring
  - Esophageal biopsies
  - Gastroesophageal scintiscan
- Endoscopy is feasible in all children, even newborns, and when indicated should be performed by an experienced examiner using a pediatric instrument.

TREATMENT APPROACH

- Acute intercurrent vomiting without serious underlying disease or significant dehydration should be treated by administering clear liquids by mouth, eg, in acute gastro-enteritis or otitis media.

- Begin with frequent small quantities of clear liquids.
  - 1 teaspoonful every few minutes for infants
  - Gradually increase volume and extension of the intervening period
- If vomiting is associated with diarrhea and dehydration, oral rehydration solution is indicated.
  - Carbonated beverages may increase vomiting.
  - Fluids that tend to slow gastric emptying and should be avoided:
    - High osmolality
    - Long-chain triglycerides
    - Anticholinergic drugs
- Antiemetic drugs
  - Should be avoided in infants, but may at times be useful in older children
  - Do not appear to have a role in the management of acute viral gastroenteritis
- For persistent vomiting, a nasoduodenal infusion may be useful.
- Patients should be monitored for signs of dehydration.
- Mild to moderate degree of dehydration may be corrected by oral hydration, even in the presence of ongoing vomiting.
- Significant vomiting that requires intravenous fluid therapy is usually associated with hypochloremic alkalosis with secondary hypokalemia.

SPECIFIC TREATMENT

Antiemetics

- Antiemetic drugs used most commonly for acute symptoms are ondansetron and promethazine.
- Trimethobenzamide may be less effective but is also used.
- Rectal suppositories are preferable to oral drugs.
  - Nausea is associated with gastric atony and unpredictable absorption.
- Dopamine-receptor antagonists are effective for chemotherapy-induced vomiting.
  - Metoclopramide
  - 5-HT_3-receptor antagonists (ondansetron) appear to have even greater efficacy and are without the risks of dystonic reactions associated with metoclopramide.
- Low-dose erythromycin has been used successfully to treat some children who have idiopathic cyclic vomiting.

Motion sickness

- H_1-receptor antagonists prevent motion sickness.
  - Diphenhydramine
  - Dimenhydrinate
  - Meclizine
  - Promethazine

- As do muscarinic cholinergic receptor antagonists
  - Scopolamine

Gastroesophageal reflux

- Management of gastroesophageal reflux must be individualized.
- The extent of treatment depends on the volume of emesis and the presence of any of the complications of reflux.
  - Esophagitis with or without esophageal stricture or intractable anemia
  - Failure to thrive
  - Respiratory manifestations
- Medical management includes thickening of feeds with cereal.
  - Standard concentration is 1 tablespoonful of cereal for each 1–2 ounces of formula.
- For a sleeping infant, the left lateral decubitus position may be helpful for reflux.
  - An infant in the first months of life should never sleep prone.
- Elevating the head of the bed remains standard therapy for older children and adults.
- Older children should also avoid snacks or liquids after dinner and agents that exacerbate esophagitis, eg, alcohol, caffeine, smoking.
- Medications can be used in an attempt to improve lower esophageal function and gastric emptying.
  - Metoclopramide
  - Low-dose erythromycin
- Medications also can be used to decrease exposure of the esophageal mucosa to acid.
  - Antacids
  - H_1-receptor blockers
  - Proton pump inhibitors
- A slurry of sucralfate is used occasionally as cytoprotective.
- Medical management may be unsatisfactory.
  - In this case, antireflux surgery, fundoplication, should be considered.
  - In these children, results of surgery are generally good when performed by an experienced surgeon and benefits can be long lasting.
  - In children who have psychomotor retardation and gastroesophageal reflux, antireflux surgery may not eliminate respiratory symptoms.
    - Other factors, such as swallowing dysfunction, may contribute to these findings.
  - Among all children undergoing a Nissen fundoplication, risk of a postoperative complication requiring further surgery may be as high as 10%.
    - Underscores the need for careful patient selection for this operation

Abdominal migraine

- The following are highly effective as prophylactic treatment for abdominal migraine.
  - Cyproheptadine
  - Amitriptyline
  - Topiramate
  - Propranolol
- Treatment success helps confirm the diagnosis.

WHEN TO REFER

- Persistent vomiting
- Recurrent episodes of vomiting
- Vomiting associated with a significant underlying process (eg, surgical abdomen, neurologic problem)

WHEN TO ADMIT

- Intractable vomiting with dehydration
- Vomiting associated with severe dehydration
- Vomiting in association with symptoms or signs of an acute abdominal process (eg, acute appendicitis, pancreatitis, cholecystitis)
- Vomiting associated with metabolic derangement
- Vomiting associated with a central nervous system abnormality, such as meningoencephalitis and tumors.

FOLLOW-UP

- All patients with vomiting should be followed carefully and monitored for weight changes, signs of dehydration, and electrolyte abnormalities.

COMPLICATIONS

- The most significant complications of vomiting include:
  - Dehydration and electrolyte imbalance, especially when the vomiting is persistent
  - Aspiration pneumonia
  - Hemorrhage from prolapse gastropathy
    - A hemorrhagic area on the posterior wall of the proximal stomach
  - Less commonly, Mallory-Weiss syndrome, a tear at the gastroesophageal junction, may occur.
  - Rupture of the esophagus, which is very uncommon in children
  - Feeding refusal may follow persistent vomiting, especially in infants.
  - Persistent vomiting may lead to failure to thrive.

PROGNOSIS

- Prognosis for vomiting depends on the cause of the vomiting.

V

Weight Loss

DEFINITION

- Clinically significant weight loss is dependent on age.
  - Newborns may lose 5–10% of birth weight in the first few days of life; losses >12% are concerning.
  - In children, weight loss >5–10% from baseline may be concerning.
  - In adolescents, in addition to weight relative to baseline, consider absolute weight in relation to ideal body weight.

EPIDEMIOLOGY

- In adolescents, planned dieting must be distinguished from an eating disorder, such as anorexia nervosa or bulimia nervosa.
  - 0.5% of female adolescents have anorexia nervosa.
  - 1–5% meet criteria for bulimia.
  - 5–10% of all cases of eating disorders occur in boys.
- As many as one-half of adolescents with eating disorders do not meet the *Diagnostic and Statistical Manual of Mental Disorders* criteria.
  - These individuals remain at risk for both physical and psychological complications from their altered eating habits.

MECHANISM

- In general, weight loss occurs when caloric intake does not meet caloric expenditure.
  - In breastfed infants, actual intake may be difficult to ascertain, given dependencies on both maternal milk production and effective feeding.
  - In children, even if enteral intake appears sufficient, there may be issues with absorption and ability to metabolize the nutrition.
- Weight loss may result from fluid losses.

HISTORY

- In all patients, records of previous body weights, allowing for differences in weighing technique, can be helpful.
- Obtain a complete history, including:
  - Diet and consumption history of child and family, with caloric assessment
  - Assess parental expectations.
  - Take a careful birth, family, past medical, and medication history.
    - Assess sick contacts/exposure to illness, and immediate past history of febrile or other illness.
    - Determine the number of urinations and bowel movements per day.
    - Review gastrointestinal/malabsorption symptoms, such as emesis, constipation, and diarrhea, and amount, frequency, and character of stools.
    - Assess other indications of feeding intolerance, including rashes.
    - Compare caloric intake with estimated caloric needs.

- For infants:
  - In general, an infant should gain 25–30 g each day in the first 3 months of life.
  - Assess feeding effort and coordination.
  - If formula-feeding:
    - Discuss the proportions in which formula is constituted.
    - Estimate total caloric intake from the volume of formula and caloric density of formula (standard is 20 kcal/oz).
    - The formula-fed newborn rarely loses >5% of birth weight in the first few days.
    - Weight less than birth weight at the age of 10 days is unusual for a formula-fed infant and indicates need for thorough evaluation.
  - If breastfeeding, assess:
    - Perceived adequacy of maternal milk production
    - Ability of infant to breastfeed
    - Typically, birth weight is regained in 10 days; consider interventions if it is unlikely to be regained in the first 2 weeks, especially with new parents.
- For children and adolescents:
  - Discuss whether eating leads to symptoms, such as pain, emesis, diarrhea, or fatigue.
  - Discuss quantity and type of stools.
  - Assess body image, social context (including family function, patient's emotional well being), and stressors.
  - Consider HEADDSSS examination and substance abuse.
  - Does the patient participate in sports where weight loss is a goal?
    - Wrestling, gymnastics, ice skating, running, swimming, diving, dancing
    - If yes, obtain a thorough dietary and supplement history.
  - For girls, obtain a menstruation history.

PHYSICAL EXAM

- The definition of significant weight loss varies by the child's age and includes acute and chronic causes.
- Subjective impressions of weight loss should be verified objectively before an evaluation is undertaken.
  - True weight loss may sometimes be difficult to differentiate from factitious weight loss.
  - Errors occur in 5–20% of all children weighed because of faulty equipment or poor technique.
- Vital signs
  - Assess temperature; consider heart rate, blood pressure, and orthostatic vital signs.

- Weigh the individual and plot on growth chart; consider serial weights for computation of growth velocities.
- With breastfed infants, consider weighing the infant before and after feedings.
- Obtain length/height.
  - In children ≥2 years, compute body mass index, body mass index percentile, and weight for length/height.
- Physical examination
  - Assess mental status.
  - Assess volume status and for anemia (eg, pale conjunctiva).
  - Examine oral mucosa for thrush and ulcerations.
    - Oral aphthous ulcers may be related to Crohn disease.
    - Discoloration of teeth may be related to purging behaviors.
  - Assess cardiorespiratory status.
  - Assess abdomen and for presence of organomegaly.
  - Look for signs of malnutrition or vitamin deficiencies (eg, lanugo).
  - Assess for toxidromes in adolescents.
- In breastfed infants, where weight loss is suspected because of inadequacy of feeding, observe the mother nursing the baby.
  - The infant should be observed to latch on to the breast correctly.
    - Note whether there is loud swallowing or occasional choking at the start of feeding.

DIFFERENTIAL DIAGNOSIS

- The differential diagnosis for weight loss is broad and varies somewhat with age.
- Of note, poverty is the greatest single risk factor for failure to thrive in the US.
  - Psychosocial factors (poor parent-child interaction, depression, rumination) often underlie poor growth and development.
  - Actual weight loss is much less common in this setting than slowdown or cessation of weight gain and linear growth.
  - Psychosocial dysfunction that results in a child's weight loss requires a prompt and thorough evaluation.
  - Eating disorders have been described in prepubertal children as young as 7 years.

Newborns and young infants

- Difficulties in establishing breastfeeding
- Inappropriate dilution or choice of formula
- Inadequate intake
  - In breastfed infants, inadequate intake at the breast is the most common reason for weight loss.

- In formula-fed infants, consider unsuccessful feeding related to parental inexperience; if this is not the case:
  - Search for an organic problem.
  - Evaluate family dynamics, support mechanisms, and adjustment to the newborn.
- Infection
- Metabolic abnormality
- Craniofacial abnormalities
- Central nervous system dysfunction
- Somnolence from maternal medications/substance abuse
- Congenital heart disease
- Maternal depression, inexperience, lack of knowledge
- Excessive losses secondary to vomiting or diarrhea
- Vomiting because of gastrointestinal malformations (eg, duodenal atresia)
- Polyuria (diabetes insipidus, renal disease)
- Diarrhea

Older infants, preschoolers, and school-age children

- Pyloric stenosis
- Gastroesophageal reflux
- Central nervous system tumors
- Vomiting
- Diarrhea
- Fever and infection
- Diabetes mellitus
- Excessive activity
- Inadequate intake
- Tuberculosis
- Surgery
- Medication effect (loss of appetite)
- Cancer
- Congenital heart disease
- Poor utilization
- Malabsorption syndromes
- Inflammatory bowel disease
- Immunodeficiency disorders, especially HIV infection
- Psychosocial dysfunction
- Neglect; nonorganic failure to thrive
- Parental depression
- Childhood depression
- Rumination
- Childhood eating disorder

Adolescents

- Dieting behavior
- Adolescent eating disorders

W

- Anorexia nervosa
  - Suspect when the adolescent is unwilling or unable to maintain body weight over a minimally normal weight for age and height.
  - Attitudes and behaviors about eating or body image are distorted; amenorrhea, emaciation, and overactivity may be described.
  - Concurrently, may have hypothyroidism, bradycardia, hypothermia, growth of lanugo-like hair on body and extremities
- Bulimia nervosa
  - Binge eating, followed by self-induced vomiting, self-starvation, overactivity, and use of cathartics or diuretics to reduce weight
    - These behaviors are practiced in secret, and the adolescent often denies them.
- Other eating disorders
- Psychiatric affective disorders, especially depression
- Cancer
- Inflammatory bowel disease
- Diabetes mellitus
- Hyperthyroidism
- Tuberculosis
- Sports-related weight loss
  - Adolescents may engage in unhealthy weight-control practices to seek advantage in their athletic activities.
    - These may include food restriction, vomiting, overexercise, diet pills, stimulants, insulin, nicotine, and voluntary dehydration.

LABORATORY EVALUATION

- Evaluation is guided by clinical suspicion.
- In infants, ensure that newborn screening has been performed.
- Studies may include:
  - Blood chemistries, kidney function tests
  - Complete blood cell count, smear
  - Erythrocyte sedimentation rate
  - Serum protein and albumin levels; serum carotene; specific tests of malabsorption
  - Tuberculosis skin test
  - Stool guaiac
  - Kidney-related tests; urinalysis, including specific gravity; urine culture
  - Please also refer to the Laboratory Evaluation section of Loss of Appetite (on anorexia).

IMAGING

- Imaging is guided by clinical suspicion.

DIAGNOSTIC PROCEDURES

- Diagnostic procedures may be performed as guided by clinical suspicion.
  - Upper endoscopy with biopsy
  - Colonoscopy
  - Sweat chloride testing
  - Esophageal motility testing
  - pH probes

TREATMENT APPROACH

- In addition to diagnostic testing, serial evaluations of weight and intake are the cornerstones of assessing weight issues.

SPECIFIC TREATMENT

- See Loss of Appetite (anorexia), Anorexia Nervosa, and Bulimia Nervosa.

Infants

- In breastfed infants with inadequate weight gain, support and education are appropriate interventions.
- Appropriate weight gain in the following few days provides evidence that the infant is well and confirms the diagnosis of initial underfeeding.
- Prematurely recommending discontinuation of breastfeeding is inappropriate.
  - The mother's motivation to breastfeed and her positive or negative feelings about the experience should be discussed.
  - Encouragement and support should be given for continuation of nursing.
  - Do not reinforce parental perceptions that the mother's milk supply is insufficient or less nutritious than formula.
  - Lactation consultants or community organizations (eg, La Leche League) may be helpful in supporting lactation efforts.
  - Infants who fail to thrive while breastfeeding require more intensive nutritional rehabilitation while still preserving breastfeeding.

WHEN TO REFER

- Refer when there is evidence or suspicion of:
  - Cancer
  - Endocrinopathy (thyroid, adrenal, pituitary)
  - Gastrointestinal disorder (eg, gastroesophageal reflux; malabsorption, including cystic fibrosis; inflammatory bowel disease)
  - Pancreatitis
  - Heart disease
  - Renal disease
  - Pulmonary disease
  - Rheumatologic condition

- Central nervous system abnormality
- Metabolic disorder
- Surgical abdominal problem (eg, pyloric stenosis, Hirschsprung disease, volvulus)
- Immunodeficiency
- Unusual infection
- Psychiatric diagnosis in child or caretaker
- Anorexia nervosa or bulimia nervosa in the child or adolescent

WHEN TO ADMIT

- A newborn, when:
  - Weight loss cannot be managed as an outpatient
  - Weight loss is >12–15% of birth weight
  - Excessive fluid loss (vomiting, diarrhea, polyuria)
  - Evidence of clinically significant dehydration or inability to maintain adequate hydration status
  - Suspicion of infection, metabolic abnormality, congenital heart disease, other conditions requiring evaluation
  - Extreme passivity of the infant, which may require tube feeding
  - Need for intensive maternal education and support
- At any age, when:
  - Weight loss is excessive (>5–10% of previous weight).
  - Excessive fluid loss from vomiting or diarrhea

- New-onset of diabetes mellitus (usually)
- Evidence of severe febrile illness (eg, pneumonia, pyelonephritis, osteomyelitis, meningitis, septic arthritis)
- Evidence of dehydration
- Physiological instability
- Severe bradycardia
- Hypotension
- Hypothermia
- Orthostatic changes
- Electrolyte abnormalities (eg, hypernatremia, hypokalemia)
- Evidence of significant psychosocial dysfunction
- An adolescent, when:
  - Eating disorder cannot be managed as an outpatient
  - Severe malnutrition, with weight <75% of ideal body weight
  - Evidence of dehydration or electrolyte abnormalities
  - Physiologic instability
  - Acute food refusal
  - Uncontrollable binge eating and purging
  - Acute medical complication of malnutrition (syncope, seizures, cardiac failure, pancreatitis)
  - Suicidal intent or ideation, or psychosis

Wheezing

DEFINITION

- Wheezing is a continuous, musical sound that represents turbulent, intrathoracic airflow.
- It may be present in both inspiration and expiration but is usually more prominent during expiration.

MECHANISM

- During the normal respiratory cycle, rhythmic expansion and contraction of the thorax leads to dynamic changes in thoracic pressures, allowing air to flow into and out of the lungs.
- On inspiration, the thoracic cavity expands, resulting in negative intrathoracic and airway pressures and allowing air to flow into the lungs.
  - Extrathoracic airway obstruction, signaled by stridor, is most likely to cause turbulent airflow during this phase.
- Expiration is accomplished by contracting the volume of the thoracic cavity, creating positive pressure in the thorax, which is transmitted to the intrathoracic airways.
  - The intrathoracic airways are more prone to obstruction leading to turbulent airflow during expiration.
- Wheezing is most commonly associated with distal airway obstruction.
- External compression of large airways may be caused by:
  - Vascular abnormalities (rings and slings)
  - Mediastinal masses
  - Infectious agents, such as lymphobronchial tuberculosis
- Intrinsic airway abnormalities may be caused by:
  - Complete tracheal rings and webs
  - Acquired obstructions, such as tracheal stenosis or granulation tissue
- Asthma exacerbations can be initiated by:
  - Vigorous activity
  - Changes in weather
  - Upper respiratory infection
  - Exposure to a triggering allergen/irritant

HISTORY

- A detailed and focused history can often provide clues to an accurate diagnosis.
- History includes:
  - Onset and frequency of wheezing
  - Recent illnesses and surgeries

PHYSICAL EXAM

- Through auscultation, determine if wheezing is bilateral or unilateral.
- Unilateral wheezing
  - Most often associated with aspiration of a foreign body
  - Can accompany unilateral bronchial compression or stenosis
- Make a detailed assessment of the auditory characteristics of the wheeze.
  - Can help determine whether the obstruction is central or peripheral
    - Wheezing that varies in pitch and can be heard throughout the chest (musical, heterophonous) typically represents small airway obstruction.
    - Wheezing that is more even in pitch (monophonic, homophonous) is typically central airway obstruction and can often be heard best in central locations, such as the sternal notch.
  - Large airway obstruction is more likely to be heard throughout the entire expiratory phase.
- Positional characteristics should be evaluated.
  - Wheezing caused by a dynamic lesion (eg, tracheomalacia) is often worse when a patient is supine.
  - Mediastinal structures, such as the heart and the great vessels:
    - Tend to fall posteriorly in the supine position and can be obstructive
    - Fall anteriorly when the patient is prone, relieving pressure on the airway and improving the wheeze
  - Wheezing caused by small airway obstruction or fixed compression of a large airway does not typically change with position.

DIFFERENTIAL DIAGNOSIS

- Any process that can cause obstruction of intrathoracic airways should be considered in the differential diagnosis.
- Viral bronchiolitis and asthma account for most wheezing.
- Pulmonary hemosiderosis can cause recurrent wheezing because blood irritates the peripheral airways.
- Wheezing after a recent surgical procedure or intubation suggests acquired obstruction.
- Asthma
  - Worse with exercise or respiratory infections
  - Responds to bronchodilators and steroids
  - Reversible obstruction on pulmonary function testing
  - Heterophonous wheeze
  - Positive broncho-provocation
- Tracheomalacia
  - Worse with activity or agitation
  - Poor response to bronchodilators and steroids
  - Homophonous wheeze
  - Airway collapse on fluoroscopy
  - Collapsible trachea on bronchoscopy

- Bronchomalacia
  - Worse with activity or agitation
  - Poor response to bronchodilators and steroids
  - Homophonous wheeze
  - Airway collapse on fluoroscopy
  - Collapsible bronchus on bronchoscopy
- Foreign body
  - Sudden onset
  - May have a history of choking
  - Differential breath sounds
  - Differential hyperinflation or collapse on radiography
- Heart failure or pulmonary edema
  - Poor response to albuterol
  - Poor growth
  - Hepatomegaly
  - Radiography showing increased fluid
  - Responds to diuresis
- Bronchiolitis
  - Infant: upper respiratory infection symptoms
  - Positive viral studies
  - Wheezing caused by viral bronchiolitis:
    - Is usually preceded by upper respiratory symptoms and fever
    - Worsens within the first few days of onset
    - Tends to improve slowly thereafter
- Vocal cord dysfunction
  - Poor response to all therapies
  - Severe distress reported
  - Pulmonary function tests: normal or with abnormal inspiratory loop
  - Laryngoscopy: vocal cord adduction during inspiration
- Cystic fibrosis
  - Poor growth, gastrointestinal (GI) symptoms
  - Recurrent pneumonias
  - Positive sweat test
- Gastroesophageal reflux and aspiration
  - Variable response to bronchodilators
  - Often worse after meals
  - Poor growth, GI symptoms
  - Recurrent pneumonias
  - Positive reflux evaluation (upper GI, nuclear scan or pH probe)
- Vascular compression
  - Central wheeze
  - No bronchodilator response

- Indentation on esophagram
- Anatomy demonstrated on thoracic magnetic resonance imaging
- Large airway abnormality (stenosis, complete rings, compression)
  - No response to therapy
  - Worse with activity
  - Stridor noted at times
  - Flattened or square flow–volume loop
  - Obstruction visible on imaging or bronchoscopy
- Wheezing that appears at birth or soon afterward should prompt an evaluation for congenital airway abnormalities, such as:
  - Tracheomalacia
  - Complete rings
  - Vascular abnormalities or compression

LABORATORY EVALUATION

- Laboratory testing may be indicated to diagnose specific clinical entities.
  - Sweat test for cystic fibrosis
  - Viral studies can identify respiratory syncytial virus or influenza.

IMAGING

- Chest radiography can be used to detect:
  - Thoracic masses that cause obstruction of airways
  - Foreign body aspiration
- Airway fluoroscopy
  - Can confirm diagnosis and help quantify the severity of tracheobronchomalacia
- Esophagraphy or upper GI series
  - Useful if a vascular abnormality is suspected
- Computed tomography or magnetic resonance imaging
  - Confirmation of vascular abnormality

DIAGNOSTIC PROCEDURES

- Pulmonary function testing
  - Can help characterize a wheeze objectively
- Direct visualization of the airway via flexible bronchoscopy
  - To characterize dynamic lesions (ie, tracheobronchomalacia)
- Rigid bronchoscopy
  - Can be useful in diagnosis and treatment of tracheal stenosis

W

TREATMENT APPROACH

- In general, when evaluating and managing the wheezing child:
  - Be aware of the various clinical entities that can produce wheezing.
  - Be able to recognize by history or physical examination patients who require further workup.
  - Initiate simple diagnostic tests.

SPECIFIC TREATMENT

Asthma and viral bronchiolitis

- See Asthma.
  - Responds to bronchodilators
  - Responds to steroids
- See Viral Bronchiolitis.
  - No evidence supports the regular use of ß-agonist therapy in viral bronchiolitis.
- Some children require hospitalization for severe respiratory distress, hypoxemia, poor feeding, or dehydration.
- Wheezing associated with failure to thrive in an infant may be a sign of significant underlying disease.

WHEN TO REFER

- Refer to appropriate subspecialty physicians children with unusual presentations or poor response to conventional therapies.
  - Persistent or recurrent wheezing in an infant <1 year
  - Apparent paradoxical response to bronchodilators
  - Poor weight gain or growth associated with chronic or recurrent wheezing
  - Repeated hospitalization or multiple courses of oral corticosteroids

WHEN TO ADMIT

- Respiratory distress unresponsive to therapy
- Hypoxemia
- Tachypnea interfering with ability to eat or drink
- Altered mental status or signs of fatigue

Formulas and Reference Range Values

Formulas and Reference Range Values

Conversion Formulas

Height (length)	
1 millimeter (mm) = 0.04 inch 1 centimeter = 0.4 inch	1 inch = 2.54 centimeter 1 meter = 39.37 inches

Weight	
60 milligrams (mg) = 1 grain 28.35 grams (g) = 1 ounce 453.6 grams = 1 pound 1000 grams (1 kilogram [kg]) = 2.2046 pounds	1 liter (L) = 1.06 quarts 1 fluid ounce (oz) = 29.57 mL 1 tablespoon = 15 mL 1 teaspoon = 5 mL

Milligram–milliequivalent conversions	
mEq/L = mg/L × valence/atomic weight Equivalent weight = atomic weight/valence	mg/L = mEq/L × atomic weight/valence

Milligram-millimole conversions
Millimoles/L (mmol/L) = mg/L ÷ molecular weight

Milliosmols
The milliequivalent (mEq) is roughly equivalent to the milliosmol (mOsm), the unit of measure of osmotic pressure or tonicity. One osmole is the amount of a substance that dissociates in solution to form one mole of osmotically active particles.

From: McInerny TK, Adam HM, Campbell DE, Kamat DM, Kelleher KJ, eds. *American Academy of Pediatrics Textbook of Pediatric Care Tools for Practice.* Elk Grove Village, IL: American Academy of Pediatrics; 2009.

Blood Pressure Nomograms for Healthy Term Infants During the First 12 Hours of Life

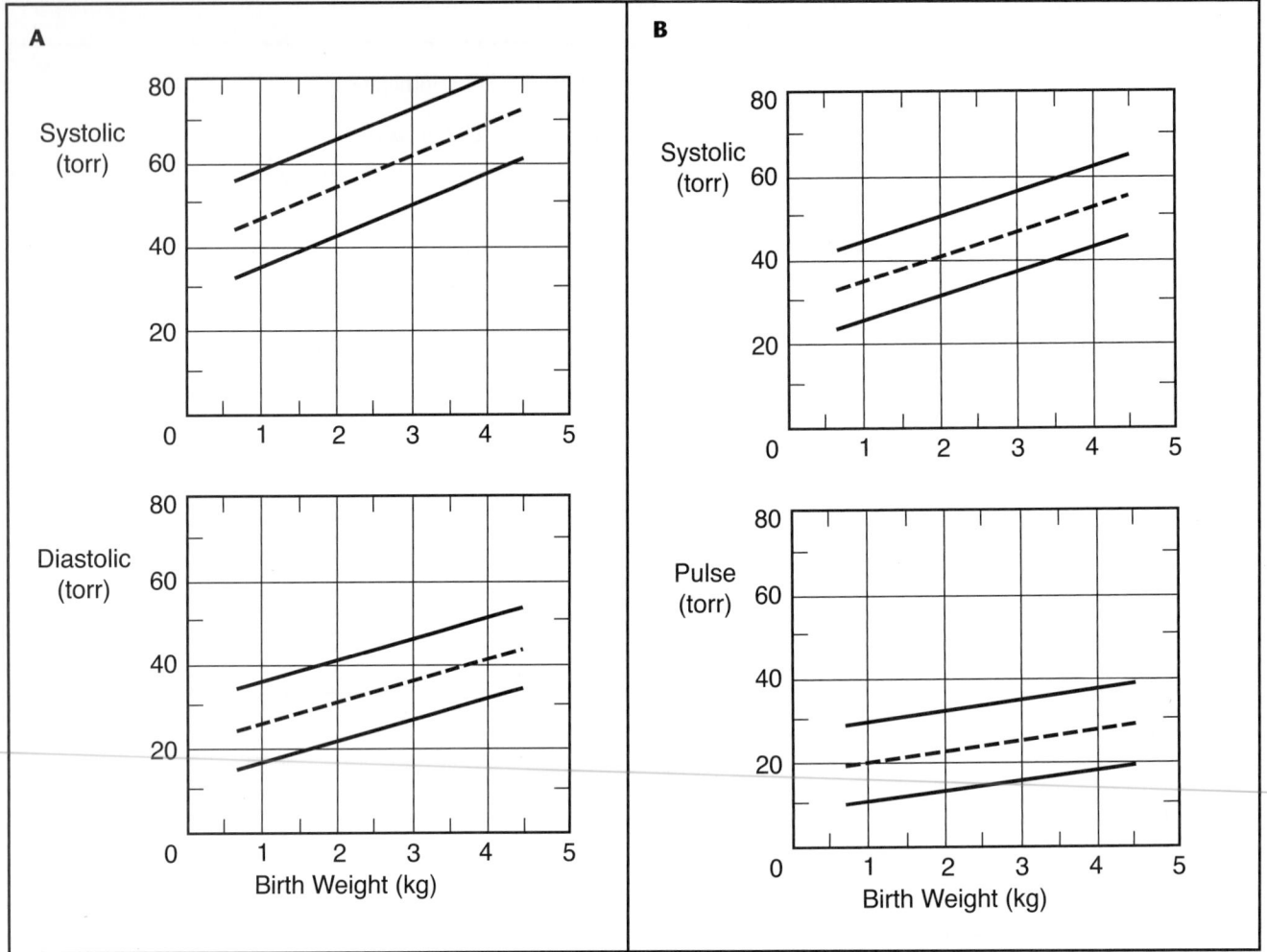

A. Linear regressions (broken lines) and 95% confidence limits (solid lines) of systolic (top) and diastolic (bottom) aortic blood pressures on birth weight in 61 healthy newborn infants during the first 12 hours after birth. For systolic pressure, $y = 7.13x + 40.45$; $r = .79$. For diastolic pressure, $y = 4.81x + 22.18$; $r = .71$. For both, $n = 413$ and $p < .001$. **B.** Linear regressions (broken lines) and 95% confidence limits (solid lines) of mean pressure (top) and pulse pressure (systolic-diastolic pressure amplitude) (bottom) on birth weight in 61 healthy newborn infants during the first 12 hours after birth. For mean pressure, $y = 5.16x + 29.80$; $n = 443$; $r = .80$. For pulse pressure, $y = 2.31x + 18.27$; $n = 413$; $r = .45$. For both, $p < .001$.

From: Versmold HT, Kitterman JA, Phibbs RH, et al. Aortic blood pressure during the first 12 hours of life in infants with birth weight 610 to 4,220 grams. *Pediatrics.* 1981;67(5):607.

Blood Pressure Nomograms for Preterm and Full-term Neonates During the First Day of Life (According to Birth Weight)

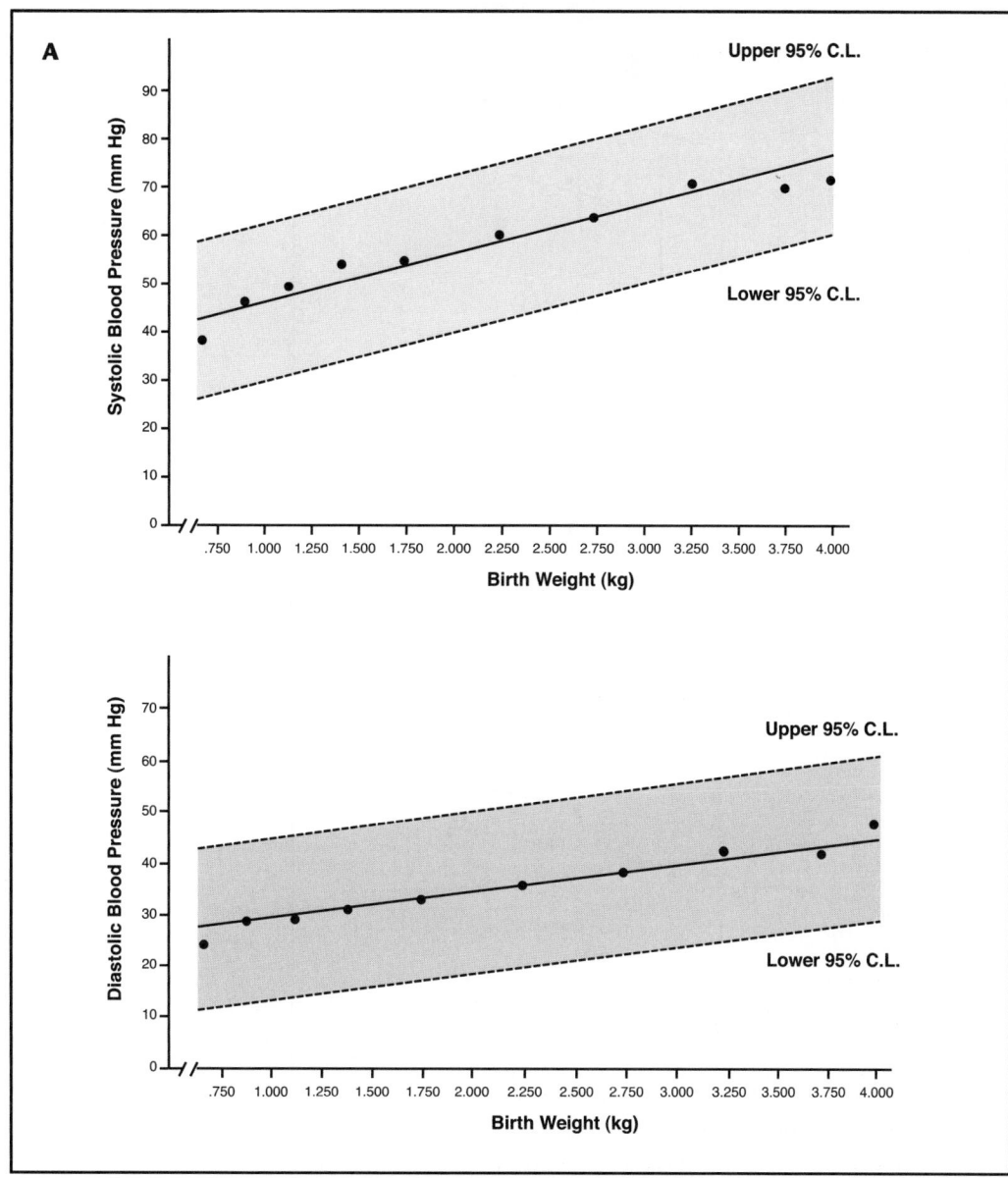

A. Linear regression of mean systolic and diastolic blood pressures by birth weight on day 1 of life, with 95% confidence limits *(upper and lower dashed lines)*.

From: Zubrow AB, Hulman S, Kushner H, et al. Determinants of blood pressure in infants admitted to neonatal intensive care units: a prospective multicenter study. *J Perinatol.* 1995;15(6):470–479. Reprinted by permission from Macmillan Publishers Ltd: *Journal of Perinatology.*

Blood Pressure Nomograms for Preterm and Full-term Neonates During the First Day of Life (According to Gestational Age)

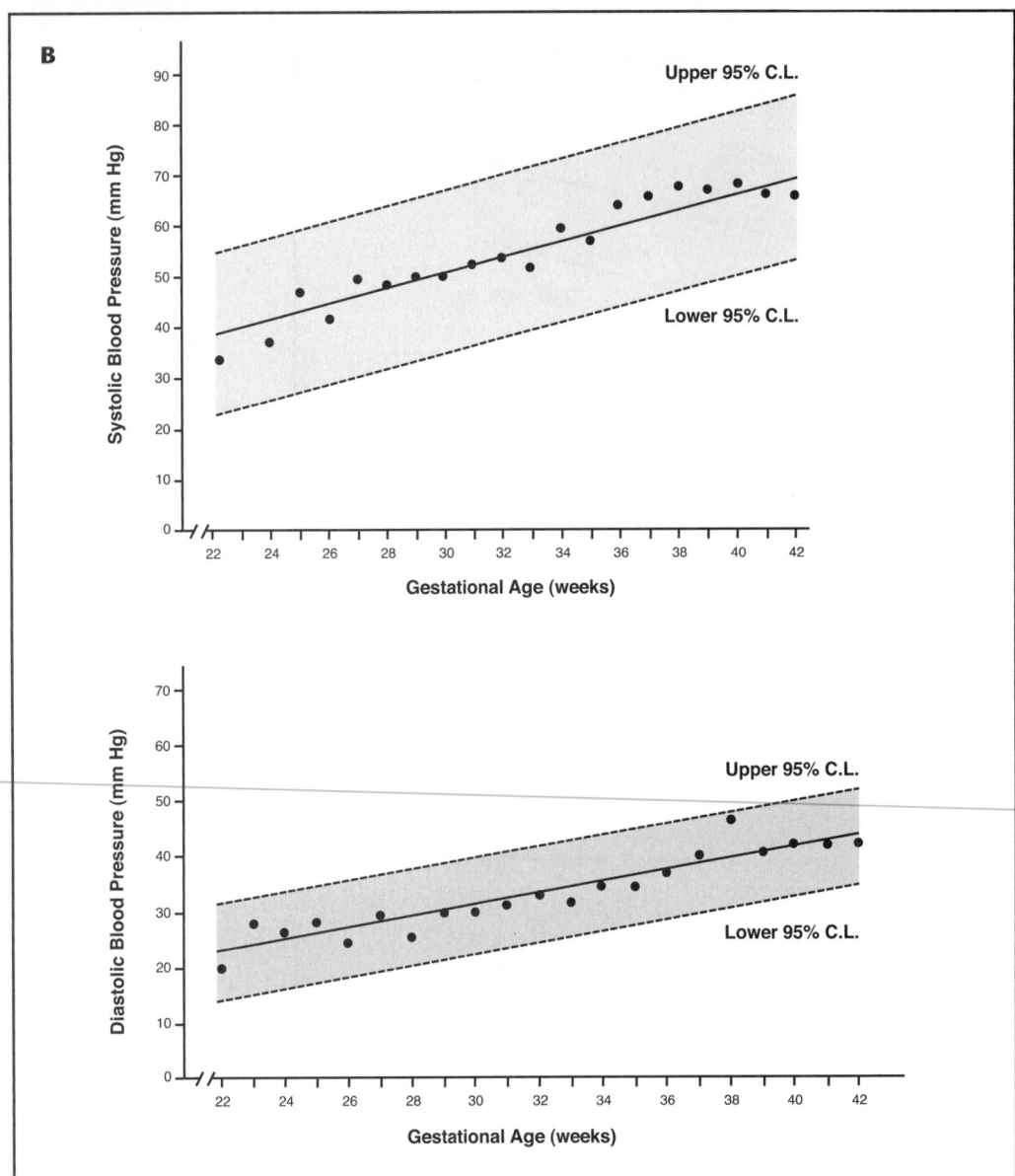

B. Linear regression of mean systolic and diastolic blood pressures by gestational age on day 1 of life, with 95% confidence limits *(upper and lower dashed lines)*.

From: Zubrow AB, Hulman S, Kushner H, et al. Determinants of blood pressure in infants admitted to neonatal intensive care units: a prospective multicenter study. *J Perinatol.* 1995;15(6):470–479. Reprinted by permission from Macmillan Publishers Ltd: *Journal of Perinatology.*

Blood Pressure Nomograms for Preterm and Full-term Neonates During the First Few Weeks of Life

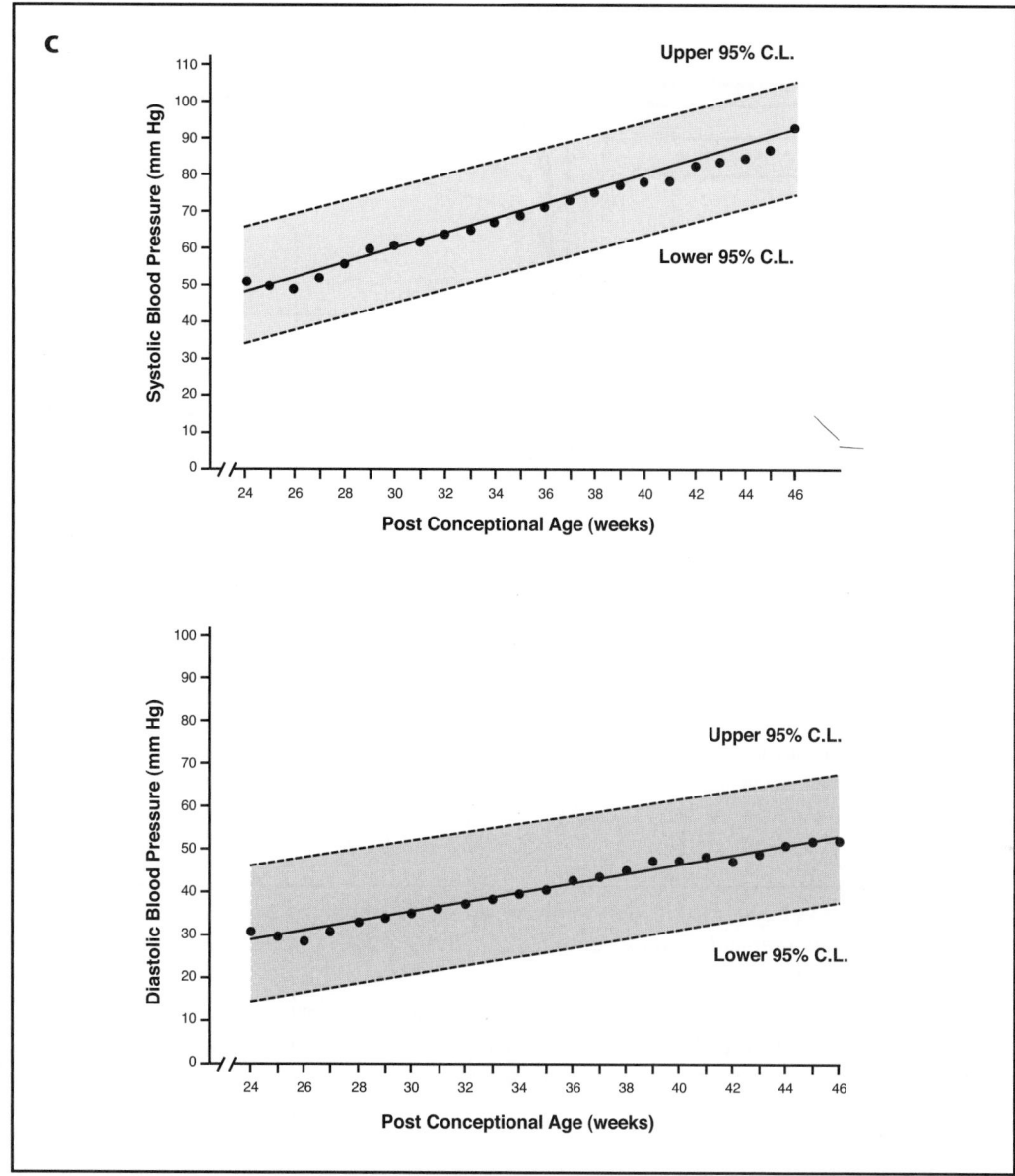

C. Linear regression of mean systolic and diastolic blood pressures by postconceptual age in weeks, with 95% confidence limits *(upper and lower dashed lines)*.

From: Zubrow AB, Hulman S, Kushner H, et al. Determinants of blood pressure in infants admitted to neonatal intensive care units: a prospective multicenter study. *J Perinatol.* 1995;15(6):470–479. Reprinted by permission from Macmillan Publishers Ltd: *Journal of Perinatology*.

Blood Pressure Nomograms for Children Younger Than 1 Year

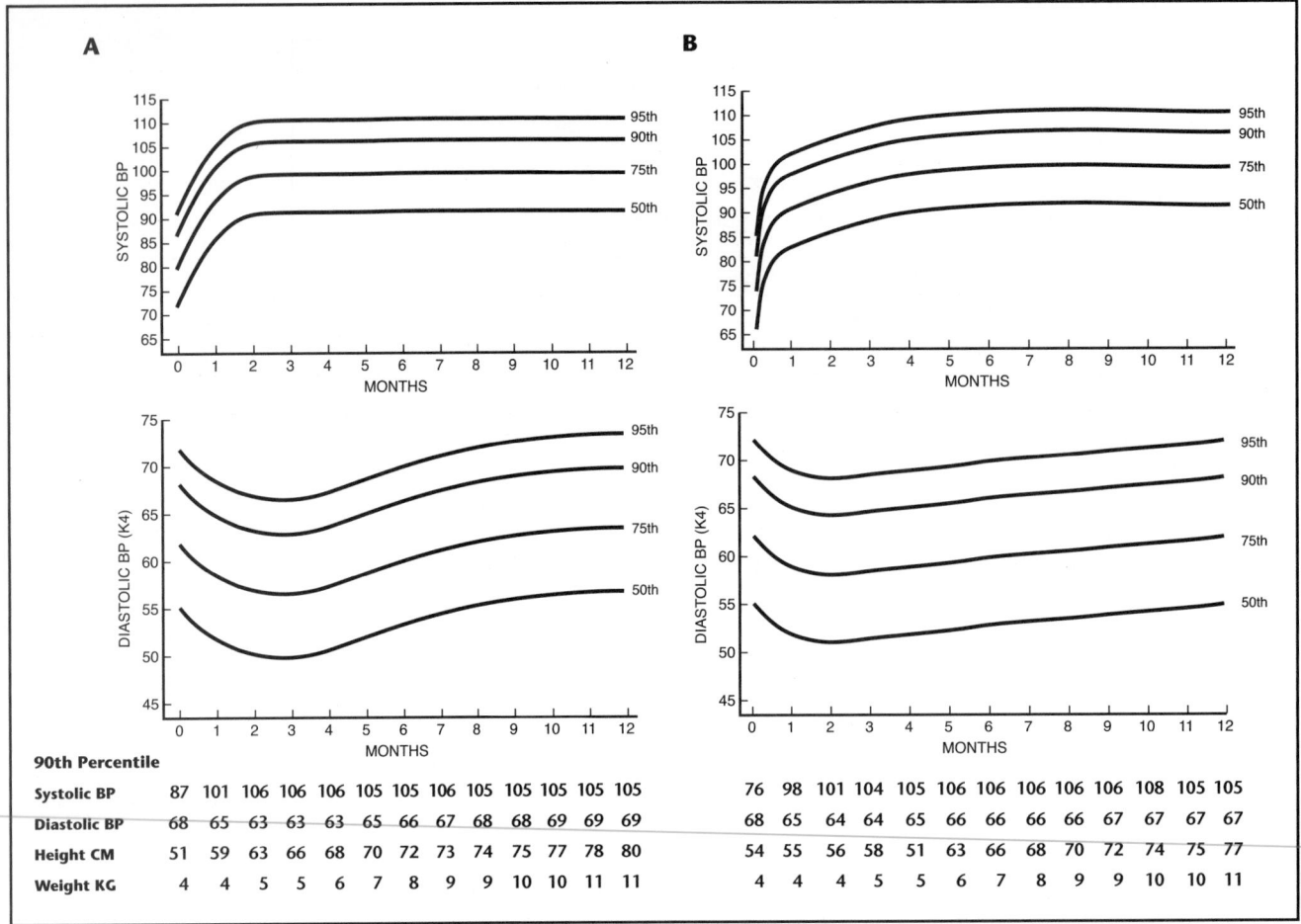

A. Age-specific percentiles of BP measurements in boys—birth to 12 months of age; Korotkoff phase IV (K4) used for diastolic BP. **B.** Age-specific percentiles of BP measurements in girls—birth to 12 months of age; Korotkoff phase IV (K4) used for diastolic BP.

From: American Academy of Pediatrics. Report of the Second Task Force on Blood Pressure Control in Children—1987. Task Force on Blood Pressure Control in Children. National Heart, Lung, and Blood Institute, Bethesda, Maryland. *Pediatrics.* 1987;79(1):1.

Blood Pressure Levels for Boys by Age and Height Percentile

Age (Year)	BP Percentile	Systolic BP (mmHg) ← Percentile of Height →								Diastolic BP (mmHg) ← Percentile of Height →						
		5th	10th	25th	50th	75th	90th	95th		5th	10th	25th	50th	75th	90th	95th
1	50th	80	81	83	85	87	88	89		34	35	36	37	38	39	39
	90th	94	95	97	99	100	102	103		49	50	51	52	53	53	54
	95th	98	99	101	103	104	106	106		54	54	55	56	57	58	58
	99th	105	106	108	110	112	113	114		61	62	63	64	65	66	66
2	50th	84	85	87	88	90	92	92		39	40	41	42	43	44	44
	90th	97	99	100	102	104	105	106		54	55	56	57	58	58	59
	95th	101	102	104	106	108	109	110		59	59	60	61	62	63	63
	99th	109	110	111	113	115	117	117		66	67	68	69	70	71	71
3	50th	86	87	89	91	93	94	95		44	44	45	46	47	48	48
	90th	100	101	103	105	107	108	109		59	59	60	61	62	63	63
	95th	104	105	107	109	110	112	113		63	63	64	65	66	67	67
	99th	111	112	114	116	118	119	120		71	71	72	73	74	75	75
4	50th	88	89	91	93	95	96	97		47	48	49	50	51	51	52
	90th	102	103	105	107	109	110	111		62	63	64	65	66	66	67
	95th	106	107	109	111	112	114	115		66	67	68	69	70	71	71
	99th	113	114	116	118	120	121	122		74	75	76	77	78	78	79
5	50th	90	91	93	95	96	98	98		50	51	52	53	54	55	55
	90th	104	105	106	108	110	111	112		65	66	67	68	69	69	70
	95th	108	109	110	112	114	115	116		69	70	71	72	73	74	74
	99th	115	116	118	120	121	123	123		77	78	79	80	81	81	82
6	50th	91	92	94	96	98	99	100		53	53	54	55	56	57	57
	90th	105	106	108	110	111	113	113		68	68	69	70	71	72	72
	95th	109	110	112	114	115	117	117		72	72	73	74	75	76	76
	99th	116	117	119	121	123	124	125		80	80	81	82	83	84	84
7	50th	92	94	95	97	99	100	101		55	55	56	57	58	59	59
	90th	106	107	109	111	113	114	115		70	70	71	72	73	74	74
	95th	110	111	113	115	117	118	119		74	74	75	76	77	78	78
	99th	117	118	120	122	124	125	126		82	82	83	84	85	86	86
8	50th	94	95	97	99	100	102	102		56	57	58	59	60	60	61
	90th	107	109	110	112	114	115	116		71	72	72	73	74	75	76
	95th	111	112	114	116	118	119	120		75	76	77	78	79	79	80
	99th	119	120	122	123	125	127	127		83	84	85	86	87	87	88
9	50th	95	96	98	100	102	103	104		57	58	59	60	61	61	62
	90th	109	110	112	114	115	117	118		72	73	74	75	76	76	77
	95th	113	114	116	118	119	121	121		76	77	78	79	80	81	81
	99th	120	121	123	125	127	128	129		84	85	86	87	88	88	89

continued

Blood Pressure Levels for Boys by Age and Height Percentile, *continued*

Age (Year)	BP Percen-tile	Systolic BP (mm Hg) ← Percentile of Height →							Diastolic BP (mm Hg) ← Percentile of Height →						
		5th	10th	25th	50th	75th	90th	95th	5th	10th	25th	50th	75th	90th	95th
10	50th	97	98	100	102	103	105	106	58	59	60	61	61	62	63
	90th	111	112	114	115	117	119	119	73	73	74	75	76	77	78
	95th	115	116	117	119	121	122	123	77	78	79	80	81	81	82
	99th	122	123	125	127	128	130	130	85	86	86	88	88	89	90
11	50th	99	100	102	104	105	107	107	59	59	60	61	62	63	63
	90th	113	114	115	117	119	120	121	74	74	75	76	77	78	78
	95th	117	118	119	121	123	124	125	78	78	79	80	81	82	82
	99th	124	125	127	129	130	132	132	86	86	87	88	89	90	90
12	50th	101	102	104	106	108	109	110	59	60	61	62	63	63	64
	90th	115	116	118	120	121	123	123	74	75	75	76	77	78	79
	95th	119	120	122	123	125	127	127	78	79	80	81	82	82	83
	99th	126	127	129	131	133	134	135	86	87	88	89	90	90	91
13	50th	104	105	106	108	110	111	112	60	60	61	62	63	64	64
	90th	117	118	120	122	124	125	126	75	75	76	77	78	79	79
	95th	121	122	124	126	128	129	130	79	79	80	81	82	83	83
	99th	128	130	131	133	135	136	137	87	87	88	89	90	91	91
14	50th	106	107	109	111	113	114	115	60	61	62	63	64	65	65
	90th	120	121	123	125	126	128	128	75	76	77	78	79	79	80
	95th	124	125	127	128	130	132	132	80	80	81	82	83	84	84
	99th	131	132	134	136	138	139	140	87	88	89	90	91	92	92
15	50th	109	110	112	113	115	117	117	61	62	63	64	65	66	66
	90th	122	124	125	127	129	130	131	76	77	78	79	80	80	81
	95th	126	127	129	131	133	134	135	81	81	82	83	84	85	85
	99th	134	135	136	138	140	142	142	88	89	90	91	92	93	93
16	50th	111	112	114	116	118	119	120	63	63	64	65	66	67	67
	90th	125	126	128	130	131	133	134	78	78	79	80	81	82	82
	95th	129	130	132	134	135	137	137	82	83	83	84	85	86	87
	99th	136	137	139	141	143	144	145	90	90	91	92	93	94	94
17	50th	114	115	116	118	120	121	122	65	66	66	67	68	69	70
	90th	127	128	130	132	134	135	136	80	80	81	82	83	84	84
	95th	131	132	134	136	138	139	140	84	85	86	87	87	88	89
	99th	139	140	141	143	145	146	147	92	93	93	94	95	96	97

BP, blood pressure

* The 90th percentile is 1.28 SD, 95th percentile is 1.645 SD, and the 99th percentile is 2.326 SD over the mean.

From: McInerny TK, Adam HM, Campbell DE, Kamat DM, Kelleher KJ, eds. *American Academy of Pediatrics Textbook of Pediatric Care Tools for Practice.* Elk Grove Village, IL: American Academy of Pediatrics; 2009.

Blood Pressure Levels for Girls by Age and Height Percentile

Age (Year)	BP Percentile	Systolic BP (mmHg) ← Percentile of Height →							Diastolic BP (mmHg) ← Percentile of Height →						
		5th	10th	25th	50th	75th	90th	95th	5th	10th	25th	50th	75th	90th	95th
1	50th	83	84	85	86	88	89	90	38	39	39	40	41	41	42
	90th	97	97	98	100	101	102	103	52	53	53	54	55	55	56
	95th	100	101	102	104	105	106	107	56	57	57	58	59	59	60
	99th	108	108	109	111	112	113	114	64	64	65	65	66	67	67
2	50th	85	85	87	88	89	91	91	43	44	44	45	46	46	47
	90th	98	99	100	101	103	104	105	57	58	58	59	60	61	61
	95th	102	103	104	105	107	108	109	61	62	62	63	64	65	65
	99th	109	110	111	112	114	115	116	69	69	70	70	71	72	72
3	50th	86	87	88	89	91	92	93	47	48	48	49	50	50	51
	90th	100	100	102	103	104	106	106	61	62	62	63	64	64	65
	95th	104	104	105	107	108	109	110	65	66	66	67	68	68	69
	99th	111	111	113	114	115	116	117	73	73	74	74	75	76	76
4	50th	88	88	90	91	92	94	94	50	50	51	52	52	53	54
	90th	101	102	103	104	106	107	108	64	64	65	66	67	67	68
	95th	105	106	107	108	110	111	112	68	68	69	70	71	71	72
	99th	112	113	114	115	117	118	119	76	76	76	77	78	79	79
5	50th	89	90	91	93	94	95	96	52	53	53	54	55	55	56
	90th	103	103	105	106	107	109	109	66	67	67	68	69	69	70
	95th	107	107	108	110	111	112	113	70	71	71	72	73	73	74
	99th	114	114	116	117	118	120	120	78	78	79	79	80	81	81
6	50th	91	92	93	94	96	97	98	54	54	55	56	56	57	58
	90th	104	105	106	108	109	110	111	68	68	69	70	70	71	72
	95th	108	109	110	111	113	114	115	72	72	73	74	74	75	76
	99th	115	116	117	119	120	121	122	80	80	80	81	82	83	83
7	50th	93	93	95	96	97	99	99	55	56	56	57	58	58	59
	90th	106	107	108	109	111	112	113	69	70	70	71	72	72	73
	95th	110	111	112	113	115	116	116	73	74	74	75	76	76	77
	99th	117	118	119	120	122	123	124	81	81	82	82	83	84	84
8	50th	95	95	96	98	99	100	101	57	57	57	58	59	60	60
	90th	108	109	110	111	113	114	114	71	71	71	72	73	74	74
	95th	112	112	114	115	116	118	118	75	75	75	76	77	78	78
	99th	119	120	121	122	123	125	125	82	82	83	83	84	85	86
9	50th	96	97	98	100	101	102	103	58	58	58	59	60	61	61
	90th	110	110	112	113	114	116	116	72	72	72	73	74	75	75
	95th	114	114	115	117	118	119	120	76	76	76	77	78	79	79
	99th	121	121	123	124	125	127	127	83	83	84	84	85	86	87

continued

Blood Pressure Levels for Girls by Age and Height Percentile, *continued*

Age (Year)	BP Percentile	Systolic BP (mm Hg) ← Percentile of Height →							Diastolic BP (mm Hg) ← Percentile of Height →						
		5th	10th	25th	50th	75th	90th	95th	5th	10th	25th	50th	75th	90th	95th
10	50th	98	99	100	102	103	104	105	59	59	59	60	61	62	62
	90th	112	112	114	115	116	118	118	73	73	73	74	75	76	76
	95th	116	116	117	119	120	121	122	77	77	77	78	79	80	80
	99th	123	123	125	126	127	129	129	84	84	85	86	86	87	88
11	50th	100	101	102	103	105	106	107	60	60	60	61	62	63	63
	90th	114	114	116	117	118	119	120	74	74	74	75	76	77	77
	95th	118	118	119	121	122	123	124	78	78	78	79	80	81	81
	99th	125	125	126	128	129	130	131	85	85	86	87	87	88	89
12	50th	102	103	104	105	107	108	109	61	61	61	62	63	64	64
	90th	116	116	117	119	120	121	122	75	75	75	76	77	78	78
	95th	119	120	121	123	124	125	126	79	79	79	80	81	82	82
	99th	127	127	128	130	131	132	133	86	86	87	88	88	89	90
13	50th	104	105	106	107	109	110	110	62	62	62	63	64	65	65
	90th	117	118	119	121	122	123	124	76	76	76	77	78	79	79
	95th	121	122	123	124	126	127	128	80	80	80	81	82	83	83
	99th	128	129	130	132	133	134	135	87	87	88	89	89	90	91
14	50th	106	106	107	109	110	111	112	63	63	63	64	65	66	66
	90th	119	120	121	122	124	125	125	77	77	77	78	79	80	80
	95th	123	123	125	126	127	129	129	81	81	81	82	83	84	84
	99th	130	131	132	133	135	136	136	88	88	89	90	90	91	92
15	50th	107	108	109	110	111	113	113	64	64	64	65	66	67	67
	90th	120	121	122	123	125	126	127	78	78	78	79	80	81	81
	95th	124	125	126	127	129	130	131	82	82	82	83	84	85	85
	99th	131	132	133	134	136	137	138	89	89	90	91	91	92	93
16	50th	108	108	110	111	112	114	114	64	64	65	66	66	67	68
	90th	121	122	123	124	126	127	128	78	78	79	80	81	81	82
	95th	125	126	127	128	130	131	132	82	82	83	84	85	85	86
	99th	132	133	134	135	137	138	139	90	90	90	91	92	93	93
17	50th	108	109	110	111	113	114	115	64	65	65	66	67	67	68
	90th	122	122	123	125	126	127	128	78	79	79	80	81	81	82
	95th	125	126	127	129	130	131	132	82	83	83	84	85	85	86
	99th	133	133	134	136	137	138	139	90	90	91	91	92	93	93

BP, blood pressure

* The 90th percentile is 1.28 SD, 95th percentile is 1.645 SD, and the 99th percentile is 2.326 SD over the mean.

From: McInerny TK, Adam HM, Campbell DE, Kamat DM, Kelleher KJ, eds. *American Academy of Pediatrics Textbook of Pediatric Care Tools for Practice.* Elk Grove Village, IL: American Academy of Pediatrics; 2009.

Determining Body Surface Area

Based on the nomogram shown in Figure C-4, a straight line joining the patient's height and weight will intersect the center column at the calculated body surface area (BSA). For children of normal height and weight, the child's weight in pounds is used, then the examiner reads across to the corresponding BSA in meters². Alternatively, Mosteller's formula can be used.

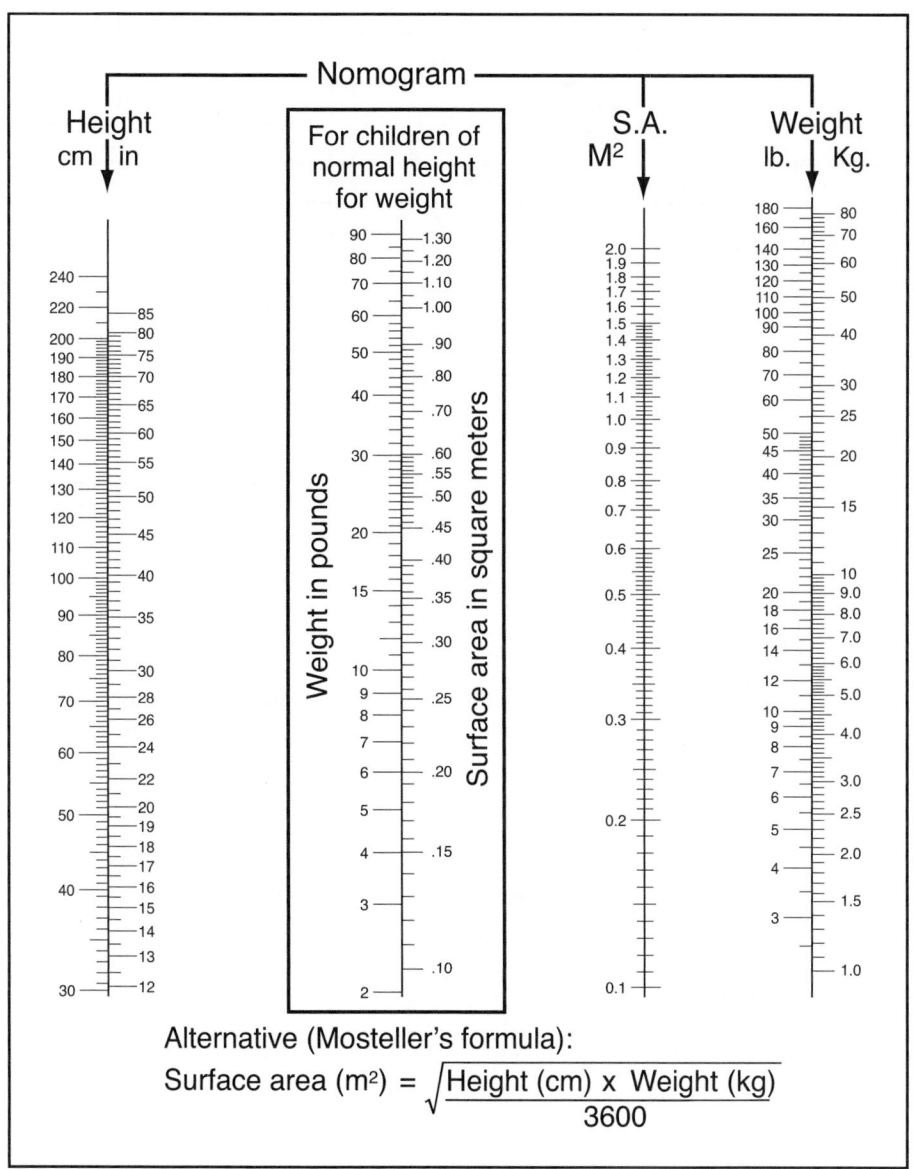

Nomogram and equation to determine body surface area.

From: Custer J, Rau R, eds. *The Harriet Lane Handbook.* 18th ed. St Louis, MO: Mosby; 2009. Copyright © Elsevier 2009. Data from: Briars GL, Bailey BJ. Surface area estimation: pocket calculator v nomogram. *Arch Dis Child.* 1994;70(3):246. With permission from BMJ Publishing Group Ltd.

Bone Age

Sontag Method

The Sontag method is used to evaluate the skeletal development of children between 1 and 60 months of age:

1. Radiographs are taken of all epiphyseal centers on the left side of the body: shoulder, elbow, wrist and hand, hip, knee (anteroposterior [AP] views before 24 months of age, lateral views after 24 months), and ankle and foot (AP views before 48 months of age, lateral views after 48 months).

2. All ossification centers in the left half of the body are counted. A center is counted as soon as it casts any shadow on the roentgenogram.

3. The number of ossification centers is compared with normal values for the patient's age (Table C 1).

Gruelich and Pyle Method

The Gruelich and Pyle method is used to evaluate the skeletal development of girls from 5 to 18 years of age and of boys from 5 to 19 years:

1. A radiograph is taken of the left hand and wrist.

2. Calculation of the skeletal development is based on the order of appearance and maturation of the epiphyseal centers. (For normal values, see Gruelich and Pyle's *Radiographic Atlas of Skeletal Development of the Hand and Wrist*.)

Mean Total Number of Centers on the Left Side of Body Ossified at Given Age Levels

Age (mos)	Boys Mean	SD	Girls Mean	SD
1	4.11	1.41	4.58	1.76
3	6.63	1.86	7.78	2.16
6	9.61	1.95	11.44	2.53
9	11.88	2.66	15.36	4.92
12	13.96	3.96	22.40	6.93
18	19.27	6.61	34.10	8.44
24	29.21	8.10	43.44	6.65
30	37.59	7.40	48.91	6.50
36	43.42	5.34	52.73	5.48
42	47.06	5.26	56.61	3.98
48	51.24	4.59	57.94	3.91
54	53.94	4.35	58.89	3.36
60	56.24	4.07	61.52	2.69

SD, standard deviation.

From: Sontag LW, Snell D, Anderson M. Rate of appearance of ossification centers from birth to the age of five years. *Am J Dis Child.* 1939;58(5):953. Copyright © 1939 American Medical Association. All rights reserved.

Acid Base Response in Respiratory Acidosis and Alkalosis

The nomogram shows confidence bands for the normal adjustment in carbon dioxide content and pH made to accommodate acute and chronic changes in arterial Pco_2).

1. The pH is determined on the nomogram from the plotted (Pco_2) and carbon dioxide content obtained from blood gas measurements.

2. If the pH value is not within confidence bands, the change in carbon dioxide content and pH is different from that expected from a pure respiratory condition; thus a metabolic abnormality is also present.

3. To estimate the effect of acute and chronic changes in Pco_2 and bicarbonate Hco_3^- on pH, the following formulas are used:

Acute change in $Paco_2$: ($\Delta\ Paco_2$) (0.008) = Δ pH
Chronic change in Pco_2: ($\Delta\ Pco_2$) (0.003) = Δ pH
Change in Hco_3^-: ($\Delta\ Hco_3^-$) (0.015) = Δ pH

Anion Gap: The gap caused by anions (other than Hco_3^- and chloride [Cl^-]) that balance the positive charge of sodium (Na^+).

Anion Gap = $Na^+ - (Cl^- + Hco_3^-)$; normal = 12 mEq/L ± 2 mEq/L

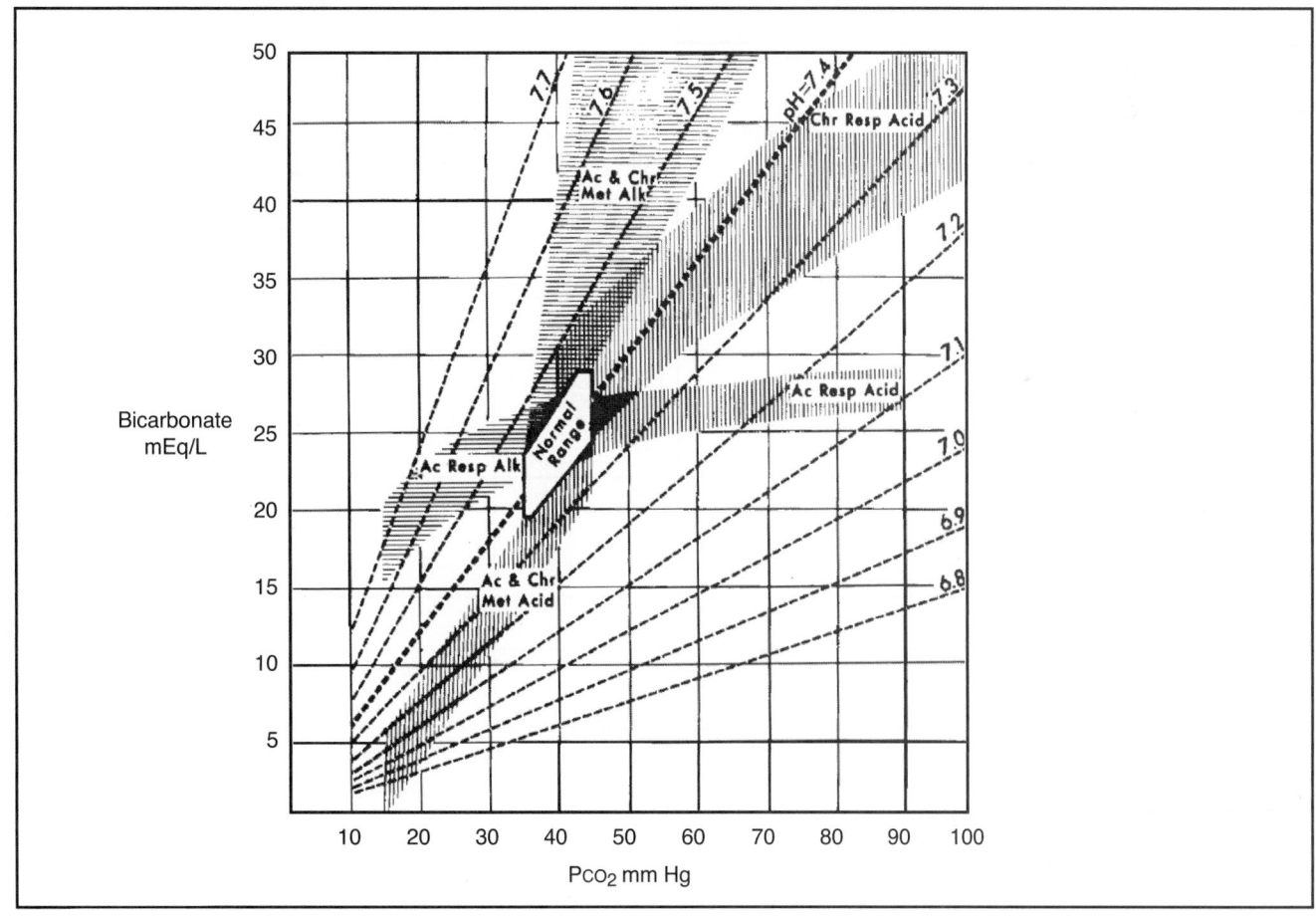

In vivo nomogram showing bands for defining a single respiratory or metabolic acid-base disturbance. Acid base response in respiratory acidosis and alkalosis.

Modified from: Arbus GS. An in vivo acid-base nomogram for clinical use. *Can Med Assoc J.* 1973;109(4):291. Copyright © Canadian Medical Association, 1973. This work is protected by copyright and the making of this copy was with the permission of Access Copyright. Any alteration of its content or further copying in any form whatsoever is strictly prohibited unless otherwise permitted by law.

Reference Range Values—Cerebrospinal Fluid

Component	Preterm Neonate	Term 1–7 Days	Term 8–30 Days	1–3 Months	4 Months– 16 Years	Adult
Color	Clear or xanthochromic	Clear or xanthochromic	Clear or xanthochromic	Clear	Clear	Clear
Red blood cells/mcL		3–23 (0–1070)[d]				
White blood cells/mcL	<25[c]–28[e]	<30[a]	<10[a]	<3	<1	<5
Polymorphonuclear cells/mcL	<20[e]–60%[c]	<38[e]–60%[a]	<10%[a]	None (36–71%)[f]	None (26–35%)[f]	None
Lymphocytes/mcL		0–20 (<24 hrs); 0–4 (7 days age)[d]	≤11	≤5	≤5	60–70%
Monocytes/mcL		<4[f] (50–99%)	≤4[f] (50–99%)	<4[f] (33–67%)	<4[f] (44–90%)	30–50%
Protein (mg/dL)	65–150[c]	<70[a] (40–120)[b]	<40[a] (20–80)[b]	15–45[b]	15–45[b]	15–45[b]
Glucose (mg/dL)	24–63 (1.3–3.5mmol/L)	>60% serum[a]	>50% serum[a] ≥38 (2.1 mmol/L)	≥45 (≥2.5 mmol/L)	45–72 (2.5–4.0 mmol/L); 60–60% serum glucose	40–85
CSF glucose/blood glucose	0.55–1.05[c]	≥0.6	≥0.6	≥0.6	≥0.6	
Lactate mmol/L	5–30 (approx × 10% serum value)[c]	<3.1 (>2 days age)	<3.1	<3.1	<2.4 (children)	
Opening pressure (mm H_2O) in lateral recumbent position		8–11	<20	<20	<20	50–180
CSF volume (mL)					60–100	100–160
Fluctuation with respiration		0.5–1.0	0.5–1.0	0.5–1.0	0.5–1.0	0.5–1.0

CSF, cerebral spinal fluid

Calculating the ratio of red blood cells (RBCs) to white blood cells (WBCs) in CSF.[a]

General rule: for every 500 RBCs in CSF, acceptable to have 1 WBC.

Normal ratio of RBCs to WBCs in peripheral blood: 1000 RBCs: 1–2 WBCs × 10^6/L.

$$\text{Number of WBCs introduced into the CSF per L} = \frac{(WBC_{[peripheral]} \times RBC_{[CSF]})}{RBC_{(peripheral)}} \times 10^6/L$$

Compare this number with the actual number of WBCs in the CSF.

1000 × 10^6/L RBCs in CSF raises CSF protein by approximately 0.015 g/L.

[a] Lipton JD, Schafermeyer RW. Evolving concepts in pediatric bacterial meningitis—part I: pathophysiology and diagnosis. *Ann Emerg Med.* 1993;22:1602; Griffith BP, Booss J. Neurologic infections of the fetus and newborn. *Neurol Clin.* 1994;12:541.

[b] Soldin JS, Brugnara C, Gunter KC, et al, eds. *Pediatric Reference Ranges.* 2nd ed. Washington, DC: AAAC Press; 1997.

[c] McMillan JA, Oski FA, Feigin RD, et al, eds. *Oski's Pediatrics: Principles and Practice.* 3rd ed. Philadelphia, PA: JB Lippincott; 1999.

[d] Naidoo BT. The cerebrospinal fluid in the healthy newborn infant. *S Afr Med J.* 1968;42:933.

[e] Nascimento-Carvalho CMC, Moreno-Carvalho OA. Normal cerebrospinal fluid values in full-term gestation and premature neonates. *Arq Neuropsiquiatr.* 1998;56(3-A):375.

[f] Ahmed A, Hickey SM, Ehrett S, et al. Cerebrospinal fluid values in the term neonate. *Pediatr Infect Dis J.* 1996;15(4):298.

[g] Biou D, Benoist J-F, Huong CN-TX, et al. Cerebrospinal fluid protein concentrations in children: age-related values in patients without disorders of the central nervous system. *Clin Chem.* 2000;46(3):399.

[h] Wong M, Schlagger BL, Buller RS, et al. Cerebrospinal fluid protein concentration in pediatric patients: defining clinically relevant reference values. *Arch Pediatr Adolesc Med.* 2000;154:827.

From: McInerny TK, Adam HM, Campbell DE, Kamat DM, Kelleher KJ. *American Academy of Pediatrics Textbook of Pediatric Care Tools for Practice.* Elk Grove Village, IL: American Academy of Pediatrics; 2009.

Reference Range Values— Clinical Chemistry

Determination	Standard Units	X Conversion Factor	SI Units
Acid phosphate			
Newborn	7.4–19.4 U/L		7.4–19.4 U/L
2–13 yr	6.4–15.2 U/L		6.4–15.2 U/L
Adult male	0.5–11.0 U/L		0.5–11.0 U/L
Adult female	0.2–9.5 U/L		0.2–9.5 U/L
Alanine aminotransferase (ALT or SGPT)			
Neonate/infant	13–45 U/L		13–45 U/L
Adult male	10–40 U/L		10–40 U/L
Adult female	7–35 U/L		7–35 U/L
Aldolase			
10–24 mos	3.4–11.8 U/L		3.4–11.8 U/L
2–6 yrs	1.2–8.8 U/L		1.2–8.8 U/L
Adult	1.7–4.9 U/L		1.7–4.9 U/L
Alkaline phosphatase			
Newborn	35–213 U/L		35–213 U/L
Infant	150–420 U/L		150–420 U/L
2–10 yrs	100–320 U/L		100–320 U/L
Male adolescent	100–390 U/L		100–390 U/L
Female adolescent	100–320 U/L		100–320 U/L
Adult	30–120 U/L		30–120 U/L
Ammonia		0.7139	
Newborn	90–150 mcg/dl		64–107 mcmol/L
0–2 wks	79–129 mcg/dl		56–92 mcmol/L
>1 mo	29–70 mcg/dl		21–50 mcmol/L
Adult	0–50 mcg/dl		0–35.7 mcmol/L
Amylase			
Newborn	5–65 U/L		5–65 U/L
Adult	27–131 U/L		27–131 U/L
Aspartate aminotransferase (AST or SGOT)			
Newborn	25–75 U/L		25–75 U/L
Infant	15–60 U/L		15–60 U/L
1–3 yrs	20–60 U/L		20–60 U/L
4–6 yrs	15–50 U/L		15–50 U/L
7–9 yrs	15–40 U/L		15–40 U/L
10–11 yrs	10–60 U/L		10–60 U/L
12–19 yrs	15–45 U/L		15–45 U/L

Determination	Standard Units	X Conversion Factor	SI Units
Bicarbonate		1	
Newborn	17–24 mEq/L		17–24 mmol/L
2 mos–2 yrs	16–24 mEq/L		16–24 mmol/L
>2 yrs	22–26 mEq/L		22–26 mmol/L
Bilirubin (Total)		17.1	
Cord			
Preterm	<2 mg/dL		<34 mcmol/L
Term	<2 mg/dL		<34 mcmol/L
0–1 day			
Preterm	<8 mg/dL		<137 mcmol/L
Term	<8.7 mg/dL		<149 mcmol/L
1–2 days			
Preterm	<12 mg/dl		<205 mcmol/L
Term	<11.5 mg/dL		<197 mcmol/L
3–5 days			
Preterm	<16 mg/dL		<274 mcmol/L
Term	<12 mg/dL		<205 mcmol/L
Older infants			
Preterm	<2 mg/dL		<34 mcmol/L
Term	<1.2 mg/dL		<21 mcmol/L
Adult	0.3–1.2 mg/dL		5–21 mcmol/L
Bilirubin (conjugated)			
Neonate	<0.6 mg/dL		<10 mcmol/L
Infant/children	<0.2 mg/dL		<3.4 mcmol/L

	pH	Pao_2 (mmHg)	$Paco_2$ (mmHg)	Hco_3- (MEq/L)
Blood Gas, Arterial (Breathing Room Air)				
Newborn (birth)	7.26–7.29	60	55	19
Newborn (>4 hr)	7.37	70	33	20
Infant (1–24 mo)	7.40	90	34	20
Child (7–19 yr)	7.39	96	37	22
Adult (>9 yr)	7.35–7.45	90–110	35–45	22–26

Note: Venous blood gases can be used to assess acid-base status, not oxygenation. Pco_2 averages 6–8 mmHg higher than $Paco_2$, and pH is slightly lower. Peripheral venous samples are strongly affected by the local circulatory and metabolic environment. Capillary blood gases correlate best with arterial pH and moderately well with $Paco_2$.

continued

Reference Range Values—Clinical Chemistry, *continued*

continued from page 1473

Determination	Standard Units	X Conversion Factor	SI Units
Calcium			
Total		0.2495	
Preterm	6.2–11 mg/dL		1.6–2.8 mmol/L
Full term <10 days	7.6–10.4 mg/dL		1.9–2.6 mmol/L
10 days–24 mos	9.0–11 mg/dL		2.3–2.8 mmol/L
2–12 yrs	8.8–10.8 mg/dL		2.2–2.7 mmol/L
Adult	8.6–10 mg/dL		2.2–2.5 mmol/L
Ionized		0.5	
Newborn <36 hrs	4.20–5.48 mg/dL		1.05–1.37 mmol/L
Newborn 36–84 hrs	4.40–5.68 mg/dL		1.10–1.42 mmol/L
1–18 yrs	4.80–5.52 mg/dL		1.20–1.38 mmol/L
Adult	4.64–5.28 mg/dL		1.16–1.32 mmol/L
Chloride (serum)		1	
Newborn	98–113 mEq/L		98–113 mmol/L
Child/adult	98–107 mEq/L		98–107 mmol/L
C-reactive protein	0–0.5mg/dl		
Creatinine kinase (creatinine phosphokinase)			
Newborn	10–200 U/L		10–200 U/L
Female	10–80 U/L		10–80 U/L
Male	15–105 U/L		15–105 U/L
Creatinine (serum)		88.4	
Cord	0.6–1.2 mg/dL		53–106 mcmol/L
Newborn	0.3–1.0 mg/dL		27–88 mcmol/L
Infant	0.2–0.4 mg/dL		18–35 mcmol/L
Child	0.3–0.7 mg/dL		27–62 mcmol/L
Adolescent	0.5–1.0 mg/dL		44–88 mcmol/L
Man	0.7–1.3 mg/dL		62–115 mcmol/L
Woman	0.6–1.1 mg/dL		53–97 mcmol/L
Erythrocyte sedimentation rate (ESR)			
Term neonate	0–4 mm/hr		
Child	4–20 mm/hr		
Adult (male)	1–15 mm/hr		
Adult (female)	4–25 mm/hr		
Ferritin		1	
Newborn	25–200 ng/mL		25–200 ng/ml
1 mo	200–600 ng/mL		200–600 ng/ml
2–5 mos	50–200 ng/mL		50–200 ng/ml
6 mos–15 yrs	7–140 ng/mL		7–140 ng/ml
Male adult	20–250 ng/mL		20–250 ng/ml
Female adult	10–120 ng/mL		10–120 ng/ml

Determination	Standard Units	X Conversion Factor	SI Units
Folate (serum)		2.266	
Newborn	150–200 ng/mL		11–147 nmol/L
Infant	15–55 ng/mL		34–125 nmol/L
2–16 yrs	5–21 ng/mL		11–48 nmol/L
>16 yrs	3–20 ng/mL		7–45 nmol/L
Folate (red blood cells)			
Newborn	150–200 ng/mL		340–453 nmol/L
Infant	75–1000 ng/mL		170–2265 nmol/L
2–16 yrs	>160 ng/mL		>362 nmol/L
>16 yrs	140–628 ng/mL		317–1422 nmol/L
Galactose		0.05551	
Newborn	0–20 mg/dL		0–1.11 mmol/L
Thereafter	<5 mg/dL		<0.28 mmol/L
γ-**Glutamyl transferase** (GGT)			
Cord	19–270 U/L		19–270 U/L
Preterm	56–233 U/L		56–233 U/L
0–3 wks	0–130 U/L		0–130 U/L
3 wks–3 mos	4–120 U/L		4–120 U/L
3–12 mos (boy)	5–65 U/L		5–65 U/L
3–12 mos (girl)	5–35 U/L		5–35 U/L
1–15 yrs	0–23 U/L		0–23 U/L
Male adult	11–50 U/L		11–50 U/L
Female adult	7–32 U/L		7–32 U/L
Glucose (serum)		0.05551	
Preterm	20–50 mg/dL		1.1–3.3 mmol/L
Newborn <1 day	40–60 mg/dL		2.2–3.3 mmol/L
Newborn >1 day	50–80 mg/dL		2.8–4.5 mmol/L
Child	60–100 mg/dL		3.3–5.6 mmol/L
>16 yrs	74–106 mg/dL		4.1–5.9 mmol/L
Haptoglobin			
Newborn	5–48 mg/dL		50–480 mg/dL
>30 days	26–185 mg/dL		260–1850 mg/dL
Hemoglobin F (mean [standard deviation (SD)] percentage of total hemoglobin)			
1 day	77.0 (7.3)		
5 days	76.8 (5.8)		
3 wks	70.0 (7.3)		
6–9 wks	52.9 (11)		
3–4 mos	23.2 (16)		
6 mos	4.7 (2.2)		
8–11 mos	1.6 (1.0)		
Adult	<2.0		

continued

Reference Range Values—Clinical Chemistry, *continued*

continued from page 1475

Determination	Standard Units	X Conversion Factor	SI Units
Iron		0.1791	
Newborn	100–250 mcg/dL		17.9–44.8 mcmol/L
Infant	40–100 mcg/dL		7.2–17.9 mcmol/L
Child	50–120 mcg/dL		9.0–21.5 mcmol/L
Male adult	65–175mc/dL		11.6–31.3 mcmol/L
Female adult	50–170 mcg/dL		9.0–30.4 mcmol/L
Ketones (Serum)			
Quantitative	0.5–3.0 mg/dL		5–30 mg/L
Lactate capillary blood			
Newborn	<27 mg/dL		0.0–3.0 mmol/L
Child	5–20 mg/dL		0.56–2.25 mmol/L
Venous	5–20 mg/dL		0.5–2.2 mmol/L
Arterial	5–14 mg/dL		0.5–1.6 mmol/L
Lactate dehydrogenase (at 37° C)			
0–4 days	290–775 U/L		290–775 U/L
4–10 days	545–2000 U/L		545–2000 U/L
10 days–24 mos	180–430 U/L		180–430 U/L
24 mos–12 yrs	110–295 U/L		110–295 U/L
>12 yrs	100–190 U/L		100–190 U/L
Lead			
Child	<10 µg/dL		<0.48 µmol/L
Lipase			
0–90 days	10–85 U/L		
3–12 mos	9–128 U/L		
1–11 yrs	10–150 U/L		
>11 yrs	10–220 U/L		
Lipids			
Cholesterol (mg/dL)	Desirable	Borderline	High
Child/adolescent	<170	170–199	>200
Adult	<200	200–239	>240
Low-density lipoprotein (mg/dL)			
Child/adolescent	<110	110–129	>130
Adult	<100	100–159	>160
High-density lipoprotein (mg/dL)			
Child/adolescent	45		
Adult	45		
Magnesium	1.3–2.0 mEq/L	0.5	0.65–1.0 mmol/L
Methemoglobin	<1.5% total Hgb		

Determination	Standard Units	X Conversion Factor	SI Units
Osmolality	275–295 mOsm/kg	1	275–295 mmol/kg
Phenylalanine			
Preterm	2.0–7.5 mg/dL		121–454 mcmol/L
Newborn	1.2–3.4 mg/dL		73–206 mcmol/L
Adult	0.8–1.8 mg/dL		45–109 mcmol/L
Phosphorus		0.3229	
Newborn	4.5–9.0 mg/dL		1.45–2.9 mmol/L
10 days–24 mos	4.5–6.7 mg/dL		1.45–2.16 mmol/L
24 mos–12 yrs	4.5–5.5 mg/dL		1.45–1.78 mmol/L
>12 yrs	2.7–4.5 mg/dL		0.87–1.45 mmol/L
Potassium		1	
Newborn	3.7–5.9 mEq/L		3.7–5.9 mmol/L
Infant	4.1–5.3 mEq/L		4.1–5.3 mmol/L
Child	3.4–4.7 mEq/L		3.4–4.7 mmol/L
Adult	3.5–5.1 mEq/L		3.5–5.1 mmol/L
Prealbumin			
Newborn	7–39 mg/dL		
1–6 mos	8–34 mg/dL		
6 mos–4 yrs	2–36 mg/dL		
4–6 yrs	12–30 mg/dL		
6–19 yrs	12–42 mg/dL		

Proteins (protein electrophoresis) (g/dL)						
Age	TP	Albumin	α-1	α-2	β	γ
Cord	4.8–8	2.2–4.0	0.3–0.7	0.4–0.9	0.4–1.6	0.8–1.6
Newborn	4.4–7.6	3.2–4.8	0.1–0.3	0.2–0.3	0.3–0.6	0.6–1.2
1 day–1 mos	4.4–7.6	2.5–5.5	0.1–0.3	0.3–1.0	0.2–1.1	0.4–1.3
1–3 mos	3.6–7.4	2.1–4.8	0.1–0.4	0.3–1.1	0.3–1.1	0.2–1.1
4–6 mos	4.2–7.4	2.8–5.0	0.1–0.4	0.3–0.8	0.3–0.8	0.1–0.9
7–12 mos	5.1–7.5	3.2–5.7	0.1–0.6	0.3–1.5	0.4 –1.0	0.2–1.2
13–24 mos	3.7–7.5	1.9–5.0	0.1–0.6	0.4–1.4	0.4 –1.4	0.4–1.6
25–36 mos	5.3–8.1	3.3–5.8	0.1–0.3	0.4–1.1	0.3–1.2	0.4–1.5
3–5 yrs	4.9–8.1	2.9–5.8	0.1–0.4	0.4–1.0	0.5–1.0	0.4–1.7
6–8 yrs	6.0–7.9	3.3–5.0	0.1–0.5	0.5–.08	0.5–0.9	0.7–2.0
9–11 yrs	6.0–7.9	3.2–5.0	0.1–0.4	0.7–0.9	0.6–1.0	0.8–2.0
12–16 yrs	6.0–7.9	3.2–5.1	0.1–0.4	0.5–1.1	0.5–1.1	0.6–2.0
Adult	6.0–8.0	3.1–5.4	0.1–0.4	0.4–1.1	0.5–1.2	0.7–1.7

continued

Reference Range Values—Clinical Chemistry, *continued*

continued from page 25

Determination	Standard Units	X Conversion Factor	SI Units
Pyruvate	0.3–0.9 mg/dL		0.3–0.10 mmol/L
Sodium			
Preterm	130–140 mEq/L		130–140 mmol/L
Older infants	133–146 mEq/L		133–146 mmol/L
Total iron-binding capacity (TIBC)		0.1791	
Infant	100–400 mcg/dL		17.9–71.6 mcmol/L
Adult	250–425 mcg/dL		44.8–76.1 mcmol/L
Transferrin		0.01	
Newborn	130–275 mg/dL		1.30–2.75 g/L
3 mos–10 yrs	203–360 mg/dL		2.03–3.6 g/L
Adult	215–380 mg/dL		2.15–3.8 g/L

Age	5th	mean	75th	90th	95th
Total triglycerides (mg/dL)					
Cord	14	34			84
1–4 yrs					
Male	29	56	68	85	99
Female	34	64	74	95	112
5–9 yrs					
Male	28	52	58	70	85
Female	32	64	74	103	126
10–14 yrs					
Male	33	63	74	94	111
Female	39	72	85	104	120
15–19 yrs					
Male	38	78	88	125	143
Female	36	73	85	112	126

Determination	Standard Units	X Conversion Factor	SI Units
Troponin-I	0–0.1 mcg/L		
Urea nitrogen		0.357	
Premature (<1 wk)	3–25 mg/dL		1.1–8.9 mmol/L
Newborn	4–12 mg/dL		1.4–4.3 mmol/L
Infant/children	5–18 mg/dL		1.8–6.4 mmol/L
Adult	6–20 mg/dL		2.1–7.1 mmol/L

Determination	Standard Units	X Conversion Factor	SI Units
Uric acid			
0–2 yrs	2.4–6.4 mg/dL		0.14–0.38 mmol/L
2–12 yrs	2.4–5.9 mg/dL		0.14–0.35 mmol/L
12–14 yrs	2.4–6.4 mg/dL		0.14–0.38 mmol/L
Male adult	3.5–7.2 mg/dL		0.20–0.43 mmol/L
Female adult	2.4–6.4 mg/dL		0.14–0.38 mmol/L
Vitamin A (retinol)		0.03491	
Preterm	13–46 mcg/dL		0.46–1.61 mcmol/L
Full term	18–50 mcg/dL		0.63–1.75 mcmol/L
1–6 yrs	20–43 mcg/dL		0.75–1.5 mcmol/L
7–12 yrs	20–49 mcg/dL		0.9–1.7 mcmol/L
13–19 yrs	26–72 mcg/dL		0.9–2.5 mcmol/L
Vitamin B_1 (thiamine)	5.3–7.9 mcg/dL		0.16–0.23 mcmol/L
Vitamin B_2 (riboflavin)	4–24 mcg/dL		106–638 nmol/L
Vitamin B_{12} (cobalamin)		0.7378	
Newborn	160–1300 pg/mL		118–959 pmol/L
Child/adult	200–835 pg/mL		148–616 pmol/L
Vitamin C (ascorbic acid)	0.4–1.5 mg/dL	56.78	23–85 mcmol/L
Vitamin D_3 (1,25-dihydroxy-vitamin D)	16–65 pg/mL		42–169 pmol/L
Vitamin E			
<11 yrs	3–15 mg/L		7.0–35 mcmol/L
>11yrs	5–20 mg/L		11.6–46.4 mcmol/L
Zinc	70–120 mg/dL		10.7–18.4 mmol/L

SGOT, serum glutamic oxaloacetic transaminase; *SGPT,* serum glutamic pyruvic transaminase.
From: Custer J, Rau R, eds. *The Harriet Lane Handbook.* 18th ed. St. Louis, MO: Mosby; 2009.
Copyright © Elsevier 2009; Young DS. Implementation of SI units for clinical laboratory data: style specifications and conversion tables. *Ann Intern Med.* 1987;106(1):114. Erratum published in *Ann Intern Med.* 1991;114(2):172.

Reference Range Values—Newborn Clinical Chemistry

Descriptive Statistics of Measured Variables in Samples Obtained From Cord and From Venous Blood at 2–4 Hours of Life

	Cord Blood			2–4 Hour Blood			
	Mean ± SD	Range of Values	95% CI	Mean ± SD	Range of Values	95% CI	P Value
pH	7.35 ± 0.05	7.19–7.42	7.25–7.45	7.36 ± 0.04	7.27–7.45	7.28–7.44	NS
P_{CO_2}	40 ± 6	24.5–56.7	28–52	43 ± 7	30–65	29–57	0.034
Hct %	48 ± 5	37–60	38–58	57 ± 5	42–67	47–67	<0.001
Hgb G/L	1.65 ± 0.16	1.29–2.06	1.33–1.97	1.90 ± 0.22	0.88–2.3	1.46–2.34	<0.001
Na+ mmol/L	138 ± 3	129–144	132–144	137 ± 3	130–142	131–143	NS
K+ mmol/L	5.3 ± 1.3	3.4–9.9	2.7–7.9	5.2 ± 0.5	4.4–6.4	4.2–6.2	NS
Cl− mmol/L	107 ± 4	100–121	99–115	111 ± 5	105–125	101–121	0.002
ICa mmol/L	1.15 ± 0.35	0.21–1.5	0.4–1.85	1.13 ± 0.08	0.9–1.3	0.97–1.29	NS
IMg mmol/L	0.28 ± 0.06	0.09–0.39	0.12–0.4	0.30 ± 0.05	0.23–0.46	0.2–0.4	0.0005
Glucose mmol/L	4.16 ± 1.05	0.16–6.66	2.05–6.27	3.50 ± 0.67	5.11–16.10	2.16–4.82	
Glucose mg/dL	75 ± 19	2.9–120	37–113	63 ± 12	29–92	39–87	0.0005
Lactate mmol/L	4.6 ± 1.9	1.1–9.6	0.8–8.4	3.9 ± 1.5	1.6–9.8	0.9–6.9	0.033
BUN mmol/L	2.14 ± 0.61	1.07–3.57	0.93–3.36	2.53 ± 0.71	1.43–4.28	1.11–3.96	
BUN mg/dL	6.0 ± 1.7	3.0–10.0	2.6–9.4	7.1 ± 2.0	4–12	3.1–11.1	0.0029

BUN, blood urea nitrogen; CI, Confidence interval; Hct, hematocrit; Hgb, hemoglobin; ICa, ionized calcium; IMg, ionized magnesium; P_{CO_2}, partial pressure of carbon dioxide.
Based on data from 100 healthy full-term newborns.
From: Dollberg S, Bauer R, Lubetzky R, et al. A reappraisal of neonatal blood chemistry reference ranges using the Nova M electrodes. *Am J Perinatol.* 2001;18(8):433–440. Reprinted with permission.

Reference Range Values—Hematology

Hematologic Values

Age	Hemoglobin (grams %) Mean (± 2 SD)	Hematocrit (%) Mean (± 2 SD)	Mean Cell Volume (fL) Mean (± 2 SD)	Mean Corpuscular Hemoglobin Concentration (grams/dL RBC) Mean (± 2 SD)	Reticulo-cytes %	WBC/I0³ Mean (± 2 SD)	Platelets (10³ mm³) Mean (± 2 SD)
26–30 wks gestation*	13.4 (11)	41.5 (34.9)	118.2 (106.7)	37.9 (30.6)	—	4.4 (2.7)	254 (180–327)
28 wks	14.5	45	120	31	5–10	—	275
32 wks	15.0	47	118	32	3–10	—	290
Term (cord)**	16.5 (13.5)	51 (42)	108 (98)	33 (30)	3–7	18.1 (9–30)	290
1–3 days	18.5 (14.5)	56 (45)	108 (95)	33 (29)	1.8-4.6	18.9 (9.4–34)	192
2 wks	16.6 (13.4)	53 (41)	105 (88)	31.4 (28.1)		11.4 (5–20)	252
1 mo	13.9 (10.7)	44 (33)	101 (91)	31.8 (28.1)	0.1–1.7	10.8 (4-19.5)	
2 mos	11.2 (9.4)	35 (28)	95 (84)	31.8 (28.3)			
6 mos	12.6 (11.1)	36 (31)	76 (68)	35 (32.7)	0.7-2.3	11.9 (6–17.5)	
6 mos–2 yrs	12.0 (10.5)	36 (33)	78 (70)	33 (30)		10.6 (6–17)	(150–350)
2–6 yrs	12.5 (11.5)	37 (34)	81 (75)	34 (31)	0.5–1.0	8.5 (5–15.5)	(150–350)
6–12 yrs	13.5 (11.5)	40 (35)	86 (77)	34 (31)	0.5–1.0	8.1 (4.5–13.5)	(150–350)
12–18 yrs							
Male	14.5 (13)	43 (36)	88 (78)	34 (31)	0.5–1.0	7.8 (4.5–13.5)	(150-350)
Female	14.0 (12)	41 (37)	90 (78)	34 (31)	0.5–1.0	7.8 (4.5–13.5)	(150-350)
Adult							
Male	15.5 (13.5)	47 (41)	90 (80)	34 (31)	0.8-2.5	7.4 (4.5–11)	(150–350)
Female	14.0 (12)	41 (36)	90 (80)	34 (31)	0.8-4.1	7.4 (4.5–11)	(150–350)

*Values are from fetal samplings.

**Under 1 mo of age, capillary hemoglobin exceeds venous hemoglobin: age 1 hr –by 3.6 g; age 5 days –by 2.2 g; age 3 wk –by 1.1 g. Mean (95% confidence limits)

Modified from: Custer J, Rau R, eds. *The Harriet Lane Handbook*. 18th ed. St. Louis, MO; Mosby; 2009. Data from: Forestier F, Daffos F, Galaktéros F, et al. Hematological values of 163 normal fetuses between 18–30 weeks of gestation. *Pediatr Res.* 1986;20:342; Oski FA, Naiman JL. *Hematological Problems in the Newborn Infant*. Philadelphia, PA: WB Saunders; 1982; Nathan D, Oski FA. *Hematology of Infancy and Childhood*. Philadelphia, PA: WB Saunders; 1998; Matoth Y, Zaizov R, Varsano I. Postnatal changes in some red cell parameters. *Acta Paediatr Scand.* 1971;60:317; and Wintrobe MM. *Clinical Hematology*. Baltimore, MD: Williams and Wilkins; 1999.

Reference Range Values—Thyroid Function Tests

Reference Ranges in Very Low Birth Weight Infants

Postnatal days	Screening T4 Levels by Birth Weight and Postnatal Age (mcg/dL)		
	VLBW (<1500 grams)	LBW (< 2500 grams)	Term
1–3	7.9 ± 3.3	11.4 ± 2.5	12 ± 1.9
4–6	6.5 ± 2.9	9.9 ± 2.5	11 ± 2.5
7–10	6.3 ± 3.0	9.5 ± 2.3	
11–14	5.7 ± 2.8	9.2 ± 2.1	
15–18	7.0 ± 2.5	9.1 ± 2.3	
29–56	7.8 ± 2.5	9.3 ± 3.3	

LBW, low birth weight; T4, thyroxine; VLBW, very low birth weight. Data expressed as ± SD.
From: Frank JE, Faix JE, Hermos RJ, et al. Thyroid function in very low birth weight infants: effects on neonatal hypothyroidism screening. *J Pediatr.* 1996;128(4):548. Copyright © Elsevier 1996.

Reference Ranges for Preterm Infants

Gestational Age	Free T4 (ng/dL)	Thyroid-Stimulating Hormone (mcU/mL)
25–27 wks	0.6–2.2	0.2–30.3
28–30 wks	0.6–3.4	0.2–20.6
31–33 wks	1.0–3.8	0.7–27.9
34–36 wks	1.2–4.4	1.2–21.6
37–42 wks (term)	2.0–5.3	1.0–39
PCA	Concentrations after the first wk of life*	
Preterm 28–40 wks	0.8–2.6	0.8–12.0
Term infants 42–60 wks	0.9–2.3	1.7–9.1

PCA, postconceptional age (gestational age + postnatal age); T4, thyroxine.
From: Adams LM, Emery JR, Clark SJ, et al. Reference ranges for newer thyroid function tests in premature infants. *J Pediatr.* 1995;126(1):122. Copyright © Elsevier 1995.
*Clark SJ, Deming DD, Emery JR, et al. Reference ranges for thyroid function tests in premature infants beyond the first week of life. *J Perinatol.* 2001;21:531.

Reference Ranges for Infants, Children, and Adults

Age	Thyroxine (mcg/dL)	Free Thyroxine (ng/dL)	Triiodothyronine (ng/dL)	Free Triiodothyronine (ng/dL)	Thyroxine-Binding Globulin (mg/dL)	Thyroid-Stimulating Hormone (mcU/mL)
Cord blood	6.6–17.5	1.03–1.73	14–86	0.09–0.36	0.7–4.7	<2.5–17.4
1–3 days	11.0–21.5	0.6–2.0 (1–10days)	100–380	0.17–0.57‡	—	<2.5–13.3
1–4 wks	8.2–16.6	0.7–1.7 (>10 days)	99–310	0.17–0.65‡	0.5–4.5	0.6–10.0
1–12 mos	7.2–15.6	0.8–1.8 (5–24 mo) †	102–264	0.24–0.65‡	1.6–3.6	0.6–6.3
1–5 yrs	7.3–15	1.0–2.1 (2–7 y) †	105–269	0.29–0.8‡	1.3–2.8	0.6–6.3
6–10 yrs	6.4–13.3	0.8–1.9 (8–20 y)†	94–241	0.34–0.72‡	1.4–2.6	
11–15 years	5.6–11.7	0.59–2.45§	83–213	0.37–0.7‡	1.4–2.6	0.6–6.3
16–20 yrs	4.2–11.8	0.54–2.23§	80–210	0.42–0.68 (16–18 yrs) ‡	1.4–2.6	0.2–7.6
21–45 yrs	4.3–12.5	0.9–2.5	70–204		1.2–2.4	0.2–7.6

* Delange F, Fisher DA. The thyroid gland. In: CGD Brook, ed. *Clinical Paediatric Endocrinology*. London, UK: Blackwell; 1995.

† Nelson JC, Clark SJ, Borut DL, et al. Age-related changes in serum free thyroxine during childhood and adolescence. *J Pediatr.* 1993;123:899.

‡ Soldin SJ, Morales A, Albalos F, et al. Pediatric reference ranges on the Abbott Imx for FSH, LH, Prolactin, TSH, T4, T3, free T4, free T3, T-uptake, IgE and Ferritin. *Clin Biochem.* 1995;28:603.

§ Zurakowski D, DiCanzio J, Majzoub JA. Pediatric reference intervals for serum thyroxine, triiodothyronine, thyrotropin and free thyroxine. *Clin Chem.* 1999;45:1087.

From: McInerny TK, Adam HM, Campbell DE, Kamat DM, Kelleher KJ, eds. *American Academy of Pediatrics Textbook of Pediatric Care Tools for Practice.* Elk Grove Village, IL: American Academy of Pediatrics; 2009.

Reference Range Values—Coagulation Tests

Reference Ranges for Coagulation Tests in the Healthy Full-term Infant During the First 6 Months of Life

Tests	Day 1 (n)	Day 5 (n)	Day 30 (n)	Day 90 (n)	Day 180 (n)	Adult (n)
PT (sec)	13.0 ± 1.43 (61)*	12.4 ± 1.46 (77)*†	11.8 ± 1.25 (67)*†	11.9 ± 1.15 (62)*	12.3 ± 0.79 (47)*	12.4 ± 0.78 (29)
aPTT (sec)	42.9 ± 5.80 (61)	42.6 ± 8.62 (76)	40.4 ± 7.42 (67)	37.1 ± 6.52 (62)*	35.5 ± 3.71 (47)*	33.5 ± 3.44 (29)
TCT (sec)	23.5 ± 2.38 (58)*	23.1 ± 3.07 (64)†	24.3 ± 2.44 (53)*	25.1 ± 2.32 (52)*	25.5 ± 2.86 (41)*	25.0 ± 2.66 (19)
Fibrinogen (g/L)	2.83 ± 0.58 (61)*	3.12 ± 0.75 (77)*	2.70 ± 0.54 (67)*	2.43 ± 0.68 (60)*†	2.51 ± 0.68 (47)*†	2.78 ± 0.61 (29)
II (U/mL)	0.48 ± 0.11 (61)	0.63 ± 0.15 (76)	0.68 ± 0.17 (67)	0.75 ± 0.15 (62)	0.88 ± 0.14 (47)	1.08 ± 0.19 (29)
V (U/Ml)	0.72 ± 0.18 (61)	0.95 ± 0.25 (76)	0.98 ± 0.18 (67)	0.90 ± 0.21 (62)	0.91 ± 0.18 (47)	1.06 ± 0.22 (29)
VII (U/mL)	0.66 ± 0.19 (60)	0.89 ± 0.27 (75)	0.90 ± 0.24 (67)	0.91 ± 0.26 (62)	0.87 ± 0.20 (47)	1.05 ± 0.19 (29)
VIII (U/mL)	1.00 ± 0.39 (60)*†	0.88 ± 0.33 (75)*†	0.91 ± 0.33 (67)*†	0.79 ± 0.23 (62)*†	0.73 ± 0.18 (47)†	0.99 ± 0.25 (29)
vWF (U/mL)	1.53 ± 0.67 (40)†	1.40 ± 0.57 (43)†	1.28 ± 0.59 (40)†	1.18 ± 0.44 (40)†	1.07 ± 0.45 (46)†	0.92 ± 0.33 (29)†
IX (U/mL)	0.53 ± 0.19 (59)	0.53 ± 0.19 (75)	0.51 ± 0.15 (67)	0.67 ± 0.23 (62)	0.86 ± 0.25 (47)	1.09 ± 0.27 (29)
X (U/mL)	0.40 ± 0.14 (60)	0.49 ± 0.15 (76)	0.59 ± 0.14 (67)	0.71 ± 0.18 (62)	0.78 ± 0.20 (47)	1.06 ± 0.23 (29)
XI (U/mL)	0.38 ± 0.14 (60)	0.55 ± 0.16 (74)	0.53 ± 0.13 (67)	0.69 ± 0.14 (62)	0.86 ± 0.24 (47)	0.97 ± 0.15 (29)
XII (U/mL)	0.53 ± 0.20 (60)	0.47 ± 0.18 (75)	0.49 ± 0.16 (67)	0.67 ± 0.21 (62)	0.77 ± 0.19 (47)	1.08 ± 0.28 (29)
PK (U/mL)	0.37 ± 0.16 (45)†	0.48 ± 0.14 (51)	0.57 ± 0.17 (48)	0.73 ± 0.16 (46)	0.86 ± 0.15 (43)	1.12 ± 0.25 (29)
HMWK (U/mL)	0.54 ± 0.24 (47)	0.74 ± 0.28 (63)	0.77 ± 0.22 (50)*	0.82 ± 0.32 (46)*	0.82 ± 0.23 (48)*	0.92 ± 0.22 (29)

Reference Ranges for Coagulation Tests in the Healthy Full-term Infant During the First 6 Months of Life, *continued*

Tests	Day 1 (n)	Day 5 (n)	Day 30 (n)	Day 90 (n)	Day 180 (n)	Adult (n)
XIIIa (U/mL)	0.79 ± 0.26 (44)	0.94 ± 0.25 (49)*	0.93 ± 0.27 (44)*	1.04 ± 0.34 (44)*	1.04 ± 0.29 (41)*	1.05 ± 0.25 (29) †
XIIIb (U/mL)	0.76 ± 0.23 (44)	1.06 ± 0.37 (47)*	1.11 ± 0.36 (45)*	1.16 ± 0.34 (44)*	1.10 ± 0.30 (41)*	0.97 ± 0.20 (29)
Plasminogen (CTA, U/mL)	1.95 ± 0.35 (44)	2.17 ± 0.38 (60)	1.98 ± 0.36 (52)	2.48 ± 0.37 (44)	3.01 ± 0.40 (47)	3.36 ± 0.44 (29)

NOTE: All factors except fibrinogen and plasminogen are expressed as units per milliliter where pooled plasma contains 1.0 U/mL. Plasminogen units are those recommended by the Committee on Thrombolytic Agents (CTA). All values are expressed as mean ± 1 standard deviation. aPTT, activated partial thromboplastin time; HMWK, high molecular–weight kininogen; PK, prekallikrein; PT, prothrombin time; TCT, thrombin clotting time; vWF, von Willebrand factor.

*Values that do not differ statistically from the adult values.

† These measurements are skewed because of a disproportionate number of high values. The lower limit that excludes the lower 2.5th percentile of the population has been given in the respective figures. The lower limit for factor VIII was 0.50 U/mL at all time points for the infant.

From: Andrew M, Paes B, Milner R, et al. Development of the human coagulation system in the full-term infant. *Blood.* 1987;70(1):165. This research was originally published in *Blood.* Copyright © American Society of Hematology.

Formulas

Preparation of Infant Formulas for Standard and Soy Formulas*

Formula Type	Caloric Concentration (kcal/oz)	Amount of Formula	Water (oz)
Liquid concentrates (40 kcal/oz)	20	13 oz	13
	24	13 oz	8.5
	27	13 oz	6.3
	30	13 oz	4.3
Powder (44 kcal/scoop)	20	1 scoop	2
	24	3 scoops	5
	27	3 scoops	4.25
	30	3 scoops	4

* Does not apply to Enfacare LIPIL, Neocate Infant, Neosure Advance, EleCare; Enfamil AR should not be concentrated greater than 24 kcal/oz. Use a packed measure for Nutramigen LIPIL and Pregestimil LIPIL; all others unpacked powder.
Modified from: Custer J, Rau R, eds. *The Harriet Lane Handbook*. 18th ed. St Louis, MO: Mosby; 2009. Copyright © Elsevier 2009.

Common Caloric Supplements*

Component		Calories
Protein	Casec	3.7 kcal/g (0.9 g protein)
		17 kcal/tbsp (4 g protein)
	Beneprotein	25 kcal/scoop (6 g protein)
	Complete Amino Acid Mix	3.28 kcal/g (0.82 g protein)
Carbohydrate	Polycose	Powder: 3.8 kcal/g, 8 kcal/tsp
		Liquid: 2.0 kcal/mL, 10 kcal/tsp
Fat	MCT oil†	7.7 kcal/mL
	Vegetable oil	8.3 kcal/mL
	Microlipid	4.5 kcal/mL
Fat and Carbohydrate	Duocal	42 kcal/tbsp (59% carbohydrates, 41% fat; 35% fat as MCT oil)

* Use these caloric supplements when you want to increase protein or when you have reached the maximum concentration tolerated and wish to further increase caloric density.
† MCT oil is unnecessary unless there is fat malabsorption.
From: Custer J, Rau R, eds. *The Harriet Lane Handbook*. 18th ed. St Louis, MO: Mosby; 2009. Copyright © Elsevier 2009.

Section 3

Tables

Tables

NEUROLOGIC

OBESITY

ORAL HEALTH

Development

Primary Teeth Eruption Chart

Primary Teeth

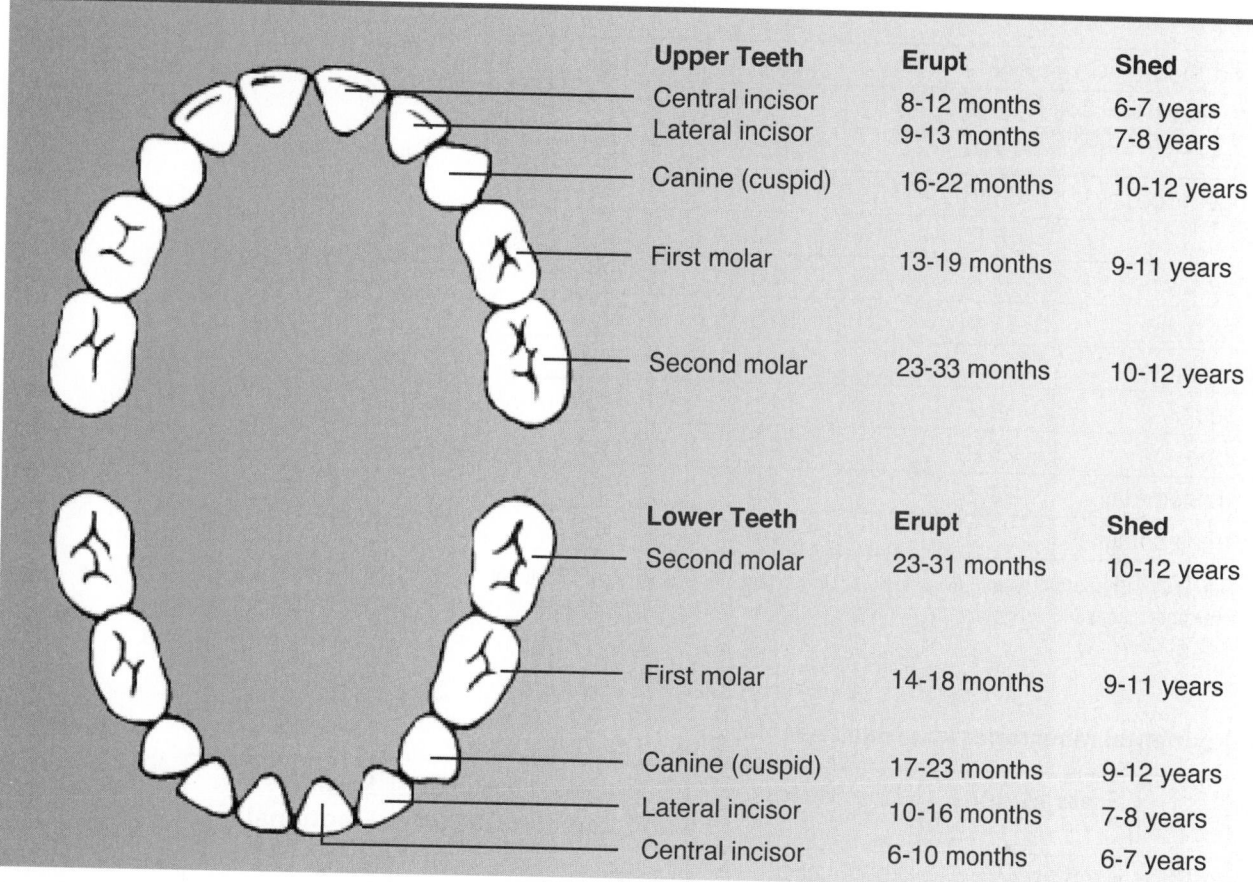

Upper Teeth	Erupt	Shed
Central incisor	8-12 months	6-7 years
Lateral incisor	9-13 months	7-8 years
Canine (cuspid)	16-22 months	10-12 years
First molar	13-19 months	9-11 years
Second molar	23-33 months	10-12 years

Lower Teeth	Erupt	Shed
Second molar	23-31 months	10-12 years
First molar	14-18 months	9-11 years
Canine (cuspid)	17-23 months	9-12 years
Lateral incisor	10-16 months	7-8 years
Central incisor	6-10 months	6-7 years

From: American Dental Association. Tooth eruption: the primary teeth. *J Am Dent Assoc.* 2005;136(11):1619.

Developmental Milestones by Age and Ethnicity, Months

Task	Anglo	Puerto Rican	Filipino
Eat solid food	8.2	10.	16.7
Use training cup	12.0	17.1	21.9
Use utensils	17.7	26.5	32.4
Eat finger foods	8.9	9.4	9.5
Wean	16.8	18.2	36.2
Sleep by self	13.8	14.6	38.8
Sleep all night	11.4	14.5	32.4
Choose clothes	31.1	44.2	33.1
Dress self	38.2	44.2	39.2
Play alone	25.0	24.8	12.3
Toilet trained (day)	31.6	29.0	20.4
Toilet trained (night)	33.2	31.8	34.2

From: Carlson VJ, Harwood RL. What do we expect? Understanding and negotiating cultural differences concerning early developmental competence: the six raisin solution. *Zero to Three*.1999;20:19–24.

Developmental Milestones at a Glance—Infancy

Age	Gross Motor	Fine Motor	Cognitive, Linguistic, and Communication	Social-Emotional
2 Months	Head up 45° Lift head	Follow past midline Follow to midline	Laugh Vocalize	Smile spontaneously Smile responsively
4 Months	Roll over Sit—head steady	Follow to 180° Grasp rattle	Turn to rattling sound Laugh	Regard own hand
6 Months	Sit—no support Roll over	Look for dropped yarn Reach	Turn to voice Turn to rattling sound	Feed self Work for toy (out of reach)
9 Months	Pull to stand Stand holding on	Take 2 cubes Pass cube (transfer)	Dada/Mama, nonspecific Single syllables	Wave bye-bye Feed self

KEY

Black Color: 50% to 90% of children pass this item.

Blue Color: More than 90% of children pass this item.

From: Frankenburg WK, Camp, BW, Van Natta PA, et al. Reliability and Stability of the Denver Developmental Screening Test. *Child Dev.* 1071;42:1315–1325.

Developmental Milestones at a Glance—Early Childhood

Age	Gross Motor	Fine Motor	Cognitive, Linguistic, and Communication	Social-Emotional
1 Year	•Stand alone •Pull to stand	•Put block in cup •Bang 2 cubes held in hands	•**Imitate vocalizations and sounds** •**Babbling*** •1 word	•**Protodeclarative pointing*** •Wave bye-bye •Imitate activities •Play pat-a-cake
15 Months	•Walk backwards •Stoop and recover •Walk well	•Scribble •Put block in cup	•**1 word*** •3 words	•Drink from cup •Wave bye-bye
18 Months	•Walk up steps •Run •Walk backwards	•Dump raisin, demonstrated •Tower of 2 cubes •Scribble	•Point to at least 1 body part •6 words •3 words	•Remove garment •Help in house
2 Years	•Throw ball overhand •Jump up •Kick ball forward •Walk up steps	•Tower of 6 cubes •Tower of 4 cubes	•Name 1 picture •Combine words •Point to 2 pictures	•Put on clothing •Remove garment
2½ Years	•Throw ball overhand •Jump up	•Imitate vertical line •Tower of 8 cubes •Tower of 6 cubes	•Know 2 actions •Speech half understandable •Point to 6 body parts •Name 1 picture	•Wash and dry hands •Put on clothing
3 Years	•Balance on each foot 1 second •Broad jump •Throw ball overhand	•Thumb wiggle •Imitate vertical line •Tower of 8 cubes •Tower of 6 cubes	•Speech all understandable •Name 1 color •Know 2 adjectives •Name 4 pictures	•Name friend •Brush teeth with help
4 Years	•Hop •Balance on each foot 2 seconds	•Draw a person with 3 parts •Tower of 8 cubes	•Define 5 words •Name 4 colors •Speech all understandable	•Copy a cross (+) •Copy a circle

continued

KEY

Black Color: 50% to 90% of children pass this item.

Blue Color: More than 90% of children pass this item.

*Absence of these milestones should trigger screening for autism.

Developmental Milestones at a Glance—Early Childhood, *continued*

1. Frankenburg WK, Dodds J, Archer P, et al: DENVER II Training Manual, 1992. Denver Developmental Materials. Denver, CO

2. Diego MA, Field T, Hart S, et al. Facial expressions and EEG in infants of intrusive and withdrawn mothers with depressive symptoms. *Depress Anxiety*. 2002;15:10–17

3. Diego MA, Field T, Hernandez-Reif M, et al. Prepartum, postpartum, and chronic depression effects on newborns. *Psychiatry*. 2004;67:63–80

4. Field T. Early interventions for infants of depressed mothers. *Pediatrics*. 1998;102(5SupplE):1305–1310

5. Bowman BT. Educating language minority children: challenges and opportunities. *Phi Delta Kappan*. 1989;71:118–120

6. Kopp CB. Antecedents of self-regulation: a developmental perspective. *Dev Psychol*. 1982;18:199–214

7. Raffaelli M, Crockett LJ, Shen YL. Developmental stability and change in self-regulation from childhood to adolescence. *J Genet Psychol*. 2005;166:54–75

8. Thiedke CC. Nocturnal enuresis. *Am Fam Physician*. 2003;67:1499–1506

9. Evans GD. *Bedwetting*. Gainesville, FL: Department of Family, Youth, and Community Sciences, Florida Cooperative Extension Service, Institute of Food and Agriculture Sciences, University of Florida; 2003. Available at: http://edis.fas.ufl.edu/pdffiles/HE/HE79400.pdf. Accessed September 13, 2007

10. Search Institute. Developmental Assets. Minneapolis, MN: Search Institute; 1997. Available at: http://www.search-institute.org/assets. Accessed September 5, 2007

11. Scales P, Leffert N, Lerner RM. *Developmental Assets: A Synthesis of the Scientific Research on Adolescent Development*. Minneapolis, MN: Search Institute; 1999

12. Biles B. Activities that promote racial and cultural awareness. *Family Child-Care Connections*. 1994;4:1-4. Available at: http://web.aces.uiuc.edu/vista/pdf_pubs/CHILDCARE.PDF. Accessed September 13, 2007

13. American Academy of Pediatrics, Committee on Psychosocial Aspects of Child and Family Health. Guidance for effective discipline. *Pediatrics*. 1998;101:723-728. Erratum in: *Pediatrics*. 1998;102–433

14. Burns MS, Griffin P, Snow CE. *Starting Out Right: A Guide to Promoting Children's Reading Success*. Washington, DC: National Academy Press; 1999

15. Podhajski B, Nathan J. Promoting early literacy through professional development for childcare providers. *Early Educ Dev*. 2005;16:1–5

16. Zuckerman BS, Klass P. Doctors Promoting Child Development with Books. Available at: http://www.ced.org/docs/report/report_ivk_zuckerman_2006.pdf. Accessed September 5, 2007

17. Glassy D, Romano J, American Academy of Pediatrics, Committee on Early Childhood, Adoption, and Dependent Care. Selecting appropriate toys for young children: the pediatrician's role. *Pediatrics*. 2003;111:911–913

18. US Department of Health and Human Services, Health Resources and Services Administration, Maternal and Child Health Bureau. *Child Health USA 2004*. Rockville, MD: US Department of Health and Human Services; 2004. Available at www.mchb.hrsa.gov/mchirc/chusa_04/-pdf/eo4.pdf. Accessed September 13, 2007

19. Capizzano J, Adams G, Sonenstein F. *Child Care Arrangements for Children Under Five: Variation Across States*. Washington, DC: Urban Institute; 2000

20. Raver CC. *Emotions Matter: Making the Case for the Role of Young Children's Emotional Development for Early School Readiness*. Ann Arbor, MI: Society for Research in Child Development; 2002

21. Rimm-Kaufman SE, Pianta RC, Cox MJ. Teachers' judgments of problems in the transition to kindergarten. *Early Child Res Q*. 2000;15:147–166

22. Rouse C, Brooks-Gunn J, McLanahan S. School readiness: closing racial and ethnic gaps: introducing the issue. *Future Child*. 2005;15:5–14

23. Farran DC, Shonkoff JP. Developmental disabilities and the concept of school readiness. *Early Educ Dev*. 1994;5:141–151

24. West J, Flanagan KD, Germino-Hausken E. *America's Kindergartners: Findings from the Early Childhood Longitudinal Study, Kindergarten Class of 1998-99 Fall 1998*. Washington, DC: US Department of Education, National Center for Education Statistics; 1998. Publication No. NCES2000070

25. Meisels SJ. Assessing readiness. In: Pianta RC, Cox MJ, eds. *The Transition to Kindergarten*. Baltimore, MD: Paul H Brookes; 1999:39–66

26. Coplan J. *Early Language Milestone Scale*. 2nd ed. Austin, TX: Pro-Ed Inc; 1993

Social and Emotional Development in Middle Childhood

Topics	Key Areas
	(Key areas in italics are especially important for children with special health care needs.)
Self	**Self-esteem:** • Experiences of success • Reasonable risk-taking behavior • Resilience and ability to handle failure • Supportive family and peer relationships **Self-image:** • Body image, *celebrating different body images* • Prepubertal changes; initiating discussion about sexuality and reproduction; *prepubertal changes related to physical care issues*
Family	**What matters at home:** • Expectation and limit setting • Family times together • Communication • Family responsibilities • Family transitions • Sibling relationships • *Caregiver relationships*
Friends	**Friendships:** • Making friends, *friendships with peers with and without special health care needs* • Family support of friendships, *family support to have typical friendship activities, as appropriate*
School	**School:** • Expectation for school performance, *school performance/ defined in the Individualized Education Program (IEP)* • Homework • Child-teacher conflicts, *building relationships with teachers* • *Parent-teacher communication* • Ability of schools to address the needs of children from diverse backgrounds • Awareness of aggression, bullying, and victimization • Absenteeism
Community	**Community strengths:** • Community organizations • Religious groups • Cultural groups **High-risk behaviors and environments:** • Substance use • Unsafe friendships • Unsafe community environments • *Particular awareness of risk-taking behaviors and unsafe environments, because children may be easily victimized*

From: Hagan JF, Shaw JS, Duncan PM, eds. *Bright Futures: Guidelines for Health Supervision of Infants, Children, and Adolescents.* 3rd ed. Elk Grove Village, IL: American Academy of Pediatrics; 2008.

Domains of Adolescent Development

	Early Adolescence (11 to 14 Years)	**Middle Adolescence** (15 to 17 Years)	**Late Adolescence** (18 to 21 Years)
Physiological	Onset of puberty, growth spurt, menarche (females)	Ovulation (females), growth spurt (males)	Growth completed
Psychological	Concrete thought, preoccupation with rapid body changes, sexual identity, questioning independence, parental controls remain strong	Competence in abstract and future thought, idealism, sense of invincibility or narcissism, sexual identity, beginning of cognitive capacity to provide legal consent	Future orientation, emotional independence, unmasking of psychiatric disorders, capacity for empathy, intimacy, and reciprocity in interpersonal relationships, self-identity, recognized as legally capable of providing consent,[64] attainment of legal age for some issues (eg, voting) but not all issues (eg, drinking alcohol)
Social	Search for same-sex peer affiliation, good parental relationships, other adults as role models; transition to middle school, involvement in extracurricular activities; sensitivity to differences between home culture and culture of others	Beginning emotional emancipation, increased power of peer group, conflicts over parental control, interest in sexual relationships, initiation of driving, risk-taking behavior, transition to high school, reduced involvement in extracurricular activities, possible cultural conflict as adolescent navigates between family's values and values of broader culture and peer culture	Individual over peer relationships; transition in parent-child relationship, transition out of home; may begin preparation for further education, career, marriage, and parenting
Potential Problems	Delayed puberty; acne; orthopedic problems; school problems; psychosomatic concerns; depression; unintended pregnancy; initiation of tobacco, alcohol, or other drug use	Experimentation with health risk behaviors (eg, sex, drinking, drug use, smoking), auto crashes, menstrual disorders, unintended pregnancy, acne, short stature (males), conflicts with parents, overweight, physical inactivity, poor eating behaviors, eating disorders (eg, purging, binge eating, and anorexia nervosa)	Eating disorders, depression, suicide, auto crashes, unintended pregnancy acne, smoking, alcohol or drug dependence

From: Hagan JF, Shaw JS, Duncan PM, eds. *Bright Futures: Guidelines for Health Supervision of Infants, Children, and Adolescents.* 3rd ed. Elk Grove Village, IL: American Academy of Pediatrics; 2008.

Feeding and Nutrition

Degree of Dehydration

PARAMETER	DEGREE OF DEHYDRATION		
	MILD	MODERATE	SEVERE
Weight loss (%)—infants	5	10	15
Weight loss (%)—children	3	6	>9
Skin color	Pale	Gray	Mottled
Skin turgor	May be normal	Decreased	Tenting
Mucous membranes	Slightly dry	Dry	Dry, parched, collapse of sublingual veins
Eyes	Normal	Decreased tears	Sunken, absence of tears
Central nervous system	Alert but thirsty	Irritable	Lethargic, grunting, coma
Pulse	Normal and strong	Rapid and slightly weak	Significantly tachycardic and very weak to not palpable
Capillary refill	Normal (<2 sec)	2-4 sec	>4 sec
Blood pressure	No change	Orthostatic decrease	Shock
Urine	Normal to mildly reduced	Significantly reduced	Anuria
Volume of deficit—infants	50 mL/kg	60 mL/kg	150 mL/kg
Volume of deficit—children	30 mL/kg	100 mL/kg	>90 mL/kg

From: McInerny TK, Adam HM, Campbell DE, Kamat DM, Kelleher KJ. *American Academy of Pediatrics Textbook of Pediatric Care.* Elk Grove Village, IL: American Academy of Pediatrics; 2008.

Composition of Fluids Frequently Used in Oral Rehdration

Solution	Glucose/CHO, g/L	Sodium, mEq/L	HCO_3^-, mEq/L	Potassium mEq/L	Osmolality, mmol/L	CHO/Sodium
Pedialyte (Abbott Laboratories, Columbus, OH)	25	45	30	20	250	3.1
Pediatric Electrolyte (PendoPharm, Montreal, Quebec)	25	45	20	30	250	3.1
Kaolectrolyte (Pfizer, New York, NY)	20	48	28	20	240	2.4
Rehydralyte (Abbott Laboratories, Columbus, OH)	25	75	30	20	310	1.9
WHO ORS, 2002 (reduced osmolarity)	75	75	10[†]	30	224	1.0
WHO ORS, 1975, (original formulation)	111	90	10[†]	20	311	1.2
Cola*	126	2	13	0.1	750	1944
Apple juice*	125	3	0	32	730	1278
Gatorade* (Gatorade, Chicago, IL)	45	20	3	3	330	62.5

CHO indicates carbohydrate; HCO_3^-, bicarbonate; WHO, World Health Organization.

*Cola, juice, and Gatorade are shown for comparison only; they are not recommended for use.

Mainly for maintenance therapy; may be used for rehydration therapy in mildly dehydrated patients.

[†] Citrate.

From: Kleinman RE, ed. *Pediatric Nutrition Handbook.* Elk Grove Village, IL: American Academy of Pediatrics; 2009.

Fluid Therapy Chart

Degree of Dehydration	Signs	Fluids	Feeding
Mild*	Slightly dry mucous membranes, increased thirst	ORS, 50–60 mL/kg[†]	Breastfeeding, undiluted lactose-free formula, full-strength cow milk, or lactose-containing formula
Moderate	Sunken eyes, sunken fontanelle, loss of skin turgor, dry mucous membranes	ORS, 80–100 mL/kg[†]	Same as above
Severe	Signs of moderate dehydration plus one or more of the following: rapid thready pulse, cyanosis, rapid breathing, delayed capillary refill time, lethargy, coma	Intravenous or intraosseous isotonic Fluids (0.9% saline or Ringer lactate), 40 mL/kg per hour until pulse and state of consciousness return to normal, then 50–100 mL/kg of ORS based on remaining degree of dehydration[‡]	Begin after clinically improved and ORS has begun

* If no signs of dehydration are present, rehydration phase may be omitted. Proceed with maintenance therapy and replacement of ongoing losses.

[†] First 4 hours, repeat until no signs of dehydration remain. Replace ongoing stool losses and vomitus with ORS, 10 mL/kg for each diarrheal stool and 5 mL/kg for each episode of vomiting.

[‡] Although parenteral access is being sought, nasogastric infusion of ORS may be begun at 30 mL/kg per hour, provided airway protective reflexes remain intact.

From: Kleinman RE, ed. *Pediatric Nutrition Handbook.* Elk Grove Village, IL: American Academy of Pediatrics; 2008.

Selected Bioactive Factors in Human Milk

Secretory IgA	Specific antigen-targeted anti-infective action
Lactoferrin	Immunomodulation, iron chelation, antimicrobial action, anti-adhesive, trophic for intestinal growth
Lysozyme	Bacterial lysis, immunomodulation
κ-casein	Anti-adhesive, bacterial flora
Oligosaccharides	Bacterial attachment
Cytokines	Anti-inflammatory, epithelial barrier function

Growth factors
  Epidermal growth factor
  Transforming growth factor (TGF)
 	
  Nerve growth factor
	
	Luminal surveillance, repair of intestine
	Promotes epithelial cell growth (TGF-α)
	Suppresses lymphocyte function (TGF-β)
	Growth

Enzymes
  Platelet-activating factor-acetylhydrolase
  Glutathione peroxidase
	
	Blocks action of platelet activating factor
	Prevents lipid oxidation

Nucleotides	Enhance antibody responses, bacterial flora
Vitamins A, E, C	Antioxidants
Amino acids Glutamine	 Intestinal cell fuel, immune responses
Lipids	Anti-infective properties

IgA indicates immunoglobulin A.

Adapted from: American Academy of Pediatrics and American College of Obstetricians and Gynecologists. The importance of breastfeeding for infants, mothers, and society. In: *Breastfeeding Handbook for Physicians.* Elk Grove Village, IL: American Academy of Pediatrics; 2006:19–36.

Cow Milk–Based Infant Formulas: Label Claim Nutrient Contents (per L at 20 kcal/oz)

Part 1 of 3

Contents	Enfamil LIPIL*‡ (Mead Johnson, Evansville, IN)	Enfamil Gentlease LIPIL (Mead Johnson, Evansville, IN)	Enfamil LactoFree LIPIL*† (Mead Johnson, Evansville, IN)	Enfamil A.R. LIPIL* (Mead Johnson, Evansville, IN)	Nestlé Good Start*† (Nestlé, Glendale, CA)	Nestlé Good Start DHA & ARA*† (Mead Johnson, Evansville, IN)	Nestlé Good Start DHA & ARA Natural Cultures† (powder only) (Nestlé, Glendale, CA)
Energy, kcal	680	680	680	680	670	670	670
Protein, g	14.2	15.6	14.2	16.9	15	15	15
Casein, % of total protein	40	40‡	80	80	0	0	0
Whey, % of total protein	60	60‡	20	20	100‡	100‡	100‡
Fat, g Polyunsaturated, % Monounsaturated, % Saturated, % Source	36 20 37 43 Palm olein, soy, coconut, high-oleic sunflower, DHA and ARA§	36 20 37 43 Palm olein, soy, coconut, high-oleic sunflower, DHA and ARA§	36 20 37 43 Palm olein, soy, coconut, high-oleic sunflower, DHA and ARA§	34 20 37 43 Palm olein, soy, coconut, high-oleic sunflower, DHA and ARA§	34 22 33 45 Palm olein, soy, coconut, high-oleic safflower/sunflower	34 22 33 45 Palm olein, soy, coconut, high-oleic safflower/sunflower, DHA and ARA§	34 22 33 45 Palm olein, soy, coconut, high-oleic safflower/sunflower, DHA and ARA§
Carbohydrate, g	74 Lactose	73 Corn-syrup solids, lactose	74 Corn-syrup solids	74 Lactose, rice starch, and maltodextrin	75 Lactose, corn maltodextrin	75 Lactose, corn maltodextrin	75 Lactose, corn maltodextrin
Osmolality, mOsm/kg	300	220	200	230‖/240¶	260	260	260
Minerals							
Calcium, mg	530	550	550	530	449	449	449
Phosphorus, mg	290	310	310	360	255	255	255
Magnesium, mg	54	54	54	54	47	47	47
Iron, mg	12.2	12.2	12.2	12.2	10	10	10
Zinc, mg	6.8	6.8	6.8	6.8	5	5	5
Manganese, µg	101	101	101	101	101	101	101
Copper, µg	510	510	510	510	536	536	536
Iodine, µg	68	68	101	68	80	80	80
Sodium, mEq	8	9.6	8.7	11.7	8	8	8
Potassium, mEq	18.7	18.7	18.9	18.7	19	19	19
Chloride, mEq	12.1	12.1	12.7	14.4	12	12	12
Vitamins							
A, IU	2000	2000	2000	2000	2010	2010	2010
D, IU	410	410	410	410	402	402	402
E, IU	13.5	13.5	13.5	13.5	13	13	13
K, µg	54	54	54	54	54	54	54
Thiamine (B$_1$), µg	540	540	540	540	670	670	670
Riboflavin (B$_2$), µg	950	950	950	950	938	938	938

continued

Cow Milk–Based Infant Formulas: Label Claim Nutrient Contents (per L at 20 kcal/oz)

Part 1 of 3, continued

Contents	Enfamil LIPIL*‡ (Mead Johnson, Evansville, IN)	Enfamil Gentlease LIPIL (Mead Johnson, Evansville, IN)	Enfamil LactoFree LIPIL*† (Mead Johnson, Evansville, IN)	Enfamil A.R. LIPIL* (Mead Johnson, Evansville, IN)	Nestlé Good Start*† Nestlé, Glendale, CA)	Nestlé Good Start DHA & ARA*† (Mead Johnson, Evansville, IN)	Nestlé Good Start DHA & ARA Natural Cultures† (powder only) (Nestlé, Glendale, CA)
Pyridoxine, µg	410	410	410	410	503	503	503
B$_{12}$, µg	2	2	2	2	2	2	2
Niacin, mg	6.8	6.8	6.8	6.8	7	7	7
Folic acid, µg	108	108	108	108	101	101	101
Pantothenic acid, mg	3.4	3.4	3.4	3.4	3	3	3
Biotin, µg	20	20	20	20	29	29	29
C (ascorbic acid), mg	81	81	81	81	60	60	60
Choline, mg	162	162	162	81	161	161	161
Inositol, mg	41	41	41	41	40	40	40

LCPUFA indicates long-chain polyunsaturated fatty acids; DHA, docosahexaenoic acid; ARA, arachidonic acid.

* Liquid and powder.
† With nucleotides.
‡ Partially hydrolyzed.
§ From single-cell oils *Crypthecodinium cohnii* and *Mortierella alpina*, respectively.
∥ Powder form.
¶ Liquid form.
# Organic ingredients.
** Low iron.

Part 2 of 3

Contents	Similac with Iron*† (Abbott Nutrition, Columbus, OH)	Similac Advance*† (Abbott Nutrition, Columbus, OH)	Similac Organic*† (Abbott Nutrition, Columbus, OH)	Similac PM 60/40 (powder only) (Abbott Nutrition, Columbus, OH)	Similac Sensitive*† (Abbott Nutrition, Columbus, OH)
Energy, kcal	676	676	676	676	676
Protein, g	14	14	14.0#	15	14.47
Casein, % of total protein	52	52	82	40	18
Whey, % of total protein	48	48	18	60	82
Fat, g Polyunsaturated, % Monounsaturated, % Saturated, % Source	36.5 26 40 34 High-oleic safflower, soy, coconut	36.5 27 40 33 High-oleic safflower, soy, coconut, DHA and ARA§	37.1 21 44 35 High-oleic,# sunflower,# soy,# coconut,# DHA and ARA§	37.9 26 40 34 High-oleic safflower, soy, coconut	36.5 27 40 33 High-oleic safflower, soy, coconut, DHA and ARA§
Carbohydrate, g	73 Lactose	73 Lactose	71.4 Corn maltodextrin,# lactose,# sucrose#	69 Lactose	72.4 Corn maltodextrin, sucrose
Osmolality, mOsm/kg	300	300	225	280	200
Minerals					
Calcium, mg	528	528	528	379	568
Phosphorus, mg	284	284	284	189	379
Magnesium, mg	41	41	41	40.6	40.6
Iron, mg	12.2	12	12.2	4.7**	12.2

Part 2 of 3, continued

Contents	Similac with Iron*† (Abbott Nutrition, Columbus, OH)	Similac Advance*† (Abbott Nutrition, Columbus, OH)	Similac Organic*† (Abbott Nutrition, Columbus, OH)	Similac PM 60/40 (powder only) (Abbott Nutrition, Columbus, OH)	Similac Sensitive*† (Abbott Nutrition, Columbus, OH)
Zinc, mg	5.1	5.1	5.1	5.1	5.1
Manganese, µg	34	34	34	34	34
Copper, µg	609	609	609	609	609
Iodine, µg	41	41	41	41	61
Sodium, mEq	7.1	7.1	7.1	7.1	8.8
Potassium, mEq	18.2	18.2	18.1	13.8	18.5
Chloride, mEq	12.4	12.4	12.4	11.3	12.4
Vitamins					
A, IU	2029	2029	2029	2029	2029
D, IU	406	406	406	406	406
E, IU	10.1	10.1	10.1	10.1	20.3
K, µg	54	54	54	54	54
Thiamine (B_1), µg	676	676	676	676	676
Riboflavin (B_2), µg	1014	1014	1014	1014	1014
Pyridoxine, µg	406	406	406	406	406
B_{12}, µg	1.7	1.7	1.69	1.7	1.7
Niacin, mg	7.1	7.1	7.1	7.1	7.1
Folic acid, µg	101	101	101	101	101
Pantothenic acid, mg	3.04	3.04	3.04	3.04	3.04
Biotin, µg	29.8	29.8	29.8	30.4	29.8
C (ascorbic acid), mg	61	61	61	61	61
Choline, mg	108	108	108	81	108
Inositol, mg	31.8	32	31.8	162	29.1

LCPUFA indicates long-chain polyunsaturated fatty acids; DHA, docosahexaenoic acid; ARA, arachidonic acid.

* Liquid and powder.
† With nucleotides.
‡ Partially hydrolyzed.
§ From single-cell oils *Crypthecodinium cohnii* and *Mortierella alpina,* respectively.
‖ Powder form.
¶ Liquid form.
# Organic ingredients.
** Low iron.

Cow Milk–Based Infant Formulas: Label Claim Nutrient Contents (per L at 20 kcal/oz)

Part 3 of 3

Contents	Store Brand Milk-Based Formula With Iron[†] (powder only) (PBM Nutritionals, Georgia, VT)	Store Brand Milk-Based Formula With LCPUFA*[†] (PBM Nutritionals, Georgia, VT)	Store Brand Milk-Based Lactose-Free Formula With LCPUFA[†] (powder only) (PBM Nutritionals, Georgia, VT)	Store Brand Milk-Based Partially Hydrolyzed Formula With LCPUFA[‡] (powder only) (PBM Nutritionals, Georgia, VT)	Store Brand Milk-Based A.R. Formula With LCPUFA (powder only) (PBM Nutritionals, Georgia, VT)	Store Brand Organic Milk-Based Formula With LCPUFA[†] (powder only) (PBM Nutritionals, Georgia, VT)
Energy, kcal	672	668	672	672	666	672
Protein, g	15	14	15	15	17	15[#]
Casein, % of total protein	40	40	40	40	80	40
Whey, % of total protein	60	60	60	60[*]	20	60
Fat, g Polyunsaturated, % Monounsaturated, % Saturated, % Source	36 Palm olein, soy, coconut, high-oleic safflower or sunflower	36 Palm olein, soy, coconut, high-oleic safflower/ sunflower, DHA and ARA[§]	36 Palm olein, soy, coconut, high-oleic safflower/ sunflower, DHA and ARA[§]	36 Palm olein, soy, coconut, high-oleic safflower/sunflower, DHA and ARA[§]	34 Palm olein, soy, coconut, high-oleic safflower/ sunflower, DHA and ARA[§]	36 Palm or palm olein,[#] soy,[#] coconut,[#] high-oleic safflower/ sunflower[#] DHA and ARA[§]
Carbohydrate, g	72 Lactose	72 Lactose	72 Corn-syrup solids	72 Corn-syrup solids	73 Lactose, maltodextrin, rice starch	72 Lactose[#]
Osmolality, mOsm/kg	281	293	207	182		274
Minerals						
Calcium, mg	420	520	550	547	520	420
Phosphorus, mg	280	287	366	307	353	280
Magnesium, mg	45	53	45	53	53	45
Iron, mg	12	12	12	12	12	12
Zinc, mg	5	6.7	5	6.7	6.7	5
Manganese, µg	100	100	100	100	100	100
Copper, µg	470	500	470	500	500	470
Iodine, µg	60	67	60	67	67	60
Sodium, mEq	6.52	7.83	6.52	9.26	11.6	6.52
Potassium, mEq	14.34	18.72	14.34	18.43	18.43	14.34
Chloride, mEq	10.72	11.85	11.44	12.01	14.3	11.44
Vitamins						
A, IU	2000	2000	2000	2000	2000	2000
D, IU	400	400	400	400	400	400
E, IU	9.5	13	13	13	13	13
K, µg	55	53	55	53	53	55
Thiamine (B_1), µg	670	533	670	533	533	670
Riboflavin (B_2), µg	1000	933	1000	933	933	1000

Part 3 of 3, continued

Contents	Store Brand Milk-Based Formula With Iron[†] (powder only) (PBM Nutritionals, Georgia, VT)	Store Brand Milk-Based Formula With LCPUFA*[†] (PBM Nutritionals, Georgia, VT)	Store Brand Milk-Based Lactose-Free Formula With LCPUFA[†] (powder only) (PBM Nutritionals, Georgia, VT)	Store Brand Milk-Based Partially Hydrolyzed Formula With LCPUFA[‡] (powder only) (PBM Nutritionals, Georgia, VT)	Store Brand Milk-Based A.R. Formula With LCPUFA (powder only) (PBM Nutritionals, Georgia, VT)	Store Brand Organic Milk-Based Formula With LCPUFA[†] (powder only) (PBM Nutritionals, Georgia, VT)
Pyridoxine, μg	420	400	420	400	400	420
B_{12}, μg	1.3	2	1.3	2	2	1.3
Niacin, mg	5	6.7	5	6.7	6.7	5
Folic acid, μg	50	107	100	107	107	50
Pantothenic acid, mg	2.1	3.3	2.1	3.3	3.3	2.1
Biotin, μg	15	20	15	20	20	15
C (ascorbic acid), mg	55	80	55	80	80	60
Choline, mg	100	160	100	160	160	100
Inositol, mg	27	40	114	40	40	27

LCPUFA indicates long-chain polyunsaturated fatty acids; DHA, docosahexaenoic acid; ARA, arachidonic acid.

* Liquid and powder.

† With nucleotides.

‡ Partially hydrolyzed.

§ From single-cell oils *Crypthecodinium cohnii* and *Mortierella alpina*, respectively.

‖ Powder form.

¶ Liquid form.

Organic ingredients.

** Low iron.

From: Kleinman RE, ed. *Pediatric Nutrition Handbook*. Elk Grove Village, IL: American Academy of Pediatrics; 2009.

Soy-Based Infant Formulas: Label Claim Nutrient Contents (per L at 20 kcal/oz)

Part 1 of 2

Contents	Nestlé Good Start Soy DHA & ARA* (Nestlé, Glendale, CA)	Enfamil ProSobee LIPIL* (Mead Johnson, Evansville, IN)	Similac Isomil* (Abbott Nutrition Columbus, OH)	Similac Isomil Advance* (Abbott Nutrition, Columbus, OH)	Similac Isomil DF (liquid only) (Abbott Nutrition, Columbus, OH)
Energy, kcal	670	680	676	676	676
Protein, g Source	17 Soy protein† isolate and L-methionine	16.9 Soy protein isolate and L-methionine	16.55 Soy protein isolate and L-methionine	16.57 Soy protein isolate and L-methionine	17.99 Soy protein isolate and L-methionine
Fat, g Polyunsaturated, % Monounsaturated, % Saturated, % Sources	34 23 32 45 Palm olein, soy, coconut, high-oleic safflower/sunflower, DHA and ARA‡	36 20 37 43 Palm olein, soy, coconut, high-oleic sunflower, DHA and ARA‡	36.9 27 40 33 High-oleic safflower, soy, coconut	36.9 27 40 33 High-oleic safflower, soy, coconut, DHA and ARA‡	36.9 39 17 44 Soy, coconut
Carbohydrate, g	74 Corn maltodextrins, sucrose (+ cornstarch in liquids)	72 Corn-syrup solids	69.6 Corn-syrup solids and sucrose	69.7 Corn-syrup solids and sucrose	68.3 Corn-syrup solids and sucrose
Osmolality, mOsm/kg	185	170	200	200	240
Minerals					
Calcium, mg	704	710	710	710	710
Phosphorus, mg	422	470	507	507	507
Magnesium, mg	74	74	50.7	50.7	50.7
Iron, mg	12	12.2	12.2	12.2	12.2
Zinc, mg	6	8.1	5.07	5.07	5.07
Manganese, µg	168	169	169	169	169
Copper, µg	536	510	507	507	507
Iodine, µg	101	101	101	101	101
Sodium, mEq	12	10.4	12.9	12.9	12.9
Potassium, mEq	20	21	18.7	18.7	18.7
Chloride, mEq	13	15.2	11.8	11.8	11.8
Vitamins					
A, IU	2010	2000	2029	2029	2029
D, IU	402	410	406	406	406
E, IU	20	13.5	10.1	10.1	10.1
K, µg	60	54	74	74	74
Thiamine (B$_1$), µg	402	540	406	406	406
Riboflavin (B$_2$), µg	630	610	609	609	609
Pyridoxine, µg	402	410	406	406	406
B$_{12}$, µg	2	2	3.04	3.04	3.04
Niacin, mg	9	6.8	9.13	9.13	9.13

Part 1 of 2, continued

Contents	Nestlé Good Start Soy DHA & ARA* (Nestlé, Glendale, CA)	Enfamil ProSobee LIPIL* (Mead Johnson, Evansville, IN)	Similac Isomil* (Abbott Nutrition Columbus, OH)	Similac Isomil Advance* (Abbott Nutrition, Columbus, OH)	Similac Isomil DF (liquid only) (Abbott Nutrition, Columbus, OH)
Folic acid, μg	107	108	101	101	101
Pantothenic acid, mg	3	3.4	5.1	5.1	5.1
Biotin, μg	34	20	30.4	30.4	30.4
C (ascorbic acid), mg	80	81	61	61	61
Choline, mg	161	162	81	81	81
Inositol, mg	40	41	33.8	33.8	33.8

* Liquid and powder.
† Partially hydrolyzed.
‡ From single-cell oils Crypthecodinium cohnii and Mortierella alpina, respectively.
§ Organic ingredients.

Part 2 of 2

Contents	Store Brand Soy Infant Formula With Iron (powder only) (PBM Nutritionals, Georgia, VT)	Store Brand Soy Infant Formula With LCPUFA* (PBM Nutritionals, Georgia, VT)	Store Brand Soy Organic, Kosher, Vegetarian and Halal-Certified Infant Formula With LCPUFA (powder only) (PBM Nutritionals, Georgia, VT)
Energy, kcal	672	667	664
Protein, g Source	18 Soy protein isolate and L-methionine	16.7 Soy protein isolate and L-methionine	16.7 Soy protein isolate§ and L-methionine
Fat, g Polyunsaturated, % Monounsaturated, % Saturated, % Source	36 Palm olein, coconut, soy, high-oleic safflower/sunflower	35.3 Palm olein, coconut, soy, high-oleic safflower/sunflower, DHA and ARA‡	35.3 Palm olein,§ coconut,§ soy,§ high-oleic safflower/sunflower,§ DHA and ARA‡
Carbohydrate, g	69 Corn-syrup solids, sucrose	70.7 Corn-syrup solids	70 Corn-syrup solids§
Osmolality, mOsm/kg	217	162	178
Minerals			
Calcium, mg	600	700	700
Phosphorus, mg	420	553	460
Magnesium, mg	67	73	73
Iron, mg	12	12	12
Zinc, mg	5	8	8

continued

Soy-Based Infant Formulas: Label Claim Nutrient Contents (per L at 20 kcal/oz) *continued*
Part 2 of 2, continued

Contents	Store Brand Soy Infant Formula With Iron (powder only) (PBM Nutritionals, Georgia, VT)	Store Brand Soy Infant Formula With LCPUFA* (PBM Nutritionals, Georgia, VT)	Store Brand Soy Organic, Kosher, Vegetarian and Halal-Certified Infant Formula With LCPUFA (powder only) (PBM Nutritionals, Georgia, VT)
Manganese, µg	200	167	167
Copper, µg	470	500	500
Iodine, µg	60	100	100
Sodium, mEq	8.7	10.4	10.4
Potassium, mEq	17.9	20.5	20.5
Chloride, mEq	10.7	15.2	15.2
Vitamins			
A, IU	2000	2000	2000
D, IU	400	400	400
E, IU	9.5	13	13
K, µg	55	53	53
Thiamine (B$_1$), µg	670	533	533
Riboflavin (B$_2$), µg	1000	600	600
Pyridoxine, µg	420	400	400
B$_{12}$, µg	2	2	2
Niacin, mg	5	6.7	6.7
Folic acid, µg	50	107	107
Pantothenic acid, mg	3.0	3.3	3.3
Biotin, µg	35	20	20
C (ascorbic acid), mg	55	80	80
Choline, mg	85	80	160
Inositol, mg	27	40	40

* Liquid and powder.
† Partially hydrolyzed.
‡ From single-cell oils *Crypthecodinium cohnii* and *Mortierella alpina*, respectively.
§ Organic ingredients.

From: Kleinman RE, ed. *Pediatric Nutrition Handbook.* Elk Grove Village, IL: American Academy of Pediatrics; 2009.

Increasing the Caloric Density of Infant Formula

Caloric Density	Water	Concentrated Liquid	Approximate Yield
20 kcal/fl oz	13 fl oz	13 fl oz (1 can)	26 fl oz
22 kcal/fl oz	11 fl oz	13 fl oz (1 can)	24 fl oz
24 kcal/fl oz	9 fl oz	13 fl oz (1 can)	22 fl oz
27 kcal/fl oz	6 fl oz	13 fl oz (1 can)	19 fl oz
30 kcal/fl oz	4.5 fl oz	13 fl oz (1 can)	17.5 fl oz

Using Powder

Because of the variability of scoop sizes for different formulas from different manufacturers and the variability of household measures, no single set of recipes can be provided that is safe for all products. Some manufacturers provide recipes for their specific products on their Web sites. In the absence of such information, contact the manufacturer directly.

Increasing Caloric Density Using Other Additives

- Medium-chain triglyceride oil provides 7.7 kcal/mL; 1 teaspoon provides 38 kcal.
- Vegetable oils provide 40 kcal/teaspoon.
- Polycose powder (Abbott Nutrition, Columbus, OH) contains 8 kcal/teaspoon.

Note that increasing caloric density using fat and/or carbohydrate should be done with caution, because the additional energy (kcal) effectively decreases the density (amount per 100 kcal) of all other nutrients.

From: Kleinman RE, ed. *Pediatric Nutrition Handbook.* Elk Grove Village, IL: American Academy of Pediatrics; 2009.

Estimated Energy Requirements

Age	Estimated Energy Requirements*
0–3 mo	(89 × weight [kg] − 100) + 175 kcal
4–6 mo	(89 × weight [kg] − 100) + 56 kcal
7–12 mo	(89 × weight [kg] − 100) + 22 kcal
13–36 mo	(89 × weight [kg] − 100) + 20 kcal
Boys 3 through 8 y	88.5 − (61.9 × age [y]) + PA × (26.7 × weight [kg] + 903 × height [m]) + 20 kcal
Girls 3 through 8 y	135.3 − (30.8 × age [y]) + PA × (10.0 × weight [kg] + 934 × height [m]) + 20 kcal
Boys 9 through 18 y	88.5 − (61.9 × age [y]) + PA × (26.7 × weight [kg] + 903 × height [m]) + 25 kcal
Girls 9 through 18 y	135.3 − (30.8 × age [y]) + PA × (10.0 × weight [kg] + 934 × height [m]) + 25 kcal

*Total energy expenditure + energy deposition.

PA indicates the physical activity coefficient:

For boys 3 through 18 years of age:

PA = 1.00 (sedentary, estimated physical activity level 1.0–1.4)

PA = 1.13 (low active, estimated physical activity level 1.4–1.6)

PA = 1.26 (active, estimated physical activity level 1.6–1.9)

PA = 1.42 (very active, estimated physical activity level 1.9–2.5)

For girls 3 through 18 years of age:

PA = 1.00 (sedentary, estimated physical activity level 1.0–1.4)

PA = 1.16 (low active, estimated physical activity level 1.4–1.6)

PA = 1.31 (active, estimated physical activity level 1.6–1.9)

PA = 1.56 (very active, estimated physical activity level 1.9–2.5)

From: Institute of Medicine. Dietary Reference Intakes for Energy, Carbohydrate, Fiber, Fat, Fatty Acids, Cholesterol, Protein, and Amino Acids (Macronutrients). Washington, DC: The National Academies Press; 2005. Reprinted with permission from The National Academies Press, Copyright 2005, National Academy of Sciences.

American Academy of Pediatrics Recommendations Relevant to the Initiation of Complementary Foods

Nutrient/Food	Subgroups	AAP Recommendations
Human milk	Most infants	Exclusive breastfeeding for minimum of 4 but preferably 6 mo.
	Infants with unique needs or feeding patterns	Individual infants may require complementary foods as early as 4 mo of age or may be unable to accept them until about 8 mo of age.[7]
Calcium	Term infants	Recommended intakes, human milk or infant formulas: First 6 mo: 210 mg/day 7–12 mo: 270 mg/day No benefit from increasing calcium content of infant formulas above these amounts.
	Preterm infants	Have higher calcium requirements than term infants. Can meet requirements using human milk plus commercial fortifiers or preterm infant formulas enriched with calcium and vitamin D. Optimal calcium concentrations and duration of use unknown.[8]
Cholesterol	Infants younger than 2 y	No restriction of fat or cholesterol; rapid growth requires high energy intake.[9]
Fluoride	Infants 6 mo and older	Supplement with 0.25 mg/day in areas with <0.3 ppm fluoride concentration in community drinking supplies (see Chapter 48).
Iron	Breastfed infants 6–12 mo	Iron from complementary foods at 6 mo of age (see Chapters 2 and 18).
	Nonbreastfed infants younger than 12 mo	Ingest iron-fortified formula (10–12 mg/L) until weaning at 12 mo of age.
	Breastfed preterm or low birth weight infant	Oral iron supplement drops at 2 mg/kg per day, 1–12 mo of age (see Chapter 4).
	Formula-fed preterm infants	May benefit from an additional iron supplement (drops) of 1 mg/kg per day.
Lactose	Children from populations with high rates of lactose malabsorption	Unwise to discourage use of milk unless children have severe diarrhea or clear intolerance; clinical problems usually manifest at 5–7 y of age.[10]
Vitamin D	All breastfed infants and nonbreastfed infants	Should have a supplement of 400 IU/day of vitamin D beginning during first 2 mo of life through childhood and adolescence unless ingesting at least 500 mL/day of vitamin D-fortified formula or milk.[11]

American Academy of Pediatrics Recommendations Relevant to the Initiation of Complementary Foods, *continued*

Nutrient/Food	Subgroups	AAP Recommendations
Fruit juice	Infants up to 1 y of age	Should not be introduced before 6 mo of age.
		Should not be given juice in containers that allow them to consume juice easily throughout the day.
		Should not be given at bedtime.
		Should not consume unpasteurized juices.[12]
Soy protein-based formulas	Term infants whose nutritional needs are not met by human or cow milk	Isolated soy protein-based formula is a safe, effective alternative.
	Infants with documented lactose intolerance	Use is appropriate.
	Most infants with documented immunoglobulin E-mediated allergy to cow milk	Use may be appropriate.
	Preterm infants who weigh <1800 g	Use is not recommended.[13]
Water*	All infants up to 1 y of age	No data basis for minimum or maximum usual water intake recommendations; water intoxication not a discernable public health problem.
	Formula-fed infants	*During hot weather:* No recommendations.
	Infants up to 1 y of age, exclusively breastfed or partial breastfeeding eating complementary foods	Monitor for dark or decreased urine output. When present, offer solute-free water up to maximum of 225 mL/kg per day.

* AAP Committee on Nutrition advice, based on literature search pertaining to water intoxication, current recommendations from AAP materials, and opinions of pediatric nutrition experts.

From: Kleinman RE, ed. *Pediatric Nutrition Handbook.* Elk Grove Village, IL: American Academy of Pediatrics; 2009.

Dietary Reference Intakes: Recommended Intakes for Individuals, Food and Nutrition Board, Institute of Medicine

	Infants 0–6 mo	Infants 7–12 mo	Children 1–3 y	Children 4–8 y	Males 9–13 y	Males 14–18 y	Females 9–13 y	Females 14–18 y	Pregnancy 18 y	Lactation 18 y
Carbohydrate (g/day)	60*	95*	130	130	130	130	130	130	175	210
Total Fiber (g/day)	ND	ND	19*	25*	31*	38*	26*	26*	28*	29*
Fat (g/day)	31*	30*	ND	ND	ND	ND	ND	ND	ND	ND
n-6 Polyunsaturated Fatty Acids (g/day) (Linoleic Acid)	4.4*	4.6*	7*	10*	12*	16*	10*	11*	13*	13*
n-3 Polyunsaturated Fatty Acids (g/day) (α-Linolenic Acid)	0.5*	0.5*	0.7*	0.9*	1.2*	1.6*	1.0*	1.1*	1.4*	1.3*
Protein (g/kg/day)	1.52*	1.2*	1.05*	0.95*	0.95*	0.85*	0.95*	0.85*	1.1*	1.3*
Vitamin A (µg/day)[†]	400*	500*	300	400	600	900	600	700	750	1200
Vitamin C (mg/day)	40*	50*	15	25	45	75	45	65	80	115
Vitamin D (µg/day)[‡§]	5*	5*	5*	5*	5*	5*	5*	5*	5*	5*
Vitamin E (mg/day)[∥]	4*	5*	6	7	11	15	11	15	15	19
Vitamin K (µg/day)	2.0*	2.5*	30*	55*	60*	75*	60*	75*	75*	75*
Thiamin (mg/day)	0.2*	0.3*	0.5	0.6	0.9	1.2	0.9	1.0	1.4	1.4
Riboflavin (mg/day)	0.3*	0.4*	0.5	0.6	0.9	1.3	0.9	1.0	1.4	1.6
Niacin (mg/day)[¶]	2*	4*	6	8	12	16	12	14	18	17
Vitamin B$_6$ (mg/day)	0.1*	0.3*	0.5	0.6	1.0	1.3	1.0	1.2	1.9	2.0
Folate (µg/day)[#]	65*	80*	150	200	300	400	300	400**	600††	500
Vitamin B$_{12}$ (µg/day)	0.4*	0.5*	0.9	1.2	1.8	2.4	1.8	2.4	2.6	2.8
Pantothenic Acid (mg/day)	1.7*	1.8*	2*	3*	4*	5*	4*	5*	6*	7*
Biotin (µg/day)	5*	6*	8*	12*	20*	25*	20*	25*	30*	35*
Calcium (mg/day)	210*	270*	500*	800*	1300*	1300*	1300*	1300*	1300*	1300*
Choline[‡‡] (mg/day)	125*	150*	200*	250*	375*	550*	375*	400*	450*	550*
Chromium (µg/day)	0.2*	5.5*	11*	15*	25*	35*	21*	24*	29*	44*
Copper (µg/day)	200*	220*	340	440	700	890	700	890	1000	1300
Fluoride (mg/day)	0.01*	0.5*	0.7*	1*	2*	3*	2*	3*	3*	3*
Iodine (µg/day)	110*	130*	90	90	120	150	120	150	220	290
Iron (mg/day)	0.27*	11	7	10	8	11	8	15	27	10
Magnesium (mg/day)	30*	75*	80	130	240	410	240	360	400	360
Manganese (mg/day)	0.003*	0.6*	1.2*	1.5*	1.9*	2.2*	1.6*	1.6*	2.0*	2.6*
Molybdenum (µg/day)	2*	3*	17	22	34	43	34	43	50	50
Phosphorus (mg/day)	100*	275*	460	500	1250	1250	1250	1250	1250	1250
Selenium (µg/day)	15*	20*	20	30	40	55	40	55	60	70
Zinc (mg/day)	2*	3	3	5	8	11	8	9	12	13
Potassium (g/day)	0.4*	0.7*	3.0*	3.8*	4.5*	4.7*	4.5*	4.7*	4.7*	5.1*
Sodium (g/day)	0.12*	0.37*	1.0*	1.2*	1.5*	1.5*	1.5*	1.5*	1.5*	1.5*
Chloride (g/day)	0.18*	0.57*	1.5*	1.9*	2.3*	2.3*	2.3*	2.3*	2.3*	2.3*

Dietary Reference Intakes: Recommended Intakes for Individuals, Food and Nutrition Board, Institute of Medicine, *continued*

This table (taken from the DRI reports; see http://www.iom.edu/CMS/3788/21370.aspx) presents Recommended Dietary Allowances (RDAs) in bold type, and Adequate Intakes (AIs) are in ordinary type followed by the symbol (*). ND indicates not determined.

* RDAs and AIs may both be used as goals for individual intake. RDAs are set to meet the needs of almost all (97%–98%) individuals in a group. For healthy breastfed infants, the AI is the mean intake. The AI for other life stage and gender groups is believed to cover needs of all individuals in the group, but lack of data or uncertainty in the data prevent being able to specify with confidence the percentage of individuals covered by this intake.

† As retinol activity equivalents (RAEs). 1 RAE = 1 μg retinol, 12 μg β-carotene, 24 μg α-carotene, or 24 μg β-cryptoxanthin in foods. The RAE for dietary provitamin A carotenoids is twofold greater than retinol equivalents (RE), whereas the RAE for preformed vitamin A is the same as RE.

‡ As cholecalciferol. 1 μg cholecalciferol = 40 IU vitamin D.

§ In the absence of adequate exposure to sunlight.

‖ As α-tocopherol. α-Tocopherol includes RRR-α-tocopherol, the only form of α-tocopherol that occurs naturally in foods, and the 2R-stereoisomeric forms of α-tocopherol (RRR-, RSR-, RRS-, and RSS-α-tocopherol) that occur in fortified foods and supplements. It does not include the 2S-stereoisomeric forms of α-tocopherol (SRR-, SSR-, SRS-, and SSS-α-tocopherol), also found in fortifi ed foods and supplements.

¶ As niacin equivalents (NEs). 1 mg of niacin = 60 mg of tryptophan; 0–6 mo = preformed niacin (not NEs).

As dietary folate equivalents (DFEs). 1 DFE = 1 μg food folate = 0.6 μg of folic acid from fortified food or as a supplement consumed with food = 0.5 μg of a supplement taken on an empty stomach.

** In view of evidence linking folate intake with neural tube defects in the fetus, it is recommended that all women capable of becoming pregnant consume 400 μg from supplements or fortified foods in addition to intake of food folate from the diet.

†† It is assumed that women will continue consuming 400 μg from supplements or fortified food until their pregnancy is confirmed and they enter prenatal care, which ordinarily occurs after the end of the periconceptional period—the critical time for formation of the neural tube.

‡‡ Although AIs have been set for choline, there are few data to assess whether a dietary supply of choline is needed at all stages of the life cycle, and it may be that the choline requirement can be met by endogenous synthesis at some of these stages.

From: Kleinman RE, ed. *Pediatric Nutrition Handbook*. Elk Grove Village, IL: American Academy of Pediatrics; 2009.

Feeding Guide for Children

Food Group	Age, y						Comments
	2–3		**4–8**		**9–12**		
	Portion Size	Daily Amounts*	Portion Size	Daily Amounts*	Portion Size	Daily Amounts*	
Milk, yogurt, and cheese	1/2 cup (4 oz)	2 cups	1/2–3/4 cup (4–6 oz)	2 cups	1/2–1 cup (4–8 oz)	3 cups	Make most choices fat free or low fat. The following may be substituted for 1/2 cup fluid milk: 1/2–¾ oz cheese, 1/2 cup low-fat yogurt, or 21/2 tbsp nonfat dry milk.
Meat, fish, poultry, dry beans, eggs, and nuts	1–2 oz	2 oz	1–2 oz	3 oz	2 oz	5 oz	Make most choices lean or low fat. The following may be substituted for 1 oz meat, fish, or poultry: 1 egg, 2 tbsp peanut butter, or 4 tbsp cooked dry beans or peas.
Vegetables Cooked Raw*	2–3 tbsp Few pieces	1 cup	3–4 tbsp Few Pieces	11/2 cups	1/4–1/2 cup Several pieces	2 cups	Include dark green and orange vegetables, such as carrots, spinach, broccoli, winter squash, or greens. Limit starchy vegetables (potatoes) to 21/2 cups weekly (11/2 cups for 2- to 3-year-olds).
Fruit Raw Canned Juice	1/2–1 small 2–4 tbsp 3–4 oz	1 cup	1/2–1 small 4–6 tbsp 4 oz	1 cup	1 medium 1/4–1/2 cup 4 oz	11/2 cups	Make less than half of total fruit choices juice.
Grains (bread, cereal, rice, and pasta) Whole-grain or enriched bread Cooked cereal Dry cereal	3 oz eq. 1/2–1 slice 1/4–1/2 cup 1/2–1 cup		4 oz eq 1 slice 1/2 cup 1 cup		5 oz eq 1 slice 1/2–1 cup 1 cup		One oz eq equals a 1-oz slice of bread. The following may be substituted for 1 slice of bread: 1/2 cup spaghetti, macaroni, noodles, or rice; 5 saltine crackers; 1/2 English muffin or bagel; 1 tortilla; corn grits; or posole. Make at least 1/2 of grain intake whole grain.

* Daily amounts are from MyPyramid Plans to meet needs for sedentary children of average size at the younger end of each age range. Amounts shown are from 1000-kcal (2- to 3-year-olds), 1200-kcal (4- to 8-year-olds), and 1600-kcal MyPyramid Plans. Active, older, and larger children would need more energy and foods from each group. A specific MyPyramid Plan for a child of a specified age, gender, and activity level can be found at http://www.mypyramid.gov/. For children 9 years and older, height and weight can also be specified in selecting a MyPyramid Plan.

† Do not give to young children until they can chew well.

From: Kleinman RE, ed. *Pediatric Nutrition Handbook.* Elk Grove Village, IL: American Academy of Pediatrics; 2009.

Interpretation of Cholesterol Concentrations for Children and Adolescents

Term	Total Cholesterol, mg/dL	LDL, mg/dL
Acceptable	<170	<110
Borderline	170–199	110–129
High	≥200	>130

From: National Cholesterol Education Program (NCEP): highlights of the report of the Expert Panel on Blood Cholesterol Levels in Children and Adolescents. *Pediatrics*. 1992;89(3):495–501.

Classification, Education, and Follow-up Based on LDL Concentration (from the NCEP)

To convert mg/dL to mmol/l, multiply by 0.02586.

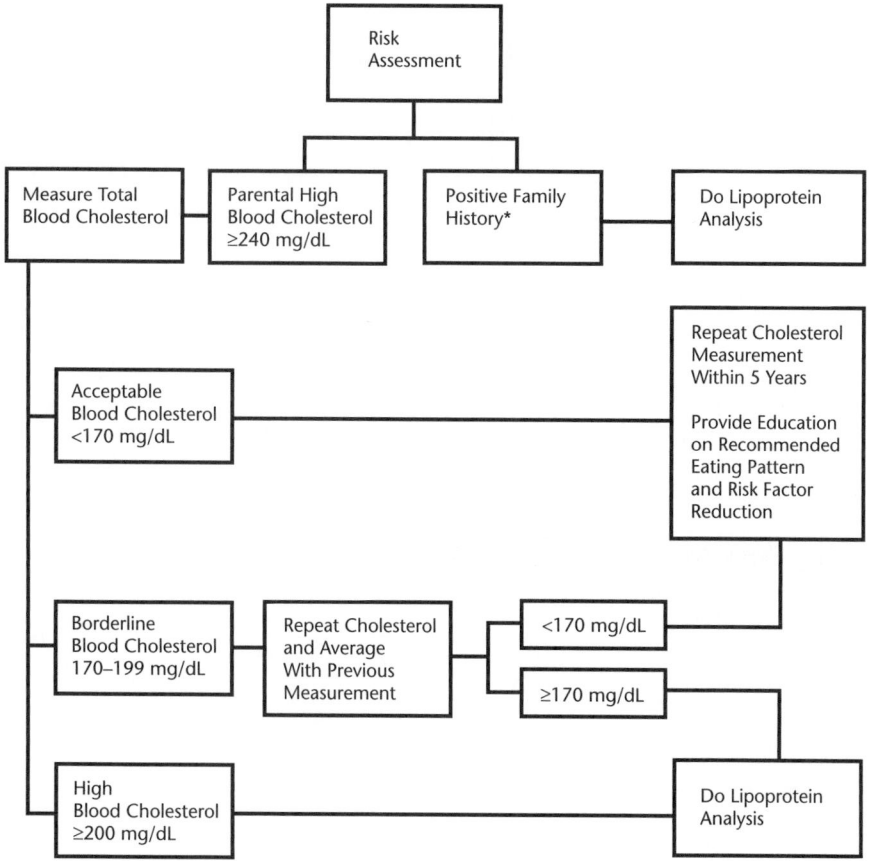

From: National Cholesterol Education Program (NCEP): highlights of the report of the Expert Panel on Blood Cholesterol Levels in Children and Adolescents. *Pediatrics*. 1992;89(3):495–501.

Growth Charts

Length for Age and Weight Percentiles: Girls, Birth to 36 Months

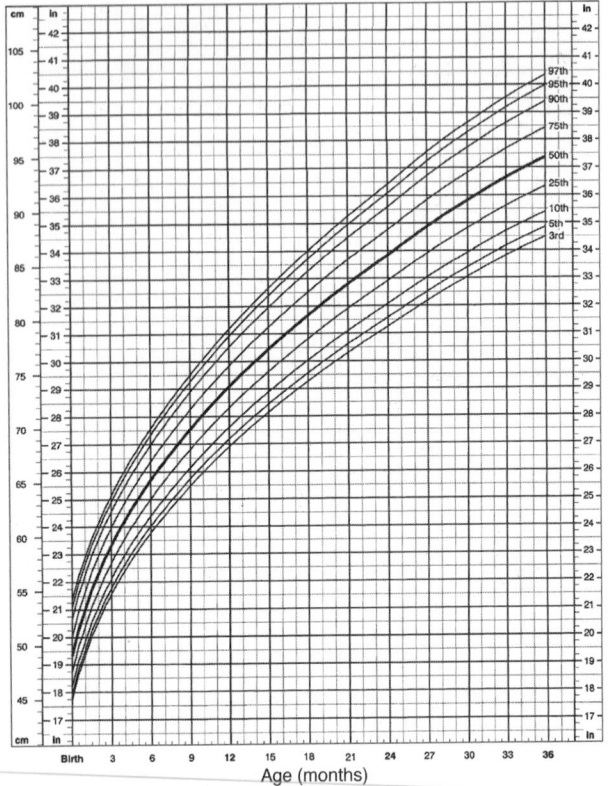

Age (months)

Head Circumference by Age and Weight by Length Percentiles: Girls, Birth to 36 Months

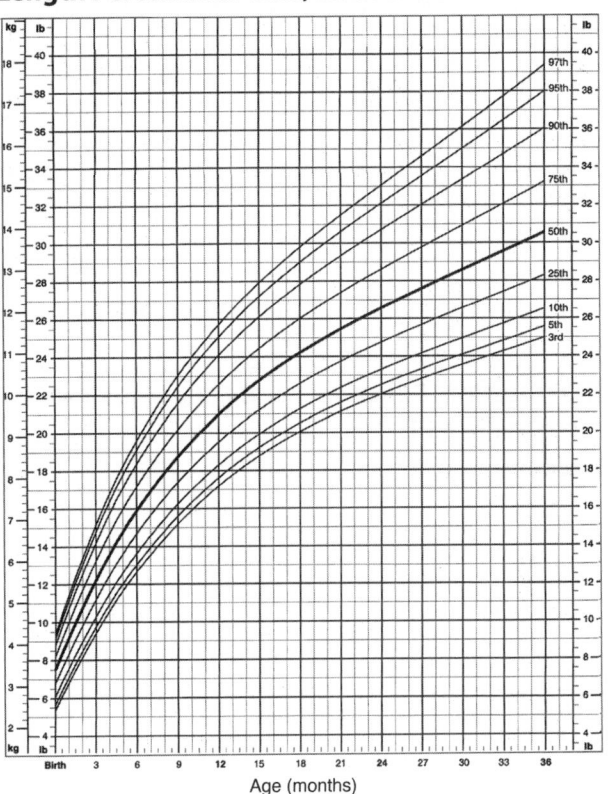

Age (months)

Stature for Age and Weight Percentiles: Girls, 2 to 20 years

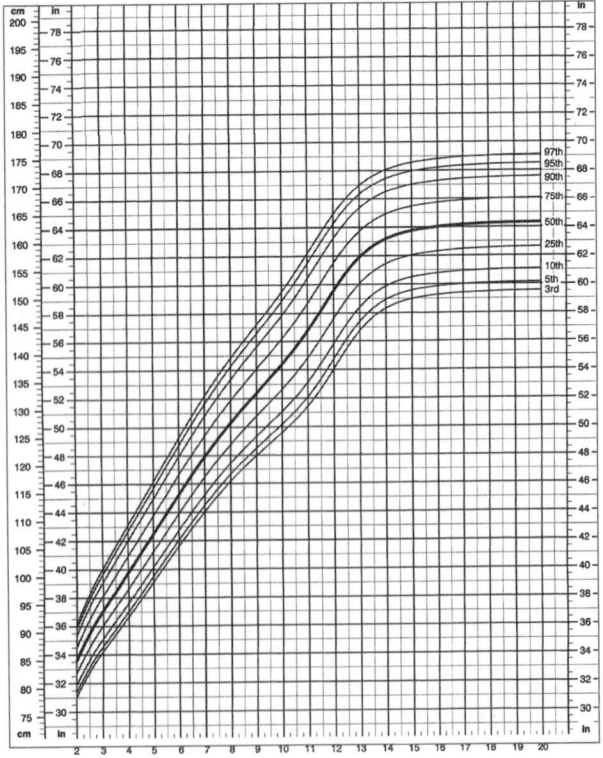

Age (years)

Developed by the National Center for Health Statistics in collaboration with the National Center for Chronic Disease Preventionand Health Promotion (2000).

Length for Age and Weight Percentiles: Boys, Birth to 36 Months

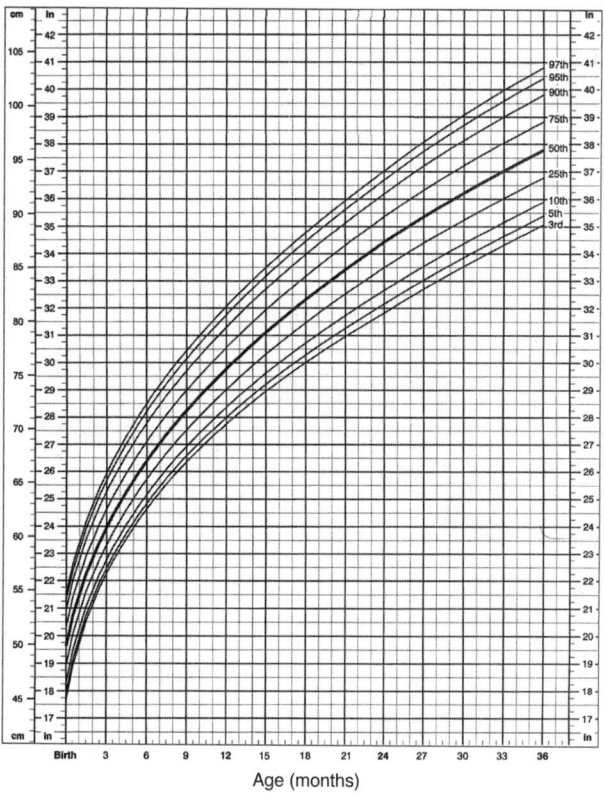

Age (months)

Head Circumference by Age and Weight by Length Percentiles: Boys, Birth to 36 Months

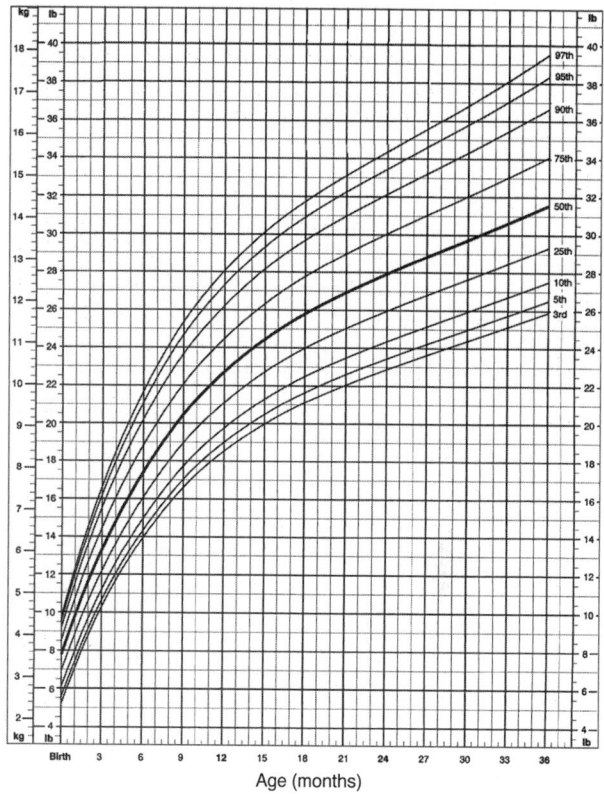

Age (months)

Length for Age and Weight Percentiles
Boys, 2 to 20 years

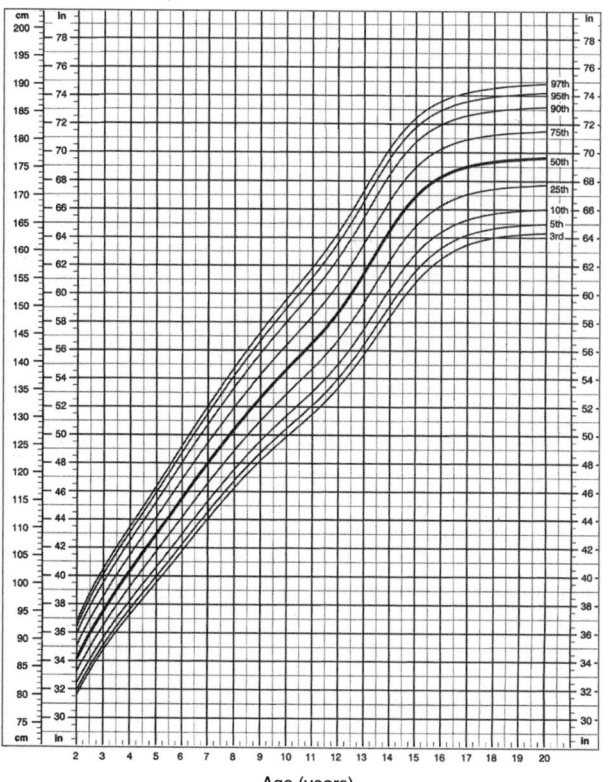

Age (years)

Developed by the National Center for Health Statistics in collaboration with the National Center for Chronic Disease Prevention and Health Promotion (2000).

IHDP Growth Percentiles: LBW Premature Girls

IHDP Growth Percentiles:
LBW Premature Girls[1,2]
(1501 to 2500 g BW, ≤37 wk GA)

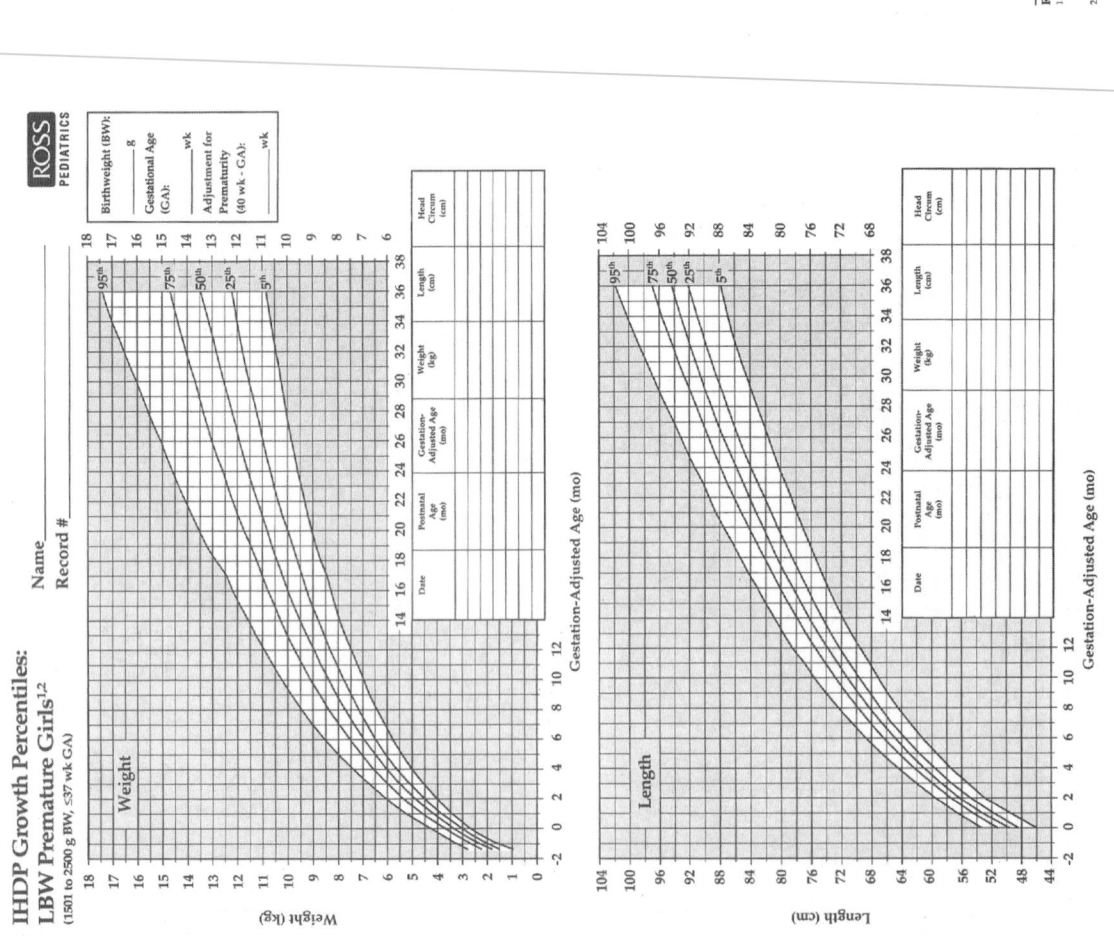

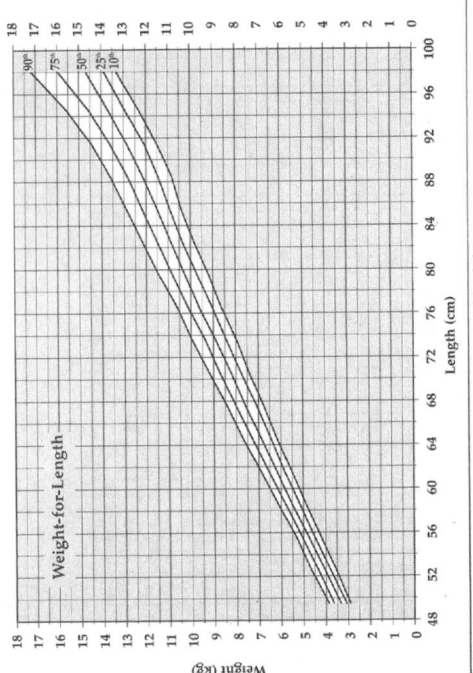

References

1. Gao SS, Roche AF, Chumlea WC, et al. Growth in weight, recumbent length, and head circumference for preterm low-birthweight infants during the first three years of life using gestation-adjusted age. *Early Hum Dev* 1997;47:305-325.

2. Gao SS, Whollihan K, Roche AF, et al. Weight-for-length reference data for preterm, low-birth-weight infants. *Arch Pediatr Adolesc Med* 1996;150:964-970. Copyright. 1996, American Medical Association.

Acknowledgment

IHDP studies were supported by grants from the Robert Wood Johnson Foundation, Pew Charitable Trusts, and the Bureau of Maternal and Child Health, US Department of Health and Human Services. The IHDP growth percentile graphs were prepared by S.S. Guo and A.F. Roche, Wright State University, Yellow Springs, Ohio. IHDP, its sponsors and the investigators do not endorse specific products.

© 1999 Abbott
A72229/MARCH 1999
LITHO IN USA

ROSS PRODUCTS DIVISION
ABBOTT LABORATORIES INC.
COLUMBUS, OHIO 43215-7254

Provided as a service of
Similac NeoSure™
Infant Formula With Iron

IHDP Growth Percentiles: LBW Premature Boys

IHDP Growth Percentiles:
LBW Premature Boys[1,2]
(1501 to 2500 g BW, ≤37 wk GA)

Name _____

Record # _____

Birthweight (BW): _____ g

Gestational Age (GA): _____ wk

Adjustment for Prematurity
(40 wk - GA): _____ wk

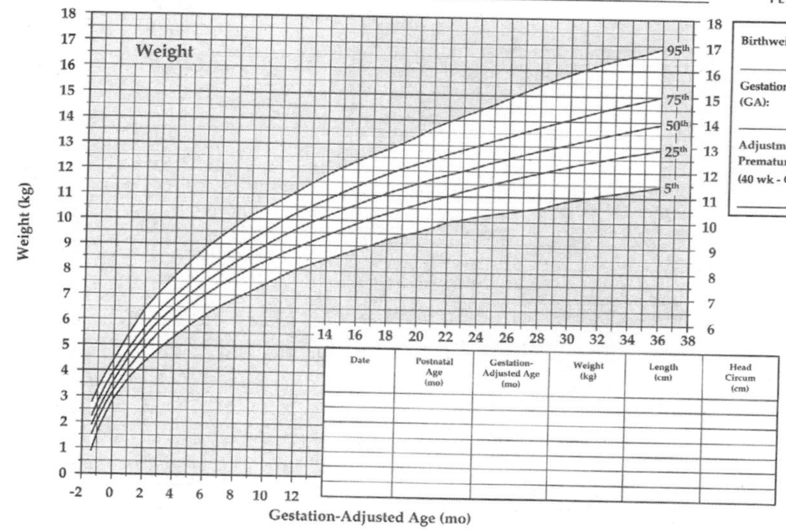

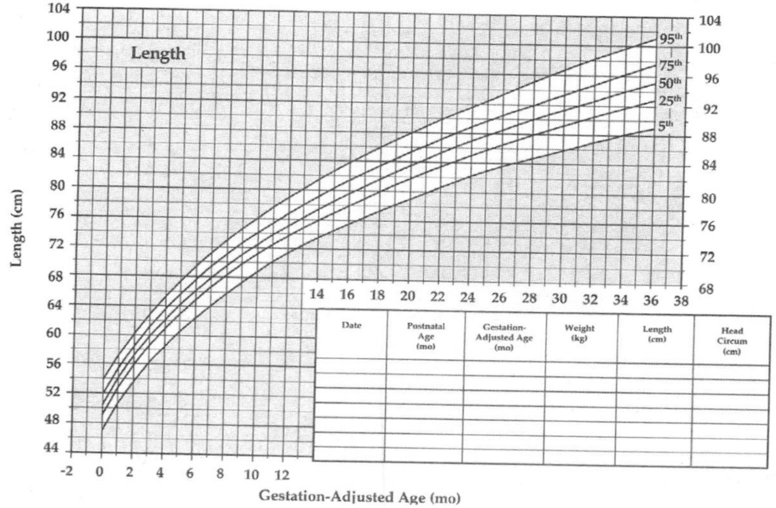

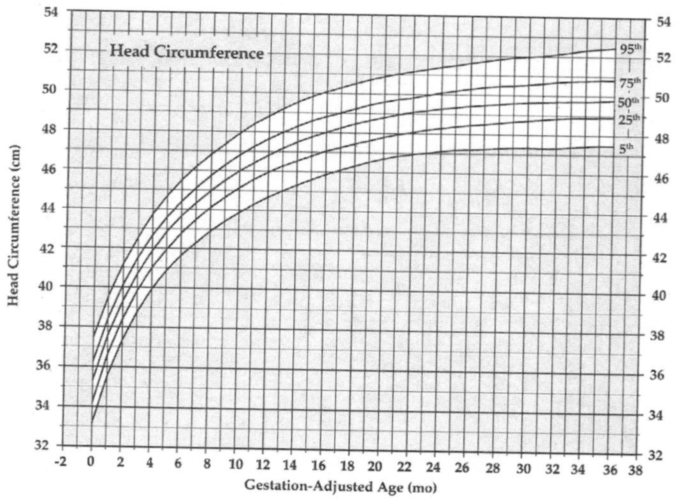

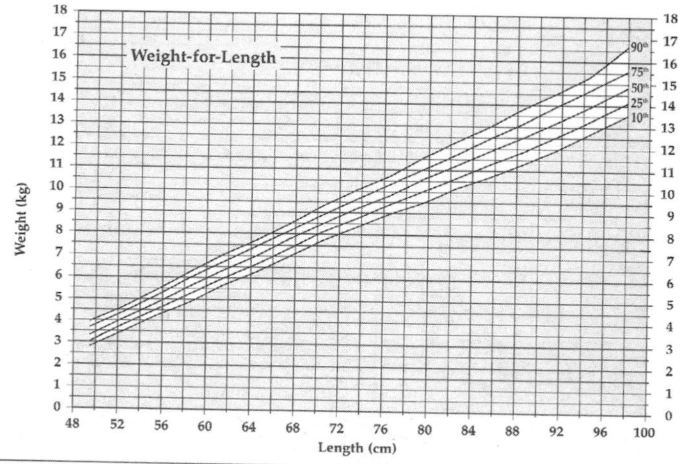

Weight — Gestation-Adjusted Age (mo)

Length — Gestation-Adjusted Age (mo)

Head Circumference — Gestation-Adjusted Age (mo)

Weight-for-Length — Length (cm)

Acknowledgment

IHDP studies were supported by grants from the Robert Wood Johnson Foundation, Pew Charitable Trusts, and the Bureau of Maternal and Child Health, US Department of Health and Human Services. The IHDP growth percentile graphs were prepared by S.S. Guo and A.F. Roche, Wright State University, Yellow Springs, Ohio. IHDP, its sponsors and the Investigators do not endorse specific products.

References
1. Guo SS, Roche AF, Chumlea WC, et al: Growth in weight, recumbent length, and head circumference for preterm low-birthweight infants during the first three years of life using gestation-adjusted ages. *Early Hum Dev* 1997;47:305-325.
2. Guo SS, Wholihan K, Roche AF, et al: Weight-for-length reference data for preterm, low-birthweight infants. *Arch Pediatr Adolesc Med* 1996;150:964-970. Copyright 1996, American Medical Association.

© 1999 Abbott
A7222/MARCH 1999
LITHO IN USA

ROSS PRODUCTS DIVISION
ABBOTT LABORATORIES INC
COLUMBUS, OHIO 43215-1724

Provided as a service of

Similac NeoSure™
Infant Formula With Iron

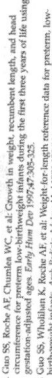

IHDP Growth Percentiles: VLBW Premature Girls

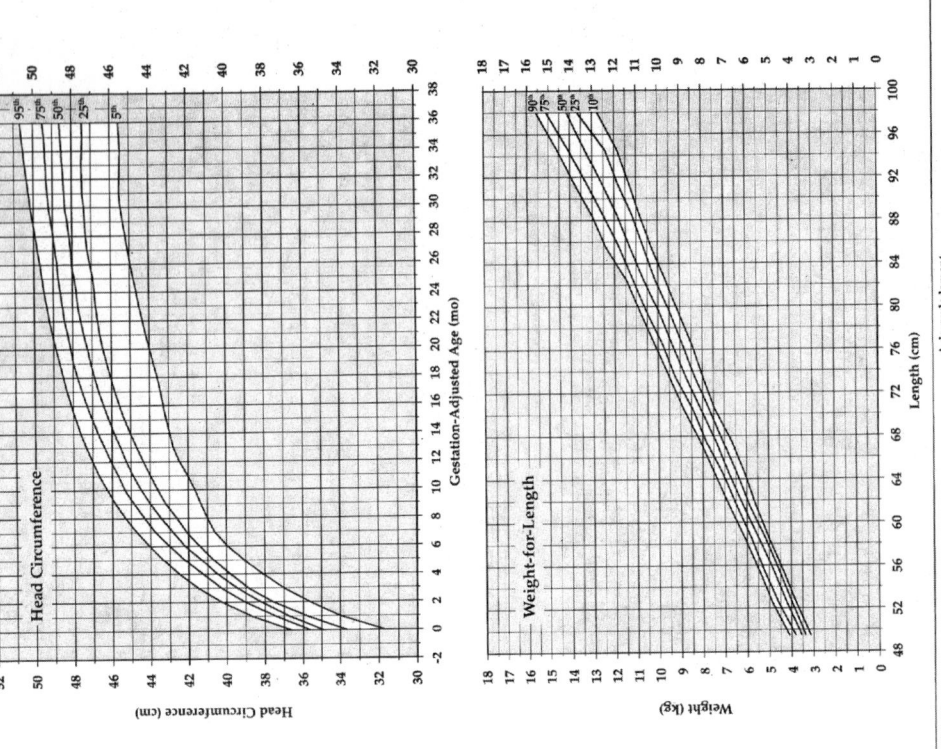

IHDP Growth Percentiles:
VLBW Premature Girls[1,2]

(≤1500 g BW, ≤37 wk GA)

References

1. Guo SS, Roche AF, Chumlea WC, et al: Growth in weight, recumbent length, and head circumference for preterm low-birthweight infants during the first three years of life using gestation-adjusted ages. *Early Hum Dev* 1997;47:305-325.

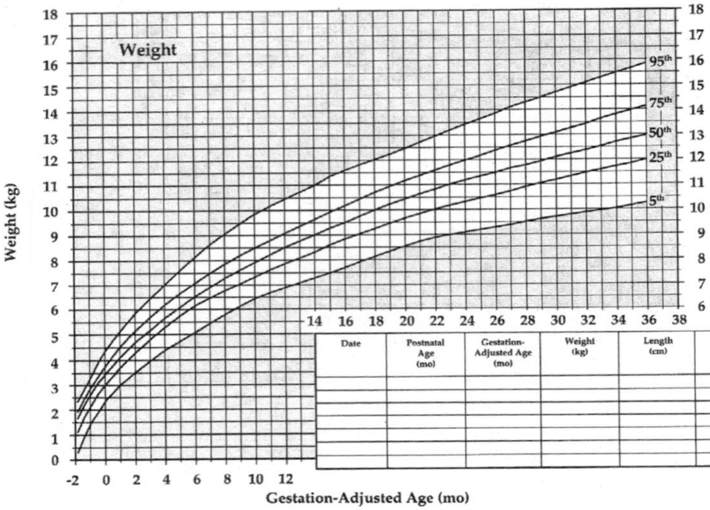

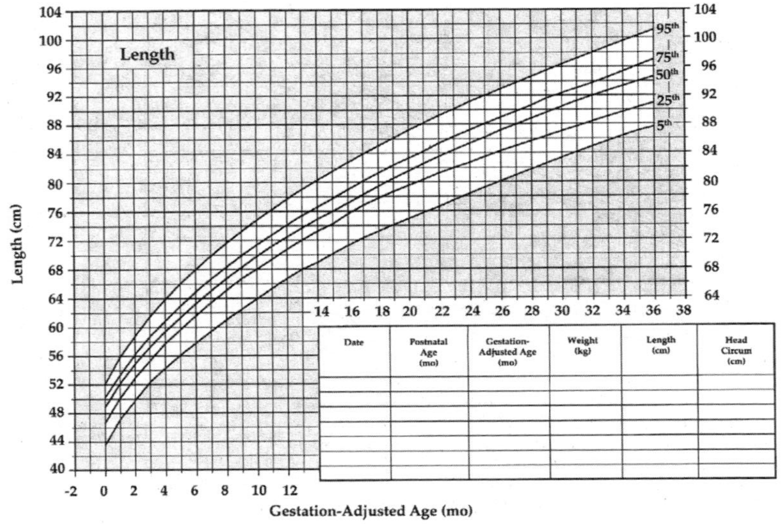

2. Guo SS, Wisahlan K, Roche AF, et al: Weight-for-length reference data for preterm, low-birth-weight infants. *Arch Pediatr Adolesc Med* 1996;150:964-970. Copyright 1996, American Medical Association.

© 1999 Abbott
A7220/MARCH 1999
LITHO IN USA

Acknowledgment

IHDP studies were supported by grants from the Robert Wood Johnson Foundation, Pew Charitable Trusts, and the Bureau of Maternal and Child Health, US Department of Health and Human Services. The IHDP growth percentile graphs were prepared by S.S. Guo and A.F. Roche, Wright State University, Yellow Springs, Ohio. IHDP, its sponsors and the investigators do not endorse specific products.

Provided as a service of
Similac NeoSure™
Infant Formula With Iron

ROSS ROSS PRODUCTS DIVISION
ABBOTT LABORATORIES INC.
COLUMBUS, OHIO 43215-1724

IHDP Growth Percentiles: VLBW Premature Boys

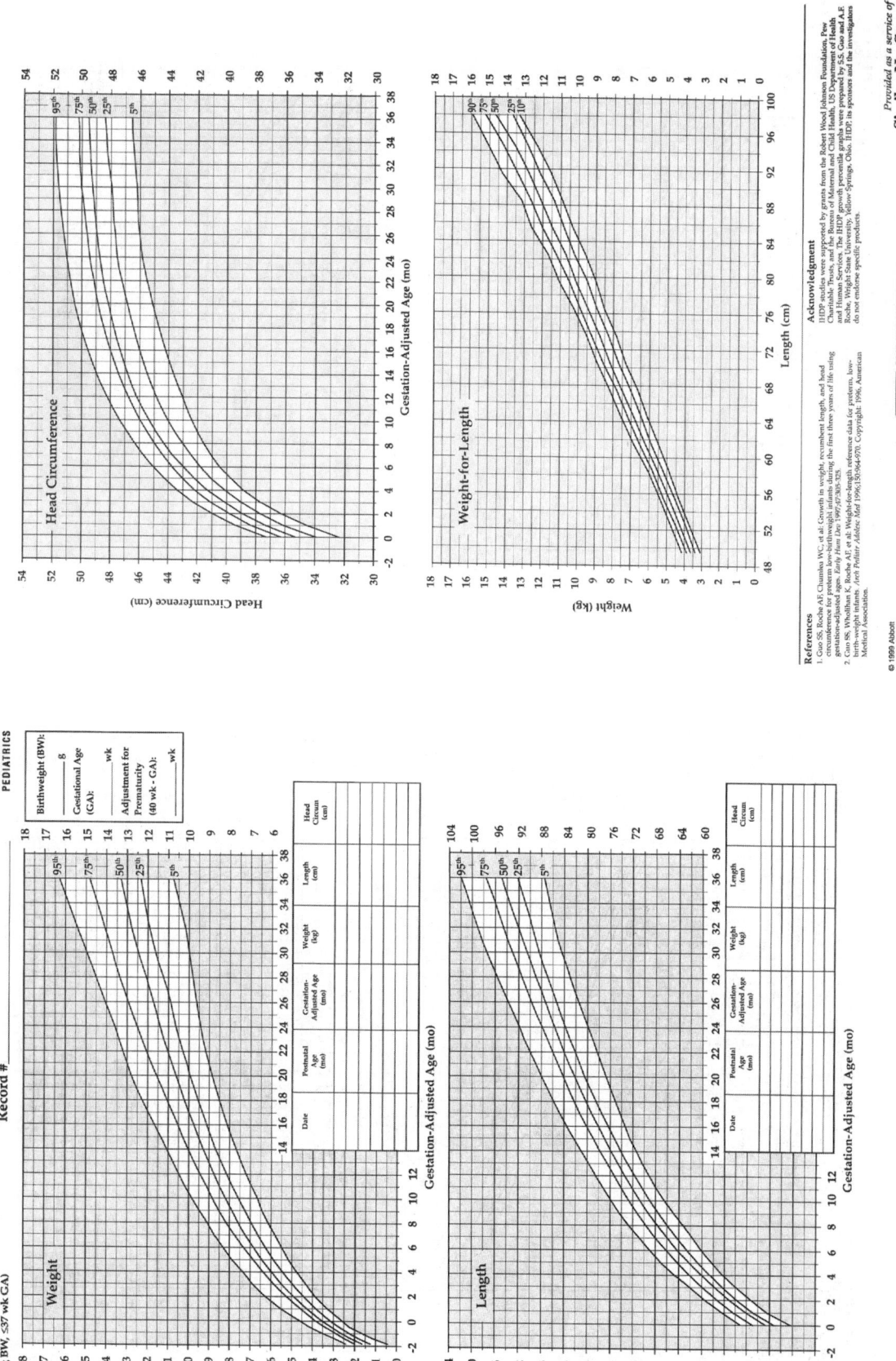

IHDP Growth Percentiles:
VLBW Premature Boys[1,2]
(≤1500 g BW, ≤37 wk GA)

References

1. Guo SS, Roche AF, Chumlea WC, et al. Growth in weight, recumbent length, and head circumference for preterm low-birthweight infants during the first three years of life using gestation-adjusted ages. *Early Hum Dev* 1997;47:305-325.

2. Guo SS, Wholihan K, Roche AF, et al. Weight-for-length reference data for preterm, low-birth-weight infants. *Arch Pediatr Adolesc Med* 1996;150:964-970. Copyright 1996, American Medical Association.

Acknowledgment

IHDP studies were supported by grants from the Robert Wood Johnson Foundation, Pew Charitable Trusts, and the Bureau of Maternal and Child Health, US Department of Health and Human Service. The IHDP growth percentile graphs were prepared by S.S. Guo and A.F. Roche, Wright State University, Yellow Springs, Ohio. IHDP, its sponsors and the investigators do not endorse specific products.

© 1999 Abbott
A7221/MARCH 1999
LITHO IN USA

Provided as a service of
Similac NeoSure™
Infant Formula With Iron

ROSS PRODUCTS DIVISION
ABBOTT LABORATORIES INC
COLUMBUS, OHIO 43215-1724

Immunization

Vaccines Licensed for Immunization and Distributed in the United States and Their Routes of Administration[a]

Vaccine	Type	Route
BCG	Live bacteria	ID (preferred) or SC
Diphtheria-tetanus (DT, Td)	Toxoids	IM
DTaP	Toxoids and inactivated bacterial components	IM
DTaP, hepatitis B, and IPV	Toxoids and inactivated bacterial components, recombinant viral antigen, inactivated virus	IM
DTaP/Hib conjugate (PRP-T[b] reconstituted with DTaP)	Toxoids and inactivated bacterial components with polysaccharide-protein conjugate	IM
DTaP-IPV	Toxoids and inactivated bacterial components, inactivated virus	IM
DTaP-IPV/Hib (PRP-T reconstituted with DTaP-IPV)	Toxoids and inactivated bacterial components, polysaccharide-protein conjugate, inactivated virus	IM
Hepatitis A	Inactivated viral antigen	IM
Hepatitis B	Recombinant viral antigen	IM
Hepatitis A-hepatitis B	Inactivated and recombinant viral antigens	IM
Hib conjugates[b]	Polysaccharide-protein conjugate	IM
Hib conjugate (PRP-OMP[b]) -hepatitis B	Polysaccharide-protein conjugate with recombinant viral antigen	IM
Human papillomavirus (HPV)	Recombinant viral antigens	IM
Influenza	Inactivated viral components	IM
Influenza	Live-attenuated viruses	Intranasal
Japanese encephalitis	Inactivated virus	SC
Meningococcal	Polysaccharide	SC
Meningococcal conjugate	Polysaccharide-protein conjugate	IM
MMR	Live-attenuated viruses	SC
MMRV	Live-attenuated viruses	SC
Pneumococcal	Polysaccharide	IM or SC
Pneumococcal conjugate	Polysaccharide-protein conjugate	IM
Poliovirus (IPV)	Inactivated viruses	SC or IM
Rabies	Inactivated virus	IM
Rotavirus	Live-attenuated virus	Oral
Tdap	Toxoids and inactivated bacterial component	IM
Tetanus	Toxoid	IM
Typhoid	Capsular polysaccharide	IM
Typhoid	Live-attenuated bacteria	Oral
Varicella	Live-attenuated virus	SC
Zoster	Live-attenuated virus	SC
Yellow fever	Live-attenuated virus	SC

BCG indicates bacille Calmette-Guérin; ID, intradermal; SC, subcutaneous; DT, diphtheria and tetanus toxoids (for children younger than 7 years of age); Td, diphtheria and tetanus toxoids (for children 7 years of age or older and adults); IM, intramuscular; DTaP, diphtheria and tetanus toxoids and acellular pertussis, adsorbed; IPV, inactivated poliovirus; Hib, *Haemophilus influenzae* type b; PRP-T, polyribosylribitol phosphate-tetanus toxoid; PRP-OMP, polyribosylribitol phosphate-meningococcal outer membrane protein; MMR, live measles-mumps-rubella; MMRV, live measles-mumps-rubella-varicella (monovalent measles, mumps, and rubella components are not being produced in the United States); Tdap, tetanus toxoid, reduced diphtheria toxoid, and acellular pertussis.

[a]Other vaccines licensed in the United States but not distributed include anthrax, smallpox, oral poliovirus (OPV), and H5N1 influenza vaccines. The FDA maintains a Web site listing currently licensed vaccines in the United States (**www.fda.gov/cber/vaccine/licvacc.htm**). The AAP maintains a Web site (**www.aapredbook.org/news/vaccstatus.dtl**) showing status of licensure and recommendations for new vaccines.

[b]See Table 3.11, p 319.

From: American Academy of Pediatrics. Active immunization. In: Pickering LK, Baker CJ, Kimberlin DW, Long SS, eds. *Red Book: 2009 Report of the Committee on Infectious Diseases*. 28th ed. Elk Grove Village, IL: American Academy of Pediatrics; 2009:10–11.

Site and Needle Length by Age for Intramuscular Immunization

Age Group	Needle Length, inches (mm)[a]	Suggested Injection Site
Newborns (preterm and term) and infants <2 mo of age	5/8 (16)	Anterolateral thigh muscle
Term infants, 2–12 mo of age	1 (25)	Anterolateral thigh muscle
Toddlers and children	5/8 (16)	Deltoid muscle of the arm
	1–1 1/4 (25–32)	Anterolateral thigh muscle
Adolescents and young adults		
Female and male, weight <60 kg	5/8 (16)	Deltoid muscle of the arm
Female, weight 60–90 kg	1 (25)	Deltoid muscle of the arm
Female, weight >90 kg	1 1/2 (38)	Deltoid muscle of the arm
Male, weight 60–118 kg	1 (25)	Deltoid muscle of the arm
Male, weight >118 kg	1 1/2 (38)	Deltoid muscle of the arm

[a]Assumes that needle is inserted fully.

From: American Academy of Pediatrics. Active immunization. In: Pickering LK, Baker CJ, Kimberlin DW, Long SS, eds. *Red Book: 2009 Report of the Committee on Infectious Diseases.* 28th ed. Elk Grove Village, IL: American Academy of Pediatrics; 2009:19.

Guidelines for Spacing of Live and Inactivated Antigens

Antigen Combination	Recommended Minimum Interval Between Doses
2 or more inactivated[a]	None; can be administered simultaneously or at any interval between doses
Inactivated and live	None; can be administered simultaneously or at any interval between doses
2 or more live[b]	28-day minimum interval if not administered at the same visit

[a]If simultaneous administration of tetanus toxoid, reduced diphtheria toxoid, and acellular pertussis (Tdap) vaccine and meningococcal conjugate vaccine (MCV4) is not feasible (ie, one of the vaccines is not available), the American Academy of Pediatrics recommends that administration be separated by at least 28 days.

[b]Some live oral vaccines (eg, Ty21a typhoid vaccine, oral poliovirus vaccine, rotavirus vaccine) can be administered simultaneously or at any interval before or after inactivated or live parenteral vaccines.

From: American Academy of Pediatrics. Active immunization. In: Pickering LK, Baker CJ, Kimberlin DW, Long SS, eds. *Red Book: 2009 Report of the Committee on Infectious Diseases.* 28th ed. Elk Grove Village, IL: American Academy of Pediatrics; 2009:22.

Recommended Immunization Schedule for Persons Aged 0 Through 6 Years—United States • 2010
For those who fall behind or start late, see the catch-up schedule

Vaccine ▼ Age ▶	Birth	1 month	2 months	4 months	6 months	12 months	15 months	18 months	19–23 months	2–3 years	4–6 years
Hepatitis B[1]	HepB	HepB				HepB					
Rotavirus[2]			RV	RV	RV[2]						
Diphtheria, Tetanus, Pertussis[3]			DTaP	DTaP	DTaP	see footnote[3]	DTaP				DTaP
Haemophilus influenzae type b[4]			Hib	Hib	Hib[4]	Hib					
Pneumococcal[5]			PCV	PCV	PCV	PCV				PPSV	
Inactivated Poliovirus[6]			IPV	IPV		IPV					IPV
Influenza[7]						Influenza (Yearly)					
Measles, Mumps, Rubella[8]						MMR	see footnote[8]				MMR
Varicella[9]						Varicella	see footnote[9]				Varicella
Hepatitis A[10]						HepA (2 doses)				HepA Series	
Meningococcal[11]										MCV	

Range of recommended ages for all children except certain high-risk groups

Range of recommended ages for certain high-risk groups

This schedule includes recommendations in effect as of December 15, 2009. Any dose not administered at the recommended age should be administered at a subsequent visit, when indicated and feasible. The use of a combination vaccine generally is preferred over separate injections of its equivalent component vaccines. Considerations should include provider assessment, patient preference, and the potential for adverse events. Providers should consult the relevant Advisory Committee on Immunization Practices statement for detailed recommendations: http://www.cdc.gov/vaccines/pubs/acip-list.htm. Clinically significant adverse events that follow immunization should be reported to the Vaccine Adverse Event Reporting System (VAERS) at http://www.vaers.hhs.gov or by telephone, 800-822-7967.

1. **Hepatitis B vaccine (HepB).** (Minimum age: birth)
   At birth:
   - Administer monovalent HepB to all newborns before hospital discharge.
   - If mother is hepatitis B surface antigen (HBsAg)-positive, administer HepB and 0.5 mL of hepatitis B immune globulin (HBIG) within 12 hours of birth.
   - If mother's HBsAg status is unknown, administer HepB within 12 hours of birth. Determine mother's HBsAg status as soon as possible and, if HBsAg-positive, administer HBIG (no later than age 1 week).
   After the birth dose:
   - The HepB series should be completed with either monovalent HepB or a combination vaccine containing HepB. The second dose should be administered at age 1 or 2 months. Monovalent HepB vaccine should be used for doses administered before age 6 weeks. The final dose should be administered no earlier than age 24 weeks.
   - Infants born to HBsAg-positive mothers should be tested for HBsAg and antibody to HBsAg 1 to 2 months after completion of at least 3 doses of the HepB series, at age 9 through 18 months (generally at the next well-child visit).
   - Administration of 4 doses of HepB to infants is permissible when a combination vaccine containing HepB is administered after the birth dose. The fourth dose should be administered no earlier than age 24 weeks.
2. **Rotavirus vaccine (RV).** (Minimum age: 6 weeks)
   - Administer the first dose at age 6 through 14 weeks (maximum age: 14 weeks 6 days). Vaccination should not be initiated for infants aged 15 weeks 0 days or older.
   - The maximum age for the final dose in the series is 8 months 0 days
   - If Rotarix is administered at ages 2 and 4 months, a dose at 6 months is not indicated.
3. **Diphtheria and tetanus toxoids and acellular pertussis vaccine (DTaP).** (Minimum age: 6 weeks)
   - The fourth dose may be administered as early as age 12 months, provided at least 6 months have elapsed since the third dose.
   - Administer the final dose in the series at age 4 through 6 years.
4. **Haemophilus influenzae type b conjugate vaccine (Hib).** (Minimum age: 6 weeks)
   - If PRP-OMP (PedvaxHIB or Comvax [HepB-Hib]) is administered at ages 2 and 4 months, a dose at age 6 months is not indicated.
   - TriHiBit (DTaP/Hib) and Hiberix (PRP-T) should not be used for doses at ages 2, 4, or 6 months for the primary series but can be used as the final dose in children aged 12 months through 4 years. See *MMWR* 1997;46(No. RR-8).
5. **Pneumococcal vaccine.** (Minimum age: 6 weeks for pneumococcal conjugate vaccine [PCV]; 2 years for pneumococcal polysaccharide vaccine [PPSV])
   - PCV is recommended for all children aged younger than 5 years. Administer 1 dose of PCV to all healthy children aged 24 through 59 months who are not completely vaccinated for their age.
   - Administer PPSV 2 or more months after last dose of PCV to children aged 2 years or older with certain underlying medical conditions, including a cochlear implant.

6. **Inactivated poliovirus vaccine (IPV)** (Minimum age: 6 weeks)
   - The final dose in the series should be administered on or after the fourth birthday and at least 6 months following the previous dose.
   - If 4 doses are administered prior to age 4 years a fifth dose should be administered at age 4 through 6 years. See *MMWR* 2009;58(30):829–30.
7. **Influenza vaccine (seasonal).** (Minimum age: 6 months for trivalent inactivated influenza vaccine [TIV]; 2 years for live, attenuated influenza vaccine [LAIV])
   - Administer annually to children aged 6 months through 18 years.
   - For healthy children aged 2 through 6 years (i.e., those who do not have underlying medical conditions that predispose them to influenza complications), either LAIV or TIV may be used, except LAIV should not be given to children aged 2 through 4 years who have had wheezing in the past 12 months.
   - Children receiving TIV should receive 0.25 mL if aged 6 through 35 months or 0.5 mL if aged 3 years or older.
   - Administer 2 doses (separated by at least 4 weeks) to children aged younger than 9 years who are receiving influenza vaccine for the first time or who were vaccinated for the first time during the previous influenza season but only received 1 dose.
   - For recommendations for use of influenza A (H1N1) 2009 monovalent vaccine see *MMWR* 2009;58(No. RR-10).
8. **Measles, mumps, and rubella vaccine (MMR).** (Minimum age: 12 months)
   - Administer the second dose routinely at age 4 through 6 years. However, the second dose may be administered before age 4, provided at least 28 days have elapsed since the first dose.
9. **Varicella vaccine.** (Minimum age: 12 months)
   - Administer the second dose routinely at age 4 through 6 years. However, the second dose may be administered before age 4, provided at least 3 months have elapsed since the first dose.
   - For children aged 12 months through 12 years the minimum interval between doses is 3 months. However, if the second dose was administered at least 28 days after the first dose, it can be accepted as valid.
10. **Hepatitis A vaccine (HepA).** (Minimum age: 12 months)
    - Administer to all children aged 1 year (i.e., aged 12 through 23 months). Administer 2 doses at least 6 months apart.
    - Children not fully vaccinated by age 2 years can be vaccinated at subsequent visits
    - HepA also is recommended for older children who live in areas where vaccination programs target older children, who are at increased risk for infection, or for whom immunity against hepatitis A is desired.
11. **Meningococcal vaccine.** (Minimum age: 2 years for meningococcal conjugate vaccine [MCV4] and for meningococcal polysaccharide vaccine [MPSV4])
    - Administer MCV4 to children aged 2 through 10 years with persistent complement component deficiency, anatomic or functional asplenia, and certain other conditions placing them at high risk.
    - Administer MCV4 to children previously vaccinated with MCV4 or MPSV4 after 3 years if first dose administered at age 2 through 6 years. See *MMWR* 2009; 58:1042–3.

The Recommended Immunization Schedules for Persons Aged 0 through 18 Years are approved by the Advisory Committee on Immunization Practices (http://www.cdc.gov/vaccines/recs/acip), the American Academy of Pediatrics (http://www.aap.org), and the American Academy of Family Physicians (http://www.aafp.org). Department of Health and Human Services • Centers for Disease Control and Prevention

Recommended Immunization Schedule for Persons Aged 7 Through 18 Years—United States • 2010

For those who fall behind or start late, see the schedule below and the catch-up schedule

Vaccine ▼ Age ▶	7–10 years	11–12 years	13–18 years	
Tetanus, Diphtheria, Pertussis[1]		Tdap	Tdap	Range of recommended ages for all children except certain high-risk groups
Human Papillomavirus[2]	see footnote 2	HPV (3 doses)	HPV series	
Meningococcal[3]	MCV	MCV	MCV	
Influenza[4]	Influenza (Yearly)			
Pneumococcal[5]	PPSV			Range of recommended ages for catch-up immunization
Hepatitis A[6]	HepA Series			
Hepatitis B[7]	Hep B Series			
Inactivated Poliovirus[8]	IPV Series			Range of recommended ages for certain high-risk groups
Measles, Mumps, Rubella[9]	MMR Series			
Varicella[10]	Varicella Series			

This schedule includes recommendations in effect as of December 15, 2009. Any dose not administered at the recommended age should be administered at a subsequent visit, when indicated and feasible. The use of a combination vaccine generally is preferred over separate injections of its equivalent component vaccines. Considerations should include provider assessment, patient preference, and the potential for adverse events. Providers should consult the relevant Advisory Committee on Immunization Practices statement for detailed recommendations: http://www.cdc.gov/vaccines/pubs/acip-list.htm. Clinically significant adverse events that follow immunization should be reported to the Vaccine Adverse Event Reporting System (VAERS) at http://www.vaers.hhs.gov or by telephone, 800-822-7967.

1. **Tetanus and diphtheria toxoids and acellular pertussis vaccine (Tdap).**
   (Minimum age: 10 years for Boostrix and 11 years for Adacel)
   - Administer at age 11 or 12 years for those who have completed the recommended childhood DTP/DTaP vaccination series and have not received a tetanus and diphtheria toxoid (Td) booster dose.
   - Persons aged 13 through 18 years who have not received Tdap should receive a dose.
   - A 5-year interval from the last Td dose is encouraged when Tdap is used as a booster dose; however, a shorter interval may be used if pertussis immunity is needed.
2. **Human papillomavirus vaccine (HPV).** (Minimum age: 9 years)
   - Two HPV vaccines are licensed: a quadrivalent vaccine (HPV4) for the prevention of cervical, vaginal and vulvar cancers (in females) and genital warts (in females and males), and a bivalent vaccine (HPV2) for the prevention of cervical cancers in females.
   - HPV vaccines are most effective for both males and females when given before exposure to HPV through sexual contact.
   - HPV4 or HPV2 is recommended for the prevention of cervical precancers and cancers in females.
   - HPV4 is recommended for the prevention of cervical, vaginal and vulvar precancers and cancers and genital warts in females.
   - Administer the first dose to females at age 11 or 12 years.
   - Administer the second dose 1 to 2 months after the first dose and the third dose 6 months after the first dose (at least 24 weeks after the first dose).
   - Administer the series to females at age 13 through 18 years if not previously vaccinated.
   - HPV4 may be administered in a 3-dose series to males aged 9 through 18 years to reduce their likelihood of acquiring genital warts.
3. **Meningococcal conjugate vaccine (MCV4).**
   - Administer at age 11 or 12 years, or at age 13 through 18 years if not previously vaccinated.
   - Administer to previously unvaccinated college freshmen living in a dormitory.
   - Administer MCV4 to children aged 2 through 10 years with persistent complement component deficiency, anatomic or functional asplenia, or certain other conditions placing them at high risk.
   - Administer to children previously vaccinated with MCV4 or MPSV4 who remain at increased risk after 3 years (if first dose administered at age 2 through 6 years) or after 5 years (if first dose administered at age 7 years or older). Persons whose only risk factor is living in on-campus housing are not recommended to receive an additional dose. See MMWR 2009;58:1042–3.

4. **Influenza vaccine (seasonal).**
   - Administer annually to children aged 6 months through 18 years.
   - For healthy nonpregnant persons aged 7 through 18 years (i.e., those who do not have underlying medical conditions that predispose them to influenza complications), either LAIV or TIV may be used.
   - Administer 2 doses (separated by at least 4 weeks) to children aged younger than 9 years who are receiving influenza vaccine for the first time or who were vaccinated for the first time during the previous influenza season but only received 1 dose.
   - For recommendations for use of influenza A (H1N1) 2009 monovalent vaccine. See MMWR 2009;58(No. RR-10)
5. **Pneumococcal polysaccharide vaccine (PPSV).**
   - Administer to children with certain underlying medical conditions, including a cochlear implant. A single revaccination should be administered after 5 years to children with functional or anatomic asplenia or an immunocompromising condition. See MMWR 1997;46(No. RR-8).
6. **Hepatitis A vaccine (HepA).**
   - Administer 2 doses at least 6 months apart.
   - HepA is recommended for children older than 23 months of age who live in areas where vaccination programs target older children or who are at increased risk for infection or for whom immunity against hepatitis A is desired.
7. **Hepatitis B vaccine (HepB).**
   - Administer the 3-dose series to those not previously vaccinated.
   - A 2-dose series (separated by at least 4 months) of adult formulation Recombivax HB is licensed for children aged 11 through 15 years.
8. **Inactivated poliovirus vaccine (IPV).**
   - The final dose in the series should be administered on or after the fourth birthday and at least 6 months following the previous dose.
   - If both OPV and IPV were administered as part of a series, a total of 4 doses should be administered, regardless of the child's current age.
9. **Measles, mumps, and rubella vaccine (MMR).**
   - If not previously vaccinated, administer 2 doses or the second dose for those who have received only 1 dose, with at least 28 days between doses.
10. **Varicella vaccine.**
   - For persons aged 7 through 18 years without evidence of immunity (see MMWR 2007;56[No. RR-4]), administer 2 doses if not previously vaccinated or the second dose if only 1 dose has been administered.
   - For persons aged 7 through 12 years, the minimum interval between doses is 3 months. However, if the second dose was administered at least 28 days after the first dose, it can be accepted as valid.
   - For persons aged 13 years and older, the minimum interval between doses is 28 days.

Catch-up Immunization Schedule for Persons Aged 4 Months Through 18 Years Who Start Late or Who Are More Than 1 Month Behind—United States • 2010

The table below provides catch-up schedules and minimum intervals between doses for children whose vaccinations have been delayed. A vaccine series does not need to be restarted, regardless of the time that has elapsed between doses. Use the section appropriate for the child's age.

PERSONS AGED 4 MONTHS THROUGH 6 YEARS

Vaccine	Minimum Age for Dose 1	Minimum Interval Between Doses			
		Dose 1 to Dose 2	Dose 2 to Dose 3	Dose 3 to Dose 4	Dose 4 to Dose 5
Hepatitis B[1]	Birth	4 weeks	8 weeks (and at least 16 weeks after first dose)		
Rotavirus[2]	6 wks	4 weeks	4 weeks[2]		
Diphtheria, Tetanus, Pertussis[3]	6 wks	4 weeks	4 weeks	6 months	6 months[3]
Haemophilus influenzae type b[4]	6 wks	4 weeks if first dose administered at younger than age 12 months / 8 weeks (as final dose) if first dose administered at age 12–14 months / No further doses needed if first dose administered at age 15 months or older	4 weeks[4] if current age is younger than 12 months / 8 weeks (as final dose)[4] if current age is 12 months or older and first dose administered at younger than age 12 months and second dose administered at younger than 15 months / No further doses needed if previous dose administered at age 15 months or older	8 weeks (as final dose) This dose only necessary for children aged 12 months through 59 months who received 3 doses before age 12 months	
Pneumococcal[5]	6 wks	4 weeks if first dose administered at younger than age 12 months / 8 weeks (as final dose for healthy children) if first dose administered at age 12 months or older or current age 24 through 59 months / No further doses needed for healthy children if first dose administered at age 24 months or older	4 weeks if current age is younger than 12 months / 8 weeks (as final dose for healthy children) if current age is 12 months or older / No further doses needed for healthy children if previous dose administered at age 24 months or older	8 weeks (as final dose) This dose only necessary for children aged 12 months through 59 months who received 3 doses before age 12 months or for high-risk children who received 3 doses at any age	
Inactivated Poliovirus[6]	6 wks	4 weeks	4 weeks	6 months	
Measles, Mumps, Rubella[7]	12 mos	4 weeks			
Varicella[8]	12 mos	3 months			
Hepatitis A[9]	12 mos	6 months			

PERSONS AGED 7 THROUGH 18 YEARS

Vaccine	Minimum Age for Dose 1	Dose 1 to Dose 2	Dose 2 to Dose 3	Dose 3 to Dose 4	
Tetanus, Diphtheria/ Tetanus, Diphtheria, Pertussis[10]	7 yrs[10]	4 weeks	4 weeks if first dose administered at younger than age 12 months / 6 months if first dose administered at 12 months or older	6 months if first dose administered at younger than age 12 months	
Human Papillomavirus[11]	9 yrs	Routine dosing intervals are recommended[11]			
Hepatitis A[9]	12 mos	6 months			
Hepatitis B[1]	Birth	4 weeks	8 weeks (and at least 16 weeks after first dose)		
Inactivated Poliovirus[6]	6 wks	4 weeks	4 weeks	6 months	
Measles, Mumps, Rubella[7]	12 mos	4 weeks			
Varicella[8]	12 mos	3 months if person is younger than age 13 years / 4 weeks if person is aged 13 years or older			

1. **Hepatitis B vaccine (HepB).**
   - Administer the 3-dose series to those not previously vaccinated.
   - A 2-dose series (separated by at least 4 months) of adult formulation Recombivax HB is licensed for children aged 11 through 15 years.
2. **Rotavirus vaccine (RV).**
   - The maximum age for the first dose is 14 weeks 6 days. Vaccination should not be initiated for infants aged 15 weeks 0 days or older.
   - The maximum age for the final dose in the series is 8 months 0 days.
   - If Rotarix was administered for the first and second doses, a third dose is not indicated.
3. **Diphtheria and tetanus toxoids and acellular pertussis vaccine (DTaP).**
   - The fifth dose is not necessary if the fourth dose was administered at age 4 years or older.
4. **Haemophilus influenzae type b conjugate vaccine (Hib).**
   - Hib vaccine is not generally recommended for persons aged 5 years or older. No efficacy data are available on which to base a recommendation concerning use of Hib vaccine for older children and adults. However, studies suggest good immunogenicity in persons who have sickle cell disease, leukemia, or HIV infection, or who have had a splenectomy; administering 1 dose of Hib vaccine to these persons who have not previously received Hib vaccine is not contraindicated.
   - If the first 2 doses were PRP-OMP (PedvaxHIB or Comvax), and administered at age 11 months or younger, the third (and final) dose should be administered at age 12 through 15 months and at least 8 weeks after the second dose.
   - If the first dose was administered at age 7 through 11 months, administer the second dose at least 4 weeks later and a final dose at age 12 through 15 months.
5. **Pneumococcal vaccine.**
   - Administer 1 dose of pneumococcal conjugate vaccine (PCV) to all healthy children aged 24 through 59 months who have not received at least 1 dose of PCV on or after age 12 months.
   - For children aged 24 through 59 months with underlying medical conditions, administer 1 dose of PCV if 3 doses were received previously or administer 2 doses of PCV at least 8 weeks apart if fewer than 3 doses were received previously.
   - Administer pneumococcal polysaccharide vaccine (PPSV) to children aged 2 years or older with certain underlying medical conditions, including a cochlear implant, at least 8 weeks after the last dose of PCV.
6. **Inactivated poliovirus vaccine (IPV).**
   - The final dose in the series should be administered on or after the fourth birthday and at least 6 months following the previous dose.
   - A fourth dose is not necessary if the third dose was administered at age 4 years or older and at least 6 months following the previous dose.
   - In the first 6 months of life, minimum age and minimum intervals are only recommended if the person is at risk for imminent exposure to circulating poliovirus (i.e., travel to a polio-endemic region or during an outbreak).
7. **Measles, mumps, and rubella vaccine (MMR).**
   - Administer the second dose routinely at age 4 through 6 years. However, the second dose may be administered before age 4, provided at least 28 days have elapsed since the first dose.
   - If not previously vaccinated, administer 2 doses with at least 28 days between doses.
8. **Varicella vaccine.**
   - Administer the second dose routinely at age 4 through 6 years. However, the second dose may be administered before age 4, provided at least 3 months have elapsed since the first dose.
   - For persons aged 12 months through 12 years, the minimum interval between doses is 3 months. However, if the second dose was administered at least 28 days after the first dose, it can be accepted as valid.
   - For persons aged 13 years and older, the minimum interval between doses is 28 days.
9. **Hepatitis A vaccine (HepA).**
   - HepA is recommended for children older than 23 months who live in areas where vaccination programs target older children, who are at increased risk for infection, or for whom immunity against hepatitis A is desired.
10. **Tetanus and diphtheria toxoids vaccine (Td) and tetanus and diphtheria toxoids and acellular pertussis vaccine (Tdap).**
    - Doses of DTaP are counted as part of the Td/Tdap series
    - Tdap should be substituted for a single dose of Td in the catch-up series or as a booster for children aged 10 through 18 years; use Td for other doses.
11. **Human papillomavirus (HPV).**
    - Administer the series to females at age 13 through 18 years if not previously vaccinated.
    - Use recommended routine dosing intervals for series catch-up (i.e., the second and third doses should be administered at 1 to 2 and 6 months after the first dose). The minimum interval between the first and second doses is 4 weeks. The minimum interval between the second and third doses is 12 weeks, and the third dose should be administered at least 24 weeks after the first dose.

Information about reporting reactions after immunization is available online at http://www.vaers.hhs.gov or by telephone, 800-822-7967. Suspected cases of vaccine-preventable diseases should be reported to the state or local health department. Additional information, including precautions and contraindications for immunization, is available from the National Center for Immunization and Respiratory Diseases at http://www.cdc.gov/vaccines or telephone, 800-CDC-INFO (800-232-4636).

Department of Health and Human Services • Centers for Disease Control and Prevention

Recommended and Minimum Ages and Intervals Between Vaccine Doses

Vaccine and Dose No.	Recommended Age for This Dose	Minimum Age for This Dose	Recommended Interval to Next Dose	Minimum Interval to Next Dose
Hepatitis B (HepB)-1[c]	Birth	Birth	1–4 mo	4 wk
HepB-2	1–2 mo	4 wk	2–17 mo	8 wk
HepB-3[d]	6–18 mo	24 wk	…	…
Diphtheria-tetanus-acellular pertussis (DTaP)-1[c]	2 mo	6 wk	2 mo	4 wk
DTaP-2	4 mo	10 wk	2 mo	4 wk
DTaP-3	6 mo	14 wk	6–12 mo	6 mo[e,f]
DTaP-4	15–18 mo	12 mo	3 y	6 mo[e]
DTaP-5	4–6 y	4 y	…	…
Haemophilus influenzae type b (Hib)-1[c,g]	2 mo	6 wk	2 mo	4 wk
Hib-2	4 mo	10 wk	2 mo	4 wk
Hib-3[h]	6 mo	14 wk	6–9 mo	8 wk
Hib-4	12–15 mo	12 mo	…	…
Inactivated poliovirus (IPV)-1[c]	2 mo	6 wk	2 mo	4 wk
IPV-2	4 mo	10 wk	2–14 mo	4 wk
IPV-3	6–18 mo	14 wk	3–5 y	4 wk
IPV-4	4–6 y	18 wk	…	…
Pneumococcal conjugate (PCV)-1[g]	2 mo	6 wk	2 mo	4 wk
PCV-2	4 mo	10 wk	2 mo	4 wk
PCV-3	6 mo	14 wk	6 mo	8 wk
PCV-4	12–15 mo	12 mo	…	…
Measles-mumps-rubella (MMR)-1[i]	12–15 mo	12 mo	3–5 y	4 wk
MMR-2[i]	4–6 y	13 mo	…	…
Varicella (Var)-1[i]	12–15 mo	12 mo	3–5 y	12 wk[j]
Var-2[i]	4–6 y	15 mo	…	…
Hepatitis A (HepA)-1	12–23 mo	12 mo	6–18 mo[e]	6 mo[e]
HepA-2	18–41 mo	18 mo	…	…
Influenza inactivated (TIV)[k]	6 mo–18 y	6 mo[l]	1 mo	4 wk
Influenza live-attenuated (LAIV)[k]	24 mo–18 y	24 mo	1 mo	4 wk
Meningococcal conjugate (MCV)	11–12 y	2 y	…	…
Meningococcal poly-saccharide (MPSV)-1	…	2 y	5 y[m]	5 y[m]
MPSV-2[n]	…	7 y	…	…
Td	11–12 y	7 y	10 y	5 y
Tdap[o]	≥11 y	10 y	…	…
Pneumococcal polysaccha-ride (PPV)-1	…	2 y	5 y	5 y
PPV-2[p]	…	7 y	…	…
Human papillomavirus (HPV)-1[q]	11–12 y	9 y	2 mo	4 wk
HPV-2	11–12 y (+2 mo)	109 mo	4 mo	12 wk[r]
HPV-3[r]	11–12 y (+6 mo)	114 mo	…	…
Rotavirus (RV)-1[s]	2 mo	6 wk	2 mo	4 wk
RV-2	4 mo	10 wk	2 mo	4 wk

continued

Recommended and Minimum Ages and Intervals Between Vaccine Doses, *continued*

Vaccine and Dose No.	Recommended Age for This Dose	Minimum Age for This Dose	Recommended Interval to Next Dose	Minimum Interval to Next Dose
RV-3[t]	6 mo	14 wk	…	…
Herpes zoster[u]	60 y	60 y	…	…

DTaP indicates diphtheria and tetanus toxoids and acellular pertussis vaccine; MMR, measles-mumps-rubella; TIV, trivalent (inactivated) influenza vaccine; LAIV, live-attenuated (intranasal) influenza vaccine; Td, tetanus and reduced diphtheria toxoids; Tdap, tetanus toxoid, reduced diphtheria toxoid, and reduced acellular pertussis vaccine.

[a] Combination vaccines are available and may be used to reduce the number of injections. When administering combination vaccines, the minimum age for administration is the oldest age for any of the individual components; the minimum interval between doses is equal to the greatest interval of any of the individual components.

[b] For travel vaccines, including typhoid, Japanese encephalitis, and yellow fever, see **www.cdc.gov/travel.**

[c] Combination vaccines containing the hepatitis B component are available (HepB-Hib, DTaP-HepB-IPV, and HepA-HepB). These vaccines should not be administered to infants younger than 6 weeks of age because of the other components (ie, Hib, DTaP, HepA, and IPV).

[d] HepB-3 should be administered at least 8 weeks after HepB-2 and at least 16 weeks after HepB-1 and should not be administered before 24 weeks of age.

[e] Calendar months.

[f] The minimum recommended interval between DTaP-3 and DTaP-4 is 6 months. However, DTaP-4 need not be repeated if administered at least 4 months after DTaP-3.

[g] For Hib and PCV, children receiving the first dose of vaccine at 7 months of age or older require fewer doses to complete the series (see Fig 1.1–1.3, p 24–28).

[h] If PRP-OMP (Pedvax-Hib) was administered at 2 and 4 months of age, a dose at 6 months of age is not required.

[i] Combination measles-mumps-rubella-varicella (MMRV) vaccine can be used for children 12 months through 12 years of age.

[j] The minimum interval from VAR-1 to VAR-2 for people beginning the series at 13 years of age or older is 4 weeks.

[k] One dose of influenza vaccine per season is recommended for most people. Children younger than 9 years of age who are receiving influenza for the first time or received only 1 dose the previous season (if it was their first immunization season) should receive 2 doses this season.

[l] The minimum age for inactivated influenza vaccine varies by vaccine manufacturer (see Influenza, p 400).

[m] Some experts recommend a second dose of MPSV 3 years after the first dose for people at increased risk of meningococcal disease (see Meningococcal Infections, p 455).

[n] A second dose of meningococcal vaccine is recommended for people previously immunized with MPSV who remain at high risk of meningococcal disease. MCV is preferred when reimmunizing people 2 through 55 years of age, but a second dose of MPSV is acceptable.

[o] Only one dose of Tdap is recommended. Subsequent doses should be given as Td. If immunization to prevent tetanus and/or diphtheria disease is required for children 7 through 9 years of age, Td should be administered (minimum age for Td is 7 years). For one brand of Tdap, the minimum age is 11 years. The preferred interval between Tdap and a previous dose of Td is 5 years. In people who have received a primary series of tetanus-toxoid containing vaccine, for management of a tetanus-prone wound, the minimum interval after a previous dose of any tetanus-containing vaccine is 5 years.

[p] A second dose of PPV is recommended for people at highest risk of serious pneumococcal infection and those who are likely to have a rapid decline in pneumococcal antibody concentration (see Pneumococcal Infections, p 524).

[q] HPV is approved only for females 9 through 26 years of age.

[r] HPV-3 should be administered at least 12 weeks after HPV-2 and at least 24 weeks after HPV-1.

[s] The first dose of RV should be administered at 6 through 14 weeks of age. The vaccine series should not be started at 15 weeks of age or older. RV should not be administered to children older than 8 calendar months of age regardless of the number of doses received between 6 weeks and 8 calendar months of age.

[t] If Rotarix is administered as age appropriate, a third dose is not necessary.

[u] Herpes zoster vaccine is approved as a single dose for people 60 years of age and older.

From: American Academy of Pediatrics. Active immunization. In: Pickering LK, Baker CJ, Kimberlin DW, Long SS, eds. *Red Book: 2009 Report of the Committee on Infectious Diseases.* 28th ed. Elk Grove Village, IL: American Academy of Pediatrics; 2009:29–31.

Combination Vaccines Licensed by the US Food and Drug Administration (FDA)

Vaccine[b]	Trade Name (Year Licensed)	FDA Licensure	
		Age Group	Recommendations
Hib-HepB	Comvax (1996)	6 wk through 71 mo	Three-dose schedule given at 2, 4, and 12 through 15 mo of age.
DTaP/Hib	TriHIBit (1996)	Fourth dose of Hib and DTaP series	15 through 18 mo of age.
Hep A-HepB	Twinrix (2001)	≥18 y	Three doses on a 0-, 1-, and 6-mo schedule.
DTaP-HepB-IPV	Pediarix (2002)	6 wk through 6 y	Three-dose series at 2, 4, and 6 mo of age.
MMRV	ProQuad (2005)	12 mo through 12 y	Two doses 28 days apart on or after first birthday.
DTaP-IPV	Kinrix (2008)	4 through 6 y	Booster for fifth dose of DTaP and fourth dose of IPV.
DTaP-IPV/Hib	Pentacel (2008)	6 wk through 4 y	Four-dose series at 2, 4, 6, and 15 through 18 mo of age.

Hib indicates *Haemophilus influenzae* type b vaccine; HepB, hepatitis B vaccine; DTaP indicates diphtheria and tetanus toxoids and acellular pertussis vaccine; HepA, hepatitis A vaccine; IPV/Hib trivalent inactivated polio vaccine and *Haemophilus influenzae* type b vaccine; MMRV, measles-mumps-rubella-varicella vaccine.

[a] Excludes measles-mumps-rubella (MMR), DTaP, Tdap, and IPV vaccines, for which individual components are not available.

[b] Dash (-) indicates products are supplied in their final form by the manufacturer and do not require mixing or reconstitution by user; slash (/) indicates products are mixed or reconstituted by user.

From: American Academy of Pediatrics. Active immunization. In: Pickering LK, Baker CJ, Kimberlin DW, Long SS, eds. *Red Book: 2009 Report of the Committee on Infectious Diseases.* 28th ed. Elk Grove Village, IL: American Academy of Pediatrics; 2009:35.

Uses of Immune Globulin Intravenous (IGIV) for Which There is Approval by the US Food and Drug Administration

Primary immunodeficiency states

Kawasaki disease

Immune-mediated thrombocytopenia

Pediatric human immunodeficiency virus infection

Secondary immunodeficiency in chronic lymphocytic leukemia

Prevention of graft-versus-host disease and infection in hematopoietic cell transplantation in adults

[a]Therapeutic differences among IGIV products from different manufacturers are likely to exist.

From: American Academy of Pediatrics. Passive immunization. In: Pickering LK, Baker CJ, Kimberlin DW, Long SS, eds. *Red Book: 2009 Report of the Committee on Infectious Diseases.* 28th ed. Elk Grove Village, IL: American Academy of Pediatrics; 2009:59.

Immunization of Children and Adolescents With Primary and Secondary Immune Deficiencies

Category	Example of Specific Immunodeficiency	Vaccine Contraindications	Effectiveness and Comments
Primary[a]			
B lymphocyte (humoral)	Severe antibody deficiencies (eg, X-linked agammaglobulinemia and common variable immunodeficiency)	OPV,[b] smallpox, LAIV, yellow fever, and live-bacteria vaccines[c]; consider measles vaccine; no data for varicella or rotavirus vaccines	Effectiveness of any vaccine dependent only on humoral response is doubtful; IGIV therapy interferes with measles and possibly varicella immune response.
	Less severe antibody deficiencies (eg, selective IgA deficiency and IgG subclass deficiencies)	OPV[b]; other live vaccines[d] appear to be safe, but caution is urged	All vaccines probably effective. Immune response may be attenuated.
T lymphocyte (cell-mediated and humoral)	Complete defects (eg, severe combined immunodeficiency, complete DiGeorge syndrome)	All live vaccines[c,d]	All vaccines ineffective.
	Partial defects (eg, most patients with DiGeorge syndrome, Wiskott-Aldrich syndrome, ataxia telangiectasia)	All live vaccines[c,d]	Effectiveness of any vaccine depends on degree of immune suppression. Recommend inactivated vaccines.
Complement	Deficiency of early components (C1, C4, C2, C3)	None	All routine vaccines probably effective. Pneumococcal and meningococcal vaccines are recommended.
	Deficiency of late components (C5–C9), properdin, factor B	None	All routine vaccines probably effective. Meningococcal and pneumococcal vaccines are recommended.
Phagocytic function	Chronic granulomatous disease, leukocyte adhesion defects, myeloperoxidase deficiency	Live-bacteria vaccines[c]	All inactivated vaccines safe and probably effective. Live-virus vaccines probably safe and effective.
Secondary[a]			
	HIV/AIDS	OPV,[b] smallpox, BCG, LAIV[d]; withhold MMR and varicella in severely immunocompromised children	MMR, varicella, rotavirus, and all inactivated vaccines, including inactivated influenza, may be effective.[e]
	Malignant neoplasm, transplantation, autoimmune disease, immunosuppressive or radiation therapy	Live-virus and -bacteria, depending on immune status[c,d]	Effectiveness of any vaccine depends on degree of immune suppression.

OPV indicates oral poliovirus; LAIV, live-attenuated influenza vaccine; IGIV, Immune Globulin Intravenous; Ig, immunoglobulin; HIV, human immunodeficiency virus; AIDS, acquired immunodeficiency syndrome; BCG, bacille Calmette-Guérin; MMR, measles-mumps-rubella.

[a] All children and adolescents should receive an annual age-appropriate inactivated influenza vaccine. LAIV is indicated only for healthy people 5 to 49 years of age.

[b] OPV vaccine no longer is recommended for routine use in the United States.

[c] Live-bacteria vaccines: BCG and Ty21a *Salmonella typhi* vaccine.

[d] Live-virus vaccines: LAIV, MMR, measles-mumps-rubella-varicella (MMRV), herpes zoster (ZOS), OPV, varicella, yellow fever, vaccinia (smallpox), and rotavirus.

[e] HIV-infected children should receive Immune Globulin after exposure to measles (see Measles, p 444) and may receive varicella vaccine if CD4+ lymphocyte count ≥15% of expected for age (see Varicella-Zoster Infections, p 714).

From: American Academy of Pediatrics. Immunization in special clinical circumstances. In: Pickering LK, Baker CJ, Kimberlin DW, Long SS, eds. *Red Book: 2009 Report of the Committee on Infectious Diseases*. 28th ed. Elk Grove Village, IL: American Academy of Pediatrics; 2009:74–75.

Schedule for Trivalent Inactivated Influenza Vaccine (TIV) Dosage by Age

Age	Dose, mL[b]	No. of Doses	Route[c]
6 through 35 mo	0.25	1–2[d]	Intramuscular
3 through 8 y	0.5	1–2[d]	Intramuscular
9 y or older	0.5	1	Intramuscular

[a]Manufacturers include sanofi pasteur (Fluzone, split-virus vaccine licensed for people 6 months of age or older), Novartis Vaccine (Fluvirin, purified surface antigen, licensed for people 4 years of age or older), CSL Biotherapies (Afluria, split-virus vaccine licensed for people 18 years of age or older), and GlaxoSmithKline Biologicals (Fluarix and FluLaval, split-virus vaccines licensed for people 18 years of age or older).

[b]Dosages are those recommended in recent years. Physicians should refer to the product circular each year to ensure that the appropriate dosage is given.

[c]For adults and older children, the recommended site of immunization is the deltoid muscle. For infants and young children, the preferred site is the anterolateral aspect of the thigh.

[d]Two doses administered at least 4 weeks apart are recommended for children younger than 9 years of age who are receiving inactivated trivalent influenza vaccine for the first time. If possible, the second dose should be administered before December.

From: American Academy of Pediatrics. Influenza. In: Pickering LK, Baker CJ, Kimberlin DW, Long SS, eds. *Red Book: 2009 Report of the Committee on Infectious Diseases.* 28th ed. Elk Grove Village, IL: American Academy of Pediatrics; 2009:406.

Schedule for Live-Attenuated Influenza Vaccine (LAIV)

Age	Dose, mL[b]	No. of Doses	Route
2 through 8 y	0.2	1–2[c]	Intranasal
9 y or older	0.2	1	Intranasal

[a]Manufacturer: MedImmune Vaccines, Inc (FluMist).

[b]Dosage is the one recommended in recent years. Physicians should refer to the product circular each year to ensure that the appropriate dosage is given.

[c]Two doses administered at least 4 weeks apart are recommended for children younger than 9 years of age who are receiving LAIV for the first time. If possible, the second dose should be administered before December.

From: American Academy of Pediatrics. Influenza. In: Pickering LK, Baker CJ, Kimberlin DW, Long SS, eds. *Red Book: 2009 Report of the Committee on Infectious Diseases.* 28th ed. Elk Grove Village, IL: American Academy of Pediatrics; 2009:407.

Suggested Intervals Between Immune Globulin Administration and Measles Immunization (MMR, MMRV, or Monovalent Measles Vaccine)

Indications or Product	Route	Dose U or mL	Dose mg IgG/kg	Interval, mo[a]
Tetanus prophylaxis (as TIG)	IM	250 U	10	3
Hepatitis A prophylaxis (as IG)				
Contact prophylaxis	IM	0.02 mL/kg	3.3	3
International travel	IM	0.06 mL/kg	10	3
Hepatitis B prophylaxis (as HBIG)	IM	0.06 mL/kg	10	3
Rabies prophylaxis (as RIG)	IM	20 IU/kg	22	4
Varicella prophylaxis (as VariZIG)	IM	125 U/10 kg (maximum 625 U)	20–40	5
Measles prophylaxis (as IG)				
Standard	IM	0.25 mL/kg	40	5
Immunocompromised host	IM	0.50 mL/kg	80	6
RSV prophylaxis (palivizumab monoclonal antibody)[b]	IM	…	15 mg/kg (monoclonal)	None
Cytomegalovirus Immune Globulin	IV	3 mL/kg	150	6
Blood transfusion				
Washed RBCs	IV	10 mL/kg	Negligible	0
RBCs, adenine-saline added	IV	10 mL/kg	10	3
Packed RBCs	IV	10 mL/kg	20–60	5
Whole blood	IV	10 mL/kg	80–100	6
Plasma or platelet products	IV	10 mL/kg	160	7
Replacement (or therapy) of immune deficiencies (as IGIV)	IV	…	300–400	8
ITP (as IGIV)	IV	…	400	8
ITP	IV	…	1000	10
ITP for Kawasaki disease	IV	…	1600–2000	11

MMR indicates measles-mumps-rubella; MMRV, measles-mumps-rubella-varicella; IgG, immunoglobulin G; TIG, Tetanus Immune Globulin; IG, Immune Globulin; IM, intramuscular; HBIG, Hepatitis B IG; RIG, Rabies IG; VariZIG, Varicella-Zoster Immune Globulin; RSV, respiratory syncytial virus; IV, intravenous; RBCs, Red Blood Cells; IGIV, IG intravenous; ITP, immune (formerly termed "idiopathic") thrombocytopenic purpura.

[a]These intervals should provide sufficient time for decreases in passive antibodies in all children to allow for an adequate response to measles vaccine. Physicians should not assume that children are fully protected against measles during these intervals. Additional doses of IG or measles vaccine may be indicated after exposure to measles (see text).

[b]Monoclonal antibodies, such as palivizumab, and tumor necrosis factor (TNF) inhibitors do not interfere with response to vaccines.

From: American Academy of Pediatrics. Measles. In: Pickering LK, Baker CJ, Kimberlin DW, Long SS, eds. *Red Book: 2009 Report of the Committee on Infectious Diseases.* 28th ed. Elk Grove Village, IL: American Academy of Pediatrics; 2009:448.

General Recommendations for Exclusion of Children in Out-of-Home Child Care

Symptom(s)	Management
Illness preventing participation in activities, as determined by child care staff	Exclusion until illness resolves and able to participate in activities
Illness that requires a need for care that is greater than staff can provide without compromising health and safety of others	Exclusion or placement in care environment where appropriate care can be provided, without compromising care of others
Severe illness suggested by fever with behavior changes, lethargy, irritability, persistent crying, difficulty breathing, progressive rash	Medical evaluation and exclusion until symptoms have resolved
Rash with fever or behavioral change	Medical evaluation and exclusion until illness is determined not to be communicable
Persistent abdominal pain (2 hours or more) or intermittent abdominal pain associated with fever, dehydration, or other systemic signs and symptoms	Medical evaluation and exclusion until symptoms have resolved
Vomiting 2 or more times in preceding 24 hours	Exclusion until symptoms have resolved, unless vomiting is determined to be caused by a noncommunicable condition and child is able to remain hydrated and participate in activities
Diarrhea or stools containing blood or mucus	Medical evaluation and exclusion until symptoms have resolved
Oral lesions	Exclusion until child or staff member is considered to be noninfectious (lesions crusted and dry)

From: American Academy of Pediatrics. Children in out-of-home child care. In: Pickering LK, Baker CJ, Kimberlin DW, Long SS, eds. *Red Book: 2009 Report of the Committee on Infectious Diseases.* 28th ed. Elk Grove Village, IL: American Academy of Pediatrics; 2009:128.

Disease- or Condition-Specific Recommendations for Exclusion of Children in Out-of-Home Child Care

Condition	Management of Case	Management of Contacts
Hepatitis A virus (HAV) infection	Serologic testing to confirm HAV infection in suspected cases. Exclusion until 1 week after onset of jaundice.	If ≥1 case confirmed in child or staff attendees or ≥2 cases in households of staff or attendees, HAV vaccine or Immune Globulin (IG) should be administered within 14 days of exposure to unimmunized staff and attendees. In centers without diapered children, HAV vaccine or IG should be given to unimmunized classroom contacts of index case. Asymptomatic IG recipients may return after receipt of IG (see Hepatitis A, p 329).
Impetigo	Exclusion until 24 hours after treatment has been initiated. Lesions on exposed skin covered with watertight dressing.	No intervention unless additional lesions develop.
Measles	Exclusion until 4 days after beginning of rash and when the child is able to participate.	Immunize exposed children without evidence of immunity within 72 hours of exposure. Children who do not receive vaccine within 72 hours or who remain unimmunized after exposure should be excluded until at least 2 weeks after onset of rash in the last case of measles. For use of IG, see Measles (p 444).
Mumps	Exclusion until 5 days after onset of parotid gland swelling.	In outbreak setting, people without documentation of immunity should be immunized or excluded. Immediate readmission may occur following immunization. Unimmunized people should be excluded for ≥26 days following onset of parotitis in last case.
Pediculosis capitis (head lice)	Treatment at end of program day and readmission on completion of first treatment.	Household and close contacts should be examined and treated if infested. No exclusion necessary.
Pertussis	Exclusion until 5 days of appropriate antimicrobial therapy course have been completed (see Pertussis, p 504).	Immunization and chemoprophylaxis should be administered as recommended for household contacts. Symptomatic children and staff should be excluded until completion of 5 days of antimicrobial therapy course. Untreated adults should be excluded until 21 days after onset of cough (see Pertussis Infections, p 504).
Rubella	Exclusion until 6 days after onset of rash for postnatal infection.	Pregnant contacts should be evaluated (see Rubella, p 579).
Salmonella serotype Typhi infection	Exclusion until diarrhea resolves. Three negative stool culture results required before readmission.	Stool cultures should be performed for attendees and staff; infected people should be excluded on the basis of age (see *Salmonella* Infections, p 584).
Non-serotype Typhi *Salmonella* infection	Exclusion until diarrhea resolves. Negative stool culture results not required for non-serotype Typhi *Salmonella* species.	Symptomatic contacts should be excluded until symptoms resolve. Stool cultures are not required for asymptomatic contacts. Antimicrobial therapy is not recommended for asymptomatic infection or uncomplicated diarrhea or for contacts.
Scabies	Exclusion until after treatment given.	Close contacts with prolonged skin-to-skin contact should have prophylactic therapy. Bedding and clothing in contact with skin of infected people should be laundered (see Scabies, p 589).
Shiga toxin-producing *Escherichia coli* (STEC), including *E coli* O157:H7, or *Shigella* infection	Exclusion until diarrhea resolves and results of 2 stool cultures are negative for these organisms, depending on state regulations.	Meticulous hand hygiene; stool cultures should be performed for contacts. Center(s) with cases should be closed to new admissions during *E coli* O157:H7 outbreak (see *Escherichia coli* diarrhea, p 294, and *Shigella* infections, p 593).
Staphylococcus aureus skin infections	Exclusion only if skin lesions are draining and cannot be covered with a watertight dressing.	Meticulous hand hygiene; cultures of contacts are not recommended.
Streptococcal pharyngitis	Exclusion until 24 hours after treatment has been initiated and the child is able to participate in activities.	Symptomatic contacts of documented cases of group A streptococcal infection should be tested and treated if test results are positive.
Tuberculosis	For active disease, exclusion until determined to be noninfectious by physician or health department authority. May return to activities after therapy is instituted, symptoms have diminished, and adherence to therapy is documented. No exclusion for latent tuberculosis infection (LTBI).	Local health department personnel should be informed for contact investigation (see Tuberculosis, p 680).
Varicella (see Varicella-Zoster Infections, p 714)	Exclusion until all lesions have dried and crusted (usually 6 days after onset of rash in immunocompetent people; may be longer in immunocompromised people).	Varicella vaccine should be administered by 3 to 5 days after exposure, and Varicella-Zoster Immune Globulin should be administered up to 96 hours after exposure when indicated.

From: American Academy of Pediatrics. Children in out-of-home child care. In: Pickering LK, Baker CJ, Kimberlin DW, Long SS, eds. *Red Book: 2009 Report of the Committee on Infectious Diseases.* 28th ed. Elk Grove Village, IL: American Academy of Pediatrics; 2009:129-130.

Antiviral Drugs for Influenza

Drug (Trade Name)	Virus	Administration	Treatment Indications[a]	Prophylaxis Indications[a]	Adverse Effects
Oseltamivir[b] (Tamiflu)	A and B	Oral	1 y of age or older	1 y of age or older	Nausea, vomiting
Zanamivir (Relenza)	A and B	Inhalation	7 y of age or older	5 y of age or older	Bronchospasm
Amantadine[c] (Symmetrel)	A	Oral	1 y of age or older	1 y of age or older	Central nervous system, anxiety, gastrointestinal
Rimantadine[c] (Flumadine)	A	Oral	13 y of age or older	1 y of age or older	Central nervous system, anxiety, gastrointestinal

[a]US Food and Drug Administration (FDA)-approved ages.
[b]High prevalence of resistance among H1N1 influenza strains.
[c]High prevalence of adamantane resistance among H3N2 and B influenza strains.

See **www.cdc.gov/flu/professionals/antivirals/index.htm** or **www.aapredbook.org/flu** for current information for use of antiviral drugs for treatment or chemoprophylaxis against influenza.

From: American Academy of Pediatrics. Influenza. In: Pickering LK, Baker CJ, Kimberlin DW, Long SS, eds. *Red Book: 2009 Report of the Committee on Infectious Diseases.* 28th ed. Elk Grove Village, IL: American Academy of Pediatrics; 2009:404.

Definitions of Positive Tuberculin Skin Test (TST) Results in Infants, Children, and Adolescents

Induration 5 mm or greater

Children in close contact with known or suspected contagious people with tuberculosis disease

Children suspected to have tuberculosis disease:
* Findings on chest radiograph consistent with active or previous tuberculosis disease
* Clinical evidence of tuberculosis disease[b]

Children receiving immunosuppressive therapy[c] or with immunosuppressive conditions, including human immunodeficiency (HIV) infection

Induration 10 mm or greater

Children at increased risk of disseminated tuberculosis disease:
* Children younger than 4 years of age
* Children with other medical conditions, including Hodgkin disease, lymphoma, diabetes mellitus, chronic renal failure, or malnutrition (see Table 3.80, p 684)

Children with likelihood of increased exposure to tuberculosis disease:
* Children born in high-prevalence regions of the world
* Children frequently exposed to adults who are HIV infected, homeless, users of illicit drugs, residents of nursing homes, incarcerated or institutionalized, or migrant farm workers
* Children who travel to high-prevalence regions of the world

Induration 15 mm or greater

Children 4 years of age or older without any risk factors

[a]These definitions apply regardless of previous bacille Calmette-Guérin (BCG) immunization (see also Interpretation of TST Results in Previous Recipients of BCG Vaccine, p 685); erythema alone at TST site does not indicate a positive test result. Tests should be read at 48 to 72 hours after placement.
[b]Evidence by physical examination or laboratory assessment that would include tuberculosis in the working differential diagnosis (eg, meningitis).
[c]Including immunosuppressive doses of corticosteroids (see Corticosteroids, p 694).

From: American Academy of Pediatrics. Tuberculosis. In: Pickering LK, Baker CJ, Kimberlin DW, Long SS, eds. *Red Book: 2009 Report of the Committee on Infectious Diseases.* 28th ed. Elk Grove Village, IL: American Academy of Pediatrics; 2009:681.

Tuberculin Skin Test (TST) Recommendations for Infants, Children, and Adolescents[a]

Children for whom immediate TST or IGRA is indicated[b]:
- Contacts of people with confirmed or suspected contagious tuberculosis (contact investigation)
- Children with radiographic or clinical findings suggesting tuberculosis disease
- Children immigrating from countries with endemic infection (eg, Asia, Middle East, Africa, Latin America, countries of the former Soviet Union), including international adoptees
- Children with travel histories to countries with endemic infection and substantial contact with indigenous people from such countries[c]

Children who should have annual TST or IGRA:
- Children infected with HIV infection (TST only)
- Incarcerated adolescents

Children at increased risk of progression of LTBI to tuberculosis disease: Children with other medical conditions, including diabetes mellitus, chronic renal failure, malnutrition, and congenital or acquired immunodeficiencies deserve special consideration. Without recent exposure, these people are not at increased risk of acquiring tuberculosis infection. Underlying immune deficiencies associated with these conditions theoretically would enhance the possibility for progression to severe disease. Initial histories of potential exposure to tuberculosis should be included for all of these patients. If these histories or local epidemiologic factors suggest a possibility of exposure, immediate and periodic TST or IGRA should be considered. **An initial TST or IGRA should be performed before initiation of immunosuppressive therapy, including prolonged steroid administration, use of tumor necrosis factor-alpha antagonists, or other immunosuppressive therapy in any child requiring these treatments.**

IGRA indicates interferon-gamma release assay; HIV, human immunodeficiency virus; LTBI, latent tuberculosis infection.
[a]Bacille Calmette-Guérin immunization is not a contraindication to a TST.
[b]Beginning as early as 3 months of age.
[c]If the child is well, the TST or IGRA should be delayed for up to 10 weeks after return.

From: American Academy of Pediatrics. Tuberculosis. In: Pickering LK, Baker CJ, Kimberlin DW, Long SS, eds. *Red Book: 2009 Report of the Committee on Infectious Diseases.* 28th ed. Elk Grove Village, IL: American Academy of Pediatrics; 2009:684.

Validated Questions for Determining Risk of LTBI in Children in the United States

- Has a family member or contact had tuberculosis disease?
- Has a family member had a positive tuberculin skin test result?
- Was your child born in a high-risk country (countries other than the United States, Canada, Australia, New Zealand, or Western European countries)?
- Has your child traveled (had contact with resident populations) to a high-risk country for more than 1 week?

LTBI indicates latent tuberculosis infection.

From: American Academy of Pediatrics. Tuberculosis. In: Pickering LK, Baker CJ, Kimberlin DW, Long SS, eds. *Red Book: 2009 Report of the Committee on Infectious Diseases.* 28th ed. Elk Grove Village, IL: American Academy of Pediatrics; 2009:685.

Management of Septic Shock Algorithm

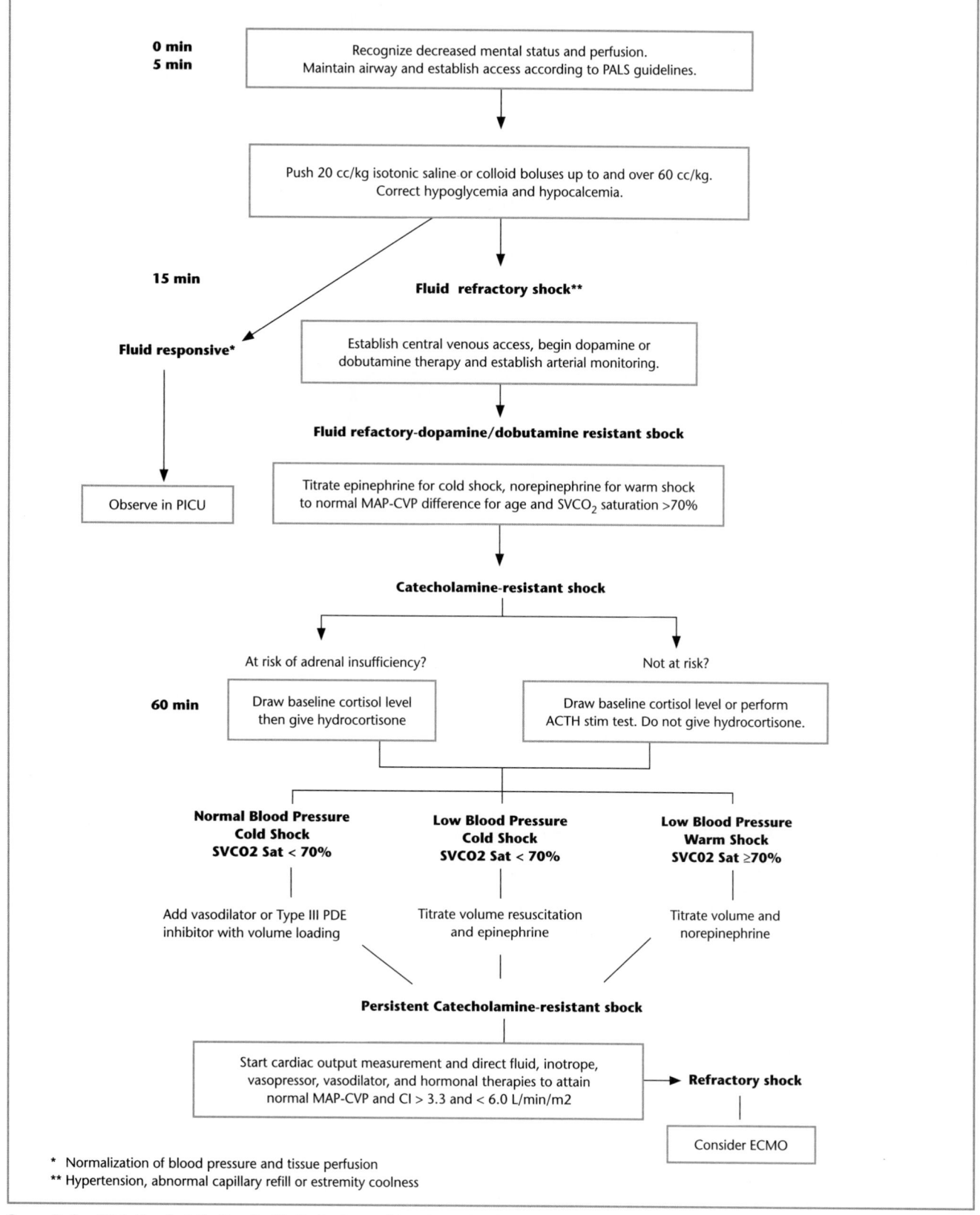

0 min
5 min
Recognize decreased mental status and perfusion.
Maintain airway and establish access according to PALS guidelines.

Push 20 cc/kg isotonic saline or colloid boluses up to and over 60 cc/kg.
Correct hypoglycemia and hypocalcemia.

15 min

Fluid refractory shock**

Establish central venous access, begin dopamine or
dobutamine therapy and establish arterial monitoring.

Fluid responsive*

Fluid refactory-dopamine/dobutamine resistant sbock

Titrate epinephrine for cold shock, norepinephrine for warm shock
to normal MAP-CVP difference for age and $SVCO_2$ saturation >70%

Observe in PICU

Catecholamine-resistant shock

At risk of adrenal insufficiency?   Not at risk?

60 min
Draw baseline cortisol level
then give hydrocortisone

Draw baseline cortisol level or perform
ACTH stim test. Do not give hydrocortisone.

Normal Blood Pressure
Cold Shock
SVCO2 Sat < 70%

Low Blood Pressure
Cold Shock
SVCO2 Sat < 70%

Low Blood Pressure
Warm Shock
SVC02 Sat ≥70%

Add vasodilator or Type III PDE
inhibitor with volume loading

Titrate volume resuscitation
and epinephrine

Titrate volume and
norepinephrine

Persistent Catecholamine-resistant sbock

Start cardiac output measurement and direct fluid, inotrope,
vasopressor, vasodilator, and hormonal therapies to attain
normal MAP-CVP and CI > 3.3 and < 6.0 L/min/m2

Refractory shock

Consider ECMO

* Normalization of blood pressure and tissue perfusion
** Hypertension, abnormal capillary refill or estremity coolness

From: Parker MM, Hazelzet JA, Carcillo JA. Pediatric considerations. *Crit Care Med.* 2004;32(11 suppl):S591-S594.

Medications

Drugs for Which Absorption Is Increased by Food

Atovaquone (administer with a high-fat meal)
Cefpodoxime
Cefuroxime
Erythromycin
Griseofulvin (administer with a high-fat meal)
Morphine sulfate (oral solution)
Nitrofurantoin
Theophylline sustained release (food may induce sudden release of sustained-release preparation)

From: Kleinman RE, ed. *Pediatric Nutrition Handbook*. Elk Grove Village, IL: American Academy of Pediatrics; 2009.

Drugs for Which Absorption May Be Delayed by Food or Milk

Medication Name	Comments
Acetaminophen	Rate may decreased by high carbohydrate load
Amitriptyline	Increased fiber may decrease effect
Ampicillin	Food decreases rate and extent of absorption
Cefaclor	Delays and decreases peak concentration
Cephalexin	Food may delay absorption
Cimetidine	Limit xanthine-containing food and beverages
Ciprofloxacin	Dairy products/minerals decrease concentration
Digoxin	Increased fiber or pectin may decrease absorption
Diltiazem	Food may increase absorption from sustained-release product
Fluoxetine	Food may delay absorption
Furosemide	Avoid acidic solutions
Glipizide	Rate of absorption, not extent, delayed by food
Lansoprazole	Food decreases bioavailability by 40%
Metronidazole	
Omeprazole	Administering with food decreases level by 50%
Penicillin	
Trazodone	Rate of absorption, not extent, delayed by food
Valproic acid	Rate of absorption, not extent, delayed by food
Zafirlukast	Food decreases absorption by 40%
Zalcitabine	

(Drugs in this category should either be administered on an empty stomach or taken consistently with regard to food.)
From: Kleinman RE, ed. *Pediatric Nutrition Handbook*. Elk Grove Village, IL: American Academy of Pediatrics; 2009.

Drugs That Should Be Administered on an Empty Stomach

Medication Name	Comments
Ampicillin	
Amprenavir	Avoid antacids and high-fat meals
Captopril	
Ceftibuten	
Cloxacillin	
Dicloxacillin	
Didanosine	
Diltiazem	
Efavirenz	
Erythromycin base	
Indinavir	
Iron	Avoid milk and antacids
Isoniazid	
Itraconazole oral solution	
Ketoconazole	Administer 2 h before antacids; may administer with food to decrease gastrointestinal distress
Lansoprazole	
Levofloxacin oral solution	
Loracarbef	
Mycophenolate	
Nifedipine	
Omeprazole	
Rifampin	May administer with food to decrease gastrointestinal distress
Tacrolimus	Separate antacids by at least 2 hours
Tetracycline	
Zafirlukast	

From: Kleinman RE, ed. *Pediatric Nutrition Handbook.* Elk Grove Village, IL: American Academy of Pediatrics; 2009.

Neurologic

Classification of Concussion

GRADE	DEFINITION	MANAGEMENT
1	Transient confusion No loss of consciousness, mental status abnormalities for < 15 min	Return to sports activities same day only if all symptoms resolve within 15 min. If a second grade-1 concussion occurs, no sports activity until asymptomatic for 1 week.
2	Transient confusion No loss of consciousness, mental status abnormalities for > 15 min	No sports activity until asymptomatic for 1 week. If a grade-2 concussion occurs on the same day as a previous grade-1 concussion, no sports activity for 2 weeks.

3	Concussion involving any loss of consciousness	No sports activity until asymptomatic for 1 week if loss of consciousness was brief (seconds).
		No sports activity until asymptomatic for 2 weeks if loss of consciousness was prolonged (minutes or longer).
		Second grade-3 concussion.
		    No sports activity until asymptomatic for 1 month.
		Any abnormality on CT or MRI.
		    No sports activity for remainder of season.
		    Patient should be discouraged from any future return to contact sports.

*Concussion symptoms: early (minutes and hours)—headache, dizziness or vertigo, lack of awareness of surroundings, nausea or vomiting. Late (days to weeks)—persistent low-grade headache, light-headedness, poor attention and concentration, memory dysfunction, easy fatigability, irritability and low frustration tolerance, intolerance to bright lights or difficulty focusing vision, intolerance of loud noises, sometimes ringing in the ears, anxiety or depressed mood, sleep disturbance. CT, Computed tomography; MRI, magnetic resonance imaging.

From: Quality Standards Committee, American Academy of Neurology. Practice parameter: the management of concussion in sports (summary statement). Neurology. 1997;48(3):581–585.

Glasgow Coma Scale

EYE-OPENING RESPONSE

SCORE	>1 YEAR	<1 YEAR
4	Spontaneous	Spontaneous
3	To verbal command	To shout
2	To pain	To pain
1	None	None

MOTOR RESPONSE

SCORE	>1 YEAR	<1 YEAR
6	Obeys commands	Spontaneous response
5	Localizes pain	Localizes pain
4	Withdraws from pain	Withdraws from pain
3	Displays abnormal flexion to pain (decorticate rigidity)	Displays abnormal flexion to pain (decorticate rigidity)
2	Displays abnormal extension to pain (decerebrate rigidity)	Displays abnormal extension to pain (decerebrate rigidity)
1	None	None

VERBAL RESPONSE

SCORE	>5 YEARS	2 TO 5 YEARS	0-23 MONTHS
5	Is oriented and converses	Uses appropriate words and phrases	Babbles, coos appropriately
4	Conversation is confused	Use inappropriate words	Cries but is consolable
3	Words are inappropriate	Cries or screams persistently to pain	Cries or screams persistently to pain
2	Sounds are incomprehensible	Grunts or moans to pain	Grunts or moans to pain
1	None	None	None

*The Glasgow Coma Scale score is the sum of best eye-opening, motor, and verbal responses. Scores range from 3 to 15. Severe indicates a score of <9; moderteate, 9-12; and mild, 13-15.

Modified from:Teasdale G, Jennett B.Assessment of coma and impaired consciousness: a practical scale. *Lancet.* 1974;304(7872):81-84. Copyright © Elsevier 1974.

Obesity

**Body Mass Index for Age Percentiles:
Girls, 2 to 20 Years**

**Body Mass Index for Age Percentiles:
Boys, 2 to 20 Years**

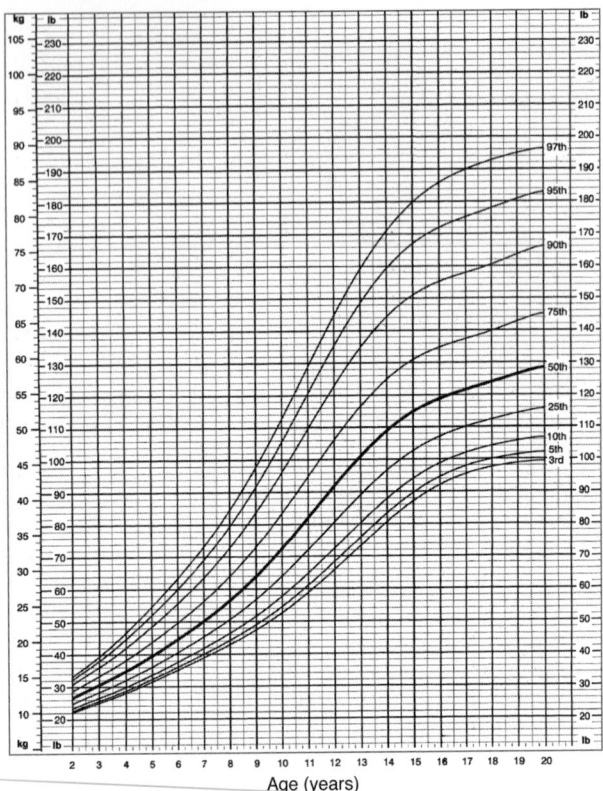

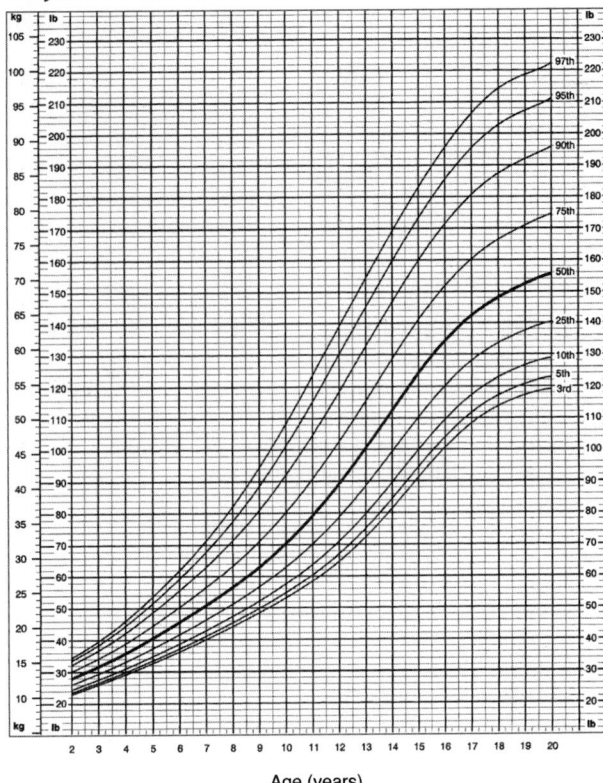

Developed by the National Center for Health Statistics in collaboration with the National Center for Chronic Disease Prevention and Health Promotion (2000).

Interpreting BMI

Growth Indicator	Anthropometric Indices	Percentile Cutoff
Underweight	Low BMI for age and gender	<5th percentile
Normal	Normal BMI for age and gender	≥5th percentile but <85th percentile
Overweight	High BMI for age and gender	≥85th percentile but <95th percentile
Obese	High BMI for age and gender	≥95th percentile

From: Hagan JF, Shaw JS, Duncan PM, eds. *Bright Futures: Guidelines for Health Supervision of Infants, Children, and Adolescents.* 3rd ed. Elk Grove Village, IL: American Academy of Pediatrics; 2008.

Percentiles for Assessing Overweight and Obesity

Percentile	Status
<85th	Normal, or healthy, weight
≥85th but <95th	Overweight
≥95th	Obese

From: Hagan JF, Shaw JS, Duncan PM, eds. *Bright Futures: Guidelines for Health Supervision of Infants, Children, and Adolescents.* 3rd ed. Elk Grove Village, IL: American Academy of Pediatrics; 2008.

Oral Health

American Academy of Pediatrics Dentistry Caries-Risk Assessment Tool (CAT)

Risk Factors to Consider	Risk Indicators		
(For each item below, circle the most accurate response found to the right under "Risk Indicators")	High	Moderate	Low
Part 1 – History (determined by interviewing the parent/primary caregiver)			
Child has special health care needs, especially any that impact motor coordination or cooperation[A]	Yes		No
Child has condition that impairs saliva (dry mouth)[B]	Yes		No
Child's use of dental home (frequency of routine dental visits)	None	Irregular	Regular
Child has decay	Yes		No
Time lapsed since child's last cavity	<12 months	12 to 24 months	>24 months
Child wears braces or orthodontic/oral appliances[C]	Yes		No
Child's parent and/or sibling(s) have decay	Yes		No
Socioeconomic status of child's parents[D]	Low	Mid-level	High
Daily between-meal exposures to sugars/cavity producing foods (includes on demand use of bottle/sippy cup containing liquid other than water; consumption of juice, carbonated beverages, or sports drinks; use of sweetened medications)[E]	>3	1 to 2	Mealtime only
Child's exposure to fluoride[F,G]	Does not use fluoridated toothpaste; drinking water is not fluoridated and is not taking fluoride supplements	Uses fluoridated toothpaste; usually does not drink fluoridated water and does not take fluoride supplements	Uses fluoridated toothpaste; drinks fluoridated water or takes fluoride supplements
Times per day that child's teeth/gums are brushed	<1	1	2-3
Part 2 – Clinical evaluation (determined by examining the child's mouth)			
Visible plaque (white, sticky buildup)	Present		Absent
Gingivitis (red, puffy gums)[H]	Present		Absent
Areas of enamel demineralization (chalky white-spots on teeth)	More than 1	1	None
Enamel defects, deep pits/fissures[I]	Present		Absent
Part 3 – Supplemental professional assessment (Optional)[J]			
Radiographic enamel caries	Present		Absent
Levels of mutans streptococci or lactobacilli	High	Moderate	Low

Each child's overall assessed risk for developing decay is based on the highest level of risk indicator circled above (ie, single risk indicator in any area of the "high risk" category classifies a child as being "high risk").

continued

American Academy of Pediatrics Dentistry Caries-Risk Assessment Tool (CAT), continued

A   Children with special health care needs are those who have a physical, developmental, mental, sensory, behavioral, cognitive, or emotional impairment or limiting condition that requires medical management, health care intervention, and/or use of specialized services. The condition may be developmental or acquired and may cause limitations in performing daily self-maintenance activities or substantial limitations in a major life activity. Health care for special needs patients is beyond that considered routine and requires specialized knowledge, increased awareness and attention, and accommodation.

B   Alteration in salivary flow can be the result of congenital or acquired conditions, surgery, radiation, medication, or age-related changes in salivary function. Any condition, treatment, or process known or reported to alter saliva flow should be considered an indication of risk unless proven otherwise.

C   Orthodontic appliances include both fixed and removable appliances, space maintainers, and other devices that remain in the mouth continuously or for prolonged time intervals and which may trap food and plaque, prevent oral hygiene, compromise access of tooth surfaces to fluoride, or otherwise create an environment supporting caries initiation.

D   National surveys have demonstrated that children in low-income and moderate-income households are more likely to have caries and more decayed or filled primary teeth than children from more affluent households. Also, within income levels, minority children are more likely to have caries. Thus, socioeconomic status should be viewed as an initial indicator of risk that may be offset by the absence of other risk indicators.

E   Examples of sources of simple sugars include carbonated beverages, cookies, cake, candy, cereal, potato chips, French fries, corn chips, pretzels, breads, juices, and fruits. Clinicians using caries-risk assessment should investigate individual exposures to sugars known to be involved in caries initiation.

F   Optimal systemic and topical fluoride exposure is based on use of a fluoride dentifrice and American Dental Association/American Academy of Pediatrics guidelines for exposure from fluoride drinking water and/or supplementation.

G   Unsupervised use of toothpaste and at-home topical fluoride products are not recommended for children unable to expectorate predictably.

H   Although microbial organisms responsible for gingivitis may be different than those primarily implicated in caries, the presence of gingivitis is an indicator of poor or infrequent oral hygiene practices and has been associated with caries progression.

I   Tooth anatomy and hypoplastic defects (eg, poorly formed enamel, developmental pits) may predispose a child to develop caries.

J   Advanced technologies such as radiographic assessment and microbiologic testing are not essential for using this tool.

From: Hagan JF, Shaw JS, Duncan PM, eds. *Bright Futures: Guidelines for Health Supervision of Infants, Children, and Adolescents.* 3rd ed. Elk Grove Village, IL: American Academy of Pediatrics; 2008.

Dietary Fluoride Supplementation Schedule

Age	<0.3 ppm F	0.3-0.6 ppm F	>0.6 ppm F
Birth-6 months	0	0	0
6 mo-3 years	0.25 mg	0	0
3-6 years	0.50 mg	0.25 mg	0
6 y up to at least 16 years	1.00 mg	0.50 mg	0

From: American Academy of Pediatric Dentistry Liaison with Other Groups Committee; American Academy of Pediatric Dentistry Council on Clinical Affairs. Guideline on fluoride therapy. *Pediatr Dent.* 2008–2009;30(7 Suppl):121–124. The Guideline on Fluoride Therapy is Copyright © 2009–10 by the American Academy of Pediatric Dentistry and is reproduced with their permission.

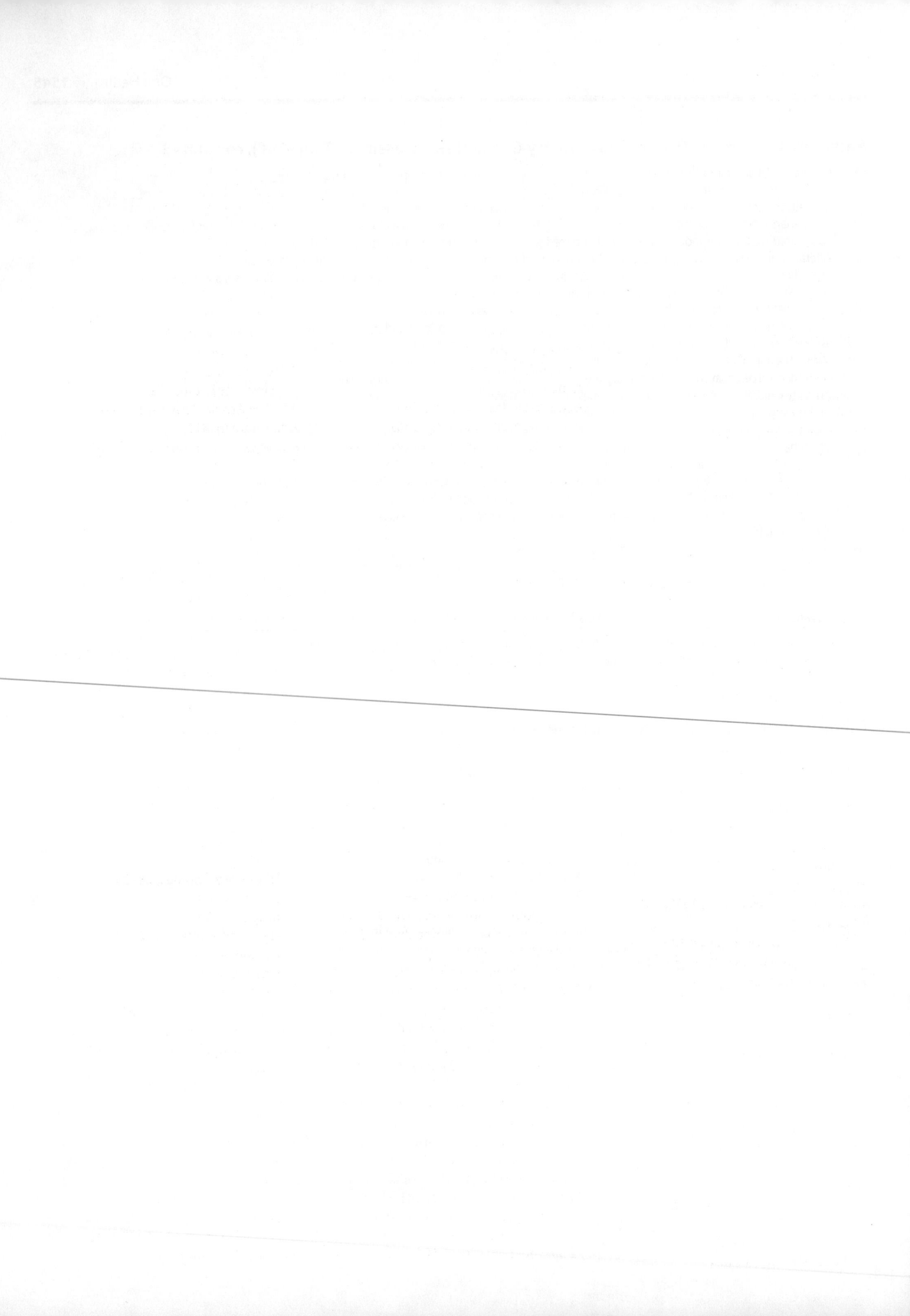

Index

Chapter 15

Changing the Social Environment to Prevent Injuries

James A. Mercy, Karin A. Mack, and
Malinda Steenkamp

15.1. INTRODUCTION

The social environment has a powerful influence on the risk of being injured. This influence is mediated through the myriad ways it shapes the lifestyles, exposures, and behaviors of individuals. The building blocks of our social environment are social interactions or the ways that people act toward, respond to, or influence one another (Robertson, 1987). These interactions are shaped by our culture, the structure of social relations as reflected in the nature of institutions such as the family and the economic order, and processes such as the socialization of children.

Although we have made great strides in modifying the physical environment as an injury prevention strategy, our understanding of how to intervene on the social environment to prevent injury remains relatively undeveloped. Part of the reason lies in the imbalance that has existed in epidemiological research on injury. This research, much like for many other areas of public health, has been dominated by an individually focused risk-factor paradigm that directs attention toward programs that are designed to help people change their behavior to lower their risk for injury or behaving violently (Stokols, 1992; Yen & Syme, 1999). A focus on the social environment shares the ultimate intention of changing individual behavior, but the focus of intervention shifts from the individual to the social environment in which people live and interact (Task Force on Community Preventive Services [TFCPS], 2003; Yen & Syme, 1999).

The purposes of this chapter are (1) to provide a conceptual framework for discussing the relationship between the social environment and injury prevention; (2) to provide illustrative evidence for a link between the social environment and injury; (3) to articulate the value of modifying the social environment for injury prevention; and (4) to describe and assess the evidence for selected injury prevention interventions, programs, or policies that are related to the social environment.

We hope this chapter will provide a basis for more fully incorporating injury prevention strategies that address the social environment into the mainstream of the injury prevention field.

15.2.   KEY DIMENSIONS OF THE SOCIAL ENVIRONMENT

Our social environment shapes our lives in multiple ways. The influence that the groups to which we belong and the social interactions that take place within these groups have on our personality, behavior, social experience, and options in life, however, is often not recognized or is taken for granted. The tendency for people everywhere is to accept their society and its customs unquestionably and to view their social environment as largely immutable. But society is, in fact, changing all of the time and is a product created by human beings and capable of being changed by them as well.

Three dimensions of the social environment that are particularly important to injury prevention are culture, social structure, and social processes. Through an understanding of these dimensions we can begin to appreciate the numerous ways that the social environment affects injury and the possibilities for changing the social environment in order to prevent injury.

15.2.1.   Culture

Unlike animals, human beings are not born with inflexible, genetically determined behavior patterns that enable them to survive in specific habitats (Robertson, 1987). Human beings must invent and learn cultural means of adapting to different environments and changing conditions (Dubos, 1980). Whereas other animals must rely on biological evolution to adapt to their environments, humans can use culture to adapt quickly to changing conditions. Culture embodies the learned ways of life that are used to adapt to our environment. It includes the shared beliefs, values, customs, symbols, communication styles, and behaviors that members of a society "use to cope with the world and with one another, and that are transmitted from generation to generation through learning" (Bates & Fratkin, 2003: pp. 3–4). Cultural context plays an important role in both contributing to injury and protecting people from injury (Vaughn, Anderson, Agran, & Winn, 2004). The difficulty of changing culture, however, should not be underestimated. Cultural beliefs, values, customs, symbols, and behaviors are often very entrenched in societies because they are rationalized by a body of shared knowledge and beliefs that most members of a society accept, sometimes without question and often unconsciously (Mercy, 2005).

15.2.2.   Social Structure

All complex things have a structure that is composed of a set of interrelated parts. Social structure is the "pattern of relationships among the basic components of a society" (Robertson, 1987: p. 90). The most important components of social structure are statuses, roles, groups, and institutions (Robertson, 1987). These components are found in every human society, although their nature and the interrelationships among them vary from society to society.

Status refers to a person's position within society. Some examples of social status include parent, elder, teacher, or poor person. Socioeconomic status is particularly relevant for understanding and preventing injury. Roles are the "set of expected behavior patterns, obligations, and privileges associated with a particular status" (Robertson, 1987: p. 91). A parent, for example, is a social status that is associated with a role or set of expectations for how a person occupying that status is expected to behave in raising his or her children. The nature of the expectations for parental behavior in a particular society, such as those associated with discipline or supervision, may have an important influence on the risks for injury faced by their children. Some of these expectations are codified in laws. Groups are "a collection of people interacting together in an orderly way on the basis of shared expectations about each others' behavior" (Robertson, 1987: p. 92). Membership in certain groups such as gangs can have a profound influence on the risk of suffering an injury or behaving violently toward another person (Esbensen & Huizinga, 1993). Institutions are "a stable cluster of values, norms, statuses, roles, and groups that are organized to address a basic social need" (Robertson, 1987: p. 93). The institution of the family provides for the care of children, economic institutions provide and distribute goods and services, and political institutions allocate and maintain power. The nature of the familial, economic, political, educational, legal, and religious institutions that make up societies can play a pivotal role in affecting the character and magnitude of injury in any society. The citizens of nations with disorganized or corrupt legal institutions, for example, are at greater risk of injuries associated with the extrajudicial use of violence to solve problems, which the police or courts are unable or unwilling to address (Mercy, 2005).

The social structure of a society also has important implications for the nature and intensity of social interactions in a society. For example, the organization of communities influences the extent to which people feel connected to, interact with, and trust other people in their community. Early sociological research on social organization has supported the idea that communities have features that "strengthen or weaken social support and social cohesion, and these have important implications for the health of residents in those areas" (Yen & Kaplan, 1999; Yen & Syme, 1999: p. 293). Building on this early research, scholars are now examining the relationship between social organization and the ability of a community to realize its own values and maintain effective social controls over violence and other antisocial behavior (Sampson, 1998; Sampson, Raudenbush & Earls, 1997).

15.2.3. Social Processes

In addition to the cultural and structural building blocks of society, there are also common patterns of social interaction that enable societies to dynamically address basic social needs. These social processes are based on clusters of values, norms, and beliefs and enacted out in the context of groups and institutions. As with social structures, these processes are found in every human society, although their nature may vary greatly from society to society. Socialization, for example, is the process of social interaction whereby people learn "the norms, values, languages, skills, beliefs and other patterns of thought and action that are essential for social living" (Robertson, 1987: p. 115). Family, schools, peers, media, and religious institutions all play a role in socialization. How children are socialized in a particular society about values related to risk taking or their role as intimate partners, caregivers, or workers may have an important influence on their risk for injury. Another social process that is particularly relevant to injury prevention is the process of conflict resolution. The extent to which violence is legitimized as a means of conflict resolution, for example, has clear implications for certain types of injury.

15.2.4. The Ecological Model

One way to illustrate the different ways that the social environment influences behavior related to injury is through the use of an ecological framework (Fig. 15.1) (Bronfenbrenner, 1992). This type of framework is useful for organizing risk and protective factors and the prevention strategies that can be used to address them. It also helps us see how the experiences and attributes of individuals that contribute to injury and its prevention are nested within and influenced by increasingly broader social contexts (Allegrante, Marks, & Hansen, 2006). The social environment encompasses those ecological contexts that surround the individual (Fig. 15.1)—that is, the relationship, community, and societal levels. The influence of culture, social structure, and social processes are evident within each of the levels of this model.

The individual level of the ecological model addresses biological and personal characteristics (e.g., gender, age, ability to swim, history of aggression) that may influence injury-related behaviors. The relationship level addresses the influence that close interpersonal relationships, such as those with family members, peers, caregivers, and intimate partners, have on the occurrence of injury and its prevention. This would include, for example, the influence of peer pressure on engaging in risky behaviors (e.g., drunk driving) or even on participating in bullying and fighting behaviors.

The community level focuses on the characteristics of communities or settings within communities (e.g., neighborhoods, schools, churches, and workplaces) that may create conditions that increase or decrease the risk of injury. For example, the extent to which the elderly are socially isolated within a community, due to the rural nature of a community or the absence of support services, may influence risk for a variety of injuries from falls to those resulting from elder abuse.

The societal level encompasses the influence of broad cultural, social, and economic factors on the risk of injury and its prevention. Included among these factors, for example, are the social norms or values imbedded in the culture, the laws and other broad social policies (e.g., welfare reform) that are adopted, and the influence of economic cycles on the risk of injury (e.g., recessions). Laws that require seat belts and air bags to be built into our cars or proscribe heavy sentences if we are convicted of assaulting another person are examples of societal-level influences because they are so broadly endorsed and enforced that their influence crosscuts

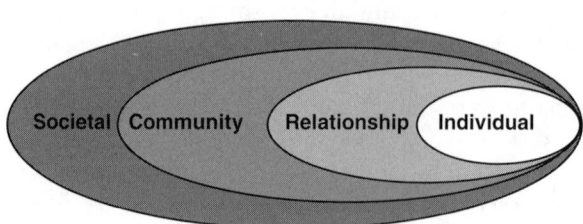

Figure 15.1. The ecological model. (Reprinted with permission from Dahlberg and Krug, 2002.)

communities in our society (Stier, Mercy, & Kohn, 2006). Each of the broader ecological niches can have an effect on the niches within it (Stokols, 1992, 1996). For example, changing societal norms about the acceptability of drinking and driving may influence the nature of key relationships and interactions between individuals such as the extent to which parents supervise their children's driving behaviors or the extent to which people intervene to prevent their friends and acquaintances from drinking and driving.

15.3.   THE SOCIAL ENVIRONMENT AND THE OCCURRENCE OF INJURY

As we have suggested, there are many ways in which the social environment is related to the risk of suffering or causing an injury. In this section we provide examples to illustrate these interconnections organized around the levels of the ecological model that make up the social environment.

15.3.1.   Relationships

Perhaps the most influential set of social relationships in any society are those we have with our family. One of the primary roles of the family is the socialization of children, and the primary actors in the socialization of children are, of course, parents. The manner in which parents carry out this role has been found to have an important effect on the likelihood that a child will behave violently later in life. Early inconsistent and harsh discipline of children younger then 5 years old by parents has consistently been found to predict behavior problems, including violence, in adolescence (Dodge & Pettit, 2003; Knutson, DeGarmo, & Reid, 2004). Aggression and antisocial behavior are commonly reported outcomes for both physically abused and neglected children (Knutson & Schartz, 1997). Parental neglect and poor supervision are thought to contribute to violent and antisocial behavior by compromising the social competence of children and, thereby, impairing their ability to form positive relationships with well-socialized peers (Dishion, Spracklen, Andrews, & Patterson, 1996; Knutson & Schartz, 1997). These children are more likely, therefore, to be rejected by well-socialized peers and form affiliations with deviant peers who encourage and model antisocial behavior.

One primary role of the parent is protecting the child or fostering socialization toward injury prevention behaviors (Peterson, Bartelstone, Kern, & Gillies, 1995). Parents, however, may believe that injuries are a natural part of growing and learning and are simply the result of careless or inattentive behavior on the part of the child. Further, parents may believe unintentional injuries are a necessary part of childhood to learn about risky situations or coping with pain (Lewis, DiLillo, & Peterson, 2004; Morrongiello & Dayler, 1996; Murphy, 2001). If the role of the family within a society is to raise independent, resilient children, there may be a greater emphasis on allowing children to "be curious" or "make mistakes" so they can learn lessons that toughen them for adulthood (Lewis et al., 2004). These beliefs make injury prevention efforts challenging. These concepts carry over beyond parental supervision and into other realms such as sports. Coaching styles, for example, may influence the extent to which pain and injury are normalized ("no pain, no gain") as part of the process of participating in some sports (Nixon, 1992).

Other relationships important to injury include those with peers. Friends and peers have an increasingly important influence on children as they move into and through adolescence (Dahlberg, 1998; Mercy, Sleet, & Doll, 2006). Although peer influences during adolescence are generally considered positive and important in shaping later interpersonal relationships, they can also have negative effects. Having delinquent friends, for example, is one of the strongest and most consistently found risk factors for violent behavior among youth (Lipsey & Derzon, 1998; Thornberry, Huizinga, & Loeber, 1995; U.S. Department of Health and Human Services [HHS], 2001).

15.3.2.   Community[1]

An important feature of communities that has implications for injury prevention is the degree, nature, and distribution of poverty that exists within their boundaries. Poverty is, in part, a consequence of broader societal influences, such as the prevailing economic system and business cycles; but the influence of poverty on the risk for injury within communities has more direct implications for prevention. Poverty is consistently found to have a strong and positive correlation with interpersonal violence, especially homicide (Wilson, 1987). However, when other community indicators of social structure distinct from, but related to, poverty are controlled, this association is substantially weakened, suggesting that the effect of poverty on interpersonal violence may be conditional on these factors. These factors include high residential mobility; concentrations of poverty; family disruption; high population density; and community disorganization, as reflected in weak intergenerational family and community ties, weak control of peer groups, and low participation in community organizations (Reiss & Roth, 1993; Sampson & Lauritsen, 1994). Another feature of a society's economic structure is the magnitude of the gap between the rich and the poor. This gap is typically measured by examining economic inequality. Great inequality in incomes is strongly associated with higher homicides rates in cross-national comparisons (Fajnzylber, Lederman, & Loayza, 2002; Gartner, 1990).

Poorer communities and their residents appear to be most vulnerable to interpersonal violence when exposed to fundamental economic and population changes that contribute to community disorganization and, ultimately, to a community's ability to control violent behavior. In the United States, for example, it has been argued that the shift from goods-producing industries to service-producing industries—and the associated relocation of manufacturing industries out of the inner cities that began in the 1960s—caused many inner-city communities to become increasingly isolated islands of poverty as middle- and working-class residents moved out of impoversihed communities into areas with better housing and job opportunities (Unnithan & Whitt, 1992). The exodus of more economically stable families from inner cities undermined the viability of basic community institutions, such as churches and schools, as social buffers against violence. The resulting concentration of poverty isolated primarily racial and ethnic minority (e.g., African-Americans and Hispanics) inner-city residents from job networks, available marriage partners, quality schools, and conventional role models. This led to a high concentration of the very factors that appear to mediate the relationship between poverty and interpersonal violence—residential instability, family disruption, and community

---

[1]Parts of this section were taken with minor revision from Mercy (2005).

disorganization (Reiss & Roth, 1993; Sampson & Lauritsen, 1994; Wilson, 1987). Recent research has supported the theory that the concentration of poverty and the imbalance between concentrations of affluence and poverty in a neighborhood are important predictors of community variations in interpersonal violence (Morenoff, Sampson, & Raudenbush, 2001).

Poverty has also been shown to be associated with increased risk of unintentional injuries (Cubbin & Smith, 2002; Durkin, Davidson, Kuhn, O'Connor, & Barlow, 1994; Lindqvist, Timpka, & Karlsson, 2004; Williams, Currie, Wright, Elton, & Beattie, 1996). Research efforts are now being directed at explaining this association by examining the cause of injuries and the location of injury events. Thus while some studies find no overall gradient in total incidence of medically attended injuries and socioeconomic status, there is evidence that some specific kinds of injuries have a strong relationship to poverty (Anderson et al., 1994; Williams et al., 1996). For example, low family affluence has been found to be predictive of injuries occurring in the home and on the roads, and high family affluence is predictive of a high incidence of injuries in schools and sports (Williams et al., 1996). Children eligible for Aid to Families with Dependent Children (AFDC) have been found to die at a higher rate than children not enrolled in AFDC from exogenous causes such as fires, drowning, firearms, and motor-vehicle crashes (Nelson, 1992). In addition, socioeconomic instability and ethnic diversity appear to have a protective effect on the risk of traffic- and sports-related injuries among boys but an aggravating one in the case of injuries from falls (Laflamme & Eilert-Petersson, 2001).

A characteristic of the social structure of communities that is closely related to the issues around poverty and that has received greater attention in recent years is social capital. Social capital has been defined as "those features of social organization—such as networks of secondary association, high levels of interpersonal trust and norms of mutual aid and reciprocity—which act as resources for individuals and facilitate collective action" (Lochner, Kawachi, & Kennedy, 1999, p. 260). It has been hypothesized that communities with low social capital would lack sufficient capacity to maintain or establish norms or social controls that reduce violence (Sampson & Wilson, 1995). Several studies have found low social capital to be associated with higher rates of homicide in states and neighborhoods in the United States (Galea, Karpati, & Kennedy, 2002; Kennedy, Kawachi, Prothrow-Stith, Lochnev, & Gupta, 1998; Sampson et al., 1997). High social capital has also been found to help explain children's well-being and healthy development in high-risk communities and, consequently, may also be associated with lower risk of maltreatment and unintentional injury among children (Runyan et al., 1998).

Another aspect of social structure that is associated with injury and is related to the concept of social captial is the degree to which people feel connected to other people and the institutions in their community. Students who feel connected to their school, for example, are less likely to experience emotional distress and suicidal thoughts; are less likely to drink alcohol, carry weapons, or engage in other delinquent behaviors; and are more likely to wear seat belts and bicycle helmets and use prosocial skills (e.g., cooperation, conflict resolution, and helping others) (Battistich & Hom, 1997; Hawkins & Lam, 1987; Nutbeam, Smith, Moore, & Bauman, 1993; Resnick et al., 1997). Students who feel connected to school also tend to perform better in school, and poor school performance is an early risk factor for violence (O'Donnell, Hawkins, Catalano, Abbott, & Day, 1995; USDHHS, 2001; Voelkl, 1995). One strategy that has been suggested for increasing feelings of connectedness to school is to foster the development of prosocial norms, skills, and behaviors (e.g., social competence, problem solving, autonomy, and role modeling) throughout the school environment—among faculty, staff members, and students. (Centers for Disease Control and Prevention [CDC], 2001).

15.3.3.   Societal[2]

One of the most important dimensions of the societal level of the ecological model is culture. Perhaps the most common way that culture influences injury is in the way it shapes our attitudes and beliefs toward other people. Injuries from violence, for example, can result from cultural beliefs and attitudes that foster negative stereotypes. A form of violence that is associated with negative or stereotypical attitudes and beliefs has come to be known as hate violence. Hate violence consists of acts of interpersonal or collective violence that are directed toward other people, property, or organizations because of the group to which they belong or identify with (American Psychological Association [APA], 1998). These forms of violence are most commonly perpetrated against individuals or groups based on race, ethnicity, religion, and sexual orientation.

Hate violence has a long tradition in the United States. It is perhaps best exemplified by the lynching of African Americans by both organized groups, such as the Ku Klux Klan, and unorganized lynch mobs, which escalated after the Civil War and Reconstruction (Brown, 1979). But other groups have also been targets of hate-related violence in the United States. Surveys conducted between 1988 and 1991 indicated that from 9% to 24% of gay respondents reported that they had been punched, hit, or kicked because of their sexual orientation (Berrill, 1992). Moreover, between 37% and 45% of gay respondents reported they had received threats of physical violence because of their sexual orientation (Berrill, 1992). In the 10 days after the terrorist attacks on September 11, 2001, violent attacks on people of Middle Eastern descent or those perceived to be of Middle Eastern descent escalated dramatically in the United States (Swahn et al., 2003).

Cultural norms about the status and role of men and women that we see in many parts of the world have an important influence on the nature and degree of violence that occurs between the genders. Cultural traditions that favor male over female children, early marriage for girls, male sexual entitlement, and female "purity," for example, place women and girls in a subordinate position relative to men and make them highly vulnerable to violent victimization (Bennet, Manderson, & Astbury, 2000; Hayward, 2000). More subtle cultural attitudes and beliefs about female roles may also contribute to violence and exist, to varying degrees, in every part of the world (Dobash & Dobash, 1979). An ethnographic study of wife beating in 90 societies concluded that it occurs most often in societies in which men hold the household economic and decision-making power, divorce is difficult for women to obtain, and violence is a common conflict-resolution tactic (Levinson, 1989). Rape is also more common in societies in which cultural traditions favoring male superiority are strong (Sanday, 1981).

Culturally proscribed gender roles and expectations have implications for risk of unintentional injuries as well. While there is little in the injury prevention literature focused on gender differences in injury risk and prevention, development of profiles of how risk-taking behaviors among men or women are generated by

---

[2]Parts of this section were taken with minor revision from Mercy (2005).

the social environment are being discussed (Mack, 2004; Moller, 1995; Nathanson, 1977), especially as they relate to the health of men (Courtenay, 2000; White, 2002). Morrongiello & Hogg (2004, p. 103) note that one of the "most robust epidemiological findings is that boys are at greater risk of injury than girls." Boys engage in more risk taking and in activities that pose greater risk for injury (Coppens & Gentry, 1991; Kontos, 2004; Spady, Saunders, Schopflocher, & Svenson, 2004). Gendered risk taking continues into adulthood as males define their roles to include heroic and risky behavior (Korllos, 1993; McCutcheon, Curtis, & White, 1997; Nathanson, 1977). This may be especially apparent in the area of sports, beyond that which can be accounted for by increased exposure. Injury prevention activities need to be planned to assist with the development of competence in sports but also consider, or in some cases mediate, gender role expectations.

15.4.   INTERVENING IN THE SOCIAL ENVIRONMENT TO PREVENT INJURY

Although examples of the association between the social environment and injury abound, examples of effective strategies for intervening in the social environment to prevent injury are harder to find, particularly at the community and societal levels. Nevertheless, there are some compelling examples that illustrate the potential that modifying the social environment has for injury prevention (Table 15.1). In this section we review knowledge about selected programs and policies that target the social environment as a means of preventing injury at each of the social levels of the ecological model.

15.4.1.   Relationship

There is a substantial body of work on interventions that target the social relationship between parents and children as a means of reducing childhood unintentional injuries, child maltreatment, and youth violence. Other chapters in this book more fully discuss these interventions (see Chapters 8, 9, and 18). Some of the most promising for the prevention of childhood injury include nurse home-

Table 15.1. Injury Prevention Strategies and Modifiable Factors by Ecological Context

Ecological Context	Modifiable Factors	Intervention Strategies
Relationship	Child-rearing practices; parenting skills; presence of a positive adult role; peer pressure	Parenting-training programs; mentoring programs; home visitation programs
Community	Community organization; economic inequalities; concentration of poverty; social capital; social cohesion or connectedness	Social support networks; poverty deconcentration; promotion of social integration among conflicting groups; building trust and engagement in community institutions
Societal	Social norms, beliefs, values, stereotypes; absence of deterrents for risky behavior	Health communication and social marketing campaigns; laws that provide sanctions for risky behavior (e.g., drinking & driving)

visitation programs and programs that provide comprehensive home-safety train-ing for parents. Programs that focus on the internal dynamics of families and their ability to manage external pressures appear to be the most successful for addressing child maltreatment and youth violence (Dahlberg and Butchart, 2005). In general, the earlier in a child's life these programs are delivered, the greater the benefits (Yoshikawa, 1995).

There is some evidence that positive adult role models for adolescents provided through mentoring programs many be protective for violent behavior (Thornton, Craft, Dahlberg, Lynch, & Baer, 2000). However, participation in mentoring pro-grams by both mentors and youth can be uneven, and negative effects of these programs have been reported (Dahlberg & Butchart, 2005; Grossman & Rhodes, 2002).

15.4.2. Community

There is some evidence that policies that reduce the concentration of poverty in urban communities may be effective in reducing both violent behavior by youth and the violent victimization of families. The potential positive effect on violent behavior by adolescents was shown in an experimental evaluation of a housing voucher program called Moving to Opportunity (MTO), conducted in Baltimore, Maryland (Ludwig, Duncan, & Hirschfield, 2001). In this study, families living in public housing in high-poverty neighborhoods were randomly divided into three groups: (1) families that received rental vouchers, counseling, and other assistance to move to communities with lower levels of poverty; (2) families that received only rental vouchers and had no restrictions on where they could move; and (3) families that had no special assistance. The study found that adolescents in the families that received vouchers and moved to communities with lower levels of poverty were significantly less likely to engage in violent behavior. An extension of this study into five cities (Baltimore, Boston, Chicago, Los Angeles, and New York) where the MTO experiment was conducted generally supported the finding of the earlier study that violent crime arrests were lower for those in the experimental group then those in the control (Kling, Ludwig, & Katz, 2005). Although these findings were consistent for females, the reductions in violent crime arrests for males were offset by increases in the experimental group relative to the controls for property crime offenses. The authors argue that because violent crime imposes substantially higher costs on society than property crime, the net increase in prop-erty crime appears to be more than offset by reductions in violent crime. In addi-tion to this research, a systematic review of evaluations of the effects of housing voucher programs found them also to be effective in reducing violent victimization and property crime (TFCPS, 2003). Efforts to reduce extreme concentrations of poverty may be a powerful strategy for preventing the violence that plagues many inner-city communities.

An example of a successful effort to reduce injury in a broad community is provided by a suicide-prevention project implemented by the U.S. Air Force (Knox, Litts, Talcott, Feig, & Caine, 2003). After significant increases in suicide rates among African American and white men aged 24–35 years in the Air Force, a multilayered intervention with a population-orientated risk-reduction approach was adopted. The intervention was aimed at changing social norms to decrease stigma around help-seeking behavior, enhancing supportive social networks, and increasing understanding of mental-health issues throughout the Air Force. To accomplish these aims, the Air Force incorporated suicide-prevention education into the courses for squadron commanders, other professional military personnel, and for nonprofessional personnel. They also established an integrated delivery system for human services prevention activities, established a multidisciplinary team to respond to traumatic events that could trigger suicide, and enhanced the availability of staff for community-based mental-health services at Air Force mental-health centers. It is very important that they took steps to establish and reinforce psychotherapist–patient privilege for individuals at risk of suicide to promote help-seeking behavior. The program was associated over time with a 33% risk reduction for completed suicide. Moreover, the program also resulted in significant risk reductions for unintentional injury deaths, homicide, and moderate to severe family violence (Knox et al., 2003).

15.4.3. Societal

Cultural norms undergo change, which can be promoted and even accelerated. Norms associated with the acceptability of smoking in the United States, for example, have undergone substantial changes over the past several decades. The effects of normative influences on drug use in general (Tobler, 1986) and alcohol use in particular (Kafka & London, 1991; Kandel & Andrews, 1987; La Greca, Prinstein, & Fetter, 2001; Urberg, Degirmencioghu, & Pilgrim, 1997) are well documented. Social norms have been found to influence compliance with physical modifications, such as smoke alarms (McLoughlin, Marchone, Hanger, German, & Baker, 1985). Social marketing and approaches to influencing social norms that are based on reinforcing sentiments or beliefs within a population that run counter to a harmful norm have been successful in reducing alcohol abuse on college campuses and have been suggested for addressing sexual assault (Berkowitz, 1998; Mattern & Neighbors, 2004; Perkins & Craig, 2002; see also Chapter 24). Injury prevention messages repeated in different forms and contexts can facilitate the development of a "culture of safety" within communities (Lund & Aaro, 2004; Towner & Dowswell, 2002), although evidence of sustainability is lacking.

Efforts to curb alcohol-impaired driving and prevent crashes have taken on many parts of the social environment, but perhaps most visibly in the area of norms. Media campaigns promote positive social norms but also seek to portray the alcohol impaired drivers as dangerous. These campaigns typically work on desired outcomes through intermediate variables, such as social norms and peer influences (Elder et al., 2004). The strongest evidence of effectiveness in reducing risk for alcohol-impaired driving is found for interventions that focus on retailers, alcohol taxation, reducing alcohol availability, training servers of alcohol, and legal strategies (such as sobriety checkpoints, lower blood alcohol concentration (BAC) laws, and minimum legal drinking age laws) (Howat, Sleet, Elder, & Maycock, 2004; see also Chapter 16). Elder et al. (2004), however, also found strong evidence that, under certain conditions, mass media campaigns were effective in reducing alcohol-impaired driving and alcohol-related crashes. Greenfield and Room (1997) documented the norm shift in the 1990s regarding drinking and driving, showing a trend toward overall reduced social acceptance of drinking and driving.

Another example in which health messages have affected norms is in the area of helmet use while riding a bicycle. Laws requiring helmets, especially for younger riders, have increased use; nevertheless, barriers to use remain strong. Recent work has shown that the barrier to use is not necessarily a question of effectiveness or of having access to a helmet but rather peer use of helmets and issues around comfort and style (Finnoff, Laskowski, Altman, & Diehl, 2001; Forjuoh,

Schuchmann, Fiesinger, & Mason 2003; Liller, Morissette, Noland, McDermott, 1998). Thus, while educating the public on the effectiveness of bike helmets in reducing the severity of head injury, interventions must also consider incorporating elements of use by peers and parents as well as concerns for comfort and fashion (Finnoff et al., 2001; Thompson, Sleet, & Sacks, 2002).

15.5.   RESEARCH RECOMMENDATIONS

The scientific literature suggests that many aspects of the social environment are associated with the risk of injury and violent behavior. Less is known about the effectiveness of interventions that target the social environment as a means of preventing injuries, but the potential is evident. There are four general directions that would help strengthen this research base.

First, research in this area has focused largely on demonstrating associations between the social characteristics of a geographic area and injury, primarily using cross-sectional study designs and aggregate population data. More research is needed that helps us identify the causal pathways or mechanisms that help explain these associations (Yen & Syme, 1999). Prospective studies will be essential for identifying these causal pathways. Prospective studies that address outcomes associated with unintentional injury or violence should incorporate key measures of the social environment. The development of theoretical models that clearly conceptualize the social factors and their relationships will also be important in guiding the research into these mechanisms. Understanding these mechanisms will be extremely useful in the development of programs and policies to prevent injury through intervening on the social environment.

Second, in research to identify causal pathways and to evaluate the effects of social interventions on injury outcomes, the use of multilevel or hierarchical modeling techniques is strongly advised (Yen & Syme, 1999). The application of these techniques will allow researchers to disentangle the influence individual characteristics have on injury from those attributable to the social environment in which that individual lives and interacts (e.g., schools, census tracts, neighborhoods). These analytic approaches are increasingly being used in epidemiologic research (Von Korff, Koepsell, Curry, & Diehr, 1992; Yen & Syme, 1999).

Third, additional research and more sophisticated methodologies are needed to evaluate the efficacy, effectiveness, and efficiency of interventions that address the social environment as a means of preventing injury. In particular, the effectiveness of social marketing or social norms campaigns is rarely evaluated in a rigorous way. In addition, multifaceted community programs that include at least one component addressing the social environment are rarely evaluated in a satisfactory way. Given the expectation that ultimately the most effective approach to injury prevention will combine programs and policies targeting the social and physical environment with those focusing on individual behavior change, it will be important to understand and be able to disentangle the effects of these potentially complementary approaches in multifaceted programs.

Fourth, successful dissemination and implementation of effective injury and violence-prevention strategies will be enhanced by research that helps us understand how the social environment influences the diffusion of innovations. Research is needed to bridge the gap between research and everyday practice by building a knowledge base about how scientifically based evidence is integrated into specific practice settings. Understanding the role of the social environment will be critical to filling this research gap. For example, regardless of whether an effective intervention focuses on the individual or social environment, we need to understand how specific cultural norms, attitudes, and beliefs may hinder or enhance the adoption of an innovation, what the existing organizational and community capacity is to engage in injury prevention, how that capacity can be enhanced, and how broader political or social processes affect the dissemination and implementations of an innovation. Although we did not review dissemination and implementation research related to the social environment in this chapter, this is an important priority for future research (see Chapter 28).

15.6.   IMPLICATIONS FOR PRACTITIONERS

The importance of addressing the social environment in injury prevention programs is reinforced by what we are learning about effective prevention programs for a variety of health problems. We are learning that the involvement of parents in prevention programs that target children and adolescents is a component of many successful plans (Dryfoos, 1990). We are also learning that effective programs tend to include multiple interventions addressing an array of important risk and protective factors, settings, and systems associated with the target problem (Nation et al., 2003). Addressing community or school norms related to problem behaviors, for example, appears to be a particularly important dimension of effective programs (Center for Substance Abuse Prevention, 1996; Janz, Zimmerman, Wren, & Israel, 1996). In addition, matching the program to local community norms and cultural beliefs and practices appears to be critical for producing positive outcomes by increasing the relevance of the program for participants (Nation et al., 2003). Addressing the social environment helps maintain and reinforce positive changes in individual behaviors by influencing the ecological niches in which individuals interact. The effectiveness of injury prevention programs will be enhanced so they are able to create conditions in which individuals' safe behavior and lifestyle are supported in their key relationships with parents and peers and reinforced by the social norms in the settings in which they regularly participate (e.g., school, work, church) as well as by predominant cultural beliefs and values.

The most common way of addressing the social environment in injury prevention programs is through programs that use multiple interventions targeting multiple settings. Practitioners may want to look at the World Health Organization's (WHO's) Safe Community program as an example of this type of approach to injury prevention. The WHO program has been described in detail elsewhere (Coggan & Bennett, 2004; Hanson, Vardon, & Lloyd, 2002), but generally it uses an ecological paradigm to intervene at a community level to reduce the risk of unintentional injury and increase safety. The intent is that multiple activities are used as interventions to empower a community to change. These activities have included, for example, education programs, physical environment modifications, and subsidies for safety equipment. A recent Cochrane review notes that there is some evidence that the model does reduce injuries in communities (Spinks, Turner, Nixon, & McClure, 2005). It is unclear, however, from published reports whether social environmental changes and effects can be disentangled to understand the relative importance of each activity and the applicability or usefulness of the programs in other settings.

15.7. CONCLUSIONS

In sum, the social environment can have a profound effect on the risk of being injured or causing injury through violent behavior. We need more information, however, on the causal mechanisms that help explain these associations. While interventions that include modifications of the social environment are being fielded, much more work needs to be done in measuring social environmental change and in evaluating programs that target the social environment. New programs and policies that are based on the emerging evidence should continue to develop. Understanding the role of the social environment in injury causation and prevention opens up new and exciting possibilities for injury prevention. We can study the influence of such issues as cultural norms, socialization, concentration of poverty, economic inequalities, and social capital on injury and its prevention independent of the individual risk and protective factors involved. But we do not always need to wait for a complete understanding of the causal mechanisms to advance understanding of prevention in this area. There are often natural experiments that arise out of a community's desire to address social issues for reasons other than injury prevention that provide the opportunity to understand the social environment and its relation to injury. For example, do poverty-reduction or job-training programs also prevent injury? Do efforts to provide social support to parents reduce unintentional childhood injury and maltreatment? Studying the effect of programs and policies such as these can also inform our understanding of the causal mechanisms connecting the social environment and injury. Modifications of the social environment hold the potential to reduce the risk for injury across broader populations and for longer periods of time then interventions targeted at individuals. Research and programmatic development in this area can lead to new discoveries, paradigms, and theories that hold great potential for advancing the goal of reducing morbidity and mortality from injuries.

REFERENCES

Allegrante, J., Marks, R., & Hansen, D. W. (2006). Ecological models for the prevention and control of unintentional injury. In A. C. Glelen, D. A. Sleet, & R. DiClemente (Eds.), *Injury and violence prevention: Behavior change theories, methods, and applications* (pp. 105–126). San Francisco: Jossey-Bass.

American Psychological Association. (1998). *Hate crimes today: An age-old foe in modern dress.* Washington, DC: American Psychological Association.

Anderson, R., Dearwater, S. R., Olsen, T., Aaron, D. J., Kriska, A. M., & LaPorte, R. E. (1994). The role of socioeconomic status and injury morbidity risk in adolescents. *Archives of Pediatrics & Adolescent Medicine, 148,* 245–249.

Bates, D. G., & Fratkin, E. M. (2003). *Cultural anthropology* (pp. 3–4). New York: Allyn & Bacon.

Battistich, V., & Hom, A. (1997). The relationship between students' sense of their school as a community and their involvement in problem behaviors. *American Journal of Public Health, 87,* 1997–2001.

Bennet, L., Manderson, L., & Astbury, J. (2000). *Mapping a global pandemic: Review of current literature on rape, sexual assault and sexual harassment of women.* Melbourne, Australia: University of Melbourne.

Berkowitz, A. D. (1998). *How can we prevent sexual harassment and sexual assault. Educators guide to controlling sexual harassment.* Washington, DC: Greenwood Press.

Berrill, K. T. (1992). Anti-gay violence and victimization in the United States: An overview. In G. M. Herek, & K. T. Berrill (Eds.), *Hate crimes: Confronting violence against lesbians and gay men* (pp. 19–45). Newbury Park, CA: Sage.

Bronfenbrenner, U. (1992). Ecological systems theory. In R. Vasta (Ed.), *Six theories of child development* (pp. 187–250). London: Jessica Kingsley.

Brown, R. M. (1979). The American vigilante tradition. In H. D. Graham, & T. R. Gurr (Eds.), *Violence in America: Historical and comparative perspectives* (pp. 153–185). Beverly Hills, CA: Sage.

Center for Substance Abuse Prevention. (1996). *A review of alternative activities and alternatives in youth-oriented prevention.* Washington, DC: Center for Substance Abuse Prevention.

Centers for Disease Control and Prevention. (2001). School health guidelines to prevent unintentional injuries and violence. *Morbidity & Mortality Weekly Report, Recommendations & Reports 50* (RR-22), 1–73.

Coggan, C., & Bennett, S. (2004). Community-based injury prevention programs. In R. McClure, M. Stevenson, S. McEvoy (Eds.) *The scientific basis of injury prevention and control* (pp. 347–358). Melbourne, Australia: IP Communications.

Coppens, N. M., & Gentry, L. K. (1991). Video analysis of playground injury-risk situations. *Research in Nursing & Health, 14* (2), 129–136.

Courtenay, W. (2000). Constructions of masculinity and their influence on men's well-being: A theory of gender and health. *Social Science & Medicine, 50,* 1385–1401.

Cubbin, C., & Smith, G. S. (2002). Socioeconomic inequalities in injury: Critical issues in design and analysis. *Annual Review of Public Health, 23,* 349–375.

Dahlberg, L. L. (1998). Youth violence in the United States: Major trends, risk factors, and prevention approaches. *American Journal of Preventive Medicine, 14,* 259–272.

Dahlberg, L. L., & Butchart, A. (2005). State of the science: Violence prevention efforts in developing and developed countries. *International Journal of Injury Control & Safety Promotion, 12* (2), 93–104.

Dahlberg, L. L., & Krug, E. G. (2002). Violence—A global public health problem. In E. Krug, L. L. Dahlberg, J. A. Mercy, A. B. Zwi, & R. Lozano (Eds.), *World report on violence and health* (pp. 147–181). Geneva: World Health Organization.

Dishion, T. J., Spracklen, K. M., Andrews, D. W., & Patterson, G. R. (1996). Deviancy training in male adolescent friendships. *Behavioral Therapy, 27,* 373–390.

Dobash, R. E., & Dobash, R. P. (1979). *Violence against wives: A case against the patriarchy.* New York: Free Press.

Dodge, K. A., & Pettit, G. S. (2003). A biopsychosocial model of the development of chronic conduct problems in adolescence. *Developmental Psychology, 39* (2), 349–371.

Dryfoos, J. G. (1990). *Adolescents at risk: Prevalence and prevention.* New York: Oxford University Press.

Dubos, R. (1980). *Man adapting.* New Haven, CT: Yale University Press.

Durkin, M. S., Davidson, L. L., Kuhn, L., O'Connor, P., & Barlow, B. (1994). Low income neighborhoods and the risk of severe pediatric injury: A small-area analysis in northern Manhattan. *American Journal of Public Health, 84,* 587–592.

Elder, R. W., Shults, R. A., Sleet, D. A., Nichols, J. L., Thompson, R. S., Rajab, W., & Task Force on Community Preventive Services. (2004). Effectiveness of mass media campaigns for reducing drinking and driving and alcohol-involved crashes: A systematic review. *American Journal of Preventive Medicine, 27* (1), 57–65.

Esbensen, F., & Huizinga, D. (1993). Gangs, drugs, and delinquency in a survey of urban youth. *Criminology, 31* (4), 565–589.

Fajnzylber, P., Lederman, D., & Loayza, N. (2002). Inequality and violent crime. *Journal of Law & Economics, 45,* 1–40.

Finnoff, J. T., Laskowski, E. R., Altman, K. L., & Diehl, N. N. (2001). Barriers to bicycle helmet use. *Pediatrics, 108* (1), E4.

Forjuoh, S. N., Schuchmann, J. A., Fiesinger, T., & Mason, S. (2003). Parent-child concordance on reported barriers to helmet use by children. *Medical Science Monitor, 9* (10), CR436–441.

Galea, S., Karpati, A., & Kennedy, B. (2002). Social capital and violence in the United States, 1974–1993. *Social Science & Medicine, 55,* 1373–1383.

Gartner, R. (1990). The victims of homicide: A temporal and cross-national comparison. *American Sociological Review, 55,* 92–106.

Greenfield, T., & Room, R. (1997). Situational norms for drinking and drunkenness: Trends in the US adult population, 1979–1990. *Addition, 92* (1), 33–47.

Grossman, J. P., & Rhodes, J. E. (2002). The test of time: Predictors and effects of duration in youth mentoring programs. *American Journal of Community Psychology, 30,* 199–206.

Hanson, D., Vardon, P., & Lloyd, J. (2002). Safe communities: An ecological approach to safety promotion. In R. Muller (Ed.), *Reducing injuries in Mackay, North Queensland* (pp. 17–34). Warwick, Queensland, Australia: Warwick Educational Publishing.

Hawkins, J. D., & Lam, T. (1987). Teacher practices, social development, and delinquency. In J. D. Burchard, & S. N. Burchard (Eds.), *Prevention of delinquent behavior* (pp. 241–274). Newbury Park, CA: Sage.

Hayward, R. F. (2000). Breaking the Earthenware Jar: Lessons from South Asia to End Violence Against Women and Girls. Kathmandu, Nepal: UNICEF.

Howat, P., Sleet, D., Elder, R., & Maycock, B. (2004). Preventing alcohol-related traffic injury: A health promotion approach. *Traffic Injury Prevention, 5* (3), 208–219.

Janz, N. K., Zimmerman, M. A., Wren, P. A., & Israel, B. A. (1996). Evaluation of 37 AIDS prevention projects: Successful approaches and barriers to program effectiveness. *Health Education Quarterly, 23*, 80–97.

Kafka, R., & London, P. (1991). Communication in relationships and adolescent substance use: The influence of parents and friends. *Adolescence, 26*, 587–597.

Kandel, D., & Andrews, K. (1987). Processes of adolescent socialization by parents and peers. *International Journal of the Addictions, 22*, 319–342.

Kennedy, B. P., Kawachi, I., Prothrow-Stith, D., Lochner, K., & Gupta, V. (1998). Social capital, income inequality, and firearm violent crime. *Social Science & Medicine, 47* (1), 7–17.

Kling, J. R., Ludwig, J., & Katz, L. F. (2005). Neighborhood effects on crime for female and male youth: Evidence from a randomized housing voucher experiment. *Quarterly Journal of Economics, 120* (1), 87–130.

Knox, K. L., Litts, D. A., Talcott, G. W., Feig, J. C., & Caine, E. D. (2003). Risk of suicide and related adverse outcomes after exposure to a suicide prevention programme in the US Air Force: Cohort study. *British Medical Journal, 327* (7428), 1376–1380.

Knutson, J. F., DeGarmo, D. S., & Reid, J. B. (2004). Social disadvantage and neglectful parenting as precursors to the development of antisocial and aggressive child behaviour: Testing a theoretical model. *Aggressive Behavior, 30*, 187–205.

Knutson, J. F., & Schartz, H. A. (1997). Physical abuse and neglect of children. In T. A. Widiger, A. J. Frances, H. A. Pincus, R. Ross, M. B. First, & W. Davis (Eds.), *DSM-IV sourcebook* (pp. 713–804, Vol. 3). Washington, DC: American Psychiatric Association.

Kontos, A. P. (2004). Perceived risk, risk taking, estimation of ability and injury among adolescent sport participants. *Journal of Pediatric Psychology, 29* (6), 447–455.

Korllos, T. S. (1993). Theoretical perspectives on the nature of accidents. *Sociological Viewpoints, 9*, 43–54.

Laflamme, L., & Eilert-Petersson, E. (2001). Injury risks and socioeconomic groups in different settings: Differences in morbidity between men and between women at working ages. *European Journal of Public Health, 11* (3), 309–313.

La Greca, A., Prinstein, M., & Fetter, M. (2001). Adolescent peer crowd affiliation: Linkages with health-risk behaviors and close friendships. *Journal of Pediatric Psychology, 26*, 131–143.

Lewis, T., DiLillo, D., & Peterson, L. V. (2004). Parental beliefs regarding developmental benefits of childhood injuries. *American Journal of Health Behavior, 28* (Supplement 1), S61–68.

Levinson, D. (1989). *Family violence in a cross-cultural perspective.* Thousand Oaks, CA: Sage.

Liller, K. D., Morissette, B., Noland, V., & McDermott, R. J. (1998). Middle school students and bicycle helmet use: Knowledge, attitudes, beliefs, and behaviors. *Journal of School Health, 68* (8), 325–328.

Lindqvist, K., Timpka, T., & Karlsson, N. (2004). Impact of social standing on injury prevention in a World Health Organization Safe Community—Intervention outcome by household employment contract. *International Journal of Epidemiology, 33*, 605–611.

Lipsey, M. W., & Derzon, J. H. (1998). Predictors of violent or serious delinquency in adolescence and early adulthood: A synthesis of longitudinal research. In R. Loeber, & D. P. Farrington (Eds.), *Serious and violent juvenile offenders: Risk factors and successful interventions* (pp. 86–105). Thousand Oaks, CA: Sage.

Lochner, K., Kawachi, I., & Kennedy, B. P. (1999). Social capital: A guide to its measurement. *Health & Place, 5*, 259–270.

Ludwig, J., Duncan, G. J., & Hirschfield, P. (2001). Urban poverty and juvenile crime: Evidence from a randomized housing-mobility experiment. *Quarterly Journal of Economics, 16*, 655–680.

Lund, J., & Aaro, L. (2004). Accident prevention. Presentation of a model placing emphasis on human, structural and cultural factors. *Safety Science, 42*, 271–324.

Mack, K. (2004). Unintentional injuries in adult women. *Journal of Women's Health, 13* (7), 754–763.

Mattern, J. L., & Neighbors, C. (2004). Social norms campaigns: Examining the relationship between changes in perceived norms and changes in drinking levels. *Journal of Studies on Alcohol, 65* (4), 489–493.

McCutcheon, T. I., Curtis, J. E., & White, P. G. (1997). The socioeconomic distribution of sport injuries: Multivariate analyses using Canadian national data. *Sociology of Sport Journal, 14* (1), 57–72.

McLoughlin, E., Marchone, M., Hanger, L., German, P., & Baker, S. (1985). Smoke detector legislation: Its effect on owner-occupied homes. *American Journal of Public Health, 75* (8), 858–862.

Mercy, J. A. (2005). Assaultive violence and war. In B. S. Levy, & V. W. Sidel (Eds.), *Social injustice and public health*. New York: Oxford University Press.

Mercy, J. A., Sleet, D. A., & Doll, L. (2006). Applying a developmental and ecological framework to injury and violence prevention. In K. Liller (Ed.). *Injury prevention for children and adolescents: Research, practice and advocacy* (pp. 1–14). Washington, D.C.: American Public Health Association.

Moller, J. (1995). *Injury among 15 to 29 year old males* (Australian Injury Prevention Bulletin 11). Adelaide: National Injury Surveillance Unit.

Morenoff, J., Sampson, R. J., & Raudenbush, S. W. (2001). Neighborhood inequality, collective efficacy, and the spatial dynamics of urban violence. *Criminology, 39*, 517–560.

Morrongiello, B., & Dayler, L. (1996). A community based study of parents knowledge, attitudes and beliefs related to childhood injuries. *Canadian Journal of Public Health, 87* (6), 383–388.

Morrongiello, B. A., & Hogg, K. (2004). Mother's reactions to children's misbehaving in ways that can lead to injury: Implications for gender differences in children's risk taking and injuries. *Sex Roles, 50*, 103–118.

Murphy, L. B. (2001). Adolescent mothers' beliefs about parenting and injury prevention. *Journal of Pediatric Health Care, 15*, 194–199.

Nathanson, C. (1977). Sex roles as variables in preventive health behavior. *Journal of Community Health, 3* (2), 142–155.

Nelson, M. (1992). Socioeconomic status and childhood mortality in North Carolina. *American Journal of Public Health, 82*, 1131–1133.

Nixon, H. (1992). A social network analysis of influence on athletes to play with pain and injury. *Journal of Sport & Social Issues, 16* (2), 127–135.

Nation, M., Crusto, C., Wandersman, A., Kumpfer, K. L., Seybolt, D., Morrissey-Kane, E., & Davino, K. (2003). What works in prevention: Principles of effective prevention programs. *American Psychologist, 58* (6/7), 449–456.

Nutbeam, D., Smith, C., Moore, L., & Bauman, A. (1993). Warning! Schools can damage your health: Alienation from school and its impact on health behavior. *Journal of Paediatrics & Child Health, 29* (Supplement 1), S25–S30.

O'Donnell, J., Hawkins, J. D., Catalano, R. F., Abbott, R. D., & Day, L. E. (1995). Preventing school failure, drug use, and delinquency among low-income children: Long-term intervention in elementary schools. *American Journal of Orthopsychiatry, 65*, 87–100.

Perkins, H. W., & Craig, D. W. (2002). *A multifaceted social norms approach to reduce high-risk drinking*. Newton, MA: The Higher Education Center for Alcohol and Other Drug Prevention.

Peterson, L., Bartelstone, J., Kern, T., & Gillies, R. (1995). Parents' socialization of children's injury prevention: description and some initial parameters. *Child Development, 66* (1), 224–235.

Reiss, A. J., & Roth, J. A. (Eds.). (1993). *Understanding and preventing violence*. Washington, DC: National Academy Press.

Resnick, M. D., Bearman, P. S., Blum, R. W., Bauman, K. E., Harris, K. M., Jones, J., Tabor, J., Beuhring, T., Sieving, R. E., Shew, M., Ireland, M., Bearinger, L. H., & Udry, J. R. (1997). Protecting adolescents from harm: Findings from the National Longitudinal Study on Adolescent Health. *Journal of the American Medical Association, 278*, 823–832.

Robertson, I. (1987). *Sociology* (3rd ed.). New York: Worth Publishers.

Runyan, D. K., Hunter, W. M., Socolar, R. R. S., Amaya-Jackson, L., English, D., Landsverk, J., Dubowitz, H., Browne, D. H., Bangdiwala, S. I., & Mathew, R. M. (1998). Children who prosper in unfavorable environments: The relationship to social capital. *Pediatrics, 101* (1), 12–18.

Sampson, R. J. (1998). What "community" supplies. In R. Ferguson, & W. Dickens (Eds.), *The future of community development: A social science synthesis*. (pp. 241–292). Washington, DC: Brookings Institution.

Sampson, R. J., & Lauritsen, J. L. (1994). Violent victimization and offending: Individual-, situational-, and community-level risk factors. In A. J. Reiss, & J. A. Roth (Eds.), *Understanding and preventing violence. Volume 3: Social influences* (pp. 1–114). Washington, DC: National Academy Press.

Sampson, R. J., Raudenbush, S. W., & Earls, F. (1997). Neighborhoods and violent crime: A multilevel study of collective efficacy. *Science, 277*, 918–924.

Sampson, R. J., & Wilson, W. J. (1995). Toward a theory of race, crime, and urban inequality. In J. Hagan, & R. D. Peterson (Eds.), *Crime & inequality* (pp. 37–56). Stanford: Stanford University Press.

Sanday, P. (1981). The socio-cultural context of rape: A cross-cultural study. *Journal of Social Issues, 37*, 5–27.

Spady, D. W., Saunders, D. L., Schopflocher, D. P., & Svenson, L. W. (2004). Patterns of injury in children: A population-based approach. *Pediatrics, 113*, 522–529.

Spinks, A., Turner, C., Nixon, J., & McClure, R. (2005). The 'WHO Safe Communities' model for the prevention of injury in whole populations. *The Cochrane Database of Systematic Reviews, 2*, CD004445.

Stier, D., Mercy, J. A., & Kohn, M. (In press). Injury prevention and the law. In R. A. Goodman, M. A. Rothstein, R. E. Hoffman, W. Lopez, & G. W. Matthews (Eds.), *Law in public health practice*. New York: Oxford.

Stokols, D. (1992). Establishing and maintaining healthy environments. *American Psychologist, 47* (1), 6–22.

Stokols, D. (1996). Translating social ecological theory into guidelines for community health promotion. *American Journal of Health Promotion, 10* (4), 282–298.

Swahn, M. H., Mahendra, R. R., Paulozzi, L. J., Winston, R. L., Shelley, G. A., Taliano, J., Frazier, L., & Saul, J. R. (2003). Violent attacks on Middle Easterners in the United States during the month following the September 11, 2001 terrorist attacks. *Injury Prevention, 9*, 187–189.

Task Force on Community Preventive Services. (2003). Recommendations to promote healthy social environments. *American Journal of Preventive Medicine, 24* (3S), 21–24.

Thompson, N., Sleet, D. A., & Sacks, J. (2002). Increasing the use of bicycle helmets: Lessons from behavioral science. *Patient Education and Counseling, 46* (3): 191–197.

Thornberry, T. P., Huizinga, D., & Loeber, R. (1995). The prevention of serious delinquency and violence: Implications from the program of research on the causes and correlates of delinquency. In J. C. Howell, B. Krisberg, J. D. Hawkins, & J. J. Wilson (Eds.), *Sourcebook on serious, violent, and chronic juvenile offenders* (pp. 213–237). Thousand Oaks, CA: Sage.

Thornton, T. N., Craft, C. A., Dahlberg, L. L., Lynch, B. S., & Baer, K. (2000). *Best practices of youth violence prevention: A sourcebook of community action*. Atlanta, GA: Centers for Disease Control and Prevention, National Center for Injury Prevention and Control.

Tobler, N. (1986). Meta-analysis of 143 adolescent drug prevention programs: Quantitative outcome results of program participants compared to a control or comparison group. *Journal of Drug Issues, 16* (4), 537–567.

Towner, E., & Dowswell, T. (2002). Community-based childhood injury prevention interventions: What works? *Health Promotion International, 17* (3), 273–284.

U.S. Department of Health and Human Services. (2001). *Youth violence: A report of the surgeon general*. Rockville, MD: U.S. Department of Health and Human Services; Centers for Disease Control and Prevention, National Center for Injury Prevention and Control; Substance Abuse and Mental Health Services Administration, Center for Mental Health Services; and National Institutes of Health, National Institute of Mental Health.

Unnithan, N. P., & Whitt, H. P. (1992). Inequality, economic development and lethal violence: A cross-national analysis of suicide and homicide. *International Journal of Comparative Sociology, 33* (3–4), 182–196.

Urberg, K., Degirmencioglu, S., & Pilgrim, C. (1997). Close friend and group influence on adolescent cigarette smoking and alcohol use. *Developmental Psychology, 33*, 834–844.

Vaughan, E., Anderson, C., Agran, P., & Winn, D. (2004). Cultural differences in young children's vulnerability to injuries: A risk and protection perspective. *Health Psychology, 23* (3), 289–298.

Voelkl, K. E. (1995). School warmth, student participation, and achievement. *Journal of Experimental Education, 63*, 127–138.

Von Korff, M., Koepsell, T., Curry, S., & Diehr, P. (1992). Multi-level analysis in epidemiologic research on health behaviors and outcomes. *American Journal of Epidemiology, 135*, 1077–1082.

White, R. (2002). Social and political aspects of men's health. *Health: An Interdisciplinary Journal for the Social Study of Health, Illness & Medicine, 6* (3), 267–485.

Williams, J. M., Currie, C. E., Wright, P., Elton, R. A., & Beattie, T. F. (1996). Socioeconomic status and adolescent injuries. *Social Science & Medicine, 44*, 1881–1891.

Wilson, W. J. (1987). *The truly disadvantaged: The inner city, the underclass, and public policy*. Chicago: University of Chicago Press.

Yen, I. H., & Kaplan, G. (1999). Neighborhood social environment and risk of death: Multilevel evidence from the Alameda County study. *American Journal of Epidemiology, 149* (1), 898–907.

Yen, I. H., & Syme, S. L. (1999). The social environment and health: A discussion of the epidemiologic literature. *Annual Review of Public Health, 20*, 287–308.

Yoshikawa, H. (1995). Long-term effects of early childhood programs on social outcomes and delinquency. *Future of Children, 4*, 51–75.

Chapter **16**

Interventions to Prevent Alcohol-Related Injuries

Ralph W. Hingson, Monica H. Swahn, and David A. Sleet

16.1. INTRODUCTION

Alcohol, the most commonly used drug among adults and adolescents (Substance Abuse and Mental Health Services Administration [SAMHSA], 2004), is related to many adverse health outcomes, including injuries and deaths (Room, Babor, & Rehm, 2005). In 2001, excessive alcohol use was associated with approximately 75,000 deaths and 2.3 million years of potential life lost (about 30 years of life lost per death) (Centers for Disease Control and Prevention [CDC], 2004). While the magnitude of alcohol-related injury mortality is similar to alcohol-related chronic disease mortality, far more years of life are lost as a result of injuries because the injury deaths occur at a younger age (CDC 2004; Lunetta & Smith 2005). In addition, alcohol use and alcohol-related consequences among adolescents are associated with significant costs to society, as much as $58 billion per year, with the three most costly domains consisting of violent crime ($36 billion), traffic crashes ($18 billion), and suicide attempts ($1.5 billion) (Levy, Stewart, & Wilbur, 1999). Although the magnitude and costs of alcohol-related negative consequences such as injuries and violence have been well defined and described, much less is known about the most effective prevention and intervention efforts for reducing alcohol-related injuries and violence. However, a number of evidence-based prevention efforts are available. Some of the most effective options are increasing alcohol taxes, restricting alcohol availability, and laws and programs to reduce the occurrence of drinking and driving (Room et al., 2005).

This chapter briefly describes the magnitude of alcohol-related injuries in the United States, the mechanisms linking alcohol use and injuries, and the primary and secondary prevention strategies to reduce and prevent alcohol use and alcohol-related injuries. More emphasis will be given to alcohol-related traffic crashes and interventions because there is much more information available in this area.

16.2. ALCOHOL-RELATED INJURIES: MAGNITUDE OF THE PROBLEM

In 2001, there were 40,933 injury deaths associated with excessive alcohol use or binge drinking (CDC, 2004). Binge drinking, is typically defined as the consumption of 5 or more alcoholic drinks on a single occasion over a 2-hour period for a man or 4 or more drinks on a single occasion over a 2-hr period for a woman (National Institute on Alcohol Abuse and Alcoholism [NIAAA], 2004). Of these, 26,359 were unintentional deaths (13,878 traffic deaths and 12,233 nontraffic deaths) and 14,821 were violence-related (6,995 suicides and 7,826 homicides). In addition to the injury deaths for which alcohol was involved in 2002, an estimated 8 million people were treated in emergency departments for alcohol-related injuries (McDonald, Wang, & Camouge, 2004). Another study indicates that 7% of the 20 million emergency department injury admissions annually are alcohol related (Gentilello, Ebel, Wickizer, Salkever, & Rivara, 2005). A recent case crossover study (in which patients served as their own controls) showed that there is a 9-fold increase in the odds of injury among patients who reported consuming five to six drinks during a 6-hour period before the injury and a 17-fold increase among patients consuming seven or more drinks before the injury (Vinson, Maclure, Reidinger, & Smith, 2003). Moreover, a recent international study of injured patients in emergency departments found that patients with a blood alcohol concentration (BAC) of 0.08 g/dL (the physiologic definition of binge drinking in the United States; NIAAA, 2004) were at least three times more likely to experience a violent injury than an unintentional injury; the study noted a significant does–response relationship between the amount of alcohol consumed and the risk of violent injury (MacDonald et al., 2005).

16.2.1. Mechanisms of Alcohol and Injury Risk

In a review of alcohol and injury research, Lunetta and Smith (2005) described several ways that alcohol can increase risk of injury. It can have a direct biological effect through the impairment of human performance by slowing the decision-making process, reducing visual acuity and adaptation to brightness and glare, dividing one's attention, changing perceptions, and increasing reaction time. It may also have indirect effects by increasing the sense of confidence, inhibiting self-control, and reducing the perception of and response to hazards. The link between alcohol use and involvement in violent behavior is seen in the disinhibition of norms and behavior in certain situations and contexts. This plausibly explains why some interpersonal interactions and disputes escalate to violent behavior when alcohol is involved (Parker, 2004). Under the influence of alcohol, people may be more prone to risk taking, which can increase the likelihood of injury and the likelihood that disagreements between people escalate to violent acts. Alcohol may also hamper decision making regarding safety (such as the use of seat belts, floatation devices, child car seats, and helmets) and assessing dangerous situations or places. For example, alcohol may affect judgment, leading swimmers and boaters into more dangerous situations and making it less likely they will wear floatation devices.

Alcohol may impair natural defense against hypothermia in cold climates and water, and depresses the cough reflex, increasing the risk of choking and aspiration—a frequent contributor to alcohol overdose deaths. Alcohol also contributes to fall injury through its effects on postural control, balance, and gait. Under the influence of alcohol, people who fall may have less effective reflexes and thus may be unable to avoid head injury. Alcohol also increases drowning risk by increasing the likelihood of falling into water. Once in the water, the capacity to swim and resist cold temperatures can be reduced. Alcohol contributes to fire risk if an intoxicated person falls asleep while smoking. Also, people who have been drinking may be less likely to hear a smoke alarm or fire alarm (Lunetta & Smith 2005).

16.2.2. Alcohol-Related Violence

Each year, an estimated 2.7 million people are victims of a violent crime in which the perpetrators had been drinking, which represents one out of four of all violent crimes (Greenfeld, 1998). Alcohol use is common during the commission of violent crimes among probationers, jail inmates, and state prisoners who had been arrested for different types of violent offenses (Greenfeld, 1998; Roizen, 1997). Studies have generally found that the more serious the crime, the more likely alcohol was involved. Greenfeld (1998) reported that 15% of robberies, 26% of aggravated and simple assaults, and 37% of rapes and sexual assaults are perpetrated by drinking offenders. Leonard and Quigley (1999) found that physical domestic violence episodes, were four times more likely to involve a husband's drinking than were verbal aggression episodes.

Other research of emergency room populations, which more likely reflect the experiences of victims rather than of perpetrators of violence, show that the attributable risk of injury is greater for drinking before the injury event than for a particular pattern of drinking and that the risk is higher for violence-related injuries than for other types of injuries (Cherpitel, Ye, & Bond, 2005). Likewise, research on adolescent trauma patients shows that alcohol use is associated with injuries due to assault (Spain et al., 1997). For example, in 2001, there were an estimated 244,331 alcohol-related emergency department visits in the United States among young people aged 13–25 years; 58,136 visits were assaults, 21,065 visits were self-harm, and 163,537 visits were due to unintentional/unknown injuries (Elder, Shults, Swahn, & Strife, 2004d). However, visits due to assaults were over three times more likely to be alcohol related than were visits for unintentional/unknown injuries.

Research on high school students shows that frequent or heavy alcohol use increases the odds of involvement in physical fights, resulting in injuries to self and to others (Swahn, Simon, Hamming, & Guerrero, 2004). Relatively few studies have specifically examined co-occurring alcohol use and violence in community samples of adolescents. In particular, one study reported that among drinkers, 11% of boys and 6% of girls were involved in alcohol-related fighting in the past year (Bonomo et al., 2001).

Alcohol use is also linked with completed suicides (10–69%) and suicide attempts (10–73%) (Cherpitel, Borges, & Wilcox, 2004). It seems that the strongest link between alcohol use and suicidal behavior pertains mostly to acute use (within 6 hours of the attempt) (Borges et al., 2004). However, as with the link between alcohol use and interpersonal violence, the mechanism by which alcohol use facilitates suicidal behavior is not well understood.

16.2.3.   Alcohol-Related Unintentional Injuries

Excessive alcohol is a contributing factor to deaths from many different types of injuries. According to the Alcohol-Related Disease Impact Software (ARDI), based on 2001 data, the alcohol attributable fractions are high for a number of acute causes of death (CDC, 2004). For example, the alcohol attributable fractions for deaths due to falls are 0.32, for fire-related injury deaths 0.42, for firearm injury deaths 0.18, hypothermia deaths 0.42, occupational- and machine-related injury deaths 0.18, poisoning deaths (not including alcohol) 0.29, and water transport deaths 0.18. However, because of the more comprehensive alcohol testing among fatally injured drivers, there is much more information about the epidemiology of alcohol-related motor-vehicle injuries than deaths from other types of injuries (CDC, 2005a).

Worldwide, alcohol is implicated in one quarter to two thirds of the 1.2 million road traffic fatalities annually (Peden et al., 2004). In the United States, traffic crashes are the leading cause of death for people aged 1–34 years (CDC, 2005b). According to the National Highway Traffic Safety Administration (NHTSA) (2003b), 41% of motor-vehicle crash deaths were alcohol-related (i.e., those in which a driver or pedestrian had a BAC greater than 0), and 35% were in crashes involving someone with a BAC of 0.08% or higher. Of the total number of people injured in traffic crashes, 9% were injured in alcohol–related crashes.

Of all alcohol-related crashes in 2002, 4% resulted in a death, and 42% percent in an injury (NHTSA, 2003b). In contrast, of the crashes that did not involve alcohol, 0.6% resulted in a death, and 31% in an injury. Many people other than drinking drivers are killed in crashes involving drinking drivers. In 2002, of those who died in traffic crashes involving a drinking driver with a BAC of 0.01% or higher, 44% were people other than the drinking driver: 7% were other drivers in vehicles struck by drinking drivers, 22% were passengers in vehicles with drinking drivers or that were struck by drinking drivers, 13% were pedestrians, and 2% were bicyclists (NHTSA, 2003b). In 2002, a total of 573 children younger than age 16 years died in crashes involving drinking drivers. Overall most child passenger victims were in the same vehicle driven by the impaired driver (Quinlan, Brewer, Sleet, & Dellinger, 2000).

In 2002, about 84% of the drivers who had been drinking and were involved in fatal crashes had a BAC at or above 0.08% (NHTSA, 2003b). Currently 0.08% is the legal blood alcohol limit for noncommercial adult drivers in all U.S. states. Impairment in driving skills begins with any departure from 0% BAC, and virtually all drivers exhibit some impairment on some critical driving measure by the time they reach a BAC of 0.08% (Moskowitz & Fiorentino, 2000). Experimental laboratory studies have reported several physical deficits experienced with a 0.08% BAC and below, including reduced peripheral vision, poor recovery from glare, poor performance in complex visual tracking, and reduced divided attention performance (i.e., the simultaneous performance of two or more tasks, such as tracking, visual search, number monitoring, and detection of auditory stimuli) (Moskowitz & Fiorentino, 2000; Howat, Sleet, & Smith, 1991). However, driver simulation and road course studies have revealed poorer parking performance, poorer driver performance at slow speeds, and steering inaccuracy at BACs of 0.05% and higher, and roadside observational studies have identified increased deterioration of speeding and breaking performance (Hingson & Winter, 2003).

Alcohol involvement in fatal crashes is disproportionately higher among males, Native Americans, some Hispanics (Mexican Americans), and people younger than age 44 years (NHTSA, 2003a). Alcohol is also disproportionately a factor in single-vehicle crashes, at night and on weekends. Moreover, impaired drivers are more likely to have prior driving while intoxicated (DWI) arrests, to have been speeding, and to be less likely to wear a safety belt (Hingson & Winter, 2003; NHTSA, 2003a, 2003b).

16.3.   INTERVENTIONS TO REDUCE ALCOHOL-RELATED INJURIES

It is beyond the scope of this review to outline all the different individual and environmental factors that can reduce alcohol-related injuries and deaths. We, however, focus on interventions that can influence individual behavior and reduce involvement in violence-related or unintentional injuries. While most of the interventions listed pertain specifically to reducing alcohol-related motor-vehicle crashes (see also Chapter 4), we note which of the interventions have been found to also reduce other types of alcohol-related injuries and deaths (see Table 16.1). Five types of interventions are discussed:

- Individually oriented interventions to change knowledge, attitudes, and behaviors.
- Environmental interventions to reduce alcohol availability and to deter drinking and driving.
- Laws to deter alcohol-related injuries.
- Enforcement and education.
- Comprehensive community interventions designed to reduce alcohol availability and drinking and driving behaviors.

16.3.1.   Individually Oriented Interventions

Alcoholism screening, treatment, and brief interventions are promising tools to prevent alcohol-impaired driving. Many, if not most, drinking drivers involved in alcohol-related fatal crashes are alcohol dependent or abusers (Hingson, Heeren, Winter, & Wechsler, 2005a). Currently, 32 states have laws that require people convicted of drinking and driving to be assessed for alcohol abuse or dependence and to attend alcohol treatment (Mothers Against Drunk Driving [MADD], 2002). Independent evaluations of mandated treatment of convicted drinking and driving offenders revealed that treatment reduces the incidence of repeat offences up to 9% more than standard sanctions, such as license suspension, revocations, and fines (Wells-Parker, Bangert-Drowns, McMillen, & Williams, 1995). Treatment strategies that combined punishment and group or individual therapy were more effective than any single approach for first-time and repeat offenders (Wells-Parker et al., 1995).

A review of alcoholism treatment studies in the United States concluded that alcohol problems (e.g., alcohol-related injury or job loss) among alcohol-dependent people who receive pharmaceutical treatment and/or counseling are reduced by two thirds and the consumption of alcohol is cut in half, (Miller, Walters, & Bennett, 2001). Reducing consumption and alcohol treatment have

Table 16.1. Interventions to Reduce Alcohol Related Problems[a]

Intervention	Motor-Vehicle Injury	Non-Motor-Vehicle Unintentional Injury	Homicides	Suicides	Other Violent Injury
Individually oriented interventions					
Alcoholism treatment–drinking driving offenders	E				
Alcoholism treatment—general population	E	P		P	P
Trauma center, emergency department—brief intervention	P	P			
School-based interventions	P				
Environmental interventions					
Increased legal minimum drinking age	E			P	P
Zero tolerance—under 21 years	E				
Increased price of alcohol	E		P	P	P
Reduced outlet density					
Alcohol sales ban					P
Dram shop laws	P				
Keg registration	P				
Responsible beverage service	P				
Off-premise monopoly	E				
Server training	E				
Drinking driving laws					
Administrative license revocation criminal per se	E				
0.08% legal blood alcohol concentration	E				
Lower blood alcohol concentration of convicted offenders	E				
Impounding vehicles or license plates	E				
Ignition interlocks	E				
Sobriety checkpoints	E				
Mass media campaigns	E				
Comprehensive community programs	E				P

[a]E = effective; P = promising; *empty cell* = insufficient evidence.

also been associated with reduction in drunk driving offenses, suicide attempts, domestic violence, falls, drinking-related injuries, and hospitalizations (Dinh-Zarr, Diguiseppi, Heitman, & Roberts, 1999).

Trauma center and emergency department studies of screening and brief intervention counseling among people presenting with an alcohol-related injury have shown reductions in alcohol consumption and alcohol-related injuries (Gentilello et al., 1999; Longabaugh et al., 2001; Mello et al., 2005). These are important populations for interventions because research shows that trauma patients who test positive for alcohol on admission have a twofold elevated risk of subsequent injury death than those not testing positive for alcohol (Dischinger, Mitchell, Kufera, Soderstorm, & Lowenfels, 2001). Moreover, screening and brief intervention for alcohol problems in trauma patients is a cost-effective intervention (Gentilello et al., 2005).

Larimer and Cronce (2002) reviewed individually oriented strategies to reduce problematic alcohol consumption by college students and found that several skills-based interventions, including self-monitoring, self-assessment, and brief motivational interventions, resulted in reductions in alcohol consumption. Another review (Elder et al., 2005) found that school-based programs that provided information to students about the risks of drinking and driving, life-skills development, and refusal skills reduced riding with a drinking driver but not drinking and driving itself.

16.3.2.   Environmental Interventions

Environmental interventions seek to reduce or eliminate the availability of alcohol or to directly deter, through environmental means, specific alcohol-related behaviors such as impaired driving.

16.3.2.1.   Reducing Availability

In Barrow, Alaska, during a 33-month period, a citizen referendum imposed a total ban on alcohol sales, then withdrew it, then reimposed it. There were significant decreases in emergency room visits for assaults when alcohol was banned and increases in assaults when the ban was lifted (Chiu, Perez, & Parker, 1997). Other research also shows that reducing alcohol use and availability is linked to reductions in violent behavior (Parker, 2004). Primarily, alcohol consumption and alcohol-related problems can be affected by restricting the hours and days when alcohol can be purchased and by reducing the number and types of alcohol outlets (Room et al., 2005). Moreover, alcohol server's liability for damage seems effective for reducing both rates of traffic fatalities and homicides (Room et al., 2005).

16.3.2.2.   Legal Minimum Drinking Age and Zero Tolerance

The increase in the age of legal sales of alcohol has been the most successful intervention to date in reducing drinking and alcohol-related crashes among people under age 21 years (Shults et al., 2001; Wagenaar & Toomey, 2002). NHTSA (2005) estimates that a legal drinking age of 21 saves 700–1,000 lives annually and that more than 22,000 traffic deaths have been prevented by such laws since 1976. Approximately half the people who die in crashes involving drinking drivers under age 21 years are not the drinking driver, and more than one third of them are older than age 21 (NHTSA, 2005). Raising the drinking age to 21 also saves other people's lives. One national study indicated that individuals who grew up in states with a drinking age of 21 not only drank less when they were 21 but also drank less at ages 21–25 years (O'Malley & Wagenaar, 1991). A large review of empirical studies that examined the effects of the minimum drinking age law on fighting, assaults, and injury deaths (including drowning, homicides, and suicides) concluded that although there is some evidence that higher legal drinking ages reduce rates of other health and social problems, results are not as consistent as they are for traffic crashes (Wagenaar & Toomey, 2002).

Zero-tolerance laws, which make it illegal for people under 21 years old to drive after any drinking, have also contributed to declines in driving after drinking and alcohol-related traffic deaths among people younger than 21 (Shults et al., 2001; Voas, Tippetts, & Fell 2003; Wagenaar, O'Malley, & LaFond, 2001). Stepped-up enforcement of alcohol purchase laws aimed at sellers and buyers can reduce sales and consumption by underage drinkers (Bonnie & O'Connell, 2003; Wagenaar et al., 2000).

16.3.2.3.   Price of Alcohol

Research clearly shows that increasing the price of alcoholic beverages reduces drinking, heavy drinking, and alcohol-related problems (Chaloupka, Grossman, & Saffer 2002). Price increases can also reduce violence and crime (Babor et al., 2003). Cook and Moore (1993a, 1993b); Chaloupka, Shaffer, & Grossman (1993b); Markowitz and Grossman (2000); and Ruhm (1996) all found that raising taxes on alcohol reduces alcohol-related harm, including suicide, homicide, rape, robbery, assault, motor-vehicle theft, domestic violence, and child abuse. For example, a 10% increase in the tax on beer could reduce the probability of any child abuse by 1.2% and of severe child abuse by 2.1%. (Markowitz & Grossman, 2000). Among moderate drinkers, a 1% price increase has been associated with a 1.19% decrease in consumption (Manning, Blumberg, & Moulton, 1995). Hollingworth et al. (2006) concluded that a 17% increase in the price of alcohol could reduce deaths from harmful drinking by 1,490.

16.3.2.4.   Alcohol Outlet Density and Hours of Sale

Alcohol outlet density has been associated with higher levels of community violence (Parker, 2004), and reducing density may prevent alcohol-related problems. Grube and Stewart (2004) identified six prospective studies of changes in outlet density. Effect sizes were small and inconsistent. Likewise, findings from studies of reducing hours of alcohol sale have also been mixed (Grube & Stewart, 2004). Research in the United Kingdom found no significant changes in alcohol-related or assault hospital admissions as a result of restricting hours of sales. A temporary extension of sale hours in Australia was not associated with increases in maximum consumption (McLaughlin & Harrison-Stewart, 1992). However, Smith (1988) found a 12% increase in traffic injury crashes after pub closing hours were extended from 6 to 10 P.M., Monday through Saturday in Victoria, Australia.

16.3.2.5.   Responsible Beverage Service and Dram Shop Laws

Alcohol purchase surveys indicate that 40–90% of outlets will sell alcohol to underage people. Responsible beverage service (RBS) requires all servers to be above age 21 years, to not sell alcohol to individuals who are under-age, to check identification and verify age, to train managers to identify false credentials, and to monitor drinks consumed by patrons. Lang, Stockwell, Rydan, and Beel (1998) and Saltz and Stanghetta (1997) found little effect of RBS on car crashes. Others (Forster et al., 1994; Grube, 1997) found that RSB can reduce car crashes. Shults et al. (2001) found that server training programs were effective in reducing car crashes if they involved face-to-face instruction and strong management support. Dram shop laws, which enable injured individuals to recover damages from the retailer who sold alcohol to the individual causing the injury, have been estimated to reduce traffic fatalities among underage drinkers by 3–4% (Chaloupka, Saffer, & Grossman, 1993a).

16.3.2.6.   Keg Registration, Social Host Liability, and Alcohol Licensing

Cohen, Mason, and Scribner (2001) reported that keg registration (where each keg purchased can be traced back to its buyer) is negatively correlated with traffic fatality rates. Unfortunately, no other studies of this intervention have been reported (Grube & Stewart, 2004). Grube and Stewart (2004) were able to identify one study (Whetten-Goldstein, Sloan, Stout, & Liang, 2000) that found social host liability laws were associated with lower alcohol-related motor-vehicle crash deaths. This effect was found among adults but not minors. There is strong evidence that sales monopoly systems, such as state- or government-owned, -operated, and -controlled liquor outlets, can limit both alcohol consumption and related problems. Total consumption generally increases when government-owned outlets are replaced by privately owned ones (Howat, Sleet, Elder, & Maycock, 2004).

16.3.3.   Laws to Deter Drinking and Driving

16.3.3.1.   Administrative License Revocation

Enactment and enforcement of administrative license revocation (ALR) laws, allow police to immediately seize the drivers license of anyone operating a motor vehicle while above the legal blood alcohol limit. These laws, in place in 40 states, have been associated with 6–12% declines in alcohol-related traffic deaths, (Tippetts, Voas, Fell, & Nichols, 2005; Voas, Tippetts, & Taylor, 2000).

16.3.3.2.   Blood Alcohol Concentration Limit

By 2004, all U.S. states had set the legal BAC limit for drivers to 0.08%. This legal limit has been repeatedly associated with significant declines in alcohol-related crashes and fatalities (Bernat, Dunsmuir & Wagenaar, 2004, Hingson, Heeren, & Winter, 2000; Shults et al., 2001, Tippetts et al., 2005, Voas et al., 2000).

16.3.3.3.   Laws for Convicted DWI Offenders

In 1988, Maine lowered its legal BAC limit for people with prior convictions from 0.10% to 0.05%. This new limit resulted in a 25% reduction in the proportion of fatal crashes involving drivers with prior convictions (Hingson, Heeren, & Winter, 1998). Impounding vehicles or license plates of previously convicted DWI offenders (Voas, Tippets, & Taylor, 1997, 1998), and mandated use of ignition interlocks (Beck, Rooch, & Baker, 1999) have also reduced recidivism.

16.3.4.   Enforcement and Education

Passage of a law does not by itself ensure reduction in injuries or deaths (Shaw & Ogolla, 2006). The extent to which these laws are enforced will influence their effect. The process of informing the public about new laws, their rationale, and that laws will be enforced is critical to success (Howat et al., 2004).

16.3.4.1.   Sobriety Checkpoints

Sobriety checkpoints are a highly effective enforcement intervention (Elder et al., 2002; Shults et al., 2001) and have yielded declines of 18%–24% in alcohol-related fatal crashes (Fell, Lacey, & Voas, 2004). Checkpoints conducted by as few as 3–5 officers can be just as effective as checkpoints conducted by 15 or more officers.

16.3.4.2. Mass Media Campaigns

Elder et al. (2004) found a median decrease in injury crashes of 10% in their systematic review of the effectiveness of some mass media educational campaigns. The effects were similar for messages focused on legal consequences and on health consequences. They concluded that carefully planned, well-executed media campaigns, that attain adequate audience exposure and are implemented in conjunction with other ongoing prevention activities are effective in reducing alcohol-impaired driving and alcohol-related crashes. Additional support for media effects comes from a study demonstrating alcohol advertising has a direct link to alcohol consumption among underage drinkers (Snyder, Milici, Slater, Sun, & Strizhakova, 2006).

16.3.5. Comprehensive Community Programs

Several carefully conducted community-based initiatives have had particular success in reducing drinking and/or related alcohol problems among young people (Hingson & Howland 2002). Often multiple intervention strategies are incorporated into the programs, including school-based programs involving students, peer leaders, and parents; media advocacy; community organizing and mobilization; environmental policy change to reduce alcohol availability to youth; and heightened enforcement of laws regulating sales and distribution of alcohol and laws reducing alcohol-related traffic injuries and deaths.

Comprehensive community programs that have shown significant reductions in alcohol problems include Communities Mobilizing for Change Program (Wagenaar et al., 2000), Community Trials Program (Holder et al., 2000), Saving Lives Program (Hingson et al., 1996), Matter of Degree Program (Weitzman, Nelon, Lee, & Wechsler, 2004), Fighting Back Program (Hingson et al., 2005a) and a college community intervention (Clapp et al., 2005). Compared to controls, the Communities Mobilizing for Change communities noted the following changes: 17% more alcohol outlets checked the age identification of youthful-looking customers, sales by bars and restaurants to potential underage purchasers decreased by 24%, the proportion of 18- to 20- year-olds seeking to buy alcohol decreased by 25%, the proportion of older teens who provided alcohol to younger teens decreased by 17%, and the number of underage respondents who drank alcohol in the past 30 days decreased by 7%. (Wagenaar et al., 2000)

In the Saving Lives program (Hingson et al., 1996), the proportion of drivers younger than 20 years who reported driving after drinking declined from 19% to 9% in 5 years. Fatal crashes declined 25%, and alcohol-related crashes declined 42% relative to the rest of Massachusetts.

In the Community Trials program, nighttime injury crashes declined by 10%, crashes in which the driver had been drinking declined by 6%, and assault injuries observed in emergency departments declined by 43% (Holder et al., 2000).

The Matter of Degree Program, a college and community partnership showed significant reductions in heavy and frequent drinking, driving after drinking, alcohol-related injury, and other alcohol-related problems (Weitzman et al., 2004). Significant reductions were also observed in the proportion of students who reported being assaulted by another drinking college student.

The Fighting Back program, in which five communities augmented environmental interventions to reduce alcohol availability with increased substance abuse treatment, found a 22% decline in alcohol-related fatal crashes at 0.01% BAC or higher, a 20% decline at 0.08% BAC or higher, and a 17% decline at 0.15% BAC or higher during a 10-year period (Hingson et al., 2005b). A recent systematic review of community-based programs to reduce alcohol-impaired driving found positive results on a number of outcome measures. (Elder, Shults, Sleet, Compton, & Nichols, in press)

16.4.   CONCLUSION

Research has identified a variety of strategies that can prevent alcohol-related injuries and deaths either by reducing individuals' level of alcohol consumption or by restricting people who have been drinking from engaging in behaviors that may pose a risk to themselves or others (e.g., driving a car).

By far, the most extensive literature on reducing alcohol-related injuries is in the arena of reducing motor-vehicle deaths. The interventions that have produced the greatest decline in alcohol-related traffic deaths are raising the legal drinking age to 21 years and general and specific deterrence laws (e.g., criminal per se laws, ALR, lowering of legal blood alcohol limits for adult drivers, zero-tolerance laws for underage drivers, and mandatory screening and treatment for drivers convicted of driving while intoxicated).

The progress made over the last two decades in reducing alcohol-related traffic crash deaths is attributable in part to the high and consistent level of testing for alcohol in drivers fatally injured in crashes. This has facilitated the evaluation of interventions designed to reduce alcohol-related traffic deaths. Unfortunately, alcohol testing of people who die from other injury deaths (e.g., falls, drownings, burns, poisonings, homicides, and suicides) has not been as comprehensive or consistent. Consequently, it is much more difficult to monitor the effect of interventions that seek to reduce other types of injury deaths. However, the implementation of the new National Violent Death Reporting System (NVDRS) by the CDC will facilitate the study of alcohol involvement in violent deaths. The NVDRS is a population-based system that collects information about violent deaths related to suicide, homicides, undetermined intent, legal intervention, and unintentional firearm injury (Paulozzi, Mercy, Frazier, & Annest, 2004). In addition, to improve surveillance of alcohol-related injury, every unnatural death in the United States should be tested for alcohol. The average cost of such testing would be approximately $50 per deceased person or an annual cost of $7.2 million, if all people who die from injuries annually (about 140,000) were tested for alcohol impairment.

Despite the lack of comprehensive alcohol testing of people who die from homicide, suicide, and unintentional injuries, the research literature indicates that individually oriented treatment and brief intervention counseling can reduce alcohol-related traffic deaths, suicide attempts, domestic violence, and other unintentional injuries. Screening and brief counseling for alcohol problems is also effective in reducing heavy alcohol use (Babor et al., 2003) and has been shown to be cost effective among trauma patients (Gentilello et al., 2005). Likewise, environmental interventions have been associated with reduction in alcohol-related injuries. In particular, increasing the price of alcohol has been associated with reductions in alcohol-related traffic deaths, suicides, homicides, domestic violence, child abuse, rapes, robberies, and assaults. Moreover, raising the legal drinking age has reduced alcohol-related traffic deaths, suicide, fighting, and assault.

There are several promising areas for future research. In particular, additional efforts to further delay the initiation of alcohol use among minors are warranted and can build on current knowledge showing that the earlier youth begin to drink, the more likely they will experience unintentional injuries, motor-vehicle crashes, and physical fights after drinking both as adolescents and as adults (Hingson, Heeren, Jamanka & Howland, 2000; Hingson, Heeren, Zakocs, 2001; Hingson, Heeren, Levenson, Jamanka & Voas, 2002). Moreover, cross-cutting efforts that seek to reduce and measure a range of alcohol-related injuries are warranted. Rather than focusing on one type of injury, intervention efforts should examine multiple outcomes. In addition, there is a need to examine the potential role of the use of other substances and injuries. This chapter focused exclusively on alcohol use and injuries. Many alcohol consumers also use other substances, often concurrently with their alcohol use, which can potentially increase their risk for injury. However, little information is available about the injury risk among those who use multiple substances or about appropriate prevention strategies.

Research in trauma centers and emergency departments indicates screening and brief interventions in those settings can reduce alcohol-related problems. According to the Alcoholism Alcohol Policy Information System, there are laws currently in place in 28 states and the District of Columbia (NIAAA, 2005) that allow insurance companies to deny medical reimbursement for treatment of people who have been injured under the influence of alcohol or impairing drugs. Clearly, these laws serve as disincentives for diagnosing alcohol problems in these settings. Whether repeal of those insurance laws will result in more emergency department patients being screened and offered alcohol counseling and whether that, in turn, will reduce alcohol-related injuries and deaths at the population level warrant research attention.

Grassroots organizations such as MADD have played a pivotal role in stimulating passage of laws to reduce injuries related to alcohol. But, as this chapter indicates, both education and enforcement are needed for these laws to succeed. A growing number of evaluations of comprehensive community interventions indicate that education, reducing alcohol availability, and enforcement of alcohol-control and drinking and driving laws (particularly using sobriety check points at the community level) can further reduce alcohol-related traffic injuries and death. Ecological and health promotion approaches that focus on using multidisciplinary and multisector strategies are also needed (Hingson & Sleet, 2006). These programs may also have the potential to reduce nontraffic alcohol-related injuries. A key question is how to mobilize actions at the community level to motivate policy makers, city planners, and advocacy groups to work together to reduce all injuries related to alcohol.

ACKNOWLEDGMENTS. We acknowledge Bob Brewer, MD, Ruth Shults, RN, PhD, Ann Dellinger, MPH, PhD, and Randy Elder, PhD, from the Centers for Disease Control and Prevention for their helpful comments.

REFERENCES

Babor, T. F., Caetano, R., Casswell, S., Edwards, G., Giesbrecht, N., Graham K., Grube, J., Gruenewald, P., Hill, L., Holder, H., Homel, R., Österberg, E., Rehm, J., Room, R., & Rossow, I. (2003). Alcohol: No ordinary commodity—research and public policy. (pp. 106–116) New York: Oxford University Press.

Beck, K., Rooch, W. J., & Baker, E. (1999). Effects of ignition interlock license restrictions on drivers with multiple alcohol offenses: A randomized trial in Maryland. *American Journal of Public Health, 89* (11), 1646–1700.

Bernat, D. H., Dunsmuir, W. T., & Wagenaar, A. (2004). Effects of lowering the legal BAC to 0.08 on single-vehicle-nighttime fatal traffic crashes in 19 juristictions. *Accident Analysis & Prevention, 36*, 1089–1097.

Bonnie, R. J., & O'Connell, M. E. (Eds.). (2003). *Reducing underage drinking: A collective responsibility.* Washington, DC: National Academy of Sciences.

Bonomo, Y., Coffey, C., Wolfe, R., Lynskey, M., Bowes, G., & Patton, G. (2001). Adverse outcomes of alcohol use in adolescents. *Addiction, 96*, 1485–1496.

Borges, G., Cherpitel, C. J., MacDonald, S., Giesbrecht, N., Stockwell, T., & Wilcox, H. C. (2004). A case-cross-over study of acute alcohol use and suicide attempt. *Journal of Studies on Alcohol, 65*, 708–714.

Centers for Disease Control and Prevention, National Center for Chronic Disease Prevention and Health Promotion. (2004). Alcohol attributable deaths and years of potential life lost—United States 2001. *Morbidity & Mortality Weekly Report, 53* (37), 866–870.

Centers for Disease Control and Prevention. (2005a). Alcohol-related disease impact software (ARDI). Retrieved December 8, 2005, from www.cdc.gov/alcohol.

Centers for Disease Control and Prevention. (2005b). National Center for Injury Prevention and Control. Web-based Injury Statistics Query and Reporting System (WISQARS). Retrieved December 8, 2005, from www.cdc.gov/ncipc/wisqars.

Chaloupka, F., Grossman, M., & Saffer, H. (2002). The effects of price on alcohol consumption on alcohol related problems. *Alcohol Research & Health, 26* (1), 22–33.

Chaloupka, F. J., Saffer, H., & Grossman, M. (1993a). Alcohol control policies and motor vehicle fatalities. *Journal of Law & Economics, 22*, 161–186.

Chaloupka, F. J., Saffer, H., & Grossman, M. (1993b). Effects of price on the consequences of alcohol use and abuse. In M. Galanter (Ed.). *Recent developments in alcoholism. The consequences of alcoholism* (vol. 14) (pp. 331–346). New York: Plenum Press.

Cherpitel, C. J., Borges, G. L., & Wilcox, H. C. (2004). Acute alcohol use and suicidal behavior: A review of the literature. *Alcoholism: Clinical & Experimental Research, 28* (5, suppl.), 18s–28s.

Cherpitel, C. J., Ye, Y., & Bond, J. (2005). Attributable risk of injury associated with alcohol use: Cross-national data from the emergency room collaborative alcohol analysis project. *American Journal of Public Health, 95* (2), 266–272.

Chiu, A. Y., Perez, P. E., & Parker, R. N. (1997). Impact of banning alcohol on outpatient visits in Barrow, Alaska. *Journal of the American Medical Association, 278* (21), 1775–1777.

Clapp, J. D., Johnson, M., Voas, R. B., Lange, J. E., Shillington, A., & Russell, C. (2005). Reducing DUI among U.S. college students: Results of an environmental prevention trial. *Addiction, 100*, 327–334.

Cohen, D. A., Mason, K., & Scribner, R. A. (2001). The population consumption model, alcohol control practices, and alcohol-related traffic fatalities. *Preventive Medicine, 34*, 187–197.

Cook, P. J., & Moore, M. J. (1993a). *Economic perspectives on reducing alcohol-related violence. Alcohol and interpersonal violence: Fostering multidisciplinary perspectives. NIAAA Research Monograph 24* (NIH Pub 93-3496). (pp 193–212). Washington, DC.: National Institute on Alcohol Abuse and Alcoholism.

Cook, P. J., & Moore, M. J. (1993b). Taxation on alcoholic beverages. In M. E. Hilton & G. Bloss (Eds.), *Economics and the prevention of alcohol-related problems* (NIH Publication 93-3513), (pp. 33–58). Rockville, MD: National Institute on Alcohol Abuse and Alcoholism.

Dinh-Zarr, T., Diguiseppi, C., Heitman, E., & Roberts, I. (1999). Preventing injuries through interventions for problem drinking: A systematic review of randomized controlled trials. *Alcohol & Alcoholism, 34*, 609–621.

Dischinger, P. C., Mitchell, K. A., Kufera, J. A., Soderstrom, C. A., & Lowenfels, A. B. (2001). A longitudinal study of former trauma center patients: The association between toxicology status and subsequent injury mortality. *Journal of Trauma: Injury; Infection & Critical Care, 51* (5), 877–886.

Elder, R. W., Nichols, J. L., Shults, R. A., Sleet, D. A., Barrios, L.C., Compton, R. & Task Force on Community Preventive Services. (2005). Effectiveness of school-based programs for reducing drinking and driving and riding with drinking drivers: A systematic review. *American Journal of Preventive Medicine, 28* (5S), 288–304.

Elder, R. W., Shults, R. A., Sleet, D. A., Compton, R., & Nichols, J. (In press). Systematic review of multi-component interventions with community mobilization to reduce alcohol-impaired driving. *American Journal Preventive Medicine.*

Elder, R., Shults, R., Sleet, D., Nichols, J. L., Thompson, R., & Rajab, W. (2004b). Effectiveness of mass media campaigns for reducing drinking and driving and alcohol involved crashes. *American Journal of Preventive Medicine, 27* (1), 57–65.

Elder, R. W., Shults, R. A., Sleet, D. A., Nichols, J. L., Zaza, S., & Thompson, R. S. (2002). Effectiveness of sobriety checkpoints for reducing alcohol-involved crashes. *Traffic Injury Prevention, 3,* 266–274.

Elder, R. W., Shults, R. A., Swahn, M. H., & Strife, B. J. (2004a). Alcohol-related emergency department visits among 13–25 year-olds. *Journal of Studies on Alcohol, 65* (3), 297–300.

Fell, S., Lacey, J., & Voas, R. (2004). Sobriety checkpoints: Evidence of effectiveness is strong, but use is limited. *Traffic Injury Prevention, 5* (3), 220–227.

Forster, J. L., McGovern, P. G., Wagenaar, A. C., Wolfson, M., Perry, C. L., & Anstine, P. S. (1994). The ability of young people to purchase alcohol without age identification in northeastern Minnesota, USA. *Addiction, 89,* 699–705.

Gentilello, L. M., Ebel, B. E., Wickizer, T. M., Salkever, D. S., & Rivara, F. P. (2005). Alcohol interventions for trauma patients treated in emergency departments and hospitals: a cost benefit analysis. *Annals of Surgery, 241* (4), 541–550.

Gentilello, L. M., Rivara, F. P., Donovan, D. M., Jurkovich, G. J., Daranciang, E., Dunn, C. W., Villaveces, A., Copass, M., & Ries, R. R. (1999). Alcohol intervention in a trauma center as a means of reducing the risk of injury recurrence. *Annals of Surgery, 230* (4), 473–483.

Greenfeld, L. A. (1998) *Alcohol and crime: An analysis of national data on the prevalence of alcohol involvement in crime* (Bureau of Justice Statistics: Report Prepared for the Assistant Attorney General's National Symposium on Alcohol and Crime). Retrieved Dec. 8, 2005 from www.ojp.usdoj.gov/bjs/pub/pdf/ac.pdf.

Grube, J. W. (1997). Preventing sales of alcohol to minors: Results from a community trial. *Addiction, 92* (S2), S251–S260.

Grube, J., & Stewart, K. (2004). Preventing impaired driving using alcohol policy traffic. *Injury Prevention, 5* (4), 199–207.

Hingson, R. W., Heeren, T., Jamanka, A., & Howland, J. (2000). Age medical of drinking onset and unintentional injury involvement after drinking. *Journal of the American Medical Association, 284,* 1527–1533.

Hingson, R., Heeren, T., Levenson, S., Jamanka, A., & Voas, R. (2002). Age of drinking onset, driving after drinking, and involvement in alcohol-related motor-vehicle crashes. *Accident Analysis & Prevention, 34,* 85–92.

Hingson, R., Heeren, T., & Winter, M. (1998). Effects of Maine's 0.05% legal blood alcohol level for drivers with DWI convictions. *Public Health Reports, 113,* 440–446.

Hingson, R., Heeren, T., & Winter, M. (2000). Effects of recent 0.08% legal blood alcohol limits on fatal crash involvement. *Injury Prevention, 6,* 109–114.

Hingson, R., Heeren, T., Winter, M., & Wechsler, H. (2005d). Magnitude of alcohol-related mortality and morbidity among U.S. college students ages 18–24: Changes from 1998 to 2001. *Annual Review of Public Health, 26* (24), 1–24.

Hingson, R., Heeren, T., & Zakocs, R. (2001). Age of drinking onset and involvement in physical fights after drinking. *Pediatrics, 108,* 872–877.

Hingson, R., & Howland, J. (2002). Comprehensive community interventions to promote health: Implications for college-age drinking problems. *Journal of Studies on Alcohol, 14* (S), 226–240.

Hingson, R., McGovern, T., Howland, J., Heeren, T., Winter, M., & Zakocs, R. (1996). Reducing alcohol impaired driving in Massachusetts: The Saving Lives program. *American Journal of Public Health, 86,* 791–797.

Hingson, R., & Sleet, D. A. (2006). Modifying alcohol use to reduce motor vehicle injury. In A. C. Gielen, D. A. Sleet, R., Clemente (Eds). *Injury and violence prevention: Behavior change theories, methods and applications.* (pp 234–256). San Francisco, CA: Jossey-Bass.

Hingson, R., & Winter, M. (2003). Epidemiology and consequences of drinking and driving. *Alcohol Research & Health, 27* (1), 63–78.

Hingson, R., Zakocs, R., Heeren, T., Winter, M., Rosenbloom, D., & DeJong W. (2005b). Effects on alcohol-related fatal crashes of a community based initiative to increase substance abuse treatment and reduce alcohol availability. *Injury Prevention, 11,* 84–90.

Holder, H., Gruenewald, P. J., Ponicki, W. R., Treno, A. J., Grube, J. W., Saltz, R. F., Voas, R. B., Reynolds, R., Davis, J., Sanchez, L., Gaumont, G., & Roeper, P. (2000). Effects of community-based interventions on high risk driving and alcohol-related injuries. *Journal of the American Medical Association, 284* (18), 2341–2347.

Hollingsworth, W., Ebel, B., McCarthy, C. A., Garrison, M., Christakis, D., & Rivara, F. (2006). Prevention of deaths from harmful drinking in the United States: The potential effects of tax increases and advertising bans on young drinkers. *Journal of Studies on Alcohol, 67,* 1–9.

Howat, P., Sleet, D. A., & Smith, D. I. (1991). Alcohol and Driving: Is the 0.05% blood alcohol concentration limit justified? *Drug & Alcohol Review (Australia), 10* (1), 151–166.

Howat, P., Sleet, D., Elder, R., & Maycock, B. (2004). Preventing alcohol related traffic injury: A health promotion approach. *Traffic Injury Prevention, 5* (3), 199–208.

Lang, E., Stockwell, T., Rydon, P., & Beel, A. (1998). Can training bar staff in responsible serving practices reduce alcohol-related harm? *Drug & Alcohol Review, 17,* 39–50.

Larimer, M., & Cronce, J. (2002). Identification prevention treatment: A review of individually-focused strategies to reduce problematic alcohol consumption by college students. *Journal of Studies on Alcohol, 14* (Supplement), 148–163.

Levy, D. T., Stewart, K., & Wilbur, P. M. (1999). Costs of underage drinking. Retrieved June 23, 2000, from www.pire.org/udetc/documents/costs.pdf.

Leonard, K. E., & Quigley, B. M. (1999). Drinking and marital aggression in newlyweds: An event based analyses of drinking and the occurrence of husband marital aggression. *Journal of Studies on Alcohol, 60,* 537–545.

Longabaugh, R., Woolard, R., Nirenberg, T., Minugh, A. P., Becker, B., Clifford, P. R., Carty, K., Licsw, Sparadeo, F., & Gogineni, A. (2001). Evaluating the effects of a brief motivational intervention for injured drinkers in the emergency department. *Journal of Studies on Alcohol, 62,* 806–816.

Lunetta, P., & Smith, G. S. (2005). The role of alcohol in injury deaths. In R. Preedy, R. Watson, (Eds.), *Comprehensive handbook of alcohol related pathology,* Vol I, (pp 147–164). New York: Academic Press.

Macdonald, S., Cherpitel, C. J., Borges, G., DeSouza, A., Giesbrecht, N., & Stockwell, T. (2005). The criteria for causation of alcohol in violent injuries based on emergency room data from six countries. *Addictive Behaviors, 30* (1), 103–113.

Manning, W. G., Blumberg, L., & Moulton, L. H. (1995). The demand for alcohol: The differential response to price. *Journal Health Economics, 14* (2), 123–148.

Markowitz, S., & Grossman, M. (2000). The effects of beer taxes on child abuse. *Journal Health Economics, 19* (2), 271–282.

McDonald, A., Wang, N., & Camouge, L. (2004). Emergency department visits for alcohol related diseases and injuries between 1992 and 2000. *Archives of Internal Medicine, 164* (5), 531–537.

McLaughlin, K. L., & Harrison-Stewart, A. J. (1992). The effect of temporary period of relaxing licensing laws on the alcohol consumption of young male drinkers. *International Journal of the Addictions, 27,* 409–423.

Mello, M. J., Nirenberg, T. D., Longabaugh, R., Woolard, R., Minugh, A., Becker, B., Baird, J., & Stein, L. (2005). Emergency department brief motivational interventions for alcohol with motor vehicle crash patients. *Annals of Emergency Medicine, 45* (6), 620–625.

Miller, W. R., Walters, S. T., & Bennett, M. E. (2001). How effective is alcoholism treatment in the U.S.? *Journal of Studies on Alcohol, 67,* 211–220.

Moskowitz, H., & Fiorentino, D. (2000). *Review of the literature on the effects of doses of alcohol on driving related skills* (Report No. DOT HS 809-028) Washington, DC.: U.S. Department of Transportation, National Highway Safety Administration.

Mothers Against Drunk Driving. (2002). *Rating the states: An assessment of the nation's attention to the problem of drunk driving and underage drinking.* Irving, TX: Author.

National Highway Traffic Safety Administration. (2003b). *Traffic safety facts 2002.* Retrieved December 8, 2005, from www-nrd.nhtsa.dot.gov/pdf/nrd-30/NCSA/TSFAnn/TSF2002Final.pdf.

National Highway Traffic Safety Administration, National Center for Statistics and Analysis. (2003a). *2002 annual assessment of motor vehicle crashes based on the Fatality Analysis Reporting System, the National Accident Sampling System and the General Estimates System.* Washington, DC: U.S. Department of Transportation.

National Highway Traffic Safety Administration (2005). Traffic safety facts 2003. Retrieved Dec. 8, 2005, from www-nrd.nhtsa.dot.gov/pdf/nrd-30/NCSA/TSFAnn/TSF2003F.pdf.

National Institute on Alcohol Abuse and Alcoholism (2004). *NIAAA Newsletter.* No. 3. Retrieved December 9, 2005, from http://pubs.niaaa.nih.gov/publications/Newletter/winter2004/Newsletter_Number3.pdf.

National Institute on Alcohol Abuse and Alcoholism (2005). Alcohol policy information system (APIS) Website. Retrieved December 8, 2005, from www.alcoholpolicy.niaaa.nih.gov.

O'Malley, P., & Wagenaar, A. (1991). Effects of minimum drinking age laws on alcohol use, related behavior and traffic crash involvement among American youth. *Journal of Studies on Alcohol, 52,* 478–491.

Parker, R. N. (2004). Alcohol and violence: Connections, evidence, and possibilities for prevention. *Journal of Psychoactive Drugs, 2,* 157–163.

Paulozzi, L. J., Mercy, J., Frazier Jr, L., & Annest J. L. (2004). CDC's National Violent Death Reporting System: background and methodology. *Injury Prevention, 10,* 47–52.

Peden, M., Scurfield, R., Sleet, D., Mohan, D., Hyder, A. A., Jarowan, E., & Mathers, C. (Eds). (2004). *World report on road traffic injury prevention.* Geneva: World Health Organization.

Quinlan, K. P., Brewer, R. D., Sleet, D. A., & Dellinger A. M. (2000). Characteristics of child passenger deaths and injuries involving drinking drivers. *Journal of the American Medical Association, 283,* 2249–2252.

Roizen, J. (1997). Epidemiological issues in alcohol-related violence. *Recent Developments in Alcoholism, 13,* 7–40.

Room, R., Babor, T., & Rehm, J. (2005). Alcohol and public health. *Lancet, 365,* 519–530.

Ruhm, C. J. (1996). Alcohol policies and highway vehicle fatalities. *Journal of Health Economics, 15* (4), 435–454.

Saltz, R. F., & Stanghetta, P. (1997). A community-wide responsible beverage service program in three communities: Early findings. *Addiction, 92* (S2), S237–S249.

Shaw, F. E., & Ogolla, C. P. (2006). Law, behavior and injury prevention. In Gielen, A., Sleet, D. A., & DiClemente, R. (Eds.). *Injury and violence prevention: Behavioral science theories, methods and applications.* San Francisco: Jossey-Bass.

Shults, R. A., Elder, R. W., Sleet, D. A., Nichols, J. L., Alao, M. O., & Carande-Kulis, V, G., Zasa, S., Sosin, D. M., Thompson, R. S., & Task Force on Community Preventive Services (2001). Reviews of evidence regarding interventions to reduce alcohol-impaired driving. *American Journal of Preventive Medicine, 21* (S4), 66–88.

Smith, D. I. (1988). Effect of casualty traffic accidents of the introduction of 10 p.m. Monday to Saturday hotel closing in Victoria. *Drug & Alcohol Review,* (Australia), *7,* 163–166.

Snyder, L. B., Milici, F. F., Slater, M., Sun, H., & Strizhakova, Y. (2006). Effects of alcohol advertising exposure on drinking among youth. *Archives of Pediatric & Adolescent Medicine, 160,* 18–24.

Spain, D. A., Boaz, P. W., Davidson, D. J., Miller, F. B., Carrillo, E. H., & Richardson, J. D. (1997). Risk-taking behaviors among adolescent trauma patients. *Journal of Trauma, 43* (2), 423–426.

Substance Abuse and Mental Health Services Administration. (2004). Results from the 2003 national survey on drug use and health: National findings (Office of Applied Studies). Retrieved December 8, 2005, from http://oas.samhsa.gov/nhsda/2k3nsduh/2k3Overview.htm#toc.

Swahn, M. H., Simon, T. R., Hammig, B. J., & Guerrero, J. L. (2004). Alcohol consumption behaviors and risk for physical fighting and injuries among adolescent drinkers. *Addictive Behaviors, 29* (5), 959–963.

Tippetts, A. S., Voas, R. B., Fell, J. C., & Nichols, J. L. (2005). A meta-analysis of 0.08 BAC laws in 19 juristictions in the U.S. *Accident Analysis & Prevention, 37,* 149–161.

Vinson, D. C., Maclure, M., Reidinger, C., & Smith, G. S. (2003). A population-based case-crossover and case-control study of alcohol and the risk of injury. *Journal of Studies on Alcohol, 64,* 358–366.

Voas, R. B., Tippetts, A., & Fell, J. (2003). Assessing the effectiveness of minimum legal drinking age and zero tolerance laws in the United States. *Accident Analysis & Prevention, 35* (4), 579–587.

Voas, R. B., Tippetts, A., & Taylor, E. (1997). Temporary vehicle immobilization: Evaluation of a program in Ohio. *Accident Analysis & Prevention, 29* (5), 635–642.

Voas, R. B., Tippetts, A., & Taylor, E. (1998). Temporary vehicle impoundment in Ohio: A replication and confirmation. *Accident Analysis & Prevention, 30* (5), 651–656.

Voas, R., Tippetts, A., & Taylor, E. (2000). The relationship of alcohol safety laws to drinking drivers in fatal crashes. *Accident Analysis & Prevention, 32,* 483–492.

Wagenaar, A. C., Murray, D. M., Gehan, J. P., Wolfson, M., Forster, J., Toomey, T., & Perry, C. L. (2000). Communities mobilized for change on alcohol: effects of a randomized trail on arrests and traffic crashes. *Addiction, 95,* 209–217b.

Wagenaar, A. C., O'Malley, P. M., & LaFond, C. (2001). Lowered legal blood alcohol limits for young drivers: Effects on drinking, driving and driving after drinking behaviors in 30 states. *American Journal of Public Health, 91,* 801–804.

Wagenaar, A. C., & Toomey, T. L. (2002). Effects of minimum drinking age laws: Review and Analysis of the Literature from 1960–2000. *Journal of Studies on Alcohol, 14* (suppl.), 206–226.

Weitzman, E. R., Nelon, T. F., Lee, H., & Wechsler, H. (2004). Reducing drinking and related harms in college: Evaluation of the matter of degree program. *American Journal of Preventive Medicine, 27,* 187–196.

Wells-Parker, E., Bangert-Drowns, R., McMillen, R., & Williams, M. (1995). Final results from a meta-analysis of remedial intervention with drink/drive offenders. *Addiction, 90,* 907–926.

Whetten-Goldstein, K., Sloan, F. A., Stout, E., & Liang, L. (2000). Civil liability, criminal law, and other policies and alcohol-related motor vehicle fatalities in the United States: 1984–1995. *Accident Analysis & Prevention, 32* (6), 723–733.

Chapter 17

Reducing the Misuse of Firearms

Frederick P. Rivara and Arthur L. Kellermann

17.1 INTRODUCTION

Firearm injuries, by virtue of the number of deaths, years of life lost, and cost to society, represent an important and persistent public health problem. It is also a problem that crosses several disciplines, particularly public health, clinical medicine, mental health, criminology, and criminal justice. Approaches to controlling injuries due to guns involve all of these disciplines and include many strategies that have been effective for other injury control problems. In 2005, the U.S. Task Force on Community Preventive Services published a systematic review of gun laws and effects on homicide and suicide (Hahn et al., 2005). That review contains detailed tables about the effect of a variety of laws. The National Academies was recently asked to assess "the strengths and limitations of the existing research and data on gun violence." Their report (National Research Council, 2005) provides another comprehensive review, with detailed tables, weighing the evidence for various interventions. Due to space constraints, neither document can be summarized here. The intended audience and the goals of these two reports differ from those of this chapter. The National Research Council (NRC) report was targeted at researchers, and its recommendations were directed at stimulating a stronger evidence base for gun policy through rigorous research. The Task Force report was narrowly focused on legislative approaches and, similar to the NRC report, was directed at assessing the quality of the current research evidence on gun policy. This chapter, on the other hand, is directed at public health practitioners and policy makers—individuals who must base their actions and decisions on the evidence that is available now.

Although the total fluctuates from year to year, firearms consistently rank second only to motor vehicle crashes as a cause of fatal injury in the United States. More than 95% of fatal firearm injuries are the result of self-directed or interpersonal violence (Figs. 17.1 and 17.2). Data on deaths and injuries from firearms can be obtained from a number of sources. Deaths are almost completely captured by the vital statistics systems. While complete, these data provide no information

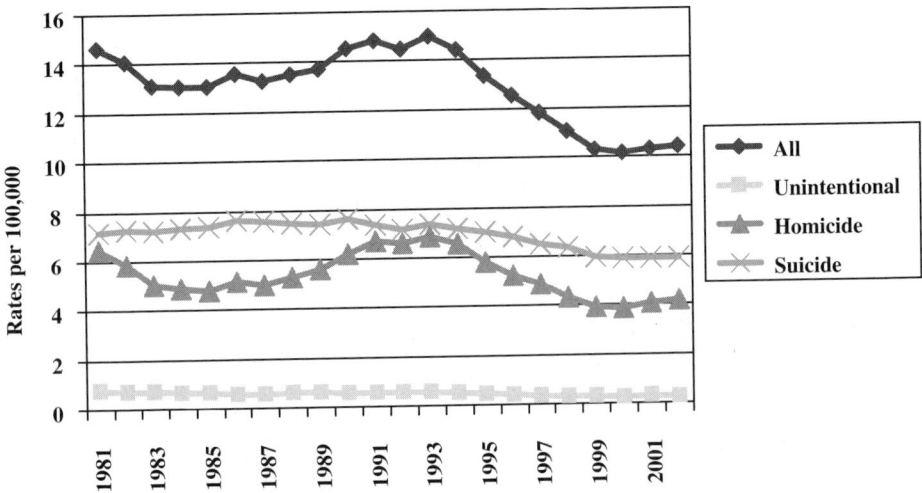

Figure 17.1. Changing rates of firearm-related fatality rates by intent, 1981–2002.

on the identity or characteristics of the perpetrator, make or model of gun, or circumstances of the shooting. The Uniform Crime Reports have more detailed information on the circumstances of firearm homicides but are part of a voluntary system, often incomplete, and provide no information about suicides or unintentional shootings.

A more promising source of data is the National Violent Death Reporting System (NVDRS) established by the Centers for Disease Control and Prevention (CDC) in 2002 (Paulozzi, Mercy, Frazier, & Annest, 2004). Modeled after the Fatality Analysis Reporting System of the National Highway Traffic Safety Administration (NHTSA) for motor-vehicle crash-related injuries, this data set is intended to provide more detailed, uniform information on all violent deaths, regardless of method, including suicides and unintentional shootings. Nonfatal injuries are most often treated in hospital emergency departments; however, few states have any systematic data on nonadmitted patients. Local surveillance systems can be developed

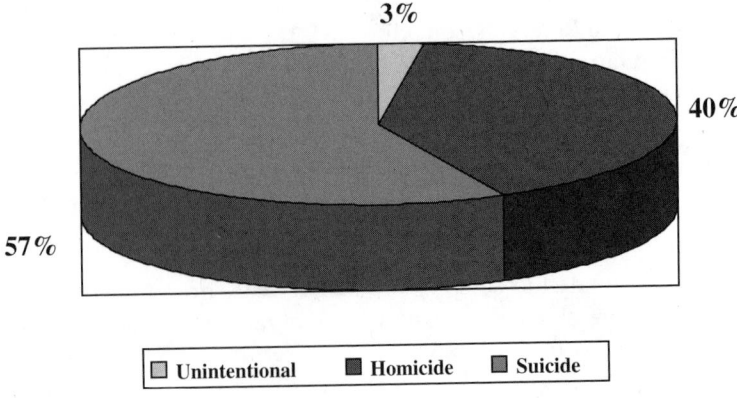

Figure 17.2. Percentage of deaths caused by gun suicides, homicides, and unintentional injuries in 2002.

and can be used to guide intervention efforts (Kellermann, Bartolomeos, Fuqua-Whitley, Sampson, & Parramore, 2001). Hospitalized injuries can be captured by statewide hospital discharge databases, many of which are available through the Agency for Healthcare Research and Quality (2005) in its Healthcare Cost and Utilization Project (HCUP).

The available data demonstrate that firearm injuries continue to be a major cause of mortality in the United States, producing approximately 30,000 deaths per year. In 2002, more than half of these deaths were suicides, a fact that has been neglected by much of the public health community and largely outside the scope of criminal justice efforts to decrease firearm misuse. Firearm deaths from suicide have decreased by only 17% since 1981, whereas homicide deaths have decreased by 35% and unintentional deaths by 65%. Thus interventions to reduce firearm-related mortality must consider suicides as well as homicides and unintentional deaths.

Gun injuries have a very high case-fatality ratio, especially self-inflicted gunshot wounds. In a large population-based study, self-inflicted gunshot wounds had a case fatality ratio of 0.86 and assault-related firearm injuries had a case fatality ratio of 0.16 (Kellermann et al., 1996). Many of these individuals were pronounced dead on the scene or died before or shortly after reaching a hospital. Because the case-fatality ratio for firearm injuries is so high, they are not as great a cause of hospitalizations (relative to their contribution to deaths) as are falls or motor-vehicle crashes (Wadman, Muelleman, Coto, & Kellermann, 2003) (Figs. 17.3 and 17.4).

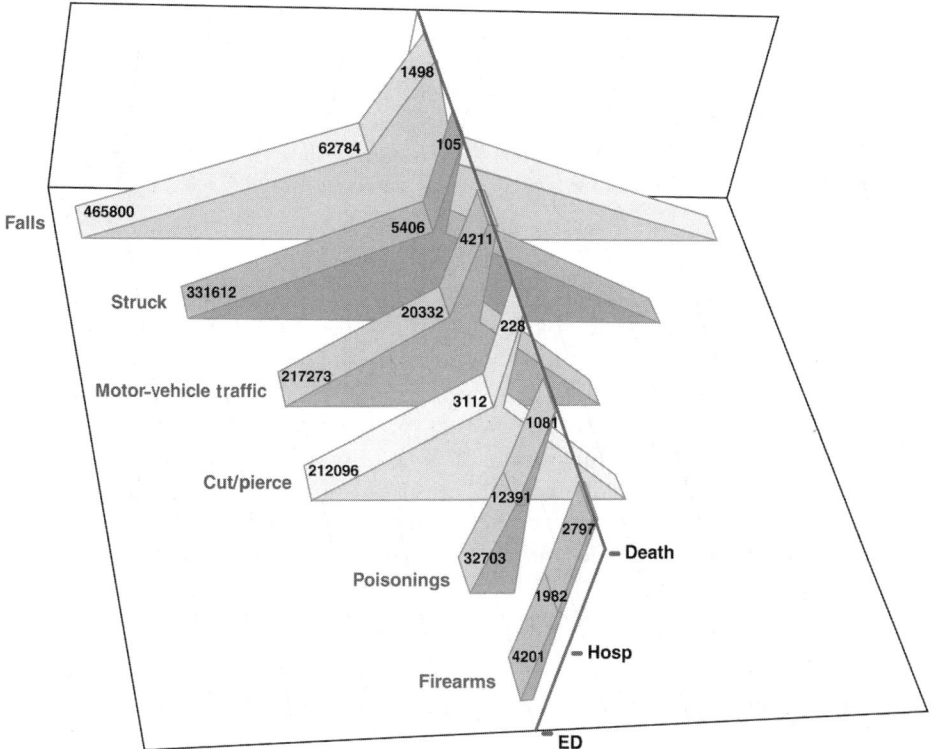

Figure 17.3. The pyramid of injury for all causes of injury—Missouri and Nebraska, 1996–1998. The base represents emergency department visits (*ED*), the middle third represents hospitalizations (*Hosp*), and the apex represents fatalities (*Death*).

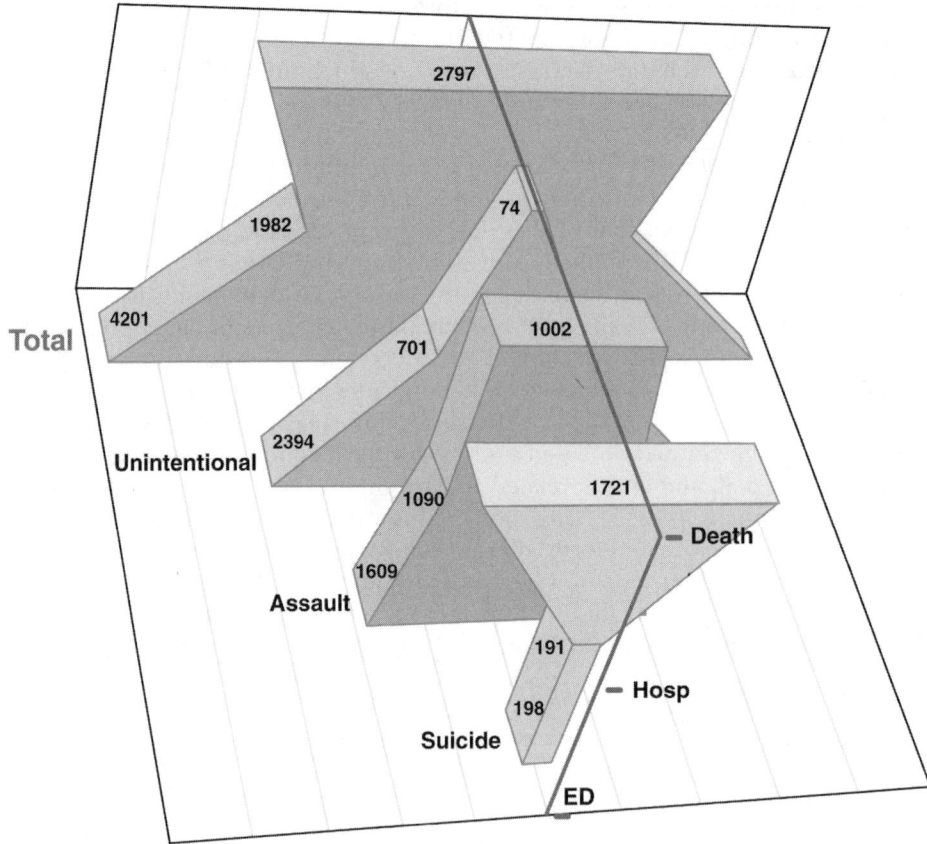

Figure 17.4. The pyramid of injury for firearm injuries—Missouri and Nebraska, 1996–1998. The base represents emergency department visits (*ED*), the middle third represents hospitalizations (*Hosp*), and the apex represents fatalities (*Death*).

The long-term consequences of firearm injury can be substantial. In one study of hospitalized gunshot victims, health status (measured by the Short-Form (SF)-36) 6–12 months after injury was significantly worse than before the event. In addition to physical disabilities, more than one third of individuals studied reported symptoms of posttraumatic stress disorder (Greenspan & Kellermann, 2002).

Another measure of the magnitude of the gun problem and its importance for society are the costs of gun violence. Recently, Cook and Ludwig (2000) conducted an extensive analysis of these costs. Their approach considered not only the costs stemming from gunshot injuries but also "the costs of all the efforts to deter shootings or protect against them" (p. 49). They estimate that the costs of gun violence in the United States are on the order of $116 billion per year (in 2004 dollars).

17.2.   HISTORY OF PUBLIC HEALTH PREVENTION EFFORTS

Public health efforts to prevent firearm injuries have been relatively limited. Most have consisted of educational efforts, which, as reviewed below, have not proven to be very effective. Some efforts have been made to promote safe storage of guns, an intervention now resting on firmer ground with the publication of recent data.

In contrast to the limited efforts of public health, police and the criminal justice community have made extensive efforts to combat the gun violence problem. Concern about gun violence intensified during the crack cocaine–induced homicide epidemic of the mid-1980s to early 1990s, a surge driven almost entirely by gun homicides (Blumstein, Rivara, & Rosenfeld, 2000). Some of the efforts implemented in response to this challenge appear to have been successful, although not without controversy (NRC, 2005).

No injury control problem in America is more politically contentious than injuries resulting from the use or misuse of firearms. The political passions that surround any discussion of "gun control" have seriously hindered efforts to adopt broad-based, public health approaches to firearm injury (Kellermann, 1997).

17.3.   REVIEW OF INTERVENTIONS (TABLE 17.1)

17.3.1.   Educational Interventions

The vast majority of educational efforts specifically designed to prevent firearm injuries are focused on youth and the prevention of unintentional shootings. Some interventions are directed at parents, some at youth, and some at both. This literature was extensively reviewed by the NRC (2005). Of the more than 80 programs disseminated in the United States, the NRC identified formal evaluations for 11. No evidence of effects on real-life behavior or on shootings was found. The experience of the two decades since the publication of *Injury in America* (NRC, 1985) has taught us that evaluation of educational interventions *must* extend beyond measuring changes in knowledge, attitudes, and self-reported behaviors or even observed behavior in laboratory settings. It has been repeatedly shown that such measures correlate poorly with actual behavior in the real world, much less reductions in the incidence or severity of injuries.

Despite numerous studies and stories of firearm injuries involving children, many gun-owning parents still have an unrealistic notion of how responsibly their child would behave around a loaded firearm (Farah, Simon, & Kellermann, 1999). In one study, covert observation of 8- to 12-year-old boys playing in a room where a specially instrumented firearm was placed revealed that boys this age cannot be trusted to behave safely around firearms if no adult is present. This was true even among boys previously taught about firearm safety (Jackman, Farah, Kellermann, & Simon, 2001). No education intervention program has yet been shown to change this pattern of behavior. In the absence of such studies, there is no evidence to support the effectiveness (or lack of effectiveness) of educational programs aimed at reducing firearm injuries. When educational programs directed at young children have been implemented to prevent other kinds of injuries, results have been mixed (NRC, 2005). In light of these facts, we cannot endorse large-scale implementation of child gun safety programs, unless they are done as part of a well-designed prospective study.

Although little is known about how to teach children to behave safely around guns, even less is known about how to prevent mishaps at the other end of the age spectrum, when cognitive decline can pose significant danger to gun owners (Green & Kellerman, 1996). Suicide among individuals with declining health

Table 17.1. Potential Interventions to Prevent Injuries and Deaths from Firearms

Educational interventions
- Educational interventions for youth and their parents
- School-based suicide-prevention programs
- Educational programs to help families of depressed individuals
- Education to promote safe storage of guns in the home

Youth violence prevention programs
- Nurse home visiting
- Early childhood education
- Multisystemic therapy
- Therapeutic foster parents

Engineering interventions
- Gun locks, lock boxes, and other safe storage technology
- Redesigning guns to reduce the risk of unintended discharge
  ○ Grip safeties
  ○ Loaded chamber indicators
  ○ Magazine disconnect devices
  ○ Drop safeties
  ○ Child-resistant designs
  ○ Personalized guns
- Nonlethal adjuncts for self-defense and law enforcement
- Designing environments to reduce the potential for gun violence
  ○ Metal detector technology
  ○ Bulletproof partitions in cabs, all-night gas stations, and convenience stores
  ○ Crime prevention through environmental design
  ○ Surveillance cameras

Enforcement of laws to reduce illegal carrying and/or use of firearms
- Right-to-carry laws
- Enhanced sentences for crimes committed with a firearm
- Increasing legal sanctions for unlawful carrying of a firearm
- Problem-oriented policing
- Directed patrols to identify and arrest illegal firearm carriers

Decreasing the supply of firearms
- Regulating firearm sales
- Restrictive licensing of would-be purchasers
- Banning the sale of all firearms in a jurisdiction
- Firearm buyback programs
- Background checks of firearm purchasers
- Restrict access by perpetrators of intimate partner violence
- Increased oversight of firearm dealers
- Systematic tracing of firearms seized from criminals to identify scofflaw dealers and/or straw purchasers

status is another concern. As America's population ages, these issues will grow in importance.

The vast majority of educational interventions implemented to date are mostly focused on unintentional injuries, which account for a relatively small fraction of the firearm-injury problem in the United States (Fig. 17.2). Several educational programs have been implemented to prevent suicides, but none has specifically focused on suicides with guns. Some states mandate school-based suicide-prevention programs (Metha, Weber, & Webb, 1998) in hopes of increasing awareness; promoting identification of students at high risk of suicide attempts and suicide; enhancing the coping abilities of teenagers; and providing information to students, teachers, and parents on the availability of mental health resources for those who need them. Evaluations of these programs indicate potentially beneficial effects but all use weak study designs (Kalaft, 1997; Metha et al., 1998; Zenere & Lazarus, 1997).

Conversely, educational interventions to encourage family members or next-of-kin to remove guns from the homes of depressed people have not proven to be successful. In one study involving parents of depressed adolescents, 26.9% of families heeded the advice of their physicians to remove guns from the home. Unfortunately, another 17.1% actually acquired one or more guns during the 2-year follow-up period (Brent, Baugher, Birmaher, Kolko, & Bridge, 2000).

17.3.2. Engineering Measures

17.3.2.1. Safe Storage

Families that are unwilling to consider removing guns from the home are generally more receptive to the idea of safe storage, using a variety of technologies, reviewed below. The idea of safe storage appears to be particularly acceptable to gun owners with small children in their homes. Most organizations, regardless of their position in the larger gun control debate, endorse the idea that guns and ammunition in the home should be stored safely.

There are good reasons to adopt this strategy. A population-based study of shootings in three United States cities found that 73% of unintentional shootings and 87% of firearm suicides occurred in a home, most often the home of the victim (Kellermann et al., 1996). Safe storage of firearms by a variety of means—including use of gun locks, lock boxes, or a gun safe—has the potential to reduce unintentional shootings; some gun suicides; and, by preventing thefts, perhaps some homicides as well. Studies of the relationship between readily accessible firearms and the risk of unintentional shootings or suicide in the home have found varying degrees of association (Brent et al., 1991, 1988, 1993; Conwell et al., 2002; Kellermann et al., 1992; Shah, Hoffman, Wake, & Marine, 2000). A recent case-control study demonstrated that locking guns up is associated with a 73% decrease in the risk of a youth gun suicide or unintentional gun death (Grossman et al., 2005). Another recent case-control study examined the effect of safe storage on suicide risk, stratifying by the degree of the individual's intent to die (Shenassa, Rogers, Spalding, & Roberts, 2004). Safe storage appeared to prevent suicide among those with low or medium intention to die but was not protective for those with a high intent to die.

Despite the potential benefits of this strategy, it is unclear whether programs that promote safe storage of guns are effective. A systematic review of seven evaluations of efforts to promote safe storage yielded mixed results (McGee, Coyne-Beasley, & Johnson, 2003). Only one of these studies was a randomized controlled trial; it showed no effect (Grossman et al., 2000).

Another argument marshaled in support of safe storage of guns is prevention of theft—an important source of guns used in crime. Cook, Molliconi, & Cole (1995) estimate that as many as 500,000 guns are stolen each year in the United States. As many as 10% of guns that are not acquired legally from federally licensed dealers are stolen (Alcohol, Tobacco, and Firearms [ATF], 2000). In theory, there could be adverse effects from promoting gun locks, if this impaired access to a gun when urgently needed for self-defense. Estimates of the annual incidence of defensive gun use vary widely, from 100,000 per year (McDowall & Wiersema, 1994) to 2.5 million or more per year (Kleck & Gertz, 1995). However, at least one study suggests that firearms are infrequently used to resist home invasion crime. In a study of 198 such incidents, the victim used a gun to successfully resist the intruder in only 3 (1.5%). However, six victims lost their firearm to the intruder(s) (Kellermann, Westphal, Fischer, & Harvard, 1995). Unfortunately, the gun that is kept loaded and within easy reach for protection may also be reached by a curious child, an angry spouse, or a depressed grandparent. The odds that the firearm kept in the home will be involved in the death or injury of a member of the household substantially outweigh the odds that it will be used to injure or kill an intruder (Kellermann, Somes, Rivara, Lee, & Banton, 1998).

One compromise that provides a measure of safety yet allows quick access is use of a lockbox or safe with a push-button lock or user-specific sensor. These devices allow almost instantaneous access to the gun. Unfortunately, there are no data on whether safe storage of guns with these devices increases or decreases important outcomes, such as the rate of home invasions, burglary, or firearm theft.

17.3.2.2. Safer Firearms

The science of injury control has repeatedly demonstrated that one of the most effective methods to prevent unintentional injuries or decrease their severity is by building safety into the device itself. The number of motor-vehicle crash deaths per million miles driven has steadily declined over the last four decades due in great part to changes in the vehicle itself: collapsible steering wheels, side-impact protection, padded dashes, laminated windshields, antilock brakes, and other changes. Conversely, most changes made to guns over the same time period, such as changing the most prevalent design from low-capacity revolvers with a relatively slow rate of fire to high-capacity pistols with faster rates of fire, have increased their lethality (Wintemute, 1996).

Meanwhile, manufacturers have done little to make their products less prone to inadvertent or unauthorized discharge. As many as one third of fatal and nonfatal firearm shootings may be attributed to lack of basic safety features and other shortcomings in gun design (Ismach et al., 2003). A number of simple and readily available devices can reduce unintentional shootings; these include grip safeties, loaded chamber indicators, and magazine-disconnect devices. Grip safeties require that the firearm be held properly and with a certain amount of strength, thereby preventing careless users and young children from inadvertently discharging the firearm. Loaded chamber indicators show the user that the gun has a bullet in the chamber, even if the magazine has been removed. A magazine disconnect device can prevent the firearm from being discharged once the magazine is removed. This is important because one third of U.S. adults believe that a firearm cannot be shot if the magazine is removed (Vernick, Meisel, Teret, Milne, & Hargarten, 1999).

More technologically sophisticated options could be easily adopted as well (Teret & Culross, 2002; Teret, DeFransecco, Hargarten, & Robinson, 1998). One idea that has been insufficiently explored is to design firearms to meet a certain standard of child resistance. Although this approach was employed to great effect to develop child-resistant containers for pharmaceuticals and other poisons, it has not been attempted to decrease child injuries from firearms. Polls show that the idea has strong public support, even among gun owners. (Ismach et al., 2003; Karlson & Hargarten, 1997; Teret et al., 1998). Yet another option is the idea of personalizing guns to prevent an unauthorized user, be it a child or another adult, from using the gun. Personalization of guns could involve requiring the owner to wear a programmable electronic or magnetic ring on the hand that grips the gun or equipping the firearm with a device that recognizes the fingerprints of the authorized user. Use of personalizing technology could have a major effect on the 500,000 stolen guns entering the secondary market each year because stolen guns with this feature would be useless to criminals (Cook & Ludwig, 2000).

Currently, imported handguns must meet AFT (AFT, 1983) designer and performance criteria; domestically manufactured guns do not. These criteria provide importers with a modest incentive to include certain gun safety features in their products, but they aren't required to do so. An examination of 755 different handgun models made or imported into the United States revealed that all of the imported handguns but only 66% of the domestic models met the ATF's criteria However, no handgun, whether imported or domestically manufactured, contained all four desirable safety devices: a loaded chamber indicator, grip safety, magazine safety, and a firing pin block. Many did not include even one of these (Milne, Hargarten, Kellermann, & Wintemute, 2003).

Unfortunately, none of these technological options has been evaluated in large-scale studies to determine if they reduce unintended shootings. Although there are strong theoretical reasons to support the adoption of engineering countermeasures to reduce unintended shootings, there are no empirical studies to prove the validity of this approach. The NRC (2005, p. 215) report concluded that in the absence of such data, arguments on both sides of the issue of gun technology "are largely speculative."

17.3.3.   Enforcement Measures

17.3.3.1.   Child Access Prevention Laws

Sometimes, individuals can be persuaded to adopt a desired injury prevention behavior under the force of law. In response to public concern about unintended shootings of children, several states adopted child access prevention (CAP) laws that make it a crime if a child is shot with an adult's gun. The goal of CAP laws is to promote the safe storage of guns.

Evaluations of CAP laws have produced conflicting results. Lott and Whitley (2002) found no effect of CAP laws on unintentional injuries or suicides among youth but reported a net increase in violent crime. In contrast, Cummings, Grossman, Rivara, and Koepsell (1997) found that CAP laws were associated with a 23% reduction in unintentional shooting deaths among children under the age of 15 years. State-level declines in homicide and suicide rates were noted as well, but these differences were not statistically significant. Webster, Vernick, Zeoli, and Manganello (2004) evaluated CAP laws and found that their enactment was associated with an 11% decrease in firearm suicides and no compensatory increase in nonfirearm suicides among 14- to 17-year-olds. They found a similar effect on both gun and nongun suicides for 18- to 20-year-olds as well. Thus CAP laws may represent an important intervention for prevention of youth suicides, especially suicides with a firearm.

17.3.3.2.   Increased Likelihood of Arrest and Punishment

Illegal acquisition and illegal carrying of guns can be reduced by increasing the likelihood of arrest and the legal consequences of proscribed possession. Firearms, even illegally acquired firearms, can be approached as a commodity using

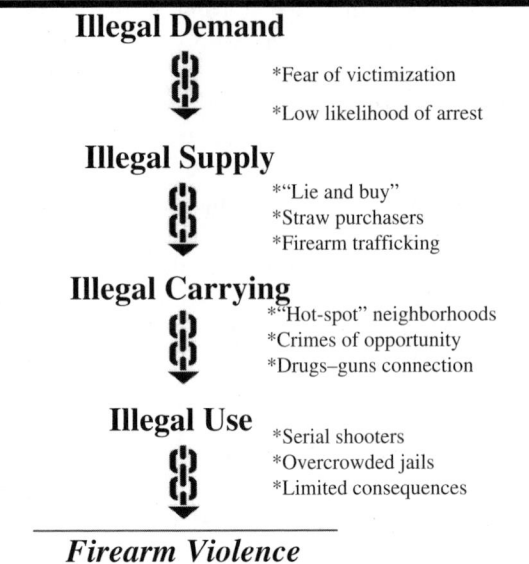

Illegal Demand

*Fear of victimization

*Low likelihood of arrest

Illegal Supply

*"Lie and buy"
*Straw purchasers
*Firearm trafficking

Illegal Carrying

*"Hot-spot" neighborhoods
*Crimes of opportunity
*Drugs–guns connection

Illegal Use

*Serial shooters
*Overcrowded jails
*Limited consequences

Firearm Violence

Figure 17.5. The chain of events leading to firearm violence.

the economic principles of supply and demand. Decreasing illegal demand for firearms among criminals or reducing illegal supply and/or the illegal carrying of firearms could potentially break the chain of events that leads to gun violence and thereby reduce the incidence of gun assaults and homicides (Fig. 17.5). Most of the research on the effectiveness of various strategies to reduce illegal acquisition, use, or carrying of firearms has been conducted by researchers in criminal justice and criminology and thus may be unfamiliar to public health professionals. Because legislation and enforcement are important components of injury control, it is important to examine the evidence of potential benefit from efforts directed at decreasing illegal use of guns.

17.3.3.3.   Right-to-Carry Laws

According to the NRC (2005), 34 states have current laws (also known as shall issue laws) allowing individuals who do not meet certain disqualifying criteria (primarily criminal record, mental illness, or domestic violence offender) to carry concealed handguns. The effect of these laws on crime and murder has been hotly debated in the literature. Some analyses indicate that these laws reduce crime and violence (Lott, 2000; Lott & Mustard, 1997). However, other analyses have reached the opposite conclusion (Ayres & Donohue, 2003a, 2003b) Still other evaluations have found no significant effect one way or the other (Duggan, 2001). The most recent study indicates that right-to-carry laws are associated with an 8% increase in homicide (Relative Risk (RR): 1.08; 95% confidence interval [CI]: 0.99–1.17) (Rosengart et al., 2005). What is clear is that the results are very sensitive to the analytic model employed and the variables used. The NRC (2005, p. 121) concluded (although not without dissent) that "it is impossible to draw strong conclusions from the existing literature on the causal impact of these laws."

17.3.3.4.   Enhanced Sentences for Firearm Crimes

Judicial interventions to decrease demand for criminal use of guns have centered on stiffening sentences for crimes committed with guns and on incarcerating individuals, especially juveniles, for unlawfully carrying a gun. Perhaps the most well known of the sentence-enhancement efforts for firearm-related crimes is Richmond's Project Exile, begun in 1997. The core of the program was transferring prosecution for selected felonies committed while in possession of a gun from state to federal courts, which do not allow parole and therefore result in much longer sentences.

Project Exile was widely touted as a great success, but subsequent analyses suggest that its effect may have been less than originally thought (Raphael & Ludwig, 2003). Project Exile was implemented at a time when firearm homicide and overall homicide rates were dropping substantially in many cities across the country. In addition, because Richmond experienced a surge in firearm crime immediately before implementing Project Exile, the subsequent decline may be due at least in part to regression to the mean. Once these factors are taken into consideration, the effect of Project Exile appears to be modest at best.

17.3.3.5.   Unlawful Carrying

Another strategy to reduce criminal use of guns is to directly target the unlawful carrying or use of firearms. The best-known example of this strategy is the Bartley-Fox law, which was implemented in Massachusetts in 1975. This law mandated a minimum 1 year of incarceration for unlawful carrying of a firearm. Actual implementation of the law was marked by the use of lesser possession charges, and potentially fewer gun arrests. Analyses of the Bartley-Fox law produced mixed results, suggesting unclear effects (Beha, 1977; Deutsch & Alt, 1977; Pierce & Bowers, 1981). Other countries have attempted to discourage illegal carrying in their own way. Responding to skyrocketing rates of firearm homicide, the mayors of Cali and Bogotá, Colombia, established a ban on the carrying of firearms on weekends after a payday and on holidays, times of particularly high homicide rates. Under this ordinance, police had authority to stop and search any citizen on the street. Even in a country as violent as Colombia, enforcement of the ban was associated with a 13–14% lower rate of homicide during these periods compared to times when gun carrying was allowed (Villaveces et al., 2000).

17.3.3.6.   Effect of Policing Policies

Although such an indiscriminant policing strategy as used in Colombia could not pass constitutional muster in the United States, other tactics can be legally employed to break the chain of illegal acts before a violent crime occurs (Fig. 17.5). Policing strategies can take a number of different forms, but most fall under the rubric of "problem-oriented policing" in which police focus on areas of the community or individuals associated with high rates of gun crime (NRC, 2005). These policies are based on a large body of data that have consistently found that a small proportion of the population is responsible for a large portion of violent crime in a community (Farrington, 1996; Farrington, Langan, & Tonry, 2004; Loeber et al., 1999; Moffitt, 2003).

Several problem-oriented policing strategies have been subjected to rigorous examination for their effect on homicide. The most well known of these programs is the Kansas City Gun Project, in which extra proactive police patrols were used to target illegal gun carrying in a small area of Kansas City with a homicide rate 20 times the national average. These patrols increased the detection of gun carrying though car checks, pedestrian checks, searches associated with other arrests, and car stops for traffic violations. Although the effort produced a modest increase in the number of guns seized, the results were dramatic—the intervention area showed a 49% decrease in gun crimes compared to the control area, which had no decrease (Sherman & Rogan, 1995).

This program was subsequently replicated in Indianapolis. There, police focused on detecting illegal gun carrying by searching the cars of suspicious individuals during traffic stops. The effort resulted in a 50% increase in the number of illegal guns seized and significantly decreased the gun homicide rate in the target area (McGarrell, Chermak, Weiss, & Wilson, 2001).

In 1998, Pittsburgh implemented stepped-up police patrols to detect illegal gun carrying by suspicious persons in two areas of the city with historically high rates of gun crime. To maximize its effect, the operation was focused on particularly dangerous days of the week ("high risk places at high risk times") (Cohen & Ludwig, 2003). A rigorous analysis of the program found that it produced a 71% reduction in gunshot injuries from assault in the intervention areas on patrol days compared to control areas (Cohen & Ludwig, 2003).

Could similar strategies be employed to reduce illegal gun carrying by juveniles? One study of incarcerated juvenile offenders in Fulton County, Georgia, revealed that more than 80% of gun carriers acquired their first gun before the age of 15 years. A total of 40% of those who carried a gun reported that they did so to feel safer; another 40% felt more "energized" or excited by carrying a gun. However, 34% reported anxiety, mainly due to fear of being caught. Almost all of the respondents reported that guns were widely available from a variety of sources (Ash, Kellermann, Fuqua-Whitley, & Johnson, 1996). Findings like these suggest that interventions designed to reduce juveniles' fear of crime, and therefore their perceived need to carry a gun for protection, and measures that increase fear of arrest could reduce levels of juvenile gun carrying (Ash et al., 1996).

A somewhat different approach was used by the Boston Gun Project to combat the high juvenile murder rate in that city during the late 1980s and early 1990s. Working together, an interdisciplinary group of police agencies, prosecutors, community groups, and academics implemented Operation Ceasefire—an highly coordinated effort to reduce gang violence by telling gangs that violence would not be tolerated and that violent acts by a gang would result in an immediate, severe, and sustained response. Gangs that challenged the prohibition quickly learned that the threat was real. Unlike the other programs described earlier, evaluation was built into the planning process. After implementation of Operation Ceasefire, the monthly total of homicides declined 63%, a trend significantly different from that in other cities during the same time frame (Braga, Kennedy, Piehl, & Waring, 2001a, 2001b; NRC, 2005).

17.3.4. Reducing Firearm Availability

It may also be possible, through a variety of tactics, to reduce gun violence by decreasing the illegal supply of firearms and/or reducing diversion of firearms from legal to illegal markets.

17.3.4.1.   Regulating Firearm Sales

Only federally licensed dealers can legally receive interstate shipments of guns, and these guns can be legally sold only after a background check on the purchaser. The requirement for a background check and a 5-day waiting period was mandated by Congress in the Brady Bill of 1994. In 1998, the law was modified to allow "instant" background checks, and it was extended from handguns to cover the purchase of long guns as well. Despite the intuitive appeal of this strategy, and the political struggle that surrounded its enactment, evaluations showed that the law had no *overall* effect on homicide or suicide rates (Ludwig & Cook, 2000). However, in the subset of states that instituted and maintained a waiting period, the rate of firearm suicides involving people ages 55 years of age and older substantially declined. The value of a background check is supported by a study from California, which revealed that during the first week after purchase of a handgun, purchasers have a firearm suicide rate 57-fold higher than the general population (Wintemute, Parham, Beaumont, Wright, & Drake, 1999)

There are other data supporting the practice of conducting background checks and denying proscribed individuals the right to purchase a handgun may decrease firearm injuries and fatalities. For example, studies by Wintemute and colleagues (Wintemute, Wright, Drake, & Beaumont, 2001; Wright, Wintemute, & Rivara, 1999) of individuals denied handgun purchase in California indicate that denial was associated with subsequent decreases in the rate of arrest for gun offences and violent crimes.

Prohibition of sales of particular types of guns have been part of the federal effort to decrease gun injuries since 1934, when Congress outlawed the sale of machine guns and sawed-off shotguns (Vernick & Hepburn, 2003). This was subsequently expanded to include Saturday night specials in some states, assault-type semiautomatic weapons in 1994 (Vernick & Hepburn, 2003), and a few types of ammunition (e.g., exploding bullets). A study of the Maryland law banning Saturday night specials found no immediate effect of the law but possibly a delayed effect, with a 6.8–11.5% lower rate of gun homicides in subsequent years (Webster, Vernick, & Hepburn, 2002). A more recent analysis of the law found no net effect on firearm homicides or suicides (Rosengart et al., 2005). Faced with conflicting accounts of its effect and the powerful political opposition to its continuation, the assault weapons ban was allowed to expire on September 13, 2004.

Another tactic to reduce illegal supply of guns involves limiting the number of guns that can be bought at a single time by any one individual. The idea behind this policy is to discourage straw purchasing—the legal acquisition of guns followed by rapid resale of the guns to legally proscribed individuals, such as felons or juveniles. After a "one gun a month" law was implemented in Virginia, the number of crime guns that could be traced back to purchases in Virginia decreased by 36% (Weil & Knox, 1996). There was also a 66% reduction in crime guns along the I-95 corridor to the northeast United States that could be traced back to Virginia after enactment of the law. However, another evaluation of Virginia's law and a similar law in Maryland found no net effect on either state's rate of gun homicides or suicides (Rosengart et al., 2005). This suggests that any shortfall in supply was offset by guns from states with lax gun laws, such as Georgia and Alabama.

Canada has long adopted a restrictive approach to firearms, particularly handguns. Two retrospective cohort studies designed to assess the effect of Canada's approach to gun control compared rates of crime, violence, homicide, and suicide by method in Vancouver, British Columbia, to those of Seattle, Washington, a

U.S. city of similar characteristics. Although the two cities had very similar rates of criminal activity and assault during the 7-year study interval (1980–1986), the rate of homicide in Seattle was 63% higher than in Vancouver. Virtually all of this excess risk was attributable to a 4.8-fold higher rate of handgun homicide in Seattle (Sloan et al., 1988). It is interesting that when the effects of Canadian-style gun control on suicide rates in King County, Washington, and the Vancouver metro area were examined a different pattern emerged. This study revealed that firearms were used to commit suicide in King County more than twice as often as guns were used to commit suicide in Vancouver. Handguns were used more than five times more often in King County. However, the higher rate of gun suicide in King County was entirely offset by a proportionately higher rate of firearm suicides in Vancouver. The only age group in which a higher rate of gun suicides in King County was not entirely offset by a higher rate of nongun suicides in Vancouver was among 15- to 24-year-olds, a group thought to make more impulsive suicide attempts (Sloan, Rivara, Reay, Ferris, & Kellermann, 1990).

To the best of our knowledge, there are no studies of the effect of bans of specific types of ammunition. Ammunition bans were not covered in the NRC (2005) report or in recent systematic review of firearm laws by the Task Force on Community Preventive services (Hahn et al., 2005).

17.3.4.2.   Banning the Sale of All Firearms

For understandable reasons, banning the sale of all guns has rarely been tried. In 1976, Washington, D.C., banned the purchase, sale, transfer, or possession of handguns by any civilian in the District. Loftin, McDowall, Wiersema, and Cottey (1991) compared the homicide and suicide rate in the District to that in the adjacent metropolitan areas of Maryland and Virginia over the following 9 years. During that time interval, the authors found that the law was associated with a 25% decrease in gun homicides, a 23% decrease in gun suicides, and with no increase in nongun homicides or suicides. Others have examined the effect of the D.C. handgun ban and reached different conclusions. One reported that homicide rates in D.C. increased compared to Baltimore (Britt, Bordua, & Kleck, 1996). Because handgun bans are controversial, studies of their effect should be conducted in other cities that have enacted such policies. For example, Chicago banned the sale of handguns in 1982, although the prohibition does not extend to the city's numerous (and nearby) suburbs.

17.3.4.3.   Gun Buy-back Programs

One way that has been suggested to decrease the pool of available guns is to buy them back from individuals, with no questions asked. The largest such program was instituted in Australia after the massacre of 35 people at Port Arthur in 1996 by an individual wielding a semiautomatic rifle. This led to a government prohibition of self-loading rifles and self-loading and pump-action shotguns and an offer to buy back those that were already in circulation, resulting in an estimated 50–90% of these weapons being taken out of circulation. The net result of this policy was removal of approximately 20% of all firearms in Australia (Reuter & Mouzos, 2003). Following this gun buyback, firearm homicides and suicides sharply declined, but there was no significant change in Australia's overall homicide and suicide rates (Reuter & Mouzos, 2003). It is important to note, however, that guns were never the dominant means of homicide or suicide in Australia. Even a 50% reduction in long-gun homicides would decrease the overall homicide rate in the nation by only 5%. Buy-back programs in the United States are popular, but they have never been shown to be effective. (Callahan, Rivara, & Koepsell, 1994; Sherman, 2001). The concept of gun buybacks in the United States is probably inherently flawed, because the guns turned in are almost all low-risk guns, rather than guns most likely to be used in assaults (Kuhn et al., 2002).

17.3.4.4. *Preventing Access by Intimate Partner Violence Offenders*

In the United States, about 11% of murder victims are killed by an intimate partner; among females, this is as high as one third of murders (Fox & Zawitz, 2001; Kellermann & Heron, 1999). More than twice as many women are shot and killed by their spouse or an intimate acquaintance than are murdered by strangers using a gun, knife, or any other means (Kellermann & Mercy, 1992). An abusive male having access to a gun has been associated with a 7.6 fold increased risk of intimate partner femicide (Campbell et al., 2003). In one large case-control study of gun ownership as a risk factor for homicide in the home, keeping a gun in the home was associated with a 2.7-fold increased risk. Virtually all of this risk was due to homicide at the hands of a family member or intimate acquaintance (Kellermann, Rivara, & Rushforth, 1993).

In response to the problem, federal and state laws were enacted to prevent individuals convicted of intimate partner misdemeanors, as well as those under a current protection order, from purchasing or owning a gun (Vigdor & Mercy, 2003). Convicted felons, regardless of offense, are already prohibited from legally purchasing or owning a gun. State laws directed at preventing individuals with an active protection order from owning a gun appear to be associated with a 9% reduction in both overall and firearm-related intimate partner homicide. In contrast, laws prohibiting gun ownership by individuals convicted of past intimate partner violence misdemeanors have no appreciable effect. Similar results were found for federal laws; there did not appear to be an additive effect when a jurisdiction had both a federal and state law (Vigdor & Mercy, 2003).

17.3.4.5. *Regulating Firearm Dealers*

Just as a small proportion of individuals account for the majority of crimes, so do a small proportion of federal firearms licensees account for the majority of the sales of guns subsequently used for assault and homicide (ATF, 2000). By systematically tracing all crime guns seized within a geographical area, law-enforcement agencies can readily determine if any federally licensed gun dealers are disproportionately involved in the sale of guns that are subsequently used to commit crimes. A California study of crime guns used by youth under 25 years identified 812 federal firearm licensed dealers who were involved with the sale of at least one traced gun. However, 13 dealers, representing only 1.6% of all dealers involved with traced guns, sold 16.6% of these crime guns in California (Wintemute, Romero, Wright, & Grassel, 2004). Tightening of licensing requirements and increasing the fees charged for a federal firearms license reduced the number of federally licensed dealers from a high of 286,000 in April 1993 to a low of 102,020 in March 2000 (ATF, 2004). Whether this reduction contributed to the decline in gun homicide that occurred during this interval is unknown.

17.4.   DISCUSSION

One of the basic premises of injury control is that specific injury problems should be addressed by specific countermeasures. Public health–based efforts to reduce firearm injuries and fatalities can be done only by considering the three basic types of firearm injuries separately: interpersonal violence (including firearm assaults and homicides), self-directed violence (attempted and completed suicides), and unintentional shootings.

Compared with suicides and homicides, the problem of unintentional firearm injuries is small but nevertheless important, especially for children. In contrast to the other two causes of firearm injury, it should be readily amenable to prevention. Most parents overestimate their child's ability to be safe around guns (Jackman et al., 2001). Unfortunately, the few educational programs tested to date have not shown to be effective. Faced with extravagant claims, but no empirical evidence of benefit, many parents may falsely conclude that it is no longer necessary to store their firearms in a safe and secure manner. In light of new evidence of the importance of safe storage of guns and ammunition, an effective public health effort to promote safe storage might prevent many unintentional shootings and perhaps a few suicides. Unfortunately, no public education campaign has yet been shown to increase safe storage of guns (Sidman et al., 2005). This does not mean that such efforts are futile. Well-implemented, multifaceted community campaigns have been found to be effective in promoting other safety behaviors, such as bike helmet use (Rivara et al., 1994) and car seat use (Ebel, Koepsell, Bennett, & Rivara, 2003).

Changing product design offers the greatest hope for prevention of unintentional gun injuries, just as they have been effective with other types of unintentional injuries, such as motor-vehicle crash-related injuries. On this point, the NRC (2005, p. 217) seriously erred when it declared that engineering approaches are ineffective. This is a fruitful avenue for exploration.

There is clear evidence that the type of weapon matters in determining whether a criminal assault will end in serious injury or death. Criminologists refer to this as an "instrumentality effect." This instrumentality of violence suggests that measures aimed at reducing illegal supply, acquisition, carrying, or use of firearms could contribute to an overall decrease in gun violence, including gun homicides (Fig. 17.5).

There is no evidence to date that traditional public health approaches are effective for preventing intentional firearm injuries. However, two avenues are available that may allow public health practitioners to address this problem. One is to attack the underlying causes of violence. Recent reviews and decision models (Ebel et al., 2005) indicate that early childhood and adolescent interventions such as home visiting (Bilukha et al., 2005), early childhood education (Schweinhart, Barnes, & Weikart, 1993), multisystemic therapy (Borduin et al., 1995), and therapeutic foster care (Hahn et al., 2004) can prevent violent behavior among youth. Because there is strong continuity in behavior over time (Farrington, 1996) and because most murders are committed by individuals with a history of violence dating back to childhood, interventions implemented in early life may reduce gun homicides later on.

The other avenue for public health practitioners is to actively collaborate with police and criminal justice agencies in addressing firearm carrying and firearm violence. The St. Louis, Kansas City, and Boston projects indicate that targeted interventions on high-risk individuals and behaviors can potentially reduce firearm violence in a community. Public health professionals, and particularly acute-care clinicians such as trauma surgeons, emergency physicians and emergency nurses, can play an active role in supporting law-enforcement agencies in identifying victims, collecting spent projectiles for ballistics analysis, conducting population-based firearm injury surveillance, and evaluating the impact of community-based gun violence countermeasures (Kellermann, 2004; Kellermann et al., 2001).

The evidence for instrumentality effects of guns is even stronger for suicide than for homicide (NRC, 2005). The treatment of depression is beyond the scope of our chapter and is not reviewed here. The strategies discussed here for unintentional injuries, including safe storage and changes in gun design, also have the potential to have an effect on rates of firearm suicide, the most common method of suicide in the United States. Strategies like these are solidly within the public health purview.

17.5.   RESEARCH NEEDS

The recommendations in the NRC (2005) report addressed research needs to inform public policy around guns and are not to be repeated here. Nevertheless, there are some specific recommendations for the public health community that we can make. While randomized community intervention trials are difficult, they are necessary to understand accurately what works and what does not (Koepsell et al., 1992; Koepsell, Diehr, Cheadle, & Kristal, 1995) Because of confounding by different individual and community characteristics, observational studies cannot address many important issues of program efficacy; these can be resolved only by conducting large-sale, randomized studies.

Unfortunately, it is difficult to convince policymakers to fund evaluation research, particularly on an issue as controversial as gun control. Responding to pressure from political interest groups in the first half of the 1990s, Congress has curtailed funding for firearm injury prevention research (Kassirer, 1995, 1998; Kellermann, 1997). The resulting lack of experimental evidence has hampered the development of sound public policies and public health interventions to decrease deaths and injuries from firearms. Notwithstanding these difficulties, it is clear that we are reaching the limits of what can be accomplished with prehospital care, trauma surgery, and rehabilitation. If we want to save more lives from firearm injuries, we must do a better job of prevention.

REFERENCES

Agency for Healthcare Research and Quality. (2005). *Healthcare cost and utilization project.* Retrieved January 31, 2005, from www.ahrq.gov/data/hcup/.

Alcohol, Tobacco, and Firearms. (1983). *Factoring criteria for weapons* (No. Form 4590 [5330.5]). Washington, DC: Department of the Treasury.

Alcohol, Tobacco, and Firearms. (2000). *ATF regulatory actions: Report to the Secretary on firearm initiative.* Washington, DC: Department of the Treasury.

Alcohol, Tobacco, and Firearms. (2004). *Firearms commerce in the United States—2001/2002.* Washington, DC: Department of the Treasury.

Ash, P., Kellermann, A. L., Fuqua-Whitley, D., & Johnson, A. (1996). Gun acquisition and use by juvenile offenders. *Journal of the American Medical Association, 275* (22), 1754–1758.

Ayres, I., & Donohue, J. J. III (2003a). The latest misfires in the "more guns, less crime" hypothesis. *Stanford Law Review, 55,* 1371–1398.

Ayres, I., & Donohue, J. J. III (2003b). Shooting down the "more guns, less crime" hypothesis. *Stanford Law Review, 55,* 1193.

Beha, J. A. (1977). "And nobody can get you out." The impact of a mandatory prison sentence for the illegal carrying of a firearm on the use of firearms and on the administration of criminal justice in Boston. *Boston University Law Review, 57,* 96–146, 289–333.

Bilukha, O., Hahn, R. A., Crosby, A., Fullilove, M. T., Liberman, A., Moscicki, E., Snyder, S., Tuma, F., Corso, P., & Schofield, A. (2005). The effectiveness of early childhood home visitation in preventing violence: A systematic review. *American Journal of Preventive Medicine, 28* (2 suppl. 1), 11–39.

Blumstein, A., Rivara, F. P., & Rosenfeld, R. (2000). The rise and decline of homicide—And why. *Annual Review of Public Health, 21,* 505–541.

Borduin, C. M., Mann, B. J., Cone, L. T., Henggeler, S. W., Fucci, B. R., Blaske, D. M., & Williams, R. A. (1995). Multisystemic treatment of serious juvenile offenders: Long-term prevention of criminality and violence. *Journal of Consulting and Clinical Psychology, 63* (4), 569–578.

Braga, A. A., Kennedy, D. M., Piehl, A. M., & Waring, E. J. (2001a). Problem-oriented policing, deterrence and youth violence: An evaluation of Boston's Operation Ceasefire. *Journal of Research on Crime & Delinquency, 38* (3), 195–225.

Braga, A. A., Kennedy, D. M., Piehl, A. M., & Waring, E. J. (2001b). *Reducing gun violence: The Boston Gun Project's Operation Ceasefire.* Washington, DC: National Institute of Justice.

Brent, D. A., Baugher, M., Birmaher, B., Kolko, D. J., & Bridge, J. (2000). Compliance with recommendations to remove firearms in families participating in a clinical trial for adolescent depression. *Journal of American Academy of Child & Adolescent Psychiatry, 39* (10), 1220–1226.

Brent, D. A., Perper, J. A., Allman, C. J., Moritz, G. M., Wartella, M. E., & Zelenak, J. P. (1991). The presence and accessibility of firearms in the homes of adolescent suicides. A case-control study. *Journal of the American Medical Association, 266* (21), 2989–2995.

Brent, D. A., Perper, J. A., Goldstein, C. E., Kolko, D. J., Allan, M. J., Allman, C. J., & Zelenak, J. P. (1988). Risk factors for adolescent suicide. A comparison of adolescent suicide victims with suicidal inpatients. *Archive of General Psychiatry, 45* (6), 581–588.

Brent, D. A., Perper, J. A., Moritz, G., Baugher, M., Schweers, J., & Roth, C. (1993). Firearms and adolescent suicide. A community case-control study. *American Journal of Diseases in Children, 147* (10), 1066–1071.

Britt, C., Bordua, D. J., & Kleck, G. (1996). A reassessment of the D. C. gun law: Some cautionary notes on the use of interrupted time series design for policy impact assessment. *Law & Society Review, 30,* 361–380.

Callahan, C. M., Rivara, F. D., & Koepsell, T. D. (1994). Money for guns: Evaluation of the Seattle gun buy-back program. *Public Health Reports, 109* (4), 472–477.

Campbell, J. C., Webster, D., Koziol-McLain, J., Block, C., Campbell, D., Curry, M. A., et al., (2003). Risk factors for femicide in abusive relationships: Results from a multisite case control study. *American Journal of Public Health, 93* (7), 1089–1097.

Cohen, J., & Ludwig, J. (2003). Policing crime guns. In J. Ludwig & P. J. Cook (Eds.), *Evaluating gun policy: Effects on crime & violence* (pp. 217–239). Washington, DC: Brookings Institution Press.

Conwell, Y., Duberstein, P. R., Connor, K., Eberly, S., Cox, C., & Caine, E. D. (2002). Access to firearms and risk for suicide in middle-aged and older adults. *American Journal of Geriatric Psychiatry, 10* (4), 407–416.

Cook, P. J., & Ludwig, J. (2000). *Gun violence: The real costs.* New York: Oxford University Press.

Cook, P. J., Molliconi, S., & Cole, T. (1995). Regulating gun markets. *Journal of Criminal Law and Criminology, 86,* 59–82.

Cummings, P., Grossman, D. C., Rivara, F. P., & Koepsell, T. D. (1997). State gun safe storage laws and child mortality due to firearms. *Journal of the American Medical Association, 278* (13), 1084–1086.

Deutsch, S. J., & Alt, F. B. (1977). The effect of Massachusetts' gun control law on gun-related crimes in the city of Boston. *Education Quarterly, 1,* 543–568.

Duggan, M. (2001). More guns, more crime. *Journal of Political Economy, 109* (4), 1086–1114.

Ebel, B. E., Koepsell, T. D., Bennett, E. E., & Rivara, F. P. (2003). Use of child booster seats in motor vehicles following a community campaign: A controlled trial. *Journal of the American Medical Association, 289,* 879–884.

Ebel, B. E., Loeber, R., McCarty, C. A., Garrison, M. M., Farrington, D. P., Christakis, D. A., Hawkins, J. D., & Rivara, F. P. (2005). *Prevention of deaths from violence in the US: The role of interventions during childhood and adolescence.* Manuscript submitted for publication.

Farah, M. M., Simon, H. K., & Kellermann, A. L. (1999). Firearms in the home: Parental perceptions. *Pediatrics, 104* (5 Pt 1), 1059–1063.

Farrington, D. P. (1996). *Understanding and preventing youth crime.* York, UK: Joseph Rowntree Foundation.

Farrington, D. P., Langan, P. A., & Tonry, M. (2004). *Cross-national studies in crime and justice* (No. NCJ 200988.). Washington, DC: Department of Justice, Office of Justice Programs, Bureau of Justice Statistics.

Fox, J. A., & Zawitz, M. W. (2001). *Homicide trends in the United States.* Washington, DC: Department of Justice.

Green, R. C., & Kellerman, A. L. (1996). Grandfather's gun: When should we intervene? *Journal of the American Geriatrics Society, 44* (4), 467–469.

Greenspan, A. I., & Kellermann, A. L. (2002). Physical and psychological outcomes 8 months after serious gunshot injury. *Journal of Trauma, 53* (4), 709–716.

Grossman, D. C., Cummings, P., Koepsell, T. D., Marshall, J., D'Ambrosio, L., Thompson, R. S., & Mack, R. S. (2000). Firearm safety counseling in primary care pediatrics: A randomized, controlled trial. *Pediatrics, 106* (1 Pt 1), 22–26.

Grossman, D. C., Mueller, B. A., Riedy, C., Dowd, M. D., Villaveces, A., Prodzinski, J., Nakagawara, J., Howard, J., Thiersch, N., & Harruff, R. (2005). Gun storage practices and risk of youth suicide and unintentional firearm injuries. *Journal of the American Medical Association, 293,* 707–714.

Hahn, R. A., Bilukha, O., Crosby, A., Fullilove, M. T., Liberman, A., Moscicki, E., Snyder, S., Tuma, F., & Briss, P. A. (2005). Firearms laws and the reduction of violence: A systematic review. *American Journal of Preventive Medicine, 28* (2 suppl. 1), 40–71.

Hahn, R. A., Lowy, J., Bilukha, O., Snyder, S., Briss, P., Crosby, A., Fullilove, M. T., Tuman, F., Moscicki, E. K., Lieberman, A., Schofield, A., & Corso, P. S., & CDC Task Force on Community Preventive Services (2004). Therapeutic foster care for the prevention of violence: A report on recommendations of the Task Force on Community Preventive Services. *MMWR Recommendation and Reports, 53* (RR-10), 1–8.

Ismach, R. B., Reza, A., Ary, R., Sampson, T. R., Bartolomeos, K., & Kellermann, A. L. (2003). Unintended shootings in a large metropolitan area: An incident-based analysis. *Annals of Emergency Medicine, 41* (1), 10–17.

Jackman, G. A., Farah, M. M., Kellermann, A. L., & Simon, H. K. (2001). Seeing is believing: What do boys do when they find a real gun? *Pediatrics, 107* (6), 1247–1250.

Kalaft, J. (1997). Prevention of youth suicide. *Healthy Children 2010: Enhancing children's wellness, 8,* 175–213.

Karlson, I., & Hargarten, S. W. (1997). *Reducing firearm injury and death: A public health sourcebook.* New Brunswick, NJ: Rutgers.

Kassirer, J. P. (1995). A partisan assault on science—The threat to the CDC. *New England Journal of Medicine, 333* (12), 793–794.

Kassirer, J. P. (1998). Private arsenals and public peril. *New England Journal of Medicine, 338* (19), 1375–1376.

Kellermann, A., & Heron, S. (1999). Firearms and family violence. *Emergency Medicine Clinics of North America, 17* (3), viii, 699–716.

Kellermann, A. L. (1997). Comment: Gunsmoke—Changing public attitudes toward smoking and firearms. *American Journal of Public Health, 87* (6), 910–913.

Kellermann, A. L. (2004). Treating gun violence before the 911 call. *Annals of Emergency Medicine, 43* (6), 743–745.

Kellermann, A. L., Bartolomeos, K., Fuqua-Whitley, D., Sampson, T. R., & Parramore, C. S. (2001). Community-level firearm injury surveillance: Local data for local action. *Annals of Emergency Medicine, 38* (4), 423–429.

Kellermann, A. L., & Mercy, J. A. (1992). Men, women, and murder: Gender-specific differences in rates of fatal violence and victimization. *Journal of Trauma, 33* (1), 1–5.

Kellermann, A. L., Rivara, F. P., Lee, R. K., Banton, J. G., Cummings, P., Hackman, B. B., & Somes, G. (1996). Injuries due to firearms in three cities. *New England Journal of Medicine, 335* (19), 1438–1444.

Kellermann, A. L., Rivara, F. P., & Rushforth, N. B. (1993). Gun ownership as a risk factor for homicide in the home. *New England Journal of Medicine, 329,* 1084–1091.

Kellermann, A. L., Rivara, F. P., Somes, G., Reay, D. T., Francisco, J., Banton, J. G., Prodzinski, J., Fligner, C., & Hackman, B. B. (1992). Suicide in the home in relation to gun ownership. *New England Journal of Medicine, 327* (7), 467–472.

Kellermann, A. L., Somes, G., Rivara, F. P., Lee, R. K., & Banton, J. G. (1998). Injuries and deaths due to firearms in the home. *Journal of Trauma, 45* (2), 263–267.

Kellermann, A. L., Westphal, L., Fischer, L., & Harvard, B. (1995). Weapon involvement in home invasion crimes. *Journal of the American Medical Association, 273* (22), 1759–1762.

Kleck, G., & Gertz, M. (1995). Armed resistance to crime: The prevalence and nature of self-defense with a gun. *Journal of Criminal Law and Criminology, 86,* 150–187.

Koepsell, T. D., Diehr, P. H., Cheadle, A., & Kristal, A. (1995). Invited commentary: Symposium on community intervention trials. *American Journal of Epidemiology, 142* (6), 594–599.

Koepsell, T. D., Wagner, E. H., Cheadle, A. C., Patrick, D. L., Martin, D. C., Diehr, P. H., Perrin, E. B., Kristal, A. R., Allan-Andrida, C. H., & Dey, L. L. (1992). Selected methodological issues in evaluating community-based health promotion and disease prevention programs. *Annual Review of Public Health, 13,* 31–57.

Kuhn, E. M., Nie, C. L., O'Brien, M. E., Withers, R. L., Wintemute, G. J., & Hargarten, S. W. (2002). Missing the target: A comparison of buyback and fatality related guns. *Injury Prevention, 8* (2), 143–146.

Loeber, R., DeLamatre, M., Tita, G., Cohen, J., Stouthamer-Loeber, M., & Farrington, D. P. (1999). Gun injury and mortality: The delinquent backgrounds of juvenile victims. *Violence & Victims, 14* (4), 339–352.

Loftin, C., McDowall, D., Wiersema, B., & Cottey, T. J. (1991). Effects of restrictive licensing of handguns on homicide and suicide in the District of Columbia. *New England Journal of Medicine, 325* (23), 1615–1620.

Lott, J. R. (2000). *More guns, less crime: Understanding crime and gun-control laws.* Chicago: University of Chicago Press.

Lott, J. R., & Mustard, J. E. (1997). Crime, deterrence, and right-to-carry concealed handguns. *Journal of Legal Studies, 26* (1), 1–68.

Lott, J. R., & Whitley, J. E. (2002). Safe storage gun laws: Accidental deaths, suicide, and crime. *Journal of Law & Economics, 44* (1), 659–689.

Ludwig, J., & Cook, P. J. (2000). Homicide and suicide rates associated with implementation of the Brady Handgun Violence Prevention Act. *Journal of the American Medical Association, 284* (5), 585–591.

McDowall, D., & Wiersema, B. (1994). The incidence of defensive firearm use by U.S. crime victims, 1987 through 1990. *American Journal of Public Health, 84* (12), 1982–1984.

McGarrell, E., Chermak, S., Weiss, A., & Wilson, J. (2001). Reducing firearm violence through directed police patrol. *Criminology & Public Policy, 1,* 119–148.

McGee, K. S., Coyne-Beasley, T., & Johnson, R. M. (2003). Review of evaluations of educational approaches to promote safe storage of firearms. *Injury Prevention, 9* (2), 108–111.

Metha, A., Weber, B., & Webb, L. D. (1998). Youth suicide prevention: A survey and analysis of policies and efforts in the 50 states. *Suicide & Life-Threatening Behavior, 28* (2), 150–164.

Milne, J. S., Hargarten, S. W., Kellermann, A. L., & Wintemute, G. J. (2003). Effect of current federal regulations on handgun safety features. *Annuals of Emergency Medicine, 41* (1), 1–9.

Moffitt, T. E. (2003). Life-course-persistent and adolescent-limited antisocial behavior: A 10-year research review and a research agenda. In B. B. Lahey & T. E. Moffitt (Eds.), *Causes of conduct disorder and juvenile delinquency* (pp. 49–75). New York: Guilford Press.

National Research Council. (1985). *Injury in America.* Washington, DC: National Academy Press.

National Research Council. (2005). *Firearms and violence: A critical review.* Washington, DC: National Academies Press.

Paulozzi, L. J., Mercy, J., Frazier, L. Jr., & Annest, J. L. (2004). CDC's National Violent Death Reporting System: Background and methodology. *Injury Prevention, 10* (1), 47–52.

Pierce, G. L., & Bowers, W. J. (1981). The Bartley-Fox gun law's short-term impact on crime in Boston. *Annals of the American Academy of Political Social Science, 455,* 120–137.

Raphael, S., & Ludwig, J. (2003). Prison sentence enhancements: The case of Project Exile. In J. Ludwig & P. J. Cook (Eds.), *Evaluating gun policy: Effects on crime and violence* (pp. 251–277). Washington, DC: Brookings Institution Press.

Reuter, P., & Mouzos, J. (2003). Australia: A massive buyback of low-risk guns. In J. Ludwig & P. J. Cook (Eds.), *Evaluating gun policy: Effects on crime and violence.* (pp. 121–142). Washington, DC: Brookings Institution Press.

Rivara, F. P., Thompson, D. C., Thompson, R. S., Rogers, L. W., Alexander, B., Felix, D., & Bergman, A. B. (1994). The Seattle children's bicycle helmet campaign: Changes in helmet use and head injury admissions. *Pediatrics, 93,* 567–569.

Rosengart, M. R., Cummings, P., Nathens, A. B., Heagerty, P., Maier, R. V., & Rivara, F. P. (2005). An evaluation of state firearm regulations and homicide and suicide deaths. *Injury Prevention, 11,* 77–83.

Schweinhart, L. J., Barnes, H. V., & Weikart, D. P. (1993). *Significant benefits: The High-Scope Perry preschool study through age 27.* Ypsilanti, MI: High/Scope Press.

Shah, S., Hoffman, R. E., Wake, L., & Marine, W. M. (2000). Adolescent suicide and household access to firearms in Colorado: Results of a case-control study. *Journal of Adolescent Health, 26* (3), 157–163.

Shenassa, E. D., Rogers, M. L., Spalding, K. L., & Roberts, M. B. (2004). Safer storage of firearms at home and risk of suicide: A study of protective factors in a nationally representative sample. *Journal of Epidemiology & Community Health, 58* (10), 841–848.

Sherman, L. W. (2001). *Reducing gun violence: What works, what doesn't, what's promising.* Paper presented at the Perspectives on Crime and Justice: 1999–2001 Lecture Series, Washington, DC.

Sherman, L. W., & Rogan, D. (1995). Effects of gun seizures on gun violence: "Hot spots" patrol in Kansas City. *Justice Quarterly, 12* (4), 673–694.

Sidman, E. A., Grossman, D. C., Koepsell, T., D'Ambrosio, L., Britt, J., Simpson, E. S., Rivara, F. P., & Bergman, A. B. (2005). Evaluation of a community-based handgun safe-storage campaign. *Pediatrics, 115,* e654–e661.

Sloan, J. H., Kellermann, A. L., Reay, D. T., Ferris, J. A., Koepsell, T., Rivara, F. P., Rice, C., Gray, L., & LoGerfo, J. (1988). Handgun regulations, crime, assaults, and homicide. A tale of two cities. *New England Journal of Medicine, 319* (19), 1256–1262.

Sloan, J. H., Rivara, F. P., Reay, D. T., Ferris, J. A., & Kellermann, A. L. (1990). Firearm regulations and rates of suicide. A comparison of two metropolitan areas. *New England Journal of Medicine, 322* (6), 369–373.

Teret, S. P., & Culross, P. L. (2002). Product-oriented approaches to reducing youth gun violence. *Future of Children, 12* (2), 118–131.

Teret, S. P., DeFransecco, S., Hargarten, S. W., & Robinson, K. D. (1998). Making guns safer. *Issues in Science & Technology, Summer,* 37–40.

Teret, S. P., Webster, D. W., Vernick, J. S., Smith, T. W., Leff, D., Wintemute, G. J., Cook, P. J., Hawkins, D. F., Kellermann, A. L., Sorensen, S. B., & Defrancesco, S. (1998). Support for new policies to regulate firearms. Results of two national surveys. *New England Journal of Medicine, 339* (12), 813–818.

Vernick, J. S., & Hepburn, L. M. (2003). State and federal gun laws: Trends for 1970–1999. In J. Ludwig & P. J. Cook (Eds.), *Evaluating gun policy: Effects on crime and violence.* (pp. 345–402). Washington, DC: Brookings Institution Press.

Vernick, J. S., Meisel, Z. F., Teret, S. P., Milne, J. S., & Hargarten, S. W. (1999). "I didn't know the gun was loaded": An examination of two safety devices that can reduce the risk of unintentional firearm injuries. *Journal of Public Health Policy, 20* (4), 427–440.

Vigdor, E. R., & Mercy, J. A. (2003). Disarming batterers: The impact of domestic violence firearm laws. In J. Ludwig & P. J. Cook (Eds.), *Evaluating gun policy: Effects on crime and violence* (pp. 157–204). Washington, DC: Brookings Institution Press.

Villaveces, A., Cummings, P., Espitia, V. E., Koepsell, T. D., McKnight, B., & Kellermann, A. L. (2000). Effect of a ban on carrying firearms on homicide rates in 2 Colombian cities. *Journal of the American Medical Association, 283* (9), 1205–1209.

Wadman, M. C., Muelleman, R. L., Coto, J. A., & Kellermann, A. L. (2003). The pyramid of injury: Using Ecodes to accurately describe the burden of injury. *Annals of Emergency Medicine, 42* (4), 468–478.

Webster, D. W., Vernick, J. S., & Hepburn, L. M. (2002). Effects of Maryland's law banning "Saturday night special" handguns on homicides. *American Journal of Epidemiology, 155* (5), 406–412.

Webster, D. W., Vernick, J. S., Zeoli, A. M., & Manganello, J. A. (2004). Association between youth-focused firearm laws and youth suicides. *Journal of the American Medical Association, 292* (5), 594–601.

Weil, D. S., & Knox, R. C. (1996). Effects of limiting handgun purchases on interstate transfer of firearms. *Journal of the American Medical Association, 275* (22), 1759–1761.

Wintemute, G. J. (1996). The relationship between firearm design and firearm violence. Handguns in the 1990s. *Journal of the American Medical Association, 275* (22), 1749–1753.

Wintemute, G. J., Parham, C. A., Beaumont, J. J., Wright, M., & Drake, C. (1999). Mortality among recent purchasers of handguns. *New England Journal of Medicine, 341,* 1583–1589.

Wintemute, G. J., Romero, M. P., Wright, M. A., & Grassel, K. M. (2004). The life cycle of crime guns: A description based on guns recovered from young people in California. *Annals of Emergency Medicine, 43* (6), 733–742.

Wintemute, G. J., Wright, M. A., Drake, C. M., & Beaumont, J. J. (2001). Subsequent criminal activity among violent misdemeanants who seek to purchase handguns: Risk factors and effectiveness of denying handgun purchase. *Journal of the American Medical Association, 285* (8), 1019–1026.

Wright, M. A., Wintemute, G. J., & Rivara, F. P. (1999). Effectiveness of denial of handgun purchase to persons believed to be at high risk for firearm violence. *American Journal of Public Health, 89* (1), 88–90.

Zenere, F. J. III, & Lazarus, P. J. (1997). The decline of youth suicidal behavior in an urban, multicultural public school system following the introduction of a suicide prevention and intervention program. *Suicide & Life-Threatening Behavior, 27* (4), 387–402.

Chapter **18**

Parenting and the Prevention of Childhood Injuries

Ronald J. Prinz

18.1. INTRODUCTION

Injuries in childhood represent a serious public health problem in the United States. Unintentional injury is the most common cause of death and disability for children. For example, injuries are the cause of half the deaths that occur for children 1–4 years of age. Over 600,000 children are hospitalized annually for injuries, and approximately 16 million children yearly are seen in emergency rooms as a result of injury (Centers for Disease Control and Prevention [CDC], 1990). Injuries that are clearly unintentional are not the only sources of the problem. Child maltreatment adds to the number of injury-based fatalities, disabilities, and medical treatments. For example, in 2001 an estimated 903,000 children were confirmed by child protective agencies in the United States to have been maltreated (i.e., abuse and/or neglect), and an estimated 1,300 children died from abuse or neglect (a rate of 1.81 per 100,000 children in the population). Many more children suffered from nonfatal injuries (U.S. Department of Health and Human Services [HHS], 2003).

Prevention of both unintentional and maltreatment-based injuries in childhood is obviously of utmost importance. This chapter focuses on parenting-related interventions aimed at the prevention of childhood injury. Parents and other family caregivers are logical contributors to prevention of childhood injuries, in part because the injuries often occur in the home or in close proximity to a parent. This chapter focuses only on the preadolescent age group (children from infancy to 12 years of age) and does not consider injury prevention among adolescents.

Two isolated areas of unintentional injury and child maltreatment have grown up side by side with little interaction between the two. The boundaries between inadvertent (unintentional) injuries and injuries attributable to child maltreatment are somewhat blurred and artificial. Peterson (1994) and others have argued that the commonalities between the two areas outnumber the differences and that it is

333

often difficult to reliably classify childhood injuries as either unintentional or not. With respect to parenting-based preventive interventions, the boundaries between prevention of unintentional injury and prevention of child maltreatment are even more blurred because many of the parenting strategies and intervention methods are of generic utility.

18.2. PRELIMINARY CONSIDERATIONS

Three lines of parenting-based intervention research potentially relate to the prevention of childhood injuries. The first line of work involves preventive interventions that are aimed at preventing childhood injuries in the general population and reducing risk in selected populations (e.g., economically disadvantaged groups, families already having experienced a child injury). The second line examines interventions aimed at preventing child maltreatment (physical abuse, neglect, or both), with the possible additional goal (either explicit or implicit) of reducing risk for childhood injury. The third line of research focuses on interventions aimed at strengthening parenting efficacy, mainly applied to parents of children with behavioral or emotional problems but also includes preventative strategies (Taylor & Biglan, 1998).

Some of the parenting-based approaches to prevention of childhood injuries target only one domain (e.g., the use of smoke alarms in the home or the prevention of scalding from hot tap water), whereas other approaches target multiple domains. Because preventive interventions that concentrate on only one domain involve relatively lower prevalence rates, a large segment of the population must be tested to detect effects on injury reduction. By contrast, preventive interventions with a broader focus have higher cross-injury rates and thus the effects can be detected in a smaller sample; however, a more comprehensive program would be needed to measure these effects. There is a trade-off between maximizing the number of target domains to produce a wide effect and the extent of programming coverage needed.

Descriptive research on parenting strategies and home-safety practices in the general population provides some clues about potentially effective methods to prevent childhood injuries (Morrongiello & House, 2004; Morrongiello & Kiriakou, 2004; Morrongiello, Ondejko, & Littlejohn, 2004; Peterson, DiLillo, Lewis, & Sher, 2002). Parents use a mixture of strategies to prevent child injury, depending on the child's developmental level, the particular location of the home or environment (e.g., living room versus child's play area), the parent's goal in the situation, and the parent's perception of risk (Morrongiello & Lasenby, 2006). Space does not permit coverage of the rich details from this important line of descriptive research. Some of the observations, however, provide an appropriate backdrop to the review of interventions. It appears that caregivers who are efficacious at preventing childhood injury (1) use active strategies of monitoring and supervision that change as a function of child age, activity, and setting; (2) have a broad repertoire of strategies for use with their children; (3) are not completely consistent in adopting and enforcing every possible safeguard and precaution; and (4) usually have rationales for their prevention/action responses that they communicate in age-appropriate ways to their children so that the children acquire self-regulation skills over time.

All of the interventions reviewed in this chapter involve parents in some way. Interventions that involve only interventionist contact with the children (e.g., in some of the work on latchkey children) were excluded. Nonetheless, the interventions vary considerably in terms of goals and targets. The reviewed interventions focus on parental knowledge about specific injury risks (e.g., hot water scalding, bicycle riding without a helmet), safe caregiver practices in the home, parental involvement and supervision, elimination of neglectful or unhealthy conditions, promotion of noncoercive parenting practices, or some combination of these. The parent/caregiver role in interventions also varies along a passive–active continuum—for example, from simply receiving information or materials to interacting with program staff to receiving high levels of coaching and consultation.

18.3.   INTERVENTIONS AND EXTENT OF EVIDENCE

The interventions involving parents and parenting cut across a wide array of strategies and approaches. Some of the intervention studies come from research on prevention of unintentional injury in the general population, whereas others are from research on prevention of child maltreatment in high-risk groups. Both domains are considered. Interventions from the general parent-training literature are briefly considered as well.

18.3.1.   Interventions from Unintentional Injury Research

18.3.1.1.   Safety Counseling and Education with Parents

There is some evidence that brief, focused parent education about a specific topic such as smoke alarm use or burn prevention can yield positive results. A number of studies have found that parent education about scald burns and prevention resulted in significantly greater likelihood that parents tested and lowered their home tap-water temperature (Katcher, Landry, & Shapiro, 1989; Kelly, Sein, & McCarthy, 1987; Thomas, Hassanein, & Christophersen, 1984).

Parent education via brief consultation or home visits, supplemented by free safety items, such as smoke alarms, safety latches, outlet plugs, and poison stickers, appears to have some promise in promoting home safety. Gallagher, Hunter, and Guyer (1985) tested a home-injury prevention program that involved parent education about safety hazards, installation of safety devices, and notification about changes in legal requirements for safety standards. They found that safety counseling plus provision of safety supplies resulted in significantly better home safety behaviors than safety counseling alone. Similar decreases in home hazards were found by Paul, Sanson-Fisher, Redman, and Carter (1994) and by Bablouzian, Freeman, Wolski, and Fried (1997), although improvements found in the latter study occurred only in those domains for which safety materials were distributed. A research group in Canada found that parent education plus provision of low-cost helmets produced increased children's bicycle helmet use compared to both parent education and control conditions (Morris & Trimble, 1991).

DiGuiseppi and Roberts (2000) reviewed parenting-related interventions to increase smoke alarm use in homes and found that those involving small parenting classes or safety counseling with individual parents were more effective if smoke alarms were provided to families at a discounted price. An exception was a brief intervention that involved 15 minutes of safety education from a physician plus an information sheet but did not include financial incentives (Kelly et al., 1987):

the intervention group showed greater acquisition of smoke alarms compared to the control group. A wide-scale educational campaign that included provision of smoke alarms produced a decrease in fatality rates from home fires in Oklahoma City (Mallonee et al., 1996), suggesting, at least for the increased use of smoke alarms, that parenting interventions might not be essential but provision of free or cheap alarms is critical.

Burn-prevention programs aimed at encouraging parents to test and lower tap-water temperatures have been tested and shown to be successful. A 1-hour well-child parenting class about burn prevention, hot water equipment, and water thermometers found that 44% of participating parents, compared to 29% of control parents, lowered their tap-water temperature at home (Barone, 1988). Similar effects were found in a study aimed at teaching parents about scald burns (Corrarino, Walsh, & Nadel, 2001). In a pediatric clinic, Katcher et al. (1989) found that brief advice about tap-water temperature and a free thermometer led to 44% of parents testing their home tap water (compared with 23% of control parents) and 14% (compared with 9%) lowering the water temperature. What is not clear is whether this intervention (and the interventions in the aforementioned studies) ultimately led to a lower incidence of child scald burns. Finally, a study by Thomas et al. (1984), testing a parent-education intervention aimed at lowering hot water temperature settings and encouraging installation of smoke alarms, demonstrated that a significant proportion of parents lowered their hot water heater temperatures but did not install smoke alarms at a significantly greater rate than controls.

18.3.1.2.   Brief Home Visitation by Safety Inspectors

Another strategy of potential utility is brief home visitation by safety inspectors. A cogent example of this was tested by King et al. (2001) using a randomized controlled trial with a case-control study. The key sample included families with a child under 8 years of age (median age 8 years) who had presented at a hospital emergency room for one of the targeted injuries (i.e., tap-water scald, burn from a fire in the home, poisoning or other dangerous ingestion, choking from ingestion of a foreign object, injury from a fall, bicycle-related head injury). Home inspections were conducted for households in both the intervention and the control conditions. Parents in the intervention condition received a detailed information packet on injury prevention, review of findings from the home inspection, instructions on how to correct home safety deficiencies, detailed instruction regarding prevention of each of the targeted injuries, discount coupons for purchase of recommended safety devices, demonstration of the appropriate use of the safety devices, and follow-up telephone calls 4 and 8 months after the initial home visit. The investigators found that despite lack of intervention effects on parental awareness and knowledge about childhood injury risk and prevention, there was a lower rate of reported medical visits for child injury by families in the intervention condition (King et al., 2001).

In a study with Head Start families, Johnston, Britt, D'Ambrosio, Mueller, and Rivara (2000) deployed a safety home visiting protocol that included a baseline home inspection, a prevention-knowledge assessment, three monthly home visits, safety information for parents in areas identified as safety concerns, and safety items for the families (e.g., smoke alarm, batteries for smoke alarms, syrup of ipecac, a booster car seat). Home visits were conducted by family service case workers. It was not clear from the published report how the home visitors interacted with parents in terms of process. Families in the intervention condition differed from the comparison families at the 3-month follow-up in terms of being more likely to have a smoke detector, a car seat, or syrup of ipecac and less likely to have poisonous substances in the home.

In an injury prevention program conducted within an urban African American community, Schwarz, Grisso, Miles, Homes, and Sutton (1993) made use of safety inspectors who helped parents identify home hazards, modeled how to correct the problems, and provided low-cost materials. The investigators found that intervention parents, compared with control parents, created significantly safer homes with respect to the less challenging safety issues (e.g., maintaining functional smoke alarms and keeping medications away from children) but not with respect to more difficult problems (e.g., poor lighting or major floor repairs). Although the inspectors modeled safety-promoting behaviors for the parents to emulate, they did not appear to provide concerted opportunities for parents to engage in specific preventive actions and receive feedback.

18.3.1.3. Use of Rewards for Parents and Children

Roberts and Turner (1986) demonstrated that rewarding parents if their children were buckled in car seats or seat belts when arriving at daycare produced a higher use of car safety restraints. The rewards were lottery tickets that could be redeemed for various prizes. Foss (1989) conducted a similar study and essentially replicated the results; other investigators distributed lottery tickets for rewards (e.g., coloring books, pizzas, stickers) if everyone in the family car was buckled up when the child arrived at school also with favorable results (Roberts & Fanurik, 1986; Roberts, Fanurik, & Wilson 1988). Other studies have found that systematic implementation of reward-based behavioral training with parents produced greater short-term and to some extent long-term use of child safety restraints (Liberator, Eriacho, Schmiesing, & Krump, 1989; Stuy, Green, & Doll, 1993). Britt, Silver, and Rivara (1998) used similar principles with low-income parents to increase children's use of bicycle helmets. In a systematic review of the literature, Zaza et al. (2001) found that incentives plus education increased the use of child safety seats.

18.3.1.4. Training Parents as Safety Instructors

Peterson, Mori, Selby, and Rosen (1988) conducted a series of small studies examining the viability of training parents to serve as "safety-skills instructors" for their 8- to 10-year-old children. They found that the parents were reasonably good at acquiring the necessary training skills, but there was only a modest effect on the children's acquisition of safe behaviors. Subsequent injury prevention with the small samples was not assessed. Despite the low cost of the procedures, the intensity of the intervention apparently was not high enough to produce sufficient positive effects on the children.

18.3.2. Interventions from Research on Prevention of Child Maltreatment

18.3.2.1. Comprehensive Home-Safety Training for Parents

By far the most intensive and one of the best examples of training parents in home safety is Project 12-Ways (Gershater-Molko, Lutzker, & Sherman, 2002; Lutzker,

Bigelow, Doctor, Gershater, & Greene, 1998; Lutzker, Campbell, Newman, & Harrold, 1989; Lutzker, Frame, & Rice, 1982; Lutzker & Rice, 1984, 1987; Lutzker, Wesch, & Rice, 1984; Wesch & Lutzker, 1991). A derivative program is Project SafeCare (Gershater-Molko, Lutzker, & Wesch, 2002, 2003; Lutzker et al., 1998; Metchikian, Mink, Bigelow, Lutzker, & Doctor, 1999; Taban & Lutzker, 2001). These programs were designed primarily for parents who have entered the child protective services system for child neglect and other forms of child maltreatment and are mandated to participate in safety training and parenting improvement. Project 12-Ways and Project SafeCare are both delivered in the home using an ecobehavioral framework for assessment and programming. Project 12-Ways involves selected intervention components based on needs identified in an in-depth assessment of each family and home. Services components include basic skills training related to child toilet training and general hygiene, home safety, health maintenance, nutrition, parent–child interactions, and stress reduction, and provides training related to money management, job finding, and practical problem solving. Project SafeCare, which is a distillation of Project 12-Ways, focuses only on child health care, parent–child interactions (and the associated parenting skills), and safety (i.e., home safety and injury prevention). Data from multiple studies support the utility and efficacy of this overall approach in improving household safety and hygiene, reducing child neglect, reducing coercive parenting practices, increasing positive strategies, and reducing referrals for child maltreatment. The approach is particularly noteworthy because it is focused, easy for parents to understand and accept, practical in terms of parenting actions, and researchable because the elements are replicable and readily documented.

18.3.2.2.   Home Visitation

A popular modality of intervention in child maltreatment is home visitation, particularly for high-risk caregivers with very young children (i.e., infants and toddlers). Most home visitation programs have multiple facets that address, for example, child health and development, basic infant care, parent–child interaction, strategies for prevention of child abuse and neglect, adjustment of the caregiver, and broader family issues. Home visitation programs for the prevention of child maltreatment were extensively reviewed by the Task Force on Community Preventive Services (convened by the CDC and other agencies) and are summarized by Bilukha et al. (2005). Of the 20 studies reviewed that examined child abuse and neglect as an outcome, only 6 demonstrated a positive effect of home visitation. Only 5 home visitation studies examined childhood injury as an outcome, and none of these showed a positive effect in reducing or preventing child injury. The field is conflicted about the value and preventive effect of home visitation on child abuse and neglect (Chaffin, 2004).

Worthy of special note as one of the more extensive strategies for prevention of childhood injury and child maltreatment is the Olds home visitation program (Olds et al., 1999). Focused primarily on young economically disadvantaged mothers giving birth for the first time, the Olds home visitation program involves recurring visits by nurses beginning in the prenatal period and continuing throughout the first 2 years of the child's life. The visits last 75–90 minutes, and the nurses make eight prenatal visits on average per mother (up to 18 visits) and 25 visits per family (up to 71 visits) from birth to the child's second birthday. In a randomized controlled trial, the Olds research team was able to demonstrate that children of the mothers receiving the nurse visitation program showed significantly lower rates of injury during the first 2 years of life compared with children of mothers providing usual care (Kitzman et al., 1997). The impressive aspect of this work is that the investigators were able to demonstrate actual preventive benefits in terms of reductions in injury rates. This approach relies heavily on enhancement of social support, confidence building with the mothers, and general assistance related to health and daily living. From an injury prevention standpoint, it is not clear how to tease out which facets of parenting and which elements of the intervention are critical to the reduced rate of childhood injuries. Given that the intervention accrued benefits in other areas as well (e.g., employment, mental health, unintentional injury), this approach seems quite promising for the selected population (i.e., young economically disadvantaged single first-time mothers) and developmental period (i.e., first 2 years of the children's lives).

18.3.2.3. *Cognitive-Behavioral Parent Training*

A promising cognitive-behavioral approach to prevention of child maltreatment was developed by Peterson, Tremblay, Ewigman, & Saldana (2003) and tested in a randomized controlled trial with high-risk mothers. The program included modeling, role-playing, interactive (Socratic-style) dialogue, home practice, and home visits (with observation and feedback). Intervention effects were demonstrated in the seven target areas: parenting skills, developmentally appropriate parenting responses, acquisition of developmentally appropriate beliefs about their children, regulation of negative affect, acceptance of responsibility for parent role, acceptance of nurturing role, and self-efficacy. Gains were maintained at follow-up. There was not sufficient power to detect reductions in subsequent referrals for child maltreatment, but the participating mothers did show reductions in coercive parenting practices and maladaptive beliefs.

A study by Sanders and colleagues (2004) demonstrated that retraining parental attributions and undergoing anger management as part of a parenting intervention called Triple P—Positive Parenting Program—can positively effect parents at risk for maltreatment of their preschool-age children. The investigators found that Pathways Triple P (a variant of the well-tested Triple P system) reduced coercive parenting practices, negative parental attributions, unrealistic parental expectations, potential for child maltreatment, and child behavioral problems; the gains were maintained at the 6-month follow-up. Although subsequent child maltreatment referrals and child injuries were not examined, the Pathways Triple P program shows promise as a relatively efficient and focused intervention for the prevention of the physical abuse of children and the reduction of risk for maltreatment-related childhood injuries.

18.3.3. Generic Behavioral Training for Parents and Children

There is a large area of research on interventions aimed at improving parenting skills and reducing or preventing child behavioral and emotional problems without being tied specifically to the prevention of either unintentional childhood injury or child maltreatment (Chronis, Chacko, & Fabiano, 2004; Griest & Wells, 1983; Kazdin, 2003; Miller & Prinz, 1990; Prinz & Dumas, 2003; Prinz & Jones, 2003; Sanders, Turner, & Markie-Dadds, 2003). Nonetheless, to the extent that children with behavioral and emotional problems (e.g., ADHD, oppositional-defiant disorder) are at heightened risk for injury during childhood and adolescence, effective parenting interventions that mitigate the behavioral and emotional problems have the potential to reduce risk for injury. Some evidence supports an association between childhood behavioral and emotional problems and greater risk for injury, although the data are not consistent. There are a number of ways in which parenting interventions might conceivably contribute to injury prevention. Young children with high rates of wild and reckless behavior place themselves in dangerous situations, and effective parenting interventions can assist parents in strategies to reduce the problematic behaviors. Increased supervision and monitoring of children and, perhaps, adolescents might afford parents opportunities to prevent some injuries (e.g., from playing with matches, getting into the medicine cabinet, climbing to unsafe heights, playing in the street, getting into unsafe environments). Despite the potential for this large category of parenting interventions with respect to prevention and reduction of childhood injury, there have been no published population-level studies of this proposition to date.

18.3.4.   Summary of Findings for Interventions

Each of the interventions discussed here was rated in terms of effectiveness based on the available scientific evidence and summarized using a 5-point scale: *5*, effective; *4*, promising; *3*, insufficient evidence; *2*, not effective, and *1*, iatrogenic (Table 18.1). The summary focuses on two types of outcomes. The first is childhood injury; some of the intervention studies did not assess childhood injury directly, whereas others found no preventive effects on childhood injury. The second outcome is risk reduction, which typically includes improvement in parental safety practices, parent knowledge about injury prevention, and parenting practices or lower rate of referral for child maltreatment. The assumption behind the risk-reduction category is that these variables are clearly linked to risk for child injury.

Table 18.1. Summary of Effectiveness for Parenting-Based Interventions Aimed at Preventing Child Injury[a]

Intervention	Injury Prevention	Risk Reduction
Drawn from unintentional injury research		
Safety counseling and education with parents	3	4
Safety counseling and education with parents plus provision of safety materials	4	4
Brief home visitation by safety inspectors	3	3
Use of rewards for parents and children	Unknown	4
Training parents as safety instructors	Unknown	3
Drawn from child-maltreatment prevention research		
Comprehensive home-safety training	4	5
Home visitation (general approaches)	3	4
Nurse home visitation model	4	5
Cognitive-behavioral parent training	3	5
Generic Parent Training	Unknown	5

[a]The scale is as follows: *5*, effective (supported by two or more well designed studies); *4*, promising (supported by one well-designed study); *3*, insufficient (not enough evidence or mixed evidence); *2*, not effective (no effect found in two or more well-designed studies); *1*, iatrogenic (potentially harmful effect supported by two or more well-designed studies); *unknown*, no studies found.

18.4.   IMPLICATIONS AND LIMITATIONS FOR PUBLIC HEALTH PRACTICE

Taking into account prevention research on both childhood injury in the general population and child maltreatment in high-risk samples, some common themes emerged that have implications for public health practice:

- The more successful interventions emphasize active parental involvement, specific parenting practices, concrete actions that parents can readily take, and program implementation in naturalistic settings (i.e., primarily in the home).
- Providing safety items such as car seats, smoke alarms, and tap-water thermometer for free or at reduced cost seems to add significantly to the effect of preventive interventions. A number of factors may account for this. Providing these items to families with limited financial resources frees parents from having to choose between paying for subsistence and housing and purchasing safety materials. Providing safety items at reduced or no cost to other families facilitates the process of acquisition and perhaps gives a built-in incentive to act. The latter point is consistent with data on safety interventions involving provision of explicit incentives for parents and children.
- Programming delivered in the home makes ecological sense but does not in and of itself ensure effectiveness. Home visitation programs and other home-delivered interventions vary in effect. Process and content of home-delivered programs and fidelity of implementation clearly are important facets to consider, even though the huge variation in actual substance is masked by the catch-all term *home visitation*.

Some of the interventions are predicated on the assumption that educating, or at least informing, parents on what to do and how to do it is sufficient to prevent child injury. The evidence for this is minimal. Some parents might benefit from information about smoke alarms; seat belt arrangements for infants, toddlers, and children; safe tap-water temperatures; bicycle helmets; and safety-proofing the home for infants and toddlers. However, it is not clear how different methods of providing this information (e.g., via media, pamphlets, brief primary care explanation) affect the success of such interventions. What is clear is that it is important to have parents take action and practice with feedback or consultation, rather than just learn cognitively about the topic. This is apparent from home inspections, which help parents figure out what they need to change. The advantages of this approach over just providing information to parents are relatively obvious. First, the safety inspectors can see what parents are actually doing (or not doing) at home that needs to be augmented or changed. Second, parents can ask questions in the context of actual rather than hypothetical conditions. And third, the interventionists can tailor their actions to meet each family's situation and needs. On the downside, some parents may find the visits intrusive or may balk because they fear the possibility of involvement by child protective services.

What seems to be missing or at least underspecified in most of the reviewed interventions is how parents might interact with their children to optimize safe conditions. Parents could benefit from coaching, skill building, practice feedback, and tips on how to enlist the cooperation of their children in implementing safe practices. For example, depending on the age of the children in the home, parents could benefit from learning how to get children to respond appropriately if a smoke alarm goes off. On a related issue, interventions need to better address the processes of parent–child interactions and parents' parenting practices, which may play into how safe or unsafe the home and family are for the children. An exception to this limitation is found in Project 12-Ways and Project SafeCare, which are exemplars of how to address parenting practices in an explicit manner within an injury prevention approach. These programs accomplish multiple goals through home visits that are structured, practical, and oriented to problem solving. These two programs were designed primarily for parents who have entered the child protective service system because of child neglect. It might be possible to draw critical elements from this approach (e.g., skills training, application in an ecological context, positive action orientation) and adapt them to a broader segment of the population.

To increase cost effectiveness and effect at a population level, it is necessary to combine goals in the design of intervention programs. For example, programs for parenting in which safety and injury reduction are but one part make sense and are more likely to be adopted. The prime examples of this are Project 12-Ways, Project SafeCare, and the Olds home visitation program. Project 12-Ways and Project SafeCare pursue multiple goals related to parental functioning, including but not restricted to home safety and hygiene. This type of program is a model for child protective services intervention with neglectful families. The Olds home visitation program, which has shown some long-term prevention of childhood injuries, is geared toward a particular segment of the population—namely, young economically disadvantaged single mothers during the first 2 years of their children's lives. Given the level of intensity and the associated cost, this approach does not lend itself readily to universal application to the general population. Nonetheless, the promise of this intervention model suggests that a consolidated version might prove useful for the general population of first-time parents, a concept that will require further testing. When considering the broader population, policymakers should consider programming for parents that similarly pursues multiple goals but is invoked without the requirements of entry into the social-services system or the initial childbirth of a young single mother living in poverty.

An example of a population approach that has potential utility for multiple goals is found in the Triple P system of interventions (Sanders et al., 2003). Triple P is a multitiered system of interventions of increasing intensity; it consists of flexible delivery formats based on a unifying set of parenting principles and a broad array of positive parenting strategies. The Triple P system, which has a large evidence base supporting it (to date, 25 clinical trials), has program levels that can be applied universally in a cost-effective manner (e.g., in primary care and early childhood educational settings), and other levels that provide more intensive programming for parents facing greater challenges, including risk for child maltreatment. This population approach can provide an integrated framework that potentially addresses multiple goals, including promotion of effective parenting practices, reduction or prevention of child behavioral and emotional problems, risk reduction for child maltreatment, and risk reduction for childhood injuries (across the continuum of intentionality).

18.5.   RESEARCH GAPS

It is not clear to what extent improvements in intermediary goals ultimately lead to prevention or reduction of childhood injuries. Examples of intermediary goals include awareness of a safety issue (e.g., risk of scalding from hot tap water), knowledge of safe practices (e.g., installing and checking smoke alarms, making medicines and household cleaners inaccessible to young children), and implementation of safe practices. It is possible to have made significant changes in parental awareness, knowledge, and implementation practices and yet still have not produced positive changes in injury prevalence rates at a population level. Part of the difficulty lies in the research samples being studied. Most of the samples are too small to test population effects on the low-rate childhood injuries being addressed because the effects would not be detectable or the outcome measure not sufficiently reliable. A related problem is that some of the interventions are too intensive and expensive to implement at a population level.

Researchers need to test the extent to which programming for effective parenting can be implemented in a cost-effective manner, addressing injury prevention and child-welfare promotion simultaneously and evaluating the effect at a population level. This approach is consistent with the surgeon general's recent call for a national strategic plan aimed simultaneously at preventing child maltreatment and optimizing (promoting) healthy child development.

18.6.   CONCLUSIONS

Parents obviously can and do play a large role in moderating (or not moderating) childhood risk of injury. Preventive interventions that actively promote proactive efforts on the part of parents have promise to reduce childhood injury. The more effective strategies emphasize parent–child interaction, knowledge of safety practices linked to specific actions, in vivo practice and implementation, use of feedback and incentives, and provision of safety materials such as car seats and smoke alarms. The field needs to focus on dissemination methods that combine goals, both across injury domains and with respect to other areas (e.g., promotion of noncoercive parenting, strengthening of parental involvement) and that demonstrate population-level benefits in terms of reduced injury rates.

REFERENCES

Bablouzian, L., Freeman, E. S., Wolski, K. E., & Fried, L. E. (1997). Evaluation of a community based childhood injury prevention program. *Injury Prevention, 3*, 14–16.

Barone, B. J. (1988). *An analysis of well-child parenting classes: The extent of parent compliance with health care recommendations to decrease potential injury of their toddlers.* Lawrence, KS: University of Kansas. Unpublished doctoral dissertation, Lawrence.

Bilukha, O., Hahn, R., Crosby, A., Fullilove, M., Liberman, A., Moscicki, E., Snyder, S., Tuma, F., Corso, P., & Schofield, A. (2005). The effectiveness of early childhood home visitation in preventing violence: A systematic review. *American Journal of Preventive Medicine, 28*, 11–39.

Britt, J., Silver, I., & Rivara, F. P. (1998). Bicycle helmet promotion among low-income preschool children. *Injury Prevention, 4*, 238–283.

Centers for Disease Control and Prevention. (1990). Childhood injuries in the United States. *American Journal of Diseases in Children, 144*, 627–646.

Chaffin, M. (2004). Is it time to rethink healthy start/healthy families? *Child Abuse & Neglect, 28,* 589–595.

Chronis, A. M., Chacko, A., & Fabiano, G. A. (2004). Enhancements to the behavioral parent training paradigm for families of children with ADHD: Review and future directions. *Clinical Child & Family Psychology Review, 7,* 1–27.

Corrarino, J. E., Walsh, P. J., & Nadel, E. (2001). Does teaching scald burn prevention to families of young children make a difference? A pilot study. *Journal of Pediatric Nursing, 16,* 256–262.

DiGuiseppi, C., & Roberts, I. G. (2000). Individual-level injury prevention strategies in the clinical setting. *Future of Children, 10,* 53–82.

Foss, R. (1989). Evaluation of a community-wide incentive program to promote safety restraint use. *American Journal of Public Health, 79,* 304–306.

Gallagher, S., Hunter, P., & Guyer, B. (1985). A home injury prevention program for children. *Pediatric Clinics of North America, 1,* 95–112.

Gershater-Molko, R. M., Lutzker, J. R., & Sherman, J. A. (2002). Intervention in child neglect: An applied behavioral perspective. *Aggression & Violent Behavior, 7,* 103–124.

Gershater-Molko, R. M., Lutzker, J. R., & Wesch, D. (2002). Using recidivism data to evaluate Project SafeCare: Teaching bonding, safety, and health care skills to parents. *Journal of the American Professional Society on the Abuse of Children, 7,* 277–285.

Gershater-Molko, R. M., Lutzker, J. R., & Wesch, D. (2003). Project SafeCare: Improving health, safety, and parenting skills in families reported for and at risk for child maltreatment. *Journal of Family Violence, 18,* 377–386.

Griest, D. L., & Wells, K. C. (1983). Behavioral family therapy with conduct disorders in children. *Behavior Therapy, 14,* 37–53.

Johnston, B. D., Britt, J., D'Ambrosio, D., Mueller, B. A., & Rivara, F. P. (2000). A preschool program for safety and injury prevention delivered by home visitors. *Injury Prevention, 6,* 305–309.

Katcher, M. L., Landry, G. L., & Shapiro, M. M. (1989). Liquid-crystal thermometer use in pediatric office counseling about tap water burn prevention. *Pediatrics, 83,* 766–771.

Kazdin, A. E. (Ed.). (2003). *Evidence-based psychotherapies for children and adolescents.* New York: Guilford.

Kelly, B., Sein, C., & McCarthy, P. L. (1987). Safety education in a pediatric primary care setting. *Pediatrics, 79,* 818–824.

King, W. J., Klassen, T. P., LeBlanc, J., Bernard-Bonnin, C., Robitaille, Y., Pham, B., Coyle, D., Tenenbein, M., & Pless, I. B. (2001). The effectiveness of a home visit to prevent childhood injury. *Pediatrics, 108,* 382–388.

Kitzman, H., Olds, D. L., Henderson, C. R., Hanks, C., Cole, R., Tatelbaum, R., McConnochie, K. M., Sidora, K., Luckey, D. W., Shaver, D., Engelhardt, K., James, D., & Barnard, K. (1997). Effect of prenatal and infancy home visitation by nurses on pregnancy outcomes, childhood injuries, and repeated childbearing: A randomized controlled trial. *Journal of the American Medical Association, 278,* 644–652.

Liberator, C. P., Eriacho, B., Schmiesing, J., & Krump, M. (1989). Safesmart safety seat intervention project: A successful program for the medically indigent. *Patient Education & Counseling, 13,* 161–170.

Lutzker, J. R., Bigelow, K. M., Doctor, R. M., Gershater, R. M., & Greene, B. F. (1998). An ecobehavioral model for the prevention and treatment of child abuse and neglect: History and applications. In J. R. Lutzker (Ed.), *Handbook of child abuse research and treatment* (pp. 239–266). New York: Plenum.

Lutzker, J. R., Campbell, R. V., Newman, M. R., & Harrold, M. (1989). Ecobehavioral interventions for abusive, neglectful, and high-risk families. In G. H. S. Singer & L. K. Irvin (Eds.), *Support for caregiving families: Enabling positive adaptation to disability* (pp. 313–326). Baltimore: Brookes.

Lutzker, J. R., Frame, R. E., & Rice, J. M. (1982). Project 12-Ways: An ecobehavioral approach to the treatment and prevention of child abuse and neglect. *Education & Treatment of Children, 5,* 141–155.

Lutzker, J. R., & Rice, J. M. (1984). Project 12-Ways: Measuring outcome of a large in-home service for treatment and prevention of child abuse and neglect. *Child Abuse & Neglect, 8,* 519–524.

Lutzker, J. R., & Rice, J. M. (1987). Using recidivism data to evaluate Project 12-Ways: An ecobehavioral approach to the treatment and prevention of child abuse and neglect. *Journal of Family Violence, 2,* 283–290.

Lutzker, J. R., Wesch, D., & Rice, J. M. (1984). A review of Project 12-Ways: An ecobehavioral approach to the treatment and prevention of child abuse and neglect. *Advances in Behaviour Research & Therapy, 6,* 63–73.

Mallonee, S., Istre, G., Rosenburg, M., Reddish-Douglas, M., Jordan, F., Silverstein, P., & Tunnell, W. (1996). Surveillance and prevention of residential-fire injuries. *New England Journal of Medicine, 335,* 27–31.

Metchikian, K. L., Mink, J. M., Bigelow, K. M., Lutzker, J. R., & Doctor, R. M. (1999). Reducing home safety hazards in the homes of parents reported for neglect. *Child & Family Behavior Therapy, 21,* 23–34.

Miller, G. E., & Prinz, R. J. (1990). The enhancement of social learning family interventions for childhood conduct disorder. *Psychological Bulletin, 108,* 291–307.

Morris, B. P., & Trimble, N. E. (1991). Promotion of bicycle helmet use among schoolchildren: A randomized clinical trial. *Canadian Journal of Public Health, 82,* 92–94.

Morrongiello, B. A., & House, K. (2004). Measuring parent attributes and supervision behaviors relevant to child injury risk: Examining the usefulness of questionnaire measures. *Injury Prevention, 10,* 114–118.

Morrongiello, B. A., & Kiriakou, S. (2004). Mothers' home-safety practices for preventing six types of childhood injuries: What do they do, and why? *Journal of Pediatric Psychology, 29,* 285–297.

Morrongiello, B. A., & Lasenby, J. (2006). Supervision as a behavioral approach to reducing child-injury risk. Chapter 18. In A. C. Gielen, D. A. Sleet, & R. DiClemente (Eds). *Injury and violence prevention: Behavior change theories, methods and applications* (pp 395–418). San Francisco, CA: Jossey-Bass.

Morrongiello, B. A., Ondejko, L., & Littlejohn, A. (2004). Understanding toddlers' in-home injuries: II. Examining parental strategies, and their efficacy for managing child injury risk. *Journal of Pediatric Psychology, 29,* 433–446.

Olds, D. L., Henderson, C. R., Kitzman, H. J., Eckenrod, J. J., Cole, R. E., & Tatelbaum, R. C. (1999). Prenatal and infancy home visitation by nurses: Recent findings. *The Future of Children, 9,* 44–65.

Paul, C., Sanson-Fisher, R., Redman, S., & Carter, S. (1994). Preventing accidental injury to young children in the home using volunteers. *Health Promotion International, 9,* 241–249.

Peterson, L. (1994). Child injury and abuse-neglect: Common etiologies, challenges, and courses toward prevention. *Current Directions in Psychological Science, 3,* 116–120.

Peterson, L., DiLillo, D., Lewis, T., & Sher, K. (2002). Improvement in quantity and quality of prevention measurement of toddler injuries and parental interventions. *Behavior Therapy, 33,* 271–297.

Peterson, L., Mori, L., Selby, V., & Rosen, B. N. (1988). Community interventions in children's injury prevention: Differing costs and differing benefits. *Journal of Community Psychology, 16,* 188–204.

Peterson, L., Tremblay, G., Ewigman, B., & Saldana, L. (2003). Multilevel selected primary prevention of child maltreatment. *Journal of Consulting and Clinical Psychology, 71,* 601–612.

Prinz, R. J., & Dumas, J. E. (2003). Prevention of oppositional-defiant disorder and conduct disorder in children and adolescents. In P. Barrett & T. H. Ollendick (Eds.), *Handbook of interventions that work with children and adolescents: From prevention to treatment* (pp. 475–488). West Sussex, Great Britain: Wiley.

Prinz, R. J., & Jones, T. L. (2003). Family-based interventions. In C. A. Essau (Ed.), *Conduct and oppositional defiant disorders: Epidemiology, risk factors, and treatment* (pp. 279–298). Mahwah, NJ: Erlbaum.

Roberts, M. C., & Fanurik, D. (1986). Rewarding elementary school children for their use of safety belts. *Health Psychology, 5,* 185–196.

Roberts, M. C., Fanurik, D., & Wilson, D. (1988). A community program to reward children's use of seat belts. *American Journal of Community Psychology, 16,* 395–407.

Roberts, M. C., & Turner, D. S. (1986). Rewarding parents for their children's use of safety seats. *Journal of Pediatric Psychology, 11,* 25–36.

Sanders, M. R., Pidgeon, A. M., Gravestock, F., Connors, M. D., Brown, S., & Young, R. W. (2004). Does parental attributional retrainng and anger management enhance the effects of the Triple P–Positive parenting program with parents at risk of child maltreatment? *Behavior Therapy, 35,* 513–535.

Sanders, M. R., Turner, K. M. T., & Markie-Dadds, C. (2003). The development and dissemination of the Triple P—Positive Parenting Program: A multilevel, evidence-based system of parenting and family support. *Prevention Science, 3,* 173–189.

Schwarz, D. F., Grisso, J. A., Miles, C., Homes, J., & Sutton, R. (1993). An injury prevention program in an urban African American community. *American Journal of Public Health, 83,* 675–680.

Stuy, M., Green, M., & Doll, J. (1993). Child care centers: A community resource for injury prevention. *Journal of Developmental & Behavioral Pediatrics, 14,* 224–229.

Taban, N., & Lutzker, J. R. (2001). Consumer evaluation of an ecobehavioral program for prevention and intervention of child maltreatment. *Journal of Family Violence, 16,* 323–330.

Taylor, T. K., & Biglan, A. (1998). Behavioral family interventions for improving child-rearing: A review of the literature for clinicians and policy makers. *Clinical Child & Family Psychology Review, 1,* 41–60.

Thomas, K. A., Hassanein, R. S., & Christophersen, E. R. (1984). Evaluation of group well-child care for improving burn prevention practices in the home. *Pediatrics, 74,* 879–882.

U.S. Department of Health and Human Services. (2003). *Child maltreatment 2001.* Washington, DC: Administration on Children, Youth and Families.

Wesch, D., & Lutzker, J. R. (1991). A comprehensive 5-year evaluation of Project 12-Ways: An ecobe-havioral program for treating and preventing child abuse and neglect. *Journal of Family Violence, 6,* 17–35.

Zaza, S., Sleet, D. A., Thompson, R. S., Sosin, D. M., & Bolen, J. C. (2001). Task Force on Community Preventive Services. Reviews of evidence regarding interventions to increase the use of child safety seats. *American Journal of Preventive Medicine, 21* (4S), 31–47.

Chapter **19**

Building Resilience to Mass Trauma Events

Betty J. Pfefferbaum, Dori B. Reissman, Rose L. Pfefferbaum, Richard W. Klomp, and Robin H. Gurwitch

19.1. INTRODUCTION

Terrorist attacks and continuing threats coupled with frequent disasters of natural and accidental origin compel the attention of professionals involved in injury and violence prevention interventions. Potential psychosocial consequences associated with terrorism and disasters include distress, changed attitudes and behavior, and psychiatric morbidity. Although psychiatric morbidity, including but not limited to posttraumatic stress disorder (PTSD), is generally confined to individuals directly affected or endangered by an incident or those with close ties to victims and survivors, less severe reactions may be pervasive and extend to people outside the immediate vicinity of an event. These reactions can be addressed on an individual basis or in small groups (such as within families, in the workplace, or in school classrooms) and through a variety of medical and psychosocial interventions before, during, and after the disaster. Another approach—one that complements attention to individual needs—is for elected, appointed, or informal leaders, in concert with a diverse mixture of community coalitions, to prevent or reduce adverse psychological, health, and social outcomes through building community resilience. This may also be a more comprehensive health protection strategy. This chapter provides a preliminary framework for examining community resilience in relation to mass trauma events.

19.2. TERMS AND CONCEPTS

A number of terms—including community, community disaster, terrorism, and resilience—warrant definition to set the stage for a discussion of building community resilience to avert or reduce the harmful physical, social, and mental health consequences of mass trauma.

19.2.1.   Community

Communities traditionally have been viewed as being made up of individuals sharing origin, history, culture, values, laws, and geographic proximity, though there may be considerable diversity among individual members and groups. A community includes the organizations and structures within its boundaries, a sense of relatedness, and common health risks and conditions. Community members live and work in the same dynamic environment and are affected by similar social, economic, and physical risk factors. Communities reflect perceptions, beliefs, and attitudes that influence behavior. The potential for interaction among members is essential because without it, values and norms cannot be shared. The social system associated with a community provides services and addresses problems including those of its own making (Institute of Medicine [IOM], 2003; Issel, 2004; Jerusalem, Kaniasty, Lehman, Ritter, & Turnbull, 1995; Kulig, 2000). Traditional notions of community must be broadened in light of modern technology, which fosters networks that transcend conventional limits of physical proximity and boundaries, networks that place the community within a larger suprasystem of heterogeneous communities linked by a common social order or applied technology.

19.2.2.   Community Disaster

Disasters result from endogenous or exogenous forces, of natural or human origin, which overwhelm the resources of a community. They include floods, hurricanes, earthquakes, airplane crashes, chemical leaks, major urban power outages, school shootings, violent rampages, and suicide bombings. Community disasters are characterized by mass destruction of such severity as to warrant assistance from outside the community (Yahmed & Koob, 1996). Often of sudden and unexpected onset, disasters frequently kill and maim those in the way, damage property and deplete resources, disrupt routines, generate physical and emotional reactions, and alter social networks and processes. Disasters change a community by altering, at least temporarily, the way individuals relate to each other, social roles, the rules governing behavior, the social organization, and the allocation and use of resources, thus threatening the functioning of the community (Eränen & Liebkind, 1993; Sjoberg, 1962). The ensuing emotional, physical, and communal injuries associated with events of this magnitude potentially interfere with productive interactions that could reestablish coactive existence. Social support can be mobilized or may deteriorate after a disaster, depending in part on the characteristics of the community, its members, and the disaster itself (Jerusalem et al., 1995).

The Buffalo Creek flood of 1972 provides an example of utter devastation wrought by disaster. The mining community was decimated when a dam broke, unleashing a torrent of water and sludge that destroyed homes and the countryside, killing many residents, and severing the emotional bonds and mutual concern that had characterized Buffalo Creek. A community unusually rich in social capital—born of common heritage and tradition; a shared history of physical, economic, and social adversity; and individual emotional investment in public welfare—was torn asunder by the flood. Contributing factors exacerbated the situation, leaving residents fearful, isolated, apathetic, and demoralized (Erikson, 1976).

19.2.3. Terrorism

Terrorism is a type of community disaster that involves the illegal or threatened use of force to coerce societies or governments by inducing fear and mistrust in their populations. Terrorism is an extreme form of violence directed at more than the individual; it is an attack on the will of a people. Typically motivated by ideology and politics, terrorism is "primarily a psychological assault that erodes our sense of safety and sense of security, two of the most basic human needs" (IOM, 2004, p. 24). The intended consequences of terrorism extend beyond the death and injury of those in the immediate path of an attack, the grief of loved ones, the ruin of property, the disruption of government and commerce, and the chaos and confusion that lie in its wake. The consequences include, as evidenced by the word itself, the terror that infests an environment and the emotional repercussions that result.

The emotional, behavioral, and attitudinal consequences of terrorism are designed to undermine political and social structures. The terrorist target is the community, in its broadest sense, not simply the geographic space or even the individuals themselves but rather that which binds them: their culture, values, mores, government, and laws; their sense of belonging and relatedness; and their systems for addressing problems and delivering services. The psychological effects (emotional, behavioral, and cognitive changes and psychiatric disorders) on the population at large are a primary concern (IOM, 2004). True psychiatric morbidity is likely to occur only in those most directly affected by an incident or those who have close relationships with victims and survivors. Other reactions include anger, mistrust, a sense of isolation, feelings of personal vulnerability, recognition of one's own mortality, a lost sense of control over one's environment, and a shattered worldview (Difede, Apfeldorf, Cloitre, Spielman, & Perry, 1997; Ofman, Mastria, & Steinbery, 1995).

19.2.4. Resilience

Resilience is the ability to execute efficient and effective adjustment processes to alleviate stress and restore equilibrium in the face of trauma, tragedy, and threat (Steinberg & Ritzmann, 1990). Resilience is an ongoing process—involving attitudes, beliefs, behaviors, and even physical functioning—that must be sustained over time and support growth. Resources and skills associated with resilience can be cultivated and practiced (American Psychological Association [APA], 2005; Reissman, Klomp, Kent, & Pfefferbaum, 2004).

19.3. COMMUNITY RESILIENCE

Community resilience is grounded in the ability of community members to take meaningful, deliberate, collective action to remedy the effect of a problem, including the ability to interpret the environment, intervene, and move on. More than the ability of members to cope individually, community resilience involves interactions as a collective unit. It serves a community by fortifying it against a host of social concerns such as violence, crime, and poverty as well as terrorism and other disasters. Community resilience also addresses behavioral and functional problems at the individual level such as abuse, absenteeism, excessive risk taking, and injuries. Consisting of both reactive and proactive elements, community resilience couples recovery from adversity with efforts by individuals and groups to transform their environments to mitigate future events. As such, community resilience is not simply returning to homeostasis; it entails the potential to grow from the crisis (Brown & Kulig, 1996–1997; Kulig, 2000). These transformational characteristics are part of what distinguishes community resilience from social capital. Community resilience includes, but is more than, a web of relationships or network of accessible resources.

Multiple disciplines including health and public health, sociology, and psychology are beginning to recognize community resilience as a preparedness strategy for mass casualty events and as a mechanism to prevent adverse psychological, psychosomatic, and social consequences associated with terrorism and other disasters (Friedman, 2005). The concept of community resilience, still new to the lexicon, is related to community health and associated concepts such as community capacity, competence, cohesion, mobilization, and empowerment. For example, the community capacity and competence literature has identified factors that can be used to characterize community resilience (Cottrell, 1976; Gibbon, Labonte, & Laverack, 2002; Goeppinger & Baglioni, 1985; Goodman et al., 1998; Labonte & Laverack, 2001). We drew on this literature to identify seven interrelated factors associated with community resilience. These factors were endorsed by a panel of experts convened by the Centers for Disease Control and Prevention (CDC) and the Terrorism and Disaster Branch (TDB) of the National Center for Child Traumatic Stress: connectedness, commitment, and shared values; participation; structure, roles, and responsibilities; resources; support and nurturance; critical reflection and skill building; and communication. This preliminary set of factors awaits empirical examination and validation in relation to community resilience, terrorism, and disasters. Literature and research from an array of related topics in community development may suggest additional factors and help formulate activities to enhance their development.

19.3.1. Connectedness, Commitment, and Shared Values

Community membership implies connection to a place and a group of people with shared history, laws, and social mores. The sense of belonging may be strengthened if members perceive their personal well-being as deriving from and their needs fulfilled through affiliation with the community. A strong commitment to the community and relationships characterized by mutual concern and benefit should contribute to consensus building and collaboration. Communities that embrace diversity among members may be better able to address their needs in the face of adversity.

19.3.2. Participation

Participation may strengthen the sense of belonging. Communities that foster and facilitate member involvement in activities and organizations may be better able to identify and address issues through local cooperation and civic engagement. Opportunities for involvement should be sensitive to the diversity, ability, and interests of members. When participation is deemed important, members are likely to derive increased benefit from involvement, thus helping the community address needs and problems that arise in conjunction with disasters as well as those that occur more commonly.

19.3.3.   Structure, Roles, and Responsibilities

Communities include individuals, groups, and organizations with reciprocal links that form overlapping networks. In communities characterized by resilience, interactions are frequent, supportive, and collaborative, with individuals and groups identifying and addressing common concerns. Solutions may emerge from new associations that form to resolve issues. Communities with strong and responsive leadership; able teamwork; clear organizational structures; and well-defined roles, responsibilities, and lines of authority can further adaptation and recovery. Community resilience appears to be enhanced when differences in roles and responsibilities reflect an appreciation for equity rather than discrimination and when community standards, rules, and procedures facilitate social interaction and governance. Communities must manage relations with the larger society, accepting, working with, and supporting other communities.

19.3.4.   Resources

A community's resources include those belonging to its members and those that are attached to the community itself. In addition to land and raw materials, communities have physical capital, which creates an infrastructure and tools for the community, and human resources, which provide a workforce and expertise and leadership for development. The relationships and support systems within a community along with characteristics such as cohesion constitute social resources. Communities characterized by resilience acquire, mobilize, allocate, and use resources effectively. Resilience is likely to necessitate ongoing investment in physical, human, and social capital, such as improvements in schools and health facilities, job training, and neighborhood development.

19.3.5.   Support and Nurturance

Support and nurturance are important in enhancing resilience at the community and individual levels. Supportive and nurturing communities attend to the needs of their members and help them achieve goals and overcome problems. Supportive and nurturing communities provide opportunities for members to be heard, promote member well-being, instill hope, and empower individuals and groups. Communities should become more resilient through the process of providing support and nurturance. Support and nurturance may be enhanced when communities become more adept at identifying, acquiring, and equitably distributing resources within community boundaries and with the larger society.

19.3.6.   Critical Reflection and Skill Building

Resilient communities are characterized by the ability to identify and address issues, needs, and problems; establish structures to collect, analyze, and use information; and develop the means to plan, manage, and evaluate activities and programs. Critical reflection about values, the community's history, and the experiences of others, should enable local leaders to reason, set goals, make decisions, and develop and implement strategies for the betterment of the population. Learning, accommodation, and growth may lead to a sense of self-determination and enhanced capacity.

19.3.7. Communication

Community resilience is reinforced by effective, clear, and accurate communication among members and across boundaries. Effective communication requires common meanings and understandings and the perception of openness and honesty. Members and groups should have opportunities to articulate their needs, views, and attitudes, especially if diversity is to be addressed and supported. Open and productive communication can further the community's trust in leadership, increasing the likelihood of participation and compliance with directives in the face of disasters.

The operating assumption is that communities with higher levels of the seven factors will be more effective at mitigating negative emotional responses to a community disaster during and after the event. Community resilience–building activities need not focus directly on disaster-related issues to accomplish the desired reduction in adverse emotional reactions to mass trauma.

19.4. PREDICTORS OF INDIVIDUAL EMOTIONAL OUTCOME

Developing community resilience with respect to the mental health consequences of terrorism and disasters requires an understanding of the factors that influence individual outcomes. An ecological approach to health recognizes the importance of interconnectedness among biological, behavioral, physical, and socioenvironmental domains. A population's health is determined by micro influences (e.g., gender and age differences in susceptability to a disease) and by macro influences (e.g., social, economic, cultural, and environmental conditions and policies) (IOM, 2003). For terrorism and disasters, each person's reactions are influenced by individual characteristics, the nature of the event, individual exposure, and aspects of the recovery environment.

19.4.1. Predisposing Individual Characteristics

Demographic characteristics and preexisting psychiatric conditions are among the individual factors that have been examined in relation to disaster trauma (Bromet & Dew, 1995; Norris, Friedman, & Watson, 2002; Norris et al., 2002). Disaster studies that have examined gender have typically found women more likely than men to report stress, distress, and PTSD symptoms. Gender may also interact with other factors such as culture and appraisal of the event to produce adverse outcomes. Age effects are less clear and may depend on social, cultural, and economic factors. Although ethnic minorities may experience greater adverse outcomes to disasters, these may reflect differential exposure and more fragile surroundings rather than greater inherent vulnerability. Preexisting emotional problems also influence post-disaster outcomes (Norris, Friedman, & Watson, 2002; Norris et al., 2002).

19.4.2. Characteristics of the Disaster and Exposure

Although human-caused disasters have been described as more pathogenic than natural disasters to the extent that culpability can be established (Weisaeth & Tønnessen, 2003), this conclusion is not universally supported (Rubonis &

Bickman, 1991). Other aspects of disasters—such as casualty rates and the horror associated with an experience—may be more important than whether the disaster is natural or human made (Reissman, Spencer, Tanielian, & Stein, 2005). Differences in methodology and timing of studies make it difficult to compare outcomes across disasters. Using a consistent approach to examine the survivors of natural disasters, technological accidents, and deliberate human-caused events, North and colleagues demonstrated greater psychiatric morbidity associated with human-caused events (McMillen, North, & Smith, 2000; North et al., 1999; North & Smith, 1990; North, Smith, McCool, & Lightcap, 1989; North, Smith, McCool, & Shea, 1989; North, Smith, & Spitznagel, 1994). After an extensive review of the disaster mental health literature, these researchers also concluded that severe emotional impairment was more likely in mass violence than in technological or natural disasters (Norris, Friedman, & Watson, 2002; Norris et al., 2002).

Qualitative and quantitative aspects of disaster exposure are important determinants of psychological outcome. In the case of terrorism, distinctions in exposure deserve special attention because the intended and potential targets extend beyond those physically present at an attack site (North & Pfefferbaum, 2004; Pfefferbaum, 2003). Direct exposure occurs in individuals physically present at a disaster site and those infected or contaminated by a hazardous agent. Eyewitnesses to an event, especially those in close enough proximity to experience potential danger, are considered directly exposed even if they did not sustain obvious physical injury. Less direct forms of exposure occur through interpersonal relationships with victims and survivors and through secondary negative consequences of an event such as disruption of daily life. Remotely affected segments of the population, those located outside the community where an event occurs, are affected through membership in the greater society (North & Pfefferbaum, 2004; Pfefferbaum, 2003).

Quantitative aspects of disaster exposure may be described with reference to a dose response measured in physical proximity, sensory effects (such as seeing, hearing, or feeling), number of specific stressors associated with an incident, injury, loss and grief, property damage, financial burden, and duration and recurrence of exposure. For biological, chemical, nuclear, and radiological incidents, dose, lethality, and spread of the agent are key considerations. The relative importance of these and other factors are likely to differ in accordance with the event and qualitative aspects of exposure (Reissman et al., 2005).

19.4.3.   Aspects of the Recovery Environment

The recovery environment and characteristics of the community in which a disaster occurs also contribute to emotional outcomes of community members. A community with a well-organized response that provides prompt health and medical assessment and intervention, communicates accurate and necessary information, reestablishes social roles, and returns to known sources of social support can reduce harm and facilitate recovery for community members and the community as a whole (Holloway, Norwood, Fullerton, Engel, & Ursano, 1997). The recovery environment not only affects outcomes, but may be changed by the event via secondary sequelae (e.g., enduring disruption and chaos, possible dislocation and relocation of community members, and economic hardship) (Becker, 2001).

19.4.4.   A Caveat

Community resilience is not simply derived from a collection of resilient residents; the whole is more than the sum of the parts. The fallacies of composition and division caution that it is erroneous to assume that what is true of the parts is also necessarily true of the whole and, the reverse, that what is true of the whole is necessarily true of the units making it up (Holowchak, 2004). A collection of resilient individuals does not guarantee resilience in the community, nor does resilience at the community level ensure that all individuals are resilient.

One cannot easily divorce the individual from his or her community for they are durably entwined—especially, it would seem, in the case of resilience. Individual resilience is fostered through, among other things, supportive relationships and connectedness (APA, 2005; Reissman et al., 2004), which are at the heart of community. For the most part, therefore, one might expect positive externalities to be associated with increased individual resilience. Thus increased individual resilience may benefit both others in the community and the community as a whole.

19.5.   DEVELOPING COMMUNITY RESILIENCE: PUBLIC HEALTH LEADERSHIP'S ROLE

Community resilience building is a population-based prevention approach with implications for individuals and groups within the community. Population-based prevention strategies recognize that disease risk occurs on a continuum, that the majority of a population falls in the middle of the continuum rather than at the extremes, and that individual risk cannot be considered in isolation from population risk. A universal population-based prevention intervention would focus on modifying risk for the entire population rather than on individuals at especially high risk (IOM, 2003; Rose, 1981), thus creating what has been termed the *prevention paradox* because significant benefits accrue to the community at large rather than to each individual member (Rose, 1981). Selective and indicated prevention interventions focus, respectively, on individuals with elevated risk and those who are symptomatic. While indicated preventive measures are usually provided within the context of clinical practice, selective and indicated interventions could be used in conjunction with or integrated into a community resilience building approach.

Various sectors in a community—such as business, education, health, mental health, local government, and faith- and community-based organizations—have common and unique functions in developing, maintaining, and enhancing community resilience. These functions can be addressed in relationship to the seven community resilience factors described earlier. First responders, for example, can participate in community activities and help develop local resources while working, as many already do, with schools, local businesses, and other community groups to increase awareness of hazards, teach safety, and describe roles and responsibilities associated with emergency response. Businesses can partner with local organizations in advancing community goals and can participate in disaster preparedness and continuity planning. In addition to developing specialized skills in disaster mental health, mental health professionals can work with others in the community to de-stigmatize mental health service use.

All sectors must learn about the roles, responsibilities, and resources associated with each sector. Partnering within and across sectors in mental health preparedness can enhance connectedness, participation, and communication and can facilitate the integration of mental health in the daily lives of community members. Efforts to become culturally proficient typically require critical reflection and communication, thus buttressing those skills while fostering the development of support and nurturance. Motivated community leaders can appoint advisory groups with diverse membership to identify practical interventions for their local environment. Participation and connectedness can be exercised as a community comes together to inform its members about threats, vulnerabilities, potential outcomes, effective preparedness, and response strategies. To a large extent, community resilience is built, resources are enhanced, and roles and responsibilities are defined by making all factors operational.

Turning Point, launched in 1997 as an initiative of the Robert Wood Johnson Foundation and the W. K. Kellogg Foundation, employs concepts associated with community resilience building to transform and strengthen the nation's public health system by making it more community based and collaborative. Recognizing that the underlying causes of poor health are related to social issues too complex to be addressed solely by disease models of intervention, Turning Point links public health agencies and their partners to other sectors within a community (such as education, criminal justice, faith communities, and business) and brings health-conscious people and organizations together to address the community's health. In doing so, Turning Point helps communities take meaningful, deliberate, collective action to improve the public's health, thereby fostering community resilience. Local Turning Point partners collaborate to gather data, develop consensus about local priority health issues, mobilize local resources, create action plans to address health priorities, communicate local needs and priorities, and inform the development of effective health policy (Turning Point, 2003).

The Federal Emergency Management Agency approach to disaster response also illustrates concepts in community resilience in its reliance on local resources to address problems at the closest possible organizational and jurisdictional level while providing national capability to address broader regional and national issues. In the aftermath of a disaster, many people experience disruption and loss but most do not see themselves as needing mental health services (Substance Abuse and Mental Health Services Administration, 2005). A federal mental health response is initiated in presidentially declared disasters, when state and local resources are inadequate to address the need. Services include outreach and public education, crisis intervention, and support services for common reactions that arise after disaster's (rather than traditional mental health treatment for psychiatric illnesses). The federal response relies on local providers and networks to create a system that includes triage and referral and that promotes access by using programs with a local cultural base. The response builds on the strength of the community, reinforcing services as necessary during the early stages of recovery. By training and using local providers in disaster response, this approach contributes to community capacity building, fosters community participation and cohesion, and promotes a sense of community efficacy and empowerment—all of which enhance and strengthen community resilience.

Although community resilience building is within the scope of activities of all stakeholders, it is a particularly appropriate function of public health. As part of an illness prevention and community wellness agenda, public health can foster preparedness planning and practice drills as the norm at all levels and across all sectors, encouraging ongoing review and revision of plans based on new threats and emerging methods for responding to them. Working with emergency management, public health can assist community volunteers and neighborhood organizations to improve local disaster response capabilities. Depending on context, public health can help redefine first responders to include health care workers, business people, school personnel, essential service workers, and community members. Public health can also assist first responder organizations in reviewing and establishing lines of authority and responsibility within and across bureaucratic boundaries, facilitate cooperative relationships, and promote joint training and cross-training.

As part of public health education strategies for community resilience building, community members can be trained in psychological first aid. Individuals can be taught personal resilience building skills that can be reinforced in times of disaster. Public health can join with mental health in the essential effort to destigmatize mental health problems. Communities can be sensitized to the cultural and ethnic diversity of their members and come to value that diversity for the potential it creates. Media, an essential community partner, can be engaged in developing public service announcements based on principles of effective risk communication.

With its command of public resources, limited as they may be, and connections to nongovernmental organizations, public health is in a position to help identify, inventory, and map resources and to develop plans for resource allocation and deployment. Public health can serve an organizing and integrating function, linking mental health programs to other services including health care and social services; businesses and schools; and neighborhood, faith-based, and cultural organizations. Public health can also foster leadership and community development, civic engagement, and attention to health in public and private policies across the full spectrum of social concerns, including communication, commerce, transportation, education, and social welfare (IOM, 2003).

The investigation of community resilience is still in its infancy; but clearly, it holds promise as a construct for and approach to preventing adverse mental health outcomes associated with terrorism and disasters. Factors in community resilience, which warrant further examination and clarification, can guide development of specific prevention interventions in community resilience building.

REFERENCES

American Psychological Association. (2005). *Fostering resilience in response to terrorism: A fact sheet for psychologists working with adults.* Retrieved May 14, 2005, from www.apahelpcenter.org/featuredtopics/feature.php?id=6.

Becker, S. M. (2001). Psychosocial effects of radiation accidents. In I. A. Gusev, A. K. Guskova, & F. A. Mettler (Eds.), *Medical management of radiation accidents* (pp. 519–525, 2nd ed.). Boca Raton, FL: CRC Press.

Bromet, E., & Dew, M. A. (1995). Review of psychiatric epidemiologic research on disasters. *Epidemiologic Reviews, 17* (1), 113–119.

Brown, D. D., & Kulig, J. C. (1996–1997). The concept of resiliency: Theoretical lessons from community research. *Health & Canadian Society, 4* (1), 29–50.

Cottrell, L. S., Jr. (1976). The competent community. In B. H. Kaplan, R. N. Wilson, & A. H. Leighton (Eds.), *Further explorations in social psychiatry* (pp. 195–209). New York: Basic Books.

Difede, J., Apfeldorf, W. J., Cloitre, M., Spielman, L. A., & Perry, S. W. (1997). Acute psychiatric responses to the explosion at the World Trade Center: A case series. *Journal of Nervous & Mental Disease, 185* (8), 519–522.

Eränen, L., & Liebkind, K. (1993). Coping with disaster: The helping behavior of communities and individuals. In J. P. Wilson & B. Raphael (Eds.), *International handbook of traumatic stress syndromes* (pp. 957–964). New York: Plenum Press.

Erikson, K. T. (1976). *Everything in its path: Destruction of community in the Buffalo Creek flood.* New York: Simon & Schuster.

Friedman, M. J. (2005). Toward a public mental health approach for survivors of terrorism. *Journal of Aggression, Maltreatment & Trauma, 10* (1–2), 527–539.

Gibbon, M., Labonte, R., & Laverack, G. (2002). Evaluating community capacity. *Health & Social Care in the Community, 10* (6), 485–491.

Goeppinger, J., & Baglioni, A. J. Jr. (1985). Community competence: A positive approach to needs assessment. *American Journal of Community Psychology, 13* (5), 507–523.

Goodman, R. M., Speers, M. A., McLeroy, K., Fawcett, S., Kegler, M., Parker, E., Smith, S. R., Sterling, T. D., & Wallerstein, N. (1998). Identifying and defining the dimensions of community capacity to provide a basis for measurement. *Health Education & Behavior, 25* (3), 258–278.

Holloway, H. C., Norwood, A. E., Fullerton, C. S., Engel, C. C., Jr., & Ursano, R. J. (1997). The threat of biological weapons: Prophylaxis and mitigation of psychological and social consequences. *Journal of the American Medical Association, 278* (5), 425–427.

Holowchak, M. A. (2004). *Critical reasoning and philosophy: A concise guide to reading, evaluating, and writing philosophical works.* Lanham, MD: Rowman & Littlefield.

Institute of Medicine (2003). *The future of the public's health in the 21ˢᵗ century.* Washington, DC: National Academies Press.

Institute of Medicine (2004). *Preparing for the psychological consequences of terrorism: A public health strategy.* Washington, DC: National Academies Press.

Issel, L. M. (2004). *Health program planning and evaluation: A practical, systematic approach for community health.* Boston: Jones & Bartlett.

Jerusalem, M., Kaniasty, K., Lehman, D. R., Ritter, C., & Turnbull, G. J. (1995). Individual and community stress: Integration of approaches at different levels. In S. E. Hobfoll & M. W. de Vries (Eds.), *Extreme stress and communities: Impact and intervention* (pp. 105–129). Dordrecht, Netherlands: Kluwer Academic.

Kulig, J. C. (2000). Community resiliency: The potential for community health nursing theory development. *Public Health Nursing, 17* (5), 374–385.

Labonte, R., & Laverack, G. (2001). Capacity building in health promotion, Part 1: For whom? And for what purpose? *Critical Public Health, 11* (2), 111–127.

McMillen, J. C., North, C. S., & Smith, E. M. (2000). What parts of PTSD are normal: Intrusion, avoidance, or arousal? Data from the Northridge, California, earthquake. *Journal of Traumatic Stress, 13* (1), 57–75.

Norris, F. H., Friedman, M. J., & Watson, P. J. (2002). 60,000 Disaster victims speak: Part II. Summary and implications of the disaster mental health research. *Psychiatry, 65* (3), 240–260.

Norris, F. H., Friedman, M. J., Watson, P. J., Byrne, C. M., Diaz, E., & Kaniasty, K. (2002). 60,000 Disaster victims speak: Part I. An empirical review of the empirical literature, 1981–2001. *Psychiatry, 65* (3), 207–239.

North, C. S., Nixon, S. J., Shariat, S., Mallonee, S., McMillen, J. C., Spitznagel, E. L., & Smith, E. M. (1999). Psychiatric disorders among survivors of the Oklahoma City bombing. *Journal of the American Medical Association, 282* (8), 755–762.

North, C. S., & Pfefferbaum, B. (2004). The state of research on the mental health effects of terrorism. *Epidemiologia e Psichiatria Sociale, 13* (1), 4–9.

North, C. S., & Smith, E. M. (1990). Post-traumatic stress disorder in disaster survivors. *Comprehensive Therapy, 16* (12), 3–9.

North, C. S., Smith, E. M., McCool, R. E., & Lightcap, P. E. (1989). Acute postdisaster coping and adjustment. *Journal of Traumatic Stress, 2* (3), 353–360.

North, C. S., Smith, E. M., McCool, R. E., & Shea, J. M. (1989). Short-term psychopathology in eyewitnesses to mass murder. *Hospital & Community Psychiatry, 40* (12), 1293–1295.

North, C. S., Smith, E. M., & Spitznagel, E. L. (1994). Posttraumatic stress disorder in survivors of a mass shooting. *American Journal of Psychiatry, 151* (1), 82–88.

Ofman, P. S., Mastria, M. A., & Steinberg, J. (1995). Mental health response to terrorism: The World Trade Center bombing. *Journal of Mental Health Counseling, 17* (3), 312–320.

Pfefferbaum, B. (2003). Victims of terrorism and the media. In A. Silke (Ed.), *Terrorists, victims and society: Psychological perspectives on terrorism and its consequences.* (pp. 175–187) West Sussex, UK: Wiley.

Reissman, D. B., Klomp, R. W., Kent, A. T., & Pfefferbaum, B. (2004). Exploring psychological resilience in the face of terrorism. *Psychiatric Annals, 33* (8), 626–632.

Reissman, D. B., Spencer, S., Tanielian, T. L., & Stein, B. D. (2005). Integrating behavioral aspects into community preparedness and response systems. *Journal of Aggression, Maltreatment & Trauma, 10* (3–4), 707–720.

Rose, G. (1981). Strategy of prevention: Lessons from cardiovascular disease. *British Medical Journal, 282,* 1847–1851.

Rubonis, A. V., & Bickman, L. (1991). Psychological impairment in the wake of disaster: The disaster-psychopathology relationship. *Psychological Bulletin, 109* (3), 384–399.

Sjoberg, G. (1962). Disasters and social change. In G. W. Baker & D. W. Chapman (Eds.), *Man and society in disaster* (pp. 356–384). New York: Basic Books.

Steinberg, A., & Ritzmann, R. F. (1990). A living systems approach to understanding the concept of stress. *Behavioral Science, 35,* 138–146.

Substance Abuse and Mental Health Services Administration. (2005). *Federal Emergency Management Agency (FEMA) mental health training manual.* Retrieved May 14, 2005, from www.mentalhealth.samhsa.gov/cmhs/EmergencyServices/.

Turning Point. (2003). *Turning Point: Collaborating for a new century in public health.* Retrieved June 21, 2005, from www.turningpointprogram.org/Pages/New_TP_brochure.pdf.

Weisaeth, L., & Tønnessen, A. (2003). Responses of individuals and groups to consequences of technological disasters and radiation exposure. In R. J. Ursano, C. S. Fullerton, & A. E. Norwood (Eds.), *Terrorism and disaster* (pp. 209–235). Cambridge, UK: Cambridge University Press.

Yahmed, S. B., & Koob, P. (1996). Health sector approach to vulnerability reduction and emergency preparedness. *World Health Statistics Quarterly, 49,* 172–178.

Chapter **20**

Trends and Challenges in Intervention Research Methods

Brian F. Oldenburg and Alison M. Brodie

20.1. INTRODUCTION

Community interventions offer a promising option for reducing both intentional and unintentional injuries in children and adults as a result of their potential to influence and achieve widespread, long-term change in a large number of individuals from the population(s) at risk. Community interventions can positively influence individuals' behavior(s) while they facilitate positive and health-enhancing changes to people's living environments. They can also have a long-term and sustainable influence on societal norms that are relevant to safety and related behaviours (Oldenburg & Burton, 2004).

Community-based interventions and public health interventions do not aim to lower the injury or harm risk of single individuals but aim to reduce the average level of risk in a large group of individuals or population subgroup by delivering interventions or programs in settings such as schools, workplaces, and other public settings. Typically, such an approach uses a broad array of strategies that may include educational/behavioural, engineering/technology, and legislation/ enforcement components (Klassen, MacKay, Moher, Walker, & Jones, 2000; Sleet & Gielen, 2004). Educational/behavioural strategies aim to increase the awareness of injury risk and the importance of risk-reducing behaviors and include media broadcasts, public service announcements, classroom instruction, written material, incentives, negative feedback, behavioral change strategies, and modeling (Klassen et al., 2000). The goal of engineering/technology interventions is to alter the physical environment (such as by placing speed humps on streets or installing smoke detectors in homes) or modify the design of safety devices (such as bicycle helmets or child passenger seats). Finally, legislation/enforcement interventions involve the passage and enforcement of new laws or the increased enforcement of existing laws (Klassen et al., 2000).

Generally speaking, the particular strategies used differ among the communities in which they are applied due to differences in population characteristics, setting, composition, and the nature of the problem being addressed. The following statement by Moller (1991, p. 52) nicely summarizes the importance and potential for the concept of *community* being incorporated into the design, implementation, and evaluation of intervention strategies in relation to injury control:

> The community-based model for injury prevention is an explicit approach to achieving reductions in the incidence of injury at the population level by application of multiple countermeasures, and multiple strategies in the context of community-defined problems, and community-owned solutions.

Since the first well-evaluated community intervention trials for cardiovascular disease prevention were conducted almost 30 years ago (Maccoby, Farquhar, Wood, & Alexander, 1977; Puska et al., 1979), a lot of progress has been made in the conceptualization, understanding, implementation, and evaluation of such approaches. For example, in recent years, the World Health Organization (WHO) Safe Communities Model has provided a contemporary framework for conceptualizing community-based interventions relevant to injury control and prevention, which has now been embraced globally by more than 90 communities (Lindqvist, Timpka, Schelp, & Risto, 2002). However, when these first community intervention trials were conducted during the 1970s, the intervention strategies and the methods used to evaluate them often did not take into account the unique attributes or characteristics of communities or the ways in which they operated.

A lot has been learned about the conduct and evaluation of such interventions trials over the past 25 years. There has been much progress made in understanding the implications of the community as a unit of randomization, the importance of the interactions and networks among individuals within the same community, and the special analytical techniques required for evaluating interventions that are conducted in particular community settings or in the community as a whole.

Despite this progress in knowledge and understanding of community intervention trials, evaluation of these trials is still challenged by issues related to reliability, validity, and objectivity (Israel, Schultz, Parker, & Becker, 1998), which can make it problematic to identify the "real" effects of any given intervention (Thompson, Coronado, Snipes, & Puschel, 2003). The purpose of this chapter is to:

- Review current issues and challenges with respect to the development, implementation, and evaluation of community interventions.
- Review intervention methods and evaluation approaches in the injury control field.
- Identify the strengths and weaknesses of this body of research.
- Identify trends and challenges for future research.

20.2.   CURRENT ISSUES IN THE DEVELOPMENT, IMPLEMENTATION, AND EVALUATION OF COMMUNITY INTERVENTIONS

A number of authors have reviewed the intervention and evaluation challenges posed by community interventions (see also Chapters 21 and 27). An important review carried out by Sorensen, Emmons, Hunt, and Johnson (1998) focused primarily on the results of population-level interventions conducted in entire communities and community settings, such as worksites and schools. They considered how the results obtained might be strengthened and made more sustainable in the future. Thompson et al. (2003) considered the methodological and other advances of community-based health promotion programs conducted in more recent years. Both of these reviews make a number of recommendations and highlight some of the key challenges for the next generation of community interventions. The authors cite evidence indicating that attention to these issues will lead to more effective and more sustainable interventions. Nine important issues or recommendations were highlighted in either or both of those reviews.

- *Designing interventions based on a good theory.* An intervention designed around a theoretical model recognizes the influence of a wide range of factors— from intrapersonal and interpersonal factors to institutional- and community-level factors as well as societal-level factors such as public policy—on behavior and develops a framework for implementing strategies aimed at these multiple levels of influence.
- *Using multifaceted interventions.* Multifaceted interventions are those that use more than one mode of strategy delivery, such as by combining educational activities with environmental modifications or policy initiatives. Depending on the breadth and different components of the intervention, these may be delivered selectively to various subgroups within the target population.
- *Community involvement in program planning and implementation.* The degree and type of community involvement in program development, implementation, and evaluation can vary significantly from one program to another. In some programs, a community may simply approve or sanction what researchers have already planned and designed. In more recent years though, it has become common for a community to participate fully in the planning and design of a health-promotion initiative and furthermore, it might also be involved in monitoring, implementing, and evaluating the program.
- *Tailoring of interventions.* Interventions may be tailored to address the unique needs and cultures of communities, such as variations in literacy levels, race, or locale. This may involve methodological flexibility, which improves acceptability and therefore uptake in the community.
- *Addressing social inequalities and disadvantage.* Interventions that address social inequalities respond to the influence of socioeconomic position on the availability of social and material resources that have long-lasting effects on health. Targeting inequalities may therefore involve researching and/or instituting structural changes and broad-based policy initiatives designed to reduce social and other disparities.
- *Using rigorous study designs.* Improvements in study design come from the prudent selection and use of a well-designed research methodology. Such methodology should address the diverse needs for scientific rigor, appropriateness to research questions, acceptability to the community, and feasibility in terms of cost and setting.
- *Improving process evaluation and implementation measurement.* Process and implementation evaluation involves the measurement of "dose" or intensity of intervention strategies, an assessment of the extent to which the intervention was delivered as planned, and a measurement of program coverage and participation. This knowledge helps elucidate whether the

population targeted for behavior change is receiving the right messages, leading the members to make health changes.

- *Assessing the durability and sustainability of interventions.* The durability of an intervention is its likelihood of being sustainable in the community after external funding has ended. Durability allows time for any small positive effects resulting from an intervention to become larger ones and thereby facilitates long-term population-based change in behavior.
- *Economic evaluation.* An economic evaluation of a community trial assesses its "value for money" and is based on an analysis of thorough and accurate substantiating data, such as start-up costs, overhead costs, and statements of benefits.

In the following section we use these nine issues as criteria for considering the quality of intervention trials that have been conducted in the injury control field; the major focus is on those interventions that have been conducted in the general community or particular settings in the community.

20.3.   OVERVIEW OF INTERVENTION AND EVALUATION METHODS IN THE INJURY CONTROL FIELD

We conducted a narrative evaluation of the major published systematic reviews of injury interventions, assessing the quality of interventions in the injury control field in relation to the nine quality issues, and identifying the aspects that might benefit from more systematic attention. A search of the Web of Science database (using the keywords "injury" AND "intervention" or "program*" AND "systematic review") and the Cochrane Database of Systematic Reviews (Cochrane Injuries Group) identified 30 relevant review articles published between 1998 and early 2005 (Table 20.1). Oldenburg, Ffrench, and Sallis (2000) and Oldenburg, Sallis, Ffrench, and Owen (1999) used such an approach to assess the quantity and quality of published health promotion intervention trials. Salient issues from these articles are considered and discussed in this chapter. Here, we consider only the information and details available in the 30 systematic reviews listed in Table 20.1; we have not reviewed in detail the more than 600 individual studies that were examined in those articles.

20.3.1.   Key Findings Arising from the Quality Review

Most of the major categories of nonintentional injury were reflected in the 30 reviews of interventions and health promotion programs, including injuries caused by a moving vehicle (motor vehicle, motorcycle, bicycle) to another vehicle, vehicle occupant, or pedestrian (10 reviews); occupational injury, including farm injuries, falls, needlestick, eye injuries, and injuries due to shiftwork and other workplace accidents (7 reviews); injuries to children, including poisoning, burns and scalds, and drowning (5 reviews); fall-related injuries in older people (3 reviews); home hazards, including promotion of smoke alarms and modification of home environment (2 reviews); sport and recreational injuries (2 reviews); and general community-based interventions (1 review). The number of individual studies considered in each systematic review varied from 3 to 117 (an average of 19); therefore, the majority of the 30 reviews were based on a moderate to large number of individual studies.

Table 20.1. Summary of Reviews of Community Intervention Trials

Reference	Study Field	Studies Reviewed (Target Group)	Study Setting	Study Design
Nixon et al. (2004)	Poisoning in children	4 (children 0–15 years)	Community	• 2 RCTs • 2 historical before/after • 7 Non-RCTs
Spinks et al. (2004)	All injuries for children	9 (children 0–14 years)	Community	• 2 historical before/after
Thompson and Rivara (1998)	Pool fencing for prevention of drowning	3 (children 0–14 years with pools)	Community (pool owners)	Population-based case-control studies
Towner and Dowsell (2002)	Childhood injury prevention	10 (all ages)	Home/school and community	• 9 Non-RCTs • 1 before/after study
Turner et al. (2004)	Burns/scalds in children	3 (children 0–14 years)	School and community (libraries, fire/police, day care)	Controlled before-and-after interventions
Carter et al. (2001)	Falls in older people	13 (adults aged 60 years and over)	Community and aged-care institutions	RCTs
Chang et al. (2004)	Falls in older people	40 (adults aged 65 years and older)	Seniors centers and nursing homes, community	RCTs
Hartling et al. (2004)	Fall-related injuries in older people	5 (adults aged 65 years and older)	Community	Controlled, population-based interventions
Di Guiseppi and Higgins (2001)	Smoke alarm ownership and function	26 (all ages, people living at home)	Clinical/hospital; home/school	• 13 RCTs • 13 Non-RCTs
Lyons et al. (2003)	Home hazard modification	28 (all ages, people living at home)	Home/nursing home; clinics/hospital; kindergarten	• 13 RCTs • 14 Non-RCTs • 1 Controlled before/after study
Dinh-Zarr et al. (2001)	Increasing safety-belt use via safety belt laws, primary enforcement laws (seat belts), and enhanced enforcement	19 (children over 5 years, adolescents, adults)	Community	• 7 time series with comparison • 4 time series/no comparison • Cross-sectional

Table 20.1. *Continued*

Reference	Study Field	Studies Reviewed (Target Group)	Study Setting	Study Design
Zaza, Sleet, et al.,	Increasing safety seat use via safety seat laws, communitywide information and enhanced enforcement campaigns, distribution and education programs, and incentives and education	14	Community	• 2 RCTs • 3 Non-RCT • 2 time series, no comparison • 2 before/after, no comparison • 2 Non-random individual trials • 1 cross-sectional
Duperrex et al. (2002)	Prevention of pedestrian injury	14 (pedestrians of all ages)	School; community	RCTs
Ker et al. (2003)	Prevention of road traffic crashes	24 (all ages, drivers with valid licence)	Driving school	RCTs
Kwan and Mapstone (2002)	Prevention of death and injury to pedestrians and cyclists	37 (volunteers and observers, paid and unpaid)	Driving school/driving laboratory	• 2 randomized participants only • 3 randomized participants and visibility aids • 14 randomized aids only • 18 balanced/counterbalanced
Roberts et al. (2001)	Prevention of traffic crashes	3 (unlicensed drivers aged 15–24 years)	Driving school	RCTs
Liu et al. (2003)	Helmets for preventing injury in motorcycle riders	53 (motorcycle riders)	Community	Retrospective cross-sectional studies
Shults et al. (2001)	Reduction of alcohol-impaired driving	66	Community	• 26 time series with concurrent comparison • 16 time series no concurrent comparison • 26 before/after with concurrent comparison

Table 20.1. *Continued*

Reference	Study Field	Studies Reviewed (Target Group)	Study Setting	Study Design
Thompson et al. (1999)	Helmets for preventing injuries in bicyclists	5 (bicyclists of all ages involved in a bike crash or fall)	Community	Case-control studies
MacKay et al. (2004)	Sport and recreational injury among children and youth	117 (children/youth involved in baseball, basketball, cycling, football, ice hockey, rugby, alpine skiing, or soccer)	Community sports grounds and laboratory settings	• Prospective cohort (30%) • 1 group pretest/posttest (20%) • RCTs (16%) • Retrospective cohort, case-control, time-series
Olsen et al. (2004)	Soccer-related injuries	4 (all ages, professional and amateur soccer players)	Community/college sports club	• 1 RCT • 2 time series • 1 nonequivalent control
De Roo and Rautiainen (2000)	Farm safety interventions	25 (farmers and farm operators)	Farm/community	Mainly pretest and posttest design
Hartling, Brison et al. (2004)	Childhood farm injuries	23 (children)	Schools; farms; community	• 1 RCT • 4 RCTs • 5 controlled trials • 14 quasi-experimental or observational studies
Keifer (2000)	Pesticide overexposure and poisonings	17 (people working with pesticide)	Workplace (multiple)	• 7 different study designs • No RCTs
Rivara and Thompson 2000(a)	Prevention of falls in the construction industry	3 (any age, construction workers)	Workplace (construction industry)	• 2 Before/after comparisons • 1 ecological study
Rogers and Goodno (2000)	Needlestick injuries in health-care occupations	11 (health care workers)	Workplace (hospital)	RCTs
Lipscomb (2000)	Work-related eye injuries	7 (manufacturing, construction, or agricultural workers)	Workplace (multiple)	• 5 before/after study • 1 Non-RCT • 1 case-control study
Frank (2000)	Injuries related to shiftwork	7 (fixed and/or rotating shift workers)	Workplace (manufacturing industry)	• 7 different study designs • No RCTs
Segui-Gomez (2000)	Promoting safety belts at the work site	44 (workers driving at work and/or to and from work)	Workplace (white and blue collar)	• 1 RCT • 26 quasi-experimental • 18 ecologic time series
Klassen et al. (2000)	Community-based injury prevention interventions	28 (variety of ages and populations)	Schools/preschool; home/community	• 6 RCTs • 22 nonrandomized RCTS

The populations targeted for the interventions varied in accordance with the type of injury being studied; however, in the majority of the reviews, a specific group (e.g., motor vehicle drivers, farm workers, or shift workers) was selected, rather than the whole community. When the target population was defined by age, it was typically either the very young or older adults (children 14 years or younger and, adults 60 years or older). One review (Roberts, Kwan, & the Cochrane Injuries Group Driver Education Reviewers, 2001) focused on unlicensed drivers between 15 and 24 years.

20.3.1.1. Use of Theory

Few individual studies made a reference to a theoretical framework supporting either the choice of strategy or the mode of delivery of the interventions. Two reviews—Dinh-Zarr et al. (2001) and Zaza, Carande-Kulis et al. (2001)—described a conceptual approach developed by the reviewers to inform and frame their reviews.

20.3.1.2. Use of Multifaceted Interventions

The majority of reviewed interventions used multiple strategies, which commonly involved an educational component in addition to environmental/regulatory/economic strategies. Four reviews described education-only interventions; two reviews described environmental-only interventions (such as wearing protective clothing), and six reviews considered regulatory/legislative initiatives that examined the effectiveness of laws (such as the wearing of seat belts to reduce injury in motor-vehicle crashes). Interventions were delivered either to specific target groups (such as drivers who had previously been involved in a road crash; $n = 18$), to the general population on a community-wide basis (such as legislation to prevent drinking and driving; $n = 17$), or to a combination of these. No reviews focused exclusively on individual-level intervention strategies; however, eight reviews described interventions targeted at a combination of individuals as well as groups and communities. The choice of settings for the interventions depended on the nature of the injury topic and the target population. For example, interventions targeting occupational injury in the community were delivered at the worksite, and interventions targeting sports injuries typically took place at sports fields or sports laboratories.

20.3.1.3. Community or Consumer Involvement in Program Planning and Implementation

In the majority of the reviews, community participation was neither discussed in the text of the review nor featured as a major descriptor in the summary table of interventions. Three reviews implied some community involvement in one or more of the studies considered (Ker et al., 2003; Klassen et al., 2000; Lyons et al., 2003); however, no further details of this involvement were discussed. Community participation (ranging from community planning workshops to the development of community interagency collaborations) was a featured descriptor in three higher quality reviews, all of which were related to prevention of injuries in children (Spinks, Turner, McClure, & Nixon, 2004; Towner & Dowsell, 2002; Turner, Spinks, McClure, & Nixon, 2004), however the precise nature of this involvement and other details were not described.

20.3.1.4.   Tailoring of Interventions

No explicit information was provided on the tailoring of interventions in any of the reviews.

20.3.1.5.   Addressing Social Inequalities

Minimal attention was given to social inequalities in any of the reviews.

20.3.1.6.   Study Design Factors

The methodological quality of papers in the reviews varied significantly, depending on the source from which the reviews were taken. Cochrane reviews, by definition, select for the highest quality research in their field, and this was evidenced by the higher percentage of Cochrane (compared to non-Cochrane) papers that consisted either entirely or primarily of randomized control trials (RCTs). A total of 5 reviews (3 Cochrane) examined RCTs only, and 2 large Cochrane studies contained 50% RCTs (Di Guiseppi & Higgins, 2001; Lyons et al., 2003). Exactly half (15) of the reviews had at least one RCT among their reviewed studies, however, in 4 of these reviews, RCTs made up only a small percentage of the studies considered. The remaining 15 reviews that did not contain any RCTs were made up primarily of nonrandomized control trials (which were mostly quasi-experimental studies) or time series studies, with and without comparison groups.

The majority of reviews contained studies of only one or two designs; however nine reviews described three or more study designs among their group, and two reviews described seven (including time series with and without a comparison group, non-RCTs, quasi-experimental, before-and-after comparisons, prospective cross-sectional, and ecological studies). There was one review (examining the effectiveness of helmets in preventing head injuries in motorcyclists) in which only retrospective cross-sectional studies were described (Liu, Ivers, Norton, Blows, & Lo, 2003). In two reviews (one studying pool fencing for preventing drowning in children and another examining the effectiveness of helmets in preventing facial injuries in cyclists) all studies were case control studies (Thompson & Rivara, 1998; Thompson, Rivara, & Thompson, 1999).

20.3.1.7.   Outcome and Process Measurement

Across the reviews, there was a wide variety of injury, behavioral and other outcomes measured. These included specific injury incidence rates (such as incidence and severity of burns and falls); change in injury prevention knowledge, attitude, or behavior (self-reported and observed); and use of protective device (such as seat belt or bicycle helmet). Also examined were hospital or emergency department attendance, days off work through injury, workers' compensation claims, observation of hazards, measurement of skin levels of toxins, and (in one instance) community involvement. The majority of reviews contained at least some studies that employed multiple measures of outcome. A total of 3 reviews reported only a single measure of outcome across all studies examined, whereas 6 reviews noted two outcomes, 12 measured three outcomes, and 9 measured four or more outcomes. Process evaluation was specifically mentioned in only 2 reviews: De Roo and Rautiainen (2000) described an intervention that used some nonspecific measure of process to examine implementation; Towner and Dowswell (2002) described an intervention that used process data from health planners as well as a diverse (unspecified) range of process measures.

20.3.1.8. *Durability and Duration of Intervention and Follow-Up*

Brief and nonspecific details of follow-up were described in just over half of the reviews ($n = 18$). The period of follow-up ranged from a minimum of 2 weeks in a strategy to increase smoke alarm ownership and function (DiGuiseppi & Higgins, 2001), to a maximum of 14.4 years in an intervention to reduce alcohol-impaired driving (Shults et al., 2001). The most common time for follow-up was 12 months. In 12 studies, follow-up was not described in either the text or the table summaries.

20.3.1.9. *Economic Evaluation*

One review (Shults et al., 2001) described interventions with economic evaluations. Three reviews (Dinh-Zarr et al., 2001; Zaza, Sleet, Thompson, Sosin, & Bolen, 2001; Nixon et al., 2004) used economic evaluation as one of the descriptors, but the authors did not find any interventions that evaluated it. There were no other reviews in which economic evaluation was described.

20.4. STRENGTHS AND WEAKNESSES OF THE INJURY CONTROL EVIDENCE BASE

The previous section demonstrates that there is an impressive and expanding evidence base of more than 600 studies in the injury control field that contribute to an understanding of community interventions; however, there are several ways in which this field of research can be improved on. Before considering these points though, there are a couple of important limitations in relation to the approach we have adopted in carrying out this review of reviews. Without reviewing in detail all of the original 680 papers contained in the 30 systematic reviews, it is impossible to be certain whether the original studies adequately and sufficiently considered the nine quality issues (described earlier). The authors of systematic reviews typically select and summarize the methodological and other issues that they regard as being most salient in terms of the effectiveness, effect, and outcomes of relevant interventions. Given that we have reviewed only the systematic reviews and not the original studies themselves, it is possible that this chapter has not adequately reflected other information contained in the original papers that might be relevant to the nine quality issues that are the focus of this chapter.

These shortcomings notwithstanding, we are confident that the findings of this review of reviews do highlight a number of important intervention design, implementation, and evaluation issues that warrant more attention in the future. There are two particular issues that stand out. First, although a variety of study designs are being used in research in the injury control field, it is still common for the authors of systematic reviews to lament a relative paucity of high-quality research from which evidence on effectiveness can be obtained. Indeed, a number of these authors have expressed the need for more well designed research and the appropriate use of relevant study designs, even when a controlled trial design was not appropriate or possible (MacKay et al., 2004; Rivara & Thompson, 2000a). Other methodological issues that were raised in more than one of the reviews included inadequate sample size, lack of use of a multifactorial study design, small uptake rates and large attrition rates, poor or nonexistent control for confounders, short-term follow-up, inappropriate or poorly chosen measures of outcome, poor timing of outcome assessment with no long-term follow-up, and inability to identify which components of a multicomponent program were the effective ones.

Second, even acknowledging the limitations associated with the methods used in this chapter, it is still rather surprising that some key issues that have been identified as being important to the design, implementation, and evaluation of interventions in the community have received so little attention. For example, we found a lack of the use of theory. Furthermore little attention was given to the concept of community and community participation; social inequalities and disadvantages; and durability, sustainability, and measurement of interventions. Finally, methods of economic evaluation were generally missing.

20.5. FUTURE TRENDS AND CHALLENGES IN THE EVALUATION OF COMMUNITY-BASED INTERVENTIONS

While our review shows that some excellent progress has been made in the design, implementation, and evaluation of community-based interventions in recent years, there are still a number of important areas in which progress can be made.

20.5.1. Designing Interventions That Target Multiple Levels of Influence and That Are Guided by a Good Theoretical Model

More than a decade ago, Koepsell et al. (1992) noted that the theoretical model underlying many community interventions was often unclear. They advocated an approach that carefully articulated how an intervention strategy should be underpinned by a clearly identified theory or model. In their approach, studies should also identify how the measurements of process, effect, and outcome are linked to the model and the different intervention components. Sleet and Gielen (see Chapter 22) reinforce this notion, outlining specific theoretical frameworks for designing and evaluation injury interventions. Thompson et al. (2003) in their review of methodological advances and challenges in community-based health promotion programs, noted that, even though the vast majority of studies do not indicate use of a particular theory, only a small number (in this case, 20%) specifically identify how the theory was used to develop an intervention strategy. An even smaller number of studies report what strategies were used to interact with the target population to establish the most appropriate and acceptable intervention strategies for that population.

This finding has also been confirmed by Trifiletti, Gielen, Sleet, & Hopkins (2005), who conducted a recent review of the published literature on behavioral and social science theory models as they apply specifically to unintentional injury problems. The authors concluded that the use of theories and models in unintentional injury prevention research is only marginally represented in the mainstream, peer-reviewed literature and that several important theories have never been applied to unintentional injury prevention. The paper provides some useful examples of the way that models and theories have already been applied by some researchers to specific injury topics and in what way they have been used to guide program design or implementation or to develop evaluation measures. Specific applications of behavior change theories and methods to injury prevention were summarized by Gielen and Sleet (2003), and are elaborated on in more detail by Gielen, Sleet, & DiClemente (2006).

Several tools exist to aid our current understanding and to facilitate the development of theory-based, multilevel interventions. For example, a logic model is a graphic display or map of the relationship among a program's resources, activities, and underlying theory and assumptions (McLaughlin & Jordan, 1999; Renger & Titcomb, 2002). Use of a logic model guides program planners in applying the scientific method—of articulating a clear hypothesis or objective to be tested—to the development, implementation, and monitoring of their program. In recent years, it has become common for program funders to require community-based initiatives to develop logic models as part of the grant application and as part of the on-going monitoring, reporting, and evaluation. Kaplan and Garrett (2005) examine this process in three community programs. They describe the benefits and challenges of using logic models to help build consensus, foster collaboration within a community coalition, strengthen the program design (by assessing underlying assumptions held by program planners); and facilitate internal and external communication. As an alternative to logic modeling, intervention mapping provides a framework for applying theory to the development of community interventions and has been used extensively in many different areas of health promotion around the world (Bartholomew, Parcel, & Kok, 1998).

20.5.2. Using Multifaceted Interventions

It has become increasingly common for community trials to implement and attempt to evaluate multiple intervention strategies at the individual, group, system, and community levels in the quest to move beyond purely individual-level intervention strategies. While this is consistent with a population health approach, a major limitation of such a method is that the different intervention components can often be poorly implemented and evaluated, so that it remains difficult to ascertain which components might have contributed to overall program effectiveness. It is thus important for such interventions to have an evaluation and framework that identify which intervention activities were related to outcomes to maximize the generalizability of the findings to other settings and communities.

20.5.3. Involving Communities in Program Planning and Implementation

It is generally assumed that sustainable behavior change is more likely to occur when the people affected by a problem are involved in defining and finding solutions for the problem. It follows, therefore, that a program defined by a community and that allows for flexibility in response to community priorities would be well suited to its particular audience, thereby increasing participation and program effectiveness compared to other programs. Indeed, a review of the WHO Safe Communities Model shows that community participation has been positively associated with perceptions of ownership and subsequent commitment to engage in injury prevention initiatives (Coggan & Bennett, 2004). In addition, evidence indicates interventions that are not community driven and initiated (but that are driven and initiated by external professionals) have the potential to foster community dependency and do not achieve sustainability (Hanson, Vardon, & Lloyd, 2002).

The next generation of researchers has much to learn from research conducted in recent years on empowerment, self-efficacy, social support, social networks, and community psychology for identifying ways to improve community health through community organization and community building. However, the Sorensen, Emmous, Hurt, and Johnston (1998) and Thompson, Coronado, Snipes, and Puschel (2003) reviews raise some important issues when considering how best to incorporate community participation into a research study design:

- If an RCT is involved, should randomization occur before or after community consultation? Early community involvement fosters a more balanced power distribution by which community members can suggest many intervention activities, and evaluation measures.
- New methods need to be developed to incorporate rigorous assessment of study outcomes while enhancing intervention effectiveness by increasing community participation and input.
- Sufficient time must be allowed for trials to work with community partners to build interventions and devise evaluation plans for the mutual benefit of both sides. Current time frames for interventions involving community participation are too short to allow for more than a cursory understanding of the communities that might wish to be involved.

South, Fairfax, and Green (2005) describe the development of a self-assessment tool for evaluating community involvement that was designed for organizations to assess their progress and identify areas for improvement. They also discuss some of the methodological challenges that pertain to the measurement of community involvement.

20.5.4. Using Rigorous Process Evaluation

Most population-based community trials rely on active participation and community involvement to promote and sustain change. To determine if the population targeted for behavior change is receiving the right messages and/or the right activities to lead them to making health changes, it is important to conduct early formative process evaluation by measuring indicators such as (variations in) intervention "dose" or intensity (amount, length, and timing of intervention delivered and received by community members), fidelity (the extent to which the intervention was delivered as planned), and program coverage and participation. This topic is addressed in detail in an excellent book (Steckler & Linnan, 2002). Qualitative research methods, such as interviews and focus groups, have an important role in eliciting information for process evaluation.

20.5.5. Addressing Social Inequalities in Disease and Injury Risk

Socioeconomic position can have a substantial influence on the availability and quality of important social and material resources and thus a profound and long-lasting influence on all aspects of health. Although inequalities should not necessarily be a focus in all trials, unless programs specifically and proactively address social inequalities, then there is likely to be minimal benefit for disadvantaged population subgroups. To address such disparities, community interventions need to respond to differences in socioeconomic position by focusing on the more "upstream" influences of such disparities, which have historically been poorly addressed by most community-level efforts. Of course, to address these influences often requires consideration of more structural, institutional, or broad-based policy initiatives, which can be designed to reduce social inequalities.

20.5.6. Incorporating Approaches for Tailoring Interventions to the Population Level

Research has shown that health communication programs that succeed in making information relevant to their intended audience, by tailoring it to a specific individual (based on literacy level, race, or locale), are generally more effective than those that do not (Kreuter and Wray, 2003) (see Chapter 24). Tailored communication differs from targeted communication, which is intended to reach a population subgroup based on characteristics presumed to be shared by all members of that group. In contrast, tailored communication is intended to reach a specific individual (most commonly through print communication or through telephone counseling) based on the characteristics of that person. For this reason, tailored interventions have commonly been applied in health care settings in which individual-level data have already been obtained.

Research has shown that tailoring has specific advantages over targeting (or nontailoring) when the members of the audience differ significantly on key outcome determinants, such as knowledge, beliefs, and behaviors (Kreuter & Wray, 2003). However, although tailoring is a proven approach for enhancing message relevance, it is not the only approach; and under some circumstances, such as when nontailored messages happen to be a good fit for a given individual or when the general level of awareness of the health problem in the community is low (as in some lower socioeconomic groups), it may not be the preferred choice. Interventions that have been individually tailored have often omitted to study social contextual changes that are crucial for disadvantaged groups to effect changes in health behavior, and as such, alternative strategies (such as using peer health advisers to deliver the intervention in various settings) should be considered to expand the potential benefit of this approach (Sorensen et al., 1998).

20.5.7. Using the Appropriate Study Design

While it is clearly the case that RCTs are the gold standard of research design in clinical trials, this is often not the case for more community-based research. Aside from their sometimes prohibitive cost, an RCT necessitates treating a whole community as the unit of randomization and taking into consideration a complex number of activities. Randomization can even present challenges that may affect the interaction between the intervention and the community, resulting in an attenuation of the intervention's effectiveness. When an intervention or program is being delivered to a whole community but the data are collected from individuals, cluster randomization, in which a community or another large unit is the unit of randomization, is often advocated. Cluster randomization helps minimize treatment contamination between intervention and control participants, which is an issue in some control trials in which participants from different groups might be in regular contact with each other. Because cluster trials are usually much larger than individually randomized trials and can be susceptible to recruitment bias, they are often warranted only when expected contamination is likely to exceed 30% (Torgerson, 2001). For a more detailed overview of methodological issues in study design, see

Atienza and King (2002); Rychetnik, Frommer, Hawe, and Shiell (2002); and Hawe, Shiell, and Riley (2004).

When a particular program is using program or intervention components that have already been scientifically evaluated under similar conditions and demonstrated to influence long-term behavioral and/or injury outcomes, the emphasis of the evaluation should be on measuring implementation and process. It is, therefore, important to consider a study design that is appropriate to the specific question being asked in relation to the available evidence base for answering it. As Sorensen et al. (1998) argue, research being conducted to generate hypotheses or develop methods will generally require a different study or evaluation design from a program in which the major focus is on achieving sustainability or durability.

20.5.8. Assessing the Durability of an Intervention or Program

Until recently, relatively little attention in the research literature has been given to methods and approaches for achieving long-term sustainability or durability of program effects in the community after the external project funding has ended (Oldenburg & Parcel, 2002). Pluye, Potvin, Denis, Pelletier, & Mannoni (2005), argue that the process of implementation and planning for sustainability should occur simultaneously from the beginning of a program, aided by the development of routinized activities. The authors present eight program events that are associated with the presence or absence of routinized activities and hence with sustainability:

- Stabilization of resources (by the renewal of material resources when needed, the turnover of key personnel after the appropriate period of time, the widespread use of the new activities in the organization, and the incorporation of program activity financing into the core funding of an organization).
- Organizational risk taking (leading to confidence building in program staff).
- Provision of incentives (such as promotions of personnel into positions of greater responsibility).
- Adaptation of activities according to the local circumstances or environment.
- Fitting of program objectives with the values of the organization and staff.
- Transparent or open communication and the sharing of values, beliefs, and feelings between the program and the organization.
- Incorporation of program rules into the organization's rules, the investment of adequate resources to complete the activities.
- Practical compatibility of the activities with those of the organization.

The authors suggest that health promoters should plan for program sustainability from the commencement of program implementation and that application of the eight principles may be able to influence the long-term sustainability of a program.

20.5.9. Economic Evaluation of Interventions

By their very nature, most community trials tend to have small effects. These small effects notwithstanding, it is still quite unusual for such trials to conduct an economic evaluation to identify whether the changes have provided value for money. Economic evaluation involves a comparative analysis of the costs and consequences of alternative courses of action (Drummond, O'Brien, Stoddart, & Torrance, 1997). Conducting thorough and high-quality economic evaluations provides crucial information to help program and policy managers choose the best interventions from the large pool of effective methods and help allocate resources in a way that provides the greatest return on investment (Finkelstein, Corso, & Miller, 2000).

Contrary to clinical trials, few community interventions are evaluated in terms of their cost-effectiveness. When this has been attempted, the validity of the findings is often questionable due to the complexity and the amount of data required. According to Miller (2001), another factor contributing to the dearth of economic analyses in the literature on community interventions is that published program descriptions and effectiveness evaluations almost never report costs of program implementation or replication. Thus, it is important to ensure that peer reviewers and journal editors push for cost data, perhaps even by making program cost a category in structured abstracts describing interventions.

Hendrie and Miller (2004) give a thorough overview of the various types of economic evaluations and the framework under which they can be conducted. In summary, the steps involved are as follows:

- Defining the intervention to be evaluated (including its objectives, the target population and setting, the time frame over which the costs and outcomes will be calculated, and the type of evaluation).
- Determining the perspectives of the analysis (e.g., a societal perspective).
- Adjusting for differential timing by using costs incurred in a common base year.
- Estimating the costs of alternative options (minus the costs common to all interventions).
- Selecting the relevant outcome measures (depending on the type of economic evaluation, the intervention being evaluated, and the availability of effectiveness data).
- Estimating the effectiveness and calculating the outcomes of alternative options (through epidemiological studies, existing research, or professional opinion).
- Computing the cost-outcome measure (e.g., by a comparing of the additional costs that one alternative imposes over another, against additional benefits).
- Describing any unqualified costs and benefits (e.g., those that might occur outside of the time frame of the analysis, affect other than the target population, or result from more widespread adoption of an intervention).
- Analyzing who pays and who benefits.
- Conducting a sensitivity analysis that tests whether plausible changes in the values of the main study variables affect the results of the analysis.

20.6.   THE WHO SAFE COMMUNITIES MODEL

The WHO Safe Communities Model is a contemporary model for conceptualizing community-based interventions relevant to injury control and prevention, which emphasizes a social-ecological perspective and the building of local partnerships as a foundation for all intervention strategies. There is a current network of safe communities that now extends globally and includes more than 90 designated member safe communities in over 19 countries. The intervention and evaluation model for a safe community includes the following components (Lindqvist et al., 2002):

- An infrastructure based on partnership and collaborations, governed by a cross-sectional group that is responsible for safety promotion in the community.
- Long-term, sustainable programs covering both genders and all ages, environments, and situations.
- Programs that target high-risk groups and environments and programs that promote safety for vulnerable groups.
- Programs that document the frequency and causes of injuries.
- Evaluation measures to assess programs, processes, and the effects of change.
- Ongoing participation in national and international safe communities networks.

Any safe community is characterized by having the following four essential characteristics:

- Use of multiple sources of data to identify community injury problems.
- Citizen involvement.
- Expanded partnerships.
- A comprehensive and integrated injury control system.

A review of the WHO Safe Communities Model for the prevention of injury (Spinks, McClure, Nixon, & Turner, 2005) suggests that where this approach has been implemented, it has been effective in reducing injuries in whole populations. However, methodological limitations and a lack of reported detail in relation to many of the criteria already outlined in this chapter do not allow for strong conclusions to be drawn about generalizability to other communities. The authors describe a need for more high-quality, methodologically strong evaluations of the model in a range of diverse communities (including developing countries) as well as detailed reporting of implementation processes.

Incorporating a number of the elements of a safe community, the Childhood Injury Prevention Project (ChIPP) is a community-based program targeting the major causes of accidents and injuries among children aged 4 years or younger, which is being implemented in two rural and remote centers in Queensland, Australia, over a 3- to 5-year period, beginning in 2004 (Injury Prevention and Control Australia, 2003; Yorkston, Turner, Schluter, & McClure, 2005). The ChIPP project is regarded as a demonstration project; its focus is on translating the efficacious strategies that have been devised by other studies (many of which are described in this chapter) into an effective community intervention program. The strategies used in this project include the following:

- Multiagency collaboration (as witnessed by joint project's sponsorship between two state government agencies and a multiagency steering committee).
- A community development approach to planning, which aims to develop links and networks of organizations in the community to develop an injury prevention agenda.
- Continuous community involvement through local working groups that help monitor and implement the program in addition to providing specific local input.

- A multistrategy approach to implementation, using education, environmental, and legislative strategies.
- A controlled design to compare two intervention communities with two matched control communities.
- Methodological flexibility in response to locally identified issues.
- Clear, well-defined outcomes and goals.
- Use of process logs to document and monitor project activities on a daily basis.
- Use of up-to-date local injury surveillance data.
- Rigorous process, effect, and outcome evaluation.
- Whole community involvement but with a focus on particular at-risk groups (such as the local indigenous population).
- Articulation of strategies to encourage durability/sustainability of the program.
- A commitment to economic evaluation.

Although only at the halfway point of implementation and evaluation, this strongly evidence-based approach to the development, implementation, and evaluation of a complex multilevel community program has certainly achieved excellent implementation and results.

The crucial factor in planning and developing effective community interventions, however, is that there is sufficient understanding of their unique dynamics to enable methods to be effectively applied in any setting regardless of material resources. In light of this, Moller (2004, p. 3) calls for the need for research literature to stimulate discussion regarding the "definitions, values, and principles of community-based prevention," including development, testing, and evaluation of new methods; the measurement of efficacy and effectiveness; and a critical analysis of common problems and solutions. In other words, it is important that there is a redefinition of what is considered by reviewers as being high-quality intervention research. Future research would benefit by having reports published despite there being insufficient evidence of effectiveness and/or when study design factors such as sample size, control group, and data quality are the best possible (even though not ideal). By this means, learning through the critical sharing of evidence becomes possible.

In the words of Fortmann et al. (1995, p. 583), "Perhaps the most important lesson we have learned about communities is that there is much we do not know." In light of this, the evaluation of past evidence in conjunction with the application of new knowledge and approaches represents an important step toward improving our understanding of the complexity of communities and how best to address this from an injury prevention perspective.

20.7. KEY CHALLENGES FOR THE NEXT GENERATION OF COMMUNITY INTERVENTIONS

Key challenges and issues for the future include the following:

- To design, implement, and evaluate interventions based on comprehensive theoretical frameworks, and to identify what theories and models work best for specific types of intentional and unintentional injuries.

- To use multifaceted interventions and to develop an evaluation framework that can identify which intervention activities are related to outcomes.
- To involve the community in program planning and implementation.
- To tailor interventions to the unique characteristics of the community.
- To better address social inequalities and disadvantage by addressing more upstream influences on health disparities.
- To use traditional RCTs or cluster randomized trials when possible and appropriate but also to consider alternative study designs that meet the needs for scientific rigor, appropriateness to research questions, and feasibility in terms of cost and setting.
- To improve process evaluation and implementation measurement.
- To assess the durability and sustainability of interventions and to begin planning for sustainability at the commencement of implementation.
- To conduct more thorough and high-quality economic evaluations of interventions.

REFERENCES

Atienza, A. A., & King, A. C. (2002). Community-based health intervention trials: An overview of methodological issues. *Epidemiologic Reviews, 24*, 72–79.

Bartholomew, L. K., Parcel, G. S., & Kok, G. (1998). Intervention mapping: A process for developing theory- and evidence-based health education programs. *Health Education & Behavior, 25* (5), 545–563.

Carter, N., Kannus, P., & Khan, K. (2001). Exercise in the prevention of falls in older people: A systematic literature review examining the rationale and the evidence. *Sports Medicine, 31*, 427–438.

Chang, J. T., Morton, S. C., Rubenstein, L. Z., Mojica, W. A., Maglione, M., Suttorp, R. J., Roth, E. A., Shekelle, P. G. (2004). Interventions for the prevention of falls in older adults: systematic review and meta-analysis of randomised clinical trials. *British Medical Journal, 328* (7441), 680–683.

Coggan, C., & Bennett, S. (2004). Community-based injury prevention programs. In R. McClure, M. Stevenson, & S. McEvoy (Eds.), *The scientific basis of injury prevention and control* (pp. 347–358). Melbourne, Australia: IP Communications.

DeRoo, L. A., & Rautiainen, R. H. (2000). A systematic review of farm safety interventions. *American Journal of Preventive Medicine, 18*, 51–62.

DiGuiseppi C., & Higgins, J. P. T. (2001). Interventions for promoting smoke alarm ownership and function (CD002246. DOI: 10.1002/14651858.CD002246). *Cochrane Database of Systematic Reviews*, (2). First published online 23 Apr 2001 in Issue 2, 2001.

Dinh-Zarr, T. B., Sleet, D. A., Shults, R. A., Zaza, S., Elder, R. W., Nichols, J. L., Thompson, R. S., & Sosin, D. M. (2001). Reviews of evidence regarding interventions to increase the use of safety belts. *American Journal of Preventive Medicine, 21*, 48–65.

Drummond, M. F., O'Brien, B., Stoddart, G. L., & Torrance, G. W. (1997). *Methods for the economic evaluation of health care programmes* (2nd ed.). Oxford, UK: Oxford University Press.

Duperrex, O., Bunn, F., & Roberts, I. (2002). Safety education of pedestrians for injury prevention: A systematic review of randomised controlled trials. *British Medical Journal, 24*, 1129–1131.

Finkelstein E., Corso P., & Miller T. (2000). *The incidence and economic burden of injuries in the U.S.* New York: Oxford University Press.

Fortmann, S. P., Flora, J. A., Winkleby, M. A., Schooler, C., Taylor, C. B., & Farquhar, J. W. (1995). Community intervention trials: Reflections on the Stanford Five-City Project experience. *American Journal of Epidemiology, 142*, 576–586.

Frank, A. L. (2000). Injuries related to shiftwork. *American Journal of Preventive Medicine, 18*, 33–36.

Gielen, A. C., & Sleet, D. A. (2003). Application of behaviour change theories and methods to injury prevention. *Epidemiologic Reviews, 25*, 65–76.

Gielen, A. C., Sleet, D. A., & DiClemente, R. J. (2006). *Injury and violence prevention: Behavioral science theories, methods and applications.* San Francisco: Jossey-Bass.

Hanson, D., Vardon, P., & Lloyd, J. (2002). Becoming Queensland's first Safe Community: Considering sustainability from the outset. In R. Muller (Ed.), *Reducing injuries in Mackay, North Queensland* (pp. 35–52). Warwick, Australia: Warwick Educational.

Hartling, L., Brison, R. J., Crumley, E. T., Klassen, T. P., & Pickett, W. (2004). A systematic review of interventions to prevent childhood farm injuries. *Pediatrics, 114*, E483–E496.

Hartling, L., Wiebe, N., Russell, K., Petruk, J., Spinola, C., & Klassen, T. (2004). Graduated driver licensing for reducing motor vehicle crashes among young drivers. (DOI: 10.1002/14651858.CD003300. pub2.) *Cochrane Database of Systematic Reviews 2004*, Issue 2, Art. No. CD003300.

Hawe, P., Shiell, A., & Riley, T. (2004). Complex interventions: how "out of control" can a randomised controlled trial be? *British Medical Journal, 328*, 1561–1563.

Hendrie, D., & Miller, T. (2004). Economic evaluation. In R. McClure, M. Stevenson, & S. McEvoy (Eds.), *The scientific basis of injury prevention and control* (pp. 372–390). Melbourne, Australia: IP Communications.

Injury Prevention and Control Australia (2005). *Evaluation of CEO's child injury prevention project*. Retrieved July 2005, from www.ipca.com.au/www/index.aspx?itemID=29.

Israel, B. A., Schultz, A. J., Parker, E. A., & Becker, A. B. (1998). Review of community-based research: Assessing partnership approaches to improve public health. *Annual Review of Public Health, 19*, 173–202.

Kaplan, S. A., & Garrett, K. E. (2005). The use of logic models by community-based initiatives. *Evaluation and Program Planning, 28*, 167–172.

Keifer, M. C. (2000). Effectiveness of interventions in reducing pesticide overexposure and poisonings. *American Journal of Preventive Medicine, 18*, 80–89.

Ker, K., Roberts, I., Collier, T., Beyer, F., Bun, F., & Frost, C. (2003). Post-licence driver education for the prevention of road traffic crashes. (CD003734. DOI: 10.1002/14651858.CD003734). *Cochrane Database of Systematic Reviews*, (3).

Klassen, T. P., MacKay, J. M., Moher, D., Walker, A., & Jones, A. L. (2000). Community-based injury prevention interventions. *Future of Children, 10*, 83–110.

Koepsell, T. D., Wagner, E. H., Cheadle, A. C., Patrick, D. L., Martin, D. C., Diehr, P. H., Perrin, E. B., Kristal, A. R., Allan-Andrilla, C. H., & Dey, L. J. (1992). Selected methodological issues in evaluating community-based health promotion and disease prevention programs. *Annual Review of Public Health, 13*, 31–57.

Kreuter, M. W., & Wray, R. J. (2003). Tailored and targeted health communication: Strategies for enhancing information relevance. *American Journal of Health Behavior, 27*, S227–S232.

Kwan, I., & Mapstone, J. (2002). Interventions for increasing pedestrian and cyclist visibility for the prevention of death and injuries. (CD003438. DOI: 10.1002/14651858.CD003438). *Cochrane Database of Systematic Reviews*, (2).

Lindqvist, K., Timpka, T., Schelp, L., & Risto, O. (2002). Evaluation of a child safety program based on the WHO Safe Community Model. *Injury Prevention, 8*, 23–26.

Lipscomb, H. J. (2000). Effectiveness of interventions to prevent work-related eye injuries. *American Journal of Preventive Medicine, 18*, 27–32.

Liu, B., Ivers, R., Norton, R., Blows, S., & Lo, S. K. (2003). Helmets for preventing injury in motorcycle riders (CD004333. DOI: 10.1002/14651858.CD004333.pub2). *Cochrane Database of Systematic Reviews*, (4).

Lyons, R. A., Sander, L. V., Weightman, A. L., Patterson, J., Jones, S. A., Lannon, S., Rolfe, B., Kemp, A., & Johansen, A. (2003). Modification of the home environment for the reduction of injuries (CD003600. DOI: 10.1002/14651858.CD003600). *Cochrane Database of Systematic Reviews*, (4).

Maccoby, N., Farquhar, J. W., Wood, P. D., & Alexander, J. (1977). Reducing the risk of cardiovascular disease: Effects of a community-based campaign on knowledge and behaviour. *Journal of Community Health, 3*, 110–114.

MacKay, M., Scanlan, A., Olsen, L., Reid, D., Clark, M., McKim, K., & Raina, P. (2004). Looking for the evidence: A systematic review of prevention strategies addressing sport and recreational injury among children and youth. *Journal of Science & Medicine in Sport, 7*, 58–73.

McLaughlin, J. A., & Jordan, G. B. (1999). Logic models: A tool for telling your program's performance story. *Evaluation and Program Planning, 22*, 65–72.

Miller, T. R. (2001). The effectiveness review trials of Hercules and some economic estimates for the stables. *American Journal of Preventive Medicine, 21* (Supplement 4), 9–12.

Moller, J. (1991). Community-based interventions: An emerging dimension of injury control models. *Health Promotion Journal of Australia, 1* (2), 51–54.

Moller, J. (2004). Reconsidering community based interventions. *Injury Prevention, 10*, 2–3.

Nixon, J., Spinks, A., Turner, C., & McClure, R. (2004). Community based programs to prevent poisoning in children 0–15 years. *Injury Prevention, 10*, 43–46.

Oldenburg, B., & Burton, N. W. (2004). Social and environmental strategies. In J. Kerr, R. Weitkunat, & M. Moretti (Eds.), *ABC of behaviour change: A guide to successful disease prevention and health promotion*. Edinburgh, UK: Elsevier.

Oldenburg, B., Ffrench, M., & Sallis, J. (2000). Health behavior research: The quality of the evidence base. *American Journal of Health Promotion, 14*, 253–257.

Oldenburg, B., & Parcel, G. (2002). Diffusion of health promotion and health education innovations. In K. Glanz, F. Lewis, & B. Rimer (Eds.), *Health behavior and health education: Theory, research and practice* (pp. 312–334, 3rd ed.). San Francisco: Jossey-Bass.

Oldenburg, B., Sallis, J., Ffrench, M., & Owen, N. (1999). Health promotion research and the diffusion and institutionalization of interventions. *Health Education Research, 14*, 121–130.

Olsen, S., Scanlan, A., MacKay, M., Babul, S., Reid, D., Clark, M., & Raina, P. (2004). Strategies for prevention of soccer related injuries: a systematic review. *British Journal of Sports Medicine, 38*, 89–94.

Pluye, P., Potvin, L., Denis, J.-L., Pelletier, J., & Mannoni, C. (2005). Program sustainability begins with the first events. *Evaluation and Program Planning, 28*, 123–137.

Puska, P., Tuomilehto, J., Salonen, J., Neittaanmaki, L., Maki, J., Virtamo, J., Nissinen, A., Koskela, K., & Takalo, T. (1979). Changes in coronary risk factors during a comprehensive five-year community programme to control cardiovascular diseases (North Karelia project). *British Medical Journal, 2*, 1173–1178.

Renger, R., & Titcomb, A. (2002). A three-step approach to teaching logic models. *American Journal of Evaluation, 23* (4), 493–503.

Rivara, F. P., & Thompson, D. C. (2000a). Prevention of falls in the construction industry: Evidence for program effectiveness. *American Journal of Preventive Medicine, 18*, 23–26.

Rivara, F. P., & Thompson, D. C. (2000b). Systematic reviews of injury prevention strategies for occupational injuries: An overview. *American Journal of Preventive Medicine, 18*, 1–3.

Roberts, I., Kwan, I., & the Cochrane Injuries Group Driver Education Reviewers. (2001). School based driver education for the prevention of traffic crashes. (CD003201. DOI: 10.1002/14651858. CD003201). *Cochrane Database of Systematic Reviews*, (3).

Rogers, B., & Goodno, L. (2000). Evaluation of interventions to prevent needlestick injuries in health care occupations. *American Journal of Preventive Medicine, 18*, 90–98.

Rychetnik, L., Frommer, M., Hawe, P., & Shiell, A. (2002). Criteria for evaluating evidence on public health interventions. *Journal of Epidemiology & Community Health, 56*, 119–127.

Segui-Gomez, M. (2000). Evaluating worksite-based interventions that promote safety belt use. *American Journal of Preventive Medicine, 18*, 11–22.

Shults, R. A., Elder, R. W., Sleet, D. A., Nichols, J. L., Alao, M. O., Carande-Kulis, V. G., Zaza, S., Sosin, D. M., & Thompson, R. S. (2001). Reviews of evidence regarding interventions to reduce alcohol-impaired driving. *American Journal of Preventive Medicine, 21*, 66–88.

Sleet, D. A., & Gielen, A. C., (2004). Behavioral approaches to injury prevention. In R. McClure, M. Stevenson, & S. McEvoy (Eds.) *The scientific basis of injury prevention and control*, (pp. 214–232), Melbourne: Australia: IP Communications.

Sorensen, G., Emmons, K., Hunt, M. K., & Johnston, D. (1998). Implications of the results of community intervention trials. *Annual Review of Public Health, 19*, 379–416.

South, J., Fairfax, P., & Green, E. (2005). Developing an assessment tool for evaluating community involvement. *Health Expectations, 8*, 64–73.

Spinks, A., Turner, C., McClure, R., & Nixon, J. (2004). Community based prevention programs targeting all injuries for children. *Injury Prevention, 10*, 180–185.

Spinks, A., McClure, R., Nixon, J., & Turner, C. (2005). The WHO Safe Communities Model for the prevention of injury in whole populations. (DOI: 10.1002/14651858.CD004445.pub2.) Cochrane Database of Systematic Reviews 2005, Issue 2. Art. No.: CD004445.

Steckler, A., & Linnan, L. (Eds.). (2002). *Process evaluation for public health interventions and research*. San Francisco: Jossey-Bass.

Thompson, B., Coronado, G., Snipes, S. A., & Puschel, K. (2003). Methodologic advances and ongoing challenges in designing community-based health promotion programs. *Annual Review of Public Health, 24*, 315–340.

Thompson, D. C., & Rivara, F. P. (1998). Pool fencing for preventing drowning in children (CD001047. DOI: 10.1002/14651858.CD001047). *Cochrane Database of Systematic Reviews*, (1).

Thompson, D. C., Rivara, F. P., & Thompson, R. (1999). Helmets for preventing head and facial injuries in bicyclists (CD001855. DOI: 10.1002/14651858.CD001855). *Cochrane Database of Systematic Reviews*, (4).

Torgerson, D. J. (2001). Contamination in trials: Is cluster randomisation the answer? *British Medical Journal, 322* (7282), 355–357.

Towner, E., & Dowswell, T. (2002). Community-based childhood injury prevention interventions: What works? *Health Promotion International, 17,* 273–284.

Trifiletti, L. B., Gielen, A. C., Sleet, D. A., & Hopkins, K. (2005). Behavioral and social sciences theories and models: Are they used in unintentional injury prevention research? *Health Education Research, 20* (3), 298–307.

Turner, C., Spinks, A., McClure, R., & Nixon, J. (2004). Community-based interventions for the prevention of burns and scalds in children (CD004335. DOI: 10.1002/14651858.CD004335.pub2). *Cochrane Database of Systematic Reviews,* (2).

Yorkston, E., Turner, C., Schluter, P., & McClure, R. (2005). Validity and reliability of responses to a self-report home safety survey designed for use in a community-based childhood injury prevention program. *Injury Control & Safety Promotion, 12* (3): 193–196.

Zaza, S., Carande-Kulis, V. G., Sleet, D. A., Sosin, D. M., Elder, R. W., Shults, R. A., Dinh-Zarr, T. B., Nichols, J. L., & Thompson, R. S. (2001). Methods for conducting systematic reviews of the evidence of effectiveness and economic efficiency of interventions to reduce injuries to motor vehicle occupants. *American Journal of Preventive Medicine, 21,* 23–30.

Zaza, S., Sleet, D. A., Thompson, R. S., Sosin, D. M., & Bolen, J. C. (2001). Reviews of evidence regarding interventions to increase use of child safety seats. *American Journal of Preventive Medicine, 21,* 31–47.

Part IV

Interventions in the Field

Interpreting Evidence of Effectiveness: How Do You Know When a Prevention Approach Will Work for Your Community?

Corinne L. Peek-Asa and Sue Mallonee

21.1. INTRODUCTION

Many valuable lessons have been learned from injury prevention programs that have been implemented and evaluated. When thinking about implementing a program in your community, literature about program effectiveness can be a powerful tool in your decision making throughout the design, implementation, and evaluation of your program.

Existing evidence can help you identify the most promising approaches for your specific injury focus and community characteristics and can be helpful in steering you away from programs that have not worked well in the past. Existing evidence can help you gain support for your project because securing community support or resources for your project will be much more successful if you can demonstrate that the approach has already been effective. Existing evidence can also help focus the design and implementation of your project and help you understand what measures to include in your evaluation.

This chapter helps you find the existing evidence, understand what factors are important when reading this evidence, and understand other factors that are important when translating a program to your community.

21.2.   FINDING EVIDENCE OF EFFECTIVENESS

A wealth of evaluation studies have been published in the peer-reviewed literature, and these studies can be accessed by various search databases. MEDLINE, the most widely used, is the U.S. National Library of Medicine's bibliographic database covering the fields of medicine, nursing, dentistry, veterinary medicine, health care systems, and the preclinical sciences. It provides access to abstracts of articles and citations from more than 4000 biomedical journals published worldwide. A list of available Internet MEDLINE searching services (e.g., PubMed, OVID), including the dates covered, if registration is required for access, and whether or not the service is free, can be found at http://omni.ac.uk/medline. Other search engines, such as Google Scholar (http://scholar.google.com), search MEDLINE and non-medical journals (e.g., criminal justice, architectural, engineering) and books. Because injury evidence exists in a number of different fields, this wider search can be very helpful.

When examining the peer-reviewed literature, be aware that there is a publication bias toward studies with statistically significant results (Dickersin & Min, 1993; Easterbrook, Berlin, Gopalan, & Matthews, 1991). The presence of significant findings often outweighs considerations about the quality of the study, so many published studies do not have strong study designs (Dickersin & Min, 1993; Elvik, 1998; Easterbrook et al., 1991). Thus the pool of published literature must be read with caution, and we present some of these cautions later in this chapter.

Systematic reviews and meta-analyses synthesize information from existing evaluation studies on a specific topic, and these are useful for determining effectiveness (Cooper & Hedges, 1994). Systematic reviews identify and summarize the best available research by considering all available literature and applying rigorous scientific criteria. Meta-analysis is a quantitative method for combining and summarizing the results of different studies into single estimates of effectiveness (Cook, Sackett, & Spitzer, 1994). *The Guide to Community Preventive Services: Systematic Reviews and Evidence-Based Recommendations* (the *Guide*), developed by the Task Force on Community Preventive Services (TFCPS), is one source for systematic reviews (Pappaioanou & Evans, 1998; The Guide to Community Preventive Services). The *Guide*'s recommendations are primarily based on evidence of effectiveness, including the suitability of the study design, but they also assess the applicability of the intervention to other populations or settings, the economic effect, barriers observed in implementing the interventions, and if the intervention had other beneficial or harmful effects (Briss et al., 2000). The *Guide* then provides a recommendation as to whether the approach is "strongly recommended," "recommended," has "insufficient evidence," or is "discouraged" (Table 21.1). The *Guide* has evaluated the use of child safety seats and safety belts, reducing alcohol-impaired driving, therapeutic foster care for the prevention of violence, early childhood home visitation programs, and firearm laws; these recommendations can be found at www.thecommunityguide.org (The Guide to Community Preventive Services).

The Cochrane Collaboration provides scientific evidence-based reviews of health care interventions through the Cochrane Library (Bero & Rennie, 1995). Although a subscription is necessary to access these reviews, many academic institutions are subscribers and can partner with you to find relevant information. The reviews follow internationally accepted guidelines and are peer reviewed by independent panels (Alderson, Green, & Higgins, 2004). The reviews also attempt

Table 21.1. Assessing the Strength of a Body of Evidence on Effectiveness of Population-Based Interventions in the *Guide to Community Preventive Services*[a]

Evidence of effectiveness[b]	Execution (good or fair)[c]	Design Suitability (greatest, moderate, or least)	Number of Studies	Consistent[d]	Effect Size[e]	Expert Opinion[f]
Strong	Good	Greatest	At least 2	Yes	Sufficient	Not used
	Good	Greatest or moderate	At least 5	Yes	Sufficient	Not used
	Good or fair	Greatest	At least 5	Yes	Sufficient	Not used
	Meet design, execution, number and consistency criteria for sufficient but not strong evidence				Large	Not used
Sufficient	Good	Greatest	1	Not applicable	Sufficient	Not used
	Good or fair	Greatest or moderate	At least 3	Yes	Sufficient	Not used
	Good or fair	Greatest, moderate, or least	At least 5	Yes	Sufficient	Not used
Expert opinion	Varies	Varies	Varies	Varies	Sufficient	Supports a recommendation
Insufficient[a]						

[a]Reprint from: Briss et al. (2000).
[b]The categories are not mutually exclusive; a body of evidence meeting criteria for more than one of these should be categorized in the highest possible category.
[c]Studies with limited execution are not used to assess effectiveness.
[d]Generally consistent in direction and size.
[e]Sufficient and large effect sizes are defined on a case-by-case basis and are based on task force opinion.
[f]Expert opinion will not be routinely used in the *Guide* but can affect the classification of a body of evidence as shown.
[g]Reasons for determining that evidence is insufficient is described as follows: A, insufficient designs or executions; B, too few studies; C, inconsistent; D, effect size too small; E, expert opinion not used. These categories are not mutually exclusive and one or more of these will occur when a body of evidence fails to meet the criteria for strong or sufficient evidence.

to overcome publication bias by searching for unpublished studies and include a summary of implications for both practice and research.

The Cochrane Injuries Group has published 57 reviews on the prevention, treatment, and rehabilitation of traumatic injuries. There are 13 reviews of general injury prevention interventions, including fall-related injuries to older persons, pool fencing to prevent drowning in children, and interventions for promoting smoke alarm ownership and function. There are 16 reviews of prevention strategies to reduce traffic injuries, including graduated driver's licensing, increasing pedestrian and cyclist visibility to prevent crashes, and safety education of pedestrians. A list of reviews conducted by the Cochrane Injuries Group can be found at: www.cochrane-injuries.lshtm.ac.uk/Review%20links.htm (The Cochrane Collaboration, 2004)

21.3.   EVALUATING THE SCIENTIFIC EVIDENCE

The most desirable prevention strategies have been studied in a number of different settings, have undergone rigorous evaluation, and have easily available information about the populations and conditions in which they are effective. Although there are some programs that have such strong evidence, it is far from the usual case.

Research, especially evaluation research, is a slow process. The absence of a strong body of evidence for a specific approach is not reason enough to dismiss it as a promising program. However, if evidence suggests that the program has not been effective in previous settings or has led to unintended harmful consequences, the program is not likely to perform better in a new setting for which it was not originally designed. The next section discusses several criteria that should be considered when evaluating evidence that measures program effectiveness.

21.3.1.   Criteria to Evaluate Evidence

The first step in evaluating evidence is to determine the strength of the evaluation studies that have been conducted. A growing focus on evidence-based public health has led to several frameworks on which to assess the rigor of the available research. One of the most widely cited is the hierarchy of evidence, which places a stronger weight on evidence that comes from more rigorous study designs (Popay & Williams, 1998).

However, there is growing recognition that this hierarchy is not a sufficient framework to weigh all of the information needed to decide if an intervention approach is appropriate for a community (Petticrew & Roberts, 2003; Rychetnic, Frommer, Hawe, & Shiell, 2002; Tang, Ehsani, & McQueen, 2003). New models of evidence-based public health recognize that each study design can contribute important information (Petticrew & Roberts, 2003). For example, a randomized control trial might be the best method to identify if an educational program led to increased knowledge and safety behaviors and decreased injury rates. It is not, however, the most efficient design to decide how well participants liked the program or how to identify effective protocols to implement the program. Additional concerns that should be considered in typologies of evidence include the program repeatability, potential for compliance, timing, and predictability (Tang et al., 2003). Following are some examples of standard designs used in evaluation studies and how they can contribute to existing evidence.

21.3.1.1. Experimental Designs

21.3.1.1.1. Randomized Control Trials. The randomized control trial (RCT) is the most rigorous evaluation design because it allows direct control of who does and does not get the intervention. Such studies usually randomize individuals into treatment groups, which helps create comparable groups. Day et al. (2002) used this design to evaluate the effects of group-based exercise, home hazard management, and vision improvement on reducing falls in the elderly. They identified elderly individuals who lived in their own homes; after recruiting a sufficient sample size, the researchers randomized the subjects into one of the three treatment groups. They followed the three groups to estimate fall incidence and found that exercise and balance programs had the strongest effect on reducing falls.

There are a number of variations to the RCT. One variation occurs when an agency or group is randomized, rather than an individual. This type of design is especially effective when the intervention occurs at the group level, such as a classroom education program. For these programs, there are concerns about how individuals receiving the intervention might affect the outcome of those not receiving it, perhaps by sharing knowledge or influencing behaviors. To avoid randomizing students within one class, which could lead to contamination and might also be infeasible for the teachers, the randomization can occur by classroom or by school.

It is important to note that randomization does not guarantee comparability among groups. Evaluations should provide additional evidence that groups were comparable, such as by comparing groups by age, gender, race/ethnicity, or socioeconomic status.

21.3.1.1.2. Quasi-Experimental Studies. There are many variations of experimental designs used for evaluations, and the usefulness of these varies widely. For example, some evaluations describe only outcomes after an intervention. Without baseline data or a comparison group, these studies cannot determine if any changes are actually due to the intervention. Many studies use baseline data to compare outcomes in the intervention group before and after the intervention to show changes.

Even when studies have some baseline or preintervention data, it can still be difficult to determine if the program was effective. For example, consider an evaluation of a peer-mediation program to reduce delinquency and physical fighting among high-risk youth. A before-and-after comparison of students in the program shows that delinquency and fights actually increased after the program. With just these data, it would appear that the program was not only ineffective but potentially harmful. But, what if additional data showed that delinquency and fighting among students who were not in the program increased even more? Now the results are interpreted very differently. When evaluating quasi-experimental designs, the quality of the study and the comparisons made are important considerations.

21.3.1.2. Nonexperimental Studies

Nonexperimental studies are often called observational, and in these studies the allocation of the intervention is not controlled by the investigator. These study designs include cohort, case-control, case-crossover, cross-sectional, and ecological.

21.3.1.2.1. Cohort Studies.   A cohort study follows a defined population over time to determine the distribution of exposure and outcomes. Cohort studies can be of varying quality, depending on how they are implemented. Well-designed cohort studies can be valuable for identifying how an intervention works in an observed population. For example, investigators could identify a cohort of homes in a small city, some of which had functioning smoke alarms and some of which did not. They could then compare reported fires and fire-related injuries to see if the smoke alarms led to reductions in these outcomes. The only difference between this cohort study and a RCT is that the investigators did not decide which homes had smoke alarms. In this cohort study, there could be systematic differences in the homes that did and did not have smoke alarms that are unrelated to the effectiveness of the smoke alarm. For example, if all the homes with smoke alarms are of high socioeconomic status, they might not be comparable to homes without smoke alarms.

21.3.1.2.2. Case-Control Studies.   In case-control studies, a series of individuals who have experienced a health outcome are identified as cases, and then a group of people who have not experienced the outcome are identified as controls. Cases and controls are then compared based on the exposure of interest, such as the use of an injury prevention approach. Case-control studies are useful for identifying the protective effect of safety strategies. For example, Grossman et al. (2005) identified a series of children and adolescents in several states who had committed suicide, made a suicide attempt, or had unintentionally injured someone with a firearm (cases). The researchers next identified homes in which children lived or visited and that had firearms but that had not experienced a shooting (controls). They compared reported safe storage practices of firearms between homes that did and did not have a shooting and found that homes without a shooting were much more likely to have stored firearms using safe storage practices.

21.3.1.2.3. Ecological Studies.   Ecological studies involve measurements on groups rather than individuals. Ecological studies can be useful for evaluating population-level outcomes, such as legislation and policy changes, and can be helpful for measuring changes due to several simultaneous interventions. For example, Ozanne-Smith, Ashby, Newstead, Stathakis, and Clapperton (2004) measured changes in state firearm regulations and their relation to firearm death rates. Although the authors did not know if each specific firearm death was related to specific changes in the regulations, they did note population-level decreases.

21.3.1.2.4. Qualitative Studies.   Qualitative data have an important role in evaluation evidence. Qualitative data are particularly useful in the formative, process, and effect phases of program evaluation and can be an efficient approach for identifying issues such as community readiness, acceptance, compliance, appropriateness, and satisfaction. Although this information is rarely included in published manuscripts, it is useful for designing and implementing interventions. Azeredo and Stephens-Stidham (2003) evaluated an elementary-school safety curriculum and described the collection of qualitative data, which included measures of receptiveness, satisfaction, and methods for negotiating school protocols. As systematic reviews place a greater emphasis on information pertaining to program implementation, published manuscripts will, we hope, begin to include more of this information.

21.3.1.3.   Example of Weighing the Evidence

A number of different evaluations of childhood safety education programs have been conducted. Think First, a multi-topic elementary school education program, is an example. The majority of published evaluations show that knowledge and attitudes changes among participants, but the quality of this evidence varies. Hall-Long, Schell, and Corrigan (2001) evaluated knowledge gain among 140 students who underwent the curriculum. They found a knowledge gain but had no control group to show that this was due to the curriculum. Greene et al. (2002) and Wesner (2003) also found knowledge increases, but they used control groups to show that knowledge gain was differentially higher among children who received the curriculum than in controls. However, these studies did not randomize classrooms into the intervention. Wesner (2003) matched intervention to control classrooms on age, grade, and socioeconomic background, and this step increases the weight of evidence. Finally, Gresham et al. (2001) conducted an RTC in which participating schools were randomly assigned to the intervention group. This study, which found increased knowledge and decreased reported risk behaviors, provides the strongest evidence because of the well-controlled study design.

21.3.1.4.   Frequently Used Measures of Association

Statistical tests are commonly used to determine whether or not study results are meaningful, and results are often reported through a p value. Statistical p values less than .05 are typically considered significant, which indicates that we are 95% certain that the measured change was due to the intervention and not found by chance alone. A p value of .003 for example, suggests the probability that results found had a 3 in 1000 chance of not being related to the intervention. However, many factors affect the p value, and results should not be disregarded simply because the p value was greater than .05. Similarly, a significant p value is not all that meaningful if the study design was weak. The p value measures only the likelihood of random error and does not account for other weaknesses, such as the presence of selection bias, poor measurement of the exposures or outcomes, or comparisons of groups that are not similar.

Many studies report findings through risk ratios (RRs) or odds ratios (ORs). While the theory and correct estimation of these measures is complex, a simple understanding of the terms can be helpful for interpreting the literature. Basically, RRs and ORs both measure how an outcome, such as an injury rate, is affected by an exposure, such as an intervention program. If the exposure had no effect on the outcome (e.g., the intervention program had no effect on injury rates), then the OR (or RR) will be equal to 1. If the OR is greater than 1, then the exposure led to an increase in the outcome. Similarly, if the OR is less than 1, then the exposure led to a decrease in the outcome.

The OR alone is not sufficient to determine effectiveness of the intervention; the OR should be accompanied by a confidence interval (CI). Most studies use a 95% CI, which means that we are 95% certain that the true estimate lies within the limits of the confidence interval. However, other confidence intervals (90% or even 80%) can be used.

A confidence interval that spans 1, the null value, is often interpreted as being nonsignificant from a statistical perspective, somewhat like the p value. However, a confidence interval is much more than a test of significance. The confidence interval also shows precision, so that a narrow confidence interval (e.g., 0.5–0.8) is much more helpful than a wide one (e.g., 0.1–5.1). For example, compare two programs that both had an OR of 0.92 when evaluating the effects of an intervention program on a community's injury rate. This OR would be interpreted as "the odds of an injury were 8% lower in the intervention than in the nonintervention group." However, one confidence interval was 0.1–0.99, and the other was 0.8–1.01. Even though the second confidence interval spans 1, it provides stronger support of the program than the first interval because it expresses a more precise estimate.

21.3.2.   Other Criteria to Consider When Evaluating Evidence

Other criteria that are important when reviewing existing evidence include strength of the intervention effects, knowledge of how the program works, integration with other injury prevention activities, generalization, feasibility, acceptability, and equity (Runyan, 1998).

21.3.2.1.   *Strength of the Evidence*

Many injury prevention approaches have strong supportive research. However, many evaluations do not show strong support, and these findings must be considered carefully.

If published evaluations indicate weak performance, it does not necessarily mean that the approach is ineffective. Many studies fail to measure a significant outcome because they used small sample sizes and did not have sufficient power to detect differences between intervention groups. In other circumstances, the findings are weak because the program was not implemented properly. When deciding to implement a program with weak support, it is important to make sure the evidence suggesting some effect is of high quality, that there is information about how best to implement the program, and that the program is not likely to have adverse unintended consequences.

Prevention programs are often continued even when there is sufficient evidence that they are ineffective and potentially even harmful. For example, Neighborhood Watch programs were developed from community policing theories, and they involve organizing community members to conduct surveillance (watch the neighborhood) and share information about crime and crime prevention (Rosenbaum, 1987). The goals were to reduce crime and fear of crime. Repeated evaluations, however, have found that these programs have a negligible to no effect on crime and actually increase fear of crime (Darian-Smith, 1993; Rosenbaum, 1987; Sherman et al., 1997). Why? The high-crime neighborhoods most in need of crime prevention were unable to mobilize and sustain a community policing effort (Hope, 1995; Sherman et al., 1997). Law-enforcement involvement, which is a tenet of the program, was difficult because residents were distrustful of police and police did not actively engage community members (Rosenbaum, 1987). In contrast, neighborhoods with low crime rates were able to implement and sustain programs, but they had very little to gain from crime prevention efforts. Over time, programs led to increased fear of crime and distrust of visitors or strangers in the community (Sherman et al., 1997).

Why would a community continue to use an ineffective program? One reason is failure to examine existing evaluation evidence. Another might be strong community support for a program, which may stem from a particular event or an individual's experience. Reviewing existing evidence can help alleviate the risk of implementing a program that has proven ineffective.

21.3.2.2.   Knowledge of Why the Program Worked

The most helpful evaluations document not only that the program worked but also why it worked (Tang et al., 2003). This type of information can sometimes be found in reviews of evaluation studies that assess how the program performed in different settings.

In general, the question about why a program worked is best answered if the evaluation included process, effect, and outcome components. For example, reviews of programs to reduce robbery and associated injury in retail businesses have identified that strategies including cash control, good lighting and visibility, employee training, and safety signage are effective (Casteel & Peek-Asa, 2000). These evaluations compared robberies or assaults before and after program implementation but included no effect evaluation—they did not actually measure changes made by the individual businesses. Thus it was difficult to attribute crime reductions to the program elements. A more recent evaluation measured differential changes in violent crimes based on the number and types of strategies implemented by each business (Peek-Asa, Casteel, Mineschian, Erickson, & Kraus, 2004). This evaluation found crime reductions among businesses that implemented all or most of the program elements but no reductions among businesses that had low implementation. Because this evaluation included an effect component, it is much stronger in supporting the effectiveness of the program and in explaining why the program worked.

A recent review of mass-media campaigns to reduce alcohol-impaired driving identified a median crash decrease of 13% (Elder et al., 2004). However, success depended on the program being carefully planned and executed, with pretested messages, adequate audience exposure, and coordination with other ongoing prevention activities. In contrast, programs that failed to use the mainstream media; devoted minimal resources to craft, test, and deliver messages; and did not identify a specific audience were likely to fail. From this review, we know that similar programs will work only when implemented a certain way.

21.3.2.3.   Integration with Other Injury Prevention Activities

The review of mass-media campaigns discussed above also identified that mass-media campaigns worked best in conjunction with increased enforcement efforts, grassroots activities, and other messages related to drinking and driving (Elder et al., 2004). In fact, the mass-media campaigns may have been unsuccessful without them. This is an example of programs that are effective only when integrated with broader efforts.

Coordination of activities is also critical for sobriety checkpoints to reduce impaired driving. Sobriety checkpoints, which can occur through either randomized or selective breath testing, result in a median fatal crash decrease of 22% (Elder et al., 2002). However, the range in success rates varies widely, with some evaluations finding no real effects. Systematic reviews of these evaluations show that program success depends on several factors, including the coexistence of programs that publicize the checkpoint activities (Elder et al., 2002; Fell, Ferguson, Williams, & Fields, 2003; Peek-Asa, 1999). Public campaigns have also been important in enforcement efforts to increase seat belt use, in some states called Click-it or Ticket programs (Shults, Nichols, Dinh-Zarr, Sleet, & Elder, 2004; Solomon, Ulmer, & Pruesser, 2002; Williams, Lund, Preusser, & Blomberg, 1987). The coordination of public-awareness campaigns with enforcement activities are effective because the campaigns reach a broader audience, support the public message, and increase the perception that violators will be caught.

21.3.2.4.   *Generalizability to Your Community*

Effective prevention programs are designed for specific populations, and evidence that they work in one community does not necessarily mean they will work for yours.

One of the most important issues to consider when reading the literature is whether or not the demographic characteristics of your community are similar to those of the community in which the program was evaluated. These characteristics are age, gender, race/ethnicity/culture, socioeconomic status (particularly educational status), and population density. If these characteristics differ, then you must determine if there are fundamental differences between your community and the one that has been evaluated that could make the program ineffective. For example, nationwide Safe Routes to School programs involve community-wide multicomponent efforts to encourage children to walk or ride their bicycles to school and to ensure that they are safe when doing so. Evaluations have shown program success. (Appleyard 2003; National Highway Traffic Safety Administration [NHTSA], 2002). However, these programs are not likely to work in communities in which children live too far from their schools to bicycle or walk, such as in rural areas and cities that use long-distance busing.

21.3.2.5.   *Equity*

Successful prevention programs should not create inequities among participants or their communities. In the Safe Routes to School programs, there could potentially be deleterious consequences if some children cannot participate in the program because they are among a minority who live too far from school to participate. If a segment of the children are selectively excluded from participating, they will also be excluded from rewards or recognition that goes to program participants. This type of inequity is important to consider for all programs but is rarely measured in evaluations. Although it is difficult to create programs that are entirely equitable, the potential for inequity and methods to cope with necessary inequity should be considered in program development.

21.3.2.6.   *Feasibililty*

Just because a program is accepted and integrated into one community does not mean it will be feasible in another. For example, universal helmet use laws have strong evidence of effectiveness, yet they have been a topic of great legislative controversy. Most states that have enacted a universal law have had repeated attempts for repeal, often successful. Efforts to enact a motorcycle helmet use law in a state that does not have an effective political climate will likely be ineffective. For policy efforts, it is important to find key supporters that can help carry the policy through; often, even with support, such efforts take many years.

21.3.2.7. *Acceptability*

Prevention programs should be acceptable to at least some portion of the community, especially if the program is community based. Some programs are not acceptable due to political or legal issues. For example, random breath testing has been shown to be more effective than selective breath testing, the latter of which is conducted in the United States (Elder et al., 2002; Peek-Asa, 1999). However, random testing is not acceptable under the U.S. legal system, which has constitutional protections against unwarranted search and seizure (NHTSA, 1990).

Although many of these criteria seem obvious, failure to consider them can derail an otherwise carefully planned program. Some of this information will be available in existing evaluations or can be gleaned from evaluations of similar programs.

21.4. CONCLUSION

Beginning a literature search to evaluate existing evidence can be a daunting task. A systematic review is the best place to start, and the best places to find reviews are described in this chapter. If you find a review or reviews that support your proposed program, then it is important to consider how the program will translate to your community. If a review is not available, next look for individual studies that evaluate your proposed approach. Studies that evaluate programs or approaches similar to yours can provide relevant information. Studies that explain why the program was successful or that describe how programs are best implemented are especially helpful. The best way to start is to dive in—do not be intimidated—and to encourage lively discussion about what you are learning as you read the literature.

When reviewing the scientific literature and making decisions about a prevention approach, assembling a collaborative team can be beneficial. The team can include practitioners who have experience with a specific prevention approach, community members who know the intended audience well, and academicians who have experience with research and/or program evaluation methodologies. Experienced practitioners can be identified in state or local public health injury programs by contacting the State and Territorial Injury Prevention Director's Association www.stipda.org). Academicians may be found in local colleges, universities, or teaching hospitals, especially those that have injury or violence research programs. One resource for identifying injury researchers is the Society for the Advancement of Violence and Injury Research (formerly the National Association of Injury Control Research Centers) (www.savirweb.org). Although individuals you contact will have time limitations, they may be able to answer focused questions about the scientific literature or the prevention approach you are considering and may be interested in collaborating.

Existing evidence is important to inform decisions about prevention activities, but it can never replace the expertise of prevention practitioners. To help the injury prevention community continue to grow and improve, it is important to communicate the lessons you have learned when implementing your programs.

ACKNOWLEDGMENTS. We would like to thank Christy Cechman, contract reference librarian with the National Center for Injury Prevention and Control, for her invaluable help in identifying and retrieving citations.

REFERENCES

Alderson, P., Green, S., & Higgins, J. P. T. (Eds.). (2004). *Cochrane Reviewers' Handbook 4.2.2.* Retrieved February 22, 2005, from www.cochrane.org/resources/handbook/hbook.htm.

Appleyard, B. S. (2003). Planning safe routes to school. *Planning, 69* (5), 34–37.

Azeredo, R., & Stephens-Stidham, S. (2003). Design and implementation of injury prevention curricula for elementary schools: Lessons learned. *Injury Prevention, 9,* 274–278.

Bero, L., & Rennie, D. (1995). The Cochrane Collaboration. Preparing, maintaining, and disseminating systematic reviews of the effects of health care. *Journal of the American Medical Association, 274,* 1935–1938.

Briss, P. A., Zaza, S., Pappaioanou, M., Fielding, J., Wright-De Aguero, L., Truman, B. I., Hopkins, D. P., Hennessy, M. H., Sosin, D. M., Anderson, L., Carande-Kulis, V. G., Teutch, S. M., & Pappaioanou, M. (2000). Developing an evidence-based *Guide to Community Preventive Services*—Methods. *American Journal of Preventive Medicine, 19* (1S), 35–43.

Casteel, C., & Peek-Asa, C. (2000). The effectiveness of Crime Prevention through Environmental Design (CPTED) in reducing robberies. *American Journal of Preventive Medicine, 18* (4S), 99–115.

The Cochrane Collaboration. (2004). Retrieved December 9, 2005, from www.cochrane.org/index0.htm.

Cook, D. J., Sackett, D. L., & Spitzer, W. O. (1994). Methodological guidelines for systematic reviews of randomized control trials in health care for the Potsdam Consultation on Meta-Analysis. *Journal of Clinical Epidemiology, 48,* 167–171.

Cooper, H., & Hedges, L. V., (Eds.). (1994). *The handbook of research synthesis.* New York: Russell Sage Foundation.

Darian-Smith, E. (1993). Neighborhood Watch—Who watches whom? Reinterpreting the concept of neighborhood. *Human Organizations, 52* (1), 83–88.

Day, L., Fildes, B., Gordon, I., Fitzharris, M., Flamer, H., & Lord, S. (2002). Randomized factorial trial of falls prevention among older people living in their own homes. *British Medical Journal, 325,* 128–133.

Dickersin, K., & Min, Y. I. (1993). Publication bias: The problem that won't go away. *Annals of the New York Academy of Sciences, 703* (1), 135–146.

Easterbrook, P. J., Berlin, J. A., Gopalan, R., & Matthews, D. R. (1991). Publication bias in clinical research. *Lancet, 337,* 868–872.

Elder, R. W., Shults, R. A., Sleet, D. A., Nichols, J. L., Thompson, R. S., & Rajat, W. (2004). Effectiveness of mass media campaigns for reducing drinking and driving and alcohol-involved crashes: A systematic review. *American Journal of Preventive Medicine, 27* (1), 57–65.

Elder, R. W., Shults, R. A., Sleet, D. A., Nichols, J. L., Zaza, S., & Thompson, R. S. (2002). Effectiveness of sobriety checkpoints for reducing alcohol-involved crashes. *Traffic Injury Prevention, 3,* 266–274.

Elvik, R. (1998). Are road safety evaluation studies published in peer reviewed journals more valid than similar studies not published in peer reviewed journals? *Accident Analysis & Prevention, 30,* 101–118.

Fell, J. C., Ferguson, S. A., Williams, A. F., & Fields, M. (2003). Why are sobriety checkpoints not widely adopted as an enforcement strategy in the United States? *Accident Analysis & Prevention, 35,* 897–902.

Greene, A., Barnett, P., Crossen, J., Sexton, G., Ruzicka, P., & Neuwelt, E. (2002). Evaluation of the Think First for Kids injury prevention curriculum for primary students. *Injury Prevention, 8,* 257–258.

Gresham, L. S., Zirkle, D. L., Tolchin, S., Jones, C., Maroufi, A., & Miranda, J. (2001). Partnering for injury prevention: Evaluation of a curriculum-based intervention program among elementary school chidren. *Journal of Pediatric Nursing, 16* (2), 79–87.

Grossman, D. C., Mueller, B. A., Riedy, C., Dowd, M. D., Villaveces, A., Prodzinski, J., Nakagawara, J., Howard, J., Thiersch, N., & Harruff, R. (2005). Gun storage practices and risk of youth suicide and unintentional firearm injuries. *Journal of American Medical Association, 293,* 171–714.

Guide to Community Preventive Services. Systematic Reviews and Evidence Based Recommendations. Retrieved December 9, 2005, from www.thecommunityguide.org.

Hall-Long, B. A., Schell, K., & Corrigan, V. (2001). Youth safety education and injury prevention program. *Pediatric Nursing, 27* (2), 141–146.

Hope, T. (1995). Community crime prevention. In M. Tonry, & D. P. Farrington (Eds.). *Building a safer society. Crime and Justice* (pp. 216–228, vol. 19). Chicago: University of Chicago Press.

National Highway Traffic Safety Administration. (1990). *The use of sobriety checkpoints for impaired driving enforcement* (Report DOT HS-807 656). Washington, DC: Author.

National Highway Traffic Safety Administration. (2002). *Safe routes to school* (Report HS-809 497). Washington, DC: Author.

Ozanne-Smith, J., Ashby, K., Newstead, S., Stathakis, V. Z., & Clapperton, A. (2004). Firearm related deaths: The impact of regulatory reform. *Injury Prevention, 10* (5), 280–286.

Pappaioanou, M., & Evans, C., Jr. (1998). Development of *The Guide to Community Preventive Services*: A U.S. Public Health Service initiative. *Journal of Public Health Management & Practice, 4* (S2), 48–54.

Peek-Asa, C. (1999). The effect of random alcohol screening in reducing motor vehicle crash injuries. *American Journal of Preventive Medicine, 16* (1S), 57–67.

Peek-Asa, C., Casteel, C. H., Mineschian, L., Erickson, R., & Kraus, J. F. (2004). Implementation of a workplace robbery and violence prevention program in small retail businesses. *American Journal of Preventive Medicine, 4*, 276–283.

Petticrew, M., & Roberts, H. (2003). Evidence, hierarchies, and typologies: Horses for courses. *Journal of Epidemiology & Community Health, 57*, 527–529.

Popay, J., & Williams, G. (1998). Qualitative research and evidence-based healthcare. *Journal of the Royal Society of Medicine, 91* (S35), 32–37.

Rosenbaum, D. (1987). The theory and research behind Neighborhood Watch: Is it a sound fear and crime reduction strategy? *Crime & Delinquency, 33* (1), 103–134.

Runyan, C. W. (1998). Using the Haddon Matrix: Introducing the third dimension. *Injury Prevention, 4*, 302–307.

Rychetnic, L., Frommer, M., Hawe, P., & Shiell, A. (2002). Criteria for evaluating evidence on public health interventions. *Journal of Epidemiology & Community Health, 56*, 119–127.

Sherman, L. W., Gottfredson, D., MacKenzie, D., Eck, J., Reuter, P., & Bushway, S. (1997). *Preventing crime: What works, what doesn't, and what's promising? A Report to the United States Congress* (8-1 to 8-58). Washington, DC: National Institute of Justice.

Shults, R. A., Nichols, J. L., Dinh-Zarr, T. B., Sleet, D. A., & Elder, R. W. (2004). Effectiveness of primary enforcement safety belt laws and enhanced enforcement of safety belt laws: A summary of the *Guide to Community Preventive Services* systematic review. *Journal of Safety Research, 35*, 189–196.

Solomon, M. G., Ulmer, R. G., & Pruesser, D. F. (2002). *Evaluation of Click-it or Ticket model programs* (Report No HS-809 498). Washington, DC: National Highway Traffic Safety Administration.

Tang, K. C., Ehsani, J. P., McQueen, D. V. (2003). Evidence based health promotion: Recollections, reflections, and reconsiderations. *Journal of Epidemiology & Community Health, 57*, 841–843.

Wesner, M. L. (2003). An evaluation of Think First Saskatchewan: A head and spinal cord injury prevention program. *Canadian Journal of Public Health, 94* (2), 115–120.

Williams, A. F., Lund, A. K., Preusser, D. F., & Blomberg, R. D. (1987). Results of a seat belt use law enforcement and publicity campaign in Elmira, New York. *Accident Analysis & Prevention, 19*, 243–249.

Chapter 22

Behavioral Interventions for Injury and Violence Prevention*

David A. Sleet and Andrea Carlson Gielen

22.1. INTRODUCTION

Behavioral science has made a wide range of contributions to developing and sustaining public health. Behavioral, psychosocial and sociocultural factors associated with lifestyle behaviors are major contributors to morbidity and mortality. Efforts to control behaviors contributing to obesity, heart disease, diabetes, cancer, and HIV have successfully used behavioral and sociocultural strategies to reduce risks and improve the prospects for prevention (Green, 1999; Holtgrave, Doll, Harrison, 1997). Injury control can benefit from this legacy. It has only been recently that researchers and practitioners have recognized the value of using behavioral approaches for injury prevention and control (Gielen & Girasek, 2001; Gielen & Sleet, 2003).

Whether by violent or unintentional means, injury exacts a large toll on individuals, families, workplaces, and the community. Yet behaviors that give rise to injury and violence are amenable to preventive interventions. Experts in the behavioral and social sciences can help by documenting behavioral and social risk factors, developing and evaluating interventions, influencing social norms, assisting in postinjury recovery from psychological harm, and shaping individual and community preventive behaviors (Sleet, Hammond, Jones, Thomas, & Whitt, 2004).

However, the models, theories, and behavior change strategies so successful in addressing other public health problems have been sorely underrepresented in the injury literature (Trifilitti, Gielen, Sleet, & Hopkins, 2005). This chapter highlights the significance of taking a behavioral approach to the growing problem of injuries in public health and demonstrates how behavioral science strategies can contribute to solutions. As examples, we address the role of behavior change in injury prevention and provide further examples of applying behavioral and social-psychological

*Portions of this chapter were excerpted with permission from Oxford University Press from Gielen, A. C., and Sleet, D. (2003). Application of behavior-change theories and methods to injury prevention, *Epidemiologic Review, 25*, 65–76.

theory and methods to injury prevention. Other chapters in this book address sociological theories and discuss social science applications (see Chapter 15).

22.2.   BEHAVIORAL SCIENCE AND INJURY PREVENTION

It is rarely feasible to achieve injury reduction without some element of behavior change. Behavioral change is integral to any comprehensive approach to injury prevention. We define *behavioral interventions* as the development and application of behavioral science theory, knowledge, strategies, and techniques to the understanding and modification of injury risk behaviors and harms. Behavioral science applications have lagged behind other approaches to injury prevention, despite repeated calls for more behavioral science research in injury prevention (Bonnie, Fulco, & Liverman, 1999; National Committee on Injury Prevention and Control, 1989). Historically, little scholarly attention has been paid to understanding determinants of injury-related behaviors or how to initiate and sustain injury behavior changes. In the past, interventions to change injury behaviors were often based on simplistic assumptions that changing individuals' awareness about an injury problem would lead to changes in behavior. We know the process is more complex than this and that behavior change strategies cannot rely on information and education alone. Yet many practitioners in public health still approach behavioral change with this assumption in mind.

Many authors have noted the need to improve behavioral interventions by using better empirical data about behavioral determinants and by employing modern health behavior change theories and frameworks (Runyan, 1993; Thompson, Sleet, & Sacks, 2002; Geller et al., 1990). A growing body of work is emerging that demonstrates the positive effect of using behavioral science approaches to understand and reduce injury risk behaviors (Gielen, Sleet, & DiClemente, 2006; Sleet & Hopkins, 2004).

22.3.   THE NEED FOR BEHAVIORAL CHANGE

Although the rationale for using structural or environmental interventions to change injury patterns might seem straightforward, there is rarely an environmental change that does not require behavioral adaptation. For every technological advance, there are behavioral components that need to be addressed. Children need to wear helmets while bicycling; parents need to correctly install child safety seats and booster seats; home owners need to check their smoke alarms and change the batteries; parents with four-sided fences around their backyard pool need to ensure that the gate to the pool is always closed; occupants alerted by a smoke alarm still need to find their way to safety. Even the more passive approach to poison prevention through the use of child-resistant closures—one of the great successes in injury control—requires active individual effort in replacing lids correctly (DiLillo, Peterson, & Farmer, 2002; Shields, 1997).

Integrating knowledge about behavioral science into the mainstream of injury prevention research and practice will help avoid the false dichotomy between active and passive strategies and reduce the tendency to choose one over the other. In Haddon's (1980) epidemiological approach to injury, the host's role in injury reflects only personal risk at the level of the individual. Much of the research on injury behavior change has been on individuals whose behavior puts them at risk, such as the drinking driver (Geller, Elder, Hovell, & Sleet, 1991) or the child pedestrian (Cross, Hall, & Howat, 2003). However, because so many of the effective injury countermeasures are policy oriented in nature, practitioners may find behavioral change strategies useful for modifying injury prevention policy at the community level (Gielen, 1992; Gielen & Girasek, 2001; Runyan, 1998). Finding effective ways to activate individuals to become advocates for safer products, policies, and environments represents a new opportunity for behavioral change to contribute to injury prevention (DeFrancesco et al., 2003).

Safer products and environments require behavior change, too, on the part of manufacturers (such as toy makers) and environmental designers (such as city planners) as well as policy makers who regulate exposure to hazards and those who mandate and enforce safety behaviors (such as legislators, judges, and police) (McGinnis, Williams-Russo, & Knickman, 2002; Shaw & Ogolla, 2006). Cataldo et al. (1986, p. 233) emphasised this point when they said "Ultimately, injury control must entail some degree of behavior change, requiring the establishment and maintenance of appropriate safety behavior—by parents, legislators, judges and juries, police, health educators, physicians, reporters and the like."

In the following sections, we discuss theories and examples that can help facilitate the change process among individuals at risk as well as among those in a position to influence policy and environmental change.

22.4. THEORIES FROM BEHAVIORAL SCIENCE

In the last few years there has been growing national interest in the contributions of theoretical models from the behavioral sciences to public health (Glanz, Rimer, & Lewis, 2002; Rutter & Quine, 2002). The limited success of behavioral change efforts in modifying injury related behaviors, however, can be traced, in part, to failure to apply these theories to develop and implement effective injury prevention interventions (Liller & Sleet, 2004). Theories are important not simply because they help us understand causes of problems but because they also allow us to identify mechanisms of change, determine why programs succeed or fail, and perhaps most important guide us to build better prevention programs (DiClemente, Crosby, & Kegler, 2002). Selecting the most appropriate theory is situation specific and depends on the specific audience, the setting, and the characteristics of the behavior to be changed (Rimer & Glanz, 2005).

22.4.1. Ecological Models

What has emerged recently in public health is the importance of taking an ecological perspective for understanding and intervening on contemporary public health problems such as injury (Allegrante, Marks, & Hanson, 2006). The report *Promoting Health* (Smedley & Syme, 2000, pp. 9, 2) summarized it this way:

> Perhaps the most significant contribution of behavioral and social sciences to health research is the development of strong theoretical models for interventions.
>
>   The committee . . . found an emerging consensus that research and intervention efforts should be based on an ecological model.

The ecological model states that health and well-being are affected by a dynamic interaction among biology, behavior, and the environment and this interaction changes over the life course (Committee on Health and Behavior, 2001; Schneiderman, Speers, Silva, Tomes, & Gentry, 2001). This definition conveys the notion of multiple levels of influence on health and makes clear the importance of both individual level and community level factors in shaping health-related behaviors. Reductions in motor-vehicle-related deaths and homicide are examples of improving population health through interventions at multiple levels of influence (see Chapters 4, 15, 16, and 17). Legislative policies, educational programs, and changes in the physical and social environment all contribute to changes in injury and injury risks. Thus an ecological model has utility in both describing influencing factors and developing prevention programs (Green, Richard, & Potvin, 1996).

22.4.2. Influencing Change

In translating an ecological model to action programs, Rimer & Glanz (2005) describe three levels of influence for change. (1) Intrapersonal change refers to influencing an individual's knowledge, attitudes, or beliefs about his or her behavior. Theories of cognition, perception, and motivation are relevant here. (2) Interpersonal change refers to the influence of significant others such as families, friends, and co-workers. Relevant here is the modifying effect of social influence and social norms on individual behavior. (3) Community-level change includes the influence of organizational settings (such as workplaces, schools, and religious institutions such as churches, synagoges, and mosques, and their influence on behavior. On a larger societal level, there are the influences of social and health policies (e.g., those related to welfare reform) and other influences such as poverty and disenfranchisement that affect injury risk behaviors.

Examples of models applied to the community level are community mobilization, organizational change, and intersectoral action. Theories and models can help explain community and individual change processes in an ecological context. For example, simple changes in community zoning and urban planning can dramatically affect injury-related behaviors, ranging from less youth violence and crime to more cycling and walking. Community-level change strategies are described in other chapters this book.

Different intervention strategies and methods are available when working with individuals and with communities (Bartholomew, Parcel, Kok, & Gottlieb, 2001; Bensley & Brookins-Fisher, 2003). For example, at the individual level, the typical intervention strategies include a variety of behavioral, educational, counseling, skills-development, and training methods. Innovative new technologies such as computer-tailored messaging and behavioral prescriptions, Web-based learning, and motivational interviewing are promising approaches to strengthen the effect of individual level injury prevention interventions (Dunn, DeRoo, & Rivara, 2001; Kreuter, Jacobsen, McDonald, & Gielen, 2003). When interventions focus on organizations, communities, and policies, the use of social marketing, mass media, and media advocacy are important (Wallack, Dorfman, Jernigan, & Themba, 1993) as are coalition building, social planning, and community development (Bracht, Kingbury, & Rissel, 1999).

22.5. APPLICATION OF HEALTH BEHAVIOR THEORY TO INJURY PREVENTION

A complete enumeration of the theories used in the field of health behavior change is beyond the scope of this chapter, although interested readers are referred to relevant textbooks (DiClemente et al., 2002; Rimer & Glanz, 2005) and reports

(Committee on Health and Behavior, 2001; Smedley & Syme, 2000). Behavioral change theories, methods, and applications in injury prevention have been described by Gielen et al. (2006). Here, we describe several examples of well-respected behavior change theories or models that have been applied to injury problems.

22.5.1. Individual Level Theories and Models

The Health Belief Model (HBM), Theory of Reasoned Action (TRA), Stages of Change (SOC), and applied behavioral analysis (ABA) have extensive literature supporting their utility. Each has been used for understanding injury problem. In this section, we briefly describe the key constructs of each of these models and provide an example of their application to an injury problem.

22.5.1.1. Health Belief Model

The Health Belief Model says that preventive behaviors are a function of individuals' beliefs about their susceptibility to the health problem in question, the severity of the health problem, and the benefits versus costs of adopting the preventive behavior, as well as experiencing a cue to action (Janz & Becker, 1984). In recent years, the concept of self-efficacy was added to the model. Self-efficacy, a concept originally from Bandura's (1989) work, refers to one's confidence in his or her ability to perform a specific behavior. An illustration of this model in injury prevention comes from Peterson, Farmer, & Kashani's (1990) study of the beliefs and safety practices of 198 parents of 8- to 17-year-old children. They used the HBM to predict how parents' attitudes might influence their injury prevention teaching and environmental modifications. Parents were generally not very worried about injuries to their child (i.e., low perceived susceptibility). The HBM constructs most strongly associated with parental safety efforts were beliefs that their actions would be effective (benefits), a realistic appraisal of the costs of action (costs), and feeling knowledgeable and competent to perform the behaviors (efficacy). In this case, the authors suggest that practitioners use interventions influencing parents' beliefs about their child's susceptibility to injury through education, while increasing parents' competency to intervene through specific behavior change strategies. Health education methods and strategies might include direct communications to address susceptibility and skills training and improved access to safety products to address competence.

22.5.1.2. Theory of Reasoned Action

The Theory of Reasoned Action model describes behavior as a function of behavioral intention, subjective norms, and attitudes (Fishbein & Ajzen, 1975). The model focuses on the individual's intention to perform a behavior as predictive of their actual behavior. Intention is a function of attitudes and subjective norms. Ajzen (1991) later modified the TRA, renaming it the Theory of Planned Behavior, to include the concept of perceived behavioral control, which reflects how easy or difficult the individual perceives the behavior.

In practical use, the TRA was used as the conceptual framework for a survey of parents' beliefs and practices regarding car safety seat usage (Gielen, Eriksen, Daltroy, & Rost, 1984). Attitude toward car seat use was found to be the single best variable for distinguishing between car seat users and nonusers. This variable consisted of responses to six items measuring beliefs about the consequences of the behavior (e.g., using a car seat would be a hassle; your child would be better behaved in a car seat). Respondents who believed that their spouse would approve of using a car seat (a measure of subjective norm) were also more likely to report using one. These results can help practitioners develop public and patient education materials using salient messages with credible spokespersons. For example, media messages might communicate the ease with which car seat use becomes a habit with positive consequences, such as child comfort and spouse approval.

22.5.1.3. Stages of Change

The Stages of Change (SOC) model is also called the Transtheoretical Model because it incorporates constructs from several older models (Prochaska & DiClemente, 1983). This model conceptualizes behavior change as a dynamic rather than static process, acknowledging that individuals differ in their readiness to change a behavior, and changes occur in discrete steps over time. There are typically five stages in the SOC model: (1) precontemplative, not thinking about changing; (2) contemplative, aware and thinking about changing; (3) preparation, taking steps necessary for changing; (4) action, making the change for a short period of time; and (5) maintenance, having successfully changed the behavior, usually measured as 6 months or longer. This model includes the possibility of relapse to earlier stages, noting that maintained behavior change often occurs after a cyclical process of progressing and relapsing, as in smoking control. The SOC model has been used to describe men's ability to change their abusive behaviors (Daniels & Murphy, 1997) and to describe abused women's safety behaviors and their ability to end their abuse (Burke, Gielen, McDonnell, O'Campo, & Maman, 2001). In Burke et al.'s (2001) study of women's descriptions of how they coped with and ended their abuse, there were clear examples of women moving from precontemplation (e.g., not considering their partner's behavior toward them as a problem or not labeling their experiences as abuse), to action (e.g., recognizing the abuse as a problem and taking some protective action, such as calling a shelter, contacting legal assistance, moving out), to maintenance (e.g., having experienced no abuse or having been away from the partner for 6 months or more). Identifying an individual's stage of change allows the practitioner to select and apply the most appropriate, stage-matched intervention. For example, increasing knowledge and awareness may help someone progress from the precontemplation to the contemplation stage. To move someone from contemplation to preparation and action may require identifying, providing, and facilitating access to and use of the necessary resources.

22.5.1.4. Applied Behavior Analysis

The term *applied behavior analysis* (ABA) is a specific subfield within psychology that uses the technology of behavior modification and operant conditioning to facilitate change. Behavior is viewed as learned, and principles of stimulus control, feedback, reinforcement, and punishment shape the acquisition, maintenance, and extinction of behavior (Hovell, Elder, Blanchard, & Sallis, 1986). Applied behavior analysis or behavioral safety addresses the ABCs of behavior by manipulating the antecedents, behaviors, and consequences associated with behavior. Antecedents occur before the behavior (such as cues in the environment), behaviors include the context in which the behavior occurs, and consequences are those things that follow the behavior.

Understanding the ABCs that control a behavior can help the practitioner intervene by shaping the behavior and the environment to bring about change. Forbidding roadside billboards that remind drivers of drinking, increasing prompts and cues in the drinking environment that discourage drinking and driving, and selecting a designated driver are all ways that might modify the antecedents of drinking and driving. Slowing the rate of alcohol consumption, learning drinking or binge drinking refusal skills, promoting server interventions in the drinking environment, and providing feedback from blood alcohol consumption meters might be used to modify the drinking behavior. Social and peer support for not drinking and driving, positive feedback, incentives or rewards from bartenders or friends, and punishment for being caught for drinking and driving can be used to modify consequences (Geller et al., 1991; Girasek, Gielen, & Smith, 2002; Sleet & Lonero, 2002).

In traffic safety, applications of applied behavior analysis have effectively increased the use of safety belts (Streff & Geller, 1986) and child restraints (Cataldo et al., 1986; Sleet, Hollenbach, & Hovell, 1986), reduced vehicle speeding (Ragnarsson & Bjorgvinsson, 1991), and improved bicycle helmet use (Thompson, Sleet, & Sacks, 2002). In other areas of injury prevention, applied behavior analysis has been used to reduce children's fall-related behavior on playgrounds (Heck, Collins, & Peterson, 2001) and to change safety behaviors in a fire in public buildings (Leslie, 2001).

This approach also has a strong history of use and success in promoting occupational health and safety (Margolis & Kroes, 1975) and has been successfully applied to increase the use of personal protection devices such as hard hats and ear protection, to reduce injuries on the job, and to increase worker productivity and morale (Krause, Hidley, & Hodson, 1990).

22.5.1.5. Integrating Individual Level Models

In 1991, the National Institute of Mental Health convened a theorists' workshop to bring together creators of behavioral theory to develop a unifying framework to facilitate health behavior change (Fishbein et al., 1991). Their discussions led to an enumeration of five theories that, taken together, contain virtually all the variables that have been used in attempts to understand and change human behaviors: The Health Belief Model, Social Cognitive Theory, Theory of Reasoned Action, Theory of Self-Regulation and Self-Control, (Kanfer & Kanfer, 1991), and Theory of Subjective Culture and Interpersonal Relations (Triandis, 1980). Considering all five theories and their many variables, eight variables appear to account for most of the variations in health-related behaviors: intentions, environmental barriers, skills, outcome expectancies (or attitudes), social norms, self-standards, emotional reactions, and self-efficacy. It is likely that these same eight variables might also regulate and predict change in injury risk behavior (M. Fishbein, personal communication, January 23, 2003).

Translating this guidance to action, Fishbein et al. (2001) concluded that, generally speaking, for a person to perform a given behavior, one or more of the following must be present:

- The person forms a strong positive intention or makes a commitment to perform the behavior.
- There are no environmental barriers that make it *impossible* to perform the behavior.
- The person possesses the skills necessary to perform the behavior.
- The person believes that the advantages of performing the behavior outweigh the disadvantages.
- The person perceives more normative pressure to perform than not to perform the behavior.
- The person perceives that performance of the behavior is consistent with his or her self-image or values.
- The person's emotional reaction to performing the behavior is more positive than negative.
- The person perceives that he or she has the capabilities to perform the behavior under different circumstances.

The first three factors are viewed as necessary and sufficient for producing any behavior, and the remaining five are viewed as modifying variables, influencing the strength and direction of intentions. By way of a hypothetical example, we can apply these notions to the injury control behavior of testing the functionality of a residential smoke alarms. If a homeowner is committed to testing the smoke alarms every month, has access to the alarms in the home, and has the skills necessary to successfully test the alarms, we would predict that there is a high probability he or she will perform the behavior. The probability that the individual will test the smoke alarms monthly would be predicted to increase even more if the homeowner also believes that testing is worth the time and trouble, knows that neighbors all test their alarms, believes that testing is consistent with his or her values as a responsible homeowner, has no negative emotional reaction to testing, and can test the alarms under different conditions in the home. According to this notion, the probability of testing monthly would be predicted to reach nearly 100% under these conditions. In practice, this integrated model has not been applied to this or any other injury related behavior but holds promise as an innovative approach to program development, at least until such time as sufficient research is available on specific theories as they related to injury and violence prevention.

22.5.2.   Community Level Theories and Models

Community-based injury prevention occurs when people and organizations collaborate as communities to design and implement strategies to keep citizens safe (Coggan & Bennett, 2004). A community can be defined either geographically or on the basis of common interests. Community organization and mobilization and community-based participatory research focus on the active participation and development of the community to enable members to better evaluate and solve their own health and social problems (Minkler & Wallerstein, 1997).

Gielen and Collins (1993) and McLoughlin, Vince, Lee, & Crawford (1982) described the difference between community-wide interventions and community-based programs, highlighting the importance of treating the community as the source and not simply the site of prevention programs. Green & Kreuter (1991), p. 261 described the necessary components of community interventions this way:

> Given reasonable resources, the chances are that a community intervention will succeed if the practitioner (1) builds from a base of com-

munity ownership of the problems and the solution, (2) plans carefully, (3) uses sound theory, meaningful data and local experience as a basis for problem decisions, (4) knows what types of interventions work best for specific populations and circumstances, and (5) has an organizational and advocacy plan to orchestrate multiple intervention strategies into a complementary cohesive program.

Among the more successful applications of community level theories and models in injury prevention is the safe community movement, initiated in Sweden in the 1980s (Svanstrom, 1999). The program combining top-down with bottom-up strategies was developed in eight steps: (1) epidemiological mapping, (2) selection of risk groups and hazardous environments, (3) forming coalitions or interdisciplinary workgroups, (4) joint action planning with many sectors involved, (5) implementation, (6) evaluation, (7) program modification from feedback, and (8) transfer of program success to others. In the United States, the safe community model has been applied mostly to the traffic safety sector; it was officially adopted by the National Highway Traffic Safety Administration (NHTSA) as a part of its support to the Governor's Offices of Highway Safety Programs in many parts of the country.

Sweden, Norway, Australia, New Zealand, Canada and many other countries have implemented a number of injury prevention projects based on the safe community model (Coggan & Bennett, 2004; Moller, 1995) In each project, the community, which ranged from large suburban areas to small country towns, was involved in developing a series of injury prevention strategies. Multidisciplinary lay-professional coalitions were formed to develop and implement the strategies.

In the United States, Hingson et al. (1996) describe a community-based program to reduce drinking and driving in which intervention cities reduced fatal crashes by 25% and fatal crashes involving alcohol by 42%, relative to the rest of the state of Massachusetts during the 5 years of the program and in comparison to the previous 5 years without the program. This community level approach is attracting much interest among injury prevention practitioners worldwide and efforts are under way to evaluate its impact (Spinks, Turner, McClure, Acton, & Nixon, 2005).

22.5.2.1. *Community Action*

Community action for injury prevention benefits from community organization and mobilization, defined as efforts to involve community members in activities ranging from defining needs for prevention to obtaining community support for a predesigned prevention program. Mobilization emphasizes changing the social and economic structures that influence injury risk. Treno and Holder (1997) note that mobilization can include elements of both grassroots efforts and leader-initiated strategies. In the former, the community members define the problems and decide the solutions, and in the latter outside experts (external or self-appointed community leaders) decide. Because community leaders understand their local culture, politics, and traditions better than outsiders, their participation is essential for tailoring prevention programs to local needs.

In the Community Trials Project to reduce alcohol-involved trauma (Treno & Holder, 1997), a community-research partnership was formed to focus on changes in the social and structural contexts of alcohol use. They worked to implement prevention policies and activities that were evidence based and asked communities to customize and prioritize their initiatives based on local concerns and interests.

Specific components of the mobilization effort were directed toward responsible beverage service, drinking and driving, underage drinking, and alcohol access. Coalitions, task forces, and media advocacy were used to raise awareness and support for effective policies with the public and decision makers. An evaluation of the effect of the mobilization efforts demonstrated significant reductions in the following indicators: 6% in the reported quantity of alcohol consumed, 51% in driving over the legal alcohol limit, 10% in nighttime injury crashes, 6% in alcohol related crashes, and 43% in alcohol-related assault injuries seen in emergency departments (Holder et al., 2000).

22.5.2.2.   *Community-Based Participatory Research*

Community-based participatory research (CBPR) is a collaborative approach to research that equitably involves all partners in the research process and recognizes the unique strengths that each brings. CBPR begins with a research topic of importance to the community with the aim of combining knowledge and action for social change to improve community health and eliminate health disparities (Green & Mercer, 2001; Minkler & Wallerstein, 2003). It contains elements of both community organization and mobilization. While participatory research is increasingly being advocated for dealing with a multitude of public health problems, it is perhaps especially important for problems that relate to individual behavior. To implement and evaluate policies and programs that attempt to change personal behavior requires extreme sensitivity to the ethical issues surrounding the protection of individual autonomy. By engaging communities in needs assessment and decision making about program design and evaluation, for example, the strategies that result are more likely to be consistent with the core values of the community and society (see Chapter 27).

For practitioners, these theories at both the individual and the community levels should help clarify assumptions on which interventions are selected; when used in conjunction with thorough needs assessments these theories should contribute to building successful injury prevention programs.

22.6.   CONCLUSIONS

The use of behavioral theories and methods has been critical to progress in improving public health and injury prevention. Behavioral interventions can complement structural approaches and environmental change efforts and can facilitate the work of law makers and product designers in ways that can ultimately protect whole populations.

This brief review of behavioral approaches should enable practitioners and researchers in injury and violence prevention to more easily identify potentially useful strategies for many injury problems. Researchers and policy makers have highlighted the need for more effective educational approaches and behavioral change applications to injury control (Gielen et al., 2006; Grossman & Johnston, 2004; Zaza & Thompson, 2001; Sleet & Hopkins, 2004), and some scholarly journals have dedicated whole issues to this topic (Gielen, 2002; Liller and Sleet, 2004; Ludwig, Geller, & Mawhinney, 2000; Schwartz, 2003; Sleet & Bryn, 2003).

Because of the wide range of types of injury, preventive behaviors, and various target groups and community characteristics, there remains a great need for additional research using behavioral theories and models. More attention must also be paid to the issues of training researchers and practitioners in the application of relevant theories. Training more behavioral scientists in the epidemiology of injury and the science of injury control is an urgent first step. Likewise, enhancing the behavioral science training of injury practitioners and researchers is essential.

Theoretical research is needed to clarify the mechanisms by which change occurs across levels of ecological models. Applied research can help us understand and modify risk perceptions, social norms, and other psychosocial factors associated with behavior and improve behavior change programs (Buckley & Sheehan, 2004). Developmental research is needed to reduce child and adolescent injuries. Community level research is necessary to understand mechanisms for influencing large populations through behavioral and environmental strategies. Evidence from a single study can provide useful information for practitioners about what variables to target and, in some cases, about program efficacy—but only a preponderance of research conducted for each injury preventive behavior and in many population groups can provide the kind of evidence needed to develop best practices. Ultimately, what is needed is substantial research on both the determinants of behavior and the efficacy of program approaches so that recommendations can be made to practitioners about the most important strategies (Sleet, Trifilitti, Simons-Morton, & Gielen, 2006). We believe these are important steps for strengthening the application of behavioral science to injury control, which in turn can contribute to changing individual behaviors, environmental conditions, and social structures in ways that prevent injuries.

REFERENCES

Ajzen, I. (1991). The theory of planned behavior. *Organizational Behavior & Human Decision Processes, 50,* 179–211.

Allegrante, J. P., Marks, R., & Hanson, D. (2006). Ecological approaches to unintentional injury prevention. In A. Gielen, D. A. Sleet, & R. A. DiClemente (Eds.), *Injury and violence prevention: Behavioral science theories, methods and applications.* San Francisco: Jossey-Bass.

Bandura, A. (1989). Perceived self-efficacy in the exercise of personal agency. *Psychological Bulletin of British Psychological Society, 10,* 411–424.

Bartholomew, L. K., Parcel, G. S., Kok, G., & Gottlieb, N. H. (2001). *Intervention mapping book.* Mountain View, CA: Mayfield.

Bensley, R. J., & Brookins-Fisher, J. (2003). *Community health education methods: A practical guide* (2nd ed.). Boston: Jones and Bartlett.

Bonnie, R. J., Fulco, C. E., & Liverman, C. T. (Eds.). (1999). *Reducing the burden of injury: Advancing prevention & treatment.* Washington, DC: National Academy Press.

Bracht, N., Kingsbury, L., & Rissel, C. (1999). A Five-stage community organization model for health promotion, empowerment and partnership strategies. In N. Bracht, (Ed.), *Health promotion at the community level* (2nd ed.) (pp. 83–104). Thousand Oaks, CA: Sage Publications.

Buckley, L., & Sheehan, M. (2004). Behavior change programs. In R. McClure, M. Stevenson, & S. McEvoy (Eds.), *The scientific basis of injury prevention and control.* (pp. 334–346). Melbourne, Australia: ISA Press.

Burke, J. G., Gielen, A. C., McDonnell, K. A., O'Campo, P., & Maman, S. (2001). The process of ending abuse in intimate relationships: A qualitative exploration of the transtheoretical model. *Violence against Women, 7* (10), 1144–1163.

Cataldo, M. F., Dershewitz, R. A., Wilson, M., Christophersen, E. R., Finney, J. W., Fawcett, W. S. B., & Seekins, T. (1986). Childhood injury control. In N. A. Krasnegor, J. D. Arasteh, & M. F. Cataldo (Eds.), *Child health behavior: A behavioral pediatrics perspective.* (p. 233). New York: Wiley.

Coggan, C., & Bennett, S. (2004). Community-based injury prevention programs. In R. McClure, M. Stevenson, & S. McEvoy (Eds.), *The scientific basis of injury prevention and control* (pp. 347–358). Melbourne, Australia: ISA Press.

Committee on Health and Behavior. (2001). *Health & behavior: The interplay of biological, behavioral and societal influences.* Washington, DC: National Academy Press.

Cross, D., Hall, M., & Howat, P. (2003). Using theory to guide practice in children's pedestrian safety education. *American Journal of Health Education* (Supplement), *34* (5), S42–S47.

Daniels, J. W., & Murphy, C. M. (1997). Stages of processes of change in batterers' treatment. *Cognitive & Behavioral Practice, 4,* 123–145.

DiClemente, R. J., Crosby, R. A., & Kegler, M. C. (Eds.). (2002). *Emerging theories in health promotion practice and research.* San Francisco: Jossey-Bass.

DeFrancesco, S., Gielen A. C., Bishai, D., Mahoney, P., Ho, S., & Guyer, B. (2003). Parents as advocates for child pedestrian injury prevention: What do they believe about the efficacy of prevention strategies and about how to create change? *American Journal of Health Education* (Supplement), *34* (5), S48–S53.

DiLillo, D., Peterson, L., & Farmer, J. (2002). Injury and poisoning. In T. J. Boll, S. B. Johnson, N. W. Perry, R. H. Rozensky (Eds.), *Handbook of clinical health psychology. Vol 1, Medical disorders and behavioral applications* (pp. 555–582). Washington, DC: American Psychological Association.

Dunn, C., DeRoo, L., & Rivara, F. (2001). The use of brief interventions adapted from motivational interviewing across behavioral domains: A systematic review. *Addiction, 96,* 1725–1742.

Fishbein, M., & Ajzen, I. (1975). *Belief, attitude, intention, & behavior: An introduction to theory and research.* Reading, MA: Addison-Wesley.

Fishbein, M., Bandura, A., Triandis, H. C., Kanfer, F. H., Becker, M. H., & Middlestadt, S. E. (1991). *Factors influencing behavior and behavior change. Final Report—theorists workshop.* Washington, DC: National Institute of Mental Health.

Fishbein, M., Triandis, H. C., Kanfer, F. H., Becker, M., Middlestadt, S. E., & Eichler, A. (2001). Factors influencing behavior and behavior change. In A. Baum, T. A. Revenson, & J. E. Singer (Eds.), *Handbook of health psychology* (pp. 3–17). Mahwah, NJ: Erlbaum.

Geller, E. S., Berry, T., Ludwig, T. D., Evans, R. E., Gilmore, M. R., & Clarke, S. W. (1990). A conceptual framework for developing and evaluating behavior change interventions for injury control. *Health Education Research, 5* (2), 125–137.

Geller, E. S., Elder, J. P., Hovell, M. F., & Sleet, D. A. (1991). Behavior change approaches to deterring alcohol-impaired driving. *Advances in Health Education & Promotion, 3,* 45–68.

Gielen, A. C. (1992). Health education and injury control: Integrating approaches. *Health Education Quarterly, 19,* 203–218.

Gielen, A. C. (Ed.). (2002). Injury and domestic violence prevention [Special issue]. *Patient Education and Counseling, 46* (3), 161–232.

Gielen, A. C., & Collins, B. (1993). Community-based interventions for injury prevention. *Family & Community Health, 15,* 1–11.

Gielen, A. C., Eriksen, M. P., Daltroy, L. H., & Rost, K. (1984). Factors associated with the use of child restraint devices. *Health Education Quarterly, 11* (2), 195–206.

Gielen, A. C., & Girasek, D. C. (2001). Integrating perspectives on the prevention of unintentional injuries. In N. Schneiderman, M. A. Speers, J. M. Silva, H. Tomes, & J. H. Gentry (Eds.), *Integrating behavioral and social sciences with public health* (pp. 203–230). Washington, DC: American Psychological Association.

Gielen, A. C., & Sleet, D. A. (2003). Application of behavior-change theories and methods to injury prevention. *Epidemiologic Reviews, 25,* 65–76.

Gielen, A. C., Sleet, D. A., & DiClemente, R. (2006). Injury and violence prevention: Behavioral science theories, methods and applications. San Francisco: Jossey-Bass.

Girasek, D. C., Gielen, A. C., & Smith, G. S. (2002). Alcohol's contribution to fatal injuries: A report on public perceptions. *Annals of Emergency Medicine, 39,* 622–652.

Glanz, K., Rimer, B., & Lewis, F. (Eds.) (2002). *Health behavior and health education: Theory, research and practice* (3rd ed.). San Francisco: Jossey-Bass.

Green, L. W. (1999). Health education's contribution to public health in the twentieth century: A glimpse through health promotion's rear-view mirror. *Annual Review of Public Health, 20,* 67–88.

Green, L. W., & Kreuter, M. W. (1991). *Health promotion planning: An educational and environmental approach* (2nd ed.) (p. 261). Mountain View: CA: Mayfield.

Green, L. W., & Mercer, S. L. (2001). Can public health researchers and agencies reconcile the push from funding bodies and the pull from communities? Community-based participatory research. *American Journal of Public Health, 91* (12), 1926–1943.

Green, L. W., Richard, L., & Potvin, L. (1996). Ecological foundation of health promotion. *American Journal of Health Promotion, 10* (4), 270–281.

Grossman, D., & Johnston, B. (Eds.) (2004). *Behavioral approaches to injury control. Participant's notebook and workshop materials.* Seattle: Harborview Injury Prevention and Research Center. Retrieved March 10, 2006, from www.hiprc.gov.

Haddon, W. (1980). Advance in the epidemiology of injuries as a basis for public policy. *Public Health Reports, 95,* 411–421.

Hingson, R., McGovern, T., Howland, J., Heeren, T., Winter, M., & Zakocs, R. (1996). Reducing alcohol-impaired driving in Massachusetts: The Saving Lives Program. *American Journal of Public Health, 86,* 791–797.

Heck, A., Collins, J., & Peterson, L. (2001). Decreasing children's risk taking on the playground. *Journal of Applied Behavior Analysis, 34,* 349–352.

Holder, H. D., Gruenewald, P. J., Ponicki, W. R., Treno, A. J., Grube, J. W., Saltz, R. F., Voas, R. B., Reynolds, R., Davis, J., Sanchez, L., Gaumont, G., & Roeper, P. (2000). Effect of community-based interventions on high-risk drinking and alcohol related injuries, *Journal of American Medical Association, 284* (18), 2341–2347.

Holtgrave, D. R., Doll, L. S., & Harrison, J. (1997). Influence of behavioral and social science on public health policy making. *American Psychologist, 52,* 154–166.

Hovell, M. F., Elder, J. P., Blanchard, J., & Sallis, J. F. (1986). Behavior analysis and public health perspectives: Combining paradigms to effect prevention. *Education & Treatment of Children, 9* (4), 287–306.

Janz, N. K., & Becker, M. H. (1984). The health belief model: A decade later. *Health Education, 11,* 1–47.

Kanfer, R., & Kanfer, F. H. (1991). Goals and self-regulation: Applications of theory to work settings. In M. L. Machr, & P. R. Pintrich (Eds.), *Advances in motivation & achievement* (pp. 287–326, vol. 7). Greenwich, CT: JAI Press.

Krause, T. R., Hidley, J. H., & Hodson, S. J. (1990). *The behavior-based safety process,* New York: Van Nostrand Reinhold.

Kreuter, M. W., Jacobsen, H. A., McDonald, E. M., & Gielen, A. C. (2003). *Developing computerised tailored health messages in community health education methods: A practical guide* (2nd ed.). Boston: Jones and Bartlett.

Leslie, J. (2001). Behavioral safety: Extending the principles of applied behavioral analysis to safety in fires in public buildings. In Proceedings of the 2nd international symposium on Human Behavior in fire. MIT, Cambridge, MA. Interscience Communications, Ltd., pp. 1–10.

Liller, K. D., & Sleet, D. A. (Eds.). (2004). Injury prevention [Special issue]. *American Journal of Health Education, 28* (Supplement 1), S1–S72.

Ludwig, T. D., Geller, E. S., & Mawhinney, T. C. (2000). Intervening to improve the safety of occupational driving: A behavior-change model and review of empirical evidence. *Journal of Organizational Behavior Management, 19* (4), 1–124.

Margolis, B. L., & Kroes, W. H. (Eds.). (1975). *The human side of accident prevention: Psychological concepts and principles which bear on industrial safety.* Springfield, IL: Charles C. Thomas.

McGinnis, J. M., Williams-Russo, P., & Knickman, J. R. (2002). The case for more active policy attention to health promotion, *Health Affairs, 21,* 78–93.

McLoughlin, E., Vince, C., Lee, A., & Crawford, J. (1982). Project burn prevention: Outcome and implications. *American Journal of Public Health, 72,* 241–247.

Minkler, M., & Wallerstein, N. (1997). Improving health through community organization and community building. In K. Glanz, F. M. Lewis, & B. K. Rimer (Eds.), *Health behavior and health education: Theory, research, and practice* (pp. 241–269, 2nd ed.). San Francisco: Jossey-Bass.

Minkler, M., & Wallerstein, N. (2003). *Community-based participatory research for health.* San Francisco: Jossey-Bass.

Moller, J. (1995). An Introduction to community-based injury prevention. In J. Ozanne-Smith, & F. Williams (Eds.), *Injury research and prevention: a text* (pp. 210–220). Victoria, Australia: Monash University Accident Research Center.

National Committee for Injury Prevention and Control. (1989). Injury prevention: Meeting the challenge. Supplement to the *American Journal of Preventive Medicine, 5,* vol 5 (3). New York: Oxford University Press.

Peterson, L., Farmer, J., & Kashani, J. H. (1990). Parental injury prevention endeavors: A function of health beliefs? *Health Psychology, 9* (2), 177–191.

Prochaska, J. O., & DiClemente, C. C. (1983). Stages and processes of self-change of smoking: Toward an integrative model of change, *Journal of Consulting and Clinical Psychology, 51,* 390–395.

Ragnarsson, R. S., & Bjorgvinsson, T. (1991). Effects of public posting on driving speed in Icelandic traffic. *Journal of Applied Behavior Analysis, 24*, 53–58.

Rimer, B. K., & Glanz, K. (2005). *Theory at a glance: A guide for health promotion practice.* Washington, D.C.: U.S. Department of Health and Human Services. Publication No. 05-3896.

Runyan, C. W. (1993). Progress and potential in injury control. *American Journal of Public Health, 83* (5), 637–639.

Runyan, C. W. (1998). Using the Haddon Matrix: Introducing the third dimension, *Injury Prevention, 4* (4), 302–307.

Rutter, D., & Quine, L. (2002). *Changing health behavior.* Philadelphia: Open University Press.

Schneiderman, N., Speers, M. A., Silva, J. M., Tomes, H., & Gentry, J. H. (Eds.) (2001). *Integrating behavioral & social sciences with public health.* Washington, DC: American Psychological Association.

Schwartz, R. (Ed.). (2003). Focal point issue: Injury prevention and control. *Health Promotion Practice, 4*, 85–196.

Shaw, F. E., & Ogolla, C. P. (2006). Injury prevention behavior and the law. In A. Gielen, D. A. Sleet, & R. Diclemente (Eds.), *Injury & violence prevention: behavioral science theories, methods and applications.* San Francisco: Jossey-Bass.

Shields, J. (1997). Have we become so accustomed to being passive that we've forgotten to be active? *Injury Prevention, 3*, 243–246.

Sleet, D. A., & Bryn, S. (Eds.). (2003). Injury prevention for children and youth [Special issue]. *American Journal of Health Education, 34* (5), (Supplement 1), S1–S64.

Sleet, D. A., Hammond, W. R., Jones, R. T., Thomas, N., & Whitt, B. (2004). Injury and violence prevention in the community. In R. H. Rozensky, N. G. Johnson, C. D. Goodheart, & W. R. Hammond (Eds.), *Building healthy communities: Psychology's role in public health* (pp. 185–216). Washington, DC: American Psychological Association.

Sleet, D. A., Hollenbach, K., & Hovell, M. (1986). Applying behavioral principles to motor vehicle occupant protection. *Education & Treatment of Children, 9* (4), 320–333.

Sleet, D., & Hopkins, K. (Eds.). (2004). *Bibliography on behavioral science research and unintentional injury prevention* [CD-ROM]. Atlanta, GA: Centers for Disease Control and Prevention. National Center for Injury Prevention and Control.

Sleet, D. A., & Lonero, L. (2002). Behavioral strategies for reducing traffic crashes. In L. Breslow (Ed.), *Encyclopedia of Public Health* (pp. 105–107). New York: Macmillan.

Sleet, D. A., Trifiletti, L. B., Simons-Morton, B., & Gielen, A. C. (2006). Individual level models: Applications of behavioral theory. In A. C. Gielen, D. A. Sleet, & R. DiClemente (Eds.), *Injury and violence prevention: Behavior change theories, methods and applications.* San Francisco: Jossey-Bass.

Smedley, B. D., & Syme, S. L. (Eds.). (2000). *Promoting health: Intervention strategies from social and behavioral research.* Washington, DC: National Academy Press.

Spinks, A., Turner, C., McClure, R., Acton, C., & Nixon, J. (2005). Community-based programmes to promote use of bicycle helmets in children aged 0–14 years: A systematic review. *International Journal of Injury Control & Safety Promoton, 12* (3), 131–143.

Streff, F. M., & Geller, E. S. (1986). Strategies for motivating safety belt use: The application of applied behavior analysis. *Health Education Research, 1*, 47–59.

Svanstrom, L. (1999). Building safe communities—a safety promotion movement entering 2000. In *Best Practices; Quality and effectiveness of health promotion.* Proceeding of 4th European CIUHPE Conference, Helsinki and Tallinn, 1999, pp. 102–112.

Thompson, N. J., Sleet, D., & Sacks, J. J. (2002). Increasing the use of bicycle helmets: Lessons from behavioral science. *Patient Education and Counseling, 46* (3), 191–197.

Treno, A. J., & Holder, H. D. (1997). Community mobilization: Evaluation of an environmental approach to local action, *Addiction, 92* (Supplement 2), 173–187.

Triandis, H. C. (1980). Values, attitudes and interpersonal behavior. In H. E. Howe, & M. M. Page (Eds.), *Nebraska symposium on motivation 1979* (pp. 197–259). Lincoln: University of Nebraska Press.

Trifiletti L. B., Gielen A. C., Sleet D. A., & Hopkins K. (2005). Behavioral and social sciences theories and models: Are they used in unintentional injury prevention research? *Health Education Research, 20* (3), 298–307.

Wallack, L., Dorfman, L., Jernigan, D., & Themba, M. (1993). *Media advocacy and public health: Power for prevention.* Thousand Oaks, CA: Sage.

Zaza, S., & Thompson R. S. (Eds.). (2001). The guide to community preventive services: Reducing injuries to motor vehicle occupants: Systematic reviews of evidence, recommendations from the Task Force on Community Preventive Services, and expert commentary. *American Journal of Preventive Medicine, 21* (4S), 1–90.

Chapter 23

Developing Interventions When There Is Little Science

Carol W. Runyan and Kimberley E. Freire

23.1. INTRODUCTION

Injury control practice would be easy if only there were packaged programs that were sure to work in any setting and that all one had to do was open them up, implement them and—*Voilá*—watch the rates of injury decline. It would be like having a simple cake mix that works anywhere with only the addition of water. But this is not the case. Few highly successful packaged programs exist. And even when evidence of success exists, it can be hard to know which program components were the active "ingredients" responsible for the outcomes. There is often no clear recipe for exactly replicating the intervention. Plus, no two settings are completely alike, requiring careful adaptation to the particular environmental and cultural characteristics of different populations. Program development is not as straightforward as taking a new medical procedure from one hospital to the next. Injury and the prevention of injury, as with other complex public health problems, result from the interplay of complicated social dynamics that must be accommodated.

Consequently, successful injury interventions rely on sound planning to determine which strategies to implement and which injury risks to change. Interventions can include one or more strategies that address injury risks at different levels and different approaches to program and policy. For example intervention strategies may include policies intended to change environments (e.g., changes in playground design), policies intended to modify behaviors (e.g., seat belt laws), and efforts at the organizational level (e.g., changes in the safety climate within a workplace or screening procedures within a health care facility). Interventions may also include strategies directed at modifying behaviors of individuals at risk (e.g., pedestrian education), caregivers (e.g., appropriate discipline of children), and those who make or enforce policy decisions (e.g., legislator's consideration of smoke alarm legislation, school coaching practices or law enforcement of speed limits).

This chapter is designed to help practitioners develop strategies for intervention development that uses available and appropriate evidence when it does exist and facilitates progress even when scientific evidence has not been well developed. It addresses what planners need to consider in assessing an injury problem and structuring an intervention by applying a systematic approach to planning that relies on critical thinking skills. In addition, this chapter includes questions for practitioners to consider and suggests important areas for professional development.

23.2. PRINCIPLES UNDERLYING INTERVENTION PLANNING

In an analysis of successful interventions for substance abuse, risky sexual behaviors, delinquency and violence, and school failure, published in the 1990s, Nation et al. (2003) reviewed 35 interventions and cataloged the characteristics of effective programs. This analysis identified program elements critical to success. First, the more comprehensive programs had greater effect. This included both programs that employ multiple interventions (e.g., information and awareness interventions and interventions focused on skill development) and interventions that engaged with multiple settings (e.g., clinical and school settings). In addition, the authors noted that programs that used varied teaching methods were more effective as were those that incorporated a sufficient dosage of intervention, were theory driven, promoted positive relationships, were appropriately timed, were tailored to the sociocultural norms of the community, included outcome evaluation, and were conducted by well-trained staff.

Although Nation et al. (2003) focused on interventions that addressed educational strategies and a limited range of behavioral problems, the list of characteristics associated with successful programs highlights the kinds of issues that injury planners need to consider—for example, the importance of tackling problems at multiple levels and relying on more than one method, with adequate dose or intensity over sufficient time periods for the intervention to effect change. Extending from this is the essential process of carefully considering what other interventionists have done and learning from their successes and failures through the use of sound evidence-based approaches.

As described in other chapters, evidence-based planning increasingly is recommended for public health, health promotion, and injury prevention interventions, drawing on the lessons from evidence-based medicine (Brownson, Baker, Leet, & Gillespie, 2003; Glasgow, Lichtenstein, & Marcus, 2003; Rychetnik & Wise, 2004) An evidence-based approach emphasizes the importance of applying sound scientific principles to understanding problems and designing solutions. However, public health interventions, including those designed to address injury problems, can be complex and require components addressing multiple interacting levels within a social-ecological framework (Bronfenbrenner, 1979; Stokols, 1992). A social-ecological perspective to injury prevention argues that practitioners should pay attention to risk and protective factors at the level of the individual who is at risk (i.e., the intrapersonal level) as well as factors at the interpersonal level (i.e., the interactions among the individual at risk and other individuals with whom he or she associates, such as friends, colleagues, and family members) (Runyan, 2003). Another level addresses organizational issues, including the various institutions with which the person interacts, such as schools, workplaces, and religious organizations; and finally the sociocultural level made up of the social customs and norms as well as governmental policies, laws, and regulations that affect all the other levels.

Varied types of intervention strategies are available. One relatively simple typology can help the practitioner think through some of the possible approaches along two continua. One continuum, from mandatory to voluntary, addresses the extent to which interventions rely on mandatory (e.g., passing and enforcing laws that require certain behaviors) to coercive (e.g., using insurance incentives), to persuasive strategies (e.g., education encouraging voluntary behavior change). The other dimension refers to the extent to which the strategy is active (i.e., requiring individuals to take steps to effect change) vs. passive (i.e., strategies that are engineered into the environment). Examples are given in Table 23.1 (Runyan, Fischer, Moore, Waller, & Hooten, 1993).

Deciding among intervention strategies should, ideally, rely on sound evidence so as to enhance the probability of program success. Unfortunately, in a young field like injury prevention, there is not an extensive base of evidence on which to build. Furthermore, programs that have been effective for one group may not work for other groups—for example, different cultural groups, adults vs. children or boys vs. girls. Consequently, the practitioner faces a major challenge of deciding what evidence is good enough when making decisions about how to most judiciously use scarce resources to design and deliver the best interventions in a manner that is socially acceptable and culturally appropriate. Practitioners can partner with university and other institutional collaborators to learn where to find scientific evidence and how to evaluate its quality. In addition, they can partner with other stakeholders to collect, interpret, and apply lessons from informal data sources, such as intended audiences, community leaders, and practitioner colleagues. A challenge for all practitioners is making the transition from the established evidence to an intervention that works in their own settings and then contributing back to the field by critically examining these efforts through careful observation and evaluation and by making the results of the work accessible to others. Even more difficult is the need to build a sound approach to addressing a particular injury problem when there is little scientific evidence about what does and does not work. This chapter helps with these challenges.

Table 23.1. Continuum of Intervention Approaches

Approach	Active	Passive
Voluntary	Interventions that rely on repeated voluntary actions (wearing bike helmets, driving safely, providing adequate supervision of children, storing guns safely)	Interventions that rely on voluntary action to put in place a passive intervention (requesting plumbers to set hot water heaters at a safe level on installation, encouraging families to install a fence around swimming pools, encouraging families to buy only personalized guns)
Mandatory	Interventions that mandate individual action (requiring seat belt or child restraint use, requiring use of motorcycle helmets, requiring safe storage of firearms in homes with children)	Passive interventions that are required by law (requiring air bags in all cars, requiring pool fencing, requiring that only personalized firearms be sold)

23.3.   A SYSTEMATIC APPROACH TO INTERVENTION PLANNING

Sound interventions require careful planning. Figure 23.1 provides a model for planning developed by Freire and Runyan (2006) that represents a combination of a standard program-planning approach, the PRECEDE-PROCEED model

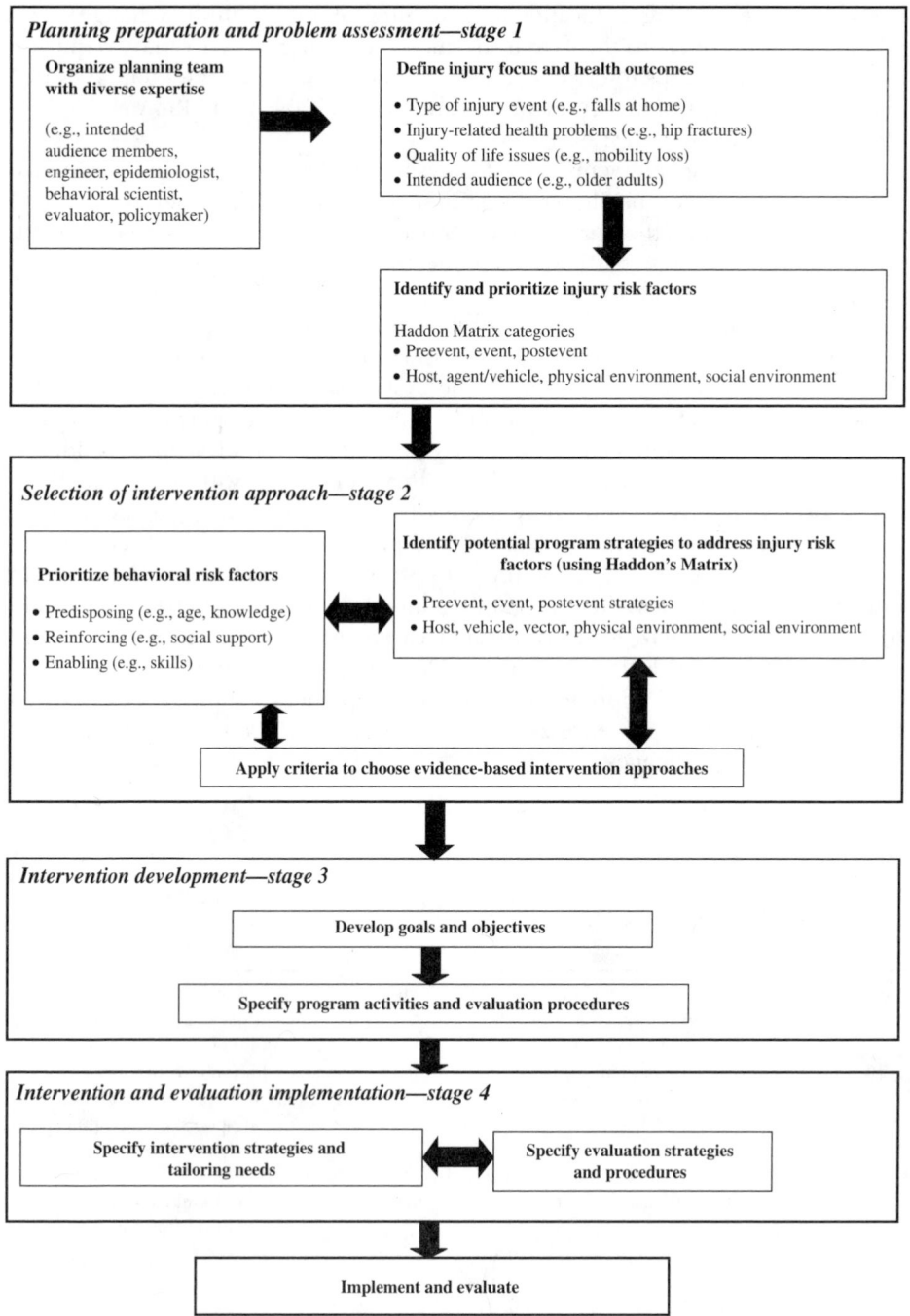

Figure 23.1. Planning process. (Reprinted with permission from Freire & Runyan [2006]).

(Green & Kreuter, 2005), with the Haddon Matrix (Haddon, 1972, 1980; Runyan, 1998). Throughout the planning process multiple types of evidence are necessary. Problem assessment requires both surveillance data and other information about the affected population or community. Other types of evidence address what risk factors can be modified through interventions, what interventions work in what situations, and what evaluation approaches have been successful. At each stage, practitioners need to assess what evidence already is available and what is possible to collect to inform planning. The chapter describes four stages of a process, with emphasis on selecting an intervention approach.

23.3.1. Stage 1—Planning Preparation and Problem Assessment

In stage 1 (Fig. 23.1), planners should begin program development with a clear understanding of the injury problem they will address—it's nature, scope, and magnitude in the given population. Once the problem is clarified, planners can judge whether the problem is important and how it fits within their organization's mission and scope of work. Planners must make choices among priorities within the context of scarce resources while balancing professional judgments, community interests, and community will. Some problems have high incidence but lower severity (e.g., minor sprains/strains encountered during sports), whereas others are of lower incidence but high severity (e.g., concussions or amputations). Though difficult to balance these two factors, especially when resources are limited, the planner must make such judgments. As part of this process, one also needs to consider the extent to which the problem is preventable (Green & Kreuter, 2005). Although progress will never be made if hard problems are avoided, there may be advantages to starting with important (by incidence and severity) problems that can be addressed successfully, then tackling harder problems building on a history of success.

This process also requires considering both one's professional wisdom and that of the community. Without community buy-in, even the best intervention may have limited success. On the other hand, relying solely on community perspectives and not applying what trained professionals know is equally unwise. Learning to balance these influences in helping a community arrive at its own decisions about what topics and issues to tackle and how to tackle them requires finesse and experience. There is a growing literature on community participatory action research that provides guidance about these issues (Leung, Yen, & Minkler, 2004; Minkler, 2000).

It is also helpful to affirm that tackling a given problem is within the mission of the organization and to consider whether and how affiliating with other groups would strengthen the organization's capabilities, recognizing that no one organization can do everything (Box 23.1).

A practitioner cannot accurately assess how a program affected an injury problem unless the problem can be clearly defined. Therefore, if it is not possible to clearly define the problem or if the problem is of limited importance, one should consider moving on to other issues. If the problem is important but not fully within the scope of the organization, carefully assess partnership opportunities. And, if the problem is important, but the evidence is of limited availability or quality, one should develop the foundation more fully before proceeding. This argues for a team of people having expertise in epidemiology and surveillance as well as other forms of needs assessment who can help interpret data. Consider the issues identified with stage 1 in Figure 23.1 as part of defining the injury focus and health outcome of interest and prioritizing the risk factors to address.

Box 23.1. *Questions to Consider at Stage 1*

- *Have you clearly defined the problem?*
- *What additional information do you need to define the problem?*
- *Are the incidence and severity of the problem sufficient to warrant attention?*
- *How important is the problem relative to other priorities from the perspective of the community (i.e., those affected) and the professionals responsible for addressing the problem in the community?*
- *Does tackling this problem fall within the scope of your organization, collaborating groups, and resources?*
- *What additional resources can you obtain to tackle the most important problems?*
- *What evidence exists about the problem in peer-reviewed journals to help you understand and prioritize what risk or protective factors to address with an intervention? Specifically, consider the following:*
  - *How much evidence is there?*
  - *How good is the quality of the evidence?*
  - *How applicable is it to your situation?*

The Haddon Matrix can be used here as a means of helping identify risk factors (an example is given in Table 23.2). The matrix combines the time element inherent in the process of an injury (the rows) with elements that are either modifiable risk factors or protective factors consistent with the social-ecological framework (the columns). The rows define the preevent phase (before the person comes in contact with the injury producing energy), the event phase (during the time when the energy is causing injury), and the postevent phase (after an injury has occurred but while it is still possible to influence the severity of injury or the outcome). The risk factors are classified in terms of individual (host) factors particular to the biology or behavior of the at-risk person; factors associated with the mechanism by which the energy is delivered (inanimate vehicles such as particular products or animate vectors such as assailants), and the characteristics of the physical environment (workplace design, home construction) and social environment (laws, policies, social climate, norms) that influence and are influenced by all other risk and protective factors. Information from Chapters 1–20 about specific injury problems and cross-cutting issues helps with this process.

23.3.2.   Stage 2—Selecting an Intervention Approach

Once the risk and protective factors are understood, the process requires selecting an intervention approach. The majority of this chapter focuses on this aspect.

Three elements are included in stage 2 (Fig. 23.1). One can start in different places within this step and work through each element and will likely need to cycle through the process more than once. Ultimately, the goal at this stage is to decide who will be the intended audience(s) of the intervention and what specific strategies or combination of strategies will be applied.

Table 23.2. Haddon Matrix Used to Identify Risk Factors: Poisoning

Phase[a]	Risk Factors That Influence Injury Process			
	Host (child and caregiver)	Agent/Vehicle/Vector (energy source and means of transmitting—e.g., chemical products and packaging)	Physical Environment (general environment)	Social Environment (interpersonal, organizational, cultural)
Pre-event (before ingestion)	• Child's developmental factors (e.g., curiosity, lack of judgment) • Parent's characteristics (e.g., distractedness, lack of knowledge of poison hazards, poison storage behaviors, literacy)	• Ease with which the package can be opened • Attractiveness of the substance • Lack of visibility and/or understandability of warning labels (e.g., poorly placed, not visible, not clear, not in language of the reader)	• Absence of locking devices on cabinets • Cupboards where poisons stored in places easy for young child to reach	• Lack of regulations (e.g., marketing of substances in containers that look like food)
Event (during ingestion)	• Child's secrecy about ingesting (e.g., hiding) • Parent's ability to notice unusual behavior on part of child who is ingesting	• Chemical composition of the poison • Substance easy to swallow in sufficient quantities to do harm	• Presence of hiding places where young child could ingest substances and not be noticed	• Inaccessible health care system that deters parents from seeking guidance about potential ingestion
Postevent (after ingestion)	• Child's ability to communicate with adults about what was ingested • Parent's ability to access and communicate with poison-control resources	• Chemical agent that does not have antidote	• Lack of accessibility for emergency vehicles	• Lack of a poison-control facility or emergency medical care • Poor publicity of poison-control resources and how to access them

[a]At which the risk factor has influence.

23.3.2.1.   Consider Behavioral Elements

During this stage, behavior or behavior-related components are considered, including predisposing, enabling, and reinforcing factors (Green & Kreuter, 2005). Sometimes these will focus on the behavior of the individual affected by the injury risk; other times it may be a caregiver (e.g., parent, teacher, health care provider) and other times people who make decisions about design of the physical environment or products (e.g., engineers, architects) or about policies (e.g., legislators, corporate executives). Predisposing factors are individual characteristics such as developmental stage, knowledge, attitudes, and values, all of which affect how individuals perceive an intervention and the intended behavior change. Enabling factors are the skills and resources necessary to facilitate behavioral and environmental change (e.g., access to funding, appropriately trained staff, political will). Reinforcing factors provide negative and positive feedback that affect behavior maintenance. They include such elements as social relationships and the structural factors (e.g., workplace safety climate) that facilitate adherence to worker safety policies (Barling & Frone, 2004; Hofman & Tetrick, 2003). To learn more about these concepts see Green and Kreuter (2005) and Freire and Runyan (2006).

23.3.2.2.   Develop Intervention Ideas

At this stage of the planning process, it is useful to apply the Haddon Matrix in the more traditional way it is used—that is, to generate ideas about interventions. The model (Table 23.3.) facilitates the consideration of a range of strategies to address interventions within the social-ecological framework, helping planners identify strategies directed not only at the person at risk but also at the mechanisms through inanimate vehicles (e.g., consumer products) or animate vectors (e.g., assailants) that transmit injury-producing energy. This could include redesigning potentially dangerous products such as toys, cars, household appliances, and firearms that serve as the vehicles by which the energy is transferred. In addition, one can address behavioral changes in the vector that transmits energy (e.g., intervening with perpetrators to prevent violence-related events). In addition, developing interventions aimed at changing the physical environment might include strategies related to architectural or engineering designs of the home, school, workplace, playground, or highway, such as installation of fencing on bridges to prevent suicides, speed humps on roads, smoke alarms in homes, and improved playground surfacing. The model also highlights the social environment, which may include strategies directed at altering systems, policies, and norms within the institutional or organizational context (e.g., work hours and staffing patterns in a factory, how protocols for diagnosing and reporting child maltreatment are applied in a given health care facility, and how schools monitor playgrounds and crosswalks) as well as broader social and cultural norms. This could be policies that are designed explicitly to affect injuries (e.g., controls on the sale of hazardous consumer products, bike helmet ordinances, required fencing around swimming pools) and social policies that may be designed for broader purposes but have an influence on injury (e.g., policies that affect availability of jobs, welfare programs, or taxes on alcoholic beverages). Social norms also are powerful influences on behavior and on injury prevention. Examples are norms about parenting, child discipline, and supervision; the availability or storage of firearms; the consumption of alcohol; and the use of designated drivers.

Table 23.3. Haddon Matrix Applied to The Problem of Preventing Childhood Poison Ingestion

	Factors to Be Altered by the Intervention			
Phases[a]	Host (child and caregiver)	Agent/Vehicle/Vector (energy source and means of transmitting—e.g., chemical products and packaging)	Physical Environment (general environment)	Social Environments (interpersonal, organizational, cultural)
Pre-event (before ingestion)	• Teach child to avoid poisonous substances	• Childproof packaging of medicines and toxins • Clear labeling of toxic products	• Ensure that homes are built with locked cabinets for storing medicines and other toxins • Encourage stocking and marketing of locking cabinets by home-building stores	• Counseling by pharmacists and physicians about toxicity of chemicals and safe storage • Alter pharmacist dispensing to nonlethal doses in package • Regulate availability of toxic substances that are easily mistaken for edible items
Event (during ingestion)	• Improve parent–child communication to help in responding to questions and describing ingested material • Teach parents how to identify unusual behavior on part of child	• Ensure that drugs are packaged by manufacturer in amounts too small to cause serious consequences even if all are ingested	• Household sound or video-monitoring systems to assist in monitoring child behavior when in another room	• Ready access to poison-control centers
Postevent (after ingestion)	• Teach parents how to contact and communicate effectively with poison-control facility	• Package in containers that are easily stored to reduce temptation to repackage in ways in which substance is not easily identified	• Clear directions, marking of residence to facilitate access by emergency personnel	• Good-quality, affordable emergency medical care available

[a]At which the intervention has its effect.

The other dimension of the matrix facilitates consideration of interventions at various phases of the injury process. Examples of interventions having their effects at different phases are those that prevent a potentially injury-producing event from occurring (e.g., improved brakes to reduce likelihood of a crash), those that reduce the likelihood of injury during an event (e.g., seat belts protecting against injury during a crash), and those that facilitate rescue and recovery (e.g., in-car global positioning devices to facilitate location of wrecks by rescue personnel).

23.3.2.3. *Choosing Interventions*

The other part of stage 2 (Fig. 23.1) is the application of the third dimension of the Haddon Matrix which provides planners with assistance in weighing decisions about which program, among multiple options, to select (Runyan, 1998). This dimension, derived from literature on policy analysis (Haskins & Gallagher, 1981; McRae & Wilde, 1979; Patton & Sawicki, 1993), suggests a variety of value criteria that a planner might want to consider in judging the relative merits of different intervention ideas. Each of these types of criteria relies on different types of evidence either gathered by the planner or derived from other sources. In some cases, the evidence will be directly relevant to the injury problem at hand. In other cases, one may have to rely on information collected for other purposes and make judgments about the applicability to the injury intervention being considered (e.g., parental acceptance of guidance from pediatricians about diet and exercise may provide clues to the extent to which they will be receptive to guidance about discipline or use of child car seats). However, assuming that responses to all problems or solutions are similar should be done with caution, given the complexities of human behavior.

First and foremost is the issue of program effectiveness, which relies on prior intervention evaluations and documentation of the extent to which an intervention worked in other settings. In considering effectiveness, all the issues associated with finding, assessing, and critiquing available scientific evidence and its applicability to the given situation are essential, as discussed more extensively in Chapter 21.

Another important factor to consider is the extent to which a given intervention option is compatible with the preferences, wishes, and cultural beliefs of the affected population. The extent to which the affected community's views and cultural perspective can be addressed will often greatly affect the likelihood of intervention effectiveness. This is important not only to determine which intervention to apply, as it closely relates to the political feasibility of the intervention as well as to issues of cultural sensitivity, but also to ensure that the implementation strategies put into place are culturally appropriate, as discussed below.

In addition, planners also need to consider other criteria such as the costs of doing the intervention (e.g., implementation costs) balanced against the costs of not doing it (e.g., medical care expenses, lost wages). Another consideration is equity. There are two types of equity. Vertical equity concerns equalizing risk through unequal treatment of certain groups so as to make the groups more equal (e.g., car seat giveaway programs for low-income families). Horizontal equity is often addressed by providing universal interventions or services that affect everyone equally (e.g., development and enforcement of building codes for all types of dwellings). For many types of interventions, particularly those that involve mandated changes, there are issues involving restriction of personal freedoms. In this case, it is important to consider how much and what type of restriction on freedom is associated with the intervention and whose freedom is affected. An intervention to

Box 23.2. *Criteria to Consider at Stage 2*

- *Effectiveness*
- *Preferences*
- *Cost*
- *Equity*
- *Freedom*
- *Stigmatization*
- *Feasibility*
- *Others suited to the situation*

protect one group (e.g., freedom of children to walk safely to school) may come into conflict with the freedoms of another group (e.g., drivers wanting to drive faster on certain roadways). Freedom issues often create intense public discourse as in the case of efforts to limit access to certain types of firearms or to require motorcycle helmets. Variations in culture often relate to acceptance of specific safety measures that may restrict freedom.

Another delicate issue is that of stigmatization, a value sometimes considered in intervention planning from the standpoint of avoiding stigmatizing individuals who have some distinguishing characteristic (e.g., poverty, disability, and mental health problems) but is sometimes deliberate (e.g., identifying prior sex offenders in a community). Often stigmatization issues affect the most vulnerable populations, so it requires careful attention.

Finally, once other features of the intervention have been considered, it is important to examine technological and political feasibility. These two factors are often related to effectiveness and equity and freedom issues. As noted above, political feasibility relates to the preferences of the affected community and to many political forces that affect how decisions are made. Again, input from intended audience members can help planners determine how politically feasible selected strategies will be within a given community. To be applied, an intervention must also be technologically feasible (e.g., the technology for intelligent vehicle design has enabled new safety approaches not available a decade ago). Though feasibility issues may present obstacles, they often can be overcome if other criteria all point toward adopting a particular intervention. In addition, any given situation may require consideration of additional or different factors. These should be identified at the outset, with evidence about how much each option does or doesn't achieve the desired criterion considered along with the other criteria suggested here (Box 23.2).

Runyan (1998) describes a process for using this framework to guide planning that includes defining which criteria are important and identifying evidence to address the concerns. The planner needs to decide, with guidance from other stakeholders and community members, how much to emphasize each of these or other criteria in making choices among interventions.

23.3.2.4. *Finding Alternative Sources of Evidence*

In stage 2, it is important to search widely for available evidence about prior interventions to understand effectiveness and value criteria (e.g., cost, political feasibility, community views). The first step is to look for articles published in peer-reviewed journals. The purpose of the peer-review process it to allow critical reviewers to consider a manuscript with a skeptical eye and ask the author to respond to detailed questions before it is determined that the paper is of high enough quality to merit publication. Information indicating if a given journal is peer reviewed is usually found in the section of the journal or journal Web site providing information for authors or by asking a librarian.

Another consideration at this stage is to think about the consistency of results across multiple studies. It is important to examine the whole body of evidence, not just one or two reports. If there are multiple evaluations of the same intervention all pointing in the same direction, even though none is perfect, the weight of the evidence as a whole can be used to help make a judgment. The more there is consistency in the success or failure of trying a given intervention implemented in multiple places, the more likely the result can be successfully generalized to other settings. This does not mean that an intervention tried in only one place is not helpful. But an intervention having been tried in multiple places with consistent findings can strengthen one's confidence in replicating it. On the other hand, taking this too literally may squelch innovation when, in fact, new ideas are needed.

Practitioners must be skeptical but recognize that there may well be successful interventions for which no published report exists. This could be for a variety of reasons. Some who conduct interventions do not do thorough evaluations or do evaluations but never publish their results. It is also important to remember that getting published takes time, so information about newer interventions may take longer than a year to be published. This emphasizes the value of maintaining networks of practitioners who can provide direct information about their experiences and indicate when new findings are being released. In addition, useful information does appear in places other than the peer-reviewed literature.

23.3.2.5. Other Sources

Gray literature describes project reports, technical reports, and monographs. These are written documents that are often filed with funding agencies but have not undergone review by a peer-reviewed journal. Sometimes technical reports can be an excellent source of data on injury incidence and trends as well as local and state injury prevention efforts. Agency collaborators, such as program officers and evaluators, can help practitioners discern the quality of program data by providing a context for data collection and reporting limitations.

There is an increasing amount of information available on the Internet but little or no quality control. Good information can be found on the Web sites of relevant federal agencies (Centers for Disease Control and Prevention, National Highway Traffic Safety Administration, Department of Labor) and many reputable nongovernmental organizations (Insurance Institute for Highway Safety, State and Territorial Injury Prevention Directors Association, the Society for the Advancement of Violence and Injury Research) or via electronic versions of peer-reviewed journals. Lists of research studies in the peer-reviewed literature are updated regularly online at www.safetylit.org.

Starting with searches on reputable Web sites is a good way to get a feel for who is working on an injury problem and which strategies have been implemented. However, it is important to remember that just because it looks slick does not mean it is of high quality. In addition, groups use terms such as "*best*" and "*promising*" practice in different ways and may not apply the same standards of evidence review discussed in this book. Another aspect of this search is to identify whether there are interventions that are considered strong by reputation—that is, known by practitioners to work even if the evidence is not yet available. The use of gray literature or reliance on reputationally strong programs should never substitute for trying to find peer-reviewed literature but is an appropriate addition to the search process and sometimes is the only option available.

23.3.2.6.   *Judging the Evidence*

There are numerous factors to consider in assessing evidence. It is important to consider whether the studies match the problem at hand. This is where having a clear understanding of the problem, derived from careful surveillance and needs assessment is useful. It is also important to assess whether the evidence available can be generalized to the particular setting in which it will be adopted. What "plays in Peoria" may not be equally applicable in Miami or in rural New Mexico. In doing this, consider the specific social and cultural elements of the problem being addressed and the aspects of the interventions as they have been previously applied. Imagine applying this exact intervention in your setting. Does it seem like it would be culturally appropriate and effective or is something off about it? Behavior is complex to understand and to change, and no two situations are exactly alike. Hence it is best to rely on information with some degree of similarity to the situation at hand and make educated guesses about the transferability of the findings. Although this approach is not as good as evidence from a highly similar setting, with a very similar population to address the same problem, useful information often can be gleaned and is far better than starting without benefit of others' experiences. Often this requires subtle judgments that can benefit from discussion among several people knowledgeable about the problem, the setting, and program planning. This is another argument for a team approach that brings varied expertise to the planning process.

Depending on one's success in finding evidence to help structure an intervention, practitioners may be faced with the decision of starting fresh vs. deciding whether to wait until more of a scientific base is developed before tackling the issue. Another consideration is that of thinking through the potential that, by addressing the problem without tested methods, one could actually do harm. For example, screening women to identify domestic violence without a plan for what to do when abuse is discovered may be more harmful than helpful if revealing the abuse puts women at risk with their partners or endangers their children.

23.3.2.7.   *Developing an Intervention Strategy*

As with any public health issue, injury problems can be approached through a wide range of intervention options. There are two key elements to consider. One is to determine what needs to be changed and how that change will result in the desired outcome. For example, the desired change may alter the injury-causing product, the physical environment, social norms, or the behavior of individuals or some combination of these. Two, there needs to be thought given to what is going to be done to bring about this change. For example, if individual behavior change is the key, then understanding issues of knowledge, attitudes, beliefs and behaviors is critical, and interventions might be devised to address any and all of these. If, on the other hand, the focus of the intervention is determined to require changes in the physical environment (e.g., the design of a new playground), then it is critical to determine what is required (e.g., hire a playground designer, change a playground maintenance policy, find funds to purchase new equipment, educate the school board or county commissioners about the need to make the playground safer, and/or raise the awareness of parents about the lack of safety in the playground). In both these examples, the construction of a logic model, as described below, is helpful to clarify the relationships among the factors that need to change to achieve the desired effect (Gielen & McDonald, 2002). As a consequence, one can then disentangle the elements of the problem and the solution and decide where and how to target the intervention—for example, a mass-media campaign to change community awareness, an educational campaign to change individual behaviors, an advocacy strategy to alter policy or raise resources, or an engineering approach to redesign the equipment.

23.3.3.   Stage 3—Intervention Development

23.3.3.1.   Adopting and Adapting Interventions

If sound evidence demonstrates that a given intervention is effective, or at least promising, then it is wise to consider either adopting the intervention or adapting it to your setting rather than starting over. A number of questions are suggested below to help you think about this. Do not underestimate the value of learning from others who have attempted to address the same problem and/or implemented the intervention before. Be sure to ask people to share their experiences of program failures and successes.

   If the evidence does not fit the circumstances in which new planning is taking place, no matter how high the quality, it may be helpful to look at other literatures on related problems and/or similar settings so as to consider whether to adapt information from other domains to the problem at hand. For example, if one is thinking of an initiative to increase use of carbon monoxide detectors, it could be helpful to look at smoke alarm distribution efforts as a close parallel. Likewise, an effort to improve use of fall-protection devices (i.e., harnesses) by young construction workers might benefit from literature on efforts to increase use of protective devices among similarly aged athletes (e.g., football helmets or knee braces). Interventions for the same population aimed at changing other behaviors may also be informative (e.g., efforts to increase construction worker's use of steel-toed boots or adherence to protocols for operating equipment near power lines). Finally, it may be useful to consider the transferability of intervention strategies that have been successful with a different health or injury problem. For example, examining how media campaigns have been successful in reducing tobacco initiation among teens (Hopkins et al., 2001) or alcohol-impaired driving (Elder, Shults, & Sleet, 2004) may be helpful in thinking about the applicability of using media strategies to intervene on specific types of injury or violence problems. Given that public health approaches to injury control are not as longstanding as attempts to address other problems, there is much to be learned from other areas of public health (e.g., infectious or chronic diseases, reproductive issues). However, any of these efforts to transfer experiences from one population, topic, setting, or strategy to another must be done with both caution and careful judgment. Even with a peer-

---

Box 23.3. *Questions to Consider in Adopting or Adapting an Existing Intervention*

- *What types of evidence are available (peer reviewed, gray literature)?*
- *Are there interventions that have a reputation of being good (reputationally strong programs)? What can you learn from these programs?*
- *What is the quality of the evidence from these sources?*
- *How much evidence is there?*
- *How consistent are the results across studies and settings?*
- *How well did the intervention(s) work?*
- *Do the results generalize to your setting?*
    - *How similar to the current population is the population from which the evidence was derived (age distribution, gender distribution, ethnic variations, cultural traditions, injury risk factors, or receptivity)?*
    - *To what extent might these differences between the populations used in other intervention studies make a difference in how the intervention would work in the new setting?*
    - *How similar is the setting to your setting?*
    - *Who carried out the successful intervention (specific types of professionals vs. community members or volunteers)?*
        - *Can the same kind of person or group carry out the intervention in your setting? Would it be culturally appropriate to do so?*
        - *How will the setting affect program implementation?*
        - *What changes would need to be made in the way the intervention is delivered (sequence and timing issues or the general approach)*
        - *What other things about the approach would need to vary (did the other program have a well-known community leader recruit the participants, but you have no such leader)?*
        - *How likely are any of these kinds of factors to alter how the intervention works in the new setting?*
        - *What, if any, elements of the original intervention are not feasible to implement in your setting and how much difference will this make?*
        - *What, specifically, do you need to do to adapt this to your setting?*
- *Are there interventions from parallel literatures (about similar problems in the same or similar populations) from which you can extrapolate?*

---

reviewed paper, it is often wise to contact those who have done the intervention before to learn about their experiences and how it may or may not be transferable to a new locale (Box 23.3).

23.3.3.2. Developing New Interventions

In developing new interventions, a critical stage of planning involves the development of clear goals and objectives. A *goal* articulates the overall purpose of the intervention including what change will occur and who or what will experience the change. Two examples are to reduce mortality from drowning among children age 3 years and younger (injury goal) and to increase use of fall-protection devices by construction workers (behavioral goal). Objectives are more specific, defining more concretely what will be accomplished by whom within a specific time frame.

Ideally, practitioners should be able to link program objectives to specific evalua-tion measures to demonstrate their program's affect. Therefore, objectives should be specific, measurable, achievable, relevant, and time bound (i.e., "SMART") (Green & Kreuter, 2005). Examples of specific objectives are to decrease the rate of drowning among residents of North Carolina by 10% within the first 3 years of the program (injury objective) and during the first year of the program, to increase safety harness use nationally among construction workers by 30% from baseline. It should be very clear from an objective what the criteria of success are and what sources of information are needed to measure success.

In addition to developing goals and objectives, planners can create a logic model to illustrate how program activities relate to changes in risk and protec-tive factors and injury outcomes (W. K. Kellogg Foundation, 2004). Logic models can help planners consider the causal pathway through which an injury process may occur and where in the chain of events an intervention serves to interrupt the process and create new pathways to the desired end. They can also help plan-ners identify obvious gaps in resources, activities or risk factors that will influence program implementation, and injury events. Hence a good logic model helps plan-ners articulate the "theory of change" behind the program.

23.3.4.   Stage 4—Intervention and Evaluation Implementation

As discussed in Chapters 26 and 28, fidelity to the original intervention is criti-cally important when replicating someone else's intervention. Unfortunately, many reports of effective programs often have brief descriptions of program implementa-tion and little discussion of lessons learned. Practitioners can usually contact the original program developers to learn more about the process and potential pitfalls and to get advice about how to adhere to the protocol. It can be useful to ask for copies of forms that have been used to monitor program delivery, participation, or other attributes of process because they can facilitate more precise replication. The interview questions suggested in Box 23.4 can be helpful here as well. Practitioners should understand how any changes or omissions to the original program might

---

Box 23.4. *Suggested Interview Questions*

- *What worked well in carrying out this intervention and what didn't go as planned?*
- *Did some elements of the intervention work better than others? Which ones and why?*
- *What positive or negative unanticipated consequences did you discover?*
- *If you could do the intervention over again, what would you do differently this time around? Be specific about any and all elements that might need revision or refinement.*
- *What aspects do you think are absolutely critical to keep the way you did them? Why is that?*
- *What challenges can I expect if I try to carry this out in my setting (describe your setting)? Can you give me advice about overcoming these challenges?*
- *Do you know others who have tried this same intervention, or one very similar to it, from whom I might learn about their experiences?*

effect desired changes in program outcomes. Some adaptation is likely. The trick is to figure out how much adaptation is appropriate without changing the intervention so much that the prior evaluation results are invalid. This is a judgment call, best considered by a multidisciplinary team experienced in program design. Once adapted, fidelity to the plan established for the new setting is critical.

The purpose of process evaluation is to learn about how the program was carried out. This is particularly important for programs that are not as successful as hoped. It allows the planner to consider whether the program was inherently limited in design or if the problem was in the area of program implementation. If someone has conducted a new intervention, it is hoped that they have documented exactly what constituted the intervention, who carried it out, what they did, and how it may have been modified along the way for any of a variety of reasons. For example if one designs an intervention in which coaches are to encourage their soccer players to voluntarily use shin guards, it is important to know exactly what the coaches did (e.g., made a rule, created incentives, told the players they would lose playing time if they didn't wear them, gave a handout to players about the benefits of shin guards, asked parents to buy shin guards, reminded players to use the shin guards before every game). Perhaps it is clear that the intervention was a reminder to all players before every game. Did this actually get done or did the coach forget to remind players at away games? Did the coach do the reminding at some games and the trainer other times? Was the reminder done in such a way that the players were sure to hear it or was it simply written on the board in the locker room? Any of these variations could potentially affect the outcome of the intervention. If the intervention fails, it is critical to know what was actually done so proper corrective action can be taken rather than to assume the intervention has no worth. Likewise, if the intervention succeeded, it is important to know what was done so that others who want to replicate it will know exactly what the intervention contained.

Unfortunately, process information often is not included in reports of program evaluations. In the absence of process data, the intervention has little meaning and is merely a black box. This would be akin to a surgeon telling another doctor how to do a new type of open-heart surgery by merely saying, "take the patient to the operating room and perform surgery" instead of describing the procedure in detail. In addition to contacting the person who carried out the program and interviewing him or her about process issues, one might consider inviting someone from the prior project's operational team to serve as a consultant.

The extent of adaptation required often is determined by responses to the kinds of questions listed above. If extensive change is envisioned, it may be wise to plan for and conduct a formative evaluation as part of the adaptation process. Issues to think about in adapting an intervention include similarity of the settings in which the intervention has been applied before and the situation in which new application is planned, considering what adjustments for culture, language, or historical changes might be in order. In addition, one should always consider carefully whether certain types of changes may alter the intervention too much. As always, effort should be made to measure any changes made via careful process documentation and evaluation. This will not only help keep the adaptation on target but also permit interpretation of differences in effect compared to the setting in which the interventions were originally implemented. Finally, careful conduct and publication of the process and outcome of your own evaluation is critical to the further development of the field.

23.4.   MAINTAINING SKILLS IN INJURY PREVENTION PRACTICE

Developing, conducting, and evaluating interventions, regardless of the presence of prior evidence, require skills that improve with experience. To help identify the basic competencies for injury control practitioners, the National Training Initiative for Injury and Violence Prevention (NTI) has developed a set of core competencies, drawing on the expertise and input of a national panel of experts. (NTI, 2005) Also of importance are skills in critical thinking, getting help from others, and contributing to the knowledge base in the field.

23.4.1.   Developing Basic Competency in Injury Prevention Practice

Nine core competencies have been defined by the NTI (Table 23.4). For each there are multiple specific objectives outlined for achieving the competency (available at: www.injuryed.org) (NTI, 2005). These core competencies may be achieved by any individual at any level of proficiency, depending on his or her role and the setting in which he or she works. Many of these skill areas are discussed elsewhere in this book. These are intended to help guide individuals' professional development as well as help organizations assemble teams with complementary expertise.

23.4.2.   Critical Thinking

Also important to good science and good practice is asking questions with a skeptical eye, making careful observations, systematically approaching problems, and carefully recording information about what is observed and learned, and sharing that information with others. One needs a certain degree of skepticism when considering what others have done, not trusting information at face value but rather carefully examining its merits and applicability (as discussed above). Also important is a willingness to identify one's own assumptions and biases about how things work and be sure they are based on evidence and not just beliefs without basis in fact. It is often useful to ask: How do I know this? Am I sure I know this? Do I need to

Table 23.4. Core Competencies for Injury and Violence Prevention[a]

- Ability to describe and explain injury and/or violence as a major social and health problem
- Ability to access, interpret, use, and present injury and/or violence data
- Ability to design and implement injury and/or violence prevention activities
- Ability to evaluate injury and/or violence prevention activities
- Ability to build and manage an injury and/or violence prevention program
- Ability to disseminate information related to injury and/or violence prevention to the community, other professionals, key policy makers, and leaders through diverse communication networks
- Ability to stimulate change related to injury and/or violence prevention through policy, enforcement, advocacy, and education
- Ability to maintain and further develop competency as an injury and/or violence prevention professional
- Demonstrate the knowledge, skills, and best practices necessary to address at least one specific injury and/or violence topic (e.g., motor-vehicle occupant injury, intimate partner violence, fire and burns, suicide, drowning, child injury) and be able to serve as a resource regarding that area

---

[a]Developed by the SAVIR-STIPDA Joint Committee on Infrastructure Development (2005). (SAVIR was formerly the National Association of Injury Control Research Centers.)

gather more information to be confident that my assumptions are true? Likewise, be sure you question other people's assumptions—don't take anything as gospel just because someone told you or it is printed in a report. As a general principle: Always question assumptions, especially your own.

23.4.3.   Getting Help

A critical skill is knowing when and how to get extra help from outsiders. Depending on the circumstances, one solution is to find a collaborator and/or seek consultation and technical assistance on specific aspects of the program. In so doing, it is important to consider what aspects of program development, implementation, and evaluation are suited to an individual's own skills and setting and what needs supplementation from outsiders. If ongoing help is needed, it may be helpful to add a collaborator who can invest in the project in the long term. For example, it may be wise to add a collaborator with skills in instrument design, data collection, or program evaluation—elements required at different points in the project. On the other hand, if the need is more short term, requiring someone to help make sense of existing data or to conduct a specific set of focus groups, this might be easily handled by employing a consultant.

Once it is clear what is needed, it is prudent to get advice from more than one person about where to find help. Most university faculty and agency staff are receptive to email or telephone communication from people seeking help, provided the question is focused and that the person asking has done his or her homework and has prepared the request based on careful thought and review of existing resources. Calling with a very broad question such as "I want to develop a program to reduce child injury in my community; where should I start?" is too vague. In contrast, a question such as "I am developing a smoke alarm giveaway program and need help identifying a good instrument for evaluating its effects" is a more easily handled request.

When engaging with a consultant or new collaborator, it is always a good idea to be clear about the scope of help required as well as the timing of work and any deadlines that may exist. For example, calling someone for help with developing an evaluation instrument that needs to be in the field in a week is very different from contacting them as one works toward a deadline in 6 months. Be sure expectations are both realistic and clear. In negotiating this strategy, it may be helpful to explore with the individual what types of barriers or facilitators impinge on his or her ability to assist. For example, faculty often have restricted time schedules associated with the academic calendar but may also be very receptive to consulting work during the summer months and/or be more eager if there are opportunities to collaborate on publications or involve their students.

In addition, be sure to understand any payment (consulting fees, travel) or payback (authorship on publications, access to data) that a consultant may require or expect. It is always best to clarify these kinds of obligations at the outset.

23.4.4.   Sharing Results

Often it is assumed that publishing results of interventions is reserved for academics, yet most interventions do not take place in academic settings. Consequently, it is critical to advancing the science of injury control for practitioners to engage in the process of sharing evidence with the field at large. This requires not only skill development but also a commitment to participating as a member of a community of scholars exchanging experiences and ideas and participating in a scholarly approach to injury control. Though beyond the scope of this chapter, there are resources for learning to prepare and publish papers about practice experience in the peer-reviewed literature (Rivara & Cummings, 2001).

23.5.   CONCLUSION

This chapter has explained a systematic process to program planning, including integration of evidence of various types and at various stages in the planning process. The chapter introduces readers to a range of issues related to finding and evaluating various types of evidence and possible intervention approaches. Many of these topics are addressed more fully in other chapters of this volume and in other sources.

Systematically developing and implementing interventions are critical components of the quest to reduce injury. The science base to support this work is multidisciplinary and multifaceted, requiring clear and collaborative thinking to be successful. More important than any of the specific guidance offered is taking a perspective that injuries are preventable, that no one approach is likely to solve any problem, and that change takes a long time. But change is possible with careful thinking and perseverance.

ACKNOWLEDGMENTS.   This chapter has benefited from critical review and helpful suggestions from reviewers of earlier drafts: Dr. Corinne Peek-Asa, Dr. Lynda Doll, Dr. Renee Johnson, Ms. Janet Place, and Dr. Desmond Runyan. This work was supported, in part, by funding from the National Center for Injury Prevention and Control to the University of North Carolina Injury Prevention Research Center (Grant number 1R49/CE000196-01) and by a R. J. Reynolds Faculty Leave from the University of North Carolina at Chapel Hill to Dr. Runyan.

REFERENCES

Barling, J., & Frone, M. (2004). *The psychology of workplace safety.* Washington, DC: American Psychological Association.

Bronfenbrenner, U. (1979). *The ecology of human development.* Cambridge, MA: Harvard University Press.

Brownson, R. C., Baker, E. A., Leet, T. L., & Gillespie, K. N. (2003). *Evidence Based Public Health.* New York: Oxford Press.

Elder, R. W., Shults, R. A., & Sleet, D. A. (2004). Effectiveness of mass media campaigns in reducing alcohol-impaired driving: A systematic review. *American Journal of Preventive Medicine, 25,* 57–65.

Freire, K., & Runyan, C. W. (2006). Planning models: PRECEDE/PROCEED and Haddon Matrix. In A. C. Gielen, D. Sleet, & R. J. DiClemente (Eds.), *Injury prevention: Behavior change theories, methods and applications.* San Francisco: Jossey-Bass.

Gielen, A. C., & McDonald, E. M. (2002). Using the PRECEDE-PROCEED planning model to apply health behavior theories. In K. Glanz, B. K. Rimer, & F. M. Lewis (Eds.), *Health behavior and health education: theory, research and practice* (pp. 409–436, 3rd ed.). San Francisco: Jossey-Bass.

Glasgow, R. E., Lichtenstein, E., Marcus, A. C. (2003). Why don't we see more translation of health promotion research to practice? Rethinking the efficacy-to-effectiveness transition. *American Journal of Public Health, 93* (8), 1261–1267.

Green, L. W., & Kreuter, M. W. (2005). *Health program planning: An educational and ecological approach* (4th ed.). New York: McGraw-Hill.

Haddon, W. (1972). A logical framework for categorizing highway safety phenomena and activity. *Journal of Trauma, 12,* 193–207.

Haddon, W. (1980). Advances in the epidemiology of injuries as a basis for public policy. *Public Health Reports, 95,* 411–421.

Haskins, R., & Gallagher, J. (1981). *Models for social policy analysis: An introduction.* Norwood, NJ: Ablex Press.

Hofman, D. A., & Tetrick, L. E. (2003). *Health and safety in organizations: A multilevel perspective.* San Francisco: Jossey-Bass.

Hopkins, D. P., Briss, P. A., Ricard, C. J., Husten, C. G., Carande-Kulis, V. G., Fielding, J. E., Alao, M. O., McKenna, J. W., Sharp, D. J., Harris, J. R., Woollery, T. A., Harris, K. W., & Task Force on Community Preventive Services. (2001). Reviews of evaluations regarding interventions to reduce tobacco use and environmental exposure to tobacco smoke. *American Journal of Preventive Medicine, 20* (2S), 16–66.

Leung, M. W., Yen, I. H., & Minkler, M. (2004) Community based participatory research: A promising approach to increasing epidemiology's relevance in the 21st century. *International Journal of Epidemiology, 33* (3), 499–506.

McRae, D., & Wilde, J. (1979). *Policy analysis for public decisions.* Belmont, CA: Duxbury Press.

Minkler, M. (2000). Using participatory action research to build health communities. *Public Health Reports, 115* (2–3), 191–197.

Nation, M., Crusto, C., Wandersman, A., Kumpfer, K. L., Seybolt, D., Morissey-Kane, E., & Davino, K. (2003). What works in prevention. Principles of effective prevention programs. *American Psychologist, 58* (6–7), 449–456.

National Training Initiative for Injury and Violence Prevention (NTI) (2005). Retrieved March 1, 2006, from www.injuryed.org.

Patton, C. V., & Sawicki, D. S. (1993). *Basic models of policy analysis and planning.* Englewood Cliffs, NJ: Prentice Hall.

Rivara, F. P., & Cummings, P. (2001). Writing for publication in *Archives of Pediatrics and Adolescent Medicine. Archives of Pediatric and Adolescent Medicine, 155,* 1090–1092.

Runyan, C. W. (1998). Using the Haddon Matrix: Introducing the third dimension. *Injury Prevention, 4,* 302–307.

Runyan, C. W. (2003). Introduction: Back to the future—Revisiting Haddon's conceptualization of injury epidemiology and prevention. *Epidemiologic Reviews, 25,* 60–64.

Runyan, C. W., Fischer, P., Moore, J., Waller, P., & Hooten, E. (1993). Attempting to change local injury policy. *Family & Community Health, 5* (4), 6–74.

Rychetnik, L., & Wise, M. (2004). Advocating evidence-based health promotion: reflections and a way forward. *Health Promotion International, 19* (2), 247–257.

Stokols, D. (1992). Establishing and maintaining healthy environments: Toward a social ecology of health promotion. *American Psychologist, 47,* 6–22.

W. K. Kellogg Foundation. (2004). *Logic model development guide: Using logic models to bring together planning, evaluation and action.* Retrieved August 5, 2005, from www.wkkf.org.

Chapter 24

Developing and Implementing Communication Messages

Nadine Henley, Rob J. Donovan, and
Mark J. Francas

24.1. INTRODUCTION

Creating effective communication messages involves a two-step process: "getting the right message" and "getting the message right" (Egger, Donovan, & Spark, 1993, p. 79). The first step requires understanding how people can be motivated to try to change behavior (e.g., install back seat passenger restraints) or to initiate an intermediate behavior (e.g., ask about the efficacy of such restraints and their cost of installation) through changing attitudes and beliefs. We identify a number of principles to apply when designing communication messages for social change and demonstrate the importance of formative research methods in this process, such as in-depth interviews with key stakeholders and focus groups with members of the target audience. The second step in creating effective communication messages, "getting the message right," involves generating alternative ways of communicating the identified motivators and pretesting these executions with appropriate target audiences.

A case study will be used throughout this chapter to illustrate theory and process. The case study is the innovative Western Australian Freedom From Fear campaign to prevent domestic violence by targeting male perpetrators of intimate partner violence to voluntarily call the Men's Domestic Violence Helpline to seek help to stop their violence (Donovan, Francas, Paterson, & Zappelli, 2000; Donovan, Paterson & Francas, 1999). The principles illustrated here can apply to any unintentional injury campaign; hence occasional reference is made to other injury prevention campaigns.

It should also be emphasized that communication campaigns by themselves are not expected to bring about long-established, habitual, or addicted behavior change. However, they can by themselves initiate intermediate behaviors such as calling a helpline or asking for advice, which requires that these elements also be present and efficacious. For example, the decision to make a call to the Men's Domestic Violence Helpline requires some courage on the part of the caller, and the act of calling often follows a period of indecision. For some men, there is only a small window of opportunity when the perpetrator actually makes the call, usually in the remorse phase of what is known as the cycle of abuse (Roberts, 1984). Hence it is important that sufficient staff are always on hand to receive and act on calls.

In most cases then, the role of media components is to sensitize people to other program elements by maintaining salience and motivating people to respond to program components when opportunities are presented (Egger et al., 1993; Donovan & Henley, 2003). This case study is about motivating an intermediate behavior: calling the Men's Domestic Violence Helpline or seeking professional assistance to reduce violent behavior.

As far as we are aware, this campaign is a unique initiative, being the first government-funded, mass-media, nonpunitive campaign targeted primarily toward male perpetrators of domestic violence (men who have committed violent acts against their partner) and potential perpetrators (men who have subjected their partner to nonphysical forms of abuse because this behavior is often a precursor to physical violence). Rather than threatening imprisonment and other legal sanctions, the campaign asked them to voluntarily seek help to change by amplifying feelings of guilt and remorse in perpetrators and by emphasizing the effects of violence on children. This message was universally relevant. Primary target audience members who did not have children still responded to this message, many of them recalling their own experience of violence as children.

The secondary target audience included all men, given that attitudes of men in general toward violence against women provides a social context for such violence. Further target audiences included professionals who may come into contact with members of the primary target audience, victims and their families, and the community in general.

Mass-media advertising was used to create and maintain awareness of the Men's Domestic Violence Helpline and to encourage violent and potentially violent men to call the helpline, which was staffed by qualified, experienced male violence counselors. The primary aim of the helpline counselors was to refer as many qualified callers as possible into no-fee government-funded counseling programs provided primarily by private-sector organizations. Traditionally, programs aimed at a reduction of abuse have been based around the criminal justice system, targeting both police and the judiciary. In Australia, women no longer have to lodge a complaint before police can charge the perpetrator with assault (thus removing one of the major barriers to women reporting incidents). A major target with the judiciary has been to obtain mandatory treatment programs for offenders (Healey & Smith, 1998). Where public education components have accompanied such campaigns, these have aimed at increasing the public's (and perpetrators') perception that domestic violence is a crime (Buchanan, 1996). Such campaigns generally encourage women to report incidents and, where necessary, to leave the family home and to take out civil protection (or restraining) orders against violent partners.

Although the incarceration of violent men and the issuing of protection orders are necessary components of domestic violence prevention interventions, and do alleviate some violence (Keilitz, Davis, Efkeman, Flango, & Hannaford, 1998), they do not—and cannot—remove the fear women experience in terms of the man reappearing some time, some place, often with tragic consequences (De Becker, 1998). Furthermore, many women do not want to leave the relationship, nor do they want the man incarcerated; they simply want the violence to stop. The Freedom From Fear campaign acknowledges these factors and aims to reduce women's (and children's) fear by encouraging perpetrators and potential perpetrators to voluntarily attend counseling (perpetrator or batterer programs). These programs vary in their approach (Jukes 1999; Lee, Sebold, & Uken, 2003); and although the results of the programs are mixed and many are not evaluated in the longer term, the overall finding is that they can be effective in reducing short-term and long-term violence, especially where a co-existing problem such as alcohol or drug abuse is dealt with concurrently (Gondolf, 2002).

Getting the right message involves identifying what message(s) will motivate the target audience to adopt the recommended action (what advertising agency people call the hot buttons to push). Developing the right messages takes into account the target audience's initial knowledge, beliefs, and attitudes and has the capacity to shift beliefs, attitudes, and behavior in the desired direction.

In this context a *belief* can be defined as a perception that a certain state of affairs exists or is true (regardless of whether it is or not), and an *attitude* can be defined as the extent to which positive or negative feelings are held toward a state of affairs. A state of affairs can include references to objects, persons, behaviors, or ideas. The *salience* of a belief refers to the readiness with which a belief comes to mind when the person's attention is drawn to the issue. In many cases, an expressed attitude will depend on what beliefs come to mind when a person is asked about a particular issue (Donovan & Henley, 2003).

When implementing a communication campaign to create awareness of and positive attitudes toward a concept, issue, or behavior, whether face to face or mass mediated, the first step should focus on issues for which there is most agreement between the desired end point and the target audience's existing attitudes and beliefs. In many cases, existing areas of agreement may have low salience (i.e., rarely thought about), or are weakly held. Beginning the communication process from a point of common agreement also builds source credibility and trust. This provides a favorable context within which to neutralize negative attitudes and beliefs and to create positive attitudes and beliefs. Once a platform of credibility is established, strategies such as attaching a negative belief to a positive belief to increase the likelihood of acceptance of the negative belief can be used.

In the Freedom From Fear campaign, the primary communication objectives for all audiences—perpetrators, victims, counselors, and the wider community—were that the perpetrator, not the victim, is responsible for the violence and that there are no circumstances in which violence is justified. For members of the primary target audience (male perpetrators and potential perpetrators), the main communication objectives were to increase awareness that nonpunitive, anonymous help was available and to stimulate motivations and intentions to seek help. The intermediate behavioral objective was that they should call the helpline for assistance or seek assistance from some credible source. The final behavioral objectives—particularly after counseling—were a reduction in violent incidents, both physical and nonphysical, among perpetrators and the prevention of violence among potential perpetrators.

Formative research was conducted to establish what would motivate violent and potentially violent men to seek help.

24.2.   OBJECTIVES

The broad objectives of the first phase of research were to:

- Gain some understanding of perpetrators' beliefs and attitudes, and hence assess whether reaching and affecting the primary target group was viable via mass-media advertising.
- Examine the awareness, knowledge, attitudes, perceptions, and behaviors of men in general, with respect to domestic violence.
- Assess the effectiveness of five potential message themes for a community education campaign: criminal sanctions, community intervention, social disapproval, consequences, and help is available; these themes were derived from the literature and talking with stakeholders.

24.3.   SAMPLES FOR FORMATIVE RESEARCH

24.3.1.   Perpetrators

Three group discussions, arranged through organizations providing counseling programs, were held with violent men. All participants were in treatment programs, some voluntarily and others court mandated. Their participation in the group discussions was voluntary. Counselors were on hand to debrief the men if issues were raised that needed attention, and a criminologist assisted in the planning and moderating of the initial groups.

Because these men were in counseling programs for various lengths of time, the groups contained a mix of men in the various stages of change (Prochaska & DiClemente, 1984). The stages of change concept has been recommended for social marketing programs (Andreasen, 1995; Donovan & Owen, 1994) and was used in an evaluation of the Milwaukee Women's Center's perpetrator interventions (National Center for Injury Prevention and Control [NCIPC], 1999). The men's statements allowed identification of their stage status (e.g., statements with respect to responsibility and blame; whether the violence was deserved; empathy for the victim; attitude to the treatment program). One aim of the qualitative research was to identify and assess the appropriate motivators for men in the contemplation stage because contemplators are considered the most likely to respond to any mass-media-driven public health/injury prevention campaign. Participants in the perpetrator groups were obviously not blind to the topic of discussion, hence a warm-up discussion, common to most focus groups, was superfluous. Instead, the moderators got straight to the point of what sort of communication campaign could prevent men's violence against their partners.

24.3.2.   General-Population Males

A total of 15 focus groups were conducted with general-population males aged 18–40 years, stratified by age and social economic status. Of these 9 groups were conducted in the metropolitan area of the state's capital and 6 groups were held in four regional towns. The groups were recruited by a professional recruiting agency. It was assumed that these groups would include a number of potentially (or actually) violent men, although group participants were not asked this directly.

In order not to sensitize participants to the issue of domestic violence (which might have resulted in violent or potentially violent men or those with positive attitudes to partner violence excluding themselves), all group participants at recruitment were told only that the groups would be discussing some important social issues. The issue of violence in society was introduced at the start of the discussion. This allowed the issue of domestic violence to arise spontaneously in discussion (which it invariably did), and hence allowed the moderator to focus on this area without being seen to impose the topic on the group.

The moderator probed men's general beliefs and attitudes about intimate partner violence (perceived causes, definitions, awareness of and reaction to previous campaigns), and attempted to elicit examples of physical or verbal/emotional abuse in participants' current or previous relationship(s) or in their friends' and relatives' relationships.

Domestic violence was perceived by men in general as an important issue, and they generally had an understanding that domestic violence incorporated not just physical violence but included emotional and verbal abuse, social isolation, and financial deprivation. Hence there was seen to be little need for a campaign to deal just with identifying these behaviors as domestic violence.

Three important points emerged from the research with perpetrators:

- The first time (i.e., the first act of physical violence) is a critical event that facilitates subsequent violence. Hence the campaign needed to attract potentially violent men to seek help before this first act of violence occurred.
- Many perpetrators expressed shame and guilt about their behavior, yet were unaware of where or how to seek help without legal implications. Hence the primary target audience and the underlying rationale of the campaign were confirmed.
- Many perpetrators exhibited a siege mentality and felt persecuted. They considered the allocation of 100% blame for domestic violence to men as being grossly unfair. This highlighted that messages would need to avoid an accusatory or blaming tone to avoid being rejected by perpetrators.

24.4.   POTENTIAL MESSAGE THEMES

24.4.1.   Criminal Sanctions

Criminal sanctions were not seen as a significant deterrent or as entirely credible by perpetrators or males in general. Perpetrators with considerable experience with the criminal justice system commented that legal sanctions were often not particularly severe and therefore had little deterrent effect: "The first couple of times you'd probably just get probation . . . it wouldn't make you stop doing it." Furthermore, many perpetrators had seen men getting away with domestic violence over the course of many years.

24.4.2.   Community Intervention

The theme of encouraging people to report or intervene in suspected cases of domestic violence was largely rejected by perpetrators (and males in general) because it was deemed inconsistent with social norms (i.e., there is a culture in Australia that it is not acceptable to dob in [inform on] people to legal authorities). Furthermore, no doubt reinforced by their own experiences, the theme lacked credibility in that perpetrators felt other people would be reluctant to get involved—and in general did express such reluctance.

24.4.3.   Social Disapproval

Men in general reacted favorably to the theme that violent behavior toward a female is unacceptable for a man and that men who engage in such behavior should be rejected by their peers. Perpetrators, however, doubted the credibility of such an approach, and several of them reacted angrily to the peer rejection message; it seemed to exacerbate the siege mentality alluded to earlier. As perpetrators were the primary target audience, this message was not deemed potentially efficacious.

24.4.4.   Consequences

Two separate themes were tested with perpetrators and men in general: damage to partner and damage to children. Men in general doubted that perpetrators cared sufficiently about the damage to their partners for this approach to be effective. They considered that perpetrators' violent behavior was self-evident proof that this would not be a motivating factor. Furthermore, most perpetrators in our groups provided little indication that such an appeal would motivate them to seek help, even when they admitted that their behavior caused harm. It appears that for many, their partner's resilience may have lessened an appreciation of the physical harm caused, with little appreciation of psychological harm. Evidence suggests that many violent men have an inability to empathize with the harm caused to their victims (Jukes 1993, 1999). Hence, rather than being a motivator to take action, the development of such an empathy is the task of perpetrator counseling programs.

In contrast, damage to children was a powerful motivator among perpetrators, whether they had children or not. Those with children expressed strong feelings for their children, with some recalling that their children's reactions to specific instances of domestic violence had a very vivid impact on them. Both men with and without children also responded that this approach stimulated recall of their own feelings in violent family situations when they were children. Furthermore, the damage to children theme was also accepted by precontemplator perpetrators and hence had potential to move this group toward contemplation. This theme was also considered to be an effective theme by men in general and was selected as the key motivating strategy for the initial phase of the campaign.

24.4.5.   Help Is Available

The theme that help is available was universally endorsed by perpetrators because it was seen as a positive message that addressed the siege mentality syndrome and because many were aware that they needed help but did not know how to go about getting it. The view of most perpetrators was that the focus should be on access to formal help (e.g., counseling programs, treatment programs) rather than informal help. This theme was also strongly endorsed by men in general. There was broad support for a media campaign to publicize this assistance.

Overall then, the formative research confirmed the viability of reaching violent and potentially violent men via a mass-media campaign that was nonjudgemental, offered formal assistance, and emphasized the damage to children that men's violence caused. The specific communication objectives were (1) children are adversely affected by domestic violence and (2) help is available. The specific behavioral objective was Call the Helpline.

24.5. MESSAGE ACCEPTANCE

Donovan and Henley (2003) identified the following tactics that increase message acceptance in high involvement controversial areas such as domestic violence prevention:

- Link the desired belief to an already accepted belief or one that cannot easily be refuted. In Freedom From Fear, violent men may not readily accept that their violence harms their partner, but they will readily accept that exposure to violence adversely affects their or their partner's children.
- Stay within the target audience's latitude of acceptance—that is, the claimed threat and/or promised benefit must not be exaggerated. In Freedom From Fear, the depiction of an adverse effect on children should be credible; help can be realistically depicted as available right now (but it would not be realistic to guarantee that change will inevitably follow).
- Leave the target audience members to draw their own conclusions rather than telling them to adopt the promoted stance (often labeled cool rather than hot messages). In Freedom From Fear, it is left to the perpetrator to see the effect on children, and help is offered rather than urged.

The selected motivating strategy and the research on which the strategy was based were then explored in individual interviews with key stakeholders, including victims, women's refuge operators, women's advocacy groups, and counselors and other health professionals. All accepted that the strategy could be effective and gave approval to proceed.

Getting the message right entails presenting the message in a way that attracts attention, is believable, is relevant, is able to be understood, arouses appropriate emotions, and does not lead to counterargument (Donovan, 1991). In Freedom From Fear, it means executing the message in a language and style that violent men will pay attention to, understand, and find believable. At the same time, the execution must not be seen to either condemn or condone their violence because either of these perceptions would lead to them rejecting the ad's request for them to seek help. Furthermore, it was important that the message execution would not be seen by victims and other stakeholders to be condoning or excusing the men's violence and that it did not make victims of domestic violence feel responsible, guilty, or more helpless.

24.5.1. Pretesting

The effects of domestic violence on children can be depicted in a variety of scenarios. Pretesting the ad was essential to ensure message understanding and credibility as well as ensuring that the perceived tone of the ad did not antagonize men. Even with the right message, a poorly executed ad not only could be ineffective but could have negative unintended effects on the target audience and other audiences exposed to the campaign messages.

The pretesting was conducted in two stages: a qualitative concept screening stage and a quantitative animatic testing phase.

Six concepts based on the findings of the qualitative research were tested in storyboard form with perpetrators, general-population males and females, victims, various stakeholder representatives, and children exposed to domestic violence. A total of 17 focus groups and eight individual interviews were conducted in Perth, Western Australia, and country areas. Individual written reaction to the concepts was obtained before any group discussion using a modified ADTEST® questionnaire (see below), based on standard advertising pretest measures (Rossiter & Percy, 1997). In the perpetrator groups, counselors were on hand to assist nonliterate men complete the questionnaires and to deal with issues that required attention. The major focus of this stage was on the credibility of the concept message, the realism of the depicted situation, and the capacity of the message to stimulate violent men to think about seeking help to stop their violence.

As the key element of the message strategy was a focus on consequences for children, most of the concepts portrayed small children being exposed to domestic violence. However, it was crucial that the ads, although scheduled to be run only at adult times, did not trigger clinical stress symptoms in children, especially children of victims, and that children did not misunderstand the ads and think *they* were being asked to call the helpline or that they should ask their father or mother's partner to call the helpline. Groups of children at selected women's refuges were exposed to the advertising materials while a child psychologist observed and assessed the children's reactions.

It is important that none of the perpetrators—or any others exposed to the concepts—indicated that the ads made them think that they should simply be sure that the violence was not in front of the children. As indicated above, even those without children saw the message as the violence per se needing to stop.

Following the above, three concepts considered potentially most effective were developed as animatics for testing among men in general:

- "Nightmare": depicted a child tossing and turning in his bed against a shadowy background and the sound effects of a man abusing a woman; the ad ended with the caption "This child is not having a nightmare, he is living one."
- "Horror Movie": two children are watching television against a similar background as above; the caption stated that the children are "Not watching a horror movie, they are living one."
- "Back Seat": a child's view, from the back seat of a car, of a male verbally abusing a woman in the front seat.

The ADTEST procedure, based on published advertising pretest measures (Rossiter & Percy, 1997) was used to test the animatics among men in general. This procedure has been used extensively in pretesting health and social issues advertising (Donovan, Jalleh, & Henley, 1999). Potential respondents were intercepted in the city center, screened for age and socioeconomic status, invited to the research agency's test center, and randomly allocated to view one of the three animatics. The ad was exposed twice so that respondents had ample opportunity to understand what was going on in the ad and to make a judgment about its intended message (Donovan et al., 1999; Rossiter & Percy, 1997) Respondents were exposed to the animatic in groups of two to four, then took a self-completion questionnaire (to facilitate frankness in responding), followed by a face-to-face, interviewer-administered questionnaire on the less sensitive aspects of their reactions (e.g., likes/dislikes about the ad's execution). A total of 302 interviews was conducted with 18- to 40-year-old males, of whom 24% indicated they had come close to hitting their partner on at least one occasion.

All three animatics performed acceptably on all the crucial ADTEST measures; the diagnostic data suggested several ways to increase their effectiveness. Selected results (combined across all three ads) were as follows (Donovan Research, 1998):

- All respondents correctly understood the ads' messages (effect on children, help is available, call the helpline).
- Cognitive response measures indicated high acceptance of the ads' messages and minimal counterarguing.
- Approximately 90% stated that the ads made them feel concerned for the children in the animatics.
- Approximately half thought "a lot" or "somewhat" that the ads suggested that men must take responsibility for their violent behavior.
- Approximately 7% thought the ads communicated that "women who get beaten deserve it."
- Almost 99% found the ads believable (45% "very," 44% "fairly").
- Approximately half thought "a lot" or "somewhat" that the ads would make violent men think they should do something about their behavior.
- There was overwhelming approval for an advertising campaign to encourage violent and potentially violent men to call a helpline.

Appropriate modifications were then made to the ads before final production. All finished ads were shown to stakeholders for final approval before going to air.

We identify a number of overall principles relevant to conducting successful communication campaigns—that is, campaigns that meet their communication and behavioral objectives (Egger et al., 1993; Office of National Drug Control Policy [ONDCP], 1997). Members of the audience are active participants in the communication process. Preexisting beliefs, attitudes, experiences, and knowledge affect attending to, interpretation of, and acceptance of messages. This is particularly important in sensitive, controversial, and core values areas, for which existing attitudes often screen out incoming messages that contradict the individual's existing beliefs and attitudes. Hence particular care is needed when constructing messages aimed at those antagonistic to or sceptical of the proposed idea or behavior. In Freedom From Fear, formative research indicated that male perpetrators' preexisting beliefs would lead to them rejecting messages overtly accusing violent men of inexcusable behavior and threatening criminal sanctions but would support messages appealing to concern for their children. It was possible to draw on the motivating factor (children) without conveying any overt condemnation of their violent behavior. At the same time, it was important not to reinforce any beliefs they had that their behavior was justified—that is, condone their behavior. Similarly, in the unintentional injury context of falls prevention, elderly people will not respond to falls-prevention campaigns when they do not believe that they are at risk of falling (Henley, 2004). Hence a first stage must confront this belief by highlighting hazards and visually modeling how these contribute to falls.

Target audiences must be segmented by beliefs and attitudes before the development of targeted messages. In Freedom From Fear, the primary target audience was defined (and confirmed in formative research) as male perpetrators and potential perpetrators in Prochaska & DiClemente's (1984) contemplation, ready for action, and action stages with respect to doing something about their violence or potential violence. Although these men may still minimize and deny (at some level or on some occasions) full responsibility for their behavior, they are reachable through mass media because they do accept some responsibility. Hard-core perpetrators still in a strong state of denial (Eisikovits & Buchbinder, 1997) were not part of the primary target audience for this campaign. Likewise, road-safety campaigns usually target drivers, but there may also be benefits in targeting passengers to influence the driver's behavior. Furthermore, some drivers are motivated to drive safely by a desire to avoid harm to others, whereas others might be motivated to avoid damage to their valued and valuable vehicle.

Given the importance of existing beliefs and attitudes affecting message processing, formative research is essential to gain an understanding of each target audience's beliefs and attitudes on the issue to be addressed. Also following from the above, it is crucial that messages be pretested against target audiences to ensure correct message understanding and that minimal counterarguing occurs. Pretesting is also necessary to ensure that messages aimed at primary target audiences do not have unintended negative effects on secondary audiences.

In Freedom From Fear, extensive formative research ensured that the ad messages would not adversely affect victims and children, especially victims' children. Child psychologists were used in testing the ad concepts with victims and their children. Although the ads were to be scheduled in adult time, it was still regarded as crucial that any child who saw the ad would not experience clinical stress. The concepts were also tested to ensure that children did not take away the message that they should encourage the perpetrator to call the helpline, as this might put children in greater danger. Other checks included assessing the extent to which the ads appeared to be an unwarranted attack on men in general and whether the ads appeared to condone violence toward women under any circumstances.

In a smoke alarms campaign in New South Wales, the message "Smoke alarms wake you up if there's a fire" was far more understandable and motivating among those of a non-English-speaking background than the generally used slogan "Smoke alarms save lives" (Camit, 2005).

24.5.2. Theoretical Framework

Campaigns that have been guided by theoretical frameworks are more successful than those that have not. A full analysis of all the models relevant to communication theory is beyond the scope of this chapter; but in this section we present a number of factors derived from some of the important models of attitude and behavior change, such as the Health Belief Model (HBM), Protection Motivation Theory, Theory of Reasoned Action (TRA), and the Theory of Trying (Donovan & Henley, 2003).

Most of these models are based on the assumption that an individual's beliefs about some person, group, issue, object, or behavior will determine the individual's attitude and intentions with respect to that person, group, issue, object, or behavior. These intentions, in turn, subject to environmental facilitators and inhibitors, will predict how the individual actually acts with respect to that person, group, issue, object, or behavior. An understanding of knowledge-attitude-behavior models provides us with directions for setting communication objectives and for generating message strategies and executions to achieve these objectives. These processes depend on a thorough understanding of the sorts of beliefs that influence attitudes toward the recommended behavior, how these beliefs and other facilitators and inhibitors influence intentions to behave, and when and how intentions are fulfilled or not fulfilled.

24.5.2.1. Likelihood, Imminence, and Severity

Three attitude factors are the individual's perception of the likelihood of the threat occurring if nothing changes, the perceived imminence of the threat occurring if nothing changes, and the perceived severity of the threat if it does occur. In Freedom From Fear, formative research indicated that male perpetrators of intimate partner violence were aware that (1) there was a high likelihood that children would be affected by their violent actions (many of them remembered being affected as children); (2) the threat was imminent—it would occur at the same time as the violence; and (3) the threat was severe—that is, it could have serious long-term consequences. For most unintentional injury prevention campaigns, these are crucial factors. For example, for road-safety interventions to decrease speeding to be effective, they must increase the perception that getting caught if speeding is likely, that it could occur on any road, and that penalties for transgression are severe.

The efficacy factor has two parts: solution efficacy, the perceived likelihood of the threat being averted if the recommended behavior is adopted, and self-efficacy, the perceived ability to adopt the recommended behavior.

In Freedom From Fear, the recommended behavior was simply to call the helpline for help. There was an explicit promise that help was available and an implicit promise that the help could be effective in helping the perpetrator control his behavior. Smoke alarm promoters must ensure that the target audience sees them as effective; drivers are more likely to wear a seat belt if they consider them effective in reducing injury.

24.5.2.2. Attitude Toward Adopting Recommended Behavior

An important factor relates to the perceived barriers and constraints that may inhibit adoption of the recommended behavior. These barriers may be psychological (the perceived benefits of the undesired behavior may outweigh the perceived losses—for example, perceptions that smoking is necessary to alleviate stress), social (the individual may value the social connection provided by the undesired behavior—for example, binge drinking behavior may provide adolescents with social cohesion), or environmental (it may be physically difficult to perform the desired behavior—for example, to find somewhere to exercise safely). In Freedom From Fear, it was recognized that a 1-minute or 30-second advertisement would be unable to address the complexity of preventing domestic violence. The recommended behavior was not, therefore, to stop being violent but rather call the helpline. Helplines have a number of advantages: they allow dissemination of information to large numbers of self-selected people, yet they can also provide a highly personalized service; they are convenient and private (almost everyone has easy and affordable access to a telephone, and helplines are often free of charge); they can be staffed 24 hours; and they are personal, yet they also offer a degree of anonymity (Anderson, Duffy, & Hallett, 1992). Confidentiality was a major issue in this case; many of the callers to the helpline were admitting a criminal act. Anonymity was ensured and callers were not pressed to give their name. When a referral to counseling was not possible, the helpline counselors asked the caller to provide an address to which they could send educational self-help booklets and audiocassettes.

24.5.3.   Sources of Information and Influence

The individual may be motivated to act by receiving information from influential sources, social interactions, and perceived social norms. In Freedom From Fear, the helpline advertising was not branded to the police department as many campaigns are, and the content of the advertising was clearly nonpunitive and communicated the simple clear message that help was available to violent (and potentially violent) men. Social norms and the perceived behavior of others are powerful influences. Swimmers are unlikely to heed warnings to swim between the flags if they arrive at the beach and see many people swimming outside the flags.

24.5.4.   Supportive Environment

It was also important to create and reinforce positive community attitudes to the counseling of violent men as a legitimate domestic violence-prevention strategy (complementary to police arrest and sentencing, and mandatory referral into counseling by courts) and hence worthy of government funding.

There was a need to address the potential criticism that the campaign helped the perpetrator at the expense of the victim and that these resources would be better used in providing help for victims and their children. This was done by keeping the focus on the ultimate aim of the women's need to be free from the fear of violence by providing counseling to the perpetrator as distinct from legal sanctions such as restraining orders, which do not necessarily reduce the fear. New counseling programs for women and children were also funded by the state government.

24.5.5.   Successful Campaigns

Successful campaigns are comprehensive in their reach. The Freedom From Fear program is provided in 12 locations throughout Western Australia, 6 of them in regional areas. Given the state's geography, it was recognized that access to counseling programs would necessarily be limited in remote areas but it is hoped to extend access in later phases of the campaign. Meanwhile, self-help materials can be sent to any location. Access to programs is provided in nonworking hours, and the helpline is staffed both day and night. It was decided that all materials and programs would be provided free to ensure that no financial barrier existed or could be rationalized as existing at any income level. The focus was on the victim; it was important that victims of low-income perpetrators would not be disadvantaged.

Communication campaigns must be coordinated with other environmental and on-the-ground strategies to ensure attitudinal and behavioral success. This factor relates to the aspects of the environment that might facilitate or inhibit adoption. For example, will government policy makers be willing to act in ways that facilitate the adoption?

In Freedom From Fear, directing resources toward male perpetrator programs is generally viewed negatively by female victim support organizations. Hence it was crucial to gain such organizations'—and female victims'—support for the program in principle and then ensure their continued support for the various program materials as they were produced. This required an initial acceptance that prevention of violence via perpetrators' and potential perpetrators' voluntary entry to counseling was a legitimate and potentially effective violence-prevention strategy. Updating of developments and clearing of materials with these groups was continued through to final production. It was required that this sector be reassured that targeting perpetrators and funding perpetrator programs was consistent with feminist philosophy with respect to domestic violence prevention—that is, that victim safety is paramount and that directing services toward men must ultimately be about victim safety and freedom from fear.

The referral process involves cooperation between two government departments and all (competing) service providers for the system to work. This cooperation was gained only after extensive consultation and interpersonal networking. When the caller accepts a referral, the counselor takes details from the caller and completes a referral form, which is faxed to the appropriate service provider the same day. Service providers are required to contact callers within 2 days (most attempt to do so within 24 hours) to make an appointment for an assessment interview.

Similarly in an area such as road safety, the police, driving instructors, road engineers, car manufacturers, local governments, hospital emergency departments and ambulance operators, insurance companies, and licensed entertainment venue operators must all cooperate and coordinate activities for maximal effect on preventing crashes and minimizing injury when they do occur. There is no point in road-safety advertising if there is no visible police enforcement of regulations, and vice versa, police enforcement has more effect when accompanied by related advertising.

Communication campaigns involving a number of message delivery channels and more than one source appear more successful than those that do not (Lefebvre, Olander, & Levine, 2000). In Freedom From Fear, police were encouraged to promote perpetrators' use of the telephone counseling service when called to "domestics" and particularly when no charges could or would be laid. Radio was used to supplement the television ads, along with posters and merchandise, such as drink coasters, that provided the helpline number. Publicity is a major additional channel for communication campaigns, especially when individuals representative of the target group recount their experiences and reinforce the "it could happen to you" message. Although these sorts of opportunities are more limited for domestic violence prevention campaigns, they can be widely used in other injury prevention areas in which victims or their loved ones talk about the incidents and the aftermath. At the same time, publicity that feeds back information about the success of campaigns (e.g., reductions in road toll; reductions in alcohol-related injuries) not only reinforces public support for such campaigns but reinforces those target group members who have responded to the campaign.

Communication campaigns must be sustained to achieve and maintain success. In sensitive areas such as domestic violence, it would be unethical to raise hopes and motivation to change unless sufficient resources were available and accessible over a sufficient time period. Freedom From Fear is nominally a 10-year campaign, receiving substantial funding from the state government. With successive governments, further interpersonal networking is necessary to promote continued support for this campaign. The success of road-safety campaigns in Australia since the 1980s is undoubtedly due to the sustained effort over a variety of areas, including the communication components.

24.6.   CONCLUSIONS

This chapter identified key principles for developing and implementing communication messages and illustrated their application through the Western Australian Freedom From Fear campaign. Formative research has been shown to be essential to the process of getting the right message—that is, identifying attitudes, beliefs, and possible motivations for change. Pretesting of possible ad executions has been shown to be essential for getting the message right—that is, identifying an execution that the target audiences will believe, understand, and respond to and that will not have an adverse effect on any unintended audiences.

A full evaluation of the Freedom From Fear campaign is beyond the scope of this chapter. However, from August 1998 to January 2005, the campaign received over 21,000 calls, almost 13,000 of which were from the target group. Of these, 8,200 men identified themselves as perpetrators and 3,800 voluntarily entered counseling. Self-report evaluation instruments indicate that men who complete the program say they are less likely to use physical violence and more likely to accept that they, and not their partners or their children, are responsible for the violence (Cant, Downie, Fisher, Henry, & Froyland, 2002). One man with a long history of abusive behavior told this story in his 23rd counseling session (Cant et al., 2002, p. 38):

> We were working in the garden, and my 7-year old son was playing about with the outside tap that was obviously not properly fastened to the wall, he must have been swinging on it. Suddenly there was a scream and water spraying everywhere. I jumped up and swung around and in that split second saw the look of absolute terror on the faces of my wife and four children. I went to my son, told him it was OK and said I would show him how to turn the water off at the mains.

When asked how he would have reacted a year ago he said: "I would have picked up the broken pipe and beaten him with it, my wife would have tried to stop me and I would have beaten her with it too." The following week, he told the group that the family had again spent time together at the house, "My four children all climbed on my knee and cuddled me. They wanted to be there. It was the first time I had ever felt like a father."

REFERENCES

Anderson, D. M., Duffy, K., & Hallett, C. (1992). Cancer prevention counseling on telephone helplines. *Public Health Reports, 107,* 278–283.

Andreasen, A. (1995). *Marketing social change: Changing behavior to promote health, social development, and the environment.* San Francisco: Jossey-Bass.

Buchanan, F. (1996). Zero tolerance in South Australia: A statewide community initiative. *Australian Journal of Primary Health-Interchange, 2* (1), 107–112.

Camit, M. (2005). *Smoke alarms wake you up if there is a fire: A smoke alarm campaign targeting Arabic, Chinese and Vietnamese communities in New South Wales, Australia.* Paper presented at the Second Social Marketing Downunder Conference, Wellington, New Zealand.

Cant, R., Downie, R., Fisher, C., Henry, P., & Froyland, I. (2002). *Evaluation of perpetrator programs for mandated and voluntary participants in Western Australia.* Perth, Australia: Centre for Research on Women. Family and Domestic Violence Unit.

De Becker, G. (1998). *A gift of fear: survival signals that protect us from violence.* New York: Dell.

Donovan, R. J. (1991). Public health advertising: Execution guidelines for health promotion professionals. *Health Promotion Journal of Australia, 1,* 40–45.

Donovan, R. J., Francas, M., Paterson, D., & Zappelli, R. (2000). Formative research for mass media-based campaigns: Western Australia's "Freedom From Fear" campaign targeting male perpetrators of intimate partner violence. *Health Promotion Journal of Australia, 10* (2), 78–83.

Donovan, R., & Henley, N. (2003). *Social marketing: Principles and practice.* Melbourne, Australia: IP Communications.

Donovan, R. J., Jalleh, G., & Henley, N. (1999). Effective road safety advertising: Are big production budgets necessary? *Accident Analysis & Prevention, 31,* 243–252.

Donovan, R. J., & Owen, N. (1994). Social marketing and population interventions. In R. K. Dishman (Ed.), *Advances in exercise adherence* (pp. 249–290, 2nd ed.). Champaign, IL: Human Kinetics.

Donovan, R. J., Paterson, D., & Francas, M. (1999). Targeting male perpetrators of intimate partner violence: Western Australia's "Freedom from Fear" campaign. *Social Marketing Quarterly, 5* (3), 127–143.

Donovan Research (1998). *Concept screening and ADTEST®* (Reports to Domestic Violence Prevention Unit). Perth, Western Australia: Author.

Egger, G., Donovan, R. J., & Spark, R. (1993). *Health and the media: Principles and practice for health promotion.* Sydney, Australia: McGraw-Hill.

Eisikovits, Z., & Buchbinder, E. (1997). Talking violent: A phenomenological study of metaphors battering men use. *Violence Against Women, 3* (5), 482–498.

Gondolf, E. W. (2002). *Batterer intervention systems: Issues, outcomes and recommendations.* Newbury Park, CA: Sage.

Healey, K. M., & Smith, C. (1998). *Batterer programs: What criminal justice agencies need to know* (Research in Action). National Institute of Justice. Retrieved December 15, 2005, from www.ojp.usdoj.gov/nij/pubs-sum/171683.htm,

Henley, N. (2004). Social marketing: "Selling" injury prevention. In R. McClure, M. Stevenson, & S. McEvoy (Eds.), *The scientific basis of injury prevention and control* (pp. 318–333). Melbourne, Australia: IP Communications.

Jukes, A. (1993). *Why men hate women.* London: Free Association Books.

Jukes, A. (1999). *Men who batter women.* London: Routledge.

Keilitz, S. L., Davis, C., Efkeman, H. S., Flango, C., & Hannaford, P. L. (1998). *Civil protection orders: Victims' views on effectiveness* (Research review). *National Institute of Justice.* Retrieved December 15, 2005, from www.ojp.usdoj.gov/nij/pubs-sum/171683.htm.

Lee, M. Y., Sebold, J., & Uken, A. (2003). *Solution-focused treatment of domestic violence offenders.* Oxford, UK: Oxford University Press.

Lefebvre, C., Olander, C., & Levine, E. (2000). The impact of multiple channel delivery of nutrition messages on student knowledge, motivation and behavior: Results from the Team Nutrition pilot study. *Social Marketing Quarterly, 5* (3), 90–98.

National Center for Injury Prevention and Control. (1999). *Family and intimate violence prevention program: Multifaceted community-based projects.* Retrieved December 15, 2005, from www.cdc.gov/ncipc/factsheets/ipvfacts.htm.

Office of National Drug Control Policy. (1997). *National youth anti-drug media campaign.* Washington, DC: Author.

Prochaska, J. O., & DiClemente, C. C. (1984). *The transtheoretical approach: Crossing the traditional boundaries of therapy.* Irwin, IL: Dow-Jones/Irwin.

Roberts, A. R. (Ed.). (1984). *Battered women and their families: Intervention strategies and treatment programs.* New York: Springer.

Rossiter, J. R., & Percy, L. (1997). *Advertising communications and promotion management* (2nd ed). New York: McGraw-Hill.

Chapter 25

Cultural Appropriateness in Interventions for Racial and Ethnic Minorities

Sharyn E. Parks and Matthew W. Kreuter

25.1. INTRODUCTION

Eliminating racial and ethnic disparities in health is one of the two overarching goals of Healthy People 2010 and injuries are a leading cause of death for all Americans and the leading cause for those aged 1–44 years (U.S. Department of Health and Human Services [HHS], 2000). Significant disparities exist in rates of both intentional and unintentional injury; racial and ethnic population subgroups usually bear an excess burden of morbidity and/or mortality. The most highly publicized of these disparities has been violence victimization. Homicide is the leading cause of death for African Americans aged 15–34 years (Centers for Disease Control and Prevention [CDC], 2003/2004), the second leading cause of death for Hispanics aged 10–24 years, and the third leading cause of death for American Indians/Alaskan Natives and Asian/Pacific Islanders aged 10–24 (Anderson & Smith, 2003). Overall, American Indian/Alaska Native women and men report more violent victimization than any other racial/ethnic group. American Indians/ Alaska Natives aged 15–24 also have the highest rates of suicide of any group in the United States (CDC, 2003/2004).

Although comparatively less attention has been paid to disparities in unintentional injury, the pattern of population effect is similar. For example, African American and Native American populations are at greater risk than other groups for fire-related injuries and deaths, and African Americans have a 1.4–2.6 times greater risk of drowning compared to white Americans (CDC, 2003/2004). Across all age categories, African Americans have a fatality rate from pedestrian injuries that is almost twice that of white Americans and greater risks of spinal cord injury and death from traumatic brain injury than any other racial or ethnic group (CDC, 2003/2004). Disparities also exist in behaviors that can prevent or reduce harm from unintentional injuries. For example, African American students are less likely to wear seat-belts when driving or riding in a motor vehicle, which increases the risk of death or disability in a crash (CDC, 2003).

While many studies have been carried out to document and describe these injury disparities, far fewer have explored the effectiveness of injury prevention and control programs that are designed specifically for the groups experiencing disparities. Furthermore, little is known about how, if at all, intervention approaches are adapted for different population subgroups, and to what effect. By better understanding how to intervene effectively with diverse populations, we can build an evidence base of injury prevention and control programs that can be applied with confidence to a range of groups and can help eliminate disparities in injury morbidity and mortality.

This chapter reports results from a systematic literature review of injury prevention and control interventions in racial and ethnic population subgroups. Using a recently proposed typology of strategies to enhance cultural appropriateness in health promotion programs (Kreuter, Lukwago, Bucholtz, Clark, & Sanders-Thompson, 2003), we examined studies for their use of five distinct approaches: peripheral, evidential, linguistic, constituent involving, and sociocultural (see next section). The chapter describes the extent to which and how each approach is used and provides recommendations for applying these findings to injury prevention and control research in racial and ethnic population subgroups.

25.2.   FIVE APPROACHES TO ACHIEVING CULTURAL APPROPRIATENESS

Although it is widely accepted that health-promotion efforts (including injury prevention) should consider cultural factors when addressing the needs of racial and ethnic population subgroups, there is surprisingly little evidence that doing so enhances effectiveness. In its 2002 report *Speaking of Health,* the Institute of Medicine concluded that "there is little evidence available as to whether diversity strategies contribute to success" (pp. 8–7). It also identified as "urgent" the need for comparative effectiveness studies and field tests of different strategies to address diversity.

To help facilitate such research, Kreuter, Lukwago et al. (2003) identified commonly used strategies for enhancing the relevance and appropriateness of interventions designed for different population subgroups, and classified them into five types of approaches: peripheral, evidential, linguistic, constituent involving, and sociocultural (Table 25.1). Given the newness of this conceptualization of approaches, it is not yet clear how, if at all, different approaches may influence reactions to or effectiveness of injury prevention intervention. However, having a typology to guide the formulation of research questions and study designs may help accelerate research progress in this area. The five categories are intended primarily to provide conceptual clarity and are not necessarily mutually exclusive. In both research and practice, it is common for more than one approach to be used in the same intervention or program. Each of the five strategies is described below.

Table 25.1. Summary of Five Approaches to Cultural Appropriateness

Approach to Cultural Appropriateness	Description
Peripheral	Using colors, images, fonts, pictures or images of group members, or declarative titles that overtly convey relevance to those in the group
Evidential	Providing evidence, often in the form of data, that a given problem affects members of the group
Linguistic	Making program activities and/or materials more accessible by providing them in the dominant or native language of the group
Constituent involving	Drawing on the experience and knowledge of the group's members when planning and/or delivering programs or interventions
Sociocultural	Integrating cultural norms, values, beliefs, and behaviors of the group into program activities and/or materials

25.2.1.   Peripheral Approaches

Peripheral approaches include using colors, images, fonts, or pictures of group members that overtly convey relevance to those in the group. Giving injury prevention programs or materials the appearance of cultural appropriateness is thought to increase their appeal to the targeted group and/or the amount of attention the group's members pay the program. Resnicow, Baranowski, Ahluwalia, and Braithwaite (1999) suggested that matching materials to "surface" characteristics of a target population may also enhance how accepting the group is to information being presented. Such approaches are referred to as "peripheral" in reference to Petty and Cacioppo's (1981) explanation of how information processing and persuasion can sometimes be influenced by such factors. When the visual style of injury prevention program materials reflects the social and cultural world of an intended audience, the materials will seem familiar and comfortable (Bechtel & Davidhizar, 2000). This language of pictures, colors, and images can be perceived almost immediately (Schiffman, 1995). Elements of design such as these can gain attention and/or create interest, establish credibility, and set the tone for related injury prevention content (Moriarty, 1995).

25.2.2.   Evidential Approaches

Injury prevention programs may seek to enhance the perceived relevance of a given problem for a given group by providing evidence of its effect on that group. In most cases, the "evidence" provided takes the form of epidemiological data about the effect of the problem for that population. For example, evidential approaches to cultural appropriateness for violence prevention among African American teenagers might include statements such as "Homicide is the leading cause of death for African Americans your age." Statements and facts such as this are intended to raise awareness, concern, and/or perceived susceptibility to violent victimization by showing that it affects other people like you. Research based on Weinstein and Sandman's (1992) Precaution Adoption Model (Orlandi, Landers, Weston, & Haley, 1990) has shown that individuals who perceive a problem as affecting others who are like them may think more about the problem, decide to take preventive action, and make plans to do so.

25.2.3.   Linguistic Approaches

Injury prevention programs and materials can also be made more accessible by providing them in the dominant or native language of the target group. Because language is fundamental to effective communication, Rogler, Malgady, Costantino, and Blumenthal (1987, p. 566) have called linguistic accessibility "the lowest common denominator of cultural sensitivity." Although linguistic approaches include translating program information from one language to another, this is just a small part of linguistic appropriateness. Without considering how an injury prevention program's content, approach or delivery fits within a culture's norms and values, using linguistic strategies alone can result in increased access to and use of a program or service that is culturally inappropriate (Rogler et al., 1987).

25.2.4.   Constituent-Involving Approaches

Health educators have long understood the importance of drawing on the experience and knowledge of a target group's members when planning programs or interventions. Constituent-involving approaches include hiring staff members indigenous to the population served, training paraprofessionals or "natural helpers" drawn from the target group (Altpeter, Earp, Bishop, & Eng, 1999; "Lay Health Advisors," 1997; Thomas, Eng, Clark, Robinson, & Blumenthal, 1998), and following principles of participation (Green & Kreuter, 1999) in identifying substantive roles for lay community members. Involving constituents in this way can also strengthen linguistic approaches described earlier and can provide valuable insights into cultural characteristics and how they may be associated with specific injury prevention beliefs or behaviors.

25.2.5.   Sociocultural Approaches

Injury prevention topics may seem more relevant to a given group when presented in the context of broader social and/or cultural values shared by the group's members. Resnicow et al. (1999) refer to sociocultural characteristics as the "deep structure" of cultural sensitivity and propose that they convey salience to a target group when incorporated in health-promotion programs. Using this approach, a group's cultural values, beliefs, and behaviors are recognized, reinforced, and built on to provide context and meaning to information, messages, or program activities around a given health problem or behavior. Sociocultural approaches will reflect an understanding of culturally normative practices and beliefs—the inner workings of culture rather than just outward appearances.

In a study of cancer prevention and control among African American women, Kreuter et al. (2005) compared the effects of a series of magazines that were tailored on either behavioral constructs only (the conventional approach), cultural constructs only (a sociocultural approach), or a combination of behavioral and cultural constructs. The cultural constructs—religiosity, collectivism, racial pride, and time orientation—were measured by brief scales administered to each participant (Lukwago, Kreuter, Bucholtz, Holt, & Clark, 2001). Women's scores on the cultural construct scales were associated with cancer knowledge and beliefs (Lukwago et al., 2003) and reactions to the magazines (Kreuter, Steger-May et al., 2003), and women who received magazines tailored on a combination of behavioral and cultural constructs were most likely to report getting mammograms and to have increased fruit and vegetable consumption at an 18-month follow-up (Kreuter et al., 2005). These findings suggest that presenting health information in the context of both individual (i.e., behavior) and group (i.e., culture) characteristics may enhance program effectiveness.

25.3.   METHODS

To determine the extent to which the five approaches to cultural appropriateness have been used in injury prevention interventions evaluated to date, we identified and reviewed published articles reporting on injury prevention activities conducted among racial and ethnic population subgroups.

25.3.1.   Search Strategy and Data Sources

The goal of the literature search was to identify studies in which a program or intervention seeking to prevent or control injuries was delivered to a population composed primarily or exclusively of members of a racial or ethnic population subgroup. Intervention studies published from 1966 through March 2004 were identified through electronic database searches in PubMed, MEDLINE, PsychInfo, and the Cumulative Index to Nursing and Allied Health Literature. In general, the search strategy examined the intersection of three domains: problem (e.g., injury), solution (e.g., prevention), and population (e.g., racial or ethnic group). Selected search terms were employed in various combinations with Boolean operators to form 10 search strings. The terms used were intervention, education, evaluation studies, intervention studies, injury prevention, accident prevention, primary prevention, race, ethnicity, injury, prevention, accident, black, African American, Hispanic, Latino, Native American, American Indian, Asian, immigrant, motor-vehicle crash, burn, poisoning, fall, and choking.

25.3.2.   Study Selection

For inclusion in this review, articles had to describe an actual intervention focused on primary or secondary prevention of intentional or unintentional injury. From this initial pool, we selected articles that specifically targeted a racial or ethnic population subgroup for intervention. Multiple levels of targeting were allowed; for instance, interventions could be targeted to individuals in a specific age category within a race or ethnic group. Articles were selected if they reported results of a systematic evaluation of an existing intervention or described an intervention currently being implemented and/or evaluated. Medical interventions, systematic reviews, meta-analyses, and organization-level programs (e.g., state health department injury prevention initiatives and occupational-injury prevention programs) and those whose target population was defined only by age or gender, but not race or ethnicity were excluded.

The initial database search yielded 482 articles. After eliminating duplicates and articles not meeting the study selection criteria, the list was reduced to 37 articles. We independently reviewed each of the 37 articles. After this review, an additional 19 articles were excluded because they either did not describe a specific intervention or did not address a specific racial or ethnic group. Decisions on the final sample of 18 articles included in the study were made through discussion and agreement between us.

25.3.3.   Review Criteria

Each of us independently reviewed the 18 eligible articles and determined whether peripheral, evidential, linguistic, constituent involving, and/or sociocultural approaches were used based on descriptions of each provided in the original source (Kreuter, Lukwago et al., 2003). Articles were also examined to determine the target audience for the intervention and the type of injury or injuries being addressed.

25.3.4.   Interreviewer Agreement

After completing independent reviews of the 18 eligible articles, we compared ratings. There were a total of 90 possible ratings (18 articles times 5 possible approaches to enhance cultural appropriateness used in each). Overall, the rate of agreement between us was 79%. Approach-specific rates of agreement were as follows: 78% peripheral, 83% evidential, 89% linguistic, 61% constituent involving, and 83% sociocultural. When ratings were discrepant, we jointly reexamined the article in question and came to a consensus rating. The final ratings are shown in Table 25.2.

25.4.   FINDINGS

The types of injury addressed, primary population subgroups targeted, and use of the five approaches to cultural appropriateness are described below and summarized in Table 25.2.

25.4.1.   Type of Injury Addressed

Selected articles addressed both violence and unintentional injury prevention. Of the 18 articles, 8 (44%) addressed violence outcomes only, 6 (33%) addressed unintentional injury only, and 4 articles (22%) addressed both violence and unintentional injuries.

25.4.2.   Targeted Population Subgroups

A total of 6 articles (33%) described interventions conducted in primarily or exclusively African American populations, 4 (22%) described interventions for native populations (e.g., American Indians, Maori populations in New Zealand), and 3 (17%) addressed Hispanic populations. We found 5 articles (28%) that described interventions that addressed more than one racial or ethnic subgroup, most commonly African American and Hispanic populations.

25.4.3.   Approaches to Cultural Appropriateness

Most articles ($n = 15$; 83%) described using at least one of the five approaches to achieving cultural appropriateness. Constituent-involving approaches were used

Table 25.2. Summary of Articles Reviewed

Reference	Audience Targeted[a]	Area of injury[b]	Strategy for targeting Peripheral	Evidential	Linguistic	Constituent-Involving	Sociocultural
Zaloshnja et al. (2003)	Native Americans	U/V				X	X
Wiist et al. (1996)	AA and Hispanic youth	V	X		X	X	X
Schwarz et al. (1993)	AA, low income, urban	U				X	
Orpinas et al. (1995)	AA and Hispanic, sixth grade	V		X		X	
Orpinas et al. (2000)	Hispanic and AA, sixth to eighth grade	V				X	X
Nansel et al. (2002)	AA parents	U	X	X			
Hendrickson (1984)	Hispanic, low income, fourth grade	U		X	X		
Farrell et al. (1996)	AA, sixth grade	V				X	
Davidson et al. (1994)	Harlem, ages 5–16 year	U/V	X			X	
Coggan et al. (2000)	Pakeha and European, Maori	U/V				X	
Campbell et al. (2001)	Hispanic adolescent	U			X		
Cardenas & Simons-Morton (1993)	Hispanic mothers	U	X		X		
Brewin & Coggan (2002)	Maori	U				X	X
Brewin & Coggan (2004)	Maori	U/V	X		X	X	X
Becker et al. (2004)	Violently injured youth	V		X		X	

[a]Predominant race or ethnicities represented in the study sample. AA, African American.
[b]U, unintentional; V, violence.

most often (n = 11; 61%), followed by peripheral, linguistic, and sociocultural approaches, each described in 5 articles (28% each). Evidential approaches were described in 4 articles (22%). A total of 11 articles described using a combination of at least two different approaches, but only 2 of these described using three or more approaches. Findings for each of the five approaches are described separately below.

25.4.3.1.   Peripheral Approaches

Peripheral approaches, which seek to give programs or materials the appearance of cultural appropriateness by including certain colors, images, fonts, pictures of group members, or declarative titles that overtly convey relevance to a given population subgroup, were used in five of the interventions described. For example, in an intervention designed to prevent pediatric tap-water burns among Hispanics in Texas, Cardenas and Simons-Morton (1993) used printed educational materials in which core prevention content was delivered by Hispanic cartoon characters. Nansel et al. (2002) used tailored print materials delivered to parents of young children in a primary-care setting to reduce child injury risks in the home and in automobiles. These materials were personalized with each child's name, which is a peripheral approach based on individual rather than group characteristics. Other peripheral approaches included intervention materials given declarative titles that connote race or ethnicity (e.g., Effective Black Parenting and Padres Con Poder) (Wiist et al., 1996), mural painting in parks and playgrounds (Davidson et al., 1994), and promotional materials for a road-safety program (e.g., fact sheets, flyers, posters, balloons, T-shirts) that were designed to appeal to the target population of Maori in the Ngati Porou community (Brewin & Coggan, 2004).

25.4.3.2.   Evidential Approaches

Evidential approaches were the least commonly used approach in this review, with only 4 of the 18 articles describing this as part of the intervention. Evidential approaches are design to enhance the perceived relevance of a given problem for a given group by providing evidence of its effect on that group. The most creative example of this was provided by Becker, Hall, Ursic, Jain, and Calhoun (2004), who used "living evidence" to illustrate the effect of violence to youth. The program's peer staff member—many of whom had been previously incarcerated or disabled from a violent injury—were all from the same communities as the youth participants. In other articles reviewed, the evidence provided to intervention recipients was less likely to be framed as relevant "for your racial or ethnic group" than framed as relevant "for people like you." This is understandable given the homogeneity of study populations in most articles. In other words, if all intervention recipients belong to the same racial or ethnic group, framing the evidence as relevant for your racial or ethnic group may seem redundant. Examples from these articles include providing evidence of the magnitude of violence as a societal program in a middle school based violence-prevention program (Orpinas et al., 1995), children discussing how a head injury could change a person's life after watching a video about bicycle helmet use (Hendrickson & Becker, 1998), and personal injury risk profiles for young children to their parents (Nansel et al., 2002).

25.4.3.3.   Linguistic Approaches

Linguistic approaches incorporate the dominant or native language of the target group(s) into the intervention. In five of the articles, intervention materials and/ or activities were delivered in both English and another language. For example, because 27% of the study population in Hendrickson and Becker's (1998) school-based bicycle injury prevention program were Hispanic, all print and video materials were available in Spanish (Henkrickson & Becker, 1998; Orpinas et al., 2000). The Ngati Porou Community Injury Prevention Project (Brewin & Coggan, 2004) addressed an indigenous Maori population and thus used educational and promotional materials that were presented in both Maori and English (Brewin & Coggan, 2004). In a program to prevent household injuries among migrant Hispanic adolescents, Campbell et al. (2001) used Red Cross training course materials that were modified and delivered by bilingual group leaders. Cardenas and Simons-Morton's (1993) hot tap water burn-prevention program also used a linguistic approach. Its target audience of low socioeconomic status Hispanics in Houston, Texas, were provided educational cartoons and questionnaires in both English and Spanish. Wiist et al.'s (1996) school-based youth violence-prevention intervention also used a linguistic approach to help reach its target population of Hispanic and African American students. The program involved parent- and student-directed interventions, both of which were delivered by bilingual (English/Spanish) staff members.

25.4.3.4.   Constituent-Involving Approaches

Constituent involving approaches, which draw on the experience and knowledge of a target group's members in planning and delivering interventions, were the most commonly used approach to achieving cultural appropriateness—described in 11 of the 18 articles. Most of the constituent-involving approaches were found in school-based interventions ($n = 6$) in which at least one component of an intervention was delivered by trained peer educators or peer leaders (Becker et al., 2004; Farrell et al., 1996; Orpinas et al., 2000; Orpinas et al., 1995; Wiist et al., 1996; Zaloshnja et al., 2003). The other interventions using constituent-involving approaches were community based. In these articles, community members were described as assisting in various aspects of planning and delivery of injury prevention intervention. For example, in Davidson et al.'s (1994) report on the Safe Kids/Healthy Neighborhood Injury Prevention Program in Harlem, coalitions of community groups and local agencies were formed to plan and support program activities. Similarly, Brewin and Coggan (2002, 2004) describe how community volunteers and local business worked together to increase the availability of injury prevention devices (e.g., child car restraints) and/or educational programs (Coggan et al., 2000). In another article, individuals who were similar to the target population were hired from within the same community to deliver the injury prevention intervention (Schwarz et al., 1993).

25.4.3.5.   Sociocultural Approaches

Using sociocultural approaches, injury prevention information and activities are integrated in the context of social and/or cultural values that are important to the target audience. Such approaches were described in one third of the 18 articles

($n = 6$). These articles provided many excellent examples of how culture can be integrated into injury prevention for special populations. For example, Zaloshnja et al. (2003) describe how a culturally appropriate message suggested by tribal elders was effective in reducing deaths from drowning in a population of Alaska Natives. Specifically, program developers learned that community members believed that falling in the local river would be fatal whether or not you were wearing a floatation device (i.e., the cold temperatures alone could not be survived). It was not surprising that efforts to promote use of floatation devices that focused on their effectiveness as a form of drowning prevention failed. Tribal elders pointed out that when someone drowns, community members must drag the river for their body—a difficult and time-consuming task. The elders suggested that a more effective way to promote use of floatation jackets would be to note that if you were wearing one and fell in the river, your body would float and therefore be much easier for the community to recover. This culturally aware message appeared to increase demand for flotation jackets and reduce drowning, without the risk and challenge of trying to change a culturally held belief.

Sociocultural approaches were also described in interventions developed for Maori populations in New Zealand (Brewin & Coggan, 2002, 2004). Although injury prevention was the objective of each program, cultural ideology and values such as love, assistance, support, and prayer were central themes underlying the intervention activities. The authors described this approach as a "collaborative, holistic Maori framework." Similarly, in a school-based violence prevention program, Wiist et al. (1996) included a peer-education component whose goals included strengthening social support and cultural pride. Finally, Orpinas et al. (1995), considered the culture of middle school students in designing the Students for Peace violence-prevention program. A peer-mediator component of the intervention specifically addressed issues such as name calling, rumors, and threats, all of which had been identified as important in the culture of middle school students at the target schools.

25.5. DISCUSSION

Despite compelling data on injury disparities by race and ethnicity and a national call for eliminating disparities from the U.S. Department of Health and Human Services, we found fewer published articles reporting on injury prevention interventions among minority populations. Of these, even fewer addressed unintentional injuries or U.S. populations other than African Americans and Hispanics. Establishing an evidence-based collection of injury prevention interventions shown to be effective in diverse communities should help in eliminating injury disparities. This may require developing new programs or adapting existing ones and evaluating their effectiveness in different population subgroups. Either way, ensuring cultural appropriateness of the interventions will likely be an important ingredient in program success.

In this review, we found that most injury prevention interventions targeting racial and/or ethnic population subgroups used at least one of five types of approaches to achieving cultural appropriateness, but only a handful of interventions used multiple strategies. Thus, although there appears to be general recognition of the importance of considering culture in intervention planning and delivery among developers, there is also room for expanding the scope of these efforts.

Although the typology of approaches to cultural appropriateness is not presented as a hierarchy, we and others (Resnicow et al., 1999) would generally argue that certain approaches (i.e., constituent involving and sociocultural) require a greater understanding of more complex population characteristics than do other approaches (i.e., peripheral and evidential) and have greater potential for stimulating higher order (i.e., behavioral) changes related to injury prevention. In this review, constituent-involving approaches—long a staple of health-promotion program planning—were used in over half of the articles reviewed. However, no other approach, including sociocultural, was used in more than a third of articles.

25.5.1.   Limitations

While this review provides a snapshot of which approaches to cultural appropriateness have been used to date in injury prevention and control interventions for racial and ethnic population subgroups, it has several limitations and it leaves many interesting and important questions unanswered. First, the review was based on only that information provided in the published articles. Due to space constraints in journals and editorial decisions of authors and editors, the level of detail in which interventions are described can vary considerably. Thus it is possible that some of the interventions actually included additional approaches to cultural appropriateness that were not coded in our review because they were not described in the article. Accordingly, the findings reported in this chapter should probably be considered a conservative estimate of how frequently the cultural appropriateness approaches are used.

Second, all of the articles included in this review were from the published literature. We did not explicitly exclude nonresearch articles; however, the nature of most electronic databases and the publications included therein results in an underrepresentation of nonresearch reports. While we feel the breadth of approaches incorporated in our review was representative of the current state of injury prevention research we cannot be certain that culturally appropriate interventions that use one or more of our five suggested strategies for tailoring effectively are not being implemented outside of the research realm.

Third, as noted earlier in the chapter, it is not yet known whether these five approaches enhance the effectiveness of injury prevention programs for diverse populations and whether different approaches work through different mechanisms or have different effects. Nor do we know whether using two or more of these approaches in combination produces synergy or dose effects. These are important empirical questions, but cannot be answered by this study. The small number of total articles found, diverse outcomes of interest across articles, wide-ranging levels of methodological rigor (e.g., inclusion of comparison groups in the study design), and different stages of evaluation (e.g., process vs. outcome) prevent making meaningful comparisons at this time, either anecdotal or statistical.

25.5.2.   Recommendations

This chapter has identified many unmet needs in the injury prevention intervention literature. There is clearly a need for more studies providing a rigorous evaluation of injury prevention and control interventions designed or adapted specifically for racial and ethnic population subgroups. Such studies might also examine the relative and combined effects of using different approaches to achieving cultural appropriateness. In the absence of strong evidence to guide decisions about how best to integrate culture into injury prevention programs, intervention planners and practitioners should rely on theories and theory-based hypotheses, established processes for planning, and the successful experiences of others.

For example, this chapter reports that several health-promotion scholars have proposed that peripheral approaches to achieving cultural appropriateness may be most useful in capturing the attention of a specific group or making information or materials more appealing to its members. Recognizing this, as well as the hypothesized effects of other approaches to cultural appropriateness, can help in strategically selecting different methods to reach different injury prevention program objectives. Applying established processes for program planning should have the same effects. Specifically, every component of an intervention—including different approaches to cultural appropriateness—should be linked directly to some outcome of interest. By explicitly stating that "Approach A is included to achieve Outcome B" and knowing how and why Outcome B will enhance the likelihood of injury prevention behaviors or beliefs, arbitrary application of cultural appropriateness approaches will be avoided.

Finally, it is essential that intervention developers and researchers learn from the experiences of one another. Although the articles reviewed in this chapter are small in number, they are rich in examples and ideas about how the five approaches to cultural appropriateness can be applied in actual intervention settings. We strongly encourage readers to examine these studies, starting with Wiist et al. (1996) and Brewin and Coggan (2004), both of which provide excellent examples of multiple approaches.

REFERENCES

Altpeter, M., Earp, J., Bishop, C., & Eng, E. (1999). Lay health advisor activity levels: Definitions from the field. *Health Education & Behavior, 26* (4), 495–512.

Anderson, R., & Smith, B. (2003). Deaths: Leading causes for 2001. *National Vital Statistics Report, 52* (9), 1–85.

Bechtel, G., & Davidhizar, R. (2000). Integrating cultural diversity in patient education. *Seminars in Nurse Management, 7* (4), 193–197.

Becker, M., Hall, J., Ursic, C., Jain, S., & Calhoun, D. (2004). Caught in the crossfire: The effects of a peer-based intervention program for violently injured youth. *Journal of Adolescent Health, 34* (3), 177–183.

Brewin, M., & Coggan, C. (2002). Evaluation of a New Zealand indigenous community injury prevention project. *Injury Control & Safety Promotion, 9* (2), 83–88.

Brewin, M., & Coggan, C. (2004). Evaluation of the Ngati Porou Community Injury Prevention Project. *Ethnicity & Health, 9* (1), 11–15.

Campbell, N., Ayala, G., Litrownik, A., Slymen, D., Zavala, F., & Elder, J. (2001). Evaluation of a first aid and home safety program for Hispanic migrant adolescents. *American Journal of Preventive Medicine, 20* (4), 258–265.

Cardenas, M., & Simons-Morton, B. (1993). The effect of anticipatory guidance on mothers' self-efficacy and behavioral intentions to prevent burns caused by hot tap water. *Patient Education and Counseling, 21* (3), 117–123.

Centers for Disease Control and Prevention. Youth Risk Behavior Surveillance—United States, 2003. (2005). National Center for Chronic Disease Prevention and Health Promotion (producer). Retrieved April 26, 2005, from apps.nccd.cdc.gov/yrbss/CategoryQuestions.asp?cat=1%desc=Unintentional%20Injuries%20and%20Violence.

Centers for Disease Control and Prevention, National Centers for Injury Prevention and Control. (2003/2004). Web-based injury statistics query and reporting system (WISQARS). Retrieved April 26, 2005, from www.cdc.gov/ncipc/wisqars.

Coggan, C., Patterson, P., Brewin, M., Hooper, R., & Robinson, E. (2000). Evaluation of the Waitakere Community Injury Prevention Project. *Injury Prevention, 6* (2), 130–134.

Davidson, L., Durkin, M., Kuhn, L., O'Conner, P., Barlow, B., & Heagarty, M. (1994). The impact of the Safe Kids/Healthy Neighborhoods Injury Prevention Program in Harlem, 1988 through 1991. *American Journal of Public Health, 84* (4), 580–586.

Farrell, A., Meyer, A., & Dahlberg, L. (1996). Richmond Youth Against Violence: A school-based program for urban adolescents. *American Journal of Preventive Medicine, 12* (5 supplement), 13–21.

Green, L., & Kreuter, M. (1999). *Health promotion planning: An educational and ecological approach* (3rd ed.). Mountain View, CA: Mayfield.

Hendrickson, S., & Becker, H. (1998). Impact of a theory based intervention to increase bicycle helmet use in low income children. *Injury Prevention, 4* (2), 126–131.

Institute of Medicine. (2002). *Speaking of health: Assessing health communication strategies for diverse populations.* Washington, DC: National Academies Press.

Kreuter, M., Lukwago, S., Bucholtz, D., Clark, E., & Sanders-Thompson, V. (2003). Achieving cultural appropriateness in health promotion programs: Targeted and tailored approaches. *Health Education & Behavior, 30* (2), 133–146.

Kreuter, M., Steger-May, K., Bobra, S., Booker, A., Holt, C., Lukwgo, S., & Skinner, C. (2003). Sociocultural characteristics and responses to cancer education materials among African American women. *Cancer Control, 10* (5 supplement), 69–80.

Kreuter, M., Sugg-Skinner, C., Holt, C., Clark, E., Haire-Joshu, D., Fu, Q., Booker, A., Steger-May, K., & Bucholtz, D. (2005). Cultural tailoring for mammography and fruit and vegetable intake among low-income African American women in urban public health centers. *Preventive Medicine, 41* (1), 53–62.

Lay health advisors: A critical link to community capacity building [Special Issue]. (1997). *Health Education & Behavior, 24*, 407–510.

Lukwago, S., Kreuter, M., Bucholtz, D., Holt, C., & Clark, E. (2001). Development and validation of brief scales to measure collectivism, religiosity, racial pride, and time orientation in urban African American women. *Family & Community Health, 24* (3), 63–71.

Lukwago, S., Kreuter, M., Holt, C., Steger-May, K., Bucholtz, D., & Skinner, C. (2003). Sociocultural correlates of breast cancer knowledge and screening in urban African American women. *American Journal of Public Health, 93* (8), 1271–1274.

Moriarty, S. (1995). Visual communication as primary system. *Journal of Visual Literacy, 14* (2), 11–21.

Nansel, T., Weaver, N., Donlin, M., Jacobsen, H., Kreuter, M., & Simons-Morton, B. (2002). Baby, be safe: The effect of pediatric injury prevention tailored communications provided in a primary care setting. *Patient Education and Counseling, 46* (3), 175–190.

Orlandi, M., Landers, C., Weston, R., & Haley, N. (1990). Diffusion of health promotion innovations. In K. Glanz, F. Lewis, & B. Rimer (Eds.), *Health behavior and health education: Theory, research, and practice* (pp. 288–313). San Francisco: Jossey-Bass.

Orpinas, P., Kelder, S., Frankowski, R., Murray, N., Zhang, Q., & McAlister, A. (2000). Outcome evaluation of a multi-component violence-prevention program for middle schools: The Students for Peace Project. *Health Education Research, 15* (1), 45–58.

Orpinas, P., Parcel, G., McAlister, A., & Frankowski, R. (1995). Violence prevention in middle schools: A pilot evaluation. *Journal of Adolescent Health, 17* (6), 360–371.

Petty, R., & Cacioppo, J. (1981). *Attitudes and persuasion: Classic and contemporary approaches.* Dubuque, IA: Brown.

Resnicow, K., Baranowski, T., Ahluwalia, J., & Braithwaite, R. (1999). Cultural sensitivity in public health: Defined and demystified. *Ethnicity & Disease, 9* (1), 10–21.

Rogler, L., Malgady, R., Costantino, G., & Blumenthal, R. (1987). What do culturally sensitive mental health services mean? *American Psychologist, 42* (6), 565–570.

Schiffman, C. (1995). Ethnovisual and sociovisual elements of design: Visual dialect as a basis for creativity in public service graphic design. *Journal of Visual Literacy, 14* (2), 23–39.

Schwarz, D., Grisso, J., Miles, C., Holmes, J., & Sutton, R. (1993). An injury prevention program in an urban African-American community. *American Journal of Public Health, 83* (5), 675–680.

Thomas, J., Eng, E., Clark, M., Robinson, J., & Blumenthal, C. (1998). Lay health advisors: Sexually transmitted disease prevention through community involvment. *American Journal of Public Health, 88* (8), 1252–1253.

U.S. Department of Health and Human Services. (2000). *Healthy People 2010* (vol. 1). Washington, DC: U.S. Government Printing Office.

Weinstein, N., & Sandman, P. (1992). A model of the precaution adoption process: Evidence from home radon testing. *Health Psychology, 11* (3), 170–180.

Wiist, W., Jackson, R., & Jackson, K. (1996). Peer and community leader education to prevent youth violence. *American Journal of Preventive Medicine, 12* (5 supplement), 56–64.

Zaloshnja, E., Miller, T., Galbraith, M., Lawrence, B., DeBruyn, L., Bill, N., Hicks, K., Keiffer, M., & Perkins, R. (2003). Reducing injuries among Native Americans: Five cost-outcome analyses. *Accident Analysis & Prevention, 35* (5), 631–639.

Chapter 26

Evaluating Fidelity and Effectiveness of Interventions

Lawrence R. Berger and David C. Grossman

26.1. INTRODUCTION

The implementation and dissemination of injury control interventions in community settings often follows the publication of findings from formal research trials. In the absence of strong evidence for an intervention, public health administrators must decide to solve problems by creating new solutions or implementing interventions that appear to be promising and model current public health best practice. In either scenario, program officers need to understand if the decision to implement the intervention led to an important public health effect in their community setting. The evaluation of the effectiveness of an intervention or program is particularly important if there are few previous studies of the program's effectiveness in real-world settings because the future diffusion of the program to other sites depends on its demonstrated effectiveness. The evaluation of the fidelity of the program implementation process is also an important task for program officials. *Fidelity* is defined as the accuracy or exactness of the replication of an intervention, based on the prototype model. Program administrators must be careful to monitor the fidelity of the program components as they have been developed in previous research models. Failure to monitor the quality of implementation of the intervention procedures could lead to reduced effectiveness of the program.

The purpose of this chapter is to review approaches toward the evaluation of program effectiveness and fidelity. The intended audience for this chapter is primarily injury control and public health program administrators and their staff. In this chapter, we describe two specific scenarios frequently faced by program administrators. The first is the development of an evaluation section of a funding proposal from a state government department of health to disseminate an injury prevention intervention. The second involves planning for a site visit to evaluate an injury prevention program in a state or local health department. Both require extensive preparation and coordination of people and activities. Both require careful attention to program implementation and evaluation strategies. We believe that the execution of these scenarios illustrates some of the practical principles regarding the evaluation of program fidelity and effectiveness.

26.2. PLANNING A GRANT APPLICATION FOR A PROGRAM

26.2.1. The Rationale for Well-Developed Evaluation Plans

Imagine yourself as the director of an injury control program for a state or provincial health department, and you have just spotted a request for funding proposals from a federal agency to disseminate an injury prevention program in your area. Given the needs of your community, the expertise of your staff, and your budget, you decide to apply for funding to increase the proportion of households that have functional smoke alarms in two poor, rural counties in your state. Your long-term goal is to reduce the rates of death and hospitalization from house fires, which are known to be disproportionately high in those two counties. Having done some review of the topic, you decide to conduct this intervention by distributing and installing photoelectric smoke alarms with 10-year lithium batteries (Lee, 2002). You are aware of some recent evidence from a randomized controlled trial in the United Kingdom that the distribution of alarms in poor urban areas did not lead to a reduction in fire injuries in that setting (DiGuiseppi et al., 2002). But that same trial found that predictors of functional alarms included the use of long-life lithium batteries and that a major disappointing outcome of the trial was that many of the alarms were not installed. Furthermore, you are also aware of an intervention in the state of Oklahoma that demonstrated a substantial decrease in the rate of fire deaths after a smoke alarm distribution program (Mallonee et al., 1996). Knowing that there is strong evidence for the effectiveness of alarms, reasonable and plausible evidence for the use of lithium batteries, conflicting evidence regarding the effect of distribution programs, and conflicting evidence regarding the value of ionization or photoelectric alarms (Fazzini, Perkins, & Grossman, 2000), you decide to develop a new solution by building on this knowledge base. You propose a new program that distributes and installs photoelectric alarms with long-life lithium batteries.

Not long after hatching this concept, your colleagues challenge you regarding the need for an evaluation. They ask, "Why evaluate this program when the evaluation funds could be used to provide more households with alarms?" Your response should emphasize that your proposed approach is relatively novel and that it will provide new information about the effectiveness of this general intervention. Unlike having to redemonstrate the protective value of well-proven interventions, such as a bike helmet distribution programs, this program has some untested features and is based on some conflicting evidence. Your funding agency's requirement to have an evaluation will also be persuasive to your colleagues.

26.2.1.1. Evaluation Goals

The preparation of the evaluation section for your grant application will need to include a carefully crafted statement of the goals of the evaluation. These goals should translate to specific objectives and the action steps necessary to realize them.

Furthermore, the evaluation goals should stem from the specific aims of the entire proposal. For example, the major long-term aim of the proposed program is to reduce the rate of house fire deaths among residents of two poor, rural counties by increasing the proportion of households in those counties with functional smoke alarm systems. Distributing and systematically installing smoke alarms, along with a brief behavioral intervention, is your proposed strategy. In this instance, your evaluation section should address how you propose to measure the effectiveness of the program with regard to the long-term aim and the process by which you propose to achieve that aim.

26.2.1.2.   Stakeholders

Who are the stakeholders for the evaluation and how should they be included in your plan? Even if this intervention does not meet the strict definitions of community-based participatory research, the leadership of the communities touched by this intervention should have a clear stake in its outcome and assist with its design. Your funding agency is another clear stakeholder and may want to have an explicit role in the design and implementation of the evaluation if your award is a cooperative agreement. Other potential stakeholders could be the fire departments and brigades from the counties in question as well as the local health departments.

26.2.1.3.   Formative Evaluation Planning

As you write the evaluation section, it occurs to you that you know little about the acceptability of the proposed intervention plans to the target households. Ideally, you would have some preliminary data demonstrating the wisdom of your proposed approach to have public safety personnel conduct the intervention and of your approach to remove and replace existing smoke alarms that do not use lithium batteries. A "formative evaluation" assesses the feasibility and acceptability of intervention components (including messages, materials, and delivery channels) to both target audiences and program deliverers during the planning and early intervention stages of a program (Christoffel & Scavo Gallagher, 1999). For example, if you held focus groups of county senior citizens, you may find that they would allow entry for uniformed personnel working out of official vehicles but not for off-duty personnel in civilian clothing.

26.2.1.4.   Fidelity Measurement

Your evaluation plan should also include a section regarding how you would measure the fidelity of the intervention implementation, as it is described in the grant. You realize that you will be working with 10 different public safety agencies to install these alarms and that your staff will be training each agency individually. To measure the fidelity of your implementation strategy, you will need to identify the key components (e.g., training, notification of households, identification of households eligible for alarms, delivery/installation of alarms) and specify the delivery mechanism (e.g., public safety personnel). In some types of fidelity evaluations, your staff will need to pay close attention to the dosing and frequency of the intervention, if these parameters are specified. In this example, your staff may find that the installers were successful with the installation of the first alarm, but often missed the need to replace other alarms in the house. If repeat visits are needed, how will you measure if they occurred? Your plan also specifies that staff will accompany and observe a random number of verbal interactions with the homeowners. This provides some assurance that the messaging about fire safety and alarm maintenance is delivered consistently, regardless of the agency or person involved.

26.2.1.5.   Outcome and Measurement Issues

Assessing the health effect of some injury prevention interventions can often prove difficult if the outcome of interest is rare, or if the population affected by the intervention is relatively small. In cases in which the association of the intervention and the health outcome have been demonstrated, such as the use of seat belts to prevent occupant injuries, the measurement of an intermediate outcome yields persuasive evidence of the program's effect. Even when health effect outcomes are used, measurement of intermediate outcomes can provide insight into the potential reasons for the failure of a program. In your program, you are certain that you wish to measure an intermediate outcome, such as the presence of a functional alarm in the home. You decide to define a *functional* smoke alarm as one that alarms when a test dose of artificial smoke is introduced near the detector. Nonfunctional smoke alarms may have dead batteries, may have been disconnected, or are otherwise broken. You choose this intermediate outcome because it is the main pathway by which you believe your intervention will succeed. There may be other potential pathways by which this intervention could prove successful (e.g., by activating residents to take other fire safety precautions). You also cannot simply assume that, because agencies distributed and installed the alarms, the alarms are still present in the houses. Residents could remove the smoke alarm because of nuisance alarms, remove the valuable battery for other uses, or even sell the alarm.

What exactly will you measure, how will you measure it, and where will you conduct the measurements? Your staff attempts to persuade you to perform random digit dial telephone calls to the county residents asking them if they have a functional smoke alarm. They argue that this efficient strategy could save money by not requiring travel. You discover, however, that the evidence regarding the validity of self-reports of smoke alarm functional status is not very good (Douglas, Mallonee, & Istree, 1999) and disagree with this suggestion. Instead, you propose to identify a random sample of households in the two targeted counties and in two control counties at two different time intervals, before and after the intervention. You propose to have your staff visit these homes and inspect them for at least one functional alarm (by spraying some artificial smoke into the alarm). A biostatistician confirms that you can afford to visit enough households to be able to demonstrate an important and statistically significant difference in the rates of homes with functional smoke alarms between the test counties and the control counties. Given that several studies have already confirmed the effectiveness of smoke alarms, the results of your evaluation of smoke alarm prevalence and functionality could prove to be very powerful, even without direct evidence of health effect.

Measurement of intermediate outcomes can be either quantitative or qualitative (Broughton, 1991). Though this program evaluation would appear to rest primarily on quantitative data, qualitative data can also add an important dimension to our understanding of how and why interventions succeed or fail. The main distinction between qualitative and quantitative data is the format of data collection. Qualitative assessments are based on asking open-ended questions. The data are the narrative responses one receives. If your evaluation relied only on the presence or absence of a functional alarm and a few close-ended questions about problems with the smoke alarm, then you may miss important explanatory information that would help explain why so many lithium batteries were missing from the recently installed alarms. Your assumption may be that they were removed because of nuisance alarms. If you had planned to routinely and systematically ask the following open-ended question to all homeowners who had nonfunctional smoke alarms: "Why is the battery missing?" you may uncover an explanation that did not occur to you at the time you created the follow-up questionnaire. The commonly heard theme is that batteries were removed after a rumor swept through the community that lithium batteries were associated with adverse health effects.

Ultimately, your staff and stakeholders would like to know if the program demonstrated an effect on the public's health. Every injury prevention intervention proposal should attempt to address this question in the evaluation section of the proposal. However, this goal is not always possible to achieve. For example, measuring the success of suicide prevention programs on adolescent mortality can be exceedingly difficult given the relatively rare frequency of the outcome. If mortality effect cannot be assessed, then consider the measurement of the effect of the intervention on rates of hospital admissions, emergency department visits, or even emergency medical system responses. Aside from health effects, other important domains for evaluation are costs, community awareness and satisfaction, and a feasibility assessment for diffusion of the program into other counties. Community demonstration programs provide more realistic estimates of the implementation costs than research trials. Though the fiscal costs of the program will be of interest to your colleagues in state government, ideally you would like to demonstrate some type of cost analysis that helps pinpoint the value of the program. Though sophisticated cost-effectiveness and cost-utility analyses may be beyond the scope of your program evaluation, a crude estimate of the cost to benefit ratio (measured as the costs in dollars of the intervention, divided by the savings in dollars that resulted from the program) can be persuasive to policy makers, especially if there are net savings. This program might result in a heightened community awareness and activation level about house fire prevention that extends beyond the goals of the original program. A local philanthropic group or person, in an enthusiastic response to your program, may decide to augment the program by providing free fire extinguishers to county residents. The image of public safety officers in the community may be enhanced significantly through their participation in the program as intervention agents. These are important elements to capture and help affirm the success of the program's ability to leverage community support.

Your evaluation plan for the proposal should also assess potential negative ramifications of the intervention plan. Some of these negative consequences cannot be anticipated but should be collected and reported as potential outcomes. The public appears to have much lower tolerance for serious adverse effects from preventive interventions, compared to interventions to correct a known problem.

26.2.1.6. *Oversight and Governance*

Your evaluation plan should also include a proposal for oversight of the evaluation. Research studies that use controlled clinical trial study designs are usually required to have a data safety monitoring board to monitor the progress and safety of a study. Though the accountability of the success of the program usually resides with the principal investigator (PI) of a grant, the PI needs to specify the role of oversight boards in the evaluation phase of the program, particularly if there could be potential adverse effects of the intervention. In this study, you may wish to include community members and other stakeholders on a formal oversight board.

Though this chapter focuses on program evaluation, most program interventions that are developed with the specific intention of generating new knowledge should be reviewed by an institutional review board (IRB), which reviews proposals to ensure ethical treatment of human subjects in research. IRBs are responsible for reviewing and monitoring the conduct of most research activities and should be consulted in the early stages of proposal development for a judgment regarding the need for review. IRBs may use the intention to publish peer-reviewed publications as one proxy for defining an activity as research. An explicit intention to publish the results of this program should provoke a decision as to whether an IRB review is necessary. You have nearly completed the program evaluation section for your grant. Before you send it in, you remember to have two colleagues review it, critique it, and provide feedback. Now you're set to get your grant.

26.2.2. Summary

The preparation of an evaluation section in a funding proposal requires considerable attention and advanced planning. The proposal authors must clarify the goals of the evaluation and how they relate to the goals of the overall project. Ideally, stakeholders are identified early in the process and included in the planning of the project and its evaluation. Some formative evaluation may be required to assess the acceptability and optimal delivery method of the intervention to the target population. The fidelity of the program delivery requires careful assessment to ensure that the intervention was received as intended. Finally, the choice of appropriate intermediate outcome or health effect measures for the evaluation is a critical component of any evaluation proposal. The success of any public health project evaluation can be enhanced by the formation of an oversight body consisting of internal advisers and external stakeholders.

26.3. IMPLEMENTATION EVALUATION

Another role in which program managers require evaluation skills is when serving as external program reviewers. A program review (also referred to as interim evaluation, program monitoring, and implementation evaluation) assesses a program during its implementation phase.

Consider the following scenario: You agree to participate in a site visit to an injury prevention program in another city. This community-based program, titled Healthy Children, Healthy Families (HCHF), has a goal of reducing injuries and deaths from child maltreatment in Nosuch County. It uses home visitation, coordination of family services, and community-based strategies to promote optimal child growth and development. The county has a population of 30,000. The program began a year ago with a 5-year grant from the Benevolent Foundation. Most of the grant funds are used to support a program coordinator, four nurse home visitors, and a community-awareness campaign.

Even for a program as focused as this, the components of implementation that can be evaluated are virtually limitless. It is, therefore, imperative to have priorities that can be balanced against time, data availability, local expertise, and other constraints. In an approach to evaluation variously called action, participatory, utilization focused, and empowerment evaluation, program stakeholders (program managers, staff, clients, community members) are active participants in identifying key components, setting priorities, and determining the evaluative approaches likely to be most useful and most feasible to implement (Crump & Letourneau, 2002; Doll, Bartenfeld, & Binder, 2003; Quinn Patton, 2002). Funding agencies are usually interested in ensuring financial and programmatic accountability and maximizing the effect of their funds by improving program performance. Except when they are specifically funding research initiatives, their primary intent is not to generate new, potentially generalizable insights into program implementation. The latter goal usually requires more rigorous, intensive, and expensive evaluation efforts.

The usual methods for collecting information during a site visit are to review written materials—the original grant, work plans, budgets, funding agency reports—and to interview the program coordinator and key staff. Summary statistics of quantitative process measures for the Nosuch program might include the number of home visits, families served, and referrals made/completed to specific agencies. Examples of evaluation documents relevant to the community awareness and involvement activities of the program appear in Table 26.1.

An external evaluator can also schedule meetings with members of the program's advisory committee or oversight board and with community members or program participants. With sufficient lead time, a site-visit team can request that specific assessment instruments be completed, such as a customer satisfaction survey or the Partnership Self-Assessment Tool (discussed later in this chapter). There is also the option of creating an e-mail survey, with or without the help of a no-cost or low-cost Internet survey service (e.g., SurveyMonkey and SurveyConsole).

Preparing a checklist or matrix is a useful approach for organizing a program review. A typical matrix includes a list of program components (such as fidelity, budget/finances, marketing efforts, sustainability, training), selected indicators, and performance criteria (Crump & Letourneau, 2002; State and Territorial Injury Prevention Directors' Association, 2003). Here is an example for the Nosuch HCHF program:

- *Component:* data collection and analysis
- *Evaluation indicators:* types of data collected, sources of data, data quality (comparability, relevance, completeness, accuracy, timeliness), accessibility of data for analyses and reports
- *Criteria for advanced performance:* a data form is completed for every attempted home visit; at least 20% of participant feedback forms are received and analyzed; there are data-sharing agreements with key agencies, including No such child protection services, the community hospital, and the Nosuch police department; a community survey of residents' recall and understanding of media messages is conducted annually; an annual program report, including maltreatment-related hospitalizations and mortality data, is distributed to key stakeholders (police chief, service providers, legislators, funders), and the community

A much more comprehensive example of an evaluation matrix was published by Crump and Letourneau (2002). Also, the web site of the Evaluation Center of Western Michigan University (2005) (a center that focuses primarily on education

Table 26.1. Documenting Community Implementation Components[a]

Implementation Activities	Types of Records
Community coalition or community development meetings	Meeting announcement/flyer; agenda and minutes; list of issues of concern; recommendations for action; participant sign-in sheets
Community recruitment: phone calls, personal contacts, letters, visits to organizations or agencies to solicit support	List of outreach activities: date, organization, individual contacted, outcome; sample letters and/or materials as appropriate
Community informational meetings/presentations	Agenda or presentation outline; list of presentations: location, date, time, name of presenter, number in attendance; materials distributed; participant sign-in sheets
Community events: special events, such as festivals, rodeos, pageants, health fairs, holiday or cultural celebrations	Description: activity, location, date, time, population served, estimated number of participants, brief explanation of how prevention issues were promoted
Conduct trainings: education and training activities for professionals or community members with a predetermined curriculum	Training agenda: dates, location, names of trainers; training materials; participant sign-in sheets; evaluation summary for each training event; list of trainings conducted by participants, if train-the-trainer
Provide technical assistance	List of technical assistance activities: date, organization, individual contacted, nature of technical assistance provided, outcome; sample materials
Serve as a member of a committee convened by another agency or organization	List of meetings attended: name of committee, agency or organization, date, location, brief statement of contributions made and benefits derived from participation; agenda and minutes
Media activities	Media plan; list of media venues: type, location, play dates; copies of print media, posters, audio/video scripts; news conference materials: event plan, announcement, tapes of audio or video productions; surveys to assess exposure, penetration, recall, and understanding

[a]Adapted from V. Foster, personal communication (2001).

and human services evaluations) maintains a database of evaluation checklists, including the Checklists Development Checklist (Quinn Patton, 2002).

The following sections address some key issues for implementation evaluation: financial accountability, program progress, fidelity and adaptation, collaborations, sustainability, and reporting.

26.3.1. Financial Accountability

When a project officer for a child passenger safety grant was asked what evaluation questions she most wanted answered, she replied: "I want to know that they actually purchased the car seats." (personal communication, anonymous) Financial accountability is a priority for all funding sources and a midcourse review of a program's budget, financial status, and estimated cost-per-unit-of-service can be very revealing. The purpose of the review is to ensure that funds are being expended and accounted for appropriately, to detect problematic expenditures before they overwhelm the program, to maximize resource allocation decisions, and to confirm that essential cost information is being recorded for future outcome evaluation. A program coordinator or manager should be able to provide a budget with amounts expended to date, obligated funds, and funds remaining for each line item along with service statistics, such as the number of program participants, list of activities conducted, and staff time sheets.

The budgetary review might identify line items with large unexpended funds, suggesting that program components are not being fully implemented or key personnel were not hired when they should have been. Conversely, line items with excessive expenditures might indicate unanticipated or inappropriate expenses (such as paying home visitors for non-program-related activities).

Even a crude cost estimate can suggest multiple avenues to improving program effectiveness. Suppose the Nosuch HCHF program spends $10,000 in a 3-month period when only 20 home visits were completed. The crude average of $500/visit seems excessive, and the program managers might ask the following:

- Are the data collection methods accurate and complete, both for costs and number of home visits?
- Is there a less costly way to conduct the home visits, such as scheduling visits to minimize transportation costs?
- Is there a way to increase the home visit completion rate, such as making telephone calls or mailing reminders to families of scheduled visits?
- Is the program in fact cost effective—for example, because the expenditures for that quarter included one-time media development costs in addition to the home visits?

More rigorous economic evaluations (such as cost–benefit and cost-effectiveness analyses) can be both complex and controversial. Sophisticated cost analyses are likely to require the services of a consultant to identify all the direct costs, determine which costs are fixed and which are variable, allocate indirect costs, define appropriate units of service and outcomes, and conduct sensitivity analyses (Aos, Lieb, Mayfield, Miller, & Pennucci, 2004; Pietrazak, Ramler, Renner, Ford, & Gilbert, 1990; Plotnick & Deppman, 1999; Sewell & Marczak, 1998).

26.3.2.   Program Progress

Essential questions for any interim evaluation are the following: To what extent is the program fulfilling its original objectives and action plan? Have certain project activities been ignored or abandoned? Has all the key staff been hired? For service delivery programs, what has been the pace of subject recruitment and dropout? Comparing the activities and timeline described in the original proposal with progress to date can reveal challenges to effective program implementation, such as staff turnover and competing agency priorities. It is also important to identify challenges to outcome evaluation. Are there secular trends or historical factors (changing economic conditions, new laws, other heightened enforcement procedures) that might influence the effect of the program?

Other essential questions are: What have been the consequences of implementing the program so far? What are the program's accomplishments and successes? Have there been any negative consequences? An example of an unanticipated negative consequence might be political pressure to end sobriety checkpoints resulting from the arrest of a legislator at a checkpoint.

26.3.3.   Fidelity and Adaptation

Fidelity of implementation is another aspect of program accountability. Are all the components considered vital for success by the developers of the intervention being implemented (Center for the Study and Prevention of Violence, 2005.) The Nosuch home visitation program was designed to replicate the success of the Nurse-Family Partnership (NFP) program, founded by Olds (Nurse-Family Partnership, 2005b; Olds, et al., 2004). Key aspects of the NFP program include:

- Provide services to low-income, first-time parents and their children.
- Have registered nurses conduct the home visits.
- Require that home visitors complete 60 hours of instruction from the NFP professional development team.
- For each family served, aim to complete 14 visits during pregnancy, 28 during infancy, and 22 during toddlerhood.
- Provide services to a sufficient number of families (generally 100) to benefit from basic operational efficiencies.
- Limit caseloads to 25 families.
- Use visit guidelines that "focus on the mother's personal health, quality of care giving, and life-course development" (Nurse-Family Partnership, 2005a).
- Begin making visits before 28 weeks of gestation of pregnancy.
- Continue visits through the first 2 years of the child's life.
- Involve family and community support systems.
- Use a clinical information system to record family characteristics, needs, services, and progress toward goals.

Of course, every program will require adaptations based on local circumstances and needs. Before the Nosuch program was implemented, what kinds of formative evaluation (focus groups, interviews, surveys) were conducted and what were the results? How were the results used to modify or redesign the interventions? For the Nosuch HCHF program, questions might have included:

- How widespread is support for a nurse home visitation program within the community and among existing service providers, such as child protective service workers, social workers, and child-care providers?
- What are the concerns/arguments against implementing a home visitation program? Are there any obstacles to implementation, such as cultural barriers, lack of qualified staff, confidentiality issues, legal or financial constraints, competing priorities, or visitor safety?
- How might these arguments and concerns be addressed to best meet the needs of families?

When it comes to fidelity and adoption, the urgent evaluation question is, Do deviations from the original intervention design represent enhancements (such as the translation of materials into other languages) or changes that might seriously compromise program effectiveness (such as substituting non-nurse home visitors for nurses to reduce program costs)?

26.3.4.   Collaborations, Partnerships, and Public Participation

The Nosuch HCHF program includes a community coalition; informal, collaborative relationships with Nosuch social services, law enforcement, counseling services, and other agencies; and a commitment to maximize public participation in its community-based efforts. Quantitative process measures (such as the number of people participating in a coalition meeting and the number of public presentations) can document the nature and level of these activities. However, qualitative approaches provide deeper insights into how effectively these activities are being conducted. Two useful instruments that elicit feedback from partnership participants are the Collaboration Factor Inventory Score (CFIS) sheet (Amherst H. Wilder Foundation, 2005) and the Partnership Self-Assessment Tool (PSAT) (Center for the Advancement of Collaborative Strategies in Health, 2004). Both assess key areas of partnership functioning, such as leadership, communication, conflict resolution, administration and management, adequacy of resources, decision making, satisfaction with participation, and synergy (by working together, how well are the partners able to solve problems, develop goals, and respond to the needs of the community?). The Nosuch program coordinator or chairperson of the HCHF coalition could distribute the CFIS or register the coalition with the PSAT web site (participants are given 30 days to complete the survey). The feedback report and recommendations could be made available to the coalition members and discussed at the site visit.

A conceptual framework for public participation (Fig. 26.1) (International Association for Public Participation (IAP2), 2005) suggests important questions for implementation evaluation: What is the program's public participation goal—inform, consult, involve, collaborate, or empower? What tools are being used to foster public participation? To improve the program's effectiveness and visibility, should the program be promoting an increased level of public participation? IAP2 offers a toolbox that summarizes techniques for sharing information (fact sheets to technical reports), compiling input, providing feedback (information hotlines to web-based meetings), and bringing people together (tours to citizen juries).

26.3.5. Sustainability

Is a program effective if it is not sustainable? One should ask, "What will happen when the grant funding ends?" well in advance of the termination date. Reviewing a program's approach to sustainability can be a valuable contribution of an interim evaluation. Having a mechanism, such as a resource development committee, to create both a business plan and a marketing plan can greatly enhance the likelihood of long-term sustainability. The marketing plan should address external marketing (how the program is made visible to the community) and internal marketing (how the program is made visible within the agency or organization). Distributing newsletters, creating e-mail mailing lists, and nurturing "program champions" (middle- to upper-level administrators who can serve as program advocates) (Center for Civic Partnerships [CCP], 2001) are examples of internal marketing techniques. Publicizing program activities via mass media (articles and editorial pieces in magazines, newspapers, and professional journals; public service announcements; radio and television interviews) is one avenue of external marketing. Other methods are to create and distribute slide sets, software, training manuals, newsletters, annual reports, brochures, and videotapes; make presentations to the public, political leaders, agency staff, and professional colleagues; and establish a web site.

A narrow definition of *sustainability* is the ability to continue program activities in the face of major changes in funding. It may not be necessary or advisable to

INCREASING LEVEL OF PUBLIC IMPACT

INFORM	CONSULT	INVOLVE	COLLABORATE	EMPOWER
Public Participation Goal:	Public Participation Goal:	Public Participation Goal:	Public Participation Goal:	Public Participation Goal:
To provide the public with balanced and objective information to assist the public in understanding the problem, alternatives, opportunities and/or solutions.	To obtain public feedback on analysis, alternatives and/or decisions.	To work directly with the public throughout the process to ensure that public concerns and aspirations are consistently understood and considered.	To partner with the public in each aspect of the decision including the development of alternatives and the identification of the preferred solution.	To place final decision-making in the hands of the public.
Promise to the Public:	Promise to the Public:	Promise to the Public:	Promise to the Public:	Promise to the Public:
We will keep you informed.	We will keep you informed, listen to and acknowledge concerns and aspirations, and provide feedback on how public input influenced the decision.	We will work with you to ensure that your concerns and aspirations are directly reflected in the alternatives developed and provide feedback on how public input influenced the decision.	We will look to you for direct advice and innovation in formulating solutions and incorporate your advice and recommendations into the decisions to the maximum extent possible.	We will implement what you decide.
Example Techniques to Consider:	Example Techniques to Consider:	Example Techniques to Consider:	Example Techniques to Consider:	Example Techniques to Consider:
• Fact sheets • Web sites • Open houses	• Public comment • Focus groups • Surveys • Public meetings	• Workshops • Deliberate polling	• Citizen Advisory Committees • Consensus-building • Participatory decision-making	• Citizen juries • Ballots • Delegated decisions

Figure 26.1. IAP2 Public Participation Spectrum, developed by the International Association for Public Participation. © 2005 International Association for Public Participation. All rights reserved.

continue all of a program's components. Among the approaches to maintaining activities of the Nosuch program are to:

- *Seek grants and contracts:* Funding sources for child maltreatment prevention programs include both government agencies (e.g., Children's Bureau) and private foundations (e.g., Doris Duke Charitable Foundation, Freddie Mac, Annie E. Casey and Robert Wood Johnson Foundations).
- *Become a line item in an existing budget (institutionalization):* Form a home visitation unit within the Nosuch Health Department.
- *Persuade another organization to continue all or part of an effort:* Have the Nosuch Safe Kids Coalition adopt the community-awareness activities of the HCHF program.
- *Acquire public funding:* Create a dedicated fund for child maltreatment prevention activities by increasing marriage license fees (state Children's

Trust Funds) or by obtaining Community Development Block Grant funding.

- *Request in-kind support:* Ask local radio and TV stations for help creating public service announcements and providing air time.
- *Find free or low-cost personnel resources:* Recruit volunteers to assist HCHF program families by providing transportation for medical appointments, locating child care, and tutoring; involve student interns to help write news releases and editorial pieces.

Programs with a wide community base and that provide direct services to individuals can consider other approaches, such as sharing resources among organizations, conducting fund-raising events, seeking private contributions, requiring fees for specific services, or establishing membership fees and dues (CCP, 2001; Nagy, 2003).

CCP (2001) defines sustainability more broadly as "the continuation of community health or quality of life benefits over time." In this broader perspective, obtaining continuation funding or institutionalizing existing programs are but two options. Other methods for maintaining program benefits long term are to establish new policies and procedures (e.g., establish a state-funded home visitation program for all new parents) and to build the "capacity of individuals, agencies, and organizations to own the problem and maintain involvement in the process" (CCP, 2001)—for example, conduct information sessions for local news reporters on effective strategies for promoting child well-being.)

26.3.6.   Summarizing the Interim Evaluation

The final report of the site visit should summarize the purpose and methods of the evaluation, key findings related to the program's strengths and weaknesses, and recommendations. The recommendations should address at least these two questions:

- With existing resources, how can the program maximize its effectiveness in the realms of administration, data collection, and implementation of core components?
- If the program had more resources, what activities (direct services, educational efforts, partnerships/collaboration, and advocacy) would most enhance program effectiveness?

The findings and recommendations can be formatted in multiple ways for presentation to different audiences. Preparing not only a complete report, but also an executive summary and *Power Point* presentation, for example, can help attract additional funding, improve collaboration, and enhance program effectiveness.

26.4.   CONCLUSION

A great deal of program evaluation is aimed at answering four questions:

- What activities has the program implemented (or not implemented)? (fidelity)
- How much of each activity has occurred? (fidelity)
- Who have been the recipients of the interventions? (fidelity)

- What have been the consequences (short and long term, positive and negative)? (effectiveness)

An outcome evaluation needs to address all four questions. A grant application needs to answer these questions in anticipation of future implementation. An evaluation of an existing program can assess short- but not long-term consequences.

The best evaluations are the result of collaborative planning, performance, and analysis among key stakeholders: evaluators, funding sources, service providers, and program participants. They result in enhanced knowledge of what works and what does not, improved program functioning, and better allocation of scarce resources to improve health and well-being.

REFERENCES

Amherst H. Wilder Foundation. (2005). *The Wilder collaboration factors inventory.* Retrieved September 13, 2005, from surveys.wilder.org/public_cfi/index.php.

Aos, S., Lieb, R., Mayfield, J., Miller, M., & Pennucci, A. (2004). *Benefits and costs of prevention and early intervention programs for youth.* Olympia: Washington State Institute for Public Policy.

Broughton, W. (1991). Qualitative methods in program evaluation. *American Journal of Health Promotion, 5,* 461–465.

Center for the Advancement of Collaborative Strategies in Health. (2004). *Partnership self-assessment tool.* Retrieved September 13, 2005, from www.PartnershipTool.net/overview.htm.

Center for Civic Partnerships. (2001). *Sustainability toolkit.* Retrieved September 13, 2005, from http://www.civicpartnerships.org/.

Center for the Study and Prevention of Violence. (2005). *Blueprints for violence prevention.* Retrieved September 13, 2005, from www.colorado.edu/cspv/blueprints.

Christoffel, T., & Scavo Gallagher, S. (1999). *Injury prevention and public health.* Gaithersburg, MD: Aspen Publishers.

Crump, C. E., & Letourneau, R. J. (2002). Developing a process to evaluate a national injury prevention program: The Indian Health Service injury prevention program. In A. Steckler & L. Linnan (Eds.), *Process evaluation for public health interventions* (pp. 321–357). San Francisco: Josey-Bass.

DiGuiseppi, C., Roberts, I., Wade, A., Sculpher, M., Edwards, P., Godward, C., Pan, H., & Slater, S. (2002). Incidence of fires and related injuries after giving out free smoke alarms: Cluster randomised controlled trial. *British Medical Journal, 325,* 995.

Doll, L., Bartenfeld, T., & Binder, S. (2003). Evaluation of interventions designed to prevent and control injuries. *Epidemiologic Reviews, 25,* 51–59.

Douglas, M. R., Mallonee, S., & Istre, G. R. (1999). Estimating the proportion of homes with functioning smoke alarms: A comparison of telephone survey and household survey results. *American Journal of Public Health, 89,* 1112–1114.

The Evaluation Center of Western Michigan University. (2005). *Evaluation checklists.* Retrieved September 13, 2005, from www.wmich.edu/evalctr/checklists/checklistmenu.htm.

Fazzini, T. M., Perkins. R., & Grossman D. (2000). Ionization and photoelectric smoke alarms in rural Alaskan homes. *Western Journal of Medicine, 173,* 89–92.

International Association for Public Participation. Public participation spectrum. Retrieved December 15, 2005, from iap2.org/practitionertools/spectrum.pdf.

International Association for Public Participation. IAP2 Home page. Retrieved December 15, 2005, from www.iap2.org.

Lee, A. (2002). *Preliminary test results on lithium batteries used in residential smoke alarms.* Retrieved September 13, 2005, from www.cpsc.gov/LIBRARY/FOIA/FOIA02/os/LithiumFinal.pdf.

Mallonee, S., Istre, G.R., Rosenberg, M., Reddish-Douglas, M., Jordan, F., Silverstein, P., & Tunnell, W. (1996). Surveillance and prevention of residential-fire injuries. *New England Journal of Medicine, 335,* 27–31.

Nagy, J. (2003). *Getting grants and financial resources: Developing a plan for financial sustainability.* Retrieved September 13, 2005, from ctb.ku.edu/tools/en/chapter_1042.htm.

Nurse-Family Partnership. (2005a). Fact sheet: Overview of nurse-family partnership. Retrieved September 3, 2005, from www.nursefamilypartnership.org/resources/files/PDF/Fact_Sheets/NFPOverview.pdf.

Nurse-Family Partnership. (2005b). Nurse-Family Partnership Home page. Retrieved September 3, 2005, from www.nursefamilypartnership.org.

Olds, D. L., Kitzman, H., Cole, R., Robinson, J., Sidora, K., Luckey, D. W., Henderson, C. R. J., Houks, C., Bondy, J., & Holmberg, J. (2004). Effects of nurse home-visiting on maternal life course and child development: Age 6 follow-up results of a randomized trial. *Pediatrics, 114,* 1550–1559.

Pietrazak, J., Ramler, M., Renner, T., Ford, L., & Gilbert, N. (1990). *Practical program evaluation: Examples from child abuse prevention.* Thousand Oaks, CA: Sage.

Plotnick, R., & Deppman, L. (1999). Using benefit-cost analysis to assess child abuse prevention and intervention programs. *Child Welfare, 78,* 381–407.

Quinn Patton, M. (2002). *Utilization-focused evaluation checklist.* Retrieved September 13, 2005, from www.wmich.edu/evalctr/checklists/ufechecklist.htm.

Sewell, M., & Marczak, M. S. (1998). *Using cost analysis in evaluation.* Retrieved September 3, 2005, from ag.arizona.edu/fcs/cyfernet/cyfar/Costben2.htm.

State and Territorial Injury Prevention Directors' Association. (2003). *Safe States,* 2003 edition. Atlanta, GA: Author.

Other Resources

Centers for Disease Control and Prevention. (2000). *Demonstrating your program's worth: A primer on evaluation for programs to prevent unintentional injury.* Retrieved September 13, 2005, from www.cdc.gov/ncipc/pub-res/demonstr.htm.

Milstein, B., Wetterhall S., & CDC Evaluation Working Group. (2003). *Introduction to evaluation: A framework for program evaluation: A gateway to tools.* Retrieved September 13, 2005, from http://ctb.ku.edu/tools/en/chapter_1036.htm.

National Highway Traffic Safety Administration, Department of Transportation. (1999). *The art of appropriate evaluation: A guide for highway safety program managers* (NHTSA, DOT HS 808–894). Washington, DC: National Highway Traffic Safety Administration.

University of Texas-Houston Health Science Center. (2000). *Practical evaluation of public health programs: PHTN course VC-0017 workbook.* Retrieved September 13, 2005, from www.cdc.gov/eval/workbook.PDF.

Chapter **27**

Involving the Community in Injury Prevention: An Approach Using Community Readiness Interviews

Lorann Stallones and Sallie R. Thoreson

27.1. INTRODUCTION

27.1.1. Community Participation

In 1998, Margolis and Runyan published an article describing barriers that exist in the collaboration between academics, collaborating agencies, and community organizations (Margolis & Runyan, 1998). The barriers listed were differences in approaches to defining and prioritizing problems and strategies for solutions, values and requirements for career advancement, work styles, time demands, and approaches to using information. This list provides a good point to begin to understand what issues arise when trying to develop and maintain injury interventions in communities. Although the authors addressed these issues in regard to academics, communities, and agencies only, these barriers exist equally within organizations. Furthermore, the emphasis on understanding individual risk factors and the application of interventions targeting individuals tends to obscure the contribution of social and environmental conditions to adoption or rejection of specific interventions (Israel, Schulz, Parker, & Becker, 1998).

There have also been calls for more community involvement and control in the development of research and public health programs (Israel et al., 1998). One approach that has been used to address the needed changes in practice is discussed in the case studies later in this chapter. Renewed interest in community-based approaches in research and public health practice has provided new opportunities for integration of community members in collaboration with professionals to design, implement, evaluate, and maintain programs (Green, Daniel, & Novick, 2001). Green et al. (2001) include a wide number of groups in the definition of community partners, including local, state, and national government offices; voluntary agencies; hospitals; community health centers; self-help groups; and universities. A fundamental characteristic of community-based research is the emphasis on the participation and influence of nonacademic researchers in the process of creating knowledge (Israel et al., 1998).

Community-based research recognizes community members as having a sense of identification with one another and of shared values, norms, and mutual influence. It also builds on strengths and resources in the community; facilitates collaborative partnerships in all phases of research; integrates knowledge and action for mutual benefit of all partners; promotes an empowering process that attends to social inequalities; and involves an iterative process that includes partnership development, community assessment, problem definition, develop of methodologies, data collection and analysis, interpretation of data, determination of action, dissemination of results, taking appropriate action, and establishing sustainability (Israel et al., 1998).

Community-based interventions have gone from being viewed as one among many approaches for reducing injuries to the view that that they are an accepted injury control strategy (Spinks, Turner, McClure, & Nixon, 2004) and are currently actively promoted in injury prevention (Nixon, Spinks, Turner, McClure, 2004).

27.1.2.   Community Readiness

Communities vary greatly in their interest and willingness to try new prevention strategies (Aniskiewicz & Wysong, 1990; Bukaski & Amsel, 1994). The adoption of programs is often independent of the leading injury rates in the community; rather it is based on perceived risk or on the presence of an active advocacy group. This is in marked contrast to the scientific research model that would suggest that the rates of injury will be the driving force in developing prevention programs, a view that tends to ignore the social and political environment and competing concerns that may be more pressing for community leaders. An understanding of the social, cultural, and political environments in which programs take place must be incorporated for programs to continue and to grow.

To address these issues, the Colorado Injury Control Research Center (CICRC) has developed as an organization that uses a participatory action research theoretical model to drive community-based interactions in the development of research and programs. To facilitate the participatory action approach, programs within the CICRC have used the Community Readiness Model (Edwards, Jumper-Thurman, Plested, Oetting, & Swansom, 2000) as a tool to establish community contacts, to guide the development of prevention strategies, and to help injury coalitions better understand community perspectives.

The Community Readiness Model was developed using two research traditions: psychological readiness for treatment and community development (Edwards et al., 2000). A number of theoretical models have been developed to describe individual readiness to adopt new behaviors or to comply with treatment regimens. One of the most widely used in public health was developed by Prochaska, DiClemente, & Norcross (1992). This model includes five stages of psychological readiness in which individuals engage in prevention activities: precontemplation (involves minimal awareness of a problem and consequently no intent to invest in change), contemplation (includes awareness but no commitment to action), preparation (involves clear recognition of the problem and exploration of options), action (involves implementation of proposed changes in behavior), and maintenance (includes both consolidation and relapse prevention).

In keeping with the need to incorporate the role of the community in the process of adoption of innovation, several other theories were incorporated, such as the innovation decision-making process (Rogers, 1983) and the social action process (Warren, 1978). Rogers's stages for the innovation decision-making process include knowledge (first awareness of an innovation), persuasion (changing attitudes), decision (adopting the idea), implementation (trying it out), and confirmation (when it is used again or discontinued after initial trial). This provides a community-based parallel approach to the stages of change of the individual suggested by Prochaska et al. (1992). Warren's social action approach parallels these stages, focusing on group processes. The stages include stimulation of interest (recognition of need), initiation (development of problem definition and alternative solutions among community members, who first propose new programs), legitimization (in which local leaders accept the need for action), decision to act (developing specific plans that involve a wider set of community members), and action (or implementation).

Community Readiness interviews are designed to address six dimensions: community efforts in prevention programming, community knowledge about the prevention efforts, community leadership, community climate to support prevention of the issue, knowledge about the magnitude of the problem as an issue in the community, and resources available to address the issue (Edwards et al., 2000). A key informant survey technique is used to assess readiness because the planning, funding, and implementation of prevention programs often lie in the hands of community leaders and because they are the ones most likely to know about activities in their community (Edwards et al., 2000).

The Community Readiness Scale, which is derived from responses of the key informants, results in a single score that represents the stage of readiness for prevention and intervention efforts in the specific problem area and a score for each of the six dimensions (Edwards et al., 2000). Table 27.1 contains a detailed description of the stages of readiness that have been developed. Practical suggestions for activities to move a community to the next stage of readiness are included in the table.

Case Study 1 describes the first attempt made to use Community Readiness in a scientific research project related to traumatic brain injury prevention and the reorientation that occurred among the researchers related to community involvement in the development of injury prevention programs. Case Study 2 describes the use of the Community Readiness Model to help target prevention messages intended to increase the use of child booster seats in a community with a strong traffic safety coalition. Case Study 3 provides a description of how the Community Readiness Model served to increase cohesion in a new rural injury prevention coalition in which the activity related to increasing seat belt use through increased law enforcement.

Table 27.1. Stages, Scores, Stage Definition, and Proposed Activities to Increase Readiness for the Nine Stages in the Community Readiness Model[a]

Stage	Score	Stage Definition	Activities to Increase Readiness Stage
No awareness	0–1.9	Behavior/problem tolerated by community leaders	One-on-one meetings with community leaders and small groups
Denial	2.0–2.9	Behavior/problem regarded as a general problem, not a local problem	Continue visits with community leaders; discuss local experiences related to the issue; engage health and education programs with flyers, posters, brochures
Vague awareness	3.0–3.9	Behavior/problem regarded as a local problem and something should be done but no motivation evident to do anything	Present information at local community events; post flyers and posters; initiate community events; conduct informal surveys; write editorials
Preplanning	4.0–4.9	Clear recognition of a local problem by some community leaders but an absence of focused or detailed efforts	Introduce information through media and presentations; visit community leaders; review existing programs; conduct local focus groups to discuss issues; use public service announcements
Preparation	5.0–5.9	General information on the behavior/problem available focused on practical details but no formally collected data at a local level	Conduct formal surveys; sponsor a community event to kick off program activities; use community leaders to speak to groups and participate in local television or radio talk shows
Initiation	6.0–6.9	Trained staff and enthusiasm among community leaders, actions and policies justified	Conduct in-service training for professionals; plan publicity events; conduct consumer interviews to identify service gaps; search for funding and resources
Stabilization	7.0–7.9	One or two programs for behavior/problem running with support by administrators or community decision makers	Introduce program evaluation; conduct training for community members; conduct regular meetings to review progress and modify programs; prepare newspaper articles detailing progress
Confirmation/ expansion	8.0–8.9	Standard programs, policies, and activities in place for behavior/problem, support for expanding and improving programs	Develop formal network; prepare community-specific risk profile; publish local services directory; develop speakers bureau; initiate policy change through local officials; conduct media outreach on local data trends
Professionalism	9.0+	Detailed knowledge regarding behavior/problem, some efforts targeted at specific risk groups, effective evaluation used to modify existing programs and policies	Engage local businesses and solicit financial support; provide more advanced training of professionals; continue reassessment of programs and issue; use external evaluation and feedback for program modification; track outcome data for use in future grants

[a]From Edwards et al. (2000).

27.2. CASE STUDY 1: ENGAGING RESEARCHERS TO INVOLVE THE COMMUNITY IN INJURY PREVENTION—TRAUMATIC BRAIN INJURY PREVENTION

27.2.1. Study Objectives

The long-term goal of the study was to develop a strategy for involving communities in a traumatic brain injury (TBI) prevention program.

27.2.2. Methods

Four counties (Summit, Montrose, Conejos, and Morgan) in Colorado were selected for participation in the study based on a priori selection criteria. Traumatic brain injury rates for each county were obtained from a TBI surveillance system operated by the Colorado Department of Public Health and Environment (CDPHE) injury epidemiology staff. The study was conducted using before and after telephone interviews with key informants to determine the stage of community readiness for conducting brain injury prevention programs. Prevention activities were to be developed by staff at the CICRC and implemented and evaluated using postintervention Community Readiness Interviews.

27.2.3. Community Readiness Interviews

All questions in this study targeted TBIs. Specific questions related to TBI were developed to represent prevention programs, community knowledge about prevention efforts, leadership, community climate, community knowledge about TBI, and resources for prevention of traumatic brain injuries. Semistructured interviews were conducted by telephone with a minimum of four key informants per county by trained staff. Key informants were identified as being community leaders involved in the traumatic head injury field and included representatives from public health, human services, schools and hospitals, law enforcement, mental health, and the outdoor recreation industries in the counties. Each interview took between 30 and 45 minutes. Interviews were transcribed and sent to staff at the Tri-Ethnic Center for Prevention at Colorado State University for scoring. Baseline interviews were conducted during 1999–2000; follow-up interviews were conducted within a year of the original interviews, during 2000–2001. Key informants selected for the interviews are not targeted individuals but rather individuals who represent specific segments of the community; therefore, before and after interviews were not always conducted with the same individuals.

27.2.4. Community-Initiated Prevention Activities

In the first county in which key informants were contacted, several individuals immediately asked if there were funds available for specific TBI prevention activities. At this point in the study, CICRC staff decided to approach the intervention portion of the study in a different way. Rather than using the Community Readiness Model to develop prevention programs in the study communities, the intervention approach shifted to a model of providing assistance to communities in which community leaders expressed a need for financial or technical assistance.

27.2.5.   Results

The community leaders in Summit County took a formal approach to prevention, consistent with the preparation stage of community readiness. In Summit County the following three prevention activities were undertaken by several community organizations: acquisition of bicycle and ski helmets for youth in the county, teaching junior high students (12–14 years of age) about the importance and effect of brain injuries, and upgrading data-collection capabilities in the local community. In Conejos County, one community leader requested technical assistance. Traumatic brain injury educational materials in Spanish were located by CICRC staff and provided to the community. Conejos County was at the denial stage of awareness and providing educational information about the general topic of TBI prevention was an appropriate activity to bring the county farther along the readiness continuum. The postactivity interviews indicated there had been a change to vague awareness of the issue. In Morgan and Montrose Counties, key informants did not request any funding or technical assistance. Morgan County did not experience any change in the overall stage of readiness. Montrose County scored in the denial stage in the preactivity interviews and in the vague awareness stage in the postactivity interviews.

27.2.6.   Conclusions

When the community had an active program and a group of concerned community leaders, it could identify the specific needs which would expand its capacity to prevent TBIs. In communities in which there was little or no awareness of the problem, the prevention needs were not recognized by key informants or they were minimal and related to basic information. Community Readiness Interviews served to reorient the CICRC staff to the need for flexibility in the implementation of community-based intervention projects when the philosophy espoused is one of community-based participation. The research led to a long-term program of funding for community-initiated requests related to injury prevention activities. This decision resulted in the development of the community-based participatory approach at the CICRC and the establishment of our Community Initiated Program, which has been used to fund numerous requests from community advocates and leaders to support injury prevention programs. These requests provide further opportunities for collaborative research on new injury problems and assistance with the evaluation of ongoing programs.

27.3.   CASE STUDY 2: ENGAGING COMMUNITY ADVOCATES IN SYSTEMATIC PREVENTION EFFORTS—CHILD BOOSTER SEATS

27.3.1.   Purpose

The purpose of the program was to increase the use of child booster seats in one community in Colorado.

27.3.2.   Methods

Observational studies of booster seat use were conducted to determine preintervention and postintervention use of child booster seats over a 3-year period in an intervention and a comparison community. Community Readiness Interviews were conducted among key informants in both communities. A total of 18 questions were asked in relation to community knowledge about prevention: 4 questions were asked about leadership, 3 questions were asked about community climate, 3 questions were asked about knowledge about the problem, and 8 questions were asked about community resources for prevention efforts. Key informants included elected officials, school personnel, police, health department staff, physicians, and local merchants. The interview results in the intervention community were used to define target population groups, to refine the educational and media messages, and to develop strategies for delivering the intervention information. Focus groups were conducted in the intervention community to further understand issues related to low use of child booster seats. In addition, in several locations, parents were asked to provide information about knowledge, attitudes, and behaviors related to booster seat use.

27.3.3.   Results

Five key informant Community Readiness Interviews were completed in the intervention and in the control community. Table 27.2 shows the Community Readiness scores before and after the intervention. The intervention community was at the preplanning stage before initiation of the intervention program. According to the Community Readiness Model, the program strategy was to move all community dimensions to preplanning and then move the community to the next stages of preparation and initiation. This entailed improving community leadership knowledge of the booster seat issue and increasing community knowledge of the benefits of booster seats for children ages 4–8. This was accomplished through the media; by working with parents through the schools, child-care providers, physicians, and groups that serve low-income clients; by involving community leaders in the program; and by identifying additional strategies from focus

Table 27.2. Community Readiness Scores before and after Child Booster Seat Intervention in Two Communities, Colorado 2001–2003

Dimension	Preintervention, 2001 (score)	Postintervention, 2003 (score)
Intervention community		
Community efforts	Preparation (5.8)	Preparation (5.7)
Community knowledge—efforts	Vague awareness (3.4)	Preplanning (4.1)
Leadership	Vague awareness (3.3)	Preplanning (4.3)
Community climate	Vague awareness (3.8)	Preplanning (4.2)
Community knowledge—issue	Vague awareness (3.8)	Preplanning (4.5)
Resources	Preparation (5.0)	Preparation (5.4)
Overall score	Preplanning (4.4)	Preplanning (4.7)
Booster Seat usage	11%	46%
Control community		
Community efforts	Preparation (5.0)	Preparation (5.8)
Community knowledge—efforts	Denial (2.5)	Preplanning (4.1)
Leadership	Denial (2.8)	Preplanning (4.7)
Community climate	Denial (2.8)	Vague awareness (3.9)
Community knowledge—issue	Vague awareness (3.2)	Preplanning (4.3)
Resources	Denial (2.0)	Preplanning (4.7)
Overall score	Vague awareness (3.0)	Preplanning (4.6)
Booster seat usage	2.5%	13%

groups and parent surveys. The researchers at CICRC and the CDPHE assisted the local traffic safety coalition in applying the Community Readiness Model to define target groups (physicians, parents, community leaders) and refine educational messages (emphasizing protective benefits of booster seat use, letting parents know children would accept booster seats, and providing information about the cost of child booster seats) and enhance the current strategies (using media, using children as messengers, and showing older children in child booster seats).

During the 3-year campaign, 1,390 child booster seats were distributed at community and school events. Mass-media campaigns included 17 radio stations, reaching approximately 340,000 people per week, that aired child booster seat messages; 13 billboards and 12 bus shelters that displayed child booster seat messages; more than 35,000 informational brochures in English and Spanish that were distributed; and information that was provided to local physicians. Booster seat use in the community increased from 11% to 46%.

The intervention community remained at the preplanning stage of community readiness, but the local coalition made great strides in improving community knowledge, leadership, and climate. The increase in booster seat use in the control community (2.5% to 13%) over the study period may have resulted from a national booster seat media campaign, statewide media about the passage of a new state booster seat law in 2002, and local health department educational efforts.

27.3.4. Conclusions

The local traffic safety coalition gained skills in how to apply a research-based model to a specific public health problem. The group also understood the basis for moving their community to the next stages of readiness to ensure the continued increase in booster seat use. In addition, the revitalized health department program in the control community had some principles to use in developing an effective booster seat program.

27.4. CASE STUDY 3: USING COMMUNITY READINESS IN INJURY COALITION BUILDING—ENHANCED ENFORCEMENT OF SEATBELT LAWS

27.4.1. Purpose

The purpose of this ongoing program is to increase seatbelt use by 10% in two rural counties using newly developed community coalitions to implement an enhanced enforcement program of increasing the enforcement of seatbelt and child restraint laws and using the media to inform the community of these important efforts.

27.4.2. Methods

CDPHE staff is currently working with two rural counties to develop specific enhanced enforcement coalitions and campaigns. Staff at the CICRC conducted key informant interviews in the communities to determine initial Community Readiness for an enhanced enforcement program. The Community Readiness Interview used in this study addressed two separate issues related to seatbelt use: education programs and enforcement programs. Although the initial design called for interviews in two intervention counties and three comparison counties, the newly formed coalition members in one of the counties were concerned that there were significant differences in communities within their county. Therefore, that county was segmented into the four separate communities (suggested by the coalition), and interviews were done separately for each of the four areas. Seatbelt observations were also conducted in the four communities within the county.

27.4.3.   Results

The first barrier encountered was a resistance to the idea of enhanced enforcement among the coalition members. Many members wanted to increase educational programs, especially in the schools, and to distribute more educational materials. The group felt that enhanced enforcement was punitive and that the community would not accept more enforcement. Community Readiness Scores presented to the coalition indicated that the four communities interviewed were similar in their readiness to accept enhanced enforcement. All communities had vague awareness related to enforcement of seatbelt laws. The seatbelt surveys also showed the coalition that current seatbelt use was consistently low in all four communities.

27.4.4.   Conclusions

The results of the Community Readiness Interviews and the seatbelt observation, in addition to a presentation by CDPHE staff on the success of enhanced enforcement in other rural counties in Colorado, helped create acceptance of this approach by the newly formed coalition. In addition, the coalition learned how a research-based approach could assist local efforts in designing and implementing a program. In 18 months, through the coalition efforts, the county moved to participation of all law-enforcement agencies in seatbelt enforcement with community support, the implementation of a media campaign, and the formation of a countywide child passenger safety program.

27.5.   CONCLUDING REMARKS

Community Readiness Interviews elucidated important issues in the case studies that were helpful in targeting injury prevention activities. In Case Study 1, the interviews themselves resulted in specific requests for assistance in two of four communities and provided the impetus for the CICRC to implement a program of community-initiated funds consistent with the philosophy of community-based participatory action research. In Case Study 2, the results were used to develop specific aspects of an intervention program and to monitor changes in the readiness of the intervention and control communities. In Case Study 3, Community Readiness results assisted the group in recognizing similarities in the communities they had viewed as very different and assisted in the development of shared goals among the group.

Community Readiness is one tool that has been used in a variety of ways to design, initiate, and evaluate injury prevention programs in which the involvement of community leaders is critical. Community Readiness Interviews help identify where the key leaders in a community stand on a particular issue and provide a starting point for a community group to begin to target prevention activities, as shown in Case Study 2. The maintenance of programs is far more problematic and deserves further attention. Stages of change theories provide a means to consider baseline commitment to programs and may provide a starting point for predicting the sustainability of injury prevention programs.

The most difficult aspect of the process of developing injury prevention programs is in the ability to maintain them. Programs that receive funding for a particular period may disappear when the external funding is terminated. For programs to continue, the involvement of individuals from the local community is absolutely necessary. In the course of working with community partners, one commitment that needs to be explicit is the development of necessary skills to continue or modify the prevention activities as the needs and resources in the local area change. Recognition that the only way to maintain interest is by adopting issues that have high salience to the committed individuals is key to the continuation of injury prevention programs. The committed group of individuals involved is likely to change over time, thereby altering the salience of specific topics, and may explain why some programs are maintained while others are not. The Community Readiness Model addresses this in the transition stages described here. When the community has programs in place that are well integrated into local organizational activities, there is less likelihood that a change of individuals will result in the demise of a program.

A significant factor in the maintenance of injury prevention programs and research in Colorado has been the outstanding established programs in prevention and epidemiology in existence at the CDPHE. The CDPHE Injury and Suicide Prevention and Injury Epidemiology programs have been in existence since 1989. These programs have been maintained, in part, through the active collaboration among the staff at the CDPHE, local health departments, traffic safety, occupational safety, fire safety, medical-care providers, consumer-protection agencies, insurance and risk management companies, community-based organizations, and local universities (University of Colorado Health Sciences Center; the University of Colorado at Boulder; the University of Northern Colorado in Greeley; and Colorado State University, which houses CICRC, established in 1995). The Injury Epidemiology program has maintained injury-related surveillance systems since 1991. The availability of these data has provided unique opportunities to design and evaluate injury prevention programs.

Nonetheless, maintenance of specific injury prevention programs in the small communities in Colorado continues to depend on the presence of a group of committed individuals. There are no development tools that can provide that ingredient, and it remains the role of the academics and the professional injury prevention specialists to identify such individuals and to work with them to maintain and develop new community-based programs through a coalition or the leadership of one or more local organizations. The development of programs and of coalitions should not be viewed as a fixed target that can be reached with any one approach but rather as an ongoing process.

REFERENCES

Aniskiewicz, R., & Wysong, E. (1990). Evaluating DARE: Drug education and the multiple meanings of success. *Policy Studies Review, 9,* 727–747.

Bukaski, W., & Amsel, Z. (Eds.). (1994). *Drug abuse prevention: Sourcebook on strategies and research.* Westport, CT: Greenwood.

Edwards, R., Jumper-Thurman, P., Plested, B., Oetting, E., & Swansom, L. (2000). Community readiness: Research to practice. *Journal of Community Psychology, 28*(3), 291–307.

Green, L., Daniel, M., & Novick, L. (2001). Partnerships and coalitions for community-based research. *Public Health Reports, 116,* 20–31.

Israel, B. A., Schulz, A. J., Parker, E. A., & Becker, A. B. (1998). Review of community-based research: Assessing partnership approaches to improve public health. *Annual Review of Public Health, 19,* 173–202.

Margolis, L. H., & Runyan, C. W. (1998). Understanding and reducing barriers to collaboration by academics with agencies and community organizations: A commentary. *Injury Prevention, 4,* 132–134.

Nixon, J., Spinks, A., Turner, C., & McClure, R. (2004). Community based programs to prevent poisoning in children 0–15. *Injury Prevention, 10,* 43–46.

Prochaska, J., DiClemente, C., & Norcross, J. (1992). In search of how people change: Applications to addictive behaviors. *American Psychologist, 47*(2), 1102–1114.

Rogers, E. (1983). *Diffusion of innovations* (3rd ed.). New York: Free Press.

Spinks, J., Turner, C., McClure, R., & Nixon, J. (2004). Community based prevention programs targeting all injuries for children. *Injury Prevention, 10,* 180–185.

Warren, R. (1978). *The community in America* (3rd ed.). Chicago: Rand-McNally.

Part V

Dissemination and Adoption of Effective Interventions and Policies

Dissemination, Implementation, and Widespread Use of Injury Prevention Interventions

Ellen D. Sogolow, David A. Sleet, and Janet Saul

28.1. INTRODUCTION

Despite the existence of many effective interventions, including those described throughout this handbook, more than 160,000 injury- and violence-related deaths occurred in the United States in 2002 (Centers for Disease Control and Prevention [CDC], 2005). In addition, in 2003, there were nearly 30 million nonfatal injuries requiring emergency department care (CDC, 2005). Too often, science-based interventions existed to prevent these injuries and deaths, but they were not available or were not used by providers and consumers.

This situation is equivalent to developing a life-saving medication but not telling physicians or patients that it is available, not packaging the product for public use, not having skilled pharmacists to dispense the medication, and not providing guidance about the management of its effects. This gap between research and practice, and between discovery and delivery, is large and continues to impede our progress in preventing and controlling injuries and violence (Sleet, Hopkins, & Olson, 2003).

For example, we know that the installation and maintenance of smoke alarms save lives, yet about half of the injuries from residential fires occur in homes where there are no smoke alarms (Ahrens, 2004). Furthermore, where smoke alarms are installed in homes, 20% are not functional (Smith, 1994). (See more on fires in Chapter 6.) To save more lives, consumers and providers need information about effective interventions, but more important, they need support for adopting, using, and maintaining interventions over time. For maximum impact, effective interventions require widespread, sustained use.

These issues are the focus of this chapter. Specifically, we emphasize the importance of diffusion of effective interventions to injury prevention and suggest activities that may strengthen the capacity to deliberately spread the use of science-based interventions. We emphasize the need for specific research related to this process that would strengthen practice applications and discuss barriers to and strategies for moving from evidence of effectiveness to widespread practice. We close with strategies for diffusion research in injury prevention, lessons learned from diffusion research at CDC, and additional needs in the field.

28.2.   THE IMPORTANCE OF DIFFUSION TO INJURY PREVENTION

Diffusion is the process of moving an innovation—an idea, product, or practice—into widespread use. The process includes dissemination, or spreading the word about a product, practice, or idea; implementation—that is, adopting and using it; and promotion of its widespread use. In injury prevention, we stress the importance of dissemination, implementation, and widespread use because the best interventions have little chance of achieving a public health impact if they don't end up in practice or aren't translated into policy.

For many years, injury prevention researchers have assumed that an intervention deemed efficacious in an experimental setting will easily (or often automatically) be translated to the field of practice. Unfortunately, this is not the case. The limited empirical base for diffusion research was documented by Oldenburg, Sallis, French, & Owen (1999), who reviewed 1,210 articles in 12 public health and health promotion journals published in 1994 and discovered that less than 1% were characterized as diffusion research and only 5% as policy implementation research. Only 8 articles in the entire database of 1,210 were related to injury, and virtually none had focused on diffusion research.

In injury prevention, as in other areas of public health, many factors determine whether an individual or a community will use a particular intervention, even when it has been found effective (Backer, David, & Soucy, 1995; Canadian Conference on Dissemination Research, 1996; Elliott et al., 2003; National Center for Injury Prevention and Control (NCIPC), 2002). As indicated in this chapter, we could strengthen dissemination, implementation, and widespread use of effective interventions by building in a few additional steps before, during, and after intervention development and by overcoming some of the barriers that hinder the translation process. Typically, little time or effort is dedicated to taking these steps and even less to researching effectiveness afterward.

A fundamental shift in the concept of intervention research is under way—a recognition that research doesn't end when a study demonstrates an intervention is effective (Grunfeld et al., 2004; Institute of Medicine, 2001; Kerner, Rimer, & Emmons, 2005; Lenfant, 2003; NCIPC, 2002; President's Cancer Panel, 2005). The scientific language and intervention protocols used by the original research team must be translated into everyday terms for use by practitioners, and materials must be developed to help guide the end users (e.g., health departments and community-based organizations) in adopting and implementing the intervention.

In this view, researchers remain essential to the process. They understand best what made the intervention effective, know the training and technical assistance provided to their staff, and can provide guidance on the range of modifications that would be appropriate (or inappropriate) in practice. Because translation activities can involve curriculum development and multimedia formats to support training and implementation, the original researchers may not be the best persons to undertake these translation tasks, but they can be important consultants to the process. This is why collaboration between researchers and policy makers, advocates, media experts, and social marketers is often necessary to achieve success in moving the science into practical use (Fielding et al., 2002).

We acknowledge the complexity and effort involved in the process of taking interventions to scale. Often a variety of stakeholders is involved (especially researchers, administrators, end users, and policy makers), and the intervention is introduced in a range of organizational and social settings. A new intervention may call for individuals, organizations, and communities to change their own behaviors, policies, or norms. It may be met with user resistance, result in personal or organizational delay, or generate rejection. These and other barriers can occur whether you are introducing a new style of bicycle helmet, installing a four-sided swimming pool fence, starting a falls-reduction exercise program, or changing the built environment to reduce violence (See Chapter 14). We need to anticipate this possible range of responses as we plan for activities associated with dissemination, implementation, and widespread use of injury prevention interventions.

We also need to recognize that new interventions may compete with existing programs for scarce public health resources. Therefore, in planning activities to accelerate dissemination, implementation, and widespread use, it is important to provide the rationale, materials, and other information administrators or other decision makers need as they contemplate how to manage the process. These "gatekeepers" often decide whether and how an organization will adopt the new intervention and, if so, whether new staff are needed to integrate the intervention into existing programs and manage the implementation effort.

28.3. ACTIVITIES TO FACILITATE DISSEMINATION AND IMPLEMENTATION AND TO ACHIEVE WIDESPREAD USE

Research on dissemination, implementation, and widespread use (i.e., diffusion research) intends to bridge the gap between experimental research and everyday practice by building a knowledge base about how injury prevention ideas, products, and practices are translated and transmitted for use by individuals and communities. The public health model identifies four stages in the progression from research to application, or from discovery to delivery: (a) defining the problem, (b) identifying risk factors, (c) developing and testing interventions, and (d) widespread use (Mercy, Rosenberg, Powell, Broome, & Roper, 1993; Sogolow et al., 2000). Although this model provides a logical sequence of events, the progression from defining the problem to widespread use is by no means automatic. Each stage must consist of its own planned and sequential activities, and in each stage, researchers and practitioners must be prepared to address external factors that may introduce barriers.

Once an intervention is successfully developed and tested, researchers may improve its perceived value and likelihood of adoption if they plan for dissemination, implementation, and widespread use by engaging in deliberate activities that fall within the public health model approximately between "developing and testing an intervention" and "widespread use" (Glasgow, Lichtenstein, & Marcus, 2003; Parcel, et al., 1989; President's Cancer Panel, 2005). These activities include

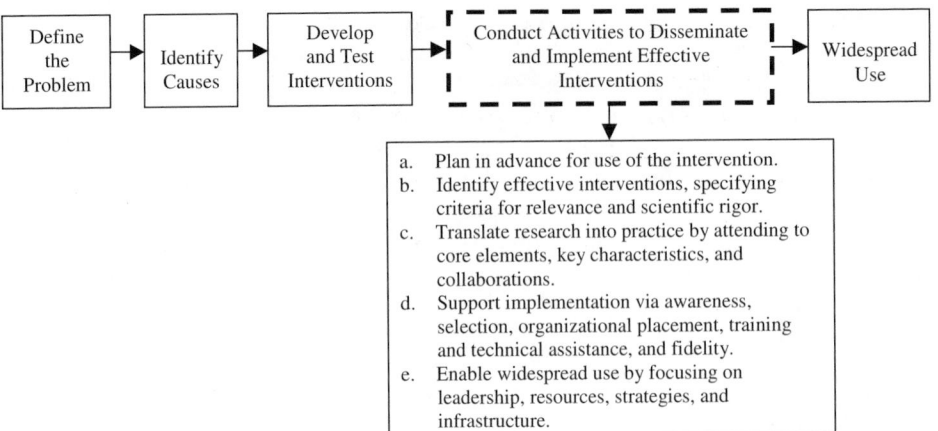

Figure 28.1. Extending the public health model.

(a) planning in advance to use the intervention with end users; (b) identifying and selecting effective interventions based on relevance and scientific rigor; (c) translating the intervention from research to practice by attending to core elements, key characteristics, and collaborations needed; (d) supporting implementation through awareness and selection of the most effective interventions, organizational placement, training and technical assistance, and establishment and maintenance of fidelity; and (e) enabling widespread use by focusing on leadership, resources, strategies, and infrastructure. These activities comprise the extended public health model (Figure 28.1). Without focusing deliberately on these activities, even effective interventions may not be translated for real-world use and, consequently, widespread use will not be attained.

28.3.1. Plan in Advance

There are many examples of rigorous, expensive, multiyear trials that identified effective interventions that were not feasible to execute in practice. An injury prevention program for schools, for example, may have worked in experimental trials, but the 2 hours per week necessary to teach the lessons simply may not be available in the school's curriculum.

Researchers who involve the end users during the early phases of study design and implementation of the intervention will learn what is feasible to implement and, therefore, what is likely to be adopted if the intervention proves effective. For example, focus groups with end users, including gatekeepers and other decision makers, might suggest which components of the intervention would be appealing and what barriers might exist in their systems to prevent implementation with fidelity. Interviews with administrators might reveal the availability of resources (time, settings, staff, materials)—or lack thereof—to implement the intervention. In a clinic setting, end users might be staff implementers and/or patients. In a school, planning in advance might involve the views of principals or department chairs, parents, and students.

28.3.2.   Identify Effective Interventions

Because resources for injury prevention are scarce, it is important to avoid wasting time and effort on interventions that do not work. Two criteria guide the process of identifying effective interventions for dissemination, implementation, and widespread use. The first criterion is *relevance,* including the specific outcomes measured to determine effectiveness. For instance, a fall prevention-related intervention that reduces the fear of falling may not be relevant to programs trying to reduce fall rates (Gillespie et al., 2004). The second criterion is the scientific or methodologic *rigor* of the intervention, the degree to which the study design permits the determination of a valid casual relationship. The more rigorous the design, the more confidence one has that the observed outcomes are attributable to the intervention (Campbell & Stanley, 1966; Cook & Campbell, 1979; Mulrow, Langhorne, & Grimshaw, 1997; Wortman, 1983). Many injury and violence prevention effectiveness studies have used rigorous research methods and, thus, engender confidence that the intervention works. Numerous examples of such studies exist for interventions to prevent falls (Southern California Evidence-Based Practice Center, 2003) and to reduce intimate partner violence in young people (Foshee et al., 2004).

Randomized control trials are considered the gold standard of rigor in clinical research, but they are not always feasible or desirable. Where rigorous studies are not available to inform evidence-based practice, quasi-experimental studies and practice-based evidence may be collected and reviewed by a panel of experts and practitioners to identify and describe effective interventions (Green, 2004).

28.3.3.   Translate Research into Practice

Published research on effective interventions is often not written to facilitate dissemination, implementation, and widespread use (Berwick, 2003; Kelly, Sogolow, & Neumann, 2000). Published intervention research typically does not address implementation issues such as staff requirements, space needs, training, and financial resources necessary to succeed. Also frequently lacking are details about intervention delivery and standardization of the delivery protocol, elements of the intervention essential to its effectiveness, and adjustments made for particular audiences or circumstances (Kraft, Mezoff, Sogolow, Neumann, & Thomas, 2000). These weaknesses or omissions hinder the ability to translate research results into practice.

Several translation activities can improve this situation. One central requirement is that the original researcher should identify the core elements or aspects of the intervention that are thought to be responsible for its success. Once identified, these elements should be implemented "as is" in the field, rather than modified or adapted for convenience (Sogolow et al., 2000). Where research showed, for example, that smoke alarm installation programs succeeded in reducing fire deaths in rural homes, simply giving away smoke alarms to residents would be insufficient and not expected to succeed (Ballesteros, Jackson, & Martin, 2005). Furthermore, the original researcher (as well as local end user) may have insights about key characteristics of the intervention—that is, the activities and delivery methods for conducting an intervention—that may be tailored to different local settings and populations (Kelly et al., 2000). The researcher may have replicated the study in other settings and can provide guidance on the range of issues likely to arise and suggest strategies for resolving them. Kelly et al. (2000) worked with original researchers to explain the notion of core elements and key characteristics for a series of HIV/AIDS intervention replications and offered the following (p. 90):

> The notion of core elements, and the process of distinguishing the core elements and the key characteristics of an intervention, is analogous to making chocolate-chip cookies. The core elements in a recipe, such as flour, sugar, and chocolate chips, are essential to the identity and successful production of chocolate-chip cookies. If any ingredients are omitted, substituted, or measured inaccurately, the product would not be recognizable as a chocolate-chip cookie. On the other hand, the cookie preparation, or key characteristics, can be adapted to the kitchen and the cook. Using a mixer or a spoon, baking in a gas or an electric oven, and shaping the dough into bite-sized or plate-sized pieces would still produce recognizable chocolate-chip cookies.

All of the researcher-generated information provides a foundation for other experts who can develop curricula or other protocols and field-oriented materials. These experts may include health educators, graphic designers, video technicians, communication experts, manufacturers and/or distributors, and marketing advisors. A range of approaches to translation can be seen in packaged programs (interventions in a box), such as those available from the Substance Abuse and Mental Health Services Administration's National Registry of Effective Programs and Practices (2005) and the *Blueprints* document for the prevention of violence (Center for the Study and Prevention of Violence, 2005).

28.3.4. Support Implementation

The quality of intervention implementation is a critical determinant of prevention success. When interventions found effective in an experimental setting are taken to scale in the field, they often do not work the same or do not work at all. Some point to "implementation failure" as the cause. Implementation of an injury intervention, product, or service can be considered a failure if it does not perform technically as well as expected, it is not integrated into a system, or it does not deliver the benefits originally expected. Several theorists and researchers have laid out conceptual models of effective implementation that include from two to six steps, stages, or tasks (Elliott & Mihalic, 2004; Fixsen, Naoom, Blase, Friedman, & Wallace, 2005; Frambach & Schillewaert, 2002; Greenhalgh, Robert, MacFarlane, Bate, & Kyriakidou, 2004; Rogers, 2003; Wandersman, Imm, Chinman, & Kafterian, 2000). Successful implementation includes awareness and selection of an effective intervention, organizational placement, training and technical assistance, and fidelity.

28.3.4.1. *Awareness and Selection of an Effective Intervention*

Practitioners must know about effective interventions and have ready access to them. Public health communication and information systems (e.g., journals and websites) and knowledge-management resources (such as Cochrane Collaboration) can help practitioners learn about interventions and, where possible, relevant information about effectiveness, cost-effectiveness, generalizability, and relative harm (Zaza, Briss, & Harris, 2005). If a service provider believes that current practices work, then persuasive communications must stress why the recommended intervention will work better. Current practices have the advantage of being familiar. Researchers must work with communicators to transmit evidence-based knowledge in ways that resonate with practitioners. Information about interventions should allow practitioners to answer the question, "Why is this new intervention better than what I do now?" (Dirksen, Ament, & Go, 1996; Greenhalgh et al., 2004; Mansfield, 1993; Marshall, 1990; Rogers, 2003).

In selecting an intervention to implement, Fixsen et al. (2005) and others (Frambach & Schillewaert, 2002; Greenhalgh et al., 2004; Meyer, Johnson, & Ethington, 1997) emphasize the importance of considering the *risk of implementing the intervention.* This view recognizes that risk is inherent in doing something new and different, and staff or program administrators may be unwilling to take the risk when the results are unknown. There could be unanticipated financial costs and the need to sacrifice other resources for the new intervention. These perceived risks are real and can be addressed using some social marketing and risk management strategies (Fisher & Price, 1992; Kotler, 1998).

28.3.4.2.   Organizational Placement of the Intervention

Supporting the transfer of a science-based intervention to the field does not end when a decision is made to adopt the intervention. Management and organizational support are necessary. Key decisions are needed regarding who will implement the intervention. Fixsen et al. (2005) suggest that a logical approach may be to focus staff selection or assignment on skills that staff already possess. For example, Olds et al. (2002) in a study of the effectiveness of home visitation programs to prevent child abuse found that nurses were more successful at implementing the intervention than were other staff who had to be trained to implement it. In a review of literature on adoption of innovations within organizations, Frambach and Schillewaert (2002) state three critical marketing factors to increase organizational adoption: (a) engaging those most likely to be the early adopters, (b) communicating in a way to affect attitudes toward adoption, and (c) using marketing strategies that encourage adoption (e.g., making the intervention affordable).

Another factor supporting implementation is the alignment of the intervention with the philosophy and values of the potential adopter (Greenhalgh et al., 2004; Rogers, 2003). If these are at odds, adoption will be less likely. Developing a partnership with social marketers and collaborating with the intended audience will help avoid this potential barrier.

28.3.4.3.   Training and Technical Assistance

Based on their review of meta-analyses and experimental studies, Fixsen et al. (2005) conclude that effective training for practice purposes requires a mix of didactic presentation of information, skills demonstrations, and opportunity for skills mastery. Supplying information alone, and even pairing information with training are not sufficient for successful implementation (Azocar, Cuffel, Goldman, & McCarter, 2003; Azocar, Cuffel, Goldman, & McCulloch, 2001; Ellis et al., 2003; Fine et al., 2003). Rather, to sustain changes in practitioner behavior requires ongoing technical assistance, sometimes called follow-up consultation or coaching (Dansereau & Dees, 2002; Davis, 1995; Kelly et al., 2000). For youth violence prevention, the *Blueprints* program has developed a cadre of certified trainers who provide consultation on implementation of model programs (Center for the Study and Prevention of Violence, 2005).

28.3.4.4. Fidelity

Implementing an intervention so that fidelity is established calls for using the same strategies as the original intervention that was found effective. Optimally, all core elements—that is, those aspects of the intervention that are thought to be essential to effectiveness—would be replicated, and key characteristics of the intervention would be adopted or tailored so that the intervention was appropriate to the audience and setting. Concern with maintaining fidelity recognizes that new patterns of behavior may fade or circumstances (staff, resources, audiences, social norms) may change over time, so that ongoing fidelity to the core elements may require continuing education or other renewal. At the same time, to be responsive to local needs, additional tailoring of the key characteristics may be required for the intervention to remain relevant.

Controversy exists about whether strict fidelity is necessary or if it is wiser to allow some local adaptation to increase relevance. Generally, the more a program is adapted, the less likely it is to retain its original level of effectiveness (Battistich, Schaps, Watson, Soloman, & Lewis, 1996; Blakely et al., 1987; Center for Substance Abuse Prevention, 2001; Fuchs & Fuchs, 1989; Gottfredson, 2001; Gray, Emshoff, Jakes, & Blakely, 2000). Findings from these studies did not, however, distinguish between core elements essential for effectiveness and key characteristics that may be tailored without compromising outcomes.

Less is known about long-term sustainability of injury interventions, even when they are implemented with fidelity. Change theories predict that initial motivations can dissipate rather quickly. As Nguyen, Gauvin, Martineau, and Grignon (2005) point out, a number of factors can influence participation in any health improvement program, and interventions may need to change over time to increase adherence without losing fidelity.

28.3.5. Enable Widespread Use

Widespread use of effective interventions does not occur spontaneously. Once an intervention has been implemented and found effective in one setting or population, it must be made available or modified for other audiences. Sometimes called "going to scale," this effort involves integrating the intervention within existing social systems, such as within an entire community, in healthcare settings, or in schools (Brink, Levenson-Gingiss, & Gottlieb, 1991; Bryant, 1996; Green & Johnson, 1996; Solarz, 2001). For example, a suicide prevention program found effective in military settings is now being prepared for widespread use in civilian populations (Knox, Litts, Talcott, Feig, & Caine, 2004). To enable widespread use of effective injury and violence prevention interventions, leadership, resources, strategies, and infrastructure are necessary.

28.3.5.1. Leadership

Stimulating widespread use requires leadership. Berwick (2003, p. 1969) discusses the Institute of Medicine (2001) report on the chasm between the "health care we have and the health care we could have" and suggests that the first rule, after identifying effective interventions, is to find and support innovators. When a respected organization is an early adopter, others may be more likely to follow.

28.3.5.2. Resources

Financial and human resources are necessary to increase awareness about effective interventions and to promote adoption throughout systems. Leveraging media through collaborative private and public resources can accelerate diffusion (Agency for Healthcare Policy and Quality, 2003). Sometimes costs related to implementing the intervention on a wider scale can be recovered through user fees (Nguyen et al., 2005). Determination of the costs and resources necessary to implement injury interventions can be part of the initial research protocols. A decision maker (or decision-making team) that is fully informed at the time of adopting the intervention may experience fewer challenges and resistance later.

28.3.5.3. Strategies

Even public health changes that seem spontaneous may be the result of more deliberate efforts when examined closely. For example, efforts to reduce alcohol-impaired driving in the United States required strategic planning and direct action on many fronts simultaneously: enforcement, education, research evidence, advocacy, victim testimony, and community action (see Chapter 16). Mandatory pool fencing has become the norm in some regions (Quan & Gomez, 1990) because of actions taken by parents who lost a child from a pool drowning. Advocacy for self-extinguishing cigarettes (those less likely to cause smoldering fires) has begun to pay off with specific legislation after years of strategic action (McGuire, 2005). Conversely, in 1975, more than 47 states had mandatory motorcycle helmet laws; in 2004, there were just 20 (National Highway Traffic Safety Association (NHTSA), 2006). Many states revoked or modified their helmet laws, bowing to deliberate efforts by those opposed to the policies (Shaw & Ogolla, 2006). Approaches that increase awareness can help people and social systems prepare for change (Prochaska & DiClemente, 1983). Strategies that employ a multifaceted approach to encouraging widespread use of effective interventions may have the greatest likelihood of success (Howat, Sleet, Elder, & Maycock, 2004; Preston, Baranowski, & Higginbotham, 1988).

28.3.5.4. Infrastructure

Efforts to increase widespread use can benefit from national infrastructures such as in government agencies like CDC, the National Institutes of Health (NIH), and the Agency for Healthcare Research and Quality (AHRQ); in research centers, including the CDC-sponsored, university-based Prevention Research Centers (PRC) and Injury Control Research Centers (ICRC); and in nongovernment organizations, with some focused on promoting replications of injury and violence prevention programs, and others oriented more toward advocacy. Regardless of affiliation, the infrastructure needs to have a clear focus to be effective in achieving widespread use of effective interventions. It may be dedicated to training implementers, or to facilitating end users' access to science-based services, or to evaluating health outcomes.

Health departments at the state and local level are also essential. For instance, they may dedicate personnel to state- and local-level dissemination and implementation activities. Such personnel may serve as role models, trainers, and consultants until a critical mass of implementers is established.

In addition, the infrastructures in place in strong, well-organized injury and violence prevention coalitions are vital resources. Some may be intermediaries, linking evidence and advocacy to legislation. Others may set priorities and direct funds to support a network of providers (e.g., the Coalition to Prevent Violence Against Women or Area Agencies on Aging) who conduct dissemination and implementation activities nationwide.

28.4.   RESEARCH ON MOVING EFFECTIVE INTERVENTIONS INTO PRACTICE

Research focused on how science-based interventions become prevalent in practice involves the study of processes that lead to improved dissemination, implementation, and widespread use. For too long, injury and violence prevention researchers have assumed that an intervention found efficacious or effective through clinical trials, in the laboratory, or from experimental studies will be transmitted easily to the field. This has not been the case (Gielen, Sleet, & Green, 2006). Whereas many interventions, such as those catalogued in this volume, demonstrate effectiveness to prevent a variety of injuries and violence, most have not been translated from research to lay language; tailored to be responsive to diverse cultural and societal norms; or implemented in communities and evaluated for feasibility, fit with local needs, and fidelity with the core elements. Consequently, they have not been candidates for widespread acceptance and use.

Research related to dissemination, implementation, and widespread use is a high priority at CDC, NIH, AHRQ, and other federal agencies that are committed to bridging science and service, discovery and delivery, and research and practice. Mark Rosenberg, former director of CDC's National Center for Injury Prevention and Control, once reminded his staff: "We took penicillin and delivered it in programs to control VD; we took Pap smears and mammograms, and we delivered cancer prevention programs; we took biological and behavioral science findings and delivered programs to reduce smoking" (note to staff following NIH Director Harold Varmus's 1996 Harvard Commencement speech, June 6, 1996). Injury prevention, too, can bridge science and programs not only to make discoveries . . . but to make discoveries work.

28.4.1.   Types of Diffusion Research

Research procedures in any field include specifying the research questions (hypotheses), developing a rationale for the study, selecting an appropriate study design and methods (e.g., pre-post, cohort, randomized control trial), developing a plan for analyzing data, and anticipating the impact of the research on practice. These are the same procedures for diffusion research, whether focused on dissemination, implementation, or widespread use.

28.4.1.1.   Dissemination-Related Research

Dissemination-related studies address the extent to which the intervention and its core elements are available, adopted or used, or ignored. Such research might examine mechanisms to promote use or overcome resistance to adoption, and the role of media, communications science, and the marketplace in these processes. A subset of such research might be the channels and strategies employed to increase the use of injury prevention products and technologies, such as helmets, hip protectors, pool fences, and injury surveillance systems.

28.4.1.2.   Implementation-Related Research

Implementation research examines how various characteristics of the intervention, the user, and the context affect successful implementation and, thus, the ultimate outcome of the intervention. Research can uncover issues such as message penetration and cultural sensitivity. For example, environmental and ecological factors may lead to uneven delivery, weak participation, or even drop out—such implementation challenges would make it difficult to achieve the expected changes in behaviors or health outcomes. Implementation-related research may address training content and methods, the use of technical assistance to improve competence and implementation with fidelity, ways that local organizational climate and management policies affect use of the intervention, and the potential for norms and laws to facilitate or hinder implementation.

28.4.1.3.   Research Related to Widespread Use

The achievement of nationwide use of effective interventions across many different settings and/or populations and maintaining fidelity while tailoring to the community's needs is no simple undertaking. Little is known about how and under what circumstances widespread use of an intervention or innovative practice can be predicted. Research in this area would include, for instance, studies to examine which factors influence and accelerate organizational and societal norms for selecting and adopting effective interventions; which methods facilitate the deliberate spread of injury prevention technologies, and how these may vary by characteristics of the intervention, audience, and setting; how communication channels and systems contribute to diffusion; how to achieve the best fit between marketing strategies and adoption of interventions, again for types of interventions, populations, and settings; which mechanisms opinion leaders use to pave the way for others; and how local and state policies and laws can be influenced to make populations safer. Also, studies might focus on people and organizations at various stages in the implementation process and examine factors that support entry to different stages, such as early adoption.

28.5.   BARRIERS AND POSSIBLE FACILITATORS

Injury researchers and practitioners have been challenged by funders and government organizations to translate what is learned in research into practice. Such translation is more difficult than it appears, and it is important to learn not only about possible facilitators for this process, but also about barriers to translating effectiveness research into programs and policies in real-world settings (Michie et al., 2005; Zapka, Goins, Pbert, & Ockene, 2004.

One important barrier is lack of communication about what diffusion research is, why it is important, and how to do it. Agencies and organizations need to consider ways to make key research findings, as well as funding opportunities for research on dissemination, implementation, and widespread use, widely available to others. One such opportunity is the launch of the new journal *Implementation Science*, now available at www.implementation science.com, which focuses on research examining methods to accelerate the implementation of evidence-based practices in routine healthcare settings. The obvious successes we have realized in injury prevention from the development of innovative products (e.g., child-resistant packaging, smoke alarms, bicycle helmets), programs (e.g., nurse home visitation and parent training programs for child maltreatment prevention), and policies (e.g., 0.08 BAC laws) point to the importance of conducting research on how to ensure these life-saving interventions get used.

In this section, we propose possible strategies for promoting dissemination, implementation, and widespread use of effective interventions in injury prevention, with an emphasis on diffusion research that supports accelerating the process of moving interventions into practice.

Progress in public health research could be measured not only by the development and testing of interventions, but by how well these interventions are translated into programs that end users will choose and can integrate readily into self-sustaining components of clinic practice, school curricula, or community programs. Future research should be directed at identifying efficient mechanisms to accomplish this translation and integration.

Many constraints on dissemination, implementation, and widespread use can be linked to the "relative newness" of an intervention, inadequate planning and preparation for practice, implementation failure, or lack of adequate funding to enable adoption and to take the intervention to scale. A fundamental barrier to removing these constraints is lack of scientific knowledge about the diffusion process and how effective injury prevention practices can be readily adopted and maintained. Overcoming this barrier will require focused diffusion research.

Injury and violence prevention generally lack a dedicated infrastructure to support dissemination and implementation research and the study of efforts to promote widespread use of interventions that work. Wherever an investment is being made in the development and testing of interventions, a parallel investment needs to be made in disseminating and implementing the intervention in other settings and with other audiences. Sufficient fiscal and staff resources must be made available within the infrastructure to accomplish these goals and the related research that will lead to effective diffusion.

Mechanisms need to be developed and supported to facilitate translation of effective programs into replicable model programs. Understanding the core elements and key characteristics of what made the intervention work will require guidance from the original researchers. Supplemental funding could be made available for this purpose to enable the researchers to shift immediately from intervention research to the activities that facilitate dissemination and implementation and the related research that is needed to achieve widespread use.

Coalitions, advocacy groups, public interest groups, citizens, and professional organizations have an important role to play in promoting a culture of safety in civil societies. They can be primary change agents, convening and leading stakeholders, using their own networks to promote dissemination and implementation activities, and serving as opinion leaders in many communities nationwide. Another key role is as "linkage agents," facilitating the smooth implementation of programs by providing resources to help translate and disseminate effective interventions, developing and providing training, and troubleshooting adoption and maintenance problems (Oldenburg, Hardcastle, & Kok, 1997). Research is needed to better understand the strategies such groups and organizations can use to mobilize for this purpose.

Costs and cost-effectiveness research on effective interventions is lacking. Knowledge about costs would inform the dissemination and implementation process and assist approaches to achieving nationwide use. Collecting or modeling implementation cost information would help practitioners and end users as well, as they contemplate adoption and use of new policies, practices, or products. Those who fund intervention effectiveness studies could include, at a minimum, collection and estimation of implementation cost data (excluding costs associated with the research per se) as a component of the study.

Many of these possible strategies for improving widespread use of effective interventions include or depend on system-level change (Nguyen et al., 2005; Valdiserri, 1996). Such change is likely to be evolutionary and may encounter resistance along the way. Still, looking at the progress many fields have made already, such change appears to be ultimately welcomed and worthwhile.

28.6.   LESSONS LEARNED AND FUTURE DIRECTIONS

Both the *CDC Injury Research Agenda* (NCIPC, 2002) and the *Health Protection Research Guide* (CDC, 2006) emphasize the need for research that will build knowledge about methods, structures, and processes to disseminate, implement, and encourage widespread use of effective interventions. Other agencies at NIH (National Institute of Mental Health, 1999; President's Cancer Panel, 2004–2005) and AHRQ (2003) have invested heavily in research translation activities and policies. Successful translation in injury prevention can benefit from the guidelines, theoretical constructs, and approaches already developed in other areas of public health (Sleet & Sogolow, 2004; Svanstrom, Boleslav, & Grivna, 2004).

To further this aim, in 2002–2004, NCIPC issued Requests for Applications for research to evaluate strategies for the dissemination and implementation of effective interventions to prevent unintentional injuries (such as injuries at home and in the community, from alcohol-impaired driving, and from older adult falls) and to prevent violence (such as intimate partner violence, sexual violence, child maltreatment, suicide, and youth violence). The goals of the research announcement were to encourage injury researchers to work with interdisciplinary teams to advance our understanding of practices that maximize the adoption, use, and maintenance of injury prevention "best practices" and policies. We sought proposals to design and test theory-based strategies for disseminating and implementing effective interventions and studies that would accurately measure the outcomes of using these strategies. An objective peer review of these proposals revealed that many investigators lacked training and/or experience in diffusion research and were unfamiliar with the relevant literature. Many of the applications we received proposed dissemination and implementation of untested, unproven interventions and presented programs that were, in effect, dissemination/implementation activities, but not research.

From this experience, we underscore the need to familiarize the injury research community with the important scientific work on diffusion research in chronic and infectious disease, where theories and rigor have been applied. While we could not find any examples where these concepts and principles had been rigorously applied to injury prevention programs and technology transfer, examples abound in cancer, HIV, heart disease, exercise, mental health, and smoking prevention (King, Hawe, & Wise, 1996; National Institute of Mental Health, 2005; Oldenburg et al., 1997).

28.6.1. Future Directions

What we need in the future are

- Collaborations among injury researchers and those in other areas of public health in which investments in dissemination, implementation, and widespread use have been more substantial.
- Training in methods used in diffusion research, especially for investigators in the social, behavioral, and communications sciences.
- Increased funding for research on diffusion of innovations in injury prevention and on methods to increase dissemination, implementation, and widespread use of effective interventions.
- Creation of infrastructures at national, state, and local levels to further the progression of science-based interventions into everyday practice.
- Publications addressing issues of moving research into practice for injury prevention, including the importance of research on dissemination, implementation, and widespread use of effective interventions, methods, and strategies for conducting this research, and case studies of success.

With such steps, we expect there will be less confusion about what constitutes effectiveness; greater clarity about what is meant by dissemination, implementation, and widespread use; and improved understanding about research that will be most helpful in the future.

Federal institutions can and must be catalysts in initiating and sustaining diffusion research in injury prevention. This leadership may take the form of training injury researchers or sponsoring interdisciplinary meetings, workshops, and conferences where researchers and practitioners—in injury and other disciplines—can share their approaches to research. Through the process of grants, cooperative agreements, and contracts, federal and private agencies can convene, integrate, and advocate for dissemination and implementation activities to propel widespread use of effective injury and violence prevention strategies and technologies.

Kok and Green (1990, p. 305) cite the findings from the Dutch Smoking Prevention Program for adolescents as an example of what can happen if we don't pay attention to these needs: "After 4 years of careful and internationally respected research and development, deVries and co-workers presented their programme to be implemented nationwide. Now, almost 2 years later, absolutely nothing has happened."

Injury prevention can learn from this example and invest in specific activities to ensure that dissemination, implementation, and widespread use of effective interventions occur.

REFERENCES

Agency for Healthcare Research and Quality. (2003). *Diffusion and dissemination of evidence-based cancer control interventions, Summary.* Evidence report/technology assessment number 79 (AHRQ Publication No. 03-E032). Retrieved January 20, 2006, from www.ahrq.gov/clinic/epcsums/canconsum.htm.

Ahrens, M. (2004). *U.S. experience with smoke alarms and other fire detection/alarm equipment.* Quincy, MA: National Fire Protection Association.

Azocar, F., Cuffel, B. D., Goldman, W., & McCarter, L. (2003). The impact of evidence-based guideline dissemination for the assessment and treatment of major depression in managed behavioral health care organizations. *Journal of Behavioral Health Services & Research, 30* (1), 109–118.

Azocar, F., Cuffel, B. D., Goldman, W., & McCulloch, J. (2001). Best practices: Dissemination of guidelines for the treatment of major depression in a managed behavioral health care network. *Psychiatric Services, 52* (8), 1014–1016.

Backer, T. E., David, S. L., & Soucy, C. (1995). *Reviewing the behavioral science knowledge base on technology transfer.* National Institute on Drug Abuse [NIDA], Research Monograph Series, 155 (Pub. No. 95-4035). Retrieved December 20, 2005, from www.nida.nih.gov/pdf/monographs/155.pdf.

Ballesteros, M. F., Jackson, M. L., & Martin, M. W. (2005). Working towards the elimination of residential fire deaths: CDC's Smoke Alarm Installation and Fire Safety Education (SAIFE) Program. *Journal of Burn Care & Rehabilitation, 26* (5), 434–439.

Battistich, V., Schaps, E., Watson, M., Solomon, D., & Lewis, C. (1996). Prevention effects of the child development project: Early findings from an ongoing multisite demonstration trial. *Journal of Adolescent Research, 11,* 12–35.

Berwick, D. (2003). Disseminating interventions in health care. *Journal of the American Medical Association, 289* (15), 1969–1975.

Blakely, C., Mayer, J., Gottschalk, R., Schmitt, N., Davidson, W., Roitman, D., & Emshoff, J. G. (1987). The fidelity-adaptation debate: Implications for the implementation of public sector social programs. *American Journal of Community Psychology, 15,* 253–268.

Brink, S. G., Levenson-Gingiss, P., & Gottlieb, N. H. (1991). An evaluation of the effectiveness of a planned diffusion process: The smoke-free class of 2000 project in Texas. *Health Education Research, 6* (3), 353–362.

Bryant, H. (1996). Breast cancer screening in Canada: Climbing the diffusion curve. *Canadian Journal of Public Health, 87* (Suppl. 2), S60–S62.

Canadian Conference on Dissemination Research (1996). Strengthening health promotion and disease prevention. *Canadian Journal of Public Health, 87* (Suppl. 2), 27–29.

Campbell, D. T., & Stanley, J. C. (1966). *Experimental and quasi-experimental designs for research.* Chicago: Rand-McNally.

Centers for Disease Control and Prevention, National Center for Injury Prevention and Control. (2005). Web-based Injury Statistics Query and Reporting System (WISQARS) [online]. Retrieved August 30, 2005, from www.cdc.gov/ncipc/wisqars.

Centers for Disease Control and Prevention. *Health protection research guide, 2006–2015.* (2006). Atlanta: Centers for Disease Control and Prevention and the Agency for Toxic Substances and Disease Registry, U.S. Department of Health and Human Services.

Center for the Study and Prevention of Violence. (2005). *Blueprints for violence prevention.* Retrieved July 1, 2005, from www.colorado.edu/cspv/blueprints/index.html.

Center for Substance Abuse Prevention. (2001). *Finding the balance: Program fidelity and adaptation in substance abuse.* Rockville, MD: Substance Abuse and Mental Health Services Administration.

Cook, T. D., & Campbell, D. T. (1979). *Quasi-experimentation: Design & analysis issues for field settings.* Chicago: Rand-McNally.

Dansereau, D. F., & Dees, S. M. (2002). Mapping training: The transfer of a cognitive technology for improving counseling. *Journal of Substance Abuse Treatment, 22,* 219–230.

Davis, D. A. (1995). Changing physician performance: A systematic review of the effect of continuing medical education strategies. *Journal of the American Medical Association, 274* (9), 700–705.

Dirksen, C. D., Ament, A. J., & Go, P. M. (1996). Diffusion of six surgical endoscopic procedures in the Netherlands: Stimulating and restraining factors. *Health Policy, 37* (2), 91–104.

Elliott, D. S., & Mihalic, S. (2004). Issues in disseminating and replicating effective prevention programs. *Prevention Science, 5* (1), 47–53.

Elliott, S. J., O'Loughlin, J., Robinson, K., Eyles, J., Cameron, R., Harvey, D., Raine, K., & Gelskey, D. (2003). Conceptualizing dissemination research and activity: The case of the Canadian heart health initiative. *Health Education & Behavior, 30* (3), 267–282.

Ellis, P., Robinson, P., Ciliska, D., Armour, T., Raina, P., Brouwers, M., O'Brien, M.A., Gould, M., & Baldassarre, F. (2003). *Diffusion and dissemination of evidence-based cancer control interventions.* Evidence report/technology assessment number 79. (AHRQ Publication No. 03-E033). Rockville, MD: Agency for Healthcare Research and Quality.

Fielding, J. E., Marks, J. S., Meyers, B. W., Nolan, P. A., Raswon, R. D., & Toomey, K. E. (2002). How do we translate science into public health policy and law? *Journal of Law, Medicine, & Ethics, 30* (Suppl. 3), 22–32.

Fine, M. J., Stone, R. A., Lave, J. R., Hough, L. J., Obrosky, D. S., Mor, M. K., & Kapoor, W. N. (2003). Implementation of an evidence-based guideline to reduce duration of intravenous antibiotic therapy and length of stay for patients hospitalized with community-acquired pneumonia: A randomized controlled trial. *American Journal of Medicine, 115* (5), 343–35l.

Fisher, R. L., & Price, L. L. (1992). An investigation into the social context of early adoption behavior. *Journal of Consumer Research, 19,* 477–487.

Fixsen, D. L., Naoom, S. F., Blase, K. A., Friedman, R. M., & Wallace, F. (2005). *Implementatian research: A review* (FMHI Publication #231). Tampa, FL: University of South Florida, Louis de la Parte Florida Mental Health Institute, the National Implementation Research Network.

Foshee, V., Bauman, S., Ennett, S., Linder, G., Benefield, T., & Suchindran, C. (2004). Assessing the long-term effects of the Safe Dates program and a booster in preventing and reducing adolescent dating violence victimization and perpetration. *American Journal of Public Health, 94,* 619–624.

Frambach, R. T., & Schillewaert, N. (2002). Organizational innovation adoption: A multi-level framework of determinants and opportunities for future research. *Journal of Business Research, 55,* 163–176.

Fuchs, D., & Fuchs, L. (1989). Exploring effective and efficient preferential interventions: A component analysis of behavioral consultation. *School Psychology Review, 18,* 260–283.

Gielen, A. C., Sleet, D. A., & Green, L. W. (2006). Community models and approaches for interventions. In A. C. Gielen, D. A. Sleet, & R. J. DiClemente (Eds). *Injury and violence prevention: Behavioral science theories, methods, and applications* (pp. 65–82). San Francisco: Jossey-Bass.

Gillespie, L. D., Gillespie, W. J., Robertson, M. C., Lamb, S. E., Cumming, R. G., & Rowe, B. H. (2004). Interventions for preventing falls in elderly people (Cochrane Review). In *The Cochrane Library,* Issue 3. Chichester, UK: John Wiley & Sons, Ltd.

Glasgow, R. E., Lichtenstein, E., & Marcus, A. C. (2003). Why don't we see more translation of health promotion research to practice? Rethinking the efficacy-to-effectiveness transition. *American Journal of Public Health, 93* (8), 1261–1267.

Gottfredson, D. (2001). *Schools and delinquency.* Cambridge, UK: Cambridge University Press.

Gray, D., Emshoff, J., Jakes, S., & Blakely, C. (2000). *ESID and dissemination research: A case study and critique of a change model's fidelity.* College Station, TX: Texas A&M University.

Green, L. W., & Johnson, J. L. (1996). Dissemination and utilization of health promotion and disease prevention knowledge: Theory, research, and experience. *Canadian Journal of Public Health, 87* (Suppl.), S12–S17.

Green, L. W. (2004). From evidence-based practice to practice-based evidence: The role of participatory research. Keynote address, 21st Annual Oregon Rural Health Conference, Portland, Oregon.

Greenhalgh, T., Robert, G., MacFarlane, F., Bate, P., & Kyriakidou, O. (2004). Diffusion of innovations in service organizations: Systematic review and recommendations. *Milbank Quaterly, 82* (4), 581–629.

Grunfeld, E., Zitzelsberger, L., Evans, W. K., Cameron, R., Hayter, C., Berman, N., & Stern, H. (2004). Better knowledge translation for effective cancer control: A priority for action. *Cancer Causes & Control, 15,* 503–510.

Howat, P., Sleet, D. A., Elder, R., & Maycock, B. (2004). Preventing alcohol-related traffic injury: A health promotion approach. *Traffic Injury Prevention, 5* (3), 208–219.

Institute of Medicine (2001). Crossing the quality chasm: A new health system for the 21st century. Washington, DC: National Academy Press.

Kelly, J. A., Sogolow, E. D., & Neumann, M. S. (2000). Future directions and emerging issues in technology transfer between HIV prevention researchers and community-based service providers. Turning HIV prevention research into practice. *AIDS Education and Prevention, 12* (Suppl. 5), 126–141.

Kerner, J., Rimer, B., & Emmons, K. (2005). Dissemination research and research dissemination: How can we close the gap? [Introduction to special section]. *Health Psychology, 24* (5), 443–500.

King, L., Hawe, P., & Wise, M. (1996). From research into practice in health promotion: A review of the literature on dissemination. Sydney, Australia: National Center for Heath Promotion.

Knox, K. L., Litts, D. A., Talcott, G. W., Feig, J. C., & Caine, E. D. (2004). Risk of suicide and related adverse outcomes after exposure to a suicide prevention programme in the U.S. Air Force: Cohort study. *British Medical Journal, 327,* 1379–1380.

Kok, G., & Green, L. W. (1990). Research to support health promotion in practice: A plea for increased cooperation. *Health Promotion International, 5,* 173–179.

Kotler, P. (1998). *Marketing management, analysis, planning, implementation, and control.* Englewood Cliffs, NJ: Prentice-Hall.

Kraft, J. M., Mezoff, J. S., Sogolow, E. D., Neumann, M. S., & Thomas, P. A. (2000). A technology transfer model for effective HIV/AIDS interventions: Science and practice. *AIDS Education and Prevention, 12* (Suppl. A), 7–20.

Lenfant, C. (2003). Clinical research to clinical practice—lost in translation? *New England Journal of Medicine*, *9* (9), 868–874.

Mansfield, E. (1993). The diffusion of flexible manufacturing systems in Japan, Europe, and the United States. *Management Science*, *39*, 149–159.

Marshall, J. G. (1990). Diffusion of innovation theory and end-user searching. *Library & Information Science Research*, *6* (1), 55–69.

McGuire, A. (2005). To burn or not to burn: An advocate's report from the field. *Injury Prevention*, *11*, 264–266.

Mercy, J. A., Rosenberg, M. L., Powell, K. E., Boome, C. V., Roper, W. L. (1993). Public health policy for preventing violence. *Health Affairs*, *12* (4), 7–29.

Meyer, M., Johnson, D., & Ethington, C. (1997). Contrasting attributes of preventive health innovations. *Journal of Communication*, *47*, 112–131.

Michie, S., Johnston, M., Abraham, C., Lawton, R., Parkter, D., & Walker, A. on behalf of the "Psychological Theory" group (2005). Making psychological theory useful for implementing evidence based practice: a consensus approach. *Quality & Safety in Health Care* (14), 26–33.

Mulrow, C. D., Langhorne, P., & Grimshaw, J. (1997). Integrating heterogeneous pieces of evidence in systemic reviews. *Annals of Internal Medicine*, *127*, 989–995.

National Center for Injury Prevention and Control (NCIPC). (2002). *CDC injury research agenda*. Atlanta, GA: Centers for Disease Control and Prevention. (www.cdc.gov/ncipc/pub-res/research_agenda/agenda.htm)

National Highway Traffic Safety Association (NHTSA) (2006). Traffice Safety Facts. Motorcycles. National Center for Statistics and Analysis, Washington, D.C.: US Department of Transportation.

National Institute of Mental Health. (1999). *Translating behavioral science into action. Report of the National Advisory Mental Health Council Behavioral Science Workgroup. Final Report.* Bethesda, MD: National Institutes of Health.

National Institute of Mental Health. (2005). Program announcement on dissemination and implementation research in mental health. (PA #02-131& PA #99-068). Bethesda, MD: National Institutes of Health.

Nguyen, M-N., Gauvin, L., Martineau, I., & Grignon, R. (2005). Sustainability of the impact of a public health intervention: Lessons learned from the Laval Walking Clubs Experience. *Health Promotion Practice*, *6* (1), 44–52.

Oldenburg, B., Hardcastle, D. M., & Kok, G. (1997). Diffusion of innovation. In K. Glanz, F.M. Lewis, & B. K. Rimer (Eds.), *Health behavior and health education* (pp. 270–286). San Francisco: Jossey-Bass.

Oldenburg, B. F., Sallis, J. F., French, M. L., & Owen, N. (1999). Health promotion research and the diffusion and institutionalization of interventions. *Health Education Research*, *14* (1), 121–130.

Olds, D. L., Robinson, J., O'Brien, R., Luckey, D. W., Pettitt, L. M., Henderson, C. R., Jr., Ng, R. K., Sheff, K. L., Korfmacher, J., Hiatt, S., & Talmi, A. (2002). Home visiting by paraprofessionals and by nurses: A randomized control trial. *Pediatrics*, *110* (3), 486–496.

Parcel, G. S., Taylor, W. C., Brink, S. G., Gottlieb, N., Engquist, K., O'Hara, N. M., & Eriksen, M. (1989). Translating theory into practice: Intervention strategies for the diffusion of a health promotion innovation. *Family & Community Health*, *12* (3), 1–13.

President's Cancer Panel. (2005). *Translating research into cancer care: Delivering on the promise. 2004–2005 annual report.* Bethesda, MD: National Cancer Institute, National Institutes of Health.

Preston, M. A., Baranowski, T., & Higginbotham, J. C. (1988). Orchestrating the points of community intervention: Enhancing the diffusion process. *International Quarterly of Community Health Education*, *9* (1), 11–34.

Prochaska, J. O., & DiClemente, C. C. (1983). Stages and processes of self-change in smoking: Toward an integrative model of change. *Journal of Consulting and Clinical Psychology*, (51), 390–395.

Quan, L., & Gomez, A. (1990). Swimming pool safety: An effective submersion prevention program. *Journal of Environmental Health*, *52* (6), 344–346.

Rogers, E. M. (2003). *Diffusion of innovations* (5th ed.). New York, Simon & Schuster.

Shaw, F. E., & Ogolla, C. P. (2006). Law, behavior, and injury prevention. In A. C. Gielen, D. A. Sleet, & R. J. DiClemente (Eds.), *Injury and violence prevention: Behavioral science theories, methods and applications* (pp 442–466). San Francisco: Jossey-Bass.

Sleet, D. A., Hopkins, K. N., & Olson, S. J. (2003). From discovery to delivery: Injury prevention at CDC. *Health Promotion Practice*, *4* (2), 98–102.

Sleet, D. A., & Sogolow, E. (2004). Translation from science to practice: An essential link in injury prevention. Presentation to the New South Wales Health Department, Sydney, Australia.

Solarz, A. L. (2001). Investing in children, families, and communities: Challenges for an interdivisional public policy collaboration. *American Journal of Community Psychology*, *29* (1), 1–14.

Smith, C. (1994). *Smoke detector operability survey-report on findings.* Bethesda, MD: U.S. Consumer Product Safety Commission.

Sogolow, E., Kay, L., Doll, L., Neumann, M. S., Mezoff, J., Eke, A., Semaan, S., & Anderson, J. R. (2000). Strengthening HIV prevention: Application of a research-to-practice framework. *AIDS Education and Prevention, 12* (Suppl. A), S21–32.

Southern California Evidence-Based Practice Center. (2003). *Evidence report and evidence-based recommendations: Fall prevention interventions in the Medicare population.* Rand Report. (Contract No. 500-98-281).

Substance Abuse and Mental Health Services Administration. (2005). *SAMHSA model programs: SAMHSA's National Registry of Evidence-based Programs and Practices* (NREPP). Retrieved July 1, 2005, from www.modelprograms.samhsa.gov.

Svanstrom, L., Boleslav, J., & Grivna, M. (2004). *Sustainability within safe communities.* Prague: Centrum Urazove Prevence.

Valdiserri, R. O. (1996). Managing system-wide change in HIV prevention programs: A CDC perspective. *Public Administration & Review, 56* (6), 545–553.

Wandersman, A., Imm, P., Chinman, M., & Kafterian, S. (2000). Getting to outcomes: A results-based approach to accountability. *Evaluation and Program Planning, 23* (3), 389–395.

Wortman, P. M. (1983). Evaluation research: A methodological perspective. *Annual Review Psychology, 34,* 223–260.

Zapka, J., Goins, K. V., Pbert, L., & Ockene, J. K. (2004). Translating efficacy research to effectiveness studies in practice: Lessons from research to promote smoking cessation in community health centers. *Health Promotion Practice, 5* (3), 245–255.

Zaza, S., Briss, P., & Harris, K. (Eds). (2005). *The guide to community preventive services: What works to promote health?* New York: Oxford University Press.

Chapter **29**

Encouraging Adoption of Science-Based Interventions: Organizational and Community Issues

Renée F. Wilson-Simmons and Lydia N. O'Donnell

29.1. INTRODUCTION

Communities nationwide are under increasing pressure to adopt evidence-based interventions to address a range of public health problems, including intentional and unintentional injuries. This pressure is the result of a remarkable shift over the last decade in the number and stringency of requirements that practitioners are expected to meet when seeking funds for the implementation of new programs. The need for greater fiscal and programmatic accountability at federal, state, and local levels has resulted in new policies, chief among them, that local decision making and services be based on solid evidence of what works. However, local agencies and practitioners face considerable challenges when they attempt to implement evidence-based strategies and obtain the desired reductions in morbidity and mortality.

The accumulated experience of an array of research-to-practice initiatives has shown that communities often find it difficult to adopt and sustain innovations that may have worked in research or other less-than-real-world settings. As a result, investigators whose previous efforts have focused on developing and evaluating interventions are being called on to direct similar attention to the process of implementation (Forgatch, 2003; National Institute on Drug Abuse [NIDA], 2003). In addition, they are being urged by funders to work collaboratively with communities not only to better understand problems associated with implementation but also to replace the unidirectional science-to-practice model with a practice-to-science-to-practice framework.

Developing innovations that are feasible, effective, and sustainable requires that significant attention be devoted to the technology transfer process, which is not only complex but also resource and time intense. For example, the violence-prevention field has made significant progress in its attempts to develop and implement scientific tests of interventions and summarize the literature on effectiveness. However, those are only the first steps in the technology transfer process. Practitioners must be provided with some level of support in their efforts to adopt science-based interventions, not only via documentation but also through training and technical assistance (Holtgrave, 2004). Still, even when technology transfer does take place, multiple studies have illustrated that implementation success is often modest and hampered by numerous obstacles (Mihalic & Irwin, 2003). Not the least among these impediments is the need for a long-term commitment of funds to sustain programs and determine their true level of effectiveness. Such financial support is often unattainable, despite an organization's best efforts. Given these barriers, some now question whether best practice requirements, including the formation of community-based coalitions to engage a broad constituency in prevention efforts, will produce hoped-for results without the longer-term commitments of both technical assistance and funding (Embry, 2004).

In their discussion of barriers to the implementation of a middle school social skills training program, Rotheram-Borus, Bickford, and Milburn (2001) make a point that is helpful to keep in mind when discussing the process of adoption of innovation: As much public health research has revealed, most people who attempt a behavior change, even when a significant personal health risk is involved, fail—often multiple times—before achieving success. The same is the case for organizations, for which the complexity of individual behaviors is further complicated by group norms, values, practices, and expectations. Clearly, adopting proven programs entails changing multiple behaviors of many individuals, whether the undertaking appears to be relatively simple, such as the use of safer needle devices by hospitals (Sinclair, 2002), or multilayered, such as efforts to establish community coalitions to address a public health problem (Butterfoss, 2004). Having both funding sources and local providers acknowledge this reality of establishing goals and timelines is critical for setting reasonable expectations and encouraging the continued application of prevention science, even in the face of initial failures or setbacks.

Indeed, whether a transfer of technology effort is viewed as a success or a failure depends on one's perspective. In two large studies of the transfer of science-based HIV interventions, one domestic and one global, Kelly and colleagues (2000, 2004) report on the successes and challenges experienced by the agencies asked to implement new programs. Whether domestic or international, those agencies that received greater training and technical assistance were more successful in program adoption than those that received implementation packages alone. What is also notable, however, is that a majority of international agencies and a substantial proportion of domestic ones did not adopt programs, even with the maximum level of support.

That some agencies successfully implemented science-based interventions with technology transfer support services is an important advance. However, while such technical assistance is clearly a good investment, for some agencies, more is needed. Furthermore, when programs are required to demonstrate successful implementation—as well as positive outcomes of their new efforts—such failure rates are problematic. On the one hand, proof of success may be a legitimate screening criterion for determining which agencies merit continued funding; on the other hand, community providers, quite reasonably, are concerned that funders, in their zeal to move to science-based practices, will forget the importance of local adaptations and promising practices, as well as understate the trial-and-error learning process involved in adopting an innovation. An empirical and theoretical understanding of community and organizational issues that must be addressed throughout the process of implementing and sustaining an intervention is essential for the continued adoption of science-based injury and violence prevention programs.

29.2. THE COMPLEXITY OF LOCAL ADOPTION OF SCIENCE-BASED PROGRAMS: A COMPOSITE CASE

To illustrate the multiplicity of issues that communities must address when adopting a new intervention—and the sequence of steps that make up the local adoption process—the following hypothetical example of Claremont is offered. In constructing this case, we drew on our experience both as researchers and as providers of training and support services to state and local agencies and organizations attempting to adopt evidence-based interventions. Our work in the latter area began in 1991 with a review of the state of adolescent violence prevention commissioned by the Carnegie Corporation (Wilson-Brewer, Cohen, O'Donnell, & Goodman, 1991), which led to our development of the National Network of Violence Prevention Practitioners, a membership organization that was made up of practitioners dedicated to preventing youth violence. This work continued during operation of the Children's Safety Network Adolescent Violence Prevention Resource Center, funded by the Maternal and Child Health Bureau to provide state agencies with information, resources, and technical assistance to facilitate the development of new programs and the improvement of current efforts to promote safety and prevent violence. Today, our understanding of the issues that must be addressed to successfully encourage the adoption of science-based interventions is enhanced via our operation of the National Center for Mental Health Promotion and Youth Violence Prevention. Funded by the Substance Abuse and Mental Health Services Administration (SAMHSA) to provide training and technical assistance to school districts and communities that receive SAMHSA grants, the center is supporting grantees in their efforts to create and expand coalitions to prevent youth violence, suicide, substance abuse, and other behavioral as well as mental health problems. Although the case presented here is hypothetical, it is a conceptual whole composed from our experiences working with diverse communities across the nation.

29.2.1. Violence Prevention in Claremont

Claremont, a mid-size city of 200,000 residents, is proud of its diversity and strong neighborhood roots. Despite experiencing an overall downward trend in violence in 2004 that mirrored state and national statistics, Claremont was recently the site of several incidents of serious and highly publicized youth violence. At its largest middle school, a cafeteria fight resulted in serious injuries to more than 20 students, and in a neighborhood with a history of interstreet rivalries, several acts of predatory violence and interpersonal conflict, some involving weapons, had occurred among young people. In response, the Claremont Community Coalition, a group brought together by the mayor's office about 5 years ago, voted to make youth violence prevention a priority. The coalition is composed of representatives from the mayor's office, the school department, the police department, a youth council, and community-based agencies providing direct health and social services to young people and their families. At their last meeting, coalition members agreed to move forward, but wanted additional information about what strategies are likely to be most effective and what similar communities have done.

Two committee members were charged with reviewing science-based youth violence prevention programs. Their research led them to numerous web sites, some sponsored by federal agencies, some by program developers, and others by advocacy groups. They also made calls to the directors of youth violence prevention programs in their state to determine what interventions had been employed and with what results. Because the coalition had conducted similar research in the past, some of its members had experience making sense of terms such as *promising, science based, evidence based, effective,* and *proven* as well as other program descriptors (e.g., *comprehensive, coordinated, multilevel, key elements, replication packages*). The review team found that most of the programs it identified had been evaluated with populations different from Claremont's and in communities with higher or lower rates of youth violence. However, the review team was able to identify several programs made up of interventions that seemed applicable to their community.

The review team presented the best fits to the coalition, providing written details on several that seemed most appropriate. After reviewing the information, asking questions of the members charged with conducting the review, and discussing and debating the issues, the coalition agreed to select a multilevel, multiintervention program with evidence of effectiveness. Members also discussed how they would monitor implementation and determine program success, which they acknowledged were critical for securing ongoing funding. They set criteria to guide the coalition's decision, agreeing that cost must be a major factor.

At the next coalition meeting, the list of possible programs was narrowed, and each member was asked to obtain input from his or her agency regarding which strategies seemed most feasible and would build on, but not duplicate, current efforts. An open meeting of the city's residents was scheduled and well publicized via major media outlets as well as community channels. Special invitations were sent to teachers and other school staff, students, and parents from the middle school where the cafeteria fight took place as well as those residing in the neighborhoods surrounding the school. The meeting was also publicized most aggressively in the neighborhood where the interstreet violence was taking place.

The coalition was pleased by the number of residents who attended the meeting and contributed to the discussion. However, because so many questions were raised about the interventions being suggested, a final decision was delayed until more information could be obtained about implementation requirements, including agency and staff training needs and whether technical assistance is available—and at what price. After obtaining the missing information, talking with the directors of the interventions on its short list, and determining which ones met Claremont's needs and available funding from the mayor's office, the coalition members voted to adopt an antiviolence program made up of both school and community components. This vote was taken after the coalition held meetings with police and school department leaders as well as the directors of several community-based agencies. During those meetings, the identified interventions were discussed and the coalition obtained assurances that staff would be available for an orientation meeting where all groups would come together, as well as for training and implementation of the program and that all parties would remain involved for as long as required to determine the program's effectiveness.

Selected staff members from settings where the program was to be implemented were designated as the implementation team. They attended a 3-day national training session led by the program developers that emphasized the importance of adhering to the core elements of the intervention. There they also learned about an online discussion board in which program users shared their experiences and could interact with, learn from, and be supported by others. On the last day of training, they met their assigned technical assistance provider and were assured that she had practical experience working with cities and agencies much like their own.

Back home, those trained quickly initiated the preimplementation steps covered during the training. However, those steps took somewhat longer than planned. A teacher training on the new curriculum that would be part of the school-based program had to be scheduled and the teachers' next professional development day had already been set, resulting in a delay of 2 months. In addition, although the training provided information about how to conduct the teacher training, the process for selecting teachers to be trained had not been explained. So, with assistance from the program's technical assistance provider, the team developed a list of selection criteria and presented it to the school for review and approval. The police department's community policing commander was to be the community program's primary contact person. However, the department was still recruiting for the position a month after the intervention was to begin. Despite these delays, all preimplementation steps were eventually accomplished, including the interagency collection and sharing of data on youth violence and the assignment of a person from the mayor's office to house and regularly update the information.

Because a solid foundation of community and organizational support had been laid, implementation proceeded relatively smoothly. As planned, teachers were trained and delivered the violence-prevention curriculum; school climate changes were implemented and supported by school administration and by parents via a parental involvement component. The police department piloted its community policing intervention in two neighborhoods and the identified community-based organizations implemented a mentoring program in the same two areas. The implementation team monitored progress and ensured that all evaluation activities were completed and data forwarded to the mayor's office. Adaptations were made to some program components, but the team ensured that fidelity to core elements was maintained, with assistance from the technical assistance provider.

As promised, every quarter, the implementation team provided an update to the coalition. The program was publicized and praised via a range of media, and more students and parents became involved. After the program had been running for about 9 months, it became clear to the coalition that there was sufficient support to keep it going but that additional funds would be required to maintain staff positions after the special 2-year budget allocation from the mayor's office was depleted. The coalition prepared and submitted to the mayor a budget request for continued funding, one that requested a line item in the city budget. The amount of funding requested was slightly higher than the original amount provided, because program leaders, including newly hired staff, would need to attend a refresher course and the cost of program materials had increased. Given promising evidence that some forms of youth violence—especially fighting at the middle school—had declined slightly, the budget request was approved.

As the program became embedded in the community and as Claremont's youth profile changed, additional adaptations to the program's interventions were made. The implementation team felt that its changes made the program more user friendly and strengthened it. The team shared its modifications with the technical assistance provider who, in turn, reported them to the program developers. The program developers agreed that the adaptations were useful and did not alter any essential components of the program. At the coalition's annual presentation to the mayor's office, the initiative was praised and the implementation team was commended. Several city department directors noted that, in addition to producing data that supported program effectiveness, there had been increased communication and collaboration about youth violence prevention among city agencies and with community-based organizations, which were additional and unexpected benefits of the initiative.

29.2.2.   Lessons Learned

Sounds good, doesn't it? It is, however, far from what most communities could ever expect to accomplish, especially given the fact that violence prevention is only one of multiple health and social issues that compete for resources, stakeholders, and goodwill. By illustrating the adoption process the coalition used, it is easy to understand why it rarely proceeds so smoothly, given the number of steps that must be taken, the levels of collaboration that are needed, the coordination of resources that is required, and the amount of effort that is involved. Even in this almost-idyllic situation, issues like staff turnover, delays in implementation, budgetary concerns, and adaptation needs emerged.

Admittedly, it may be tempting to discount this example because of the complexity of problems being addressed and the multi-level interventions chosen to address it. However, Dahlberg and Potter (2001), among many others, argue that such a comprehensive approach is necessary to address youth violence and that intensive interventions are more likely to be successful. In this respect, the field of youth violence prevention is not unique: Other interventions in intentional and unintentional injuries also call for multilevel interventions that target changes at individual, organization, and community levels. Choosing, initiating, and sustaining an innovation is challenging, whether the community in question is defined geographically (e.g., a city attempting to adopt a program to prevent youth violence, promote seatbelt or bicycle helmet use, or reduce access to firearms) or as a community of practice (e.g., emergency room providers seeking to address intimate partner violence or nursing home directors trying to reduce falls among the elderly).

As more is learned about what it takes to achieve the adoption of science-based practices in public health, many overly simplistic assumptions about the process of technology transfer are being overturned. For example:

- Researchers who once assumed that adoption of interventions was accomplished through the dissemination of research findings in academic journals now develop manuals and packages to replicate their evaluated programs.
- Program developers who once thought that manuals and replication packages would be sufficient to support local adoption of their science-based programs have learned that even beautiful materials get shelved—or

adapted beyond recognition—by organizations that are not trained to implement or sustain a program and become discouraged by the poor results their efforts produce.

- Agencies that once believed one-time implementation training would result in programs and materials being used effectively have learned that organizational leadership is needed to ensure that institutional support is in place and technical assistance is provided throughout the adoption process.
- Trainers and technical assistance providers are reporting to funders and developers that technology transfer is not a one-way street from science-to-practice, and that greater community input is required to identify problems and strategies for addressing them.

The injury and violence prevention fields are slowly but surely gaining a better theoretical and empirical understanding of how communities adopt new initiatives and what supports help overcome barriers that are typically encountered. Here, we summarize strategies that encourage communities to adopt science-based interventions.

29.3. CONCEPTUAL FRAMEWORK FOR ENCOURAGING COMMUNITY ADOPTION OF INNOVATION

Many communities are clear about the need to implement prevention policies and programs that address a range of injury and violence risks. However, it is unlikely that the practitioners within these communities will adopt science-based interventions simply because such strategies are "better." The factors that facilitate—or impede—the adoption and implementation of science-based interventions are based, in large part, on the extent to which the needs of practitioners and the contexts and constraints within which they operate are addressed.

Lessons learned by those working in the substance abuse prevention field are important to consider here. For example, the Center for Substance Abuse Prevention's (CSAP) (2001) six regional Centers for the Application of Prevention Technologies (CAPTs) focus on bringing research to practice by providing materials, training, and technical assistance that *motivate* the field to embrace a science-based approach to prevention planning, implementation, and evaluation; *promote* the application of science-based strategies; and *support* the implementation of science in prevention practice (Center for Substance Abuse Prevention [CSAP], 2001). In their efforts to narrow the gap between research and practice, the regional centers have learned a great deal that has been captured and synthesized into lessons learned. With few exceptions, these lessons are applicable to the injury and violence prevention fields. They highlight the importance of (1) diffusion activities that enable science-based interventions to stand out from the surrounding "noise"; (2) the regionalization of technical assistance that facilitates responses to regional challenges; (3) serving as a *Consumer Reports* for practitioners and policymakers, helping them make well-informed decisions and avoid aggressively marketed interventions that lack scientific evidence of effectiveness; (4) providing science-based prevention information in terms that are not oversimplified but are grounded in the realities facing communities; and (5) acknowledging the existence of a digital divide among some practitioners by using a range of channels to reach those without electronic access (Center for Substance Abuse Prevention, 2001). These lessons have been learned by those working in the injury and violence prevention fields as well, although they have not been as widely disseminated and discussed, perhaps because a similar CAPT system does not exist. The CAPTs or CAPT centers work with states, jurisdictions, and local communities to transfer research from a range of federal agencies to prevention providers through a customized, proactive technology transfer process. This process is employed to produce systemic change not only at the state level but also at the community level with prevention providers—a population that is also of vital importance in injury and violence prevention efforts. The need to understand how to promote community-level change is essential to this work.

29.3.1. Promoting Community-Level Change

Three broad conceptual frameworks inform attempts to promote community-level change: community-level models, diffusion of innovation, and organizational theory (National Cancer Institute, 2005). Community-level models emphasize the importance of participatory approaches in creating capacity and fostering collective empowerment to address health and social problems (Bracht, 1990). Diffusion of innovation theory, first described by Rogers (1995), is widely used to both guide dissemination efforts and help understand how a new idea or intervention is spread. Organizational theory recognizes not only that community agencies charged with adopting science-based interventions are complex social systems, with unique structures, cultures, roles, and norms, but also that change is accomplished through multiple stages (Steckler, Goodman, & Kegler, 2002).

As depicted in our example, the Claremont Community Coalition represents a cross-section of key city leaders, agencies, and community representatives who share the common mission of promoting the health of citizens, young and old. With a social planning and action agenda, it took collective action by setting priorities and developing a timetable that supported innovation. Committee members were prepared to gather the information needed to make informed decisions and share responsibility for choosing a new program that addressed an identified priority, was relevant to target populations, and fit local needs and resources. A community-level model is especially important when the innovation to be adopted is multilevel (i.e., it involves multiple agencies or internal divisions in coordinated efforts to address the identified complex problem of youth violence).

Complementing community participatory models, diffusion of innovation calls attention to innovation characteristics that influence whether or not it can be easily adopted and to the social systems and distribution channels that can support dissemination. Interventions with the greatest potential to be successfully adopted share similar characteristics that program developers and communities making decisions about what interventions to adopt should consider. They are more likely to be perceived as better than what is currently being employed and have clear benefits (relative advantage), are compatible with the target populations' norms and values (compatibility), are relatively easy to understand and use (complexity), are available to try out before a commitment to adopt is made (trialability), and have visible and tangible results (observability). The multilevel program that Claremont adopted was complex, which is a drawback. However, it was also judged by the coalition to be an improvement over current practice, and community members were asked to provide input on its compatibility. Efforts were made to obtain observable results, which proved to be useful in securing ongoing funding.

In addition to focusing on intervention characteristics, diffusion of innovation theory views communication as a two-way process in which opinion leaders at the local level influence what decisions are made, as well as how successful adoption efforts will be. Interventions are also more likely to be adopted if they are actively promoted by their innovators and channels for ongoing communication between early innovators and new users are developed and encouraged (Tenaski & Mohrman, 1995). In our example, the coalition had multiple opportunities—some of which it took—to apply these theoretical constructs in its deliberations. Criteria were set based on relative advantage (e.g., cost factors, ongoing efforts) and observability, among others, and they also tried to obtain input from key leaders and members of the community.

The final conceptual model informing adoption is drawn from theories of organizational change. These recognize that the community agencies charged with adopting science-based interventions are complex social systems, with unique structures, cultures, roles, and norms. Change is accomplished through multiple stages, beginning with building awareness about a problem and choosing a new strategy for addressing it and proceeding through preimplementation, implementation, and maintenance or institutionalization. There is a growing awareness that organizations need support through each of these stages, even though the types and levels of support might change. The Claremont coalition, for example, recognized the need for involving school and police leadership in decision making, carefully selecting staff within these departments to carry out implementation, and providing refresher training. Given evidence that the program was making a difference, institutionalization was supported through the request for line funding in the city budget. Perhaps most important, the coalition recognized that its job was not done once the program had been chosen; it continued to monitor and support all program components, at least in the short-term that our snapshot provides.

29.4.   ENCOURAGING ADOPTION OF SCIENCE-BASED INTERVENTIONS: A FOCUS ON IMPLEMENTATION

While the number of interventions termed *model*, *exemplary*, or *promising* continues to rise, organizational and community issues inhibit progress in the adoption and implementation of science-based interventions. We still know little about the process of program implementation, how to measure it, the factors that influence it, and the relationship between the quality of implementation and outcomes obtained (Greenberg, Domitrovich, Graczyk, & Zins, 2001, 2003). Although the importance of understanding program implementation as a next step in advancing the field of prevention programming has been acknowledged by researchers from a range of disciplines, sufficient attention has yet to be placed on delineating the factors that influence the quality of implementation for different types of programs or determining ways to ensure that such factors are preserved when programs are replicated. For example, in a review of more than 1,200 published prevention studies, Durlak (1997) found that program implementation data were provided for less than 5%, and an examination of school-based behavioral interventions determined that only 14.9% measured implementation integrity (Gresham, Gansle, Noell, Cohen, & Rosenbaum, 1993). A recent extensive literature review of the diffusion of innovation in service organizations commissioned by the UK Department of Health underscores the dearth of empirical studies on the processes through which innovations are implemented and sustained in local contexts, leaving many unanswered questions about how these processes can be enhanced (Greenhalgh, Robert, MacFarlane, Bate, & Kyriakidou, 2004).

29.4.1.   Practitioner/Staff Development

There are no clear guidelines readily available for use in determining which prevention program is most appropriate for a specific population or how to gain the support and training needed to implement it. A frequently expressed concern in the current literature on school personnel training has been the ineffectiveness of traditional approaches to staff development (Richardson, 2003). For example, despite well-established research regarding significant differences in adult learning styles, school districts seldom offer staff development programs that are sufficient in length and depth to engage teachers in a learning process that results in an increase in knowledge and the acquisition of skills that produce significant changes in practice.

"One size fits all" methods of preparing the implementers of interventions tend to be brief events, and rarely is adequate follow-up technical assistance available. Those being trained are not given sufficient time to raise important questions and have them answered convincingly, express doubts about certain aspects of a program, and engage in discussions that result in their concerns being addressed satisfactorily or practice new or difficult techniques and obtain feedback that builds skills and creates confidence.

Those who are truly engaged in a learning process are actively involved in meaningful inquiry, reflection, and problem solving (Jones, Valdez, Nowakowski, & Rasmussen, 1994). However, in attempting to engage adults in the adoption of new programming, it is essential to acknowledge that they bring their accumulated life experiences to this process, making them practical problem solvers. Their experiences represent the richest resource for learning, and thus must be capitalized on. Adult learners must be provided with opportunities for self-direction and taking responsibility for the learning process (Cantor, 1992; Hiemstra & Brockett, 1994; Knowles, 1990; Tennant, 1997). We also know that adults are relevancy oriented; it is essential that they understand why they are being asked to learn something *and* perceive that what is being taught is of immediate value to them. The fact that an intervention is evidence based is not sufficient grounds for adoption and implementation.

This knowledge of adult learners has resulted in the development of important principles that should be applied in the effective training of intervention implementers. These principles, well articulated by Loucks-Horsley (1995) in relation to teachers and other school staff, are also applicable efforts to prepare potential implementers: The process of preparation must be driven by a well-defined image of effective learning and teaching, provide opportunities for those being trained to build knowledge and skills, use/model the strategies that will be employed with the target population, build a learning community, instruct and support implementers in ways that will enable them to serve in leadership roles, illustrate and provide access to links to other parts of the system in which the intervention is being implemented, and be improved on through an assessment process to maintain relevancy.

Clearly, process and context must be taken into account along with content. Process standards include providing a framework for relating an intervention to the organization's mission and needs; using a variety of approaches to prepare the implementers; following up to ensure improvement in practice; using stages of group development to build effective, collegial teams; and promoting collaborative skills among implementers.

The importance of colleague collaboration is also supported by a National Center for Education Statistics survey of teacher preparation and staff development. Teachers who participated in regularly scheduled collaboration with other teachers, networking with teachers outside the school, and mentoring of another teacher in a formal relationship were more likely than those who did not participate in any of these activities to report feeling very well prepared for the demands of their classroom assignments (Parsad, Lewis, & Farris, 2001).

29.4.2.   Institutional Readiness

In terms of context, although the majority of training efforts focus exclusively on individuals, almost without exception, barriers to improved outcomes are related to an institution's structure and processes. Therefore, it is necessary to understand the range of individual- and organizational-level factors that can inhibit or facilitate successful intervention implementation to address them. Chief among these factors are the degree of responsiveness to change among staff (Gingiss, Gottlieb, & Brink, 1994; Gottfredson, 1997), the level of shared involvement and ownership (Backer, David, & Soucy, 1995), commitment of time and/or resources (Saunders, 1998), administrative support for intervention implementation (Zetlin, 1998), and willingness/ability to take a leadership role to mobilize intervention support (Lowenthal, 1996). And so, just as training must address the individual's needs in relation to the change process, it must also consider the change process within an organization. The delicate balance between the need for both top-down and bottom-up involvement must be handled correctly to build and sustain programming (Sparks & Loucks-Horsey, 1990). Top-down efforts are needed to set general directions and to communicate expectations regarding performance. Bottom-up efforts are necessary to fully engage all staff in the implementation process, involving them in the planning process in meaningful ways while still ensuring intervention fidelity.

To generate both top-down and bottom-up approaches, all members of an organization or community where implementation will take place must be provided with a framework for understanding how the intervention can be integrated effectively into the organizational structure and programming and how it can contribute to the organization's mission. Without a framework for integrating programmatic changes, intervention implementation will be fragmented, coordination with existing activities will not be achieved, and changes will not be sustained.

29.4.3.   Broad-Based Support

No matter the science-based intervention to be implemented, broad-based support will be achieved only if representatives from all constituencies within a community where implementation will take place participate in training. Although some types of interventions require that larger numbers of some constituencies participate in the training process, garnering cooperation and support is achieved only when a collaborative model is employed that engages all stakeholders in the process of implementation. Such a model also supports collaborative problem solving and consensus-building.

It also is vital to build a strong base of support among those both directly and indirectly responsible for program implementation. However, doing so requires time and effort. In addition to needing a team and a strong leader, sites must have sufficient time to plan for implementation, educating staff at all levels and gaining support. This team approach not only improves communication, a major factor promoting successful implementation; it also produces "many champions of the program who could carry the program forward even if other key individuals left" (Blueprints for Violence Prevention, 2000, pp. 1–2).

29.5. RECOMMENDATIONS

Our recommendations for effective ways to encourage the adoption of science-based interventions are based on all of the factors described above. We also draw on the research on change, conducted by Fullan and Stiegelbauer (1991), which has been valuable in our technology transfer work. Each stage of change—intervention introduction, implementation, and institutionalization—requires different support mechanisms. During *introduction/preadoption*, implementers need clear information and support to spread the message of change. In the *implementation phase*, strong support that uses such research-based strategies as coaching and support groups are needed to help implementers institute new practices in their settings and to increase their feelings of self-efficacy and commitment to the intervention. However, while expert training is crucial for an intervention to be implemented with fidelity, high-quality training alone is not sufficient. Follow-up technical assistance that extends the training experience to the real world and provides support for intervention implementation and maintenance are also required (Elias, 1997; Gottfredson, Fink, Skroban, & Gottfredson, 1997; McCormick, Steckler, & McLeroy, 1995). Finally, because successful intervention *institutionalization depends* in large part on the intervention's connectedness to the setting where it is being implemented, this stage is achieved, at least in part, by planning for integration of the intervention into the existing structures during the initiation phase and providing the levels of training and technical assistance that will enable communities to implement the intervention with fidelity, thus increasing the likelihood of obtaining the desired outcomes and engaging program implementers and advocates after the funding period has ended. However, all of these phases—from introduction/preadoption to implementation to institutionalization—cannot be accomplished without strong institutional vision and leadership. Such leadership builds the conditions for reflection, open dialogue, mutual respect for ideas, and both professional and institutional growth (MacBeath, Moos, & Riley, 1998).

In addition to keeping these phases of change in mind to work effectively with organizations and communities, we offer these additional recommendations:

- Encourage the National Institutes of Health, the Centers for Disease Control and Prevention, and other major funders of public health innovations to support the development and evaluation of interventions that are informed by community practice and implementation research that clearly shows the importance of factors such as feasibility, adaptability, sustainability, resource intensity, and cost-effectiveness.
- Recognize the academic as well as the pragmatic contributions of empirical studies of how innovative interventions are implemented and sustained in

local contexts and encourage the use of rigorous, in-depth, mixed methodology studies (Greenhalgh et al., 2004).

- Provide support to community agencies that encounter and document barriers to implementation, acknowledging that first attempts may be unsuccessful but yield important lessons that contribute to later success.
- Draw from private-enterprise models that place an emphasis on the acceptability of an innovation's design features to consumers and use marketing strategies to tailor and adapt designs for different subgroups (Rotheram-Borus & Duan, 2003).

Expectations that interventions adopted by communities would be similar—and achieve similar results—to those observed in research settings remain relatively untested and need to be supported by additional evidence gathered through systematic research on the implementation process. Supporting the conduct of "blended research," as Botvin (2004) has termed the collaborative investigations of prevention scientists and practitioners, is sorely needed if we are to encourage the adoption of science-based interventions.

REFERENCES

Backer, T. E., David, S. L., & Soucy, G. (1995). The challenge of technology transfer. In T. E. Backer, S. L. David, & G. Soucy (Eds.), *Reviewing the behavioral science knowledge base on technology transfer* (pp. 1–20). Washington, DC: National Institute on Drug Abuse.

Blueprints for Violence Prevention, Center for the Study and Prevention of Violence. (2000) Assessment and planning for implementation. *Blueprints News 1* (3), 1–2.

Botvin, G. J. (2004). Advancing prevention science and practice: Challenges, critical issues, and future directions. *Prevention Science, 5* (1), 69–72.

Bracht, N. (Ed.). (1990). *Health promotion at the community level.* Newbury Park, CA.: Sage.

Butterfoss, F. D. (2004). The coalition technical assistance and training framework: Helping community coalitions help themselves. *Health Promotion Practice, 5* (2), 118–126.

Cantor, J. A. (1992). *Delivering instruction to adult learners.* Toronto: Wall & Emerson.

Center for Substance Abuse Prevention. (2001). *Closing the gap between research and practice: Lessons of the first three years of CSAP's National CAPT System 1997–2000* (National Research Conference ed.). Washington, DC: Author.

Dahlberg, L. L., & Potter, L. B. (2001). Youth violence: Developmental pathways and prevention challenges. *American Journal of Preventive Medicine, 20,* 3–14.

Durlak, J. (1997). *Successful prevention programs for children.* New York: Plenum Press.

Elias, M. (1997). Reinterpreting dissemination of prevention programs as widespread implementation with effectiveness and fidelity. In R. P. Weisberg, T. P. Gullotta, R. L. Hampton, B. A. Ryan, & G. R. Adams (Eds.), *Healthy Children 2010: Enhancing children's wellness* (pp. 253–289). Thousand Oaks, CA: Sage.

Embry, D. D. (2004). Community-based prevention using simple, low-cost, evidence-based kernels and behavior vaccines. *Journal of Community Psychology, 32,* 575–591.

Forgatch, M. S. (2003). Implementation as a second stage in prevention research. *Prevention & Treatment, 6,* 24 (c).

Fullan, M. G., & Stiegelbauer, S. M. (1991). *The new meaning of educational change.* New York: Teachers College Press.

Gingiss, P., Gottlieb, N. H., & Brink, S. G. (1994). Measuring cognitive characteristics associated with adoption and implementation of health innovations in schools. *American Journal of Health Promotion, 8* (4), 294–301.

Gottfredson, D. C. (1997). School-based crime prevention. In L. W. Sherman, D. C. Gottfredson, D. Mackenzie, J. Eck, P. Reuter, & S. Bushway (Eds.), *Preventing crime: What works, what doesn't, what's promising: A report to the United States Congress* (NCJ 171676, pp. 125–182). Washington, DC: U.S. Department of Justice, Office of Justice Programs.

Gottfredson, D. C., Fink, C. M., Skroban, S., & Gottfredson, G. D. (1997). Making prevention work. In R. P. Weissberg (Ed.), *Issues in children's and families' lives (Vol. 4): Healthy Children 2010: Establishing preventive services* (pp. 219–252). Thousand Oaks, CA: Sage.

Greenberg, M. T., Domitrovich, C. E., Graczyk, P., & Zins, J. (2001). *A conceptual model of implementation for school-based preventive interventions: Implications for research, practice, and policy* (Report to the Center for Mental Health Services, Substance Abuse and Mental Health Services Administration). Rockville, MD: U.S. Department of Health and Human Services.

Greenberg, M. T., Domitrovich, C. E., Graczyk, P., & Zins, J. (2003). *The study of implementation in school-based preventive interventions: Theory, practice, and research.* Washington, DC: Center for Mental Health Services, Substance Abuse and Mental Health Services Administration.

Greenhalgh T., Robert, G., Macfarlance, F., Bate, P., & Kyriakidou, O. (2004). Diffusion of innovatioins in service organizations: Systematic review and recommendations. *Milbank Quarterly, 82* (4), 1–31.

Gresham, F. M., Gansle, K. A., Noell, G. H., Cohen, S., & Rosenbaum, S. (1993). Treatment integrity of school-based behavioral intervention studies. *School Psychology Review, 22,* 254–272.

Hiemstra, R., & Brockett, R. (1994). From behaviorism to humanism: Incorporating self-direction in learning concepts into the instructional design process. In H. B. Long & Associates, *New ideas about self-directed learning* (pp. 59–80). Norman: Oklahoma Research Center for Continuing Professional and Higher Education, University of Oklahoma.

Holtgrave, D. R. (2004). The role of quantitative policy analysis in HIV prevention technology transfer. *Public Health Reports, 119* (1), 19–22.

Jones, B., Valdez, G., Nowakowski, J., & Rasmussen, C. (1994). *Designing learning and technology for educational reform.* Oak Brook, IL: North Central Regional Educational Laboratory.

Kelly, J. A., Somlai, A. M., Benotsch, E. G., McAuliffe, T. L., Amirkhanian, Y. A., Brown, K. D., Stevenson, L. Y., Fernandez, M. I., Sitzler, C., Gore-Felton, C., Pinkerton, S. D., Weinhardt, L. S., & Opgenorth, K. M. (2004). Distance communication transfer of HIV prevention interventions to service providers. *Science, 305,* 1953–1955.

Kelly, J. A., Somlai, A. M., DiFranceisco, W. J., Otto-Salaj, L. L., McAuliffe, T. L., Hackl, K. L., Heckman, T. G., Holtgrave, D. R., & Rompa, D. (2000). Bridging the gap between the science and service of HIV prevention: Transferring effective research-based HIV prevention interventions to community AIDS service providers, *American Journal of Public Health, 90,* 1082–1088.

Knowles, M. S. (1990). *The adult learner: A neglected species* (4th ed.) Houston, TX: Gulf.

Loucks-Horsley, S. (1995). Professional development and the learner centered school. *Theory into Practice, 34* (4), 265–271.

Lowenthal, B. (1996). Integrated school services for children at risk: Rationale, models, barriers, and recommendations for implementation. *Intervention in Schools & Clinic, 31* (3), 154–157.

MacBeath, J., Moos, L., & Riley, K. (1998). Time for a change. In J. MacBeath, (Ed.), *Effective school leadership: Responding to change* (pp. 20–31). Thousand Oaks, CA: Sage.

McCormick, L. K., Steckler, A. B., & McLeroy, K. R. (1995). Diffusion of innovations in schools: A study of adoption and implementation of school-based tobacco prevention curricula. *American Journal of Health Promotion, 9* (3), 210–219.

Mihalic, S. F., & Irwin, K. (2003). Blueprints for violence prevention: From research to real-world settings—Factors influencing successful replication of model programs. *Youth Violence and Juvenile Justice, 1,* 307–329.

National Cancer Institute. (2005). *Theory at a glace: A guide for health promotion practice* (2nd ed.) Rockville, MD: U.S. Department of Health and Human Services, National Institutes of Health, February 2, 2005.

National Institute of Drug Abuse. (2003). *Clinical trials network.* Retrieved February 3, 2005, from www.drugabuse.gov/CTN/about.html.

Parsad, B., Lewis, L., & Farris, E. (2001). *Teacher preparation and professional development: 2000.* Washington, DC: National Center for Education Statistics.

Richardson, V. (2003). The dilemmas of professional development. *Phi Delta Kappan, 84* (5), 401–406.

Rogers, R. E. (1995). *Diffusion of innovations* (4th ed.). New York: Free Press.

Rotheram-Borus, M. J., Bickford, B., & Milburn, N. G. (2001). Implementing a classroom-based social skills training program in middle childhood. *Journal of Educational and Psychological Consultation, 12,* 91–110.

Rotheram-Borus, M. J., & Duan, N. (2003). Next generation of preventive interventions. *Journal of the American Academy of Child & Adolescent Psychiatry, 42* (5), 518–526.

Saunders, T. (1998). School-linked services in action: Results in an implementation project. *Social Work in Education, 21* (1), 37–47.

Sinclair, R. C. (2002). Prevalence of safer needle devices and factors associated with their adoption: Results of a national hospital survey. *Public Health Reports, 117,* 340–349.

Sparks, D., & Loucks-Horsey, S. (1990). *Five models of staff development.* Oxford, OH: National Staff Development Council.

Steckler, A., Goodman, R. M., & Kegler, M. C. (2002). Mobilizing organizations for health enhancement: Theories of organizational change. In K. Glanz, B. K. Rimer, & F. M. Lewis (Eds.), *Health behavior and health education: Theory, research and practice* (pp. 335–360, 3rd ed.). San Francisco: Jossey-Bass.

Tenkasi, R. V., & Mohrman, S. A. (1995). Technology transfer as collaborative learning. In T. E. Backer, S. L. David, & G. Soucy (Eds.), *Reviewing the behavioral science knowledge base on technology transfer,* (pp. 147–167). Rockville, MD: U.S. Department of Health and Human Services, Public Health Service, National Institutes of Health.

Tennant, M. (1997). *Psychology and adult learning* (2nd ed.). London: Routledge.

Wilson-Brewer, R., Cohen, S., O'Donnell, L., & Goodman, I. (1991). *Violence prevention for young adolescents: A survey of the state of the art* (ERIC Document Reproduction Service No. ED356442). Washington, DC: Carnegie Council on Adolescent Development, Carnegie Corporation of New York.

Zetlin, A. G. (1998). *Lesson learned about integrating services* (Publication Series No. 4. Mid-Atlantic Laboratory for Student Success). Philadelphia: National Research Center on Education in the Inner Cities.

Appendices

Appendix 1

Key Injury and Violence Prevention Resources*

Compiled by Christy L. Cechman

A1.1. GENERAL INJURY

Baker, S. P., O'Neill, B., Ginsburg, M. J., & Li, G. (1992). *The injury fact book* (2nd ed.). New York: Oxford University Press.

Barss, P., Smith, G. S., Baker, S. P., & Mohan, D. (1998). *Injury prevention: An international perspective: Epidemiology, surveillance and policy.* New York: Oxford University Press.

Berger, L. R., & Mohan, D. (1996). *Injury control: A global view.* New York: Oxford University Press.

Bergman, A. B. (1992). *Political approaches to injury control at the state level.* Seattle: University of Washington Press.

Bonnie, R. J., Fulco, C. E., & Liverman, C. T. (1999). *Reducing the burden of injury: Advancing prevention and treatment.* Washington, DC: National Academy Press.

Bracht, N. F. (1999). *Health promotion at the community level 2: New advances* (2nd ed.). Thousand Oaks, CA: Sage.

Centers for Disease Control and Prevention. (2001). School health guidelines to prevent unintentional injuries and violence [Electronic version]. *MMWR Recommendations & Reports, 50* (No. RR-22). www.cdc.gov/mmwr/indrr_2001html

Christoffel, K. K., & Runyan, C. W. (1995). *Adolescent injuries: Epidemiology and prevention.* Philadelphia: Hanley & Belfus.

Christoffel, T. (1993). *Protecting the public: Legal issues in injury prevention.* New York: Oxford University Press.

Christoffel, T., & Gallagher, S. S. (2006). *Injury prevention and public health: Practical knowledge, skills, and strategies* (2nd ed.). Sudbury, MA: Jones & Bartlett.

Committee on Trauma Research. (1985). *Injury in America: A continuing public health problem.* Washington, DC: National Academy Press.

DiClemente, R. J., Crosby, R. A., & Kegler, M. C. (2002). *Emerging theories in health promotion practice and research: Strategies for improving public health.* San Francisco: Jossey-Bass.

Finkelstein, E. A., Corso, P. S., & Miller, T. R. (2006). *The incidence and economic burden of injuries in the United States, 2000.* New York: Oxford University Press.

Gielen, A. C. (Ed.). (2002). Injury and domestic violence prevention [Special issue]. *Patient Education & Counseling, 46* (3).

Gielen, A., Sleet, D. A., & DiClemente, R. (2006). *Injury and violence prevention: Behavioral science theories, methods and applications.* San Francisco: Jossey-Bass.

*Inclusion in this list does not necessarily represent the official policies and views of or endorsement by the federal government, U.S. Department of Health and Human Services, or the Centers for Disease Control and Prevention, and none should be inferred.

Glanz, K., Rimer, B. K., & Lewis, F. M. (2002). *Health behavior and health education: Theory, research, and practice* (3rd ed.). San Francisco: Jossey-Bass.

Goldsmith, S. K. (2002). *Reducing suicide: A national imperative.* Washington, DC: National Academies Press.

Goodman, R. A., Rothstein, M. A., Hoffman, R. E., Lopez, W., & Matthews, G. W. (In press). *Law in public health practice* (2nd ed.). New York: Oxford University Press.

Gregg, M. B. (2002). *Field epidemiology* (2nd ed.). New York: Oxford University Press.

Haddix, A. C., Teutsch, S. M., & Corso, P. S. (2003). *Prevention effectiveness: A guide to decision analysis and economic evaluation* (2nd ed.). New York: Oxford University Press.

Hale, A. R. & Glendon, A. I. (1987). *Individual behavior in the control of danger.* New York: Elsevier.

Holder, Y., Peden, M., Krug, E., Lund, J., Gururaj, G., & Kobusingye, O. (2001). *Injury surveillance guidelines.* www.who.int/violence_injury_prevention/publications/surveillance/surveillance_guidelines/en/.

Hornik, R. C. (2002). *Public health communication: Evidence for behavior change.* Mahwah, NJ: Lawrence Erlbaum Associates.

Institute of Medicine. (2002). *Speaking of health: Assessing health communication strategies for diverse populations.* Washington, DC: National Academies Press.

Karlson, T. A., & Hargarten, S. W. (1997). *Reducing firearm injury and death: A public health sourcebook on guns.* New Brunswick, NJ: Rutgers University Press.

Liller, K. (2006). *Injury prevention in children and youth.* Washington, DC: American Public Health Association.

Liller, K. D., & Sleet, D. A. (Eds.). (2004). Special issue on injury prevention [Special issue]. *American Journal of Health Behavior, 28* (suppl. 1).

McClure, R., Stevenson, M., & McEvoy, S. (2004). *The scientific basis of injury prevention and control.* Melbourne, Australia: IP Communications.

Mohan, D., & Tiwari, G. (2000). *Injury prevention and control.* New York: Taylor & Francis.

National Center for Injury Prevention and Control. (2002). *CDC injury research agenda.* Atlanta, GA: Centers for Disease Control and Prevention, National Center for Injury Prevention and Control. www.cdc.gov/ncipc/pub-res/research-agenda/agenda.htm

National Committee for Injury Prevention and Control. (1989). *Injury prevention: Meeting the challenge.* New York: Oxford University Press.

National Safety Council. (1999–). *Injury facts.* Itasca, IL: Author.

National Safety Council. (March 13, 2006). *Report on injuries in America, 2005.* Retrieved May 20, 2003, from www.nsc.org/library/report_injury_usa.htm

Ozanne-Smith, J., & Williams, F. (1995). *Injury research and prevention.* Victoria, Australia: Monash University Accident Research Centre.

Rice, D. P., & Mackenzie, E. J. (1989). *Cost of injury in the United States: A report to Congress, 1989.* San Francisco: Institute for Health & Aging, University of California, San Francisco Baltimore: Injury Prevention Center, School of Hygiene and Public Health, The Johns Hopkins University.

Rivara, F. P., Cummings, P., Koepsell, T. D., Grossman, D. C., & Maier, R. V. (2001). *Injury control: A guide to research and program evaluation.* New York: Cambridge University Press.

Roberts, M. C., & Brooks, P. H. (Eds.). (1987). Children's injuries: Prevention and public policy [Special issue]. *Journal of Social Issues, 43* (2).

Robertson, L. S. (1998). *Injury epidemiology* (2nd ed.). New York: Oxford University Press.

Schneiderman, N. (2001). *Integrating behavioral and social sciences with public health.* Washington, DC: American Psychological Association.

Sethi, D., Habibula, S., McGee, K., Peden, M., Bennett, S., Hyder, A. A., Klevens, J., Odero, W., & Suriyawongpaisal, P. (2004). *Guidelines for conducting community surveys on injuries and violence.* http://whqlibdoc.who.int/publications/2004/9241546484.pdf.

Sleet, D. A., & Bryn, S. (Eds.). (2003). Injury prevention for children and youth [Special issue]. *American Journal of Health Education, 34* (5).

Swartz, R. (Ed.). (2003). Focal point issue: Injury prevention and control. *Health Promotion Practice, 4* (2).

Thacker, S. B., & MacKenzie, E. J. (Eds.). (2003). Injury Prevention and Control. *Epidemiologic Reviews, 25.*

Waller, J. A. (1985). *Injury control: A guide to the causes and prevention of trauma.* Lexington, MA: Lexington Books.

Ward, J. (Ed.). (2006). *A safer, healthier America: The advancement of public health in the 20th Century.* New York: Oxford University Press.

Widome, M. D. (1997). *Injury prevention and control for children and youth* (3rd ed.). Elk Grove Village, IL: American Academy of Pediatrics.

Wilson, M. H., Baker, S. P., Teret, S. P., Shock, S. S., & Garbarina, J. (1991). *Saving children: A guide to injury prevention.* New York: Oxford University Press.

World Health Organization. (2002). *Injury chart book: A graphical overview of the global burden of injuries.* http://whqlibdoc.who.int/publications/924156220X.pdf.

World Health Organization. (2002). *Injury: A leading cause of the global burden of disease, 2000.* www.who.int/violence_injury_prevention/publications/other_injury/injury/en/.

Zaza, S., Briss, P. A., Harris, K. W., & Task Force on Community Preventive Services. (2005). *The guide to community preventive services: What works to promote health?* New York: Oxford University Press.

A1.2.   UNINTENTIONAL INJURY

Behrman, R. E. (Ed.). (2000). Unintentional injuries in childhood. *Future of Children, 10* (1).

Branche, C. M., Dellinger, A. M., Sleet, D. A., Gilchrist, J., & Olson, S. J. (2004). Unintentional injuries: The burden, risks, and preventive strategies to address diversity. In I. L. Livingston (Ed.), *Praeger handbook of black American health: Policies and issues behind disparities in health* (pp. 317–327). Westport, CT: Praeger.

Elvik, R., & Vaa, T. (2004). *The handbook of road safety measures.* Boston: Elsevier.

Evans, L. (2004). *Traffic safety.* Bloomfield Hills, MI: Science Serving Society.

Fletemeyer, J. R., & Freas, S. J. (1999). *Drowning: New perspectives on intervention and prevention.* Boca Raton, FL: CRC Press.

Geller, E. S. (Ed.). (1991). Road safety: International perspectives [Special issue]. *Journal of Applied Behavior Analysis, 24* (1).

Holt, D. J. (2004). *Pedestrian safety.* Warrendale, PA: SAE International.

Liverman, C. T., Altevogt, B. M., Joy, J. E., & Johnson, R. T. (2005). *Spinal cord injury: Progress, promise and priorities.* Washington, DC: National Academies Press.

Nantulya, V. M., & Sleet, D. A. (Eds.). (2003). The global challenge of road traffic injuries [Special issue]. *Injury Control & Safety Promotion, 10* (1–2).

Parra, E. K., & Stevens, J. A. (2002). *U.S. fall prevention programs for seniors.* Atlanta, GA: Centers for Disease Control and Prevention, National Center for Injury Prevention and Control.

Peden, M., Scurfield, R., Sleet, D., Mohan, D., Hyder, A. A., Jarawan, E., & Mathers, C. (2004). *World report on road traffic injury prevention.* www.who.int/world-health-day/2004/infomaterials/world_report/en/index.html.

Posner, M. (2000). *Preventing school injuries.* New Brunswick, NJ: Rutgers University Press.

Rothe, J. P. (2002). *Driving lessons: Exploring systems that make traffic safer.* Edmonton, Alberta: University of Alberta Press.

Rothengatter, T., & Carbonell, E. (1997). *Traffic and transport psychology: Theory and application.* New York: Pergamon.

Seiffert, U., & Wech, L. (2003). *Automotive safety handbook.* Warrendale, PA: SAE International.

Shults, R., & Harvey, P. (1996). *Efforts to increase smoke detector use in U.S. households.* Atlanta, GA: Centers for Disease Control and Prevention, National Center for Injury Prevention and Control.

Sleet, D. A., & Hopkins, K. (Eds.). (2004). *Bibliography of behavioral science research in unintentional injury prevention* [CD-ROM]. Atlanta, GA: Centers for Disease Control and Prevention, National Center for Injury Prevention and Control.

Sleet, D. A., Wagenaar, A., & Waller, P. (Eds.). (1989). Drinking, driving and health promotion [Special issue]. *Health Education Quarterly, 16* (3).

Tennstedt, S. L. (Ed.). (2002–2003). Falls and fall-related injuries. *Generations: Journal of the American Society on Aging, XXVI* (4).

Transportation Research Board. (2003). *Implementing impaired driving countermeasures: Putting research into action* (Transportation Research E-Circular, E-C072), from http://trb.org/publications/circulars/ec072.pdf.

Zaza, S., Briss, P. A., Harris, K. W., & Task Force on Community Preventive Services. (2005). The guide to community preventive services! What works to promote health? New York: Oxford University Press.

A1.3.   VIOLENCE-RELATED INJURY

Basile, K. C., & Saltzman, L. E. (2002). *Sexual violence surveillance: Uniform definitions and recommended data elements, version 1.0.* www.cdc.gov/ncipc/pub-res/sv_surveillance/sv.htm.

Bonnie, R. J., & Wallace, R. B. (2003). *Elder mistreatment: Abuse, neglect, and exploitation in an aging America.* Washington, DC: National Academy Press.

Chalk, R., & King, P. (1998). *Violence in families: Assessing prevention and treatment programs*. Washington, DC: National Academy Press.

Cohn, F., Salmon, M. E., & Stobo, J. D. (2002). *Confronting chronic neglect: The education and training of health professionals on family violence*. Washington, DC: National Academies Press.

Crosson-Tower, C. (2004). *Understanding child abuse and neglect* (6th ed.). Boston: Allyn & Bacon.

Dahlberg, L. L., Toal, S. B., & Behrens, C. B. (2005). *Measuring violence-related attitudes, behaviors, and influences among youths: A compendium of assessment tools* (2nd ed.). www.cdc.gov/ncipc/pub-res/measure.htm.

Elliott, D. S., Hamburg, B. A., & Williams, K. R. (1998). *Violence in American schools: A new perspective*. Cambridge, UK: Cambridge University Press.

Finkelhor, D. (1986). *A sourcebook on child sexual abuse*. Beverly Hills, CA: Sage.

Goldsmith, S. K. (2002). *Reducing suicide: A national imperative*. Washington, DC: National Academies Press.

Ikeda, R. M., & Dodge, K. A. (Eds.). (2001). Youth violence prevention: The science of moving research to practice [Special issue]. *American Journal of Preventive Medicine, 20* (suppl. 1).

Klein, E., Campbell, J. C., Soler, E., & Ghez, M. (1997). *Ending domestic violence: Changing public perceptions/halting the epidemic*. Thousand Oaks, CA: Sage.

Krug, E. G., Dahlberg, L. L., Mercy, J. A., Zwi, A. B., & Lozano, R. (2002). *World report on violence and health*. www.who.int/violence_injury_prevention/violence/world_report/en/index.html.

Mills, L. G. (2003). *Insult to injury: Rethinking our responses to intimate abuse*. Princeton, NJ: Princeton University Press.

Moore, M. H. (2003). *Deadly lessons: Understanding lethal school violence*. Washington, DC: National Academy Press.

National Research Council Panel of Research on Child Abuse and Neglect. (1993). *Understanding child abuse and neglect*. Washington, DC: National Academy Press.

Reiss, A. J., & Roth, J. A. (1993). *Understanding and preventing violence*. Washington, DC: National Academy Press.

Reyes, C., Rudman, W. J., & Hewitt, C. R. (2002). *Domestic violence and health care: Policies and prevention*. New York: Haworth Medical Press.

Roberts, A. R. (2002). *Handbook of domestic violence intervention strategies: Policies, programs, and legal remedies*. New York: Oxford University Press.

Rosenberg, M. L. & Fenley, M. A. (1991). *Violence in America: A public health approach*. New York: Oxford University Press.

Saltzman, L. E., Fanslow, J. L., McMahon, P. M., & Shelley, G. A. (1999). *Intimate partner violence surveillance: Uniform definitions and recommended data elements, version 1.0*. www.cdc.gov/ncipc/pub-res/ipv_surveillance/intimate.htm.

Thornton, T. N., Craft, C. A., Dahlberg, L. L., Lynch, B. S., & Baer, K. (2002). *Best practices of youth violence prevention: A sourcebook for community action* (rev. ed.). www.cdc.gov/ncipc/dvp/bestpractices.htm.

Towner, E., Downswell, T., Simpson, G., & Jarvis, S. (1996). *Health promotion in childhood and young adolescence for the prevention of unintentional injuries*. London: Health Education Authority.

U.S. Department of Health and Human Services. (2001). *National strategy for suicide prevention: Goals and objectives for action*. www.mentalhealth.samhsa.gov/publications/allpubs/SMA01-3517/.

U.S. Department of Health and Human Services. (2001). *Youth violence: A report of the Surgeon General*. www.surgeongeneral.gov/library/youthviolence/toc.html.

Wellford, C. F., Pepper, J. V., & Petrie, C. V. (2005). Firearms and violence: A critical review. Washington, DC: National Academies Press.

A1.4.   INTERVENTION FUNDAMENTALS

Barnett, D. W., Bell, S. H., & Carey, K. T. (1998). *Designing preschool interventions: A practitioner's guide*. New York: Guilford Press.

Bartholomew, L. K., Parcel, G. S., Kok, G., & Gottlieb, N. H. (2001). *Intervention mapping: Designing theory- and evidence-based health promotion programs*. Mountain View, CA: Mayfield.

Bensley, R. J., & Brookins-Fisher, J. (2003). *Community health education methods: A practical guide* (2nd ed.). Sudbury, MA: Jones & Bartlett.

CDC/ATSDR, Committee on Community Engagement. (1997). *Principles of community engagement*. www.cdc.gov/phppo/pce/.

Erickson, M. F., & Kurz-Riemer, K. (1999). *Infants, toddlers, and families: A framework for support and intervention.* New York: Guilford Press.

Green, L. W., & Kreuter, M. W. (2005). *Health program planning: An educational and ecological approach* (4th ed.). New York: McGraw-Hill.

Guttman, N. (2000). *Public health communication interventions: Values and ethical dilemmas.* Thousand Oaks, CA: Sage.

Rathvon, N. (1999). *Effective school interventions: Strategies for enhancing academic achievement and social competence.* New York: Guilford Press.

Rutter, D. R., & Quine, L. (2002). *Changing health behaviour: Intervention and research with social cognition models.* Philadelphia: Open University Press.

Schneiderman, N., Speers, M. A., Silva, J. M., Tomes, H., & Gentry, J. H. (2001). *Integrating behavioral and social sciences with public health.* Washington, DC: American Psychological Association.

Smedley, B. D., & Syme, S. L. (2000). *Promoting health: Intervention strategies from social and behavioral research.* Washington, DC: National Academy Press.

A1.5. CRISIS AND TRAUMA

Dattilio, F. M., & Freeman, A. M. (2000). *Cognitive-behavioral strategies in crisis intervention* (2nd ed.). New York: Guilford Press.

France, K. (1996). *Crisis intervention: A handbook of immediate person-to-person help* (3rd ed.). Springfield, IL: Thomas.

Hutchison, S. B. (2005). *Effects of and interventions for childhood trauma from infancy through adolescence: Pain unspeakable.* New York: Haworth Maltreatment & Trauma Press.

Litz, B. T. (2004). *Early intervention for trauma and traumatic loss.* New York: Guilford Press.

Osofsky, J. D. (2004). *Young children and trauma: Intervention and treatment.* New York: Guilford Press.

Roberts, A. R. (2005). *Crisis intervention handbook: Assessment, treatment, and research* (3rd ed.). New York: Oxford University Press.

Wainrib, B. R., & Bloch, E. L. (1998). *Crisis intervention and trauma response: Theory and practice.* New York: Springer.

A1.6. TRAUMATIC BRAIN INJURY

National Center for Injury Prevention and Control. (2003). *Heads up: Brain injury in your practice.* Atlanta, GA: Centers for Disease Control and Prevention, National Center for Injury Prevention and Control. Available online: www.cdc.gov/ncipc/pub-res/tbi_toolkit/physicians/introduction.htm

National Center for Injury Prevention and Control. (2005). *Heads up: Concussion in high school sports.* Atlanta, GA: Centers for Disease Control and Prevention, National Center for Injury Prevention and Control. Available online: www.cdc.gov/ncipc/tbi/Coaches_Tool_Kit.htm

Semrud-Clikeman, M. (2001). *Traumatic brain injury in children and adolescents: Assessment and intervention.* New York: Guilford Press.

A1.7. UNINTENTIONAL INJURY

Branche, C. M., Dellinger, A. M., Sleet, D. A., Gilchrist, J., & Olson, S. J. (2004). Unintentional injuries: The burden, risks, and preventive strategies to address diversity. In I. L. Livingston (Ed.), *Praeger handbook of black American health: Policies and issues behind disparities in health* (pp. 317–327). Westport, CT: Praeger.

Christoffel, T., & Gallagher, S. S. (In press). *Injury prevention and public health: Practical knowledge, skills, and strategies* (2nd ed.). Sudbury, MA: Jones & Bartlett.

Fletemeyer, J. R., & Freas, S. J. (1999). *Drowning: New perspectives on intervention and prevention.* Boca Raton, FL: CRC Press.

Gielen, A., Sleet, D. A., & DiClemente, R. (2006). *Injury and violence prevention: Behavioral science theories, methods and applications.* San Francisco: Jossey-Bass.

Parra, E. K., & Stevens, J. A. (2002). *U.S. fall prevention programs for seniors.* Atlanta, GA: Centers for Disease Control and Prevention, National Center for Injury Prevention and Control. www.cdc.gov/ncipc/falls/default.htm

Posner, M. (2000). *Preventing school injuries.* New Brunswick, NJ: Rutgers University Press.

Shults, R., & Harvey, P. (1996). *Efforts to increase smoke detector use in U.S. households.* Atlanta, GA: Centers for Disease Control and Prevention, National Center for Injury Prevention and Control.

Sleet, D. A., & Hopkins, K. (Eds.). (2004). *Bibliography of behavioral science research in unintentional injury prevention* [CD-ROM]. Atlanta, GA: Centers for Disease Control and Prevention, National Center for Injury Prevention and Control.

Zaza, S., Briss, P. A., Harris, K. W., & Task Force on Community Preventive Services. (2005). *The guide to community preventive services: What works to promote health?* New York: Oxford University Press.

A1.8.   VIOLENCE-RELATED INJURY

Aldarondo, E., & Mederos, F. (2002). *Programs for men who batter: Intervention and prevention strategies in a diverse society.* Kingston, NJ: Civic Research Institute.

Burton, J. E., Rasmussen, L. A., Bradshaw, J., Christopherson, B. J., & Huke, S. C. (1998). *Treating children with sexually abusive behavior problems: Guidelines for child and parent intervention.* New York: Haworth Maltreatment & Trauma Press.

Center for the Study and Prevention of Violence, University of Colorado at Boulder. (1998–2004). *Blueprints for violence prevention series.* Boulder, CO: Author.

Chalk, R., & King, P. (1998). *Violence in families: Assessing prevention and treatment programs.* Washington, DC: National Academy Press.

Christoffel, T., & Gallagher, S. S. (In press). *Injury prevention and public health: Practical knowledge, skills, and strategies* (2nd ed.). Sudbury, MA: Jones & Bartlett.

Cohen, J. J., & Fish, M. C. (1993). *Handbook of school-based interventions: Resolving student problems and promoting healthy educational environments.* San Francisco: Jossey-Bass.

Corcoran, M. H., & Cawood, J. S. (2003). *Violence assessment and intervention: The practitioner's handbook.* Boca Raton, FL: CRC Press.

Dishion, T., & Kavanagh, K. (2003). *Intervening in adolescent problem behavior: A family-centered approach.* New York: Guilford Press.

Eisikovits, Z., & Buchbinder, E. (2000). *Locked in a violent embrace: Understanding and intervening in domestic violence.* Thousand Oaks, CA: Sage.

Faller, K. C. (1999). *Maltreatment in early childhood: Tools for research-based intervention.* New York: Haworth Maltreatment & Trauma Press.

Fawcett, B., Featherston, B., Hearn, J., & Toft, C. (1996). *Violence and gender relations: Theories and interventions.* Thousand Oaks, CA: Sage.

Geffner, R., Jaffe, P. G., & Sudermann, M. (2000). *Children exposed to domestic violence: Current issues in research, intervention, prevention, and policy development.* New York: Haworth Maltreatment & Trauma Press.

Geffner, R., Loring, M. T., & Young, C. (2001). *Bullying behavior: Current issues, research, and interventions.* New York: Haworth Maltreatment & Trauma Press.

Geffner, R., & Rosenbaum, A. (2002). *Domestic violence offenders: Current interventions, research, and implications for policies and standards.* New York: Haworth Press.

Gielen, A., Sleet, D. A., & DiClemente, R. (2006). *Injury and violence prevention: Behavioral science theories, methods and applications.* San Francisco: Jossey-Bass.

Goldstein, A. P., Glick, B., & Gibbs, J. C. (1998). *Aggression replacement training: A comprehensive intervention for aggressive youth* (rev. ed.). Champaign, IL: Research Press.

Goldstein, S. L. (1998). *The sexual exploitation of children: A practical guide to assessment, investigation, and intervention* (2nd ed.). Boca Raton, FL: CRC Press.

Graham-Bermann, S. A., & Edleson, J. L. (2001). *Domestic violence in the lives of children: The future of research, intervention, and social policy.* Washington, DC: American Psychological Association.

Greenwald, R. (2002). *Trauma and juvenile delinquency: Theory, research, and interventions.* New York: Haworth Maltreatment & Trauma Press.

Gullotta, T. P., Adams, G. R., & Montemayor, R. (1998). *Delinquent violent youth: Theory and interventions.* Thousand Oaks, CA: Sage.

Gullotta, T. P., & McElhaney, S. J. (1999). *Violence in homes and communities: Prevention, intervention, and treatment.* Thousand Oaks, CA: Sage.

Hamberger, L. K., & Phelan, M. B. (2004). *Domestic violence screening and intervention in medical and mental healthcare settings.* New York: Springer.

Kendall-Tackett, K. A., & Giacomoni, S. M. (2005). *Child victimization: Maltreatment, bullying and dating violence, prevention and intervention.* Kingston, NJ: Civic Research Institute.

Koenig, L. J., Doll, L., O'Leary, A., & Pequegnat, W. (2004). *From child sexual abuse to adult sexual risk: Trauma, revictimization, and intervention.* Washington, DC: American Psychological Association.

Loeber, R. (1998). *Serious and violent juvenile offenders: Risk factors and successful interventions.* Thousand Oaks, CA: Sage.

Loeber, R. & Farrington, D. P. (2001). *Child delinquents: Development, intervention, and service needs.* Thousand Oaks, CA: Sage.

Lutzker, J. R. (2005). *Preventing violence: Research and evidence-based intervention strategies.* Washington, DC: American Psychological Association.

Mills, L. G. (1998). *The heart of intimate abuse: New interventions in child welfare, criminal justice, and health settings.* New York: Springer.

Moghaddam, F. M., & Marsella, A. J. (2004). *Understanding terrorism: Psychosocial roots, consequences, and interventions.* Washington, DC: American Psychological Association.

O'Carroll, P. W., & Potter, L. B. (1994). Suicide contagion and the reporting of suicide: Recommendations from a national workshop. *MMWR Recommendations & Reports, 43* (No. RR-6), 9–18.

O'Carroll, P. W., Potter, L. B., & Mercy, J. A. (1994). Programs for the prevention of suicide among adolescents and young adults. *MMWR Recommendations & Reports, 43* (No. RR-6), 1–7.

Quinn, M. J., & Tomita, S. K. (1997). *Elder abuse and neglect: Causes, diagnosis, and intervention strategies* (2nd ed.). New York: Springer.

Reid, J. B., Patterson, G. R., & Snyder, J. J. (2002). *Antisocial behavior in children and adolescents: A developmental analysis and model for intervention.* Washington, DC: American Psychological Association.

Roberts, A. (1998). *Battered women and their families: Intervention strategies and treatment programs* (2nd ed.). New York: Springer.

Roberts, A. R. (2002). *Handbook of domestic violence intervention strategies: Policies, programs, and legal remedies.* New York: Oxford University Press.

Schewe, P. A. (2002). *Preventing violence in relationships: Interventions across the life span.* Washington, DC: American Psychological Association.

Smith, P. K., Pepler, D. J., & Rigby, K. (2004). *Bullying in schools: How successful can interventions be?* New York: Cambridge University Press.

Zaza, S., Briss, P. A., Harris, K. W., & Task Force on Community Preventive Services. (2005). *The guide to community preventive services: What works to promote health?* New York: Oxford University Press.

Appendix **2**

Key Evaluation Resources*

Compiled by Christy L. Cechman

Bablouzian, L., Freedman, E. S., Wolski, K. E., & Fried, L. E. (1997). Evaluation of a community based childhood injury prevention program. *Injury Prevention, 3*, 14–16.

Backer, T. E. (2003). *Evaluating community collaborations.* New York: Springer.

Boulmetis, J., & Dutwin, P. (2005). *The ABCs of evaluation: Timeless techniques for program and project managers* (2nd ed.). San Francisco: Jossey-Bass.

Centers for Disease Control and Prevention. (1999). Framework for program evaluation in public health. www.cdc.gov/mmwr/preview/mmwrhtml/rr4811a1.htm.

Centers for Disease Control and Prevention Evaluation Workgroup. (2005). *Introduction to program evaluation for public health programs: A self-study guide.* www.cdc.gov/eval/evalguide.pdf.

Chen, H. T. (2004). *Practical program evaluation: Assessing and improving planning, implementation, and effectiveness.* Thousand Oaks, CA: Sage.

Cohen, M. A., & Miller, T. R. (1998). The cost of mental health care for victims of crime. *Journal of Interpersonal Violence, 13*, 93–110.

Dale, R. (1998). *Evaluation frameworks for development programmes and projects.* Thousand Oaks, CA: Sage.

Davidson, E. J. (2005). *Evaluation methodology basics: The nuts and bolts of sound evaluation.* Thousand Oaks, CA: Sage.

Drummond, M. F., Sculper, M. J., Torrance, G. W., O'Brien, B. J., & Stoddart, G. L. (2005). *Methods for the economic evaluation of health care programmes* (3rd ed.). New York: Oxford University Press.

Fetterman, D. A. (2001). *Foundations of empowerment evaluation.* Thousand Oaks, CA: Sage.

Fetterman, D. A., Kaftarian, S. J., & Wandersman, A. (1996). *Empowerment evaluation: Knowledge and tools for self-assessment and accountability.* Thousand Oaks, CA: Sage.

Fetterman, D. A., & Wandersman, A. (2004). *Empowerment evaluation principles in practice.* New York: Guilford Press.

Fink, A. (2005). *Evaluation fundamentals: Insights into the outcomes, effectiveness, and quality of health programs* (2nd ed.). Thousand Oaks, CA: Sage.

Finkelstein, E. A., Corso, P. S., & Miller, T. R. (2006). *The incidence and economic burden of injuries in the United States, 2000.* New York: Oxford University Press.

Fisher, D., Imm, P., Wandersman, A., & Chinman, M. (In press). *Getting to outcomes with developmental assets: Ten steps to measuring success in youth programs and communities.* Minneapolis, MN: Search Institute.

Foss, R. D. (1989). Evaluation of a community-wide incentive program to promote safety restraint use. *American Journal of Public Health, 79*, 304–306.

Fromm, S. (2001). *Total estimated cost of child abuse and neglect in the United States: Statistical evidence.* www.preventchildabuse.org/learn_more/research_docs/cost_analysis.pdf.

*Inclusion in this list does not necessarily represent the official policies and views of or endorsement by the federal government, U.S. Department of Health and Human Services, or the Centers for Disease Control and Prevention, and none should be inferred.

Gold, R. S., Green, L. W., & Kreuter, M. W. (1998). *EMPOWER: Enabling methods of planning and organizing within everyone's reach.* Sudbury, MA: Jones & Bartlett.

Grembowski, D. (2001). *Practice of health program evaluation.* Thousand Oaks, CA: Sage.

Haddix, A. C., Mallonee, S., Waxweiler, R., & Douglas, M. R. (2001). Cost effectiveness analysis of a smoke alarm giveaway program in Oklahoma City, Oklahoma. *Injury Prevention, 7,* 276–281.

Haddix, A. C., Teutsch, S. M., & Corso, P. S. (2002). *Prevention effectiveness: A guide to decision analysis and economic evaluation* (2nd ed.). New York: Oxford University Press.

Kushner, S. (2000). *Personalizing evaluation.* Thousand Oaks, CA: Sage.

Lazenbatt, A. (2002). *The evaluation handbook for health professionals.* New York: Routledge.

Mark, M. M., Henry, G. T., & Julnes, G. (2002). *Evaluation: An integrated framework for understanding, guiding, and improving policies and programs.* San Francisco: Jossey-Bass.

McLaughlin, J. A. & Jordan, G. B. (1999). Logic models: A tool for telling your program's performance story. *Evaluation & Program Planning, 22,* 65–72.

Muennig, P., & Khan, K. (2002). *Designing and conducting cost-effectiveness analyses in medicine and health care.* San Francisco: Jossey-Bass.

Owen, J. (1999). *Program evaluation: Forms and approaches.* Thousand Oaks, CA: Sage.

Patton, M. Q. (1997). *Utilization-focused evaluation: The new century text* (3rd ed.). Thousand Oaks, CA: Sage.

Patton, M. Q. (2002). *Qualitative research and evaluation methods* (3rd ed.). Thousand Oaks, CA: Sage.

Pietrzak, J., Ramler, M., Renner, T., Ford, L., & Gilbert, N. (1990). *Practical program evaluation: Examples from child abuse prevention.* Thousand Oaks, CA: Sage.

Posavac, E. J., & Carey, R. G. (2002). *Program evaluation: Methods and case studies* (6th ed.). Upper Saddle River, NJ: Prentice Hall.

Riger, S., Bennett, L., Wasco, S. M., Schewe, P. A., Frohmann, L., Camacho, J. M., & Campbell, R. (2002). *Evaluating services for survivors of domestic violence and sexual assault.* Thousand Oaks, CA: Sage Publications.

Rivara, F. P., Cummings, P., Koepsell, T. D., Grossman, D. C., & Maier, R. V. (2001). *Injury control: A guide to research and program evaluation.* New York: Cambridge University Press.

Rootman, I. (2001). *Evaluation in health promotion: Principles and perspectives.* www.euro.who.int /InformationSources/Publications/Catalogue/20010911_43.

Rossi, P. H., Freeman, H. E., & Lipsey, M. W. (2004). *Evaluation: A systematic approach* (7th ed.). Thousand Oaks, CA: Sage.

Schalock, R. L. (2001). *Outcome-based evaluation* (2nd ed.). New York: Kluwer Academic/Plenum Publishers.

Steckler, A., & Linnan, L. (2002). *Process evaluation for public health interventions and research.* San Francisco: Jossey-Bass.

Thompson, N. J., & McClintock, H. O. (2000). *Demonstrating your program's worth* (2nd ed.). www.cdc.gov/ncipc/pub-res/demonstr.htm.

Thorogood, M., & Coombes, Y. (2004). *Evaluating health promotion: Practice and methods* (2nd ed.). New York: Oxford University Press.

Valente, T. W. (2002). *Evaluating health promotion programs.* New York: Oxford University Press.

Veale, J. R., Morley, R. E., & Erickson, C. L. (2002). *Practical evaluation for collaborative services: Goals, processes, tools, and reporting systems for school-based programs.* Thousand Oaks, CA: Corwin Press.

Ward, S. K., & Finkelhor, D. (2000). *Program evaluation and family violence research.* New York: Haworth Maltreatment & Trauma Press.

Wholey, J. S., Hatry, H. P., & Newcomer, K. E. (2004). *Handbook of practical program evaluation* (2nd ed.). San Francisco: Jossey-Bass.

Windsor, R. A., Clark, N., Boyd, N. R., & Goodman, R. M. (2003). *Evaluation of health promotion, health education, and disease prevention programs* (3rd ed.). New York: McGraw-Hill.

Worthen, B. R., Sanders, J. R., & Fitzpatrick, J. L. (2003). *Program evaluation: Alternative approaches and practical guidelines* (3rd ed.). Boston: Allyn & Bacon.

Appendix 3

Key Injury and Violence Data Resources*

Joseph L. Annest, Christy L. Cechman, and Kimberly E. Brice

A3.1. ALCOHOL AND DRUG ABUSE DATA

Alcohol-Related Disease Impact (ARDI)

- Affiliation: National Center for Chronic Disease Prevention and Health Promotion (CDC-NCCDPHP)
- Frequency: periodic
- URL: http://apps.nccd.cdc.gov/ardi/Homepage.aspx

ARDI was released in 2004 as a tool for estimating alcohol-related deaths and years of potential life lost for the general population at the state and national levels. Acute causes of death resulting from alcohol abuse include those related to motor-vehicle incident, drowning, falls, fires, homicide and suicide.

Drug Abuse Warning Network (DAWN)

- Affiliation: Substance Abuse and Mental Health Services Administration (SAMHSA)
- Frequency: ongoing
- URL: www.dawninfo.samhsa.gov

DAWN is a public health surveillance system that monitors drug-related hospital emergency department visits and drug-related deaths to track the impact of drug use, misuse, and abuse in the United States. Recent changes have expanded the

*Inclusion in this list does not necessarily represent the official policies and views of or endorsement by the federal government, U.S. Department of Health and Human Services, or the Centers for Disease Control and Prevention, and none should be inferred.

scope of DAWN to help communities identify emerging problems, improve patient care, and manage resources.

Health Behavior in School-Aged Children (HBSC) Series

- Affiliation: Substance Abuse and Mental Health Data Archive (SAMHDA)
- Frequency: periodic
- URL: http://webapp.icpsr.umich.edu/cocoon/SAMHDA-SERIES/00195.xml

HBSC Series has been sponsored by the World Health Organization Regional Office for Europe since 1982. Information is collected from school-aged children in as many as 30 participating countries, including the United States, and is meant to help researchers monitor and understand health-risk behaviors and attitudes in youth, including drug and alcohol use, fighting, and bringing weapons to school.

Monitoring the Future (MTF) Series

- Affiliation: Substance Abuse and Mental Health Data Archive (SAMHDA)
- Frequency: annual
- URL: http://webapp.icpsr.umich.edu/cocoon/SAMHDA-SERIES/00035.xml

MTF surveys, conducted annually since 1975, were designed to examine changes in values, behaviors, and lifestyle orientations of contemporary American youth and to attempt to explain the relationships and trends observed. Information regarding drug use, demographics, and attitudes toward a variety of subjects (e.g., parental influences, drug education, and violence and crime) are collected from nationally representative samples of 8th-, 10th-, and 12th-grade students in the United States.

Monitoring the Future Survey (MTFS)

- Affiliation: National Institute on Drug Abuse (NIDA)
- Frequency: annual
- URL: www.nida.nih.gov/DrugPages/mtf.html

MTFS is conducted by the University of Michigan's Institute for Social Research and funded by the National Institute on Drug Abuse. MTFS surveys almost 50,000 students from over 400 schools nationwide about illicit drug use and attitudes toward drugs. Students from 8th, 10th, and 12th grade are asked about their lifetime use, past year use, past month use, and daily use of drugs, alcohol, cigarettes, and smokeless tobacco. Results from the survey are released each fall.

National Longitudinal Survey of Youth (NLSY97)

- Affiliation: U.S Department of Labor, Bureau of Labor Statistics
- Frequency: ongoing
- URL: www.bls.gov/nls/nlsy97.htm

NLSY97 involved interviewing a sample of approximately 9000 youths who were 12–16 years old as of December 31, 1996, as well as one of that youth's parents.

Youth were then interviewed on a yearly basis thereafter. Data were released in June and October of 2005. The survey was designed to document the transition from school to work and into adulthood. In addition to education and work-related experiences, the survey also gathered information on criminal behavior and alcohol and drug use.

National Survey on Drug Use and Health (NSDUH) (formerly the National Household Survey on Drug Abuse [NHSDA])

- Affiliation: Substance Abuse and Mental Health Services Administration (SAMHSA)
- Frequency: annual
- URL: www.oas.samhsa.gov/nhsda.htm

NSDUH collects data on drug and alcohol use and abuse by the civilian noninstitutionalized population, aged 12 years and over, in the United States. Data are collected on illegal drug use, the nonmedical use of legal drugs, and the use of alcohol and tobacco products. Periodically, the survey also collects data on special topics such as criminal behavior and mental health issues. The purpose of the survey is to produce estimates on the incidence and prevalence of drug and alcohol use and abuse in the United States.

National Youth Survey (NYS) Series

- Affiliation: Substance Abuse and Mental Health Data Archive (SAMHDA)
- Frequency: periodic
- URL: http://webapp.icpsr.umich.edu/cocoon/SAMHDA-SERIES/00088.xml

NYS data were gathered from interviews with parents and youth about behavior by youths. Information collected includes demographic data, disruptive events in the home, neighborhood problems, attitudes toward deviance in adults and juveniles, parental discipline, community involvement, drug and alcohol use, victimization, pregnancy, and spouse violence by respondent and partner.

Youth Risk Behavior Surveillance System (YRBSS)

- Affiliation: National Center for Chronic Disease Prevention and Health Promotion (CDC-NCCDPHP)
- Frequency: biennial
- URL: www.cdc.gov/nccdphp/dash/yrbs/index.htm

YRBSS was developed to monitor health risk behaviors among youth and adults in the United States. Health risk behaviors (e.g., tobacco, alcohol, other drug abuse; suicide attempt; weapon carrying; and physical fighting) are often established during childhood and early adolescence and can contribute highly to the leading causes of death, disability, and social problems among Americans. YRBSS was intended to help determine the prevalence of health risk behaviors and assess behavior trends over time and among populations. The survey includes data from national, state, and local school-based samples of 9th- through 12th-grade students and is conducted every 2 years.

A3.2.   BEHAVIORAL RISK FACTORS

Behavioral Risk Factor Survey System (BRFSS)

- Affiliation: National Center for Chronic Disease Prevention and Health Promotion (CDC-NCCDPHP)
- Frequency: annual
- URL: www.cdc.gov/brfss

BRFSS uses telephone surveys to track health risk behavior in the United States to improve the health of the American people. All 50 states, the District of Columbia, and 3 territories participate in the survey. Questions are asked to determine actual behaviors, such as smoking, physical activity, and seat belt use, rather than attitudes toward or knowledge of health-related behavior. Annual reports are published to track major health risks among Americans, giving states and territories the information they need to create policies and initiatives to meet health-related goals and track their successes.

Health Behavior in School-aged Children (HBSC) Series

See "A3.1. Alcohol and Drug Abuse Data."

Injury Control and Risk Surveys (ICARIS-1, ICARIS-2)

- Affiliation: National Center for Injury Prevention and Control (CDC-NCIPC)
- Frequency: periodic
- URL: No Web site available at this time.

ICARIS-1 and ICARIS-2 were conducted as national random digit dial telephone surveys of the noninstitutionalized English- and Spanish-speaking population aged 18 and older in the 50 states and the District of Columbia. The purpose of these surveys was to collect data on injuries and injury risk factors. ICARIS-1 was conducted in 1994 and covered 11 modules, including respondent demographics and a variety of unintentional and intentional injury topics. Data were collected on more than 5,000 respondents. ICARIS-2, conducted from July 23, 2001, to February 7, 2003, collected data from almost 10,000 respondents. Besides repeating a number of questions asked in the initial survey, additional questions and additional modules were added. Both sets of survey data were weighted to adjust for selection probabilities and nonresponse and were poststratified to the most recent population data by age, gender, and race. These surveys provide national estimates of selected types of injuries and injury-related risk factors.

Monitoring the Future (MTF) Series

See "A3.1. Alcohol and Drug Abuse Data."

National Health Interview Survey (NHIS)

- Affiliation: National Center for Health Statistics (CDC-NCHS)
- Frequency: annual
- URL: www.cdc.gov/nchs/nhis.htm

NHIS collects current statistical information on the health of the civilian noninstitutionalized population of the United States, including data on illness and disability and the services rendered for or because of such conditions. The information
gathered by the NHIS can be used by the public health community to monitor
trends in injuries, illnesses, and disability, track progress in achieving national
health objectives, determine barriers to health care access, and evaluate federal
health-care programs. The NHIS surveys over 43,000 households per year to collect
demographic and socioeconomic data as well basic indicators of health status and
use of health-care services.

National Youth Survey (NYS) Series

See "A3.1. Alcohol and Drug Abuse Data."

Youth Risk Behavior Surveillance System (YRBSS)

See "A3.1. Alcohol and Drug Abuse Data."

A3.3.   CRIME AND VICTIMIZATION DATA

Census of Juveniles in Residential Placement (CJRP)

- Affiliation: Office of Juvenile Justice and Delinquency Prevention (OJJDP)
- Frequency: periodic
- URL: http://ojjdp.ncjrs.org/ojstatbb/cjrp

The CJRP data book contains tables detailing the characteristics (age, sex, race/
ethnicity, offense, type of facility, and placement status) of juvenile offenders in
residential placement facilities.

Law Enforcement Officers Killed and Assaulted (LEOKA)

- Affiliation: Federal Bureau of Investigation (FBI)
- Frequency: annual
- URL: www.fbi.gov/ucr/ucr.htm

LEOKA is one of several reporting systems of the Uniform Crime Reporting Program
of the FBI. LEOKA addresses crimes the murder, assault, and accidental deaths of
law-enforcement officers occuring in the line of duty. Data include information on
weapons used, use of body armor, and circumstances surrounding murders and
assaults of officers.

Monitoring the Future (MTF) Series

See "A3.1. Alcohol and Drug Abuse Data."

National Child Abuse and Neglect Data System (NCANDS)

- Affiliation: National Clearinghouse on Child Abuse and Neglect (NCCAN)
- Frequency: annual
- URL: www.ndacan.cornell.edu/NDACAN/Datasets/Abstracts/DatasetAbstract_NCANDS_General.html

Each year, data are collected for NCANDS by the Children's Bureau, Administration on Children, Youth and Families in the Administration for Children and Families, U.S. Department of Health and Human Services. The resulting *Child Maltreatment Report* is published annually and presents national data about child abuse and neglect in the United States. The Child Abuse Prevention and Treatment Act (CAPTA) requires all states that receive funds from the basic state grant program to provide specific data, to the extent practicable, on children who have been maltreated.

National Crime Victimization Survey (NCVS)

- Affiliation: Bureau of Justice Statistics (BJS)
- Frequency: annual
- URL: www.ojp.usdoj.gov/bjs/cvict.htm

NCVS is the chief source of criminal victimization information in the United States. Data are gathered annually from a sample of 42,000 households, including nearly 76,000 people, on the frequency, characteristics, and consequences of criminal victimization. The purpose of the survey is to enable BJS to estimate the likelihood of victimization of individuals 12 years of age or older by rape, sexual assault, robbery, assault, theft, household burglary, and motor-vehicle theft for the population as a whole as well as for segments of the population such as women, the elderly, members of various racial groups, city dwellers, and other groups.

National Incidence Study of Child Abuse and Neglect (NIS)

- Affiliation: National Clearinghouse on Child Abuse and Neglect (NCCAN)
- Frequency: periodic
- URL: http://nccanch.acf.hhs.gov

The NIS has been conducted three times since 1980, most recently in 1993. The congressionally mandated study seeks to provide information on the extent of child abuse and neglect in the United States and measure changes that have occurred since the previous study. The NIS-3 study, published in 1996, sampled over 5600 professionals nationwide and includes cases investigated by child protective service agencies as well as children seen by other professionals, such as police departments, schools, hospitals and public health departments. Therefore, the NIS results are more comprehensive than official statistics reported by child protective services.

National Incident-Based Reporting System (NIBRS)

- Affiliation: Federal Bureau of Investigation (FBI)
- Frequency: ongoing
- URL: www.fbi.gov/hq/cjisd/ucr.htm

NIBRS was created from the Uniform Crime Reporting (UCR) Program to enhance the crime data collection abilities of law enforcement, improve methods for analyzing and publishing crime data, and provide more details about the circumstances of the incident. Over 17,000 local, state, and federal law enforcement agencies nationwide contribute statistics on crime in the United States.

National Violence Against Women Survey (NVAW)

- Affiliation: National Institute of Justice (NIJ) and National Center for Injury Prevention and Control (CDC-NCIPC)
- Frequency: conducted only once, in 1995–1996
- URL: www.ncjrs.org/pdffiles1/nij/181867.pdf; www.ncjrs.org/pdffiles1/nij/183781.pdf; www.ncjrs.org/pdffiles/169592.pdf; www.ncjrs.org/pdffiles/172837.pdf

NVAW was conducted in 1995–1996 and presents findings from 8000 women and 8000 men in the United States about their experiences as victims of intimate partner violence. The respondents answered questions about their lifetime experiences of intimate partner violence, including frequency, injuries received, treatment sought, and use of the criminal justice system. Findings are available in PDF format.

National Violent Death Reporting System (NVDRS)

- Affiliation: National Center for Injury Prevention and Control (CDC-NCIPC)
- Frequency: 17 states currently report to this system (AK, CA, CO, GA, KY, MA, MD, NC, NJ, NM, OK, OR, RI, SC, UT, VA, WI)
- URL: www.cdc.gov/ncipc/profiles/nvdrs/facts.htm

NVDRS was created to provide accurate and timely violent death-related information to inform decision makers about the magnitude and characteristics of the problem in the United States and to provide a tool for evaluation of state-based violence prevention programs and policies. NVDRS is designed to fill in the gaps created by the lack of certain death certificate data, such as the link between victim and perpetrator. The goals of NVDRS include helping identify risk factors for multiple homicide or homicide-suicide occurrences, to provide more timely information about violent deaths, and to provide characteristics about perpetrators and their relationships to victims.

National Youth Survey (NYS) Series

See "A3.1. Alcohol and Drug Abuse Data."

School Survey on Crime and Safety (SSOCS)

- Affiliation: National Center for Education Statistics (NCES)
- Frequency: annual
- URL: http://nces.ed.gov/surveys/ssocs/ [info]; available on CD-ROM by request: http://nces.ed.gov/pubsearch/pubsinfo.asp?pubid=2004306

SSOCS contains information from a sample of the U.S. public elementary, middle, secondary schools designed to provide estimates of school crime, discipline, disorder, programs and policies. The survey is administered to over 3000 school principals each year and asks questions about a variety of topics relating to school crime and safety, including policies and procedures, school violence prevention programs, and frequency of criminal, hate-related and gang-related incidents at school.

A3.4.   INJURY DEATHS

Alcohol-Related Disease Impact (ARDI)

See "A3.1. Alcohol and Drug Abuse Data."

Census of Fatal Occupational Injuries (CFOI)

- Affiliation: Bureau of Labor Statistics (BLS)
- Frequency: annual
- URL: www.bls.gov/iif/oshfat1.htm

CFOI is a federal–state cooperative program producing comprehensive statistics regarding fatal work injuries. CFOI is implemented in all 50 states and the District of Columbia. Multiple sources, such as death certificates and worker's compensation records, are cross-referenced to identify, verify, and profile fatal worker injuries. Data from the preceding year are issued annually.

Drug Abuse Warning Network (DAWN)

See "A3.1. Alcohol and Drug Abuse Data."

Fatality Analysis Reporting System (FARS)

- Affiliation: National Highway Traffic Safety Administration (NHTSA)
- Frequency: ongoing
- URL: www-fars.nhtsa.dot.gov

FARS annually tracks national statistics regarding motor-vehicle crash deaths occurring on a public roadway. NHTSA provides an interactive query system that allows users to access FARS data on the Internet regarding crash details, specifics of the people involved, vehicle type, and driver characteristics. Results may be shown for one or more states, and several report format options are available.

Injuries, Illnesses and Fatalities (IIF)

- Affiliation: Bureau of Labor Statistics (BLS)
- Frequency: annual
- URL: www.bls.gov/iif/home.htm

IIF provides information on injuries and illness on the job and data on worker fatalities.

Law Enforcement Officers Killed and Assaulted (LEOKA)

See "A3.3. Crime and Victimization Data."

National Mortality Followback Survey—1993 (NMFS93)

- Affiliation: National Center for Health Statistics (CDC-NCHS)
- Frequency: periodic
- URL: www.cdc.gov/nchs/about/major/nmfs/nmfs.htm

NMFS collects information for a sample of U.S. residents from the next of kin or another person familiar with the decedent's life history to supplement death certificate information. This information provides a unique opportunity to study the cause of disease, demographic trends in mortality, and other health issues. The 1993 survey samples individuals from 49 states, aged 15 years or over, who died in 1993 and emphasizes deaths due to homicide, suicide, and unintentional injury. The 1993 NMFS focuses on five subject areas: socioeconomic differentials in mortality; associations between risk factors and cause of death; disability; access and use of health care facilities in the last year of life; and reliability of certain items reported on the death certificate.

National Traumatic Occupational Fatality Surveillance System (NTOF)

- Affiliation: National Institute for Occupational Safety and Health (CDC-NIOSH)
- Frequency: no longer active with new data
- URL: www.cdc.gov/niosh/injury

NTOF is a nationwide surveillance system for occupation injury deaths. Death certificates are the source of data for NTOF and are estimated to include over 80% of all occupation deaths in the United States. NTOF data are available for the years 1980–1995 for civilian workers and 1980–1993 for active military personnel. Statistics are included for demographic and injury characteristics and can be used to develop prevention strategies and identify the leading causes of workplace injury and death.

National Violent Death Reporting System (NVDRS)

See "A3.3. Crime and Victimization Data."

National Vital Statistics System (NVSS)

- Affiliation: National Center for Health Statistics (CDC-NCHS)
- Frequency: ongoing
- URL: www.cdc. gov/nchs/nvss.htm

NVSS collects and disseminates the official vital statistics collected from the 50 states and 5 territories (Puerto Rico, the Virgin Islands, Guam, American Samoa, and the Commonwealth of the Northern Mariana Islands). Data are obtained from birth, marriage, divorce, and death certificates collected from various official registries. Standard procedures for vital statistics registration and data collection are developed by NCHS as well as training and instructional materials. Data can be obtained electronically through Vital Statistics of the United States, National Vital Statistics Reports, and other reports.

Web-Based Injury Statistics Query and Reporting System (WISQARS)

- Affiliation: National Center for Injury Prevention and Control (CDC-NCIPC)
- Frequency: ongoing
- URL: www.cdc.gov/ncipc/wisqars

WISQARS is an interactive database that provides injury-related data for both fatal and nonfatal injuries. WISQARS Fatal uses death data from the National Vital Statistics System and can be used to create reports that provide number of injury deaths and death rates for specific external causes of injuries. For example, leading causes of death reports provide the number of injury-related deaths relative to the number of other leading causes of death in the United States or in individual states. WISQARS Nonfatal uses injury data from the National Electronic Injury Surveillance System All Injury Program and provides national estimates of nonfatal injuries treated in U.S. hospital emergency departments and allows access to charts that rank leading causes of nonfatal injuries by selected demographic characteristics of those who died from an injury in the United States.

Work-Related Injury Statistics Query System (Work-RISQS)

- Affiliation: National Institute for Occupational Safety and Health (CDC-NIOSH)
- Frequency: ongoing
- URL: www2.cdc.gov/risqs/default.asp

Work-RISQS is a public-access database containing national estimates and rates for nonfatal occupational injuries and illnesses treated in U.S. hospital emergency departments. This Web-based interactive system allows queries based on demographic characteristics, nature of injury/illness, and incident circumstances for the years 1998 and 1999; more years will be added.

A3.5.   INJURY INCIDENCE

Behavioral Risk Factor Survey System (BRFSS)

See "A3.2. Behavioral Risk Factors."

Healthcare Cost and Utilization Project Online Statistics (HCUPnet)

- Affiliation: Agency for Healthcare Research and Quality (AHRQ)
- Frequency: ongoing
- URL: http://hcup.ahrq.gov/HCUPnet.asp

HCUPnet is an on-line query system that allows the user to generate tables and graphs using statistics from national, regional and some state community hospitals in the United States, including injury and poisoning data. HCUPnet generates statistics using data from HCUP's Nationwide Inpatient Sample (NIS), the Kids' Inpatient Database (KID), and the State Inpatient Databases (SID).

Injury Control and Risk Surveys (ICARIS-1, ICARIS-2)

See "A3.2. Behavioral Risk Factors."

International Collaborative Effort (ICE) on Injury Statistics

- Affiliation: National Center for Health Statistics (CDC-NCHS)
- Frequency: Annual/biennial meetings and proceedings
- URL: www.cdc.gov/nchs/advice.htm

ICE on Injury Statistics is one of several international activities sponsored by the Centers for Disease Control and Prevention's National Center for Health Statistics. The goal is to provide a forum for international exchange and collaboration among injury researchers who develop and promote international standards in injury data collection and analysis. A secondary goal is to produce products of the highest quality to facilitate the comparability and improved quality of injury data.

National Health Interview Survey (NHIS)

See "A3.2. Behavioral Risk Factors."

Youth Risk Behavior Surveillance System (YRBSS)

See "A3.1. Alcohol and Drug Abuse Data."

A3.6.   INJURY MORBIDITY DATA

Healthcare Cost and Utilization Project (HCUP)

- Affiliation: Agency for Healthcare Research and Quality (AHRQ)
- Frequency: ongoing
- URL: www.ahrq.gov/data/hcup

The goal of HCUP is to bring together data collected from state data organizations, hospital associations, private data organizations, and the federal government to create a national collection of patient-level health care databases and software tools. This broad spectrum of data is available to public and private users to enable research on health care issues at the national, state, and local market levels.

Indian Health Service (IHS) Division of Program Statistics Website

- Affiliation: Indian Health Service (IHS)
- Frequency: ongoing
- URL: www.ihs.gov/nonmedicalprograms/ihs%5Fstats

The IHS Division of Program Statistics collects and compiles demographic and patient-care information about the American Indian and Alaska Native populations from several sources, including the U.S. Census, birth and death certificates, and hospital discharge and ambulatory medical services data. Its objective is to present trends in key health status indicators over time for the American Indian and Alaska Native populations compared to all U.S. populations and regional differences in Indian health, comparing key health status indicators among the 12 IHS Areas/ Regions and the total U.S. population.

National Ambulatory Medical Care Survey (NAMCS)

- Affiliation: National Center for Health Statistics (CDC-NCHS)
- Frequency: annual
- URL: www.cdc.gov/nchs/about/major/ahcd/ahcd1.htm

NAMCS is designed to provide information about the provision and use of ambulatory medical care services in the United States. Data are collected during 1-week reporting periods for a random sample of visits to private, office-based physicians who are primarily engaged in direct patient care. Data are obtained on patients' symptoms, physicians' diagnoses, medications ordered or provided, diagnostic procedures, patient management, planned future treatment and demographic characteristics of patients. The survey was conducted annually from 1973 to 1981, in 1985, and annually since 1989.

National Electronic Injury Surveillance System (NEISS)

- Affiliation: U.S. Consumer Product Safety Commission (CPSC)
- Frequency: ongoing
- URL: www.cpsc.gov/library/neiss.html; www.cpsc.gov/cpscpub/pubs/3002. html

NEISS uses data collected from a sample of selected U.S. hospital emergency department visits involving an injury associated with consumer products to estimate the total number of product-related injuries treated in hospital emergency rooms nationwide. Web access to NEISS allows certain estimates to be retrieved on-line and can be customized by setting one or more variables for date, product, sex, age, diagnosis, disposition, locale, or body part.

National Hospital Ambulatory Medical Care Survey (NHAMCS)

- Affiliation: National Center for Health Statistics (CDC-NCHS)
- Frequency: annual
- URL: www.cdc.gov/nchs/about/major/ahcd/ahcd1.htm

NHAMCS is designed to provide information on the use and provision of ambulatory care services in hospital emergency and outpatient departments in the United States. Data are collected from a systematic random sample of patient visits to the emergency departments and outpatient departments of noninstitutional general and short-stay hospitals during a 4-week reporting period. Information obtained includes patient demographics, payment, patients' complaints, physicians' diagnoses, services and procedures, causes of injury where applicable, and hospital characteristics.

National Hospital Discharge Survey (NHDS)

- Affiliation: National Center for Health Statistics (CDC-NCHS)
- Frequency: annual
- URL: www.cdc.gov/nchs/about/major/hdasd/nhds.htm

NHDS is a national probability survey that annually gathers information on characteristics of inpatients discharged from nonfederal, short-stay hospitals in the United States. The survey collects data from a national sample of approximately 270,000 inpatient records acquired from approximately 500 hospitals. Patient demographics and administrative information, such as length of stay and discharge status, are collected manually by the hospital's staff or by staff of the U.S. Bureau of the Census on behalf of NCHS, or through an automated system using machine-readable medical record data purchased from commercial organizations, state data systems, hospitals, or hospital associations.

Outcome and Assessment Information Set (OASIS)

- Affiliation: Centers for Medicare and Medicaid Services (CMS)
- Frequency: ongoing
- URL: www.cms.hhs.gov/oasis

OASIS is a component of Medicare's home health care industry created to measure and assess home health care outcomes in adult (nonmaternity) patients. Data about selected attributes of health service use are collected as well as information on sociodemographics, health status, and functional status of home care patients.

Web-Based Injury Statistics Query and Reporting System (WISQARS)

See "A3.4. Injury Deaths."

Work-Related Injury Statistics Query System (Work-RISQS)

See "A3.4. Injury Deaths."

A3.7.   MOTOR-VEHICLE-RELATED BEHAVIORAL INJURY DATA

Alcohol-Related Disease Impact (ARDI)

See "A3.1. Alcohol and Drug Abuse Data."

Motor Vehicle Occupant Safety Survey (MVOSS)

- Affiliation: National Highway Traffic Safety Administration (NHTSA)
- Frequency: biennial
- URL: www.nhtsa.dot.gov/people/injury/research/occu_protection.html

MVOSS is conducted biennially by national telephone surveys. The survey is administered to a randomly selected national sample of about 6000 individuals age

16 years or older and collects information concerning attitudes, knowledge, and behavior in different occupant protection and highway safety issues. Areas of interest include seatbelts, child safety seats, air bags, (bicyclist and motorcyclist) helmet use, emergency medical services, and crash injury experiences.

National Occupant Protection Use Survey (NOPUS)

- Affiliation: National Highway Traffic Safety Administration (NHTSA)
- Frequency: periodic
- URL: www-nrd.nhtsa.dot.gov/departments/nrd-01/summaries/4313ga. html

NOPUS was created to estimate safety belt and child restraint use in the United States. Data were collected by observation from over 2000 intersections with traffic lights or stop signs. The goal of NOPUS is to promote a better understanding of occupant safety protection use to evaluate current restraint use programs and develop new programs.

A3.8. MOTOR-VEHICLE-RELATED INJURY DATA

Fatality Analysis Reporting System (FARS)

See "A3.4. Injury Deaths."

National Automotive Sampling System-Crashworthiness Data System (NASS-CDS)

- Affiliation: National Highway Traffic Safety Administration (NHTSA)
- Frequency: annual
- URL: www-nrd.nhtsa.dot.gov/departments/nrd-30/ncsa/cds.html

Each year, NASS-CDS provides information on thousands of minor, serious, and fatal crashes across the country involving passenger cars, light trucks, vans, and utility vehicles. Data are collected by researchers who investigate crash sites, examine the vehicles involved, interview crash victims, and review medical records to determine the nature and severity of the injuries. The data are used by NHTSA to identify existing and potential traffic safety problems; assess vehicle crash performance, safety systems, and design; increase knowledge about the nature of crash injuries and the relationship between crash characteristics and the resultant injuries; and evaluate traffic safety programs and the effect of changes in traffic flow, such as increased large truck traffic.

National Automotive Sampling System-General Estimates System (NASS-GES)

- Affiliation: National Highway Traffic Safety Administration (NHTSA)
- Frequency: annual
- URL: www-nrd.nhtsa.dot.gov/departments/nrd-30/ncsa/ges.html

NASS-GES was created to identify traffic safety problem areas and to answer motor vehicle safety questions for the regulatory community, researchers and consumers.

Data are obtained from police reported crashes involving at least one motor vehicle traveling on a roadway way, resulting in property damage, injury, or death. The information from about 50,000 crashes per year is used to estimate the number and type of motor vehicle crashes and what happens when they occur. *Traffic Safety Facts* is published annually for nonfatal crashes and information on fatal crashes is contained in the Fatal Analysis Reporting System.

Special Crash Investigation (SCI)

- Affiliation: National Highway Traffic Safety Administration (NHTSA)
- Frequency: ongoing
- URL: www-nrd.nhtsa.dot.gov/departments/nrd-30/ncsa/sci.html; cases shown as being "available" can be found at: www-nass.nhtsa.dot.gov/BIN/logon.exe/airmislogon

SCI was created to examine the safety impact of new, emerging, and rapidly changing technology (such as air bags and alternative fuel systems) and to explore alleged or potential vehicle defects. SCI provides detailed crash investigation information from routine police and insurance crash reports and special reports by professional crash investigation teams for over 200 crashes each year. Data elements collected include those related to the vehicle, occupants, injury mechanisms, roadway, and safety systems involved. Data collected by SCI are intended to provide information that is useful for understanding crash circumstances or outcomes from an engineering perspective.

TransStats: The Intermodal Transportation Database

- Affiliation: Bureau of Transportation Statistics (BTS)
- Frequency: ongoing
- URL: www.transtats.bts.gov

TranStats is designed to simplify the search for transportation data for researchers and analysts by grouping many different transportation research tools into one place. TranStats features a searchable index of over 100 transportation-related databases across every mode of transportation, and includes important social and demographic data. Users can search for information by mode or subject area, such as bike/pedestrian and safety. Data are downloadable, and several interactive tools allow researchers to create statistical summaries, time series, cross-tabulations, and graphs.

A3.9.   OCCUPATIONAL INJURY DATA

Census of Fatal Occupational Injuries (CFOI)

- Affiliation: Bureau of Labor Statistics (BLS)
- Frequency: annual
- URL: www.bls.gov/iif/oshfat1.htm

CFOI is a federal–state cooperative program producing comprehensive statistics regarding fatal work injuries. CFOI is implemented in all 50 states and the District of Columbia. Multiple sources, such as death certificates and worker's compensation records, are cross-referenced to identify, verify, and profile fatal worker injuries. Data from the preceding year are issued annually.

Injuries, Illnesses and Fatalities (IIF)

See "A3.4. Injury Deaths."

National Traumatic Occupational Fatality Surveillance System (NTOF)

See "A3.4. Injury Deaths."

Work-Related Injury Statistics Query System (Work-RISQS)

See "A3.4. Injury Deaths."

A3.10.   OTHER INJURY DATA

Medicare Provider Analysis and Review (MEDPAR) File and 5% Sample Standard Analysis File (SAF)

- Affiliation: Health Care Finance Administration (HCFA)
- Frequency: ongoing
- URL: www.cms.hhs.gov/statistics/medpar/default.asp

MEDPAR File and SAF both provide Medicare claims information. MEDPAR provides national and state claims data for short-stay hospital inpatient services, including total charges, covered charges, Medicare reimbursement, total days, number of discharges, and average total days of stay. SAF provides information on final action claims data for a 5% sample of Medicare beneficiaries.

National Fire Incident Reporting System (NFIRS)

- Affiliation: United States Fire Administration (USFA)
- Frequency: annual
- URL: www.usfa.fema.gov/nfirs

NFIRS was created to gather and analyze information on the nature and causes of injuries, deaths, and property loss resulting from fires in the United States and to develop uniform data reporting methods that can be used to more accurately assess and subsequently combat the fire problem at a national level. Over 11,000 fire departments from 49 states and the District of Columbia voluntarily report an average of four million incidents each year. The NFIRS database includes roughly one third of all reported fires that occur annually.

United States Eye Injury Registry (USEIR)

- Affiliation: American Society of Ocular Trauma (ASOT)
- Frequency: ongoing
- URL: www.useironline.org

USEIR collects data from state eye injury registries, documenting serious eye injuries or those that have a likelihood of resulting in permanent damage. The goals of USEIR include the promotion of descriptive epidemiology of eye injuries to facilitate research and development of preventive strategies and the dissemination of information about eye injury prevention to the public and the professional community.

A3.11.   POISONING DATA

Healthcare Cost and Utilization Project online statistics (HCUPnet)

See "A3.5. Injury Incidence."

Toxic Exposure Surveillance System (TESS)

- Affiliation: American Association of Poison Control Centers (AAPCC)
- Frequency: annual
- URL: www.aapcc.org/poison1.htm

TESS monitors poisoning in the United States. The TESS database contains detailed toxicological information on more than 24 million poison exposures reported to U.S. poison centers since 1983. The data can be used to identify hazards, determine prevention education and training, guide clinical research, and detect potential chemical or bioterrorism incidents. TESS is an important tool used to initiate product reformulation and repackaging and recalls and also as a postmarketing surveillance of pharmaceuticals.

A3.12.   TRAUMA CARE

National Trauma Data Bank (NTDB)

- Affiliation: American College of Surgeons (ACS)
- Frequency: ongoing
- URL: www.facs.org/trauma/ntdb.html

NTDB contains trauma registry data collected from over one million records from 405 U.S. trauma centers. NTDB is designed to provide information to the medical community, the public and decision makers about issues affecting care for injured people in the United States. Areas of interest in the data bank include epidemiology, injury control, research, education, acute care, and resource allocation.

Toxic Exposure Surveillance System (TESS)

See "A3.11. Poisoning Data."

United States Eye Injury Registry (USEIR)

See "A3.10. Other Injury Data."

A3.13.   VIOLENT DEATH DATA

Drug Abuse Warning Network (DAWN)

See "A3.1. Alcohol and Drug Abuse Data."

Law Enforcement Officers Killed and Assaulted (LEOKA)

See "A3.3. Crime and Victimization Data."

National Incident Based Reporting System (NIBRS)

See "A3.3. Crime and Victimization Data."

National Violent Death Reporting System (NVDRS)

See "A3.3. Crime and Victimization Data."

A3.14.   YOUTH-RELATED DATA

Census of Juveniles in Residential Placement (CJRP)

See "A3.3. Crime and Victimization Data."

Health Behavior in School-aged Children (HBSC) Series

See "A3.1. Alcohol and Drug Abuse Data."

Monitoring the Future (MTF) Series

See "A3.1. Alcohol and Drug Abuse Data."

Monitoring the Future Survey (MTFS)

See "A3.1. Alcohol and Drug Abuse Data."

Motor Vehicle Occupant Safety Survey (MVOSS)

See "A3.7. Motor-Vehicle-Related Behavioral Injury Data."

National Child Abuse and Neglect Data System (NCANDS)

See "A3.3. Crime and Victimization Data."

National Incidence Study of Child Abuse and Neglect (NIS)

See "A3.3. Crime and Victimization Data."

National Longitudinal Survey of Youth (NLSY97)

See "A3.1. Alcohol and Drug Abuse Data."

National Occupant Protection Use Survey (NOPUS)

See "A3.7. Motor-Vehicle-Related Behavioral Injury Data"

National Youth Survey (NYS) Series

See "A3.1. Alcohol and Drug Abuse Data."

School Survey on Crime and Safety (SSOCS)

See "A3.3. Crime and Victimization Data."

Youth Risk Behavior Surveillance System (YRBSS)

See "A3.1. Alcohol and Drug Abuse Data."

Key Injury and Violence Web Resources*

Compiled by Christy L. Cechman

A4.1. FEDERAL AGENCIES

Health Resources and Services Administration (HRSA)
www.hrsa.gov

Indian Health Service (IHS) Injury Prevention Program
www.ihs.gov/MedicalPrograms/InjuryPrevention

National Center for Health Statistics (NCHS)
www.cdc.gov/nchs

National Center for Injury Prevention and Control (NCIPC)
www.cdc.gov/injury

National Clearinghouse on Families and Youth (NCFY)
www.ncfy.com

National Highway Traffic Safety Administration (NHTSA)
www.nhtsa.dot.gov

National Institute for Occupational Safety and Health (NIOSH)
www.cdc.gov/niosh

National Institute of Child Health and Human Development (NICHD)
www.nichd.nih.gov

National Institute of Justice (NIJ)
www.ojp.usdoj.gov/nij

National Institute of Mental Health (NIMH)
www.nimh.nih.gov

*Inclusion in this list does not necessarily represent the official policies and views of or endorsement by the federal government, U.S. Department of Health and Human Services, or the Centers for Disease Control and Prevention, and none should be inferred.

National Institute on Alcohol Abuse and Alcoholism (NIAAA)
www.niaaa.nih.gov

National Institute on Disability and Rehabilitation Research (NIDRR)
www.ed.gov/about/offices/list/osers/nidrr

National Strategy for Suicide Prevention (NSSP)
www.mentalhealth.samhsa.gov/suicideprevention/strategy.asp

Safe Communities
www.nhtsa.dot.gov/safecommunities

Substance Abuse and Mental Health Services Administration (SAMHSA)
www.samhsa.gov

U.S. Consumer Product Safety Commission (CSPC)
www.cpsc.gov

U.S. Fire Administration (USFA)
www.usfa.fema.gov

A4.2. ASSOCIATIONS AND ORGANIZATIONS

AAA Foundation for Traffic Safety
www.aaafoundation.org

American Academy of Pediatrics (AAP)
www.aap.org

American Association of Poison Control Centers (AAPCC)
www.aapcc.org

American Association of Suicidology (AAS)
www.suicidology.org

American College of Emergency Physicians (ACEP)
www.acep.org

American College of Surgeons Trauma Programs
www.facs.org/trauma

American Public Health Association (APHA) Injury Control and Emergency Health Services Section (ICEHS)
www.icehs.org

American Trauma Society (ATS)
www.amtrauma.org

Association for the Advancement of Automotive Medicine (AAAM)
www.carcrash.org

Association of Schools of Public Health (ASPH) Injury Prevention and Control
www.asph.org/document.cfm?page=828

Association of State and Territorial Health Officials (ASTHO)
www.astho.org

Brain Injury Association of America (BIAA)
www.biausa.org

Children's Safety Network (CSN)
www.childrenssafetynetwork.org

Council of State and Territorial Epidemiologists (CSTE)
www.cste.org

Directors of Health Promotion and Education (DHPE)
www.astdhpphe.org

Emergency Medical Services for Children (EMSC)
www.ems-c.org

Family Violence Prevention Fund (FVPF)
http://endabuse.org

Governors Highway Safety Association (GHSA)
www.naghsr.org

HELP Network
www.helpnetwork.org

Home Safety Council (HSC)
www.homesafetycouncil.org

Injury Free Coalition for Kids (IFCK)
www.injuryfree.org

Insurance Institute for Highway Safety (IIHS)
www.highwaysafety.org

National Alliance to End Sexual Violence
www.naesv.org

National Association of County and City Health Officials (NACCHO) Injury Prevention
www.naccho.org/topics/HPDP/injuryprevention.cfm

National Association of EMS Physicians (NAEMSP)
www.naemsp.org

National Association of State EMS Directors (NASEMSD)
www.nasemsd.org

National Center on Child Fatality Review (NCFR)
www.ican-ncfr.org

National Council on the Aging (NCOA)
www.ncoa.org

National Fire Protection Association (NFPA)
www.nfpa.org

National Network to End Domestic Violence (NNEDV)
www.nnedv.org

National Online Resource Center on Violence Against Women (VAWnet)
www.vawnet.org

National Organizations for Youth Safety (NOYS)
www.noys.org

National Program for Playground Safety (NPPS)
www.uni.edu/playground

National Resource Center for Safe Aging (NRCSA)
www.safeaging.org

National Safety Council (NSC)
www.nsc.org

National Sexual Violence Resource Center (NSVRC)
www.nsvrc.org

National Youth Violence Prevention Resource Center (NYVPRC)
www.safeyouth.org

Operation Lifesaver (OL)
www.oli.org

Prevent Child Abuse America
http://preventchildabuse.org

Safe Kids Worldwide
www.safekids.org

SafeUSA
www.safeusa.org

SmartRisk (Canada)
www.smartrisk.ca

Stop It Now! The Campaign to Prevent Child Sexual Abuse
www.stopitnow.org

Society for Advancement of Violence and Injury Research (SAVIR)
www.savirweb.org

Society for Public Health Education (SOPHE)
www.sophe.org

State and Territorial Injury Prevention Directors Association (STIPDA)
www.stipda.org

Suicide Prevention Action Network USA (SPAN-USA)
www.spanusa.org

Suicide Prevention Resource Center (SPRC)
www.sprc.org

ThinkFirst National Injury Prevention Foundation
www.thinkfirst.org

United Tribes Technical College Injury Prevention Program http://catalog.
unitedtribestech.com/courses/distance/onlineipp.asp

World Health Organization (WHO) Department of Injuries and Violence Prevention
www.who.int/violence_injury_prevention/en

A4.3.   RESEARCH RESOURCES

APHA Injury Control and Emergency Health Services Section Newsletter
www.icehs.org/news.htm

Children's Safety Network CSNDiscuss
www.childrenssafetynetwork.org/resources/csndiscusspost.asp

Cochrane Injuries Group
www.cochrane-injuries.lshtm.ac.uk/Review%20links.htm

End Violence against Women eNewsletter
www.endvaw.org/enewsletter.php

EU Injury Prevention Programme Newsletter   http://europa.eu.int/comm/health/horiz_newsletter_en.htm#3

Family Violence Prevention and Health Practice
http://endabuse.org/health/ejournal/about/

Guide to Community Preventive Services
www.thecommunityguide.org

Healthy People 2010 Information Access Project Injury and Violence Prevention
http://phpartners.org/hp/injuryandviolenceprevention.html

Healthy People 2010 Objectives Injury Prevention
www.safetypolicy.org/hp2010/hp2010.htm

Injury-L Electronic Mailing List
listserv@listserv.wvu.edu to subscribe

International Classification of Diseases, Tenth Revision (ICD-10)
www.who.int/classifications/icd/en

International Classification of Diseases, Tenth Revision, Clinical Modification (ICD-10-CM)
www.cdc.gov/nchs/about/otheract/icd9/abticd10.htm

National Center for Injury Prevention and Control Announcement Electronic Mailing List
www.cdc.gov/ncipc/email_list.htm to subscribe

SafetyLit
www.safetylit.org

SAVIR Member Research Project DataBank
www.quickbase.com/db/6tejwf5t

A4.4.   JOURNALS

Accident Analysis and Prevention
www.elsevier.com/locate/aap

Aggression and Violent Behavior
www.elsevier.com/locate/aggviobeh

Annals of Emergency Medicine
www.annemergmed.com

Child Abuse and Neglect
www.elsevier.com/wps/product/cws_home/586

Crisis: The Journal of Crisis Intervention and Suicide Prevention
www.hhpub.com/journals/crisis

Disability and Rehabilitation
www.tandf.co.uk/journals/titles/09638288.asp

Disaster Management and Response
www.disastermgmt.com

Emergency Medicine Journal
www.emjonline.com

Homicide Studies
www.sagepub.com/journal.aspx?pid=74

Injury
www.elsevier.com/locate/injury

Injury Prevention
www.injuryprevention.com

International Journal of Disaster Medicine
www.tandf.co.uk/journals/titles/15031438.asp

International Journal of Injury Control and Safety Promotion
www.tandf.co.uk/journals/titles/17457300.asp

Journal of Aggression, Maltreatment and Trauma
www.haworthpressinc.com/web/JAMT

Journal of Child Sexual Abuse
www.haworthpressinc.com/web/JCSA

Journal of Elder Abuse and Neglect
www.haworthpressinc.com/web/JEAN

Journal of Family Violence
www.springeronline.com/sgw/cda/frontpage/0,11855,4-10126-70-35608912-0,00.
html

Journal of Head Trauma Rehabilitation
www.lww.com/product/?08859701

Journal of Interpersonal Violence
http://jiv.sagepub.com

Journal of Safety Research
www.nsc.org/lrs/res/jsr.htm

Journal of School Violence
www.haworthpressinc.com/web/JSV

Journal of Trauma
www.jtrauma.com

Prehospital Emergency Care
www.naemsp.org/publications-pec.asp

Safety + Health
www.nsc.org/shnews

Sexual Abuse: A Journal of Research and Treatment
www.atsa.com/pubJrnl.html

Suicide and Life-Threatening Behavior
www.guilford.com/cgi-bin/cartscript.cgi?page=periodicals/jnsl.htm&cart_id=

Traffic Injury Prevention
www.tandf.co.uk/journals/titles/15389588.asp

Transportation Research Part F: Traffic Psychology and Behaviour
www.elsevier.com/locate/trf

Trauma, Violence, and Abuse
http://tva.sagepub.com

Violence Against Women
http://vaw.sagepub.com

INDEX